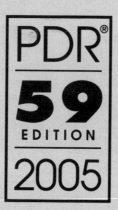

PDR® 59 EDITION 2005

PHYSICIANS' DESK REFERENCE®

Supplement A

For important errata, turn the page.

IMPORTANT NOTICE

ERRATA

PDR 2005

Lilly ICOS LLC

On page 1907, under the Description section for **Cialis**, the structural formula is incorrect. The correct structural formula is as follows:

Paddock Laboratories, Inc.

In the **Manufacturers' Index** on page 11, the "Other Products Available" section should have appeared as follows:

Aluminum Paste
Aquabase
Aspirin Suppositories 300 mg, 600 mg
Aspirin Tablets, Enteric-Coated 325 mg
Belladonna and Opium Suppositories 16.2 mg/30 mg and
    16.2 mg/60 mg CII
Benzoin Compound Tincture USP
Bisacodyl Suppositories USP 10 mg
Bisacodyl Tablets USP 5 mg
Castor Oil USP
Colistimethate for Injection, USP 150 mg Colistin Base
Colistin Sulfate USP Powder
Colloidon, Flexible USP
Compro (Prochlorperazine Suppositories), USP 25 mg
Cyclosporine Injection, USP 250 mg/5 mL
Dermabase
Dexamethasone Sodium Phosphate USP Powder
Dihydroergotamine Mesylate Injection, USP 1 mg/mL
Docusate Sodium Capsules USP 100 mg, 250 mg
Encort (Hydrocortisone Acetate Suppositories) 30 mg
Fattibase
Ferrous Gluconate Tablets USP 324 mg
Ferrous Sulfate Tablets 324 mg
Flavoxate HCl 100 mg Tablets
Glutol
Glycerin USP Liquid
Hydrocortisone USP Micronized Powder
Hydrocortisone Acetate USP Micronized Powder
Hydrocortisone Acetate Suppositories 25 mg
Hydrocream Base
Hydromorphone HCl USP non-sterile Powder CII
Hydromorphone HCl Suppositories 3 mg CII
Ipecac Syrup USP
Lanolin USP (Anhydrous)
Liqua-Gel
Milk of Magnesia USP
Morphine Sulfate USP Powder CII
Morphine Sulfate Suppositories 5 mg, 10 mg, 20 mg, 30 mg CII
Norepinephrine Bitartrate Injection, USP 4 mg/4 mL
Ora-Plus
Ora-Sweet
Ora-Sweet SF
Phenadoz (Promethazine Suppositories) 12.5 mg, 25 mg
Polybase
Prednisolone Sodium Phosphate, USP Oral Solution 5 mg/5 mL
Progesterone USP Micronized Powder
Progesterone USP Wettable Microcrystalline Powder
Promethazine Hydrochloride Injection, USP 25 mg/mL
Sorbitol Solution USP 70%
Suspendol-S
Testosterone USP Micronized non-sterile Powder CIII
Testosterone Propionate USP Micronized non-sterile Powder CIII
Triamcinolone Acetonide USP Micronized Powder
Trimethobenzamide HCl Suppositories 100 mg, 200 mg
Zincate Capsules 220 mg

Romark Pharmaceuticals

Alinia Tablets should appear in the following indices: **Manufacturers' Index**, on page 14 under Romark Pharmaceuticals; **Brand and Generic Name Index**, on page 102 under the brand name heading ALINIA TABLETS, and on page 117, under the generic name heading NITAZOXANIDE; and the **Product Category Index**, on page 205 under the main/subheading ANTI-INFECTIVE AGENTS, SYSTEMIC/ MISCELLANEOUS ANTI-INFECTIVES.

TaroPharma

On page 16 of the **Manufacturers' Index**, first column, "Topicort LP .05% Gel" should read **Topicort LP .05% Cream**.
On page 124 of the **Brand and Generic Name Index**, first column, "Topicort LP .05% Gel" should read **Topicort LP .05% Cream**.

NEW AND REVISED PRODUCT LISTINGS INDEX

Listed below are new *PDR* listings first appearing in 2005 *PDR Supplement A*, as well as listings that have been revised since the publication of the main 2005 edition. New listings are in **bold type** and include comprehensive descriptions of new pharmaceutical products, new dosage forms of previously described products, and existing products not described in the main 2005 edition. Revised listings are in light type and may include new research data or clinical findings of importance.

NEW PRODUCT LISTINGS

This section contains comprehensive descriptions of new pharmaceutical products introduced since publication of the 2005 *PDR*, new dosage forms of products already described, and existing pharmaceutical products not described in the 2005 *PDR*.

AstraZeneca LP
WILMINGTON, DE 19850-5437

For Product Full Prescribing Information, Business Information, Medical Information, Adverse Drug Experiences, and Customer Service:

Information Center
1-800-236-9933

For Product Ordering:

Trade Customer Service
1-800-842-9920

For Product Full Prescribing Information:
Internet: www.astrazeneca-us.com

NEXIUM® I.V.   ℞
[něx'sē-um]
(esomeprazole sodium)
for Injection
Rx only

DESCRIPTION

The active ingredient in NEXIUM® I.V. (esomeprazole sodium) for Injection is (*S*)-5-methoxy-2[[(4-methoxy-3,5-dimethyl-2-pyridinyl)-methyl]sulfinyl]-1 *H*-benzimidazole sodium a compound that inhibits gastric acid secretion. Esomeprazole is the S-isomer of omeprazole, which is a mixture of the S- and R- isomers. Its empirical formula is $C_{17}H_{18}N_3O_3SNa$ with molecular weight of 367.4 g/mol (sodium salt) and 345.4 g/mol (parent compound). Esomeprazole sodium is very soluble in water and freely soluble in ethanol (95%). The structural formula is:

NEXIUM I.V. for Injection is supplied as a sterile, freeze-dried, white to off-white, porous cake or powder in a 5 mL vial, intended for intravenous administration after reconstitution with 0.9% Sodium Chloride Injection, USP; Lactated Ringer's Injection, USP or 5% Dextrose Injection, USP. NEXIUM I.V. for Injection contains esomeprazole sodium 21.3 mg or 42.5 mg equivalent to esomeprazole 20 mg or 40 mg, edetate disodium 1.5 mg and sodium hydroxide q.s. for pH adjustment. The pH of reconstituted solution of NEXIUM I.V. for Injection depends on the reconstitution volume and is in the pH range of 9 to 11. The stability of esomeprazole sodium in aqueous solution is strongly pH dependent. The rate of degradation increases with decreasing pH.

CLINICAL PHARMACOLOGY
Pharmacokinetics
Absorption
The pharmacokinetic profile of NEXIUM I.V. for Injection 20 mg and 40 mg was determined in 24 healthy volunteers for the 20 mg dose and 38 healthy volunteers for the 40 mg dose following once daily administration of 20 mg and 40 mg of NEXIUM I.V. for Injection by constant rate over 30 minutes for five days. The results are shown in the following table:

Pharmacokinetic Parameters of NEXIUM Following I.V. Dosing for 5 days		
Parameter	NEXIUM I.V. 20 mg	NEXIUM I.V. 40 mg
AUC	5.11	16.21
(µmol*h/L)	(3.96:6.61)	(14.46:18.16)
C_{max}	3.86	7.51
(mmol/L)	(3.16:4.72)	(6.93:8.13)
$t_{1/2}$ (h)	1.05	1.41
	(0.90:1.22)	(1.30:1.52)

Values represent the geometric mean (95% CI)

Distribution
Esomeprazole is 97% bound to plasma proteins. Plasma protein binding is constant over the concentration range of 2-20 µmol/L. The apparent volume of distribution at steady state in healthy volunteers is approximately 16 L.
Metabolism
Esomeprazole is extensively metabolized in the liver by the cytochrome P450 (CYP) enzyme system. The metabolites of esomeprazole lack antisecretory activity. The major part of esomeprazole's metabolism is dependent upon the CYP2C19 isoenzyme, which forms the hydroxy and desmethyl metabolites. The remaining amount is dependent on CYP3A4 which forms the sulphone metabolite. CYP2C19 isoenzyme exhibits polymorphism in the metabolism of esomeprazole, since some 3% of Caucasians and 15-20% of Asians lack CYP2C19 and are termed Poor Metabolizers. At steady state, the ratio of AUC in Poor Metabolizers to AUC in the rest of the population (Extensive metabolizers) is approximately 2.
Following administration of equimolar doses, the S- and R-isomers are metabolized differently by the liver, resulting in higher plasma levels of the S- than of the R-isomer.
Excretion
Esomeprazole is excreted as metabolites primarily in urine but also in feces. Less than 1% of parent drug is excreted in the urine. Esomeprazole is completely eliminated from plasma and there is no accumulation during once daily administration. The plasma elimination half-life of intravenous esomeprazole is approximately 1.1 to 1.4 hours and is prolonged with increasing dose of intravenous esomeprazole.
Special Populations
Investigation of age, gender, race, renal, and hepatic impairment and metabolizer status have been made previously with oral esomeprazole. The pharmacokinetics of esomeprazole is not expected to be affected differently by intrinsic or extrinsic factors after intravenous administration compared to oral administration. The same recommendations for dose adjustment in special populations are suggested for intravenous esomeprazole as for oral esomeprazole.
Geriatric
In oral studies, the AUC and C_{max} values were slightly higher (25% and 18%, respectively) in the elderly as compared to younger subjects at steady state. Dosage adjustment based on age is not necessary.
Pediatric
The pharmacokinetics of esomeprazole have not been studied in patients < 18 years of age.
Gender
In oral studies, the AUC and C_{max} values were slightly higher (13%) in females than in males at steady state. Similar differences have been seen for intravenous administration of esomeprazole. Dosage adjustment based on gender is not necessary.
Hepatic Insufficiency
In oral studies, the steady state pharmacokinetics of esomeprazole obtained after administration of 40 mg once daily to 4 patients each with mild (Child Pugh A), moderate (Child Pugh Class B), and severe (Child Pugh Class C) liver insufficiency were compared to those obtained in 36 male and female GERD patients with normal liver function. In patients with mild and moderate hepatic insufficiency, the AUCs were within the range that could be expected in patients with normal liver function. In patients with severe hepatic insufficiency the AUCs were 2 to 3 times higher than in the patients with normal liver function. No dosage adjustment is recommended for patients with mild to moderate hepatic insufficiency (Child Pugh Classes A and B). However, in patients with severe hepatic insufficiency (Child Pugh Class C) a dose of 20 mg once daily should not be exceeded. (See **DOSAGE AND ADMINISTRATION**).
Renal Insufficiency
The pharmacokinetics of esomeprazole in patients with renal impairment are not expected to be altered relative to healthy volunteers as less than 1% of esomeprazole is excreted unchanged in urine.
Pharmacodynamics
Mechanism of Action
Esomeprazole is a proton pump inhibitor that suppresses gastric acid secretion by specific inhibition of the H^+/K^+-ATPase in the gastric parietal cell. The S- and R-isomers of omeprazole are protonated and converted in the acidic compartment of the parietal cell forming the active inhibitor, the achiral sulphenamide. By acting specifically on the proton pump, esomeprazole blocks the final step in acid production, thus reducing gastric acidity. This effect is dose-related up to a daily dose of 20 to 40 mg and leads to inhibition of gastric acid secretion.
Antisecretory Activity
The effect of intravenous esomeprazole on intragastric pH was determined in two separate studies. In the first study, 20 mg of NEXIUM I.V. for Injection was administered intravenously once daily at constant rate over 30 minutes for 5 days. Twenty-two healthy subjects were included in the study. In the second study, 40 mg of NEXIUM I.V. for Injection was administered intravenously once daily at constant rate over 30 minutes for 5 days. Thirty-eight healthy were included in the study.

Effect of NEXIUM I.V. for Injection on Intragastric pH on Day 5		
	Esomeprazole 20 mg (n=22)	Esomeprazole 40 mg (n=38)
% Time Gastric pH>4	49.5	66.2
(95% CI)	41.9-57.2	62.4-70.0

Gastric pH was measured over a 24-hour period

Serum Gastrin Effects
In oral studies, the effect of NEXIUM on serum gastrin concentrations was evaluated in approximately 2,700 patients in clinical trials up to 8 weeks and in over 1,300 patients for up to 6-12 months. The mean fasting gastrin level increased in a dose-related manner. This increase reached a plateau within two to three months of therapy and returned to baseline levels within four weeks after discontinuation of therapy.
Enterochromaffin-like (ECL) Cell Effects
There are no data available on the effects of intravenous esomeprazole on ECL cells.
In 24-month carcinogenicity studies of oral omeprazole in rats, a dose-related significant occurrence of gastric ECL cell carcinoid tumors and ECL cell hyperplasia was observed in both male and female animals (see **PRECAUTIONS, Carcinogenesis, Mutagenesis, Impairment of Fertility**). Carcinoid tumors have also been observed in rats subjected to fundectomy or long-term treatment with other proton pump inhibitors or high doses of H_2-receptor antagonists.

Continued on next page

Nexium I.V.—Cont.

Human gastric biopsy specimens have been obtained from more than 3,000 patients treated orally with omeprazole in long-term clinical trials. The incidence of ECL cell hyperplasia in these studies increased with time; however, no case of ECL cell carcinoids, dysplasia, or neoplasia has been found in these patients.

In over 1,000 patients treated with NEXIUM (10, 20 or 40 mg/day) up to 6-12 months, the prevalence of ECL cell hyperplasia increased with time and dose. No patient developed ECL cell carcinoids, dysplasia, or neoplasia in the gastric mucosa.

Endocrine Effects

NEXIUM had no effect on thyroid function when given in oral doses of 20 or 40 mg for 4 weeks. Other effects of NEXIUM on the endocrine system were assessed using omeprazole studies. Omeprazole given in oral doses of 30 or 40 mg for 2 to 4 weeks had no effect on carbohydrate metabolism, circulating levels of parathyroid hormone, cortisol, estradiol, testosterone, prolactin, cholecystokinin or secretin.

Clinical Studies

Acid Suppression in Gastroesophageal Reflux Disease (GERD)

Four multicenter, open-label, two-period crossover studies were conducted to compare the pharmacodynamic efficacy of the intravenous formulation of esomeprazole (20 mg and 40 mg) to that of NEXIUM delayed-release capsules at corresponding doses in patients with symptoms of GERD, with or without erosive esophagitis. The patients (n=206, 18 to 72 years old; 112 female; 110 Caucasian, 50 Black, 10 Oriental, and 36 Other Race) were randomized to receive either 20 or 40 mg of intravenous or oral esomeprazole once daily for 10 days (Period 1), and then were switched in Period 2 to the other formulation for 10 days, matching their respective dose level from Period 1. The intravenous formulation was administered as a 3-minute injection in two of the studies, and as a 15-minute infusion in the other two studies. Basal acid output (BAO) and maximal acid output (MAO) were determined 22-24 hours post-dose on Period 1, Day 11; on Period 2, Day 3; and on Period 2, Day 11. BAO and MAO were estimated from 1-hour continuous collections of gastric contents prior to and following (respectively) subcutaneous injection of 6.0 μg/kg of pentagastrin.

In these studies, after 10 days of once daily administration, the intravenous dosage forms of NEXIUM 20 mg and 40 mg were similar to the corresponding oral dosage forms in their ability to suppress BAO and MAO in these GERD patients (see table below).

There were no major changes in acid suppression when switching between intravenous and oral dosage forms.

[See table below]

INDICATIONS AND USAGE

NEXIUM I.V. for Injection is indicated for the short-term treatment (up to 10 days) of GERD patients with a history of erosive esophagitis as an alternative to oral therapy in patients when therapy with NEXIUM Delayed-Release Capsules is not possible or appropriate.

When oral therapy is possible or appropriate, intravenous therapy with NEXIUM I.V. for Injection should be discontinued and the therapy should be continued orally.

CONTRAINDICATIONS

NEXIUM is contraindicated in patients with known hypersensitivity to any component of the formulation or to substituted benzimidazoles.

PRECAUTIONS

General

Symptomatic response to therapy with NEXIUM does not preclude the presence of gastric malignancy.

Atrophic gastritis has been noted occasionally in gastric corpus biopsies from patients treated long-term with omeprazole, of which NEXIUM is an enantiomer.

Treatment with NEXIUM I.V. for Injection should be discontinued as soon as the patient is able to resume treatment with NEXIUM Delayed-Release Capsules.

Drug Interactions

Esomeprazole is extensively metabolized in the liver by CYP2C19 and CYP3A4.

In vitro and *in vivo* studies have shown that esomeprazole is not likely to inhibit CYPs 1A2, 2A6, 2C9, 2D6, 2E1 and 3A4. No clinically relevant interactions with drugs metabolized by these CYP enzymes would be expected. Drug interaction studies have shown that esomeprazole does not have any clinically significant interactions with phenytoin, warfarin, quinidine, clarithromycin or amoxicillin. Post-marketing reports of changes in prothrombin measures have been received among patients on concomitant warfarin and esomeprazole therapy. Increases in INR and prothrombin time may lead to abnormal bleeding and even death. Patients treated with proton pump inhibitors and warfarin concomitantly may need to be monitored for increases in INR and prothrombin time.

Esomeprazole may potentially interfere with CYP2C19, the major esomeprazole metabolizing enzyme. Coadministration of esomeprazole 30 mg and diazepam, a CYP2C19 substrate, resulted in a 45% decrease in clearance of diazepam. Increased plasma levels of diazepam were observed 12 hours after dosing and onwards. However, at that time, the plasma levels of diazepam were below the therapeutic interval, and thus this interaction is unlikely to be of clinical relevance.

Coadministration of oral contraceptives, diazepam, phenytoin, or quinidine did not seem to change the pharmacokinetic profile of esomeprazole.

Studies evaluating concomitant administration of esomeprazole and either naproxen (non-selective NSAID) or rofecoxib (COX-2 selective NSAID) did not identify any clinically relevant changes in the pharmacokinetic profiles of esomeprazole or these NSAIDs.

Esomeprazole inhibits gastric acid secretion. Therefore, esomeprazole may interfere with the absorption of drugs where gastric pH is an important determinant of bioavailability (eg, ketoconazole, iron salts and digoxin).

Carcinogenesis, Mutagenesis, Impairment of Fertility

The carcinogenic potential of esomeprazole was assessed using omeprazole studies. In two 24-month oral carcinogenicity studies in rats, omeprazole at daily doses of 1.7, 3.4, 13.8, 44.0 and 140.8 mg/kg/day (about 0.7 to 57 times the human dose of 20 mg/day expressed on a body surface area basis) produced gastric ECL cell carcinoids in a dose-related manner in both male and female rats; the incidence of this effect was markedly higher in female rats, which had higher blood levels of omeprazole. Gastric carcinoids seldom occur in the untreated rat. In addition, ECL cell hyperplasia was present in all treated groups of both sexes. In one of these studies, female rats were treated with 13.8 mg omeprazole/kg/day (about 5.6 times the human dose on a body surface area basis) for 1 year, then followed for an additional year without the drug. No carcinoids were seen in these rats. An increased incidence of treatment-related ECL cell hyperplasia was observed at the end of 1 year (94% treated vs 10% controls). By the second year the difference between treated and control rats was much smaller (46% vs 26%) but still showed more hyperplasia in the treated group. Gastric adenocarcinoma was seen in one rat (2%). No similar tumor was seen in male or female rats treated for 2 years. For this strain of rat no similar tumor has been noted historically, but a finding involving only one tumor is difficult to interpret. A 78-week oral mouse carcinogenicity study of omeprazole did not show increased tumor occurrence, but the study was not conclusive.

Esomeprazole was negative in the Ames mutation test, in the *in vivo* rat bone marrow cell chromosome aberration test, and the *in vivo* mouse micronucleus test. Esomeprazole, however, was positive in the *in vitro* human lymphocyte chromosome aberration test. Omeprazole was positive in the *in vitro* human lymphocyte chromosome aberration test, the *in vivo* mouse bone marrow cell chromosome aberration test, and the *in vivo* mouse micronucleus test.

The potential effects of esomeprazole on fertility and reproductive performance were assessed using omeprazole studies. Omeprazole at oral doses up to 138 mg/kg/day in rats (about 56 times the human dose on a body surface area basis) was found to have no effect on reproductive performance of parental animals.

Pregnancy

Teratogenic Effects. Pregnancy Category B

Teratology studies have been performed in rats at oral doses up to 280 mg/kg/day (about 57 times the human dose on a body surface area basis) and in rabbits at oral doses up to 86 mg/kg/day (about 35 times the human dose on a body surface area basis) and have revealed no evidence of impaired fertility or harm to the fetus due to esomeprazole. There are, however, no adequate and well-controlled studies in pregnant women. Because animal reproduction studies are not always predictive of human response, this drug should be used during pregnancy only if clearly needed.

Teratology studies conducted with omeprazole in rats at oral doses up to 138 mg/kg/day (about 56 times the human dose on a body surface area basis) and in rabbits at doses up to 69 mg/kg/day (about 56 times the human dose on a body surface area basis) did not disclose any evidence for a teratogenic potential of omeprazole. In rabbits, omeprazole in a dose range of 6.9 to 69.1 mg/kg/day (about 5.5 to 56 times the human dose on a body surface area basis) produced dose-related increases in embryo-lethality, fetal resorptions, and pregnancy disruptions. In rats, dose-related embryo/fetal toxicity and postnatal developmental toxicity were observed in offspring resulting from parents treated with omeprazole at 13.8 to 138.0 mg/kg/day (about 5.6 to 56 times the human doses on a body surface area basis). There are no adequate and well-controlled studies in pregnant women. Sporadic reports have been received of congenital abnormalities occurring in infants born to women who have received omeprazole during pregnancy.

Nursing Mothers

The excretion of esomeprazole in milk has not been studied. However, omeprazole concentrations have been measured in breast milk of a woman following oral administration of 20 mg. Because esomeprazole is likely to be excreted in human milk, because of the potential for serious adverse reactions in nursing infants from esomeprazole, and because of the potential for tumorigenicity shown for omeprazole in rat carcinogenicity studies, a decision should be made whether to discontinue nursing or to discontinue the drug, taking into account the importance of the drug to the mother.

Pediatric Use

Safety and effectiveness in pediatric patients have not been established.

Geriatric Use

Of the total number of patients who received oral NEXIUM in clinical trials, 1,459 were 65 to 74 years of age and 354 patients were ≥75 years of age.

No overall differences in safety and efficacy were observed between the elderly and younger individuals, and other reported clinical experience has not identified differences in responses between the elderly and younger patients, but greater sensitivity of some older individuals cannot be ruled out.

ADVERSE REACTIONS

Safety Experience with Intravenous NEXIUM

The safety of intravenous esomeprazole is based on results from clinical trials conducted in three different populations including patients having symptomatic GERD with or without a history of erosive esophagitis (n=206), patients with erosive esophagitis (n=246) and healthy subjects (n=204).

Adverse experiences occurring in >1% of patients treated with intravenous esomeprazole (n=359) in trials irrespective of the relationship to NEXIUM are listed below by body system:

Skin and appendages disorders: pruritus (1.1%); ***Central and peripheral nervous system disorders:*** dizziness (2.5%), headache (10.9%); ***Gastrointestinal system disorders:*** abdominal pain (5.8%), constipation (2.5%), diarrhea (3.9%), dyspepsia (6.4%), flatulence (10.3%), mouth dry (3.9%), nausea (6.4%); ***Respiratory system disorders:*** respiratory infection (1.1%), sinusitis (1.7%); ***Body as a whole – general disorders:*** AE associated with test procedure (23.1%); and ***Application site disorders:*** application site reaction (1.7%) (including mild focal erythema and pruritus at IV insertion site).

Intravenous treatment with esomeprazole 20 and 40 mg administered as an injection or as an infusion was found to have a safety profile similar to that of oral administration of esomeprazole 20 and 40 mg.

Safety Experience with Oral NEXIUM

The safety of oral NEXIUM was evaluated in over 15,000 patients (aged 18-84 years) in clinical trials worldwide including over 8,500 patients in the United States and over 6,500 patients in Europe and Canada. Over 2,900 patients were treated in long-term studies for up to 6-12 months.

The safety in the treatment of healing of erosive esophagitis was assessed in four randomized comparative clinical trials, which included 1,240 patients on NEXIUM 20 mg, 2,434 patients on NEXIUM 40 mg, and 3,008 patients on omeprazole 20 mg daily. The most frequently occurring adverse events (≥1%) in all three groups was headache (5.5, 5.0, and 3.8, respectively) and diarrhea (no difference among the three groups). Nausea, flatulence, abdominal pain, constipation, and dry mouth occurred at similar rates among patients taking NEXIUM or omeprazole.

Additional adverse events that were reported as possibly or probably related to NEXIUM with an incidence <1% are listed below by body system:

Body as a Whole: abdomen enlarged, allergic reaction, asthenia, back pain, chest pain, chest pain substernal, facial edema, peripheral edema, hot flushes, fatigue, fever, flu-like disorder, generalized edema, leg edema, malaise, pain, rigors; ***Cardiovascular:*** flushing, hypertension, tachycardia; ***Endocrine:*** goiter; ***Gastrointestinal:*** bowel irregularity, constipation aggravated, dyspepsia, dysphagia, dysplasia GI, epigastric pain, eructation, esophageal disorder, frequent stools, gastroenteritis, GI hemorrhage, GI symptoms not otherwise specified, hiccup, melena, mouth disorder, pharynx disorder, rectal disorder, serum gastrin increased, tongue disorder, tongue edema, ulcerative stomatitis, vomiting; ***Hearing:*** earache, tinnitus; ***Hematologic:*** anemia, anemia hypochromic, cervical lymphoadenopathy, epistaxis, leukocytosis, leukopenia, thrombocytopenia; ***Hepatic:*** bilirubinemia, hepatic function abnormal, SGOT increased, SGPT increased; ***Metabolic/Nutritional:*** glycosuria, hyperuricemia, hyponatremia, increased alkaline phosphatase, thirst, vitamin B12 deficiency, weight increase, weight decrease; ***Musculoskeletal:*** arthralgia, arthritis aggravated, arthropathy, cramps, fibromyalgia syndrome, hernia, poly-

Mean (SD) BAO and MAO measured 22-24 hours post-dose following once daily oral and intravenous administration of esomeprazole for 10 days in GERD patients with or without a history of erosive esophagitis

Study	Dose in mg	Intravenous Administration Method	BAO in mmol H^+/h		MAO in mmol H^+/h	
			Intravenous	Oral	Intravenous	Oral
1 (N=42)	20	3-minute injection	0.71 (1.24)	0.69 (1.24)	5.96 (5.41)	5.27 (5.39)
2 (N=44)	20	15-minute infusion	0.78 (1.38)	0.82 (1.34)	5.95 (4.00)	5.26 (4.12)
3 (N=50)	40	3-minute injection	0.36 (0.61)	0.31 (0.55)	5.06 (3.90)	4.41 (3.11)
4 (N=47)	40	15-minute infusion	0.36 (0.79)	0.22 (0.39)	4.74 (3.65)	3.52 (2.86)

myalgia rheumatica; ***Nervous System/Psychiatric:*** anorexia, apathy, appetite increased, confusion, depression aggravated, dizziness, hypertonia, nervousness, hypoesthesia, impotence, insomnia, migraine, migraine aggravated, paresthesia, sleep disorder, somnolence, tremor, vertigo, visual field defect; ***Reproductive:*** dysmenorrhea, menstrual disorder, vaginitis; ***Respiratory:*** asthma aggravated, coughing, dyspnea, larynx edema, pharyngitis, rhinitis, sinusitis; ***Skin and Appendages:*** acne, angioedema, dermatitis, pruritus, pruritus ani, rash, rash erythematous, rash maculo-papular, skin inflammation, sweating increased, urticaria; ***Special Senses:*** otitis media, parosmia, taste loss, taste perversion; ***Urogenital:*** abnormal urine, albuminuria, cystitis, dysuria, fungal infection, hematuria, micturition frequency, moniliasis, genital moniliasis, polyuria; ***Visual:*** conjunctivitis, vision abnormal.

Endoscopic findings that were reported as adverse events include: duodenitis, esophagitis, esophageal stricture, esophageal ulceration, esophageal varices, gastric ulcer, gastritis, hernia, benign polyps or nodules, Barrett's esophagus, and mucosal discoloration.

The incidence of treatment-related adverse events during 6-month maintenance treatment was similar to placebo. There were no differences in types of related adverse events seen during maintenance treatment up to 12 months compared to short-term treatment.

Two placebo-controlled studies were conducted in 710 patients for the treatment of symptomatic gastroesophageal reflux disease. The most common adverse events that were reported as possibly or probably related to NEXIUM were diarrhea (4.3%), headache (3.8%), and abdominal pain (3.8%).

Postmarketing Reports – There have been spontaneous reports of adverse events with postmarketing use of esomeprazole. These reports have included rare cases of anaphylactic reaction and severe dermatologic reactions, including toxic epidermal necrolysis (TEN, some fatal), Stevens-Johnson syndrome, and erythema multiforme, and pancreatitis. Other adverse events not observed with NEXIUM, but occurring with omeprazole can be found in the omeprazole package insert, **ADVERSE REACTIONS** section.

Laboratory Events

The following potentially clinically significant laboratory changes in clinical trials, irrespective of relationship to NEXIUM, were reported in ≤1% of patients: increased creatinine, uric acid, total bilirubin, alkaline phosphatase, ALT, AST, hemoglobin, white blood cell count, platelets, serum gastrin, potassium, sodium, thyroxine and thyroid stimulating hormone (see **CLINICAL PHARMACOLOGY**, *Endocrine Effects* for further information on thyroid effects). Decreases were seen in hemoglobin, white blood cell count, platelets, potassium, sodium, and thyroxine.

OVERDOSAGE

The minimum lethal dose of esomeprazole sodium in rats after bolus administration was 310 mg/kg (about 62 times the human dose on a body surface area basis). The major signs of acute toxicity were reduced motor activity, changes in respiratory frequency, tremor, ataxia and intermittent clonic convulsions.

There have been some reports of overdosage with oral esomeprazole. Reports have been received of overdosage with oral omeprazole in humans. Doses ranged up to 2,400 mg (120 times the usual recommended clinical dose). Manifestations were variable, but included confusion, drowsiness, blurred vision, tachycardia, nausea, diaphoresis, flushing, headache, dry mouth, and other adverse reactions similar to those seen in normal clinical experience (see omeprazole package insert - **ADVERSE REACTIONS**). No specific antidote for esomeprazole is known. Since esomeprazole is extensively protein bound, it is not expected to be removed by dialysis. In the event of overdosage, treatment should be symptomatic and supportive.

As with the management of any overdose, the possibility of multiple drug ingestion should be considered. For current information on treatment of any drug overdose, a certified Regional Poison Control Center should be contacted. Telephone numbers are listed in the Physicians' Desk Reference (PDR) or local telephone book.

DOSAGE AND ADMINISTRATION

GERD with a history of Erosive Esophagitis

The recommended adult dose is either 20 or 40 mg esomeprazole given once daily by intravenous injection (no less than 3 minutes) or intravenous infusion (10 to 30 minutes). NEXIUM I.V. for Injection should not be administered concomitantly with any other medications through the same intravenous site and or tubing. The intravenous line should always be flushed with either 0.9% Sodium Chloride Injection, USP, Lactated Ringer's Injection, USP or 5% Dextrose Injection, USP both prior to and after administration of NEXIUM I.V. for Injection.

Treatment with NEXIUM I.V. for Injection should be discontinued as soon as the patient is able to resume treatment with NEXIUM Delayed-Release Capsules.

Safety and efficacy of NEXIUM I.V. for Injection as a treatment of GERD patients with a history of erosive esophagitis for more than 10 days have not been demonstrated (see **INDICATIONS AND USAGE**).

Special Populations

Geriatric: No dosage adjustment is necessary. (See **CLINICAL PHARMACOLOGY, Pharmacokinetics.**)

Renal Insufficiency: No dosage adjustment is necessary. (See **CLINICAL PHARMACOLOGY, Pharmacokinetics.**)

Hepatic Insufficiency: No dosage adjustment is necessary in patients with mild to moderate liver impairment (Child Pugh Classes A and B). For patients with severe liver impairment (Child Pugh Class C), a dose of 20 mg of NEXIUM should not be exceeded (See **CLINICAL PHARMACOLOGY, Pharmacokinetics.**)

Gender: No dosage adjustment is necessary. (See **CLINICAL PHARMACOLOGY, Pharmacokinetics.**)

Preparations for use:

Intravenous Injection (20 or 40 mg) over no less than 3 minutes

The freeze-dried powder should be reconstituted with 5 mL of 0.9% Sodium Chloride Injection, USP. Withdraw 5 mL of the reconstituted solution and administer as an intravenous injection over no less than 3 minutes.

The reconstituted solution should be stored at room temperature up to 30°C (86°F) and administered within 12 hours after reconstitution. No refrigeration is required.

Intravenous Infusion (20 or 40 mg) over 10 to 30 minutes

A solution for intravenous infusion is prepared by first reconstituting the contents of one vial with 5 mL of 0.9% Sodium Chloride Injection, USP, Lactated Ringer's Injection, USP or 5% Dextrose Injection, USP and further diluting the resulting solution to a final volume of 50 mL. The solution (admixture) should be administered as an intravenous infusion over a period of 10 to 30 minutes.

The admixture should be stored at room temperature up to 30°C (86°F) and should be administered within the designated time period as listed in the Table below. No refrigeration is required.

Diluent	Administer within:
0.9% Sodium Chloride Injection, USP	12 hours
Lactated Ringer's Injection, USP	12 hours
5% Dextrose Injection, USP	6 hours

NEXIUM I.V. for Injection should not be administered concomitantly with any other medications through the same intravenous site and or tubing. The intravenous line should always be flushed with either 0.9% Sodium Chloride Injection, USP, Lactated Ringer's Injection, USP or 5% Dextrose Injection, USP both prior to and after administration of NEXIUM I.V. for Injection.

Parenteral drug products should be inspected visually for particulate matter and discoloration prior to administration, whenever solution and container permit.

HOW SUPPLIED

NEXIUM I.V. for Injection is supplied as a freeze-dried powder containing 20 mg or 40 mg of esomeprazole per single-use vial.

NDC 0186-6020-01 one carton containing 10 vials of NEXIUM I.V. for Injection (each vial contains 20 mg of esomeprazole).

NDC 0186-6040-01 one carton containing 10 vials of NEXIUM I.V. for Injection (each vial contains 40 mg of esomeprazole).

Storage

Store at 25°C (77°F); excursions permitted to 15°-30°C (59°-86°F). [See USP Controlled Room Temperature]. Protect from light. Store in carton until time of use.

NEXIUM is a registered trademark of the AstraZeneca group of companies

AstraZeneca LP
Wilmington, DE 19850
808628-00 Rev. 03/05

AstraZeneca

To keep your **PDR** up to date throughout the year, note these revisions on the corresponding pages of the annual volume. Simply write **"See Supplement A"** next to the product heading.

AstraZeneca Pharmaceuticals LP

1800 CONCORD PIKE
WILMINGTON, DE 19850-5437 USA

For Product Full Prescribing Information, Business Information, Medical Information, Adverse Drug Experiences, and Customer Service:

Information Center
1-800-236-9933

For Product Ordering:

Trade Customer Service
1-800-842-9920

For Product Full Prescribing Information:

Internet: www.astrazeneca-us.com

ZOMIG® ℞
[*zō' mig*]
(zolmitriptan)
TABLETS
ZOMIG-ZMT®
ZOLMITRIPTAN
ORALLY DISINTEGRATING TABLETS

DESCRIPTION

ZOMIG® (zolmitriptan) Tablets and ZOMIG-ZMT® (zolmitriptan) Orally Disintegrating Tablets contain zolmitriptan, which is a selective 5-hydroxytryptamine $_{1B/1D}$ ($5\text{-HT}_{1B/1D}$) receptor agonist. Zolmitriptan is chemically designated as (S)-4-[[3-[2-(dimethylamino)ethyl]-1H-indol-5-yl]methyl]-2-oxazolidinone and has the following chemical structure:

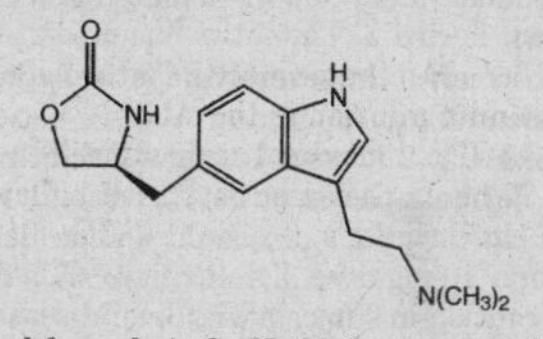

The empirical formula is $C_{16}H_{21}N_3O_2$, representing a molecular weight of 287.36. Zolmitriptan is a white to almost white powder that is readily soluble in water. ZOMIG Tablets are available as 2.5 mg (yellow) and 5 mg (pink) film coated tablets for oral administration. The film coated tablets contain anhydrous lactose NF, microcrystalline cellulose NF, sodium starch glycolate NF, magnesium stearate NF, hydroxypropyl methylcellulose USP, titanium dioxide USP, polyethylene glycol 400 NF, yellow iron oxide NF (2.5 mg tablet), red iron oxide NF (5 mg tablet), and polyethylene glycol 8000 NF.

ZOMIG-ZMT® Orally Disintegrating Tablets are available as 2.5 mg and 5.0 mg white uncoated tablets for oral administration. The orally disintegrating tablets contain mannitol USP, microcrystalline cellulose NF, crospovidone NF, aspartame NF, sodium bicarbonate USP, citric acid anhydrous USP, colloidal silicon dioxide NF, magnesium stearate NF and orange flavor SN 027512.

CLINICAL PHARMACOLOGY

Mechanism of Action: Zolmitriptan binds with high affinity to human recombinant 5-HT_{1D} and 5-HT_{1B} receptors. Zolmitriptan exhibits modest affinity for 5-HT_{1A} receptors, but has no significant affinity (as measured by radioligand binding assays) or pharmacological activity at 5-HT_2, 5-HT_3, 5-HT_4, $alpha_1$-, $alpha_2$- or $beta_1$-adrenergic; H_1, H_2, histaminic; muscarinic; $dopamine_1$, or $dopamine_2$ receptors. The N-desmethyl metabolite also has high affinity for $5\text{-HT}_{1B/1D}$ and modest affinity for 5-HT_{1A} receptors.

Current theories proposed to explain the etiology of migraine headache suggest that symptoms are due to local cranial vasodilatation and/or to the release of sensory neuropeptides (vasoactive intestinal peptide, substance P and calcitonin gene-related peptide) through nerve endings in the trigeminal system. The therapeutic activity of zolmitriptan for the treatment of migraine headache can most likely be attributed to the agonist effects at the $5\text{-HT}_{1B/1D}$ receptors on intracranial blood vessels (including the arterio-venous anastomoses) and sensory nerves of the trigeminal system which result in cranial vessel constriction and inhibition of pro-inflammatory neuropeptide release.

Clinical Pharmacokinetics and Bioavailability:

Absorption: Zolmitriptan is well absorbed after oral administration for both the conventional tablets and the orally disintegrating tablets. Zolmitriptan displays linear kinetics over the dose range of 2.5 to 50 mg.

The AUC and C_{max} of zolmitriptan are similar following administration of ZOMIG Tablets and ZOMIG-ZMT Orally Disintegrating Tablets, but the T_{max} is somewhat later with ZOMIG-ZMT, with a median T_{max} of 3 hours for the orally disintegrating tablet compared with 1.5 hours for the conventional tablet. The AUC, C_{max}, and T_{max} for the active N-desmethyl metabolite are similar for the two formulations.

During a moderate to severe migraine attack, mean AUC_{0-4} and C_{max} for zolmitriptan, dosed as a conventional tablet, were decreased by 40% and 25%, respectively, and mean T_{max} was delayed by one-half hour compared to the same patients during a migraine free period.

Continued on next page

Zomig/Zomig ZMT—Cont.

Food has no significant effect on the bioavailability of zolmitriptan. No accumulation occurred on multiple dosing.
Distribution: Mean absolute bioavailability is approximately 40%. The mean apparent volume of distribution is 7.0 L/kg. Plasma protein binding of zolmitriptan is 25% over the concentration range of 10-1000 ng/mL.
Metabolism: Zolmitriptan is converted to an active N-desmethyl metabolite such that the metabolite concentrations are about two thirds that of zolmitriptan. Because the $5HT_{1B/1D}$ potency of the metabolite is 2 to 6 times that of the parent, the metabolite may contribute a substantial portion of the overall effect after zolmitriptan administration.
Elimination: Total radioactivity recovered in urine and feces was 65% and 30% of the administered dose, respectively. About 8% of the dose was recovered in the urine as unchanged zolmitriptan. Indole acetic acid metabolite accounted for 31% of the dose, followed by N-oxide (7%) and N-desmethyl (4%) metabolites. The indole acetic acid and N-oxide metabolites are inactive.
Mean total plasma clearance is 31.5 mL/min/kg, of which one-sixth is renal clearance. The renal clearance is greater than the glomerular filtration rate suggesting renal tubular secretion.
Special Populations
Age: Zolmitriptan pharmacokinetics in healthy elderly non-migraineur volunteers (age 65–76 yrs) were similar to those in younger non-migraineur volunteers (age 18-39 yrs).
Gender: Mean plasma concentrations of zolmitriptan were up to 1.5-fold higher in females than males.
Renal Impairment: Clearance of zolmitriptan was reduced by 25% in patients with severe renal impairment (Clcr ≥ 5 ≤ 25 mL/min) compared to the normal group (Clcr > = 70 mL/min); no significant change in clearance was observed in the moderately renally impaired group (Clcr ≥ 26 ≤ 50 mL/min).
Hepatic Impairment: In severely hepatically impaired patients, the mean C_{max}, T_{max}, and $AUC_{0-\infty}$ of zolmitriptan were increased 1.5, 2 (2 vs 4 hr), and 3-fold, respectively, compared to normals. Seven out of 27 patients experienced 20 to 80 mm Hg elevations in systolic and/or diastolic blood pressure after a 10 mg dose. Zolmitriptan should be administered with caution in subjects with liver disease, generally using doses less than 2.5 mg (see WARNINGS and PRECAUTIONS).
Hypertensive Patients: No differences in the pharmacokinetics of zolmitriptan or its effects on blood pressure were seen in mild to moderate hypertensive volunteers compared to normotensive controls.
Race: Retrospective analysis of pharmacokinetic data between Japanese and Caucasians revealed no significant differences.
Drug Interactions: All drug interaction studies were performed in healthy volunteers using a single 10 mg dose of zolmitriptan and a single dose of the other drug except where otherwise noted.
Fluoxetine: The pharmacokinetics of zolmitriptan, as well as its effect on blood pressure, were unaffected by 4 weeks of pretreatment with oral fluoxetine (20 mg/day).
MAO Inhibitors: Following one week of administration of 150 mg bid moclobemide, a specific MAO-A inhibitor, there was an increase of about 25% in both C_{max} and AUC for zolmitriptan and a 3-fold increase in the C_{max} and AUC of the active N-desmethyl metabolite of zolmitriptan (see CONTRAINDICATIONS and PRECAUTIONS).
Selegiline, a selective MAO-B inhibitor, at a dose of 10 mg/day for 1 week, had no effect on the pharmacokinetics of zolmitriptan and its metabolite.
Propranolol: C_{max} and AUC of zolmitriptan increased 1.5-fold after one week of dosing with propranolol (160 mg/day). C_{max} and AUC of the N-desmethyl metabolite were reduced by 30% and 15%, respectively. There were no interactive effects on blood pressure or pulse rate following administration of propranolol with zolmitriptan.
Acetaminophen: A single 1 g dose of acetaminophen does not alter the pharmacokinetics of zolmitriptan and its N-desmethyl metabolite. However, zolmitriptan delayed the T_{max} of acetaminophen by one hour.
Metoclopramide: A single 10 mg dose of metoclopramide had no effect on the pharmacokinetics of zolmitriptan or its metabolites.
Oral Contraceptives: Retrospective analysis of pharmacokinetic data across studies indicated that mean plasma concentrations of zolmitriptan were generally higher in females taking oral contraceptives compared to those not taking oral contraceptives. Mean C_{max} and AUC of zolmitriptan were found to be higher by 30% and 50%, respectively, and T_{max} was delayed by one-half hour in females taking oral contraceptives. The effect of zolmitriptan on the pharmacokinetics of oral contraceptives has not been studied.
Cimetidine: Following the administration of cimetidine, the half-life and AUC of a 5 mg dose of zolmitriptan and its active metabolite were approximately doubled (see PRECAUTIONS).
Clinical Studies: The efficacy of ZOMIG Tablets in the acute treatment of migraine headaches was demonstrated in five randomized, double-blind, placebo controlled studies, of which 2 utilized the 1 mg dose, 2 utilized the 2.5 mg dose and 4 utilized the 5 mg dose; all studies used the marketed formulation. In study 1, patients treated their headaches in a clinic setting. In the other studies, patients treated their headaches as outpatients. In study 4, patients who had previously used sumatriptan were excluded, whereas in the other studies no such exclusion was applied. Patients enrolled in these 5 studies were predominantly female (82%) and Caucasian (97%) with a mean age of 40 years (range 12-65). Patients were instructed to treat a moderate to severe headache. Headache response, defined as a reduction in headache severity from moderate or severe pain to mild or no pain, was assessed at 1, 2, and, in most studies, 4 hours after dosing. Associated symptoms such as nausea, photophobia, and phonophobia were also assessed. Maintenance of response was assessed for up to 24 hours postdose. A second dose of ZOMIG Tablets or other medication was allowed 2 to 24 hours after the initial treatment for persistent and recurrent headache. The frequency and time to use of these additional treatments were also recorded. In all studies, the effect of zolmitriptan was compared to placebo in the treatment of a single migraine attack.
In all five studies, the percentage of patients achieving headache response 2 hours after treatment was significantly greater among patients receiving ZOMIG Tablets at all doses (except for the 1 mg dose in the smallest study) compared to those who received placebo. In the two studies that evaluated the 1 mg dose, there was a statistically significant greater percentage of patients with headache response at 2 hours in the higher dose groups (2.5 and/or 5 mg) compared to the 1 mg dose group. There were no statistically significant differences between the 2.5 and 5 mg dose groups (or of doses up to 20 mg) for the primary end point of headache response at 2 hours in any study. The results of these controlled clinical studies are summarized in Table 1.
Comparisons of drug performance based upon results obtained in different clinical trials are never reliable. Because studies are conducted at different times, with different samples of patients, by different investigators, employing different criteria and/or different interpretations of the same criteria, under different conditions (dose, dosing regimen, etc.), quantitative estimates of treatment response and the timing of response may be expected to vary considerably from study to study.

Table 1: Percentage of Patients with Headache Response (Mild or no Headache) 2 Hours Following Treatment (n=number of patients randomized)

	Placebo	ZOMIG 1.0 mg	ZOMIG 2.5 mg	ZOMIG 5 mg
Study 1[a]	16% (n=19)	27% (n=22)	NA	60%*# (n=20)
Study 2	19% (n=88)	NA	NA	66%* (n=179)
Study 3	34% (n=121)	50%* (n=140)	65%*# (n=260)	67%*# (n=245)
Study 4[b]	44% (n=55)	NA	NA	59%* (n=491)
Study 5	36% (n=92)	NA NA	62%* (n=178)	NA

* p<0.05 in comparison with placebo.
\# p<0.05 in comparison with 1 mg.
a This was the only study in which patients treated the headache in a clinic setting.
b This was the only study where patients were excluded who had previously used sumatriptan.
NA - not applicable

The estimated probability of achieving an initial headache response by 4 hours following treatment is depicted in Figure 1.

Figure 1: Estimated Probability of achieving initial headache response within 4 hours*

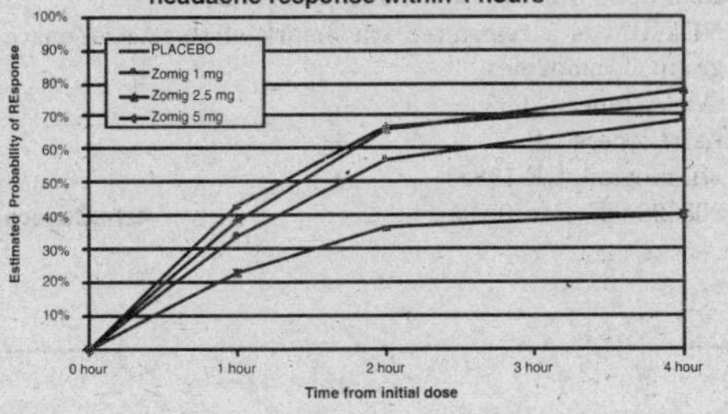

*Figure 1 shows the Kaplan-Meier plot of the probability over time of obtaining headache response (no or mild pain) following treatment with zolmitriptan. The averages displayed are based on pooled data from 3 placebo-controlled, outpatient trials providing evidence of efficacy (Trials 2, 3 and 5). Patients not achieving headache response or taking additional treatment prior to 4 hours were censored to 4 hours.
For patients with migraine associated photophobia, phonophobia, and nausea at baseline, there was a decreased incidence of these symptoms following administration of ZOMIG as compared to placebo.
Two to 24 hours following the initial dose of study treatment, patients were allowed to use additional treatment for pain relief in the form of a second dose of study treatment or other medication. The estimated probability of patients taking a second dose or other medication for migraine over the 24 hours following the initial dose of study treatment is summarized in Figure 2.

Figure 2: The Estimated Probability Of Patients Taking A Second Dose Or Other Medication For Migraines Over The 24 Hours Following The Initial Dose Of Study Treatment*

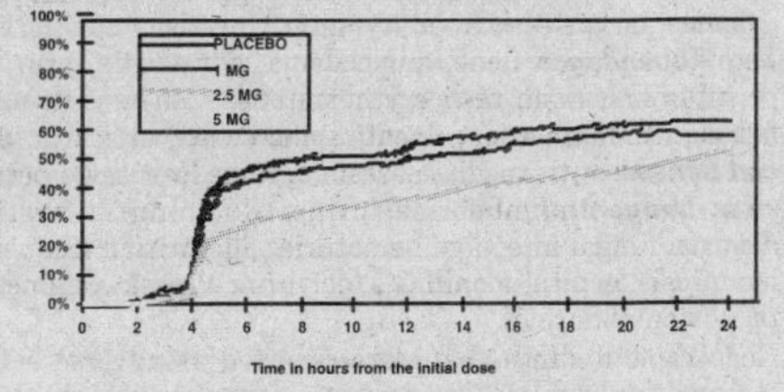

*This Kaplan-Meier plot is based on data obtained in 3 placebo controlled clinical trials (Study 2, 3 and 5). Patients not using additional treatments were censored at 24 hours. The plot includes both patients who had headache response at 2 hours and those who had no response to the initial dose. It should be noted that the protocols did not allow remedication within 2 hours postdose.

The efficacy of ZOMIG was unaffected by presence of aura; duration of headache prior to treatment; relationship to menses; gender, age, or weight of the patient; pretreatment nausea or concomitant use of common migraine prophylactic drugs.
ZOMIG-ZMT Orally Disintegrating Tablets
The efficacy of ZOMIG-ZMT 2.5 mg was demonstrated in a randomized, placebo-controlled trial that was similar in design to the trials of ZOMIG Tablets. Patients were instructed to treat a moderate to severe headache. Of the 471 patients treated in the study, 87% were female and 97% were Caucasian, with a mean age of 41 years (range 18-62). At 2 hours post-dosing response rates in patients treated with ZOMIG-ZMT 2.5 mg were 63% compared to 22% in the placebo group. The difference was statistically significant. The estimated probability of achieving an initial headache response by 2 hours following treatment with ZOMIG-ZMT Tablets is depicted in Figure 3.

Figure 3: Estimated Probability of Achieving Initial Headache Response by 2 Hours

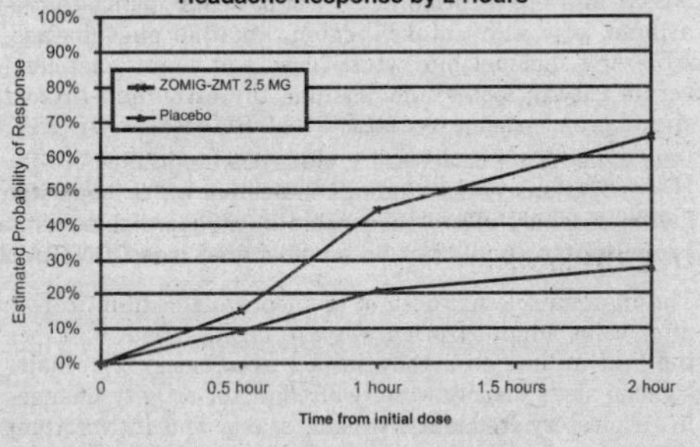

Figure 3 shows the Kaplan-Meier plot of the probability over time of obtaining headache response (no or mild pain) following treatment with ZOMIG-ZMT Tablets or placebo. Patients taking additional treatment or not achieving headache response prior to 2 hours were censored at 2 hours.
For patients with migraine-associated photophobia, phonophobia and nausea at baseline, there was a decreased incidence of these symptoms following administration of ZOMIG-ZMT as compared to placebo.
Two to 24 hours following the initial dose of study treatment, patients were allowed to use additional treatment in the form of a second dose of study treatment or other medication. The estimated probability of patients taking a second dose or other medication for migraine over the 24 hours following the initial dose of study treatment is summarized in Figure 4.

Figure 4: The Estimated Probability of Patients Taking a Second Dose or Other Medication for Migraines Over the 24 Hours Following The Initial Dose of Study Treatment

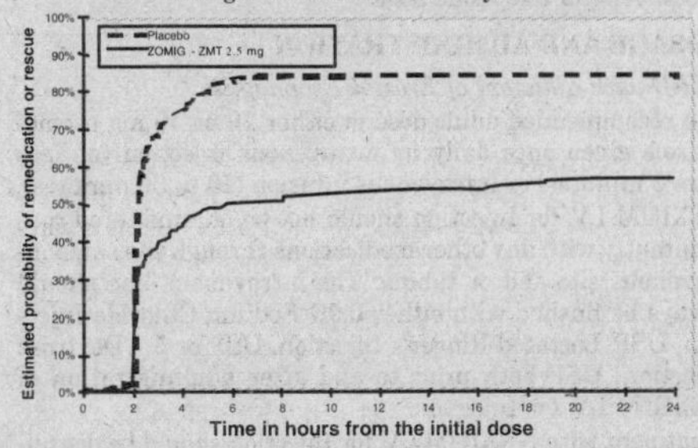

In this Kaplan-Meier plot, patients not using additional treatments were censored at 24 hours. The plot includes both patients who had headache response at 2 hours and those who had no response to the initial dose. Remedication was allowed 2 hours post-dose, and unlike the conventional tablet, remedication prior to 4 hours was not discouraged.

INDICATIONS AND USAGE

ZOMIG is indicated for the acute treatment of migraine with or without aura in adults.
ZOMIG is not intended for the prophylactic therapy of migraine or for use in the management of hemiplegic or basi-

lar migraine (see CONTRAINDICATIONS). Safety and effectiveness of ZOMIG have not been established for cluster headache, which is present in an older, predominantly male population.

CONTRAINDICATIONS

ZOMIG should not be given to patients with ischemic heart disease (angina pectoris, history of myocardial infarction, or documented silent ischemia) or to patients who have symptoms or findings consistent with ischemic heart disease, coronary artery vasospasm, including Prinzmetal's variant angina, or other significant underlying cardiovascular disease (see WARNINGS).

Because ZOMIG may increase blood pressure, it should not be given to patients with uncontrolled hypertension (see WARNINGS).

ZOMIG should not be used within 24 hours of treatment with another 5-HT$_1$ agonist, or an ergotamine-containing or ergot-type medication like dihydroergotamine or methysergide.

ZOMIG should not be administered to patients with hemiplegic or basilar migraine.

Concurrent administration of MAO-A inhibitors or use of zolmitriptan within 2 weeks of discontinuation of MAO-A inhibitor therapy is contraindicated (see CLINICAL PHARMACOLOGY: Drug Interactions and PRECAUTIONS: Drug Interactions).

ZOMIG is contraindicated in patients who are hypersensitive to zolmitriptan or any of its inactive ingredients.

WARNINGS

ZOMIG should only be used where a clear diagnosis of migraine has been established.

Risk of Myocardial Ischemia and/or Infarction and Other Adverse Cardiac Events: ZOMIG should not be given to patients with documented ischemic or vasospastic coronary artery disease (see CONTRAINDICATIONS). It is strongly recommended that zolmitriptan not be given to patients in whom unrecognized coronary artery disease (CAD) is predicted by the presence of risk factors (e.g., hypertension, hypercholesterolemia, smoker, obesity, diabetes, strong family history of CAD, female with surgical or physiological menopause, or male over 40 years of age) unless a cardiovascular evaluation provides satisfactory clinical evidence that the patient is reasonably free of coronary artery and ischemic myocardial disease or other significant underlying cardiovascular disease. The sensitivity of cardiac diagnostic procedures to detect cardiovascular disease or predisposition to coronary artery vasospasm is modest, at best. If, during the cardiovascular evaluation, the patient's medical history, electrocardiographic or other investigations reveal findings indicative of, or consistent with, coronary artery vasospasm or myocardial ischemia, zolmitriptan should not be administered (see CONTRAINDICATIONS). For patients with risk factors predictive of CAD, who are determined to have a satisfactory cardiovascular evaluation, it is strongly recommended that administration of the first dose of zolmitriptan take place in the setting of a physician's office or similar medically staffed and equipped facility unless the patient has previously received zolmitriptan. Because cardiac ischemia can occur in the absence of clinical symptoms, consideration should be given to obtaining on the first occasion of use an electrocardiogram (ECG) during the interval immediately following ZOMIG, in these patients with risk factors.

It is recommended that patients who are intermittent long-term users of ZOMIG and who have or acquire risk factors predictive of CAD, as described above, undergo periodic interval cardiovascular evaluation as they continue to use ZOMIG.

The systematic approach described above is intended to reduce the likelihood that patients with unrecognized cardiovascular disease will be inadvertently exposed to zolmitriptan.

Cardiac Events and Fatalities: Serious adverse cardiac events, including acute myocardial infarction, have been reported within a few hours following administration of zolmitriptan. Life-threatening disturbances of cardiac rhythm, and death have been reported within a few hours following the administration of other 5-HT$_1$ agonists. Considering the extent of use of 5-HT$_1$ agonists in patients with migraine, the incidence of these events is extremely low.

ZOMIG can cause coronary vasospasm; at least one of these events occurred in a patient with no cardiac disease history and with documented absence of coronary artery disease. Because of the close proximity of the events to ZOMIG use, a causal relationship cannot be excluded. In the cases where there has been known underlying coronary artery disease, the relationship is uncertain.

Patients with symptomatic Wolff-Parkinson-White syndrome or arrhythmias associated with other cardiac accessory conduction pathway disorders should not receive ZOMIG.

Premarketing experience with zolmitriptan: Among the more than 2,500 patients with migraine who participated in premarketing controlled clinical trials of ZOMIG Tablets, no deaths or serious cardiac events were reported.

Postmarketing experience with zolmitriptan: Serious cardiovascular events have been reported in association with the use of ZOMIG Tablets, and in very rare cases, these events have occurred in the absence of known cardiovascular disease. The uncontrolled nature of postmarketing surveillance, however, makes it impossible to determine definitively the proportion of the reported cases that were actually caused by zolmitriptan or to reliably assess causation in individual cases.

Cerebrovascular Events and Fatalities with 5-HT$_1$ agonists: Cerebral hemorrhage, subarachnoid hemorrhage, stroke, and other cerebrovascular events have been reported in patients treated with 5-HT$_1$ agonists; and some have resulted in fatalities. In a number of cases, it appears possible that the cerebrovascular events were primary, the agonist having been administered in the incorrect belief that the symptoms experienced were a consequence of migraine, when they were not. It should be noted that patients with migraine may be at increased risk of certain cerebrovascular events (e.g., stroke, hemorrhage, transient ischemic attack).

Other Vasospasm-Related Events: 5-HT$_1$ agonists may cause vasospastic reactions other than coronary artery vasospasm such as peripheral and gastrointestinal vascular ischemia. As with other serotonin 5-HT$_1$ agonists, very rare gastrointestinal ischemic events including ischemic colitis and gastrointestinal infarction or necrosis have been reported with ZOMIG Tablets; these may present as bloody diarrhea or abdominal pain.

Increase in Blood Pressure: As with other 5-HT$_1$ agonists, significant elevations in systemic blood pressure have been reported on rare occasions with ZOMIG Tablet use, in patients with and without a history of hypertension; very rarely these increases in blood pressure have been associated with significant clinical events. Zolmitriptan is contraindicated in patients with uncontrolled hypertension. In volunteers, an increase of 1 and 5 mm Hg in the systolic and diastolic blood pressure, respectively, was seen at 5 mg. In the headache trials, vital signs were measured only in the small inpatient study and no effect on blood pressure was seen. In a study of patients with moderate to severe liver disease, 7 of 27 experienced 20 to 80 mm Hg elevations in systolic and/or diastolic blood pressure after a dose of 10 mg of zolmitriptan (see CONTRAINDICATIONS).

An 18% increase in mean pulmonary artery pressure was seen following dosing with another 5-HT$_1$ agonist in a study evaluating subjects undergoing cardiac catheterization.

PRECAUTIONS

General: As with other 5-HT$_{1B/1D}$ agonists, sensations of tightness, pain, pressure, and heaviness have been reported after treatment with ZOMIG Tablets in the precordium, throat, neck and jaw. Because zolmitriptan may cause coronary artery vasospasm, patients who experience signs or symptoms suggestive of angina following dosing should be evaluated for the presence of CAD or a predisposition to Prinzmetal's variant angina before receiving additional doses of medication, and should be monitored electrocardiographically if dosing is resumed and similar symptoms recur. Similarly, patients who experience other symptoms or signs suggestive of decreased arterial flow, such as ischemic bowel syndrome or Raynaud's syndrome following the use of any 5-HT$_1$ agonist are candidates for further evaluation (see WARNINGS).

Zolmitriptan should also be administered with caution to patients with diseases that may alter the absorption, metabolism, or excretion of drugs, such as impaired hepatic function (see CLINICAL PHARMACOLOGY).

For a given attack, if a patient does not respond to the first dose of zolmitriptan, the diagnosis of migraine headache should be reconsidered before administration of a second dose.

Binding to Melanin-Containing Tissues: When pigmented rats were given a single oral dose of 10 mg/kg of radiolabeled zolmitriptan, the radioactivity in the eye after 7 days, the latest time point examined, was still 75% of the value measured after 4 hours. This suggests that zolmitriptan and/or its metabolites may bind to the melanin of the eye. Because there could be accumulation in melanin rich tissues over time, this raises the possibility that zolmitriptan could cause toxicity in these tissues after extended use. However, no effects on the retina related to treatment with zolmitriptan were noted in any of the toxicity studies. Although no systematic monitoring of ophthalmologic function was undertaken in clinical trials, and no specific recommendations for ophthalmologic monitoring are offered, prescribers should be aware of the possibility of long-term ophthalmologic effects.

Phenylketonurics: Phenylketonuric patients should be informed that ZOMIG-ZMT contain phenylalanine (a component of aspartame). Each 2.5 mg orally disintegrating tablet contains 2.81 mg phenylalanine. Each 5 mg orally disintegrating tablet contains 5.62 mg phenylalanine.

Information for Patients: See PATIENT INFORMATION at the end of this labeling for the text of the separate leaflet provided for patients.

ZOMIG-ZMT Orally Disintegrating Tablets

The orally disintegrating tablet is packaged in a blister. Patients should be instructed not to remove the tablet from the blister until just prior to dosing. The blister pack should then be peeled open, and the orally disintegrating tablet placed on the tongue, where it will dissolve and be swallowed with the saliva.

Laboratory Tests: No monitoring of specific laboratory tests is recommended.

Drug Interactions: Ergot-containing drugs have been reported to cause prolonged vasospastic reactions. Because there is a theoretical basis that these effects may be additive, use of ergotamine-containing or ergot-type medications (like dihydroergotamine or methysergide) and zolmitriptan within 24 hours of each other should be avoided (see CONTRAINDICATIONS).

MAO-A inhibitors increase the systemic exposure of zolmitriptan. Therefore, the use of zolmitriptan in patients receiving MAO-A inhibitors is contraindicated (see CLINICAL PHARMACOLOGY and CONTRAINDICATIONS).

Concomitant use of other 5-HT$_{1B/1D}$ agonists within 24 hours of ZOMIG treatment is not recommended (see CONTRAINDICATIONS).

Following administration of cimetidine, the half-life and AUC of zolmitriptan and its active metabolites were approximately doubled (see CLINICAL PHARMACOLOGY).

Selective serotonin reuptake inhibitors (SSRIs) (eg, fluoxetine, fluvoxamine, paroxetine, sertraline) have been reported, rarely, to cause weakness, hyperreflexia, and incoordination when coadministered with 5-HT$_1$ agonists. If concomitant treatment with zolmitriptan and an SSRI is clinically warranted, appropriate observation of the patient is advised.

Drug/Laboratory Test Interactions: Zolmitriptan is not known to interfere with commonly employed clinical laboratory tests.

Carcinogenesis, Mutagenesis, Impairment of Fertility:

Carcinogenesis: Carcinogenicity studies by oral gavage were carried out in mice and rats at doses up to 400 mg/kg/day. Mice were dosed for 85 weeks (males) and 92 weeks (females). The exposure (plasma AUC of parent drug) at the highest dose level was approximately 800 times that seen in humans after a single 10 mg dose (the maximum recommended total daily dose). There was no effect of zolmitriptan on tumor incidence. Control, low dose and middle dose rats were dosed for 104-105 weeks; the high dose group was sacrificed after 101 weeks (males) and 86 weeks (females) due to excess mortality. Aside from an increase in the incidence of thyroid follicular cell hyperplasia and thyroid follicular cell adenomas seen in male rats receiving 400 mg/kg/day, an exposure approximately 3000 times that seen in humans after dosing with 10 mg, no tumors were noted.

Mutagenesis: Zolmitriptan was mutagenic in an Ames test, in 2 of 5 strains of S. typhimurium tested, in the presence of, but not in the absence of, metabolic activation. It was not mutagenic in an *in vitro* mammalian gene cell mutation (CHO/HGPRT) assay. Zolmitriptan was clastogenic in an *in vitro* human lymphocyte assay both in the absence of and the presence of metabolic activation; it was not clastogenic in an *in vivo* mouse micronucleus assay. It was also not genotoxic in an unscheduled DNA synthesis study.

Impairment of Fertility: Studies of male and female rats administered zolmitriptan prior to and during mating and up to implantation have shown no impairment of fertility at doses up to 400 mg/kg/day. Exposure at this dose was approximately 3000 times exposure at the maximum recommended human dose of 10 mg/day.

Pregnancy: Pregnancy Category C: There are no adequate and well controlled studies in pregnant women; therefore, zolmitriptan should be used during pregnancy only if the potential benefit justifies the potential risk to the fetus.

In reproductive toxicity studies in rats and rabbits, oral administration of zolmitriptan to pregnant animals was associated with embryolethality and fetal abnormalities. When pregnant rats were administered oral zolmitriptan during the period of organogenesis at doses of 100, 400 and 1200 mg/kg/day, there was a dose-related increase in embryolethality which became statistically significant at the high dose. The maternal plasma exposures at these doses were approximately 280, 1100 and 5000 times the exposure in humans receiving the maximum recommended total daily dose of 10 mg. The high dose was maternally toxic, as evidenced by a decreased maternal body weight gain during gestation. In a similar study in rabbits, embryolethality was increased at the maternally toxic doses of 10 and 30 mg/kg/day (maternal plasma exposures equivalent to 11 and 42 times exposure in humans receiving the maximum recommended total daily dose of 10 mg), and increased incidences of fetal malformations (fused sternebrae, rib anomalies) and variations (major blood vessel variations, irregular ossification pattern of ribs) were observed at 30 mg/kg/day. Three mg/kg/day was a no effect dose (equivalent to human exposure at a dose of 10 mg). When female rats were given zolmitriptan during gestation, parturition, and lactation, an increased incidence of hydronephrosis was found in the offspring at the maternally toxic dose of 400 mg/kg/day (1100 times human exposure).

Nursing Mothers: It is not known whether zolmitriptan is excreted in human milk. Because many drugs are excreted in human milk, caution should be exercised when zolmitriptan is administered to a nursing woman. Lactating rats dosed with zolmitriptan had milk levels equivalent to maternal plasma levels at 1 hour and 4 times higher than plasma levels at 4 hours.

Pediatric Use: Safety and effectiveness of ZOMIG in pediatric patients have not been established therefore, ZOMIG is not recommended for use in patients under 18 years of age.

Postmarketing experience with other triptans includes a limited number of reports that describe pediatric patients who have experienced clinically serious adverse events that are similar in nature to those reported rarely in adults.

Geriatric Use: Although the pharmacokinetic disposition of the drug in the elderly is similar to that seen in younger adults, there is no information about the safety and effectiveness of zolmitriptan in this population because patients over age 65 were excluded from the controlled clinical trials. (see CLINICAL PHARMACOLOGY: Special Populations)

ADVERSE REACTIONS

Serious cardiac events, including myocardial infarction, have occurred following the use of ZOMIG Tablets. These events are extremely rare and most have been reported in

Continued on next page

Zomig/Zomig ZMT—Cont.

patients with risk factors predictive of CAD. Events reported, in association with drugs of this class, have included coronary artery vasospasm, transient myocardial ischemia, myocardial infarction, ventricular tachycardia, and ventricular fibrillation (see CONTRAINDICATIONS, WARNINGS, and PRECAUTIONS).

Incidence in Controlled Clinical Trials: Among 2,633 patients treated with ZOMIG Tablets in the active and placebo controlled trials, no patients withdrew for reasons related to adverse events, but as patients treated a single headache in these trials, the opportunity for discontinuation was limited. In a long-term, open label study where patients were allowed to treat multiple migraine attacks for up to 1 year, 8% (167 out of 2,058) withdrew from the trial because of adverse experience. The most common events were paresthesia, asthenia, nausea, dizziness, pain, chest or neck tightness or heaviness, somnolence and warm sensation.

Table 2 lists the adverse events that occurred in ≥ 2% of the 2,074 patients in any one of the ZOMIG 1 mg, ZOMIG 2.5 mg or ZOMIG 5 mg Tablets dose groups of the controlled clinical trials. Only events that were more frequent in a ZOMIG Tablets group compared to the placebo groups are included. The events cited reflect experience gained under closely monitored conditions of clinical trials in a highly selected patient population. In actual clinical practice or in other clinical trials, these frequency estimates may not apply, as the conditions of use, reporting behavior, and the kinds of patients treated may differ.

Several of the adverse events appear dose related, notably paresthesia, sensation of heaviness or tightness in chest, neck, jaw, and throat, dizziness, somnolence, and possibly asthenia and nausea.

[See table 2 below]

ZOMIG is generally well tolerated. Across all doses, most adverse reactions were mild and transient and did not lead to long-lasting effects. The incidence of adverse events in controlled clinical trials was not affected by gender, weight, or age of the patients; use of prophylactic medications; or presence of aura. There were insufficient data to assess the impact of race on the incidence of adverse events.

Other Events: In the paragraphs that follow, the frequencies of less commonly reported adverse clinical events are presented. Because the reports include events observed in open and uncontrolled studies, the role of ZOMIG in their causation cannot be reliably determined. Furthermore, variability associated with adverse event reporting, the terminology used to describe adverse events, etc., limit the value of the quantitative frequency estimates provided. Event frequencies are calculated as the number of patients who used ZOMIG Tablets (n=4,027) and reported an event divided by the total number of patients exposed to ZOMIG Tablets. All reported events are included except those already listed in the previous table, those too general to be informative, and those not reasonably associated with the use of the drug. Events are further classified within body system categories and enumerated in order of decreasing frequency using the following definitions: infrequent adverse events are those occurring in 1/100 to 1/1,000 patients and rare adverse events are those occurring in fewer than 1/1,000 patients.

Atypical sensations: Infrequent was hyperesthesia.

General: Infrequent were allergy reaction, chills, facial edema, fever, malaise and photosensitivity.

Cardiovascular: Infrequent were arrhythmias, hypertension and syncope. Rare were bradycardia, extrasystoles, postural hypotension, QT prolongation, tachycardia and thrombophlebitis.

Digestive: Infrequent were increased appetite, tongue edema, esophagitis, gastroenteritis, liver function abnormality and thirst. Rare were anorexia, constipation, gastritis, hematemesis, pancreatitis, melena, and ulcer.

Hemic: Infrequent was ecchymosis. Rare were cyanosis, thrombocytopenia, eosinophilia and leukopenia.

Metabolic: Infrequent was edema. Rare were hyperglycemia and alkaline phosphatase increased.

Musculoskeletal: Infrequent were back pain, leg cramps and tenosynovitis. Rare were arthritis, asthenia, tetany and twitching.

Neurological: Infrequent were agitation, anxiety, depression, emotional lability and insomnia. Rare were akathisia, amnesia, apathy, ataxia, dystonia, euphoria, hallucinations, cerebral ischemia, hyperkinesia, hypotonia, hypertonia and irritability.

Respiratory: Infrequent were bronchitis, bronchospasm, epistaxis, hiccup, laryngitis, and yawn. Rare were apnea and voice alteration.

Skin: Infrequent were pruritus, rash and urticaria.

Special Senses: Infrequent were dry eye, eye pain, hyperacusis, ear pain, parosmia, and tinnitus. Rare were diplopia and lacrimation.

Urogenital: Infrequent were hematuria, cystitis, polyuria, urinary frequency, urinary urgency. Rare were miscarriage and dysmenorrhea.

The adverse experiences profile seen with ZOMIG-ZMT Tablets was similar to that seen with ZOMIG Tablets.

Postmarketing Experience with ZOMIG Tablets: The following section enumerates potentially important adverse events that have occurred in clinical practice and which have been reported spontaneously to various surveillance systems. The events enumerated represent reports arising from both domestic and non-domestic use of oral zolmitriptan. The events enumerated include all except those already listed in the ADVERSE REACTIONS section above or those too general to be informative. Because the reports cite events reported spontaneously from worldwide postmarketing experience, frequency of events and the role of zolmitriptan in their causation cannot be reliably determined.

Cardiovascular: Coronary artery vasospasm; transient myocardial ischemia, angina pectoris, and myocardial infarction.

Digestive: Very rare gastrointestinal ischemic events including splenic infarction, ischemic colitis, and gastrointestinal infarction or necrosis have been reported; these may present as bloody diarrhea or abdominal pain (see WARNINGS).

Neurological: As with other acute migraine treatments including other 5-HT$_1$ agonists, there have been rare reports of headache.

General: As with other 5-HT$_{1B/1D}$ agonists, there have been very rare reports of anaphylaxis or anaphylactoid reactions in patients receiving ZOMIG. There have been rare reports of hypersensitivity reactions, including angioedema.

DRUG ABUSE AND DEPENDENCE

The abuse potential of ZOMIG has not been assessed in clinical trials.

OVERDOSAGE

There is no experience with clinical overdose. Volunteers receiving single 50 mg oral doses of zolmitriptan commonly experienced sedation.

The elimination half-life of ZOMIG is 3 hours (see CLINICAL PHARMACOLOGY), and therefore monitoring of patients after overdose with ZOMIG should continue for at least 15 hours or while symptoms or signs persist.

There is no specific antidote to zolmitriptan. In cases of severe intoxication, intensive care procedures are recommended, including establishing and maintaining a patent airway, ensuring adequate oxygenation and ventilation, and monitoring and support of the cardiovascular system.

It is unknown what effect hemodialysis or peritoneal dialysis has on the plasma concentrations of zolmitriptan.

DOSAGE AND ADMINISTRATION

ZOMIG Tablets

In controlled clinical trials, single doses of 1, 2.5 and 5 mg of ZOMIG Tablets were effective for the acute treatment of migraines in adults. A greater proportion of patients had headache response following a 2.5 or 5 mg dose than following a 1 mg dose (see Table 1). In the only direct comparison of 2.5 and 5 mg, there was little added benefit from the larger dose but side effects are generally increased at 5 mg (see Table 2). Patients should, therefore, be started on 2.5 mg or lower. A dose lower than 2.5 mg can be achieved by manually breaking the scored 2.5 mg tablet in half.

If the headache returns, the dose may be repeated after 2 hours, not to exceed 10 mg within a 24-hour period. Controlled trials have not adequately established the effectiveness of a second dose if the initial dose is ineffective.

The safety of treating an average of more than three headaches in a 30-day period has not been established.

ZOMIG-ZMT Orally Disintegrating Tablets

In a controlled clinical trial, a single dose of 2.5 mg of ZOMIG-ZMT Tablets was effective for the acute treatment of migraines in adults.

If the headache returns, the dose may be repeated after 2 hours, not to exceed 10 mg within a 24-hour period. Controlled trials have not adequately established the effectiveness of a second dose if the initial dose is ineffective.

The safey of treating an average of more than three headaches in a 30-day period has not been established.

Administration with liquid is not necessary. The orally disintegrating tablet is packaged in a blister. Patients should be instructed not to remove the tablet from the blister until just prior to dosing. The blister pack should then be peeled open, and the orally disintegrating tablet placed on the tongue, where it will dissolve and be swallowed with the saliva. It is not recommended to break the orally disintegrating tablet.

Hepatic Impairment: Patients with moderate to severe hepatic impairment have decreased clearance of zolmitriptan and significant elevation in blood pressure was observed in some patients. Use of a low dose with blood pressure monitoring is recommended (see CLINICAL PHARMACOLOGY AND WARNINGS).

HOW SUPPLIED

2.5 mg Tablets—Yellow, biconvex, round, film-coated, scored tablets containing 2.5 mg of zolmitriptan identified with "ZOMIG" and "2.5" debossed on one side are supplied in cartons containing a blister pack of 6 tablets (NDC 0037-7210-20).

2.5 mg Orally Disintegrating Tablets—White, flat faced, uncoated, bevelled tablet containing 2.5 mg of zolmitriptan identified with a debossed "Z" on one side are supplied in cartons containing a blister pack of 6 tablets (NDC 0037-7209-20).

5 mg Tablets—Pink, biconvex, film-coated tablets containing 5 mg of zolmitriptan identified with "ZOMIG" and "5" debossed on one side are supplied in cartons containing a blister pack of 3 tablets (NDC 0037-7211-25).

5 mg Orally Disintegrating Tablets—White, flat faced, round, uncoated, bevelled tablet containing 5.0 mg of zolmitriptan identified with a debossed "Z" and "5" on one side and plain on the other are supplied in cartons containing a blister pack of 3 tablets (NDC 0037-7213-21).

Store both ZOMIG Tablets and ZOMIG-ZMT Tablets at controlled room temperature, 20-25°C (68-77°F) [see USP]. Protect from light and moisture.

PATIENT INFORMATION

The following wording is contained in a separate leaflet provided for patients.

ZOMIG® (zolmitriptan) Tablets
ZOMIG-ZMT® (zolmitriptan) Orally Disintegrating Tablets
Patient Information about ZOMIG (Zo-mig) for Migraines
Generic Name: zolmitriptan (zol-mi-trip-tan)
Information for the Consumer on ZOMIG (zolmitriptan) Tablets: Please read this leaflet carefully before you administer ZOMIG Tablets. This provides a summary of the information available on your medicine. Please do not throw away this leaflet until you have finished your medicine. You may need to read this leaflet again. This leaflet does not contain all the information on ZOMIG Tablets. For further information or advice, ask your doctor or pharmacist.

Information About Your Medicine: The name of your medicine is ZOMIG Tablets. It can be obtained only by prescription from your doctor. The decision to use ZOMIG Tablets is one that you and your doctor should make jointly, taking into account your individual preferences and medical circumstances. If you have risk factors for heart disease (such as high blood pressure, high cholesterol, obesity, diabetes, smoking, strong family history of heart disease, or you are postmenopausal or a male over the age of 40), you should tell your doctor, who should evaluate you for heart disease in order to determine if ZOMIG Tablets are appropriate for you.

1. The Purpose of Your Medicine: ZOMIG Tablets are intended to relieve your migraine, but not to prevent or reduce the number of attacks you experience. Use ZOMIG Tablets only to treat an actual migraine attack.

2. Important Questions to Consider Before Using ZOMIG Tablets: If the answer to any of the following questions

Table 2: Adverse Experience Incidence in Five Placebo-Controlled Migraine Clinical Trials: Events Reported By ≥ 2% Patients Treated With ZOMIG Tablets

Adverse Event Type	Placebo (n=401)	ZOMIG 1 mg (n=163)	ZOMIG 2.5 mg (n=498)	ZOMIG 5 mg (n=1012)
ATYPICAL SENSATIONS	6%	12%	12%	18%
Hypesthesia	1%	1%	1%	2%
Paresthesia (all types)	2%	5%	7%	9%
Sensation warm/cold	4%	6%	5%	7%
PAIN AND PRESSURE SENSATIONS	7%	13%	14%	22%
Chest-pain/tightness/pressure and/or heaviness	1%	2%	3%	4%
Neck/throat/jaw-pain/tightness/pressure	3%	4%	7%	10%
Heaviness other than chest or neck	1%	1%	2%	5%
Pain-location specified	1%	2%	2%	3%
Other-Pressure/tightness/heaviness	0%	2%	2%	2%
DIGESTIVE	8%	11%	16%	14%
Dry mouth	2%	5%	3%	3%
Dyspepsia	1%	3%	2%	1%
Dysphagia	0%	0%	0%	2%
Nausea	4%	4%	9%	6%
NEUROLOGICAL	10%	11%	17%	21%
Dizziness	4%	6%	8%	10%
Somnolence	3%	5%	6%	8%
Vertigo	0%	0%	0%	2%
OTHER				
Asthenia	3%	5%	3%	9%
Palpitations	1%	0%	<1%	2%
Myalgia	<1%	1%	1%	2%
Myasthenia	<1%	0%	1%	2%
Sweating	1%	0%	2%	3%

is **YES** or if you do not know the answer, then you must discuss it with your doctor before you use ZOMIG Tablets.

- Do you have any chest pain, heart disease, shortness of breath, or irregular heartbeats? Have you had a heart attack?
- Do you have risk factors for heart disease (such as high blood pressure, high cholesterol, obesity, diabetes, smoking, strong family history of heart disease, or you are postmenopausal or a male over the age of 40)?
- Do you have high blood pressure?
- Are you pregnant? Do you think you might be pregnant? Are you trying to become pregnant? Are you not using adequate contraception? Are you breast feeding an infant?
- If you are taking ZOMIG-ZMT®, are you sensitive to phenylalanine (a component of the artificial sweetener aspartame)?
- Have you ever had to stop taking this or any other medication because of an allergy or other problems?
- Are you taking any other migraine medications, including 5-HT$_1$ agonists (triptans) or migraine medications containing ergotamine, dihydroergotamine, or methysergide?
- Are you taking any medication for depression (monoamine oxidase inhibitors or selective serotonin reuptake inhibitors [SSRIs])?
- Are you taking cimetidine for gastrointestinal symptoms?
- Have you had, or do you have, any disease of the liver or kidney?
- Have you had, or do you have, epilepsy or seizures?
- Is this headache different from your usual migraine attacks?

Remember, if you answered YES to any of the above questions, then you must discuss it with your doctor.

3. **The Use of ZOMIG Tablets During Pregnancy:** Do not use ZOMIG Tablets if you are pregnant, think you might be pregnant, are trying to become pregnant, or are not using adequate contraception, unless you have discussed this with your doctor.

4. **How to Use ZOMIG Tablets and ZOMIG-ZMT Orally Disintegrating Tablets:** Adults should be started on a 2.5 mg dose or lower administered by mouth. A dose lower than 2.5 mg can be achieved by manually breaking the conventional film-coated, scored 2.5 mg tablet in half. It is not recommended to break the ZOMIG-ZMT Tablet. If your headache comes back after your initial dose, a second dose may be administered anytime after 2 hours of administering the dose. For any attack where you have no response to the first dose, do not take a second dose without first consulting with your doctor. Do not administer more than a total of 10 mg of ZOMIG in any 24-hour period. Discard any unused tablets or its portion that have been removed from the blister packaging. Do not take ZOMIG with any other drug in the same class (triptans) within 24 hours or within 24 hours of taking ergotamine-type medications such as ergotamine, dihydroergotamine or methysergide to treat your migraine.
Additionally for ZOMIG-ZMT Tablets, the blister pack should be peeled open and the orally disintegrating tablet placed on the tongue, where it will dissolve and be swallowed with the saliva.

5. **Side Effects to Watch For:**
- Some patients experience pain or tightness in the chest or throat, including muscle aches and pains, when using ZOMIG. If this happens to you, then discuss it with your doctor before using any more ZOMIG. If the chest pain is severe or does not go away, call your doctor immediately. As with other drugs in this class (triptans), there have been very rare reports of heart attack occurring in patients with and without risk factors for heart and blood vessel disease.
- Some people experience: alterations of heart rate; temporary increase in blood pressure; sudden and severe stomach pain.
- Shortness of breath; wheeziness; heart throbbing; swelling of eyelids, face, or lips; or a skin rash, skin lumps, or hives happens rarely. If it happens to you, then tell your doctor immediately. Do not take any more ZOMIG unless your doctor tells you to do so.
- Some people may have feelings of dry mouth, tingling, heat, heaviness or pressure after treatment with ZOMIG. A few people may feel drowsy, dizzy, tired, or sick. Tell your doctor immediately if you have symptoms that you do not understand.

6. **What To Do If An Overdose Is Taken:** If you have taken more medication than you have been told, contact either your doctor, hospital emergency department, or nearest poison control center immediately. This medicine was prescribed for your particular condition and should not be used by others or for any other condition.

7. **Storing Your Medicine:** Keep your medicine in a safe place where children cannot reach it. It may be harmful to children. Store your medication away from light and moisture, and at a controlled room temperature. If your medication has expired (the expiration date is printed on the treatment pack), throw it away as instructed. If your doctor decides to stop your treatment, do not keep any leftover medicine unless your doctor tells you to. Throw away your medicine as instructed. Be sure that discarded tablets are out of the reach of children.

ZOMIG and ZOMIG-ZMT are trademarks of the AstraZeneca group of companies.
© AstraZeneca 2003

ZOMIG® (zolmitriptan) Tablets
Manufactured for:
AstraZeneca Pharmaceuticals LP
Wilmington, DE 19850
By: IPR Pharmaceuticals, Inc.
Carolina, PR 00984
ZOMIG-ZMT® (zolmitriptan) Orally Disintegrating Tablets
Manufactured for:
AstraZeneca Pharmaceuticals LP
Wilmington, DE 19850
By: CIMA Labs, Inc.
Eden Prairie, MN 55344
Distributed by:
MedPointe Pharmaceuticals
MedPointe Healthcare Inc.
Somerset, New Jersey 08873
64209-00
Rev 10/03

ZOMIG® NASAL SPRAY   ℞
[zō-mǐg]
(zolmitriptan)
FOR NASAL USE ONLY

DESCRIPTION

ZOMIG® (zolmitriptan) Nasal Spray contains zolmitriptan, which is a selective 5-hydroxytryptamine $_{1B/1D}$ (5-HT$_{1B/1D}$) receptor agonist. Zolmitriptan is chemically designated as (S)-4-[[3-[2-(dimethylamino)ethyl]-1H-indol-5-yl]methyl]-2-oxazolidinone and has the following chemical structure:

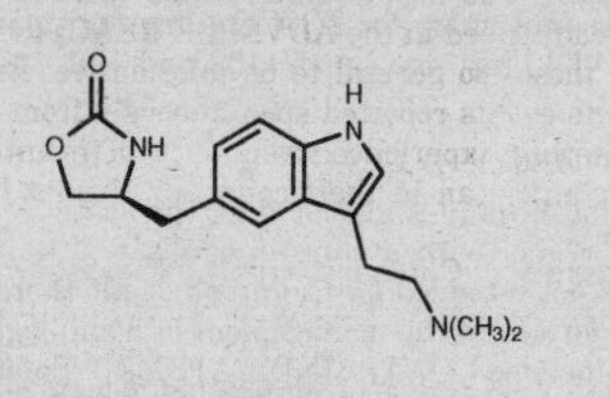

The empirical formula is $C_{16}H_{21}N_3O_2$, representing a molecular weight of 287.36. Zolmitriptan is a white to almost white powder that is readily soluble in water. ZOMIG Nasal Spray is supplied as a clear to pale yellow solution of zolmitriptan, buffered to a pH 5.0. Each ZOMIG Nasal Spray contains 5 mg of zolmitriptan in a 100-μL unit dose aqueous buffered solution containing citric acid, anhydrous, USP, disodium phosphate dodecahydrate USP and purified water USP.
ZOMIG Nasal Spray is hypertonic. The osmolarity of ZOMIG Nasal Spray 5 mg is 420 to 470 mOsmol.

CLINICAL PHARMACOLOGY
Mechanism of Action
Zolmitriptan binds with high affinity to human recombinant 5-HT$_{1D}$ and 5-HT$_{1B}$ receptors. Zolmitriptan exhibits modest affinity for 5-HT$_{1A}$ receptors, but has no significant affinity (as measured by radioligand binding assays) or pharmacological activity at 5-HT$_2$, 5-HT$_3$, 5-HT$_4$, alpha$_1$-, alpha$_2$- or beta$_1$-adrenergic; H$_1$, H$_2$, histaminic; muscarinic; dopamine$_1$, or dopamine$_2$ receptors. The N-desmethyl metabolite also has high affinity for 5-HT$_{1B/1D}$ and modest affinity for 5-HT$_{1A}$ receptors.
Current theories proposed to explain the etiology of migraine headache suggest that symptoms are due to local cranial vasodilatation and/or to the release of sensory neuropeptides (vasoactive intestinal peptide, substance P and calcitonin gene-related peptide) through nerve endings in the trigeminal system. The therapeutic activity of zolmitriptan for the treatment of migraine headache can most likely be attributed to the agonist effects at the 5-HT$_{1B/1D}$ receptors on intracranial blood vessels (including the arterio-venous anastomoses) and sensory nerves of the trigeminal system which result in cranial vessel constriction and inhibition of pro-inflammatory neuropeptide release.

Clinical Pharmacokinetics and Bioavailability
Absorption:
Zolmitriptan nasal spray is rapidly absorbed via the nasopharynx as detected in a Photon Emission Tomography (PET) study using ^{11}C zolmitriptan. Zolmitriptan was detected in plasma by 5 minutes and peak plasma concentration generally was achieved by 3 hours. The time at which maximum plasma concentrations were observed was similar after single (1 day) or multiple (4 day) nasal dosing. Plasma concentrations of zolmitriptan are sustained for 4 to 6 hours after dosing. Zolmitriptan displays linear kinetics after multiple doses of 2.5 mg, 5 mg, or 10 mg. The mean relative bioavailability of the nasal spray formulation is 102%, compared to the oral tablet.
Zolmitriptan and its active metabolite display dose proportionality after single or multiple dosing. Dose proportional increases in zolmitriptan and N-desmethyl metabolite C$_{max}$ and AUC were observed for 2.5 and 5 mg nasal spray doses. The pharmacokinetics for elimination of zolmitriptan and its active N-desmethyl metabolite are similar for all nasal spray dosages. The N-desmethyl metabolite is detected in plasma by 15 minutes and peak plasma concentration is generally achieved by 3 hours after administration.
Food has no significant effect on the bioavailability of zolmitriptan.

Distribution:
Plasma protein binding of zolmitriptan is 25% over the concentration range of 10-1000 ng/mL. The mean (±SD) apparent volume of distribution for zolmitriptan nasal spray formulation is 8.6±3.3 L/kg.
Metabolism:
Zolmitriptan is converted to an active N-desmethyl metabolite such that the metabolite concentrations are about two-thirds that of zolmitriptan. Because the 5HT$_{1B/1D}$ potency of the metabolite is 2 to 6 times that of the parent compound, the metabolite may contribute a substantial portion of the overall effect after zolmitriptan administration.
Excretion:
The mean elimination half-life for zolmitriptan and its active N-desmethyl metabolite following nasal spray administration are approximately 3 hours, which is similar to the half-life values seen after oral tablet administration. The half-life values were similar for zolmitriptan and the N-desmethyl metabolite after single (1 day) and multiple (4 day) nasal dosing.
Mean total plasma clearance is 25.9 mL/min/kg, of which one-sixth is renal clearance. The renal clearance is greater than the glomerular filtration rate suggesting renal tubular secretion.
Special Populations:
Geriatric:
The pharmacokinetics of oral zolmitriptan in healthy elderly non-migraineur volunteers (age 65-76 yrs) was similar to those in younger non-migraineur volunteers (age 18-39 yrs).
Gender:
Mean plasma concentrations of orally administered zolmitriptan were up to 1.5-fold higher in females than males.
Renal Impairment:
The effect of renal impairment on the pharmacokinetics of zolmitriptan nasal spray has not been evaluated. After orally dosing zolmitriptan, renal clearance was reduced by 25% in patients with severe renal impairment (Clcr ≥ 5 ≤ 25 mL/min) compared to the normal group (Clcr ≥ 70 mL/min); no significant change in renal clearance was observed in the moderately renally impaired group (Clcr ≥ 26 ≤ 50 mL/min).
Hepatic Impairment:
The effect of hepatic disease on the pharmacokinetics of zolmitriptan nasal spray has not been evaluated. In severely hepatically impaired patients, the mean C$_{max}$, T$_{max}$, and AUC$_{0-\infty}$ of zolmitriptan dosed orally were increased 1.5, 2, and 3-fold, respectively, compared to normals. Seven out of 27 patients experienced 20 to 80 mm Hg elevations in systolic and/or diastolic blood pressure after a 10 mg dose. Because of the similarity in exposure, zolmitriptan tablets and nasal spray should have similar dosage adjustments and should be administered with caution in subjects with liver disease, generally using doses less than 2.5 mg. Doses lower than 5 mg can only be achieved through the use of an oral formulation (see WARNINGS and PRECAUTIONS).
Hypertensive Patients:
No differences in the pharmacokinetics of oral zolmitriptan or its effects on blood pressure were seen in mild to moderate hypertensive volunteers compared to normotensive controls.
Race:
Retrospective analysis of pharmacokinetic data between Japanese and Caucasians revealed no significant differences for orally dosed zolmitriptan.

Drug Interactions
All drug interaction studies were performed in healthy volunteers using a single 10 mg dose of zolmitriptan and a single dose of the other drug except where otherwise noted. Eight drug interaction studies have been performed with zolmitriptan tablets and one study (xylometazoline) was performed with nasal spray.
Xylometazoline:
An *in vivo* drug interaction study with ZOMIG Nasal Spray indicated that 1 spray (100μL dose) of xylometazoline (0.1% w/v), a decongestant, administered 30 minutes prior to a 5 mg nasal dose of zolmitriptan did not alter the pharmacokinetics of zolmitriptan.
Fluoxetine:
The pharmacokinetics of zolmitriptan, as well as its effect on blood pressure, were unaffected by 4 weeks of pretreatment with oral fluoxetine (20 mg/day).
MAO Inhibitors:
Following one week of administration of 150 mg bid moclobemide, a specific MAO-A inhibitor, there was an increase of about 25% in both C$_{max}$ and AUC for zolmitriptan and a 3-fold increase in the C$_{max}$ and AUC of the active N-desmethyl metabolite of zolmitriptan (see CONTRAINDICATIONS and PRECAUTIONS).
Selegiline, a selective MAO-B inhibitor, at a dose of 10 mg/day for 1 week, had no effect on the pharmacokinetics of zolmitriptan and its metabolite.
Propranolol:
C$_{max}$ and AUC of zolmitriptan increased 1.5-fold after one week of dosing with propranolol (160 mg/day). C$_{max}$ and AUC of the N-desmethyl metabolite were reduced by 30% and 15%, respectively. There were no interactive effects on blood pressure or pulse rate following administration of propranolol with zolmitriptan.

Continued on next page

Zomig Nasal Spray—Cont.

Acetaminophen:
A single 1 g dose of acetaminophen does not alter the pharmacokinetics of zolmitriptan and its N-desmethyl metabolite. However, zolmitriptan delayed the T_{max} of acetaminophen by one hour.
Metoclopramide:
A single 10 mg dose of metoclopramide had no effect on the pharmacokinetics of zolmitriptan or its metabolites.
Oral Contraceptives:
Retrospective analysis of pharmacokinetic data across studies indicated that mean plasma concentrations of zolmitriptan were generally higher in females taking oral contraceptives compared to those not taking oral contraceptives. Mean C_{max} and AUC of zolmitriptan were found to be higher by 30% and 50%, respectively, and T_{max} was delayed by one-half hour in females taking oral contraceptives. The effect of zolmitriptan on the pharmacokinetics of oral contraceptives has not been studied.
Cimetidine:
Following the administration of cimetidine, the half-life and AUC of a 5 mg dose of zolmitriptan and its active metabolite were approximately doubled (see PRECAUTIONS).

Clinical Studies

The efficacy of ZOMIG Nasal Spray 0.5, 1, 2.5 and 5 mg in the acute treatment of migraine headache with or without aura was demonstrated in a randomized, outpatient, double-blind, placebo-controlled trial.

Patients were instructed to treat a moderate to severe headache. Headache response, defined as a reduction in headache severity from moderate or severe pain to mild or no pain, was assessed 15, 30, 45 minutes and 1, 2, and 4 hours after dosing. Pain free response rates and associated symptoms such as nausea, photophobia, and phonophobia were also assessed. A dose of escape medication was allowed 4 to 24 hours after the initial treatment for persistent and recurrent headache.

Of the 1372 patients treated in the study, 83% were female and 99% were Caucasian, with a mean age of 40.6 years (range 18 to 65 years).

The two hour headache response rates in patients treated with ZOMIG Nasal Spray were statistically significant among patients receiving ZOMIG Nasal Spray at all doses compared to placebo. There was a greater percentage of patients with a headache response at 2 hours in the higher dose groups. The headache response efficacy endpoints of the controlled clinical study, analyzed from the first attack data, are shown in Table 1.

[See table 1 below]

The estimated probability of achieving an initial headache response by 4 hours following treatment with ZOMIG Nasal Spray is depicted in Figure 1.

FIGURE 1: Estimated probability of achieving an initial headache response within 4 hours of initial treatment

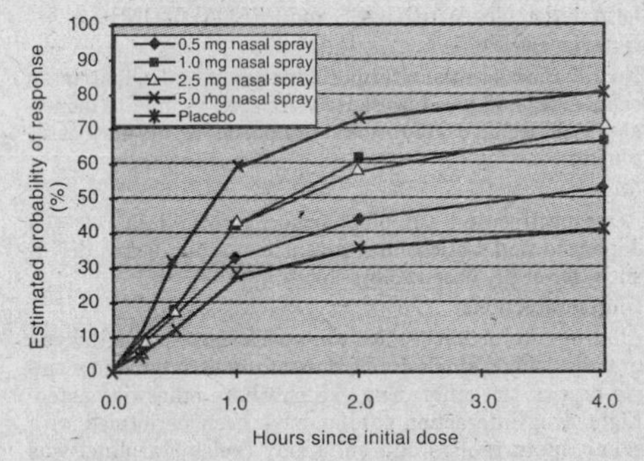

Note: Figure 1 shows the Kaplan-Meier plot of the probability over time of obtaining headache response (moderate or severe headache improving to mild or no pain) following treatment with zolmitriptan nasal spray. The averages displayed are based on a placebo controlled, outpatient trial providing evidence of efficacy. Patients not achieving headache response or taking additional treatment prior to 4 hours were censored to 4 hours.

For patients with migraine associated photophobia, phonophobia, and nausea at baseline, there was a decreased incidence of these symptoms following administration of ZOMIG Nasal Spray as compared to placebo.

Four to 24 hours following the initial dose of study treatment, patients were allowed to use additional treatment for pain relief in the form of a second dose of study treatment or other medication. The estimated probability of patients taking a second dose or other medication for migraine over the 24 hours following the initial dose of study treatment is summarized in Figure 2.

FIGURE 2: Estimated probability of patients taking an escape medication within the 24 hours following the initial dose of study treatment

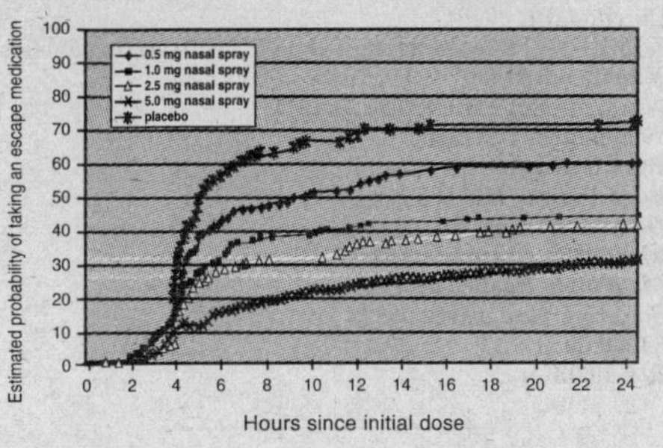

*This Kaplan-Meier plot is based on data obtained from the placebo controlled clinical trial. Patients not using additional treatments were censored at 24 hours. The plot includes both patients who had headache response at 2 hours and those who had no response to the initial dose. It should be noted that the protocol did not allow remedication within 4 hours post dose.

The efficacy of ZOMIG was unaffected by presence of aura; presence of headache upon awakening, relationship to menses; gender, age or weight of the patient; or presence of pretreatment nausea.

The efficacy of ZOMIG Nasal Spray 5 mg was further supported by an interim analysis of another similarly designed trial. The 2 hour headache response rates for the first 210 subjects in that study for ZOMIG 5 mg and placebo were 70% and 47%, respectively (N=108 and 102, respectively, p=0.0006).

INDICATIONS AND USAGE

ZOMIG Nasal Spray is indicated for the acute treatment of migraine with or without aura in adults.

ZOMIG is not intended for the prophylactic therapy of migraine or for use in the management of hemiplegic or basilar migraine (see CONTRAINDICATIONS). Safety and effectiveness of ZOMIG have not been established for cluster headache, which is present in an older, predominantly male population.

CONTRAINDICATIONS

ZOMIG should not be given to patients with ischemic heart disease (angina pectoris, history of myocardial infarction, or documented silent ischemia) or to patients who have symptoms or findings consistent with ischemic heart disease, coronary artery vasospasm, including Prinzmetal's variant angina, or other significant underlying cardiovascular disease (see WARNINGS).

ZOMIG should not be given to patients with cerebrovascular syndromes including (but not limited to) stroke of any type as well as transient ischemic attacks.

Because ZOMIG may increase blood pressure, it should not be given to patients with uncontrolled hypertension (see WARNINGS).

ZOMIG should not be used within 24 hours of treatment with another 5-HT_1 agonist, or an ergotamine-containing or ergot-type medication like dihydroergotamine or methysergide.

ZOMIG should not be administered to patients with hemiplegic or basilar migraine.

Concurrent administration of MAO-A inhibitors or use of zolmitriptan within 2 weeks of discontinuation of MAO-A inhibitor therapy is contraindicated (see CLINICAL PHARMACOLOGY: Drug Interactions and PRECAUTIONS: Drug Interactions).

ZOMIG is contraindicated in patients who are hypersensitive to zolmitriptan or any of its inactive ingredients.

WARNINGS

ZOMIG should only be used where a clear diagnosis of migraine has been established.

Risk of Myocardial Ischemia and/or Infarction and Other Adverse Cardiac Events:

ZOMIG should not be given to patients with documented ischemic or vasospastic coronary artery disease (see CONTRAINDICATIONS). It is strongly recommended that zolmitriptan not be given to patients in whom unrecognized coronary artery disease (CAD) is predicted by the presence of risk factors (eg, hypertension, hypercholesterolemia, smoker, obesity, diabetes, strong family history of CAD, female with surgical or physiological menopause, or male over 40 years of age) unless a cardiovascular evaluation provides satisfactory clinical evidence that the patient is reasonably free of coronary artery and ischemic myocardial disease or other significant underlying cardiovascular disease. The sensitivity of cardiac diagnostic procedures to detect cardiovascular disease or predisposition to coronary artery vasospasm is modest, at best. If, during the cardiovascular evaluation, the patient's medical history, electrocardiographic or other investigations reveal findings indicative of, or consistent with, coronary artery vasospasm or myocardial ischemia, zolmitriptan should not be administered (see CONTRAINDICATIONS). For patients with risk factors predictive of CAD, who are determined to have a satisfactory cardiovascular evaluation, it is strongly recommended that administration of the first dose of zolmitriptan take place in the setting of a physician's office or similar medically staffed and equipped facility unless the patient has previously received zolmitriptan.

Because cardiac ischemia can occur in the absence of clinical symptoms, consideration should be given to obtaining on the first occasion of use an electrocardiogram (ECG) during the interval immediately following ZOMIG, in these patients with risk factors.

It is recommended that patients who are intermittent long-term users of ZOMIG and who have or acquire risk factors predictive of CAD, as described above, undergo periodic interval cardiovascular evaluation as they continue to use ZOMIG.

The systematic approach described above is intended to reduce the likelihood that patients with unrecognized cardiovascular disease will be inadvertently exposed to zolmitriptan.

Cardiac Events and Fatalities:

Serious adverse cardiac events, including acute myocardial infarction, have been reported within a few hours following administration of zolmitriptan. Life-threatening disturbances of cardiac rhythm, and death have been reported within a few hours following the administration of other 5-HT_1 agonists. Considering the extent of use of 5-HT_1 agonists in patients with migraine, the incidence of these events is extremely low.

ZOMIG can cause coronary vasospasm; at least one of these events occurred in a patient with no cardiac disease history and with documented absence of coronary artery disease. Because of the close proximity of the events to ZOMIG use, a causal relationship cannot be excluded. In the cases where there has been known underlying coronary artery disease, the relationship is uncertain.

Patients with symptomatic Wolff-Parkinson-White syndrome or arrhythmias associated with other cardiac accessory conduction pathway disorders should not receive ZOMIG.

Premarketing experience with zolmitriptan:

Among the more than 2,500 patients with migraine who participated in premarketing controlled clinical trials of ZOMIG Tablets, no deaths or serious cardiac events were reported. In a premarketing controlled clinical trial of ZOMIG Nasal Spray, more than 1,300 patients participated and there were no deaths or serious cardiac events to report.

Postmarketing experience with zolmitriptan:

Serious cardiovascular events have been reported in association with the use of ZOMIG Tablets, and in very rare cases, these events have occurred in the absence of known cardiovascular disease. The uncontrolled nature of postmarketing surveillance, however, makes it impossible to determine definitively the proportion of the reported cases that were actually caused by zolmitriptan or to reliably assess causation in individual cases.

Cerebrovascular Events and Fatalities with 5-HT_1 agonists:

Cerebral hemorrhage, subarachnoid hemorrhage, stroke, and other cerebrovascular events have been reported in patients treated with 5-HT_1 agonists; and some have resulted in fatalities. In a number of cases, it appears possible that the cerebrovascular events were primary, the agonist having been administered in the incorrect belief that the symptoms experienced were a consequence of migraine, when they were not. It should be noted that patients with migraine may be at increased risk of certain cerebrovascular events (eg, stroke, hemorrhage, transient ischemic attack).

Other Vasospasm-Related Events:

5-$HT1_1$ agonists may cause vasospastic reactions other than coronary artery vasospasm such as peripheral and gastrointestinal vascular ischemia. As with other serotonin 5HT_1 agonists, very rare gastrointestinal ischemic events including ischemic colitis and gastrointestinal infarction or necrosis have been reported with ZOMIG Tablets; these may present as bloody diarrhea or abdominal pain.

Increase in Blood Pressure:

As with other 5-HT_1 agonists, significant elevations in systemic blood pressure have been reported on rare occasions with ZOMIG Tablet use, in patients with and without a history of hypertension; very rarely these increases in blood pressure have been associated with significant clinical events. Zolmitriptan is contraindicated in patients with uncontrolled hypertension. In volunteers, an increase of 1 and 5 mm Hg in the systolic and diastolic blood pressure, respectively, was seen at 5 mg. In the headache trials, vital signs were measured only in the small inpatient study and no effect on blood pressure was seen. In a study of patients with moderate to severe liver disease, 7 of 27 experienced 20 to 80 mm Hg elevations in systolic and/or diastolic blood pressure after a dose of 10 mg of zolmitriptan (see CONTRAINDICATIONS).

An 18% increase in mean pulmonary artery pressure was seen following dosing with another 5-HT_1 agonist in a study evaluating subjects undergoing cardiac catheterization.

Table 1: First Attack Data: Percentage of Patients with Headache Response to ZOMIG Nasal Spray (Mild or No Headache) 2 Hours Following Treatment (N = number of randomized patients treating a migraine attack). The 2 hour headache response was the primary end-point

	PLACEBO	ZOMIG 0.5 mg	ZOMIG 1.0 mg	ZOMIG 2.5 mg	ZOMIG 5 mg
N	(226)	(221)	(236)	(224)	(235)
2 hours	31%	40%*	59%‡	55%‡	69%‡

*p <0.05 in comparison with placebo
‡p <0.0001 in comparison with placebo

Local Adverse Reactions:
Among 922 patients using the zolmitriptan nasal spray to treat 2311 attacks in the controlled clinical study who were exposed, across all doses (0.5 to 5 mg), approximately 3% noted local irritation or soreness at the site of administration. Adverse events of any kind, perceived in the nasopharynx (which may include systemic effects of triptans) were severe in about 1 % of patients and approximately 60% resolved in 1 hour. Nasopharyngeal examinations, in a subset of patients participating in two long term trials of up to one year duration, failed to demonstrate any clinically significant changes with repeated use of ZOMIG Nasal Spray.
All nasopharyngeal adverse events with an incidence of ≥2% of patients in any zolmitriptan nasal spray dose groups are included in ADVERSE REACTIONS Table 2.

PRECAUTIONS

General:
As with other 5-$HT_{1B/1D}$ agonists, sensations of tightness, pain, pressure, and heaviness have been reported after treatment with ZOMIG Tablets in the precordium, throat, neck, and jaw. Because zolmitriptan may cause coronary artery vasospasm, patients who experience signs or symptoms suggestive of angina following dosing should be evaluated for the presence of CAD or a predisposition to Prinzmetal's variant angina before receiving additional doses of medication, and should be monitored electrocardiographically if dosing is resumed and similar symptoms recur. Similarly, patients who experience other symptoms or signs suggestive of decreased arterial flow following the use of any 5-HT agonist, such as ischemic bowel syndrome or Raynaud's syndrome, are candidates for further evaluation (see WARNINGS).
Zolmitriptan should also be administered with caution to patients with diseases that may alter the absorption, metabolism, or excretion of drugs, such as impaired hepatic function (see CLINICAL PHARMACOLOGY).
For a given attack, if a patient does not respond to the first dose of zolmitriptan, the diagnosis of migraine headache should be reconsidered before administration of a second dose.

Binding to Melanin-Containing Tissues:
When pigmented rats were given a single oral dose of 10 mg/kg of radiolabeled zolmitriptan, the radioactivity in the eye after 7 days, the latest time point examined, was still 75% of the value measured after 4 hours. This suggests that zolmitriptan and/or its metabolites may bind to the melanin of the eye. Because there could be accumulation in melanin rich tissues over time, this raises the possibility that zolmitriptan could cause toxicity in these tissues after extended use. However, no effects on the retina related to treatment with zolmitriptan were noted in any of the toxicity studies including those conducted by the nasal route. Although no systematic monitoring of ophthalmologic function was undertaken in clinical trials, and no specific recommendations for ophthalmologic monitoring are offered, prescribers should be aware of the possibility of long-term ophthalmologic effects.

Information for Patients:
See PATIENT INFORMATION at the end of this labeling for the figures and text of the separate leaflet provided for patients.
The ZOMIG Nasal Spray device is packaged in a carton and is a blue colored plastic device with a gray protection cap, labeled to indicate the nominal dose. Patients should be cautioned to not remove the gray protection cap until prior to dosing. The ZOMIG Nasal Spray device is placed in a nostril and actuated to deliver a single dose. **Patients should be cautioned to avoid spraying the contents of the device in their eyes.**

Laboratory Tests:
No monitoring of specific laboratory tests is recommended.

Drug Interactions:
Ergot-containing drugs have been reported to cause prolonged vasospastic reactions. Because there is a theoretical basis that these effects may be additive, use of ergotamine-containing or ergot-type medications (like dihydroergotamine or methysergide) and zolmitriptan within 24 hours of each other should be avoided (see CONTRAINDICATIONS).
MAO-A inhibitors increase the systemic exposure of zolmitriptan. Therefore, the use of zolmitriptan in patients receiving MAO-A inhibitors is contraindicated (see CLINICAL PHARMACOLOGY and CONTRAINDICATIONS).
Concomitant use of other 5-$HT_{1B/1D}$ agonists within 24 hours of ZOMIG treatment is not recommended (see CONTRAINDICATIONS).
Following administration of cimetidine, the half-life and AUC of zolmitriptan and its active metabolites were approximately doubled (see CLINICAL PHARMACOLOGY).
Selective serotonin reuptake inhibitors (SSRIs) (eg, fluoxetine, fluvoxamine, paroxetine, sertraline) have been reported, rarely, to cause weakness, hyperreflexia, and incoordination when coadministered with 5-HT_1 agonists. If concomitant treatment with zolmitriptan and an SSRI is clinically warranted, appropriate observation of the patient is advised.

Drug/Laboratory Test Interactions:
Zolmitriptan is not known to interfere with commonly employed clinical laboratory tests.

Carcinogenesis, Mutagenesis, Impairment of Fertility:
Carcinogenesis:
Carcinogenicity studies by oral gavage were carried out in mice and rats at doses up to 400 mg/kg/day. Mice were dosed for 85 weeks (males) and 92 weeks (females). The exposure (plasma AUC of parent drug) at the highest dose level was approximately 800 times that seen in humans after a single 10 mg dose (the maximum recommended total daily dose). There was no effect of zolmitriptan on tumor incidence. Control, low dose, and middle dose rats were dosed for 104-105 weeks; the high dose group was sacrificed after 101 weeks (males) and 86 weeks (females) due to excess mortality. Aside from an increase in the incidence of thyroid follicular cell hyperplasia and thyroid follicular cell adenomas seen in male rats receiving 400 mg/kg/day, an exposure approximately 3000 times that seen in humans after dosing with 10 mg, no tumors were noted.
Mutagenesis:
Zolmitriptan was mutagenic in an Ames test, in 2 of 5 strains of *S. typhimurium* tested, in the presence of, but not in the absence of, metabolic activation. It was not mutagenic in an *in vitro* mammalian gene cell mutation (CHO/HGPRT) assay. Zolmitriptan was clastogenic in an *in vitro* human lymphocyte assay both in the absence of and the presence of metabolic activation. Zolmitriptan was not clastogenic in *in vivo* mouse and rat micronucleus assays. Zolmitriptan was not genotoxic in an unscheduled DNA synthesis study.
Impairment of Fertility:
Studies of male and female rats administered zolmitriptan prior to and during mating and up to implantation have shown no impairment of fertility at doses up to 400 mg/kg/day. Exposure at this dose was approximately 3000 times exposure at the maximum recommended human dose of 10 mg/day.

Pregnancy:
Pregnancy Category C:
There are no adequate and well controlled studies in pregnant women; therefore, zolmitriptan should be used during pregnancy only if the potential benefit justifies the potential risk to the fetus.
In reproductive toxicity studies in rats and rabbits, oral administration of zolmitriptan to pregnant animals was associated with embryolethality and fetal abnormalities. When pregnant rats were administered oral zolmitriptan during the period of organogenesis at doses of 100, 400, and 1200 mg/kg/day, there was a dose-related increase in embryolethality which became statistically significant at the high dose. The maternal plasma exposures at these doses were approximately 280, 1100, and 5000 times the exposure in humans receiving the maximum recommended total daily dose of 10 mg. The high dose was maternally toxic, as evidenced by a decreased maternal body weight gain during gestation. In a similar study in rabbits, embryolethality was increased at the maternally toxic doses of 10 and 30 mg/kg/day (maternal plasma exposures equivalent to 11 and 42 times exposure in humans receiving the maximum recommended total daily dose of 10 mg), and increased incidences of fetal malformations (fused sternebrae, rib anomalies) and variations (major blood vessel variations, irregular ossification pattern of ribs) were observed at 30 mg/kg/day. Three mg/kg/day was a no effect dose (equivalent to human exposure at a dose of 10 mg). When female rats were given zolmitriptan during gestation, parturition, and lactation, an increased incidence of hydronephrosis was found in the offspring at the maternally toxic dose of 400 mg/kg/day (1100 times human exposure).

Nursing Mothers:
It is not known whether zolmitriptan is excreted in human milk. Because many drugs are excreted in human milk, caution should be exercised when zolmitriptan is administered to a nursing woman. Lactating rats dosed with zolmitriptan had levels in milk equivalent to maternal plasma levels at 1 hour and 4 times higher than plasma levels at 4 hours.

Pediatric Use:
Safety and effectiveness of ZOMIG in pediatric patients have not been established therefore ZOMIG is not recommended for use in patients under 18 years of age.
Postmarketing experience with other triptans includes a limited number of reports that describe pediatric patients who have experienced clinically serious adverse events that are similar in nature to those reported rarely in adults.

Geriatric Use:
Although the pharmacokinetic disposition of the drug in the elderly is similar to that seen in younger adults, there is no information about the safety and effectiveness of zolmitriptan in this population because patients over age 65 were excluded from the controlled clinical trials (see CLINICAL PHARMACOLOGY: Special Populations).

ADVERSE REACTIONS

Serious cardiac events, including myocardial infarction, have occurred following the use of ZOMIG Tablets. These events are extremely rare and most have been reported in patients with risk factors predictive of CAD. Events reported, in association with drugs of this class, have included coronary artery vasospasm, transient myocardial ischemia, myocardial infarction, ventricular tachycardia, and ventricular fibrillation (see CONTRAINDICATIONS, WARNINGS, and PRECAUTIONS).

Incidence in Controlled Clinical Trials:
Among 1383 patients treating 3398 attacks with zolmitriptan nasal spray in a blinded placebo controlled trial, there was a low withdrawal rate related to adverse events: 5 mg (1.3%), 2.5 mg (0%), 1 mg (0.8%), 0.5 mg (0.4%), and placebo (0.4%). None of the withdrawals were due to a serious event. One patient was withdrawn due to abnormal ECG changes from baseline that were incidentally found 23 days after the last dose of ZOMIG Nasal Spray. The most common adverse events in clinical trials for ZOMIG Nasal Spray were: unusual taste, paresthesia, hyperesthesia, and dizziness. The incidence of adverse events appeared to be dose-related, especially the nasopharyngeal events.
Table 2 lists the adverse events that occurred in ≥ 2% of the 1383 patients in any one of the zolmitriptan nasal sprays for the 0.5, 1, 2.5, or 5 mg dose groups of the controlled clinical trial.
[See table 2 above]

Table 2:
Adverse events with an incidence of ≥2% of patients in any zolmitriptan nasal spray treatment group by body system.

Body System and Adverse event[a]	Placebo (N=228)	Zolmitriptan nasal spray 0.5 mg (N=224)	1.0 mg (N=238)	2.5 mg (N=224)	5.0 mg (N=236)
ATYPICAL SENSATIONS					
Hyperesthesia	0%	0%	1%	1%	5%
Paraesthesia	6%	5%	7%	5%	10%
Sensation warm	2%	0%	0%	4%	0%
EAR/NOSE/THROAT					
Disorder/Discomfort of nasal cavity	2%	1%	3%	1%	3%
PAIN AND PRESSURE SENSATIONS					
Pain Location Specified	1%	0%	2%	2%	4%
Pain Throat	1%	1%	0%	4%	4%
Tightness Throat	1%	0%	1%	0%	2%
DIGESTIVE					
Dry Mouth	0%	1%	2%	3%	2%
Nausea	1%	1%	2%	0%	4%
NEUROLOGICAL					
Dizziness	4%	2%	4%	6%	3%
Somnolence	2%	0%	1%	1%	4%
Unusual Taste	3%	5%	10%	17%	21%
OTHER					
Asthenia	1%	0%	1%	3%	3%
Palpitation	0%	1%	2%	1%	1%
Reaction Aggravation[a]	2%	1%	0%	1%	2%

[a] Includes increases in nausea, vomiting, headache, somnolence and migraine associated stomach pain.

Adverse clinical events occurring in ≥ 1% and < 2% of patients in all attacks of the controlled clinical trial were pain abdominal, pressure throat, vomiting, headache, tightness chest, dysphagia, and insomnia.
ZOMIG is generally well tolerated. Across all doses, most adverse reactions were mild and transient and did not lead to long-lasting effects. The incidence of adverse events in controlled clinical trials was not affected by gender, weight, or age of the patients (18-39 vs. 40-65 years of age), or presence of aura. There were insufficient data to assess the impact of race on the incidence of adverse events.

Other Events:
In the paragraphs that follow, the frequencies of less commonly reported adverse clinical events are presented. Because the reports include events observed in open and uncontrolled studies, the role of ZOMIG in their causation cannot be reliably determined. Furthermore, variability associated with adverse event reporting, the terminology used to describe adverse events, etc., limit the value of the quantitative frequency estimates provided. Event frequencies are calculated as the number of patients who used ZOMIG Nasal Spray and reported an event divided by the total number of patients exposed to ZOMIG Nasal Spray (n=3059). All reported events are included except those already listed in the previous table, those too general to be informative, and those not reasonably associated with the use of the drug. Events are further classified within body system categories and enumerated in order of decreasing frequency using the following definitions: infrequent adverse events are those occurring in 1/100 to 1/1,000 patients and rare adverse events are those occurring in fewer than 1/1,000 patients.

Continued on next page

Zomig Nasal Spray—Cont.

Body:
Infrequent was allergic reaction, back pain, chills, cyst, flu syndrome, infection, jaw pain, pressure other, jaw tightening, edema of the face, abnormal laboratory test, neck pain, neoplasm, and neck tightness, chest heaviness, chest pain, and chest pressure. Rare were cellulitis, fever, jaw pressure, and neck heaviness.
Cardiovascular:
Infrequent were arrhythmias, hypertension, syncope, thrombophlebitis, and tachycardia. Rare were angina pectoris, bradycardia, atrial fibrillation, myocardial infarct, vasodilation, and vascular disorder.
Digestive:
Infrequent were diarrhea, dyspepsia, tongue edema, gastrointestinal disorder, increased saliva, and thirst. Rare were increased appetite, colitis, constipation, eructation, gastritis, gastrointestinal carcinoma, gingivitis, hepatic neoplasia, intestinal obstruction, jaundice, sialadenitis, and stomatitis.
Endocrine System:
Rare were hyperthyroidism and thyroid edema.
Hemic:
Infrequent was cyanosis. Rare were ecchymosis, lymphadenopathy and leukopenia.
Metabolic Nutritional:
Rare were increased weight, dehydration, and peripheral edema.
Musculoskeletal:
Infrequent were arthralgia, joint disorder, and myalgia. Rare were bone pain, osteoporosis, tenosynovitis and twitching.
Nervous System:
Infrequent were agitation, amnesia, anxiety, ataxia, abnormal coordination, confusion, depersonalization, depression, hypertonia, insomnia, nervousness, speech disorder, abnormal thinking, tremor, vertigo, and circumoral paresthesia. Rare were apathy, convulsions, abnormal dreams, euphoria, hypertonia, irritability tardive dyskinesia, manic reaction, neuropathy, and psychosis.
Respiratory:
Infrequent were bronchitis, increased cough, dyspnea, epistasis, laryngeal edema, pharyngitis, rhinitis, sinusitis, throat discomfort, and voice alteration. Rare was hiccup, hyperventilation, laryngitis, pneumonia, increased sputum, and yawning.
Skin:
Infrequent was pruritus, rash, skin disorder, and sweating. Rare were eczema, erythema, erythema multiform, hair disorder, and neoplasm.
Special Senses:
Infrequent were amblyopia, disorder of lacrimation, ear pain, eye pain, parosmia and tinnitus. Rare were conjunctivitis, dry eye, photophobia, and visual field defect.
Urogenital:
Infrequent was polyuria and menorrhagia. Rare were breast carcinoma, dysmenorrhea, metrorrhagia, breast neoplasm, unintended pregnancy, suspicious PAP smear, uterine disorder, enlarged uterine fibroids, fibrocytic breast, vaginitis, urogenital neoplasm, cystitis, urinary tract infection, kidney pain, pyelonephritis, urinary frequency, urine impaired, and urinary tract disorder.
The adverse experience profile seen with ZOMIG Nasal Spray is similar to that seen with ZOMIG tablets and Zomig-ZMT tablets except for the occurrence of local adverse effects from the nasal spray (see ZOMIG Tablet Prescribing information).

Postmarketing Experience with ZOMIG Tablets:
The following section enumerates potentially important adverse events that have occurred in clinical practice and which have been reported spontaneously to various surveillance systems. The events enumerated represent reports arising from both domestic and non-domestic use of oral zolmitriptan. The events enumerated include all except those already listed in the ADVERSE REACTIONS section above or those too general to be informative. Because the reports cite events reported spontaneously from worldwide postmarketing experience, frequency of events and the role of zolmitriptan in their causation cannot be reliably determined.
Cardiovascular:
Coronary artery vasospasm, transient myocardial ischemia, angina pectoris, and myocardial infarction.
Digestive:
Very rare gastrointestinal ischemic events including splenic infarction, ischemic colitis and gastrointestinal infarction or necrosis have been reported; these may present as bloody diarrhea or abdominal pain. (See WARNINGS.)
Neurological:
As with other acute migraine treatments including other $5HT_1$ agonists, there have been rare reports of headache.
General:
As with other $5\text{-}HT_{1B/1D}$ agonists, there have been very rare reports of anaphylaxis or anaphylactoid reactions in patients receiving ZOMIG. There have been rare reports of hypersensitivity reactions, including angioedema.

DRUG ABUSE AND DEPENDENCE

The abuse potential of ZOMIG has not been assessed in clinical trials.

OVERDOSAGE

There is no experience with clinical overdose. Volunteers receiving single 50 mg oral doses of zolmitriptan commonly experienced sedation.
The elimination half-life of ZOMIG is 3 hours (see CLINICAL PHARMACOLOGY) and therefore monitoring of patients after overdose with ZOMIG should continue for at least 15 hours or while symptoms or signs persist.
There is no specific antidote to zolmitriptan. In cases of severe intoxication, intensive care procedures are recommended, including establishing and maintaining a patent airway, ensuring adequate oxygenation and ventilation, and monitoring and support of the cardiovascular system.
It is unknown what effect hemodialysis or peritoneal dialysis has on the plasma concentrations of zolmitriptan.

DOSAGE AND ADMINISTRATION

Administer one dose of ZOMIG Nasal Spray 5 mg for the treatment of acute migraine. If the headache returns the dose may be repeated after 2 hours. The maximum daily dose should not exceed 10 mg in any 24-hour period.
In controlled clinical trials, single doses of 0.5, 1, 2.5 and 5 mg of zolmitriptan nasal spray were administered into one nostril and were effective for the treatment of acute migraines in adults. Efficacy improved with increasing dosage of zolmitriptan nasal spray and a greater proportion of patients had 2 hour headache response following a 5 mg dose than following a 0.5, 1, or 2.5 mg dose (see Table 1). A dose dependent increase in side effects was also seen with higher incidence of side effects at the 5 mg dose. This increase was attributed mainly to increased nasopharyngeal side effects, the majority of which were mild to moderate and transient.
Individuals may vary in response to ZOMIG Nasal Spray. The pharmacokinetics of a 5 mg nasal spray dose is similar to the 5 mg oral formulations. Doses lower than 5 mg can only be achieved through the use of an oral formulation. The choice of dose, and route of administration should therefore be made on an individual basis, weighing the possible benefit of the 5 mg dose with the potential for increased incidence of adverse events. The effectiveness of a second dose has not been established in placebo-controlled trials.
The safety of treating an average of more than four headaches in a 30 day period has not been established.

Hepatic Impairment:
Patients with moderate to severe hepatic impairment have decreased clearance of zolmitriptan and significant elevation in blood pressure was observed in some patients. Use of a lower dose of an alternate formulation with blood pressure monitoring is recommended (see CLINICAL PHARMACOLOGY AND WARNINGS).

HOW SUPPLIED

The ZOMIG Nasal Spray device is a blue colored plastic device with a gray protection cap, labeled to indicate the nominal dose. Each ZOMIG Nasal Spray device administers a single dose of ZOMIG.
ZOMIG Nasal Spray is supplied as a clear to pale yellow solution of zolmitriptan, buffered to a pH 5.0. Each ZOMIG Nasal Spray device contains 5 mg of zolmitriptan in a 100-μL unit dose aqueous buffered solution containing citric acid, anhydrous, USP, disodium phosphate dodecahydrate USP and purified water USP.
5 mg ZOMIG® Nasal Spray is supplied in boxes of 6 single use nasal spray units. (NDC 0037-7208-60).
Each ZOMIG® Nasal Spray single dose unit spray supplies 5 mg of zolmitriptan. The ZOMIG® Nasal Spray unit must be discarded after use.

Storage:
Store at controlled room temperature, 20-25°C (68-77°F) [see USP].

PATIENT SUMMARY OF INFORMATION

ZOMIG® Nasal Spray
(zolmitriptan)

Please read this information before you start taking ZOMIG® Nasal Spray and each time you renew your prescription just in case anything has changed. Remember, this summary does not take the place of discussions with your doctor. You and your doctor should discuss ZOMIG Nasal Spray when you start taking your medication and at regular checkups.

What is ZOMIG Nasal Spray?
ZOMIG Nasal Spray is a prescription medication used to treat migraine headaches in adults. ZOMIG Nasal Spray is not for other types of headaches. The safety and efficacy of ZOMIG in patients under 18 have not been established.

What is a Migraine Headache?
Migraine is an intense, throbbing headache. You may have pain on one or both sides of your head. You may have nausea and vomiting, and be sensitive to light and noise. The pain and symptoms of a migraine headache can be worse than a common headache. Some women get migraines around the time of their menstrual period. Some people have visual symptoms before the headache, such as flashing lights or wavy lines, called an aura.

How does ZOMIG Nasal Spray work?
Treatment with ZOMIG Nasal Spray reduces swelling of blood vessels surrounding the brain. This swelling is associated with the headache pain of a migraine attack. ZOMIG Nasal Spray blocks the release of substances from nerve endings that cause more pain and other symptoms like nausea, and sensitivity to light and sound. It is thought that these actions contribute to relief of your symptoms by ZOMIG Nasal Spray.

Who should not take ZOMIG Nasal Spray?
Do not take ZOMIG Nasal Spray if you:
- Have heart disease or a history of heart disease
- Have uncontrolled high blood pressure
- Have hemiplegic or basilar migraine (if you are not sure about this, ask your doctor)
- Have or had a stroke or problems with your blood circulation
- Have serious liver problems
- Have taken any of the following medicines in the last 24 hours: other "triptans" like almotriptan (Axert®), eletriptan (Relpax®), frovatriptan (Frova™), naratriptan (Amerge®), rizatriptan (Maxalt®), sumatriptan (Imitrex®); ergotamines like Bellergal-S®, Cafergot®, Ergomar®, Wigraine®; dihydroergotamine like D.H.E. 45® or Migranal®; or methysergide (Sansert®). These medications have side effects similar to ZOMIG Nasal Spray.
- Have taken monoamine oxidase (MAO) inhibitors such as phenelzine sulfate (Nardil®) or tranylcypromaine sulfate (Parnate®) for depression or other conditions, or if it has been less than 2 weeks since you stopped taking a MAO inhibitor.
- Are allergic to ZOMIG Nasal Spray or any of its ingredients. The active ingredient is zolmitriptan. The inactive ingredients are listed at the end of this leaflet.

Tell your doctor about all the medicines you take or plan to take, including prescription and nonprescription medicines, supplements, and herbal remedies. Your doctor will decide if you can take ZOMIG Nasal Spray with your other medicines.
Tell your doctor if you know that you have any of the following: risk factors for heart disease like high cholesterol, diabetes, smoking, obesity (overweight), menopause, or a family history of heart disease or stroke.
Tell your doctor if you are pregnant, planning to become pregnant, breast feeding, planning to breast feed, or not using effective birth control.

How should I take ZOMIG NASAL Spray?
The ZOMIG Nasal Spray device is a blue colored plastic sprayer device with a gray protection cap, labeled to indicate the dose. For adults, the usual dose is a single nasal spray taken into one nostril. If your headache comes back after your first dose, you may take a second dose anytime after 2 hours of taking the first dose. For any attack where the first dose didn't work, do not take a second dose without talking with your doctor. Do not take more than a total of 10 mg of ZOMIG (tablets or spray combined) in any 24-hour period. If you take too much medicine, contact your doctor, hospital emergency department, or poison control center right away.
The ZOMIG Nasal Spray device consists of the following parts:

A. **The Tip:** This is the part that you put into your nostril. The medicine comes out of a tiny hole in the top.
B. **The Protective Cap:** This covers the tip to protect it. Do not remove the protective cap until just before you are ready to take your ZOMIG Nasal Spray.
C. **The Finger-grip:** This is the part that you hold when you use the sprayer.
D. **The Plunger:** This is the part that you press when you put the tip into your nostril. This sprayer works only once.

Steps for using ZOMIG Nasal Spray (Please read all steps before using for the first time):

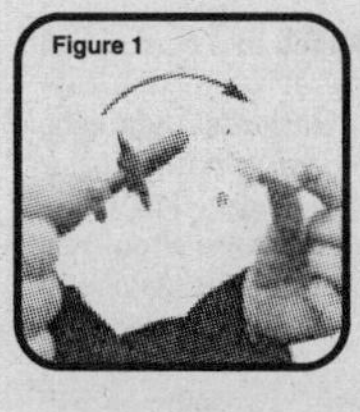
Figure 1

1. Blow your nose gently before use. Remove the protective cap (B) (Figure 1). Hold the nasal sprayer device gently with your fingers and thumb as shown in the picture to the right (Figure 2). Do not press the plunger until you have put the tip into your nostril or you will lose the dose.

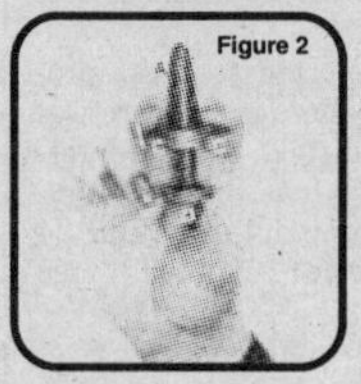
Figure 2

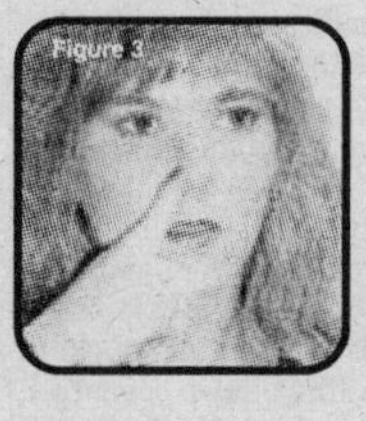
Figure 3

2. Block one nostril by pressing firmly on the side of your nose (Figure 3). Either nostril can be used. Put the tip (A) of the sprayer device into the other nostril as far as feels comfortable and tilt your head slightly as shown in the picture to the right (Figure 4).
Do not press the plunger yet.
Do not spray the contents of the device in your eyes.

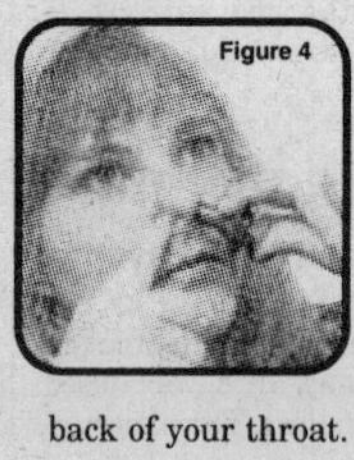
Figure 4

3. Breathe in gently through your nose and at the same time press the plunger (D) firmly with your thumb. The plunger may feel stiff and you may hear a click. Keep your head slightly tilted back and remove the tip from your nose. Breathe gently through your mouth for 5-10 seconds. You may feel liquid in your nose or the back of your throat. This is normal and will soon pass.

What are the possible side effects of ZOMIG Nasal Spray?
ZOMIG Nasal Spray is generally well tolerated. As with any medicine, people taking ZOMIG Nasal Spray may have side effects. The side effects are usually mild and do not last long.
The most common side effects of ZOMIG Nasal Spray are:
- unusual taste, dry mouth
- tingling sensation, skin sensitivity, especially around the nose
- pain, pressure, and tightness sensations (eg, in the nose, throat, or chest)
- drowsiness, weakness, dizziness
- nausea

In very rare cases, patients taking triptans may experience serious side effects, such as heart attacks, high blood pressure, stroke, or serious allergic reactions. Extremely rarely, patients have died. **Call your doctor right away if you have any of the following problems after taking ZOMIG Nasal Spray:**
- **severe tightness, pain, pressure or heaviness in your chest, throat, neck, or jaw**
- **shortness of breath or wheezing**
- **sudden or severe stomach pain**
- **hives; tongue, mouth, or throat swelling**
- **problems seeing**
- **unusual weakness or numbness**

This is not a complete list of side effects. Talk to your doctor if you develop any symptoms that concern you.
What to do in case of an overdose?
Call your doctor or poison control center or go to the ER.
General advice about ZOMIG Nasal Spray
Medicines are sometimes prescribed for conditions that are not mentioned in patient information leaflets. Do not use ZOMIG Nasal Spray for a condition for which it was not prescribed. Do not give ZOMIG Nasal Spray to other people, even if they have the same symptoms as you. People may be harmed if they take medicines that have not been Hold the nasal sprayer device gently with your fingers and thumb as shown in the picture to the right (Figure 2). Do not press the plunger until you have put the tip into your nostril or you will lose the dose.prescribed for them.
This leaflet summarizes the most important information about ZOMIG Nasal Spray. If you would like more information about ZOMIG Nasal Spray, talk to your doctor. You can ask your doctor or pharmacist for information on ZOMIG Nasal Spray that is written for health professionals. You can also call 1-800-236-9933 or visit our web site at www.ZOMIG.com.
What are the Ingredients in ZOMIG Nasal Spray?
Active ingredient: zolmitriptan
Inactive ingredients: anhydrous citric acid, dibasic sodium phosphate, and purified water
Store your medication at controlled room temperature, 20–25°C (68–77°F), and away from children. Discard after use or when it expires.

ZOMIG is a trademark of the AstraZeneca group.
© AstraZeneca 2003

Manufactured for:
AstraZeneca Pharmaceuticals LP
Wilmington, Delaware 19850
By: AstraZeneca UK Limited, Macclesfield,
Cheshire UK

Made in the United Kingdom
Rev 04/04   28573-02

Boehringer Ingelheim
Pharmaceuticals, Inc.

A subsidiary of Boehringer Ingelheim
900 RIDGEBURY ROAD
POST OFFICE BOX 368
RIDGEFIELD, CT 06877-0368
u.s.boehringer-ingelheim.com

For Medical Information Contact:
1–800–542–6257
or email:
druginfo@rdg.boehringer-ingelheim.com

ATROVENT® HFA   ℞
[ä′trō″vĕnt]
(ipratropium bromide HFA)
Inhalation Aerosol
For Oral Inhalation Only
Prescribing Information

DESCRIPTION
The active ingredient in ATROVENT® HFA (ipratropium bromide HFA) Inhalation Aerosol is ipratropium bromide. It is an anticholinergic/bronchodilator chemically described as 8-azoniabicyclo (3.2.1)-octane, 3-(3-hydroxy-1-oxo-2-phenyl-propoxy)-8-methyl-8-(1-methylethyl), bromide, monohydrate (endo,syn)-,(±)-: a synthetic quaternary ammonium compound, chemically related to atropine. The structural formula for ipratropium bromide is:

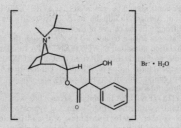

C$_{20}$H$_{30}$BrNO$_3$•H$_2$O   ipratropium bromide   Mol. Wt. 430.4

Ipratropium bromide is a white to off-white crystalline substance, freely soluble in water and methanol and sparingly soluble in ethanol and insoluble in lipophilic solvents such as ether, chloroform, and fluorocarbons.
ATROVENT HFA Inhalation Aerosol is a pressurized metered-dose aerosol unit for oral inhalation that contains a solution of ipratropium bromide. The net weight of each canister is 12.9 grams and provides 200 inhalations. After priming, each actuation of the inhaler delivers 21 mcg of ipratropium bromide from the valve in 56 mg of solution and delivers 17 mcg of ipratropium bromide from the mouthpiece. The actual amount of drug delivered to the lung may depend on patient factors, such as the coordination between the actuation of the device and inspiration through the delivery system. The excipients are HFA-134a (1,1,1,2-tetrafluoroethane) as propellant, purified water, dehydrated alcohol, and anhydrous citric acid. This product does not contain chlorofluorocarbons (CFCs) as a propellant. ATROVENT HFA Inhalation Aerosol should be primed before using for the first time by releasing 2 test sprays into the air away from the face. In cases where the inhaler has not been used for more than 3 days, prime the inhaler again by releasing 2 test sprays into the air away from the face.

CLINICAL PHARMACOLOGY
Mechanism of Action
Ipratropium bromide is an anticholinergic (parasympatholytic) agent which, based on animal studies, appears to inhibit vagally mediated reflexes by antagonizing the action of acetylcholine, the transmitter agent released at neuromuscular junctions in the lung. Anticholinergics prevent the increases in intracellular concentration of cyclic guanosine monophosphate (cyclic GMP) which are caused by interaction of acetylcholine with the muscarinic receptor on bronchial smooth muscle.

Pharmacodynamic Properties
Controlled clinical studies have demonstrated that ATROVENT (ipratropium bromide HFA) Inhalation Aerosol CFC does not alter either mucociliary clearance or the volume or viscosity of respiratory secretions.

Pharmacokinetics and Metabolism
Most of an administered dose is swallowed as shown by fecal excretion studies. Ipratropium bromide is a quaternary amine. It is not readily absorbed into the systemic circulation either from the surface of the lung or from the gastrointestinal tract as confirmed by blood level and renal excretion studies.
Autoradiographic studies in rats have shown that ipratropium bromide does not penetrate the blood-brain barrier. The half-life of elimination is about 2 hours after inhalation or intravenous administration. Ipratropium bromide is minimally bound (0 to 9% in vitro) to plasma albumin and α_1-acid glycoprotein. It is partially metabolized to inactive ester hydrolysis products. Following intravenous administration, approximately one-half of the dose is excreted unchanged in the urine.
A pharmacokinetic study with 29 chronic obstructive pulmonary disease (COPD) patients (48-79 years of age) demonstrated that mean peak plasma ipratropium concentrations of 59±20 pg/mL were obtained following a single administration of 4 inhalations of ATROVENT HFA Inhalation Aerosol (84 mcg). Plasma ipratropium concentrations rapidly declined to 24±15 pg/mL by six hours. When these patients were administered 4 inhalations QID (16 inhalations/day=336 mcg) for one week, the mean peak plasma ipratropium concentration increased to 82±39 pg/mL with a trough (6 hour) concentration of 28±12 pg/mL at steady state.

Special Populations
Geriatric Patients
In the pharmacokinetic study with 29 COPD patients, a subset of 14 patients were >65 years of age. Mean peak plasma ipratropium concentrations of 56±24 pg/mL were obtained following a single administration of 4 inhalations (21 mcg/puff) of ATROVENT HFA Inhalation Aerosol (84 mcg). When these 14 patients were administered 4 inhalations QID (16 inhalations/day) for one week, the mean peak plasma ipratropium concentration only increased to 84±50 pg/mL indicating that the pharmacokinetic behavior of ipratropium bromide in the geriatric population is consistent with younger patients.

Renally Impaired Patients
The pharmacokinetics of ATROVENT HFA Inhalation Aerosol have not been studied in patients with renal insufficiency.

Hepatically Impaired Patients
The pharmacokinetics of ATROVENT HFA Inhalation Aerosol have not been studied in patients with hepatic insufficiency.

CLINICAL STUDIES
Conclusions regarding the efficacy of ATROVENT HFA (ipratropium bromide HFA) Inhalation Aerosol were derived from two randomized, double-blind, controlled clinical studies. These studies enrolled males and females ages 40 years and older, with a history of COPD, a smoking history of >10 pack-years, an FEV$_1$ <65% and an FEV$_1$/FVC <70%. One of the studies was a 12-week randomized, double-blind active and placebo controlled study in which 505 of the 507 randomized COPD patients were evaluated for the safety and efficacy of 42 mcg (n=124) and 84 mcg (n=126) ATROVENT HFA Inhalation Aerosol in comparison to 42 mcg (n=127) ATROVENT Inhalation Aerosol CFC and their respective placebos (HFA n=62, CFC n=66). Data for both placebo HFA and placebo CFC were combined in the evaluation.
Serial FEV$_1$ (shown in Figure 1, below, as means adjusted for center and baseline effects on test day 1 and test day 85 (primary endpoint)) demonstrated that 1 dose (2 inhalations/21 mcg each) of ATROVENT HFA Inhalation Aerosol produced significantly greater improvement in pulmonary function than placebo. During the six hours immediately post-dose on day 1, the average hourly improvement in adjusted mean FEV$_1$ was 0.148 liters for ATROVENT HFA Inhalation Aerosol (42 mcg) and 0.013 liters for placebo. The mean peak improvement in FEV$_1$, relative to baseline, was 0.295 liters, compared to 0.138 liters for placebo. During the six hours immediately post-dose on day 85, the average hourly improvement in adjusted mean FEV$_1$ was 0.141 liters for ATROVENT HFA Inhalation aerosol (42 mcg) and 0.014 liters for placebo. The mean peak improvement in FEV$_1$, relative to baseline, was 0.295 liters, compared to 0.140 liters for placebo.
ATROVENT HFA Inhalation Aerosol (42 mcg) was shown to be clinically comparable to ATROVENT Inhalation Aerosol CFC (42 mcg).

Figure 1   Day 1 and Day 85 (Primary Endpoint) Results

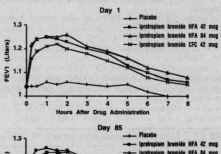
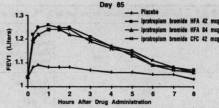

In this study, both ATROVENT HFA Inhalation Aerosol and ATROVENT Inhalation Aerosol CFC formulations were equally effective in patients over 65 years of age and under 65 years of age.
The median time to improvement in pulmonary function (FEV$_1$ increase of 15% or more) was within approximately 15 minutes, reached a peak in 1-2 hours, and persisted for 2 to 4 hours in the majority of the patients. Improvements in Forced Vital Capacity (FVC) were also demonstrated.
The other study was a 12-week, randomized, double-blind, active-controlled clinical study in 174 adults with COPD, in which ATROVENT HFA Inhalation Aerosol 42 mcg (n=118) was compared to ATROVENT Inhalation Aerosol CFC 42 mcg (n=56). Safety and efficacy of HFA and CFC formulations were shown to be comparable.
The bronchodilatory efficacy and comparability of ATROVENT HFA Inhalation Aerosol vs. ATROVENT Inhalation Aerosol CFC were also studied in a one-year open-label safety and efficacy study in 456 COPD patients. The safety and efficacy of HFA and CFC formulations were shown to be comparable.

INDICATIONS AND USAGE
ATROVENT HFA (ipratropium bromide HFA) Inhalation Aerosol is indicated as a bronchodilator for maintenance treatment of bronchospasm associated with chronic obstructive pulmonary disease, including chronic bronchitis and emphysema.

CONTRAINDICATIONS
ATROVENT HFA (ipratropium bromide HFA) Inhalation Aerosol is contraindicated in patients with a history of hypersensitivity to ipratropium bromide or other ATROVENT HFA Inhalation Aerosol components. ATROVENT Inhalation Aerosol is also contraindicated in patients who are hypersensitive to atropine or its derivatives.

WARNINGS
ATROVENT HFA (ipratropium bromide HFA) Inhalation Aerosol is a bronchodilator for the maintenance treatment

Continued on next page

Atrovent HFA—Cont.

of bronchospasm associated with COPD and is not indicated for the initial treatment of acute episodes of bronchospasm where rescue therapy is required for rapid response.

Immediate hypersensitivity reactions may occur after administration of ipratropium bromide, as demonstrated by rare cases of urticaria, angioedema, rash, bronchospasm, anaphylaxis and oropharyngeal edema.

Inhaled medicines, including ATROVENT HFA (ipratropium bromide HFA) Inhalation Aerosol, may cause paradoxical bronchospasm. If this occurs, treatment with ATROVENT HFA (ipratropium bromide HFA) Inhalation Aerosol should be stopped and other treatments considered.

PRECAUTIONS

General

ATROVENT HFA (ipratropium bromide HFA) Inhalation Aerosol should be used with caution in patients with narrow-angle glaucoma, prostatic hypertrophy or bladder-neck obstruction.

Information for Patients

Appropriate and safe use of ATROVENT HFA Inhalation Aerosol includes providing the patient with the information listed below and an understanding of the way it should be administered (see **Patient's Instructions for Use**).

Patients should be advised that ATROVENT HFA (ipratropium bromide HFA) Inhalation Aerosol is a bronchodilator for the maintenance treatment of bronchospasm associated with COPD and is not indicated for the initial treatment of acute episodes of bronchospasm where rescue therapy is required for rapid response.

Patients should be cautioned to avoid spraying the aerosol into their eyes and be advised that this may result in precipitation or worsening of narrow-angle glaucoma, mydriasis, eye pain or discomfort, temporary blurring of vision, visual halos or colored images in association with red eyes from conjunctival and corneal congestion. Patients should also be advised that should any combination of these symptoms develop, they should consult their physician immediately.

The action of ATROVENT HFA Inhalation Aerosol should last 2-4 hours. Patients should be advised not to increase the dose or frequency of ATROVENT HFA Inhalation Aerosol without patients consulting their physician. Patients should also be advised to seek immediate medical attention if treatment with ATROVENT HFA Inhalation Aerosol becomes less effective for symptomatic relief, their symptoms become worse, and/or patients need to use the product more frequently than usual.

Patients should be advised on the use of ATROVENT HFA® Inhalation Aerosol in relation to other inhaled drugs.

Patients should be reminded that ATROVENT HFA Inhalation Aerosol should be used consistently as prescribed throughout the course of therapy.

Patients should be advised that although the taste and inhalation sensation of ATROVENT HFA Inhalation Aerosol may be slightly different from that of the CFC (chlorofluorocarbon) formulation of ATROVENT Inhalation Aerosol, they are comparable in terms of safety and efficacy.

Drug Interactions

ATROVENT HFA Inhalation Aerosol has been used concomitantly with other drugs, including sympathomimetic bronchodilators, methylxanthines, oral and inhaled steroids, that may be used in the treatment of chronic obstructive pulmonary disease. With the exception of albuterol, there are no formal studies fully evaluating the interaction effects of ATROVENT and these drugs with respect to effectiveness.

Anticholinergic agents: Although ipratropium bromide is minimally absorbed into the systemic circulation, there is some potential for an additive interaction with concomitantly used anticholinergic medications. Caution is therefore advised in the co-administration of ATROVENT HFA Inhalation Aerosol with other anticholinergic-containing drugs.

Carcinogenesis, Mutagenesis, Impairment of Fertility

In two-year oral carcinogenicity studies in rats and mice ipratropium bromide at oral doses up to 6 mg/kg (approximately 240 and 120 times the maximum recommended daily inhalation dose in adults on a mg/m^2 basis) showed no carcinogenic activity. Results of various mutagenicity studies (Ames test, mouse dominant lethal test, mouse micronucleus test and chromosome aberration of bone marrow in Chinese hamsters) were negative.

Fertility of male or female rats at oral doses up to 50 mg/kg (approximately 2000 times the maximum recommended daily inhalation dose in adults on a mg/m^2 basis) was unaffected by ipratropium bromide administration. At an oral dose of 500 mg/kg (approximately 20,000 times the maximum recommended daily inhalation dose in adults on a mg/m^2 basis), ipratropium bromide produced a decrease in the conception rate.

Pregnancy

Teratogenic Effects, *Pregnancy Category B*

Oral reproduction studies were performed at doses of 10 mg/kg/day in mice, 1,000 mg/kg in rats and 125 mg/kg/day in rabbits. These doses correspond, in each species, respectively, to approximately 200, 40,000 and 10,000 times the maximum recommended daily inhalation dose in adults on a mg/m^2 basis. Inhalation reproduction studies were conducted in rats and rabbits at doses of 1.5 and 1.8 mg/kg (approximately 60 and 140 times the maximum recommended daily inhalation dose in adults on a mg/m^2 basis). These

studies demonstrated no evidence of teratogenic effects as a result of ipratropium bromide. At oral doses of 90 mg/kg and above in rats (approximately 3600 times the maximum recommended daily inhalation dose in adults on a mg/m^2 basis) embryotoxicity was observed as increased resorption. This effect is not considered relevant to human use due to the large doses at which it was observed and the difference in route of administration. There are, however, no adequate and well-controlled studies in pregnant women. Because animal reproduction studies are not always predictive of human response, ATROVENT HFA Inhalation Aerosol should be used during pregnancy only if clearly needed.

Nursing Mothers

It is not known whether the active component, ipratropium bromide, is excreted in human milk. Although lipid-insoluble quaternary cations pass into breast milk, it is unlikely that ipratropium bromide would reach the infant to an important extent, especially when taken by aerosol. However, because many drugs are excreted in human milk, caution should be exercised when ATROVENT HFA Inhalation Aerosol is administered to a nursing woman.

Pediatric Use

Safety and effectiveness in the pediatric population have not been established.

Geriatric Use

In the pivotal 12-week study, both ATROVENT HFA Inhalation Aerosol and ATROVENT Inhalation Aerosol CFC formulations were equally effective in patients over 65 years of age and under 65 years of age.

Of the total number of subjects in clinical studies of ATROVENT HFA Inhalation Aerosol, 57% were ≥65 years of age. No overall differences in safety or effectiveness were observed between these subjects and younger subjects.

ADVERSE REACTIONS

The adverse reaction information concerning ATROVENT HFA (ipratropium bromide HFA) Inhalation Aerosol is derived from two 12-week, double-blind, parallel group studies and one open-label, parallel group study that compared ATROVENT HFA Inhalation Aerosol, ATROVENT Inhalation Aerosol CFC, and placebo (in one study only) in 1,010 COPD patients. The following table lists the incidence of adverse events that occurred at a rate of greater than or equal to 3% in any ipratropium bromide group. Overall, the incidence and nature of the adverse events reported for ATROVENT HFA Inhalation Aerosol, ATROVENT Inhalation Aerosol CFC, and placebo were comparable.

[See table 1 below]

In the one open label controlled study in 456 COPD patients, the overall incidence of adverse events was also similar between ATROVENT HFA Inhalation Aerosol and ATROVENT Inhalation Aerosol CFC formulations.

Overall, in the above mentioned studies, 9.3% of the patients taking 42 mcg ATROVENT HFA Inhalation Aerosol and 8.7% of the patients taking 42 mcg ATROVENT Inhalation Aerosol CFC reported at least one adverse event that was considered by the investigator to be related to the study drug. The most common drug-related adverse events were dry mouth (1.6% of ATROVENT HFA Inhalation Aerosol and 0.9% of ATROVENT Inhalation Aerosol CFC patients), and taste perversion (bitter taste) (0.9% of ATROVENT HFA Inhalation Aerosol and 0.3% of ATROVENT Inhalation Aerosol CFC patients).

As an anticholinergic drug, cases of precipitation or worsening of narrow-angle glaucoma, mydriasis, acute eye pain, hypotension, urinary retention, tachycardia, constipation, bronchospasm, including paradoxical bronchospasm have been reported.

Allergic-type reactions such as skin rash, angioedema of tongue, lips and face, urticaria (including giant urticaria), laryngospasm and anaphylactic reaction have been reported (see **CONTRAINDICATIONS**).

Post-Marketing Experience

Post-marketing experience with ATROVENT Inhalation Aerosol CFC in a 5-year placebo-controlled study, found that hospitalizations for supraventricular tachycardia and atrial fibrillation occurred with an incidence rate of 0.5% in patients receiving ATROVENT Inhalation Aerosol CFC.

Allergic-type reactions such as skin rash, angioedema of tongue, lips and face, urticaria (including giant urticaria), laryngospasm and anaphylactic reactions have been reported, with positive rechallenge in some cases. Many of the patients had a history of allergies to other drugs and/or foods, including soybean.

Additionally, urinary retention, mydriasis, and bronchospasm, including paradoxical bronchospasm, have been reported during the post-marketing period with use of ATROVENT Inhalation Aerosol CFC.

OVERDOSAGE

Acute overdose by inhalation is unlikely since ipratropium bromide is not well absorbed systemically after inhalation or oral administration. Oral median lethal doses of ipratropium bromide were greater than 1000 mg/kg in mice (approximately 20,000 times the maximum recommended daily inhalation dose in adults on a mg/m^2 basis); 1,700 mg/kg in rats (approximately 68,000 times the maximum recommended daily inhalation dose in adults on a mg/m^2 basis); and 400 mg/kg in dogs (approximately 53,000 times the maximum recommended daily inhalation dose in adults on a mg/m^2 basis).

DOSAGE AND ADMINISTRATION

Patients should be instructed on the proper use of their inhaler (see **Patient's Instructions for Use**).

TABLE 1   Adverse Experiences Reported in ≥ 3% of Patients in any Ipratropium Bromide Group

	Placebo-controlled 12 week Study 244.1405 and Active-controlled 12 week Study 244.1408			Active-controlled 1-year Study 244.2453	
	Atrovent HFA (N=243) %	Atrovent CFC (N=183) %	Placebo (N=128) %	Atrovent HFA (N=305) %	Atrovent CFC (N=151) %
Total With Any Adverse Event	63	68	72	91	87
BODY AS A WHOLE - GENERAL DISORDERS					
back pain	2	3	2	7	3
headache	6	9	8	7	5
influenza-like symptoms	4	2	2	8	5
CENTR & PERIPH NERVOUS SYSTEM DISORDERS					
dizziness	3	3	2	3	1
GASTRO-INTESTINAL SYSTEM DISORDERS					
dyspepsia	1	3	1	5	3
mouth dry	4	2	2	2	3
nausea	4	1	2	4	4
RESPIRATORY SYSTEM DISORDERS					
bronchitis	10	11	6	23	19
COPD exacerbation	8	14	13	23	23
coughing	3	4	6	5	5
dyspnea	8	8	4	7	4
rhinitis	4	2	4	6	2
sinusitis	1	4	3	11	14
upper resp tract infection	9	10	16	34	34
URINARY SYSTEM DISORDERS					
urinary tract infection	2	3	1	10	8

Patients should be advised that although ATROVENT HFA (ipratropium bromide HFA) Inhalation Aerosol may have a slightly different taste and inhalation sensation than that of an inhaler containing ATROVENT Inhalation Aerosol, they are comparable in terms of the safety and efficacy. ATROVENT HFA Inhalation Aerosol is a solution aerosol that does not require shaking. However, as with any other metered dose inhaler, some coordination is required between actuating the canister and inhaling the medication. Patients should "prime" or actuate ATROVENT HFA Inhalation Aerosol before using for the first time by releasing 2 test sprays into the air away from the face. In cases where the inhaler has not been used for more than 3 days, prime the inhaler again by releasing 2 test sprays into the air away from the face. Patients should avoid spraying ATROVENT HFA Inhalation Aerosol in their eyes.

The usual starting dose of ATROVENT HFA Inhalation Aerosol is two inhalations four times a day. Patients may take additional inhalations as required; however, the total number of inhalations should not exceed 12 in 24 hours. Each actuation of ATROVENT HFA Inhalation Aerosol delivers 17 mcg of ipratropium bromide from the mouthpiece.

HOW SUPPLIED

ATROVENT HFA (ipratropium bromide HFA) Inhalation Aerosol is supplied in a 12.9 g pressurized stainless steel canister as a metered-dose inhaler with a white mouthpiece that has a clear, colorless sleeve and a green protective cap (NDC 0597-0087-17).

The ATROVENT HFA Inhalation Aerosol canister is to be used only with the accompanying ATROVENT HFA Inhalation Aerosol mouthpiece. This mouthpiece should not be used with other aerosol medications. Similarly, the canister should not be used with other mouthpieces. Each actuation of ATROVENT HFA Inhalation Aerosol delivers 21 mcg of ipratropium bromide from the valve and 17 mcg from the mouthpiece. Each 12.9 gram canister provides sufficient medication for 200 inhalations. The canister should be discarded after the labeled number of actuations has been used. The amount of medication in each actuation cannot be assured after this point, even though the canister is not completely empty.

Store at 25°C (77°F). Excursions permitted to 15-30°C (59-86°F) [see USP Controlled Room Temperature]. For optimal results, the canister should be at room temperature before use.

Patients should be reminded to read and follow the accompanying "Instructions for Use", which should be dispensed with the product.

Contents Under Pressure: Do not puncture. Do not use or store near heat or open flame. Exposure to temperatures above 120°F may cause bursting. Never throw the inhaler into a fire or incinerator.

Warning: Keep out of children's reach. Avoid spraying in eyes.

Rx only

Manufactured for:
Boehringer Ingelheim Pharmaceuticals, Inc.
Ridgefield, CT 06877 USA
By:
3M Pharmaceuticals
St. Paul, MN 55144 USA
Licensed from:
Boehringer Ingelheim International GmbH
© Copyright Boehringer Ingelheim International GmbH
2004, ALL RIGHTS RESERVED
Revised November 17, 2004
IT1902
10003001/US/1
U.S. Patent No. 6,739,333

PATIENT'S INSTRUCTIONS FOR USE

Atrovent® HFA
(ipratropium bromide HFA)
Inhalation Aerosol
Read all of the instructions carefully before using.
Important Points to Remember About Using ATROVENT HFA Inhalation Aerosol

Although ATROVENT HFA Inhalation Aerosol may taste and feel different when breathed in compared to your ATROVENT Inhalation Aerosol CFC inhaler, they contain the same medicine.

You do not have to shake the **ATROVENT HFA** Inhalation Aerosol canister before using it.

ATROVENT HFA Inhalation Aerosol should be "primed" two times before taking the first dose from a new inhaler or when the inhaler has not been used for more than three days. To prime, push the canister against the mouthpiece (see Figure 1), allowing the medicine to spray into the air. **Avoid spraying the medicine into your eyes while priming ATROVENT HFA Inhalation Aerosol.**

Ask your doctor how to use other inhaled medicines with **ATROVENT HFA Inhalation Aerosol.**

Use ATROVENT HFA Inhalation Aerosol exactly as prescribed by your doctor. Do not change your dose or how often you use **ATROVENT HFA** Inhalation Aerosol without talking with your doctor. Talk to your doctor if you have questions about your medical condition or your treatment.

Instructions

1. Insert the metal canister into the clear end of the mouthpiece (see Figure 1). Make sure the canister is fully and firmly inserted into the mouthpiece. The **ATROVENT HFA** Inhalation Aerosol canister is for use only with the **ATROVENT HFA** Inhalation Aerosol mouthpiece. Do not use the **ATROVENT HFA** Inhalation Aerosol canister with

other mouthpieces. This mouthpiece should not be used with other inhaled medicines.

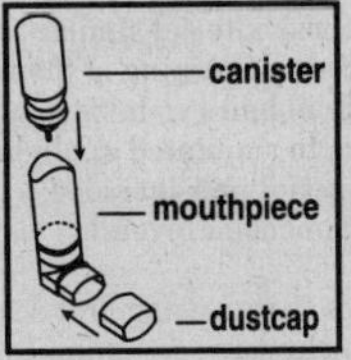

Figure 1

2. Remove the **green** protective **dust** cap. If the cap is not on the mouthpiece, make sure there is nothing in the mouthpiece before use. For best results, the canister should be at room temperature before use.
3. **Breathe out (exhale) deeply** through your mouth. Hold the canister upright as shown in Figure 2, between your thumb and first 2 fingers. Put the mouthpiece in your mouth and close your lips. Keep your eyes closed so that no medicine will be sprayed into your eyes. **ATROVENT HFA** Inhalation Aerosol can cause blurry vision, narrow-angle glaucoma or worsening of this condition or eye pain if the medicine is sprayed into your eyes.

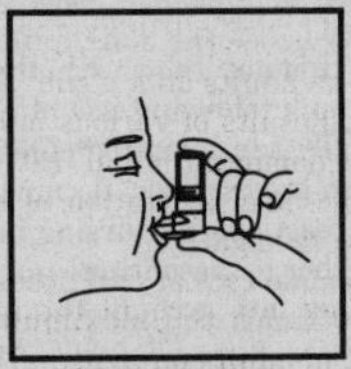

Figure 2

4. **Breathe in (inhale) slowly** through your mouth and at the same time firmly press once on the canister against the mouthpiece as shown in Figure 3. Keep breathing in deeply.

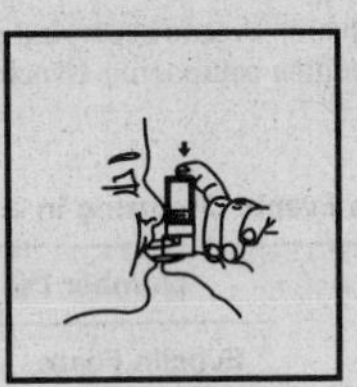

Figure 3

5. **Hold your breath** for ten seconds and then remove the mouthpiece from your mouth and breathe out slowly, as in Figure 4. **Wait at least 15 seconds and repeat steps 3 to 5 again.**

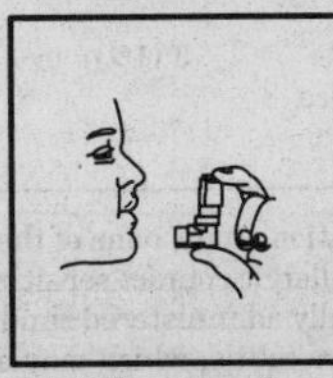

Figure 4

6. Replace the green protective dust cap after use.
7. **Keep the mouthpiece clean.** It is very important to keep the mouthpiece clean. At least once a week, wash the mouthpiece, shake it to remove excess water and let it air dry all the way (see the instructions below).

Mouthpiece Cleaning Instructions:
Step A. Remove and set aside the canister and dust cap from the mouthpiece (see Figure 1).
Step B. Wash the mouthpiece through the top and bottom with warm running water for at least 30 seconds (see Figure 5). Do not use anything other than water to wash the mouthpiece.

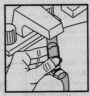

Figure 5

Step C. Dry the mouthpiece by shaking off the excess water and allow it to air-dry all the way.
Step D. When the mouthpiece is dry, replace the canister. Make sure the canister is fully and firmly inserted into the mouthpiece.
Step E. Replace the green protective dust cap.
If the mouthpiece becomes blocked, and little or no medicine comes out of the mouthpiece, wash the mouthpiece as described in Steps A to E under the "**Mouthpiece Cleaning Instructions**".

8. **Keep track of the number of sprays used. Discard the canister after 200 sprays.** Even though the canister is not empty, you cannot be sure of the amount of medicine in each spray after 200 sprays.

This product does not contain any chlorofluorocarbon (CFC) propellants.

The contents of **ATROVENT HFA** Inhalation Aerosol are under pressure. Do not puncture the canister. Do not use or store near heat or open flame. Exposure to temperatures above 120°F may cause bursting. Never throw the container into a fire or incinerator.

Keep **ATROVENT HFA** Inhalation Aerosol and all medicines out of the reach of children.

Avoid spraying into eyes.

Store at 25°C (77°F). Excursions permitted to 15-30°C (59-86°F). For best results, store the canister at room temperature before use.

Rx only

Manufactured for:
Boehringer Ingelheim Pharmaceuticals, Inc.
Ridgefield, CT 06877 USA
By:
3M Pharmaceuticals
St. Paul, MN 55144 USA
Licensed from:
Boehringer Ingelheim International GmbH
© Copyright Boehringer Ingelheim International GmbH
2004, ALL RIGHTS RESERVED
Revised November 17, 2004
IT1902
10003001/US/1
U.S. Patent No. 6,739,333

Connetics Corporation
3160 PORTER DRIVE
PALO ALTO, CA 94304

Direct Inquiries to:
(650) 843-2800
FAX: (650) 843-2899
www.connetics.com

For Medical Information Contact:
Medical Information Department
(877) 821-5337
FAX: (510) 595-8183
E-mail: medicalaffairs@connetics.com

EVOCLIN™ ℞
[ĕ-vō-klĭn]
(clindamycin phosphate) Foam, 1%
Rx Only
FOR TOPICAL USE ONLY. NOT FOR OPHTHALMIC, ORAL, OR INTRAVAGINAL USE.

DESCRIPTION

Evoclin (clindamycin phosphate) Foam, 1%, a topical antibiotic in a foam vehicle, contains clindamycin phosphate, USP, at a concentration equivalent to 10 mg clindamycin per gram in a vehicle consisting of cetyl alcohol, dehydrated alcohol (ethanol 58%), polysorbate 60, potassium hydroxide, propylene glycol, purified water, and stearyl alcohol, pressurized with a hydrocarbon (propane/butane) propellant. Chemically, clindamycin phosphate is a water-soluble ester of the semi-synthetic antibiotic produced by a 7 (S)-chloro-substitution of the 7 (R)-hydroxyl group of the parent antibiotic, lincomycin, and has the structural formula represented below:

Figure 1: Structural Formula

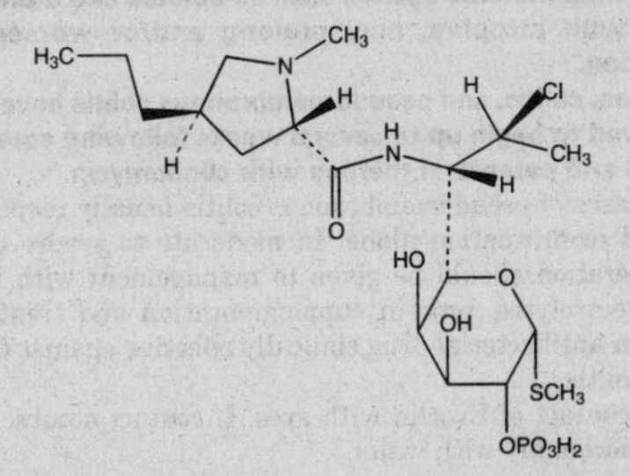

The chemical name for clindamycin phosphate is methyl 7-chloro-6,7,8-trideoxy-6-(1-methyl-*trans*-4-propyl-L-2-pyrrolidinecarboxamido)-1-thio-L-*threo*-α-D-*galacto*-octopyranoside 2-(dihydrogen phosphate).

CLINICAL PHARMACOLOGY

Pharmacokinetics: In an open label, parallel group study in 24 patients with acne vulgaris, 12 patients (3 male and 9 female) applied 4 grams of Evoclin Foam once-daily for five days, and 12 patients (7 male and 5 female) applied 4 grams of Clindagel® (clindamycin phosphate) Topical Gel, 1%, once daily for five days. On Day 5, the mean C_{max} and AUC(0-12)

Continued on next page

Evoclin—Cont.

were 23% and 9% lower, respectively, for Evoclin Foam than for Clindagel®.

Following multiple applications of Evoclin Foam less than 0.024% of the total dose was excreted unchanged in the urine over 12 hours on Day 5.

Microbiology: The clindamycin component has been shown to have in vitro activity against *Propionibacterium acnes*, an organism which is associated with acne vulgaris; however, the clinical significance of this activity against *P. acnes* was not examined in clinical trials with this product. Cross-resistance between clindamycin and erythromycin has been demonstrated.

CLINICAL STUDIES

In one multicenter, randomized, double-blind, vehicle-controlled clinical trial patients with mild to moderate acne vulgaris used Evoclin (clindamycin phosphate) Foam, 1% or the vehicle foam once daily for twelve weeks. Treatment response, defined as the proportion of patients clear or almost clear, based on the Investigator Static Global Assessment (ISGA), and the mean percent reductions in lesion counts at the end of treatment in this study are shown in the following table:

Efficacy Parameters	Evoclin Foam N=386	Vehicle Foam N=127
Treatment response (ISGA)	31%	18%*
Percent reduction in lesion counts		
Inflammatory Lesions	49%	35%*
Noninflammatory Lesions	38%	27%*
Total Lesions	43%	31%*

*P< 0.05

INDICATIONS AND USAGE

Evoclin is indicated for topical application in the treatment of acne vulgaris. In view of the potential for diarrhea, bloody diarrhea and pseudomembranous colitis, the physician should consider whether other agents are more appropriate. (See CONTRAINDICATIONS, WARNINGS, and ADVERSE REACTIONS.)

CONTRAINDICATIONS

Evoclin is contraindicated in individuals with a history of hypersensitivity to preparations containing clindamycin or lincomycin, a history of regional enteritis or ulcerative colitis, or a history of antibiotic-associated colitis.

WARNINGS

Orally and parenterally administered clindamycin has been associated with severe colitis, which may result in patient death. Use of the topical formulation of clindamycin results in absorption of the antibiotic from the skin surface. Diarrhea, bloody diarrhea, and colitis (including pseudomembranous colitis) have been reported with the use of topical and systemic clindamycin.

Studies indicate a toxin(s) produced by *Clostridia* is one primary cause of antibiotic-associated colitis. The colitis is usually characterized by severe persistent diarrhea and severe abdominal cramps and may be associated with the passage of blood and mucus. Endoscopic examination may reveal pseudomembranous colitis. Stool culture for *Clostridium difficile* and stool assay for *C. difficile* toxin may be helpful diagnostically.

When significant diarrhea occurs, the drug should be discontinued. Large bowel endoscopy should be considered to establish a definitive diagnosis in cases of severe diarrhea. Antiperistaltic agents, such as opiates and diphenoxylate with atropine, may prolong and/or worsen the condition.

Diarrhea, colitis, and pseudomembranous colitis have been observed to begin up to several weeks following cessation of oral and parenteral therapy with clindamycin.

Mild cases of pseudomembranous colitis usually respond to drug discontinuation alone. In moderate to severe cases, consideration should be given to management with fluids and electrolytes, protein supplementation and treatment with an antibacterial drug clinically effective against *C. difficile* colitis.

Avoid contact of Evoclin with eyes. If contact occurs, rinse eyes thoroughly with water.

PRECAUTIONS

General: Evoclin should be prescribed with caution in atopic individuals.

Drug Interactions: Clindamycin has been shown to have neuromuscular blocking properties that may enhance the action of other neuromuscular blocking agents. Therefore, it should be used with caution in patients receiving such agents.

Carcinogenesis, Mutagenesis, Impairment of Fertility

The carcinogenicity of a 1% clindamycin phosphate gel similar to Evoclin was evaluated by daily application to mice for two years. The daily doses used in this study were approximately 3 and 15 times higher than the human dose of clindamycin phosphate from 5 milliliters of Evoclin, assuming

complete absorption and based on a body surface area comparison. No significant increase in tumors was noted in the treated animals.

A 1% clindamycin phosphate gel similar to Evoclin caused a statistically significant shortening of the median time to tumor onset in a study in hairless mice in which tumors were induced by exposure to simulated sunlight.

Genotoxicity tests performed included a rat micronucleus test and an Ames Salmonella reversion test. Both tests were negative.

Reproduction studies in rats using oral doses of clindamycin hydrochloride and clindamycin palmitate hydrochloride have revealed no evidence of impaired fertility.

Pregnancy: Teratogenic effects - Pregnancy Category B

Reproduction studies have been performed in rats and mice using subcutaneous and oral doses of clindamycin phosphate, clindamycin hydrochloride and clindamycin palmitate hydrochloride. These studies revealed no evidence of fetal harm. The highest dose used in the rat and mouse teratogenicity studies was equivalent to a clindamycin phosphate dose of 432 mg/kg. For a rat, this dose is 84 fold higher, and for a mouse 42 fold higher, than the anticipated human dose of clindamycin phosphate from Evoclin based on a mg/m² comparison. There are, however, no adequate and well-controlled studies in pregnant women. Because animal reproduction studies are not always predictive of human response, this drug should be used during pregnancy only if clearly needed.

Nursing Mothers: It is not known whether clindamycin is excreted in human milk following use of Evoclin. However, orally and parenterally administered clindamycin has been reported to appear in breast milk. Because of the potential for serious adverse reactions in nursing infants, a decision should be made whether to discontinue nursing or to discontinue the drug, taking into account the importance of the drug to the mother.

Pediatric Use: Safety and effectiveness of Evoclin in children under the age of 12 have not been studied.

Geriatric Use: The clinical study with Evoclin did not include sufficient numbers of patients aged 65 and over to determine if they respond differently than younger patients.

ADVERSE REACTIONS

The incidence of adverse events occurring in ≥1% of the patients in clinical studies comparing Evoclin and its vehicle is presented below:

Selected Adverse Events Occurring in ≥1% of Subjects

Adverse Event	Number (%) of Subjects	
	Evoclin Foam N = 439	Vehicle Foam N = 154
Headache	12 (3%)	1 (1%)
Application site burning	27 (6%)	14 (9%)
Application site pruritus	5 (1%)	5 (3%)
Application site dryness	4 (1%)	5 (3%)
Application site reaction, not otherwise specified	3 (1%)	4 (3%)

In a contact sensitization study, none of the 203 subjects developed evidence of allergic contact sensitization to Evoclin. Orally and parenterally administered clindamycin has been associated with severe colitis, which may end fatally.

Cases of diarrhea, bloody diarrhea, and colitis (including pseudomembranous colitis) have been reported as adverse reactions in patients treated with oral and parenteral formulations of clindamycin and rarely with topical clindamycin (see WARNINGS). Abdominal pain and gastrointestinal disturbances, as well as gram-negative folliculitis, have also been reported in association with the use of topical formulations of clindamycin.

OVERDOSAGE

Topically applied Evoclin may be absorbed in sufficient amounts to produce systemic effects (see WARNINGS).

DOSAGE AND ADMINISTRATION

Apply Evoclin once daily to affected areas after the skin is washed with mild soap and allowed to fully dry. Use enough to cover the entire affected area.

To Use Evoclin:

1. Do not dispense Evoclin directly onto your hands or face, because the foam will begin to melt on contact with warm skin.

2. Remove the clear cap. Align the black mark with the nozzle of the actuator.

3. Hold the can at an upright angle and then press firmly to dispense. Dispense an amount directly into the cap or onto a cool surface. Dispense an amount of Evoclin that will cover the affected area(s). If the can seems warm or the foam seems runny, run the can under cold water.

4. Pick up small amounts of Evoclin with your fingertips and gently massage into the affected areas until the foam disappears.

Throw away any of the unused medicine that you dispensed out of the can.

Avoid contact of Evoclin with eyes. If contact occurs, rinse eyes thoroughly with water.

HOW SUPPLIED

Evoclin containing clindamycin phosphate equivalent to 10 mg clindamycin per gram, is available in the following sizes: 100 gram can - NDC 63032-061-00 and 50 gram can - NDC 63032-061-50

STORAGE AND HANDLING

Store at controlled room temperature 20°-25°C (68°-77°F). **FLAMMABLE. AVOID FIRE, FLAME OR SMOKING DURING AND IMMEDIATELY FOLLOWING APPLICATION.**

Contents under pressure. Do not puncture or incinerate. Do not expose to heat or store at temperature above 120°F (49°C).

Keep out of reach of children.

Manufactured for
Connetics Corporation
Palo Alto, CA 94304
USA

Printed in USA
November 2004

For additional information:
1-888-500-DERM or visit
www.evoclin.com
AW No: AW-0317-r4
U.S. Patent Pending
DELIVERED IN VersaFoam®
Evoclin, and the interlocking C design are trademarks, and VersaFoam and Connetics are registered trademarks of Connetics Corporation.
© 2004 Connetics Corporation

CoTherix, Inc.
5000 SHORELINE COURT, SUITE 101
SOUTH SAN FRANCISCO, CA 94080

Direct Inquires to:
Phone: 650-808-6500
Fax: 650-808-6899
Website: www.cotherix.com
For medical information:
Phone: 1-877-483-6828
Fax: 1-510-595-8183
website: www.4ventavis.com

VENTAVIS®

[vĕn-tă-vĭs]
(iloprost) Inhalation Solution
℞ Only

DESCRIPTION

Ventavis (iloprost) Inhalation Solution is a clear, colorless, sterile solution containing 10 mcg/mL iloprost formulated for inhalation via the Prodose® AAD® (Adaptive Aerosol Delivery) System, a pulmonary drug delivery device. Each single-use glass ampule contains 2 mL (20 mcg) of the solution to be added to the Prodose® AAD® System medication chamber. Each mL of the aqueous solution contains 0.01 mg iloprost, 0.81 mg ethanol, 0.121 mg tromethamine, 9.0 mg sodium chloride, and approximately 0.51 mg hydrochloric acid (for pH adjustment to 8.1) in water for injection. The solution contains no preservatives.

The chemical name for iloprost is (E)-(3aS,4R,5R,6aS)-hexahydro-5-hydroxy-4-[(E)-(3S,4RS)-3-hydroxy-4-methyl-1-octen-6-ynyl]-$\Delta^{2(1H),\Delta}$-pentalenevaleric acid. Iloprost consists of a mixture of the 4R and 4S diastereomers at a ratio of approximately 53:47. Iloprost is an oily substance, which is soluble in methanol, ethanol, ethyl acetate, acetone and pH 7 buffer, sparingly soluble in buffer pH 9, and very slightly soluble in distilled water, buffer pH 3, and buffer pH 5.

The molecular formula of iloprost is $C_{22}H_{32}O_4$. Its relative molecular weight is 360.49. The structural formula is shown below:

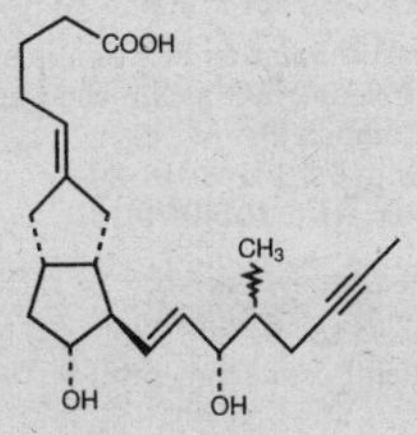

CLINICAL PHARMACOLOGY

General

Iloprost is a synthetic analogue of prostacyclin PGI_2. Iloprost dilates systemic and pulmonary arterial vascular beds. It also affects platelet aggregation but the relevance of this effect to the treatment of pulmonary hypertension is unknown. The two diastereoisomers of iloprost differ in their potency in dilating blood vessels, with the 4S isomer substantially more potent than the 4R isomer.

Pharmacokinetics

General

In pharmacokinetic studies in animals, there was no evidence of interconversion of the two diastereoisomers of iloprost. In human pharmacokinetic studies, the two diastereoisomers were not individually assayed.

Iloprost administered intravenously has linear pharmacokinetics over the dose range of 1 to 3 ng/kg/min. The half-life of iloprost is 20 to 30 minutes. Following inhalation of iloprost (5.0 mcg) patients with pulmonary hypertension have iloprost peak serum levels of approximately 150 pg/mL. Iloprost was generally not detectable in the plasma 30 minutes to 1 hour after inhalation.

Absorption and Distribution

The absolute bioavailability of inhaled iloprost has not been determined.

Following intravenous infusion, the apparent steady-state volume of distribution was 0.7 to 0.8 L/kg in healthy subjects. Iloprost is approximately 60% protein-bound, mainly to albumin, and this ratio is concentration-independent in the range of 30 to 3000 pg/mL.

Metabolism and Excretion

Clearance in normal subjects was approximately 20 mL/min/kg. Iloprost is metabolized principally via β-oxidation of the carboxyl side chain. The main metabolite is tetranor-iloprost, which is found in the urine in free and conjugated form. In animal experiments, tetranor-iloprost was pharmacologically inactive.

In vitro studies reveal that cytochrome P450-dependent metabolism plays only a minor role in the biotransformation of iloprost.

A mass-balance study using intravenously and orally administered $[^3H]$-iloprost in healthy subjects (n=8) showed recovery of total radioactivity over 14 hours post-dose was 81%, with 68% and 12% recoveries in urine and feces, respectively.

Special Populations

Liver Function Impairment

Inhaled iloprost has not been evaluated in subjects with impaired hepatic function. However, in an intravenous iloprost study in patients with liver cirrhosis, the mean clearance in Child Pugh Class B subjects (n=5) was approximately 10 mL/min/kg (half that of healthy subjects). Following oral administration, the mean $AUC_{0\text{-}8h}$ in Child Pugh 2 Class B subjects (n=3) was 1725 pg*h/mL compared to 117 pg*h/mL in normal subjects (n=4) receiving the same oral iloprost dose. In Child Pugh Class A subjects (n=5), the mean $AUC_{0\text{-}8h}$ was 639 pg*h/mL. Although exposure increased with hepatic impairment, there was no effect on half-life.

Renal Function Impairment

Inhaled iloprost has not been evaluated in subjects with impaired renal function. However, in a study with intravenous infusion of iloprost in patients with end-stage renal failure requiring intermittent dialysis treatment (n=7), the mean $AUC_{0\text{-}4h}$ was 230 pg*h/mL compared to 54 pg*h/mL in patients with renal failure (n=8) not requiring intermittent dialysis and 48 pg*h/mL in normals. The half-life was similar in both groups. The effect of dialysis on iloprost exposure has not been evaluated.

Clinical Trials

A randomized, double-blind, multi-center, placebo-controlled trial was conducted in 203 adult patients (inhaled iloprost: n=101; placebo: n=102) with NYHA Class III or IV pulmonary arterial hypertension (PAH, WHO Group I; idiopathic in 53%, associated with connective tissue disease, including CREST and scleroderma, in 17%, or associated with anorexigen use in 2%) or pulmonary hypertension related to chronic thromboembolic disease (WHO Group IV; 28%). Inhaled iloprost (or placebo) was added to patients' current therapy, which could have included anticoagulants, vasodilators (e.g. calcium channel blockers), diuretics, oxygen, and digitalis, but not PGI_2 (prostacyclin or its analogues) or endothelin receptor antagonists. Patients received 2.5 or 5.0 mcg of iloprost by repeated inhalations 6 to 9 times per day during waking hours. The mean age of the entire study population was 52 years and 68% of the patients were female. The majority of patients (59%) were NYHA Class III. The baseline 6-minute walk test values reflected a moderate exercise limitation (the mean was 332 meters for the iloprost group and 315 meters for the placebo group). In the iloprost group, the median daily inhaled dose was 30 mcg (range of 12.5 to 45 mcg/day). The mean number of inhalations per day was 7.3. Ninety percent of patients in the iloprost group never inhaled study medication during the nighttime.

Table 1 Treatment Effects by Subgroup among PAH Patients (WHO Group I)

	Composite Clinical Endpoint				6-Minute Walk*			
	n	Ventavis	n	Placebo	n	Ventavis (mean ± SD)	n	Placebo (mean ± SD)
All Subjects with PAH	68	13 (19%)	78	3 (4%)	64	31 ± 76	65	−9 ± 79
NYHA III	40	7 (18%)	47	2 (4%)	39	24 ± 72	43	−16±86
NYHA IV	28	6 (21%)	31	1 (3%)	25	43 ± 82	22	6±63
Male	23	5 (22%)	24	0 (0%)	21	37 ± 81	21	−22 ± 77
Female	45	8 (18%)	54	3 (6%)	43	29 ± 74	44	−2 ± 81
Age ≤55	41	6 (15%)	40	2 (5%)	39	24 ± 79	32	−5 ± 78
Age >55	27	7 (26%)	38	1 (3%)	25	42 ± 71	33	−13 ± 81

*Change from baseline to 12 Weeks with measurement 30 minutes after dosing, based on all available data.

The primary efficacy endpoint was clinical response at 12 weeks, a composite endpoint defined by: a) improvement in exercise capacity (6-minute walk test) by at least 10% versus baseline evaluated 30 minutes after dosing, b) improvement by at least one NYHA class versus baseline, and c) no death or deterioration of pulmonary hypertension. Deterioration required two or more of the following criteria: 1) refractory systolic blood pressure < 85 mmHg, 2) worsening of right heart failure with cardiac edema, ascites, or pleural effusion despite adequate background therapy, 3) rapidly progressive cardiogenic hepatic failure (e.g. leading to an increase of GOT or GPT to >100 U/L, or total bilirubin ≥5 mg/dL), 4) rapidly progressive cardiogenic renal failure (e.g. decrease of estimated creatinine clearance to 99 ≤50% of baseline), 5) decrease in 6-minute walking distance by ≥30% of baseline value, 6) new long-term need for i.v. catecholamines or diuretics, 7) cardiac index 100 101 ≤1.3 L/min/m^2, 8) CVP ≥22 mmHg despite adequate diuretic therapy, and 9) SVO_2 ≤45% despite nasal O_2 therapy. Although effectiveness was seen in the full population (response rates for the primary composite endpoint of 17% and 5%; p=0.007), there was inadequate evidence of benefit in patients with pulmonary hypertension associated with chronic thromboembolic disease (WHO Group IV); the results presented are therefore those related to patients with PAH (WHO Group I). The response rate for the primary efficacy endpoint among PAH patients was 19% for the iloprost group, compared with 4% for the placebo group (p=0.0033). All three components of the composite endpoint favored iloprost (Figure 1).

Figure 1 Composite Primary Endpoint for PAH Patients (WHO Group I)

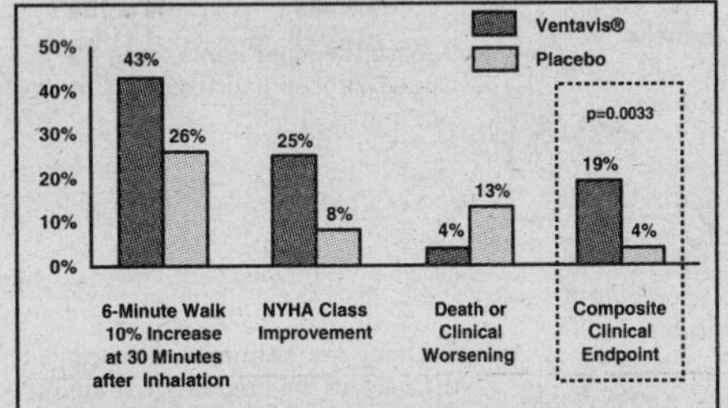

The absolute change in 6-minute walk distance (Figure 2) measured (using all available data and no imputation) 30 minutes after inhalation among patients with PAH was greater in the iloprost group compared to the placebo group at all time points. At Week 12, the placebo-corrected difference was 40 meters (p<0.01). When walk distance was measured immediately prior to inhalation, the improvement compared to placebo was approximately 60% of the effect seen at 30 minutes after inhalation.

Figure 2 Change (Mean ± SEM) in 6-Minute Walk Distance 30 Minutes post Inhalation in PAH Patients (WHO Group I).

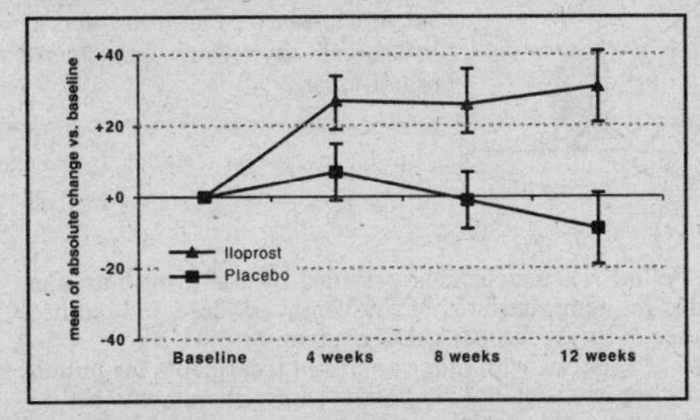

The effect of Ventavis® in various subgroups is shown in Table 1.

[See table 1 above]

Treatment-related effects on hemodynamic measures (e.g. PVR, mPAP, CO, SVO_2) have not been demonstrated.

INDICATIONS AND USAGE

Ventavis® is indicated for the treatment of pulmonary arterial hypertension (WHO Group I) in patients with NYHA Class III or IV symptoms. In controlled trials, it improved a composite endpoint consisting of exercise tolerance, symptoms (NYHA Class), and lack of deterioration (see **CLINICAL PHARMACOLOGY, Clinical Trials**). Ventavis has not been adequately studied with concomitant use of other approved therapies for pulmonary arterial hypertension.

CONTRAINDICATIONS

There are no known contraindications.

WARNINGS

Ventavis is intended for inhalation administration only via the Prodose® AAD® System, a pulmonary drug delivery device (See **DOSAGE AND ADMINISTRATION**). It has not been studied with any other nebulizers.

Because of the risk of syncope, vital signs should be monitored while initiating Ventavis. In patients with low systemic blood pressure, care should be taken to avoid further hypotension. Ventavis should not be initiated in patients with systolic blood pressure less than 85 mmHg. Physicians should be alert to the presence of concomitant conditions or drugs that might increase the risk of syncope. Syncope can also occur in association with pulmonary arterial hypertension, particularly in association with physical exertion. The occurrence of exertional syncope may reflect a therapeutic gap or insufficient efficacy, and the need to adjust dose or change therapy should be considered.

Should signs of pulmonary edema occur when inhaled iloprost is administered in patients with pulmonary hypertension, the treatment should be stopped immediately. This may be a sign of pulmonary venous hypertension.

PRECAUTIONS

General

Ventavis® solution should not be allowed to come into contact with the skin or eyes; oral ingestion of Ventavis solution should be avoided.

Direct mixing of Ventavis with other medications in the Prodose® AAD® System has not been evaluated.

Ventavis has not been evaluated in patients with chronic obstructive pulmonary disease (COPD), severe asthma, or with acute pulmonary infections.

Information for Patients

Patients receiving Ventavis should be advised to use the drug only as prescribed with the Prodose® AAD® System, a pulmonary drug delivery device, following the manufacturer's instructions (see **DOSAGE AND ADMINISTRATION**). Patients should be trained in proper administration techniques including dosing frequency, ampule dispensing, Prodose® AAD® System operation, and equipment cleaning.

Patients should be advised that they may have a fall in blood pressure with Ventavis, so they may become dizzy or even faint. They should stand up slowly when they get out of a chair or bed. If fainting gets worse, patients should consult their physicians about dose adjustment.

Patients should be advised that Ventavis should be inhaled at intervals of not less than 2 hours and that the acute benefits of Ventavis may not last 2 hours.

Drug Interactions

In studies in normal volunteers, there was no pharmacodynamic interaction between intravenous iloprost and either nifedipine, diltiazem, or captopril. However, iloprost has the potential to increase the hypotensive effect of vasodilators and antihypertensive agents. Since iloprost inhibits platelet function, there is a potential for increased risk of bleeding, particularly in patients maintained on anticoagulants. During clinical trials, iloprost was used concurrently with anticoagulants, diuretics, cardiac glycosides, calcium channel blockers, analgesics, antipyretics, nonsteroidal anti-inflammatories, corticosteroids, and other medications. Intravenous infusion of iloprost had no effect on the pharmacokinetics of digoxin. Acetylsalicylic acid did not alter the clearance (pharmacokinetics) of iloprost. Although clinical studies have not been conducted, in vitro studies of iloprost indicate that no relevant inhibition of cytochrome P450 drug metabolism would be expected.

Carcinogenesis, Mutagenesis, Impairment of Fertility

Iloprost was not mutagenic in bacterial and mammalian cells in the presence or absence of extrinsic metabolic activation. Iloprost did not cause chromosomal aberrations *in vitro* in human lymphocytes and was not clastogenic *in vivo* in NMRI/SPF mice. There was no evidence of a tumorigenic effect of iloprost clathrate (13% iloprost by weight) in Sprague-Dawley rats dosed orally for up to 8 months at doses of up to 125 mg/kg/day (Cmax of 45 ng/mL serum), followed by 16 months at 100 mg/kg/day, or in Crl:CD-1®(ICR)BR albino mice dosed orally for up to 24 months at doses of up to 125 mg/kg/day (Cmax of 156 ng/mL serum). The recommended clinical dosage regimen for iloprost (5.0 mcg) affords a serum Cmax of 0.16 ng/mL. Fertility of males or females was not impaired in Han-Wistar rats at intravenous doses up to 1 mg/kg/day.

Continued on next page

Ventavis—Cont.

Pregnancy

Pregnancy Category C. In developmental toxicity studies in pregnant Han-Wistar rats, continuous intravenous administration of iloprost at a dosage of 0.01 mg/kg daily (serum levels not available) led to shortened digits of the thoracic extremity in fetuses and pups. In comparable studies in pregnant Sprague-Dawley rats which received iloprost clathrate (13% iloprost by weight) orally at dosages of up to 50 mg/kg/day (Cmax of 90 ng/mL), in pregnant rabbits at intravenous dosages of up to 0.5 mg/kg/day (Cmax of 86 ng/mL), and in pregnant monkeys at dosages of up to 0.04 mg/kg/day (serum levels of 1 ng/mL), no such digital anomalies or other gross-structural abnormalities were observed in the fetuses/pups. However, in gravid Sprague-Dawley rats, iloprost clathrate (13% iloprost) significantly increased the number of non-viable fetuses at a maternally toxic oral dosage of 250 mg/kg/day and in Han-Wistar rats was found to be embryolethal in 15 of 44 litters at an intravenous dosage of 1 mg/kg/day. There are no adequate and well-controlled studies in pregnant women. Ventavis should be used during pregnancy only if the potential benefit justifies the potential risk to the fetus.

Nursing Mothers

It is not known whether Ventavis is excreted in human milk. In studies with Han-Wistar rats, higher mortality was observed in pups of lactating dams receiving iloprost intravenously at 1 mg/kg daily. In Sprague-Dawley rats, higher mortality was also observed in nursing pups at a maternally toxic oral dose of 250 mg/kg/day of iloprost clathrate (13% iloprost by weight). It is not known whether this drug is excreted in human milk. Because many drugs are excreted in human milk and because of the potential for serious adverse reactions in nursing infants from Ventavis® , a decision to discontinue nursing should be made, taking into account the importance of the drug to the mother.

Pediatric Use

Safety and efficacy in pediatric patients have not been established.

Geriatric Use

Clinical studies of Ventavis did not include sufficient numbers of subjects age 65 and older to determine whether they respond differently than younger subjects. Other reported clinical experience has not identified differences in responses between the elderly and younger patients. In general, dose selection for an elderly patient should be cautious, usually starting at the low end of the dosing range, reflecting the greater frequency of decreased hepatic, renal, or cardiac function and of concomitant disease or other drug therapy.

Hepatic or Renal Impairment

Ventavis has not been studied in patients with pulmonary hypertension and hepatic or renal impairment, both of which increase mean AUC in otherwise normal subjects (see **CLINICAL PHARMACOLOCY, Special Populations**).

ADVERSE REACTIONS

Safety data on Ventavis® were obtained from 215 patients with pulmonary arterial hypertension receiving iloprost in two 12-week clinical trials and two long-term extensions. Patients received inhaled Ventavis for periods from 1 day to more than 3 years. The median number of weeks of exposure was 15 weeks. Forty patients completed 12 months of open-label treatment with iloprost.

The following table shows adverse events reported by at least 4 iloprost patients and reported at least 3% more frequently for iloprost patients than placebo patients in the 12-week placebo-controlled study.

Table 2 Adverse Events in Phase 3 Clinical Trial

Adverse Event	Iloprost n=101	Placebo n=102	Placebo subtracted %
Vasodilation (flushing)	27	9	18
Cough increased	39	26	13
Headache	30	20	10
Trismus	12	3	9
Insomnia	8	2	6
Nausea	13	8	5
Hypotension	11	6	5
Vomiting	7	2	5
Alk phos increased	6	1	5
Flu syndrome	14	10	4
Back pain	7	3	4
Abnormal lab test	7	3	4
Tongue pain	4	0	4
Palpitations	7	4	3
Syncope	8	5	3
GGT increased	6	3	3
Muscle cramps	6	3	3
Hemoptysis	5	2	3
Pneumonia	4	1	3

Serious adverse events reported with the use of inhaled iloprost and not shown in Table 2 include congestive heart failure, chest pain, supraventricular tachycardia., dyspnea, peripheral edema, and kidney failure.

Adverse events with higher doses

In a study in healthy volunteers (n=160), inhaled doses of iloprost solution were given every 2 hours, beginning with 5.0 mcg and increasing up to 20 mcg for a total of 6 dose inhalations (total cumulative dose of 70 mcg) or up to the highest dose tolerated in a subgroup of 40 volunteers. There were 13 subjects (32%) who failed to reach the highest scheduled dose (20 mcg). Five were unable to increase the dose because of (mild to moderate) transient chest pain/discomfort/tightness, usually accompanied by headache, nausea, and dizziness. The remaining 8 subjects discontinued for other reasons.

OVERDOSAGE

In clinical trials of Ventavis®, no case of overdose was reported. Signs and symptoms to be anticipated are extensions of the dose-limiting pharmacological effects, including hypotension, headache, flushing, nausea, vomiting, and diarrhea. A specific antidote is not known. Interruption of the inhalation session, monitoring, and symptomatic measures are recommended.

DOSAGE AND ADMINISTRATION

Ventavis is intended to be inhaled using the Prodose® AAD® System, a pulmonary drug delivery device. The first inhaled dose should be 2.5 mcg (as delivered at the mouthpiece). If this dose is well tolerated, dosing should be increased to 5.0 mcg and maintained at that dose. Ventavis should be taken 6 to 9 times per day (no more than every 2 hours) during waking hours, according to individual need and tolerability. The maximum daily dose evaluated in clinical studies was 45 mcg (5.0 mcg 9 times per day).

Direct mixing of Ventavis with other medications in the Prodose® AAD® System has not been evaluated. To avoid potential interruptions in drug delivery due to equipment malfunctions, the patient should have easy access to a back-up Prodose® AAD® System.

Each inhalation treatment requires one single-use ampule. Each single-use ampule delivers 20 mcg/2 mL to the medication chamber of the Prodose® AAD® System, and delivers a nominal dose of either 2.5 mcg or 5.0 mcg to the mouthpiece.

For each inhalation session, the entire contents of one opened ampule of Ventavis® should be transferred into the Prodose® AAD® System medication chamber immediately before use. After each inhalation session, any solution remaining in the medication chamber should be discarded. Use of the remaining solution will result in unpredictable dosing. Patients should follow the manufacturer's instructions for cleaning the Prodose® AAD® System components after each dose administration.

Preparation

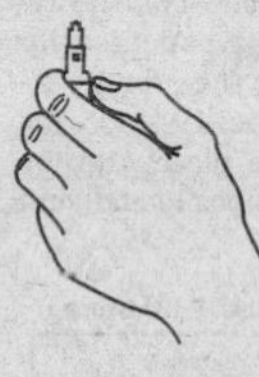

1. With one hand, hold the bottom of the ampule with the blue dot facing away from your body.

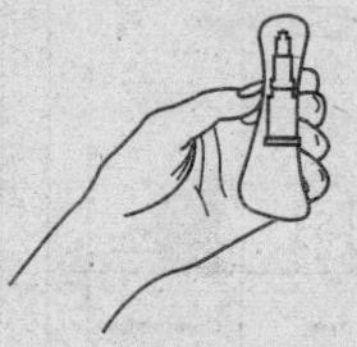

2. With the other hand, wrap the included rubber pad around the entire ampule.

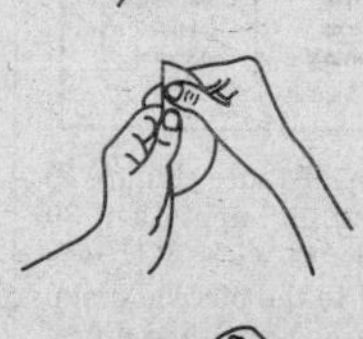

3. Using your thumbs, break open the neck of the ampule by snapping the top towards you.

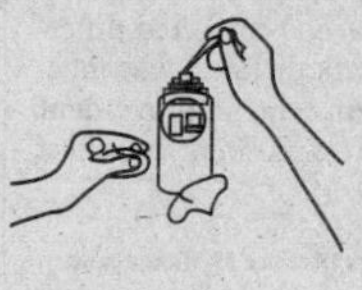

4. Transfer the entire contents of the ampule into the medication chamber of the Prodose® AAD® System.

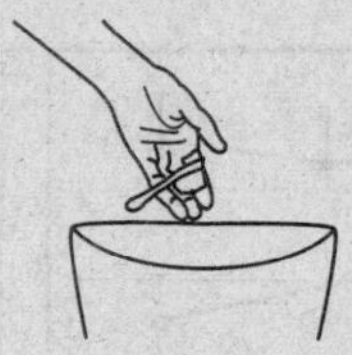

5. Safely dispose of the open ampule out of the reach of children and as instructed by your healthcare practitioner.

6. Follow the instructions provided by the drug manufacturer for administration of the Ventavis® dose and maintenance of the Prodose® AAD® System.

Use of Ventavis with other approved treatments for pulmonary hypertension has not been studied. Should patients deteriorate on this treatment, alternative treatments should be considered. Several patients whose status deteriorated while on Ventavis were successfully switched to intravenous epoprostenol.

Dosage and Administration in Hepatic Impairment

Because iloprost elimination is reduced in patients with impaired liver function (see **CLINICAL PHARMACOLOGY** and **PRECAUTIONS**), caution should be exercised during iloprost therapy in patients with at least Child Pugh Class B hepatic impairment.

Dosage and Administration in Renal Impairment

Dose adjustment is not required in patients not on dialysis. The effect of dialysis on iloprost is unknown. Use caution in treating patients on dialysis (see **CLINICAL PHARMACOLOGY** and **PRECAUTIONS**).

HOW SUPPLIED

Ventavis® (iloprost) Inhalation Solution is supplied in cartons of 30 or 100 clear glass single-use ampules (20 mcg iloprost per 2 mL ampule):

30 ampule cartons: NDC 10148-101-30

100 ampule cartons: NDC 10148-101-01

STORAGE

Store at 20 - 25 °C (68 - 77 °F)

Excursions permitted to 15 - 30 °C (59 - 86 °F)

[See USP Controlled Room Temperature]

Distributed by:

CoTherix™, Inc.

5000 Shoreline Court, Ste. 101

South San Francisco, CA 94080 12

Eisai Inc.

500 FRANK W. BURR BOULEVARD
TEANECK, NJ 07666

Direct Inquiries to:

Eisai Medical Services

1 (888) 274-2378 (888) Aricept

FAX: (201) 287-9744

Medical Emergency Contact:

Medical Emergencies:

24 hours/day, 7 days/week

1 (888) 274-2378 (888) Aricept

ARICEPT® ODT ℞

[ă'rĭ-sĕpt]

(donepezil hydrochloride)

Orally Disintegrating Tablets

DESCRIPTION

ARICEPT® (donepezil hydrochloride) is a reversible inhibitor of the enzyme acetylcholinesterase, known chemically as (±)-2,3-dihydro-5,6-dimethoxy-2-[[1-(phenylmethyl)-4-piperidinyl]methyl]-1*H*-inden-1-one hydrochloride. Donepezil hydrochloride is commonly referred to in the pharmacological literature as E2020. It has an empirical formula of $C_{24}H_{29}NO_3HCl$ and a molecular weight of 415.96. Donepezil hydrochloride is a white crystalline powder and is freely soluble in chloroform, soluble in water and in glacial acetic acid, slightly soluble in ethanol and in acetonitrile and practically insoluble in ethyl acetate and in n-hexane.

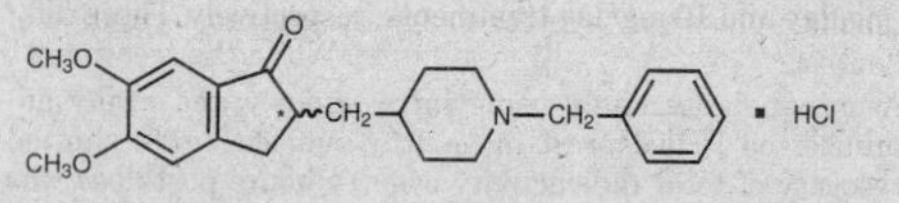

ARICEPT® ODT tablets are available for oral administration. Each ARICEPT® ODT tablet contains 5 or 10 mg of donepezil hydrochloride. Inactive ingredients are carrageenan, mannitol, colloidal silicon dioxide and polyvinyl alcohol. Additionally, the 10 mg tablet contains ferric oxide (yellow) as a coloring agent.

CLINICAL PHARMACOLOGY

Current theories on the pathogenesis of the cognitive signs and symptoms of Alzheimer's Disease attribute some of them to a deficiency of cholinergic neurotransmission.

Donepezil hydrochloride is postulated to exert its therapeutic effect by enhancing cholinergic function. This is accomplished by increasing the concentration of acetylcholine through reversible inhibition of its hydrolysis by acetylcholinesterase. If this proposed mechanism of action is correct, donepezil's effect may lessen as the disease process advances and fewer cholinergic neurons remain functionally intact. There is no evidence that donepezil alters the course of the underlying dementing process.

Clinical Trial Data

The effectiveness of ARICEPT® as a treatment for Alzheimer's Disease is demonstrated by the results of two randomized, double-blind, placebo-controlled clinical investigations in patients with Alzheimer's Disease (diagnosed by NINCDS and DSM III-R criteria, Mini-Mental State Examination ≥ 10 and ≤ 26 and Clinical Dementia Rating of 1 or 2). The mean age of patients participating in ARICEPT® trials was 73 years with a range of 50 to 94. Approximately 62% of patients were women and 38% were men. The racial distribution was white 95%, black 3% and other races 2%.

Study Outcome Measures: In each study, the effectiveness of treatment with ARICEPT® was evaluated using a dual outcome assessment strategy.

The ability of ARICEPT® to improve cognitive performance was assessed with the cognitive subscale of the Alzheimer's Disease Assessment Scale (ADAS-cog), a multi-item instrument that has been extensively validated in longitudinal cohorts of Alzheimer's Disease patients. The ADAS-cog examines selected aspects of cognitive performance including elements of memory, orientation, attention, reasoning, language and praxis. The ADAS-cog scoring range is from 0 to 70, with higher scores indicating greater cognitive impairment. Elderly normal adults may score as low as 0 or 1, but it is not unusual for non-demented adults to score slightly higher.

The patients recruited as participants in each study had mean scores on the Alzheimer's Disease Assessment Scale

(ADAS-cog) of approximately 26 units, with a range from 4 to 61. Experience gained in longitudinal studies of ambulatory patients with mild to moderate Alzheimer's Disease suggest that they gain 6 to 12 units a year on the ADAS-cog. However, lesser degrees of change are seen in patients with very mild or very advanced disease because the ADAS-cog is not uniformly sensitive to change over the course of the disease. The annualized rate of decline in the placebo patients participating in ARICEPT® trials was approximately 2 to 4 units per year.

The ability of ARICEPT® to produce an overall clinical effect was assessed using a Clinician's Interview Based Impression of Change that required the use of caregiver information, the CIBIC plus. The CIBIC plus is not a single instrument and is not a standardized instrument like the ADAS-cog. Clinical trials for investigational drugs have used a variety of CIBIC formats, each different in terms of depth and structure.

As such, results from a CIBIC plus reflect clinical experience from the trial or trials in which it was used and cannot be compared directly with the results of CIBIC plus evaluations from other clinical trials. The CIBIC plus used in ARICEPT® trials was a semi-structured instrument that was intended to examine four major areas of patient function: General, Cognitive, Behavioral and Activities of Daily Living. It represents the assessment of a skilled clinician based upon his/her observations at an interview with the patient, in combination with information supplied by a caregiver familiar with the behavior of the patient over the interval rated. The CIBIC plus is scored as a seven point categorical rating, ranging from a score of 1, indicating "markedly improved," to a score of 4, indicating "no change" to a score of 7, indicating "markedly worse." The CIBIC plus has not been systematically compared directly to assessments not using information from caregivers (CIBIC) or other global methods.

Thirty-Week Study
In a study of 30 weeks duration, 473 patients were randomized to receive single daily doses of placebo, 5 mg/day or 10 mg/day of ARICEPT®. The 30-week study was divided into a 24-week double-blind active treatment phase followed by a 6-week single-blind placebo washout period. The study was designed to compare 5 mg/day or 10 mg/day fixed doses of ARICEPT® to placebo. However, to reduce the likelihood of cholinergic effects, the 10 mg/day treatment was started following an initial 7-day treatment with 5 mg/day doses.

Effects on the ADAS-cog: Figure 1 illustrates the time course for the change from baseline in ADAS-cog scores for all three dose groups over the 30 weeks of the study. After 24 weeks of treatment, the mean differences in the ADAS-cog change scores for ARICEPT® treated patients compared to the patients on placebo were 2.8 and 3.1 units for the 5 mg/day and 10 mg/day treatments, respectively. These differences were statistically significant. While the treatment effect size may appear to be slightly greater for the 10 mg/day treatment, there was no statistically significant difference between the two active treatments.

Following 6 weeks of placebo washout, scores on the ADAS-cog for both the ARICEPT® treatment groups were indistinguishable from those patients who had received only placebo for 30 weeks. This suggests that the beneficial effects of ARICEPT® abate over 6 weeks following discontinuation of treatment and do not represent a change in the underlying disease. There was no evidence of a rebound effect 6 weeks after abrupt discontinuation of therapy.

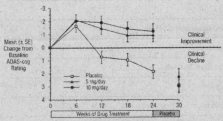

Figure 1. Time-course of the Change from Baseline in ADAS-cog Score for Patients Completing 24 Weeks of Treatment.

Figure 2 illustrates the cumulative percentages of patients from each of the three treatment groups who had attained the measure of improvement in ADAS-cog score shown on the X axis. Three change scores, (7-point and 4-point reductions from baseline or no change in score) have been identified for illustrative purposes and the percent of patients in each group achieving that result is shown in the inset table.

The curves demonstrate that both patients assigned to placebo and ARICEPT® have a wide range of responses, but that the active treatment groups are more likely to show the greater improvements. A curve for an effective treatment would be shifted to the left of the curve for placebo, while an ineffective or deleterious treatment would be superimposed upon or shifted to the right of the curve for placebo, respectively.

[See figure 2 at top of next column]

Effects on the CIBIC plus: Figure 3 is a histogram of the frequency distribution of CIBIC plus scores attained by patients assigned to each of the three treatment groups who completed 24 weeks of treatment. The mean drug-placebo differences for these groups of patients were 0.35 units and 0.39 units for 5 mg/day and 10 mg/day of ARICEPT®, respectively. These differences were statistically significant.

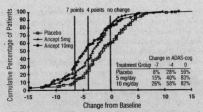

Figure 2. Cumulative Percentage of Patients Completing 24 Weeks of Double-blind Treatment with Specified Changes from Baseline ADAS-cog Scores. The Percentages of Randomized Patients who Completed the Study were: Placebo 80%, 5 mg/day 85% and 10 mg/day 68%.

There was no statistically significant difference between the two active treatments.

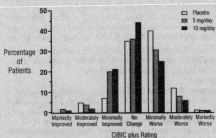

Figure 3. Frequency Distribution of CIBIC plus Scores at Week 24

Fifteen-Week Study
In a study of 15 weeks duration, patients were randomized to receive single daily doses of placebo or either 5 mg/day or 10 mg/day of ARICEPT® for 12 weeks, followed by a 3-week placebo washout period. As in the 30-week study, to avoid acute cholinergic effects, the 10 mg/day treatment followed an initial 7-day treatment with 5 mg/day doses.

Effects on the ADAS-Cog: Figure 4 illustrates the time course of the change from baseline in ADAS-cog scores for all three dose groups over the 15 weeks of the study. After 12 weeks of treatment, the differences in mean ADAS-cog change scores for the ARICEPT® treated patients compared to the patients on placebo were 2.7 and 3.0 units each, for the 5 and 10 mg/day ARICEPT® treatment groups respectively. These differences were statistically significant. The effect size for the 10 mg/day group may appear to be slightly larger than that for 5 mg/day. However, the differences between active treatments were not statistically significant.

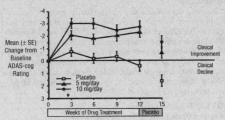

Figure 4. Time-course of the Change from Baseline in ADAS-cog Score for Patients Completing the 15-week Study.

Following 3 weeks of placebo washout, scores on the ADAS-cog for both the ARICEPT® treatment groups increased, indicating that discontinuation of ARICEPT® resulted in a loss of its treatment effect. The duration of this placebo washout period was not sufficient to characterize the rate of loss of the treatment effect, but, the 30-week study (see above) demonstrated that treatment effects associated with the use of ARICEPT® abate within 6 weeks of treatment discontinuation.

Figure 5 illustrates the cumulative percentages of patients from each of the three treatment groups who attained the measure of improvement in ADAS-cog score shown on the X axis. The same three change scores, (7-point and 4-point reductions from baseline or no change in score) as selected for the 30-week study have been used for this illustration. The percentages of patients achieving those results are shown in the inset table.

As observed in the 30-week study, the curves demonstrate that patients assigned to either placebo or to ARICEPT® have a wide range of responses, but that the ARICEPT® treated patients are more likely to show the greater improvements in cognitive performance.

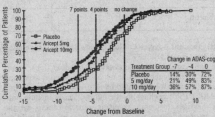

Figure 5. Cumulative Percentage of Patients with Specified Changes from Baseline ADAS-cog Scores. The Percentages of Randomized Patients Within Each Treatment Group Who Completed the Study Were: Placebo 93%, 5 mg/day 90% and 10 mg/day 82%.

Effects on the CIBIC plus: Figure 6 is a histogram of the frequency distribution of CIBIC plus scores attained by pa-

tients assigned to each of the three treatment groups who completed 12 weeks of treatment. The differences in mean scores for ARICEPT® treated patients compared to the patients on placebo at Week 12 were 0.36 and 0.38 units for the 5 mg/day and 10 mg/day treatment groups, respectively. These differences were statistically significant.

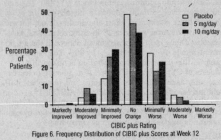

Figure 6. Frequency Distribution of CIBIC plus Scores at Week 12

In both studies, patient age, sex and race were not found to predict the clinical outcome of ARICEPT® treatment.

Clinical Pharmacokinetics
ARICEPT® ODT is bioequivalent to ARICEPT® Tablets. Donepezil is well absorbed with a relative oral bioavailability of 100% and reaches peak plasma concentrations in 3 to 4 hours. Pharmacokinetics are linear over a dose range of 1-10 mg given once daily. Neither food nor time of administration (morning vs. evening dose) influences the rate or extent of absorption of ARICEPT® Tablets. A food effect study has not been conducted with ARICEPT® ODT; however, the effect of food with ARICEPT® ODT is expected to be minimal. ARICEPT® ODT can be taken without regard to meals.

The elimination half life of donepezil is about 70 hours and the mean apparent plasma clearance (Cl/F) is 0.13 L/hr/kg. Following multiple dose administration, donepezil accumulates in plasma by 4-7 fold and steady state is reached within 15 days. The steady state volume of distribution is 12 L/kg. Donepezil is approximately 96% bound to human plasma proteins, mainly to albumins (about 75%) and alpha$_1$-acid glycoprotein (about 21%) over the concentration range of 2-1000 ng/mL.

Donepezil is both excreted in the urine intact and extensively metabolized to four major metabolites, two of which are known to be active, and a number of minor metabolites, not all of which have been identified. Donepezil is metabolized by CYP 450 isoenzymes 2D6 and 3A4 and undergoes glucuronidation. Following administration of ^{14}C-labeled donepezil, plasma radioactivity, expressed as a percent of the administered dose, was present primarily as intact donepezil (53%) and as 6-O-desmethyl donepezil (11%), which has been reported to inhibit AChE to the same extent as donepezil *in vitro* and was found in plasma at concentrations equal to about 20% of donepezil. Approximately 57% and 15% of the total radioactivity was recovered in urine and feces, respectively, over a period of 10 days, while 28% remained unrecovered, with about 17% of the donepezil dose recovered in the urine as unchanged drug.

Special Populations:
Hepatic Disease: In a study of 10 patients with stable alcoholic cirrhosis, the clearance of ARICEPT® was decreased by 20% relative to 10 healthy age and sex matched subjects.
Renal Disease: In a study of 11 patients with moderate to severe renal impairment ($Cl_{Cr} < 18$ mL/min/1.73 m^2) the clearance of ARICEPT® did not differ from 11 age and sex matched healthy subjects.
Age: No formal pharmacokinetic study was conducted to examine age related differences in the pharmacokinetics of ARICEPT®. However, mean plasma ARICEPT® concentrations measured during therapeutic drug monitoring of elderly patients with Alzheimer's Disease are comparable to those observed in young healthy volunteers.
Gender and Race: No specific pharmacokinetic study was conducted to investigate the effects of gender and race on the disposition of ARICEPT®. However, retrospective pharmacokinetic analysis indicates that gender and race (Japanese and Caucasians) did not affect the clearance of ARICEPT®.

Drug-Drug Interactions
Drugs Highly Bound to Plasma Proteins: Drug displacement studies have been performed *in vitro* between this highly bound drug (96%) and other drugs such as furosemide, digoxin, and warfarin. ARICEPT® at concentrations of 0.3-10 μg/mL did not affect the binding of furosemide (5 μg/mL), digoxin (2 ng/mL), and warfarin (3 μg/mL) to human albumin. Similarly, the binding of ARICEPT® to human albumin was not affected by furosemide, digoxin and warfarin.
Effect of ARICEPT® on the Metabolism of Other Drugs: No *in vivo* clinical trials have investigated the effect of ARICEPT® on the clearance of drugs metabolized by CYP 3A4 (e.g. cisapride, terfenadine) or by CYP 2D6 (e.g. imipramine). However, *in vitro* studies show a low rate of binding to these enzymes (mean K_i about 50-130 μM), that, given the therapeutic plasma concentrations of donepezil (164 nM), indicates little likelihood of interference.
Whether ARICEPT® has any potential for enzyme induction is not known.
Formal pharmacokinetic studies evaluated the potential of ARICEPT® for interaction with theophylline, cimetidine,

Continued on next page

Aricept ODT—Cont.

warfarin, digoxin and ketoconazole. No effects of ARICEPT® on the pharmacokinetics of these drugs were observed.

Effect of Other Drugs on the Metabolism of ARICEPT®: Ketoconazole and quinidine, inhibitors of CYP450, 3A4 and 2D6, respectively, inhibit donepezil metabolism *in vitro*. Whether there is a clinical effect of quinidine is not known. In a 7-day crossover study in 18 healthy volunteers, ketoconazole (200mg q.d.) increased mean donepezil (5mg q.d.) concentrations (AUC_{0-24} and C_{max}) by 36%. The clinical relevance of this increase in concentration is unknown.

Inducers of CYP 2D6 and CYP 3A4 (e.g., phenytoin, carbamazepine, dexamethasone, rifampin, and phenobarbital) could increase the rate of elimination of ARICEPT®.

Formal pharmacokinetic studies demonstrated that the metabolism of ARICEPT® is not significantly affected by concurrent administration of digoxin or cimetidine.

INDICATIONS AND USAGE

ARICEPT® is indicated for the treatment of mild to moderate dementia of the Alzheimer's type.

CONTRAINDICATIONS

ARICEPT® is contraindicated in patients with known hypersensitivity to donepezil hydrochloride or to piperidine derivatives.

WARNINGS

Anesthesia: ARICEPT®, as a cholinesterase inhibitor, is likely to exaggerate succinylcholine-type muscle relaxation during anesthesia.

Cardiovascular Conditions: Because of their pharmacological action, cholinesterase inhibitors may have vagotonic effects on the sinoatrial and atrioventricular nodes. This effect may manifest as bradycardia or heart block in patients both with and without known underlying cardiac conduction abnormalities. Syncopal episodes have been reported in association with the use of ARICEPT®.

Gastrointestinal Conditions: Through their primary action, cholinesterase inhibitors may be expected to increase gastric acid secretion due to increased cholinergic activity. Therefore, patients should be monitored closely for symptoms of active or occult gastrointestinal bleeding, especially those at increased risk for developing ulcers, e.g., those with a history of ulcer disease or those receiving concurrent nonsteroidal anti-inflammatory drugs (NSAIDS). Clinical studies of ARICEPT® have shown no increase, relative to placebo, in the incidence of either peptic ulcer disease or gastrointestinal bleeding.

ARICEPT®, as a predictable consequence of its pharmacological properties, has been shown to produce diarrhea, nausea and vomiting. These effects, when they occur, appear more frequently with the 10 mg/day dose than with the 5 mg/day dose. In most cases, these effects have been mild and transient, sometimes lasting one to three weeks, and have resolved during continued use of ARICEPT®.

Genitourinary: Although not observed in clinical trials of ARICEPT®, cholinomimetics may cause bladder outflow obstruction.

Neurological Conditions: Seizures: Cholinomimetics are believed to have some potential to cause generalized convulsions. However, seizure activity also may be a manifestation of Alzheimer's Disease.

Pulmonary Conditions: Because of their cholinomimetic actions, cholinesterase inhibitors should be prescribed with care to patients with a history of asthma or obstructive pulmonary disease.

PRECAUTIONS

Drug-Drug Interactions (see Clinical Pharmacology: Clinical Pharmacokinetics: Drug-drug Interactions)

Effect of ARICEPT® on the Metabolism of Other Drugs: No *in vivo* clinical trials have investigated the effect of ARICEPT® on the clearance of drugs metabolized by CYP 3A4 (e.g. cisapride, terfenadine) or by CYP 2D6 (e.g. imipramine). However, *in vitro* studies show a low rate of binding to these enzymes (mean K_i about 50-130 μM), that, given the therapeutic plasma concentrations of donepezil (164 nM), indicates little likelihood of interference.

Whether ARICEPT® has any potential for enzyme induction is not known.

Formal pharmacokinetic studies evaluated the potential of ARICEPT® for interaction with theophylline, cimetidine, warfarin, digoxin and ketoconazole. No effects of ARICEPT® on the pharmacokinetics of these drugs were observed.

Effect of Other Drugs on the Metabolism of ARICEPT®: Ketoconazole and quinidine, inhibitors of CYP450, 3A4 and 2D6, respectively, inhibit donepezil metabolism *in vitro*. Whether there is a clinical effect of quinidine is not known. In a 7-day crossover study in 18 healthy volunteers, ketoconazole (200mg q.d.) increased mean donepezil (5mg q.d.) concentrations (AUC_{0-24} and C_{max}) by 36%. The clinical relevance of this increase in concentration is unknown.

Inducers of CYP 2D6 and CYP 3A4 (e.g., phenytoin, carbamazepine, dexamethasone, rifampin, and phenobarbital) could increase the rate of elimination of ARICEPT®.

Formal pharmacokinetic studies demonstrated that the metabolism of ARICEPT® is not significantly affected by concurrent administration of digoxin or cimetidine.

Use with Anticholinergics: Because of their mechanism of action, cholinesterase inhibitors have the potential to interfere with the activity of anticholinergic medications.

Use with Cholinomimetics and Other Cholinesterase Inhibitors: A synergistic effect may be expected when cholinesterase inhibitors are given concurrently with succinylcholine, similar neuromuscular blocking agents or cholinergic agonists such as bethanechol.

Carcinogenesis, Mutagenesis, Impairment of Fertility

No evidence of a carcinogenic potential was obtained in an 88-week carcinogenicity study of donepezil hydrochloride conducted in CD-1 mice at doses up to 180 mg/kg/day (approximately 90 times the maximum recommended human dose on a mg/m² basis), or in a 104-week carcinogenicity study in Sprague-Dawley rats at doses up to 30mg/kg/day (approximately 30 times the maximum recommended human dose on a mg/m² basis).

Donepezil was not mutagenic in the Ames reverse mutation assay in bacteria, or in a mouse lymphoma forward mutation assay *in vitro*. In the chromosome aberration test in cultures of Chinese hamster lung (CHL) cells, some clastogenic effects were observed. Donepezil was not clastogenic in the *in vivo* mouse micronucleus test and was not genotoxic in an *in vivo* unscheduled DNA synthesis assay in rats.

Donepezil had no effect on fertility in rats at doses up to 10 mg/kg/day (approximately 8 times the maximum recommended human dose on a mg/m² basis).

Pregnancy

Pregnancy Category C: Teratology studies conducted in pregnant rats at doses up to 16 mg/kg/day (approximately 13 times the maximum recommended human dose on a mg/m² basis) and in pregnant rabbits at doses up to 10 mg/kg/day (approximately 16 times the maximum recommended human dose on a mg/m² basis) did not disclose any evidence for a teratogenic potential of donepezil. However, in a study in which pregnant rats were given up to 10 mg/kg/day (approximately 8 times the maximum recommended human dose on a mg/m² basis) from day 17 of gestation through day 20 postpartum, there was a slight increase in still births and a slight decrease in pup survival through day 4 postpartum at this dose; the next lower dose tested was 3 mg/kg/day. There are no adequate or well-controlled studies in pregnant women. ARICEPT® should be used during pregnancy only if the potential benefit justifies the potential risk to the fetus.

Nursing Mothers

It is not known whether donepezil is excreted in human breast milk. ARICEPT® has no indication for use in nursing mothers.

Pediatric Use

There are no adequate and well-controlled trials to document the safety and efficacy of ARICEPT® in any illness occurring in children.

Geriatric Use

Alzheimer's disease is a disorder occurring primarily in individuals over 55 years of age. The mean age of patients enrolled in the clinical studies with ARICEPT® was 73 years; 80% of these patients were between 65 and 84 years old and 49% of patients were at or above the age of 75. The efficacy and safety data presented in the clinical trials section were obtained from these patients. There were no clinically significant differences in most adverse events reported by patient groups ≥ 65 years old and < 65 years old.

ADVERSE REACTIONS

Adverse Events Leading to Discontinuation

The rates of discontinuation from controlled clinical trials of ARICEPT® due to adverse events for the ARICEPT® 5 mg/day treatment groups were comparable to those of placebo-treatment groups at approximately 5%. The rate of discontinuation of patients who received 7-day escalations from 5 mg/day to 10 mg/day, was higher at 13%.

The most common adverse events leading to discontinuation, defined as those occurring in at least 2% of patients and at twice the incidence seen in placebo patients, are shown in Table 1.

Table 1. Most Frequent Adverse Events Leading to Withdrawal from Controlled Clinical Trials by Dose Group

Dose Group	Placebo	5 mg/day ARICEPT®	10 mg/day ARICEPT®
Patients Randomized	355	350	315
Event/ % Discontinuing			
Nausea	1%	1%	3%
Diarrhea	0%	<1%	3%
Vomiting	<1%	<1%	2%

Most Frequent Adverse Clinical Events Seen in Association with the Use of ARICEPT®

The most common adverse events, defined as those occurring at a frequency of at least 5% in patients receiving 10 mg/day and twice the placebo rate, are largely predicted by ARICEPT®'s cholinomimetic effects. These include nausea, diarrhea, insomnia, vomiting, muscle cramp, fatigue and anorexia. These adverse events were often of mild intensity and transient, resolving during continued ARICEPT® treatment without the need for dose modification.

There is evidence to suggest that the frequency of these common adverse events may be affected by the rate of titration. An open-label study was conducted with 269 patients who received placebo in the 15 and 30-week studies. These patients were titrated to a dose of 10 mg/day over a 6-week period. The rates of common adverse events were lower than those seen in patients titrated to 10 mg/day over one week in the controlled clinical trials and were comparable to those seen in patients on 5 mg/day.

See Table 2 for a comparison of the most common adverse events following one and six week titration regimens.

Table 2. Comparison of rates of adverse events in patients titrated to 10 mg/day over 1 and 6 weeks

	No titration		One week titration	Six week titration
Adverse Event	**Placebo (n=315)**	**5 mg/day (n=311)**	**10 mg/day (n=315)**	**10 mg/day (n=269)**
Nausea	6%	5%	19%	6%
Diarrhea	5%	8%	15%	9%
Insomnia	6%	6%	14%	6%
Fatigue	3%	4%	8%	3%
Vomiting	3%	3%	8%	5%
Muscle cramps	2%	6%	8%	3%
Anorexia	2%	3%	7%	3%

Adverse Events Reported in Controlled Trials

The events cited reflect experience gained under closely monitored conditions of clinical trials in a highly selected patient population. In actual clinical practice or in other clinical trials, these frequency estimates may not apply, as the conditions of use, reporting behavior, and the kinds of patients treated may differ. Table 3 lists treatment emergent signs and symptoms that were reported in at least 2% of patients in placebo-controlled trials who received ARICEPT® and for which the rate of occurrence was greater for ARICEPT® assigned than placebo assigned patients. In general, adverse events occurred more frequently in female patients and with advancing age.

Table 3. Adverse Events Reported in Controlled Clinical Trials in at Least 2% of Patients Receiving ARICEPT® and at a Higher Frequency than Placebo-treated Patients

Body System/ Adverse Event	Placebo (n=355)	ARICEPT® (n=747)
Percent of Patients with any Adverse Event	72	74
Body as a Whole		
Headache	9	10
Pain, various locations	8	9
Accident	6	7
Fatigue	3	5
Cardiovascular System		
Syncope	1	2
Digestive System		
Nausea	6	11
Diarrhea	5	10
Vomiting	3	5
Anorexia	2	4
Hemic and Lymphatic System		
Ecchymosis	3	4
Metabolic and Nutritional Systems		
Weight Decrease	1	3
Musculoskeletal System		
Muscle Cramps	2	6
Arthritis	1	2
Nervous System		
Insomnia	6	9
Dizziness	6	8
Depression	<1	3
Abnormal Dreams	0	3

Somnolence	<1	2
Urogenital System		
Frequent Urination	1	2

Other Adverse Events Observed During Clinical Trials

ARICEPT® has been administered to over 1700 individuals during clinical trials worldwide. Approximately 1200 of these patients have been treated for at least 3 months and more than 1000 patients have been treated for at least 6 months. Controlled and uncontrolled trials in the United States included approximately 900 patients. In regards to the highest dose of 10 mg/day, this population includes 650 patients treated for 3 months, 475 patients treated for 6 months and 116 patients treated for over 1 year. The range of patient exposure is from 1 to 1214 days.

Treatment emergent signs and symptoms that occurred during 3 controlled clinical trials and two open-label trials in the United States were recorded as adverse events by the clinical investigators using terminology of their own choosing. To provide an overall estimate of the proportion of individuals having similar types of events, the events were grouped into a smaller number of standardized categories using a modified COSTART dictionary and event frequencies were calculated across all studies. These categories are used in the listing below. The frequencies represent the proportion of 900 patients from these trials who experienced that event while receiving ARICEPT®. All adverse events occurring at least twice are included, except for those already listed in Tables 2 or 3, COSTART terms too general to be informative, or events less likely to be drug caused. Events are classified by body system and listed using the following definitions: *frequent adverse events* - those occurring in at least 1/100 patients; *infrequent adverse events* - those occurring in 1/100 to 1/1000 patients. These adverse events are not necessarily related to ARICEPT® treatment and in most cases were observed at a similar frequency in placebo-treated patients in the controlled studies. No important additional adverse events were seen in studies conducted outside the United States.

Body as a Whole: *Frequent:* influenza, chest pain, toothache; *Infrequent:* fever, edema face, periorbital edema, hernia hiatal, abscess, cellulitis, chills, generalized coldness, head fullness, listlessness.

Cardiovascular System: *Frequent:* hypertension, vasodilation, atrial fibrillation, hot flashes, hypotension; *Infrequent:* angina pectoris, postural hypotension, myocardial infarction, AV block (first degree), congestive heart failure, arteritis, bradycardia, peripheral vascular disease, supraventricular tachycardia, deep vein thrombosis.

Digestive System: *Frequent:* fecal incontinence, gastrointestinal bleeding, bloating, epigastric pain; *Infrequent:* eructation, gingivitis, increased appetite, flatulence, periodontal abscess, cholelithiasis, diverticulitis, drooling, dry mouth, fever sore, gastritis, irritable colon, tongue edema, epigastric distress, gastroenteritis, increased transaminases, hemorrhoids, ileus, increased thirst, jaundice, melena, polydipsia, duodenal ulcer, stomach ulcer.

Endocrine System: *Infrequent:* diabetes mellitus, goiter.

Hemic and Lymphatic System: *Infrequent:* anemia, thrombocythemia, thrombocytopenia, eosinophilia, erythrocytopenia.

Metabolic and Nutritional Disorders: *Frequent:* dehydration; *Infrequent:* gout, hypokalemia, increased creatine kinase, hyperglycemia, weight increase, increased lactate dehydrogenase.

Musculoskeletal System: *Frequent:* bone fracture; *Infrequent:* muscle weakness, muscle fasciculation.

Nervous System: *Frequent:* delusions, tremor, irritability, paresthesia, aggression, vertigo, ataxia, increased libido, restlessness, abnormal crying, nervousness, aphasia; *Infrequent:* cerebrovascular accident, intracranial hemorrhage, transient ischemic attack, emotional lability, neuralgia, coldness (localized), muscle spasm, dysphoria, gait abnormality, hypertonia, hypokinesia, neurodermatitis, numbness (localized), paranoia, dysarthria, dysphasia, hostility, decreased libido, melancholia, emotional withdrawal, nystagmus, pacing.

Respiratory System: *Frequent:* dyspnea, sore throat, bronchitis; *Infrequent:* epistaxis, post nasal drip, pneumonia, hyperventilation, pulmonary congestion, wheezing, hypoxia, pharyngitis, pleurisy, pulmonary collapse, sleep apnea, snoring.

Skin and Appendages: *Frequent:* pruritus, diaphoresis, urticaria; *Infrequent:* dermatitis, erythema, skin discoloration, hyperkeratosis, alopecia, fungal dermatitis, herpes zoster, hirsutism, skin striae, night sweats, skin ulcer.

Special Senses: *Frequent:* cataract, eye irritation, vision blurred; *Infrequent:* dry eyes, glaucoma, earache, tinnitus, blepharitis, decreased hearing, retinal hemorrhage, otitis externa, otitis media, bad taste, conjunctival hemorrhage, ear buzzing, motion sickness, spots before eyes.

Urogenital System: *Frequent:* urinary incontinence, nocturia; *Infrequent:* dysuria, hematuria, urinary urgency, metrorrhagia, cystitis, enuresis, prostate hypertrophy, pyelonephritis, inability to empty bladder, breast fibroadenosis, fibrocystic breast, mastitis, pyuria, renal failure, vaginitis.

Postintroduction Reports

Voluntary reports of adverse events temporally associated with ARICEPT® that have been received since market introduction that are not listed above, and that there is inadequate data to determine the causal relationship with the drug include the following: abdominal pain, agitation, cholecystitis, confusion, convulsions, hallucinations, heart block (all types), hemolytic anemia, hepatitis, hyponatremia, neuroleptic malignant syndrome, pancreatitis, and rash.

OVERDOSAGE

Because strategies for the management of overdose are continually evolving, it is advisable to contact a Poison Control Center to determine the latest recommendations for the management of an overdose of any drug.

As in any case of overdose, general supportive measures should be utilized. Overdosage with cholinesterase inhibitors can result in cholinergic crisis characterized by severe nausea, vomiting, salivation, sweating, bradycardia, hypotension, respiratory depression, collapse and convulsions. Increasing muscle weakness is a possibility and may result in death if respiratory muscles are involved. Tertiary anticholinergics such as atropine may be used as an antidote for ARICEPT® overdosage. Intravenous atropine sulfate titrated to effect is recommended: an initial dose of 1.0 to 2.0 mg IV with subsequent doses based upon clinical response. Atypical responses in blood pressure and heart rate have been reported with other cholinomimetics when co-administered with quaternary anticholinergics such as glycopyrrolate. It is not known whether ARICEPT® and/or its metabolites can be removed by dialysis (hemodialysis, peritoneal dialysis, or hemofiltration).

Dose-related signs of toxicity in animals included reduced spontaneous movement, prone position, staggering gait, lacrimation, clonic convulsions, depressed respiration, salivation, miosis, tremors, fasciculation and lower body surface temperature.

DOSAGE AND ADMINISTRATION

The dosages of ARICEPT® shown to be effective in controlled clinical trials are 5 mg and 10 mg administered once per day.

The higher dose of 10 mg did not provide a statistically significantly greater clinical benefit than 5 mg. There is a suggestion, however, based upon order of group mean scores and dose trend analyses of data from these clinical trials, that a daily dose of 10 mg of ARICEPT® might provide additional benefit for some patients. Accordingly, whether or not to employ a dose of 10 mg is a matter of prescriber and patient preference.

Evidence from the controlled trials indicates that the 10 mg dose, with a one week titration, is likely to be associated with a higher incidence of cholinergic adverse events than the 5 mg dose. In open label trials using a 6 week titration, the frequency of these same adverse events was similar between the 5 mg and 10 mg dose groups. Therefore, because steady state is not achieved for 15 days and because the incidence of untoward effects may be influenced by the rate of dose escalation, treatment with a dose of 10 mg should not be contemplated until patients have been on a daily dose of 5 mg for 4 to 6 weeks.

ARICEPT® ODT should be taken in the evening, just prior to retiring.

Allow ARICEPT® ODT to dissolve on the tongue and follow with water.

ARICEPT® ODT can be taken with or without food.

HOW SUPPLIED

ARICEPT® ODT is supplied as tablets containing either 5 mg or 10 mg of donepezil hydrochloride.

The 5 mg orally disintegrating tablets are white. The strength, in mg (5), is embossed on one side and ARICEPT is embossed on the other side.

The 10 mg orally disintegrating tablets are yellow. The strength, in mg (10), is embossed on one side and ARICEPT is embossed on the other side.

5 mg (White)	Unit Dose Blister Package 30 (10×3) (NDC# 62856-831-30)
10 mg (Yellow)	Unit Dose Blister Package 30 (10×3) (NDC# 62856-832-30)

Storage: Store at controlled room temperature, 15°C to 30°C (59°F to 86°F).

℞ only

ARICEPT® is a registered trademark of Eisai Co., Ltd.

Manufactured and Marketed by Eisai Inc., Teaneck, NJ 07666
Marketed by
Pfizer Inc, New York, NY 10017
© 2004 Eisai Inc
Printed in U.S.A.
200400 Revised December 2004

In the PDR annual,
the **Brand and Generic Name Index**
(PINK section)
alphabetizes drugs under both
brand and generic names.

Forest Pharmaceuticals, Inc.

(Subsidiary of Forest Laboratories, Inc.)
13600 SHORELINE DRIVE
ST. LOUIS, MO 63045

Direct Inquiries to:
Professional Affairs Department
13600 Shoreline Drive
St. Louis, MO 63045
(800) 678-1605

COMBUNOX™ Ⓒ ℞

[*kŏm-bew-nŏks*]

(Oxycodone HCl and Ibuprofen) Tablets
5 mg/400 mg
Rx only

DESCRIPTION

Each combination Combunox™ tablet contains:
Oxycodone HCl, USP 5 mg
Ibuprofen, USP 400 mg

Combunox is supplied in a fixed combination tablet form for oral administration and combines the opioid analgesic agent, oxycodone HCl, with the nonsteroidal anti-inflammatory (NSAID) agent, ibuprofen.

Oxycodone HCl is a centrally acting semisynthetic opioid analgesic. Its chemical name is 4,5α-Epoxy-14-hydroxy-3-methoxy-methylmorphinan-6-one hydrochloride. Its chemical formula is $C_{18}H_{21}NO_4$ HCl and molecular weight is 351.83. Its structural formula is:

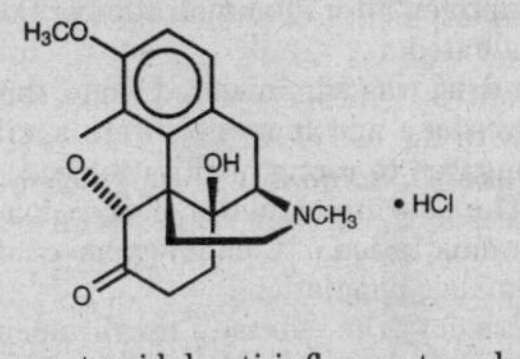

Ibuprofen is a nonsteroidal anti-inflammatory drug with analgesic and antipyretic properties. Its chemical name is (±)-2-(p-isobutylphenyl) propionic acid. Its chemical formula is $C_{13}H_{18}O_2$ and molecular weight is 206.29. Its structural formula is:

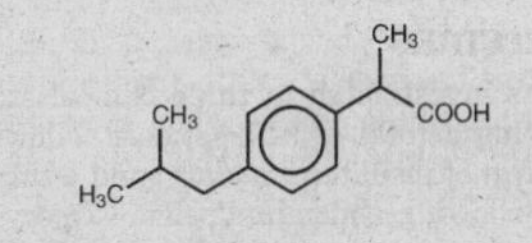

Inactive ingredients in Combunox tablets include: sodium starch glycolate, microcrystalline cellulose, colloidal silicon dioxide, stearic acid, calcium stearate, carboxymethylcellulose, povidone, Opadry® II White, Y-22 7719 coloring agent. Opadry® II White, Y-22 7719 coloring agent consists of titanium dioxide, polydextrose, hypromellose, triacetin and polyethylene glycol 8000.

CLINICAL PHARMACOLOGY

Oxycodone HCl component:

Oxycodone HCl is a semisynthetic opioid analgesic with multiple actions which involve the central nervous system and smooth muscle. The mechanism of action of oxycodone is not known but is thought to be related to its binding to opiate receptors in the central nervous system. In addition to analgesia, opioids may produce sedation and respiratory depression.

Ibuprofen component:

Ibuprofen is a nonsteroidal anti-inflammatory agent that possesses analgesic and antipyretic activities. Its mode of action, similar to other NSAIDs, is not completely understood, but is thought to be related to its inhibition of cyclooxygenase activity and prostaglandin synthesis. Ibuprofen is a peripherally acting analgesic. Ibuprofen does not have any known effects on opiate receptors.

Pharmacokinetics:

Absorption:

Oxycodone is rapidly absorbed after single dose administration of Combunox. Maximum concentrations (C_{max}) of oxycodone, ranging from 9.8 ng/mL to 11.7 ng/mL, are obtained within 1.3 hr to 2.1 hr after administration of Combunox. Repeated administration of Combunox every 6 hours results in approximately 50-65% increase in C_{max}. In the presence of food, the bioavailability of oxycodone is slightly (25%) increased.

Ibuprofen is rapidly absorbed after oral administration of Combunox. C_{max} values range from 18.5 mcg/mL to 34.3 mcg/mL and are reached 1.6 hr to 3.1 hr after oral administration of Combunox. Repeated administration of Combunox every 6 hours does not result in any accumulation of ibuprofen. The bioavailability of ibuprofen is not altered in the presence of food.

Distribution:

Oxycodone binding to protein in serum is approximately 45%.

Ibuprofen is extensively bound to plasma proteins (99%).

Continued on next page

Combunox—Cont.

Metabolism:
Oxycodone is metabolized in the liver by means of N-demethylation and O-demethylation, 6-ketoreduction and glucuronidation. The major circulating metabolite is noroxycodone, which possesses weak analgesic activity.
Oxymorphone, the end product of O-demethylation, has analgesic activity but is present in the plasma at low concentrations. Metabolism of oxycodone to oxymorphone occurs via CYP2D6.
Ibuprofen is present as a racemate and following absorption, it undergoes interconversion in the plasma from the R-isomer to the S-isomer.
Both the R- and S-isomers are metabolized to two primary metabolites: (+)-2-4′-(2-hydroxy-2-methyl-propyl) phenyl propionic acid and (+)-2-4′-(2-carboxypropyl) phenyl propionic acid, both of which circulate in the plasma at low levels relative to the parent.
Elimination:
Oxycodone is eliminated from the systemic circulation with half life ($T_{1/2}$) values ranging from 3.1 hr to 3.7 hr after single dose administration of Combunox. Urinary excretion of unchanged oxycodone amounts to approximately 4% of the administered oxycodone dose.
Ibuprofen is eliminated from the systemic circulation with half life ($T_{1/2}$) values ranging from 1.8 hr to 2.6 hr after single dose administration of Combunox. Urinary excretion of unchanged ibuprofen is minimal (less than 0.2% of administered ibuprofen dose).

Special Populations:
Gender: There are no gender effects on the pharmacokinetics of oxycodone or ibuprofen after administration of Combunox.
Age: The effects of age on the pharmacokinetics of oxycodone and ibuprofen after administration of Combunox have not been evaluated.
When either drug was administered alone, the pharmacokinetics of oxycodone and ibuprofen were similar in elderly subjects, compared to young healthy subjects.
Pediatrics: The pharmacokinetics of oxycodone and ibuprofen after administration of Combunox have not been evaluated in a pediatric population.
Renal Impairment: The effects of renal impairment on the pharmacokinetics of oxycodone and ibuprofen after administration of Combunox have not been evaluated.
Hepatic Impairment: The effects of hepatic impairment on the pharmacokinetics of oxycodone and ibuprofen after administration of Combunox have not been evaluated. (See PRECAUTIONS; Hepatic Effects)

CLINICAL STUDIES

Combunox was investigated in three clinical studies. Two studies involving a total of 949 patients following dental surgery (removal of ipsilateral molars) and a third study of 456 patients following abdominal/pelvic surgery were conducted. In the three studies patients were administered a single dose of the Combunox, ibuprofen alone, oxycodone HCl alone or placebo for acute, moderate to severe pain.
In these single dose studies, Combunox produced greater efficacy than placebo and each of Combunox's individual components as measured by the magnitude of pain relief and the reduction in pain intensity through six hours. No multiple dose efficacy studies have been performed with Combunox.

INDICATIONS AND USAGE

Combunox tablet is indicated for the short term (no more than 7 days) management of acute, moderate to severe pain.

CONTRAINDICATIONS

Combunox should not be administered to patients who have previously exhibited hypersensitivity to oxycodone HCl, ibuprofen, or any of Combunox's components, or in any situation where opioids are contraindicated. This includes patients with significant respiratory depression (in unmonitored settings or the absence of resuscitative equipment) and patients with acute or severe bronchial asthma or hypercarbia. Combunox is contraindicated in any patient who has or is suspected of having paralytic ileus. Combunox should not be given to patients who have experienced asthma, urticaria, or allergic-type reactions after taking aspirin or other NSAIDs. Severe anaphylactoid reactions to NSAIDs, some of which were fatal, have been reported in such patients (see WARNINGS - Anaphylactoid Reactions, and PRECAUTIONS - Pre-existing Asthma). Patients known to be hypersensitive to other opioids may exhibit cross-sensitivity to oxycodone.

WARNINGS

Misuse Abuse and Diversion of Opioids
Combunox contains oxycodone, which is an opioid agonist, and a Schedule II controlled substance. Opioid agonists have the potential for being abused and are sought by abusers and people with addiction disorders, and are subject to diversion.
Combunox can be abused in a manner similar to other opioid agonists, legal or illicit. This should be considered when prescribing or dispensing Combunox in situations where the physician or pharmacist is concerned about an increased risk of misuse, abuse or diversion (see DRUG ABUSE AND DEPENDENCE).
Respiratory Depression
Oxycodone may produce dose-related respiratory depression by acting directly on the brain stem respiratory centers. Oxycodone HCl also affects the center that controls respiratory rhythm, and may produce irregular and periodic breathing. Respiratory depression occurs most frequently in elderly or debilitated patients, usually following large initial doses in non-tolerant patients, or when opioids are given in conjunction with other agents that depress respiration. Combunox should be used with extreme caution in patients with significant chronic obstructive pulmonary disease or cor pulmonale, and in patients having substantially decreased respiratory reserve, hypoxia, hypercapnia, or pre-existing respiratory depression. In such patients, even usual therapeutic doses of Combunox may decrease respiratory drive to the point of apnea.

Hypotensive Effect
Combunox, like all opioid analgesics, may cause severe hypotension in an individual whose ability to maintain blood pressure has been compromised by a depleted blood volume, or after concurrent administration with drugs such as phenothiazines or other agents which compromise vasomotor tone. Combunox may produce orthostatic hypotension in ambulatory patients. Combunox, like all opioid analgesics, should be administered with caution to patients in circulatory shock, since vasodilatation produced by the drug may further reduce cardiac output and blood pressure.

Head Injury and Increased Intracranial Pressure
The respiratory depressant effects of opioids and their capacity to elevate cerebrospinal fluid pressure may be markedly exaggerated in the presence of head injury, intracranial lesions or a pre-existing increase in intracranial pressure. Furthermore, opioids produce adverse reactions that may obscure the clinical course of patients with head injuries.

Acute Abdominal Conditions
The administration of opioids may obscure the diagnosis or clinical course of patients with acute abdominal conditions.

Gastrointestinal (GI) Effects
Serious gastrointestinal toxicity, such as inflammation, bleeding, ulceration, and perforation of the stomach, small intestine or large intestine, can occur at any time, with or without warning symptoms, in patients treated with nonsteroidal anti-inflammatory drugs (NSAIDs) such as ibuprofen. Minor upper GI problems, such as dyspepsia, are common and may also occur at any time during NSAID therapy. Therefore, physicians and patients should remain alert for ulceration and bleeding even in the absence of previous GI tract symptoms. Even short term therapy is not without risk.
NSAIDs should be prescribed with extreme caution in those with a prior history of ulcer disease or gastrointestinal bleeding. Most spontaneous reports of fatal GI events are in elderly or debilitated patients and, therefore, special care should be taken in treating this population. To minimize the potential risk for an adverse GI event the treatment period should be of the shortest possible duration. For high risk patients, alternate therapies that do not involve NSAIDs should be considered.
In addition to a past history of ulcer disease, pharmacoepidemiological studies have identified several other co-therapies or co-morbid conditions that may increase the risk for GI bleeding such as: treatment with oral corticosteroids, treatment with anticoagulants, longer duration of NSAID therapy, smoking, and alcoholism.

Anaphylactoid Reactions
Anaphylactoid reactions may occur in patients without known prior exposure to Combunox. Combunox should not be given to patients with the aspirin triad or a history of angioedema. The triad typically occurs in asthmatic patients who experience rhinitis with or without nasal polyps, or who exhibit severe, potentially fatal bronchospasm after taking aspirin or other NSAIDs. Fatal reactions to NSAIDs have been reported in such patients (see CONTRAINDICATIONS and PRECAUTIONS - Pre-existing Asthma). Emergency help should be sought when anaphylactoid reaction occurs.

Advanced Renal Disease
In patients with advanced kidney disease, treatment with Combunox is not recommended. However, if Combunox therapy must be initiated, due to the NSAID component, close monitoring of the patient's kidney function is advisable (see PRECAUTIONS - Renal Effects). If NSAID therapy, however, must be initiated, close monitoring of the patient's kidney function is advisable (see PRECAUTIONS - Renal Effects).

Pregnancy
As with other NSAID-containing products, Combunox should be avoided in late pregnancy because it may cause premature closure of the ductus arteriosus.

Interactions with Alcohol and Drugs of Abuse
Oxycodone may be expected to have additive effects when used in conjunction with alcohol, other opioids, or illicit drugs that cause central nervous system depression.

PRECAUTIONS
General
Special Risk Patients
As with any opioid analgesic agent, Combunox tablets should be used with caution in elderly or debilitated patients, and those with severe impairment of hepatic, pulmonary or renal function, hypothyroidism, Addison's disease, acute alcoholism, convulsive disorders, CNS depression or coma, delirium tremens, kyphoscoliosis associated with respiratory depression, toxic psychosis, prostatic hypertrophy or urethral stricture. The usual precautions should be observed and the possibility of respiratory depression, postural hypotension, and altered mental states should be kept in mind.

Use in Pancreatic/Biliary Tract Disease
Combunox may cause spasm of the sphincter of Oddi and should be used with caution in patients with biliary tract disease, including acute pancreatitis. Opioids like Combunox may cause increases in the serum amylase level.

Cough Reflex
Oxycodone suppresses the cough reflex; as with other opioid containing products, caution should be exercised when Combunox is used postoperatively and in patients with pulmonary disease.

Effect on Diagnostic Signs
The antipyretic and anti-inflammatory activity of ibuprofen may reduce fever and inflammation, thus diminishing their utility as diagnostic signs in detecting complications of presumed noninfectious, noninflammatory painful conditions.

Hepatic Effects
As with other NSAIDs, ibuprofen has been reported to cause borderline elevations of one or more liver enzymes; this may occur in up to 15% of patients. These abnormalities may progress, may remain essentially unchanged, or may be transient with continued therapy. Notable (3 times the upper limit of normal) elevations of SGPT (ALT) or SGOT (AST) occurred in controlled clinical trials in less than 1% of patients. A patient with symptoms and/or signs suggesting liver dysfunction, or in whom an abnormal liver test has occurred, should be evaluated for evidence of the development of more severe hepatic reactions while on therapy with Combunox. Severe hepatic reactions, including jaundice and cases of fatal hepatitis, have been reported with ibuprofen as with other NSAIDs. Although such reactions are rare, if abnormal liver tests persist or worsen, if clinical signs and symptoms consistent with liver disease develop, or if systemic manifestations occur (e.g. eosinophilia, rash, etc.), Combunox should be discontinued.

Renal Effects
Caution should be used when initiating treatment with Combunox in patients with considerable dehydration. It is advisable to rehydrate patients first and then start therapy with Combunox. Caution is also recommended in patients with pre-existing kidney disease (see WARNINGS - Advanced Renal Disease).
As with other NSAIDs, long-term administration of ibuprofen has resulted in renal papillary necrosis and other renal pathologic changes. Renal toxicity has also been seen in patients in which renal prostaglandins have a compensatory role in the maintenance of renal perfusion. In these patients, administration of a nonsteroidal anti-inflammatory drug may cause a dose-dependent reduction in prostaglandin formation and, secondarily, in renal blood flow, which may precipitate overt renal decompensation. Patients at greatest risk of this reaction are those with impaired renal function, heart failure, liver dysfunction, those taking diuretics and ACE inhibitors, and the elderly. Discontinuation of nonsteroidal anti-inflammatory drug therapy is usually followed by recovery to the pretreatment state.
Ibuprofen metabolites are eliminated primarily by the kidneys. The extent to which the metabolites may accumulate in patients with renal failure has not been studied. Patients with significantly impaired renal function should be more closely monitored.

Hematological Effects
Ibuprofen, like other NSAIDs, can inhibit platelet aggregation but the effect is quantitatively less and of shorter duration than that seen with aspirin. Ibuprofen has been shown to prolong bleeding time in normal subjects. Because this prolonged bleeding effect may be exaggerated in patients with underlying hemostatic defects, Combunox should be used with caution in persons with intrinsic coagulation defects and those on anticoagulant therapy. Anemia is sometimes seen in patients receiving NSAIDs, including ibuprofen. This may be due to fluid retention, GI loss, or an incompletely described effect upon erythropoiesis.

Fluid Retention and Edema
Fluid retention and edema have been reported in association with ibuprofen; therefore, the drug should be used with caution in patients with a history of cardiac decompensation, hypertension or heart failure.

Pre-existing Asthma
Patients with asthma may have aspirin-sensitive asthma. The use of aspirin in patients with aspirin-sensitive asthma has been associated with severe bronchospasm, which may be fatal. Since cross-reactivity between aspirin and other NSAIDs has been reported in such aspirin-sensitive patients, Combunox should not be administered to patients with this form of aspirin sensitivity and should be used with caution in patients with pre-existing asthma.

Aseptic Meningitis
Aseptic meningitis with fever and coma has been observed on rare occasions in patients on ibuprofen therapy. Although it is probably more likely to occur in patients with systemic lupus erythematosus and related connective tissue diseases, it has been reported in patients who do not have an underlying chronic disease. If signs or symptoms of meningitis develop in a patient on Combunox, the possibility of its being related to ibuprofen should be considered.

Information for Patients
Combunox, similar to other opioid-containing analgesics, may impair mental and/or physical abilities required for the performance of potentially hazardous tasks such as driving a car or operating machinery; patients should be cautioned accordingly.
The combination of this product with alcohol and other CNS depressants may produce an additive CNS depression and should be avoided.

Combunox can be abused in a manner similar to other opioid agonists, legal or illicit. Patients should take the drug only for as long as it is prescribed, in the amounts prescribed, and no more frequently than prescribed.
Combunox, like other drugs containing ibuprofen, is not free of side effects. The side effects of these drugs can cause discomfort and, rarely, there are more serious side effects, such as gastrointestinal bleeding, which may result in hospitalization and even fatal outcomes. Patients should be instructed to report any signs or symptoms of gastrointestinal bleeding, blurred vision or other eye problems, skin rash, weight gain, or edema.

Laboratory Tests

A decrease in hemoglobin may occur during Combunox therapy, and elevations of liver enzymes may be seen in a small percentage of patients during Combunox therapy (see PRECAUTIONS - Hematological Effects and PRECAUTIONS - Hepatic Effects).
In patients with severe hepatic or renal disease, effects of therapy should be monitored with liver and/or renal function tests.

Drug Interactions

Oxycodone

Oxycodone is metabolized in part to oxymorphone via the cytochrome P_{450} isoenzyme CYP2D6. While this pathway may be blocked by a variety of drugs (e.g., certain cardiovascular drugs and antidepressants), such blockade has not yet been shown to be of clinical significance with this agent. However, clinicians should be aware of this possible interaction.
Anticholinergics: The concurrent use of anticholinergics with oxycodone preparations may produce paralytic ileus.
CNS Depressants: Patients receiving narcotic analgesics, general anesthetics, phenothiazines, other tranquilizers, sedative-hypnotics or other CNS depressants (including alcohol) concomitantly with oxycodone may exhibit an additive CNS depression. Interactive effects resulting in respiratory depression, hypotension, profound sedation, or coma may result if these drugs are taken in combination with the usual dosage of oxycodone. When such combined therapy is contemplated, the dose of one or both agents should be reduced.
Mixed Agonist/Antagonist Opioid Analgesics: Agonist/antagonist analgesics (i.e., pentazocine, nalbuphine, butorphanol and buprenorphine) should be administered with caution to patients who have received or are receiving a course of therapy with a pure opioid agonist analgesic such as oxycodone. In this situation, mixed agonist/antagonist analgesics may reduce the analgesic effect of oxycodone and/or may precipitate withdrawal symptoms in these patients.
Monoamine Oxidase Inhibitors (MAOIs): MAOIs have been reported to intensify the effects of at least one opioid drug causing anxiety, confusion and significant depression of respiration or coma. The use of oxycodone is not recommended for patients taking MAOIs or within 14 days of stopping such treatment.
Neuromuscular Blocking Agents: Oxycodone, as well as other opioid analgesics, may enhance the neuromuscular blocking action of skeletal muscle relaxants and produce an increased degree of respiratory depression.

Ibuprofen

ACE-Inhibitors: Reports suggest that NSAIDs may diminish the antihypertensive effect of ACE-inhibitors. This interaction should be given consideration in patients taking Combunox concomitantly with ACE-inhibitors.
Aspirin: As with other products containing NSAIDs, concomitant administration of Combunox and aspirin is not generally recommended because of the potential of increased adverse effects.
Diuretics: Ibuprofen has been shown to reduce the natriuretic effect of furosemide and thiazides in some patients. This response has been attributed to inhibition of renal prostaglandin synthesis. During concomitant therapy with Combunox the patient should be observed closely for signs of renal failure (see PRECAUTIONS - Renal Effects), as well as diuretic efficacy.
Lithium: Ibuprofen has been shown to elevate plasma lithium concentration and reduce renal lithium clearance. This effect has been attributed to inhibition of renal prostaglandin synthesis by ibuprofen. Thus, when Combunox and lithium are administered concurrently, patients should be observed for signs of lithium toxicity.
Methotrexate: Ibuprofen, as well as other NSAIDs, has been reported to competitively inhibit methotrexate accumulation in rabbit kidney slices. This may indicate that ibuprofen could enhance the toxicity of methotrexate. Caution should be used when Combunox is administered concomitantly with methotrexate.
Warfarin: The effects of warfarin and NSAIDs on GI bleeding are synergistic, such that users of both drugs together have a greater risk of serious GI bleeding than users of either drug alone.

Carcinogenicity, Mutagenicity and Impairment of Fertility

Studies to evaluate the potential effects of the combination of oxycodone and ibuprofen on carcinogenicity, mutagenicity or impairment of fertility have not been conducted.

Pregnancy

Teratogenic Effects

Pregnancy Category C

Animal studies to assess the potential effects of the combination of oxycodone and ibuprofen on embryo-fetal development were conducted in the rat and rabbit model.
Pregnant rats were treated by oral gavage with combination doses of oxycodone:ibuprofen mg/kg/day (0.25:20, 0.5:40, 1.0:80, or 2.0:160) on days 7-16 of gestation. There was no evidence for developmental toxicity or teratogenicity at any dose, although maternal toxicity was noted at doses of 0.5:40 and above. The highest dose tested in the rat (2.00:160 mg/kg/day) is equivalent to the maximum recommended human daily dose (20:1600 mg/day) on a body surface area (mg/m^2) basis. This dose was associated with maternal toxicity (death, clinical signs, decreased BW).
Pregnant rabbits were treated by oral gavage with combination doses of oxycodone/ibuprofen (0.38:30, 0.75:60, 1.50:120 or 3.00:240 mg/kg/day) on gestation days 7-19. Oxycodone/ibuprofen treatment was not teratogenic under the conditions of the assay. Maternal toxicity was noted at doses of 1.5:120 (reduced body weight and food consumption) and 3:240 mg/kg/day (mortality). The NOAEL for maternal toxicity, 0.75:60 mg/kg/day, is 0.75 fold the proposed maximum daily human dose based upon the body surface area. Developmental toxicity, as evidenced by delayed ossification and reduced fetal body weights, was noted at the highest dose, which is approximately 3 times the MRHD on a mg/m^2 basis, and is likely due to maternal toxicity. The fetal no adverse effect level (NOAEL) of 1.50:120 mg/kg/day is approximately 1.5 times the MRHD on a mg/m^2 basis.
There are no adequate and well-controlled studies in pregnant women. Combunox should be used during pregnancy only if the potential benefit justifies the potential risk to the fetus. Because of the ibuprofen component, Combunox should not be used during the third trimester of pregnancy because it could cause problems in the unborn child (premature closure of the ductus arteriosus and pulmonary hypertension in the fetus/neonate).

Labor and Delivery

Combunox should not be used during the third trimester of pregnancy due to the potential for ibuprofen to inhibit prostaglandin synthetase which may prolong pregnancy and inhibit labor. Oxycodone is not recommended for use in women during and immediately prior to labor and delivery because oral opioids may cause respiratory depression in the newborn.

Nursing Mothers

Ibuprofen is not transferred to breast milk in significant quantities. The American Academy of Pediatrics classified ibuprofen as compatible with breastfeeding. In studies using a 1 mcg/mL assay, ibuprofen was not detected in the milk of lactating mothers. Oxycodone is excreted in human milk. Withdrawal symptoms and/or respiratory depression have been observed in neonates whose mothers were taking narcotic analgesics during pregnancy. Although adverse effects in the nursing infant have not been documented, withdrawal can occur in breast-feeding infants when maternal administration of an opioid analgesic is discontinued.
Because of the potential for serious adverse reactions in nursing infants from the oxycodone present in Combunox, a decision should be made whether to discontinue nursing or to discontinue the drug, taking into account the importance of the drug to the mother.

Pediatric Use

In the placebo-controlled, clinical studies of pain following dental surgery, 109 patients between the ages of 14 and 17 years were administered a single dose of Combunox. No apparent differences were noted in the safety of Combunox in patients below and above 17 years of age. Combunox has not been studied in patients under 14 years of age.

Geriatric Use

Of the total number of subjects in clinical studies of Combunox, 89 patients were 65 and over, while 37 patients were 75 and over. No overall differences in safety were observed between these subjects and younger subjects, and other reported clinical experience has not identified differences in responses between the elderly and younger patients, but greater sensitivity of some older individuals cannot be ruled out.
However, because the elderly may be more sensitive to the renal and gastrointestinal effects of nonsteroidal anti-inflammatory agents as well as possible increased risk of respiratory depression with opioids, extra caution should be used when treating the elderly with Combunox.

ADVERSE REACTIONS

Listed below are the adverse event incidence rates from single dose analgesia trials in which a total of 2437 patients received either Combunox, ibuprofen (400 mg), oxycodone HCl (5 mg), or placebo. Adverse event information is also provided from an additional 334 patients who were exposed to Combunox in a multiple dose analgesia trial, without placebo or active component comparison arms, given up to four times daily for up to 7 days.
[See table above]

Adverse Events Which Occurred at a Frequency of ≥ 1% and at a Higher Incidence than in the Placebo Group in Single Dose Studies

	5/400 mg (n=923)	400 mg Ibuprofen (n=913)	5 mg Oxycodone HCl (n = 286)	Placebo (n=315)
Digestive				
Nausea	81 (8.8%)	44 (4.8%)	46 (16.1%)	21 (6.7%)
Vomiting	49 (5.3%)	16 (1.8%)	30 (10.5%)	10 (3.2%)
Flatulence	9 (1.0%)	7 (0.8%)	3 (1.0%)	0
Nervous System				
Somnolence	67 (7.3%)	38 (4.2%)	12 (4.2%)	7 (2.2%)
Dizziness	47 (5.1%)	21 (2.3%)	17 (5.9%)	8 (2.5%)
Skin and Appendages				
Sweat	15 (1.6%)	7 (0.8%)	4 (1.4%)	1 (0.3%)

Adverse events that were reported by at least 1% of patients taking Combunox but were observed at a greater incidence in the placebo treated patients were fever, headache and pruritus.
Adverse events that occurred in less than 1% and in at least two Combunox treated patients in **Single Dose** studies not listed above include the following: **Body as Whole:** abdominal pain, asthenia, chest pain, enlarged abdomen. **Cardiovascular System:** hypotension, syncope, tachycardia, vasodilation. **Digestive System:** constipation, dry mouth, dyspepsia, eructation, ileus. **Hemic and Lymphatic System:** anemia. **Metabolic and Nutritional Disorders:** edema. **Nervous System:** euphoria, insomnia, nervousness. **Respiratory System:** hypoxia, lung disorder, pharyngitis. **Urogenital System:** urinary retention.
Adverse events that occurred in the **Multiple Dose** study in at least 2% of patients treated with Combunox include the following: **Body as Whole:** asthenia (3.3%), fever (3.0%), headache (10.2%). **Cardiovascular System:** vasodilation (3.0%). **Digestive System:** constipation (4.5%), diarrhea (2.1%), dyspepsia (2.1%), nausea (25.4%), vomiting (4.5%). **Nervous System:** dizziness (19.2%), somnolence (17.4%).
Adverse events that occurred in less than 2% of and at least two Combunox treated patients in the **Multiple Dose** study not listed previously include the following: **Body as Whole:** back pain, chills, infection. **Cardiovascular System:** thrombophlebitis. **Hemic and Lymphatic System:** ecchymosis. **Metabolic and Nutritional Disorders:** hypokalemia. **Musculoskeletal System:** arthritis. **Nervous System:** abnormal thinking, anxiety, hyperkinesia, hypertonia. **Skin and Appendages:** rash. **Special Senses:** amblyopia, taste perversion. **Urogenital System:** urinary frequency.

DRUG ABUSE AND DEPENDENCE

Combunox contains oxycodone, which is a mu-opioid agonist with an abuse liability similar to other opioid agonists and is a Schedule II controlled substance. Combunox, and other opioids used in analgesia, can be abused and are subject to criminal diversion.
Addiction is a primary, chronic, neurobiologic disease, with genetic, psychosocial, and environmental factors influencing its development and manifestations. It is characterized by behaviors that include one or more of the following: impaired control over drug use, compulsive use, continued use despite harm, and craving. Drug addiction is a treatable disease utilizing a multidisciplinary approach, but relapse is common.
"Drug seeking" behavior is very common in addicts and drug abusers. Drug-seeking tactics include emergency calls or visits near the end of office hours, refusal to undergo appropriate examination, testing or referral, repeated "loss" of prescriptions, tampering with prescriptions and reluctance to provide prior medical records or contact information for other treating physician(s). "Doctor shopping" to obtain additional prescriptions is common among drug abusers and people suffering from untreated addiction.
Abuse and addiction are separate and distinct from physical dependence and tolerance. Physical dependence usually assumes clinically significant dimensions after several days to weeks of continuous opioid use. Tolerance, in which increasingly large doses are required in order to produce the same degree of analgesia, is manifested initially by a shorter duration of analgesic effect, and subsequently by a decrease in the intensity of analgesia. The rate of development of tolerance varies among patients. Physicians should be aware that abuse of opioids can occur in the absence of true addiction and is characterized by misuse for non-medical purposes, often in combination with other psychoactive substances. Combunox, like other opioids, may be diverted for non-medical use. Record-keeping of prescribing information, including quantity, frequency, and renewal requests is strongly advised.

Continued on next page

Combunox—Cont.

Proper assessment of the patient, proper prescribing practices, periodic re-evaluation of therapy, and proper dispensing and storage are appropriate measures that help to limit abuse of opioid drugs.

OVERDOSAGE

Following an acute overdosage, toxicity may result from oxycodone and/or ibuprofen.

Signs and Symptoms:

Acute overdosage with oxycodone may be manifested by respiratory depression, somnolence progressing to stupor or coma, skeletal muscle flaccidity, cold and clammy skin, constricted pupils, bradycardia, or hypotension. In severe cases death may occur.

The toxicity of ibuprofen overdose is dependent on the amount of drug ingested and the time elapsed since ingestion, although individual response may vary, necessitating individual evaluation of each case. Although uncommon, serious toxicity and death have been reported in the medical literature with ibuprofen overdose. The most frequently reported symptoms of ibuprofen overdose include abdominal pain, nausea, vomiting, lethargy, and drowsiness. Other central nervous system symptoms include headache, tinnitus, CNS depression, and seizures. Cardiovascular toxicity, including hypotension, bradycardia, tachycardia, and atrial fibrillation, have also been reported.

Treatment:

In the treatment of opioid overdosage, primary attention should be given to the re-establishment of a patent airway and institution of assisted or controlled ventilation. Supportive measures (including oxygen and vasopressors) should be employed in the management of circulatory shock and pulmonary edema accompanying overdose, as indicated. Cardiac arrest or arrhythmias may require cardiac massage or defibrillation. The narcotic antagonist naloxone hydrochloride is a specific antidote against respiratory depression, which may result from overdosage or unusual sensitivity to narcotics including oxycodone. An appropriate dose of naloxone hydrochloride should be administered intravenously with simultaneous efforts at respiratory resuscitation. Since the duration of action of oxycodone may exceed that of the naloxone, the patient should be kept under continuous surveillance and repeated doses of the antagonist should be administered as needed to maintain adequate respiration. Management of hypotension, acidosis and gastrointestinal bleeding may be necessary. In cases of acute overdose, the stomach should be emptied through ipecac-induced emesis or gastric lavage. Orally administered activated charcoal may help in reducing the absorption and reabsorption of ibuprofen. Emesis is most effective if initiated within 30 minutes of ingestion. Induced emesis is not recommended in patients with impaired consciousness or overdoses greater than 400 mg/kg of the ibuprofen component in children because of the risk for convulsions and the potential for aspiration of gastric contents.

DOSAGE AND ADMINISTRATION

For the management of acute moderate to severe pain, the recommended dose of Combunox is one tablet.

Dosage should not exceed 4 tablets in a 24-hour period and should not exceed 7 days.

HOW SUPPLIED

Combunox are capsule shaped, white to off-white, film-coated tablets with "F" bisect "P" on one side and "5400" on the other side.

Bottles of 100-NDC #0456-5200-01

Storage:

Store at 25°C (77°F); excursions permitted to 15° to 30°C (59° to 86°F).

A Schedule CII Narcotic

Forest Pharmaceuticals, Inc.

Subsidiary of Forest Laboratories, Inc.

St. Louis, MO 63045 USA

11/04

©2004 Forest Laboratories, Inc.

To keep your **PDR** up to date throughout the year, note these revisions on the corresponding pages of the annual volume. Simply write **"See Supplement A"** next to the product heading.

GATE Pharmaceuticals

Div. of TEVA Pharmaceuticals USA
650 CATHILL ROAD
SELLERSVILLE, PA 18960

Direct Inquiries to:
1090 Horsham Road
P. O. Box 1090
North Wales, PA 19454
(800) 292-4283

TEV-TROPIN™   ℞

[těv-trōpĭn]

somatropin (rDNA origin) for injection
5 mg (15 IU)
℞ **only**

DESCRIPTION

TEV-TROPIN™ (somatropin, rDNA origin, for injection), a polypeptide of recombinant DNA origin, has 191 amino acid residues and a molecular weight of about 22,124 daltons. It has an amino acid sequence identical to that of human growth hormone of pituitary origin. TEV-TROPIN™ is synthesized in a strain of *Escherichia coli* modified by insertion of the human growth hormone gene.

TEV-TROPIN™ is a sterile, white, lyophilized powder, intended for subcutaneous administration, after reconstitution with bacteriostatic 0.9% sodium chloride injection, USP, (normal saline) (benzyl alcohol preserved). The quantitative composition of the lyophilized drug per vial is:

5 mg (15 IU) vial:

Somatropin	5 mg (15 IU)
Mannitol	30 mg

The diluent contains bacteriostatic 0.9% sodium chloride injection, USP, (normal saline), 0.9% benzyl alcohol as a preservative, and water for injection. A 5 mL vial of the diluent will be supplied with each dispensed vial of TEV-TROPIN™.

TEV-TROPIN™ is a highly-purified preparation. Reconstituted solutions have a pH in the range of 7.0 to 9.0.

CLINICAL PHARMACOLOGY

Clinical trials have demonstrated that TEV-TROPIN™ is equivalent in its therapeutic effectiveness and in its pharmacokinetic profile to those of human growth hormone of pituitary origin (somatropin). TEV-TROPIN™ stimulates linear growth in children who lack adequate levels of endogenous growth hormone. Treatment of growth hormone-deficient children with TEV-TROPIN™ produces increased growth rates and IGF-1 (Insulin-Like Growth Factor/Somatomedin-C) concentrations that are similar to those seen after therapy with human growth hormone of pituitary origin.

Both TEV-TROPIN™ and somatropin have also been shown to have other actions including:

A. *Tissue Growth*
  1. Skeletal Growth. TEV-TROPIN™ stimulates skeletal growth in patients with growth hormone deficiency. The measurable increase in body length after administration of TEV-TROPIN™ results from its effect on the epiphyseal growth plates of long bones. Concentrations of IGF-1, which may play a role in skeletal growth, are low in the serum of growth hormone-deficient children but increase during treatment with TEV-TROPIN™. Mean serum alkaline phosphatase concentrations are increased.
  2. Cell Growth. It has been shown that there are fewer skeletal muscle cells in short statured children who lack endogenous growth hormone as compared with normal children. Treatment with somatropin results in an increase in both the number and size of muscle cells.
  3. Organ Growth. Somatropin influences the size of internal organs and it also increases red cell mass.

B. *Protein Metabolism*
  Linear growth is facilitated, in part, by increased cellular protein synthesis. Nitrogen retention, as demonstrated by decreased urinary nitrogen excretion and serum urea nitrogen, results from treatment with somatropin.

C. *Carbohydrate Metabolism*
  Children with hypopituitarism sometimes experience fasting hypoglycemia that is improved by treatment with somatropin. Large doses of somatropin may impair glucose tolerance.

D. *Lipid Metabolism*
  Administration of somatropin to growth hormone-deficient patients mobilizes lipid, reduces body fat stores, and increases plasma fatty acids.

E. *Mineral Metabolism*
  Sodium, potassium, and phosphorous are conserved by somatropin. Serum concentrations of inorganic phosphates increased in patients with growth hormone deficiency after therapy with TEV-TROPIN™ or somatropin. Serum calcium concentrations are not significantly altered in patients treated with either somatropin or TEV-TROPIN™.

F. *Connective Tissue Metabolism*
  Somatropin stimulates the synthesis of chondroitin sulfate and collagen as well as the urinary excretion of hydroxyproline.

PHARMACOKINETICS

Following intravenous administration of 0.1 mg/kg of TEV-TROPIN™, the elimination half-life was about 0.42 hours (approximately 25 minutes) and the mean plasma clearance (± SD) was 133 (± 16) mL/min in healthy male volunteers.

In the same volunteers, after a subcutaneous injection of 0.1 mg/kg TEV-TROPIN™ to the forearm, the mean peak serum concentration (± SD) was 80 (± 50) ng/mL which occurred approximately 7 hours post-injection and the apparent elimination half-life was approximately 2.7 hours. Compared to intravenous administration, the extent of systemic availability from subcutaneous administration was approximately 70%.

INDICATION AND USAGE

TEV-TROPIN™ is indicated only for the long-term treatment of children who have growth failure due to an inadequate secretion of normal endogenous growth hormone.

CONTRAINDICATIONS

Growth hormone is contraindicated in patients with Prader-Willi syndrome who are severely obese or have severe respiratory impairment (see **WARNINGS**). Unless patients with Prader-Willi syndrome also have a diagnosis of growth hormone deficiency, TEV-TROPIN™ is not indicated for the long term treatment of pediatric patients who have growth failure due to genetically confirmed Prader-Willi syndrome.

Growth hormone should not be initiated to treat patients with acute critical illness due to complications following open heart or abdominal surgery, multiple accidental trauma or to patients having acute respiratory failure. Two placebo-controlled clinical trials in non-growth hormone-deficient adult patients (n = 522) with these conditions revealed a significant increase in mortality (41.9% vs. 19.3%) among somatropin treated patients (doses 5.3 to 8 mg/day) compared to those receiving placebo (see **WARNINGS**).

TEV-TROPIN™ should not be used in patients with closed epiphyses.

Patients with evidence of progression of an underlying intracranial lesion should not receive TEV-TROPIN™. Prior to the initiation of therapy with TEV-TROPIN™, intracranial tumors must be inactive and antitumor therapy completed.

TEV-TROPIN™ reconstituted with bacteriostatic 0.9% sodium chloride injection, USP (normal saline) (benzyl alcohol preserved) should not be administered to patients with a known sensitivity to benzyl alcohol.

WARNINGS

See **CONTRAINDICATIONS** for information on increased mortality in patients with acute critical illnesses in intensive care units due to complications following open heart or abdominal surgery, multiple accidental trauma or with acute respiratory failure. The safety of continuing growth hormone treatment in patients receiving replacement doses for approved indications who concurrently develop these illnesses has not been established. Therefore, the potential benefit of treatment continuation with growth hormone in patients having acute critical illnesses should be weighed against the potential risk.

There have been reports of fatalities after initiating therapy with growth hormone in pediatric patients with Prader-Willi syndrome who had one or more of the following risk factors: severe obesity, history of upper airway obstructions or sleep apnea, or unidentified respiratory infection. Male patients with one or more of these factors may be at greater risk than females. Patients with Prader-Willi syndrome should be evaluated for signs of upper airway obstruction and sleep apnea before initiation of treatment with growth hormone. If during treatment with growth hormone, patients show signs of upper airway obstruction (including onset of or increased snoring) and/or new onset sleep apnea, treatment should be interrupted. All patients with Prader-Willi syndrome treated with growth hormone should also have effective weight control and be monitored for signs of respiratory infection, which should be diagnosed as early as possible and treated aggressively (see **CONTRAINDICATIONS**).

Unless patients with Prader-Willi syndrome also have a diagnosis of growth hormone deficiency, TEV-TROPIN™ is not indicated for the long term treatment of pediatric patients who have growth failure due to genetically confirmed Prader-Willi syndrome.

Benzyl alcohol as a preservative in bacteriostatic normal saline, USP, has been associated with toxicity in newborns. When administering TEV-TROPIN™ to newborns, reconstitute with sterile normal saline for injection, USP. WHEN RECONSTITUTING WITH STERILE NORMAL SALINE, USE ONLY ONE DOSE PER VIAL AND DISCARD THE UNUSED PORTION.

PRECAUTIONS

Therapy with TEV-TROPIN™ should be directed by physicians who are experienced in the diagnosis and management of patients with growth hormone deficiency.

Patients with growth hormone deficiency secondary to intracranial lesion should be examined frequently for progression or recurrence of the underlying disease process.

Patients should be observed for evidence of glucose intolerance because human growth hormone may induce a state of insulin resistance.

Glucocorticoid therapy may inhibit the growth-promoting effect of human growth hormone. Patients with coexisting

ACTH deficiency should have their glucocorticoid replacement dose carefully adjusted to avoid an inhibitory effect on growth.
Hypothyroidism may become manifest during treatment with human growth hormone. Inadequate treatment of hypothyroidism may negate optimal response to human growth hormone. Therefore, patients should have periodic thyroid function tests and be treated with thyroid hormone when indicated.
Slipped capital femoral epiphysis may occur more frequently in patients with endocrine disorders. Physicians and parents should be alert to the development of a limp or complaint of hip or knee pain in patients treated with TEV-TROPIN™.
Intracranial hypertension (IH) has not been reported in any patients treated with TEV-TROPIN™. Nevertheless, IH with papilledema, visual changes, headache, nausea and/or vomiting has been reported in a small number of patients treated with other growth hormone products. Symptoms usually occurred within the first eight (8) weeks of the initiation of growth hormone therapy. In all reported cases, IH-associated signs and symptoms resolved after termination of therapy or a reduction of the growth hormone dose. Funduscopic examination of patients is recommended at the initiation and periodically during the course of growth hormone therapy.

Carcinogenesis, Mutagenesis, Impairment of Fertility
Carcinogenesis, mutagenesis and reproduction studies have not been conducted with TEV-TROPIN™ growth hormone.

Pregnancy
Pregnancy Category C
Animal reproduction studies have not been conducted with TEV-TROPIN™ growth hormone. It is not known whether TEV-TROPIN™ growth hormone can cause fetal harm when administered to a pregnant woman or can affect reproduction capacity. TEV-TROPIN™ growth hormone should be given to a pregnant woman only if clearly needed.

Nursing Mothers
There have been no studies conducted with TEV-TROPIN™ in nursing mothers. It is not known whether this drug is excreted in human milk. Because many drugs are excreted in human milk, caution should be exercised when TEV-TROPIN™ is administered to a nursing woman.

Geriatric Use
The safety and effectiveness of TEV-TROPIN™ in patients aged 65 and over has not been evaluated in clinical studies. Elderly patients may be more sensitive to the action of TEV-TROPIN™ and may be more prone to develop adverse reactions.

ADVERSE REACTIONS

Utilizing a double-antibody immunoassay, no antibodies to growth hormone could be detected in a group of 164 naïve and previously treated clinical trial patients after treatment with TEV-TROPIN™ for up to 40 months. However, utilizing the less specific polyethelene glycol (PEG) precipitation immunoassay, 27 of the 164 patient group were tested after treatment with TEV-TROPIN™ for 4 to 6 months and antibodies to growth hormone were detected in two patients (7.4%). The binding capacity of the antibodies from the two antibody positive patients was not determined.
None of the patients with anti-GH antibodies in the clinical studies experienced decreased linear growth response to TEV-TROPIN™ or any other associated adverse event. Growth hormone antibody binding capacities below 2 mg/L have not been associated with growth attenuation. In some cases, when binding capacity exceeds 2 mg/L, growth attenuation has been observed.
In studies of growth hormone-deficient children, headaches occurred infrequently. Injection site reactions (e.g., pain, bruise) occurred in 8 of the 164 treated patients.
Leukemia has been reported in a small number of patients treated with other growth hormone products. It is uncertain whether this risk is related to the pathology of growth hormone deficiency itself, growth hormone therapy, or other associated treatments such as radiation therapy for intracranial tumors.

OVERDOSAGE

The recommended dosage of up to 0.1 mg/kg (0.3 IU/kg) of body weight 3 times per week should not be exceeded. Acute overdose could cause initial hypoglycemia and subsequent hyperglycemia. Long-term repeated use of doses in excess of those recommended could result in signs and symptoms of gigantism and/or acromegaly consistent with the known effects of excess human growth hormone.

DOSAGE AND ADMINISTRATION

A dosage of up to 0.1 mg/kg (0.3 IU/kg) of body weight administered 3 times per week by subcutaneous injection is recommended. The dosage schedule for TEV-TROPIN™ should be individualized for each patient. Subcutaneous injection of greater than 1 mL of reconstituted solution is not recommended.
After the dose has been determined, each vial of TEV-TROPIN™ should be reconstituted with 1 to 5 mL of bacteriostatic 0.9% sodium chloride for injection, USP (benzyl alcohol preserved).* The stream of normal saline should be aimed against the side of the vial to prevent foaming. Swirl the vial with a GENTLE rotary motion until the contents are completely dissolved and the solution is clear. DO NOT SHAKE. Since TEV-TROPIN™ is a protein, shaking or vigorous mixing will cause the solution to be cloudy. If the resulting solution is cloudy or contains particulate matter, the contents MUST NOT be injected.

*Benzyl alcohol as a preservative in bacteriostatic normal saline, USP, has been associated with toxicity in newborns. When administering TEV-TROPIN™ to newborns, reconstitute with sterile normal saline for injection, USP.

Occasionally, after refrigeration, some cloudiness may occur. This is not unusual for proteins like TEV-TROPIN™ growth hormone. Allow the product to warm to room temperature. If cloudiness persists or particulate matter is noted, the contents MUST NOT be used.
Before and after injection, the septum of the vial should be wiped with rubbing alcohol or an alcoholic antiseptic solution to prevent contamination of the contents by repeated needle insertions. It is recommended that TEV-TROPIN™ be administered using sterile disposable syringes and needles. The syringes should be of small enough volume that the prescribed dose can be drawn from the vial with reasonable accuracy.

STABILITY AND STORAGE
Before Reconstitution – Vials of TEV-TROPIN™ are stable when refrigerated at 36° to 46°F (2° to 8°C). Expiration dates are stated on the labels.
After Reconstitution – Vials of TEV-TROPIN™ are stable for up to 14 days when reconstituted with bacteriostatic 0.9% sodium chloride (normal saline), USP, and stored in a refrigerator at 36° to 46°F (2° to 8°C). Do not freeze the reconstituted solution.

HOW SUPPLIED

TEV-TROPIN™ (somatropin, rDNA origin, for injection) is supplied as 5 mg (15 IU) of lyophilized, sterile somatropin per vial.
Each 5 mg carton contains one vial of TEV-TROPIN™ (5 mg per vial) and one vial of diluent [5 mL of bacteriostatic 0.9% sodium chloride for injection, USP (benzyl alcohol preserved)], and is supplied in single cartons or cartons of six.
Manufactured In Israel By:
BIO-TECHNOLOGY GENERAL (ISRAEL) LTD.
Rehovot, Israel
Distributed By:
GATE PHARMACEUTICALS
div. of Teva Pharmaceuticals USA
Sellersville, PA 18960
GATE

Rev. E 3/2005
0082-5008v2

GlaxoSmithKline
FIVE MOORE DRIVE
RESEARCH TRIANGLE PARK, NC 27709

For Medical Information for Healthcare Professionals and Consumers, Contact:
1-888-825-5249
www.us.gsk.com

ARIXTRA® ℞
[ə-rix' trə]
(fondaparinux sodium)
Injection

> **SPINAL/EPIDURAL HEMATOMAS**
> When neuraxial anesthesia (epidural/spinal anesthesia) or spinal puncture is employed, patients anticoagulated or scheduled to be anticoagulated with low molecular weight heparins, heparinoids or fondaparinux sodium for prevention of thromboembolic complications are at risk of developing an epidural or spinal hematoma which can result in long-term or permanent paralysis.
> The risk of these events is increased by the use of indwelling epidural catheters for administration of analgesia or by the concomitant use of drugs affecting hemostasis such as non-steroidal anti-inflammatory drugs (NSAIDs), platelet inhibitors, or other anticoagulants. The risk also appears to be increased by traumatic or repeated epidural or spinal puncture.
> Patients should be frequently monitored for signs and symptoms of neurologic impairment. If neurologic compromise is noted, urgent treatment is necessary.
> The physician should consider the potential benefit versus risk before neuraxial intervention in patients anticoagulated or to be anticoagulated for thromboprophylaxis (see also **WARNINGS: Hemorrhage** and **PRECAUTIONS: Drug Interactions**).

DESCRIPTION

ARIXTRA® (fondaparinux sodium) Injection is a sterile solution containing fondaparinux sodium. It is a synthetic and specific inhibitor of activated Factor X (Xa). Fondaparinux sodium is methyl O-2-deoxy-6-O-sulfo-2-(sulfoamino)-α-D-glucopyranosyl-(1→4)-O-β-D-glucopyranuronosyl-(1→4)-O-2-deoxy-3,6-di-O-sulfo-2-(sulfoamino)-α-D-glucopyranosyl-(1→4)-O-2-O-sulfo-α-L-idopyranuronosyl-(1→4)-2-deoxy-6-O-sulfo-2-(sulfoamino)-α-D-glucopyranoside, decasodium salt.

The molecular formula of fondaparinux sodium is $C_{31}H_{43}N_3Na_{10}O_{49}S_8$ and its molecular weight is 1728. The structural formula is provided below:

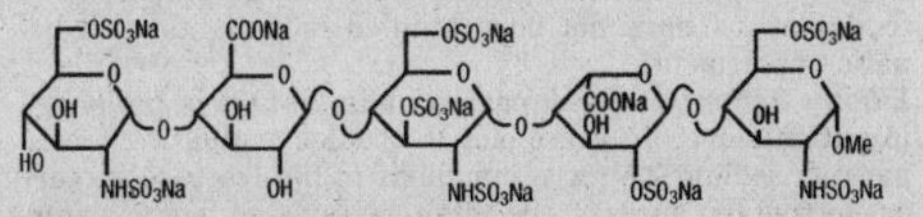

ARIXTRA is supplied as a sterile, preservative-free injectable solution for subcutaneous use.
Each single dose, prefilled syringe of ARIXTRA, affixed with an automatic needle protection system, contains 2.5 mg of fondaparinux sodium in 0.5 mL, 5.0 mg of fondaparinux sodium in 0.4 mL, 7.5 mg of fondaparinux sodium in 0.6 mL or 10.0 mg of fondaparinux sodium in 0.8 mL of an isotonic solution of sodium chloride and water for injection. The final drug product is a clear and colorless to slightly yellow liquid with a pH between 5.0 and 8.0.

CLINICAL PHARMACOLOGY

Pharmacodynamics
Mechanism of Action: The antithrombotic activity of fondaparinux sodium is the result of antithrombin III (ATIII)-mediated selective inhibition of Factor Xa. By selectively binding to ATIII, fondaparinux sodium potentiates (about 300 times) the innate neutralization of Factor Xa by ATIII. Neutralization of Factor Xa interrupts the blood coagulation cascade and thus inhibits thrombin formation and thrombus development.
Fondaparinux sodium does not inactivate thrombin (activated Factor II) and has no known effect on platelet function. At the recommended dose, fondaparinux sodium does not affect fibrinolytic activity or bleeding time.
Anti-Xa Activity: The pharmacodynamics/pharmacokinetics of fondaparinux sodium are derived from fondaparinux plasma concentrations quantified via anti-Factor Xa activity. Only fondaparinux can be used to calibrate the anti-Xa assay. (The international standards of heparin or LMWH are not appropriate for this use.) As a result, the activity of fondaparinux sodium is expressed as milligrams (mg) of the fondaparinux calibrator. The anti-Xa activity of the drug increases with increasing drug concentration, reaching maximum values in approximately 3 hours.

Pharmacokinetics
Absorption: Fondaparinux sodium administered by subcutaneous injection is rapidly and completely absorbed (absolute bioavailability is 100%). Following a single subcutaneous dose of fondaparinux sodium 2.5 mg in young male subjects, C_{max} of 0.34 mg/L is reached in approximately 2 hours. In patients undergoing treatment with fondaparinux sodium injection 2.5 mg, once daily, the peak steady-state plasma concentration is, on average, 0.39-0.50 mg/L and is reached approximately 3 hours post-dose. In these patients, the minimum steady-state plasma concentration is 0.14-0.19 mg/L. In patients with symptomatic deep vein thrombosis and pulmonary embolism undergoing treatment with fondaparinux sodium injection 5 mg (body weight <50 kg), 7.5 mg (body weight 50-100 kg) and 10 mg (body weight >100 kg) once daily, the body-weight-adjusted doses provide similar mean steady-state peaks and minimum plasma concentrations across all body weight categories. The mean peak steady-state plasma concentration is in the range of 1.20-1.26 mg/L. In these patients, the mean minimum steady-state plasma concentration is in the range of 0.46-0.62 mg/L.
Distribution: In healthy adults, intravenously or subcutaneously administered fondaparinux sodium distributes mainly in blood and only to a minor extent in extravascular fluid as evidenced by steady state and non-steady state apparent volume of distribution of 7-11 L. Similar fondaparinux distribution occurs in patients undergoing elective hip surgery or hip fracture surgery. *In vitro*, fondaparinux sodium is highly (at least 94%) and specifically bound to antithrombin III (ATIII) and does not bind significantly to other plasma proteins (including platelet Factor 4 [PF4]) or red blood cells.
Metabolism: *In vivo* metabolism of fondaparinux has not been investigated since the majority of the administered dose is eliminated unchanged in urine in individuals with normal kidney function.
Elimination: In individuals with normal kidney function fondaparinux is eliminated in urine mainly as unchanged drug. In healthy individuals up to 75 years of age, up to 77% of a single subcutaneous or intravenous fondaparinux dose is eliminated in urine as unchanged drug in 72 hours. The elimination half-life is 17-21 hours.

Special Populations
Renal Impairment: Fondaparinux elimination is prolonged in patients with renal impairment since the major route of elimination is urinary excretion of unchanged drug. In patients undergoing prophylaxis following elective hip surgery or hip fracture surgery, the total clearance of fondaparinux is approximately 25% lower in patients with mild renal impairment (creatinine clearance 50 to 80 mL/min), approximately 40% lower in patients with moderate renal impairment (creatinine clearance 30 to 50 mL/min) and approximately 55% lower in patients with severe renal impairment (<30 mL/min) compared to patients with normal renal function. A similar relationship between fondaparinux clearance and extent of renal impairment was observed in DVT treatment patients. (See **CONTRAINDICATIONS** and **WARNINGS: Renal Impairment.**)

Continued on next page

Arixtra—Cont.

Hepatic Impairment: The pharmacokinetic properties of fondaparinux have not been studied in patients with hepatic impairment.

Elderly Patients: Fondaparinux elimination is prolonged in patients over 75 years old. In studies evaluating fondaparinux sodium 2.5 mg prophylaxis in hip fracture surgery or elective hip surgery, the total clearance of fondaparinux was approximately 25% lower in patients over 75 years old as compared to patients less than 65 years old. A similar relationship between fondaparinux clearance and age was observed in DVT treatment patients.

Patients Weighing Less Than 50 kg: Total clearance of fondaparinux sodium is decreased by approximately 30% in patients weighing less than 50 kg (see **CONTRAINDICATIONS** and **DOSAGE AND ADMINISTRATION**).

Gender: The pharmacokinetic properties of fondaparinux sodium are not significantly affected by gender.

Race: Pharmacokinetic differences due to race have not been studied prospectively. However, studies performed in Asian (Japanese) healthy subjects did not reveal a different pharmacokinetic profile compared to Caucasian healthy subjects. Similarly, no plasma clearance differences were observed between Black and Caucasian patients undergoing orthopedic surgery.

Drug Interactions: see **PRECAUTIONS: Drug Interactions.**

CLINICAL STUDIES

Prophylaxis of Thromboembolic Events Following Hip Fracture Surgery

In a randomized, double-blind, clinical trial in patients undergoing hip fracture surgery, ARIXTRA (fondaparinux sodium) Injection 2.5 mg SC once daily was compared to enoxaparin sodium 40 mg SC once daily, which is not approved for use in patients undergoing hip fracture surgery. A total of 1711 patients were randomized and 1673 were treated. Patients ranged in age from 17-101 years (mean age 77 years) with 25% men and 75% women. Patients were 99% Caucasian, 1% other races. Patients with multiple trauma affecting more than one organ system, serum creatinine level more than 2 mg/dL (180 μmol/L), or platelet count less than $100,000/mm^3$ were excluded from the trial. ARIXTRA was initiated after surgery in 88% of patients (mean 6 hrs) and enoxaparin sodium was initiated after surgery in 74% of patients (mean 18 hrs). For both drugs, treatment was continued for 7 ± 2 days. The primary efficacy endpoint, venous thromboembolism (VTE), was a composite of documented deep vein thrombosis (DVT) and/or documented symptomatic pulmonary embolism (PE) reported up to Day 11. The efficacy data are provided in Table 1 below and demonstrate that under the conditions of the trial fondaparinux sodium was associated with a VTE rate of 8.3% compared with a VTE rate of 19.1% for enoxaparin sodium for a relative risk reduction of 56% (95% CI: 39%, 70%; p <0.001). Major bleeding episodes occurred in 2.2% of ARIXTRA patients and 2.3% of enoxaparin sodium patients (see Tables 7 and 8 under **ADVERSE REACTIONS: Hemorrhage**).

Table 1: Efficacy of ARIXTRA Injection in the Peri-operative Prophylaxis of Thromboembolic Events Following Hip Fracture Surgery

Endpoint	Peri-operative Prophylaxis (Day 1 to Day 7±2 post-surgery)	
	Fondaparinux Sodium 2.5 mg SC once daily[1]	Enoxaparin Sodium 40 mg SC once daily[1,2]
All Treated Hip Fracture Surgery Patients	N = 831	N = 840
All Evaluable[3] Hip Fracture Surgery Patients		
VTE[4]	52/626 8.3%[5] (6.3, 10.8)[6]	119/624 19.1% (16.1, 22.4)
All DVT	49/624 7.9%[5] (5.9, 10.2)	117/623 18.8% (15.8, 22.1)
Proximal DVT	6/650 0.9%[5] (0.3, 2.0)	28/646 4.3% (2.9, 6.2)
Symptomatic PE	3/831 0.4%[7] (0.1, 1.1)	3/840 0.4% (0.1, 1.0)

[1] ARIXTRA was initiated after surgery in 88% of patients (mean 6 hrs) and enoxaparin sodium was initiated after surgery in 74% of patients (mean 18 hrs).
[2] Not approved for use in patients undergoing hip fracture surgery.
[3] Evaluable patients were those who were treated and underwent the appropriate surgery (ie., hip fracture surgery of the upper third of the femur), with an adequate efficacy assessment up to Day 11.
[4] VTE was a composite of documented DVT and/or documented symptomatic PE reported up to Day 11.
[5] p value <0.001
[6] Numbers in parentheses indicate 95% confidence interval
[7] p value: NS

Table 3: Efficacy of ARIXTRA Injection in the Prophylaxis of Thromboembolic Events Following Hip Replacement Surgery

Endpoint	Study 1		Study 2	
	Fondaparinux Sodium 2.5 mg SC once daily[1]	Enoxaparin Sodium 30 mg SC every 12 hr[3]	Fondaparinux Sodium 2.5 mg SC once daily[2]	Enoxaparin Sodium 40 mg SC once daily[4]
All Treated Hip Replacement Surgery Patients	N = 1126	N = 1128	N = 1129	N = 1123
All Evaluable[5] Hip Replacement Surgery Patients				
VTE[6]	48/787 6.1%[7] (4.5, 8.0)[8]	66/797 8.3% (6.5, 10.4)	37/908 4.1%[10] (2.9, 5.6)	85/919 9.2% (7.5, 11.3)
All DVT	44/784 5.6%[9] (4.1, 7.5)	65/796 8.2% (6.4, 10.3)	36/908 4.0%[10] (2.8, 5.4)	83/918 9.0% (7.3, 11.1)
Proximal DVT	14/816 1.7%[7] (0.9, 2.9)	10/830 1.2% (0.6, 2.2)	6/922 0.7%[11] (0.2, 1.4)	23/927 2.5% (1.6, 3.7)
Symptomatic PE	5/1126 0.4%[7] (0.1, 1.0)	1/1128 0.1% (0.0, 0.5)	2/1129 0.2%[7] (0.0, 0.6)	2/1123 0.2% (0.0, 0.6)

[1] In Study 1, ARIXTRA was initiated after surgery in 92% of patients (mean 6.5 hrs).
[2] In Study 2, ARIXTRA was initiated after surgery in 86% of patients (mean 6.25 hrs).
[3] In Study 1, enoxaparin sodium was initiated after surgery in 97% of patients (mean 20.25 hrs).
[4] In Study 2, enoxaparin sodium was initiated before surgery in 78% of patients. The first postoperative dose was given a mean of 13 hrs after surgery.
[5] Evaluable patients were those who were treated and underwent the appropriate surgery (ie., hip replacement surgery), with an adequate efficacy assessment up to Day 11.
[6] VTE was a composite of documented DVT and/or documented symptomatic PE reported up to Day 11.
[7] p value versus enoxaparin sodium: NS.
[8] Numbers in parentheses indicates 95% confidence interval.
[9] p value versus enoxaparin sodium in study 1: <0.05.
[10] p value versus enoxaparin sodium in study 2: <0.001.
[11] p value versus enoxaparin sodium in study 2: <0.01.

Extended Prophylaxis of Thromboembolic Events Following Hip Fracture Surgery

In a noncomparative, unblinded manner, 737 patients undergoing hip fracture surgery were initially treated during the peri-operative period with ARIXTRA 2.5 mg once daily for 7 ± 1 days. Eighty one (81) of the 737 patients were not eligible for randomization into the 3-week double-blind period. Three hundred twenty six (326) patients and 330 patients were randomized to receive ARIXTRA 2.5 mg once daily or placebo, respectively, in or out of the hospital for 21 $\pm$ 2 days. Patients ranged in age from 23 to 96 years (mean age 75 years) and were 29% men and 71% women. Patients were 99% Caucasian and 1% other races. Patients with multiple traumas affecting more than one organ system or serum creatinine level more than 2 mg/dL (180 μmol/L) were excluded from the trial. The primary efficacy endpoint, venous thromboembolism (VTE), was a composite of documented deep vein thrombosis (DVT) and/or documented symptomatic pulmonary embolism (PE) reported for up to 24 days following randomization. The efficacy data are provided in Table 2 below and demonstrate that extended prophylaxis with fondaparinux sodium was associated with a VTE rate of 1.4% compared with a VTE rate of 35.0% for placebo for a relative risk reduction of 95.9% (95% CI = [98.7; 87.1], p<0.0001). Major bleeding rates during the 3-week extended prophylaxis period for ARIXTRA (2.4%) and placebo (0.6%) are provided in Tables 7 and 8 (see **ADVERSE REACTIONS: Hemorrhage**).

Table 2: Efficacy of ARIXTRA Injection in the Extended Prophylaxis of Thromboembolic Events Following Hip Fracture Surgery

Endpoint	Extended Prophylaxis (Day 8 to Day 28±2 post-surgery)	
	Fondaparinux Sodium 2.5 mg SC once daily	Placebo SC once daily
All Randomized Treated Hip Fracture Surgery Patients	N = 326	N = 330
All Randomized Evaluable Hip Fracture Surgery Patients[1]		
VTE[2]	3/208 1.4%[3] (0.3, 4.2)[4]	77/220 35.0% (28.7, 41.7)
All DVT	3/208 1.4%[3] (0.3, 4.2)	74/218 33.9% (27.7, 40.6)
Proximal DVT	2/221 0.9%[3] (0.1, 3.2)	35/222 15.8% (11.2, 21.2)
Symptomatic VTE (all)	1/326 0.3%[5] (0.0, 1.7)	9/330 2.7% (1.3, 5.1)
Symptomatic PE	0/326 0.0%[6] (0.0, 1.1)	3/330 0.9% (0.2, 2.6)

[1] Evaluable patients were those who were treated in the post-randomization period, with an adequate efficacy assessment for up to 24 days following randomization.
[2] VTE was a composite of documented DVT and/or documented symptomatic PE reported for up to 24 days following randomization.
[3] p value < 0.001.
[4] Number in parentheses indicate 95% confidence interval.
[5] p value = 0.021.
[6] p value = NS.

Prophylaxis of Thromboembolic Events Following Hip Replacement Surgery

In two randomized, double-blind, clinical trials in patients undergoing hip replacement surgery, ARIXTRA 2.5 mg SC once daily was compared to either enoxaparin sodium 30 mg SC every 12 hours (Study 1) or to enoxaparin sodium 40 mg SC once a day (Study 2). In Study 1, a total of 2275 patients were randomized and 2257 were treated. Patients ranged in age from 18 to 92 years (mean age 65 years) with 48% men and 52% women. Patients were 94% Caucasian, 4% Black, <1% Asian, and 2% others. In Study 2, a total of 2309 patients were randomized and 2273 were treated. Patients ranged in age from 24 to 97 years (mean age 65 years) with 42% men and 58% women. Patients were 99% Caucasian, and 1% other races. Patients with serum creatinine level more than 2 mg/dL (180 μmol/L), or platelet count less than $100,000/mm^3$ were excluded from both trials. In Study 1, ARIXTRA was initiated 6 ± 2 hours (mean 6.5 hrs) after surgery in 92% of patients and enoxaparin sodium was initiated 12 to 24 hours (mean 20.25 hrs) after surgery in 97% of patients. In Study 2, ARIXTRA was initiated 6 ± 2 hours (mean 6.25 hrs) after surgery in 86% of patients and enoxaparin sodium was initiated 12 hours before surgery in 78% of patients. The first post-operative enoxaparin sodium dose was given before 12 hours after surgery in 60% of patients and 12 to 24 hours after surgery in 35% of patients with a mean of 13 hrs. For both studies, both study treatments were continued for 7 ± 2 days. The efficacy data are provided in Table 3 below. Under the conditions of Study 1, fondaparinux sodium was associated with a VTE rate of 6.1% compared with a VTE rate of 8.3% for enoxaparin sodium for a relative risk reduction of 26% (95% CI: -11%, 53%; p = NS). Under the conditions of Study 2, fondaparinux sodium was associated with a VTE rate of 4.1% compared with a VTE rate of 9.2% for enoxaparin sodium for a relative risk reduction of 56% (95% CI: 33%, 73%; p<0.001). For the two studies combined, the major bleeding episodes occurred in 3.0% of ARIXTRA patients and 2.1% of enoxaparin sodium patients (see Tables 7 and 8 under **ADVERSE REACTIONS: Hemorrhage**).

[See table 3 above]

Prophylaxis of Thromboembolic Events Following Knee Replacement Surgery

In a randomized, double-blind, clinical trial in patients undergoing knee replacement surgery (i.e., surgery requiring resection of the distal end of the femur or proximal end of the tibia), ARIXTRA 2.5 mg SC once daily was compared to enoxaparin sodium 30 mg SC every 12 hours. A total of 1049 patients were randomized and 1034 were treated. Patients ranged in age from 19 to 94 years (mean age 68 years) with 41% men and 59% women. Patients were 88% Caucasian, 8% Black, <1% Asian, and 3% others. Patients with serum creatinine level more than 2 mg/dL (180 μmol/L), or platelet count less than 100,000/mm[3] were excluded from the trial. ARIXTRA was initiated 6 ± 2 hours (mean 6.25 hrs) after surgery in 94% of patients, and enoxaparin sodium was initiated 12 to 24 hours (mean 21 hrs) after surgery in 96% of patients. For both drugs, treatment was continued for 7 ± 2 days. The efficacy data are provided in Table 4 below and demonstrate that under the conditions of the trial, fondaparinux sodium was associated with a VTE rate of 12.5% compared with a VTE rate of 27.8% for enoxaparin sodium for a relative risk reduction of 55% (95% CI: 36%, 70%; p <0.001). Major bleeding episodes occurred in 2.1% of ARIXTRA patients and 0.2% of enoxaparin sodium patients (see Tables 7 and 8 under **ADVERSE REACTIONS: Hemorrhage**).

Table 4: Efficacy of ARIXTRA Injection in the Prophylaxis of Thromboembolic Events Following Knee Replacement Surgery

Endpoint	Fondaparinux Sodium 2.5 mg SC once daily[1]	Enoxaparin Sodium 30 mg SC every 12 hrs[2]
All Treated Knee Replacement Surgery Patients	N = 517	N = 517
All Evaluable[3] Knee Replacement Surgery Patients		
VTE[4]	45/361 12.5%[5] (9.2, 16.3)[6]	101/363 27.8% (23.3, 32.7)
All DVT	45/361 12.5%[5] (9.2, 16.3)	98/361 27.1% (22.6, 32.0)
Proximal DVT	9/368 2.4%[7] (1.1, 4.6)	20/372 5.4% (3.3, 8.2)
Symptomatic PE	1/517 0.2%[7] (0.0, 1.1)	4/517 0.8% (0.2, 2.0)

[1] Patients randomized to ARIXTRA 2.5 mg received the first injection 6 ± 2 hours after surgery providing that hemostasis had been achieved.

[2] Patients randomized to enoxaparin sodium received the first injection at 21 ± 2 hours after surgery closure providing that hemostasis had been achieved.

[3] Evaluable patients were those who were treated and underwent the appropriate surgery (ie., knee replacement surgery), with an adequate efficacy assessment up to Day 11.

[4] VTE was a composite of documented DVT and/or documented symptomatic PE reported up to Day 11.

[5] p value <0.001

[6] Numbers in parentheses indicates 95% confidence interval

[7] p value: NS

Treatment of Deep Vein Thrombosis and Pulmonary Embolism

Treatment of Deep Vein Thrombosis

In a randomized, double-blind, clinical trial in patients with a confirmed diagnosis of acute symptomatic DVT without PE, ARIXTRA 5 mg (body weight <50 kg), 7.5 mg (body weight 50-100 kg) or 10 mg (body weight >100 kg) SC once daily (ARIXTRA treatment regimen) was compared to enoxaparin sodium 1 mg/kg SC every 12 hours. Almost all patients started study treatment in hospital. Approximately 30% of patients in both groups were discharged home from the hospital while receiving study treatment. A total of 2205 patients were randomized and 2192 were treated. Patients ranged in age from 18-95 years (mean age 61 years) with 53% men and 47% women. Patients were 97% Caucasian, 2% Black and 1% other races. Patients with serum creatinine level more than 2 mg/dL (180 μmol/L), or platelet count less than 100,000/mm[3] were excluded from the trial. For both groups, treatment continued for a least 5 days with a treatment duration range of 7 ± 2 days, and both treatment groups received Vitamin K antagonist therapy initiated within 72 hours after the first study drug administration and continued for 90 ± 7 days, with regular dose adjustments to achieve an INR of 2-3. The primary efficacy endpoint was confirmed, symptomatic, recurrent VTE reported up to Day 97. The efficacy data are provided in Table 5 below.

Table 5: Efficacy of ARIXTRA Injection in the Treatment of Deep Vein Thrombosis

Endpoint	Fondaparinux Sodium[1] 5, 7.5 or 10 mg SC once daily (Treatment Regimen)	Enoxaparin Sodium[1] 1 mg/kg SC q 12h
All Randomized DVT Patients	N = 1098	N = 1107
Total VTE[2]	43[3] 3.9% (2.8, 5.2)[4]	45 4.1% (3.0, 5.4)
DVT only	18 1.6% (1.0, 2.6)	28 2.5% (1.7, 3.6)
Non-fatal PE	20 1.8% (1.1, 2.8)	12 1.1% (0.6, 1.9)
Fatal PE	5 0.5% (0.1, 1.1)	5 0.5% (0.1, 1.1)

[1] Patients were also treated with Vitamin K antagonists initiated within 72 hours after the first study drug administration

[2] VTE was a composite of symptomatic recurrent non fatal VTE or fatal PE reported up to Day 97

[3] The 95% confidence interval for the treatment difference for total VTE was: (-1.8% to 1.5%)

[4] Number in parentheses indicates 95% confidence interval

During the initial treatment period, 18 (1.6% of patients treated with fondaparinux sodium and 10 (0.9%) of patients treated with enoxaparin sodium had a VTE endpoint (95% CI for the treatment difference [fondaparinux sodium-enoxaparin sodium] for VTE rates: -0.2%; 1.7%).

Treatment of Pulmonary Embolism

In a randomized, open-label, clinical trial in patients with a confirmed diagnosis of acute symptomatic PE, with or without DVT, ARIXTRA 5 mg (body weight <50 kg), 7.5 mg (body weight 50-100 kg) or 10 mg (body weight >100 kg) SC once daily (ARIXTRA treatment regimen) was compared to heparin IV bolus (5000 USP units) followed by a continuous IV infusion adjusted to maintain 1.5-2.5 times aPTT control value. Patients with a PE requiring thrombolysis or surgical thrombectomy were excluded from the trial. All patients started study treatment in hospital. Approximately 15% of patients were discharged home from the hospital while receiving fondaparinux therapy. A total of 2213 patients were randomized and 2184 were treated. Patients ranged in age from 18-97 years (mean age 62 years) with 44% men and 56% women. Patients were 94% Caucasian, 5% Black and 1% other races. Patients with serum creatinine level more than 2 mg/dL (180 μmol/L), or platelet count less than 100,000/mm[3] were excluded from the trial. For both groups, treatment continued for at least 5 days with a treatment duration range 7 ± 2 days, and both treatment groups received Vitamin K antagonist therapy initiated within 72 hours after the first study drug administration and continued for 90 ± 7 days, with regular dose adjustments to achieve an INR of 2-3. The primary efficacy endpoint was confirmed, symptomatic, recurrent VTE reported up to Day 97. The efficacy data are provided in Table 6 below.

Table 6: Efficacy of ARIXTRA Injection in the Treatment of Pulmonary Embolism

Endpoint	Fondaparinux Sodium[1] 5, 7.5 or 10 mg SC once daily[1] (Treatment Regimen)	Heparin[1] aPTT adjusted IV
All Randomized PE Patients	N = 1103	N = 1110
Total VTE[2]	42[3] 3.8% (2.8, 5.1)[4]	56 5.0% (3.8, 6.5)
DVT only	12 1.1% (0.6, 1.9)	17 1.5% (0.9, 2.4)
Non-fatal PE	14 1.3% (0.7, 2.1)	24 2.2% (1.4, 3.2)
Fatal PE	16 1.5% (0.8, 2.3)	15 1.4% (0.8, 2.2)

[1] Patients were also treated with Vitamin K antagonists initiated within 72 hours after the first study drug administration

[2] VTE was a composite of symptomatic recurrent non fatal VTE or fatal PE reported up to Day 97

[3] The 95% confidence interval for the treatment difference for total VTE was: (-3.0% to 0.5%)

[4] Number in parentheses indicates 95% confidence interval

During the initial treatment period, 12 (1.1%) of patients treated with fondaparinux sodium and 19 (1.7%) of patients treated with heparin had a VTE endpoint (95% CI for the treatment difference [fondaparinux sodium-heparin] for VTE rates: -1.6%; 0.4%).

INDICATIONS AND USAGE

ARIXTRA (fondaparinux sodium) Injection is indicated for the prophylaxis of deep vein thrombosis, which may lead to pulmonary embolism:

• in patients undergoing hip fracture surgery, including extended prophylaxis;
• in patients undergoing hip replacement surgery;
• in patients undergoing knee replacement surgery.

ARIXTRA (fondaparinux sodium) Injection is indicated for:

• the treatment of acute deep vein thrombosis when administered in conjunction with warfarin sodium, and
• the treatment of acute pulmonary embolism when administered in conjunction with warfarin sodium when initial therapy is administered in the hospital.

(See **DOSAGE AND ADMINISTRATION** section for appropriate dosage regimen.)

CONTRAINDICATIONS

ARIXTRA (fondaparinux sodium) Injection is contraindicated in patients with severe renal impairment (creatinine clearance <30mL/min). ARIXTRA is eliminated primarily by the kidneys, and such patients are at increased risk for major bleeding episodes (see **WARNINGS: Renal Impairment**).

ARIXTRA prophylactic therapy is contraindicated in patients with body weight <50 kg undergoing hip fracture, hip replacement or knee replacement surgery. During the randomized clinical trials of prophylaxis in the peri-operative period following one of these procedures, occurrence of major bleeding was doubled in patients with body weight <50 kg compared with those with body weight ≥50 kg (5.4% vs. 2.1%).

The use of ARIXTRA is contraindicated in patients with active major bleeding, bacterial endocarditis, in patients with thrombocytopenia associated with a positive *in vitro* test for anti-platelet antibody in the presence of fondaparinux sodium, or in patients with known hypersensitivity to fondaparinux sodium.

WARNINGS

ARIXTRA (fondaparinux sodium) Injection is not intended for intramuscular administration.

ARIXTRA cannot be used interchangeably (unit for unit) with heparin, low molecular weight heparins or heparinoids, as they differ in manufacturing process, anti-Xa and anti-IIa activity, units, and dosage. Each of these medicines has its own instructions for use.

Renal Impairment

The risk of hemorrhage increases with increasing renal impairment. Occurrences of major bleeding in patients receiving prophylactic therapy in hip fracture, hip replacement or knee replacement surgery with normal renal function, mild renal impairment, moderate renal impairment, and severe renal impairment have been found to be 1.6% (25/1565), 2.4% (31/1288), 3.8% (19/504), and 4.8% (4/83), respectively. Occurrences of major bleeding in patients receiving therapeutic regimen in treatment of DVT and PE with normal renal function, mild renal impairment, moderate renal impairment, and severe renal impairment have been found to be 0.4% (4/1132), 1.6% (12/733), 2.2% (7/318), and 7.3% (4/55), respectively. Therefore, ARIXTRA is contraindicated in patients with severe renal impairment (creatinine clearance <30 mL/min) and should be used with caution in patients with moderate renal impairment (creatinine clearance 30-50 mL/min). (See **CLINICAL PHARMACOLOGY: Special Populations, Renal Impairment** and **CONTRAINDICATIONS.**)

Renal function should be assessed periodically in patients receiving ARIXTRA. The drug should be discontinued immediately in patients who develop severe renal impairment or labile renal function while on therapy. After discontinuation of ARIXTRA, its anticoagulant effects may persist for 2-4 days in patients with normal renal function (i.e., at least 3-5 half-lives). The anticoagulant effects of ARIXTRA may persist even longer in patients with renal impairment (see **CLINICAL PHARMACOLOGY**).

Hemorrhage

ARIXTRA Injection, like other anticoagulants, should be used with extreme caution in conditions with increased risk of hemorrhage, such as congenital or acquired bleeding disorders, active ulcerative and angiodysplastic gastrointestinal disease, hemorrhagic stroke, or shortly after brain, spinal, or ophthalmological surgery, or in patients treated concomitantly with platelet inhibitors.

Laboratory Testing

Because routine coagulation tests such as Prothrombin Time (PT) and Activated Partial Thromboplastin Time (aPTT) are relatively insensitive measures of ARIXTRA activity and international standards of heparin or LMWH are not calibrators to measure anti-Factor Xa activity of ARIXTRA, if during ARIXTRA therapy unexpected changes

Continued on next page

Arixtra—Cont.

in coagulation parameters or major bleeding occurs, ARIXTRA should be discontinued (see **PRECAUTIONS: Laboratory Tests**).

Neuraxial Anesthesia and Post-operative Indwelling Epidural Catheter Use

Spinal or epidural hematomas, which may result in long-term or permanent paralysis, can occur with the use of anticoagulants and neuraxial (spinal/epidural) anesthesia or spinal puncture. The risk of these events may be higher with post-operative use of indwelling epidural catheters or concomitant use of other drugs affecting hemostasis such as NSAIDs (see **Boxed Warning for Spinal/Epidural Hematomas**).

Thrombocytopenia: Thrombocytopenia can occur with the administration of ARIXTRA. Moderate thrombocytopenia (platelet counts between 100,000/mm^3 and 50,000/mm^3) occurred at a rate of 2.9% in patients given ARIXTRA 2.5 mg in the peri-operative hip fracture, hip replacement or knee replacement surgery clinical trials. Severe thrombocytopenia (platelet counts less than 50,000/mm^3) occurred at a rate of 0.2% in patients given ARIXTRA 2.5 mg in these clinical trials. During extended prophylaxis, no cases of moderate or severe thrombocytopenia were reported.

Moderate thrombocytopenia occurred at a rate of 0.5% in patients given the ARIXTRA treatment regimen in the DVT and PE treatment clinical trials. Severe thrombocytopenia occurred at a rate of 0.04% in patients given the ARIXTRA treatment regimen in the DVT and PE treatment clinical trials.

Thrombocytopenia of any degree should be monitored closely. If the platelet count falls below 100,000/mm^3, ARIXTRA should be discontinued.

PRECAUTIONS

General

ARIXTRA Injection should be administered according to the recommended regimen, especially with respect to the timing of the first dose after surgery. In the hip fracture, hip replacement or knee replacement surgery clinical studies, the administration of ARIXTRA before 6 hours after surgery has been associated with an increased risk of major bleeding (see ADVERSE REACTIONS: Hemorrhage and DOSAGE AND ADMINISTRATION).

ARIXTRA Injection should be used with care in patients with a bleeding diathesis, uncontrolled arterial hypertension, or a history of recent gastrointestinal ulceration, diabetic retinopathy, and hemorrhage.

ARIXTRA (fondaparinux sodium) Injection should be used with caution in elderly patients (see **PRECAUTIONS: Geriatric Use**).

ARIXTRA should be used with caution in patients with a low body weight (<50 kg) for the treatment of PE and DVT.

ARIXTRA should be used with caution in patients with a history of heparin-induced thrombocytopenia.

ARIXTRA Injection should not be mixed with other injections or infusions.

If thrombotic events occur despite ARIXTRA prophylaxis, appropriate therapy should be initiated.

Laboratory Tests

Periodic routine complete blood counts (including platelet count), serum creatinine level, and stool occult blood tests are recommended during the course of treatment with ARIXTRA Injection.

When administered at the recommended doses, routine coagulation tests such as Prothrombin Time (PT) and Activated Partial Thromboplastin Time (aPTT) are relatively insensitive measures of ARIXTRA activity, and are therefore, unsuitable for monitoring.

The anti-Factor Xa activity of fondaparinux sodium can be measured by anti-Xa assay using the appropriate calibrator (fondaparinux). Since the international standards of heparin or LMWH are not appropriate calibrators, the activity of fondaparinux sodium is expressed in milligrams (mg) of the fondaparinux and cannot be compared with activities of heparin or low molecular weight heparins (see **CLINICAL PHARMACOLOGY: Pharmacodynamics** and **Pharmacokinetics** and **WARNINGS: Laboratory Testing**).

Drug Interactions

In clinical studies performed with ARIXTRA, the concomitant use of oral anticoagulants (warfarin), platelet inhibitors (acetylsalicylic acid), NSAIDs (piroxicam), and digoxin did not significantly affect the pharmacokinetics/pharmacodynamics of fondaparinux sodium. In addition, ARIXTRA neither influenced the pharmacodynamics of warfarin, acetylsalicylic acid, piroxicam, and digoxin, nor the pharmacokinetics of digoxin at steady state.

Agents that may enhance the risk of hemorrhage should be discontinued prior to initiation of ARIXTRA therapy. If co-administration is essential, close monitoring may be appropriate.

In an *in vitro* study in human liver microsomes, inhibition of CYP2A6 hydroxylation of coumarin by fondaparinux (200 µM i.e., 350 mg/L) was 17-28%. Inhibition of the other isozymes evaluated (CYPs 2A1, 2C9, 2C19, 2D6, 3A4, and 3E1) was 0-16%. Since fondaparinux does not markedly inhibit CYP450s (CYP1A2, CYP2A6, CYP2C9, CYP2C19, CYP2D6, CYP2E1, or CYP3A4) *in vitro*, fondaparinux sodium is not expected to significantly interact with other drugs *in vivo* by inhibition of metabolism mediated by these isozymes.

Table 7: Major Bleeding Episodes[1] in Randomized, Controlled, Hip Fracture, Hip Replacement and Knee Replacement Surgery Studies

	Peri-Operative Prophylaxis (Day 1 to Day 7±1 post-surgery)		Extended Prophylaxis (Day 8 to Day 28±2 post-surgery)	
Indications	Fondaparinux Sodium 2.5 mg SC once daily	Enoxaparin Sodium[2,3]	Fondaparinux Sodium 2.5 mg SC once daily	Placebo SC once daily
Hip Fracture	18/831 (2.2%)	19/842 (2.3%)	8/327 (2.4%)[4]	2/329 (0.6%)
Hip Replacement	67/2268 (3.0%)	55/2597 (2.1%)		
Knee Replacement	11/517 (2.1%)[5]	1/517 (0.2%)		

[1] Major bleeding was defined as clinically overt bleeding that was (1) fatal, (2) bleeding at critical site (eg., intracranial, retroperitoneal, intra-ocular, pericardial, spinal or into adrenal gland), (3) associated with re-operation at operative site, or (4) with a bleeding index (BI) ≥2 calculated as [number of whole blood or packed red blood cell units transfused + [(pre-bleeding) − (post-bleeding)] hemoglobin (g/dL) values].

[2] Enoxaparin sodium dosing regimen: 30 mg every 12 hours or 40 mg once daily.

[3] Not approved for use in patients undergoing hip fracture surgery.

[4] During noncomparative, unblinded peri-operative prophylaxis, major bleeding was reported in 22/737 (3.0%) patients. Fifteen (15) of these 22 patients continued to receive ARIXTRA in extended prophylaxis. After randomization, 4/327 (1.2%) patients experienced major bleeding for the first time.

[5] p value versus enoxaparin sodium: <0.01, 95% confidence interval: (1.1%, 3.3%) in ARIXTRA group versus (0.0%, 1.1%) in enoxaparin sodium group.

Table 8: Bleeding Across Randomized, Controlled Hip Fracture, Hip Replacement and Knee Replacement Surgery Studies

	Peri-Operative Prophylaxis (Day 1 to Day 7±1 post-surgery)		Extended Prophylaxis (Day 8 to Day 28±2 post-surgery)	
	Fondaparinux Sodium 2.5 mg SC once daily	Enoxaparin Sodium[1, 2]	Fondaparinux Sodium 2.5 mg SC once daily	Placebo SC once daily
	N = 3616	N = 3956	N = 327	N = 329
Major bleeding[3]	96 (2.7%)	75 (1.9%)	8 (2.4%)[4]	2 (0.6%)
Fatal bleeding	0 (0.0%)	1 (<0.1%)	0 (0.0%)	0 (0.0%)
Non-fatal bleeding at critical site	0 (0.0%)	1 (<0.1%)	0 (0.0%)	0 (0.0%)
Re-operation due to bleeding	12 (0.3%)	10 (0.3%)	2 (0.6%)	2 (0.6%)
BI ≥ 2[5]	84 (2.3%)	63 (1.6%)	6 (1.8%)	0 (0.0%)
Minor bleeding[6]	109 (3.0%)	116 (2.9%)	5 (1.5%)	2 (0.6%)

[1] Enoxaparin sodium dosing regimen: 30 mg every 12 hours or 40 mg once daily.

[2] Not approved for use in patients undergoing hip fracture surgery.

[3] Major bleeding was defined as clinically overt bleeding that was (1) fatal, (2) bleeding at critical site (eg., intracranial, retroperitoneal, intra-ocular, pericardial, spinal, or into adrenal gland), (3) associated with re-operation at operative site, or (4) with a bleeding index (BI) ≥ 2.

[4] During non-comparative, unblinded, peri-operative prophylaxis, two fatal bleeds were reported (one in a 50 kg patient, one in a severe renal failure patient).

[5] BI ≥ 2: overt bleeding associated only with a bleeding index (BI) ≥ 2 calculated as [number of whole blood or packed red blood cell units transfused + [(pre-bleeding) − (post-bleeding)] hemoglobin (g/dL) values].

[6] Minor bleeding was defined as clinically overt bleeding that was not major.

Since fondaparinux sodium does not bind significantly to plasma proteins other than ATIII, no drug interactions by protein-binding displacement are expected.

Carcinogenesis, Mutagenesis, Impairment of Fertility

No long-term studies in animals have been performed to evaluate the carcinogenic potential of fondaparinux sodium. Fondaparinux sodium was not genotoxic in the Ames test, the mouse lymphoma cell (L5178Y/TK$^{+/-}$) forward mutation test, the human lymphocyte chromosome aberration test, the rat hepatocyte unscheduled DNA synthesis (UDS) test, or the rat micronucleus test.

At subcutaneous doses up to 10 mg/kg/day (about 32 times the recommended human dose based on body surface area), fondaparinux sodium was found to have no effect on fertility and reproductive performance of male and female rats.

Pregnancy

Teratogenic Effects

Pregnancy Category B. Reproduction studies have been performed in pregnant rats at subcutaneous doses up to 10 mg/kg/day (about 32 times the recommended human dose based on body surface area) and pregnant rabbits at subcutaneous doses up to 10 mg/kg/day (about 65 times the recommended human dose based on body surface area) and have revealed no evidence of impaired fertility or harm to the fetus due to fondaparinux sodium. There are, however, no adequate and well-controlled studies in pregnant women. Because animal reproduction studies are not always predictive of human response, this drug should be used during pregnancy only if clearly needed.

Nursing Mothers

Fondaparinux sodium was found to be excreted in the milk of lactating rats. However, it is not known whether this drug is excreted in human milk. Because many drugs are excreted in human milk, caution should be exercised when fondaparinux sodium is administered to a nursing mother.

Pediatric Use

Safety and effectiveness of ARIXTRA in pediatric patients have not been established.

Geriatric Use

ARIXTRA should be used with caution in elderly patients. Over 2300 patients, 65 years and older, have received ARIXTRA 2.5 mg in randomized clinical trials of peri-operative prophylaxis in orthopedic surgery. Over 1200 patients, 65 years and older, have received the ARIXTRA treatment regimen in the DVT and PE treatment clinical trials. The efficacy of ARIXTRA in the elderly (equal to or older than 65 years) was similar to that seen in younger patients (younger than 65 years). In the peri-operative hip fracture, hip replacement or knee replacement surgery clinical trials with patients receiving ARIXTRA 2.5 mg the risk of ARIXTRA-associated major bleeding increased with age: 1.8% (23/1253) in patients <65 years, 2.2% (24/1111) in those 65-74 years, and 2.7% (33/1227) in those ≥75 years. Serious adverse events increased with age for patients receiving ARIXTRA. In patients undergoing three weeks of extended prophylaxis following one week of peri-operative prophylaxis after hip fracture surgery, the incidence of major bleeding was: 1.9% (1/52) in patients <65 years, 1.4% (1/71) in those 65-74 years, and 2.9% (6/204) in those ≥75 years. In the DVT and PE treatment clinical trials with patients receiving the ARIXTRA treatment regimen, the risk of ARIXTRA-associated major bleeding increased with age: 0.6% (7/1151) in patients <65 years, 1.6% (9/560) in those 65-74 years, and 2.1% (12/583) in those ≥75 years. Careful attention to dosing directions and concomitant medications (especially anti-platelet medication) is advised (see **CLINICAL PHARMACOLOGY** and **PRECAUTIONS: General**). Fondaparinux sodium is substantially excreted by the kidney, and the risk of toxic reactions to ARIXTRA may be greater in patients with impaired renal function. Because elderly patients are more likely to have decreased renal function, it may be useful to monitor renal function (see **CONTRAINDICATIONS** and **WARNINGS: Renal Impairment**).

Table 9: Bleeding[1] in DVT and PE Treatment Studies

	Fondaparinux Sodium Treatment Regimen	Enoxaparin Sodium 1 mg/kg SC q 12h	Haparin aPTT adjusted IV
	(N = 2294)	(N = 1101)	(N = 1092)
Major bleeding[2]	28 (1.2%)	13 (1.2%)	12 (1.1%)
Fatal bleeding	3 (0.1%)	0 (0.0%)	1 (0.1%)
Non-fatal bleeding at a critical site	3 (0.1%)	0 (0.0%)	2 (0.2%)
Intracranial bleeding	3 (0.1%)	0 (0.0%)	1 (0.1%)
Retro-peritoneal bleeding	0 (0.0%)	0 (0.0%)	1 (0.1%)
Clinically overt bleeding with a 2 g/dl fall in hemoglobin and/or leading to transfusion of PRBC or whole blood ≥2 units	22 (1.0%)	13 (1.2%)	10 (0.9%)
Minor bleeding[3]	70 (3.1%)	33 (3.0%)	57 (5.2%)

[1] Bleeding rates are during the study drug treatment period (approximately 7 days). Patients were also treated with Vitamin K antagonists initiated within 72 hours after the first study drug administration.
[2] Major bleeding was defined as clinically overt: - and/or contributing to death – and/or in a critical organ including intracranial, retroperitoneal, intraocular, spinal, pericardial or adrenal gland – and/or associated with a fall in hemoglobin level ≥2 g/dL – and/or leading to a transfusion ≥2 units of packed red blood cells or whole blood.
[3] Minor bleeding was defined as clinically overt bleeding that was not major.

Table 10: Adverse Events Occurring in ≥ 2% of ARIXTRA, Enoxaparin Sodium or Placebo Treated Patients Regardless of Relationship to Study Drug Across Randomized, Controlled, Hip Fracture Surgery, Hip Replacement Surgery or Knee Replacement Surgery Studies

Adverse Events	Peri-Operative Prophylaxis (Day 1 to Day 7±1 post-surgery)		Extended Prophylaxis (Day 8 to Day 28±2 post-surgery)	
	Fondaparinux Sodium 2.5 mg SC once daily	Enoxaparin Sodium[1, 2]	Fondaparinux Sodium 2.5 mg SC once daily	Placebo SC once daily
	N = 3616	N = 3956	N = 327	N = 329
Anemia	707 (19.6%)	670 (16.9%)	5 (1.5%)	4 (1.2%)
Fever	491 (13.6%)	610 (15.4%)	1 (0.3%)	4 (1.2%)
Nausea	409 (11.3%)	484 (12.2%)	1 (0.3%)	4 (1.2%)
Edema	313 (8.7%)	348 (8.8%)	3 (0.9%)	2 (0.6%)
Constipation	309 (8.5%)	416 (10.5%)	6 (1.8%)	7 (2.1%)
Rash	273 (7.5%)	329 (8.3%)	2 (0.6%)	4 (1.2%)
Vomiting	212 (5.9%)	236 (6.0%)	2 (0.6%)	4 (1.2%)
Insomnia	179 (5.0%)	214 (5.4%)	3 (0.9%)	1 (0.3%)
Wound drainage increased	161 (4.5%)	184 (4.7%)	2 (0.6%)	0 (0.0%)
Hypokalemia	152 (4.2%)	164 (4.1%)	0 (0.0%)	0 (0.0%)
Urinary tract infection	136 (3.8%)	135 (3.4%)	13 (4.0%)	13 (4.0%)
Dizziness	131 (3.6%)	165 (4.2%)	2 (0.6%)	0 (0.0%)
Purpura	128 (3.5%)	137 (3.5%)	0 (0.0%)	0 (0.0%)
Hypotension	126 (3.5%)	125 (3.2%)	1 (0.3%)	0 (0.0%)
Confusion	113 (3.1%)	132 (3.3%)	4 (1.2%)	1 (0.3%)
Bullous eruption[3]	112 (3.1%)	102 (2.6%)	0 (0.0%)	1 (0.3%)
Urinary retention	106 (2.9%)	117 (3.0%)	0 (0.0%)	1 (0.3%)
Hematoma	103 (2.8%)	109 (2.8%)	7 (2.1%)	1 (0.3%)
Diarrhea	90 (2.5%)	102 (2.6%)	6 (1.8%)	8 (2.4%)
Dyspepsia	87 (2.4%)	102 (2.6%)	1 (0.3%)	2 (0.6%)
Post-operative hemorrhage	85 (2.4%)	69 (1.7%)	2 (0.6%)	2 (0.6%)
Headache	72 (2.0%)	97 (2.5%)	0 (0.0%)	2 (0.6%)
Pain	62 (1.7%)	101 (2.6%)	0 (0.0%)	0 (0.0%)
Surgical site reaction	29 (0.8%)	41 (1.0%)	5 (1.5%)	8 (2.4%)

[1] Enoxaparin sodium dosing regimen: 30 mg every 12 hours or 40 mg once daily.
[2] Not approved for use in patients undergoing hip fracture surgery.
[3] Localized blister coded as bullous eruption.

ADVERSE REACTIONS

Because clinical trials are conducted under widely varying conditions, adverse reaction rates observed in the clinical trials of a drug cannot be directly compared to rates in the clinical trials of another drug and may not reflect the rates observed in practice. The adverse reaction information from clinical trials does, however, provide a basis for identifying possible adverse events and for approximating rates. The data described below reflect exposure in 7444 patients randomized to ARIXTRA (fondaparinux sodium) Injection in controlled trials of hip fracture, hip replacement, or major knee surgeries, and DVT and PE treatment. Patients received ARIXTRA primarily in two large peri-operative dose-response trials (n = 989), four active-controlled peri-operative trials with enoxaparin sodium (n = 3616), and an extended prophylaxis trial (n = 327), a dose-response trial in DVT treatment (n = 111), an active-controlled trial with enoxaparin sodium in DVT treatment (n = 1091), and an active-controlled trial with heparin in PE treatment (n = 1092) (see CLINICAL STUDIES).

Hemorrhage
During ARIXTRA administration, the most common adverse reactions were bleeding complications (see WARNINGS).

Prophylaxis
The rates of major bleeding events reported during the hip fracture, hip replacement or knee replacement surgery clinical trials with ARIXTRA 2.5 mg Injection are provided in Tables 7 and 8 below.
[See table 7 at top of previous page]
[See table 8 on previous page]
A separate analysis of major bleeding across all randomized, controlled, peri-operative, prophylaxis clinical studies according to the time of the first injection of ARIXTRA after surgical closure was performed in patients who received ARIXTRA only post-operatively. In this analysis, the incidences of major bleeding were as follows: <4 hours was 4.8% (5/104), 4-6 hours was 2.3% (28/1196), 6-8 hours was 1.9% (38/1965). In all studies, the majority (≥75%) of the major bleeding events occurred during the first four days after surgery.

Treatment of DVT and PE
The rates of bleeding events reported during the DVT and PE clinical trials with the ARIXTRA injection treatment regimen are provided in Table 9 below.
[See table 9 at left]

Thrombocytopenia: See WARNINGS: Thrombocytopenia.

Local Reactions: Mild local irritation (injection site bleeding, rash, and pruritus) may occur following subcutaneous injection of ARIXTRA.

Elevations of Serum Aminotransferases: In the peri-operative prophylaxis randomized clinical trials of 7 ± 2 days asymptomatic increases in aspartate (AST [SGOT]) and alanine (ALT [SGPT]) aminotransferase levels greater than three times the upper limit of normal of the laboratory reference range have been reported in 1.7% and 2.6% of patients, respectively, during treatment with ARIXTRA 2.5 mg Injection versus 3.2% and 3.9%, of patients, respectively, during treatment with enoxaparin sodium 30 mg every 12 hours or 40 mg once daily enoxaparin sodium. Such elevations are fully reversible and are rarely associated with increases in bilirubin. In the extended prophylaxis clinical trial no significant differences in aspartate (AST [SGOT]) and alanine (ALT [SGPT]) aminotransferase levels between ARIXTRA 2.5 mg Injection and placebo treated patients were observed.
In the DVT and PE treatment clinical trials asymptomatic increases in aspartate (AST [SGOT]) and alanine (ALT [SGPT]) aminotransferase levels greater than three times the upper limit of normal of the laboratory reference range have been reported in 0.7% and 1.3% of patients, respectively, during treatment with the ARIXTRA injection treatment regimen. In comparison, these increases have been reported in 4.8% and 12.3%, of patients, respectively, in the DVT treatment trial during treatment with enoxaparin sodium 1 mg/kg every 12 hours, and in 2.9% and 8.7%, of patients, respectively, in the PE treatment trial during treatment with aPTT adjusted heparin.
Since aminotransferase determinations are important in the differential diagnosis of myocardial infarction, liver disease, and pulmonary emboli, elevations that might be caused by drugs like ARIXTRA should be interpreted with caution.

Other
Other adverse events that occurred during treatment with ARIXTRA, or enoxaparin sodium in clinical trials with patients undergoing hip fracture surgery, hip replacement surgery, or knee replacement surgery and that occurred at a rate of at least 2% in either treatment group, are provided in Table 10 below. Other adverse events that occurred during treatment with ARIXTRA, enoxaparin sodium or heparin in the DVT and PE treatment clinical trials and that occurred at a rate of at least 2% in any treatment group are provided in Table 11 below.
[See table 10 at left]
[See table 11 at top of next page]

OVERDOSAGE

Symptoms/Treatment
There is no known antidote for ARIXTRA (fondaparinux sodium) Injection. Overdose of ARIXTRA may lead to hemorrhagic complications. Overdosage associated with bleeding complications should lead to treatment discontinuation and initiation of appropriate therapy.
Data obtained in patients undergoing chronic intermittent hemodialysis suggest that ARIXTRA clearance can increase by 20% during hemodialysis.

DOSAGE AND ADMINISTRATION

ARIXTRA (fondaparinux sodium) Injection is administered by subcutaneous injection once daily.

Continued on next page

Table 11: Adverse Events Occurring in ≥2% of ARIXTRA, Enoxaparin Sodium or Heparin Treated Patients Regardless of Relationship to Study Drug Across VTE Treatment Studies

Adverse Events	Fondaparinux Sodium	Enoxaparin Sodium	Heparin
	(N = 2294)	(N = 1101)	(N = 1092)
Constipation	106 (4.6%)	32 (2.9%)	93 (8.5%)
Headache	104 (4.5%)	37 (3.4%)	65 (6.0%)
Insomnia	86 (3.7%)	19 (1.7%)	75 (6.9%)
Fever	81 (3.5%)	32 (2.9%)	47 (4.3%)
Nausea	76 (3.3%)	29 (2.6%)	53 (4.9%)
Urinary tract infection	53 (2.3%)	20 (1.8%)	24 (2.2%)
Coughing	48 (2.1%)	7 (0.6%)	26 (2.4%)
Diarrhea	43 (1.9%)	22 (2.0%)	27 (2.5%)
Abdominal pain	33 (1.4%)	14 (1.3%)	28 (2.6%)
Chest pain	33 (1.4%)	8 (0.7%)	26 (2.4%)
Leg pain	31 (1.4%)	10 (0.9%)	22 (2.0%)
Back pain	30 (1.3%)	11 (1.0%)	34 (3.1%)
Epistaxis	30 (1.3%)	12 (1.1%)	41 (3.8%)
Prothrombin decreased	30 (1.3%)	3 (0.3%)	34 (3.1%)
Anemia	28 (1.2%)	3 (0.3%)	23 (2.1%)
Vomiting	26 (1.1%)	14 (1.3%)	27 (2.5%)
Hypokalemia	25 (1.1%)	2 (0.2%)	23 (2.1%)
Bruise	24 (1.0%)	24 (2.2%)	14 (1.3%)
Anxiety	18 (0.8%)	8 (0.7%)	22 (2.0%)
Hepatic function abnormal	10 (0.4%)	14 (1.3%)	24 (2.2%)
Hepatic enzymes increased	7 (0.3%)	52 (4.7%)	30 (2.7%)
SGPT increased	7 (0.3%)	47 (4.3%)	8 (0.7%)
SGOT increased	4 (0.2%)	31 (2.8%)	3 (0.3%)

Arixtra—Cont.

DVT prophylaxis following hip fracture, or hip or knee replacement surgeries: In patients undergoing hip fracture, hip replacement, or knee replacement surgery, the recommended dose of ARIXTRA is 2.5 mg administered by subcutaneous injection once daily. After hemostasis has been established, the initial dose should be given 6 to 8 hours after surgery. Administration before 6 hours after surgery has been associated with an increased risk of major bleeding. The usual duration of administration is 5 to 9 days, and up to 11 days administration has been tolerated. In patients undergoing hip fracture surgery, an extended prophylaxis course of up to 24 additional days is recommended. In patients undergoing hip fracture surgery, a total of 32 days (peri-operative and extended prophylaxis) has been tolerated. (See **CLINICAL STUDIES, WARNINGS: Laboratory Testing** and **ADVERSE REACTIONS.**)

DVT and PE treatment: In patients with acute symptomatic DVT and in patients with acute symptomatic PE the recommended dose of ARIXTRA is 5 mg (body weight <50 kg), 7.5 mg (body weight 50-100 kg) or 10 mg (body weight >100 kg) by subcutaneous injection once daily (ARIXTRA treatment regimen). ARIXTRA injection treatment should be continued for a least 5 days and until a therapeutic oral anticoagulant effect is established (INR 2.0 to 3.0). Concomitant treatment with warfarin sodium should be initiated as soon as possible, usually within 72 hours. The usual duration of administration of ARIXTRA is 5 to 9 days; up to 26 days of ARIXTRA injection has been administered. (See **CLINICAL STUDIES, WARNINGS: Laboratory Testing** and **ADVERSE REACTIONS.**)

INSTRUCTIONS FOR USE
Parenteral drug products should be inspected visually for particulate matter and discoloration prior to administration.
ARIXTRA (fondaparinux sodium) Injection is provided in a single dose, prefilled syringe affixed with an automatic needle protection system. ARIXTRA is administered by subcutaneous injection. It must not be administered by intramuscular injections. ARIXTRA is intended for use under a physician's guidance. Patients may self-inject only if their physician determines that it is appropriate and with medical follow-up as necessary. Proper training in subcutaneous injection technique should be provided.
To avoid the loss of drug when using the pre-filled syringe, do not expel the air bubble from the syringe before the injection. Administration should be made in the fatty tissue, alternating injection sites (e.g., between the left and right anterolateral or the left and right posterolateral abdominal wall).

To administer ARIXTRA:
1. Wipe the surface of the injection site with an alcohol swab.
2. Twist the plunger cap and remove it.

3. Hold the syringe with either hand and use your other hand to twist the rigid needle guard (covers the needle) counter-clockwise. Pull the rigid needle guard straight off the needle.

4. Pinch a fold of skin at the injection site between your thumb and forefinger and hold it throughout the injection.
5. Hold the syringe with your thumb on the top pad of the plunger rod and your next two fingers on the finger grips on the syringe barrel. Pay attention to avoid sticking yourself with the exposed needle.

6. Insert the full length of the syringe needle perpendicularly into the skin fold held between the thumb and forefinger.
[See first figure at top of next column]
7. Push the plunger rod firmly with your thumb as far as it will go. This will ensure you have injected all the contents of the syringe.
[See second figure at top of next column]

8. When you have injected all the contents of the syringe, the plunger should be released. The plunger will then rise automatically while the needle withdraws from the skin and retracts into the security sleeve. Discard the syringe into the sharps container without replacing the rigid needle guard.
9. You will know that the syringe has worked when:
   • The needle is pulled back into the security sleeve and the white safety indicator appears above the blue upper body.
   • You may also hear or feel a soft click when the plunger rod is released fully.

HOW SUPPLIED
ARIXTRA (fondaparinux sodium) Injection is available in the following strengths and package sizes:
2.5 mg ARIXTRA in 0.5 mL single dose prefilled syringe, affixed with a 27-gauge × ½-inch needle with a blue automatic needle protection system
NDC 0007-3230-11   10 Single Unit Syringes
5 mg ARIXTRA in 0.4 mL single dose prefilled syringe, affixed with a 27-gauge × ½-inch needle with an orange automatic needle protection system
NDC 0007-3232-11   10 Single Unit Syringes
7.5 mg ARIXTRA in 0.6 mL single dose prefilled syringe, affixed with a 27-gauge x ½-inch needle with a magenta automatic needle protection system
NDC 0007-3234-11   10 Single Unit Syringes
10 mg ARIXTRA in 0.8 mL single dose prefilled syringe, affixed with a 27-gauge × ½-inch needle with a violet automatic needle protection system
NDC 0007-3236-11   10 Single Unit Syringes
Store at 25°C (77°F); excursions permitted to 15-30°C (59-86°F) [See USP Controlled Room Temperature].
Keep out of the reach of children.
Distributed by GlaxoSmithKline, Research Triangle Park, NC 27709
ARIXTRA is a registered trademark of GlaxoSmithKline.
©2004, GlaxoSmithKline. All rights reserved.
September 2004/RL-2125

BEXXAR®   ℞
[bex' ar]
**Tositumomab and
Iodine I 131 Tositumomab**

> **WARNINGS**
> **Hypersensitivity Reactions, including Anaphylaxis:** Serious hypersensitivity reactions, including some with fatal outcome, have been reported with the BEXXAR therapeutic regimen. Medications for the treatment of severe hypersensitivity reactions should be available for immediate use. Patients who develop severe hypersensitivity reactions should have infusions of the BEXXAR therapeutic regimen discontinued and receive medical attention (see **WARNINGS**).
> **Prolonged and Severe Cytopenias:** The majority of patients who received the BEXXAR therapeutic regimen experienced severe thrombocytopenia and neutropenia. The BEXXAR therapeutic regimen should not be administered to patients with >25% lymphoma marrow involvement and/or impaired bone marrow reserve (see **WARNINGS** and **ADVERSE REACTIONS**).
> **Pregnancy Category X:** The BEXXAR therapeutic regimen can cause fetal harm when administered to a pregnant woman.
> **Special requirements:** The BEXXAR therapeutic regimen (Tositumomab and Iodine I 131 Tositumomab) contains a radioactive component and should be administered only by physicians and other health care professionals qualified by training in the safe use and handling of therapeutic radionuclides. The BEXXAR therapeutic regimen should be administered only by physicians who are in the process of being or have been certified by GlaxoSmithKline in dose calculation and administration of the BEXXAR therapeutic regimen.

DESCRIPTION
The BEXXAR therapeutic regimen (Tositumomab and Iodine I 131 Tositumomab) is an anti-neoplastic radio-immunotherapeutic monoclonal antibody-based regimen

composed of the monoclonal antibody, Tositumomab, and the radiolabeled monoclonal antibody, Iodine I 131 Tositumomab.

Tositumomab

Tositumomab is a murine IgG_{2a} lambda monoclonal antibody directed against the CD20 antigen, which is found on the surface of normal and malignant B lymphocytes. Tositumomab is produced in an antibiotic-free culture of mammalian cells and is composed of two murine gamma 2a heavy chains of 451 amino acids each and two lambda light chains of 220 amino acids each. The approximate molecular weight of Tositumomab is 150 kD.

Tositumomab is supplied as a sterile, pyrogen-free, clear to opalescent, colorless to slightly yellow, preservative-free liquid concentrate. It is supplied at a nominal concentration of 14 mg/mL Tositumomab in 35 mg and 225 mg single-use vials. The formulation contains 10% (w/v) maltose, 145 mM sodium chloride, 10 mM phosphate, and Water for Injection, USP. The pH is approximately 7.2.

Iodine I 131 Tositumomab

Iodine I 131 Tositumomab is a radio-iodinated derivative of Tositumomab that has been covalently linked to Iodine-131. Unbound radio-iodine and other reactants have been removed by chromatographic purification steps. Iodine I 131 Tositumomab is supplied as a sterile, clear, preservative-free liquid for IV administration. The dosimetric dosage form is supplied at nominal protein and activity concentrations of 0.1 mg/mL and 0.61 mCi/mL (at date of calibration), respectively. The therapeutic dosage form is supplied at nominal protein and activity concentrations of 1.1 mg/mL and 5.6 mCi/mL (at date of calibration), respectively. The formulation for the dosimetric and the therapeutic dosage forms contains 4.4%-6.6% (w/v) povidone, 1-2 mg/mL maltose (dosimetric dose) or 9-15 mg/mL maltose (therapeutic dose), 0.85-0.95 mg/mL sodium chloride, and 0.9-1.3 mg/mL ascorbic acid. The pH is approximately 7.0.

BEXXAR Therapeutic Regimen

The BEXXAR therapeutic regimen is administered in two discrete steps: the dosimetric and therapeutic steps. Each step consists of a sequential infusion of Tositumomab followed by Iodine I 131 Tositumomab. The therapeutic step is administered 7–14 days after the dosimetric step. The BEXXAR therapeutic regimen is supplied in two distinct package configurations as follows:

BEXXAR Dosimetric Packaging

• A carton containing two single-use 225 mg vials and one single-use 35 mg vial of Tositumomab supplied by McKesson BioServices and
• A package containing a single-use vial of Iodine I 131 Tositumomab (0.61 mCi/mL at calibration), supplied by MDS Nordion.

BEXXAR Therapeutic Packaging

• A carton containing two single-use 225 mg vials and one single-use 35 mg vial of Tositumomab, supplied by McKesson BioServices and
• A package containing one or two single-use vials of Iodine I 131 Tositumomab (5.6 mCi/mL at calibration), supplied by MDS Nordion.

Physical/Radiochemical Characteristics of Iodine-131

Iodine-131 decays with beta and gamma emissions with a physical half-life of 8.04 days. The principal beta emission has a mean energy of 191.6 keV and the principal gamma emission has an energy of 364.5 keV (Ref 1).

External Radiation: The specific gamma ray constant for Iodine-131 is 2.2 R/millicurie hour at 1 cm. The first half-value layer is 0.24 cm lead (Pb) shielding. A range of values is shown in Table 1 for the relative attenuation of the radiation emitted by this radionuclide that results from interposition of various thicknesses of Pb. To facilitate control of the radiation exposure from this radionuclide, the use of a 2.55 cm thickness of Pb will attenuate the radiation emitted by a factor of about 1,000.

Table 1
Radiation Attenuation by Lead Shielding

Shield Thickness (Pb) cm	Attenuation Factor
0.24	0.5
0.89	10^{-1}
1.60	10^{-2}
2.55	10^{-3}
3.7	10^{-4}

The fraction of Iodine-131 radioactivity that remains in the vial after the date of calibration is calculated as follows: Fraction of remaining radioactivity of Iodine-131 after x days = $2^{-(x/8.04)}$. Physical decay is presented in Table 2.

Table 2
Physical Decay Chart: Iodine-131: Half-Life 8.04 Days

Days	Fraction Remaining
0*	1.000
1	0.917
2	0.842
3	0.772
4	0.708
5	0.650
6	0.596
7	0.547
8	0.502
9	0.460
10	0.422
11	0.387
12	0.355
13	0.326
14	0.299

* (Calibration day)

CLINICAL PHARMACOLOGY

General Pharmacology

Tositumomab binds specifically to the CD20 (human B-lymphocyte–restricted differentiation antigen, Bp 35 or B1) antigen. This antigen is a transmembrane phosphoprotein expressed on pre-B lymphocytes and at higher density on mature B lymphocytes (Ref. 2). The antigen is also expressed on >90% of B-cell non-Hodgkin's lymphomas (NHL) (Ref. 3). The recognition epitope for Tositumomab is found within the extracellular domain of the CD20 antigen. CD20 does not shed from the cell surface and does not internalize following antibody binding (Ref. 4).

Mechanism of Action: Possible mechanisms of action of the BEXXAR therapeutic regimen include induction of apoptosis (Ref. 5), complement-dependent cytotoxicity (CDC) (Ref. 6), and antibody-dependent cellular cytotoxicity (ADCC) (Ref. 5) mediated by the antibody. Additionally, cell death is associated with ionizing radiation from the radioisotope.

Pharmacokinetics/Pharmacodynamics

The phase 1 study of Iodine I 131 Tositumomab determined that a 475 mg predose of unlabeled antibody decreased splenic targeting and increased the terminal half-life of the radiolabeled antibody. The median blood clearance following administration of 485 mg of Tositumomab in 110 patients with NHL was 68.2 mg/hr (range: 30.2–260.8 mg/hr). Patients with high tumor burden, splenomegaly, or bone marrow involvement were noted to have a faster clearance, shorter terminal half-life, and larger volume of distribution. The total body clearance, as measured by total body gamma camera counts, was dependent on the same factors noted for blood clearance. Patient-specific dosing, based on total body clearance, provided a consistent radiation dose, despite variable pharmacokinetics, by allowing each patient's administered activity to be adjusted for individual patient variables. The median total body effective half-life, as measured by total body gamma camera counts, in 980 patients with NHL was 67 hours (range: 28-115 hours).

Elimination of Iodine-131 occurs by decay (see Table 2) and excretion in the urine. Urine was collected for 49 dosimetric doses. After 5 days, the whole body clearance was 67% of the injected dose. Ninety-eight percent of the clearance was accounted for in the urine.

Administration of the BEXXAR therapeutic regimen results in sustained depletion of circulating CD20 positive cells. The impact of administration of the BEXXAR therapeutic regimen on circulating CD20 positive cells was assessed in two clinical studies, one conducted in chemotherapy naïve patients and one in heavily pretreated patients. The assessment of circulating lymphocytes did not distinguish normal from malignant cells. Consequently, assessment of recovery of normal B cell function was not directly assessed. At seven weeks, the median number of circulating CD20 positive cells was zero (range: 0-490 cells/mm³). Lymphocyte recovery began at approximately 12 weeks following treatment. Among patients who had CD20 positive cell counts recorded at baseline and at 6 months, 8 of 58 (14%) chemotherapy naïve patients had CD20 positive cell counts below normal limits at six months and 6 of 19 (32%) heavily pretreated patients had CD20 positive cell counts below normal limits at six months. There was no consistent effect of the BEXXAR therapeutic regimen on post-treatment serum IgG, IgA, or IgM levels.

Radiation Dosimetry

Estimations of radiation-absorbed doses for Iodine I 131 Tositumomab were performed using sequential whole body images and the MIRDOSE 3 software program. Patients with apparent thyroid, stomach, or intestinal imaging were selected for organ dosimetry analyses. The estimated radiation-absorbed doses to organs and marrow from a course of the BEXXAR therapeutic regimen are presented in Table 3.

Table 3
Estimated Radiation-Absorbed Organ Doses

From Organ ROIs	BEXXAR mGy/MBq Median	BEXXAR mGy/MBq Range
Thyroid	2.71	1.4 - 6.2
Kidneys	1.96	1.5 - 2.5
ULI Wall	1.34	0.8 - 1.7
LLI Wall	1.30	0.8 - 1.6
Heart Wall	1.25	0.5 - 1.8
Spleen	1.14	0.7 - 5.4
Testes	0.83	0.3 - 1.3
Liver	0.82	0.6 - 1.3
Lungs	0.79	0.5 - 1.1
Red Marrow	0.65	0.5 - 1.1
Stomach Wall	0.40	0.2 - 0.8
From Whole Body ROIs		
Urine Bladder Wall	0.64	0.6 - 0.9
Bone Surfaces	0.41	0.4 - 0.6
Pancreas	0.31	0.2 - 0.4
Gall Bladder Wall	0.29	0.2 - 0.3
Adrenals	0.28	0.2 - 0.3
Ovaries	0.25	0.2 - 0.3
Small Intestine	0.23	0.2 - 0.3
Thymus	0.22	0.1 - 0.3
Uterus	0.20	0.2 - 0.2
Muscle	0.18	0.1 - 0.2
Breasts	0.16	0.1 - 0.2
Skin	0.13	0.1 - 0.2
Brain	0.13	0.1 - 0.2
Total Body	0.24	0.2 - 0.3

CLINICAL STUDIES

The efficacy of the BEXXAR therapeutic regimen was evaluated in 2 studies conducted in patients with low-grade, transformed low-grade, or follicular large-cell lymphoma. Determination of clinical benefit of the BEXXAR therapeutic regimen was based on evidence of durable responses without evidence of an effect on survival. All patients had received prior treatment without an objective response or had progression of disease following treatment. Patients were required to have a granulocyte count >1500 cells/mm³, a platelet count ≥100,000/mm³, an average of ≤25% of the intratrabecular marrow space involved by lymphoma, and no evidence of progressive disease arising in a field irradiated with >3500 cGy within 1 year of completion of irradiation.

Study 1 was a multicenter, single-arm study of 40 patients whose disease had not responded to or had progressed after at least four doses of Rituximab therapy. The median age was 57 (range: 35-78); the median time from diagnosis to protocol entry was 50 months (range: 12-170); and the median number of prior chemotherapy regimens was 4 (range: 1-11). The efficacy outcome data from this study, as determined by an independent panel that reviewed patient records and radiologic studies, are summarized in Table 4. Among the forty patients in the study, twenty-four patients had disease that did not respond to their last treatment with Rituximab, 11 patients had disease that responded to Rituximab for less than 6 months, and five patients had disease that responded to Rituximab, with a duration of response of 6 months or greater. Overall, 35 of the 40 patients met the definition of "Rituximab refractory", defined as no response or a response of less than 6 months duration. In this subset of patients the overall objective response was 63% (95% confidence interval 45%, 79%) with a median duration of 25 months (range of 4-38+ months). The complete response in this subset of patients was 29% (95% CI of 15%, 46%) with a median duration of response not yet reached (range of 4-38+ months).

Study 2 was a multicenter, single arm, open-label study of 60 chemotherapy refractory patients. The median age was 60 (range 38-82), the median time from diagnosis to protocol entry was 53 months (range: 9-334), and the median number of prior chemotherapy regimens was 4 (range 2-13). Fifty-three patients had not responded to prior therapy and 7 patients had responded with a duration of response of <6 months. The efficacy outcome data from this study, as determined by an independent panel that reviewed patient records and radiologic studies are also summarized in Table 4. Investigators continued to follow eight patients with complete response after the last independent review panel assessment. The updated duration of ongoing response as per investigators was reported to range from 42 to 85 months.

Table 4: Efficacy Outcomes in BEXXAR Clinical Studies

	Study 1 (n=40)	Study 2 (n=60)
Overall Response		
Rate	68%	47%
95% CI[a]	(51%, 81%)	(34%, 60%)
Response Duration (mos)		
Median	16	12
95% CI[a]	(10, NR[b])	(7, 47)
Range	1+ to 38+	2 to 47
Complete Response[c]		
Rate	33%	20%
95% CI[a]	(19%, 49%)	(11%, 32%)
Complete response[c] duration (mos)		
Median	NR[b]	47
95% CI[a]	(15, NR)	(47, NR)
Range	4 to 38+	9 to 47

[a] CI = Confidence Interval
[b] NR = Not reached, Median duration of follow up: Study 1 = 26 months; Study 2 = 30 months
[c] Complete response rate = Pathologic and clinical complete responses

The results of these studies were supported by demonstration of durable objective responses in three single-arm studies. In these studies, 130 patients with Rituximab-naïve follicular non-Hodgkin's lymphoma with or without transformation were evaluated for efficacy. All patients had relapsed following, or were refractory to, chemotherapy. The overall response rates ranged from 49% to 64% and the median durations of response ranged from 13 to 16 months.

Continued on next page

Bexxar—Cont.

Due to small sample sizes in the supportive studies, as in studies 1 and 2, the 95% confidence intervals for the median durations of response are wide.

INDICATIONS AND USAGE

The BEXXAR therapeutic regimen (Tositumomab and Iodine I 131 Tositumomab) is indicated for the treatment of patients with CD20 antigen-expressing relapsed or refractory, low grade, follicular, or transformed non-Hodgkin's lymphoma, including patients with Rituximab-refractory non-Hodgkin's lymphoma. Determination of the effectiveness of the BEXXAR therapeutic regimen is based on overall response rates in patients whose disease is refractory to chemotherapy alone or to chemotherapy and Rituximab. The effects of the BEXXAR therapeutic regimen on survival are not known.

The BEXXAR therapeutic regimen is not indicated for the initial treatment of patients with CD20 positive non-Hodgkin's lymphoma. (see **ADVERSE REACTIONS, Immunogenicity**)

The BEXXAR therapeutic regimen is intended as a single course of treatment. The safety of multiple courses of the BEXXAR therapeutic regimen, or combination of this regimen with other forms of irradiation or chemotherapy, has not been evaluated.

CONTRAINDICATIONS

The BEXXAR therapeutic regimen is contraindicated in patients with known hypersensitivity to murine proteins or any other component of the BEXXAR therapeutic regimen.

PREGNANCY CATEGORY X

Iodine I 131 Tositumomab (a component of the BEXXAR therapeutic regimen) is contraindicated for use in women who are pregnant. Iodine-131 may cause harm to the fetal thyroid gland when administered to pregnant women. Review of the literature has shown that transplacental passage of radioiodide may cause severe, and possibly irreversible, hypothyroidism in neonates. While there are no adequate and well-controlled studies of the BEXXAR therapeutic regimen in pregnant animals or humans, use of the BEXXAR therapeutic regimen in women of childbearing age should be deferred until the possibility of pregnancy has been ruled out. If the patient becomes pregnant while being treated with the BEXXAR therapeutic regimen, the patient should be apprised of the potential hazard to the fetus (see **BOXED WARNING, Pregnancy Category X**).

WARNINGS

Prolonged and Severe Cytopenias (see BOXED WARNINGS; ADVERSE REACTIONS, Hematologic Events): The most common adverse reactions associated with the BEXXAR therapeutic regimen were severe or life-threatening cytopenias (NCI CTC grade 3 or 4) with 71% of the 230 patients enrolled in clinical studies experiencing grade 3 or 4 cytopenias. These consisted primarily of grade 3 or 4 thrombocytopenia (53%) and grade 3 or 4 neutropenia (63%). The time to nadir was 4 to 7 weeks and the duration of cytopenias was approximately 30 days. Thrombocytopenia, neutropenia, and anemia persisted for more than 90 days following administration of the BEXXAR therapeutic regimen in 16 (7%), 15 (7%), and 12 (5%) patients respectively (this includes patients with transient recovery followed by recurrent cytopenia). Due to the variable nature in the onset of cytopenias, complete blood counts should be obtained weekly for 10-12 weeks. The sequelae of severe cytopenias were commonly observed in the clinical studies and included infections (45% of patients), hemorrhage (12%), a requirement for growth factors (12% G- or GM-CSF; 7% Epoetin alfa) and blood product support (15% platelet transfusions; 16% red blood cell transfusions). Prolonged cytopenias may also influence subsequent treatment decisions.

The safety of the BEXXAR therapeutic regimen has not been established in patients with >25% lymphoma marrow involvement, platelet count <100,000 cells/mm^3 or neutrophil count <1,500 cells/mm^3.

Hypersensitivity Reactions Including Anaphylaxis (see BOXED WARNINGS; ADVERSE REACTIONS, Hypersensitivity Reactions and Immunogenicity): Serious hypersensitivity reactions, including some with fatal outcome, were reported during and following administration of the BEXXAR therapeutic regimen. Emergency supplies including medications for the treatment of hypersensitivity reactions, e.g., epinephrine, antihistamines and corticosteroids, should be available for immediate use in the event of an allergic reaction during administration of the BEXXAR therapeutic regimen. Patients who have received murine proteins should be screened for human anti-mouse antibodies (HAMA). Patients who are positive for HAMA may be at increased risk of anaphylaxis and serious hypersensitivity reactions during administration of the BEXXAR therapeutic regimen.

Secondary Malignancies: Myelodysplastic syndrome (MDS) and/or acute leukemia were reported in 10% (24/230) of patients enrolled in the clinical studies and 3% (20/765) of patients included in expanded access programs, with median follow-up of 39 and 27 months, respectively. Among the 44 reported cases, the median time to development of MDS/leukemia was 31 months following treatment; however, the cumulative rate continues to increase.

Additional non-hematological malignancies were also reported in 54 of the 995 patients enrolled in clinical studies or included in the expanded access program. Approximately half of these were non-melanomatous skin cancers. The remainder, which occurred in 2 or more patients, included colorectal cancer (7), head and neck cancer (6), breast cancer (5), lung cancer (4), bladder cancer (4), melanoma (3), and gastric cancer (2). The relative risk of developing secondary malignancies in patients receiving the BEXXAR therapeutic regimen over the background rate in this population cannot be determined, due to the absence of controlled studies (see **ADVERSE REACTIONS**).

Pregnancy Category X: (see **BOXED WARNINGS; CONTRAINDICATIONS**).

Hypothyroidism: Administration of the BEXXAR therapeutic regimen may result in hypothyroidism (see **ADVERSE REACTIONS, Hypothyroidism**). Thyroid-blocking medications should be initiated at least 24 hours before receiving the dosimetric dose and continued until 14 days after the therapeutic dose (see **DOSAGE and ADMINISTRATION**). All patients must receive thyroid-blocking agents; any patient who is unable to tolerate thyroid-blocking agents should not receive the BEXXAR therapeutic regimen. Patients should be evaluated for signs and symptoms of hypothyroidism and screened for biochemical evidence of hypothyroidism annually.

PRECAUTIONS

Radionuclide Precautions: Iodine I 131 Tositumomab is radioactive. Care should be taken, consistent with the institutional radiation safety practices and applicable federal guidelines, to minimize exposure of medical personnel and other patients.

Renal Function: Iodine I 131 Tositumomab and Iodine-131 are excreted primarily by the kidneys. Impaired renal function may decrease the rate of excretion of the radiolabeled iodine and increase patient exposure to the radioactive component of the BEXXAR therapeutic regimen. There are no data regarding the safety of administration of the BEXXAR therapeutic regimen in patients with impaired renal function.

Immunization: The safety of immunization with live viral vaccines following administration of the BEXXAR therapeutic regimen has not been studied. The ability of patients who have received the BEXXAR therapeutic regimen to generate a primary or anamnestic humoral response to any vaccine has not been studied.

Information for Patients: Prior to administration of the BEXXAR therapeutic regimen, patients should be advised that they will have a radioactive material in their body for several days upon their release from the hospital or clinic. After discharge, patients should be provided with both oral and written instructions for minimizing exposure of family members, friends and the general public. Patients should be given a copy of the written instructions for use as a reference for the recommended precautionary actions.

The pregnancy status of women of childbearing potential should be assessed and these women should be advised of the potential risks to the fetus (see **CONTRAINDICATIONS**). Women who are breastfeeding should be instructed to discontinue breastfeeding and should be apprised of the resultant potential harmful effects to the infant if these instructions are not followed.

Patients should be advised of the potential risk of toxic effects on the male and female gonads following the BEXXAR therapeutic regimen, and be instructed to use effective contraceptive methods during treatment and for 12 months following the administration of the BEXXAR therapeutic regimen.

Patients should be informed of the risks of hypothyroidism and be advised of the importance of compliance with thyroid blocking agents and need for life-long monitoring.

Patients should be informed of the possibility of developing a HAMA immune response and that HAMA may affect the results of *in vitro* and *in vivo* diagnostic tests as well as results of therapies that rely on murine antibody technology.

Patients should be informed of the risks of cytopenias and symptoms associated with cytopenia, the need for frequent monitoring for up to 12 weeks after treatment, and the potential for persistent cytopenias beyond 12 weeks.

Patients should be informed that MDS, secondary leukemia, and solid tumors have also been observed in patients receiving the BEXXAR therapeutic regimen.

Due to lack of controlled clinical studies, and high background incidence in the heavily pretreated patient population, the relative risk of development of myelodysplastic syndrome/acute leukemia and solid tumors due to the BEXXAR therapeutic regimen cannot be determined.

Laboratory Monitoring: A complete blood count (CBC) with differential and platelet count should be obtained prior to, and at least weekly following administration of the BEXXAR therapeutic regimen. Weekly monitoring of blood counts should continue for a minimum of 10 weeks or, if persistent, until severe cytopenias have completely resolved. More frequent monitoring is indicated in patients with evidence of moderate or more severe cytopenias (see **BOXED WARNINGS** and **WARNINGS**). Thyroid stimulating hormone (TSH) level should be monitored before treatment and annually thereafter. Serum creatinine levels should be measured immediately prior to administration of the BEXXAR therapeutic regimen.

Drug Interactions: No formal drug interaction studies have been performed. Due to the frequent occurrence of severe and prolonged thrombocytopenia, the potential benefits of medications that interfere with platelet function and/or anticoagulation should be weighed against the potential increased risk of bleeding and hemorrhage.

Drug/Laboratory Test Interactions: Administration of the BEXXAR therapeutic regimen may result in the development of human anti-murine antibodies (HAMA). The presence of HAMA may affect the accuracy of the results of *in vitro* and *in vivo* diagnostic tests and may affect the toxicity profile and efficacy of therapeutic agents that rely on murine antibody technology. Patients who are HAMA positive may be at increased risk for serious allergic reactions and other side effects if they undergo *in vivo* diagnostic testing or treatment with murine monoclonal antibodies.

Carcinogenesis, Mutagenesis, Impairment of Fertility: No long-term animal studies have been performed to establish the carcinogenic or mutagenic potential of the BEXXAR therapeutic regimen or to determine its effects on fertility in males or females. However, radiation is a potential carcinogen and mutagen. Administration of the BEXXAR therapeutic regimen results in delivery of a significant radiation dose to the testes. The radiation dose to the ovaries has not been established. There have been no studies to evaluate whether administration of the BEXXAR therapeutic regimen causes hypogonadism, premature menopause, azoospermia and/or mutagenic alterations to germ cells. There is a potential risk that the BEXXAR therapeutic regimen may cause toxic effects on the male and female gonads. Effective contraceptive methods should be used during treatment and for 12 months following administration of the BEXXAR therapeutic regimen.

Pregnancy Category X: (see CONTRAINDICATIONS; WARNINGS).

Nursing Mothers: Radioiodine is excreted in breast milk and may reach concentrations equal to or greater than maternal plasma concentrations. Immunoglobulins are also known to be excreted in breast milk. The absorption potential and potential for adverse effects of the monoclonal antibody component (Tositumomab) in the infant are not known. Therefore, formula feedings should be substituted for breast feedings before starting treatment. Women should be advised to discontinue nursing.

Pediatric Use: The safety and effectiveness of the BEXXAR therapeutic regimen in children have not been established.

Geriatric Use: Clinical studies of the BEXXAR therapeutic regimen did not include sufficient numbers of patients aged 65 and over to determine whether they respond differently from younger patients. In clinical studies, 230 patients received the BEXXAR therapeutic regimen at the recommended dose. Of these, 27% (61 patients) were age 65 or older and 4% (10 patients) were age 75 or older. Across all studies, the overall response rate was lower in patients age 65 and over (41% vs. 61%) and the duration of responses was shorter (10 months vs. 16 months); however, these findings are primarily derived from 2 of the 5 studies. While the incidence of severe hematologic toxicity was lower, the duration of severe hematologic toxicity was longer in those age 65 or older as compared to patients less than 65 years of age. Due to the limited experience greater sensitivity of some older individuals cannot be ruled out.

ADVERSE REACTIONS

The most serious adverse reactions observed in the clinical trials were severe and prolonged cytopenias and the sequelae of cytopenias which included infections (sepsis) and hemorrhage in thrombocytopenic patients, allergic reactions (bronchospasm and angioedema), secondary leukemia and myelodysplasia (see **BOXED WARNINGS** and **WARNINGS**).

The most common adverse reactions occurring in the clinical trials included neutropenia, thrombocytopenia, and anemia that are both prolonged and severe. Less common but severe adverse reactions included pneumonia, pleural effusion and dehydration.

Data regarding adverse events were primarily obtained in 230 patients with non-Hodgkin's lymphoma enrolled in five clinical trials using the recommended dose and schedule. Patients had a median follow-up of 39 months and 79% of the patients were followed at least 12 months for survival and selected adverse events. Patients had a median of 3 prior chemotherapy regimens, a median age of 55 years, 60% male, 27% had transformation to a higher grade histology, 29% were intermediate grade and 2% high grade histology (IWF) and 68% had Ann Arbor stage IV disease. Patients enrolled in these studies were not permitted to have prior hematopoietic stem cell transplantation or irradiation to more than 25% of the red marrow. In the expanded access program, which included 765 patients, data regarding clinical serious adverse events and HAMA and TSH levels were used to supplement the characterization of delayed adverse events (see **ADVERSE REACTIONS, Hypothyroidism, Secondary Leukemia and Myelodysplastic Syndrome, Immunogenicity**).

Because clinical trials are conducted under widely varying conditions, adverse reaction rates observed in the clinical trials of a drug cannot be directly compared to rates in the clinical trials of another drug and may not reflect the rates observed in practice. The adverse reaction information from clinical trials does, however, provide a basis for identifying the adverse events that appear to be related to drug use and for approximating rates.

Hematologic Events: Hematologic toxicity was the most frequently observed adverse event in clinical trials with the BEXXAR therapeutic regimen (Table 6). Sixty-three (27%) of 230 patients received one or more hematologic supportive care measures following the therapeutic dose: 12% received G-CSF; 7% received Epoetin alfa; 15% received platelet transfusions; and 16% received packed red blood cell transfusions. Twenty-eight (12%) patients experienced hemorrhagic events; the majority were mild to moderate.

Infectious Events: One hundred and four of the 230 (45%) patients experienced one or more adverse events possibly related to infection. The majority were viral (e.g. rhinitis, pharyngitis, flu symptoms, or herpes) or other minor infections. Twenty of 230 (9%) patients experienced infections that were considered serious because the patient was hospitalized to manage the infection. Documented infections included pneumonia, bacteremia, septicemia, bronchitis, and skin infections.

Hypersensitivity Reactions: Fourteen patients (6%) experienced one or more of the following adverse events: allergic reaction, face edema, injection site hypersensitivity, anaphylactic reaction, laryngismus, and serum sickness. In the post-marketing setting, severe hypersensitivity reactions, including fatal anaphylaxis have been reported.

Gastrointestinal Toxicity: Eighty-seven patients (38%) experienced one or more gastrointestinal adverse events, including nausea, emesis, abdominal pain, and diarrhea. These events were temporally related to the infusion of the antibody. Nausea, vomiting, and abdominal pain were often reported within days of infusion, whereas diarrhea was generally reported days to weeks after infusion.

Infusional Toxicity: A constellation of symptoms, including fever, rigors or chills, sweating, hypotension, dyspnea, bronchospasm, and nausea, have been reported during or within 48 hours of infusion. Sixty-seven patients (29%) reported fever, rigors/chills, or sweating within 14 days following the dosimetric dose. Although all patients in the clinical studies received pretreatment with acetaminophen and an antihistamine, the value of premedication in preventing infusion-related toxicity was not evaluated in any of the clinical studies. Infusional toxicities were managed by slowing and/or temporarily interrupting the infusion. Symptomatic management was required in more severe cases. Adjustment of the rate of infusion to control adverse reactions occurred in 16 patients (7%); seven patients required adjustments for only the dosimetric infusion, two required adjustments for only the therapeutic infusion, and seven required adjustments for both the dosimetric and the therapeutic infusions. Adjustments included reduction in the rate of infusion by 50%, temporary interruption of the infusion, and in 2 patients, infusion was permanently discontinued.

Table 5 lists clinical adverse events that occurred in ≥5% of patients. Table 6 provides a detailed description of the hematologic toxicity.

Table 5
Incidence of Clinical Adverse Experiences Regardless of Relationship to Study Drug Occurring in ≥5% of the Patients Treated with BEXXAR Therapeutic Regimen[a] (N = 230)

Body System Preferred Term	All Grades	Grade 3/4
Total	**(96%)**	**(48%)**
Non-Hematologic AEs		
Body as a Whole	81%	12%
Asthenia	46%	2%
Fever	37%	2%
Infection[b]	21%	<1%
Pain	19%	1%
Chills	18%	1%
Headache	16%	0%
Abdominal pain	15%	3%
Back pain	8%	1%
Chest pain	7%	0%
Neck pain	6%	1%
Cardiovascular System	26%	3%
Hypotension	7%	1%
Vasodilatation	5%	0%
Digestive System	56%	9%
Nausea	36%	3%
Vomiting	15%	1%
Anorexia	14%	0%
Diarrhea	12%	0%
Constipation	6%	1%
Dyspepsia	6%	<1%
Endocrine System	7%	0%
Hypothyroidism	7%	0%
Metabolic and Nutritional Disorders	21%	3%
Peripheral edema	9%	0%
Weight loss	6%	<1%
Musculoskeletal System	23%	3%
Myalgia	13%	<1%
Arthralgia	10%	1%
Nervous System	26%	3%
Dizziness	5%	0%
Somnolence	5%	0%
Respiratory System	44%	8%
Cough increased	21%	1%
Pharyngitis	12%	0%
Dyspnea	11%	3%
Rhinitis	10%	0%
Pneumonia	6%	0%
Skin and Appendages	44%	5%
Rash	17%	<1%
Pruritus	10%	0%
Sweating	8%	<1%

[a] Excludes laboratory derived hematologic adverse events (see Table 6).

[b] The COSTART term for infection includes a subset of infections (e.g., upper respiratory infection). Other terms are mapped to preferred terms (e.g., pneumonia and sepsis). For a more inclusive summary see ADVERSE REACTIONS, Infectious Events.

Table 6
Hematologic Toxicity[a] (N=230)

Endpoint	Values
Platelets	
Median nadir (cells/mm^3)	43,000
Per patient incidence[a] platelets <50,000/mm^3	53% (n=123)
Median[b] duration of platelets <50,000/mm^3 (days)	32
Grade 3/4 without recovery to Grade 2, N (%)	16 (7%)
Per patient incidence[c] platelets <25,000/mm^3	21% (n=47)
ANC	
Median nadir (cells/mm^3)	690
Per patient incidence[a] ANC<1,000 cells/mm^3	63% (n=145)
Median[b] duration of ANC<1,000 cells/mm^3 (days)	31
Grade 3/4 without recovery to Grade 2, N (%)	15 (7%)
Per patient incidence[c] ANC<500 cells/mm^3	25% (n=57)
Hemoglobin	
Median nadir (gm/dL)	10
Per patient incidence[a] <8 gm/dL	29% (n=66)
Median[b] duration of hemoglobin <8.0 gm/dL (days)	23
Grade 3/4 without recovery to Grade 2, N (%)	12 (5%)
Per patient incidence[c] hemoglobin <6.5 gm/dL	5% (n=11)

[a] Grade 3/4 toxicity was assumed if patient was missing 2 or more weeks of hematology data between Week 5 and Week 9.
[b] Duration of Grade 3/4 of 1000+ days (censored) was assumed for those patients with undocumented Grade 3/4 and no hematologic data on or after Week 9.
[c] Grade 4 toxicity was assumed if patient had documented Grade 3 toxicity and was missing 2 or more weeks of hematology data between Week 5 and Week 9.

[See table 6 above]

Delayed Adverse Reactions

Delayed adverse reactions, including hypothyroidism, HAMA, and myelodysplasia/leukemia, were assessed in 230 patients included in clinical studies and 765 patients included in expanded access programs. The entry characteristics of patients included from the expanded access programs were similar to the characteristics of patients enrolled in the clinical studies, except that the median number of prior chemotherapy regimens was fewer (2 vs. 3) and the proportion with low-grade histology was higher (77% vs. 70%) in patients from the expanded access programs.

Secondary Leukemia and Myelodysplastic Syndrome (MDS): There were 44 cases of MDS/secondary leukemia reported among 995 (4.0%) patients included in clinical studies and expanded access programs, with a median follow-up of 29 months. The overall incidence of MDS/secondary leukemia among the 230 patients included in the clinical studies was 10% (24/230), with a median follow-up of 39 months and a median time to development of MDS of 34 months. The cumulative incidence of MDS/secondary leukemia in this patient population was 4.7% at 2 years and 15% at 5 years. The incidence of MDS/secondary leukemia among the 765 patients in the expanded access programs was 3% (20/765), with a median follow-up of 27 months and a median time to development of MDS of 31 months. The cumulative incidence of MDS/secondary leukemia in this patient population was 1.6% at 2 years and 6% at 5 years.

Secondary Malignancies: Of the 995 patients in clinical studies and the expanded access programs, there were 65 reports of second malignancies in 54 patients, excluding secondary leukemias. The most common included non-melanomatous skin cancers (26), colorectal cancer (7), head and neck cancer (6), breast cancer (5), lung cancer (4), bladder cancer (4), melanoma (3), and gastric cancer (2). Some of these events included recurrence of an earlier diagnosis of cancer.

Hypothyroidism: Of the 230 patients in the clinical studies, 203 patients did not have elevated TSH upon study entry. Of these, 137 patients had at least one post-treatment TSH value available and were not taking thyroid hormonal treatment upon study entry. With a median follow up period of 46 months, the incidence of hypothyroidism based on elevated TSH or initiation of thyroid replacement therapy in these patients was 18% with a median time to development of hypothyroidism of 16 months. The cumulative incidences of hypothyroidism at 2 and 5 years in these 137 patients were 11% and 19% respectively. New events have been observed up to 90 months post treatment.

Of the 765 patients in the expanded access programs, 670 patients did not have elevated TSH upon study entry. Of these, 455 patients had at least one post-treatment TSH value available and were not taking thyroid hormonal treatment upon study entry. With a median follow up period of 33 months, the incidence of hypothyroidism based on elevated TSH or initiation of thyroid replacement therapy in these 455 patients was 13% with a median time to development of hypothyroidism of 15 months. The cumulative incidences of hypothyroidism at 2 and 5 years in these patients were 9% and 17%, respectively.

Immunogenicity: One percent (11/989) of the chemotherapy-relapsed or refractory patients included in the clinical studies or the expanded access program had a positive serology for HAMA prior to treatment and six patients had no baseline assessment for HAMA. Of the 230 patients in the clinical studies, 220 patients were seronegative for HAMA prior to treatment, and 219 had at least one post-treatment HAMA value obtained. With a median observation period of 6 months, a total of 23 patients (11%) became seropositive for HAMA post-treatment. The median time of HAMA development was 6 months. The cumulative incidences of HAMA seropositivity at 6 months, 12 months, and 18 months were 6%, 17% and 21% respectively.

Of the 765 patients in the expanded access programs, 758 patients were seronegative for HAMA prior to treatment, and 569 patients had at least one post-treatment HAMA value obtained. With a median observation period of 7 months, a total of 57 patients (10%) became seropositive for HAMA post-treatment. The median time of HAMA development was 5 months. The cumulative incidences of HAMA seropositivity at 6 months, 12 months, and 18 months were 7%, 12% and 13%, respectively.

In a study of 76 previously untreated patients with low-grade non-Hodgkin's lymphoma who received the BEXXAR therapeutic regimen, the incidence of conversion to HAMA seropositivity was 70%, with a median time to development of HAMA of 27 days.

The data reflect the percentage of patients whose test results were considered positive for HAMA in an ELISA assay that detects antibodies to the Fc portion of IgG_1 murine immunoglobulin and are highly dependent on the sensitivity and specificity of the assay. Additionally, the observed incidence of antibody positivity in an assay may be influenced by several factors including sample handling, concomitant medications, and underlying disease. For these reasons, comparison of the incidence of HAMA in patients treated with the BEXXAR therapeutic regimen with the incidence of HAMA in patients treated with other products may be misleading.

OVERDOSAGE

The maximum dose of the BEXXAR therapeutic regimen that was administered in clinical trials was 88 cGy. Three patients were treated with a total body dose of 85 cGy of Iodine I 131 Tositumomab in a dose escalation study. Two of the 3 patients developed Grade 4 toxicity of 5 weeks duration with subsequent recovery. In addition, accidental overdose of the BEXXAR therapeutic regimen occurred in one patient at a total body dose of 88 cGy. The patient developed Grade 3 hematologic toxicity of 18 days duration. Patients who receive an accidental overdose of Iodine I 131 Tositumomab should be monitored closely for cytopenias and radiation-related toxicity. The effectiveness of hematopoietic stem cell transplantation as a supportive care measure for marrow injury has not been studied; however, the timing of such support should take into account the pharmacokinetics of the BEXXAR therapeutic regimen and decay rate of the Iodine-131 in order to minimize the possibility of irradiation of infused hematopoietic stem cells.

DOSAGE AND ADMINISTRATION

Recommended Dose

The BEXXAR therapeutic regimen consists of four components administered in two discrete steps: the dosimetric step, followed 7-14 days later by a therapeutic step.

Note: the safety of the BEXXAR therapeutic regimen was established only in the setting of patients receiving thyroid blocking agents and premedication to ameliorate/prevent infusion reactions (see **Concomitant Medications**).

Dosimetric step

- Tositumomab 450 mg intravenously in 50 ml 0.9% Sodium Chloride over 60 minutes. Reduce the rate of infusion by 50% for mild to moderate infusional toxicity; interrupt infusion for severe infusional toxicity. After complete resolution of severe infusional toxicity, infusion may be resumed with a 50% reduction in the rate of infusion.
- Iodine I 131 Tositumomab (containing 5.0 mCi Iodine-131 and 35 mg Tositumomab) intravenously in 30 ml 0.9% Sodium Chloride over 20 minutes. Reduce the rate of infusion by 50% for mild to moderate infusional toxicity; interrupt infusion for severe infusional toxicity. After complete resolution of severe infusional toxicity, infusion may be resumed with a 50% reduction in the rate of infusion.

Therapeutic step

Note: Do not administer the therapeutic step if biodistribution is altered (see **Assessment of Biodistribution of Iodine I 131 Tositumomab**).

Continued on next page

Bexxar—Cont.

- Tositumomab 450 mg intravenously in 50 ml 0.9% Sodium Chloride over 60 minutes. Reduce the rate of infusion by 50% for mild to moderate infusional toxicity; interrupt infusion for severe infusional toxicity. After complete resolution of severe infusional toxicity, infusion may be resumed with a 50% reduction in the rate of infusion.
- Iodine I 131 Tositumomab (see **CALCULATION OF IODINE-131 ACTIVITY FOR THE THERAPEUTIC DOSE**). Reduce the rate of infusion by 50% for mild to moderate infusional toxicity; interrupt infusion for severe infusional toxicity. After complete resolution of severe infusional toxicity, infusion may be resumed with a 50% reduction in the rate of infusion.
  - Patients with ≥150,000 platelets/mm^3: The recommended dose is the activity of Iodine-131 calculated to deliver 75 cGy total body irradiation and 35 mg Tositumomab, administered intravenously over 20 minutes.
  - Patients with NCI Grade 1 thrombocytopenia (platelet counts ≥100,000 but <150,000 platelets/mm^3): The recommended dose is the activity of Iodine-131 calculated to deliver 65 cGy total body irradiation and 35 mg Tositumomab, administered intravenously over 20 minutes.

Concomitant Medications: The safety of the BEXXAR therapeutic regimen was established in studies in which all patients received the following concurrent medications:

- Thyroid protective agents: Saturated solution of potassium iodide (SSKI) 4 drops orally t.i.d.; Lugol's solution 20 drops orally t.i.d.; or potassium iodide tablets 130 mg orally q.d. Thyroid protective agents should be initiated at least 24 hours prior to administration of the Iodine I 131 Tositumomab dosimetric dose and continued until 2 weeks after administration of the Iodine I 131 Tositumomab therapeutic dose.

  Patients should not receive the dosimetric dose of Iodine I 131 Tositumomab if they have not yet received at least three doses of SSKI, three doses of Lugol's solution, or one dose of 130 mg potassium iodide tablet (at least 24 hours prior to the dosimetric dose).
- Acetaminophen 650 mg orally and diphenhydramine 50 mg orally 30 minutes prior to administration of Tositumomab in the dosimetric and therapeutic steps.

The BEXXAR therapeutic regimen is administered via an IV tubing set with an in-line 0.22 micron filter. **THE SAME IV TUBING SET AND FILTER MUST BE USED THROUGHOUT THE ENTIRE DOSIMETRIC OR THERAPEUTIC STEP. A CHANGE IN FILTER CAN RESULT IN LOSS OF DRUG.**
Figure 1 shows an overview of the dosing schedule.

Figure 1
Dosing Schedule

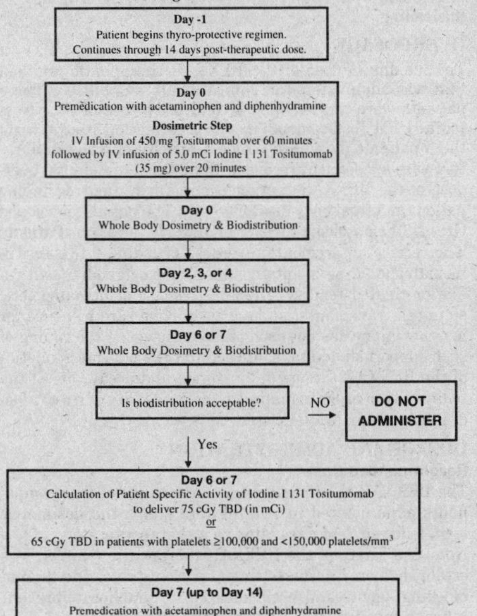

Day -1
Patient begins thyro-protective regimen.
Continues through 14 days post-therapeutic dose.
Day 0
Premedication with acetaminophen and diphenhydramine
Dosimetric Step
IV Infusion of 450 mg Tositumomab over 60 minutes followed by IV infusion of 5.0 mCi Iodine I 131 Tositumomab (35 mg) over 20 minutes
Day 0
Whole Body Dosimetry & Biodistribution
Day 2, 3, or 4
Whole Body Dosimetry & Biodistribution
Day 6 or 7
Whole Body Dosimetry & Biodistribution
Is biodistribution acceptable?
NO
DO NOT ADMINISTER
Yes
Day 6 or 7
Calculation of Patient Specific Activity of Iodine I 131 Tositumomab to deliver 75 cGy TBD (in mCi)
or
65 cGy TBD in patients with platelets ≥100,000 and <150,000 platelets/mm3
Day 7 (up to Day 14)
Premedication with acetaminophen and diphenhydramine
Therapeutic Step
IV Infusion of 450 mg Tositumomab over 60 minutes followed by prescribed therapeutic dose of Iodine I 131 Tositumomab (35 mg) over 20 minutes

PREPARATION OF THE BEXXAR THERAPEUTIC REGIMEN GENERAL

Read all directions thoroughly and assemble all materials before preparing the dose for administration.

The Iodine I 131 Tositumomab dosimetric and therapeutic doses should be measured by a suitable radioactivity calibration system immediately prior to administration. The dose calibrator must be operated in accordance with the manufacturer's specifications and quality control for the measurement of Iodine-131.

All supplies for preparation and administration of the BEXXAR therapeutic regimen should be sterile. Use appropriate aseptic technique and radiation precautions for the preparation of the components of the BEXXAR therapeutic regimen.

Waterproof gloves should be utilized in the preparation and administration of the product. Iodine I 131 Tositumomab doses should be prepared, assayed, and administered by personnel who are licensed to handle and/or administer radionuclides. Appropriate shielding should be used during preparation and administration of the product.

Restrictions on patient contact with others and release from the hospital must follow all applicable federal, state, and institutional regulations.

Preparation for the Dosimetric Step

Tositumomab Dose

Required materials not supplied:

A. One 50 mL syringe with attached 18 gauge needle (to withdraw 450 mg of Tositumomab 20 from two vials each containing 225 mg Tositumomab)
B. One 50 mL bag of sterile 0.9% Sodium Chloride for Injection, USP
C. One 50 mL syringe for drawing up 32 mL of saline for disposal from the 50 mL bag of sterile 0.9% Sodium Chloride for Injection, USP

Method:

1. Withdraw and dispose of 32 mL of saline from a 50 mL bag of sterile 0.9% Sodium Chloride for Injection, USP.
2. Withdraw the entire contents from each of the two 225 mg vials (a total of 450 mg Tositumomab in 32 mL) and transfer to the infusion bag containing 18 mL of 0.9% Sodium Chloride for Injection, USP to yield a final volume of 50 mL.
3. Gently mix the solution by inverting/rotating the bag. DO NOT SHAKE.
4. The diluted Tositumomab may be stored for up to 24 hours when stored refrigerated at 2°C-8°C (36°F-46°F) and for up to 8 hours at room temperature.

Note: Tositumomab solution may contain particulates that are generally white in nature. The product should appear clear to opalescent, colorless to slightly yellow.

Preparation of Iodine I 131 Tositumomab Dosimetric Dose

Required materials not supplied:

A. Lead shielding for preparation vial and syringe pump
B. One 30 mL syringe with 18 gauge needle to withdraw the calculated volume of Iodine I 131 Tositumomab from the Iodine I 131 Tositumomab vial. One 60 mL syringe with 18 gauge needle to withdraw the volume from the preparation vial for administration
C. One 20 mL syringe with attached needle, filled with 0.9% Sodium Chloride for Injection, USP
D. One 3 mL syringe with attached needle to withdraw Tositumomab from 35 mg vial
E. One sterile, 30 or 50 mL preparation vial
F. Two lead pots, both kept at room temperature. One pot is used to thaw the labeled antibody and the second pot is used to hold the preparation vial

Method:

1. Allow approximately 60 minutes for thawing (at ambient temperature) of the Iodine I 131 Tositumomab dosimetric vial with appropriate lead shielding.
2. Based on the activity concentration of the vial (see actual product specification sheet for the vial supplied in the dosimetric package), calculate the volume required for an Iodine I 131 Tositumomab activity of 5.0 mCi.
3. Withdraw the calculated volume from the Iodine I 131 Tositumomab vial.
4. Transfer this volume to the shielded preparation vial.
5. Assay the dose to ensure that the appropriate activity (mCi) has been prepared.
   a. If the assayed dose is 5.0 mCi (±10%) proceed with step 6.
   b. If the assayed dose does not contain 5.0 mCi (±10%) recalculate the activity concentration of the Iodine I 131 Tositumomab at this time, based on the volume and the activity in the preparation vial. Recalculate the volume required for an Iodine I 131 Tositumomab activity of 5.0 mCi. Using the same 30 mL syringe, add or subtract the appropriate volume from the Iodine I 131 Tositumomab vial so that the preparation vial contains the volume required for an Iodine I 131 Tositumomab activity of 5.0 mCi (±10%). Reassay the preparation vial and proceed with step 6.
6. Calculate the amount of Tositumomab contained in the solution of Iodine I 131 Tositumomab in the shielded preparation vial, based on the volume and protein concentration (see actual product specification sheet supplied in the dosimetric package).
7. If the shielded preparation vial contains less than 35 mg, calculate the amount of additional Tositumomab needed to yield a total of 35 mg protein. Calculate the volume needed from the 35 mg vial of Tositumomab, based on the protein concentration. Withdraw the calculated volume of Tositumomab from the 35 mg vial of Tositumomab, and transfer this volume to the shielded preparation vial. The preparation vial should now contain a total of 35 mg of Tositumomab.
8. Using the 20 mL syringe containing 0.9% Sodium Chloride for Injection, USP, add a sufficient quantity to the shielded preparation vial to yield a final volume of 30 mL. Gently mix the solutions.
9. Withdraw the entire contents from the preparation vial into a 60 mL syringe using a large bore needle (18 gauge).
10. Assay and record the activity.

Administration of the Dosimetric Step

Required materials not supplied: For questions about required materials call the BEXXAR Service Center at 1-877-423-9927.

A. IV Filter set (0.22 micron filter), 15 inch with injection site (port) and luer lock
B. One Primary IV infusion set
C. One 100 mL bag of sterile 0.9% Sodium Chloride for Injection, USP
D. Two Secondary IV infusion sets
E. One IV Extension set, 30 inch luer lock
F. One 3-way stopcock
G. One 50 mL bag of sterile 0.9% Sodium Chloride for Injection, USP
H. One Infusion pump for Tositumomab infusion
I. One Syringe Pump for Iodine I 131 Tositumomab infusion
J. Lead shielding for use in the administration of the dosimetric dose

Tositumomab Infusion:
(See Figure 1 in the **"Workbook for Dosimetry Methodology and Administration Set-Up"** for diagrammatic illustration of the configuration of the infusion set components.)

1. Attach a primary IV infusion set (Item B) to the 0.22 micron in-line filter set (Item A) and the 100 mL bag of sterile 0.9% Sodium Chloride for Injection, USP (Item C).
2. After priming the primary IV infusion set (Item B) and IV filter set (Item A), connect the infusion bag containing 450 mg Tositumomab (50 mL) via a secondary IV infusion set (Item D) to the primary IV infusion set (Item B) at a port distal to the 0.22 micron in-line filter. Infuse Tositumomab over 60 minutes.
3. After completion of the Tositumomab infusion, disconnect the secondary IV infusion set (Item D) and flush the primary IV infusion set (Item B) and the in-line IV filter set (Item A) with sterile 0.9% Sodium Chloride for Injection, USP. Discard the Tositumomab bag and secondary IV infusion set.

Iodine I 131 Tositumomab Dosimetric Infusion:
(See Figure 2 in the **"Workbook for Dosimetry Methodology and Administration Set-Up"** for diagrammatic illustration of the configuration of the infusion set components.)

1. Appropriate shielding should be used in the administration of the dosimetric dose.
2. The dosimetric dose is delivered in a 60 mL syringe.
3. Connect the extension set (Item E) to the 3-way stopcock (Item F).
4. Connect the 50 mL bag of sterile 0.9% Sodium Chloride for Injection, USP (Item G) to a secondary IV infusion set (Item D) and connect the infusion set to the 3-way stopcock (Item F). Prime the secondary IV infusion set (Item D) and the extension set (Item E). Connect the extension set (Item E) to a port in the primary IV infusion set (Item B), distal to the filter. (**Note:** You **must** use the same primary infusion set (Item B) and IV filter set (Item A) with pre-wetted filter that was used for the Tositumomab infusion. A change in filter can result in loss of up to 7% of the Iodine I 131 Tositumomab dose.)
5. Attach the syringe filled with the Iodine I 131 Tositumomab to the 3-way stopcock (Item F)
6. Set syringe pump to deliver the entire 5.0 mCi (35 mg) dose of Iodine I 131 Tositumomab over 20 minutes.
7. After completion of the infusion of Iodine I 131 Tositumomab, close the stopcock (Item F) to the syringe. Flush the extension set (Item E) and the secondary IV infusion set (Item D) with 0.9% Sodium Chloride for Injection, USP from the 50 mL bag (Item G).
8. After the flush, disconnect the extension set (Item E), 3-way stopcock (Item F) and syringe. Disconnect the primary IV infusion set (Item B) and in-line filter set (Item A). Determine the combined residual activity of the syringe and infusion set components (stopcock, extension set, primary infusion set and in-line filter set) by assaying these items in a suitable radioactivity calibration system immediately following completion of administration of all components of the dosimetric step. Calculate and record the dose delivered to the patient by subtracting the residual activity in the syringe and the infusion set components from the activity of Iodine I 131 Tositumomab in the syringe prior to infusion.
9. Discard all materials used to deliver the Iodine I 131 Tositumomab (e.g., syringes, vials, in-line filter set, extension set and infusion sets) in accordance with local, state, and federal regulations governing radioactive and biohazardous waste.

Determination of Dose for the Therapeutic Step (see Calculation of Iodine-131 Activity for Therapeutic Dose): The method for determining and calculating the patient-specific dose of Iodine-131 activity (mCi) to be administered in the therapeutic step is described below. The derived values obtained in steps 3 and 4 and calculation of the therapeutic dose as described in step 6 may be determined manually [see **"Workbook for Dosimetry Methodology and Administration Set-Up"**] or calculated automatically using the GlaxoSmithKline proprietary software program [BEXXAR Patient Management Templates]. To receive training and to obtain the "BEXXAR Patient Management Templates" call the BEXXAR Service Center at 1-877-423-9927. For assistance with either manual or automated calculations call the BEXXAR Service Center at 1-877-423-9927.

1. Following infusion of the Iodine I 131 Tositumomab dosimetric dose, obtain total body gamma camera counts and whole body images at the following timepoints:
   a. Within one hour of infusion and prior to urination
   b. 2-4 days after infusion of the dosimetric dose, following urination
   c. 6-7 days after infusion of the dosimetric dose, following urination
2. Assess biodistribution. If biodistribution is altered, the therapeutic step should not be administered.

3. Determine total body residence time (see Graph 1, "Determination of Residence Time", in the "Workbook for Dosimetry Methodology and Administration Set-Up").

4. Determine activity hours (see Table 2, "Determination of Activity Hours", in the "Workbook for Dosimetry Methodology and Administration Set-Up"), according to gender. Use actual patient mass (in kg) or maximum effective mass (in kg) whichever is lower (see Table 1, "Determination of Maximum Effective Mass", in the "Workbook for Dosimetry Methodology and Administration Set-Up").

5. Determine whether the desired total body dose should be reduced (to 65 cGy) due to a platelet count of 100,000 to <150,000 cells/mm^3.

6. Based on the total body residence time and activity hours, calculate the Iodine-131 activity (mCi) to be administered to deliver the therapeutic dose of 65 or 75 cGy. The following equation is used to calculate the activity of Iodine-131 required for delivery of the desired total body dose of radiation.

[See table above]

$$\text{Iodine-131 Activity (mCi)} = \frac{\text{Activity Hours (mCi hr)}}{\text{Residence Time (hr)}} \times \frac{\text{Desired Total Body Dose (cGy)}}{75 \text{ cGy}}$$

Preparation for the Therapeutic Step
Tositumomab Dose
Required materials not supplied:
A. One 50 mL syringe with attached 18 gauge needle (to withdraw 450 mg of Tositumomab from two vials each containing 225 mg Tositumomab)
B. One 50 mL bag of sterile 0.9% Sodium Chloride for Injection, USP
C. One 50 mL syringe for drawing up 32 mL of saline for disposal from the 50 mL bag of sterile 0.9% Sodium Chloride for Injection, USP

Method:
1. Withdraw and dispose of 32 mL of saline from a 50 mL bag of sterile 0.9% Sodium Chloride for Injection, USP.
2. Withdraw the entire contents from each of the two 225 mg vials (a total of 450 mg Tositumomab in 32 mL) and transfer to the infusion bag containing 18 mL of 0.9% Sodium Chloride for Injection, USP to yield a final volume of 50 mL.
3. Gently mix the solutions by inverting/rotating the bag. DO NOT SHAKE.
4. The diluted Tositumomab may be stored for up to 24 hours when stored refrigerated at 2°C-8°C (36°F-46°F) and for up to 8 hours at room temperature.
Note: Tositumomab solution may contain particulates that are generally white in nature. The product should appear clear to opalescent, colorless to slightly yellow.

Preparation of Iodine I 131 Tositumomab Therapeutic Dose
Required materials not supplied:
A. Lead shielding for preparation vial and syringe pump
B. One or two 30 mL syringes with 18 gauge needles to withdraw the calculated volume of Iodine I 131 Tositumomab from the Iodine I 131 Tositumomab vial(s). One or two 60 mL syringes with 18 gauge needles to withdraw the volume from the preparation vial for administration
C. One 20 mL syringe with attached needle filled with 0.9% Sodium Chloride for Injection, USP
D. One 3 mL sterile syringe with attached needle to draw up Tositumomab from the 35 mg vial
E. One sterile, 30 or 50 mL preparation vial
F. Two lead pots both kept at room temperature. One pot is used to thaw the labeled antibody, and the second pot is used to hold the preparation vial

Method:
1. Allow approximately 60 minutes for thawing (at ambient temperature) of the Iodine I 131 Tositumomab therapeutic vial with appropriate lead shielding.
2. Calculate the dose of Iodine I 131 Tositumomab required (see CALCULATION OF IODINE-131 ACTIVITY FOR THERAPEUTIC DOSE).
3. Based on the activity concentration of the vial (see actual product specification sheet for each vial supplied in the therapeutic package), calculate the volume required for the Iodine I 131 Tositumomab activity required for the therapeutic dose.
4. Using one or more 30 mL syringes with an 18-gauge needle, withdraw the calculated volume from the Iodine I 131 Tositumomab vial.
5. Transfer this volume to the shielded preparation vial.
6. Assay the dose to ensure that the appropriate activity (mCi) has been prepared.
   a. If the assayed dose is the calculated dose (±10%) needed for the therapeutic step, proceed with step 7.
   b. If the assayed dose does not contain the desired dose (±10%), re-calculate the activity concentration of the Iodine I 131 Tositumomab at this time, based on the volume and the activity in the preparation vial. Re-calculate the volume required for an Iodine I 131 Tositumomab activity for the therapeutic dose. Using the same 30 mL syringe, add or subtract the appropriate volume from the Iodine I 131 Tositumomab vial so that the preparation vial contains the volume required for the Iodine I 131 Tositumomab activity required for the therapeutic dose. Re-assay the preparation vial. Proceed to step 7.
7. Calculate the amount of Tositumomab protein contained in the solution of Iodine I 131 Tositumomab in the shielded preparation vial, based on the volume and protein concentration (see product specification sheet).
8. If the shielded preparation vial contains less than 35 mg, calculate the amount of additional Tositumomab needed to yield a total of 35 mg protein. Calculate the volume needed from the 35 mg vial of Tositumomab, based on the protein concentration. Withdraw the calcu-

lated volume of Tositumomab from the 35 mg vial of Tositumomab, and transfer this volume to the shielded preparation vial. The preparation vial should now contain a total of 35 mg of Tositumomab.
Note: If the dose of Iodine I 131 Tositumomab requires the use of 2 vials of Iodine I 131 Tositumomab or the entire contents of a single vial of Iodine I 131 Tositumomab, there may be no need to add protein from the 35 mg vial of Tositumomab.

9. Using the 20 mL syringe containing 0.9% Sodium Chloride for Injection, USP, add a sufficient volume (if needed) to the shielded preparation vial to yield a final volume of 30 mL. Gently mix the solution.
10. Withdraw the entire volume from the preparation vial into a one or more sterile 60 mL syringes using a large bore needle (18 gauge).
11. Assay and record the activity.

Administration of the Therapeutic Step
Note: Restrictions on patient contact with others and release from the hospital must follow all applicable federal, state, and institutional regulations.
Required materials not supplied: For questions about required materials call the BEXXAR Service Center at 1-877-423-9927.
A. One IV Filter set (0.22 micron, filter), 15 inch with injection site (port) and luer lock
B. One Primary IV infusion set
C. One 100 mL bag of sterile 0.9% Sodium Chloride for Injection, USP
D. Two Secondary IV infusion sets
E. One IV extension set, 30 inch luer lock
F. One 3-way stopcock
G. One 50 mL bag of sterile 0.9% Sodium Chloride for Injection, USP
H. One Infusion pump for Tositumomab infusion
I. One Syringe Pump for Iodine I 131 Tositumomab infusion
J. Lead shielding for use in the administration of the therapeutic dose

Tositumomab Infusion:
(See Figure 1 in the "Workbook for Dosimetry Methodology and Administration Set-Up" for diagrammatic illustration of the configuration of the infusion set components.)
1. Attach a primary IV infusion set (Item B) to the 0.22 micron in-line filter set (Item A) and a 100 mL bag of sterile 0.9% Sodium Chloride for Injection, USP (Item C).
2. After priming the primary IV infusion set (Item B) and filter set (Item A), connect the infusion bag containing 450 mg Tositumomab (50 mL) via a secondary IV infusion set (Item D) to the primary IV infusion set (Item B) at a port distal to the 0.22 micron in-line filter. Infuse Tositumomab over 60 minutes.
3. After completion of the Tositumomab infusion, disconnect the secondary IV infusion set (Item D) and flush the primary IV infusion set (Item B) and the IV filter set (Item A) with sterile 0.9% Sodium Chloride for Injection, USP. Discard the Tositumomab bag and secondary IV infusion set.

Iodine I 131 Tositumomab Therapeutic Infusion:
(See Figure 2 in the "Workbook for Dosimetry Methodology and Administration Set-Up" for diagrammatic illustration of the configuration of the infusion set components.)
1. Appropriate shielding should be used in the administration of the therapeutic dose.
2. The therapeutic dose is delivered in one or more 60 mL syringes.
3. Connect the extension set (Item E) to the 3-way stopcock (Item F).
4. Connect the 50 mL bag of sterile 0.9% Sodium Chloride for Injection, USP (Item G) to a secondary IV infusion set (Item D) and connect the infusion set to the 3-way stopcock (Item F). Prime the secondary IV infusion set (Item D) and the extension set (Item E). Connect the extension set (Item E) to a port in the primary IV infusion set (Item B), distal to the filter. (Note: You must use the same primary infusion set (Item B) and IV filter set (Item A) with pre-wetted filter that was used for the Tositumomab infusion. A change in filter can result in loss of up to 7% of the Iodine I 131 Tositumomab dose.)
5. Attach the syringe filled with the Iodine I 131 Tositumomab to the 3-way stopcock (Item F).
6. Set syringe pump to deliver the entire therapeutic dose of Iodine I 131 Tositumomab over 20 minutes. (Note: if more than one syringe is required, remove the syringe and repeat steps 5 and 6.)
7. After completion of the infusion of Iodine I 131 Tositumomab, close the stopcock (Item F) to the syringe. Flush the secondary IV infusion set (Item D) and the extension set (Item E) with 0.9% Sodium Chloride from the 50 mL bag of sterile, 0.9% Sodium Chloride for Injection, USP (Item G).
8. After the flush, disconnect the extension set (Item E), 3-way stopcock (Item F) and syringe. Disconnect the primary IV infusion set (Item B) and in-line filter set (Item A). Determine the combined residual activity of the syringe(s) and infusion set components (stopcock, extension set, primary infusion set and in-line filter set) by assaying these items in a suitable radioactivity calibration system immediately following completion of administration of all components of the therapeutic step. Calculate and record the dose delivered to the patient by subtracting

the residual activity in the syringe and infusion set components from the activity of Iodine I 131 Tositumomab in the syringe prior to infusion.
9. Discard all materials used to deliver the Iodine I 131 Tositumomab (e.g., syringes, vials, in-line filter set, extension set and infusion sets) in accordance with local, state, and federal regulations governing radioactive and biohazardous waste.

DOSIMETRY
The following sections describe the procedures for image acquisition for collection of dosimetry data, interpretation of biodistribution images, calculation of residence time, and calculation of activity hours. Please read all sections carefully.

IMAGE ACQUISITION AND INTERPRETATION
Gamma Camera and Dose Calibrator Procedures
Manufacturer-specific quality control procedures should be followed for the gamma camera/computer system, the collimator, and the dose calibrator. Less than 20% variance between maximum and minimum pixel count values in the useful field of view is acceptable on Iodine-131 intrinsic flood fields and variability <10% is preferable. Iodine-131-specific camera uniformity corrections are strongly recommended, rather than applying lower energy correction to the Iodine-131 window. Camera extrinsic uniformity should be assessed at least monthly using ^{99m}Tc or ^{57}Co as a source with imaging at the appropriate window.
Additional (non-routine) quality control procedures are required. To assure the accuracy and precision of the patient total body counts, the gamma camera must undergo validation and daily quality control on each day it is used to collect patient images.
Use the same setup and region of interest (ROI) for calibration, determination of background, and whole body patient studies.

Gamma Camera Set-Up
The **same** camera, collimator, scanning speed, energy window, and setup must be used for all studies. The gamma camera must be capable of whole body imaging and have a large or extra large field of view with a digital interface. It must be equipped with a parallel-hole collimator rated to at least 364 keV by the manufacturer with a septal penetration for Iodine-131 of <7%.
The camera and computer must be set up for scanning as follows:
• Parallel hole collimator rated to at least 364 keV with a septal penetration for Iodine-131 of <7%
• Symmetric window (20–25%) centered on the 364 keV photo peak of Iodine-131 (314-414 keV)
• Matrix: appropriate whole body matrix
• Scanning speed: 10–30 cm/minute

Counts from Calibrated Source for Quality Control
Camera sensitivity for Iodine-131 must be determined each day. Determination of the gamma camera's sensitivity is obtained by scanning a calibrated activity of Iodine-131 (e.g., 200-250 µCi in at least 20 mL of saline within a sealed pharmaceutical vial). The radioactivity of the Iodine-131 source is first determined using a NIST-traceable-calibrated clinical dose calibrator at the Iodine-131 setting.

Background Counts
The background count is obtained from a scan with no radioactive source. This should be obtained following the count of the calibrated source and just prior to obtaining the patient count.
If abnormally high background counts are measured, the source should be identified and, if possible, removed. If abnormally low background counts are measured, the camera energy window setting and collimator should be verified before repeating the background counts.
The counts per µCi are obtained by dividing the background-corrected source count by the calibrated activity for that day. For a specific camera and collimator, the counts per µCi should be relatively constant. When values vary more than 10% from the established ratio, the reason for the discrepancy should be ascertained and corrected and the source count repeated.

Patient Total Body Counts
The source and background counts are obtained first and the camera sensitivity (i.e., constant counting efficiency) is established prior to obtaining the patient count. The same rectangular region of interest (ROI) must be used for the whole body counts, the quality control counts of the radioactive source, and the background counts.
Acquire anterior and posterior whole body images for gamma camera counts. For any particular patient, the same gamma camera must be used for all scans. To obtain proper counts, extremities must be included in the images, and arms should not cross over the body. The scans should be centered on the midline of the patient. Record the time of the start of the radiolabeled dosimetric infusion and the time of the start of each count acquisition.
Gamma camera counts will be obtained at the three imaging time points:
• Count 1: *Within an hour of end of the infusion* of the Iodine I 131 Tositumomab dosimetric dose prior to patient voiding.

Continued on next page

Bexxar—Cont.

- **Count 2:** Two to 4 days after administration of the Iodine I 131 Tositumomab dosimetric dose and immediately following patient voiding.
- **Count 3:** Six to 7 days after the administration of the Iodine I 131 Tositumomab dosimetric dose and immediately following patient voiding.

Assessment of Biodistribution of Iodine I 131 Tositumomab

The biodistribution of Iodine I 131 Tositumomab should be assessed by determination of total body residence time and by visual examination of whole body camera images from the first image taken at the time of Count 1 (within an hour of the end of the infusion) and from the second image taken at the time of Count 2 (at 2 to 4 days after administration). To resolve ambiguities, an evaluation of the third image at the time of Count 3 (6 to 7 days after administration) may be necessary. If either of these methods indicates that the biodistribution is altered, the Iodine I 131 Tositumomab therapeutic dose should not be administered.

Expected Biodistribution

- On the first imaging timepoint: Most of the activity is in the blood pool (heart and major blood vessels) and the uptake in normal liver and spleen is less than in the heart.
- On the second and third imaging timepoints: The activity in the blood pool decreases significantly and there is decreased accumulation of activity in normal liver and spleen. Images may show uptake by thyroid, kidney, and urinary bladder and minimal uptake in the lungs. Tumor uptake in soft tissues and in normal organs is seen as areas of increased intensity.

Results Indicating Altered Biodistribution

- On the first imaging timepoint: If the blood pool is not visualized or if there is diffuse, intense tracer uptake in the liver and/or spleen or uptake suggestive of urinary obstruction the biodistribution is altered. Diffuse lung uptake greater than that of blood pool on the first day represents altered biodistribution.
- On the second and third imaging timepoints: uptake suggestive of urinary obstruction and diffuse lung uptake greater than that of the blood pool represent altered biodistribution.
- Total body residence times of less than 50 hours and more than 150 hours.

CALCULATION OF IODINE-131 ACTIVITY FOR THE THERAPEUTIC DOSE

There are two options for calculation of the Iodine-131 activity for the therapeutic dose. The derived values and calculation of the therapeutic dose may be determined manually [see **"Workbook for Dosimetry Methodology and Administration Set-Up"**] or calculated automatically using the GlaxoSmithKline proprietary software program [BEXXAR Patient Management Templates]. The following describes in greater detail the stepwise method for manual determination of the Iodine-131 activity for the therapeutic dose.

Residence Time (hr)

For each time point, calculate the background corrected total body count at each timepoint (defined as the geometric mean). The following equation is used:

$$\text{Geometric mean of counts} = \sqrt{(C_A - C_{BA})(C_P - C_{BP})}$$

In this equation, C_A = the anterior counts, C_{BA} = the anterior background counts, C_P= the posterior counts, and C_{BP} = the posterior background counts.

Once the geometric mean of the counts has been calculated for each of the 3 timepoints, the % injected activity remaining for each timepoint is calculated by dividing the geometric mean of the counts from that timepoint by the geometric mean of the counts from Day 0 and multiplying by 100.

The residence time (h) is then determined by plotting the time from the start of infusion and the % injected activity values for the 3 imaging timepoints on Graph 1 (see Worksheet **"Determination of Residence Time"** in the **"Workbook for Dosimetry Methodology and Administration Set-Up"** supplied with Dosimetric Dose Packaging). A best-fit line is then drawn from 100% (the pre-plotted Day 0 value) through the other 2 plotted points (if the line does not intersect the two points, one point must lie above the best-fit line and one point must lie below the best-fit line). The residence time (h) is read from the x-axis of the graph at the point where the fitted line intersects with the horizontal 37% injected activity line.

Activity Hours (mCi hr)

In order to determine the activity hours (mCi hr), look up the patient's maximum effective mass derived from the patient's sex and height (see Worksheet **"Determination of Maximum Effective Mass"** in the **"Workbook for Dosimetry Methodology and Administration Set- Up"** supplied with Dosimetric Dose Packaging). If the patient's actual weight is less than the maximum effective mass, the actual weight should be used in the activity hours table (see Worksheet **"Determination of Activity Hours"** in the **"Workbook for Dosimetry Methodology and Administration Set-Up"** supplied with Dosimetric Dose Packaging). If the patient's actual weight is greater than the maximum effective mass, the mass from the worksheet for **"Determination of Maximum Effective Mass"** should be used.

Calculation of Iodine-131 Activity for the Therapeutic Dose

The following equation is used to calculate the activity of Iodine-131 required for delivery of the desired total body dose of radiation.

[See table below]

HOW SUPPLIED

TOSITUMOMAB DOSIMETRIC PACKAGING

The components of the dosimetric step will be shipped **ONLY** to individuals who are participating in the certification program or have been certified in the preparation and administration of the BEXXAR therapeutic regimen. The components are shipped from separate sites; when ordering, ensure that the components are scheduled to arrive on the same day. The components of the Tositumomab Dosimetric Step include:

1. Tositumomab: Two single-use 225 mg vials (16.1 mL) and one single-use 35 mg vial (2.5 mL) of Tositumomab at a protein concentration of 14 mg/mL supplied by McKesson BioServices.
   NDC 67800-101-31
2. Iodine I 131 Tositumomab: A single-use vial of Iodine I 131 Tositumomab within a lead pot, supplied by MDS Nordion. Each single-use vial contains not less than 20 mL of Iodine I 131 Tositumomab at nominal protein and activity concentrations of 0.1 mg/mL and 0.61 mCi/mL (at calibration), respectively. (Refer to the product specification sheet for the lot-specific protein concentration, activity concentration, total activity and expiration date.)
   NDC 67800-111-10

TOSITUMOMAB THERAPEUTIC PACKAGING

The components of the therapeutic step will be shipped **ONLY** to individuals who are participating in the certification program or have been certified in the preparation and administration of the BEXXAR therapeutic regimen for an individual patient who has completed the Dosimetric Step. The components of the therapeutic step are shipped from separate sites; when ordering, ensure that the components are scheduled to arrive on the same day. The components of the Tositumomab Therapeutic Step include:

1. Tositumomab: Two single-use 225 mg vials (16.1 mL) and one single-use 35 mg vial (2.5 mL) of Tositumomab at a protein concentration of 14 mg/mL supplied by McKesson BioServices.
   NDC 67800-101-32
2. Iodine I 131 Tositumomab: One or two single-use vials of Iodine I 131 Tositumomab within a lead pot(s), supplied by MDS Nordion. Each single-use vial contains not less than 20 mL of Iodine I 131 Tositumomab at nominal protein and activity concentrations of 1.1 mg/mL and 5.6 mCi/mL (at calibration), respectively. Refer to the product specification sheet for the lot-specific protein concentration, activity concentration, total activity and expiration date.
   NDC 67800-121-10

STABILITY AND STORAGE

TOSITUMOMAB

Vials of Tositumomab (35 mg and 225 mg) should be stored refrigerated at 2°C-8°C (36°F-46°F) prior to dilution. Do not use beyond expiration date. Protect from strong light. **DO NOT SHAKE**. Do not freeze. Discard any unused portions left in the vial.

Solutions of diluted Tositumomab are stable for up to 24 hours when stored refrigerated at 2°C-8°C (36°F-46°F) and for up to 8 hours at room temperature. However, it is recommended that the diluted solution be stored refrigerated at 2°C-8°C (36°F-46°F) prior to administration because it does not contain preservatives. Any unused portion must be discarded. Do not freeze solutions of diluted Tositumomab.

IODINE I 131 TOSITUMOMAB

Store frozen in the original lead pots. The lead pot containing the product must be stored in a freezer at a temperature of –20°C or below until it is removed for thawing prior to administration to the patient. Do not use beyond the expiration date on the label of the lead pot.

Thawed dosimetric and therapeutic doses of Iodine I 131 Tositumomab are stable for up to 8 hours at 2°C-8°C (36°F-46°F) or at room temperature. Solutions of Iodine I 131 Tositumomab diluted for infusion contain no preservatives and should be stored refrigerated at 2°C-8°C (36°F-46°F) prior to administration (do not freeze). Any unused portion must be discarded according to federal and state laws.

REFERENCES

1. Weber DA, Eckman KF, Dillman LT, Ryman JC. In: MIRD: radionuclide data and decay schemes. New York: Society of Nuclear Medicine Inc. 1989:229.
2. Tedder T, Boyd A, Freedman A, Nadler L, Schlossman S. The B cell surface molecule is functionally linked with B cell activation and differentiation. J Immunol 1985;135(2):973-979.
3. Anderson, KC, Bates MP, Slaughenhoupt BL, Pinkus GS, Schlossman SF, Nadler LM. Expression of human B cell-associated antigens on leukemias and lymphomas: a model of human B cell differentiation. Blood 1984;63(6):1424-1433.
4. Press OW, Howell-Clark J, Anderson S, Bernstein I. Retention of B-cell-specific monoclonal antibodies by human lymphoma cells. Blood 1994;83:1390-7.
5. Cardarelli PM, Quinn M, Buckman D, Fang Y, Colcher D, King DJ, Bebbington C, et al. Binding to CD20 by anti-B1 antibody or F(ab')(2) is sufficient for induction of apoptosis in B-cell lines. Cancer Immunol Immunother 2002 Mar;51(1):15–24.
6. Stashenko P, Nadler LM, Hardy R, Schlossman SF. Characterization of a human B lymphocyte-specific antigen. J Immunol 1980;125:1678–85.

U.S. Lic. 1614
GlaxoSmithKline, Research Triangle Park, NC 27709
BEXXAR is a registered trademark of GlaxoSmithKline.
March 2005/RL-2179

Janssen Pharmaceutica Products, L.P.

**1125 TRENTON-HARBOURTON ROAD
P.O. BOX 200
TITUSVILLE, NJ 08560-0200**

For Medical Information Monday through Friday 9 am-5 pm EST Contact:
(800) JANSSEN
FAX: (609) 730-2461
After Hours and Weekends:
(800) JANSSEN

RAZADYNE™ ℞
(GALANTAMINE HBr)

Prescribing information for this product, which appears on pages 1739–1741 of the 2005 PDR, has been revised as follows:
The product name changed from **REMINYL®** *to* **RAZADYNE™**
The following 3 paragraphs were added to **PRECAUTIONS:** *after* **Information for Patients and Caregivers:**
Deaths in Subjects with Mild Cognitive Impairment (MCI)
In two randomized placebo controlled trials of 2 years duration in subjects with mild cognitive impairment (MCI), a total of 13 subjects on RAZADYNE™ (n=1026) and 1 subject on placebo (n=1022) died. The deaths were due to various causes which could be expected in an elderly population; about half of the RAZADYNE™ deaths appeared to result from various vascular causes (myocardial infarction, stroke, and sudden death).
Although the difference in mortality between RAZADYNE™ and placebo-treated groups in these two studies was significant, the results are highly discrepant with other studies of RAZADYNE™. Specifically, in these two MCI studies, the mortality rate in the placebo-treated subjects was markedly lower than the rate in placebo-treated patients in trials of RAZADYNE™ in Alzheimer's disease or other dementias (0.7 per 1000 person years compared to 22–61 per 1000 person years, respectively). Although the mortality rate in the RAZADYNE™-treated MCI subjects was also lower than that observed in RAZADYNE™-treated patients in Alzheimer's disease and other dementia trials (10.2 per 1000 person years compared to 23–31 per 1000 person years, respectively), the relative difference was much less. When the Alzheimer's disease and other dementia studies were pooled (n=6000), the mortality rate in the placebo group numerically exceeded that in the RAZADYNE™ group. Furthermore, in the MCI studies, no subjects in the placebo group died after 6 months, a highly unexpected finding in this population.
Individuals with mild cognitive impairment demonstrate isolated memory impairment greater than expected for their age and education, but do not meet current diagnostic criteria for Alzheimer's disease.
In **HOW SUPPLIED** *section, the following paragraph was revised:*
4 mg off-white tablet: bottles of 60 NDC 50458-396-60
8 mg pink tablet: bottles of 60 NDC 50458-397-60
12 mg orange-brown tablet: bottles of 60 NDC 50458-398-60
RAZADYNE™ (galantamine hydrobromide) 4 mg/mL oral solution (NDC 50458-490-10) is a clear colorless solution supplied in 100 mL bottles with a calibrated (in milligrams and milliliters) pipette. The minimum calibrated volume is 0.5 mL, while the maximum calibrated volume is 4 mL.
7517310
Revised March 2005
US Patent No. 4,663,318
©Janssen 2001

RAZADYNE™ ER ℞
[răz-ă-dīn ER]
galantamine HBr
EXTENDED-RELEASE CAPSULES

DESCRIPTION

RAZADYNE™ ER (galantamine hydrobromide) is a reversible, competitive acetylcholinesterase inhibitor. It is known chemically as (4aS,6R,8aS)-4a,5,9,10,11,12-hexahydro-3-methoxy-11-methyl-6H-benzofuro[3a,3,2-ef][2]benzazepin-6-ol hydrobromide. It has an empirical formula of $C_{17}H_{21}NO_3 \cdot HBr$ and a molecular weight of 368.27. Galantamine hydrobromide is a white to almost white powder and

Iodine-131 Activity (mCi)	=	$\dfrac{\text{Activity Hours (mCi hr)}}{\text{Residence Time (hr)}}$	×	$\dfrac{\text{Desired Total Body Dose (cGy)}}{75 \text{ cGy}}$

is sparingly soluble in water. The structural formula for galantamine hydrobromide is:

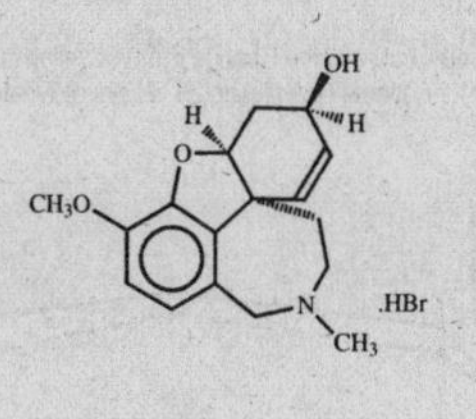

RAZADYNE™ ER is available in opaque hard gelatin extended release capsules of 8 mg (white), 16 mg (pink), and 24 mg (caramel) containing galantamine hydrobromide, equivalent to respectively 8, 16 and 24 mg galantamine base. Inactive ingredients include gelatin, diethyl phthalate, ethylcellulose, hypromellose, polyethylene glycol, titanium dioxide and sugar spheres (sucrose and starch). The 16 mg capsule also contains red ferric oxide. The 24 mg capsule also contains red ferric oxide and yellow ferric oxide.

CLINICAL PHARMACOLOGY

Mechanism of Action

Although the etiology of cognitive impairment in Alzheimer's disease (AD) is not fully understood, it has been reported that acetylcholine-producing neurons degenerate in the brains of patients with Alzheimer's disease. The degree of this cholinergic loss has been correlated with degree of cognitive impairment and density of amyloid plaques (a neuropathological hallmark of Alzheimer's disease).

Galantamine, a tertiary alkaloid, is a competitive and reversible inhibitor of acetylcholinesterase. While the precise mechanism of galantamine's action is unknown, it is postulated to exert its therapeutic effect by enhancing cholinergic function. This is accomplished by increasing the concentration of acetylcholine through reversible inhibition of its hydrolysis by cholinesterase. If this mechanism is correct, galantamine's effect may lessen as the disease process advances and fewer cholinergic neurons remain functionally intact. There is no evidence that galantamine alters the course of the underlying dementing process.

Pharmacokinetics

Galantamine is well absorbed with absolute oral bioavailability of about 90%. It has a terminal elimination half-life of about 7 hours and pharmacokinetics are linear over the range of 8–32 mg/day.

The maximum inhibition of acetylcholinesterase activity of about 40% was achieved about one hour after a single oral dose of 8 mg galantamine in healthy male subjects.

Absorption and Distribution

Galantamine is rapidly and completely absorbed with time to peak concentration about 1 hour. Bioavailability of the tablet was the same as the bioavailability of an oral solution. Food did not affect the AUC of galantamine but C_{max} decreased by 25% and T_{max} was delayed by 1.5 hours. The mean volume of distribution of galantamine is 175 L.

The plasma protein binding of galantamine is 18% at therapeutically relevant concentrations. In whole blood, galantamine is mainly distributed to blood cells (52.7%). The blood to plasma concentration ratio of galantamine is 1.2.

Metabolism and Elimination

Galantamine is metabolized by hepatic cytochrome P450 enzymes, glucuronidated, and excreted unchanged in the urine. *In vitro* studies indicate that cytochrome CYP2D6 and CYP3A4 were the major cytochrome P450 isoenzymes involved in the metabolism of galantamine, and inhibitors of both pathways increase oral bioavailability of galantamine modestly (see **PRECAUTIONS, Drug-Drug Interactions**). O-demethylation, mediated by CYP2D6 was greater in extensive metabolizers of CYP2D6 than in poor metabolizers. In plasma from both poor and extensive metabolizers, however, unchanged galantamine and its glucuronide accounted for most of the sample radioactivity.

In studies of oral ^{3}H-galantamine, unchanged galantamine and its glucuronide, accounted for most plasma radioactivity in poor and extensive CYP2D6 metabolizers. Up to 8 hours post-dose, unchanged galantamine accounted for 39–77% of the total radioactivity in the plasma, and galantamine glucuronide for 14–24%. By 7 days, 93-99% of the radioactivity had been recovered, with about 95% in urine and about 5% in the feces. Total urinary recovery of unchanged galantamine accounted for, on average, 32% of the dose and that of galantamine glucuronide for another 12% on average.

After i.v. or oral administration, about 20% of the dose was excreted as unchanged galantamine in the urine in 24 hours, representing a renal clearance of about 65 mL/min, about 20–25% of the total plasma clearance of about 300 mL/min.

RAZADYNE™ ER 24 mg extended release capsules administered once daily under fasting conditions are bioequivalent to galantamine tablets 12 mg twice daily with respect to AUC_{24h} and C_{min}. The C_{max} and T_{max} of the extended release capsules were lower and occurred later, respectively, compared with the immediate release tablets, with C_{max} about 25% lower and median T_{max} occurring about 4.5–5.0 hours after dosing. Dose-proportionality is observed for RAZADYNE™ ER extended-release capsules over the dose range of 8 to 24 mg daily and steady state is achieved within a week. There was no effect of age on the pharmacokinetics of RAZADYNE™ ER extended-release capsules. CYP2D6 poor metabolizers had drug exposures that were approximately 50% higher than for extensive metabolizers.

There are no appreciable differences in pharmacokinetic parameters when RAZADYNE™ ER extended-release capsules are given with food compared to when they are given in the fasted state.

Special Populations

CYP2D6 Poor Metabolizers

Approximately 7% of the normal population has a genetic variation that leads to reduced levels of activity of CYP2D6 isozyme. Such individuals have been referred to as poor metabolizers. After a single oral dose of 4 mg or 8 mg galantamine, CYP2D6 poor metabolizers demonstrated a similar C_{max} and about 35% AUC∞ increase of unchanged galantamine compared to extensive metabolizers.

A total of 356 patients with Alzheimer's disease enrolled in two phase 3 studies were genotyped with respect to CYP2D6 (n=210 hetero-extensive metabolizers, 126 homo-extensive metabolizers, and 20 poor metabolizers). Population pharmacokinetic analysis indicated that there was a 25% decrease in median clearance in poor metabolizers compared to extensive metabolizers. Dosage adjustment is not necessary in patients identified as poor metabolizers as the dose of drug is individually titrated to tolerability.

Hepatic Impairment:

Following a single 4 mg dose of galantamine immediate release tablets, the pharmacokinetics of galantamine in subjects with mild hepatic impairment (n=8; Child-Pugh score of 5–6) were similar to those in healthy subjects. In patients with moderate hepatic impairment (n=8; Child-Pugh score of 7–9), galantamine clearance was decreased by about 25% compared to normal volunteers. Exposure would be expected to increase further with increasing degree of hepatic impairment (see **PRECAUTIONS** and **DOSAGE AND ADMINISTRATION**).

Renal Impairment:

Following a single 8 mg dose of galantamine tablets, AUC increased by 37% and 67% in moderate and severely renal-impaired patients compared to normal volunteers. (see **PRECAUTIONS** and **DOSAGE AND ADMINISTRATION**).

Elderly:

Data from clinical trials in patients with Alzheimer's disease indicate that galantamine concentrations are 30–40% higher than in healthy young subjects.

Gender and Race:

No specific pharmacokinetic study was conducted to investigate the effect of gender and race on the disposition of galantamine, but a population pharmacokinetic analysis indicates (n=539 males and 550 females) that galantamine clearance is about 20% lower in females than in males (explained by lower body weight in females) and race (n=1029 White, 24 Black, 13 Asian and 23 other) did not affect the clearance of galantamine.

Drug-Drug Interactions

Multiple metabolic pathways and renal excretion are involved in the elimination of galantamine so no single pathway appears predominant. Based on *in vitro* studies, CYP2D6 and CYP3A4 were the major enzymes involved in the metabolism of galantamine. CYP2D6 was involved in the formation of O-desmethyl-galantamine, whereas CYP3A4 mediated the formation of galantamine-N-oxide. Galantamine is also glucuronidated and excreted unchanged in urine.

(A) Effect of Other Drugs on the Metabolism of Galantamine:

Drugs that are potent inhibitors for CYP2D6 or CYP3A4 may increase the AUC of galantamine. Multiple dose pharmacokinetic studies demonstrated that the AUC of galantamine increased 30% and 40%, respectively, during coadministration of ketoconazole and paroxetine. As coadministered with erythromycin, another CYP3A4 inhibitor, the galantamine AUC increased only 10%. Population PK analysis with a database of 852 patients with Alzheimer's disease showed that the clearance of galantamine was decreased about 25–33% by concurrent administration of amitriptyline (n = 17), fluoxetine (n = 48), fluvoxamine (n = 14), and quinidine (n = 7), known inhibitors of CYP2D6. Concurrent administration of H_2-antagonists demonstrated that ranitidine did not affect the pharmacokinetics of galantamine, and cimetidine increased the galantamine AUC by approximately 16%.

(B) Effect of Galantamine on the Metabolism of Other Drugs:

In vitro studies show that galantamine did not inhibit the metabolic pathways catalyzed by CYP1A2, CYP2A6, CYP3A4, CYP4A, CYP2C, CYP2D6 and CYP2E1. This indicated that the inhibitory potential of galantamine towards the major forms of cytochrome P450 is very low. Multiple doses of galantamine (24 mg/day) had no effect on the pharmacokinetics of digoxin and warfarin (R- and S- forms). Galantamine had no effect on the increased prothrombin time induced by warfarin.

CLINICAL TRIALS

The effectiveness of galantamine as a treatment for Alzheimer's disease is demonstrated by the results of 5 randomized, double-blind, placebo-controlled clinical investigations in patients with probable Alzheimer's disease, 4 with the immediate-release tablet, and one with the extended-release capsule [diagnosed by NINCDS-ADRDA criteria, with Mini-Mental State Examination scores that were ≥10 and ≤24]. Doses studied were 8–32 mg/day given as twice daily doses (immediate- release tablets). In 3 of the 4 studies with the immediate-release tablet, patients were started on a low dose of 8 mg, then titrated weekly by 8 mg/day to 24 or 32 mg as assigned. In the fourth study (USA 4-week Dose-Escalation Fixed-Dose Study) dose escalation of 8 mg/day occurred over 4 week intervals. The mean age of patients participating in these 4 trials was 75 years with a range of 41 to 100. Approximately 62% of patients were women and 38% were men. The racial distribution was White 94%, Black 3% and other races 3%. Two other studies examined a three times daily dosing regimen; these also showed or suggested benefit but did not suggest an advantage over twice daily dosing.

Study Outcome Measures:

In each study, the primary effectiveness of galantamine was evaluated using a dual outcome assessment strategy as measured by the Alzheimer's Disease Assessment Scale (ADAS-cog) and the Clinician's Interview Based Impression of Change that required the use of caregiver information (CIBIC-plus).

The ability of galantamine to improve cognitive performance was assessed with the cognitive sub-scale of the Alzheimer's Disease Assessment Scale (ADAS-cog), a multi-item instrument that has been extensively validated in longitudinal cohorts of Alzheimer's disease patients. The ADAS-cog examines selected aspects of cognitive performance including elements of memory, orientation, attention, reasoning, language and praxis. The ADAS-cog scoring range is from 0 to 70, with higher scores indicating greater cognitive impairment. Elderly normal adults may score as low as 0 or 1, but it is not unusual for non-demented adults to score slightly higher.

The patients recruited as participants in each study with the immediate-release tablet had mean scores on ADAS-cog of approximately 27 units, with a range from 5 to 69. Experience gained in longitudinal studies of ambulatory patients with mild to moderate Alzheimer's disease suggests that they gain 6 to 12 units a year on the ADAS-cog. Lesser degrees of change, however, are seen in patients with very mild or very advanced disease because the ADAS-cog is not uniformly sensitive to change over the course of the disease. The annualized rate of decline in the placebo patients participating in galantamine trials was approximately 4.5 units per year.

The ability of galantamine to produce an overall clinical effect was assessed using a Clinician's Interview Based Impression of Change that required the use of caregiver information, the CIBIC-plus. The CIBIC-plus is not a single instrument and is not a standardized instrument like the ADAS-cog. Clinical trials for investigational drugs have used a variety of CIBIC formats, each different in terms of depth and structure. As such, results from a CIBIC-plus reflect clinical experience from the trial or trials in which it was used and can not be compared directly with the results of CIBIC-plus evaluations from other clinical trials. The CIBIC-plus used in the trials was a semi-structured instrument based on a comprehensive evaluation at baseline and subsequent time-points of 4 major areas of patient function: general, cognitive, behavioral and activities of daily living. It represents the assessment of a skilled clinician based on his/her observation at an interview with the patient, in combination with information supplied by a caregiver familiar with the behavior of the patient over the interval rated. The CIBIC-plus is scored as a seven point categorical rating, ranging from a score of 1, indicating "markedly improved", to a score of 4, indicating "no change" to a score of 7, indicating "marked worsening". The CIBIC-plus has not been systematically compared directly to assessments not using information from caregivers (CIBIC) or other global methods.

Immediate-Release Tablets

U.S. Twenty-One-Week Fixed-Dose Study

In a study of 21 weeks duration, 978 patients were randomized to doses of 8, 16, or 24 mg of galantamine per day, or to placebo, each given in 2 divided doses (immediate release tablets). Treatment was initiated at 8 mg/day for all patients randomized to galantamine, and increased by 8 mg/day every 4 weeks. Therefore, the maximum titration phase was 8 weeks and the minimum maintenance phase was 13 weeks (in patients randomized to 24 mg/day of galantamine).

Effects on the ADAS-cog:

Figure 1 illustrates the time course for the change from baseline in ADAS-cog scores for all four dose groups over the 21 weeks of the study. At 21 weeks of treatment, the mean differences in the ADAS-cog change scores for the galantamine-treated patients compared to the patients on placebo were 1.7, 3.3, and 3.6 units for the 8, 16 and 24 mg/day treatments, respectively. The 16 mg/day and 24 mg/day treatments were statistically significantly superior to placebo and to the 8 mg/day treatment. There was no statistically significant difference between the 16 mg/day and 24 mg/day dose groups.

[See figure 1 at top of next column]

Figure 2 illustrates the cumulative percentages of patients from each of the four treatment groups who had attained at least the measure of improvement in ADAS-cog score shown on the X-axis. Three change scores (10-point, 7-point and 4-point reductions) and no change in score from baseline have been identified for illustrative purposes, and the percent of patients in each group achieving that result is shown in the inset table.

The curves demonstrate that both patients assigned to galantamine and placebo have a wide range of responses, but

Continued on next page

Razadyne ER—Cont.

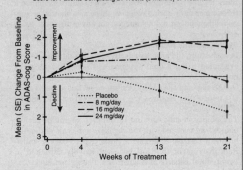

Figure 1: Time-Course of the Change From Baseline in ADAS-cog Score for Patients Completing 21 Weeks (5 Months) of Treatment

that the galantamine groups are more likely to show the greater improvements.

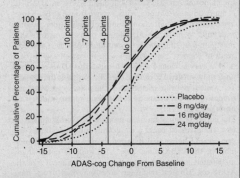

Figure 2: Cumulative Percentage of Patients Completing 21 Weeks of Double-Blind Treatment With Specified Changes From Baseline in ADAS-cog Scores. The Percentages of Randomized Patients Who Completed the Study Were: Placebo 84%, 8 mg/day 77%, 16 mg/day 78% and 24 mg/day 78%.

Effects on the CIBIC-plus:
Figure 3 is a histogram of the percentage distribution of CIBIC-plus scores attained by patients assigned to each of the four treatment groups who completed 21 weeks of treatment. The galantamine-placebo differences for these groups of patients in mean rating were 0.15, 0.41 and 0.44 units for the 8, 16 and 24 mg/day treatments, respectively. The 16 mg/day and 24 mg/day treatments were statistically significantly superior to placebo. The differences vs. the 8 mg/day treatment for the 16 and 24 mg/day treatments were 0.26 and 0.29, respectively. There were no statistically significant differences between the 16 mg/day and 24 mg/day dose groups.

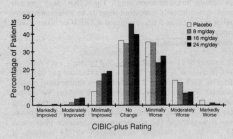

Figure 3: Distribution of CIBIC-plus Ratings at Week 21

U.S. Twenty-Six-Week Fixed-Dose Study
In a study of 26 weeks duration, 636 patients were randomized to either a dose of 24 mg or 32 mg of galantamine per day, or to placebo, each given in two divided doses (immediate release tablets). The 26-week study was divided into a 3-week dose titration phase and a 23-week maintenance phase.
Effects on the ADAS-cog:
Figure 4 illustrates the time course for the change from baseline in ADAS-cog scores for all three dose groups over the 26 weeks of the study. At 26 weeks of treatment, the mean differences in the ADAS-cog change scores for the galantamine-treated patients compared to the patients on placebo were 3.9 and 3.8 units for the 24 mg/day and 32 mg/day treatments, respectively. Both treatments were statistically significantly superior to placebo, but were not significantly different from each other.
[See figure 4 at top of next column]
Figure 5 illustrates the cumulative percentages of patients from each of the three treatment groups who had attained at least the measure of improvement in ADAS-cog score shown on the X axis. Three change scores (10-point, 7-point and 4-point reductions) and no change in score from baseline have been identified for illustrative purposes, and the percent of patients in each group achieving that result is shown in the inset table.

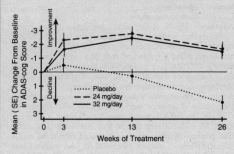

Figure 4: Time-Course of the Change From Baseline in ADAS-cog Score for Patients Completing 26 Weeks of Treatment

The curves demonstrate that both patients assigned to galantamine and placebo have a wide range of responses, but that the galantamine groups are more likely to show the greater improvements. A curve for an effective treatment would be shifted to the left of the curve for placebo, while an ineffective or deleterious treatment would be superimposed upon, or shifted to the right of the curve for placebo, respectively.

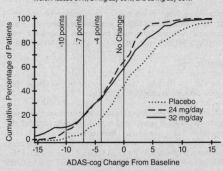

Figure 5: Cumulative Percentage of Patients Completing 26 Weeks of Double-Blind Treatment With Specified Changes From Baseline in ADAS-cog Scores. The Percentages of Randomized Patients Who Completed the Study Were: Placebo 81%, 24 mg/day 68%, and 32 mg/day 58%.

Treatment	Change in ADAS-cog			
	-10	-7	-4	0
Placebo	2.1%	5.7%	16.6%	43.9%
24 mg/day	7.6%	18.3%	33.6%	64.1%
32 mg/day	11.1%	19.7%	33.3%	58.1%

Effects on the CIBIC-plus:
Figure 6 is a histogram of the percentage distribution of CIBIC-plus scores attained by patients assigned to each of the three treatment groups who completed 26 weeks of treatment. The mean galantamine-placebo differences for these groups of patients in the mean rating were 0.28 and 0.29 units for 24 and 32 mg/day of galantamine, respectively. The mean ratings for both groups were statistically significantly superior to placebo, but were not significantly different from each other.

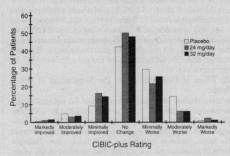

Figure 6: Distribution of CIBIC-plus Ratings at Week 26

International Twenty-Six-Week Fixed-Dose Study
In a study of 26 weeks duration identical in design to the USA 26-Week Fixed-Dose Study, 653 patients were randomized to either a dose of 24 mg or 32 mg of galantamine per day, or to placebo, each given in two divided doses (immediate release tablets). The 26-week study was divided into a 3-week dose titration phase and a 23-week maintenance phase.
Effects on the ADAS-cog:
Figure 7 illustrates the time course for the change from baseline in ADAS-cog scores for all three dose groups over the 26 weeks of the study. At 26 weeks of treatment, the mean differences in the ADAS-cog change scores for the galantamine - treated patients compared to the patients on placebo were 3.1 and 4.1 units for the 24 mg/day and 32 mg/day treatments, respectively. Both treatments were sta-

tistically significantly superior to placebo, but were not significantly different from each other.

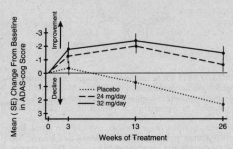

Figure 7: Time-Course of the Change From Baseline in ADAS-cog Score for Patients Completing 26 Weeks of Treatment

Figure 8 illustrates the cumulative percentages of patients from each of the three treatment groups who had attained at least the measure of improvement in ADAS-cog score shown on the X-axis. Three change scores (10-point, 7-point and 4-point reductions) and no change in score from baseline have been identified for illustrative purposes, and the percent of patients in each group achieving that result is shown in the inset table.
The curves demonstrate that both patients assigned to galantamine and placebo have a wide range of responses, but that the galantamine groups are more likely to show the greater improvements.

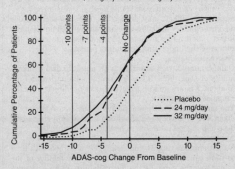

Figure 8: Cumulative Percentage of Patients Completing 26 Weeks of Double-Blind Treatment With Specified Changes From Baseline in ADAS-cog Scores. The Percentages of Randomized Patients Who Completed the Study Were: Placebo 87%, 24 mg/day 80%, and 32 mg/day 75%.

Treatment	Change in ADAS-cog			
	-10	-7	-4	0
Placebo	1.2%	5.8%	15.2%	39.8%
24 mg/day	4.5%	15.4%	30.8%	65.4%
32 mg/day	7.9%	19.7%	34.9%	63.8%

Effects on the CIBIC-plus:
Figure 9 is a histogram of the percentage distribution of CIBIC-plus scores attained by patients assigned to each of the three treatment groups who completed 26 weeks of treatment. The mean galantamine-placebo differences for these groups of patients in the mean rating of change from baseline were 0.34 and 0.47 for 24 and 32 mg/day of galantamine, respectively. The mean ratings for the galantamine groups were statistically significantly superior to placebo, but were not significantly different from each other.

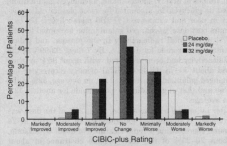

Figure 9: Distribution of CIBIC-plus Rating at Week 26

International Thirteen-Week Flexible-Dose Study
In a study of 13 weeks duration, 386 patients were randomized to either a flexible dose of 24–32 mg/day of galantamine or to placebo, each given in two divided doses (immediate release tablets). The 13-week study was divided into a 3-week dose titration phase and a 10-week maintenance phase. The patients in the active treatment arm of the study were maintained at either 24 mg/day or 32 mg/day at the discretion of the investigator.
Effects on the ADAS-cog:
Figure 10 illustrates the time course for the change from baseline in ADAS-cog scores for both dose groups over the 13 weeks of the study. At 13 weeks of treatment, the mean difference in the ADAS-cog change scores for the treated patients compared to the patients on placebo was 1.9. Galan-

tamine at a dose of 24-32 mg/day was statistically significantly superior to placebo.

Figure 10: Time-Course of the Change From Baseline in ADAS-cog Score for Patients Completing 13 Weeks of Treatment

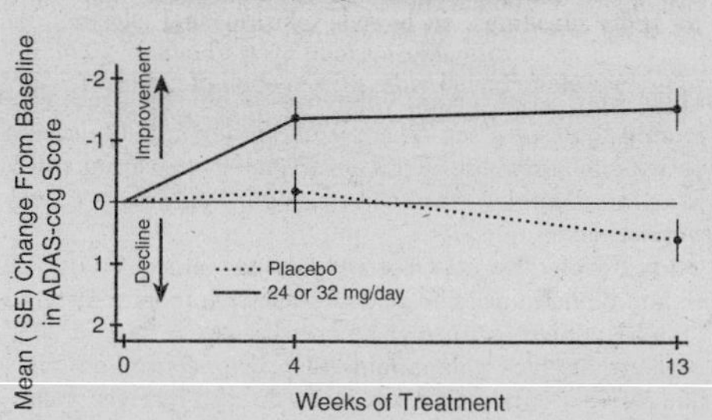

Figure 11 illustrates the cumulative percentages of patients from each of the two treatment groups who had attained at least the measure of improvement in ADAS-cog score shown on the X-axis. Three change scores (10-point, 7-point and 4-point reductions) and no change in score from baseline have been identified for illustrative purposes, and the percent of patients in each group achieving that result is shown in the inset table.

The curves demonstrate that both patients assigned to galantamine and placebo have a wide range of responses, but that the galantamine group is more likely to show the greater improvement.

Figure 11: Cumulative Percentage of Patients Completing 13 Weeks of Double-Blind Treatment With Specified Changes from Baseline in ADAS-cog Scores. The Percentages of Randomized Patients Who Completed the Study Were: Placebo 90%, 24-32 mg/day 67%.

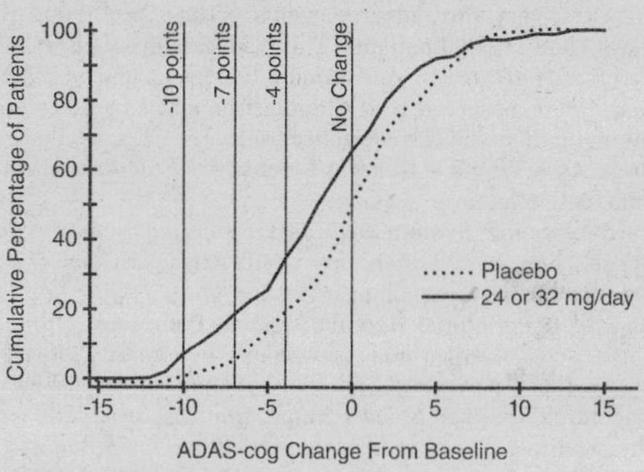

	Change in ADAS-cog			
Treatment	-10	-7	-4	0
Placebo	1.9%	5.6%	19.4%	50.0%
24 or 32 mg/day	7.1%	18.8%	32.9%	65.3%

Effects on the CIBIC-plus:

Figure 12 is a histogram of the percentage distribution of CIBIC-plus scores attained by patients assigned to each of the two treatment groups who completed 13 weeks of treatment. The mean galantamine-placebo differences for the group of patients in the mean rating of change from baseline was 0.37 units. The mean rating for the 24–32-mg/day group was statistically significantly superior to placebo.

Figure 12: Distribution of CIBIC-plus Ratings at Week 13

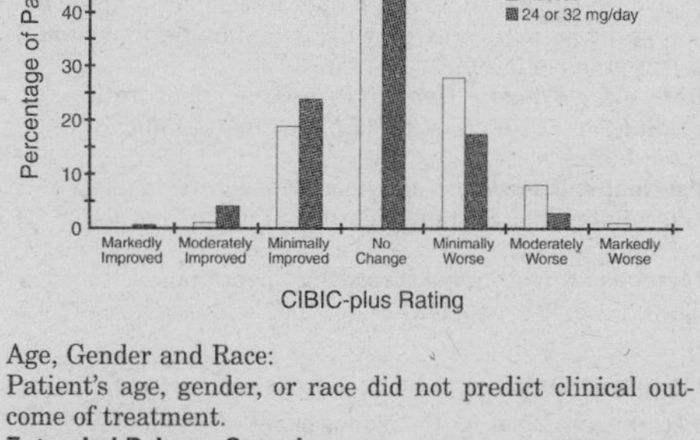

Age, Gender and Race:

Patient's age, gender, or race did not predict clinical outcome of treatment.

Extended Release Capsules

The efficacy of RAZADYNE™ ER extended-release capsules was studied in a randomized, double-blind, placebo-controlled trial which was 6 months in duration, and had an initial 4-week dose-escalation phase. In this trial, patients were assigned to one of 3 treatment groups: RAZADYNE™ ER extended-release capsules in a flexible dose of 16 to 24 mg once daily; RAZADYNE™ immediate-release tablets in a flexible dose of 8 to 12 mg twice daily; and placebo. The primary efficacy measures in this study were the ADAS-cog and CIBIC-plus. On the protocol-specified primary efficacy analysis at Month 6, a statistically significant improvement favoring RAZADYNE™ ER extended-release capsules over placebo was seen for the ADAS-cog, but not for the CIBIC-plus. RAZADYNE™ ER extended-release capsules showed a statistically significant improvement when compared with placebo on the Alzheimer's Disease Cooperative Study-Activities of Daily Living (ADCS-ADL) scale, a measure of function, and a secondary efficacy measure in this study. The effects of RAZADYNE™ ER extended release capsules and RAZADYNE™ immediate-release tablets on the ADAS-cog, CIBIC-plus, and ADCS-ADL were similar in this study.

INDICATIONS AND USAGE

RAZADYNE™ ER (galantamine hydrobromide) is indicated for the treatment of mild to moderate dementia of the Alzheimer's type.

CONTRAINDICATIONS

RAZADYNE™ ER (galantamine hydrobromide) is contraindicated in patients with known hypersensitivity to galantamine hydrobromide or to any excipients used in the formulation.

WARNINGS

Anesthesia

Galantamine, as a cholinesterase inhibitor, is likely to exaggerate the neuromuscular blocking effects of succinylcholine-type and similar neuromuscular blocking agents during anesthesia.

Cardiovascular Conditions

Because of their pharmacological action, cholinesterase inhibitors have vagotonic effects on the sinoatrial and atrioventricular nodes, leading to bradycardia and AV block. These actions may be particularly important to patients with supraventricular cardiac conduction disorders or to patients taking other drugs concomitantly that significantly slow heart rate. Postmarketing surveillance of marketed anticholinesterase inhibitors has shown, however, that bradycardia and all types of heart block have been reported in patients both with and without known underlying cardiac conduction abnormalities. Therefore all patients should be considered at risk for adverse effects on cardiac conduction.

In randomized controlled trials, bradycardia was reported more frequently in galantamine-treated patients than in placebo-treated patients, but was rarely severe and rarely led to treatment discontinuation. The overall frequency of this event was 2–3% for galantamine doses up to 24 mg/day compared with <1% for placebo. No increased incidence of heart block was observed at the recommended doses.

Patients treated with galantamine up to 24 mg/day using the recommended dosing schedule showed a dose-related increase in risk of syncope (placebo 0.7% [2/286]; 4 mg BID 0.4% [3/692]; 8 mg BID 1.3% [7/552]; 12 mg BID 2.2% [6/273]).

Gastrointestinal Conditions

Through their primary action, cholinomimetics may be expected to increase gastric acid secretion due to increased cholinergic activity. Therefore, patients should be monitored closely for symptoms of active or occult gastrointestinal bleeding, especially those with an increased risk for developing ulcers, e.g., those with a history of ulcer disease or patients using concurrent nonsteroidal anti-inflammatory drugs (NSAIDS). Clinical studies of galantamine have shown no increase, relative to placebo, in the incidence of either peptic ulcer disease or gastrointestinal bleeding.

Galantamine, as a predictable consequence of its pharmacological properties, has been shown to produce nausea, vomiting, diarrhea, anorexia, and weight loss (see **ADVERSE REACTIONS**).

Genitourinary

Although this was not observed in clinical trials with galantamine, cholinomimetics may cause bladder outflow obstruction.

Neurological Conditions

Seizures: Cholinesterase inhibitors are believed to have some potential to cause generalized convulsions. However, seizure activity may also be a manifestation of Alzheimer's disease. In clinical trials, there was no increase in the incidence of convulsions with galantamine compared to placebo.

Pulmonary Conditions

Because of its cholinomimetic action, galantamine should be prescribed with care to patients with a history of severe asthma or obstructive pulmonary disease.

PRECAUTIONS

Information for Patients and Caregivers:

Caregivers should be instructed about the recommended dosage and administration of RAZADYNE™ ER (galantamine hydrobromide). RAZADYNE™ ER extended-release capsules should be administered once daily in the morning, preferably with food (although not required).

Patients and caregivers should be advised that the most frequent adverse events associated with use of the drug can be minimized by following the recommended dosage and administration.

Patients and caregivers should be advised to ensure adequate fluid intake during treatment. If therapy has been interrupted for several days or longer, the patient should be restarted at the lowest dose and the dose escalated to the current dose.

Deaths in Subjects with Mild Cognitive Impairment (MCI)

In two randomized placebo controlled trials of 2 years duration in subjects with mild cognitive impairment (MCI), a total of 13 subjects on RAZADYNE™ (n=1026) and 1 subject on placebo (n=1022) died. The deaths were due to various causes which could be expected in an elderly population; about half of the RAZADYNE™ deaths appeared to result from various vascular causes (myocardial infarction, stroke, and sudden death).

Although the difference in mortality between RAZADYNE™ and placebo-treated groups in these two studies was significant, the results are highly discrepant with other studies of RAZADYNE™. Specifically, in these two MCI studies, the mortality rate in the placebo-treated subjects was markedly lower than the rate in placebo-treated patients in trials of RAZADYNE™ in Alzheimer's disease or other dementias (0.7 per 1000 person years compared to 22–61 per 1000 person years, respectively). Although the mortality rate in the RAZADYNE™-treated MCI subjects was also lower than that observed in RAZADYNE™-treated patients in Alzheimer's disease and other dementia trials (10.2 per 1000 person years compared to 23–31 per 1000 person years, respectively), the relative difference was much less. When the Alzheimer's disease and other dementia studies were pooled (n=6000), the mortality rate in the placebo group numerically exceeded that in the RAZADYNE™ group. Furthermore, in the MCI studies, no subjects in the placebo group died after 6 months, a highly unexpected finding in this population.

Individuals with mild cognitive impairment demonstrate isolated memory impairment greater than expected for their age and education, but do not meet current diagnostic criteria for Alzheimer's disease.

Special Populations

Hepatic Impairment

In patients with moderately impaired hepatic function, dose titration should proceed cautiously (see **CLINICAL PHARMACOLOGY** and **DOSAGE AND ADMINISTRATION**). The use of RAZADYNE™ ER in patients with severe hepatic impairment (Child-Pugh score of 10–15) is not recommended.

Renal Impairment

In patients with moderately impaired renal function, dose titration should proceed cautiously (see **CLINICAL PHARMACOLOGY** and **DOSAGE AND ADMINISTRATION**). In patients with severely impaired renal function (CL_{cr} < 9 mL/min) the use of RAZADYNE™ ER is not recommended.

Drug-Drug Interactions

Use With Anticholinergics

RAZADYNE™ ER has the potential to interfere with the activity of anticholinergic medications.

Use With Cholinomimetics and Other Cholinesterase Inhibitors

A synergistic effect is expected when cholinesterase inhibitors are given concurrently with succinylcholine, other cholinesterase inhibitors, similar neuromuscular blocking agents or cholinergic agonists such as bethanechol.

A) Effect of Other Drugs on Galantamine

In vitro

CYP3A4 and CYP2D6 are the major enzymes involved in the metabolism of galantamine. CYP3A4 mediated the formation of galantamine-N-oxide; CYP2D6 leads to the formation of O-desmethyl-galantamine. Because galantamine is also glucuronidated and excreted unchanged, no single pathway appears predominant.

In vivo

Cimetidine and Ranitidine: Galantamine was administered as a single dose of 4 mg on day 2 of a 3-day treatment with either cimetidine (800 mg daily) or ranitidine (300 mg daily). Cimetidine increased the bioavailability of galantamine by approximately 16%. Ranitidine had no effect on the PK of galantamine.

Ketoconazole: Ketoconazole, a strong inhibitor of CYP3A4 and an inhibitor of CYP2D6, at a dose of 200 mg BID for 4 days, increased the AUC of galantamine by 30%.

Erythromycin: Erythromycin, a moderate inhibitor of CYP3A4 at a dose of 500 mg QID for 4 days, affected the AUC of galantamine minimally (10% increase).

Paroxetine: Paroxetine, a strong inhibitor of CYP2D6, at 20 mg/day for 16 days, increased the oral bioavailability of galantamine by about 40%.

B) Effect of Galantamine on Other Drugs

In vitro

Galantamine did not inhibit the metabolic pathways catalyzed by CYP1A2, CYP2A6, CYP3A4, CYP4A, CYP2C, CYP2D6 or CYP2E1. This indicates that the inhibitory potential of galantamine towards the major forms of cytochrome P450 is very low.

In vivo

Warfarin: Galantamine at 24 mg/day had no effect on the pharmacokinetics of R-and-S-warfarin (25 mg single dose) or on the prothrombin time. The protein binding of warfarin was unaffected by galantamine.

Digoxin: Galantamine at 24 mg/day had no effect on the steady-state pharmacokinetics of digoxin (0.375 mg once daily) when they were coadministered. In this study, however, one healthy subject was hospitalized for 2nd and 3rd degree heart block and bradycardia.

Carcinogenesis, Mutagenesis and Impairment of Fertility

In a 24-month oral carcinogenicity study in rats, a slight increase in endometrial adenocarcinomas was observed at 10 mg/kg/day (4 times the Maximum Recommended Human Dose [MRHD] on a mg/m^2 basis or 6 times on an exposure [AUC] basis and 30 mg/kg/day (12 times MRHD on a mg/m^2 basis or 19 times on an AUC basis). No increase in neoplastic changes was observed in females at 2.5 mg/kg/day (equivalent to the MRHD on a mg/m^2 basis or 2 times on an AUC basis) or in males up to the highest dose tested of 30 mg/kg/day (12 times the MRHD on a mg/m^2 and AUC basis).

Galantamine was not carcinogenic in a 6-month oral carcinogenicity study in transgenic (P 53-deficient) mice up to 20 mg/kg/day, or in a 24-month oral carcinogenicity study in

Continued on next page

Razadyne ER—Cont.

male and female mice up to 10 mg/kg/day (2 times the MRHD on a mg/m^2 basis and equivalent on an AUC basis). Galantamine produced no evidence of genotoxic potential when evaluated in the *in vitro* Ames *S. typhimurium* or *E. coli* reverse mutation assay, *in vitro* mouse lymphoma assay, *in vivo* micronucleus test in mice, or *in vitro* chromosome aberration assay in Chinese hamster ovary cells.
No impairment of fertility was seen in rats given up to 16 mg/kg/day (7 times the MRHD on a mg/m^2 basis) for 14 days prior to mating in females and for 60 days prior to mating in males.

Pregnancy

Pregnancy Category B: In a study in which rats were dosed from day 14 (females) or day 60 (males) prior to mating through the period of organogenesis, a slightly increased incidence of skeletal variations was observed at doses of 8 mg/kg/day (3 times the Maximum Recommended Human Dose [MRHD] on a mg/m^2 basis) and 16 mg/kg/day. In a study in which pregnant rats were dosed from the beginning of organogenesis through day 21 post-partum, pup weights were decreased at 8 and 16 mg/kg/day, but no adverse effects on other postnatal developmental parameters were seen. The doses causing the above effects in rats produced slight maternal toxicity. No major malformations were caused in rats given up to 16 mg/kg/day. No drug related teratogenic effects were observed in rabbits given up to 40 mg/kg/day (32 times the MRHD on a mg/m^2 basis) during the period of organogenesis.
There are no adequate and well-controlled studies of RAZADYNE™ ER in pregnant women. RAZADYNE™ ER should be used during pregnancy only if the potential benefit justifies the potential risk to the fetus.

Nursing Mothers

It is not known whether galantamine is excreted in human breast milk. RAZADYNE™ ER has no indication for use in nursing mothers.

Pediatric Use

There are no adequate and well-controlled trials documenting the safety and efficacy of galantamine in any illness occurring in children. Therefore, use of RAZADYNE™ ER in children is not recommended.

ADVERSE REACTIONS

Pre-Marketing Clinical Trial Experience:

The specific adverse event data described in this section are based on studies of the immediate release tablet formulation. In clinical trials, once-daily treatment with RAZADYNE™ ER (galantamine hydrobromide) extended-release capsules was well tolerated and adverse events were similar to those seen with galantamine immediate-release tablets.

Adverse Events Leading to Discontinuation:

In two large scale, placebo-controlled trials of 6 months duration, in which patients were titrated weekly from 8 to 16 to 24, and to 32 mg/day, the risk of discontinuation because of an adverse event in the galantamine group exceeded that in the placebo group by about threefold. In contrast, in a 5-month trial with escalation of the dose by 8 mg/day every 4 weeks, the overall risk of discontinuation because of an adverse event was 7%, 7%, and 10% for the placebo, galantamine 16 mg/day, and galantamine 24 mg/day groups, respectively, with gastrointestinal adverse effects the principle reason for discontinuing galantamine. Table 1 shows the most frequent adverse events leading to discontinuation in this study.

Table 1: Most Frequent Adverse Events Leading to Discontinuation in a Placebo-Controlled, Double-Blind Trial With a 4-Week Dose Escalation Schedule

	4-Week Escalation		
	Placebo	16 mg/day	24 mg/day
Adverse Event	N=286	N=279	N=273
Nausea	<1%	2%	4%
Vomiting	0%	1%	3%
Anorexia	<1%	1%	<1%
Dizziness	<1%	2%	1%
Syncope	0%	0%	1%

Adverse Events Reported in Controlled Trials:

The reported adverse events in trials using galantamine immediate-release tablets reflect experience gained under closely monitored conditions in a highly selected patient population. In actual practice or in other clinical trials, these frequency estimates may not apply, as the conditions of use, reporting behavior and the types of patients treated may differ.
The majority of these adverse events occurred during the dose-escalation period. In those patients who experienced the most frequent adverse event, nausea, the median duration of the nausea was 5–7 days.
Administration of galantamine with food, the use of antiemetic medication, and ensuring adequate fluid intake may reduce the impact of these events.
The most frequent adverse events, defined as those occurring at a frequency of at least 5% and at least twice the rate on placebo with the recommended maintenance dose of either 16 or 24 mg/day of galantamine under conditions of every 4 week dose-escalation for each dose increment of 8 mg/day, are shown in Table 2. These events were primarily gastrointestinal and tended to be less frequent with the 16 mg/day recommended initial maintenance dose.

Table 2: The Most Frequent Adverse Events in the Placebo-Controlled Trial With Dose Escalation Every 4 Weeks Occurring in at Least 5% of Patients Receiving Galantamine Immediate-Release Tablets and at Least Twice the Rate on Placebo.

Adverse Event	Placebo N=286	Galantamine 16 mg/day N=279	Galantamine 24 mg/day N=273
Nausea	5%	13%	17%
Vomiting	1%	6%	10%
Diarrhea	6%	12%	6%
Anorexia	3%	7%	9%
Weight decrease	1%	5%	5%

Table 3: The most common adverse events (adverse events occurring with an incidence of at least 2% in treatment with galantamine immediate release tablets and in which the incidence was greater than with placebo treatment) are listed in Table 3 for four placebo-controlled trials for patients treated with 16 or 24 mg/day of galantamine.

Table 3: Adverse Events Reported in at Least 2% of Patients With Alzheimer's Disease Administered Galantamine Immediate-Release Tablets and at a Frequency Greater Than With Placebo

Body System Adverse Event	Placebo (N=801)	Galantamine[a] (N=1040)
Body as a whole - general disorders		
Fatigue	3%	5%
Syncope	1%	2%
Central & peripheral nervous system disorders		
Dizziness	6%	9%
Headache	5%	8%
Tremor	2%	3%
Gastrointestinal system disorders		
Nausea	9%	24%
Vomiting	4%	13%
Diarrhea	7%	9%
Abdominal pain	4%	5%
Dyspepsia	2%	5%
Heart rate and rhythm disorders		
Bradycardia	1%	2%
Metabolic and nutritional disorders		
Weight decrease	2%	7%
Psychiatric disorders		
Anorexia	3%	9%
Depression	5%	7%
Insomnia	4%	5%
Somnolence	3%	4%
Red blood cell disorders		
Anemia	2%	3%
Respiratory system disorders		
Rhinitis	3%	4%
Urinary system disorders		
Urinary tract infection	7%	8%
Hematuria	2%	3%

a: Adverse events in patients treated with 16 or 24 mg/day of galantamine in four placebo-controlled trials are included.

Adverse events occurring with an incidence of at least 2% in placebo-treated patients that was either equal to or greater than galantamine treatment were constipation, agitation, confusion, anxiety, hallucination, injury, back pain, peripheral edema, asthenia, chest pain, urinary incontinence, upper respiratory tract infection, bronchitis, coughing, hypertension, fall, and purpura.
There were no important differences in adverse event rate related to dose or sex. There were too few non-Caucasian patients to assess the effects of race on adverse event rates. No clinically relevant abnormalities in laboratory values were observed.

Other Adverse Events Observed During Clinical Trials

Galantamine immediate-release tablets were administered to 3055 patients with Alzheimer's disease. A total of 2357 patients received galantamine in placebo-controlled trials and 761 patients with Alzheimer's disease received galantamine 24 mg/day, the maximum recommended maintenance dose. About 1000 patients received galantamine for at least one year and approximately 200 patients received galantamine for two years.
To establish the rate of adverse events, data from all patients for any dose of galantamine in 8 placebo-controlled trials and 6 open-label extension trials were pooled. The methodology to gather and codify these adverse events was standardized across trials, using WHO terminology. All adverse events occurring in approximately 0.1% are included, except for those already listed elsewhere in labeling, WHO terms too general to be informative, or events unlikely to be drug caused. Events are classified by body system and listed using the following definitions: frequent adverse events - those occurring in at least 1/100 patients; infrequent adverse events - those occurring in 1/100 to 1/1000 patients; rare adverse events - those occurring in 1/1000 to 1/10000 patients; very rare adverse events – those occurring in fewer than 1/10000 patients. These adverse events are not necessarily related to galantamine treatment and in most cases were observed at a similar frequency in placebo-treated patients in the controlled studies.

Body As a Whole – General Disorders: *Frequent:* chest pain, asthenia, fever, malaise

Cardiovascular System Disorders: *Infrequent:* postural hypotension, hypotension, dependent edema, cardiac failure, myocardial ischemia or infarction

Central & Peripheral Nervous System Disorders: *Infrequent:* vertigo, hypertonia, convulsions, involuntary muscle contractions, paresthesia, ataxia, hypokinesia, hyperkinesia, apraxia, aphasia, leg cramps, tinnitus, transient ischemic attack or cerebrovascular accident

Gastrointestinal System Disorders: *Frequent:* flatulence; *Infrequent:* gastritis, melena, dysphagia, rectal hemorrhage, dry mouth, saliva increased, diverticulitis, gastroenteritis, hiccup; *Rare:* esophageal perforation

Heart Rate & Rhythm Disorders: *Infrequent:* AV block, palpitation, atrial arrhythmias including atrial fibrillation and supraventricular tachycardia, QT prolonged, bundle branch block, T-wave inversion, ventricular tachycardia; *Rare:* severe bradycardia

Metabolic & Nutritional Disorders: *Infrequent:* hyperglycemia, alkaline phosphatase increased

Platelet, Bleeding & Clotting Disorders: *Infrequent:* purpura, epistaxis, thrombocytopenia

Psychiatric Disorders: *Infrequent:* apathy, paroniria, paranoid reaction, libido increased, delirium; *Rare:* suicidal ideation; *Very rare:* suicide

Urinary System Disorders: *Frequent:* incontinence; *Infrequent:* hematuria, micturition frequency, cystitis, urinary retention, nocturia, renal calculi

Post-Marketing Experience:

Other adverse events from post-approval controlled and uncontrolled clinical trials and post-marketing experience observed in patients treated with galantamine immediate-release tablets include:

Body As a Whole – General Disorders: dehydration (including rare, severe cases leading to renal insufficiency and renal failure)

Psychiatric Disorders: aggression

Gastrointestinal System Disorders: upper and lower GI bleeding

Metabolic & Nutritional Disorders: hypokalemia

These adverse events may or may not be causally related to the drug.

OVERDOSAGE

Because strategies for the management of overdose are continually evolving, it is advisable to contact a poison control center to determine the latest recommendations for the management of an overdose of any drug.
As in any case of overdose, general supportive measures should be utilized. Signs and symptoms of significant overdosing of galantamine are predicted to be similar to those of overdosing of other cholinomimetics. These effects generally involve the central nervous system, the parasympathetic nervous system, and the neuromuscular junction. In addition to muscle weakness or fasciculations, some or all of the following signs of cholinergic crisis may develop: severe nausea, vomiting, gastrointestinal cramping, salivation, lacrimation, urination, defecation, sweating, bradycardia, hypotension, respiratory depression, collapse and convulsions. Increasing muscle weakness is a possibility and may result in death if respiratory muscles are involved.

Tertiary anticholinergics such as atropine may be used as an antidote for galantamine overdosage. Intravenous atropine sulfate titrated to effect is recommended at an initial dose of 0.5 to 1.0 mg i.v. with subsequent doses based upon clinical response. Atypical responses in blood pressure and heart rate have been reported with other cholinomimetics when coadministered with quaternary anticholinergics. It is not known whether galantamine and/or its metabolites can be removed by dialysis (hemodialysis, peritoneal dialysis, or hemofiltration). Dose-related signs of toxicity in animals included hypoactivity, tremors, clonic convulsions, salivation, lacrimation, chromodacryorrhea, mucoid feces, and dyspnea.

In one postmarketing report, one patient who had been taking 4 mg of galantamine daily for a week inadvertently ingested eight 4 mg immediate-release tablets (32 mg total) on a single day. Subsequently, she developed bradycardia, QT prolongation, ventricular tachycardia and torsades de pointes accompanied by a brief loss of consciousness for which she required hospital treatment. Two additional cases of accidental ingestion of 32 mg (nausea, vomiting, and dry mouth; nausea, vomiting, and substernal chest pain) and one of 40 mg (vomiting), resulted in brief hospitalizations for observation with full recovery. One patient who was prescribed 24 mg/day and had a history of hallucinations over the previous two years, mistakenly received 24 mg twice daily for 34 days and developed hallucinations requiring hospitalization. Another patient, who was prescribed 16 mg/day of oral solution, inadvertently ingested 160 mg (40 mL) and experienced sweating, vomiting, bradycardia, and near-syncope one hour later, which necessitated hospital treatment. His symptoms resolved within 24 hours.

DOSAGE AND ADMINISTRATION

The dosage of RAZADYNE™ ER (galantamine hydrobromide) shown to be effective in a controlled clinical trial is 16–24 mg/day.

The recommended starting dose of RAZADYNE™ ER is 8 mg/day. The dose should be increased to the initial maintenance dose of 16 mg/day after a minimum of 4 weeks. A further increase to 24 mg/day should be attempted after a minimum of 4 weeks at 16 mg/day. Dose increases should be based upon assessment of clinical benefit and tolerability of the previous dose.

RAZADYNE™ ER should be administered once daily in the morning, preferably with food.

Patients and caregivers should be advised to ensure adequate fluid intake during treatment. If therapy has been interrupted for several days or longer, the patient should be restarted at the lowest dose and the dose escalated to the current dose.

The abrupt withdrawal of RAZADYNE™ ER in those patients who had been receiving doses in the effective range was not associated with an increased frequency of adverse events in comparison with those continuing to receive the same doses of that drug. The beneficial effects of RAZADYNE™ ER are lost, however, when the drug is discontinued.

Doses in Special Populations

Galantamine plasma concentrations may be increased in patients with moderate to severe hepatic impairment. In patients with moderately impaired hepatic function (Child-Pugh score of 7–9), the dose should generally not exceed 16 mg/day. The use of RAZADYNE™ ER in patients with severe hepatic impairment (Child-Pugh score of 10–15) is not recommended.

For patients with moderate renal impairment the dose should generally not exceed 16 mg/day. In patients with severe renal impairment (creatinine clearance < 9 mL/min), the use of RAZADYNE™ ER is not recommended.

HOW SUPPLIED

RAZADYNE™ ER (galantamine hydrobromide) extended-release capsules contain white to off-white pellets.

8 mg white opaque, size 4 hard gelatin capsules with the inscription "GAL 8."

16 mg pink opaque, size 2 hard gelatin capsules with the inscription "GAL 16."

24 mg caramel opaque, size 1 hard gelatin capsules with the inscription "GAL 24."

The capsules are supplied as follows:

8 mg capsules – bottles of 30 NDC 50458-387-30

16 mg capsules – bottles of 30 NDC 50458-388-30

24 mg capsules – bottles of 30 NDC 50458-389-30

Storage and Handling

RAZADYNE™ ER extended-release capsules should be stored at 25°C (77°F); excursions permitted to 15–30°C (59–86°F) [see USP Controlled Room Temperature].

Keep out of reach of children.

RAZADYNE™ ER extended-release capsules are manufactured by:

JOLLC, Gurabo, Puerto Rico

RAZADYNE™ ER extended-release capsules are distributed by:

ORTHO-McNEIL NEUROLOGICS, INC.

Titusville, NJ 08560

10005601 Issued April 2005

US Patent No. 4,663,318

01-RM-605

ORTHO-McNEIL NEUROLOGICS, INC.

OrthoNeutrogena Division of Ortho-McNeil Pharmaceuticals, Inc.

5760 WEST 96th STREET
LOS ANGELES, CA 90045

For Medical Information Contact:
Dermatological Medical Information
(800) 426-7762

CENTANY™ ℞

[*sĕn-tă-nē*]
(mupirocin ointment), 2%
Rx only
For Dermatologic Use

DESCRIPTION

Each gram of Centany (mupirocin ointment), 2% contains 20 mg mupirocin in a soft white ointment base consisting of castor oil, oleyl alcohol, hard fat (Softisan® 378) and propylene glycol monostearate. Mupirocin is a naturally occurring antibiotic. The chemical name is (E)-(2*S*,3*R*,4*R*,5*S*)-5-[(2*S*,3*S*,4*S*,5*S*)-2,3-Epoxy-5-hydroxy-4-methylhexyl]tetrahydro-3,4-dihydroxy-β-methyl-2 *H*-pyran-2-crotonic acid, ester with 9-hydroxynonanoic acid. The molecular formula of mupirocin is $C_{26}H_{44}O_9$ and the molecular weight is 500.63. The chemical structure is:

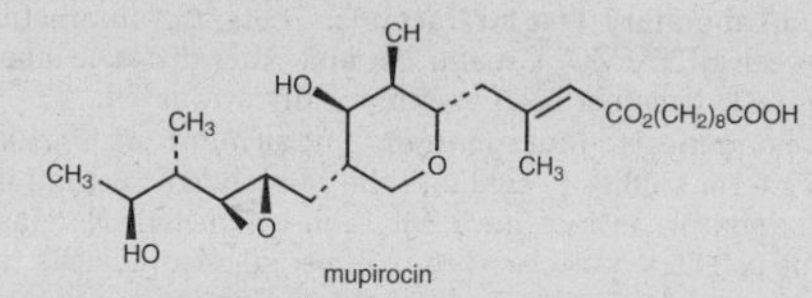

mupirocin

CLINICAL PHARMACOLOGY

Following the application of Centany (mupirocin ointment), 2% to a 400 cm^2 area on the back of 23 healthy volunteers once daily for 7 days, the mean (range) cumulative urinary excretion of monic acid over 24 hrs following the last administration was 1.25% (0.2% to 3.0%) of the administered dose of mupirocin. The monic acid concentration in urine collected at specified intervals for 24 hrs on Day 7 ranged from <0.050 to 0.637 µg/mL.

Microbiology: Mupirocin is an antibacterial agent produced by fermentation using the organism *Pseudomonas fluorescens*. Its spectrum of activity includes gram-positive baceria. It is also active, *in vitro* only, against certain gram-negative bacteria. Mupirocin inhibits bacterial protein synthesis by reversibly and specifically binding to bacterial isoleucyl transfer-RNA synthetase. Due to this unique mode of action, mupirocin does not demonstrate cross-resistance with other classes of antimicrobial agents.

When mupirocin resistance occurs, it results from the production of a modified isoleucyl-tRNA synthetase or the acquisition, by genetic transfer, of a plasmid mediating a new isoleucyl-tRNA synthetase. High-level plasmid-mediated resistance (MIC > 500 mcg/mL) has been reported in increasing numbers of isolates of *Staphylococcus aureus* and with higher frequency in coagulase-negative staphylococci. Methicillin resistance and mupirocin resistance commonly occur together in *Staphylococcus aureus* and coagulase-negative staphylococci.

Mupirocin is bactericidal at concentrations achieved by topical administration. However, the minimum bactericidal concentration (MBC) against relevant pathogens is generally eight-fold to thirty-fold higher than the minimum inhibitory concentration (MIC). In addition, mupirocin is highly protein bound (>97%), and the effect of wound secretions on the MICs of mupirocin has not been determined.

Mupirocin has been shown to be active against susceptible strains of *Staphylococcus aureus* and *Streptococcus pyogenes*, both *in vitro* and in clinical studies. (See **INDICATIONS AND USAGE.**)

INDICATIONS AND USAGE

Centany (mupirocin ointment), 2% is indicated for the topical treatment of impetigo due to: *Staphylococcus aureus* and *Streptococcus pyogenes*.

CONTRAINDICATIONS

This drug is contraindicated in individuals with a history of sensitivity reactions to any of its components.

WARNINGS

Centany (mupirocin ointment), 2% is not for ophthalmic use.

PRECAUTIONS

If a reaction suggesting sensitivity or chemical irritation should occur with the use of Centany (mupirocin ointment), 2%, treatment should be discontinued and appropriate alternative therapy for the infection instituted.

As with other antibacterial products, prolonged use may result in overgrowth of nonsusceptible organisms, including fungi. Centany (mupirocin ointment), 2% is not formulated for use on mucosal surfaces. Centany (mupirocin ointment), 2% is not intended for nasal use.

Information for Patients: Use this medication only as directed by your healthcare provider. It is for external use only. Avoid contact with the eyes. The medication should be stopped and your healthcare practitioner contacted if irritation, severe itching or rash occurs. If impetigo has not improved in 3 to 5 days, contact your healthcare practitioner.

Drug Interactions: The effect of the concurrent application of Centany (mupirocin ointment), 2% and other drug products is unknown.

Carcinogenesis, Mutagenesis, Impairment of Fertility: Long-term studies in animals to evaluate carcinogenic potential of mupirocin have not been conducted.

Results of the following studies performed with mupirocin calcium or mupirocin sodium *in vitro* and *in vivo* did not indicate a potential for genotoxicity: rat primary hepatocyte unscheduled DNA synthesis, sediment analysis for DNA strand breaks, *Salmonella* reversion test (Ames), *Escherichia coli* mutation assay, metaphase analysis of human lymphocytes, mouse lymphoma assay, and bone marrow micronuclei assay in mice.

Reproduction studies were performed in male and female rats with mupirocin adminisered subcutaneously at doses up to 14 times the human topical dose (approximately 60 mg mupirocin/day) on a mg/m^2 basis and revealed neither evidence of impaired fertility nor impaired reproductive performance attributable to mupirocin.

Pregnancy

Teratogenic Effects.

Pregnancy Category B: Reproduction studies have been performed in rats and rabbits with mupirocin administered subcutaneously at doses up to 22 and 43 times, respectively, the human topical dose (approximately 60 mg mupirocin per day) on a mg/m^2 basis and revealed no evidence of harm to the fetus due to mupirocin. There are, however, no adequate and well-controlled studies in pregnant women. Because animal studies are not always predictive of human response, this drug should be used during pregnancy only if clearly needed.

Nursing Mothers: It is not known whether this drug is excreted in human milk. Because many drugs are excreted in human milk, caution should be exercised when Centany (mupirocin ointment), 2% is administered to a nursing woman.

Pediatric Use: The safety and effectiveness of Centany (mupirocin ointment), 2% have been established in the age range of 2 months to 16 years. Use of Centany (mupirocin ointment), 2% in these age groups is supported by evidence from adequate and well-controlled studies of Centany (mupirocin ointment), 2% in impetigo in pediatric patients studied as a part of the pivotal clinical trials. (See **CLINICAL STUDIES.**)

ADVERSE REACTIONS

The following local adverse reactions have been reported in connection with the use of Centany (mupirocin ointment), 2%; application site reactions and pruritus, each in 1% of patients; contact dermatitis and furunculosis, each in 0.7% of patients; and exfoliative dermatitis and rash, each in 0.3% of patients.

DOSAGE AND ADMINISTRATION

A small amount of Centany (mupirocin ointment), 2% should be applied to the affected area three times daily. The area treated may be covered with a gauze dressing if desired. Patients not showing a clinical response within 3 to 5 days should be re-evaluated.

CLINICAL STUDIES

The efficacy of topical Centany (mupirocin ointment), 2% in impetigo was tested in one study. Patients with impetigo were randomized to receive either Centany (mupirocin ointment, 2%) or Bactroban® Ointment (mupirocin ointment, 2%) t.i.d. for 7 days. Clinical efficacy rates at the follow-up visit (one week after end of therapy) in the evaluable populations (adults and pediatric patients included) were 94% for Centany (mupirocin ointment, 2%) (n=233) and 95% for Bactroban® Ointment (mupirocin ointment, 2%) (n=242). Pathogen eradication rates at follow-up for both medications were 98%.

Pediatrics: There were 413 pediatric patients aged 2 months to 15 years in the clinical study described above. Clinical efficacy rates at follow-up in the evaluable populations were 93% for Centany (mupirocin ointment, 2%) (n=199) and 95% for Bactroban® Ointment (mupirocin ointment, 2%) (n=214).

HOW SUPPLIED

Centany (mupirocin ointment), 2% is supplied in 15 gram (NDC 0062-1610-01) and 30 gram (NDC 0062-1610-03) tubes.

Store at controlled room temperature 20° to 25°C (68° to 77°F).

OrthoNeutrogena

Distributed by: OrthoNeutrogena, Division of Ortho-McNeil Pharmaceutical, Inc.

Skillman, New Jersey 08558 ©OMP 2003 Issued May, 2003

Printed in USA

635-10-686-1 I473ONG-2

ERTACZO® ℞

[*ər'tăz-ō*]
(sertaconazole nitrate) cream, 2%
For Topical Dermatologic Use Only - Not for Oral, Ophthalmic or Intravaginal Use

DESCRIPTION

ERTACZO® (sertaconazole nitrate) Cream, 2%, contains the imidazole antifungal, sertaconazole nitrate. Sertaconazole

Continued on next page

Ertaczo—Cont.

nitrate contains one asymmetric carbon atom and exists as a racemic mixture of equal amounts of R and S enantiomers.
Sertaconazole nitrate is designated chemically as (±)-1-[2,4-dichloro-β-[(7-chlorobenzo-[*b*]thien-3-yl) methoxy]phenethyl]imidazole nitrate. It has a molecular weight of 500.8. The molecular formula is $C_{20}H_{15}Cl_3N_2OS \cdot HNO_3$, and the structural formula is as follows:

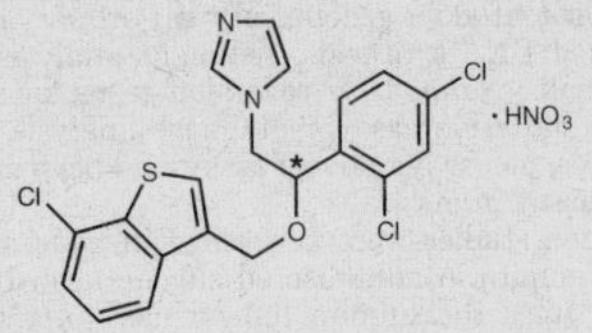

Sertaconazole nitrate is a white or almost white powder. It is practically insoluble in water, soluble in methanol, sparingly soluble in alcohol and in methylene chloride. Each gram of ERTACZO® Cream, 2%, contains 17.5 mg of sertaconazole (as sertaconazole nitrate, 20 mg) in a white cream base of ethylene glycol and polyethylene glycol palmitostearate, glyceryl isostearate, light mineral oil, methylparaben, polyoxyethylened saturated glycerides and glycolized saturated glycerides, sorbic acid and purified water.

CLINICAL PHARMACOLOGY

Pharmacokinetics: In a multiple dose pharmacokinetic study that included 5 male patients with interdigital tinea pedis (range of diseased area, 42-140 cm^2; mean, 93 cm^2), ERTACZO® Cream, 2%, was topically applied every 12 hours for a total of 13 doses to the diseased skin (0.5 grams sertaconazole nitrate per 100 cm^2). Sertaconazole concentrations in plasma measured by serial blood sampling for 72 hours after the thirteenth dose were below the limit of quantitation (2.5 ng/mL) of the analytical method used.
Microbiology: Sertaconazole is an antifungal that belongs to the imidazole class of antifungals. While the exact mechanism of action of this class of antifungals is not known, it is believed that they act primarily by inhibiting the cytochrome P450-dependent synthesis of ergosterol. Ergosterol is a key component of the cell membrane of fungi, and lack of this component leads to fungal cell injury primarily by leakage of key constituents in the cytoplasm from the cell.
Activity *In Vivo*: Sertaconazole nitrate has been shown to be active against isolates of the following microorganisms in clinical infections as described in the INDICATIONS AND USAGE section:

Trichophyton rubrum
Trichophyton mentagrophytes
Epidermophyton floccosum

CLINICAL STUDIES

In two randomized, double-blind, clinical trials, patients 12 years and older with interdigital tinea pedis applied either ERTACZO® Cream, 2%, or vehicle, twice daily for four weeks. Patients with moccasin-type (plantar) tinea pedis and/or onychomycosis were excluded from the study. Two weeks after completion of therapy (six weeks after beginning therapy), patients were evaluated for signs and symptoms related to interdigital tinea pedis.
Treatment outcomes are summarized in the table below.
[See table below]
In clinical trials, complete cure in sertaconazole treated patients was achieved in 32 of 160 (20%) patients with *Trichophyton rubrum*, in 7 of 28 (25%) patients with *Trichophyton mentagrophytes* and in 2 of 13 (15%) patients with *Epidermophyton floccosum*.

INDICATIONS AND USAGE

ERTACZO® (sertaconazole nitrate) Cream, 2%, is indicated for the topical treatment of interdigital tinea pedis in immunocompetent patients 12 years of age and older, caused by: *Trichophyton rubrum, Trichophyton mentagrophytes, and Epidermophyton floccosum* (see CLINICAL STUDIES Section).

CONTRAINDICATIONS

ERTACZO® Cream, 2%, is contraindicated in patients who have a known or suspected sensitivity to sertaconazole nitrate or any of its components or to other imidazoles.

WARNINGS

ERTACZO® Cream, 2%, is not indicated for ophthalmic, oral or intravaginal use.

PRECAUTIONS

General: ERTACZO® Cream, 2%, is for use on the skin only. If irritation or sensitivity develops with the use of ERTACZO® Cream, 2%, treatment should be discontinued and appropriate therapy instituted.
Diagnosis of the disease should be confirmed either by direct microscopic examination of infected superficial epidermal tissue in a solution of potassium hydroxide or by culture on an appropriate medium.
Physicians should exercise caution when prescribing ERTACZO® Cream, 2%, to patients known to be sensitive to imidazole antifungals, since cross-reactivity may occur.
Information for Patients: The patient should be instructed to:

1. Use ERTACZO® Cream, 2%, as directed by the physician. The hands should be washed after applying the medication to the affected area(s). Avoid contact with the eyes, nose, mouth and other mucous membranes. ERTACZO® Cream, 2%, is for external use only.
2. Dry the affected area(s) thoroughly before application, if you wish to use ERTACZO® Cream, 2%, after bathing.
3. Use the medication for the full treatment time recommended by the physician, even though symptoms may have improved. Notify the physician if there is no improvement after the end of the prescribed treatment period, or sooner, if the condition worsens.
4. Inform the physician if the area of application shows signs of increased irritation, redness, itching, burning, blistering, swelling or oozing.
5. Avoid the use of occlusive dressings unless otherwise directed by the physician.
6. Do not use this medication for any disorder other than that for which it was prescribed.

Drug/Laboratory Test Interactions: Potential interactions between ERTACZO® Cream, 2%, and other drugs or laboratory tests have not been systematically evaluated.
Carcinogenesis, Mutagenesis, Impairment of Fertility: Long-term studies to evaluate the carcinogenic potential of sertaconazole nitrate have not been conducted. No clastogenic potential was observed in a mouse micronucleus test. Sertaconazole nitrate was considered negative for sister chromatid exchange (SCE) in the *in vivo* mouse bone marrow SCE assay. There was no evidence that sertaconazole nitrate induced unscheduled DNA synthesis in rat primary hepatocyte cultures. Sertaconazole nitrate exhibited no toxicity or adverse effects on reproductive performance or fertility of male or female rats given up to 60 mg/kg/day orally by gastric intubation (16 times the maximum recommended human dose based on a body surface area comparison).
Pregnancy: Teratogenic Effects. Pregnancy Category C: Oral reproduction studies in rats and rabbits did not produce any evidence of maternal toxicity, embryotoxicity or teratogenicity of sertaconazole nitrate at an oral dose of 160 mg/kg/day (40 times (rats) and 80 times (rabbits) the maximum recommended human dose on a body surface area comparison). In an oral peri-postnatal study in rats, a reduction in live birth indices and an increase in the number of still-born pups was seen at 80 and 160 mg/kg/day.
There are no adequate and well-controlled studies that have been conducted on topically applied ERTACZO® Cream, 2%, in pregnant women. Because animal reproduction studies are not always predictive of human response, ERTACZO® Cream, 2%, should be used during pregnancy only if clearly needed.
Nursing Mothers: It is not known if sertaconazole is excreted in human milk. Because many drugs are excreted in human milk, caution should be exercised when prescribing ERTACZO® Cream, 2%, to a nursing woman.
Pediatric Use: The efficacy and safety of ERTACZO® Cream, 2%, have not been established in pediatric patients below the age of 12 years.
Geriatric Use: Clinical studies of ERTACZO® Cream, 2%, did not include sufficient numbers of subjects aged 65 and over to determine whether they respond differently from younger subjects.

ADVERSE EVENTS

In clinical trials, cutaneous adverse events occurred in 7 of 297 (2%) patients (2 of them severe) receiving ERTACZO® Cream, 2%, and in 7 of 291 (2%) patients (2 of them severe) receiving vehicle. These reported cutaneous adverse events included contact dermatitis, dry skin, burning skin, application site reaction and skin tenderness.
In a dermal sensitization study, 8 of 202 evaluable patients tested with ERTACZO® Cream, 2%, and 4 of 202 evaluable patients tested with vehicle, exhibited a slight erythematous reaction in the challenge phase. There was no evidence of cumulative irritation or contact sensitization in a repeated insult patch test involving 202 healthy volunteers.
In non-US post-marketing surveillance for ERTACZO® Cream, 2%, the following cutaneous adverse events were reported: contact dermatitis, erythema, pruritus, vesiculation, desquamation, and hyperpigmentation.

OVERDOSAGE

Overdosage with ERTACZO® Cream, 2%, has not been reported to date. ERTACZO® Cream, 2%, is intended for topical dermatologic use only. It is not for oral, ophthalmic, or intravaginal use.

DOSAGE AND ADMINISTRATION

In the treatment of interdigital tinea pedis, ERTACZO® Cream, 2%, should be applied twice daily for 4 weeks. Sufficient ERTACZO® Cream, 2%, should be applied to cover both the affected areas between the toes and the immediately surrounding healthy skin of patients with interdigital tinea pedis. If a patient shows no clinical improvement 2 weeks after the treatment period, the diagnosis should be reviewed.

HOW SUPPLIED

ERTACZO® Cream, 2%, is supplied in tubes in the following size:

30-gram tube NDC 0062-1650-03

Store at 25°C (77°F); excursions permitted to 15°-30°C (59°-86°F) [see USP Controlled Room Temperature].
Rx only.
Patent No. 5,135,943
Distributed By:
OrthoNeutrogena
DIVISION OF ORTHO-McNEIL PHARMACEUTICAL, INC.
Skillman, New Jersey 08558
Revised December 2003 128008

Treatment Outcomes as Percent (%) of Total Subjects

	Study 1		Study 2	
	Sertaconazole	Vehicle	Sertaconazole	Vehicle
Complete Cure* (Primary Efficacy Variable)	13/99 (13.1%)	3/92 (3.3%)	28/103 (27.2%)	5/103 (4.9%)
Effective Treatment**	32/99 (32.3%)	11/92 (12.0%)	52/103 (50.5%)	16/103 (15.5%)
Mycological Cure***	49/99 (49.5%)	18/92 (19.6%)	71/103 (68.9%)	20/103 (19.4%)

* Complete Cure - Patients who had complete clearing of signs and symptoms and Mycological Cure.
** Effective Treatment - Patients who had minimal residual signs and symptoms of interdigital tinea pedis and Mycological Cure.
*** Mycological Cure - Patients who had both negative microscopic KOH preparation and a negative fungal culture.

OSI Pharmaceuticals, Inc.

SUITE 110
58 SOUTH SERVICE ROAD
MELVILLE, NY 11747
(631) 962-2000

For Medical Information Contact:
(800) 572-1932
medical-information@osip.com

Or write:
Medical Information
OSI Pharmaceuticals, Inc.
2860 Wilderness Place
Boulder, CO 80301

TARCEVA™ ℞

[*tar-se-va*]
(erlotinib)
Tablets
Rx only

DESCRIPTION

TARCEVA (erlotinib) is a Human Epidermal Growth Factor Receptor Type 1/Epidermal Growth Factor Receptor (HER1/EGFR) tyrosine kinase inhibitor. Erlotinib is a quinazolinamine with the chemical name N-(3-ethynylphenyl)-6,7-bis(2-methoxyethoxy)-4-quinazolinamine. TARCEVA contains erlotinib as the hydrochloride salt which has the following structural formula:

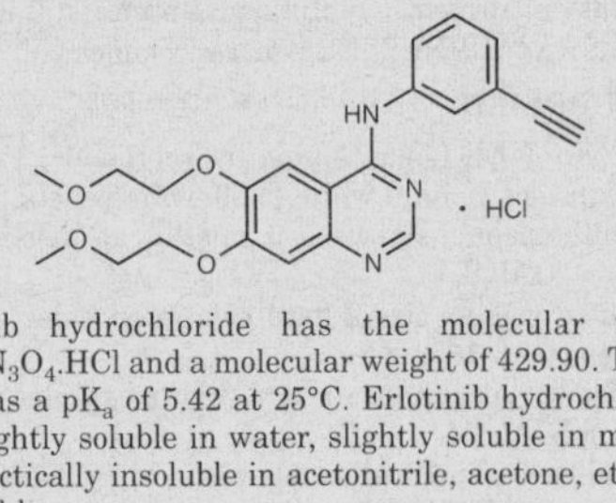

Erlotinib hydrochloride has the molecular formula $C_{22}H_{23}N_3O_4$.HCl and a molecular weight of 429.90. The molecule has a pK_a of 5.42 at 25°C. Erlotinib hydrochloride is very slightly soluble in water, slightly soluble in methanol and practically insoluble in acetonitrile, acetone, ethyl acetate and hexane.
Aqueous solubility of erlotinib hydrochloride is dependent on pH with increased solubility at a pH of less than 5 due to protonation of the secondary amine. Over the pH range of 1.4 to 9.6, maximal solubility of approximately 0.4 mg/mL occurs at a pH of approximately 2.
TARCEVA tablets are available in three dosage strengths containing erlotinib hydrochloride (27.3 mg, 109.3 mg and 163.9 mg) equivalent to 25 mg, 100 mg and 150 mg erlotinib and the following inactive ingredients: lactose monohydrate, hypromellose, hydroxypropyl cellulose, magnesium stearate, microcrystalline cellulose, sodium starch glycolate, sodium lauryl sulfate and titanium dioxide. The tablets also contain trace amounts of color additives, including FD&C Yellow #6 (25 mg only) for product identification.

CLINICAL PHARMACOLOGY

Mechanism of Action and Pharmacodynamics
The mechanism of clinical antitumor action of erlotinib is not fully characterized. Erlotinib inhibits the intracellular

phosphorylation of tyrosine kinase associated with the epidermal growth factor receptor (EGFR). Specificity of inhibition with regard to other tyrosine kinase receptors has not been fully characterized. EGFR is expressed on the cell surface of normal cells and cancer cells.

Pharmacokinetics

Erlotinib is about 60% absorbed after oral administration and its bioavailability is substantially increased by food to almost 100%. Its half-life is about 36 hours and it is cleared predominantly by CYP3A4 metabolism.

Absorption and Distribution

Bioavailability of erlotinib following a 150 mg oral dose of TARCEVA is about 60% and peak plasma levels occur 4 hrs after dosing. Food increases bioavailability substantially, to almost 100%.

Following absorption, erlotinib is approximately 93% protein bound to albumin and alpha-1 acid glycoprotein (AAG). Erlotinib has an apparent volume of distribution of 232 liters.

Metabolism and Elimination

In vitro assays of cytochrome P450 metabolism showed that erlotinib is metabolized primarily by CYP3A4 and to a lesser extent by CYP1A2, and the extrahepatic isoform CYP1A1. Following a 100 mg oral dose, 91% of the dose was recovered: 83% in feces (1% of the dose as intact parent) and 8% in urine (0.3% of the dose as intact parent).

A population pharmacokinetic analysis in 591 patients receiving single-agent TARCEVA showed a median half-life of 36.2 hours. Time to reach steady state plasma concentration would therefore be 7 – 8 days. No significant relationships of clearance to patient age, body weight or gender were observed. Smokers had a 24% higher rate of erlotinib clearance.

Special Populations

Patients with Hepatic Impairment

Erlotinib is cleared predominantly by the liver. No data are currently available regarding the influence of hepatic dysfunction and/or hepatic metastases on the pharmacokinetics of erlotinib (see **PRECAUTIONS - Patients with Hepatic Impairment, ADVERSE REACTIONS** and **DOSAGE AND ADMINISTRATION - Dose Modifications** sections).

Patients with Renal Impairment

Less than 9% of a single dose is excreted in the urine. No clinical studies have been conducted in patients with compromised renal function.

Interactions

Erlotinib is metabolized predominantly by CYP3A4, and inhibitors of CYP3A4 would be expected to increase exposure. Co-treatment with the potent CYP3A4 inhibitor ketoconazole increased erlotinib AUC by 2/3 (see **PRECAUTIONS - Drug Interactions** and **DOSAGE AND ADMINISTRATION - Dose Modifications** sections).

Pre- or co-treatment with the CYP3A4 inducer rifampicin increased erlotinib clearance by 3-fold and reduced AUC by 2/3 (see **PRECAUTIONS - Drug Interactions** and **DOSAGE AND ADMINISTRATION - Dose Modifications** sections).

CLINICAL STUDIES

TARCEVA as Monotherapy in Non-Small Cell Lung Cancer (NSCLC)

The efficacy and safety of TARCEVA was assessed in a randomized, double blind, placebo-controlled trial in 731 patients with locally advanced or metastatic NSCLC after failure of at least one chemotherapy regimen. Patients were randomized 2:1 to receive TARCEVA 150 mg or placebo (488 Tarceva, 243 placebo) orally once daily until disease progression or unacceptable toxicity. Study end points included overall survival, response rate, and progression-free survival (PFS). Duration of response was also examined. The primary endpoint was survival. The study was conducted in 17 countries. About 1/3 of the patients (238) had EGFR expression status characterized.

Table 1 summarizes the demographic and disease characteristics of the study population. Demographic characteristics were well balanced between the two treatment groups. About two-thirds of the patients were male. Approximately one-fourth had a baseline ECOG performance status (PS) of 2, and 9% had a baseline ECOG PS of 3. Fifty percent of the patients had received only one prior regimen of chemotherapy. About three quarters of these patients were known to have smoked at some time.

Table 1: Demographic and Disease Characteristics

Characteristics	TARCEVA (N = 488)		Placebo (N = 243)	
	N	(%)	N	(%)
Gender				
Female	173	(35)	83	(34)
Male	315	(65)	160	(66)
Age (years)				
< 65	299	(61)	153	(63)
≥ 65	189	(39)	90	(37)
Race				
Caucasian	379	(78)	188	(77)
Black	18	(4)	12	(5)
Asian	63	(13)	28	(12)
Other	28	(6)	15	(6)
ECOG Performance Status at Baseline*				
0	64	(13)	34	(14)
1	256	(52)	132	(54)
2	126	(26)	56	(23)
3	42	(9)	21	(9)
Weight Loss in Previous 6 Months				
< 5%	320	(66)	166	(68)
5 – 10%	96	(20)	36	(15)
> 10%	52	(11)	29	(12)
Unknown	20	(4)	12	(5)
Smoking History				
Never Smoked	104	(21)	42	(17)
Current or Ex-smoker	358	(73)	187	(77)
Unknown	26	(5)	14	(6)
Histological Classification				
Adenocarcinoma	246	(50)	119	(49)
Squamous	144	(30)	78	(32)
Undifferentiated Large Cell	41	(8)	23	(9)
Mixed Non-Small Cell	11	(2)	2	(<1)
Other	46	(9)	21	(9)
Time from Initial Diagnosis to Randomization (Months)				
< 6	63	(13)	34	(14)
6 – 12	157	(32)	85	(35)
> 12	268	(55)	124	(51)
Best Response to Prior Therapy at Baseline*				
CR/PR	196	(40)	96	(40)
PD	101	(21)	51	(21)
SD	191	(39)	96	(40)
Number of Prior Regimens at Baseline*				
1	243	(50)	121	(50)
2	238	(49)	119	(49)
3	7	(1)	3	(1)
Exposure to Prior Platinum at Baseline*				
Yes	454	(93)	224	(92)
No	34	(7)	19	(8)

* Stratification factor as documented at baseline; distribution differs slightly from values reported at time of randomization.

The results of the study are shown in Table 2.
[See table 2 at top of next page]
Survival was evaluated in the intent-to-treat population. Figure 1 depicts the Kaplan-Meier curves for overall survival. The primary survival and PFS analyses were two-sided Log-Rank tests stratified by ECOG performance status, number of prior regimens, prior platinum, best response to prior chemotherapy.
[See figure 1 at top of next column]
Note: HR is from Cox regression model with the following covariates: ECOG performance status, number of prior regimens, prior platinum, best response to prior chemotherapy. P-value is from two-sided Log-Rank test stratified by ECOG performance status, number of prior regimens, prior platinum, best response to prior chemotherapy.

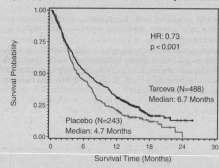

Figure 1: Kaplan–Meier Curve for Overall Survival of Patients by Treatment Group

HR: 0.73
p < 0.001

Tarceva (N=488)
Median: 6.7 Months

Placebo (N=243)
Median: 4.7 Months

A series of subsets of patients were examined in exploratory univariate analyses. The results of these analyses are shown in Figure 2. The effect of TARCEVA on survival was similar across most subsets. An apparently larger effect, however, was observed in two subsets: patients with EGFR positive tumors (HR = 0.65) and patients who never smoked (HR = 0.42). These subsets are considered further below.

Figure 2: Survival Hazard Ratio (HR) (Tarceva : Placebo) in Subgroups According to Pretreatment Characteristics

Factors	N	HR	95% CI
Tarceva : Placebo	731	0.76	0.6 – 0.9
Performance Status 0–1	486	0.73	0.6 – 0.9
Performance Status 2–3	245	0.77	0.6 – 1.0
Male	475	0.76	0.6 – 0.9
Female	256	0.80	0.6 – 1.1
Age <65	452	0.75	0.6 – 0.9
Age ≥65	279	0.79	0.6 – 1.0
Adeno Ca	365	0.71	0.6 – 0.9
Squamous Cell Ca	222	0.67	0.5 – 0.9
Other Histology	144	1.04	0.7 – 1.5
Prior Weight Loss <5%	486	0.77	0.6 – 0.9
Prior Weight Loss 5–10%	132	0.63	0.4 – 1.0
Prior Weight Loss >10%	81	0.70	0.4 – 1.1
Never Smoked	146	0.42	0.3 – 0.6
Current/Ex-Smoker	545	0.87	0.7 – 1.1
One Prior Regimen	364	0.76	0.6 – 1.0
Two+ Prior Regimens	367	0.75	0.6 – 1.0
Prior Platinum	678	0.72	0.6 – 0.9
No Prior Platinum	53	1.41	0.7 – 2.7
Prior Taxane	267	0.74	0.6 – 1.0
No Prior Taxane	464	0.78	0.6 – 1.0
Best Prior Response: CR/PR	292	0.67	0.5 – 0.9
Best Prior Response: SD	287	0.83	0.6 – 1.1
Best Prior Response: PD	152	0.85	0.6 – 1.2
<6 mos Since Diagnosis	97	0.68	0.4 – 1.1
6–12 mos Since Diagnosis	242	0.87	0.7 – 1.2
>12 mos Since Diagnosis	392	0.75	0.6 – 0.9
EGFR Positive	127	0.65	0.4 – 1.0
EGFR Negative	111	1.01	0.7 – 1.6
EGFR Unmeasured	493	0.76	0.6 – 0.9
Caucasian	567	0.79	0.6 – 1.0
Asian	91	0.61	0.4 – 1.0
Stage IV at Diagnosis	329	0.92	0.7 – 1.2
Stage <IV at Diagnosis	402	0.65	0.5 – 0.8

HR Scale: 0.00 0.50 1.00 1.50 2.00 2.50

Note: Depicted are the univariate hazard ratio (HR) for death in the TARCEVA patients relative to the placebo patients, the 95% confidence interval (CI) for the HR, and the sample size (N) in each subgroup. The hash mark on the horizontal bar represents the HR, and the length of the horizontal bar represents the 95% confidence interval. A hash mark to the left of the vertical line corresponds to a HR that is less than 1.00, which indicates that survival is better in the TARCEVA arm compared with the placebo arm in that subgroup.

Relation of Results to EGFR Protein Expression Status (as Determined by Immunohistochemistry)

Analysis of the impact of EGFR expression status on the treatment effect on clinical outcome is limited because EGFR status is known for only 238 study patients (33%). EGFR status was ascertained for patients who already had tissue samples prior to study enrollment. However, the survival in the EGFR tested population and the effects of TARCEVA were almost identical to that in the entire study population, suggesting that the tested population was a representative sample. A positive EGFR expression status was defined as having at least 10% of cells staining for EGFR in contrast to the 1% cut-off specified in the DAKO EGFR pharmDx™ kit instructions. The use of the pharmDx kit has not been validated for use in non-small cell lung cancer. TARCEVA prolonged survival in the EGFR positive subgroup (N = 127; HR = 0.65; 95% CI = 0.43 – 0.97) (Figure 3) and the subgroup whose EGFR status was unmeasured (N = 493; HR = 0.76; 95% CI = 0.61 – 0.93) (Figure 5), but did not appear to have an effect on survival in the EGFR negative subgroup (N = 111; HR = 1.01; 95% CI = 0.65 – 1.57) (Figure 4). However, the confidence intervals for the EGFR positive, negative and unmeasured subgroups are wide and overlap, so that a survival benefit due to TARCEVA in the EGFR negative subgroup cannot be excluded.

For the subgroup of patients who never smoked, EGFR status also appeared to be predictive of TARCEVA survival benefit. Patients who never smoked and were EGFR posi-

Continued on next page

Tarceva—Cont.

tive had a large TARCEVA survival benefit (N = 30; HR = 0.27; 95% CI = 0.11 – 0.67). There were too few EGFR negative patients who never smoked to reach a conclusion. Tumor responses were observed in all EGFR subgroups: 11.6% in the EGFR positive subgroup, 9.5% in the EGFR unmeasured subgroup and 3.2% in the EGFR negative subgroup. An improvement in progression free survival was demonstrated in the EGFR positive subgroup (HR = 0.49; 95% CI = 0.33 – 0.72), the EGFR unmeasured subgroup (HR = 0.56; 95% CI = 0.46 – 0.70), and less certain in the EGFR negative subgroup (HR = 0.91; 95% CI = 0.59 – 1.39).

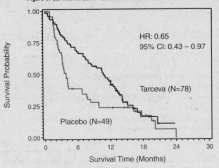

Figure 3: Survival in EGFR Positive Patients

HR: 0.65
95% CI: 0.43 – 0.97

Tarceva (N=78)

Placebo (N=49)

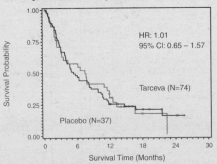

Figure 4: Survival in EGFR Negative Patients

HR: 1.01
95% CI: 0.65 – 1.57

Tarceva (N=74)

Placebo (N=37)

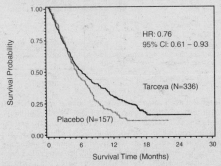

Figure 5: Survival in EGFR Unmeasured Patients

HR: 0.76
95% CI: 0.61 – 0.93

Tarceva (N=336)

Placebo (N=157)

TARCEVA Administered Concurrently with Chemotherapy in NSCLC
Results from two, multicenter, placebo-controlled, randomized, trials in over 1000 patients conducted in first-line patients with locally advanced or metastatic NSCLC showed no clinical benefit with the concurrent administration of TARCEVA with platinum-based chemotherapy [carboplatin and paclitaxel (TARCEVA, N = 526) or gemcitabine and cisplatin (TARCEVA, N = 580)].

INDICATIONS AND USAGE

TARCEVA is indicated for the treatment of patients with locally advanced or metastatic non-small cell lung cancer after failure of at least one prior chemotherapy regimen.
Results from two, multicenter, placebo-controlled, randomized, Phase 3 trials conducted in first-line patients with locally advanced or metastatic NSCLC showed no clinical benefit with the concurrent administration of TARCEVA with platinum-based chemotherapy [carboplatin and paclitaxel or gemcitabine and cisplatin] and its use is not recommended in that setting.

CONTRAINDICATIONS

None.

WARNINGS

Pulmonary Toxicity

There have been infrequent reports of serious Interstitial Lung Disease (ILD), including fatalities, in patients receiving TARCEVA for treatment of NSCLC or other advanced solid tumors. In the randomized single-agent study (see **CLINICAL STUDIES** section), the incidence of ILD (0.8%) was the same in both the placebo and TARCEVA groups. The overall incidence in TARCEVA-treated patients from all

Table 2: Efficacy Results

	Tarceva	Placebo	Hazard Ratio (1)	95% CI	p-value
Survival	Median 6.7 mo	Median 4.7 mo	0.73	0.61 – 0.86	<0.001 (2)
1-year Survival	31.2%	21.5%			
Progression-Free Survival	Median 9.9 wk	Median 7.9 wk	0.59	0.50 – 0.70	<0.001 (2)
Tumor Response (CR+PR)	8.9%	0.9%			<0.001 (3)
Response Duration	Median 34.3 wk	Median 15.9 wk			

(1) Cox regression model with the following covariates: ECOG performance status, number of prior regimens, prior platinum, best response to prior chemotherapy.
(2) Two-sided Log-Rank test stratified by ECOG performance status, number of prior regimens, prior platinum, best response to prior chemotherapy.
(3) Two-sided Fisher's exact test

studies (including uncontrolled studies and studies with concurrent chemotherapy) was approximately 0.6%. Reported diagnoses in patients suspected of having ILD included pneumonitis, interstitial pneumonia, interstitial lung disease, obliterative bronchiolitis, pulmonary fibrosis, Acute Respiratory Distress Syndrome and lung infiltration. Symptoms started from 5 days to more than 9 months (median 47 days) after initiating TARCEVA therapy. Most of the cases were associated with confounding or contributing factors such as concomitant/prior chemotherapy, prior radiotherapy, pre-existing parenchymal lung disease, metastatic lung disease, or pulmonary infections.
In the event of an acute onset of new or progressive, unexplained pulmonary symptoms such as dyspnea, cough, and fever, TARCEVA therapy should be interrupted pending diagnostic evaluation. If ILD is diagnosed, TARCEVA should be discontinued and appropriate treatment instituted as needed (see **ADVERSE REACTIONS** and **DOSAGE AND ADMINISTRATION - Dose Modifications** sections).

Pregnancy Category D

Erlotinib has been shown to cause maternal toxicity with associated embryo/fetal lethality and abortion in rabbits when given at doses that result in plasma drug concentrations of approximately 3 times those in humans (AUCs at 150 mg daily dose). When given during the period of organogenesis to achieve plasma drug concentrations approximately equal to those in humans, based on AUC, there was no increased incidence of embryo/fetal lethality or abortion in rabbits or rats. However, female rats treated with 30 mg/m^2/day or 60 mg/m^2/day (0.3 or 0.7 times the clinical dose, on a mg/m^2 basis) of erlotinib prior to mating through the first week of pregnancy had an increase in early resorptions which resulted in a decrease in the number of live fetuses. No teratogenic effects were observed in rabbits or rats.
There are no adequate and well-controlled studies in pregnant women using TARCEVA. Women of childbearing potential should be advised to avoid pregnancy while on TARCEVA. Adequate contraceptive methods should be used during therapy, and for at least 2 weeks after completing therapy. Treatment should only be continued in pregnant women if the potential benefit to the mother outweighs the risk to the fetus. If TARCEVA is used during pregnancy, the patient should be apprised of the potential hazard to the fetus or potential risk for loss of the pregnancy.

PRECAUTIONS

Drug Interactions

Co-treatment with the potent CYP3A4 inhibitor ketoconazole increases erlotinib AUC by 2/3. Caution should be used when administering or taking TARCEVA with ketoconazole and other strong CYP3A4 inhibitors such as atazanavir, clarithromycin, indinavir, itraconazole, nefazodone, nelfinavir, ritonavir, saquinavir, telithromycin, troleandomycin (TAO), and voriconazole (see **DOSAGE AND ADMINISTRATION - Dose Modifications** section).
Pre-treatment with the CYP3A4 inducer rifampicin decreased erlotinib AUC by about 2/3. Alternate treatments lacking CYP3A4 inducing activity should be considered. If an alternative treatment is unavailable, a TARCEVA dose greater than 150 mg should be considered. If the TARCEVA dose is adjusted upward, the dose will need to be reduced upon discontinuation of rifampicin or other inducers. Other CYP3A4 inducers include rifabutin, rifapentine, phenytoin, carbamazepine, phenobarbital and St. John's Wort (see **DOSAGE AND ADMINISTRATION - Dose Modifications** section).

Hepatotoxicity

Asymptomatic increases in liver transaminases have been observed in TARCEVA treated patients; therefore, periodic liver function testing (transaminases, bilirubin, and alkaline phosphatase) should be considered. Dose reduction or interruption of TARCEVA should be considered if changes in liver function are severe (see **ADVERSE REACTIONS** section).

Patients with Hepatic Impairment

In vitro and *in vivo* evidence suggest that erlotinib is cleared primarily by the liver. Therefore, erlotinib exposure may be increased in patients with hepatic dysfunction (see **CLINICAL PHARMACOLOGY - Special Populations - Patients with Hepatic Impairment** and **DOSAGE AND ADMINISTRATION - Dose Modification** sections).

Elevated International Normalized Ratio and Potential Bleeding

International Normalized Ratio (INR) elevations and infrequent reports of bleeding events including gastrointestinal bleeding have been reported in clinical studies, some associated with concomitant warfarin administration. Patients taking warfarin or other coumarin-derivative anticoagulants should be monitored regularly for changes in prothrombin time or INR (see **ADVERSE REACTIONS** section).

Carcinogenesis, Mutagenesis, Impairment of Fertility

Erlotinib has not been tested for carcinogenicity.
Erlotinib has been tested for genotoxicity in a series of *in vitro* assays (bacterial mutation, human lymphocyte chromosome aberration, and mammalian cell mutation) and an *in vivo* mouse bone marrow micronucleus test and did not cause genetic damage. Erlotinib did not impair fertility in either male or female rats.

Pregnancy

Pregnancy Category D (see **WARNINGS** and **PRECAUTIONS - Information for Patients** sections).

Nursing Mothers

It is not known whether erlotinib is excreted in human milk. Because many drugs are excreted in human milk and because the effects of TARCEVA on infants have not been studied, women should be advised against breast-feeding while receiving TARCEVA therapy.

Pediatric Use

The safety and effectiveness of TARCEVA in pediatric patients have not been studied.

Geriatric Use

Of the total number of patients participating in the randomized trial, 62% were less than 65 years of age, and 38% of patients were aged 65 years or older. The survival benefit was maintained across both age groups (see **CLINICAL STUDIES** section). No meaningful differences in safety or pharmacokinetics were observed between younger and older patients. Therefore, no dosage adjustments are recommended in elderly patients.

Information for Patients

If the following signs or symptoms occur, patients should seek medical advice promptly (see **WARNINGS**, **ADVERSE REACTIONS** and **DOSAGE AND ADMINISTRATION - Dose Modification** sections).
- Severe or persistent diarrhea, nausea, anorexia, or vomiting
- Onset or worsening of unexplained shortness of breath or cough
- Eye irritation

Women of childbearing potential should be advised to avoid becoming pregnant while taking TARCEVA (see **WARNINGS - Pregnancy Category D** section).

ADVERSE REACTIONS

Safety evaluation of TARCEVA is based on 856 cancer patients who received TARCEVA as monotherapy and 1228 patients who received TARCEVA concurrently with chemotherapy. Adverse events, regardless of causality, that occurred in at least 10% of patients treated with TARCEVA and at least 3% more often than in the placebo group in the randomized trial are summarized by NCI-CTC (version 2.0) Grade in Table 3.
There have been reports of serious ILD, including fatalities, in patients receiving TARCEVA for treatment of NSCLC or other advanced solid tumors (see **WARNINGS - Pulmonary Toxicity**, and **DOSAGE AND ADMINISTRATION - Dose Modifications** sections).
The most common adverse reactions in patients receiving TARCEVA were rash and diarrhea. Grade 3/4 rash and diarrhea occurred in 9% and 6%, respectively, in TARCEVA-treated patients. Rash and diarrhea each resulted in study discontinuation in 1% of TARCEVA-treated patients. Six percent and 1% of patients needed dose reduction for rash and diarrhea, respectively. The median time to onset of rash was 8 days, and the median time to onset of diarrhea was 12 days.
[See table 3 at top of next page]
Liver function test abnormalities (including elevated alanine aminotransferase (ALT), aspartate aminotransferase (AST) and bilirubin) have been observed. These elevations

Table 3: Adverse Events Occurring in ≥10% of TARCEVA-treated Patients
(2:1 Randomization of TARCEVA to Placebo)

NCI CTC Grade	TARCEVA N = 485			Placebo N = 242		
	Any Grade	Grade 3	Grade 4	Any Grade	Grade 3	Grade 4
MedDRA Preferred Term	%	%	%	%	%	%
Rash	75	8	<1	17	0	0
Diarrhea	54	6	<1	18	<1	0
Anorexia	52	8	1	38	5	<1
Fatigue	52	14	4	45	16	4
Dyspnea	41	17	11	35	15	11
Cough	33	4	0	29	2	0
Nausea	33	3	0	24	2	0
Infection	24	4	0	15	2	0
Vomiting	23	2	<1	19	2	0
Stomatitis	17	<1	0	3	0	0
Pruritus	13	<1	0	5	0	0
Dry skin	12	0	0	4	0	0
Conjunctivitis	12	<1	0	2	<1	0
Keratoconjunctivitis sicca	12	0	0	3	0	0
Abdominal pain	11	2	<1	7	1	<1

were mainly transient or associated with liver metastases. Grade 2 (>2.5 – 5.0 x ULN) ALT elevations occurred in 4% and <1% of TARCEVA and placebo treated patients, respectively. Grade 3 (>5.0 – 20.0 x ULN) elevations were not observed in TARCEVA-treated patients. Dose reduction or interruption of TARCEVA should be considered if changes in liver function are severe (see **DOSAGE AND ADMINISTRATION - Dose Modification** section).

Infrequent cases of gastrointestinal bleeding have been reported in clinical studies, some associated with concomitant warfarin administration (see **PRECAUTIONS - Elevated International Normalized Ratio and Potential Bleeding** section) and some with concomitant NSAID administration.

NCI-CTC Grade 3 conjunctivitis and keratitis have been reported infrequently in patients receiving TARCEVA therapy. Corneal ulcerations may also occur (see **PRECAUTIONS - Information for Patients** section).

In general, no notable differences in the safety of TARCEVA could be discerned between females or males and between patients younger or older than the age of 65 years. The safety of TARCEVA appears similar in Caucasian and Asian patients (see **PRECAUTIONS - Geriatric Use** section).

OVERDOSAGE

Single oral doses of TARCEVA up to 1,000 mg in healthy subjects and up to 1,600 mg in cancer patients have been tolerated. Repeated twice-daily doses of 200 mg in healthy subjects were poorly tolerated after only a few days of dosing. Based on the data from these studies, an unacceptable incidence of severe adverse events, such as diarrhea, rash, and liver transaminase elevation, may occur above the recommended dose of 150 mg daily. In case of suspected overdose, TARCEVA should be withheld and symptomatic treatment instituted.

DOSAGE AND ADMINISTRATION

The recommended daily dose of TARCEVA is 150 mg taken at least one hour before or two hours after the ingestion of food. Treatment should continue until disease progression or unacceptable toxicity occurs. There is no evidence that treatment beyond progression is beneficial.

Dose Modifications

In patients who develop an acute onset of new or progressive pulmonary symptoms, such as dyspnea, cough or fever, treatment with TARCEVA should be interrupted pending diagnostic evaluation. If ILD is diagnosed, TARCEVA should be discontinued and appropriate treatment instituted as necessary (see **WARNINGS - Pulmonary Toxicity** section).

Diarrhea can usually be managed with loperamide. Patients with severe diarrhea who are unresponsive to loperamide or who become dehydrated may require dose reduction or temporary interruption of therapy. Patients with severe skin reactions may also require dose reduction or temporary interruption of therapy.

When dose reduction is necessary, the TARCEVA dose should be reduced in 50 mg decrements.

In patients who are being concomitantly treated with a strong CYP3A4 inhibitor such as atazanavir, clarithromycin, indinavir, itraconazole, ketoconazole, nefazodone, nelfinavir, ritonavir, saquinavir, telithromycin, troleandomycin (TAO), or voriconazole, a dose reduction should be considered should severe adverse reactions occur.

Pre-treatment with the CYP3A4 inducer rifampicin decreased erlotinib AUC by about 2/3. Alternate treatments lacking CYP3A4 inducing activity should be considered. If an alternative treatment is unavailable, a TARCEVA dose greater than 150 mg should be considered. If the TARCEVA dose is adjusted upward, the dose will need to be reduced upon discontinuation of rifampicin or other inducers. Other CYP3A4 inducers include rifabutin, rifapentine, phenytoin, carbamazepine, phenobarbital and St. John's Wort. These too should be avoided if possible (see **PRECAUTIONS - Drug Interactions** section).

Erlotinib is eliminated by hepatic metabolism and biliary excretion. Therefore, caution should be used when administering TARCEVA to patients with hepatic impairment. Dose reduction or interruption of TARCEVA should be considered should severe adverse reactions occur (see **CLINICAL PHARMACOLOGY - Special Populations - Patients With Hepatic Impairment, PRECAUTIONS - Patients With Hepatic Impairment**, and **ADVERSE REACTIONS** sections).

HOW SUPPLIED

The 25 mg, 100 mg and 150 mg strengths are supplied as white film-coated tablets for daily oral administration.

TARCEVA™ (erlotinib) Tablets, 25 mg: Round, biconvex face and straight sides, white film-coated, printed in orange with a "T" and "25" on one side and plain on the other side. Supplied in bottles of 30 tablets (NDC 50242-062-01).

TARCEVA™ (erlotinib) Tablets, 100 mg: Round, biconvex face and straight sides, white film-coated, printed in gray with "T" and "100" on one side and plain on the other side. Supplied in bottles of 30 tablets (NDC 50242-063-01).

TARCEVA™ (erlotinib) Tablets, 150 mg: Round, biconvex face and straight sides, white film-coated, printed in maroon with "T" and "150" on one side and plain on the other side. Supplied in bottles of 30 tablets (NDC 50242-064-01).

STORAGE

Store at 25°C (77°F); excursions permitted to 15° – 30°C (59° – 86°F). See USP Controlled Room Temperature.

Manufactured for:
OSI Pharmaceuticals Inc., Melville, NY 11747

Manufactured by:
Schwarz Pharma Manufacturing, Seymour, IN 47274

Distributed by:
Genentech, Inc., 1 DNA Way, South San Francisco, CA 94080-4990

For further information please call 1-877-TARCEVA (1-877-827-2382).

Genentech   **(OSI)™ oncology**
BIOONCOLOGY

TARCEVA and **(OSI)™ oncology** are trademarks of OSI Pharmaceuticals, Inc., Melville, NY, 11747, USA.

Part No. 750165123-02
Date of Issue: December 2004

To keep your **PDR** up to date throughout the year, note these revisions on the corresponding pages of the annual volume. Simply write **"See Supplement A"** next to the product heading.

Pharmacia & Upjohn

A division of Pfizer
235 EAST 42ND STREET
NEW YORK, NY 10017-5755

For updates to the product information listed below, please check the Pfizer Web site, http://www.pfizer.com, or call (800) 438-1985. For complete product listing, please see the Manufacturers' Index.

For Medical Information, Contact:
(800) 438-1985
24 hours a day, seven days a week

Distribution:
1855 Shelby Oaks Drive North
Memphis, TN 38134
(901) 387-5200

Customer Service:
(800) 533-4535

DEPO-SUBQ PROVERA 104™   ℞
[dĕ-pŏ sub Q]
medroxyprogesterone acetate injectable suspension
104 mg/0.65 mL

> Women who use depo-subQ provera 104 may lose significant bone mineral density. Bone loss is greater with increasing duration of use and may not be completely reversible.
> It is unknown if use of depo-subQ provera 104 during adolescence or early adulthood, a critical period of bone accretion, will reduce peak bone mass and increase the risk for osteoporotic fracture in later life.
> depo-subQ provera 104 should be used long-term (e.g., longer than 2 years) only if other methods of birth control are inadequate (see WARNINGS, section 1).

Patients should be counseled that this product does not protect against HIV infection (AIDS) and other sexually transmitted diseases.

DESCRIPTION

depo-subQ provera 104 contains medroxyprogesterone acetate (MPA), a derivative of progesterone, as its active ingredient. Medroxyprogesterone acetate is active by the parenteral and oral routes of administration. It is a white to off-white, odorless crystalline powder that is stable in air and that melts between 205° and 209°C. It is freely soluble in chloroform, soluble in acetone and dioxane, sparingly soluble in alcohol and methanol, slightly soluble in ether, and insoluble in water.

The chemical name for medroxyprogesterone acetate is 17-hydroxy-6α-methylpregn-4-ene-3,20-dione 17-acetate. The structural formula is as follows:

depo-subQ provera 104 for subcutaneous (SC) injection is available in pre-filled syringes (160 mg/mL), each containing 0.65 mL (104 mg) of medroxyprogesterone acetate sterile aqueous suspension.

Each 0.65 mL contains:

Medroxyprogesterone acetate	104 mg
Methylparaben	1.040 mg
Propylparaben	0.098 mg
Sodium Chloride	5.200 mg
Polyethylene Glycol	18.688 mg
Polysorbate 80	1.950 mg
Monobasic Sodium Phosphate · H_2O	0.451 mg
Dibasic Sodium Phosphate · $12H_2O$	0.382 mg
Methionine	0.975 mg
Povidone	3.250 mg
Water for Injection	qs

When necessary, the pH is adjusted with sodium hydroxide or hydrochloric acid, or both.

CLINICAL PHARMACOLOGY

depo-subQ provera 104 (medroxyprogesterone acetate injectable suspension), when administered at 104 mg/0.65 mL to women every 3 months (12 to 14 weeks) inhibits the secretion of gonadotropins, which prevents follicular maturation and ovulation and causes endometrial thinning. These actions produce its contraceptive effect.

Supression of serum estradiol concentrations and a possible direct action of depo-subQ provera 104 on the lesions of endometriosis are likely to be responsible for the therapeutic effect on endometriosis-associated pain.

Pharmacokinetics

The pharmacokinetic parameters of medroxyprogesterone acetate (MPA) following a single SC injection of depo-subQ provera 104 are shown in Table 1 and Figure 1.

Continued on next page

depo-subQ provera 104—Cont.

[See table 1 at right]

Absorption: Following a single SC injection of depo-subQ provera 104, serum MPA concentrations reach ≥ 0.2 ng/mL within 24 hours. The mean T_{max} is attained approximately 1 week after injection.

Figure 1. Mean (SD) Serum Concentration-Time Profile of MPA after a Single Injection of depo-subQ provera 104 to Healthy Women

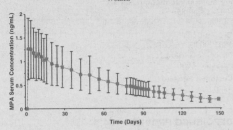

In a study to assess accumulation and the achievement of steady state following multiple SC administrations, trough concentrations of MPA were determined after 6, 12, and 24 months, and in a subset of 8 subjects, bi-weekly concentrations were determined within one dosing interval in the second year of administration. The mean (SD) MPA trough concentrations were 0.67 (0.36) ng/mL (n=157), 0.79 (0.36) ng/mL (n=144), and 0.87 (0.33) ng/mL (n=106) at 6, 12 and 24 months, respectively.

Effect of Injection Site: depo-subQ provera 104 was administered into the anterior thigh or the abdomen to evaluate effects on the MPA concentration-time profile. MPA trough concentrations (C_{min}; Day 91) were similar for the two injection locations.

Distribution: Plasma protein binding of MPA averages 86%. MPA binding occurs primarily to serum albumin. No binding of MPA occurs with sex-hormone-binding globulin (SHBG).

Metabolism: MPA is extensively metabolized in the liver by P450 enzymes. Its metabolism primarily involves ring A and/or side-chain reduction, loss of the acetyl group, hydroxylation in the 2-, 6-, and 21-positions or a combination of these positions, resulting in more than 10 metabolites.

Excretion: Residual MPA concentrations at the end of the first dosing interval (12 to 14 weeks) of depo-subQ provera 104 are generally below 0.5 ng/mL, consistent with its apparent terminal half-life of ~40 days after SC administration. Most MPA metabolites are excreted in the urine as glucuronide conjugates with only small amounts excreted as sulfates.

Linearity/Non-Linearity: Following a single SC administration of doses ranging from 50 to 150 mg, the AUC and C_{min} (Day 91) increased with higher doses of depo-subQ provera 104, but there was considerable overlap across dose levels. Serum MPA concentrations at Day 91 increased in a dose proportional manner but C_{max} did not appear to increase proportionally with increasing dose. The AUC data were suggestive of dose linearity.

Special Populations

Race: There were no significant differences in the pharmacokinetics and/or pharmacodynamics of MPA after SC administration of depo-subQ provera 104 in African-American and Caucasian women. The pharmacokinetics/pharmacodynamics of depo-subQ provera 104 were evaluated in Asian women in a separate study and also found to be similar to African-American and Caucasian women.

Effect of Body Weight: Although total MPA exposure was lower in obese women, no dosage adjustment of depo-subQ provera 104 is necessary based on body weight. The effect of body weight on the pharmacokinetics of MPA following a single dose was assessed in a subset of women (n = 42, body mass index [BMI] ranged from 18.2 to 46.7 kg/m²). The AUC_{0-91} values for MPA were 71.6, 67.9, and 46.3 ng·day/mL in women with BMI categories of ≤ 28 kg/m², >28-38 kg/m², and >38 kg/m², respectively. The mean MPA C_{max} was 1.74 ng/mL in women with BMI ≤ 28 kg/m², 1.53 ng/mL in women with BMI >28-38 kg/m², and 1.02 ng/mL in women with BMI > 38 kg/m², respectively. The MPA trough (C_{min}) concentrations had a tendency to be lower in women with BMI >38 kg/m².

Hepatic Insufficiency: No clinical studies have evaluated the effect of hepatic disease on the disposition of depo-subQ provera 104. However, steroid hormones may be poorly metabolized in patients with severe liver dysfunction (see CONTRAINDICATIONS).

Renal Insufficiency: No clinical studies have evaluated the effect of renal disease on the pharmacokinetics of depo-subQ provera 104.

Drug-Drug Interactions

See PRECAUTIONS, section 9

INDICATIONS AND USAGE

depo-subQ provera 104 is indicated for the prevention of pregnancy in women of child bearing potential.

depo-subQ provera 104 also is indicated for management of endometriosis-associated pain.

In considering use for either indication, the loss of bone mineral density (BMD) in women of all ages and the impact on peak bone mass in adolescents should be considered, along with the decrease in BMD that occurs during preg-

Table 1. Pharmacokinetic Parameters of MPA after a Single SC Injection of depo-subQ provera 104 in Healthy Women (n = 42)

	C_{max} (ng/mL)	T_{max} (day)	C_{91} (ng/mL)	AUC_{0-91} (ng·day/mL)	$AUC_{0-\infty}$ (ng·day/mL)	$t\frac{1}{2}$ (day)
Mean	1.56	8.8	0.402	66.98	92.84	43
Min	0.53	2.0	0.133	20.63	31.36	16
Max	3.08	80.0	0.733	139.79	162.29	114

C_{max} = peak serum concentration; T_{max} = time when C_{max} is observed; C_{91} = serum concentration at 91 days; AUC_{0-91} and $AUC_{0-\infty}$ = area under the concentration-time curve over 91 days or infinity, respectively; $t\frac{1}{2}$ = terminal half-life

Table 2. Percentage of Women Experiencing an Unintended Pregnancy During the First Year of Typical Use and the First Year of Perfect Use of Contraception and the Percentage Continuing Use at the End of the First Year: United States

Method	% of Women Experiencing an Unintended Pregnancy within the First Year of Use		% of Women Continuing Use at 1 Year[3]
	Typical Use[1]	Perfect Use[2]	
Chance[4]	85	85	
Spermicides[5]	26	6	40
Periodic Abstinence	25		63
Calendar		9	
Ovulation Method		3	
Symptothermal[6]		2	
Post-ovulation		1	
Cap[7]			
Parous Women	40	26	42
Nulliparous Women	20	9	56
Sponge			
Parous Women	40	20	42
Nulliparous Women	20	9	56
Diaphragm[7]	20	6	56
Withdrawal	19	4	
Condom[8]			
Female (Reality)	21	5	56
Male	14	3	61
Pill	5		71
Progestin only		0.5	
Combined		0.1	
IUD			
Progesterone T	2.0	1.5	81
Copper T 380A	0.8	0.6	78
LNg 20	0.1	0.1	81
Depo-Provera IM 150 mg	0.3	0.3	70
Norplant and Norplant-2	0.05	0.05	88
Female Sterilization	0.5	0.5	100
Male Sterilization	0.15	0.10	100

Emergency Contraceptive Pills: Treatment initiated within 72 hours after unprotected intercourse reduces the risk of pregnancy by at least 75%.[9]

Lactational Amenorrhea Method: LAM is a highly effective, temporary method of contraception.[10]

Source: Hatcher et al., 1998.[i]

[1]Among *typical* couples who initiate use of a method (not necessarily for the first time), the percentage who experience an accidental pregnancy during the first year if they do not stop use for any other reason.

[2]Among couples who initiate use of a method (not necessarily for the first time) and who use it *perfectly* (both consistently and correctly), the percentage who experience an accidental pregnancy during the first year if they do not stop use for any other reason.

[3]Among couples attempting to avoid pregnancy, the percentage who continue to use a method for 1 year.

[4]The percentages becoming pregnant in columns (2) and (3) are based on data from populations where contraception is not used and from women who cease using contraception in order to become pregnant. Among such populations, about 89% become pregnant within 1 year. This estimate was lowered slightly (to 85%) to represent the percentages who would become pregnant within 1 year among women now relying on reversible methods of contraception if they abandoned contraception altogether.

[5]Foams, creams, gels, vaginal suppositories, and vaginal film.

[6]Cervical mucus (ovulation) method supplemented by calendar in the pre-ovulatory and basal body temperature in the post-ovulatory phases.

[7]With spermicidal cream or jelly.

[8]Without spermicides.

[9]The treatment schedule is one dose within 72 hours after unprotected intercourse, and a second dose 12 hours after the first dose. The Food and Drug Administration has declared the following brands of oral contraceptives to be safe and effective for emergency contraception: Ovral (1 dose is 2 white pills), Alesse (1 dose is 5 pink pills), Nordette or Levlen (1 dose is 4 light-orange pills), Lo/Ovral (1 dose is 4 white pills), Triphasil or Tri-Levlen (1 dose is 4 yellow pills).

[10]However, to maintain effective protection against pregnancy, another method of contraception must be used as soon as menstruation resumes, the frequency or duration of breastfeeds is reduced, bottle feeds are introduced, or the baby reaches 6 months of age.

nancy and/or lactation, in the risk/benefit assessment for women who use depo-subQ provera 104 long-term (see WARNINGS, section 1).

Contraception Studies

In three clinical studies, no pregnancies were detected among 2,042 women using depo-subQ provera 104 for up to 1 year. The Pearl Index pregnancy rate in women who were less than 36 years old at baseline, based on cycles in which they used no other contraceptive methods, was 0 pregnancies per 100 women-years of use (upper 95% confidence interval = 0.25).

Pregnancy rates for various contraceptive methods are typically reported for only the first year of use and are shown in Table 2.

[See table 2 above]

Endometriosis Studies

The efficacy of depo-subQ provera 104 in the reduction of endometriosis-associated pain in women with the signs and symptoms of endometriosis was demonstrated in two active

comparator-controlled studies. Each study assessed reduction in endometriosis-associated pain over 6 months of treatment and recurrence of symptoms for 12-months post treatment. Subjects treated with depo-subQ provera 104 for 6 months received a 104 mg dose every 3 months (2 injections), while women treated with leuprolide microspheres for 6 months received a dose of 11.25 mg every 3 months (2 injections) or 3.75 mg every month (6 injections). Study 268 was conducted in the U.S. and Canada and enrolled 274 subjects (136 on depo-subQ provera 104 and 138 on leuprolide). Study 270 was conducted in South America, Europe and Asia, and enrolled 299 subjects (153 on depo-subQ provera 104 and 146 on leuprolide).

Reduction in pain was evaluated using a modified Biberoglu and Behrman scale that consisted of three patient-reported symptoms (dysmenorrhea, dyspareunia, and pelvic pain not related to menses) and two signs assessed during pelvic examination (pelvic tenderness and induration). For each category, a favorable response was defined as improvement of at least 1 unit (severity was assessed on a scale of 0 to 3) relative to baseline score (Figure 2).

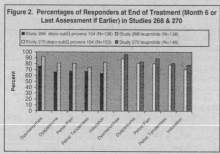

Figure 2. Percentages of Responders at End of Treatment (Month 6 or Last Assessment if Earlier) in Studies 268 & 270

■ Study 268: depo-subQ provera 104 (N=136) □ Study 268:leuprolide (N=138)
▨ Study 270:depo-subQ provera 104 (N=153) ▪ Study 270:leuprolide (N=146)

Favorable Response = reduction in severity of symptom or sign of ≥ 1 point on a scale of 0 to 3, as compared to baseline

Additionally, scores from each of the five categories were combined, with the total (composite score) considered a global measurement of overall disease improvement. For subjects with baseline scores for each of the 5 categories, a mean decrease of 4 points relative to baseline was considered a clinically meaningful improvement. Across both studies, for both treatment groups, the mean changes in the composite score met the protocol-defined criterion for improvement.

In the clinical trials, treatment with depo-subQ provera 104 was limited to six months. Data on the persistence of benefit with longer treatment are not available.

Subjects recorded daily the occurrence and severity of hot flushes. Of the depo-subQ provera 104 users, 28.6% reported experiencing moderate or severe hot flushes at baseline, 36.2% at month 3, and 26.7% at month 6. Of the leuprolide users, 32.8% reported experiencing moderate or severe hot flushes at baseline, 74.2% at month 3, and 68.5% at month 6.

CONTRAINDICATIONS
1. Known or suspected pregnancy.
2. Undiagnosed vaginal bleeding.
3. Known or suspected malignancy of breast.
4. Active thrombophlebitis, or current or past history of thromboembolic disorders, or cerebral vascular disease.
5. Significant liver disease.
6. Known hypersensitivity to medroxyprogesterone acetate or any of its other ingredients.

WARNINGS
1. Loss of Bone Mineral Density
Use of depo-subQ provera 104 reduces serum estrogen levels and is associated with significant loss of bone mineral density (BMD) as bone metabolism accommodates to a lower estrogen level. This loss of BMD is of particular concern during adolescence and early adulthood, a critical period of bone accretion. It is unknown if use of depo-subQ provera 104 by younger women will reduce peak bone mass and increase the risk for osteoporotic fracture in later life. In both adults and adolescents, the decrease in BMD appears to be at least partially reversible after depo-subQ provera 104 is discontinued and ovarian estrogen production increases. A study to assess the reversibility of loss of BMD in adolescents is ongoing.

depo-subQ provera 104 should be used long-term (e.g., longer than 2 years) only if other methods of birth control are inadequate. BMD should be evaluated when a woman needs to use depo-subQ provera 104 long-term. In adolescents, interpretation of BMD results should take into account patient age and skeletal maturity.

Other treatments should be considered in the risk/benefit analysis for the use of depo-subQ provera 104 in women with osteoporosis risk factors. depo-subQ provera 104 can pose an additional risk in patients with risk factors for osteoporosis (e.g., metabolic bone disease, chronic alcohol and/or tobacco use, anorexia nervosa, strong family history of osteoporosis or chronic use of drugs that can reduce bone mass such as anticonvulsants or corticosteroids).

Although there are no studies addressing whether calcium and Vitamin D lessen BMD loss in women using depo-subQ provera 104, all patients should have adequate calcium and Vitamin D intake.

BMD Changes in Adult Women after Long-Term Treatment for Contraception
A study comparing changes in BMD in women using depo-subQ provera 104 with women using Depo-Provera Contraceptive Injection (Depo-Provera CI, 150 mg) showed no significant differences in BMD loss between the two groups after two years of treatment. Mean percent changes in BMD in the depo-subQ provera 104 group are listed in Table 3.
[See table 3 above]
In another controlled clinical study, adult women using Depo-Provera CI (150 mg) for up to 5 years showed spine and hip BMD mean decreases of 5-6%, compared to no significant change in BMD in the control group. The decline in BMD was more pronounced during the first two years of use, with smaller declines in subsequent years. Mean changes in lumbar spine BMD of -2.86%, -4.11%, -4.89%,

Table 3. Mean Percent Change from Baseline in BMD in Women Using depo-subQ provera 104

Time on Treatment	Lumbar Spine N	Mean % Change (95% CI)	Total Hip N	Mean % Change (95% CI)	Femoral Neck N	Mean % Change (95% CI)
1 year	166	-2.7 (-3.1 to -2.3)	166	-1.7 (-2.1 to -1.3)	166	-1.9 (-2.5 to -1.4)
2 year	106	-4.1 (-4.6 to -3.5)	106	-3.5 (-4.2 to -2.7)	106	-3.5 (-4.3 to -2.6)

Table 4. Mean Percent Change from Baseline in BMD in Women Using Depo-Provera CI (150 mg) or in Control Subjects

Time in Study	Lumbar Spine Depo-Provera CI (150 mg)*	Control**	Total Hip Depo-Provera CI (150 mg)*	Control**	Femoral Neck Depo-Provera CI (150 mg)*	Control**
5 years	n=33 -5.38%	n=105 0.43%	n=21 -5.16%	n=65 0.19%	n=34 -6.12%	n=106 -0.27%
7 years	n=12 -3.13%	n=60 0.53%	n=7 -1.34%	n=39 0.94%	n=13 -5.38	n=63 -0.11%

*The treatment group consisted of women who received Depo-Provera CI (150 mg) for 5 years and were then followed for 2 years post-use.
**The control group consisted of women who did not use hormonal contraception and were followed for 7 years.

Table 5. Mean Percent Change from Baseline in BMD in Adolescents Using Depo-Provera CI (150 mg) and in Unmatched, Untreated Control Cohort Studies

Duration of Treatment Or Observation Period	Lumbar Spine Depo-Provera CI (150 mg) N	Mean % change	Control (Unmatched/ Untreated) N	Mean % change	Total Hip Depo-Provera CI (150 mg) N	Mean % change	Control (Unmatched/ Untreated) N	Mean % change	Femoral Neck Depo-Provera CI (150 mg) N	Mean % change	Control (Unmatched/ Untreated) N	Mean % change
Week 60 (1.2 yrs)	104	-2.42	171	3.47	103	-2.82	171	132	103	-3.05	171	1.87
Week 144 (2.8 yrs)	46	-2.78	111	5.41	45	-6.16	111	1.74	45	-6.01	111	2.54
Week 240 (4.6 yrs)	9	-4.17	70	5.12	9	-6.92	69	1.12	9	-6.06	69	1.45

Table 6. Mean Percent Change from Baseline in BMD after 6 Months on Therapy with depo-subQ provera 104 or Leuprolide and 6 and 12 Months after Stopping Therapy (Studies 268 and 270 Combined)

Time of Measurement	Lumbar Spine depo-subQ provera 104 N	Mean % change	Leuprolide N	Mean % change	Total Hip depo-subQ provera 104 N	Mean % change	Leuprolide N	Mean % change
Month 6 of treatment (EOT)	208	-1.20	229	-4.10	207	-0.03	227	-1.83
6 months off treatment	168	-1.06	180	-2.75	169	-0.05	181	-1.59
12 months off treatment	124	-0.54	133	-1.48	125	0.39	134	-1.15

EOT = End of Treatment

-4.93% and -5.38% after 1, 2, 3, 4 and 5 years, respectively, were observed. Mean decreases in BMD of the total hip and femoral neck were similar.

After stopping use of Depo-Provera CI (150 mg) there was partial recovery of BMD toward baseline values during the 2-year post-therapy period. Longer duration of treatment was associated with less complete recovery during this 2-year period following the last injection. Table 4 shows the extent of recovery of BMD for women who completed 5 years of treatment.
[See table 4 above]

BMD Changes in Adolescent Females (12-18 years) after Long-Term Treatment for Contraception
Preliminary results from an ongoing, open-label, self-selected, non-randomized clinical study of adolescent females (12-18 years) also showed that Depo-Provera CI (150 mg) use was associated with a significant decline in BMD from baseline (Table 5). In general, adolescents increase bone density during the period of growth following menarche, as seen in the untreated cohort. However, the two cohorts were not matched at baseline for age, gynecologic age, race, BMD and other factors that influence the

rate of acquisition of bone mineral density, with the result that they differed with respect to these demographic factors. Preliminary data from the small number of adolescents participating in the 2-year post-use observation period demonstrated partial recovery of BMD.
[See table 5 above]

BMD Changes in Adult Women after Six Months of Treatment for Endometriosis
In two clinical studies of 573 adult women with endometriosis, the BMD effects of 6 months of depo-subQ provera 104 treatment were compared to 6 months of leuprolide treatment. Subjects were then observed, off therapy, for an additional 12 months (Table 6).
[See table 6 above]

2. Bleeding Irregularities
Most women using depo-subQ provera 104 experienced changes in menstrual bleeding patterns, such as amenorrhea, irregular spotting or bleeding, prolonged spotting or bleeding, and heavy bleeding. As women continued using

Continued on next page

depo-subQ provera 104—Cont.

depo-subQ provera 104, fewer experienced irregular bleeding and more experienced amenorrhea. If abnormal bleeding is persistent or severe, appropriate investigation and treatment should be instituted.

In three contraception trials, 39.0 % of women experienced amenorrhea during month six, and 56.5% experienced amenorrhea during month 12. The changes in menstrual bleeding patterns from the three contraception trials are presented in Figures 3 and 4.

Figure 3. Percentages of depo-subQ provera 104 Treated Women with Amenorrhea per 30-Day Month in Contraception Studies (ITT Population, N=2053)

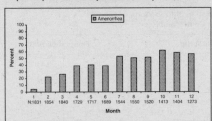

N = Number of subjects in analysis for indicated month

Figure 4. Mean (25th, 75th Percentiles) Number of Bleeding and/or Spotting Days in the Subgroup of Women with Bleeding and/or Spotting by Month for Women Treated with depo-subQ provera 104 in Contraception Studies

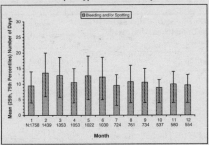

N = Number of subjects with bleeding and/or spotting during indicated month

The changes in menstrual patterns in the two endometriosis trials are presented in Figures 5 and 6.

Figure 5. Percentages of depo-subQ provera 104 Treated Women with Amenorrhea per 30-Day Month in Endometriosis Studies (Combined ITT Population, N=289)

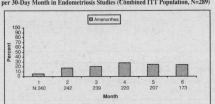

N = Number of subjects in analysis for indicated month

Figure 6. Mean (25th, 75th Percentiles) Number of Bleeding and/or Spotting Days in the Subgroup of Women with Bleeding and/or Spotting by Month for Women Treated with depo-subQ provera 104 in Endometriosis Studies Combined

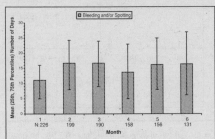

N = Number of subjects with bleeding and/or spotting during indicated month

3. Cancer Risks

Long-term, case-controlled surveillance of users of depot medroxyprogesterone acetate IM 150 mg (Depo-Provera CI, 150 mg) found slight or no increased overall risk of breast cancer and no overall increased risk of ovarian, liver, or cervical cancer, and a prolonged, protective effect of reducing the risk of endometrial cancer.

A pooled analysis[ii] from two case-control studies[iii iv] reported the relative risk (RR) of breast cancer for women who had ever used Depo-Provera CI (150 mg) as 1.1 (95% confidence interval [CI] 0.97 to 1.4). Overall, there was no increase in risk with increasing duration of use of Depo-Provera CI (150 mg). The RR of breast cancer for women of all ages who had initiated use of Depo-Provera CI (150 mg) within the previous 5 years was estimated to be 2.0 (95% CI 1.5 to 2.8). A component of the pooled analysis[iii] described above, showed an increased RR of 2.19 (95% CI 1.23 to 3.89) of breast cancer associated with use of Depo-Provera CI (150 mg) in women whose first exposure to drug was within

the previous 4 years and who were under 35 years of age. However, the overall RR for ever-users of Depo-Provera CI (150 mg) was only 1.21 (95% CI 0.96 to 1.52).

[NOTE: The value of 2.19 means that women whose first exposure to drug was within the previous 4 years and who were under 35 years of age had a 2.19-fold (95% CI 1.23 to 3.89-fold) increased risk of breast cancer relative to nonusers. The National Cancer Institute[v] reports an average annual incidence rate for breast cancer for US women, all races, age 30 to 34 years of 26.7 per 100,000. A RR of 2.19, thus, increases the possible risk from 26.7 to 58.5 cases per 100,000 women. The attributable risk, thus, is 31.8 per 100,000 women per year.]

The relative rate of invasive squamous-cell cervical cancer in women who ever used Depo-Provera CI (150 mg) was estimated to be 1.11 (95% CI 0.96 to 1.29). No trends in risk with duration of use or times since initial or most recent exposure were observed.

4. Thromboembolic Disorders

Although MPA has not been causally associated with the induction of thrombotic or thromboembolic disorders, there have been rare reports of serious thrombotic events in women using Depo-Provera CI (150 mg). Any patient who develops thrombosis while undergoing therapy with depo-subQ provera 104 should discontinue treatment unless she has no other acceptable options for birth control (see CONTRAINDICATIONS).

5. Ocular Disorders

Medication should not be re-administered pending examination if there is a sudden partial or complete loss of vision or if there is a sudden onset of proptosis, diplopia or migraine. If examination reveals papilledema or retinal vascular lesions, medication should not be re-administered.

6. Ectopic Pregnancy

Healthcare providers should be alert to the possibility of an ectopic pregnancy among women using depo-subQ provera 104 who become pregnant or complain of severe abdominal pain.

7. Anaphylaxis and Anaphylactoid Reaction

Serious anaphylactic reactions have been infrequently reported in women using Depo-Provera CI (150 mg). If an anaphylactic reaction occurs, appropriate emergency medical treatment should be instituted.

PRECAUTIONS

1. Physical Examination

It is good medical practice for all women to have annual history and physical examinations, including women using depo-subQ provera 104. The physical examination, however, may be deferred until after initiation of depo-subQ provera 104 if requested by the woman and judged appropriate by the clinician. The physical examination should include special reference to blood pressure, breasts, abdomen and pelvic organs, including cervical cytology and relevant laboratory tests. In case of undiagnosed, persistent or recurrent abnormal vaginal bleeding, appropriate measures should be conducted to rule out malignancy. Women with a strong family history of breast cancer or who have breast nodules should be monitored with particular care.

2. Fluid Retention

Because progestational drugs may cause some degree of fluid retention, conditions that might be influenced by this condition, such as epilepsy, migraine, asthma, and cardiac or renal dysfunction, require careful observation. .

3. Weight Gain

Weight gain is a common occurrence in women using depo-subQ provera 104. In three large clinical trials using depo-subQ provera 104, the mean weight gain was 3.5 lb in the first year of use. In a small, two-year study comparing depo-subQ provera 104 to Depo-Provera CI (150 mg), the mean weight gain observed for women using depo-subQ provera 104 (7.5 lb) was similar to the mean weight gain for women using Depo-Provera CI, 150 mg (7.6 lb).

Although there are no data related to weight gain beyond 2 years for depo-subQ provera 104, the data on Depo-Provera CI (150 mg) may be relevant. In a clinical study, after five years, 41 women using Depo-Provera CI (150 mg) had a mean weight gain of 11.2 lb, while 114 women using nonhormonal contraception had a mean weight gain of 6.4 lb.

4. Return to Ovulation and Fertility

Return to ovulation is likely to be delayed after stopping therapy. Among 15 women who received multiple doses of depo-subQ provera 104:

- Median time to ovulation was 10 months after the last injection
- Earliest return to ovulation was 6 months after the last injection
- 12 women (80%) ovulated within 1 year of the last injection

However, ovulation has occurred as early as 14 weeks after a single dose of depo-subQ provera 104, and therefore it is important to follow the recommended dosing schedule.

Return to fertility also is likely to be delayed after stopping therapy. Among 28 women using depo-subQ provera 104 for contraception who stopped treatment to become pregnant, 1 became pregnant within 1 year of her last injection. A second woman became pregnant 443 days after her last injection. Seven women were lost to follow-up.

5. Depression

Patients with a history of treatment for clinical depression should be carefully monitored while receiving depo-subQ provera 104.

6. Injection Site Reactions

In 5 clinical studies of depo-subQ provera 104 involving 2,325 women (282 treated for up to 6 months, 1,780 treated

for up to 1 year and 263 women treated for up to 2 years), 5% of women reported injection site reactions, and 1% had persistent skin changes, typically described as small areas of induration or atrophy.

7. Carbohydrate/Metabolism

Some patients receiving progestins may exhibit a decrease in glucose tolerance. Diabetic patients should be carefully observed while receiving such therapy.

8. Liver Function

If jaundice or any other liver abnormality develops in any woman receiving depo-subQ provera 104, treatment should be stopped while the cause is determined. Treatment may be resumed when liver function is acceptable and when the healthcare provider has determined that depo-subQ provera 104 did not cause the abnormality.

9. Drug Interactions

No drug-drug interaction studies have been conducted with depo-subQ provera 104. Aminoglutethimide administered concomitantly with depo-subQ provera 104 may significantly decrease the serum concentrations of MPA.

10. Laboratory Tests

The pathologist should be advised of progestin therapy when relevant specimens are submitted. The physician should be informed that certain endocrine and liver function tests, and blood components may be affected by progestin therapy:

(a) Plasma and urinary steroid levels are decreased (e.g., progesterone, estradiol, pregnanediol, testosterone, cortisol).
(b) Plasma and urinary gonadotropin levels are decreased (e.g., LH, FSH).
(c) SHBG concentrations are decreased.
(d) T_3-uptake values may decrease.
(e) There may be small changes in coagulation factors.
(f) Sulfobromophthalein and other liver function test values may be increased slightly.
(g) There may be small changes in lipid profiles.

11. Carcinogenesis, Mutagenesis, Impairment of Fertility

See WARNINGS, section 3 and PRECAUTIONS, section 4

12. Pregnancy

Although depo-subQ provera 104 should not be used during pregnancy, there appears to be little or no increased risk of birth defects in women who have inadvertently been exposed to medroxyprogesterone acetate injections in early pregnancy. Neonates exposed to medroxyprogesterone acetate in-utero and followed to adolescence showed no evidence of any adverse effects on their health including their physical, intellectual, sexual or social development.

13. Nursing Mothers

Although the drug is detectable in the milk of mothers receiving Depo-Provera CI (150 mg), milk composition, quality, and amount are not adversely affected. Neonates and infants exposed to medroxyprogesterone acetate from breast milk have been studied for developmental and behavioral effects through puberty, and no adverse effects have been noted.

14. Pediatric Use

depo-subQ provera 104 is not indicated before menarche. Use of depo-subQ provera 104 is associated with significant loss of bone mineral density (BMD). This loss of BMD is of particular concern during adolescence and early adulthood, a critical period of bone accretion. **In adolescents, interpretation of BMD results should take into account patient age and skeletal maturity.** It is unknown if use of depo-subQ provera 104 by younger women will reduce peak bone mass and increase the risk for osteoporotic fractures in later life. Other than concerns about loss of BMD, the safety and effectiveness are expected to be the same for postmenarchal adolescents and adult women.

15. Geriatric Use

depo-subQ provera 104 is intended for use in women with childbearing potential. Studies with depo-subQ provera 104 in geriatric women have not been conducted.

INFORMATION FOR THE PATIENT

See PATIENT LABELING.

ADVERSE REACTIONS

In five clinical studies of depo-subQ provera 104 involving 2,325 women (282 treated for up to 6 months, 1,780 treated for up to 1 year and 263 treated for up to 2 years), 9% of women discontinued treatment for adverse reactions. Among these 212 women, the most common reasons for discontinuation were:

- Uterine bleeding irregularities (35%, n=75)
- Increased weight (18%, n=39)
- Decreased libido (11%, n=23)
- Acne (10%, n=21)
- Injection site reactions (6%, n=12)

Adverse reactions reported by 5% or more of all women in these clinical trials included:

- Headache (9%)
- Intermenstrual bleeding (7%)
- Increased weight (6%)
- Amenorrhea (6%)
- Injection site reactions (5%)

Adverse reactions reported by 1% to <5% of all women in these clinical trials included:

General disorders: fatigue, injection site pain

Gastrointestinal disorders: abdominal distention, abdominal pain, diarrhea, nausea

Infections: bronchitis, influenza, nasopharyngitis, pharyngitis, sinusitis, upper respiratory tract infection, urinary tract infection, vaginal candidiasis, vaginitis, vaginitis bacterial

Investigations: abnormal cervix smear

Musculoskeletal, connective tissue, and bone disorders: arthralgia, back pain, limb pain

Nervous system disorders: dizziness, insomnia

Psychiatric disorders: anxiety, depression, irritability, decreased libido

Reproductive system and breast disorders: breast pain, breast tenderness, menometrorrhagia, menorrhagia, menstruation irregular, uterine hemorrhage, vaginal hemorrhage

Skin disorders: acne

Vascular disorders: hot flushes

Postmarketing Experience

There have been rare cases of osteoporosis including osteoporotic fractures reported postmarketing in patients taking DEPO-PROVERA Contraceptive Injection. In addition, infrequent voluntary reports of anaphylaxis and anaphylactoid reaction have been received associated with use of Depo-Provera CI (150 mg).

The following additional reactions have been reported with Depo-Provera Contraceptive Injection and may occur with use of depo-subQ provera 104:

General disorders: asthenia, axillary swelling, chills, chest pain, fever, excessive thirst

Blood and lymphatic system disorders: anemia, blood dyscrasia

Cardiac disorders: tachycardia

Gastrointestinal disorders: gastrointestinal disturbances, rectal bleeding

Hepato-biliary disorders: jaundice

Immune system disorders: allergic reaction

Infections genitourinary infections

Investigations: decreased glucose tolerance

Musculoskeletal, connective tissue, and bone disorders: loss of bone mineral density, scleroderma

Neoplasms: breast cancer, cervical cancer

Nervous system disorders: convulsions, facial palsy, fainting, paralysis, paresthesia, somnolence

Psychiatric disorders: increased libido, nervousness

Reproductive system and breast disorders: breast lumps, galactorrhea, nipple discharge or bleeding, oligomenorrhea, prevention of lactation, prolonged anovulation, unexpected pregnancy, uterine hyperplasia, vaginal cyst

Respiratory disorders: asthma, dyspnea, hoarseness

Skin disorders: angioedema, dry skin, increased body odor, melasma, pruritus, urticaria

Vascular disorders: deep vein thrombosis, pulmonary embolus, thrombophlebitis

DOSAGE AND ADMINISTRATION

CONTRACEPTION AND ENDOMETRIOSIS INDICATIONS

Route of Administration

depo-subQ provera 104 must be given by subcutaneous injection into the anterior thigh or abdomen, once every 3 months (12 to 14 weeks). depo-subQ provera 104 is not formulated for intramuscular injection. Dosage does not need to be adjusted for body weight. The pre-filled syringe of depo-subQ provera 104 must be vigorously shaken just before use to create a uniform suspension.

First Injection

Ensure that the patient is not pregnant at the time of the first injection. For women who are sexually active and having regular menses, the first injection should be given only during the first 5 days of a normal menstrual period. Women who are breast-feeding may have their first injection during or after their sixth postpartum week.

Second and Subsequent Injections

Dosing is every 12 to 14 weeks. If more than 14 weeks elapse between injections, pregnancy should be ruled out before the next injection.

IF USING FOR CONTRACEPTION AND SWITCHING FROM ANOTHER METHOD

When switching from other contraceptive methods, depo-subQ provera 104 should be given in a manner that ensures continuous contraceptive coverage. For example, patients switching from combined (estrogen plus progestin) contraceptives should have their first injection of depo-subQ provera 104 within 7 days after the last day of using that method (7 days after taking the last active pill, removing the patch or ring). Similarly, contraceptive coverage will be maintained in switching from Depo-Provera CI (150 mg) to depo-subQ provera 104, provided the next injection is given within the prescribed dosing period for Depo-Provera CI (150 mg).

IF USING FOR TREATMENT OF ENDOMETRIOSIS

Treatment for longer than two years is not recommended, due to the impact of long-term depo-subQ provera 104 on bone mineral density. If symptoms return after discontinuation of treatment, bone mineral density should be evaluated prior to retreatment.

Instructions for Administration of depo-subQ provera 104 for Subcutaneous Use

Getting ready

Ensure that the medication is at room temperature. Make sure the following components (Diagrams 1, 2, and 3) are available.

[See figure at top of next column]

depo-subQ provera 104, as with other parenteral drug products, should be inspected visually for particulate matter and discoloration prior to administration.

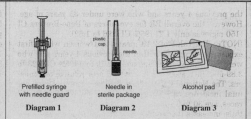

Prefilled syringe   Needle in   Alcohol pad
with needle guard   sterile package

Diagram 1   **Diagram 2**   **Diagram 3**

Step 1: Choosing and preparing the injection area.

Choose the injection area. Avoid boney areas and the umbilicus. See shaded areas (Diagram 4).

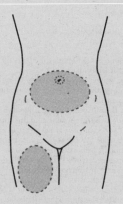

Upper thigh & Abdomen
Diagram 4

Use an alcohol pad to wipe the skin in the injection area you have chosen. Allow the skin to dry.

Step 2: Syringe preparation

Gently twist off the protective end cap from the needle to break the seal (Diagram 5). Set aside.

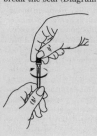

Diagram 5

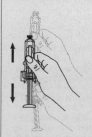

While holding the syringe firmly by the barrel pointing upward, shake it forcefully for at least 1 minute to thoroughly mix the medication (Diagram 6).

Diagram 6

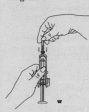

Hold the syringe barrel firmly, remove the protective tip cap from the syringe and attach the needle by pushing it onto the barrel tip (Diagram 7).

Diagram 7

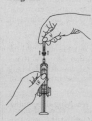

While continuing to hold the syringe barrel firmly, remove the clear protective plastic cover from the needle, making sure the needle is still firmly attached to the syringe (Diagram 8).

Diagram 8

While holding the syringe with the needle pointing upward, gently push in the plunger until the medicine is up to the top of the syringe (Diagram 9).

Diagram 9

Step 3: Injecting the dose.

Gently grasp and squeeze a large area of skin in the chosen injection area between the thumb and forefinger (Diagram 10) pulling it away from the body.

Diagram 10

Insert the needle at a 45 degree angle so that most of the needle is in the fatty tissue. The plastic hub of the needle should be nearly or almost touching the skin (Diagram 11).

Diagram 11

Inject the medication slowly until the syringe is empty (Diagram 12). This should take about 5-7 seconds.

Diagram 12

The entire dose must be given to activate the needle guard. When the entire dose is completely injected, gently pull the needle out of the skin. Remove your finger from the plunger, allowing the syringe to move up inside the device until the needle guard completely covers the exposed needle. **You will hear a 'click' when the needle guard is fully activated.** It is very important that the entire dose of depo-subQ provera 104 is given.

Use a clean cotton pad to press lightly on the injection area for a few seconds. **Do NOT rub the area.**

Following the administration of each dose, the used syringe should be discarded in a safe and proper manner.

HOW SUPPLIED

depo-subQ provera 104 for subcutaneous use (medroxyprogesterone acetate injectable suspension 104 mg/0.65 mL) is available as a pre-filled syringe, pre-assembled with an UltraSafe Passive™ Needle Guard* device, and packaged with a 26-gauge × 3/8 inch needle in the following presentation:

NDC 0009-4709-01   0.65 mL single-use, disposable syringe

Store at controlled room temperature 20° to 25° C (68° to 77°F) [see USP].

Rx only

*UltraSafe Passive™ Needle Guard is a trademark of Safety Syringes, Inc.

Distributed by
Pharmacia and Upjohn Co
Division of Pfizer Inc, NY, NY 10017
March 2005
LAB-0295-1.0

i   Trussell J. Contraceptive efficacy. In Hatcher RA, Trussell J, Stewart F, Cates W, Stewart GK, Kowel D, Guest F, Contraceptive Technology: 17th Revised Edition. New York, NY: Irvington Publishers, 1998.

ii   Skegg DCG, Noonan EA, Paul C, Spears GFS, Meirik O, Thomas DB. Depot Medroxyprogesterone Acetate and Breast Cancer: A Pooled Analysis from the World Health Organization and New Zealand Studies. JAMA. 1995; 273(10): 799-804.

iii   WHO Collaborative Study of Neoplasia and Steroid Contraceptives. Breast cancer and depot-medroxyprogesterone acetate: a multi-national study. Lancet. 1991; 338:833-838.

iv   Paul C, Skegg DCG, Spears GFS. Depot medroxyprogesterone (Depo-Provera) and risk of breast cancer. Br Med J. 1989; 299:759-762.

v   Surveillance, Epidemiology, and End Results: Incidence and Mortality Data, 1973-1977. National Cancer Institute Monograph, 57: June 1981. (NIH publication No. 81-2330).

To keep your **PDR** up to date throughout the year, note these revisions on the corresponding pages of the annual volume. Simply write **"See Supplement A"** next to the product heading.

Purdue Pharma L.P.

ONE STAMFORD FORUM
STAMFORD, CT 06901-3431

For Medical Inquiries:
888-726-7535
Adverse Drug Experiences:
888-726-7535
Customer Service:
800-877-5666
FAX 800-877-3210

PALLADONE™ Ⓒ℞

[pă'-lah-dōn]

Hydromorphone Hydrochloride Extended-Release Capsules 12 mg, 16 mg, 24 mg, 32 mg

FOR USE IN OPIOID-TOLERANT PATIENTS ONLY

WARNING

Palladone™ (hydromorphone HCl extended-release) Capsules are indicated for the management of persistent, moderate to severe pain in patients requiring continuous, around-the-clock analgesia with a high potency opioid for an extended period of time (weeks to months) or longer. Palladone™ Capsules should only be used in patients who are already receiving opioid therapy, who have demonstrated opioid tolerance, and who require a minimum total daily dose of opiate medication equivalent to 12 mg of oral hydromorphone. Patients considered opioid tolerant are those who are taking at least 60 mg oral morphine/day, or at least 30 mg of oral oxycodone/day, or at least 8 mg oral hydromorphone/day, or an equianalgesic dose of another opioid, for a week or longer. Palladone™ Capsules should be administered once every 24 hours.

Appropriate patients for treatment with Palladone Capsules include patients who require high doses of potent opioids on an around-the-clock basis to improve pain control and patients who have difficulty attaining adequate analgesia with immediate-release opioid formulations.

Palladone Capsules are contraindicated for use on an as needed basis (i.e., prn).

Palladone™ Capsules are NOT intended to be used as the first opioid product prescribed for a patient, or in patients who require opioid analgesia for a short period of time.

Palladone™ Capsules are for use in OPIOID-TOLERANT patients ONLY. Use in non-opioid-tolerant patients may lead to FATAL RESPIRATORY DEPRESSION. Overestimating the Palladone dose when converting patients from another opioid medication can result in fatal overdose with the first dose. Due to the mean apparent 18-hour elimination half-life of Palladone, patients who receive an overdose will require an extended period of monitoring and treatment that may go beyond 18 hours. Even in the face of improvement, continued medical monitoring is required because of the possibility of extended effects.

Palladone™ Capsules contain the potent Schedule II opioid agonist, hydromorphone. Schedule II opioid agonists (which include hydromorphone, fentanyl, methadone, morphine, oxycodone, and oxymorphone), have the highest risk of fatal overdoses due to respiratory depression, as well as the highest potential for abuse. Palladone can be abused in a manner similar to other opioid agonists, legal or illicit. These risks should be considered when administering, prescribing, or dispensing Palladone in situations where the healthcare professional is concerned about increased risk of misuse, abuse, or diversion.

Persons at increased risk for opioid abuse include those with a personal or family history of substance abuse (including drug or alcohol abuse or addiction) or mental illness (e.g., major depression). Patients should be assessed for their clinical risks for opioid abuse or addiction prior to being prescribed opioids. All patients receiving opioids should be routinely monitored for signs of misuse, abuse and addiction. Patients at increased risk of opioid abuse may still be appropriately treated with modified-release opioid formulations; however these patients will require intensive monitoring for signs of misuse, abuse, or addiction.

Palladone Capsules are to be swallowed WHOLE and are not to be broken, chewed, opened, dissolved or crushed. Consuming alcohol while taking Palladone™ Capsules or taking broken, chewed, dissolved, or crushed Palladone™ Capsules or its contents can lead to the rapid release and absorption of a potentially fatal dose of hydromorphone. Overestimating the Palladone dose when converting the patient from another opioid medication can result in fatal overdose with the first dose. With the long half-life of Palladone (18 hours), patients who receive the wrong dose will require an extended period of monitoring and treatment that may go beyond 18 hours. Even in the face of improvement, continued medical monitoring is required because of the possibility of extended effects.

DESCRIPTION

Palladone™ (hydromorphone HCl extended-release) Capsules are an opioid analgesic supplied in 12 mg, 16 mg, 24 mg, and 32 mg capsule strengths for oral administration. The pellet formulation is the same for all capsule strengths. The strength designation of each capsule indicates the amount of hydromorphone hydrochloride salt. The structural formula, molecular description, and molecular weight are shown below:

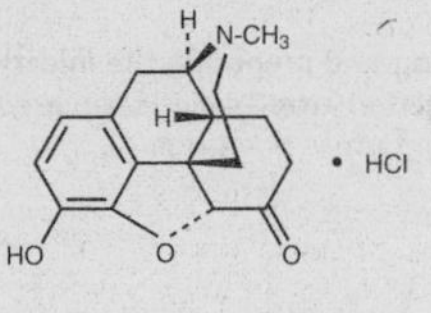

$C_{17}H_{19}NO_3 \cdot HCl$ MW 321.80

The chemical name is 4,5α-epoxy-3-hydroxy-17 methylmorphinan-6-one hydrochloride.

Hydromorphone, a fine, white (or nearly white), crystalline powder, is a semi-synthetic congener of morphine. The inactive ingredients in the pellets are ammonio methacrylate copolymer type B, ethylcellulose, and stearyl alcohol. The inactive ingredients in the capsules and the inks used to imprint them are FD&C blue #2 (24 mg strength capsule only), gelatin, red iron oxide (12 mg and 16 mg strength capsules only), synthetic black iron oxide, and titanium dioxide.

Palladone™ Capsules are based on a controlled-release melt extrusion technology in which pellets containing hydromorphone HCl and co-melted excipients release the active ingredient significantly more slowly and for a longer period than an immediate-release product. Palladone™ Capsules are designed to provide controlled delivery of hydromorphone over 24 hours. The 12 mg, 16 mg, 24 mg, and 32 mg capsules are filled with identical pellets using different fill weights to achieve different strengths.

Palladone™ Capsules are for use in opioid-tolerant patients only. Use in non-opioid-tolerant patients may lead to fatal respiratory depression.

CLINICAL PHARMACOLOGY

Hydromorphone is a pure opioid agonist whose principal therapeutic action is analgesia. Other members of the class known as opioid agonists include substances such as morphine, oxycodone, fentanyl, codeine, and hydrocodone. Pharmacological effects of opioid agonists include anxiolysis, euphoria, feelings of relaxation, respiratory depression, constipation, miosis, and cough suppression, and analgesia. Like all pure opioid agonist analgesics, with increasing doses there is increasing analgesia, unlike with mixed agonist/antagonists or non-opioid analgesics, where there is a limit to the analgesic effect with increasing doses. With pure opioid agonist analgesics, there is no defined maximum dose; the ceiling to analgesic effectiveness is imposed only by side effects, the more serious of which may include somnolence and respiratory depression.

Central Nervous System

The precise mechanism of the analgesic action is unknown. However, specific CNS opioid receptors for endogenous compounds with opioid-like activity have been identified throughout the brain and spinal cord and play a role in the analgesic effects of this drug.

Hydromorphone produces respiratory depression by direct action of brain stem respiratory centers. The respiratory depression involves both a reduction in the responsiveness of the brain stem to increases in carbon dioxide and to electrical stimulation.

Hydromorphone depresses the cough reflex by direct effect on the cough center in the medulla. Antitussive effects may occur with doses lower than those usually required for analgesia.

Hydromorphone causes miosis even in total darkness. Pinpoint pupils are a sign of opioid overdose but are not pathognomonic (e.g., pontine lesions of hemorrhagic or ischemic origin may produce similar findings). Marked mydriasis rather than miosis may be seen with hypoxia in the setting of Palladone™ Capsule overdose (see **OVERDOSAGE**).

Gastrointestinal System

Hydromorphone causes a reduction in motility associated with an increase in smooth muscle tone in the antrum of the stomach and in the duodenum. Digestion of food is delayed in the small intestine and propulsive contractions are decreased. Propulsive peristaltic waves in the colon are decreased, while tone may be increased to the point of spasm resulting in constipation. Other opioid induced-effects may include a reduction in gastric, biliary and pancreatic secretions, spasm of the sphincter of Oddi, and transient elevations in serum amylase.

Cardiovascular System

Hydromorphone may produce release of histamine with or without associated peripheral vasodilation. Manifestations of histamine release and/or peripheral vasodilation may include pruritus, flushing, red eyes, sweating, and/or orthostatic hypotension.

Endocrine System

Opioid agonists have been shown to have a variety of effects on the secretion of hormones. Opioids inhibit the secretion of ACTH, cortisol, and luteinizing hormone (LH) in humans. They also stimulate prolactin, growth hormone (GH) secretion, and pancreatic secretion of insulin and glucagon in humans and other species, rats and dogs. Thyroid stimulating hormone (TSH) has been shown to be both inhibited and stimulated by opioids.

PHARMACOKINETICS

Absorption

Administration of a single Palladone™ Capsule dose is characterized by biphasic absorption, a relatively rapid rise to an initial peak concentration, followed by a second broader peak with therapeutic plasma concentrations maintained over the 24-hour dosing interval. The absolute bioavailability of hydromorphone from Palladone™ Capsules has not been determined. Under conditions of multiple dosing, the bioavailability of a once-daily dose of Palladone™ Capsules is equivalent to the same total daily dose of immediate-release hydromorphone given in divided doses every 6 hours. Hydromorphone absorption from Palladone Capsules is pH independent but can be significantly increased in the presence of alcohol (see **DRUG INTERACTIONS**). Dose proportionality has been established in terms of C_{max} and AUC for the 12 mg and 24 mg dosage strengths. Dosage form proportionality on a dose-adjusted basis has been demonstrated for three 12 mg capsules to one 32 mg capsule.

In a study comparing 12 mg Palladone™ Capsules dosed every 24 hours to 3 mg of immediate-release hydromorphone dosed every 6 hours in healthy human subjects, the two treatments were found to be equivalent in terms of extent of absorption (AUC) (see Figure 1). The extended-release characteristics of Palladone™ Capsules resulted in lower steady-state peak levels (C_{max}), higher trough levels (C_{min}), and an approximately twofold to threefold reduction in the fluctuation seen with the immediate-release hydromorphone tablets.

FIGURE 1. Steady-State Plasma Hydromorphone Concentration-Time Curves

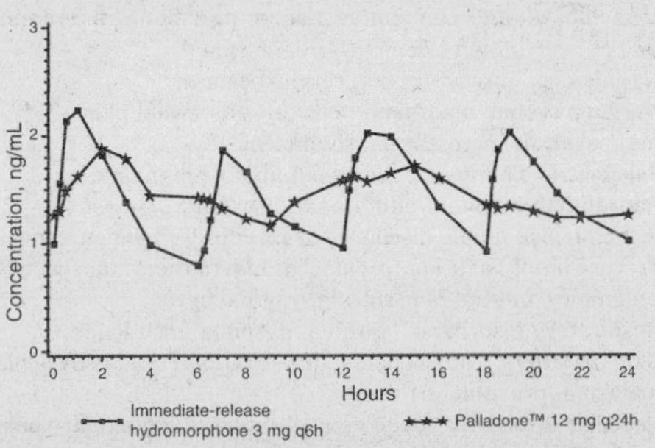

Steady-state plasma concentrations with Palladone™ Capsules were achieved within 2 to 3 days after initiation of dosing. This is consistent with the mean apparent terminal elimination half-life for Palladone™ of approximately 18.6 hours. This supports the ability to titrate every 2 to 3 days, as necessary. Hydromorphone did not accumulate significantly after multiple dosing with once-daily administration. Food had no significant effect on the peak (C_{max}), AUC or the elimination of hydromorphone from Palladone™ Capsules (See Figure 2.).

FIGURE 2. Single-Dose Palladone™ Pharmacokinetic Profiles

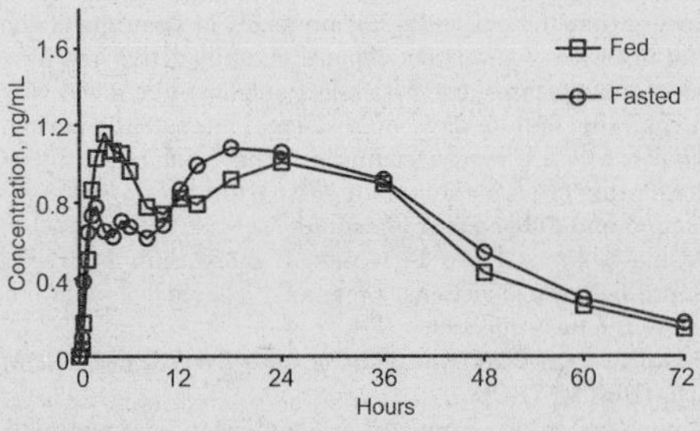

Distribution

Following intravenous administration of hydromorphone, the reported volume of distribution is 295 L (4 L/kg). Hydromorphone is approximately 20% bound to human plasma proteins.

Metabolism

Hydromorphone is metabolized by direct conjugation, or by 6-keto reduction followed by conjugation. Following absorption, hydromorphone is metabolized to the major metabolites hydromorphone-3-glucuronide, hydromorphone-3-glucoside and dihydroisomorphine-6-glucuronide. Also observed were the less prevalent metabolites, dihydroisomorphine-6-glucoside, dihydromorphine and dihydroisomorphine.

Hydromorphone metabolites have been found in plasma, urine and in human hepatocyte test systems. However, it is not known whether hydromorphone is metabolized by the cytochrome P450 enzyme system. Hydromorphone is a poor inhibitor of human recombinant CYP isoforms including CYP1A2, 2A6, 2C8, 2D6, and 3A4 with an IC50 > 50 μM. Therefore, hydromorphone is not expected to inhibit the metabolism of other drugs metabolized by these CYP isoforms.

Elimination

Full mass balance and recovery studies have not been reported for extended-release hydromorphone products. However, hydromorphone and its metabolites have been recovered in urine following the use of immediate-release hydromorphone. Following intravenous administration of hydromorphone, terminal half-life is approximately 3 hours and clearance is 1.66 L/hr. The apparent terminal half-life with controlled release hydromorphone is about 18.6 hours.

Drug Interactions

Concomitant administration of H_2 receptor blockers (cimetidine, famotidine, ranitidine) or proton pump inhibitors (omeprazole, lansoprazole) showed no significant effect on Palladone™ steady-state pharmacokinetics.

Patients taking Palladone with other opioid analgesics, general anesthetics, phenothiazines, tricyclic antidepressants or other CNS depressants may experience additional CNS depression and therefore, dose adjustments should be considered. Consuming alcohol while taking Palladone Capsules can cause significant increases in peak hydromorphone concentrations.

SPECIAL POPULATIONS

Pediatric

The safety and effectiveness of Palladone™ Capsules have not been established in patients below the age of 18.

Geriatric

Age-related increases in exposure in clinical studies were observed between geriatric and younger adult subjects. Greater sensitivity of some older individuals cannot be excluded. Dosages should be adjusted according to the clinical situation.

Gender

Pharmacokinetics of hydromorphone from Palladone™ Capsules are comparable in men and women.

Renal Impairment

In patients with mild to moderate renal impairment, based on calculated creatinine clearance, the concentrations of hydromorphone in plasma were slightly higher than in subjects with normal renal function.

Hepatic Impairment

Palladone™ Capsules were not studied in patients with severe hepatic insufficiency and are not recommended for use in such patients. Care in initial dose selection and careful observation are recommended in patients with evidence of lesser degrees of hepatic impairment.

Race

The pharmacokinetics of hydromorphone in African Americans and Caucasians in the clinical population were comparable.

CLINICAL TRIALS

The efficacy of Palladone™ Capsules was established in a double-blind, randomized, parallel group, multicenter, placebo-controlled, four-week trial of patients with pain that was present for at least one month. The majority of these patients experienced moderate to severe pain due to musculoskeletal disorders while maintained on one or more opioid analgesics, often in addition to non-opioid analgesics. Two hundred twenty-one patients with chronic moderate to severe pain were randomized to receive once daily 12 mg Palladone™ Capsules or placebo after they had demonstrated that they needed approximately 12 mg of immediate-release hydromorphone (in addition to non-opioid medication) around-the-clock to improve their pain control. Patients randomized to Palladone™ Capsules maintained adequate analgesia for a significantly longer period of time ($P<0.0001$) than patients randomized to placebo.

INDICATIONS AND USAGE

Palladone™ (hydromorphone HCl extended-release) Capsules are indicated for the management of persistent, moderate to severe pain in patients requiring continuous, around-the-clock analgesia with a high potency opioid for an extended period of time generally weeks to months or longer. Palladone™ Capsules should only be used in patients who are already receiving opioid therapy, have demonstrated opioid tolerance, and who require a minimum total daily dose of opiate medication equivalent to 12 mg of oral hydromorphone. Patients considered opioid tolerant are those who are taking at least 60 mg oral morphine/day, or at least 30 mg oral oxycodone/day, or at least 8 mg oral hydromorphone/day, or an equianalgesic dose of another opioid, for a week or longer. Appropriate patients for treatment with Palladone include patients who require high doses of potent opioids on an around-the-clock basis to improve pain control, and patients who have difficulty attaining adequate analgesia with immediate-release opioid formulations.

Palladone™ Capsules are NOT intended to be used:

- **as the first opioid product prescribed for a patient.**
- **in patients who require opioid analgesia for a short period of time.**
- **on an as needed basis (i.e., prn).**

An evaluation of the appropriateness and adequacy of immediate-release opioids is advisable prior to initiating therapy with any modified-release opioid. Prescribers should individualize treatment in every case, initiating therapy at the appropriate point along a progression from non-opioid analgesics, such as non-steroidal anti-inflammatory drugs and acetaminophen, to opioids, in a plan of pain management such as outlined by the World Health Organization, the Agency for Health Research and Quality, the Federation of State Medical Boards Model Policy, or the American Pain Society.

Patients should be assessed for their clinical risks for opioid abuse or addiction prior to being prescribed opioids. Patients receiving opioids should be routinely monitored for signs of misuse, abuse, and addiction. Persons at increased risk for opioid abuse include those with a personal or family history of substance abuse (including drug or alcohol abuse or addiction) or mental illness (e.g., major depression). Patients at increased risk may still be appropri- ately treated with modified-release opioid formulations; however these patients will require intensive monitoring for signs of misuse, abuse, or addiction.

CONTRAINDICATIONS

Palladone™ Capsules are contraindicated:

- for use on an as needed basis (i.e., prn).
- in situations of significant respiratory depression, especially in unmonitored settings where there is a lack of resuscitative equipment.
- in patients who have acute or severe bronchial asthma.
- in patients who have or are suspected of having paralytic ileus.
- in patients with known hypersensitivity to any of its components or the active ingredient, hydromorphone.

WARNINGS

Palladone Capsules are to be swallowed WHOLE and are not to be broken, chewed, opened, dissolved or crushed. Consuming alcohol while taking Palladone Capsules or taking broken, chewed, dissolved, or crushed Palladone™ Capsules or capsule contents can lead to the rapid release and absorption of a potentially fatal dose of hydromorphone.

Palladone™ Capsules are for use in OPIOID-TOLERANT patients ONLY. Use in non-opioid-tolerant patients may lead to fatal respiratory depression.

Misuse, Abuse and Diversion of Opioids

Hydromorphone is an opioid agonist of the morphine type. Such drugs are sought by drug abusers and people with addiction disorders and are subject to criminal diversion.

Like other opioid agonists, legal or illicit, hydromorphone can be abused. This should be considered when prescribing or dispensing Palladone™ Capsules in situations where the healthcare professional is concerned about an increased risk of misuse, abuse, or diversion.

Breaking, crushing, chewing, or dissolving the contents of a Palladone™ Capsule or consuming alcohol while taking Palladone Capsules can result in the uncontrolled delivery of the opioid and poses a significant risk of overdose and death (see **WARNINGS** and **DRUG ABUSE AND ADDICTION**).

Concerns about abuse, addiction, and diversion should not prevent the proper management of pain. However, all patients treated with opioids require careful monitoring for signs of abuse and addiction, since use of opioid analgesic products carries the risk of addiction even under appropriate medical use.

Healthcare professionals should contact their State Professional Licensing Board, or State Controlled Substances Authority for information on how to prevent and detect abuse or diversion of this product.

Interactions with Alcohol and Drugs of Abuse

Hydromorphone may be expected to have additive effects, when used in conjunction with alcohol, other opioids, or drugs, whether legal or illicit, which cause central nervous system depression. Additionally, consuming alcohol while taking Palladone Capsules can cause significant increases in peak hydromorphone concentrations.

Drug Abuse and Addiction

Palladone™ Capsules contain an opioid agonist (i.e., hydromorphone), that is a Schedule II controlled substance with high potential for abuse similar to fentanyl, methadone, morphine, oxycodone, and oxymorphone. Hydromorphone can be abused and is subject to criminal diversion. The high drug content in the extended-release formulation may add to the risk of adverse outcomes from abuse.

Addiction is a primary, chronic, neurobiologic disease, with genetic, psychosocial, and environmental factors influencing its development and manifestations. It is characterized by behaviors that include one or more of the following: impaired control over drug use, compulsive use, continued use despite harm, and craving. Drug addiction is a treatable disease, utilizing a multidisciplinary approach, but relapse is common.

"Drug-seeking" behavior is very common in addicts and drug abusers. Drug-seeking tactics include emergency calls or visits near the end of office hours, refusal to undergo appropriate examination, testing or referral, repeated "loss" of prescriptions, tampering with, forging or counterfeiting prescriptions and reluctance to provide prior medical records or contact information for other treating physician(s). "Doctor shopping" to obtain additional prescriptions is common among drug abusers, people suffering from untreated addiction and criminals seeking drugs to sell.

Abuse and addiction are separate and distinct from physical dependence and tolerance. Physicians should be aware that addiction may not be accompanied by concurrent tolerance and symptoms of physical dependence in all addicts. In addition, abuse of opioids can occur in the absence of addiction and is characterized by misuse for non-medical purposes, often in combination with other psychoactive substances. Since Palladone™ Capsules may be diverted for non-medical use, careful record keeping of prescribing information, including quantity, frequency, and renewal requests is strongly advised.

Proper assessment of the patient, proper prescribing practices, periodic re-evaluation of therapy, and proper dispensing and storage are appropriate measures that help to limit abuse of opioid drugs.

Palladone™ Capsules are intended for oral use only. Consumption of alcohol while taking Palladone Capsules or the use of the broken, crushed, chewed, opened, or dissolved capsule contents poses a hazard of overdose and death. This risk is increased with concurrent abuse of alcohol and other substances. Parenteral drug abuse can reasonably be expected to result in local tissue necrosis, infection, pulmonary granulomas, and increased risk of endocarditis and valvular heart injury. In addition, parenteral abuse is commonly associated with transmission of infectious diseases such as hepatitis and HIV.

Respiratory Depression

Respiratory depression is the chief hazard of opioid agonists, including hydromorphone, the active ingredient in Palladone™ Capsules. Respiratory depression is more likely to occur in elderly or debilitated patients, usually following large initial doses in non-tolerant patients, or when opioids are given in conjunction with other drugs that depress respiration.

Respiratory depression from opioids is manifested by a reduced urge to breathe and a decreased rate of respiration, often associated with the "sighing" pattern of breathing (deep breaths separated by abnormally long pauses). Carbon dioxide retention from opioid-induced respiratory depression can exacerbate the sedating effects of opioids. This makes overdoses involving drugs with sedative properties and opioids especially dangerous.

Hydromorphone should be used with extreme caution in patients with significant chronic obstructive pulmonary disease or cor pulmonale, and in patients having a substantially decreased respiratory reserve, hypoxia, hypercapnia, or pre-existing respiratory depression. In such patients, even usual therapeutic doses of hydromorphone may decrease respiratory drive to the point of apnea. In these patients, alternative non-opioid analgesics should be considered, and opioids should be employed only under careful medical supervision at the lowest effective dose.

Head Injury

The respiratory depressant effects of opioids include carbon dioxide retention and secondary elevation of cerebrospinal fluid pressure and may be markedly exaggerated in the presence of head injury, intracranial lesions, or other sources of pre-existing increased intracranial pressure. Hydromorphone produces effects on pupillary response and consciousness, which may obscure neurologic signs of further increases in intracranial pressure in patients with head injuries.

Hypotensive Effect

Palladone™ Capsules may cause severe hypotension. There is an added risk to individuals whose ability to maintain blood pressure has been compromised by a depleted blood volume or who are concurrently taking drugs such as phenothiazines or other agents which compromise vasomotor tone. Hydromorphone may produce orthostatic hypotension in ambulatory patients. Hydromorphone, like all opioid analgesics of the morphine-type, should be administered with caution to patients in circulatory shock, since vasodilation produced by the drug may further reduce cardiac output and blood pressure.

PRECAUTIONS

Palladone™ Capsules are for use in OPIOID-TOLERANT patients ONLY. Use in non-opioid-tolerant patients may lead to fatal respiratory depression (see WARNINGS).

Patients should be instructed that the use of Palladone™ by anyone other than those to whom it is prescribed is unlawful and may have serious medical consequences, including death.

General

Opioid analgesics have a narrow therapeutic index in certain patient populations, especially when combined with CNS depressant drugs, and should be reserved for cases where the benefits of opioid analgesia outweigh the known risks of respiratory depression, altered mental state, and postural hypotension.

Use of Palladone™ Capsules is associated with increased potential risks and should be used only with caution in the following conditions: alcoholism, alcohol abuse or alcohol intoxication; drug abuse; history of drug or alcohol abuse; adrenocortical insufficiency (e.g., Addison's disease); CNS depression or coma; debilitated patients; kyphoscoliosis associated with respiratory depression; myxedema or hypothyroidism; prostatic hypertrophy or urethral stricture; severe impairment of hepatic, pulmonary or renal function; and toxic psychosis.

The administration of any opioid agonist, including hydromorphone, may obscure the diagnosis or clinical course in patients with acute abdominal conditions. Hydromorphone may aggravate convulsions in patients with convulsive disorders, and all opioids may induce or aggravate seizures in some clinical settings.

Use in Pancreatic/Biliary Tract Disease

Hydromorphone may cause spasm of the sphincter of Oddi and should be used with caution in patients with biliary tract disease, including acute pancreatitis. Opioids like hydromorphone may cause increases in the serum amylase concentration.

Tolerance

Tolerance is a state of adaptation in which exposure to a drug induces changes that result in a diminution of one or more of the drug's effects over time. Tolerance may occur to both the desired and undesired effects of drugs, and may develop at different rates for different effects.

Physical Dependence

Physical dependence is a state of adaptation that is manifested by an opioid specific withdrawal syndrome that can

Continued on next page

Palladone—Cont.

be produced by abrupt cessation, rapid dose reduction, decreasing blood level of the drug, and/or administration of an antagonist.

The opioid abstinence or withdrawal syndrome is characterized by some or all of the following: restlessness, lacrimation, rhinorrhea, yawning, perspiration, chills, piloerection, myalgia, mydriasis, irritability, anxiety, backache, joint pain, weakness, abdominal cramps, insomnia, nausea, anorexia, vomiting, diarrhea, or increased blood pressure, respiratory rate, or heart rate.

In general, opioids should not be abruptly discontinued (see **DOSAGE AND ADMINISTRATION: Cessation of Therapy**).

Information for Patients/Caregivers

The healthcare professional should explain the points listed below to caregivers and patients.

1. Patients should be instructed to read the Medication Guide each time Palladone is dispensed because new information may be available. The complete text of the Medication Guide is reprinted at the end of this document.
2. Patients should be aware that Palladone™ Capsules contain hydromorphone, which is a strong pain medication similar to fentanyl, methadone, morphine, oxycodone, and oxymorphone.
3. Palladone™ Capsules are only to be swallowed whole. To prevent fatal overdose, the capsules and the pellets must not be broken, chewed, crushed, opened, or dissolved. Patients should be instructed not to consume alcohol while taking Palladone Capsules.
4. Patients should talk to their doctor if pain persists or worsens while they are taking Palladone™ Capsules. Patients who have bothersome side effects should also let their doctors know. The amount of medicine the patient takes may have to be changed.
5. Patients should NEVER change the amount of Palladone™ Capsules they take without speaking to their doctor first.
6. Palladone™ Capsules can affect a person's ability to perform activities that require a high level of attention (such as driving or using heavy machinery). Patients taking Palladone™ Capsules should be warned of these dangers and counseled accordingly.
7. Patients should NOT combine Palladone™ Capsules with alcohol or other pain medications, sleep aids, or tranquilizers except by the orders of the prescribing physician, because dangerous additive effects may occur, resulting in serious injury or death.
8. Women who become pregnant, or who plan to become pregnant, should ask their doctor about the effects that Palladone™ Capsules (or any medicine) may have on them and their unborn children.
9. Patients should be advised that if they have been receiving treatment with Palladone™ Capsules for more than a few weeks and the medicine is no longer needed, they should contact their doctor who will advise them on how to gradually decrease the medication. When Palladone™ Capsules are no longer needed, the unused capsules should be flushed down the toilet.
10. The active ingredient in Palladone™ Capsules is hydromorphone, which is a drug that some people abuse. Palladone™ Capsules should be taken only by the patient it was prescribed for, and it should be protected from theft or misuse in the work or home environment.
11. Patients should be instructed to keep Palladone™ Capsules in a secure place out of the reach of children. Children, especially small children, exposed to Palladone™ Capsules are at high risk of FATAL RESPIRATORY DEPRESSION.

Use in Drug and Alcohol Addiction

Palladone™ Capsules are not approved for use in detoxification or maintenance treatment of opioid addiction. However, the history of an addictive disorder does not necessarily preclude the use of this medication for the treatment of chronic pain. These patients will require intensive monitoring for signs of misuse, abuse, or addiction.

DRUG INTERACTIONS

CNS Depressants

Hydromorphone should be dosed with caution in patients who are concurrently taking other central nervous system depressants that may cause respiratory depression, hypotension, profound sedation or potentially result in coma. Such agents include barbiturates, other sedatives or hypnotics, general anesthetics, other opioid analgesics, phenothiazines and other neuroleptics, centrally acting antiemetics, benzodiazepines or other tranquilizers, and alcohol.

Muscle Relaxants

Hydromorphone may interact with skeletal muscle relaxants to enhance neuromuscular blocking action to increase respiratory depression.

Mixed Agonist-Antagonist Opioid Analgesics

Agonist/antagonist analgesics (i.e., pentazocine, nalbuphine, and butorphanol) should be administered with caution to a patient who has received or is receiving a course of therapy with a pure opioid agonist analgesic such as hydromorphone. In this situation, significant doses of mixed agonist/antagonist analgesics may reduce the analgesic effect of hydromorphone and/or may precipitate withdrawal symptoms in these patients.

Monoamine Oxidase Inhibitors (MAOIs)

No specific interaction between hydromorphone and monoamine oxidase inhibitors has been observed, but caution in the use of any opioid in patients taking this class of drugs is appropriate. MAOI therapy should be discontinued for at least two weeks prior to the initiation of therapy with Palladone™ Capsules.

H₂ Antagonists/Proton Pump Inhibitors

In the patients enrolled in the clinical trials, Palladone™ exposure and effects on pain were comparable when administered with or without various H₂ antagonists/proton pump inhibitors.

Drug/Laboratory Test Interactions

There is no known interference of this drug with laboratory tests.

Food

The bioavailability of Palladone™ Capsules is not significantly affected by food.

Carcinogenesis, Mutagenesis, Impairment of Fertility

No carcinogenicity studies have been conducted in animals. Hydromorphone was negative in the *in vitro* bacterial reverse mutation assay and in the *in vivo* mouse micronucleus assay. Hydromorphone was negative in the mouse lymphoma assay in the absence of metabolic activation, but was positive in the mouse lymphoma assay in the presence of metabolic activation. Morphinone, an impurity, tested as a besylate salt was negative in the *in vitro* bacterial reverse mutation assay and negative in the *in vivo* mouse micronucleus assay. Morphinone was positive in the Chinese Hamster Ovary Cell Chromosomal Aberration test in the absence and presence of metabolic activation.

Hydromorphone did not affect fertility in rats at oral doses up to 5 mg/kg which is equivalent to a 32 mg human daily oral dose on a body surface area basis.

Pregnancy

Pregnancy Category C

Hydromorphone was not teratogenic in female rats given oral doses up to 10 mg/kg or female rabbits given oral doses up to 50 mg/kg during the major period of organ development. Estimated exposures in the female rat and rabbit were approximately 3-fold and 6-fold higher than a 32 mg human daily oral dose based on exposure (AUC_{0-24h}). In a rat pre- and post-natal study, an increase in pup mortality and a decrease in pup body weight which was associated with maternal toxicity was observed at doses of 2 and 5 mg/kg/day. The maternal no effect level for hydromorphone was 0.5 mg/kg/day which is <1-fold lower than a 32 mg human daily oral dose on a body surface area. Hydromorphone had no effect on pup development or reproduction when given to female rats during the pre-natal and postnatal periods up to a dose of 5 mg/kg which is equivalent to a 32 mg human daily oral dose on a body surface area basis.

Hydromorphone administration to pregnant Syrian hamsters and CF-1 mice during major organ development revealed teratogenicity likely the result of maternal toxicity associated with sedation and hypoxia. In Syrian hamsters given single subcutaneous doses from 14 to 278 mg/kg during organogenesis (gestation days 8-10), doses ≥ 19 mg/kg hydromorphone produced skull malformations (exencephaly and cranioschisis). Continuous infusion of hydromorphone (5 mg/kg, s.c.) via implanted osmotic mini pumps during organogenesis (gestation days 7-10) produced soft tissue malformations (cryptorchidism, cleft palate, malformed ventricals and retina), and skeletal variations (supraoccipital, checkerboard and split sternebrae, delayed ossification of the paws and ectopic ossification sites). The malformations and variations observed in the hamsters and mice were at doses approximately 3-fold higher and <1-fold lower, respectively, than a 32 mg human daily oral dose on a body surface area basis.

There are no adequate and well-controlled studies in pregnant women. Hydromorphone crosses the placenta. Palladone™ Capsules should be used during pregnancy only if the potential benefit justifies the potential risk to the fetus (see **Labor and Delivery**).

Labor and Delivery

Palladone™ Capsules are not recommended to be initiated prior to or during labor or in the immediate post-partum period. Women who are taking opioids during pregnancy should not be withdrawn abruptly during labor and delivery, but maintained on their current dose of medication since abrupt withdrawal can precipitate delivery. Neonates whose mothers have been taking hydromorphone chronically may exhibit respiratory depression and/or withdrawal symptoms, at birth and/or in the post-delivery period.

Neonatal Withdrawal Syndrome

Chronic use of opioids during pregnancy can affect the fetus with subsequent withdrawal symptoms. Neonatal withdrawal syndrome presents as irritability, hyperactivity and loss of sleep pattern, abnormal crying, tremor, vomiting, diarrhea and subsequent weight loss or failure to gain weight and may result in death. The duration and severity of neonatal withdrawal syndrome varies based on the drug used, duration of use, the time and dose of last maternal use, and rate of elimination by the newborn. Use standard care as medically appropriate.

Nursing Mothers

Low concentrations of opioid analgesics have been detected in breast milk with the potential for withdrawal symptoms when administration of opioid analgesics to the mother is stopped. The distribution of hydromorphone has not been studied. It is prudent to assume that hydromorphone would also distribute into breast milk. Ordinarily, nursing should

not be undertaken while a patient is receiving Palladone™ Capsules because of the possibility of sedation and/or respiratory depression in the infant.

Pediatric Use

The safety and effectiveness of Palladone™ Capsules have not been established in patients below the age of 18 years.

Geriatric Use

Of the total number of subjects in clinical studies of Palladone™ Capsules, 22% were 65 and over, and 6% were 75 and over. Dosages should be adjusted according to the clinical situation. As with all opioids, the starting dose should be reduced to 1/3 to 1/2 of the usual dosage in debilitated patients. Respiratory depression is the chief hazard in elderly or debilitated patients, usually following large initial doses in non-tolerant patients, or when opioids are given in conjunction with other agents that depress respiration.

Laboratory Monitoring

Due to the broad range of plasma concentrations that are associated with individual daily dose requirements to achieve adequate pain relief, the varying degrees of pain, and the development of tolerance seen in patient populations, plasma hydromorphone measurements are usually not helpful in clinical management.

Hepatic Impairment

Palladone™ Capsules were not studied in patients with severe hepatic impairment and are not recommended for use in such patients. Care in initial dose selection and careful observation are recommended in patients with evidence of mild to moderate hepatic impairment.

Renal Impairment

In patients with mild to moderate renal impairment, based on calculated creatinine clearance, the concentrations of hydromorphone in plasma were slightly higher than in subjects with normal renal function. Dosages should always be adjusted according to the clinical situation.

Gender

There were no male/female differences detected for efficacy, pharmacokinetic metrics or adverse events in clinical trials.

Race

Analgesia and adverse events were similar in the various ethnic groups included in the clinical program.

ADVERSE REACTIONS

The safety of Palladone™ Capsules was evaluated in double-blind clinical trials involving 612 patients with moderate to severe pain. An open-label extension study involving 143 patients with cancer pain was conducted to evaluate the safety of Palladone™ Capsules when used for longer periods of time in higher doses than in the controlled trials. Patients were treated with doses averaging 40 to 50 mg of Palladone™ Capsules per day (ranging between 12 and 500 mg/day) for several months (range 1 to ≥ 52 weeks). Serious adverse reactions which may be associated with Palladone™ Capsules therapy in clinical use are similar to those of other opioid analgesics, including respiratory depression, apnea, respiratory arrest, and to a lesser degree, circulatory depression, hypotension, shock or cardiac arrest (see **OVERDOSAGE**).

Adverse Events Reported in Controlled Trials

Table 3 lists treatment emergent signs and symptoms that were reported in at least 2% of patients in the placebo-controlled trials for which the rate of occurrence was greater for those treated with Palladone™ 12 mg Capsules than those treated with placebo.

TABLE 3: ADVERSE EVENTS REPORTED IN THE PLACEBO-CONTROLLED CLINICAL TRIALS WITH INCIDENCE ≥ 2% IN PATIENTS RECEIVING PALLADONE™ CAPSULES FOR NONMALIGNANT PAIN

Body System/ COSTART Term	Placebo* (N = 191) Double-blind %	Palladone™* (N = 190) Double-blind %
Total percentage of patients with AEs	35.1%	49.5%
Body as a Whole	**15.7%**	**18.4%**
Headache	2.1%	4.7%
Asthenia	0.5%	3.2%
Infection	5.8%	5.3%
Digestive	**13.1%**	**27.9%**
Constipation	1.0%	15.8%
Nausea	6.3%	10.5%
Vomiting	1.6%	3.2%
Nervous	**13.1%**	**11.6%**
Somnolence	1.6%	4.7%
Skin	**5.2%**	**4.7%**
Pruritus	1.0%	2.6%

*Average exposure was 21 days for Palladone™ and 15 days for placebo.

Adverse Events Observed in Clinical Trials

Palladone™ Capsules have been administered to 785 individuals during completed clinical trials. The conditions and duration of exposure to Palladone™ varied greatly, and included open-label and double-blind studies, uncontrolled and controlled studies, inpatient and outpatient studies, fixed dose and titration studies. Untoward events associated with this exposure were recorded by clinical investigators using terminology of their own choosing.

These categories are used in the listing below. The frequencies represent the proportion of 785 patients from these trials who experienced that event while receiving Palladone™ Capsules. All adverse events included in this tabulation occurred in at least one patient. Events are classified by body system and listed using the following definitions: frequent adverse events - those occurring in at least 1/100 patients; adverse events occurring with an incidence less than 1% are considered infrequent. These adverse events are not necessarily related to Palladone™ Capsule treatment and in most cases were observed at a similar frequency in placebo-treated patients in the controlled studies.

Frequent Adverse Events
Body as a Whole: headache, asthenia, pain, abdominal pain, fever, chest pain, infection, chills, malaise, neck pain, carcinoma, accidental injury
Cardiovascular: vasodilatation, tachycardia, migraine
Digestive: nausea, constipation, vomiting, diarrhea, dyspepsia, anorexia, dry mouth, nausea and vomiting, dysphagia, flatulence
Hematologic and Lymphatic: anemia, leukopenia
Metabolic and Nutritional: peripheral edema, dehydration, edema, generalized edema, hypokalemia, weight loss
Musculoskeletal: arthralgia, bone pain, leg cramps, myalgia
Nervous: somnolence, dizziness, nervousness, confusion, insomnia, anxiety, depression, hypertonia, hypesthesia, paresthesia, tremor, thinking abnormal, hallucinations, speech disorder, agitation, amnesia, tinnitus, abnormal gait
Respiratory: dyspnea, cough increased, rhinitis, pharyngitis, pneumonia, epistaxis, hiccup, hypoxia, pleural effusion
Skin and Appendages: pruritus, sweating, rash
Special Senses: amblyopia, taste perversion
Urogenital: dysuria, urinary incontinence
Infrequent Adverse Events
Body as a Whole: face edema, ascites, allergic reaction, cellulitis, overdose, hypothermia, neoplasm, photosensitivity reaction, sepsis, flank pain
Cardiovascular: hypertension, hypotension, syncope, deep thrombophlebitis, arrhythmia, postural hypotension, atrial fibrillation, pallor, bradycardia, electrocardiogram abnormal, myocardial infarction, palpitation, angina pectoris, congestive heart failure, QT interval prolonged, supraventricular tachycardia, thrombosis, cardiomegaly, hemorrhage
Digestive: fecal impaction, intestinal obstruction, abnormal stools, fecal incontinence, hepatic failure, increased appetite, cholangitis, cholecystitis, colitis, enterocolitis, hepatomegaly, jaundice, liver function tests abnormal, biliary spasm, ileus, eructation, rectal hemorrhage, esophagitis, glossitis, melena, mouth ulceration, gastrointestinal hemorrhage, tongue edema
Endocrine: adrenal cortex insufficiency
Hematologic and Lymphatic: ecchymosis, thrombocytopenia, leukocytosis, lymphadenopathy, agranulocytosis, lymphoma like reaction, pancytopenia, petechia
Metabolic and Nutritional: hyperglycemia, hyponatremia, cachexia, hypercalcemia, hypomagnesemia, cyanosis, diabetes mellitus, gout, respiratory acidosis, elevated liver enzymes, thirst
Musculoskeletal: myasthenia
Nervous: abnormal dreams, emotional lability, paranoid reaction, sleep disorder euphoria, incoordination, stupor, ataxia, convulsion, hallucination, hostility, myoclonus, psychosis, vertigo, withdrawal syndrome, apathy, delirium, dementia, drug dependence, nystagmus, twitching, depersonalization, aphasia, cerebrovascular accident, circumoral parasthesia, seizure, hyperkinesia, hypotonia, increased salivation, neuralgia
Respiratory: hypoventilation, apnea, atelectasis, hemoptysis, asthma, hyperventilation, pulmonary embolus, laryngismus
Skin and Appendages: urticaria, maculopapular rash, alopecia
Special Senses: abnormal vision, diplopia, dry eyes, lacrimation disorder, hyperacusis
Urogenital: urinary retention, hematuria, impotence, urinary frequency, urination impaired, dysmenorrhea, creatinine increased, urinary urgency
Additional Adverse Events From Non-U.S. Experience
Addiction, blurred vision, drowsiness, dysphoria, sedation, seizure, physical dependence, biliary spasm, and ileus

OVERDOSAGE

Acute overdosage with hydromorphone can be manifested by respiratory depression, somnolence progressing to stupor or coma, skeletal muscle flaccidity, cold and clammy skin, constricted pupils, bradycardia, hypotension, and death.

The nature of extended-release hydromorphone should also be taken into account when treating the overdose. Even in the face of improvement, continued medical monitoring is required because of the possibility of extended effects. Deaths due to overdose may occur with abuse and misuse of Palladone™ Capsules.

In the treatment of hydromorphone overdosage, primary attention should be given to the re-establishment of a patent airway and institution of assisted or controlled ventilation. Supportive measures (including oxygen and vasopressors) should be employed in the management of circulatory shock and pulmonary edema accompanying overdose as indicated. Cardiac arrest or arrhythmias may require cardiac massage or defibrillation.

The pure opioid antagonists, such as naloxone or nalmefene, are specific antidotes against respiratory depression from opioid overdose. Opioid antagonists should not be administered in the absence of clinically significant respiratory or circulatory depression secondary to hydromorphone overdose. In patients who are physically dependent on any opioid agonist including Palladone™ Capsules, an abrupt or complete reversal of opioid effects may precipitate an acute abstinence syndrome. The severity of the withdrawal syndrome produced will depend on the degree of physical dependence and the dose of the antagonist administered. Please see the prescribing information for the specific opioid antagonist for details of their proper use.

DOSAGE AND ADMINISTRATION
Special Precautions
Palladone™ Capsules contain the potent Schedule II opioid agonist, hydromorphone. Schedule II opioid agonists, which include hydromorphone, fentanyl, methadone, morphine, oxycodone, and oxymorphone, have the highest risk of fatal overdoses from respiratory depression, as well as the highest potential for abuse. Hydromorphone, like morphine and other opioids used in analgesia, can be abused and is subject to criminal diversion.

Consuming alcohol while taking Palladone Capsules or taking broken, chewed, dissolved or crushed Palladone™ Capsules or its contents can lead to the rapid release and absorption of a potentially fatal dose of hydromorphone.

Overestimating the Palladone dose when converting patients from another opioid medication can result in fatal overdose with the first dose. Due to the mean apparent 18-hour elimination half-life of Palladone, patients who receive an overdose will require an extended period of monitoring and treatment that may go beyond 18 hours. Even in the face of improvement, continued medical monitoring is required because of the possibility of extended effects. Palladone™ Capsules are for use in OPIOID-TOLERANT patients only. Use in non-opioid-tolerant patients may lead to FATAL RESPIRATORY DEPRESSION.

General Principles
Palladone™ (hydromorphone HCl extended-release) Capsules are indicated for the management of persistent, moderate to severe pain in patients requiring continuous, around-the-clock analgesia with a high potency opioid for an extended period of time, generally weeks to months, or longer.

Palladone™ Capsules should only be used in patients who are already receiving opioid therapy, who have demonstrated opioid tolerance, and who require a minimum total daily dose of opiate medication equivalent to 12 mg of oral hydromorphone. Patients considered opioid tolerant are those who are taking at least 60 mg oral morphine/day, or at least 30 mg oral oxycodone/day, or at least 8 mg oral hydromorphone/day, or an equianalgesic dose of another opioid, for a week or longer. It is usually appropriate to treat a patient with only one opioid for around-the-clock therapy.

Palladone™ Capsules are not intended to be used on an as needed basis or as the first opioid product prescribed for a patient, or in patients who require opioid analgesia for a short period of time.

The extended-release nature of the formulation allows it to be administered once every 24 hours (see **CLINICAL PHARMACOLOGY**).

Physicians should individualize treatment using a progressive plan of pain management such as outlined by the World Health Organization, the American Pain Society and the Federation of State Medical Boards Model Policy. Healthcare professionals should follow appropriate pain management principles of careful assessment and ongoing monitoring (see **BOXED WARNING**).

Initiation of Therapy
Palladone™ Capsules are for use in opioid-tolerant patients ONLY.

It is critical to initiate the dosing regimen individually for each patient, taking into account the patient's prior opioid treatment. **Overestimating the Palladone dose when converting patients from another opioid medication can result in fatal overdose with the first dose. Due to the mean apparent 18-hour elimination half-life of Palladone, patients who receive an overdose will require an extended period of monitoring and treatment that may go beyond 18 hours. Even in the face of improvement, continued medical monitoring is required because of the possibility of extended effects.**

Attention should be given to:
• the patient's medical condition, past medical history, co-morbid conditions and concurrent medications;
• risk factors for abuse, addiction or diversion, including a prior history of abuse, addiction or diversion;
• the intensity, pattern, quality and expected duration of pain;
• the daily dose, potency and kind of opioid the patient has been taking;
• whether adjustments should be made to any non-opioid analgesic(s) the patient has been taking;
• the clinical variability of any conversion estimate used to calculate the dose of hydromorphone; and
• the balance between an adequate level of pain control and adverse experiences.

The total daily (24-hour) dose of the patient's previous opioid should be determined.

A) Using standard conversion ratio estimates (see Table 4 below), multiply the milligrams per day of the previous opioids by the appropriate conversion factors to obtain the equivalent total daily dose of oral hydromorphone.

The conversion ratios represent a reasonable starting point, although they have not been verified in well-controlled, multiple-dose trials.
B) Modify the dose if indicated, based primarily on considerations outlined in the 7 bulleted items listed above.
C) Round off to a dose which is appropriate for the capsule strengths available (12 mg, 16 mg, 24 mg, and 32 mg capsules).
D) Discontinue all other around-the-clock opioid analgesics when Palladone™ Capsules are initiated.

No fixed conversion ratio is likely to be satisfactory in all patients, especially patients receiving large opioid doses. The recommended doses are only a starting point, and close observation and frequent titration is indicated until a satisfactory dose is obtained on the new therapy.

TABLE 4: MULTIPLICATION FACTORS FOR CONVERTING THE DAILY DOSE OF PRIOR OPIOIDS TO THE DAILY DOSE OF ORAL HYDROMORPHONE* (MG/DAY PRIOR OPIOID X FACTOR = MG/DAY ORAL HYDROMORPHONE)

Factor PRIOR OPIOID	ORAL	PARENTERAL
Codeine	0.04	–
Hydrocodone	0.22	–
Hydromorphone	1.00	5.00
Levorphanol	1.88	3.75
Meperidine	0.02	0.10
Methadone	0.38	0.75
Morphine	0.12	0.75
Oxycodone	0.25	–

*To be used only for conversion TO oral hydromorphone.

For patients receiving high-dose parenteral opioids, a more conservative conversion is warranted. For example, for high dose parenteral morphine, use 0.38 instead of 0.75 as a multiplication factor, i.e., halve the multiplication factor.

Most patients given around-the-clock therapy with controlled-release opioids may need to have immediate-release medication available for exacerbations of pain or to treat or prevent pain that occurs predictably during certain patient activities (incident pain).

Palladone™ Capsules can be safely used concomitantly with usual doses of non-opioid analgesics and analgesic adjuvants, provided care is taken to select a proper initial dose (see **PRECAUTIONS**).

Conversion from Transdermal Fentanyl to Palladone™ Capsules
Eighteen hours following the removal of the transdermal fentanyl patch, Palladone™ Capsule treatment can be initiated. A conservative hydromorphone dose, approximately 12 mg once a day of Palladone™, should be initially substituted for each 50 µg/hr of transdermal fentanyl. The patient should be observed closely for early titration as there is very limited clinical experience with this conversion.
Conversion from Opioid Combination Drugs
Patients currently receiving around-the-clock fixed-combination-opioid analgesics, and greater than or equal to a daily dose of 45 mg of oxycodone or hydrocodone equivalents or 300 mg daily dose of codeine equivalents, may be started on 12 mg of Palladone™ Capsules once daily. The non-opioid component of the combination product may be continued as a separate drug. Alternatively, a different non-opioid analgesic may be selected.
Supplemental (Rescue) Analgesics
Most patients given around-the-clock therapy with controlled-release opioids may need to have immediate-release medication available for exacerbations of pain or to treat or prevent pain that occurs predictably during certain patient activities (incident pain).
Individualization of Dosage
Once therapy is initiated, pain relief and other opioid effects should be assessed frequently. Palladone™ Capsules should be titrated to adequate effect (generally mild or less pain with the regular use of no more than two doses of supplemental analgesics per 24 hours). Rescue medication should be available (see **Supplemental [Rescue] Analgesics**). Because steady-state plasma concentrations are achieved within approximately 2 to 3 days of therapy with Palladone™, dosage adjustment can be carried out as frequently as every two days, when clinically necessary. If more than two doses of rescue medication are needed within a 24 hour period for two consecutive days, the dose of Palladone™ should usually be titrated upward. This formulation should be administered once every 24 hours. As a guideline, the total daily hydromorphone dose (including rescue) usually can be increased by 25% to 50% of the current dose at each upward titration.

If signs of excessive opioid-related adverse experiences are observed, the dose may be reduced. If this adjustment leads to inadequate analgesia, a supplemental dose of immediate-release opioid analgesic may be given. Alternatively, non-opioid analgesic adjuvants may be administered. Dose adjustments should be made to obtain an appropriate balance between pain relief and opioid-related adverse experiences. If common opioid-related adverse events occur before the therapeutic goal of pain relief is achieved, the events should be effectively treated prior to continuing upward titration of Palladone™ Capsules. Once adverse events are under control, upward titration should continue to an acceptable level of pain control.

Continued on next page

Palladone—Cont.

During periods of changing analgesic requirements, including initial titration, frequent contact is recommended between physician, other members of the healthcare team, the patient and the caregiver/family.

Managing Expected Opioid Adverse Reactions

Many patients receiving opioids will experience adverse reactions. Frequently the adverse reactions from Palladone™ Capsules are transient, but often they require evaluation and management. Certain opioid adverse reactions such as constipation should be anticipated and effectively and prophylactically treated with a stimulant laxative and/or stool softener. Patients do not usually become tolerant to the constipating effects of opioids.

Other opioid-related adverse reactions such as sedation and nausea are usually self-limited and often do not persist beyond the first few days. If nausea persists and is unacceptable to the patient, treatment with antiemetics or other modalities may relieve these symptoms and should be considered.

Continuation of Therapy

The intent of the titration period is to establish a patient-specific daily dose that will provide adequate analgesia with acceptable side effects and minimal rescue doses (2 or less) for as long as pain relief is necessary. Should pain recur, the dose can be increased to re-establish pain control. The method of therapy adjustment outlined above should be employed to regain pain control.

During chronic around-the-clock opioid therapy, patients should be followed closely and their pain should be reassessed as clinically indicated. Patients should continue to be assessed for their clinical risks for opioid abuse or addiction, particularly with high-dose formulations.

Cessation of Therapy

When the patient no longer requires therapy with Palladone™ Capsules, doses should be tapered gradually to prevent signs and symptoms of withdrawal in the physically dependent patient. Proper disposal of unused capsules should be ensured by flushing them down the toilet.

Conversion from Palladone™ Capsules to Parenteral Opioids

To avoid overdose, conservative dose conversion ratios should be followed.

SPECIAL HANDLING AND STORAGE CONDITIONS

Palladone™ Capsules are solid dosage forms that contain hydromorphone which is a controlled substance. Like fentanyl, methadone, morphine, oxycodone, and oxymorphone, hydromorphone is controlled under Schedule II of the Federal Controlled Substances Act.

Palladone™ Capsules may be targeted for theft and diversion by criminals.

Healthcare professionals can telephone Purdue Pharma's Medical Services Department (1-888-726-7535) for information on this product.

HOW SUPPLIED

Palladone™ (hydromorphone hydrochloride extended-release) Capsules 12 mg are cinnamon-colored capsules imprinted with P-XL on the cap and 12 mg on the body. They are available in **multiple-use containers, not intended for dispensing directly to the patient.** They are supplied as follows:

NDC 59011-312-60: opaque plastic bottles of 60 capsules
NDC 59011-312-20: Unit dose packaging with 20 capsules; 10 individually numbered blister units per card: two cards per carton

Palladone™ (hydromorphone hydrochloride extended-release) Capsules 16 mg are pink capsules imprinted with P-XL on the cap and 16 mg on the body. They are available in **multiple-use containers, not intended for dispensing directly to the patient.** They are supplied as follows:

NDC 59011-313-60: opaque plastic bottles of 60 capsules
NDC 59011-313-20: Unit dose packaging with 20 capsules; 10 individually numbered blister units per card; two cards per carton

Palladone™ (hydromorphone hydrochloride extended-release) Capsules 24 mg are blue capsules imprinted with P-XL on the cap and 24 mg on the body. They are available in **multiple-use containers, not intended for dispensing directly to the patient.** They are supplied as follows:

NDC 59011-314-60: opaque plastic bottles of 60 capsules
NDC 59011-314-20: Unit dose packaging with 20 capsules; 10 individually numbered blister units per card; two cards per carton

Palladone™ (hydromorphone hydrochloride extended-release) Capsules 32 mg are white capsules imprinted with P-XL on the cap and 32 mg on the body. They are available in **multiple-use containers, not intended for dispensing directly to the patient.** They are supplied as follows:

NDC 59011-315-60: opaque plastic bottles of 60 capsules
NDC 59011-315-20: Unit dose packaging with 20 capsules; 10 individually numbered blister units per card; two cards per carton

Store at 25°C (77°F); excursions permitted to 15°-30°C (59°-86°F) [See USP Controlled Room Temperature].

Avoid temperatures above 40°C (104°F) [See USP Excessive Heat]

Dispense in a tight, light-resistant container.

CAUTION

DEA ORDER FORM REQUIRED.

©2004, Purdue Pharma L.P.

Purdue Pharma L.P.
Stamford, CT 06901-3431, USA

U.S. Patent Numbers 5,958,452; 5,965,161; 5,968,551; 6,294,195; 6,335,033; 6,706,281; 6,743,442.
November 16, 2004

MEDICATION GUIDE

PALLADONE™ (PAL-ah-doan)
(hydromorphone hydrochloride extended-release)
Capsules CII 12 mg, 16 mg, 24 mg, 32 mg

Read the Medication Guide that comes with Palladone™ before you start taking it and each time you get more Palladone. There may be new information. This information does not take the place of talking to your healthcare provider about your medical condition or your treatment. Share this important information with members of your household.

What is the most important information I should know about Palladone™?

- **Palladone is only for adults with constant (around the clock) pain that is moderate to severe and expected to last for weeks or longer.** Palladone should only be started if you are already using other narcotic medicines and your body has gotten used to them (opioid tolerant). **Palladone can cause serious side effects, including trouble breathing, which can lead to death, especially if used the wrong way.**
- **Palladone is not for occasional ("as needed") use.**
- **Palladone should not be the first opioid (narcotic) pain medicine that is prescribed for your pain.**
- **Palladone is not for patients who need opioid pain medicines for only a short time.**
- **Do not drink alcohol while taking Palladone Capsules. Do not break, crush, dissolve, chew, or open** Palladone™ **Capsules. Palladone Capsules must be swallowed whole.** Drinking alcohol while taking Palladone Capsules or taking a broken, crushed, dissolved, or chewed Palladone Capsule or its contents can release the full 24-hour dose into your body all at once. This is very dangerous. You could die from an overdose of the medicine.
- **Keep Palladone in a safe place away from children.** Accidental use by a child is a medical emergency and can result in death. If a child accidentally takes Palladone, call your local Poison Control Center or the nearest emergency room right away.
- **Palladone is an opioid (narcotic) pain medicine.** There is a chance you could get addicted to Palladone. The chance is higher if you are or have been addicted to or abused other medicines, street drugs, or alcohol, or if you have a history of mental problems.
- **Palladone™ is a Schedule II, federally controlled substance because it contains an opioid (narcotic) pain medicine** that can be a target for people who abuse prescription medicines or street drugs. Keep your Palladone in a safe place to protect it from being stolen. Never give Palladone to anyone else, even if they have the same symptoms you have. It may harm them and cause death. Selling or giving away this medicine is against the law.

What is Palladone™?

Palladone™ is a prescription medicine that contains the opioid (narcotic) pain medicine hydromorphone. Palladone™ is a very strong pain medicine. Palladone is used to treat adults (18 years of age and older) with constant (around-the-clock) pain that is moderate to severe and is expected to last for weeks or longer. Palladone should be started only after you have been taking other opioid pain medicines and your body has gotten used to them (opioid tolerant). You must stay under your healthcare provider's care while taking Palladone.

Palladone Capsules are not to be used:

- as the first opioid pain medicine prescribed for you
- if you only need opioid pain medicine for a short time
- for occasional ("as needed") use

Who should not take Palladone™?

Do Not Take Palladone if:

- your pain can be taken care of by occasional use of other pain medicines.
- you have acute (sudden) or severe asthma
- you have a stomach problem called a paralytic ileus
- you are allergic to any of the ingredients in Palladone. The active ingredient is hydromorphone. For a complete list of ingredients, see "What are the ingredients of Palladone?" at the end of this leaflet.

What should I tell my healthcare provider before starting Palladone?

Tell your healthcare provider about all of your medical and mental problems, especially the ones listed below:

- trouble breathing or lung problems such as asthma, wheezing, or shortness of breath
- a head injury
- liver or kidney problems
- seizures (convulsions or fits)
- gallbladder problems
- low thyroid (hypothyroidism)
- low blood pressure
- problems urinating
- mental problems including major depression or hallucinations (seeing or hearing things that are not there)
- adrenal gland problems such as Addison's disease
- a past or present drinking problem or alcoholism, or a family history of this problem
- a past or present drug abuse or addiction problem, or a family history of this problem

Tell your healthcare provider if you are:

- **pregnant or planning to become pregnant.** Palladone may harm your unborn baby.

- **breast feeding.** Palladone likely passes through your milk and it may cause serious harm to your baby. You and your doctor should decide whether you should take Palladone or breastfeed, but not both.

Tell your healthcare provider about all the medicines you take, including prescription and non-prescription medicines, vitamins, and herbal supplements. Some medicines may cause serious or life-threatening medical problems when taken with Palladone. Sometimes, the doses of certain medicines and Palladone need to be changed if used together. Be especially careful about other medicines that make you sleepy such as other pain medicines, sleeping pills, anxiety medicines, antihistamines, or tranquilizers. Do not start any new prescription medicine, non-prescription medicine, or herbal supplement while using Palladone until you have talked to your healthcare provider. Your healthcare provider will tell you if it is safe to take other medicines while you are using Palladone.

How should I take Palladone™?

- Take Palladone exactly as prescribed.
- **Palladone Capsules must be swallowed whole with water.** If you cannot swallow the capsule whole, tell your healthcare provider who will advise you what to do. **Do not break, chew, dissolve, crush, or open Palladone Capsules or their contents before swallowing.** Drinking alcohol while taking Palladone Capsules or taking a broken, chewed, dissolved, or crushed Palladone Capsule or its contents can release the full 24-hour dose into your body all at once. This is very dangerous. You could die from an overdose of the medicine.
- Your healthcare provider may change your dose after seeing how the medicine affects you.
- Do not change your dose unless your healthcare provider tells you to change it.
- Do not take Palladone™ more often than prescribed.
- Take Palladone once a day at the same time every day.
- If you miss a dose, take it as soon as possible. Take your next dose 24 hours later. Do not double your prescribed dose of Palladone at any time because this increases your chance of an overdose. If you are not sure what to do, call your healthcare provider.
- **If you take too much Palladone or overdose,** call your local emergency number or Poison Control Center right away, or get emergency help.
- Talk to your healthcare provider often about your pain. Your healthcare provider can decide if your dose of Palladone needs to be changed.

If you continue to have pain or side effects that worry you, call your healthcare provider.

Stopping Palladone™. You should not suddenly stop taking Palladone™. Palladone can cause physical dependence. If your healthcare provider decides you no longer need Palladone™, ask how to slowly reduce this medicine so you don't get sick with withdrawal symptoms. **Do not stop taking Palladone without talking to your healthcare provider.** Stopping Palladone suddenly can make you sick with withdrawal symptoms because your body has become used to it. After stopping Palladone according to the instructions of your healthcare provider, flush the unused capsules down the toilet.

What should I avoid while taking Palladone™?

- **Do not drive, operate heavy machinery, or do other dangerous activities** until you know how Palladone affects how alert you are. Palladone™ can make you sleepy. Ask your healthcare provider when it is okay to do these activities.
- **Do not drink alcohol while using Palladone.** It may increase your chance of getting dangerous side effects.
- **Do not take other medicines without talking to your healthcare provider.** Other medicines include prescription and non-prescription medicines, vitamins, and herbal supplements. Be especially careful about medicines that make you sleepy such as other pain medicines, sleeping pills, anxiety medicines, antihistamines, and tranquilizers.
- **Do not breast feed while using Palladone.** Palladone likely passes through your milk and it may cause serious harm to your baby. You and your doctor should decide whether you should take Palladone or breastfeed, but not both.

What are the possible or reasonably likely side effects of PALLADONE™?

Palladone can cause serious side effects including death, especially if used the wrong way. **See "What is the most important information I should know about Palladone?"**

Call your healthcare provider or get emergency medical help if you:

- have trouble breathing
- have extreme drowsiness with slowed breathing
- have shallow breathing (little chest movement with breathing)
- feel faint, dizzy, confused, or have other unusual symptoms

These can be symptoms that you have taken too much (overdose) Palladone or the dose is too high for you. These symptoms may lead to serious problems or death if not treated right away.

- **Palladone can cause your blood pressure to drop.** This can make you feel dizzy if you get up too fast from sitting or lying down.
- You can develop physical dependence on Palladone. Stopping Palladone suddenly can make you sick with withdrawal symptoms because your body has become used to it. Talk to your healthcare provider about slowly stopping Palladone.

- There is a chance you could get addicted to Palladone. The chance is higher if you are or have been addicted to or abused other medicines, street drugs, or alcohol, or if you have a history of mental problems.

The common side effects of Palladone™ are constipation, nausea, vomiting, nervousness, dizziness, drowsiness, itching, dry mouth, sweating, weakness, and headache. Constipation (not enough or hard bowel movements) is a very common side effect of opioids including Palladone and is unlikely to go away without treatment. Talk to your healthcare provider about the use of laxatives (medicines to treat constipation) and stool softeners to prevent or treat constipation while taking Palladone.

Talk to your healthcare provider about any side effect that bothers you or that does not go away.

These are not all the possible side effects of Palladone™. For a complete list, ask your healthcare provider.

How should I store Palladone?

- Store Palladone at room temperature, 59° to 86° F (15° to 30° C).
- Always keep Palladone in a safe place to protect from theft.
- Flush unused or out-of-date Palladone down the toilet.
- **Keep Palladone™ out of the reach of children. Accidental use in children is a medical emergency and can result in death. If a child accidentally takes Palladone, call your local Poison Control Center or go to the nearest emergency room right away.**

General information about the safe and effective use of Palladone

Use Palladone™ only for the pain for which it was prescribed. Do not give Palladone™ to other people, even if they have the same symptoms you have. **Palladone can harm other people and even cause death. Sharing Palladone is against the law.**

This Medication Guide summarizes the most important information about Palladone™. If you would like more information, talk with your healthcare provider. You can ask your pharmacist or other healthcare provider for information about Palladone™ that is written for health professionals or call Purdue Pharma at 1 (888)726-7535.

What are the ingredients of Palladone?

Active Ingredient: hydromorphone hydrochloride

Inactive Ingredients: Pellets - ammonio methacrylate copolymer type B, ethylcellulose, and stearyl alcohol

Capsules - FD&C blue #2 (24 mg strength capsule only), gelatin, red iron oxide (12 mg and 16 mg strength capsules only), synthetic black iron oxide, and titanium dioxide

This Medication Guide has been approved by the U.S. Food and Drug Administration.

Rx Only

Purdue Pharma L.P.
STAMFORD, CT 06901-3431, USA
OT00470D 301102-0C
November 16, 2004

The sanofi-aventis Group

300 SOMERSET CORPORATE BOULEVARD
BRIDGEWATER, NJ 08807-0977

Direct Inquiries to:
Customer Service
300 Somerset Corporate Boulevard
Bridgewater, NJ 08807-0977
(800) 207-8049

For Medical Information Contact:
Generally:
Medical Information Services
300 Somerset Corporate Boulevard
Bridgewater, NJ 08807-0977
(800) 633-1610
For Oncology Medical Information
call (866) 662-6411

ELIGARD® 45 mg ℞

[ĕl′əgärd]

(leuprolide acetate for injectable suspension)

DESCRIPTION

ELIGARD® 45 mg is a sterile polymeric matrix formulation of leuprolide acetate for subcutaneous injection. It is designed to deliver 45 mg of leuprolide acetate at a controlled rate over a six-month therapeutic period.

Leuprolide acetate is a synthetic nonapeptide analog of naturally occurring gonadotropin releasing hormone (GnRH or LH-RH) that, when given continuously, inhibits pituitary gonadotropin secretion and suppresses testicular and ovarian steroidogenesis. The analog possesses greater potency than the natural hormone. The chemical name is 5-oxo-L-prolyl-L-histidyl-L-tryptophyl-L-seryl-L-tyrosyl-D-leucyl-L-leucyl-L-arginyl-N-ethyl-L-prolinamide acetate with the following structural formula:

[See chemical structure at top of next column]

ELIGARD® 45 mg is prefilled and supplied in two separate, sterile syringes whose contents are mixed immediately prior to administration. The two syringes are joined and the single dose product is mixed until it is homogenous. ELIGARD® 45 mg is administered once every six months subcutaneously, where it forms a solid drug delivery depot.

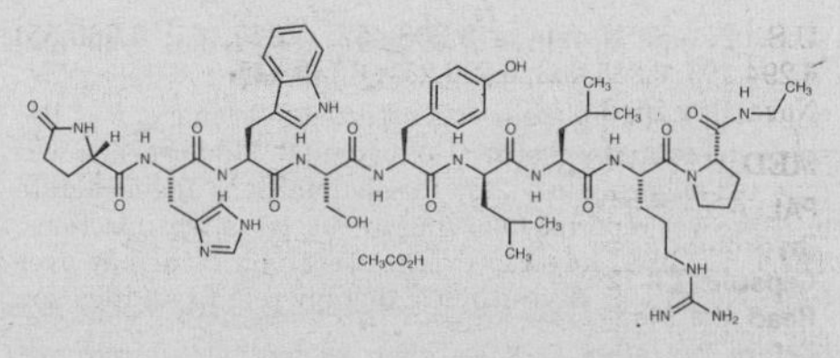

One syringe contains the ATRIGEL® Delivery System and the other contains leuprolide acetate. ATRIGEL® is a polymeric (non-gelatin containing) delivery system consisting of a biodegradable poly(DL-lactide-co-glycolide) (PLG) polymer formulation dissolved in a biocompatible solvent, *N*-methyl-2-pyrrolidone (NMP). PLG is a co-polymer with an 85:15 molar ratio of DL-lactide to glycolide with hexanediol. The second syringe contains leuprolide acetate and the constituted product is designed to deliver 45 mg of leuprolide acetate at the time of subcutaneous injection.

ELIGARD® 45 mg delivers 45 mg of leuprolide acetate (equivalent to approximately 42 mg leuprolide free base) dissolved in 165 mg *N*-methyl-2-pyrrolidone and 165 mg poly(DL-lactide-co-glycolide). The approximate weight of the administered formulation is 375 mg. The approximate injection volume is 0.375 mL.

CLINICAL PHARMACOLOGY

Leuprolide acetate, an LH-RH agonist, acts as a potent inhibitor of gonadotropin secretion when given continuously in therapeutic doses. Animal and human studies indicate that after an initial stimulation, chronic administration of leuprolide acetate results in suppression of testicular and ovarian steroidogenesis. This effect is reversible upon discontinuation of drug therapy.

In humans, administration of leuprolide acetate results in an initial increase in circulating levels of luteinizing hormone (LH) and follicle stimulating hormone (FSH), leading to a transient increase in levels of the gonadal steroids (testosterone and dihydrotestosterone in males, and estrone and estradiol in premenopausal females). However, continuous administration of leuprolide acetate results in decreased levels of LH and FSH. In males, testosterone is reduced to below castrate threshold (≤ 50 ng/dL). These decreases occur within two to four weeks after initiation of treatment.

PHARMACODYNAMICS

Following the first dose of ELIGARD® 45 mg, mean serum testosterone concentrations transiently increased, then fell to below castrate threshold (≤ 50 ng/dL) within three weeks (Figure 1). One patient at Day 1 and another patient at Day 29 were withdrawn from the study before the Month 1 blood draw. Of the 109 patients remaining in the study, 108 (99.1%) had serum testosterone levels below the castrate threshold by Month 1 (Day 28). One patient did not achieve castrate suppression and was withdrawn from the study at Day 85. Once castrate testosterone suppression was achieved, one patient (< 1%) demonstrated breakthrough (concentrations above 50 ng/dL after achieving castrate levels).

Leuprolide acetate is not active when given orally.

PHARMACOKINETICS

Absorption: The pharmacokinetics/pharmacodynamics observed during injections administered initially and at six months (ELIGARD® 45 mg) in 27 patients with advanced carcinoma of the prostate is shown in Figure 1. Mean serum leuprolide concentrations rose to 82 ng/mL and 102 ng/ml (C_{max}) at approximately 4.5 hours following the initial and second injections, respectively. After the initial increase following each injection, mean serum concentrations remained relatively constant (0.2–2.0 ng/mL). There was no evidence of significant accumulation during repeated dosing. Nondetectable leuprolide plasma concentrations have been occasionally observed during ELIGARD® 45 mg administration, but testosterone levels were maintained at castrate levels.

Figure 1 Pharmacokinetic/Pharmacodynamic Response (N = 27) to ELIGARD® 45 mg - Patients Dosed Initially and at Month 6

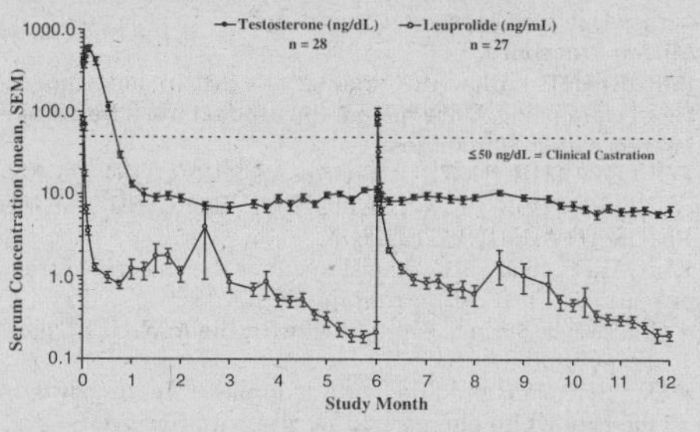

Distribution: The mean steady-state volume of distribution of leuprolide following intravenous bolus administration to healthy male volunteers was 27 L. In vitro binding to human plasma proteins ranged from 43% to 49%.

Metabolism: In healthy male volunteers, a 1 mg bolus of leuprolide administered intravenously revealed that the mean systemic clearance was 8.34 L/h, with a terminal elimination half-life of approximately three hours based on a two compartment model.[1]

No drug metabolism study was conducted with ELIGARD® 45 mg. Upon administration with different leuprolide acetate formulations, the major metabolite of leuprolide acetate is a pentapeptide (M-1) metabolite.

Excretion: No drug excretion study was conducted with ELIGARD® 45 mg.

Special Populations:

Geriatrics: The majority (72%) of the 111 patients studied in the clinical trial were age 70 and older.

Pediatrics: The safety and effectiveness of ELIGARD® 45 mg in pediatric patients have not been established (see **CONTRAINDICATIONS**).

Race: In patients studied (17 White, 7 Black, 3 Hispanic), mean serum leuprolide concentrations were similar.

Renal and Hepatic Insufficiency: The pharmacokinetics of ELIGARD® 45 mg in hepatically and renally impaired patients have not been determined.

Drug-Drug Interactions: No pharmacokinetic drug-drug interaction studies were conducted with ELIGARD® 45 mg.

CLINICAL STUDIES

In one open-label, multicenter study (AGL0205), 111 patients with advanced prostate cancer were treated with at least a single injection of study drug. Of these, 106 patients received a total of two injections of ELIGARD® 45 mg given once every six months. Five patients had Jewett stage A disease, 43 had stage B disease, 19 had stage C disease and 44 patients had stage D disease. This study evaluated the achievement and maintenance of castrate serum testosterone suppression over 12 months of therapy. A total of 103 patients completed the study.

The mean serum testosterone concentration increased from 367.7 ng/dL at Baseline to 588.6 ng/dL at Day 2 following the initial subcutaneous injection. The mean serum testosterone concentration then decreased to below Baseline by Day 14 and was 16.7 ng/dL on Day 28. At the conclusion of the study (Month 12), mean serum testosterone concentration was 12.6 ng/dL (Figure 2).

Of the original 111 patients, two were withdrawn from the study prior to the Month 1 blood draw. Serum testosterone was suppressed to below the castrate threshold (≤ 50 ng/dL) by Day 28 in 108 of 109 (99.1%) patients remaining in the study. One patient (< 1%) did not achieve castrate suppression and was withdrawn from the study on Day 85. Once testosterone suppression at or below serum concentrations of 50 ng/dL was achieved, one patient (< 1%) demonstrated breakthrough (concentration above 50 ng/dL) during the study. This patient reached castrate suppression at Day 21 and remained suppressed until Day 308 when his testosterone level rose to 112 ng/dL. At Month 12 (Day 336), his testosterone was 210 ng/dL. Of 103 evaluable patients in the study at Month 12, 102 had testosterone concentrations of ≤ 50 ng/dL.

All five non-evaluable patients who had achieved castration by Day 28 maintained castration at each timepoint, up to and including the time of withdrawal.

Figure 2 ELIGARD® 45 mg Mean Serum Testosterone Concentrations (n = 103)

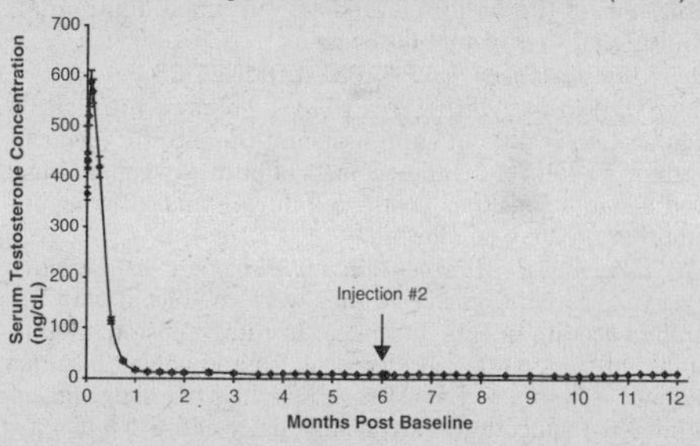

Serum PSA decreased in all patients whose Baseline values were elevated above the normal limit. Individual mean values were reduced an average of 97% from Baseline to Month 12. At Month 12, PSA levels had decreased to within normal limits in 95% of patients who presented with elevated levels at Baseline.

Other secondary efficacy endpoints evaluated included WHO performance status, bone pain, urinary pain and urinary signs and symptoms. At Baseline, 90% of patients were classified as "fully active" by the WHO performance status scale (Status=0), 7% as "restricted in strenuous activity but ambulatory and able to carry out work of a light or sedentary nature" (Status=1), and 3% as "ambulatory but unable to carry out work activities" (Status = 2). At Month 12, the percentage of fully active men increased slightly to 94%, the percentage of men classified as restricted decreased slightly to 5%, and one patient (1%) remained classified as unable to carry out work activities. At Baseline, patients experienced little bone pain, with a mean score of 1.38 (range 1-7) on a scale of 1 (no pain) to 10 (worst pain possible). At Month 12, the mean bone pain score was essentially unchanged at 1.31 (range 1-8). Urinary pain, scored on the same scale, was similarly low, with a mean of 1.22 at Baseline (range 1-8) and was essentially unchanged at Month 12, with a mean score of 1.07 (range 1-5). Urinary signs and symptoms were similarly low at Baseline and decreased modestly at Month 12. In addition, there was a reduction in patients with prostate abnormalities detected during physical exam from 89 (80%) at Screening to 60 (58%) at Month 12.

INDICATIONS AND USAGE

ELIGARD® 45 mg is indicated for the palliative treatment of advanced prostate cancer.

Continued on next page

Eligard 45 mg—Cont.

CONTRAINDICATIONS

1. ELIGARD® 45 mg is contraindicated in patients with hypersensitivity to GnRH, GnRH agonist analogs or any of the components of ELIGARD® 45 mg. Anaphylactic reactions to synthetic GnRH or GnRH agonist analogs have been reported in the literature.[2]

2. ELIGARD® 45 mg is contraindicated in women and in pediatric patients and was not studied in women or children. Moreover, leuprolide acetate can cause fetal harm when administered to a pregnant woman. Major fetal abnormalities were observed in rabbits but not in rats after administration of leuprolide acetate throughout gestation. There were increased fetal mortality and decreased fetal weights in rats and rabbits. The effects on fetal mortality are expected consequences of the alterations in hormonal levels brought about by this drug. The possibility exists that spontaneous abortion may occur.

WARNINGS

ELIGARD® 45 mg, like other LH-RH agonists, causes a transient increase in serum concentrations of testosterone during the first week of treatment. Patients may experience worsening of symptoms or onset of new signs and symptoms during the first few weeks of treatment, including bone pain, neuropathy, hematuria, or bladder outlet obstruction. Isolated cases of ureteral obstruction and/or spinal cord compression, which may contribute to paralysis with or without fatal complications, have been observed in the palliative treatment of advanced prostate cancer using LH-RH agonists (see PRECAUTIONS).

If spinal cord compression or ureteral obstruction develops, standard treatment of these complications should be instituted.

PRECAUTIONS

General: Patients with metastatic vertebral lesions and/or with urinary tract obstruction should be closely observed during the first few weeks of therapy (see WARNINGS section).

Laboratory Tests: Response to ELIGARD® 45 mg should be monitored by measuring serum concentrations of testosterone and prostate specific antigen periodically.

In the majority of patients, testosterone levels increased above Baseline during the first week, declining thereafter to Baseline levels or below by the end of the second week. Castrate levels were generally reached within two to four weeks. One patient (<1%) failed to achieve castrate levels. Once suppressed, only one patient (< 1%) experienced a testosterone breakthrough with testosterone levels exceeding 50 ng/dL.

Results of testosterone determinations are dependent on assay methodology. It is advisable to be aware of the type and precision of the assay methodology to make appropriate clinical and therapeutic decisions.

Drug Interactions: See PHARMACOKINETICS.

Drug/Laboratory Test Interactions: Therapy with leuprolide acetate results in suppression of the pituitary-gonadal system. Results of diagnostic tests of pituitary gonadotropic and gonadal functions conducted during and after leuprolide therapy may be affected.

Carcinogenesis, Mutagenesis, Impairment of Fertility: Two-year carcinogenicity studies were conducted with leuprolide acetate in rats and mice. In rats, a dose-related increase of benign pituitary hyperplasia and benign pituitary adenomas was noted at 24 months when the drug was administered subcutaneously at high daily doses (0.6 to 4 mg/kg). There was a significant but not dose-related increase of pancreatic islet-cell adenomas in females and of testicular interstitial cell adenomas in males (highest incidence in the low dose group). In mice, no leuprolide acetate-induced tumors or pituitary abnormalities were observed at a dose as high as 60 mg/kg for two years. No carcinogenicity studies have been conducted with ELIGARD® 45 mg.

Mutagenicity studies have been performed with leuprolide acetate using bacterial and mammalian systems and with ELIGARD® 7.5 mg in bacterial systems. These studies provided no evidence of a mutagenic potential.

Pregnancy, Teratogenic Effects: Pregnancy category X (see CONTRAINDICATIONS).

Pediatric Use: ELIGARD® 45 mg is contraindicated in pediatric patients and was not studied in children (see CONTRAINDICATIONS).

ADVERSE REACTIONS

The safety of ELIGARD® 45 mg was evaluated in 111 patients with advanced prostate cancer. ELIGARD® 45 mg, like other LH-RH analogs, caused a transient increase in serum testosterone concentrations during the first two weeks of treatment. Therefore, potential exacerbations of signs and symptoms of the disease during the first weeks of treatment are of concern in patients with vertebral metastases and/or urinary obstruction or hematuria. If these conditions are aggravated, it may lead to neurological problems such as weakness and/or paresthesia of the lower limbs or worsening of urinary symptoms (see WARNINGS and PRECAUTIONS).

In Study AGL0205, 111 patients were dosed with ELIGARD® 45 mg every six months for up to 12 months and injection sites were closely monitored. In all, 217 injections of ELIGARD® 45 mg were administered. Transient burning/stinging was reported at the injection site following 35 (16%) injections, with 32 of 35 (91.4%) of these events reported as mild and three of 35 (8.6%) reported as moderate. Mild pain was reported following nine (4.1%) study injections and moderate pain was reported following one (<1%) study injection (total of 2.7% of patients). Mild bruising was reported following five (2.3%) study injections and moderate bruising was reported following two (< 1%) study injections. These localized adverse events were non-recurrent over time. No patient discontinued therapy due to an injection site adverse event.

The following possibly or probably related systemic adverse events occurred during clinical trials of up to 12 months of treatment with ELIGARD® 45 mg, and were reported in ≥ 2% of patients (Table 1). Often, causality is difficult to assess in patients with metastatic prostate cancer. Reactions considered not drug-related are excluded.

Table 1 Incidence (%) of Possibly or Probably Related Systemic Adverse Events Reported by ≥ 2% of Patients (n = 111) Treated with ELIGARD® 45 mg for up to 12 Months in Study AGL0205

Body System	Adverse Event	Number	Percent
Vascular	Hot flashes*	64	57.7%
General Disorders	Fatigue	13	11.7%
	Weakness	4	3.6%
Reproductive	Testicular atrophy*	8	7.2%
	Gynecomastia*	4	3.6%
Skin	Night sweats*	3	2.7%
Musculoskeletal	Myalgia	5	4.5%
	Pain in limb	3	2.7%

In addition, the following possibly or probably related systemic adverse events were reported by 1% of the patients using ELIGARD® 45 mg in the clinical study.
General: Lethargy
Reproductive: Penile shrinkage*
Renal/Urinary: Nocturia, nocturia aggravated
Psychiatric: Loss of libido*

* Expected pharmacological consequences of testosterone suppression. In the patient population studied, a total of 89 hot flash adverse events were reported in 64 patients. Of these, 62 events (70%) were mild; 27 (30%) were moderate.

Changes in Bone Density: Decreased bone density has been reported in the medical literature in men who have had orchiectomy or who have been treated with an LH-RH agonist analog.[3] It can be anticipated that long periods of medical castration in men will have effects on bone density.

OVERDOSAGE

In clinical trials using daily subcutaneous injections of leuprolide acetate in patients with prostate cancer, doses as high as 20 mg/day for up to two years caused no adverse effects differing from those observed with the 1 mg/day dose.

DOSAGE AND ADMINISTRATION

The recommended dose of ELIGARD® 45 mg is one injection every six months. The injection delivers 45 mg of leuprolide acetate, incorporated in a polymer formulation. It is administered subcutaneously and provides continuous release of leuprolide for six months.

Once mixed, ELIGARD® 45 mg should be discarded if not administered within 30 minutes.

As with other drugs administered by subcutaneous injection, the injection site should vary periodically. The specific injection location chosen should be an area with sufficient soft or loose subcutaneous tissue. In clinical trials, the injection was administered in the upper- or mid-abdominal area. Avoid areas with brawny or fibrous subcutaneous tissue or locations that could be rubbed or compressed (i.e., with a belt or clothing waistband).

Mixing Procedure

IMPORTANT: Allow the product to reach room temperature before using. **Once mixed, the product must be administered within 30 minutes.**

FOLLOW THE INSTRUCTIONS AS DIRECTED TO ENSURE PROPER PREPARATION OF ELIGARD® 45 MG PRIOR TO ADMINISTRATION:

ELIGARD® 45 mg is packaged in either thermoformed trays or pouches. Each carton contains:
• One sterile Syringe A pre-filled with the ATRIGEL® polymer system
• One Syringe B pre-filled with leuprolide acetate powder
• One long white plunger rod for use with Syringe B
• One sterile 19-gauge, 5/8-inch needle
• Desiccant pack(s)
1. On a clean field, open all of the packages and remove the contents. Discard the desiccant pack(s).

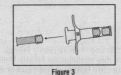

Figure 3

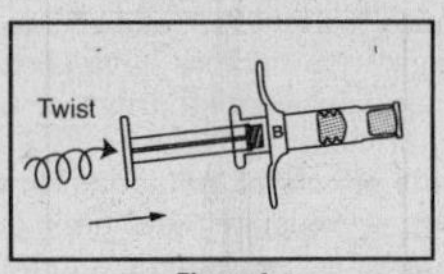

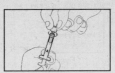

Figure 4

2. **Pull out the blue-tipped short plunger rod and attached stopper from Syringe B and discard (Figure 3).** Gently insert the long, white replacement plunger rod into the gray primary stopper remaining in Syringe B by twisting it in place (Figure 4).

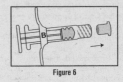

Figure 5

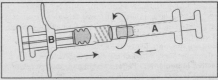

Figure 6

3. Unscrew the clear cap from Syringe A (Figure 5). Remove the gray rubber cap from Syringe B (Figure 6).

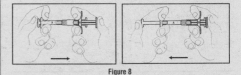

Figure 7

4. Join the two syringes together by pushing in and twisting until secure (Figure 7).

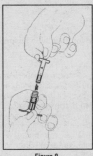

Figure 8

5. Inject the liquid contents of Syringe A into Syringe B containing the leuprolide acetate. Thoroughly mix the product by pushing the contents of both syringes back and forth between syringes (approximately 45 seconds) to obtain a uniform suspension (Figure 8). When thoroughly mixed, the suspension will appear colorless to pale yellow in color. **Please note: Product must be mixed as described; shaking will not provide adequate mixing of the product.**

6. Hold the syringes vertically with Syringe B on the bottom. The syringes should remain securely coupled. Draw the entire mixed product into Syringe B (short, wide syringe) by depressing the Syringe A plunger and slightly withdrawing the Syringe B plunger. Uncouple Syringe A while continuing to push down on the Syringe A plunger (Figure 9). **Please note: Small air bubbles will remain in the formulation - this is acceptable.**

Figure 9

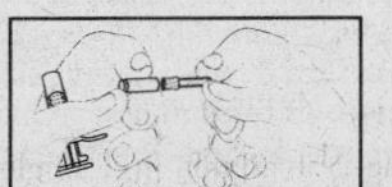

Figure 10

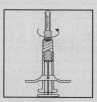

Figure 11

Figure 12

7. Hold Syringe B upright. Remove the yellow cap on the bottom of the sterile needle cartridge by twisting it (Figure 10). Attach the needle cartridge to the end of Syringe B (Figure 11) by pushing in and turning the needle until it is firmly seated. Do not twist the needle onto the syringe until it is stripped. Pull off the clear needle cartridge cover prior to administration (Figure 12).

Administration Procedure

IMPORTANT: Allow the product to reach room temperature before using. **Once mixed, the product must be administered within 30 minutes.**

1. Choose an injection site on the abdomen, upper buttocks, or anywhere with adequate amounts of subcutaneous tissue that does not have excessive pigment, nodules, lesions, or hair. Since you can vary the injection site with a subcutaneous injection, choose an area that hasn't recently been used.
2. Cleanse the injection-site area with an alcohol swab.
3. Using the thumb and forefinger of your nondominant hand, grab and bunch the area of skin around the injection site.

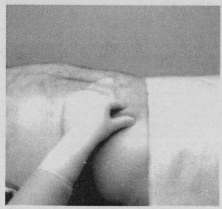

4. Using your dominant hand, insert the needle quickly. The approximate angle you use will depend on the amount and fullness of the subcutaneous tissue and the length of the needle.

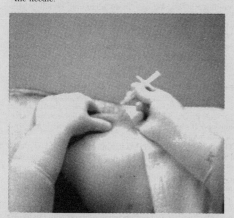

5. After the needle is inserted, release the skin with your nondominant hand.
   [See figure at top of next column]
6. Inject the drug using a slow, steady push. Press down on the plunger until the syringe is empty.
7. Withdraw the needle quickly at the same angle used for insertion.
8. Discard all components safely in an appropriate biohazard container.

HOW SUPPLIED

ELIGARD® 45 mg is available in a single use kit. The kit consists of a two-syringe mixing system, a 19-gauge 5/8-inch needle, a silicone desiccant pouch to control moisture uptake, and a package insert for constitution and administra-

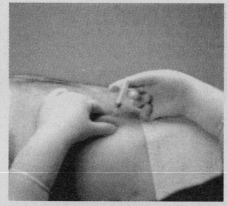

tion procedures. Each syringe is individually packaged. One contains the ATRIGEL® Delivery System and the other contains leuprolide acetate. When constituted, ELIGARD® 45 mg is administered as a single dose.
(NDC 0024-0605-45)

Rx only

Store at 2-8 °C (35.6-46.4 °F)

sanofi~synthelabo

Manufactured for Sanofi-Synthelabo Inc.
New York, NY 10016
by Atrix Laboratories, Inc.
Fort Collins, CO 80525
04318 Rev 0 12/04   Printed in USA

Revised December 2004

[1] Sennello LT et al. Single-dose pharmacokinetics of leuprolide in humans following intravenous and subcutaneous administration. J Pharm Sci 1986; 75(2): 158-160.

[2] MacLeod TL et. al. Anaphylactic reaction to synthetic luteinizing hormone releasing hormone. Fertil Steril 1987 Sept; 48(3): 500-502.

[3] Hatano T et. al. Incidence of bone fracture in patients receiving luteinizing hormone-releasing hormone agonists for prostate cancer. BJU International 2000; 86: 449-452.

Schering Corporation

a wholly-owned subsidiary of Schering-Plough Corporation
GALLOPING HILL ROAD
KENILWORTH, NJ 07033

Direct Inquiries to:
(908) 298-4000
CUSTOMER SERVICE:
(800) 222-7579
FAX: (908) 595-3729

For Medical Information Contact:
Schering Laboratories
Drug Information Services
2000 Galloping Hill Road
Kenilworth, NJ 07033
(800) 526-4099
FAX: (973) 921-7228

ASMANEX® TWISTHALER® 220 mcg   ℞

|ăs-măn-ĕcks|
(mometasone furoate inhalation powder)
FOR ORAL INHALATION ONLY

DESCRIPTION

Mōmetasone furoate, the active component of the ASMANEX TWISTHALER product, is a corticosteroid with the chemical name 9,21-dichloro-11(Beta),17-dihydroxy-16 (alpha)-methylpregna-1,4-diene-3,20-dione 17-(2-furoate) and the following chemical structure:

Mometasone furoate is a white powder with an empirical formula of $C_{27}H_{30}Cl_2O_6$, and molecular weight 521.44 Daltons.

The ASMANEX TWISTHALER 220 mcg product is a cap-activated inhalation-driven multi-dose dry powder inhaler containing mometasone furoate and anhydrous lactose (which contains milk proteins). Each actuation of the ASMANEX TWISTHALER 220 mcg inhaler provides a measured dose of 1.5 mg mometasone furoate inhalation powder, containing 220 mcg of mometasone furoate. This results in delivery of 200 mcg mometasone furoate from the mouthpiece, based on *in vitro* testing at flow rates of 30 L/min and

60 L/min with constant volume (2 L). The amount of mometasone furoate emitted from the inhaler *in vitro* did not differ significantly for flow rates ranging from 28.3 L/min to 70 L/min for fixed intervals of 2 seconds. However, the amount of drug delivered to the lung will depend on patient factors such as inspiratory flow and peak inspiratory flow through the device. In adult and adolescent patients with varied asthma severity, mean peak inspiratory flow rate through the device was 69 L/min (range 54-77 L/min).

CLINICAL PHARMACOLOGY

Mechanism of Action Mometasone furoate is a corticosteroid demonstrating potent anti-inflammatory activity. The precise mechanism of corticosteroid action on asthma is not known. Inflammation is an important component in the pathogenesis of asthma. Corticosteroids have been shown to have a wide range of inhibitory effects on multiple cell types (eg, mast cells, eosinophils, neutrophils, macrophages and lymphocytes) and mediators (eg, histamine, eicosanoids, leukotrienes, and cytokines) involved in inflammation and in the asthmatic response. These anti-inflammatory actions of corticosteroids may contribute to their efficacy in asthma. Mometasone furoate has been shown *in vitro* to exhibit a binding affinity for the human glucocorticoid receptor which is approximately 12 times that of dexamethasone, 7 times that of triamcinolone acetonide, 5 times that of budesonide, and 1.5 times that of fluticasone. The clinical significance of these findings is unknown.

In a three-way cross over study in 15 asthmatic patients receiving 50 or 100 mcg of mometasone furoate inhalation powder to placebo twice daily for two weeks, mometasone furoate inhalation powder reduced airway reactivity to adenosine monophosphate. In another study, pretreatment with the mometasone furoate inhalation powder for 5 days attenuated the early and late phase reactions following inhaled allergen challenge and also reduced allergen-induced hyperresponsiveness to methacholine. Mometasone furoate inhalation powder was also shown to attenuate the increase in inflammatory cells (total and activated eosinophils) in induced sputum following allergen and methacholine challenge. The clinical significance of these findings is unknown. Studies in asthmatic patients have demonstrated that ASMANEX TWISTHALER provides a favorable ratio of topical to systemic activity due to its primary local effect along with the extensive hepatic metabolism and the lack of active metabolites (see below).

Though highly effective for the treatment of asthma, glucocorticoids do not affect asthma symptoms immediately. However, improvement following inhaled administration of mometasone furoate can occur within 24 hours of beginning treatment, although maximum benefit may not be achieved for 1 to 2 weeks or longer after starting treatment. When glucocorticoids are discontinued, asthma stability may persist for several days or longer.

Pharmacokinetics: *Absorption:* Following a 1000 mcg inhaled dose of tritiated mometasone furoate inhalation powder to 6 healthy human subjects, plasma concentrations of unchanged mometasone furoate were shown to be very low compared to the total radioactivity in plasma. Following an inhaled single 400 mcg dose of ASMANEX TWISTHALER treatment to 24 healthy subjects, plasma concentrations for most subjects were near or below the lower limit of quantitation for the assay (50 pcg/mL). The mean absolute systemic bioavailability of the above single inhaled 400 mcg dose, compared to an intravenous 400 mcg dose of mometasone furoate, was determined to be less than 1%, with the maximum bioavailability for any subject being 4.85%. Following administration of the recommended highest inhaled dose (400 mcg twice daily) to 64 patients for 28 days, concentration-time profiles were discernible, but with large inter-subject variability. The coefficient of variation for C_{max} and AUC ranged from approximately 50-100%. The mean peak plasma concentrations at steady state ranged from approximately 94 to 114 pcg/mL and the mean time to peak levels ranged from approximately 1.0 to 2.5 hours.

Distribution: Based on the study employing a 1000 mcg inhaled dose of tritiated mometasone furoate inhalation powder in humans, no appreciable accumulation of mometasone furoate in the red blood cells was found. Following an intravenous 400 mcg dose of mometasone furoate, the plasma concentrations showed a biphasic decline, with a mean terminal half-life of about 5 hours and the mean steady-state volume of distribution of 152 liters. The *in vitro* protein binding for mometasone furoate was reported to be 98 to 99% (in a concentration range of 5 to 500 ng/mL).

Metabolism: Studies have shown that mometasone furoate is primarily and extensively metabolized in the liver of all species investigated and undergoes extensive metabolism to multiple metabolites. *In vitro* studies have confirmed the primary role of CYP 3A4 in the metabolism of this compound, however, no major metabolites were identified.

Excretion: Following an intravenous dosing, the terminal half-life was reported to be about 5 hours. Following the inhaled dose of tritiated 1000 mcg mometasone furoate, the radioactivity is excreted mainly in the feces (a mean of 74%), and to a small extent in the urine (a mean of 8%) up to 7 days. No radioactivity was associated with unchanged mometasone furoate in the urine.

Special Populations: Administration of a single inhaled dose of 400 mcg mometasone furoate to subjects with mild (n=4), moderate (n=4), and severe (n=4) hepatic impairment resulted in only 1 or 2 subjects in each group having

Continued on next page

Asmanex—Cont.

detectable peak plasma concentrations of mometasone furoate (ranging from 50 to 105 pcg/mL). The observed peak plasma concentrations appear to increase with severity of hepatic impairment, however, the numbers of detectable levels were few. The effects of renal impairment, age or gender on mometasone furoate pharmacokinetics have not been adequately investigated.

Drug-Drug Interaction: An inhaled dose of mometasone furoate 400 mcg was given to 24 healthy subjects twice daily for 9 days and ketoconazole 200 mg (as well as placebo) were given twice daily concomitantly on Days 4 to 9. Mometasone furoate plasma concentrations were <150 pcg/mL on Day 3 prior to co-administration of ketoconazole or placebo. Following concomitant administration of ketoconazole, 4 (out of 12) subjects in the ketoconazole treatment group (n=12) had peak plasma concentrations of mometasone furoate >200 pcg/mL on Day 9 (211 to 324 pcg/mL). Since mometasone furoate plasma levels appear to increase and plasma cortisol levels appear to decrease upon concomitant administration of ketoconazole, caution should be exercised in the co-administration of these drugs.

Pharmacodynamics: The potential effect of mometasone furoate on the hypothalamic-pituitary-adrenal axis was assessed in a 29-day study. A total of 64 adult patients with mild to moderate asthma were randomized to one of 4 treatment groups: ASMANEX TWISTHALER 440 mcg twice daily, ASMANEX TWISTHALER 880 mcg twice daily, oral prednisone 10 mg once daily, or placebo. Th 30-minute post-Cosyntropin stimulation serum cortisol concentration on Day 29 was 23.2 mcg/dL for the ASMANEX 440 mcg twice daily group and 20.8 mcg/dL for the ASMANEX 880 mcg twice daily group, compared to 14.5 mcg/dL for the oral prednisone 10 mg group and 25 mcg/dL for the placebo group. The difference between ASMANEX 880 mcg twice daily (twice the maximum recommended dose) and placebo was statistically significant.

Clinical Trials: The efficacy of ASMANEX TWISTHALER has been studied across a wide range of doses in double-blind placebo-controlled 12-week treatment clinical trials involving 1941 patients 12 years of age and older with asthma of varying severity.

Patients Previously Maintained on Bronchodilators Alone

ASMANEX TWISTHALER was studied in three 12-week double-blind trials in 737 patients with mild to moderate asthma (mean baseline FEV_1=2.6 L, 72% of predicted normal) who were maintained on short-acting beta-2 agonists alone. The first two trials evaluated doses of 440 mcg administered as 2 inhalations once daily in the morning and one of these studies also evaluated 200 mcg twice daily. In both trials, AM pre-dose FEV_1 was significantly improved at Endpoint (last observation) following treatment with 440 mcg ASMANEX TWISTHALER once daily in the morning as compared to placebo (14% vs. 2.5%, respectively, in one trial and 16% vs. 5.5% in the other). There was also a significant improvement in AM pre-dose FEV_1 at Endpoint following treatment with ASMANEX TWISTHALER 220 mcg twice daily. Other measures of lung function (AM and PM PEFR) also showed improvement compared to placebo. Patients receiving ASMANEX TWISTHALER treatment had reduced frequenc of beta-2 agonist rescue medication use compared to those on placebo (mean reductions at Endpoint 2.2 and 0.5 puffs per day, respectively, from a baseline of 4.1 puffs/day). Additionally, fewer patients receiving ASMANEX TWISTHALER 440 mcg once daily experienced asthma worsenings than did patients receiving placebo.

In the third trial, 195 asthmatic patients were treated with ASMANEX TWISTHALER 220 mcg once daily in the evening or placebo. The AM FEV_1 at Endpoint was significantly improved compared to placebo (mean change at Endpoint 0.43 L or 16.8% vs. 0.16 L or 6%, respectively, see Figure 1). Evening PEF increased 24.96 L/min (7%) from baseline in the ASMANEX TWISTHALER group compared to 8.67 L/min (4%) in placebo.

Figure 1: A 12-Week Trial in Patients Previously Maintained on Inhaled Beta-2 Agonists

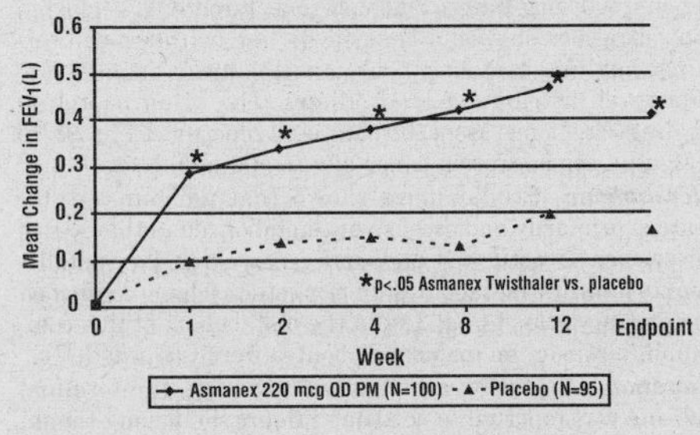
Mean Change in FEV1(L)
0.6
0.5
0.4
0.3
0.2
0.1
0
0
1
2
4
8
12
Endpoint
Week
*p<.05 Asmanex Twisthaler vs. placebo
Asmanex 220 mcg QD PM (N=100)
Placebo (N=95)

Patients Previously Maintained on Inhaled Corticosteroids

The efficacy and safety of ASMANEX TWISTHALER in doses ranging from 110 mcg twice daily to 440 mcg twice daily was evaluated in three trials in 1072 patients previously maintained on inhaled corticosteroids. In the first two trials, asthmatic patients (mean baseline FEV_1 ~2.6 L, 76% predicted) were previously on either beclomethasone dipropionate [84-1200 mcg/day], flunisolide [100-2000 mcg/day], fluticasone propionate [110-880 mcg/day], or triamcinolone acetonide [300-2400 mcg/day]. The first trial included 307 patients who were treated in an open-label fashion with ASMANEX TWISTHALER 220 mcg (110 mcg × 2 inhalations) twice daily for 2 weeks followed by 12 weeks of double-blind treatment with ASMANEX TWISTHALER 440 mcg once daily in the morning or placebo. The second trial involved 365 patients who continued on their previous dose of inhaled corticosteroids during a 2-week screening period before being switched to ASMANEX TWISTHALER 440 mcg twice daily, 220 mcg twice daily, 110 mcg twice daily, beclomethasone dipropionate 168 mcg twice daily or placebo for 12 weeks.

In the first trial, AM pre-dose FEV_1 was effectively maintained (-1.4% change from baseline to Endpoint) over the 12 weeks in the patients who were randomized to ASMANEX TWISTHALER 440 mcg once daily in the morning while decreasing 10% at Endpoint in those switched to placebo. In addition, fewer patients treated with ASMANEX TWISTHALER experienced worsenings of asthma compared to placebo.

In the second trial, AM pre-dose FEV_1 was significantly increased at Endpoint when patients were switched to ASMANEX TWISTHALER 220 mcg twice daily (7% increase) or 440 mcg twice daily (6.2% increase) as compared to a decrease of 7% when switched to placebo. Additionally, beta-2 agonist rescue medication use was decreased for patients who received ASMANEX TWISTHALER treatment relative to those on placebo (mean reduction from baseline to Endpoint 1.1 puffs/day vs. increase of 0.7 puffs/day). Fewer patients receiving ASMANEX TWISTHALER treatment experienced asthma worsenings than did patients receiving placebo.

The third trial evaluated the efficacy and safety of ASMANEX TWISTHALER compared to placebo in 400 asthmatic patients (mean FEV_1 67% predicted at baseline) previously maintained on beclomethasone dipropionate (HFA or CFC) 168-600 mcg/day, budesonide 200-1200 mcg/day, flunisolide 500-2000 mcg/day, fluticasone propionate 88-880 mcg/day or triamcinolone acetonide 400-1600 mcg/day. Following a 28-day inhaled corticosteroid dose-reduction phase, patients were randomized to ASMANEX TWISTHALER 440 mcg once daily in the evening (QD PM), 220 mcg QD PM, 220 mcg twice daily or placebo. At Endpoint, patients who received ASMANEX TWISTHALER 220 mcg QD PM, 440 mcg QD PM, or 220 mcg twice daily had a significant improvement in AM FEV_1 [0.41 L (19%), 0.49 L (22%), and 0.51 L (24%) in the 220 mcg QD PM, 440 mcg QD PM, and 220 mcg twice daily treatment group, respectively] compared to placebo [0.16 L (8%)]. (See Figure 2). Evening PEF increased 15.65 L/min (4.1%) with the 220 mcg QD PM dose, 39.26 L/min (10.7%) with the 440 mcg QD PM dose and 36.7 L/min (10.8%) with the 220 mcg twice daily dose respectively compared to a 1.4 L/min (1%) increase with placebo. Patients receiving all doses of ASMANEX TWISTHALER treatment had reduced frequency of beta agonist rescue medication use compared to those on placebo (mean reductions at Endpoint of 1.4 to 1.8 puffs/day from a baseline of more than 3 puffs/day compared to an increase in use by 0.5 puffs/day for placebo). In addition, fewer patients receiving ASMANEX TWISTHALER experienced asthma worsenings than did those on placebo.

Figure 2: A 12-Week Trial in Patients Previously Maintained on Inhaled Corticosteroids

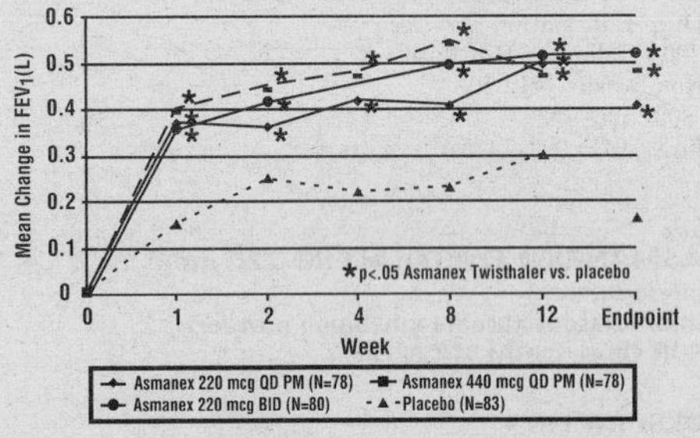
Mean Change in FEV1(L)
0.6
0.5
0.4
0.3
0.2
0.1
0
0
1
2
4
8
12
Endpoint
Week
*p<.05 Asmanex Twisthaler vs. placebo
Asmanex 220 mcg QD PM (N=78)
Asmanex 440 mcg QD PM (N=78)
Asmanex 220 mcg BID (N=80)
Placebo (N=83)

Patients Previously Maintained on Oral Corticosteroids The efficacy of ASMANEX TWISTHALER 440 mcg and 880 mcg twice daily was evaluated in one 12-week double-blind trial in patients previously maintained on oral corticosteroids. A total of 132 patients requiring oral prednisone (baseline mean daily oral prednisone requirement approximately 12 mg; baseline FEV_1 of 1.8 L, 59% of predicted normal), most of whom were also on inhaled corticosteroids (baseline inhaled steroid: beclomethasone dipropionate [168-840 mcg/day], budesonide [800-1600 mcg/day], flunisolide [1000-2000 mcg/day], fluticasone propionate [440-1760 mcg/day], or triamcinolone acetonide [400-2400 mcg/day]) were studied. Patients who received ASMANEX TWISTHALER 440 mcg twice daily had a significant reduction in their oral prednisone (46%) as compared to placebo (164% increase in oral prednisone dose). Additionally, 40% of patients on ASMANEX TWISTHALER 440 mcg twice daily were able to completely discontinue their use of prednisone, whereas 60% of patients on placebo had an increase in daily prednisone use. Patients on ASMANEX TWISTHALER had significant improvement in lung function (14% increase) compared to a 12% decrease in FEV_1 in the placebo group. Additionally, mean rescue beta-2 agonist use was reduced to approximately 3 puffs/day from a baseline of 4-5 puffs/day with ASMANEX TWISTHALER treatment, compared to an increase of 0.3 puffs/day on placebo. Patients who received ASMANEX TWISTHALER 880 mcg twice daily experienced no additional benefit beyond that seen with 440 mcg twice daily.

INDICATIONS AND USAGE

ASMANEX TWISTHALER inhaler is indicated for the maintenance treatment of asthma as prophylactic therapy in patients 12 years of age and older. The ASMANEX TWISTHALER inhaler is also indicated for asthma patients who require oral corticosteroid therapy, where adding ASMANEX TWISTHALER therapy may reduce or eliminate the need for oral corticosteroids.

ASMANEX TWISTHALER is NOT indicated for the relief of acute bronchospasm.

CONTRAINDICATIONS

ASMANEX TWISTHALER therapy is contraindicated in the primary treatment of status asthmaticus or other acute episodes of asthma where intensive measures are required. Hypersensitivity to any of the ingredients of this preparation contraindicates its use (see **DESCRIPTION**).

WARNINGS

Particular care is needed for patients who are transferred from systemically active corticosteroids to the ASMANEX TWISTHALER inhaler because deaths due to adrenal insufficiency have occurred in asthmatic patients during and after transfer from systemic corticosteroids to less systemically available inhaled corticosteroids. After withdrawal from systemic corticosteroids, a number of months are required for recovery of HPA function.

Patients who have been previously maintained on 20 mg or more per day of prednisone (or its equivalent) may be most susceptible, particularly when their systemic corticosteroids have been almost completely withdrawn. During this period of HPA suppression, patients may exhibit signs and symptoms of adrenal insufficiency when exposed to trauma, surgery or infection (particularly gastroenteritis) or other conditions associated with severe electrolyte loss. Although the ASMANEX TWISTHALER inhaler may improve control of asthma symptoms during these episodes, in recommended doses it supplies less than normal physiological amounts of glucocorticoid systemically and does NOT provide the mineralocorticoid activity necessary for coping with these emergencies.

During periods of stress or severe asthma attack, patients who have been withdrawn from systemic corticosteroids should be instructed to resume oral corticosteroids (in large doses) immediately and to contact their physicians for further instruction. These patients should also be instructed to carry a medical identification card indicating that they may need supplementary systemic corticosteroids during periods of stress or severe asthma attack.

Patients requiring oral corticosteroids should be weaned slowly from systemic corticosteroid use after transferring to ASMANEX TWISTHALER. Lung function (FEV_1 or PEF), beta agonist use, and asthma symptoms should be carefully monitored during withdrawal of oral corticosteroids. In addition to monitoring asthma signs and symptoms, patients should be observed for signs and symptoms of adrenal insufficiency such as fatigue, lassitude, weakness, nausea and vomiting, and hypotension.

Transfer of patients from systemic corticosteroid therapy to the ASMANEX TWISTHALER inhaler may unmask allergic conditions previously suppressed by the systemic corticosteroid therapy, eg, rhinitis, conjunctivitis, and eczema.

Persons who are on drugs which suppress the immune system are more susceptible to infections than healthy individuals. Chickenpox and measles, for example, can have a more serious or even fatal course in nonimmune children or adults on corticosteroids. In such children or adults who have not had these diseases or who are not properly immunized, particular care should be taken to avoid exposure. How the dose, route, and duration of corticosteroid administration affect the risk of developing a disseminated infection is not known. The contribution of the underlying disease and/or prior corticosteroid treatment to the risk is also not known. If exposed to chickenpox, prophylaxis with varicella zoster immune globulin (VZIG) may be indicated. If exposed to measles, prophylaxis with pooled intramuscular immunoglobulin (IG) may be indicated. (See the respective package inserts for complete VZIG and IG prescribing information.) If chickenpox develops, treatment with antiviral agents may be considered.

The ASMANEX TWISTHALER inhaler is not a bronchodilator and is not indicated for rapid relief of bronchospasm or other acute episodes of asthma.

As with other inhaled asthma medications, bronchospasm may occur with an immediate increase in wheezing after dosing. If bronchospasm occurs following dosing with the ASMANEX TWISTHALER inhaler, it should be treated immediately with a fast-acting inhaled bronchodilator. Treatment with the ASMANEX TWISTHALER inhaler should be discontinued and alternative therapy instituted.

Patients should be instructed to contact their physician immediately when episodes of asthma that are not responsive to bronchodilators occur during the course of treatment with the ASMANEX TWISTHALER inhaler. During such episodes, patients may require therapy with oral corticosteroids.

PRECAUTIONS

General: During withdrawal from oral corticosteroids, some patients may experience symptoms of systemically active corticosteroid withdrawal, eg, joint and/or muscular pain, lassitude, and depression, despite maintenance or even improvement of respiratory function.

The ASMANEX TWISTHALER inhaler will often improve control of asthma symptoms with less suppression of HPA function than therapeutically equivalent oral doses of prednisone. Since mometasone furoate is absorbed into the circulation and can be systemically active at higher doses, the full beneficial effects of the ASMANEX TWISTHALER inhaler in minimizing HPA dysfunction may be expected only when recommended dosages are not exceeded and individual patients are titrated to the lowest effective dose. Since individual sensitivity to effects on cortisol production exists, physicians should consider this information when prescribing the ASMANEX TWISTHALER inhaler.

Because of the possibility of systemic absorption of inhaled corticosteroids, patients treated with these drugs should be observed carefully for any evidence of systemic corticosteroid effects. Particular care should be taken in observing patients postoperatively or during periods of stress for evidence of inadequate adrenal response.

It is possible that systemic corticosteroid effects such as hypercorticism, reduced bone mineral density and adrenal suppression may appear in a small number of patients, particularly at higher doses. If such changes occur, the ASMANEX TWISTHALER inhaler dose should be reduced slowly, consistent with accepted procedures for management of asthma symptoms and for tapering of systemic steroids.

Decreases in bone mineral density (BMD) have been observed with long-term administration of products containing inhaled glucocorticoids, including mometasone furoate. The clinical significance of small changes in bone mineral density with regard to long-term outcomes is unknown. In a two-year double-blind study in 103 male and female asthma patients 18 to 50 years of age previously maintained on bronchodilator therapy (Baseline FEV_1 85-88% predicted), treatment with ASMANEX TWISTHALER 220 mcg twice daily resulted in significant reductions in lumbar spine (LS) BMD at the end of the treatment period compared to placebo. The mean change from Baseline to Endpoint in the lumbar spine BMD was -0.015 (-1.43%) for the ASMANEX TWISTHALER group compared to 0.002 (0.25%) for the placebo group. In another two-year double-blind study in 87 male and female asthma patients 18 to 50 years of age previously maintained on bronchodilator therapy (Baseline FEV_1 82-83% predicted), treatment with ASMANEX TWISTHALER 440 mcg twice daily demonstrated no statistically significant changes in lumbar spine BMD at the end of the treatment period compared to placebo. The mean change from Baseline to Endpoint in the lumbar spine BMD was -0.018 (-1.57%) for the ASMANEX TWISTHALER group compared to -0.006 (-0.43%) for the placebo group.

Patients with major risk factors for decreased bone mineral content, such as prolonged immobilization, family history of osteoporosis, or chronic use of drugs that can reduce bone mass (eg, anticonvulsants and corticosteroids) should be monitored and treated with established standards of care.

Orally inhaled corticosteroids, including mometasone furoate inhalation powder, may cause a reduction in growth velocity when administered to pediatric patients. A reduction in growth velocity in children or teenagers may occur as a result of inadequate control of asthma or from use of corticosteroids for treatment. The potential effects of prolonged treatment on growth velocity should be weighed against clinical benefits obtained and the risks associated with alternative therapies. To minimize the systemic effects of orally inhaled corticosteroids, including ASMANEX TWISTHALER, each patient should be titrated to his/her lowest effective dose. (See **PRECAUTIONS, Pediatric Use** section.)

Although patients in clinical trials have received the ASMANEX TWISTHALER inhaler on a continuous basis for periods of up to 2 years, the long-term local and systemic effects of ASMANEX TWISTHALER in human subjects are not completely known. In particular, the effects resulting from chronic use of the ASMANEX TWISTHALER inhaler on developmental or immunological processes in the mouth, pharynx, trachea, and lung are unknown.

In clinical trials with the ASMANEX TWISTHALER inhaler, localized infections with *Candida albicans* occurred in the mouth and pharynx in some patients. If oropharyngeal candidiasis develops, it should be treated with appropriate local or systemic (ie, oral) antifungal therapy while still continuing with ASMANEX TWISTHALER therapy, but at times therapy with the ASMANEX TWISTHALER inhaler may need to be temporarily interrupted under close medical supervision.

Inhaled corticosteroids should be used with caution, if at all, in patients with active or quiescent tuberculosis infection of the respiratory tract, untreated systemic fungal, bacterial, viral, or parasitic infections; or ocular herpes simplex.

Rare instances of glaucoma, increased intraocular pressure, and cataracts have been reported following the inhaled administration of corticosteroids.

Information for Patients: Patients being treated with the ASMANEX TWISTHALER inhaler should be given the following information. This information is intended to aid in the safe and effective use of the ASMANEX TWISTHALER inhaler. It is not a disclosure of all intended or possible adverse effects.

- Patients should be advised that ASMANEX TWISTHALER is not a bronchodilator and should not be used to relieve acute asthma symptoms. Acute asthma symptoms should be treated with an inhaled, short-acting beta-2 agonist such as albuterol.
- Patients should be advised to use the ASMANEX TWISTHALER inhaler at regular intervals since its effectiveness depends on regular use. Maximum benefit may not be achieved for 1 to 2 weeks or longer after starting treatment. If symptoms do not improve in that time frame or if the condition worsens, the patient should be instructed to contact the physician.
- Patients should be warned to avoid exposure to chickenpox or measles, and if they are exposed, to consult their physicians without delay.
- Patients who are at an increased risk for decreased BMD should be advised that the use of corticosteroids may pose an additional risk and should be monitored and, where appropriate, be treated for this condition.
- Patients should be advised that long-term use of inhaled corticosteroids, including ASMANEX TWISTHALER may increase the risk of some eye problems (cataracts or glaucoma).
- For the proper use of the ASMANEX TWISTHALER inhaler, and to attain maximum improvement, the patient should read and follow the accompanying Patient's Instructions for Use.

ADVERSE EVENTS WITH ≥3% INCIDENCE IN CONTROLLED CLINICAL TRIALS WITH ASMANEX TWISTHALER IN PATIENTS PREVIOUSLY ON BRONCHODILATORS AND/OR INHALED CORTICOSTEROIDS

Adverse Event	(%) of Patients			
	MF DPI			
	220 mcg BID (n=443)	440 mcg QD (n=497)	220 mcg QD PM (n=232)	Placebo (n=720)
Headache	22	17	20	20
Allergic Rhinitis	15	11	14	13
Pharyngitis	11	8	13	7
Upper Respiratory Inf.	10	8	15	7
Sinusitis	6	6	5	5
Candidiasis, oral	6	4	4	2
Dysmenorrhea[a]	9	4	4	4
Musculoskeletal Pain	8	4	4	5
Back Pain	6	3	3	4
Dyspepsia	5	3	3	3
Myalgia	3	2	3	2
Abdominal Pain	3	2	3	2
Nausea	3	1	3	2
Average Duration of Exposure (Days)	81	70	80	62

[a] Percentages are based on the number of female patients.

Patients should be instructed to record the date of pouch opening on the cap label, and discard the inhaler 45 days after opening the foil pouch or when the dose counter reads "00," whichever comes first. The inhaler should be held upright while removing the cap. The medication should be taken as directed, breathing rapidly and deeply, and patients should not breathe out through the inhaler. The mouthpiece should be wiped dry and the cap replaced immediately following each inhalation, rotated fully until the click is heard. Rinsing of mouth after inhalation is advised. Patients should store the unit as instructed. The digital dose counter displays the doses remaining. When the counter indicates zero, the cap will lock and the unit must be discarded. Patients should be advised that if the dose counter is not working correctly, the unit should not be used and it should be brought to their physician or pharmacist.

Drug Interactions: In clinical studies, the concurrent administration of the ASMANEX TWISTHALER inhaler and other drugs commonly used in the treatment of asthma was not associated with any unusual adverse events. However, ketoconazole, a potent inhibitor of cytochrome P450 3A4, may increase plasma levels of mometasone furoate during concomitant dosing.

Carcinogenesis, Mutagenesis, Impairment of Fertility: In a 2-year carcinogenicity study in Sprague Dawley rats, mometasone furoate demonstrated no statistically significant increase in the incidence of tumors at inhalation doses up to 67 mcg/kg (approximately 8 times the maximum recommended daily inhalation dose in adults on an AUC basis). In a 19-month carcinogenicity study in Swiss CD-1 mice, mometasone furoate demonstrated no statistically significant increase in the incidence of tumors at inhalation doses up to 160 mcg/kg (approximately 10 times the maximum recommended daily inhalation dose in adults on an AUC basis).

Mometasone furoate increased chromosomal aberrations in an *in vitro* Chinese hamster ovary cell assay, but did not have this effect in an *in vitro* Chinese hamster lung cell assay. Mometasone furoate was not mutagenic in the Ames test or mouse lymphoma assay, and was not clastogenic in an *in vivo* mouse micronucleus assay, a rat bone marrow chromosomal aberration assay, or a mouse male germcell chromosomal aberration assay. Mometasone furoate also did not induce unscheduled DNA synthesis *in vivo* in rat hepatocytes.

In reproductive studies in rats, impairment of fertility was not produced by subcutaneous doses up to 15 mcg/kg (approximately 6 times the maximum recommended daily inhalation dose in adults on an AUC basis).

Pregnancy: Teratogenic Effects: Pregnancy Category C: When administered to pregnant mice, rats, and rabbits, mometasone furoate increased fetal malformations. The doses that produced malformations also decreased fetal growth, as measured by lower fetal weights and/or delayed ossification. Mometasone furoate also caused dystocia and related complications when administered to rats during the end of pregnancy.

In mice, mometasone furoate caused cleft palate at subcutaneous doses of 60 mcg/kg and above (less than the maximum recommended daily inhalation dose in adults on a mcg/m^2 basis). Fetal survival was reduced at 180 mcg/kg (approximately equal to the maximum recommended daily inhalation dose in adults on a mcg/m^2 basis). No toxicity was observed at 20 mcg/kg (less than the maximum recommended daily inhalation dose in adults on a mcg/m^2 basis).

In rats, mometasone furoate produced umbilical hernia at topical dermal doses of 600 mcg/kg and above (approximately 6 times the maximum recommended daily inhalation dose in adults on a mcg/m^2 basis). A dose of 300 mcg/kg (approximately 3 times the maximum recommended daily inhalation dose in adults on a mcg/m^2 basis) produced delays in ossification, but no malformations.

In rabbits, mometasone furoate caused multiple malformations (eg, flexed front paws, gallbladder agenesis, umbilical hernia, hydrocephaly) at topical dermal doses of 150 mcg/kg and above (approximately 3 times the maximum recommended daily inhalation dose in adults on a mcg/m^2 basis). In an oral study, mometasone furoate increased resorptions and caused cleft palate and/or head malformations (hydrocephaly and domed head) at 700 mcg/kg (less than the maximum recommended daily inhalation dose in adults on an AUC basis). At 2800 mcg/kg (approximately 2 times the maximum recommended daily inhalation dose in adults on an AUC basis) most litters were aborted or resorbed. No toxicity was observed at 140 mcg/kg (less than the maximum recommended daily inhalation dose in adults on an AUC basis).

When rats received subcutaneous doses of mometasone furoate throughout pregnancy or during the later stages of pregnancy, 15 mcg/kg (approximately 6 times the maximum recommended daily inhalation dose in adults on an AUC basis) caused prolonged and difficult labor and reduced the number of live births, birth weight, and early pup survival. Similar effects were not observed at 7.5 mcg/kg (approximately 3 times the maximum recommended daily inhalation dose in adults on an AUC basis).

There are no adequate and well-controlled studies in pregnant women. The ASMANEX TWISTHALER, like other corticosteroids, should be used during pregnancy only if the potential benefits justify the potential risks to the fetus. Experience with oral corticosteroids since their introduction in pharmacologic, as opposed to physiologic, doses suggests that rodents are more prone to teratogenic effects from corticosteroids than humans. In addition, because there is a natural increase in corticosteroid production during pregnancy, most women will require a lower exogenous corticosteroid dose and many will not need corticosteroid treatment during pregnancy.

Continued on next page

Asmanex—Cont.

Nonteratogenic Effects: Hypoadrenalism may occur in infants born to women receiving corticosteroids during pregnancy. Such infants should be carefully monitored.

Nursing Mothers: It is not known if mometasone furoate is excreted in human milk. Because other corticosteroids are excreted in human milk, caution should be used when ASMANEX TWISTHALER is administered to nursing women.

Pediatric Use: The safety and effectiveness of ASMANEX TWISTHALER treatment have been established in the age group 12 to 16 years. Clinical trials in adults and adolescents included 146 patients in this age group who received ASMANEX TWISTHALER treatment. No age-related differential responses to therapy were apparent. Safety and effectiveness in pediatric patients below the age of 12 years have not been established.

Controlled clinical studies have shown that inhaled corticosteroids may cause a reduction in growth in pediatric patients. In these studies, the mean reduction in growth velocity was approximately one cm per year (range 0.3 to 1.8 per year) and appears to depend upon dose and duration of exposure. This effect was observed in the absence of laboratory evidence of hypothalamic-pituitary-adrenal (HPA) axis suppression, suggesting that growth velocity is a more sensitive indicator of systemic corticosteroid exposure in pediatric patients than some commonly used tests of HPA axis function. The long-term effects of this reduction in growth velocity associated with orally inhaled corticosteroids, including the impact on final adult height, are unknown. The potential for "catch up" growth following discontinuation of treatment with orally inhaled corticosteroids has not been adequately studied. The growth of children and adolescents (12 years of age and older) receiving orally inhaled corticosteroids, including ASMANEX TWISTHALER, should be monitored routinely (eg, via stadiometry). The potential growth effects of prolonged treatment should be weighed against clinical benefits obtained and the risks associated with alternative therapies. To minimize the systemic effects of orally inhaled corticosteroids, including ASMANEX TWISTHALER, each patient should be titrated to his/her lowest effective dose.

Geriatric Use: A total of 175 patients 65 years of age and over (23 of whom were 75 years of age and over) have been treated with ASMANEX TWISTHALER in controlled clinical trials. No overall differences in safety or effectiveness were observed between these and younger patients, and other reported clinical experience has not identified differences in responses between the elderly and younger patients, but greater sensitivity of some older individuals cannot be ruled out.

ADVERSE REACTIONS

The following incidence of common adverse experiences is based on double-blind data from ten placebo-controlled clinical trials involving a total of 2809 patients previously maintained on inhaled steroids and/or bronchodilators (1140 males, 1669 females, age 12-83 years), who were treated for up to 12 weeks with the ASMANEX TWISTHALER product, an active comparator, or placebo. Adverse events were generally mild to moderate in severity.

[See table at top of previous page]

The table above includes all events (whether considered drug-related or nondrug-related by the investigators) that occurred at a rate of ≥3% in any one mometasone furoate group and were more common than in the placebo group. In considering these data, the increased average duration of exposure for ASMANEX TWISTHALER patients should be taken into account.

The following other adverse events occurred in these clinical trials with an incidence of at least 1% but less than 3% and were more common on ASMANEX TWISTHALER therapy than on placebo:

Body as a Whole: fatigue, flu-like symptoms, fever, accidental injury, pain, post-procedure pain

Gastrointestinal: flatulence, gastroenteritis, vomiting, anorexia

Hearing, Vestibular: earache

Psychiatric: insomnia

Reproductive, Female: menstrual disorder

Resistance Mechanism: infection

Respiratory: dysphonia, epistaxis, nasal irritation, respiratory disorder, throat dry

Skin and Appendages: insect bite, skin laceration

Urinary: urinary tract infection

In a 12-week trial in adult asthmatics who previously required oral corticosteroids, the effects of ASMANEX TWISTHALER therapy administered as two 220 mcg inhalations twice daily (N=46) were compared with those of placebo (N=43). Adverse events, whether considered drug related or not by the investigators, reported in more than 3 patients in the ASMANEX TWISTHALER treatment group, and which occurred more frequently than on placebo were (ASMANEX TWISTHALER % vs. placebo %): musculoskeletal pain (22% vs. 14%), oral candidiasis (22% vs. 9%), sinusitis (22% vs. 19%), allergic rhinitis (20% vs. 5%), upper respiratory infection (15% vs. 14%), arthralgia (13% vs. 7%), fatigue (13% vs. 2%), depression (11% vs. 0%), and sinus congestion (9% vs. 0%). In considering these data, an increased duration of exposure for patients on ASMANEX TWISTHALER treatment (77 days vs. 58 days on placebo) should be taken into account.

Cases of growth suppression and decreased bone mineral density have been reported for orally inhaled corticosteroids, including mometasone furoate inhalation powder.

OVERDOSAGE

The potential for acute toxic effects following overdose with the ASMANEX TWISTHALER inhaler is low. Because of low systemic bioavailability and an absence of acute drug-related systemic findings in clinical studies, overdose is unlikely to require any treatment other than observation. If used at excessive doses for prolonged periods, systemic effects such as hypercorticism may occur. Single daily doses as high as 1200 mcg per day for 28 days were well-tolerated and did not cause a significant reduction in plasma cortisol AUC (94% of placebo AUC). Single oral doses up to 8000 mcg have been studied on human volunteers with no adverse events reported.

DOSAGE AND ADMINISTRATION

The ASMANEX TWISTHALER product should be administered by the orally inhaled route in patients 12 years of age and older. Individual patients will experience a variable time to onset and degree of symptom relief. Maximum benefit may not be achieved for 1 to 2 weeks or longer. The safety and efficacy of ASMANEX TWISTHALER when administered in excess of recommended doses have not been established.

The recommended starting doses and highest recommended daily dose for ASMANEX TWISTHALER treatment based on prior asthma therapy are provided in the table below.

RECOMMENDED DOSAGES FOR ASMANEX TWISTHALER TREATMENT

Previous Therapy	Recommended Starting Dose	Highest Recommended Daily Dose
Bronchodilators alone	220 mcg QD PM*	440 mcg**
Inhaled corticosteroids	220 mcg QD PM*	440 mcg**
Oral corticosteroids†	440 mcg BID	880 mcg

* When administered once daily ASMANEX TWISTHALER should only be taken in the PM.

** The 440 mcg daily dose may be administered in divided doses of 220 mcg twice daily or as 440 mcg once daily.

NOTE: In all patients, it is desirable to titrate to the lowest effective dose once asthma stability is achieved.

† **For Patients Currently Receiving Chronic Oral Corticosteroid Therapy:** Prednisone should be reduced no faster than 2.5 mg/day on a weekly basis, beginning after at least 1 week of ASMANEX TWISTHALER therapy. Patients should be carefully monitored for signs of asthma instability, including serial objective measures of airflow, and for signs of adrenal insufficiency (see **WARNINGS**). Once prednisone reduction is complete, the dosage of mometasone furoate should be reduced to the lowest effective dosage.

Patients should be instructed to inhale rapidly and deeply (see enclosed patient instructions). Rinsing the mouth after inhalation is advised.

HOW SUPPLIED

The ASMANEX TWISTHALER product is comprised of an assembled plastic cap-activated dosing mechanism with dose counter, drug-product storage unit, drug-product formulation (240 mg), and mouthpiece, covered by a white screw cap which bears the product label. The body of the inhaler is white and the turning grip is pink with a clear plastic window indicating the number of doses remaining. The inhaler will not deliver subsequent doses once the counter reaches zero ("00").

The ASMANEX TWISTHALER product is available as:

ASMANEX TWISTHALER 220 mcg, which delivers 200 mcg mometasone furoate from the mouthpiece: 14 inhalation units (Institutional Use Only; NDC # 0085-1341-04); 30 inhalation units (NDC # 0085-1341-03); 60 inhalation units (For more than one inhalation daily; NDC # 0085-1341-02); or 120 inhalation units (For more than 2 inhalations daily; NDC # 0085-1341-01).

Each inhaler is supplied in a protective foil pouch with Patient's Instructions for Use.

Store in a dry place at 25°C (77°F); excursions permitted to 15-30°C (59-86°F) [see USP Controlled Room Temperature].

Discard the inhaler 45 days after opening the foil pouch or when dose counter reads "00," whichever comes first.

Schering Corporation.
Kenilworth, NJ 07033 USA

AVELOX® ℞

[*ă'vĕ-lōks*]

(moxifloxacin hydrochloride) Tablets

AVELOX® I.V.

(moxifloxacin hydrochloride in sodium chloride injection)

To reduce the development of drug-resistant bacteria and maintain the effectiveness of AVELOX® and other antibacterial drugs, AVELOX should be used only to treat or prevent infections that are proven or strongly suspected to be caused by bacteria.

DESCRIPTION

AVELOX (moxifloxacin hydrochloride) is a synthetic broad spectrum antibacterial agent and is available as AVELOX Tablets for oral administration and as AVELOX I.V. for intravenous administration. Moxifloxacin, a fluoroquinolone, is available as the monohydrochloride salt of 1-cyclopropyl-7-[(S,S)-2,8-diazabicyclo[4.3.0]non-8-yl]-6-fluoro-8-methoxy-1,4-dihydro-4-oxo-3 quinoline carboxylic acid. It is a slightly yellow to yellow crystalline substance with a molecular weight of 437.9. Its empirical formula is $C_{21}H_{24}FN_3O_4$ *HCl and its chemical structure is as follows:

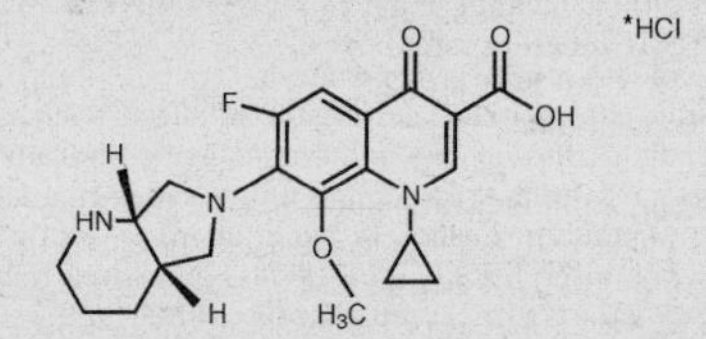

AVELOX Tablets are available as film-coated tablets containing moxifloxacin hydrochloride (equivalent to 400 mg moxifloxacin). The inactive ingredients are microcrystalline cellulose, lactose monohydrate, croscarmellose sodium, magnesium stearate, hypromellose, titanium dioxide, polyethylene glycol and ferric oxide.

AVELOX I.V. is available in ready-to-use 250 mL latex-free flexibags as a sterile, preservative free, 0.8% sodium chloride aqueous solution of moxifloxacin hydrochloride (containing 400 mg moxifloxacin) with pH ranging from 4.1 to 4.6. The appearance of the intravenous solution is yellow. The color does not affect, nor is it indicative of, product stability. The inactive ingredients are sodium chloride, USP, water for Injection, USP, and may include hydrochloric acid and/or sodium hydroxide for pH adjustment.

CLINICAL PHARMACOLOGY

Absorption

Moxifloxacin, given as an oral tablet, is well absorbed from the gastrointestinal tract. The absolute bioavailability of moxifloxacin is approximately 90 percent. Co-administration with a high fat meal (i.e., 500 calories from fat) does not affect the absorption of moxifloxacin.

Consumption of 1 cup of yogurt with moxifloxacin does not significantly affect the extent or rate of systemic absorption (AUC).

The mean (± SD) C_{max} and AUC values following single and multiple doses of 400 mg moxifloxacin given orally are summarized below.

[See first table at top of next page]

The mean (± SD) C_{max} and AUC values following single and multiple doses of 400 mg moxifloxacin given by 1 hour I.V. infusion are summarized below.

[See second table on next page]

Plasma concentrations increase proportionately with dose up to the highest dose tested (1200 mg single oral dose). The mean (± SD) elimination half-life from plasma is 12 ± 1.3 hours; steady-state is achieved after at least three days with a 400 mg once daily regimen.

Mean Steady-State Plasma Concentrations of Moxifloxacin Obtained With Once Daily Dosing of 400 mg Either Orally (n=10) or by I.V. Infusion (n=12)

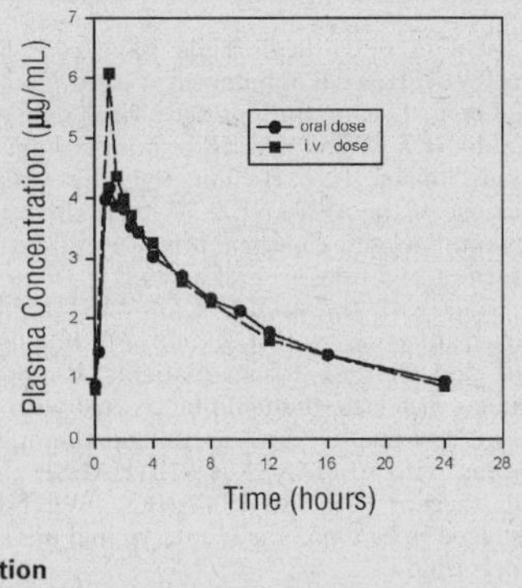

Distribution

Moxifloxacin is approximately 50% bound to serum proteins, independent of drug concentration. The volume of distribution of moxifloxacin ranges from 1.7 to 2.7 L/kg. Moxifloxacin is widely distributed throughout the body, with tissue concentrations often exceeding plasma concentrations. Moxifloxacin has been detected in the saliva, nasal and bronchial secretions, mucosa of the sinuses, skin blister fluid, and subcutaneous tissue, and skeletal muscle following oral or intravenous administration of 400 mg. Concentrations measured at 3 hours post-dose are summarized in the following table. The rates of elimination of moxifloxacin from tissues generally parallel the elimination from plasma.

[See third table at top of next page]

Metabolism

Approximately 52% of an oral or intravenous dose of moxifloxacin is metabolized via glucuronide and sulfate conjugation. The cytochrome P450 system is not involved in moxifloxacin metabolism, and is not affected by moxifloxacin. The sulfate conjugate (M1) accounts for approximately 38% of the dose, and is eliminated primarily in the feces. Approximately 14% of an oral or intravenous dose is converted to a glucuronide conjugate (M2), which is excreted exclusively in the urine. Peak plasma concentrations of M2 are approximately 40% those of the parent drug, while plasma concentrations of M1 are generally less than 10% those of moxifloxacin.

In vitro studies with cytochrome (CYP) P450 enzymes indicate that moxifloxacin does not inhibit CYP3A4, CYP2D6, CYP2C9, CYP2C19, or CYP1A2, suggesting that moxifloxacin is unlikely to alter the pharmacokinetics of drugs metabolized by these enzymes.

Excretion

Approximately 45% of an oral or intravenous dose of moxifloxacin is excreted as unchanged drug (~20% in urine and ~25% in feces). A total of 96% ± 4% of an oral dose is excreted as either unchanged drug or known metabolites. The mean (± SD) apparent total body clearance and renal clearance are 12 ± 2.0 L/hr and 2.6 ± 0.5 L/hr, respectively.

Special Populations

Geriatric

Following oral administration of 400 mg moxifloxacin for 10 days in 16 elderly (8 male; 8 female) and 17 young (8 male; 9 female) healthy volunteers, there were no age-related changes in moxifloxacin pharmacokinetics. In 16 healthy male volunteers (8 young; 8 elderly) given a single 200 mg dose of oral moxifloxacin, the extent of systemic exposure (AUC and C_{max}) was not statistically different between young and elderly males and elimination half-life was unchanged. No dosage adjustment is necessary based on age. In large phase III studies, the concentrations around the time of the end of the infusion in elderly patients following intravenous infusion of 400 mg were similar to those observed in young patients.

Pediatric

The pharmacokinetics of moxifloxacin in pediatric subjects have not been studied.

Gender

Following oral administration of 400 mg moxifloxacin daily for 10 days to 23 healthy males (19-75 years) and 24 healthy females (19-70 years), the mean AUC and C_{max} were 8% and 16% higher, respectively, in females compared to males. There are no significant differences in moxifloxacin pharmacokinetics between male and female subjects when differences in body weight are taken into consideration.

A 400 mg single dose study was conducted in 18 young males and females. The comparison of moxifloxacin pharmacokinetics in this study (9 young females and 9 young males) showed no differences in AUC or C_{max} due to gender. Dosage adjustments based on gender are not necessary.

Race

Steady-state moxifloxacin pharmacokinetics in male Japanese subjects were similar to those determined in Caucasians, with a mean C_{max} of 4.1 µg/mL, an AUC_{24} of 47 µg•h/mL, and an elimination half-life of 14 hours, following 400 mg p.o. daily.

Renal Insufficiency

The pharmacokinetic parameters of moxifloxacin are not significantly altered in mild, moderate, severe, or end-stage renal disease. No dosage adjustment is necessary in patients with renal impairment, including those patients requiring hemodialysis (HD) or continuous ambulatory peritoneal dialysis (CAPD).

In a single oral dose study of 24 patients with varying degrees of renal function from normal to severely impaired, the mean peak concentrations (C_{max}) of moxifloxacin were reduced by 21% and 28% in the patients with moderate (CL_{CR} ≥30 and ≤60 mL/min) and severe (CL_{CR} <30 mL/min) renal impairment, respectively. The mean systemic exposure (AUC) in these patients was increased by 13%. In the moderate and severe renally impaired patients, the mean AUC for the sulfate conjugate (M1) increased by 1.7-fold (ranging up to 2.8-fold) and mean AUC and C_{max} for the glucuronide conjugate (M2) increased by 2.8-fold (ranging up to 4.8-fold) and 1.4-fold (ranging up to 2.5-fold), respectively.

The pharmacokinetics of single dose and multiple dose moxifloxacin were studied in patients with $CL_{CR} < 20$ mL/min on either hemodialysis or continuous ambulatory peritoneal dialysis (8 HD, 8 CAPD). Following a single 400 mg oral dose, the AUC of moxifloxacin in these HD and CAPD patients did not vary significantly from the AUC generally found in healthy volunteers. C_{max} values of moxifloxacin were reduced by about 45% and 33% in HD and CAPD patients, respectively, compared to healthy, historical controls. The exposure (AUC) to the sulfate conjugate (M1) increased by 1.4- to 1.5-fold in these patients. The mean AUC of the glucuronide conjugate (M2) increased by a factor of 7.5, whereas the mean C_{max} values of the glucuronide conjugate (M2) increased by a factor of 2.5 to 3, compared to healthy subjects. The sulfate and the glucuronide conjugates of moxifloxacin are not microbiologically active, and the clinical implication of increased exposure to these metabolites in patients with renal disease including those undergoing HD and CAPD has not been studied.

Oral administration of 400 mg QD moxifloxacin for 7 days to patients on HD or CAPD produced mean systemic exposure (AUC_{ss}) to moxifloxacin similar to that generally seen in healthy volunteers. Steady-state C_{max} values were about 22% lower in HD patients but were comparable between CAPD patients and healthy volunteers. Both HD and CAPD removed only small amounts of moxifloxacin from the body (approximately 9% by HD, and 3% by CAPD). HD and CAPD also removed about 4% and 2% of the glucuronide metabolite (M2), respectively.

	C_{max} (mg/L)	AUC (mg•h/L)	Half-life (hr)
Single Dose Oral			
Healthy (n = 372)	3.1 ± 1.0	36.1 ± 9.1	11.5 – 15.6*
Multiple Dose Oral			
Healthy young male/female (n = 15)	4.5 ± 0.5	48.0 ± 2.7	12.7 ± 1.9
Healthy elderly male (n = 8)	3.8 ± 0.3	51.8 ± 6.7	
Healthy elderly female (n = 8)	4.6 ± 0.6	54.6 ± 6.7	
Healthy young male (n = 8)	3.6 ± 0.5	48.2 ± 9.0	
Healthy young female (n = 9)	4.2 ± 0.5	49.3 ± 9.5	

*Range of means from different studies

	C_{max} (mg/L)	AUC (mg•h/L)	Half-life (hr)
Single Dose I.V.			
Healthy young male/female (n = 56)	3.9 ± 0.9	39.3 ± 8.6	8.2 – 15.4*
Patients (n = 118)			
Male (n = 64)	4.4 ± 3.7		
Female (n = 54)	4.5 ± 2.0		
< 65 years (n = 58)	4.6 ± 4.2		
≥ 65 years (n = 60)	4.3 ± 1.3		
Multiple Dose I.V.			
Healthy young male (n = 8)	4.2 ± 0.8	38.0 ± 4.7	14.8 ± 2.2
Healthy elderly (n = 12; 8 male, 4 female)	6.1 ± 1.3	48.2 ± 0.9	10.1 ± 1.6
Patients** (n = 107)			
Male (n = 58)	4.2 ± 2.6		
Female (n = 49)	4.6 ± 1.5		
< 65 years (n = 52)	4.1 ± 1.4		
≥ 65 years (n = 55)	4.7 ± 2.7		

* Range of means from different studies
** Expected C_{max} (concentration obtained around the time of the end of the infusion)

Moxifloxacin Concentrations (mean ± SD) After Oral Dosing in Plasma and Tissues Measured 3 Hours After Dosing with 400 mg§

Tissue or Fluid	N	Plasma Concentration (µg/mL)	Tissue or Fluid Concentration (µg/mL or µg/g)	Tissue Plasma Ratio:
Respiratory				
Alveolar Macrophages	5	3.3 ± 0.7	61.8 ± 27.3	21.2 ± 10.0
Bronchial Mucosa	8	3.3 ± 0.7	5.5 ± 1.3	1.7 ± 0.3
Epithelial Lining Fluid	5	3.3 ± 0.7	24.4 ± 14.7	8.7 ± 6.1
Sinus				
Maxillary Sinus Mucosa	4	3.7 ± 1.1†	7.6 ± 1.7	2.0 ± 0.3
Anterior Ethmoid Mucosa	3	3.7 ± 1.1†	8.8 ± 4.3	2.2 ± 0.6
Nasal Polyps	4	3.7 ± 1.1†	9.8 ± 4.5	2.6 ± 0.6

§ all moxifloxacin concentrations were measured after a single 400 mg dose, except the sinus concentrations which were measured after 5 days of dosing.
† N = 5

Hepatic Insufficiency

In 400 mg single oral dose studies in 6 patients with mild (Child Pugh Class A), and 10 patients with moderate (Child Pugh Class B), hepatic insufficiency, moxifloxacin mean systemic exposure (AUC) was 78% and 102%, respectively, of 18 healthy controls and mean peak concentration (C_{max}) was 79% and 84% of controls.

The mean AUC of the sulfate conjugate of moxifloxacin (M1) increased by 3.9-fold (ranging up to 5.9-fold) and 5.7-fold (ranging up to 8.0-fold) in the mild and moderate groups, respectively. The mean C_{max} of M1 increased by approximately 3-fold in both groups (ranging up to 4.7- and 3.9-fold). The mean AUC of the glucuronide conjugate of moxifloxacin (M2) increased by 1.5-fold (ranging up to 2.5-fold) in both groups. The mean C_{max} of M2 increased by 1.6- and 1.3-fold (ranging up to 2.7- and 2.1-fold), respectively. The clinical significance of increased exposure to the sulfate and glucuronide conjugates has not been studied. No dosage adjustment is recommended for mild or moderate hepatic insufficiency (Child Pugh Classes A and B). The pharmacokinetics of moxifloxacin in severe hepatic insufficiency (Child Pugh Class C) have not been studied. (See **DOSAGE AND ADMINISTRATION**.)

Photosensitivity Potential

A study of the skin response to ultraviolet (UVA and UVB) and visible radiation conducted in 32 healthy volunteers (8 per group) demonstrated that moxifloxacin does not show phototoxicity in comparison to placebo. The minimum erythematous dose (MED) was measured before and after treatment with moxifloxacin (200 mg or 400 mg once daily), lomefloxacin (400 mg once daily), or placebo. In this study, the MED measured for both doses of moxifloxacin were not significantly different from placebo, while lomefloxacin significantly lowered the MED. (See **PRECAUTIONS Information for Patients.**)

Drug-drug Interactions

The potential for pharmacokinetic drug interactions between moxifloxacin and itraconazole, theophylline, warfarin, digoxin, atenolol, probenecid, morphine, oral contraceptives, ranitidine, glyburide, calcium, iron, and antacids has

been evaluated. There was no clinically significant effect of moxifloxacin on itraconazole, theophylline, warfarin, digoxin, atenolol, oral contraceptives, or glyburide kinetics. Itraconazole, theophylline, warfarin, digoxin, probenecid, morphine, ranitidine, and calcium did not significantly affect the pharmacokinetics of moxifloxacin. These results and the data from *in vitro* studies suggest that moxifloxacin is unlikely to significantly alter the metabolic clearance of drugs metabolized by CYP3A4, CYP2D6, CYP2C9, CYP2C19, or CYP1A2 enzymes.

As with all other quinolones, iron and antacids significantly reduced bioavailability of moxifloxacin.

Itraconazole: In a study involving 11 healthy volunteers, there was no significant effect of itraconazole (200 mg once daily for 9 days), a potent inhibitor of cytochrome P4503A4, on the pharmacokinetics of moxifloxacin (a single 400 mg dose given on the 7th day of itraconazole dosing). In addition, moxifloxacin was shown not to affect the pharmacokinetics of itraconazole.

Theophylline: No significant effect of moxifloxacin (200 mg every twelve hours for 3 days) on the pharmacokinetics of theophylline (400 mg every twelve hours for 3 days) was detected in a study involving 12 healthy volunteers. In addition, theophylline was not shown to affect the pharmacokinetics of moxifloxacin. The effect of co-administration of a 400 mg dose of moxifloxacin with theophylline has not been studied, but it is not expected to be clinically significant based on *in vitro* metabolic data showing that moxifloxacin does not inhibit the CYP1A2 isoenzyme.

Warfarin: No significant effect of moxifloxacin (400 mg once daily for eight days) on the pharmacokinetics of R- and S-warfarin (25 mg single dose of warfarin sodium on the fifth day) was detected in a study involving 24 healthy volunteers. No significant change in prothrombin time was observed. (See **PRECAUTIONS, Drug Interactions**.)

Digoxin: No significant effect of moxifloxacin (400 mg once daily for two days) on digoxin (0.6 mg as a single dose) AUC was detected in a study involving 12 healthy volunteers.

Continued on next page

Avelox—Cont.

The mean digoxin C_{max} increased by about 50% during the distribution phase of digoxin. This transient increase in digoxin C_{max} is not viewed to be clinically significant. Moxifloxacin pharmacokinetics were similar in the presence or absence of digoxin. No dosage adjustment for moxifloxacin or digoxin is required when these drugs are administered concomitantly.

Atenolol: In a crossover study involving 24 healthy volunteers (12 male; 12 female), the mean atenolol AUC following a single oral dose of 50 mg atenolol with placebo was similar to that observed when atenolol was given concomitantly with a single 400 mg oral dose of moxifloxacin. The mean C_{max} of single dose atenolol decreased by about 10% following co-administration with a single dose of moxifloxacin.

Morphine: No significant effect of morphine sulfate (a single 10 mg intramuscular dose) on the mean AUC and C_{max} of moxifloxacin (400 mg single dose) was observed in a study of 20 healthy male and female volunteers.

Oral Contraceptives: A placebo-controlled study in 29 healthy female subjects showed that moxifloxacin 400 mg daily for 7 days did not interfere with the hormonal suppression of oral contraception with 0.15 mg levonorgestrel/ 0.03 mg ethinylestradiol (as measured by serum progesterone, FSH, estradiol, and LH), or with the pharmacokinetics of the administered contraceptive agents.

Probenecid: Probenecid (500 mg twice daily for two days) did not alter the renal clearance and total amount of moxifloxacin (400 mg single dose) excreted renally in a study of 12 healthy volunteers.

Ranitidine: No significant effect of ranitidine (150 mg twice daily for three days as pretreatment) on the pharmacokinetics of moxifloxacin (400 mg single dose) was detected in a study involving 10 healthy volunteers.

Antidiabetic agents: In diabetics, glyburide (2.5 mg once daily for two weeks pretreatment and for five days concurrently) mean AUC and C_{max} were 12% and 21% lower, respectively, when taken with moxifloxacin (400 mg once daily for five days) in comparison to placebo. Nonetheless, blood glucose levels were decreased slightly in patients taking glyburide and moxifloxacin in comparison to those taking glyburide alone, suggesting no interference by moxifloxacin on the activity of glyburide. These interaction results are not viewed as clinically significant.

Calcium: Twelve healthy volunteers were administered concomitant moxifloxacin (single 400 mg dose) and calcium (single dose of 500 mg Ca^{++} dietary supplement) followed by an additional two doses of calcium 12 and 24 hours after moxifloxacin administration. Calcium had no significant effect on the mean AUC of moxifloxacin. The mean C_{max} was slightly reduced and the time to maximum plasma concentration was prolonged when moxifloxacin was given with calcium compared to when moxifloxacin was given alone (2.5 hours versus 0.9 hours). These differences are not considered to be clinically significant.

Antacids: When moxifloxacin (single 400 mg tablet dose) was administered two hours before, concomitantly, or 4 hours after an aluminum/magnesium-containing antacid (900 mg aluminum hydroxide and 600 mg magnesium hydroxide as a single oral dose) to 12 healthy volunteers there was a 26%, 60% and 23% reduction in the mean AUC of moxifloxacin, respectively. Moxifloxacin should be taken at least 4 hours before or 8 hours after antacids containing magnesium or aluminum, as well as sucralfate, metal cations such as iron, and multivitamin preparations with zinc, or VIDEX® (didanosine) chewable/buffered tablets or the pediatric powder for oral solution. (See **PRECAUTIONS, Drug Interactions** and **DOSAGE AND ADMINISTRATION**.)

Iron: When moxifloxacin tablets were administered concomitantly with iron (ferrous sulfate 100 mg once daily for two days), the mean AUC and C_{max} of moxifloxacin was reduced by 39% and 59%, respectively. Moxifloxacin should only be taken more than 4 hours before or 8 hours after iron products. (See **PRECAUTIONS, Drug Interactions** and **DOSAGE AND ADMINISTRATION**.)

Electrocardiogram: Prolongation of the QT interval in the ECG has been observed in some patients receiving moxifloxacin. Following oral dosing with 400 mg of moxifloxacin the mean (± SD) change in QTc from the pre-dose value at the time of maximum drug concentration was 6 msec (± 26) (n = 787). Following a course of daily intravenous dosing (400 mg; 1 hour infusion each day) the mean change in QTc from the Day 1 pre-dose value was 9 msec (± 24) on Day 1 (n = 69) and 3 msec (± 29) on Day 3 (n = 290). (See **WARNINGS**.)

There is limited information available on the potential for a pharmacodynamic interaction in humans between moxifloxacin and other drugs that prolong the QTc interval of the electrocardiogram. Sotalol, a Class III antiarrhythmic, has been shown to further increase the QTc interval when combined with high doses of intravenous (I.V.) moxifloxacin in dogs. Therefore, moxifloxacin should be avoided with Class IA and Class III antiarrhythmics. (See **ANIMAL PHARMACOLOGY, WARNINGS**, and **PRECAUTIONS**.)

MICROBIOLOGY

Moxifloxacin has *in vitro* activity against a wide range of Gram-positive and Gram-negative microorganisms. The bactericidal action of moxifloxacin results from inhibition of the topoisomerase II (DNA gyrase) and topoisomerase IV required for bacterial DNA replication, transcription, repair, and recombination. It appears that the C8-methoxy moiety contributes to enhanced activity and lower selection of resistant mutants of Gram-positive bacteria compared to the C8-H moiety. The presence of the bulky bicycloamine substituent at the C-7 position prevents active efflux, associated with the *NorA* or *pmrA* genes seen in certain Gram-positive bacteria.

The mechanism of action for quinolones, including moxifloxacin, is different from that of macrolides, beta-lactams, aminoglycosides, or tetracyclines; therefore, microorganisms resistant to these classes of drugs may be susceptible to moxifloxacin and other quinolones. There is no known cross-resistance between moxifloxacin and other classes of antimicrobials.

In vitro resistance to moxifloxacin develops slowly via multiple-step mutations. Resistance to moxifloxacin occurs *in vitro* at a general frequency of between 1.8×10^{-9} to $< 1 \times 10^{-11}$ for Gram-positive bacteria.

Cross-resistance has been observed between moxifloxacin and other fluoroquinolones against Gram-negative bacteria. Gram-positive bacteria resistant to other fluoroquinolones may, however, still be susceptible to moxifloxacin.

Moxifloxacin has been shown to be active against most strains of the following microorganisms, both *in vitro* and in clinical infections as described in the **INDICATIONS AND USAGE** section.

Aerobic Gram-positive microorganisms

Staphylococcus aureus (methicillin-susceptible strains only)
Streptococcus pneumoniae (including multi-drug resistant strains [MDRSP]*)
Streptococcus pyogenes

* MDRSP, Multi-drug resistant *Streptococcus pneumoniae* includes isolates previously known as PRSP (Penicillin-resistant *S. pneumoniae*), and are strains resistant to two or more of the following antibiotics: penicillin (MIC ≥ 2 µg/mL 2nd generation cephalosporins (e.g., cefuroxime), macrolides, tetracyclines, and trimethoprim/sulfamethoxazole.

Aerobic Gram-negative microorganisms

Haemophilus influenzae
Haemophilus parainfluenzae
Klebsiella pneumoniae
Moraxella catarrhalis

Other microorganisms

Chlamydia pneumoniae
Mycoplasma pneumoniae

The following *in vitro* data are available, **but their clinical significance is unknown.**

Moxifloxacin exhibits *in vitro* minimum inhibitory concentrations (MICs) of 2 µg/mL or less against most (≥90%) strains of the following microorganisms; however, the safety and effectiveness of moxifloxacin in treating clinical infections due to these microorganisms have not been established in adequate and well-controlled clinical trials.

Aerobic Gram-positive microorganisms

Staphylococcus epidermidis (methicillin-susceptible strains only)
Streptococcus agalactiae
Streptococcus viridans group

Aerobic Gram-negative microorganisms

Citrobacter freundii
Enterobacter cloacae
Escherichia coli
Klebsiella oxytoca
Legionella pneumophila
Proteus mirabilis

Anaerobic microorganisms

Fusobacterium species
Peptostreptococcus species
Prevotella species

Susceptibility Tests

Dilution Techniques: Quantitative methods are used to determine antimicrobial minimum inhibitory concentrations (MICs). These MICs provide estimates of the susceptibility of bacteria to antimicrobial compounds. The MICs should be determined using a standardized procedure. Standardized procedures are based on a dilution method[1] (broth or agar) or equivalent with standardized inoculum concentrations and standardized concentrations of moxifloxacin powder. The MIC values should be interpreted according to the following criteria:

For testing Enterobacteriaceae and *Staphylococcus* species:

MIC (µg/mL)	Interpretation	
≤ 2.0	Susceptible	(S)
4.0	Intermediate	(I)
≥ 8.0	Resistant	(R)

For testing *Haemophilus influenzae* and *Haemophilus parainfluenzae*[a]:

MIC (µg/mL)	Interpretation	
≤ 1.0	Susceptible	(S)

[a] This interpretive standard is applicable only to broth microdilution susceptibility tests with *Haemophilus influenzae* and *Haemophilus parainfluenzae* using *Haemophilus* Test Medium[1].

The current absence of data on resistant strains precludes defining any results other than "Susceptible". Strains yielding MIC results suggestive of a "nonsusceptible" category should be submitted to a reference laboratory for further testing.

For testing *Streptococcus* species including *Streptococcus pneumoniae*[b]:

MIC (µg/mL)	Interpretation	
≤ 1.0	Susceptible	(S)
2.0	Intermediate	(I)
≥ 4.0	Resistant	(R)

[b] This interpretive standard is applicable only to broth microdilution susceptibility tests using cation-adjusted Mueller-Hinton broth with 2–5% lysed horse blood.

A report of "Susceptible" indicates that the pathogen is likely to be inhibited if the antimicrobial compound in the blood reaches the concentrations usually achievable. A report of "Intermediate" indicates that the result should be considered equivocal, and, if the microorganism is not fully susceptible to alternative, clinically feasible drugs, the test should be repeated. This category implies possible clinical applicability in body sites where the drug is physiologically concentrated or in situations where a high dosage of drug can be used. This category also provides a buffer zone which prevents small uncontrolled technical factors from causing major discrepancies in interpretation. A report of "Resistant" indicates that the pathogen is not likely to be inhibited if the antimicrobial compound in the blood reaches the concentrations usually achievable; other therapy should be selected.

Standardized susceptibility test procedures require the use of laboratory control microorganisms to control the technical aspects of the laboratory procedures. Standard moxifloxacin powder should provide the following MIC values:

Microorganism		MIC (µg/mL)
Enterococcus faecalis	ATCC 29212	0.06-0.5
Escherichia coli	ATCC 25922	0.008-0.06
Haemophilus influenzae	ATCC 49247[c]	0.008-0.03
Staphylococcus aureus	ATCC 29213	0.015-0.06
Streptococcus pneumoniae	ATCC 49619[d]	0.06-0.25

[c] This quality control range is applicable to only *H. influenzae* ATCC 49247 tested by a broth microdilution procedure using *Haemophilus* Test Medium (HTM)[1].

[d] This quality control range is applicable to only *S. pneumoniae* ATCC 49619 tested by a broth microdilution procedure using cation-adjusted Mueller-Hinton broth with 2-5% lysed horse blood.

Diffusion Techniques: Quantitative methods that require measurement of zone diameters also provide reproducible estimates of the susceptibility of bacteria to antimicrobial compounds. One such standardized procedure[2] requires the use of standardized inoculum concentrations. This procedure uses paper disks impregnated with 5-µg moxifloxacin to test the susceptibility of microorganisms to moxifloxacin. Reports from the laboratory providing results of the standard single-disk susceptibility test with a 5-µg moxifloxacin disk should be interpreted according to the following criteria:

The following zone diameter interpretive criteria should be used for testing Enterobacteriaceae and *Staphylococcus* species:

Zone Diameter (mm)	Interpretation	
≥ 19	Susceptible	(S)
16-18	Intermediate	(I)
≤ 15	Resistant	(R)

For testing *Haemophilus influenzae* and *Haemophilus parainfluenzae*[e]:

Zone Diameter (mm)	Interpretation	
≥ 18	Susceptible	(S)

[e] This zone diameter standard is applicable only to tests with *Haemophilus influenzae* and *Haemophilus parainfluenzae* using *Haemophilus* Test Medium (HTM)[2].

The current absence of data on resistant strains precludes defining any results other than "Susceptible". Strains yielding zone diameter results suggestive of a "nonsusceptible" category should be submitted to a reference laboratory for further testing.

For testing *Streptococcus* species including *Streptococcus pneumoniae*[f]:

Zone Diameter (mm)	Interpretation	
≥ 18	Susceptible	(S)
15-17	Intermediate	(I)
≤ 14	Resistant	(R)

[f] These interpretive standards are applicable only to disk diffusion tests using Mueller-Hinton agar supplemented with 5% sheep blood incubated in 5% CO_2.

Interpretation should be as stated above for results using dilution techniques. Interpretation involves correlation of the diameter obtained in the disk test with the MIC for moxifloxacin.

As with standardized dilution techniques, diffusion methods require the use of laboratory control microorganisms that are used to control the technical aspects of the laboratory procedures. For the diffusion technique, the 5-µg moxifloxacin disk should provide the following zone diameters in these laboratory test quality control strains:

Microorganism		Zone Diameter (mm)
Escherichia coli	ATCC 25922	28-35
Haemophilus influenzae	ATCC 49247[g]	31-39
Staphylococcus aureus	ATCC 25923	28-35
Streptococcus pneumoniae	ATCC 49619[h]	25-31

[g] These quality control limits are applicable to only *H. influenzae* ATCC 49247 testing using *Haemophilus* Test Medium (HTM)[2].

[h] These quality control limits are applicable only to tests conducted with *S. pneumoniae* ATCC 49619 performed by disk diffusion using Mueller-Hinton agar supplemented with 5% defibrinated sheep blood.

INDICATIONS AND USAGE

AVELOX Tablets and I.V. are indicated for the treatment of adults (≥18 years of age) with infections caused by susceptible strains of the designated microorganisms in the conditions listed below. (See **DOSAGE AND ADMINISTRATION** for specific recommendations. In addition, for I.V. use see **PRECAUTIONS, Geriatric Use.**)

Acute Bacterial Sinusitis caused by *Streptococcus pneumoniae, Haemophilus influenzae,* or *Moraxella catarrhalis.*

Acute Bacterial Exacerbation of Chronic Bronchitis caused by *Streptococcus pneumoniae, Haemophilus influenzae, Haemophilus parainfluenzae, Klebsiella pneumoniae, Staphylococcus aureus,* or *Moraxella catarrhalis.*

Community Acquired Pneumonia caused by *Streptococcus pneumoniae* (including multi-drug resistant strains*), *Haemophilus influenzae, Moraxella catarrhalis, Staphylococcus aureus, Klebsiella pneumoniae, Mycoplasma pneumoniae,* or *Chlamydia pneumoniae.*

* MDRSP, Multi-drug resistant *Streptococcus pneumoniae* includes isolates previously known as PRSP (Penicillin-resistant *S. pneumoniae*), and are strains resistant to two or more of the following antibiotics: penicillin (MIC ≥2 µg/mL), 2nd generation cephalosporins (e.g., cefuroxime), macrolides, tetracyclines, and trimethoprim/sulfamethoxazole.

Uncomplicated Skin and Skin Structure Infections caused by *Staphylococcus aureus* or *Streptococcus pyogenes.*

Appropriate culture and susceptibility tests should be performed before treatment in order to isolate and identify organisms causing infection and to determine their susceptibility to moxifloxacin. Therapy with AVELOX may be initiated before results of these tests are known; once results become available, appropriate therapy should be continued.

To reduce the development of drug-resistant bacteria and maintain the effectiveness of AVELOX and other antibacterial drugs, AVELOX should be used only to treat or prevent infections that are proven or strongly suspected to be caused by susceptible bacteria. When culture and susceptibility information are available, they should be considered in selecting or modifying antibacterial therapy. In the absence of such data, local epidemiology and susceptibility patterns may contribute to the empiric selection of therapy.

CONTRAINDICATIONS

Moxifloxacin is contraindicated in persons with a history of hypersensitivity to moxifloxacin or any member of the quinolone class of antimicrobial agents.

WARNINGS

THE SAFETY AND EFFECTIVENESS OF MOXIFLOXACIN IN PEDIATRIC PATIENTS, ADOLESCENTS (LESS THAN 18 YEARS OF AGE), PREGNANT WOMEN, AND LACTATING WOMEN HAVE NOT BEEN ESTABLISHED. (SEE PRECAUTIONS-PEDIATRIC USE, PREGNANCY AND NURSING MOTHERS SUBSECTIONS.)

Moxifloxacin has been shown to prolong the QT interval of the electrocardiogram in some patients. The drug should be avoided in patients with known prolongation of the QT interval, patients with uncorrected hypokalemia and patients receiving Class IA (e.g., quinidine, procainamide) or Class III (e.g. amiodarone, sotalol) antiarrhythmic agents, due to the lack of clinical experience with the drug in these patient populations.

Pharmacokinetic studies between moxifloxacin and other drugs that prolong the QT interval such as cisapride, erythromycin, antipsychotics, and tricyclic antidepressants have not been performed. An additive effect of moxifloxacin and these drugs cannot be excluded, therefore caution should be exercised when moxifloxacin is given concurrently with these drugs. In premarketing clinical trials, the rate of cardiovascular adverse events was similar in 798 moxifloxacin and 702 comparator treated patients who received concomitant therapy with drugs known to prolong the QTc interval. Moxifloxacin should be used with caution in patients with ongoing proarrhythmic conditions, such as clinically significant bradycardia, acute myocardial ischemia. The magnitude of QT prolongation may increase with increasing concentrations of the drug or increasing rates of infusion of the intravenous formulation. Therefore the recommended dose or infusion rate should not be exceeded. QT prolongation may lead to an increased risk for ventricular arrhythmias including torsade de pointes. No cardiovascular morbidity or mortality attributable to QTc prolongation occurred with moxifloxacin treatment in over 7,900 patients in controlled clinical studies, including 223 patients who were hypokalemic at the start of treatment, and there was no increase in mortality in over 18,000 moxifloxacin tablet treated patients in a post-marketing observational study in which ECGs were not performed. (See **CLINICAL PHARMACOLOGY, Electrocardiogram**. For I.V. use see **DOSAGE AND ADMINISTRATION** and **PRECAUTIONS, Geriatric Use.**)

The oral administration of moxifloxacin caused lameness in immature dogs. Histopathological examination of the weight-bearing joints of these dogs revealed permanent lesions of the cartilage. Related quinolone-class drugs also produce erosions of cartilage of weight-bearing joints and other signs of arthropathy in immature animals of various species. (See **ANIMAL PHARMACOLOGY.**)

Convulsions have been reported in patients receiving quinolones. Quinolones may also cause central nervous system (CNS) events including: dizziness, confusion, tremors, hallucinations, depression, and, rarely, suicidal thoughts or acts. These reactions may occur following the first dose. If these reactions occur in patients receiving moxifloxacin, the drug should be discontinued and appropriate measures instituted. As with all quinolones, moxifloxacin should be used with caution in patients with known or suspected CNS disorders (e.g. severe cerebral arteriosclerosis, epilepsy) or in the presence of other risk factors that may predispose to seizures or lower the seizure threshold. (See **PRECAUTIONS: General, Information for Patients,** and **ADVERSE REACTIONS.**)

Serious anaphylactic reactions, some following the first dose, have been reported in patients receiving quinolone therapy, including moxifloxacin. Some reactions were accompanied by cardiovascular collapse, loss of consciousness, tingling, pharyngeal or facial edema, dyspnea, urticaria, and itching. Serious anaphylactic reactions require immediate emergency treatment with epinephrine. Moxifloxacin should be discontinued at the first appearance of a skin rash or any other sign of hypersensitivity. Oxygen, intravenous steroids, and airway management, including intubation, may be administered as indicated.

Severe and sometimes fatal events, some due to hypersensitivity, and some of uncertain etiology, have been reported in patients receiving therapy with all antibiotics. These events may be severe and generally occur following the administration of multiple doses. Clinical manifestations may include one or more of the following: rash, fever, eosinophilia, jaundice, and hepatic necrosis.

Pseudomembranous colitis has been reported with nearly all antibacterial agents and may range in severity from mild to life-threatening. Therefore, it is important to consider this diagnosis in patients who present with diarrhea subsequent to the administration of antibacterial agents.

Treatment with antibacterial agents alters the normal flora of the colon and may permit overgrowth of clostridia. Studies indicate that a toxin produced by *Clostridium difficile* is one primary cause of "antibiotic-associated colitis." After the diagnosis of pseudomembranous colitis has been established, therapeutic measures should be initiated. Mild cases of pseudomembranous colitis usually respond to drug discontinuation alone. In moderate to severe cases, consideration should be given to management with fluids and electrolytes, protein supplementation, and treatment with an antibacterial drug clinically effective against *C. difficile* colitis.

Peripheral neuropathy: Rare cases of sensory or sensorimotor axonal polyneuropathy affecting small and/or large axons resulting in paresthesias, hypoesthesias, dysesthesias and weakness have been reported in patients receiving quinolones.

Tendon Effects: Ruptures of the shoulder, hand, Achilles tendon or other tendons that required surgical repair or resulted in prolonged disability have been reported in patients receiving quinolones, including moxifloxacin. Post-marketing surveillance reports indicate that this risk may be increased in patients receiving concomitant corticosteroids, especially the elderly. Moxifloxacin should be discontinued if the patient experiences pain, inflammation, or rupture of a tendon. Patients should rest and refrain from exercise until the diagnosis of tendonitis or tendon rupture has been excluded. Tendon rupture can occur during or after therapy with quinolones, including moxifloxacin.

PRECAUTIONS

General: Quinolones may cause central nervous system (CNS) events, including: nervousness, agitation, insomnia, anxiety, nightmares or paranoia. (See **WARNINGS** and **Information for Patients.**)

Prescribing AVELOX in the absence of a proven or strongly suspected bacterial infection or a prophylactic indication is unlikely to provide benefit to the patient and increases the risk of the development of drug-resistant bacteria.

Information for Patients:

To assure safe and effective use of moxifloxacin, the following information and instructions should be communicated to the patient when appropriate:

Patients should be advised:

- that antibacterial drugs including AVELOX should only be used to treat bacterial infections. They do not treat viral infections (e.g., the common cold). When AVELOX is prescribed to treat a bacterial infection, patients should be told that although it is common to feel better early in the course of therapy, the medication should be taken exactly as directed. Skipping doses or not completing the full course of therapy may (1) decrease the effectiveness of the immediate treatment and (2) increase the likelihood that bacteria will develop resistance and will not be treatable by AVELOX or other antibacterial drugs in the future.
- that moxifloxacin may produce changes in the electrocardiogram (QTc interval prolongation).
- that moxifloxacin should be avoided in patients receiving Class IA (e.g. quinidine, procainamide) or Class III (e.g. amiodarone, sotalol) antiarrhythmic agents.
- that moxifloxacin may add to the QTc prolonging effects of other drugs such as cisapride, erythromycin, antipsychotics, and tricyclic antidepressants.
- to inform their physician of any personal or family history of QTc prolongation or proarrhythmic conditions such as recent hypokalemia, significant bradycardia, acute myocardial ischemia.
- to inform their physician of any other medications when taken concurrently with moxifloxacin, including over-the-counter medications.
- to contact their physician if they experience palpitations or fainting spells while taking moxifloxacin.
- that moxifloxacin tablets may be taken with or without meals, and to drink fluids liberally.
- that moxifloxacin tablets should be taken at least 4 hours before or 8 hours after multivitamins (containing iron or zinc), antacids (containing magnesium or aluminum), sucralfate, or VIDEX® (didanosine) chewable/buffered tablets or the pediatric powder for oral solution. (See **CLINICAL PHARMACOLOGY, Drug Interactions** and **PRECAUTIONS Drug Interactions.**)
- that moxifloxacin may be associated with hypersensitivity reactions, including anaphylactic reactions, even following a single dose, and to discontinue the drug at the first sign of a skin rash or other signs of an allergic reaction.
- to discontinue treatment; rest and refrain from exercise; and inform their physician if they experience pain, inflammation, or rupture of a tendon.
- that moxifloxacin may cause dizziness and lightheadedness; therefore, patients should know how they react to this drug before they operate an automobile or machinery or engage in activities requiring mental alertness or coordination.
- that phototoxicity has been reported in patients receiving certain quinolones. There was no phototoxicity seen with moxifloxacin at the recommended dose. In keeping with good medical practice, avoid excessive sunlight or artificial ultraviolet light (e.g. tanning beds). If sunburn-like reaction or skin eruptions occur, contact your physician. (See **CLINICAL PHARMACOLOGY, Photosensitivity Potential.**)
- that convulsions have been reported in patients receiving quinolones, and they should notify their physician before taking this drug if there is a history of this condition.

Drug Interactions:

Antacids, Sucralfate, Metal Cations, Multivitamins: Quinolones form chelates with alkaline earth and transition metal cations. Oral administration of quinolones with antacids containing aluminum or magnesium, with sucralfate, with metal cations such as iron, or with multivitamins containing iron or zinc, or with formulations containing divalent and trivalent cations such as VIDEX® (didanosine) chewable/buffered tablets or the pediatric powder for oral solution, may substantially interfere with the absorption of quinolones, resulting in systemic concentrations considerably lower than desired. Therefore, moxifloxacin should be taken at least 4 hours before or 8 hours after these agents. (See **CLINICAL PHARMACOLOGY, Drug Interactions** and **DOSAGE AND ADMINISTRATION.**)

No clinically significant drug-drug interactions between itraconazole, theophylline, warfarin, digoxin, atenolol, oral contraceptives or glyburide have been observed with moxifloxacin. Itraconazole, theophylline, digoxin, probenecid, morphine, ranitidine, and calcium have been shown not to significantly alter the pharmacokinetics of moxifloxacin. (See **CLINICAL PHARMACOLOGY**).

Warfarin: No significant effect of moxifloxacin on R- and S-warfarin was detected in a clinical study involving 24 healthy volunteers. No significant changes in prothrombin time were noted in the presence of moxifloxacin. Quinolones, including moxifloxacin, have been reported to enhance the anticoagulant effects of warfarin or its derivatives in the patient population. In addition, infectious disease and its accompanying inflammatory process, age, and general status of the patient are risk factors for increased anticoagulant activity. Therefore the prothrombin time, International Normalized Ratio (INR), or other suitable anticoagulation tests should be closely monitored if a quinolone is administered concomitantly with warfarin or its derivatives.

Drugs metabolized by Cytochrome P450 enzymes: *In vitro* studies with cytochrome P450 isoenzymes (CYP) indicate that moxifloxacin does not inhibit CYP3A4, CYP2D6, CYP2C9, CYP2C19, or CYP1A2, suggesting that moxifloxacin is unlikely to alter the pharmacokinetics of drugs metabolized by these enzymes (e.g. midazolam, cyclosporine, warfarin, theophylline).

Nonsteroidal anti-inflammatory drugs (NSAIDs): Although not observed with moxifloxacin in preclinical and clinical trials, the concomitant administration of a nonsteroidal anti-inflammatory drug with a quinolone may increase the risks of CNS stimulation and convulsions. (See **WARNINGS.**)

Carcinogenesis, Mutagenesis, Impairment of Fertility:

Long term studies in animals to determine the carcinogenic potential of moxifloxacin have not been performed.

Continued on next page

Avelox—Cont.

Moxifloxacin was not mutagenic in 4 bacterial strains (TA 98, TA 100, TA 1535, TA 1537) used in the Ames *Salmonella* reversion assay. As with other quinolones, the positive response observed with moxifloxacin in strain TA 102 using the same assay may be due to the inhibition of DNA gyrase. Moxifloxacin was not mutagenic in the CHO/HGPRT mammalian cell gene mutation assay. An equivocal result was obtained in the same assay when v79 cells were used. Moxifloxacin was clastogenic in the v79 chromosome aberration assay, but it did not induce unscheduled DNA synthesis in cultured rat hepatocytes. There was no evidence of genotoxicity *in vivo* in a micronucleus test or a dominant lethal test in mice.

Moxifloxacin had no effect on fertility in male and female rats at oral doses as high as 500 mg/kg/day, approximately 12 times the maximum recommended human dose based on body surface area (mg/m^2), or at intravenous doses as high as 45 mg/kg/day, approximately equal to the maximum recommended human dose based on body surface area (mg/m^2). At 500 mg/kg orally there were slight effects on sperm morphology (head-tail separation) in male rats and on the estrous cycle in female rats.

Pregnancy: Teratogenic Effects. Pregnancy Category C: Moxifloxacin was not teratogenic when administered to pregnant rats during organogenesis at oral doses as high as 500 mg/kg/day or 0.24 times the maximum recommended human dose based on systemic exposure (AUC), but decreased fetal body weights and slightly delayed fetal skeletal development (indicative of fetotoxicity) were observed. Intravenous administration of 80 mg/kg/day (approximately 2 times the maximum recommended human dose based on body surface area (mg/m^2)) to pregnant rats resulted in maternal toxicity and a marginal effect on fetal and placental weights and the appearance of the placenta. There was no evidence of teratogenicity at intravenous doses as high as 80 mg/kg/day. Intravenous administration of 20 mg/kg/day (approximately equal to the maximum recommended human oral dose based upon systemic exposure) to pregnant rabbits during organogenesis resulted in decreased fetal body weights and delayed fetal skeletal ossification. When rib and vertebral malformations were combined, there was an increased fetal and litter incidence of these effects. Signs of maternal toxicity in rabbits at this dose included mortality, abortions, marked reduction of food consumption, decreased water intake, body weight loss and hypoactivity. There was no evidence of teratogenicity when pregnant Cynomolgus monkeys were given oral doses as high as 100 mg/kg/day (2.5 times the maximum recommended human dose based upon systemic exposure). An increased incidence of smaller fetuses was observed at 100 mg/kg/day. In an oral pre- and postnatal development study conducted in rats, effects observed at 500 mg/kg/day included slight increases in duration of pregnancy and prenatal loss, reduced pup birth weight and decreased neonatal survival. Treatment-related maternal mortality occurred during gestation at 500 mg/kg/day in this study.

Since there are no adequate or well-controlled studies in pregnant women, moxifloxacin should be used during pregnancy only if the potential benefit justifies the potential risk to the fetus.

Nursing Mothers:
Moxifloxacin is excreted in the breast milk of rats. Moxifloxacin may also be excreted in human milk. Because of the potential for serious adverse reactions in infants nursing from mothers taking moxifloxacin, a decision should be made whether to discontinue nursing or to discontinue the drug, taking into account the importance of the drug to the mother.

Pediatric Use:
Safety and effectiveness in pediatric patients and adolescents less than 18 years of age have not been established. Moxifloxacin causes arthropathy in juvenile animals. (See **WARNINGS**.)

Geriatric Use:
In controlled multiple-dose clinical trials, 23% of patients receiving oral moxifloxacin were greater than or equal to 65 years of age and 9% were greater than or equal to 75 years of age. The clinical trial data demonstrate that there is no difference in the safety and efficacy of oral moxifloxacin in patients aged 65 or older compared to younger adults.

In intravenous trials in community acquired pneumonia, 45% of moxifloxacin patients were greater than or equal to 65 years of age, and 24% were greater than or equal to 75 years of age. In the pool of 491 elderly (> 65 years) patients, the following ECG abnormalities were reported in moxifloxacin vs. comparator patients: ST-T wave changes (2 events vs. 0 events), QT prolongation (2 vs. 0), ventricular tachycardia (1 vs. 0), atrial flutter (1 vs. 0), tachycardia (2 vs. 1), atrial fibrillation (1 vs. 0), supraventricular tachycardia (1 vs. 0), ventricular extrasystoles (2 vs. 0), and arrhythmia (0 vs. 1). None of the abnormalities was associated with a fatal outcome and a majority of these patients completed a full course of therapy.

ADVERSE REACTIONS

Clinical efficacy trials enrolled over 7,900 moxifloxacin orally and intravenously treated patients, of whom over 6,700 patients received the 400 mg dose. Most adverse events reported in moxifloxacin trials were described as mild to moderate in severity and required no treatment. Moxifloxacin was discontinued due to adverse reactions thought to be drug-related in 3.6% of orally treated patients and 5.7 % of sequentially (intravenous followed by oral) treated patients. The latter studies were conducted in community acquired pneumonia with, in general, a sicker patient population compared to the tablet studies.

Adverse reactions, judged by investigators to be at least possibly drug-related, occurring in greater than or equal to 3% of moxifloxacin treated patients were: nausea (7%), diarrhea (6%), dizziness (3%).

Additional clinically relevant uncommon events, judged by investigators to be at least possibly drug-related, that occurred in greater than or equal to 0.1% and less than 3% of moxifloxacin treated patients were:

BODY AS A WHOLE: headache, abdominal pain, injection site reaction, asthenia, moniliasis, pain, malaise, lab test abnormal (not specified), allergic reaction, leg pain, back pain, chest pain

CARDIOVASCULAR: palpitation, tachycardia, hypertension, peripheral edema, QT interval prolonged

CENTRAL NERVOUS SYSTEM: insomnia, nervousness, anxiety, confusion, somnolence, tremor, vertigo, paresthesia

DIGESTIVE: vomiting, abnormal liver function test, dyspepsia, dry mouth, constipation, oral moniliasis, anorexia, stomatitis, glossitis, flatulence, gastrointestinal disorder, GGTP increased

HEMIC AND LYMPHATIC: prothrombin decrease (prothrombin time prolonged/International Normalized Ratio (INR) increased), thrombocythemia, thrombocytopenia, eosinophilia, leukopenia

METABOLIC AND NUTRITIONAL: amylase increased, lactic dehydrogenase increased

MUSCULOSKELETAL: arthralgia, myalgia

RESPIRATORY: dyspnea

SKIN/APPENDAGES: rash (maculopapular, purpuric, pustular), pruritus, sweating

SPECIAL SENSES: taste perversion

UROGENITAL: vaginal moniliasis, vaginitis

Additional clinically relevant rare events, judged by investigators to be at least possibly drug-related, that occurred in less than 0.1% of moxifloxacin treated patients were: abnormal dreams, abnormal vision, agitation, amblyopia, amnesia, anemia, aphasia, arthritis, asthma, atrial fibrillation, convulsions, depersonalization, depression, diarrhea (*Clostridium difficile*), dysphagia, ECG abnormal, emotional lability, face edema, gastritis, hallucinations, hyperglycemia, hyperlipidemia, hypertonia, hyperuricemia, hypesthesia, hypotension, incoordination, jaundice (predominantly cholestatic), kidney function abnormal, parosmia, pelvic pain, prothrombin increase (prothrombin time decreased/International Normalized Ratio (INR) decreased), sleep disorders, speech disorders, supraventricular tachycardia, taste loss, tendon disorder, thinking abnormal, thromboplastin decrease, tinnitus, tongue discoloration, urticaria, vasodilatation, ventricular tachycardia

Post-Marketing Adverse Event Reports:
Additional adverse events have been reported from worldwide post-marketing experience with moxifloxacin. Because these events are reported voluntarily from a population of uncertain size, it is not always possible to reliably estimate their frequency or establish a causal relationship to drug exposure. These events, some of them life-threatening, include anaphylactic reaction, anaphylactic shock, angioedema (including laryngeal edema), hepatitis (predominantly cholestatic), pseudomembranous colitis, psychotic reaction, Stevens-Johnson syndrome, syncope, tendon rupture, and ventricular tachyarrhythmias (including in very rare cases cardiac arrest and torsade de pointes, and usually in patients with concurrent severe underlying proarrhythmic conditions).

LABORATORY CHANGES
Changes in laboratory parameters, without regard to drug relationship, which are not listed above and which occurred in ≥ 2% of patients and at an incidence greater than in controls included: increases in MCH, neutrophils, WBCs, PT ratio, ionized calcium, chloride, albumin, globulin, bilirubin; decreases in hemoglobin, RBCs, neutrophils, eosinophils, basophils, PT ratio, glucose, pO_2, bilirubin and amylase. It cannot be determined if any of the above laboratory abnormalities were caused by the drug or the underlying condition being treated.

OVERDOSAGE

Single oral overdoses up to 2.8 g were not associated with any serious adverse events. In the event of acute overdose, the stomach should be emptied and adequate hydration maintained. ECG monitoring is recommended due to the possibility of QT interval prolongation. The patient should be carefully observed and given supportive treatment. The administration of activated charcoal as soon as possible after oral overdose may prevent excessive increase of systemic moxifloxacin exposure. About 3% and 9% of the dose of moxifloxacin, as well as about 2% and 4.5% of its glucuronide metabolite are removed by continuous ambulatory peritoneal dialysis and hemodialysis, respectively.

Single oral moxifloxacin doses of 2000, 500, and 1500 mg/kg were lethal to rats, mice, and Cynomolgus monkeys, respectively. The minimum lethal intravenous dose in mice and rats was 100 mg/kg. Toxic signs after administration of a single high dose of moxifloxacin to these animals included CNS and gastrointestinal effects such as decreased activity, somnolence, tremor, convulsions, vomiting and diarrhea.

DOSAGE AND ADMINISTRATION

The dose of AVELOX is 400 mg (orally or as an intravenous infusion) once every 24 hours. The duration of therapy depends on the type of infection as described below.

Infection*	Daily Dose	Duration
Acute Bacterial Sinusitis	400 mg	10 days
Acute Bacterial Exacerbation of Chronic Bronchitis	400 mg	5 days
Community Acquired Pneumonia	400 mg	7-14 days
Uncomplicated Skin and Skin Structure Infections	400 mg	7 days

*due to the designated pathogens (See **INDICATIONS AND USAGE**.). For I.V. use see **Precautions**, **Geriatric Use**.

Oral doses of moxifloxacin should be administered at least 4 hours before or 8 hours after antacids containing magnesium or aluminum, as well as sucralfate, metal cations such as iron, and multivitamin preparations with zinc, or VIDEX® (didanosine) chewable/buffered tablets or the pediatric powder for oral solution. (See **CLINICAL PHARMACOLOGY**, **Drug Interactions** and **PRECAUTIONS**, **Drug Interactions**.)

Impaired Renal Function
No dosage adjustment is required in renally impaired patients, including those on either hemodialysis or continuous ambulatory peritoneal dialysis.

Impaired Hepatic Function
No dosage adjustment is required in patients with mild or moderate hepatic insufficiency (Child Pugh Classes A and B). The pharmacokinetics of moxifloxacin in patients with severe hepatic insufficiency (Child Pugh Class C) have not been studied. (See **CLINICAL PHARMACOLOGY**, **Hepatic Insufficiency**.)

When switching from intravenous to oral dosage administration, no dosage adjustment is necessary. Patients whose therapy is started with AVELOX I.V. may be switched to AVELOX Tablets when clinically indicated at the discretion of the physician.

AVELOX I.V. should be administered by INTRAVENOUS infusion only. It is not intended for intra-arterial, intramuscular, intrathecal, intraperitoneal, or subcutaneous administration.

AVELOX I.V. should be administered by intravenous infusion over a period of 60 minutes by direct infusion or through a Y-type intravenous infusion set which may already be in place. CAUTION: RAPID OR BOLUS INTRAVENOUS INFUSION MUST BE AVOIDED.

Since only limited data are available on the compatibility of moxifloxacin intravenous injection with other intravenous substances, additives or other medications should not be added to AVELOX I.V. or infused simultaneously through the same intravenous line. If the same intravenous line or a Y-type line is used for sequential infusion of other drugs, or if the "piggyback" method of administration is used, the line should be flushed before and after infusion of AVELOX I.V. with an infusion solution compatible with AVELOX I.V. as well as with other drug(s) administered via this common line.

AVELOX I.V. is compatible with the following intravenous solutions at ratios from 1:10 to 10:1:

0.9% Sodium Chloride Injection, USP
1M Sodium Chloride Injection
5% Dextrose Injection, USP
Sterile Water for Injection, USP
10% Dextrose for Injection, USP
Lactated Ringer's for Injection

Preparation for administration of AVELOX I.V. injection premix in flexible containers:

1. Close flow control clamp of administration set.
2. Remove cover from port at bottom of container.
3. Insert piercing pin from an appropriate transfer set (e.g. one that does not require excessive force, such as ISO compatible administration set) into port with a gentle twisting motion until pin is firmly seated.

NOTE: Refer to complete directions that have been provided with the administration set.

HOW SUPPLIED

Tablets
AVELOX (moxifloxacin hydrochloride) Tablets are available as oblong, dull red film-coated tablets containing 400 mg moxifloxacin.

The tablet is coded with the word "BAYER" on one side and "M400" on the reverse side.

Package	NDC Code
Bottles of 30:	0085-1733-01
Unit Dose Pack of 50:	0085-1733-02
ABC Pack of 5:	0085-1733-03

Store at 25°C (77°F); excursions permitted to 15-30°C (59-86°F) [see USP Controlled Room Temperature]. Avoid high humidity.

Intravenous Solution – Premix Bags
AVELOX I.V. (moxifloxacin hydrochloride in sodium chloride injection) is available in ready-to-use 250 mL latex-free flexible bags containing 400 mg of moxifloxacin in 0.8% saline. NO FURTHER DILUTION OF THIS PREPARATION IS NECESSARY.

Package	NDC Code
250 mL flexible container	0085-1737-01

Parenteral drug products should be inspected visually for particulate matter prior to administration. Samples containing visible particulates should not be used.

Since the premix flexible containers are for single-use only, any unused portion should be discarded.

Store at 25°C (77°F); excursions permitted to 15-30°C (59-86°F) [see USP Controlled Room Temperature].

DO NOT REFRIGERATE – PRODUCT PRECIPITATES UPON REFRIGERATION.

ANIMAL PHARMACOLOGY

Quinolones have been shown to cause arthropathy in immature animals. In studies in juvenile dogs oral doses of moxifloxacin ≥ 30 mg/kg/day (approximately 1.5 times the maximum recommended human dose based upon systemic exposure) for 28 days resulted in arthropathy. There was no evidence of arthropathy in mature monkeys and rats at oral doses up to 135 and 500 mg/kg, respectively.

Unlike some other members of the quinolone class, crystalluria was not observed in 6 month repeat dose studies in rats and monkeys with moxifloxacin.

No ocular toxicity was observed in a 13 week oral repeat dose study in dogs with a moxifloxacin dose of 60 mg/kg. Ocular toxicity was not observed in 6 month repeat dose studies in rats and monkeys (daily oral doses up to 500 mg/kg and 135 mg/kg, respectively). In beagle dogs, electroretinographic (ERG) changes were observed in a 2 week study at oral doses of 60 and 90 mg/kg. Histopathological changes were observed in the retina from one of four dogs at 90 mg/kg, a dose associated with mortality in this study.

Some quinolones have been reported to have proconvulsant activity that is exacerbated with concomitant use of non-steroidal anti-inflammatory drugs (NSAIDs). Moxifloxacin at an oral dose of 300 mg/kg did not show an increase in acute toxicity or potential for CNS toxicity (e.g. seizures) in mice when used in combination with NSAIDs such as diclofenac, ibuprofen, or fenbufen.

In dog studies, at plasma concentrations about five times the human therapeutic level, a QT-prolonging effect of moxifloxacin was found. Electrophysiological *in vitro* studies suggested an inhibition of the rapid activating component of the delayed rectifier potassium current (I_{Kr}) as an underlying mechanism. In dogs, the combined infusion of sotalol, a Class III antiarrhythmic agent, with moxifloxacin induced a higher degree of QTc prolongation than that induced by the same dose (30 mg/kg) of moxifloxacin alone.

In a local tolerability study performed in dogs, no signs of local intolerability were seen when moxifloxacin was administered intravenously. After intra-arterial injection, inflammatory changes involving the peri-arterial soft tissue were observed suggesting that intra-arterial administration of moxifloxacin should be avoided.

CLINICAL STUDIES

Acute Bacterial Exacerbation of Chronic Bronchitis

AVELOX Tablets (400 mg once daily for five days) were evaluated for the treatment of acute bacterial exacerbation of chronic bronchitis in a large, randomized, double-blind, controlled clinical trial conducted in the US. This study compared AVELOX with clarithromycin (500 mg twice daily for 10 days) and enrolled 629 patients. The primary endpoint for this trial was clinical success at 7-17 days post-therapy. The clinical success for AVELOX was 89% (222/250) compared to 89% (224/251) for clarithromycin.

The following outcomes are the clinical success rates at the follow-up visit for the clinically evaluable patient groups by pathogen:

PATHOGEN	AVELOX	Clarithromycin
Streptococcus pneumoniae	100% (16/16)	87% (20/23)
Haemophilus influenzae	89% (33/37)	88% (36/41)
Haemophilus parainfluenzae	100% (16/16)	100% (14/14)
Moraxella catarrhalis	85% (29/34)	100% (24/24)
Staphylococcus aureus	94% (15/16)	75% (6/8)
Klebsiella pneumoniae	90% (18/20)	91% (10/11)

The microbiological eradication rates (eradication plus presumed eradication) in AVELOX treated patients were *Streptococcus pneumoniae* 100%, *Haemophilus influenzae* 89%, *Haemophilus parainfluenzae* 100%, *Moraxella catarrhalis* 85%, *Staphylococcus aureus* 94%, and *Klebsiella pneumoniae* 85%.

Community Acquired Pneumonia

A large, randomized, double-blind, controlled clinical trial was conducted in the US to compare the efficacy of AVELOX Tablets (400 mg once daily) to that of high-dose clarithromycin (500 mg twice daily) in the treatment of patients with clinically and radiologically documented community acquired pneumonia. This study enrolled 474 patients (382 of which were valid for the primary efficacy analysis conducted at the 14-35 day follow-up visit). Clinical success for clinically evaluable patients was 95% (184/194) for AVELOX and 95% (178/188) for high dose clarithromycin.

A large, randomized, double-blind, controlled trial was conducted in the US and Canada to compare the efficacy of sequential IV/PO AVELOX 400 mg QD for 7-14 days to an IV/PO fluoroquinolone control (trovafloxacin or levofloxacin) in the treatment of patients with clinically and radiologically documented community acquired pneumonia. This study enrolled 516 patients, 362 of which were valid for the primary efficacy analysis conducted at the 7-30 day post-therapy visit. The clinical success rate was 86% (157/182) for AVELOX therapy and 89% (161/180) for the fluoroquinolone comparators.

An open-label ex-US study that enrolled 628 patients compared AVELOX to sequential IV/PO amoxicillin/clavulanate (1.2 g IV q8h/625 mg PO q8h) with or without high-dose IV/PO clarithromycin (500 mg BID). The intravenous formulations of the comparators are not FDA approved. The clinical success rate at Day 5-7 (the primary efficacy timepoint) for AVELOX therapy was 93% (241/258) and demonstrated superiority to amoxicillin/clavulanate ± clarithromycin (85%, 239/280) [95% C.I. 2.9%, 13.2%]. The clinical success rate at the 21–28 days post-therapy visit for AVELOX was 84% (216/258), which also demonstrated superiority to the comparators (74%, 208/280) [95% C.I. 2.6%, 16.3%].

The clinical success rates by pathogen across four CAP studies are presented below:

Clinical Success Rates By Pathogen (Pooled CAP Studies)

PATHOGEN	AVELOX
Streptococcus pneumoniae	94% (80/85)
Staphylococcus aureus	85% (17/20)
Klebsiella pneumoniae	92% (11/12)
Haemophilus influenzae	92% (56/61)
Chlamydia pneumoniae	93% (119/128)
Mycoplasma pneumoniae	96% (73/76)
Moraxella catarrhalis	92% (11/12)

Community Acquired Pneumonia caused by Multi-Drug Resistant *Streptococcus pneumoniae* (MDRSP)*

Avelox was effective in the treatment of community acquired pneumonia (CAP) caused by multi-drug resistant *Streptococcus pneumoniae* MDRSP* isolates. Of 37 microbiologically evaluable patients with MDRSP isolates, 35 patients (95.0%) achieved clinical and bacteriological success post-therapy. The clinical and bacteriological success rates based on the number of patients treated are shown in the table below.

* MDRSP, Multi-drug resistant *Streptococcus pneumoniae* includes isolates previously known as PRSP (Penicillin-resistant *S. pneumoniae*), and are strains resistant to two or more of the following antibiotics: penicillin (MIC ≥2 µg/mL), 2nd generation cephalosporins (e.g., cefuroxime), macrolides, tetracyclines, and trimethoprim/sulfamethoxazole. [See first table above]

Not all isolates were resistant to all antimicrobial classes tested. Success and eradication rates are summarized in the table below:

[See second table above]

Clinical and Bacteriological Success Rates for Moxifloxacin-Treated MDRSP CAP Patients (Population: Valid for Efficacy):

Screening Susceptibility	Clinical Success		Bacteriological Success	
	n/N[a]	%	n/N[b]	%
Penicillin-resistant	21/21	100%*	21/21	100%*
2nd generation cephalosporin-resistant	25/26	96%*	25/26	96%*
Macrolide-resistant**	22/23	96%	22/23	96%
Trimethoprim/sulfamethoxazole-resistant	28/30	93%	28/30	93%
Tetracycline-resistant	17/18	94%	17/18	94%

[a]n = number of patients successfully treated; N = number of patients with MDRSP (from a total of 37 patients)

[b]n = number of patients successfully treated (presumed eradication or eradication); N = number of patients with MDRSP (from a total of 37 patients)

*One patient had a respiratory isolate that was resistant to penicillin and cefuroxime but a blood isolate that was intermediate to penicillin and cefuroxime. The patient is included in the database based on the respiratory isolate.

**Azithromycin, clarithromycin, and erythromycin were the macrolide antimicrobials tested.

S. pneumoniae with MDRSP	Clinical Success	Bacteriological Eradication Rate
Resistant to 2 antimicrobials	12/13 (92.3 %)	12/13 (92.3 %)
Resistant to 3 antimicrobials	10/11 (90.9 %)*	10/11 (90.9 %)*
Resistant to 4 antimicrobials	6/6 (100%)	6/6 (100%)
Resistant to 5 antimicrobials	7/7 (100%)*	7/7 (100%)*
Bacteremia with MDRSP	9/9 (100%)	9/9 (100%)

*One patient had a respiratory isolate resistant to 5 antimicrobials and a blood isolate resistant to 3 antimicrobials. The patient was included in the category resistant to 5 antimicrobials.

Acute Bacterial Sinusitis

In a large, controlled double-blind study conducted in the US, AVELOX Tablets (400 mg once daily for ten days) were compared with cefuroxime axetil (250 mg twice daily for ten days) for the treatment of acute bacterial sinusitis. The trial included 457 patients valid for the primary efficacy determination. Clinical success (cure plus improvement) at the 7 to 21 day post-therapy test of cure visit was 90% for AVELOX and 89% for cefuroxime.

An additional non-comparative study was conducted to gather bacteriological data and to evaluate microbiological eradication in adult patients treated with AVELOX 400 mg once daily for seven days. All patients (n = 336) underwent antral puncture in this study. Clinical success rates and eradication/presumed eradication rates at the 21 to 37 day follow-up visit were 97% (29 out of 30) for *Streptococcus pneumoniae* 83% (15 out of 18) for *Moraxella catarrhalis*, and 80% (24 out of 30) for *Haemophilus influenzae*.

Uncomplicated Skin and Skin Structure Infections

A randomized, double-blind, controlled clinical trial conducted in the US compared the efficacy of AVELOX 400 mg once daily for seven days with cephalexin HCl 500 mg three times daily for seven days. The percentage of patients treated for uncomplicated abscesses was 30%, furuncles 8%, cellulitis 16%, impetigo 20%, and other skin infections 26%. Adjunctive procedures (incision and drainage or debridement) were performed on 17% of the AVELOX treated patients and 14% of the comparator treated patients. Clinical success rates in evaluable patients were 89% (108/122) for AVELOX and 91% (110/121) for cephalexin HCl.

REFERENCES

1. National Committee for Clinical Laboratory Standards, Methods for Dilution Antimicrobial Susceptibility Tests for Bacteria That Grow Aerobically-Sixth Edition. Approved Standard NCCLS Document M7-A6, Vol. 23, No. 2, NCCLS, Wayne, PA, January, 2003.
2. National Committee for Clinical Laboratory Standards, Performance Standards for Antimicrobial Disk Susceptibility Tests-Eighth Edition. Approved Standard NCCLS Document M2-A8, Vol. 23, No. 1, NCCLS, Wayne, PA, January, 2003.

Patient Information About: AVELOX®

(moxifloxacin hydrochloride)

400 mg Tablets

This section contains important information about AVELOX (moxifloxacin hydrochloride), and should be read completely before you begin treatment. This section does not take the place of discussions with your doctor or health care professional about your medical condition or your treatment. This section does not list all benefits and risks of AVELOX. The medicine described here can be prescribed only by a licensed health care professional. If you have any questions about AVELOX talk with your health care professional. Only your health care professional can determine if AVELOX is right for you.

What is AVELOX?

AVELOX is an antibiotic used to treat lung, sinus, or skin infections caused by certain germs called bacteria. AVELOX kills many of the types of bacteria that can infect the lungs and sinuses and has been shown in a large number of clinical trials to be safe and effective for the treatment of bacterial infections.

Sometimes viruses rather than bacteria may infect the lungs and sinuses (for example the common cold). AVELOX, like all other antibiotics, does not kill viruses.

You should contact your doctor if you think your condition is not improving while taking AVELOX.

AVELOX Tablets are red and contain 400 mg of active drug.

How and when should I take AVELOX?

AVELOX should be taken once a day for 5-14 days depending on your prescription. It should be swallowed and may be taken with or without food. Try to take the tablet at the same time each day.

You may begin to feel better quickly; however, in order to make sure that all bacteria are killed, you should complete the full course of medication. Do not take more than the prescribed dose of AVELOX even if you missed a dose by mistake. You should not take a double dose.

Who should not take AVELOX?

You should not take AVELOX if you have ever had a severe allergic reaction to any of the group of antibiotics known as "quinolones" such as ciprofloxacin or levofloxacin. If you develop hives, difficulty breathing, or other symptoms of a severe allergic reaction, seek emergency treatment right away. If you develop a skin rash, you should stop taking AVELOX and call your health care professional.

You should avoid AVELOX if you have a rare condition known as congenital prolongation of the QT interval. If you

Continued on next page

Avelox—Cont.

or any of your family members have this condition you should inform your health care professional. You should avoid AVELOX if you are being treated for heart rhythm disturbances with certain medicines such as quinidine, procainamide, amiodarone or sotalol. Inform your health care professional if you are taking a heart rhythm drug.

You should also avoid AVELOX if the amount of potassium in your blood is low. Low potassium can sometimes be caused by medicines called diuretics such as furosemide and hydrochlorothiazide. If you are taking a diuretic medicine you should speak with your health care professional.

If you are pregnant or planning to become pregnant while taking AVELOX, talk to your doctor before taking this medication. AVELOX is not recommended for use during pregnancy or nursing, as the effects on the unborn child or nursing infant are unknown.

AVELOX is not recommended for children.

What are the possible side effects of AVELOX?

AVELOX is generally well tolerated. The most common side effects caused by AVELOX, which are usually mild, include dizziness, nausea, and diarrhea. If diarrhea persists call your health care provider. You should be careful about driving or operating machinery until you are sure AVELOX is not causing dizziness. If you notice any side effects not mentioned in this section or you have any concerns about the side effects you are experiencing, please inform your health care professional.

In some people, AVELOX, as with some other antibiotics, may produce a small effect on the heart that is seen on an electrocardiogram test. Although this has not caused any serious problems in more than 7,900 patients who have already taken the medication in clinical studies, in theory it could result in extremely rare cases of abnormal heartbeat which may be dangerous. Contact your health care professional if you develop heart palpitations (fast beating), or have fainting spells.

Convulsions have been reported in patients receiving quinolone antibiotics. Be sure to let your physician know if you have a history of convulsions. Quinolones, including AVELOX, have been rarely associated with other central nervous system events including confusion, tremors, hallucinations, and depression.

Quinolones, including AVELOX, have been rarely associated with inflammation of tendons. If you experience pain, swelling or rupture of a tendon, you should stop taking AVELOX and call your health care professional.

What about other medicines I am taking?

Tell your doctor about all other prescription and nonprescription medicines or supplements you are taking. You should avoid taking AVELOX with certain medicines used to treat an abnormal heartbeat. These include quinidine, procainamide, amiodarone, and sotalol.

Some medicines also produce an effect on the electrocardiogram test, including cisapride, erythromycin, some antidepressants and some antipsychotic drugs. These may increase the risk of heart beat problems when taken with AVELOX.

Many antacids and multivitamins may interfere with the absorption of AVELOX and may prevent it from working properly. You should take AVELOX either 4 hours before or 8 hours after taking these products.

Remember

Take your dose of AVELOX once a day.

Complete the course of medication even if you are feeling better.

Keep this medication out of the reach of children.

This information does not take the place of discussions with your doctor or health care professional about your medical condition or your treatment.

For more complete information about AVELOX request full prescribing information from your health care professional, pharmacist, or visit our website at www.aveloxusa.com.

Manufactured by:
Bayer HealthCare
Bayer Pharmaceuticals Corporation
400 Morgan Lane
West Haven, CT 06516
Made in Germany
Distributed by:
Schering-Plough
Schering Corporation
Kenilworth, NJ 07033

AVELOX is a registered trademark of Bayer Aktiengesellschaft and is used under license by Schering Corporation.

℞ Only

08918409, R.0 10/04 12525

Printed in U.S.A.

CIPRO® I.V. ℞

[sī-prō]

(ciprofloxacin)

For Intravenous Infusion

To reduce the development of drug-resistant bacteria and maintain the effectiveness of CIPRO® I.V. and other antibacterial drugs, CIPRO I.V. should be used only to treat or prevent infections that are proven or strongly suspected to be caused by bacteria.

Steady-state Pharmacokinetic Parameter Following Multiple Oral and I.V. Doses

Parameters	500 mg q12h, P.O.	400 mg q12h, I.V.	750 mg q12h, P.O.	400 mg q8h, I.V.
AUC (μg•hr/mL)	13.7 [a]	12.7 [a]	31.6 [b]	32.9 [c]
C_{max} (μg/mL)	2.97	4.56	3.59	4.07

[a] $AUC_{0\text{-}12h}$
[b] AUC 24h=$AUC_{0\text{-}12h} \times 2$
[c] AUC 24h=$AUC_{0\text{-}8h} \times 3$

DESCRIPTION

CIPRO I.V. (ciprofloxacin) is a synthetic broad-spectrum antimicrobial agent for intravenous (I.V.) administration. Ciprofloxacin, a fluoroquinolone, is 1-cyclopropyl-6-fluoro-1,4-dihydro-4-oxo-7-(1-piperazinyl)-3-quinolinecarboxylic acid. Its empirical formula is $C_{17}H_{18}FN_3O_3$ and its chemical structure is:

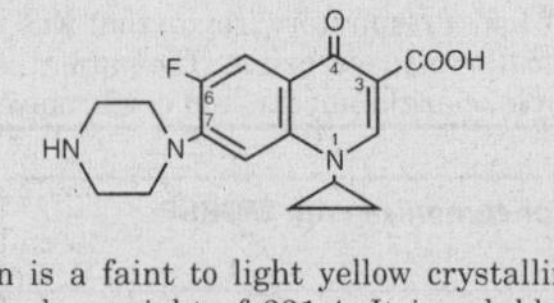

Ciprofloxacin is a faint to light yellow crystalline powder with a molecular weight of 331.4. It is soluble in dilute (0.1N) hydrochloric acid and is practically insoluble in water and ethanol. CIPRO I.V. solutions are available as sterile 1.0% aqueous concentrates, which are intended for dilution prior to administration, and as 0.2% ready-for-use infusion solutions in 5% Dextrose Injection. All formulas contain lactic acid as a solubilizing agent and hydrochloric acid for pH adjustment. The pH range for the 1.0% aqueous concentrates in vials is 3.3 to 3.9. The pH range for the 0.2% ready-for-use infusion solutions is 3.5 to 4.6.

The plastic container is latex-free and is fabricated from a specially formulated polyvinyl chloride. Solutions in contact with the plastic container can leach out certain of its chemical components in very small amounts within the expiration period, e.g., di(2-ethylhexyl) phthalate (DEHP), up to 5 parts per million. The suitability of the plastic has been confirmed in tests in animals according to USP biological tests for plastic containers as well as by tissue culture toxicity studies.

CLINICAL PHARMACOLOGY

Absorption

Following 60-minute intravenous infusions of 200 mg and 400 mg ciprofloxacin to normal volunteers, the mean maximum serum concentrations achieved were 2.1 and 4.6 μg/mL, respectively; the concentrations at 12 hours were 0.1 and 0.2 μg/mL, respectively.

Steady-state Ciprofloxacin Serum Concentrations (μg/mL) After 60-minute I.V. Infusions q12h.

Dose	Time after starting the infusion: 30 min.	1hr	3hr	6hr	8hr	12hr
200 mg	1.7	2.1	0.6	0.3	0.2	0.1
400 mg	3.7	4.6	1.3	0.7	0.5	0.2

The pharmacokinetics of ciprofloxacin are linear over the dose range of 200 to 400 mg administered intravenously. Comparison of the pharmacokinetic parameters following the 1st and 5th I.V. dose on a q 12 h regimen indicates no evidence of drug accumulation.

The absolute bioavailability of oral ciprofloxacin is within a range of 70–80% with no substantial loss by first pass metabolism. An intravenous infusion of 400-mg ciprofloxacin given over 60 minutes every 12 hours has been shown to produce an area under the serum concentration time curve (AUC) equivalent to that produced by a 500-mg oral dose given every 12 hours. An intravenous infusion of 400 mg ciprofloxacin given over 60 minutes every 8 hours has been shown to produce an AUC at steady-state equivalent to that produced by a 750-mg oral dose given every 12 hours. A 400-mg I.V. dose results in a C_{max} similar to that observed with a 750-mg oral dose. An infusion of 200 mg ciprofloxacin given every 12 hours produces an AUC equivalent to that produced by a 250-mg oral dose given every 12 hours.

[See table above]

Distribution

After intravenous administration, ciprofloxacin is present in saliva, nasal and bronchial secretions, sputum, skin blister fluid, lymph, peritoneal fluid, bile, and prostatic secretions. It has also been detected in the lung, skin, fat, muscle, cartilage, and bone. Although the drug diffuses into cerebrospinal fluid (CSF), CSF concentrations are generally less than 10% of peak serum concentrations. Levels of the drug in the aqueous and vitreous chambers of the eye are lower than in serum.

Metabolism

After I.V. administration, three metabolites of ciprofloxacin have been identified in human urine which together account for approximately 10% of the intravenous dose. The binding of ciprofloxacin to serum proteins is 20 to 40%.

Excretion

The serum elimination half-life is approximately 5–6 hours and the total clearance is around 35 L/hr. After intravenous administration, approximately 50% to 70% of the dose is excreted in the urine as unchanged drug. Following a 200-mg I.V. dose, concentrations in the urine usually exceed 200 μg/mL 0–2 hours after dosing and are generally greater than 15 μg/mL 8–12 hours after dosing. Following a 400-mg I.V. dose, urine concentrations generally exceed 400 μg/mL 0–2 hours after dosing and are usually greater than 30 μg/mL 8–12 hours after dosing. The renal clearance is approximately 22 L/hr. The urinary excretion of ciprofloxacin is virtually complete by 24 hours after dosing. Although bile concentrations of ciprofloxacin are several fold higher than serum concentrations after intravenous dosing, only a small amount of the administered dose (< 1%) is recovered from the bile as unchanged drug. Approximately 15% of an I.V. dose is recovered from the feces within 5 days after dosing.

Special Populations

Pharmacokinetic studies of the oral (single dose) and intravenous (single and multiple dose) forms of ciprofloxacin indicate that plasma concentrations of ciprofloxacin are higher in elderly subjects (> 65 years) as compared to young adults. Although the C_{max} is increased 16–40%, the increase in mean AUC is approximately 30%, and can be at least partially attributed to decreased renal clearance in the elderly. Elimination half-life is only slightly (~20%) prolonged in the elderly. These differences are not considered clinically significant. (See **PRECAUTIONS: Geriatric Use.**)

In patients with reduced renal function, the half-life of ciprofloxacin is slightly prolonged and dosage adjustments may be required. (See **DOSAGE AND ADMINISTRATION.**)

In preliminary studies in patients with stable chronic liver cirrhosis, no significant changes in ciprofloxacin pharmacokinetics have been observed. However, the kinetics of ciprofloxacin in patients with acute hepatic insufficiency have not been fully elucidated.

Following a single oral dose of 10 mg/kg ciprofloxacin suspension to 16 children ranging in age from 4 months to 7 years, the mean C_{max} was 2.4 μg/mL (range: 1.5 – 3.4 μg/mL) and the mean AUC was 9.2 μg*h/mL (range: 5.8 – 14.9 μg*h/mL). There was no apparent age-dependence, and no notable increase in C_{max} or AUC upon multiple dosing (10 mg/kg TID). In children with severe sepsis who were given intravenous ciprofloxacin (10 mg/kg as a 1-hour infusion), the mean C_{max} was 6.1 μg/mL (range: 4.6 – 8.3 μg/mL) in 10 children less than 1 year of age; and 7.2 μg/mL (range: 4.7 – 11.8 μg/mL) in 10 children between 1 and 5 years of age. The AUC values were 17.4 μg*h/mL (range: 11.8 – 32.0 μg*h/mL) and 16.5 μg*h/mL (range: 11.0 – 23.8 μg*h/mL) in the respective age groups. These values are within the range reported for adults at therapeutic doses. Based on population pharmacokinetic analysis of pediatric patients with various infections, the predicted mean half-life in children is approximately 4 - 5 hours, and the bioavailability of the oral suspension is approximately 60%.

Drug-drug Interactions: The potential for pharmacokinetic drug interactions between ciprofloxacin and theophylline, caffeine, cyclosporins, phenytoin, sulfonylurea glyburide, metronidazole, warfarin, probenecid, and piperacillin sodium has been evaluated. (See **PRECAUTIONS: Drug Interactions.**)

MICROBIOLOGY

Ciprofloxacin has *in vitro* activity against a wide range of gram-negative and gram-positive microorganisms. The bactericidal action of ciprofloxacin results from inhibition of the enzymes topoisomerase II (DNA gyrase) and topoisomerase IV, which are required for bacterial DNA replication, transcription, repair, and recombination. The mechanism of action of fluoroquinolones, including ciprofloxacin, is different from that of penicillins, cephalosporins, aminoglycosides, macrolides, and tetracyclines; therefore, microorganisms resistant to these classes of drugs may be susceptible to ciprofloxacin and other quinolones. There is no known cross-resistance between ciprofloxacin and other classes of antimicrobials. *In vitro* resistance to ciprofloxacin develops slowly by multiple step mutations.

Ciprofloxacin is slightly less active when tested at acidic pH. The inoculum size has little effect when tested *in vitro*. The minimal bactericidal concentration (MBC) generally does not exceed the minimal inhibitory concentration (MIC) by more than a factor of 2.

Ciprofloxacin has been shown to be active against most strains of the following microorganisms, both *in vitro* and in clinical infections as described in the **INDICATIONS AND USAGE** section of the package insert for CIPRO I.V. (ciprofloxacin for intravenous infusion).

Aerobic gram-positive microorganisms

Enterococcus faecalis (Many strains are only moderately susceptible.)
Staphylococcus aureus (methicillin-susceptible strains only)
Staphylococcus epidermidis (methicillin-susceptible strains only)
Staphylococcus saprophyticus
Streptococcus pneumoniae (penicillin-susceptible strains)
Streptococcus pyogenes

Aerobic gram-negative microorganisms

Citrobacter diversus
Citrobacter freundii

Enterobacter cloacae
Escherichia coli
Haemophilus influenzae
Haemophilus parainfluenzae
Klebsiella pneumoniae
Moraxella catarrhalis
Morganella morganii
Proteus mirabilis
Proteus vulgaris
Providencia rettgeri
Providencia stuartii
Pseudomonas aeruginosa
Serratia marcescens

Ciprofloxacin has been shown to be active against *Bacillus anthracis* both *in vitro* and by use of serum levels as a surrogate marker (see **INDICATIONS AND USAGE** and **IN-HALATIONAL ANTHRAX - ADDITIONAL INFORMATION**).

The following *in vitro* data are available, **but their clinical significance is unknown.**

Ciprofloxacin exhibits *in vitro* minimum inhibitory concentrations (MICs) of 1 µg/mL or less against most (≥ 90%) strains of the following microorganisms; however, the safety and effectiveness of ciprofloxacin intravenous formulations in treating clinical infections due to these microorganisms have not been established in adequate and well-controlled clinical trials.

Aerobic gram-positive microorganisms
Staphylococcus haemolyticus
Staphylococcus hominis
Streptococcus pneumoniae (penicillin-resistant strains)
Aerobic gram-negative microorganisms
Acinetobacter lwoffi
Aeromonas hydrophila
Campylobacter jejuni
Edwardsiella tarda
Enterobacter aerogenes
Klebsiella oxytoca
Legionella pneumophila
Neisseria gonorrhoeae
Pasteurella multocida
Salmonella enteritidis
Salmonella typhi
Shigella boydii
Shigella dysenteriae
Shigella flexneri
Shigella sonnei
Vibrio cholerae
Vibrio parahaemolyticus
Vibrio vulnificus
Yersinia enterocolitica

Most strains of *Burkholderia cepacia* and some strains of *Stenotrophomonas maltophilia* are resistant to ciprofloxacin as are most anaerobic bacteria, including *Bacteroides fragilis* and *Clostridium difficile*.

Susceptibility Tests

Dilution Techniques: Quantitative methods are used to determine antimicrobial minimum inhibitory concentrations (MICs). These MICs provide estimates of the susceptibility of bacteria to antimicrobial compounds. The MICs should be determined using a standardized procedure. Standardized procedures are based on a dilution method[1] (broth or agar) or equivalent with standardized inoculum concentrations and standardized concentrations of ciprofloxacin powder. The MIC values should be interpreted according to the following criteria:

For testing aerobic microorganisms other than *Haemophilus influenzae*, and *Haemophilus parainfluenzae*[a]:

MIC (µg/mL)	Interpretation
≤ 1	Susceptible (S)
2	Intermediate (I)
≥ 4	Resistant (R)

[a] These interpretive standards are applicable only to broth microdilution susceptibility tests with streptococci using cation-adjusted Mueller-Hinton broth with 2–5% lysed horse blood.

For testing *Haemophilus influenzae* and *Haemophilus parainfluenzae*[b]:

MIC (µg/mL)	Interpretation
≤ 1	Susceptible (S)

[b] This interpretive standard is applicable only to broth microdilution susceptibility tests with *Haemophilus influenzae* and *Haemophilus parainfluenzae* using Haemophilus Test Medium[1].

The current absence of data on resistant strains precludes defining any results other than "Susceptible". Strains yielding MIC results suggestive of a "nonsusceptible" category should be submitted to a reference laboratory for further testing.

A report of "Susceptible" indicates that the pathogen is likely to be inhibited if the antimicrobial compound in the blood reaches the concentrations usually achievable. A report of "Intermediate" indicates that the result should be considered equivocal, and, if the microorganism is not fully susceptible to alternative, clinically feasible drugs, the test should be repeated. This category implies possible clinical applicability in body sites where the drug is physiologically concentrated or in situations where high dosage of drug can be used. This category also provides a buffer zone, which prevents small uncontrolled technical factors from causing

major discrepancies in interpretation. A report of "Resistant" indicates that the pathogen is not likely to be inhibited if the antimicrobial compound in the blood reaches the concentrations usually achievable; other therapy should be selected.

Standardized susceptibility test procedures require the use of laboratory control microorganisms to control the technical aspects of the laboratory procedures. Standard ciprofloxacin powder should provide the following MIC values:

Organism		MIC (µg/mL)
E. faecalis	ATCC 29212	0.25 – 2.0
E. coli	ATCC 25922	0.004 – 0.015
H. influenzae[a]	ATCC 49247	0.004 – 0.03
P. aeruginosa	ATCC 27853	0.25 – 1.0
S. aureus	ATCC 29213	0.12 – 0.5

[a] This quality control range is applicable to only *H. influenzae* ATCC 49247 tested by a broth microdilution procedure using Haemophilus Test Medium (HTM)[1].

Diffusion Techniques: Quantitative methods that require measurement of zone diameters also provide reproducible estimates of the susceptibility of bacteria to antimicrobial compounds. One such standardized procedure[2] requires the use of standardized inoculum concentrations. This procedure uses paper disks impregnated with 5-µg ciprofloxacin to test the susceptibility of microorganisms to ciprofloxacin. Reports from the laboratory providing results of the standard single-disk susceptibility test with a 5-µg ciprofloxacin disk should be interpreted according to the following criteria:

For testing aerobic microorganisms other than *Haemophilus influenzae*, and *Haemophilus parainfluenzae*[a]:

Zone Diameter (mm)	Interpretation
≥ 21	Susceptible (S)
16 - 20	Intermediate (I)
≤ 15	Resistant (R)

[a] These zone diameter standards are applicable only to tests performed for streptococci using Mueller-Hinton agar supplemented with 5% sheep blood incubated in 5% CO_2.

For testing *Haemophilus influenzae* and *Haemophilus parainfluenzae*[b]:

Zone Diameter (mm)	Interpretation
≥ 21	Susceptible (S)

[b] This zone diameter standard is applicable only to tests with *Haemophilus influenzae* and *Haemophilus parainfluenzae* using Haemophilus Test Medium (HTM)[2].

The current absence of data on resistant strains precludes defining any results other than "Susceptible". Strains yielding zone diameter results suggestive of a "nonsusceptible" category should be submitted to a reference laboratory for further testing.

Interpretation should be as stated above for results using dilution techniques. Interpretation involves correlation of the diameter obtained in the disk test with the MIC for ciprofloxacin.

As with standardized dilution techniques, diffusion methods require the use of laboratory control microorganisms that are used to control the technical aspects of the laboratory procedures. For the diffusion technique, the 5-µg ciprofloxacin disk should provide the following zone diameters in these laboratory test quality control strains:

Organism		Zone Diameter (mm)
E. coli	ATCC 25922	30-40
H. influenzae[a]	ATCC 49247	34-42
P. aeruginosa	ATCC 27853	25-33
S. aureus	ATCC 25923	22-30

[a] These quality control limits are applicable to only *H. influenzae* ATCC 49247 testing using Haemophilus Test Medium (HTM)[2].

INDICATIONS AND USAGE

CIPRO I.V. is indicated for the treatment of infections caused by susceptible strains of the designated microorganisms in the conditions and patient populations listed below when the intravenous administration offers a route of administration advantageous to the patient. Please see **DOSAGE AND ADMINISTRATION** for specific recommendations.

Adult Patients:

Urinary Tract Infections caused by *Escherichia coli* (including cases with secondary bacteremia), *Klebsiella pneumoniae* subspecies *pneumoniae*, *Enterobacter cloacae*, *Serratia marcescens*, *Proteus mirabilis*, *Providencia rettgeri*, *Morganella morganii*, *Citrobacter diversus*, *Citrobacter freundii*, *Pseudomonas aeruginosa*, *Staphylococcus epidermidis*, *Staphylococcus saprophyticus*, or *Enterococcus faecalis*.

Lower Respiratory Infections caused by *Escherichia coli*, *Klebsiella pneumoniae* subspecies *pneumoniae*, *Enterobacter cloacae*, *Proteus mirabilis*, *Pseudomonas aeruginosa*, *Haemophilus influenzae*, *Haemophilus parainfluenzae*, or

Streptococcus pneumoniae. Also, *Moraxella catarrhalis* for the treatment of acute exacerbations of chronic bronchitis. NOTE: Although effective in clinical trials, ciprofloxacin is not a drug of first choice in the treatment of presumed or confirmed pneumonia secondary to *Streptococcus pneumoniae*.

Nosocomial Pneumonia caused by *Haemophilus influenzae* or *Klebsiella pneumoniae*.

Skin and Skin Structure Infections caused by *Escherichia coli*, *Klebsiella pneumoniae* subspecies *pneumoniae*, *Enterobacter cloacae*, *Proteus mirabilis*, *Proteus vulgaris*, *Providencia stuartii*, *Morganella morganii*, *Citrobacter freundii*, *Pseudomonas aeruginosa*, *Staphylococcus aureus* (methicillin susceptible), *Staphylococcus epidermidis*, or *Streptococcus pyogenes*.

Bone and Joint Infections caused by *Enterobacter cloacae*, *Serratia marcescens*, or *Pseudomonas aeruginosa*.

Complicated Intra-Abdominal Infections (used in conjunction with metronidazole) caused by *Escherichia coli*, *Pseudomonas aeruginosa*, *Proteus mirabilis*, *Klebsiella pneumoniae*, or *Bacteroides fragilis*.

Acute Sinusitis caused by *Haemophilus influenzae*, *Streptococcus pneumoniae*, or *Moraxella catarrhalis*.

Chronic Bacterial Prostatitis caused by *Escherichia coli* or *Proteus mirabilis*.

Empirical Therapy for Febrile Neutropenic Patients in combination with piperacillin sodium. (See **CLINICAL STUDIES**.)

Pediatric patients (1 to 17 years of age):

Complicated Urinary Tract Infections and Pyelonephritis due to *Escherichia coli*.

NOTE: Although effective in clinical trials, ciprofloxacin is not a drug of first choice in the pediatric population due to an increased incidence of adverse events compared to controls, including events related to joints and/or surrounding tissues. (See **WARNINGS, PRECAUTIONS, Pediatric Use, ADVERSE REACTIONS** and **CLINICAL STUDIES**.) Ciprofloxacin, like other fluoroquinolones, is associated with arthropathy and histopathological changes in weight-bearing joints of juvenile animals. (See **ANIMAL PHARMACOLOGY**.)

Adult and Pediatric Patients:

Inhalational anthrax (post-exposure): To reduce the incidence or progression of disease following exposure to aerosolized *Bacillus anthracis*.

Ciprofloxacin serum concentrations achieved in humans served as a surrogate endpoint reasonably likely to predict clinical benefit and provided the initial basis for approval of this indication.[4]

Supportive clinical information for ciprofloxacin for anthrax post-exposure prophylaxis was obtained during the anthrax bioterror attacks of October 2001. (See also, **INHALATIONAL ANTHRAX – ADDITIONAL INFORMATION**).

If anaerobic organisms are suspected of contributing to the infection, appropriate therapy should be administered.

Appropriate culture and susceptibility tests should be performed before treatment in order to isolate and identify organisms causing infection and to determine their susceptibility to ciprofloxacin. Therapy with CIPRO I.V. may be initiated before results of these tests are known; once results become available, appropriate therapy should be continued.

As with other drugs, some strains of *Pseudomonas aeruginosa* may develop resistance fairly rapidly during treatment with ciprofloxacin. Culture and susceptibility testing performed periodically during therapy will provide information not only on the therapeutic effect of the antimicrobial agent but also on the possible emergence of bacterial resistance.

To reduce the development of drug-resistant bacteria and maintain the effectiveness of CIPRO I.V. and other antibacterial drugs, CIPRO I.V. should be used only to treat or prevent infections that are proven or strongly suspected to be caused by susceptible bacteria. When culture and susceptibility information are available, they should be considered in selecting or modifying antibacterial therapy. In the absence of such data, local epidemiology and susceptibility patterns may contribute to the empiric selection of therapy.

CONTRAINDICATIONS

CIPRO I.V. (ciprofloxacin) is contraindicated in persons with history of hypersensitivity to ciprofloxacin or any member of the quinolone class of antimicrobial agents.

WARNINGS

Pregnant Women: THE SAFETY AND EFFECTIVENESS OF CIPROFLOXACIN IN PREGNANT AND LACTATING WOMEN HAVE NOT BEEN ESTABLISHED. (See **PRECAUTIONS: Pregnancy**, and **Nursing Mothers** subsections.)

Pediatrics: Ciprofloxacin should be used in pediatric patients (less than 18 years of age) only for infections listed in the **INDICATIONS AND USAGE** section. An increased incidence of adverse events compared to controls, including events related to joints and/or surrounding tissues, has been observed. (See **ADVERSE REACTIONS**.)

In pre-clinical studies, oral administration of ciprofloxacin caused lameness in immature dogs. Histopathological examination of the weight-bearing joints of these dogs revealed permanent lesions of the cartilage. Related quinolone-class drugs also produce erosions of cartilage of weight-bearing joints and other signs of arthropathy in immature animals of various species. (See **ANIMAL PHARMACOLOGY**.)

Central Nervous System Disorders: Convulsions, increased intracranial pressure and toxic psychosis have been

Continued on next page

Cipro I.V.—Cont.

reported in patients receiving quinolones, including ciprofloxacin. Ciprofloxacin may also cause central nervous system (CNS) events including: dizziness, confusion, tremors, hallucinations, depression, and, rarely, suicidal thoughts or acts. These reactions may occur following the first dose. If these reactions occur in patients receiving ciprofloxacin, the drug should be discontinued and appropriate measures instituted. As with all quinolones, ciprofloxacin should be used with caution in patients with known or suspected CNS disorders that may predispose to seizures or lower the seizure threshold (e.g. severe cerebral arteriosclerosis, epilepsy), or in the presence of other risk factors that may predispose to seizures or lower the seizure threshold (e.g. certain drug therapy, renal dysfunction). (See **PRECAUTIONS: General, Information for Patients, Drug Interaction** and **ADVERSE REACTIONS.**)

Theophylline: SERIOUS AND FATAL REACTIONS HAVE BEEN REPORTED IN PATIENTS RECEIVING CONCURRENT ADMINISTRATION OF INTRAVENOUS CIPROFLOXACIN AND THEOPHYLLINE. These reactions have included cardiac arrest, seizure, status epilepticus, and respiratory failure. Although similar serious adverse events have been reported in patients receiving theophylline alone, the possibility that these reactions may be potentiated by ciprofloxacin cannot be eliminated. If concomitant use cannot be avoided, serum levels of theophylline should be monitored and dosage adjustments made as appropriate.

Hypersensitivity Reactions: Serious and occasionally fatal hypersensitivity (anaphylactic) reactions, some following the first dose, have been reported in patients receiving quinolone therapy. Some reactions were accompanied by cardiovascular collapse, loss of consciousness, tingling, pharyngeal or facial edema, dyspnea, urticaria, and itching. Only a few patients had a history of hypersensitivity reactions. Serious anaphylactic reactions require immediate emergency treatment with epinephrine and other resuscitation measures, including oxygen, intravenous fluids, intravenous antihistamines, corticosteroids, pressor amines, and airway management, as clinically indicated.

Severe hypersensitivity reactions characterized by rash, fever, eosinophilia, jaundice, and hepatic necrosis with fatal outcome have also been reported extremely rarely in patients receiving ciprofloxacin along with other drugs. The possibility that these reactions were related to ciprofloxacin cannot be excluded. Ciprofloxacin should be discontinued at the first appearance of a skin rash or any other sign of hypersensitivity.

Pseudomembranous Colitis: Pseudomembranous colitis has been reported with nearly all antibacterial agents, including ciprofloxacin, and may range in severity from mild to life-threatening. Therefore, it is important to consider this diagnosis in patients who present with diarrhea subsequent to the administration of antibacterial agents.

Treatment with antibacterial agents alters the normal flora of the colon and may permit overgrowth of clostridia. Studies indicate that a toxin produced by *Clostridium difficile* is one primary cause of "antibiotic-associated colitis."

After the diagnosis of pseudomembranous colitis has been established, therapeutic measures should be initiated. Mild cases of pseudomembranous colitis usually respond to drug discontinuation alone. In moderate to severe cases, consideration should be given to management with fluids and electrolytes, protein supplementation, and treatment with an antibacterial drug clinically effective against *C. difficile* colitis. Drugs that inhibit peristalsis should be avoided.

Peripheral neuropathy: Rare cases of sensory or sensorimotor axonal polyneuropathy affecting small and/or large axons resulting in paresthesias, hypoesthesias, dysesthesias and weakness have been reported in patients receiving quinolones, including ciprofloxacin. Ciprofloxacin should be discontinued if the patient experiences symptoms of neuropathy including pain, burning, tingling, numbness, and/or weakness, or is found to have deficits in light touch, pain, temperature, position sense, vibratory sensation, and/or motor strength in order to prevent the development of an irreversible condition.

Tendon Effects: Ruptures of the shoulder, hand, Achilles tendon or other tendons that required surgical repair or resulted in prolonged disability have been reported in patients receiving quinolones, including ciprofloxacin. Post-marketing surveillance reports indicate that this risk may be increased in patients receiving concomitant corticosteroids, especially the elderly. Ciprofloxacin should be discontinued if the patient experiences pain, inflammation, or rupture of a tendon. Patients should rest and refrain from exercise until the diagnosis of tendonitis or tendon rupture has been excluded. Tendon rupture can occur during or after therapy with quinolones, including ciprofloxacin.

PRECAUTIONS

General: INTRAVENOUS CIPROFLOXACIN SHOULD BE ADMINISTERED BY SLOW INFUSION OVER A PERIOD OF 60 MINUTES. Local I.V. site reactions have been reported with the intravenous administration of ciprofloxacin. These reactions are more frequent if infusion time is 30 minutes or less or if small veins of the hand are used. (See **ADVERSE REACTIONS.**)

Central Nervous System: Quinolones, including ciprofloxacin, may also cause central nervous system (CNS) events, including: nervousness, agitation, insomnia, anxiety, nightmares or paranoia. (See **WARNINGS, Information for Patients,** and **Drug Interactions.**)

Crystals of ciprofloxacin have been observed rarely in the urine of human subjects but more frequently in the urine of laboratory animals, which is usually alkaline. (See **ANIMAL PHARMACOLOGY.**)

Crystalluria related to ciprofloxacin has been reported only rarely in humans because human urine is usually acidic. Alkalinity of the urine should be avoided in patients receiving ciprofloxacin. Patients should be well hydrated to prevent the formation of highly concentrated urine.

Renal Impairment: Alteration of the dosage regimen is necessary for patients with impairment of renal function. (See **DOSAGE AND ADMINISTRATION.**)

Phototoxicity: Moderate to severe phototoxicity manifested as an exaggerated sunburn reaction has been observed in some patients who were exposed to direct sunlight while receiving some members of the quinolone class of drugs. Excessive sunlight should be avoided.

As with any potent drug, periodic assessment of organ system functions, including renal, hepatic, and hematopoietic, is advisable during prolonged therapy.

Prescribing CIPRO I.V. in the absence of a proven or strongly suspected bacterial infection or a prophylactic indication is unlikely to provide benefit to the patient and increases the risk of the development of drug-resistant bacteria.

Information For Patients:

Patients should be advised:

• that antibacterial drugs including CIPRO I.V. should only be used to treat bacterial infections. They do not treat viral infections (e.g., the common cold). When CIPRO I.V. is prescribed to treat a bacterial infection, patients should be told that although it is common to feel better early in the course of therapy, the medication should be taken exactly as directed. Skipping doses or not completing the full course of therapy may (1) decrease the effectiveness of the immediate treatment and (2) increase the likelihood that bacteria will develop resistance and will not be treatable by CIPRO I.V. or other antibacterial drugs in the future.

• that ciprofloxacin may be associated with hypersensitivity reactions, even following a single dose, and to discontinue the drug at the first sign of a skin rash or other allergic reaction.

• that ciprofloxacin may cause dizziness and lightheadedness; therefore, patients should know how they react to this drug before they operate an automobile or machinery or engage in activities requiring mental alertness or coordination.

• that ciprofloxacin may increase the effects of theophylline and caffeine. There is a possibility of caffeine accumulation when products containing caffeine are consumed while taking ciprofloxacin.

• that peripheral neuropathies have been associated with ciprofloxacin use. If symptoms of peripheral neuropathy including pain, burning, tingling, numbness and/or weakness develop, they should discontinue treatment and contact their physicians.

• to discontinue treatment; rest and refrain from exercise; and inform their physician if they experience pain, inflammation, or rupture of a tendon.

• that convulsions have been reported in patients taking quinolones, including ciprofloxacin, and to notify their physician before taking this drug if there is a history of this condition.

• that ciprofloxacin has been associated with an increased rate of adverse events involving joints and surrounding tissue structures (like tendons) in pediatric patients (less than 18 years of age). Parents should inform their child's physician if the child has a history of joint-related problems before taking this drug. Parents of pediatric patients should also notify their child's physician of any joint-related problems that occur during or following ciprofloxacin therapy. (See **WARNINGS, PRECAUTIONS, Pediatric Use** and **ADVERSE REACTIONS.**)

Drug Interactions: As with some other quinolones, concurrent administration of ciprofloxacin with theophylline may lead to elevated serum concentrations of theophylline and prolongation of its elimination half-life. This may result in increased risk of theophylline-related adverse reactions. (See **WARNINGS.**) If concomitant use cannot be avoided, serum levels of theophylline should be monitored and dosage adjustments made as appropriate.

Some quinolones, including ciprofloxacin, have also been shown to interfere with the metabolism of caffeine. This may lead to reduced clearance of caffeine and prolongation of its serum half-life.

Some quinolones, including ciprofloxacin, have been associated with transient elevations in serum creatinine in patients receiving cyclosporine concomitantly.

Altered serum levels of phenytoin (increased and decreased) have been reported in patients receiving concomitant ciprofloxacin.

The concomitant administration of ciprofloxacin with the sulfonylurea glyburide has, in some patients, resulted in severe hypoglycemia. Fatalities have been reported.

The serum concentrations of ciprofloxacin and metronidazole were not altered when these two drugs were given concomitantly.

Quinolones, including ciprofloxacin, have been reported to enhance the effects of the oral anticoagulant warfarin or its derivatives. When these products are administered concomitantly, prothrombin time or other suitable coagulation tests should be closely monitored.

Probenecid interferes with renal tubular secretion of ciprofloxacin and produces an increase in the level of ciprofloxacin in the serum. This should be considered if patients are receiving both drugs concomitantly.

Renal tubular transport of methotrexate may be inhibited by concomitant administration of ciprofloxacin potentially leading to increased plasma levels of methotrexate. This might increase the risk of methotrexate associated toxic reactions. Therefore, patients under methotrexate therapy should be carefully monitored when concomitant ciprofloxacin therapy is indicated.

Non-steroidal anti-inflammatory drugs (but not acetyl salicylic acid) in combination of very high doses of quinolones have been shown to provoke convulsions in pre-clinical studies.

Following infusion of 400 mg I.V. ciprofloxacin every eight hours in combination with 50 mg/kg I.V. piperacillin sodium every four hours, mean serum ciprofloxacin concentrations were 3.02 µg/mL 1/2 hour and 1.18 µg/mL between 6–8 hours after the end of infusion.

Carcinogenesis, Mutagenesis, Impairment of Fertility: Eight *in vitro* mutagenicity tests have been conducted with ciprofloxacin. Test results are listed below:

Salmonella/Microsome Test (Negative)

E. coli DNA Repair Assay (Negative)

Mouse Lymphoma Cell Forward Mutation Assay (Positive)

Chinese Hamster V_{79}Cell HGPRT Test (Negative)

Syrian Hamster Embryo Cell Transformation Assay (Negative)

Saccharomyces cerevisiae Point Mutation Assay (Negative)

Saccharomyces cerevisiae Mitotic Crossover and Gene Conversion Assay (Negative)

Rat Hepatocyte DNA Repair Assay (Positive)

Thus, two of the eight tests were positive, but results of the following three *in vivo* test systems gave negative results:

Rat Hepatocyte DNA Repair Assay

Micronucleus Test (Mice)

Dominant Lethal Test (Mice)

Long-term carcinogenicity studies in rats and mice resulted in no carcinogenic or tumorigenic effects due to ciprofloxacin at daily oral dose levels up to 250 and 750 mg/kg to rats and mice, respectively (approximately 1.7- and 2.5-times the highest recommended therapeutic dose based upon mg/m²). Results from photo co-carcinogenicity testing indicate that ciprofloxacin does not reduce the time to appearance of UV-induced skin tumors as compared to vehicle control. Hairless (Skh-1) mice were exposed to UVA light for 3.5 hours five times every two weeks for up to 78 weeks while concurrently being administered ciprofloxacin.The time to development of the first skin tumors was 50 weeks in mice treated concomitantly with UVA and ciprofloxacin (mouse dose approximately equal to maximum recommended human dose based upon mg/m²), as opposed to 34 weeks when animals were treated with both UVA and vehicle. The times to development of skin tumors ranged from 16–32 weeks in mice treated concomitantly with UVA and other quinolones.[3]

In this model, mice treated with ciprofloxacin alone did not develop skin or systemic tumors. There are no data from similar models using pigmented mice and/or fully haired mice. The clinical significance of these findings to humans is unknown.

Fertility studies performed in rats at oral doses of ciprofloxacin up to 100 mg/kg (approximately 0.7-times the highest recommended therapeutic dose based upon mg/m²) revealed no evidence of impairment.

Pregnancy: Teratogenic Effects. Pregnancy Category C: There are no adequate and well-controlled studies in pregnant women. An expert review of published data on experiences with ciprofloxacin use during pregnancy by TERIS – the Teratogen Information System - concluded that therapeutic doses during pregnancy are unlikely to pose a substantial teratogenic risk (quantity and quality of data=fair), but the data are insufficient to state that there is no risk.[7]

A controlled prospective observational study followed 200 women exposed to fluoroquinolones (52.5% exposed to ciprofloxacin and 68% first trimester exposures) during gestation.[8] In utero exposure to fluoroquinolones during embryogenesis was not associated with increased risk of major malformations. The reported rates of major congenital malformations were 2.2% for the fluoroquinolone group and 2.6% for the control group (background incidence of major malformations is 1-5%). Rates of spontaneous abortions, prematurity and low birth weight did not differ between the groups and there were no clinically significant musculoskeletal dysfunctions up to one year of age in the ciprofloxacin exposed children.

Another prospective follow-up study reported on 549 pregnancies with fluoroquinolone exposure (93% first trimester exposures).[9] There were 70 ciprofloxacin exposures, all within the first trimester. The malformation rates among live-born babies exposed to ciprofloxacin and to fluoroquinolones overall were both within background incidence ranges. No specific patterns of congenital abnormalities were found. The study did not reveal any clear adverse reactions due to in utero exposure to ciprofloxacin.

No differences in the rates of prematurity, spontaneous abortions, or birth weight were seen in women exposed to ciprofloxacin during pregnancy.[7,8] However, these small postmarketing epidemiology studies, of which most experience is from short term, first trimester exposure, are insufficient to evaluate the risk for less common defects or to permit reliable and definitive conclusions regarding the safety

of ciprofloxacin in pregnant women and their developing fetuses. Ciprofloxacin should not be used during pregnancy unless the potential benefit justifies the potential risk to both fetus and mother (see **WARNINGS**).
Reproduction studies have been performed in rats and mice using oral doses up to 100 mg/kg (0.6 and 0.3 times the maximum daily human dose based upon body surface area, respectively) and have revealed no evidence of harm to the fetus due to ciprofloxacin. In rabbits, oral ciprofloxacin dose levels of 30 and 100 mg/kg (approximately 0.4- and 1.3-times the highest recommended therapeutic dose based upon mg/m^2) produced gastrointestinal toxicity resulting in maternal weight loss and an increased incidence of abortion, but no teratogenicity was observed at either dose level. After intravenous administration of doses up to 20 mg/kg (approximately 0.3-times the highest recommended therapeutic dose based upon mg/m^2) no maternal toxicity was produced and no embryotoxicity or teratogenicity was observed. (See **WARNINGS**.)
Nursing Mothers: Ciprofloxacin is excreted in human milk. The amount of ciprofloxacin absorbed by the nursing infant is unknown. Because of the potential for serious adverse reactions in infants nursing from mothers taking ciprofloxacin, a decision should be made whether to discontinue nursing or to discontinue the drug, taking into account the importance of the drug to the mother.
Pediatric Use: Ciprofloxacin, like other quinolones, causes arthropathy and histological changes in weight-bearing joints of juvenile animals resulting in lameness. (See **ANIMAL PHARMACOLOGY**.)
Inhalational Anthrax (Post-Exposure)
Ciprofloxacin is indicated in pediatric patients for inhalational anthrax (post-exposure). The risk-benefit assessment indicates that administration of ciprofloxacin to pediatric patients is appropriate. For information regarding pediatric dosing in inhalational anthrax (post-exposure), see **DOSAGE AND ADMINISTRATION** and **INHALATIONAL ANTHRAX – ADDITIONAL INFORMATION**.
Complicated Urinary Tract Infection and Pyelonephritis
Ciprofloxacin is indicated for the treatment of complicated urinary tract infections and pyelonephritis due to *Escherichia coli*. Although effective in clinical trials, ciprofloxacin is not a drug of first choice in the pediatric population due to an increased incidence of adverse events compared to the controls, including those related to joints and/or surrounding tissues. The rates of these events in pediatric patients with complicated urinary tract infection and pyelonephritis within six weeks of follow-up were 9.3% (31/335) versus 6.0% (21/349) for control agents. The rates of these events occurring at any time up to the one year follow-up were 13.7% (46/335) and 9.5% (33/349), respectively. The rate of all adverse events regardless of drug relationship at six weeks was 41% (138/335) in the ciprofloxacin arm compared to 31% (109/349) in the control arm. (See **ADVERSE REACTIONS** and **CLINICAL STUDIES**.)
Cystic Fibrosis
Short-term safety data from a single trial in pediatric cystic fibrosis patients are available. In a randomized, double-blind clinical trial for the treatment of acute pulmonary exacerbations in cystic fibrosis patients (ages 5-17 years), 67 patients received ciprofloxacin I.V. 10 mg/kg/dose q8h for one week followed by ciprofloxacin tablets 20 mg/kg/dose q12h to complete 10-21 days treatment and 62 patients received the combination of ceftazidime I.V. 50 mg/kg/dose q8h and tobramycin I.V. 3 mg/kg/dose q8h for a total of 10-21 days. Patients less than 5 years of age were not studied. Safety monitoring in the study included periodic range of motion examinations and gait assessments by treatment-blinded examiners. Patients were followed for an average of 23 days after completing treatment (range 0-93 days). This study was not designed to determine long term effects and the safety of repeated exposure to ciprofloxacin. Musculoskeletal adverse events in patients with cystic fibrosis were reported in 22% of the patients in the ciprofloxacin group and 21% in the comparison group. Decreased range of motion was reported in 12% of the subjects in the ciprofloxacin group and 16% in the comparison group. Arthralgia was reported in 10% of the patients in the ciprofloxacin group and 11% in the comparison group. Other adverse events were similar in nature and frequency between treatment arms. One of sixty-seven patients developed arthritis of the knee nine days after a ten day course of treatment with ciprofloxacin. Clinical symptoms resolved, but an MRI showed knee effusion without other abnormalities eight months after treatment. However, the relationship of this event to the patient's course of ciprofloxacin can not be definitively determined, particularly since patients with cystic fibrosis may develop arthralgias/arthritis as part of their underlying disease process.
Geriatric Use: In a retrospective analysis of 23 multiple-dose controlled clinical trials of ciprofloxacin encompassing over 3500 ciprofloxacin treated patients, 25% of patients were greater than or equal to 65 years of age and 10% were greater than or equal to 75 years of age. No overall differences in safety or effectiveness were observed between these subjects and younger subjects, and other reported clinical experience has not identified differences in responses between the elderly and younger patients, but greater sensitivity of some older individuals on any drug therapy cannot be ruled out. Ciprofloxacin is known to be substantially excreted by the kidney, and the risk of adverse reactions may be greater in patients with impaired renal function. No alteration of dosage is necessary for patients greater than 65 years of age with normal renal function. However, since some older individuals experience reduced renal function by virtue of their advanced age, care should be taken in dose selection for elderly patients, and renal function monitoring may be useful in these patients. (See **CLINICAL PHARMACOLOGY** and **DOSAGE AND ADMINISTRATION**.)

Findings Involving Joint or Peri-articular Tissues as Assessed by the IPSC

	Ciprofloxacin	Comparator
All Patients (within 6 weeks)	31/335 (9.3%)	21/349 (6.0%)
95% Confidence Interval*	(-0.8%, +7.2%)	
Age Group		
≥ 12 months < 24 months	1/36 (2.8%)	0/41
≥ 2 years < 6 years	5/124 (4.0%)	3/118 (2.5%)
≥ 6 years < 12 years	18/143 (12.6%)	12/153 (7.8%)
≥ 12 years to 17 years	7/32 (21.9%)	6/37 (16.2 %)
All Patients (within 1 year)	46/335 (13.7%)	33/349 (9.5%)
95% Confidence Interval*	(-0.6%, +9.1%)	

*The study was designed to demonstrate that the arthropathy rate for the ciprofloxacin group did not exceed that of the control group by more than + 6%. At both the 6 week and 1 year evaluations, the 95% confidence interval indicated that it could not be concluded that the ciprofloxacin group had findings comparable to the control group.

ADVERSE REACTIONS

Adverse Reactions in Adult Patients: During clinical investigations with oral and parenteral ciprofloxacin, 49,038 patients received courses of the drug. Most of the adverse events reported were described as only mild or moderate in severity, abated soon after the drug was discontinued, and required no treatment. Ciprofloxacin was discontinued because of an adverse event in 1.8% of intravenously treated patients.
The most frequently reported drug related events, from clinical trials of all formulations, all dosages, all drug-therapy durations, and for all indications of ciprofloxacin therapy were nausea (2.5%), diarrhea (1.6%), liver function tests abnormal (1.3%), vomiting (1.0%), and rash (1.0%).
In clinical trials the following events were reported, regardless of drug relationship, in greater than 1% of patients treated with intravenous ciprofloxacin: nausea, diarrhea, central nervous system disturbance, local I.V. site reactions, liver function tests abnormal, eosinophilia, headache, restlessness, and rash. Many of these events were described as only mild or moderate in severity, abated soon after the drug was discontinued, and required no treatment. Local I.V. site reactions are more frequent if the infusion time is 30 minutes or less. These may appear as local skin reactions which resolve rapidly upon completion of the infusion. Subsequent intravenous administration is not contraindicated unless the reactions recur or worsen.
Additional medically important events, without regard to drug relationship or route of administration, that occurred in 1% or less of ciprofloxacin patients are listed below:
BODY AS A WHOLE: abdominal pain/discomfort, foot pain, pain, pain in extremities
CARDIOVASCULAR: cardiovascular collapse, cardiopulmonary arrest, myocardial infarction, arrhythmia, tachycardia, palpitation, cerebral thrombosis, syncope, cardiac murmur, hypertension, hypotension, angina pectoris, atrial flutter, ventricular ectopy, (thrombo)-phlebitis, vasodilation, migraine
CENTRAL NERVOUS SYSTEM: convulsive seizures, paranoia, toxic psychosis, depression, dysphasia, phobia, depersonalization, manic reaction, unresponsiveness, ataxia, confusion, hallucinations, dizziness, lightheadedness, paresthesia, anxiety, tremor, insomnia, nightmares, weakness, drowsiness, irritability, malaise, lethargy, abnormal gait, grand mal convulsion, anorexia
GASTROINTESTINAL: ileus, jaundice, gastrointestinal bleeding, *C. difficile* associated diarrhea, pseudomembranous colitis, pancreatitis, hepatic necrosis, intestinal perforation, dyspepsia, epigastric pain, constipation, oral ulceration, oral candidiasis, mouth dryness, anorexia, dysphagia, flatulence, hepatitis, painful oral mucosa
HEMIC/LYMPHATIC: agranulocytosis, prolongation of prothrombin time, lymphadenopathy, petechia
METABOLIC/NUTRITIONAL: amylase increase, lipase increase
MUSCULOSKELETAL: arthralgia, jaw, arm or back pain, joint stiffness, neck and chest pain, achiness, flare up of gout, myasthenia gravis
RENAL/UROGENITAL: renal failure, interstitial nephritis, nephritis, hemorrhagic cystitis, renal calculi, frequent urination, acidosis, urethral bleeding, polyuria, urinary retention, gynecomastia, candiduria, vaginitis, breast pain. Crystalluria, cylindruria, hematuria and albuminuria have also been reported.
RESPIRATORY: respiratory arrest, pulmonary embolism, dyspnea, laryngeal or pulmonary edema, respiratory distress, pleural effusion, hemoptysis, epistaxis, hiccough, bronchospasm
SKIN/HYPERSENSITIVITY: allergic reactions, anaphylactic reactions including life-threatening anaphylactic shock, erythema multiforme/Stevens-Johnson syndrome, exfoliative dermatitis, toxic epidermal necrolysis, vasculitis, angioedema, edema of the lips, face, neck, conjunctivae, hands or lower extremities, purpura, fever, chills, flushing, pruritus, urticaria, cutaneous candidiasis, vesicles, increased perspiration, hyperpigmentation, erythema nodosum, thrombophlebitis, burning, paresthesia, erythema, swelling, photosensitivity (See **WARNINGS**.)
SPECIAL SENSES: decreased visual acuity, blurred vision, disturbed vision (flashing lights, change in color perception, overbrightness of lights, diplopia), eye pain, anosmia, hearing loss, tinnitus, nystagmus, chromatopsia, a bad taste
In several instances, nausea, vomiting, tremor, irritability, or palpitation were judged by investigators to be related to elevated serum levels of theophylline possibly as a result of drug interaction with ciprofloxacin.
In randomized, double-blind controlled clinical trials comparing ciprofloxacin (I.V. and I.V./P.O. sequential) with intravenous beta-lactam control antibiotics, the CNS adverse event profile of ciprofloxacin was comparable to that of the control drugs.
Adverse Reactions in Pediatric Patients: Ciprofloxacin, administered I.V. and /or orally, was compared to a cephalosporin for treatment of complicated urinary tract infections (cUTI) or pyelonephritis in pediatric patients 1 to 17 years of age (mean age of 6 ± 4 years). The trial was conducted in the US, Canada, Argentina, Peru, Costa Rica, Mexico, South Africa, and Germany. The duration of therapy was 10 to 21 days (mean duration of treatment was 11 days with a range of 1 to 88 days). The primary objective of the study was to assess musculoskeletal and neurological safety within 6 weeks of therapy and through one year of follow-up in the 335 ciprofloxacin- and 349 comparator-treated patients enrolled.
An Independent Pediatric Safety Committee (IPSC) reviewed all cases of musculoskeletal adverse events as well as all patients with an abnormal gait or abnormal joint exam (baseline or treatment-emergent). These events were evaluated in a comprehensive fashion and included such conditions as arthralgia, abnormal gait, abnormal joint exam, joint sprains, leg pain, back pain, arthrosis, bone pain, pain, myalgia, arm pain, and decreased range of motion in a joint. The affected joints included: knee, elbow, ankle, hip, wrist, and shoulder. Within 6 weeks of treatment initiation, the rates of these events were 9.3% (31/335) in the ciprofloxacin-treated group versus 6.0% (21/349) in comparator-treated patients. The majority of these events were mild or moderate in intensity. All musculoskeletal events occurring by 6 weeks resolved (clinical resolution of signs and symptoms), usually within 30 days of end of treatment. Radiological evaluations were not routinely used to confirm resolution of the events. The events occurred more frequently in ciprofloxacin-treated patients than control patients, regardless of whether they received I.V. or oral therapy. Ciprofloxacin-treated patients were more likely to report more than one event and on more than one occasion compared to control patients. These events occurred in all age groups and the rates were consistently higher in the ciprofloxacin group compared to the control group. At the end of 1 year, the rate of these events reported at any time during that period was 13.7% (46/335) in the ciprofloxacin-treated group versus 9.5% (33/349) comparator-treated patients.
An adolescent female discontinued ciprofloxacin for wrist pain that developed during treatment. An MRI performed 4 weeks later showed a tear in the right ulnar fibrocartilage. A diagnosis of overuse syndrome secondary to sports activity was made, but a contribution from ciprofloxacin cannot be excluded. The patient recovered by 4 months without surgical intervention.
[See table above]
The incidence rates of neurological events within 6 weeks of treatment initiation were 3% (9/335) in the ciprofloxacin group versus 2% (7/349) in the comparator group and included dizziness, nervousness, insomnia, and somnolence.
In this trial, the overall incidence rates of adverse events regardless of relationship to study drug and within 6 weeks of treatment initiation were 41% (138/335) in the ciprofloxacin group versus 31% (109/349) in the comparator group. The most frequent events were gastrointestinal: 15%

Continued on next page

Cipro I.V.—Cont.

(50/335) of ciprofloxacin patients compared to 9% (31/349) of comparator patients. Serious adverse events were seen in 7.5% (25/335) of ciprofloxacin-treated patients compared to 5.7% (20/349) of control patients. Discontinuation of drug due to an adverse event was observed in 3% (10/335) of ciprofloxacin-treated patients versus 1.4% (5/349) of comparator patients. Other adverse events that occurred in at least 1% of ciprofloxacin patients were diarrhea 4.8%, vomiting 4.8%, abdominal pain 3.3%, accidental injury 3.0%, rhinitis 3.0%, dyspepsia 2.7%, nausea 2.7%, fever 2.1%, asthma 1.8% and rash 1.8%.

In addition to the events reported in pediatric patients in clinical trials, it should be expected that events reported in adults during clinical trials or post-marketing experience may also occur in pediatric patients.

Post-Marketing Adverse Events: The following adverse events have been reported from worldwide marketing experience with quinolones, including ciprofloxacin. Because these events are reported voluntarily from a population of uncertain size, it is not always possible to reliably estimate their frequency or establish a causal relationship to drug exposure. Decisions to include these events in labeling are typically based on one or more of the following factors: (1) seriousness of the event, (2) frequency of the reporting, or (3) strength of causal connection to the drug.

Agitation, agranulocytosis, albuminuria, anosmia, candiduria, cholesterol elevation (serum), confusion, constipation, delirium, dyspepsia, dysphagia, erythema multiforme, exfoliative dermatitis, fixed eruption, flatulence, glucose elevation (blood), hemolytic anemia, hepatic failure, hepatic necrosis, hyperesthesia, hypertonia, hypesthesia, hypotension (postural), jaundice, marrow depression (life threatening), methemoglobinemia, moniliasis (oral, gastrointestinal, vaginal), myalgia, myasthenia, myasthenia gravis (possible exacerbation), myoclonus, nystagmus, pancreatitis, pancytopenia (life threatening or fatal outcome), peripheral neuropathy, phenytoin alteration (serum), potassium elevation (serum), prothrombin time prolongation or decrease, pseudomembranous colitis (The onset of pseudomembranous colitis symptoms may occur during or after antimicrobial treatment.), psychosis (toxic), renal calculi, serum sickness like reaction, Stevens-Johnson syndrome, taste loss, tendinitis, tendon rupture, torsade de pointes, toxic epidermal necrolysis (Lyell's Syndrome), triglyceride elevation (serum), twitching, vaginal candidiasis, and vasculitis. (See **PRECAUTIONS**.)

Adverse events were also reported by persons who received ciprofloxacin for anthrax post-exposure prophylaxis following the anthrax bioterror attacks of October 2001 (See also **INHALATIONAL ANTHRAX - ADDITIONAL INFORMATION**).

Adverse Laboratory Changes: The most frequently reported changes in laboratory parameters with intravenous ciprofloxacin therapy, without regard to drug relationship are listed below:

Hepatic	—	elevations of AST (SGOT), ALT (SGPT), alkaline phosphatase, LDH, and serum bilirubin
Hematologic	—	elevated eosinophil and platelet counts, decreased platelet counts, hemoglobin and/or hematocrit
Renal	—	elevations of serum creatinine, BUN, and uric acid
Other	—	elevations of serum creatine phosphokinase, serum theophylline (in patients receiving theophylline concomitantly), blood glucose, and triglycerides

Other changes occurring infrequently were: decreased leukocyte count, elevated atypical lymphocyte count, immature WBCs, elevated serum calcium, elevation of serum gammaglutamyl transpeptidase (γ GT), decreased BUN, decreased uric acid, decreased total serum protein, decreased serum albumin, decreased serum potassium, elevated serum potassium, elevated serum cholesterol. Other changes occurring rarely during administration of ciprofloxacin were: elevation of serum amylase, decrease of blood glucose, pancytopenia, leukocytosis, elevated sedimentation rate, change in serum phenytoin, decreased prothrombin time, hemolytic anemia, and bleeding diathesis.

OVERDOSAGE

In the event of acute overdosage, the patient should be carefully observed and given supportive treatment, including monitoring of renal function. Adequate hydration must be maintained. Only a small amount of ciprofloxacin (<10%) is removed from the body after hemodialysis or peritoneal dialysis.

In mice, rats, rabbits and dogs, significant toxicity including tonic/clonic convulsions was observed at intravenous doses of ciprofloxacin between 125 and 300 mg/kg.

DOSAGE AND ADMINISTRATION - ADULTS

CIPRO I.V. should be administered to adults by intravenous infusion over a period of 60 minutes at dosages described in the Dosage Guidelines table. Slow infusion of a dilute solution into a larger vein will minimize patient discomfort and reduce the risk of venous irritation. (See **Preparation of CIPRO I.V. for Administration** section.)

The determination of dosage for any particular patient must take into consideration the severity and nature of the infection, the susceptibility of the causative microorganism, the integrity of the patient's host-defense mechanisms, and the status of renal and hepatic function.

[See first table above]

ADULT DOSAGE GUIDELINES

Infection†	Severity	Dose	Frequency	Usual Duration
Urinary Tract	Mild/Moderate	200 mg	q12h	7-14 Days
	Severe/Complicated	400 mg	q12h	7-14 Days
Lower Respiratory Tract	Mild/Moderate	400 mg	q12h	7-14 Days
	Severe/Complicated	400 mg	q8h	7-14 Days
Nosocomial Pneumonia	Mild/Moderate/Severe	400 mg	q8h	10-14 Days
Skin and Skin Structure	Mild/Moderate	400 mg	q12h	7-14 Days
	Severe/Complicated	400 mg	q8h	7-14 Days
Bone and Joint	Mild/Moderate	400 mg	q12h	≥ 4-6 Weeks
	Severe/Complicated	400 mg	q8h	≥ 4-6 Weeks
Intra-Abdominal*	Complicated	400 mg	q12h	7-14 Days
Acute Sinusitis	Mild/Moderate	400 mg	q12h	10 Days
Chronic Bacterial Prostatitis	Mild/Moderate	400 mg	q12h	28 Days
Empirical Therapy in Febrile Neutropenic Patients	Severe			
	Ciprofloxacin +	400 mg	q8h	7-14 Days
	Piperacillin	50 mg/kg Not to exceed 24 g/day	q4h	
Inhalational anthrax (post-exposure)**		400 mg	q12h	60 Days

* used in conjunction with metronidazole. (See product labeling for prescribing information.)
† DUE TO THE DESIGNATED PATHOGENS (See **INDICATIONS AND USAGE**.)
Drug administration should begin as soon as possible after suspected or confirmed exposure. This indication is based on a surrogate endpoint, ciprofloxacin serum concentrations achieved in humans, reasonably likely to predict clinical benefit.[4] For a discussion of ciprofloxacin serum concentrations in various human populations, see **INHALATIONAL ANTHRAX – ADDITIONAL INFORMATION. Total duration of ciprofloxacin administration (I.V. or oral) for inhalational anthrax (post-exposure) is 60 days.

Men: Creatinine clearance (mL/min) = $\dfrac{\text{Weight (kg)} \times (140 - \text{age})}{72 \times \text{serum creatinine (mg/dL)}}$

Women: 0.85 × the value calculated for men.

PEDIATRIC DOSAGE GUIDELINES

Infection	Route of Administration	Dose (mg/kg)	Frequency	Total Duration
Complicated Urinary Tract or Pyelonephritis	Intravenous	6 to 10 mg/kg (maximum 400 mg per dose; not to be exceeded even in patients weighing > 51 kg)	Every 8 hours	10-21 days*
(patients from 1 to 17 years of age)	Oral	10 mg/kg to 20 mg/kg (maximum 750 mg per dose; not to be exceeded even in patients weighing > 51 kg)	Every 12 hours	
Inhalational Anthrax (Post-Exposure) **	Intravenous	10 mg/kg (maximum 400 mg per dose)	Every 12 hours	60 days
	Oral	15 mg/kg (maximum 500 mg per dose)	Every 12 hours	

* The total duration of therapy for complicated urinary tract infection and pyelonephritis in the clinical trial was determined by the physician. The mean duration of treatment was 11 days (range 10 to 21 days).
** Drug administration should begin as soon as possible after suspected or confirmed exposure to *Bacillus anthracis* spores. This indication is based on a surrogate endpoint, ciprofloxacin serum concentrations achieved in humans, reasonably likely to predict clinical benefit.[4] For a discussion of ciprofloxacin serum concentrations in various human populations, see **INHALATIONAL ANTHRAX – ADDITIONAL INFORMATION**.

CIPRO I.V. should be administered by intravenous infusion over a period of 60 minutes.

Conversion of I.V. to Oral Dosing in Adults: CIPRO Tablets and CIPRO Oral Suspension for oral administration are available. Parenteral therapy may be switched to oral CIPRO when the condition warrants, at the discretion of the physician. (See **CLINICAL PHARMACOLOGY** and table below for the equivalent dosing regimens.)

Equivalent AUC Dosing Regimens

CIPRO Oral Dosage	Equivalent CIPRO I.V. Dosage
250 mg Tablet q 12 h	200 mg I.V. q 12 h
500 mg Tablet q 12 h	400 mg I.V. q 12 h
750 mg Tablet q 12 h	400 mg I.V. q 8 h

Parenteral drug products should be inspected visually for particulate matter and discoloration prior to administration.

Adults with Impaired Renal Function: Ciprofloxacin is eliminated primarily by renal excretion; however, the drug is also metabolized and partially cleared through the biliary system of the liver and through the intestine. These alternative pathways of drug elimination appear to compensate for the reduced renal excretion in patients with renal impairment. Nonetheless, some modification of dosage is recommended for patients with severe renal dysfunction. The following table provides dosage guidelines for use in patients with renal impairment:

RECOMMENDED STARTING AND MAINTENANCE DOSES FOR PATIENTS WITH IMPAIRED RENAL FUNCTION

Creatinine Clearance (mL/min)	Dosage
> 30	See usual dosage.
5 - 29	200-400 mg q 18-24 hr

When only the serum creatinine concentration is known, the following formula may be used to estimate creatinine clearance:

[See second table above]

The serum creatinine should represent a steady state of renal function.

For patients with changing renal function or for patients with renal impairment and hepatic insufficiency, careful monitoring is suggested.

DOSAGE AND ADMINISTRATION - PEDIATRICS

CIPRO I.V. should be administered as described in the Dosage Guidelines table. An increased incidence of adverse events compared to controls, including events related to joints and/or surrounding tissues, has been observed. (See **ADVERSE REACTIONS** and **CLINICAL STUDIES**.)

Dosing and initial route of therapy (i.e., I.V. or oral) for complicated urinary tract infection or pyelonephritis should be determined by the severity of the infection. In the clinical trial, pediatric patients with moderate to severe infection were initiated on 6 to 10 mg/kg I.V. every 8 hours and al-

lowed to switch to oral therapy (10 to 20 mg/kg every 12 hours), at the discretion of the physician.
[See third table on previous page]
Pediatric patients with moderate to severe renal insufficiency were excluded from the clinical trial of complicated urinary tract infection and pyelonephritis. No information is available on dosing adjustments necessary for pediatric patients with moderate to severe renal insufficiency (i.e., creatinine clearance of < 50 mL/min/1.73m^2).

Preparation of CIPRO I.V. for Administration

Vials (Injection Concentrate): THIS PREPARATION MUST BE DILUTED BEFORE USE. The intravenous dose should be prepared by aseptically withdrawing the concentrate from the vial of CIPRO I.V. This should be diluted with a suitable intravenous solution to a final concentration of 1–2mg/mL. (See **COMPATIBILITY AND STABILITY**.) The resulting solution should be infused over a period of 60 minutes by direct infusion or through a Y-type intravenous infusion set which may already be in place.

If the Y-type or "piggyback" method of administration is used, it is advisable to discontinue temporarily the administration of any other solutions during the infusion of CIPRO I.V. If the concomitant use of CIPRO I.V. and another drug is necessary each drug should be given separately in accordance with the recommended dosage and route of administration for each drug.

Flexible Containers: CIPRO I.V. is also available as a 0.2% premixed solution in 5% dextrose in flexible containers of 100 mL or 200 mL. The solutions in flexible containers do not need to be diluted and may be infused as described above.

COMPATIBILITY AND STABILITY

Ciprofloxacin injection 1% (10 mg/mL), when diluted with the following intravenous solutions to concentrations of 0.5 to 2.0 mg/mL, is stable for up to 14 days at refrigerated or room temperature storage.

0.9% Sodium Chloride Injection, USP
5% Dextrose Injection, USP
Sterile Water for Injection
10% Dextrose for Injection
5% Dextrose and 0.225% Sodium Chloride for Injection
5% Dextrose and 0.45% Sodium Chloride for Injection
Lactated Ringer's for Injection

HOW SUPPLIED

CIPRO I.V. (ciprofloxacin) is available as a clear, colorless to slightly yellowish solution. CIPRO I.V. is available in 200 mg and 400 mg strengths. The concentrate is supplied in vials while the premixed solution is supplied in latex-free flexible containers as follows:

VIAL: manufactured for Bayer Pharmaceuticals Corporation by Bayer HealthCare LLC, Shawnee, Kansas.

SIZE	STRENGTH	NDC NUMBER
20 mL	200 mg, 1%	0085-1763-03
40 mL	400 mg, 1%	0085-1731-01

FLEXIBLE CONTAINER: manufactured for Bayer Pharmaceuticals Corporation by Hospira, Inc., Lake Forest, IL 60045.

SIZE	STRENGTH	NDC NUMBER
100 mL 5% Dextrose	200 mg, 0.2%	0085-1755-02
200 mL 5% Dextrose	400 mg, 0.2%	0085-1741-02

FLEXIBLE CONTAINER: manufactured for Bayer Pharmaceuticals Corporation by Baxter Healthcare Corporation, Deerfield, IL 60015.

SIZE	STRENGTH	NDC NUMBER
100 mL 5% Dextrose	200 mg, 0.2%	0085-1781-01
200 mL 5% Dextrose	400 mg, 0.2%	0085-1762-01

STORAGE

Vial: Store between 5 – 30ºC (41 – 86ºF).
Flexible Container: Store between 5 – 25ºC (41 – 77ºF).
Protect from light, avoid excessive heat, protect from freezing.

Ciprofloxacin is also available as CIPRO (ciprofloxacin HCl) Tablets 250, 500, and 750 mg and CIPRO (ciprofloxacin*) 5% and 10% Oral Suspension.

* Does not comply with USP with regards to "loss on drying" and "residue on ignition".

ANIMAL PHARMACOLOGY

Ciprofloxacin and other quinolones have been shown to cause arthropathy in immature animals of most species tested. (See **WARNINGS**.) Damage of weight bearing joints was observed in juvenile dogs and rats. In young beagles, 100 mg/kg ciprofloxacin, given daily for 4 weeks, caused degenerative articular changes of the knee joint. At 30 mg/kg, the effect on the joint was minimal. In a subsequent study in young beagle dogs, oral ciprofloxacin doses of 30 mg/kg and 90 mg/kg ciprofloxacin (approximately 1.3- and 3.5-times the pediatric dose based upon comparative plasma AUCs) given daily for 2 weeks caused articular changes which were still observed by histopathology after a treatment-free period of 5 months. At 10 mg/kg (approximately 0.6-times the pediatric dose based upon comparative plasma AUCs), no effects on joints were observed. This dose was also not associated with arthrotoxicity after an additional treatment-free period of 5 months. In another study, removal of weight bearing from the joint reduced the lesions but did not totally prevent them.

Crystalluria, sometimes associated with secondary nephropathy, occurs in laboratory animals dosed with ciprofloxacin. This is primarily related to the reduced solubility of ciprofloxacin under alkaline conditions, which predominate in the urine of test animals; in man, crystalluria is rare since human urine is typically acidic. In rhesus monkeys, crystalluria without nephropathy was noted after single oral doses as low as 5 mg/kg (approximately 0.07-times the highest recommended therapeutic dose based upon mg/m^2). After 6 months of intravenous dosing at 10 mg/kg/day, no nephropathological changes were noted; however, nephropathy was observed after dosing at 20 mg/kg/day for the same duration (approximately 0.2-times the highest recommended therapeutic dose based upon mg/m^2).

In dogs, ciprofloxacin administered at 3 and 10 mg/kg by rapid intravenous injection (15 sec.) produces pronounced hypotensive effects. These effects are considered to be related to histamine release because they are partially antagonized by pyrilamine, an antihistamine. In rhesus monkeys, rapid intravenous injection also produces hypotension, but the effect in this species is inconsistent and less pronounced.

In mice, concomitant administration of nonsteroidal anti-inflammatory drugs, such as phenylbutazone and indomethacin, with quinolones has been reported to enhance the CNS stimulatory effect of quinolones.

Ocular toxicity, seen with some related drugs, has not been observed in ciprofloxacin-treated animals.

INHALATIONAL ANTHRAX – ADDITIONAL INFORMATION

The mean serum concentrations of ciprofloxacin associated with a statistically significant improvement in survival in the rhesus monkey model of inhalational anthrax are reached or exceeded in adult and pediatric patients receiving oral and intravenous regimens. (See **DOSAGE AND ADMINISTRATION**.) Ciprofloxacin pharmacokinetics have been evaluated in various human populations. The mean peak serum concentration achieved at steady-state in human adults receiving 500 mg orally every 12 hours is 2.97 μg/mL, and 4.56 μg/mL following 400 mg intravenously every 12 hours. The mean trough serum concentration at steady-state for both of these regimens is 0.2 μg/mL. In a study of 10 pediatric patients between 6 and 16 years of age, the mean peak plasma concentration achieved is 8.3 μg/mL and trough concentrations range from 0.09 to 0.26 μg/mL, following two 30-minute intravenous infusions of 10 mg/kg administered 12 hours apart. After the second intravenous infusion patients switched to 15 mg/kg orally every 12 hours achieve a mean peak concentration of 3.6 μg/mL after the initial oral dose. Long-term safety data, including effects on cartilage, following the administration of ciprofloxacin to pediatric patients are limited. (For additional information, see **PRECAUTIONS, Pediatric Use.**) Ciprofloxacin serum concentrations achieved in humans serve as a surrogate endpoint reasonably likely to predict clinical benefit and provide the basis for this indication.[4]

A placebo-controlled animal study in rhesus monkeys exposed to an inhaled mean dose of 11 LD_{50} (~5.5 × 10^5) spores (range 5–30 LD_{50}) of *B. anthracis* was conducted. The minimal inhibitory concentration (MIC) of ciprofloxacin for the anthrax strain used in this study was 0.08 μg/mL. In the animals studied, mean serum concentrations of ciprofloxacin achieved at expected T_{max} (1 hour post-dose) following oral dosing to steady-state ranged from 0.98 to 1.69 μg/mL. Mean steady-state trough concentrations at 12 hours post-dose ranged from 0.12 to 0.19 μg/mL[5]. Mortality due to anthrax for animals that received a 30-day regimen of oral ciprofloxacin beginning 24 hours post-exposure was significantly lower (1/9), compared to the placebo group (9/10) [p=0.001]. The one ciprofloxacin-treated animal that died of anthrax did so following the 30-day drug administration period.[6]

More than 9300 persons were recommended to complete a minimum of 60 days of antibiotic prophylaxis against possible inhalational exposure to *B. anthracis* during 2001. Ciprofloxacin was recommended to most of those individuals for all or part of the prophylaxis regimen. Some persons were also given anthrax vaccine or were switched to alternative antibiotics. No one who received ciprofloxacin or other therapies as prophylactic treatment subsequently developed inhalational anthrax. The number of persons who received ciprofloxacin as all or part of their post-exposure prophylaxis regimen is unknown.

Among the persons surveyed by the Centers for Disease Control and Prevention, over 1000 reported receiving ciprofloxacin as sole post-exposure prophylaxis for inhalational anthrax. Gastrointestinal adverse events (nausea, vomiting, diarrhea, or stomach pain), neurological adverse events (problems sleeping, nightmares, headache, dizziness or lightheadedness) and musculoskeletal adverse events (muscle or tendon pain and joint swelling or pain) were more frequent than had been previously reported in controlled clinical trials. This higher incidence, in the absence of a control group, could be explained by a reporting bias, concurrent medical conditions, other concomitant medications, emotional stress or other confounding factors, and/or a longer treatment period with ciprofloxacin. Because of these factors and limitations in the data collection, it is difficult to evaluate whether the reported symptoms were drug-related.

CLINICAL STUDIES

EMPIRICAL THERAPY IN ADULT FEBRILE NEUTROPENIC PATIENTS

The safety and efficacy of ciprofloxacin, 400 mg I.V. q 8h, in combination with piperacillin sodium, 50 mg/kg I.V. q 4h, for the empirical therapy of febrile neutropenic patients were studied in one large pivotal multicenter, randomized trial and were compared to those of tobramycin, 2 mg/kg I.V. q 8h, in combination with piperacillin sodium, 50 mg/kg I.V. q 4h. Clinical response rates observed in this study were as follows:

[See first table above]

Outcomes	Ciprofloxacin/Piperacillin N = 233 Success (%)	Tobramycin/Piperacillin N = 237 Success (%)
Clinical Resolution of Initial Febrile Episode with No Modifications of Empirical Regimen*	63 (27.0%)	52 (21.9%)
Clinical Resolution of Initial Febrile Episode Including Patients with Modifications of Empirical Regimen	187 (80.3%)	185 (78.1%)
Overall Survival	224 (96.1%)	223 (94.1%)

* To be evaluated as a clinical resolution, patients had to have: (1) resolution of fever; (2) microbiological eradication of infection (if an infection was microbiologically documented); (3) resolution of signs/symptoms of infection; and (4) no modification of empirical antibiotic regimen.

Complicated Urinary Tract Infection and Pyelonephritis – Efficacy in Pediatric Patients:

NOTE: Although effective in clinical trials, ciprofloxacin is not a drug of first choice in the pediatric population due to an increased incidence of adverse events compared to controls, including events related to joints and/or surrounding tissues.

Ciprofloxacin, administered I.V. and/or orally, was compared to a cephalosporin for treatment of complicated urinary tract infections (cUTI) and pyelonephritis in pediatric patients 1 to 17 years of age (mean age of 6 ± 4 years). The trial was conducted in the US, Canada, Argentina, Peru, Costa Rica, Mexico, South Africa, and Germany. The duration of therapy was 10 to 21 days (mean duration of treatment was 11 days with a range of 1 to 88 days). The primary objective of the study was to assess musculoskeletal and neurological safety.

Clinical Success and Bacteriologic Eradication at Test of Cure (5 to 9 Days Post-Therapy)

	CIPRO	Comparator
Randomized Patients	337	352
Per Protocol Patients	211	231
Clinical Response at 5 to 9 Days Post-Treatment	95.7% (202/211)	92.6% (214/231)
	95% CI [-1.3%, 7.3%]	
Bacteriologic Eradication by Patient at 5 to 9 Days Post-Treatment*	84.4% (178/211)	78.3% (181/231)
	95% CI [-1.3%, 13.1%]	
Bacteriologic Eradication of the Baseline Pathogen at 5 to 9 Days Post-Treatment		
Escherichia coli	156/178 (88%)	161/179 (90%)

* Patients with baseline pathogen(s) eradicated and no new infections or superinfections/total number of patients. There were 5.5% (6/211) ciprofloxacin and 9.5% (22/231) comparator patients with superinfections or new infections.

Continued on next page

Cipro I.V.—Cont.

Patients were evaluated for clinical success and bacteriological eradication of the baseline organism(s) with no new infection or superinfection at 5 to 9 days post-therapy (Test of Cure or TOC). The Per Protocol population had a causative organism(s) with protocol specified colony count(s) at baseline, no protocol violation, and no premature discontinuation or loss to follow-up (among other criteria).

The clinical success and bacteriologic eradication rates in the Per Protocol population were similar between ciprofloxacin and the comparator group as shown below.

[See second table at top of previous page]

REFERENCES

1. National Committee for Clinical Laboratory Standards, Methods for Dilution Antimicrobial Susceptibility Tests for Bacteria That Grow Aerobically - Fifth Edition. Approved Standard NCCLS Document M7-A5, Vol. 20, No. 2, NCCLS, Wayne, PA, January, 2000. **2.** National Committee for Clinical Laboratory Standards, Performance Standards for Antimicrobial Disk Susceptibility Tests - Seventh Edition. Approved Standard NCCLS Document M2-A7, Vol. 20, No. 1, NCCLS, Wayne, PA, January, 2000. **3.** Report presented at the FDA's Anti-Infective Drug and Dermatological Drug Products Advisory Committee Meeting, March 31, 1993, Silver Spring, MD. Report available from FDA, CDER, Advisors and Consultants Staff, HFD-21, 1901 Chapman Avenue, Room 200, Rockville, MD 20852, USA. **4.** 21 CFR 314.510 (Subpart H – Accelerated Approval of New Drugs for Life-Threatening Illnesses). **5.** Kelly DJ, et al. Serum concentrations of penicillin, doxycycline, and ciprofloxacin during prolonged therapy in rhesus monkeys. J Infect Dis 1992; 166: 1184-7. **6.** Friedlander AM, et al. Postexposure prophylaxis against experimental inhalational anthrax. J Infect Dis 1993; 167: 1239-42. **7.** Friedman J, Polifka J. Teratogenic effects of drugs: a resource for clinicians (TERIS). Baltimore, Maryland: Johns Hopkins University Press, 2000:149-195. **8.** Loebstein R, Addis A, Ho E, et al. Pregnancy outcome following gestational exposure to fluoroquinolones: a multicenter prospective controlled study. Antimicrob Agents Chemother. 1998;42(6): 1336-1339. **9.** Schaefer C, Amoura-Elefant E, Vial T, et al. Pregnancy outcome after prenatal quinolone exposure. Evaluation of a case registry of the European network of teratology information services (ENTIS). Eur J Obstet Gynecol Reprod Biol. 1996;69:83-89.

Manufactured for:
Bayer HealthCare
Bayer Pharmaceuticals Corporation
400 Morgan Lane
West Haven, CT 06516
Distributed by:
Schering-Plough
Schering Corporation
Kenilworth, NJ 07033

CIPRO is a registered trademark of Bayer Aktiengesellschaft and is used under license by Schering Corporation.

Rx Only

08918506, R.1 2/05

EN-0706 BAYq3939
5202-4-A-U.S.-14 Printed In U.S.A.

CIPRO® XR ℞

[*sĭ'prō*]

(ciprofloxacin* extended-release tablets)

To reduce the development of drug-resistant bacteria and maintain the effectiveness of CIPRO® XR and other antibacterial drugs, CIPRO XR should be used only to treat or prevent infections that are proven or strongly suspected to be caused by bacteria.

DESCRIPTION

CIPRO XR (ciprofloxacin* extended-release tablets) contains ciprofloxacin, a synthetic broad-spectrum antimicrobial agent for oral administration. CIPRO XR tablets are coated, bilayer tablets consisting of an immediate-release layer and an erosion-matrix type controlled-release layer. The tablets contain a combination of two types of ciprofloxacin drug substance, ciprofloxacin hydrochloride and ciprofloxacin betaine (base). Ciprofloxacin hydrochloride is 1-cyclopropyl-6-fluoro-1,4-dihydro-4-oxo-7- (1-piperazinyl)-3-quinolinecarboxylic acid hydrochloride. It is provided as a mixture of the monohydrate and the sesquihydrate. The empirical formula of the monohydrate is $C_{17}H_{18}FN_3O_3 \cdot HCl \cdot H_2O$ and its molecular weight is 385.8. The empirical formula of the sesquihydrate is $C_{17}H_{18}FN_3O_3 \cdot HCl \cdot 1.5\ H_2O$ and its molecular weight is 394.8. The drug substance is a faintly yellowish to light yellow crystalline substance. The chemical structure of the monohydrate is as follows:

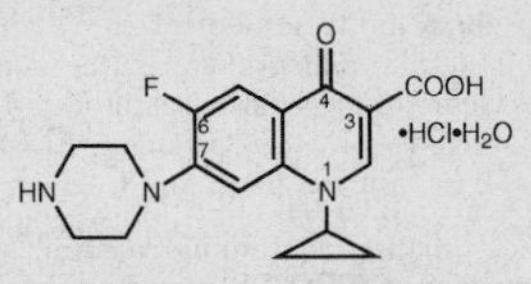

Ciprofloxacin betaine is 1-cyclopropyl-6-fluoro-1, 4-dihydro-4-oxo-7-(1-piperazinyl)-3-quinolinecarboxylic acid. As a hydrate, its empirical formula is $C_{17}H_{18}FN_3O_3 \cdot 3.5\ H_2O$ and its molecular weight is 394.3. It is a pale yellowish to light yellow crystalline substance and its chemical structure is as follows:

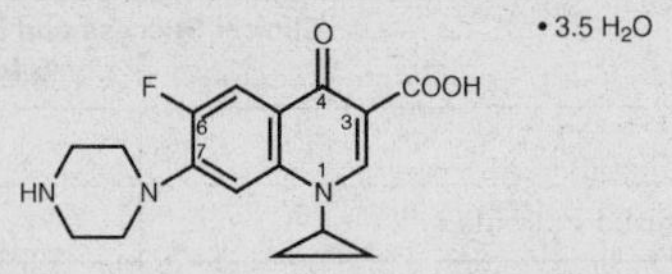

CIPRO XR is available in 500 mg and 1000 mg (ciprofloxacin equivalent) tablet strengths. CIPRO XR tablets are nearly white to slightly yellowish, film-coated, oblong-shaped tablets. Each CIPRO XR 500 mg tablet contains 500 mg of ciprofloxacin as ciprofloxacin HCl (287.5 mg, calculated as ciprofloxacin on the dried basis) and ciprofloxacin[†] (212.6 mg, calculated on the dried basis). Each CIPRO XR 1000 mg tablet contains 1000 mg of ciprofloxacin as ciprofloxacin HCl (574.9 mg, calculated as ciprofloxacin on the dried basis) and ciprofloxacin[†] (425.2 mg, calculated on the dried basis). The inactive ingredients are crospovidone, hypromellose, magnesium stearate, polyethylene glycol, silica colloidal anhydrous, succinic acid, and titanium dioxide.

* as ciprofloxacin[†] and ciprofloxacin hydrochloride
[†] does not comply with the loss on drying test and residue on ignition test of the USP monograph.

CLINICAL PHARMACOLOGY

Absorption

CIPRO XR tablets are formulated to release drug at a slower rate compared to immediate-release tablets. Approximately 35% of the dose is contained within an immediate-release component, while the remaining 65% is contained in a slow-release matrix.

Maximum plasma ciprofloxacin concentrations are attained between 1 and 4 hours after dosing with CIPRO XR. In comparison to the 250 mg and 500 mg ciprofloxacin immediate-release BID treatment, the C_{max} of CIPRO XR 500 mg and 1000 mg once daily are higher than the corresponding BID doses, while the AUCs over 24 hours are equivalent.

The following table compares the pharmacokinetic parameters obtained at steady state for these four treatment regimens (500 mg QD CIPRO XR versus 250 mg BID ciprofloxacin immediate-release tablets and 1000 mg QD CIPRO XR versus 500 mg BID ciprofloxacin immediate-release).

Ciprofloxacin Pharmacokinetics (Mean ± SD) Following CIPRO® and CIPRO XR Administration

	C_{max} (mg/L)	AUC_{0-24h} (mg•h/L)	$T_{1/2}$(hr)	T_{max}(hr)§
CIPRO XR 500 mg QD	1.59 ± 0.43	7.97 ± 1.87	6.6 ± 1.4	1.5 (1.0–2.5)
CIPRO 250 mg BID	1.14 ± 0.23	8.25 ± 2.15	4.8 ± 0.6	1.0 (0.5–2.5)
CIPRO XR 1000 mg QD	3.11 ± 1.08	16.83 ± 5.65	6.31 ± 0.72	2.0 (1–4)
CIPRO 500 mg BID	2.06 ± 0.41	17.04 ± 4.79	5.66 ± 0.89	2.0 (0.5–3.5)

§ median (range)

[See table above]

Results of the pharmacokinetic studies demonstrate that CIPRO XR may be administered with or without food (e.g. high-fat and low-fat meals or under fasted conditions).

Distribution

The volume of distribution calculated for intravenous ciprofloxacin is approximately 2.1–2.7 L/kg. Studies with the oral and intravenous forms of ciprofloxacin have demonstrated penetration of ciprofloxacin into a variety of tissues. The binding of ciprofloxacin to serum proteins is 20% to 40%, which is not likely to be high enough to cause significant protein binding interactions with other drugs. Following administration of a single dose of CIPRO XR, ciprofloxacin concentrations in urine collected up to 4 hours after dosing averaged over 300 mg/L for both the 500 mg and 1000 mg tablets; in urine excreted from 12 to 24 hours after dosing, ciprofloxacin concentration averaged 27 mg/L for the 500 mg tablet, and 58 mg/L for the 1000 mg tablet.

Metabolism

Four metabolites of ciprofloxacin were identified in human urine. The metabolites have antimicrobial activity, but are less active than unchanged ciprofloxacin. The primary metabolites are oxociprofloxacin (M3) and sulfociprofloxacin (M2), each accounting for roughly 3% to 8% of the total dose. Other minor metabolites are desethylene ciprofloxacin (M1), and formylciprofloxacin (M4). The relative proportion of drug and metabolite in serum corresponds to the composition found in urine. Excretion of these metabolites was essentially complete by 24 hours after dosing.

Elimination

The elimination kinetics of ciprofloxacin are similar for the immediate-release and the CIPRO XR tablet. In studies comparing the CIPRO XR and immediate-release ciprofloxacin, approximately 35% of an orally administered dose was excreted in the urine as unchanged drug for both formulations. The urinary excretion of ciprofloxacin is virtually complete within 24 hours after dosing. The renal clearance of ciprofloxacin, which is approximately 300 mL/minute, exceeds the normal glomerular filtration rate of 120 mL/minute. Thus, active tubular secretion would seem to play a significant role in its elimination. Co-administration of probenecid with immediate-release ciprofloxacin results in about a 50% reduction in the ciprofloxacin renal clearance and a 50% increase in its concentration in the systemic circulation. Although bile concentrations of ciprofloxacin are several fold higher than serum concentrations after oral dosing with the immediate-release tablet, only a small amount of the dose administered is recovered from the bile as unchanged drug. An additional 1% to 2% of the dose is recovered from the bile in the form of metabolites. Approximately 20% to 35% of an oral dose of immediate-release ciprofloxacin is recovered from the feces within 5 days after dosing. This may arise from either biliary clearance or transintestinal elimination.

Special Populations

Pharmacokinetic studies of the immediate-release oral tablet (single dose) and intravenous (single and multiple dose) forms of ciprofloxacin indicate that plasma concentrations of ciprofloxacin are higher in elderly subjects (> 65 years) as compared to young adults. C_{max} is increased 16% to 40%, and mean AUC is increased approximately 30%, which can be at least partially attributed to decreased renal clearance in the elderly. Elimination half-life is only slightly (~20%) prolonged in the elderly. These differences are not considered clinically significant. (See **PRECAUTIONS, Geriatric Use.**)

In patients with reduced renal function, the half-life of ciprofloxacin is slightly prolonged. No dose adjustment is required for patients with uncomplicated urinary tract infections receiving 500 mg CIPRO XR. For complicated urinary tract infection and acute uncomplicated pyelonephritis, where 1000 mg is the appropriate dose, the dosage of CIPRO XR should be reduced to CIPRO XR 500 mg q24h in patients with creatinine clearance below 30 mL/min. (See **DOSAGE AND ADMINISTRATION.**)

In studies in patients with stable chronic cirrhosis, no significant changes in ciprofloxacin pharmacokinetics have been observed. The kinetics of ciprofloxacin in patients with acute hepatic insufficiency, however, have not been fully elucidated. (See **DOSAGE AND ADMINISTRATION.**)

Drug-drug Interactions

Previous studies with immediate-release ciprofloxacin have shown that concomitant administration of ciprofloxacin with theophylline decreases the clearance of theophylline resulting in elevated serum theophylline levels and increased risk of a patient developing CNS or other adverse reactions. Ciprofloxacin also decreases caffeine clearance and inhibits the formation of paraxanthine after caffeine administration. Absorption of ciprofloxacin is significantly reduced by concomitant administration of multivalent cation-containing products such as magnesium/aluminum antacids, sucralfate, VIDEX® (didanosine) chewable/buffered tablets or pediatric powder, or products containing calcium, iron, or zinc. (See **PRECAUTIONS, Drug Interactions** and **Information for Patients**, and **DOSAGE AND ADMINISTRATION.**)

Antacids: When CIPRO XR given as a single 1000 mg dose was administered two hours before, or four hours after a magnesium/aluminum-containing antacid (900 mg aluminum hydroxide and 600 mg magnesium hydroxide as a single oral dose) to 18 healthy volunteers, there was a 4% and 19% reduction, respectively, in the mean C_{max} of ciprofloxacin. The reduction in the mean AUC was 24% and 26%, respectively. CIPRO XR should be administered at least 2 hours before or 6 hours after antacids containing magnesium or aluminum, as well as sucralfate, VIDEX® (didanosine) chewable/buffered tablets or pediatric powder, other highly buffered drugs, metal cations such as iron, and multivitamin preparations with zinc. Although CIPRO XR may be taken with meals that include milk, concomitant administration with dairy products or with calcium-fortified juices alone should be avoided, since decreased absorption is possible. (See **PRECAUTIONS, Information for Patients** and **Drug Interactions,** and **DOSAGE AND ADMINISTRATION.**)

Omeprazole: When CIPRO XR was administered as a single 1000 mg dose concomitantly with omeprazole (40 mg once daily for three days) to 18 healthy volunteers, the mean AUC and C_{max} of ciprofloxacin were reduced by 20% and 23%, respectively. The clinical significance of this interaction has not been determined. (See **PRECAUTIONS, Drug Interactions.**)

MICROBIOLOGY

Ciprofloxacin has *in vitro* activity against a wide range of gram-negative and gram-positive organisms. The bactericidal action of ciprofloxacin results from inhibition of topoisomerase II (DNA gyrase) and topoisomerase IV (both Type II topoisomerases), which are required for bacterial DNA replication, transcription, repair, and recombination. The mechanism of action of quinolones, including ciprofloxacin, is different from that of other antimicrobial agents such as beta-lactams, macrolides, tetracyclines, or aminoglycosides; therefore, organisms resistant to these drugs may be susceptible to ciprofloxacin. There is no known cross-resistance between ciprofloxacin and other classes of antimicrobials. Resistance to ciprofloxacin *in vitro* develops slowly (multiple-step mutation). Resistance to ciprofloxacin due to spontaneous mutations occurs at a general frequency of between $< 10^{-9}$ to 1×10^{-6}.

Ciprofloxacin is slightly less active when tested at acidic pH. The inoculum size has little effect when tested in vitro. The minimal bactericidal concentration (MBC) generally does not exceed the minimal inhibitory concentration (MIC) by more than a factor of 2.

Ciprofloxacin has been shown to be active against most strains of the following microorganisms, both in vitro and in clinical infections as described in the **INDICATIONS AND USAGE** section.

Aerobic gram-positive microorganisms

Enterococcus faecalis (Many strains are only moderately susceptible.)

Staphylococcus saprophyticus

Aerobic gram-negative microorganisms

Escherichia coli

Klebsiella pneumoniae

Proteus mirabilis

Pseudomonas aeruginosa

The following in vitro data are available, but their clinical significance is unknown.

Ciprofloxacin exhibits in vitro minimum inhibitory concentrations (MICs) of 1 μg/mL or less against most (≥ 90%) strains of the following microorganisms; however, the safety and effectiveness of CIPRO XR in treating clinical infections due to these microorganisms have not been established in adequate and well-controlled clinical trials.

Aerobic gram-negative microorganisms

Citrobacter koseri	Morganella morganii
Citrobacter freundii	Proteus vulgaris
Edwardsiella tarda	Providencia rettgeri
Enterobacter aerogenes	Providencia stuartii
Enterobacter cloacae	Serratia marcescens
Klebsiella oxytoca	

Susceptibility Tests

Dilution Techniques: Quantitative methods are used to determine antimicrobial minimal inhibitory concentrations (MICs). These MICs provide estimates of the susceptibility of bacteria to antimicrobial compounds. The MICs should be determined using a standardized procedure. Standardized procedures are based on a dilution method[1] (broth or agar) or equivalent with standardized inoculum concentrations and standardized concentrations of ciprofloxacin. The MIC values should be interpreted according to the following criteria:

For testing Enterobacteriaceae, Enterococcus species, Pseudomonas aeruginosa, and Staphylococcus species:

MIC (μg/mL)	Interpretation
≤ 1	Susceptible (S)
2	Intermediate (I)
≥ 4	Resistant (R)

A report of "Susceptible" indicates that the pathogen is likely to be inhibited if the antimicrobial compound in the blood reaches the concentrations usually achievable. A report of "Intermediate" indicates that the result should be considered equivocal, and, if the microorganism is not fully susceptible to alternative, clinically feasible drugs, the test should be repeated. This category implies possible clinical applicability in body sites where the drug is physiologically concentrated or in situations where high dosage of drug can be used. This category also provides a buffer zone which prevents small uncontrolled technical factors from causing major discrepancies in interpretation. A report of "Resistant" indicates that the pathogen is not likely to be inhibited if the antimicrobial compound in the blood reaches the concentrations usually achievable; other therapy should be selected.

Standardized susceptibility test procedures require the use of laboratory control microorganisms to control the technical aspects of the laboratory procedures. Standard ciprofloxacin powder should provide the following MIC values:

Microorganism		MIC Range (μg/mL)
Enterococcus faecalis	ATCC 29212	0.25 – 2.0
Escherichia coli	ATCC 25922	0.004 – 0.015
Staphylococcus aureus	ATCC 29213	0.12 – 0.5
Pseudomonas aeruginosa	ATCC 27853	0.25 – 1

Diffusion Techniques: Quantitative methods that require measurement of zone diameters also provide reproducible estimates of the susceptibility of bacteria to antimicrobial compounds. One such standardized procedure[2] requires the use of standardized inoculum concentrations. This procedure uses paper disks impregnated with 5-μg ciprofloxacin to test the susceptibility of microorganisms to ciprofloxacin. Reports from the laboratory providing results of the standard single-disk susceptibility test with a 5-μg ciprofloxacin disk should be interpreted according to the following criteria:

For testing Enterobacteriaceae, Enterococcus species, Pseudomonas aeruginosa, and Staphylococcus species:

Zone Diameter (mm)	Interpretation
≥ 21	Susceptible (S)
16–20	Intermediate (I)
≤ 15	Resistant (R)

Interpretation should be as stated above for results using dilution techniques. Interpretation involves correlation of the diameter obtained in the disk test with the MIC for ciprofloxacin.

As with standardized dilution techniques, diffusion methods require the use of laboratory control microorganisms that are used to control the technical aspects of the laboratory

procedures. For the diffusion technique, the 5-μg ciprofloxacin disk should provide the following zone diameters in these laboratory test quality control strains:

Microorganism		Zone Diameter (mm)
Escherichia coli	ATCC 25922	30 – 40
Staphylococcus aureus	ATCC 25923	22 – 30
Pseudomonas aeruginosa	ATCC 27853	25 – 33

INDICATIONS AND USAGE

CIPRO XR is indicated only for the treatment of urinary tract infections, including acute uncomplicated pyelonephritis, caused by susceptible strains of the designated microorganisms as listed below. CIPRO XR and ciprofloxacin immediate-release tablets are not interchangeable. Please see **DOSAGE AND ADMINISTRATION** for specific recommendations.

Uncomplicated Urinary Tract Infections (Acute Cystitis) caused by Escherichia coli, Proteus mirabilis, Enterococcus faecalis, or Staphylococcus saprophyticus[a].

Complicated Urinary Tract Infections caused by Escherichia coli, Klebsiella pneumoniae, Enterococcus faecalis, Proteus mirabilis, or Pseudomonas aeruginosa [a].

Acute Uncomplicated Pyelonephritis caused by Escherichia coli.

[a] Treatment of infections due to this organism in the organ system was studied in fewer than 10 patients.

THE SAFETY AND EFFICACY OF CIPRO XR IN TREATING INFECTIONS OTHER THAN URINARY TRACT INFECTIONS HAS NOT BEEN DEMONSTRATED. Appropriate culture and susceptibility tests should be performed before treatment in order to isolate and identify organisms causing infection and to determine their susceptibility to ciprofloxacin. Therapy with CIPRO XR may be initiated before results of these tests are known; once results become available appropriate therapy should be continued. Culture and susceptibility testing performed periodically during therapy will provide information not only on the therapeutic effect of the antimicrobial agent but also on the possible emergence of bacterial resistance.

To reduce the development of drug-resistant bacteria and maintain the effectiveness of CIPRO XR and other antibacterial drugs, CIPRO XR should be used only to treat or prevent infections that are proven or strongly suspected to be caused by susceptible bacteria. When culture and susceptibility information are available, they should be considered in selecting or modifying antibacterial therapy. In the absence of such data, local epidemiology and susceptibility patterns may contribute to the empiric selection of therapy.

CONTRAINDICATIONS

CIPRO XR is contraindicated in persons with a history of hypersensitivity to ciprofloxacin or any member of the quinolone class of antimicrobial agents.

WARNINGS

THE SAFETY AND EFFECTIVENESS OF CIPRO XR IN PEDIATRIC PATIENTS AND ADOLESCENTS (UNDER THE AGE OF 18 YEARS), PREGNANT WOMEN, AND NURSING WOMEN HAVE NOT BEEN ESTABLISHED. (See **PRECAUTIONS: Pediatric Use, Pregnancy,** and **Nursing Mothers** subsections.) The oral administration of ciprofloxacin caused lameness in immature dogs. Histopathological examination of the weight-bearing joints of these dogs revealed permanent lesions of the cartilage. Related quinolone-class drugs also produce erosions of cartilage of weight-bearing joints and other signs of arthropathy in immature animals of various species. (See **ANIMAL PHARMACOLOGY**.)

Convulsions, increased intracranial pressure, and toxic psychosis have been reported in patients receiving quinolones, including ciprofloxacin. Ciprofloxacin may also cause central nervous system (CNS) events including: dizziness, confusion, tremors, hallucinations, depression, and, rarely, suicidal thoughts or acts. These reactions may occur following the first dose. If these reactions occur in patients receiving ciprofloxacin, the drug should be discontinued and appropriate measures instituted. As with all quinolones, ciprofloxacin should be used with caution in patients with known or suspected CNS disorders that may predispose to seizures or lower the seizure threshold (e.g. severe cerebral arteriosclerosis, epilepsy), or in the presence of other risk factors that may predispose to seizures or lower the seizure threshold (e.g. certain drug therapy, renal dysfunction). (See **PRECAUTIONS: General, Information for Patients, Drug Interactions** and **ADVERSE REACTIONS.**)

SERIOUS AND FATAL REACTIONS HAVE BEEN REPORTED IN PATIENTS RECEIVING CONCURRENT ADMINISTRATION OF CIPROFLOXACIN AND THEOPHYLLINE. These reactions have included cardiac arrest, seizure, status epilepticus, and respiratory failure. Although similar serious adverse effects have been reported in patients receiving theophylline alone, the possibility that these reactions may be potentiated by ciprofloxacin cannot be eliminated. If concomitant use cannot be avoided, serum levels of theophylline should be monitored and dosage adjustments made as appropriate. Serious and occasionally fatal hypersensitivity (anaphylactic) reactions, some following the first dose, have been reported in patients receiving quinolone therapy. Some reactions were accompanied by cardiovascular collapse, loss of consciousness, tingling, pharyngeal or facial edema, dyspnea, urticaria, and itching. Only a few patients had a his-

tory of hypersensitivity reactions. Serious anaphylactic reactions require immediate emergency treatment with epinephrine. Oxygen, intravenous steroids, and airway management, including intubation, should be administered as indicated.

Severe hypersensitivity reactions characterized by rash, fever, eosinophilia, jaundice, and hepatic necrosis with fatal outcome have also been rarely reported in patients receiving ciprofloxacin along with other drugs. The possibility that these reactions were related to ciprofloxacin cannot be excluded. Ciprofloxacin should be discontinued at the first appearance of a skin rash or any other sign of hypersensitivity.

Pseudomembranous colitis has been reported with nearly all antibacterial agents, including ciprofloxacin, and may range in severity from mild to life-threatening. Therefore, it is important to consider this diagnosis in patients who present with diarrhea subsequent to the administration of antibacterial agents.

Treatment with antibacterial agents alters the normal flora of the colon and may permit overgrowth of clostridia. Studies indicate that a toxin produced by Clostridium difficile is one primary cause of "antibiotic-associated colitis."

If a diagnosis of pseudomembranous colitis is established, therapeutic measures should be initiated. Mild cases of pseudomembranous colitis usually respond to drug discontinuation alone. In moderate to severe cases, consideration should be given to management with fluids and electrolytes, protein supplementation, and treatment with an antibacterial drug clinically effective against C. difficile colitis. Drugs that inhibit peristalsis should be avoided.

Peripheral neuropathy: Rare cases of sensory or sensorimotor axonal polyneuropathy affecting small and/or large axons resulting in paresthesias, hypoesthesias, dysesthesias and weakness have been reported in patients receiving quinolones, including ciprofloxacin. Ciprofloxacin should be discontinued if the patient experiences symptoms of neuropathy including pain, burning, tingling, numbness, and/or weakness, or is found to have deficits in light touch, pain, temperature, position sense, vibratory sensation, and/or motor strength in order to prevent the development of an irreversible condition.

Tendon Effects: Ruptures of the shoulder, hand, Achilles tendon or other tendons that required surgical repair or resulted in prolonged disability have been reported in patients receiving quinolones, including ciprofloxacin. Post-marketing surveillance reports indicate that this risk may be increased in patients receiving concomitant corticosteroids, especially the elderly. Ciprofloxacin should be discontinued if the patient experiences pain, inflammation, or rupture of a tendon. Patients should rest and refrain from exercise until the diagnosis of tendonitis or tendon rupture has been excluded. Tendon rupture can occur during or after therapy with quinolones, including ciprofloxacin.

PRECAUTIONS

General: Crystals of ciprofloxacin have been observed rarely in the urine of human subjects but more frequently in the urine of laboratory animals, which is usually alkaline. (See **ANIMAL PHARMACOLOGY**.) Crystalluria related to ciprofloxacin has been reported only rarely in humans because human urine is usually acidic. Alkalinity of the urine should be avoided in patients receiving ciprofloxacin. Patients should be well hydrated to prevent the formation of highly concentrated urine.

Quinolones, including ciprofloxacin, may also cause central nervous system (CNS) events, including: nervousness, agitation, insomnia, anxiety, nightmares or paranoia. (See **WARNINGS, Information for Patients**, and **Drug Interactions**).

Moderate to severe phototoxicity manifested as an exaggerated sunburn reaction has been observed in patients who are exposed to direct sunlight while receiving some members of the quinolone class of drugs. Excessive sunlight should be avoided. Therapy should be discontinued if phototoxicity occurs.

Prescribing CIPRO XR in the absence of a proven or strongly suspected bacterial infection or a prophylactic indication is unlikely to provide benefit to the patient and increases the risk of the development of drug-resistant bacteria.

Information for Patients:

Patients should be advised:

• that antibacterial drugs including CIPRO XR should only be used to treat bacterial infections. They do not treat viral infections (e.g., the common cold). When CIPRO XR is prescribed to treat a bacterial infection, patients should be told that although it is common to feel better early in the course of therapy, the medication should be taken exactly as directed. Skipping doses or not completing the full course of therapy may (1) decrease the effectiveness of the immediate treatment and (2) increase the likelihood that bacteria will develop resistance and will not be treatable by CIPRO XR or other antibacterial drugs in the future.

• that CIPRO XR may be taken with or without meals and to drink fluids liberally. As with other quinolones, concurrent administration with magnesium/aluminum antacids, or sucralfate, VIDEX® (didanosine) chewable/buffered tablets or pediatric powder, other highly buffered drugs, or with other products containing calcium, iron, or zinc should be avoided. CIPRO XR may be taken two hours before or six hours after taking these products. (See

Continued on next page

Cipro XR—Cont.

CLINICAL PHARMACOLOGY, Drug-drug Interactions, DOSAGE AND ADMINISTRATION, and **PRECAUTIONS, Drug Interactions.**) CIPRO XR should not be taken with dairy products (like milk or yogurt) or calcium-fortified juices alone since absorption of ciprofloxacin may be significantly reduced; however, CIPRO XR may be taken with a meal that contains these products. (See **CLINICAL PHARMACOLOGY, Drug-drug Interactions, DOSAGE AND ADMINISTRATION**, and **PRECAUTIONS, Drug Interactions.**)

- If the patient should forget to take CIPRO XR at the usual time, he/she may take the dose later in the day. Do not take more than one CIPRO XR tablet per day even if a patient misses a dose. Swallow the CIPRO XR tablet whole. **DO NOT SPLIT, CRUSH, OR CHEW THE TABLET.**
- that ciprofloxacin may be associated with hypersensitivity reactions, even following a single dose, and to discontinue CIPRO XR at the first sign of a skin rash or other allergic reaction.
- to avoid excessive sunlight or artificial ultraviolet light while receiving CIPRO XR and to discontinue therapy if phototoxicity occurs.
- that peripheral neuropathies have been associated with ciprofloxacin use. If symptoms of peripheral neuropathy including pain, burning, tingling, numbness and/or weakness develop, they should discontinue treatment and contact their physicians.
- that if they experience pain, inflammation, or rupture of a tendon to discontinue treatment, to inform their physician, and to rest and refrain from exercise.
- that CIPRO XR may cause dizziness and lightheadedness; therefore, patients should know how they react to this drug before they operate an automobile or machinery or engage in activities requiring mental alertness or coordination.
- that CIPRO XR may increase the effects of theophylline and caffeine. There is a possibility of caffeine accumulation when products containing caffeine are consumed while taking quinolones.
- that convulsions have been reported in patients receiving quinolones, including ciprofloxacin, and to notify their physician before taking CIPRO XR if there is a history of this condition.

Drug Interactions: As with some other quinolones, concurrent administration of ciprofloxacin with theophylline may lead to elevated serum concentrations of theophylline and prolongation of its elimination half-life. This may result in increased risk of theophylline-related adverse reactions. (See **WARNINGS**.) If concomitant use cannot be avoided, serum levels of theophylline should be monitored and dosage adjustments made as appropriate.

Some quinolones, including ciprofloxacin, have also been shown to interfere with the metabolism of caffeine. This may lead to reduced clearance of caffeine and a prolongation of its serum half-life.

Concurrent administration of a quinolone, including ciprofloxacin, with multivalent cation-containing products such as magnesium/aluminum antacids, sucralfate, VIDEX® (didanosine) chewable/buffered tablets or pediatric powder, other highly buffered drugs, or products containing calcium, iron, or zinc may substantially interfere with the absorption of the quinolone, resulting in serum and urine levels considerably lower than desired. CIPRO XR should be administered at least 2 hours before or 6 hours after antacids containing magnesium or aluminum, as well as sucralfate, VIDEX® (didanosine) chewable/buffered tablets or pediatric powder, other highly buffered drugs, metal cations such as iron, and multivitamin preparations with zinc. (See **CLINICAL PHARMACOLOGY, Drug-drug Interactions, PRECAUTIONS, Information for Patients**, and **DOSAGE AND ADMINISTRATION**.)

Histamine H_2-receptor antagonists appear to have no significant effect on the bioavailability of ciprofloxacin.

Absorption of the CIPRO XR tablet was slightly diminished (20%) when given concomitantly with omeprazole. (See **CLINICAL PHARMACOLOGY, Drug-drug Interactions**.)

Altered serum levels of phenytoin (increased and decreased) have been reported in patients receiving concomitant ciprofloxacin.

The concomitant administration of ciprofloxacin with the sulfonylurea glyburide has, on rare occasions, resulted in severe hypoglycemia.

Some quinolones, including ciprofloxacin, have been associated with transient elevations in serum creatinine in patients receiving cyclosporine concomitantly.

Quinolones, including ciprofloxacin, have been reported to enhance the effects of the oral anticoagulant warfarin or its derivatives. When these products are administered concomitantly, prothrombin time or other suitable coagulation tests should be closely monitored.

Probenecid interferes with renal tubular secretion of ciprofloxacin and produces an increase in the level of ciprofloxacin in the serum. This should be considered if patients are receiving both drugs concomitantly.

Renal tubular transport of methotrexate may be inhibited by concomitant administration of ciprofloxacin potentially leading to increased plasma levels of methotrexate. This might increase the risk of methotrexate associated toxic reactions. Therefore, patients under methotrexate therapy should be carefully monitored when concomitant ciprofloxacin therapy is indicated.

Metoclopramide significantly accelerates the absorption of oral ciprofloxacin resulting in a shorter time to reach maximum plasma concentrations. No significant effect was observed on the bioavailability of ciprofloxacin.

Non-steroidal anti-inflammatory drugs (but not acetyl salicylic acid) in combination of very high doses of quinolones have been shown to provoke convulsions in pre-clinical studies.

Carcinogenesis, Mutagenesis, Impairment of Fertility: Eight *in vitro* mutagenicity tests have been conducted with ciprofloxacin, and the test results are listed below:

Salmonella/Microsome Test (Negative)
E. coli DNA Repair Assay (Negative)
Mouse Lymphoma Cell Forward Mutation Assay (Positive)
Chinese Hamster V_{79} Cell HGPRT Test (Negative)
Syrian Hamster Embryo Cell Transformation Assay (Negative)
Saccharomyces cerevisiae Point Mutation Assay (Negative)
Saccharomyces cerevisiae Mitotic Crossover and Gene Conversion Assay (Negative)
Rat Hepatocyte DNA Repair Assay (Positive)

Thus, 2 of the 8 tests were positive, but results of the following 3 *in vivo* test systems gave negative results:

Rat Hepatocyte DNA Repair Assay
Micronucleus Test (Mice)
Dominant Lethal Test (Mice)

Ciprofloxacin was not carcinogenic or tumorigenic in 2-year carcinogenicity studies with rats and mice at daily oral dose levels of 250 and 750 mg/kg, respectively (approximately 2 and 3 -fold greater than the 1000 mg daily human dose based upon body surface area).

Results from photo co-carcinogenicity testing indicate that ciprofloxacin does not reduce the time to appearance of UV-induced skin tumors as compared to vehicle control. Hairless (Skh-1) mice were exposed to UVA light for 3.5 hours five times every two weeks for up to 78 weeks while concurrently being administered ciprofloxacin. The time to development of the first skin tumors was 50 weeks in mice treated concomitantly with UVA and ciprofloxacin (mouse dose approximately equal to the maximum recommended daily human dose of 1000 mg based upon mg/m^2), as opposed to 34 weeks when animals were treated with both UVA and vehicle. The times to development of skin tumors ranged from 16-32 weeks in mice treated concomitantly with UVA and other quinolones.

In this model, mice treated with ciprofloxacin alone did not develop skin or systemic tumors. There are no data from similar models using pigmented mice and/or fully haired mice. The clinical significance of these findings to humans is unknown.

Fertility studies performed in rats at oral doses of ciprofloxacin up to 100 mg/kg (1.0 times the highest recommended daily human dose of 1000 mg based upon body surface area) revealed no evidence of impairment.

Pregnancy: Teratogenic Effects. Pregnancy Category C: There are no adequate and well-controlled studies in pregnant women. An expert review of published data on experiences with ciprofloxacin use during pregnancy by TERIS - the Teratogen Information System – concluded that therapeutic doses during pregnancy are unlikely to pose a substantial teratogenic risk (quantity and quality of data=fair), but the data are insufficient to state there is no risk.

A controlled prospective observational study followed 200 women exposed to fluoroquinolones (52.5% exposed to ciprofloxacin and 68% first trimester exposures) during gestation. In utero exposure to fluoroquinolones during embryogenesis was not associated with increased risk of major malformations. The reported rates of major congenital malformations were 2.2% for the fluoroquinolone group and 2.6% for the control group (background incidence of major malformations is 1-5%). Rates of spontaneous abortions, prematurity and low birth weight did not differ between the groups and there were no clinically significant musculoskeletal dysfunctions up to one year of age in the ciprofloxacin exposed children.

Another prospective follow-up study reported on 549 pregnancies with fluoroquinolone exposure (93% first trimester exposures). There were 70 ciprofloxacin exposures, all within the first trimester. The malformation rates among live-born babies exposed to ciprofloxacin and to fluoroquinolones overall were both within background incidence ranges. No specific patterns of congenital abnormalities were found. The study did not reveal any clear adverse reactions due to in utero exposure to ciprofloxacin.

No differences in the rates of prematurity, spontaneous abortions, or birth weight were seen in women exposed to ciprofloxacin during pregnancy. However, these small post-marketing epidemiology studies, of which most experience is from short term, first trimester exposure, are insufficient to evaluate the risk for the less common defects or to permit reliable and definitive conclusions regarding the safety of ciprofloxacin in pregnant women and their developing fetuses. Ciprofloxacin should not be used during pregnancy unless potential benefit justifies the potential risk to both fetus and mother (see **WARNINGS**).

Reproduction studies have been performed in rats and mice using oral doses up to 100 mg/kg (0.7 and 0.4 times the maximum daily human dose of 1000 mg based upon body surface area, respectively) and have revealed no evidence of harm to the fetus due to ciprofloxacin. In rabbits, ciprofloxacin (30 and 100 mg/kg orally) produced gastrointestinal disturbances resulting in maternal weight loss and

an increased incidence of abortion, but no teratogenicity was observed at either dose. After intravenous administration of doses up to 20 mg/kg, no maternal toxicity was produced in the rabbit, and no embryotoxicity or teratogenicity was observed.

Nursing Mothers: Ciprofloxacin is excreted in human milk. The amount of ciprofloxacin absorbed by the nursing infant is unknown. Because of the potential for serious adverse reactions in infants nursing from mothers taking ciprofloxacin, a decision should be made whether to discontinue nursing or to discontinue the drug, taking into account the importance of the drug to the mother.

Pediatric Use: Safety and effectiveness of CIPRO XR in pediatric patients and adolescents less than 18 years of age have not been established. Ciprofloxacin causes arthropathy in juvenile animals. (See **WARNINGS**.)

Geriatric Use: In a large, prospective, randomized CIPRO XR clinical trial in complicated urinary tract infections, 49% (509/1035) of the patients were 65 and over, while 30% (308/1035) were 75 and over. No overall differences in safety or effectiveness were observed between these subjects and younger subjects, and clinical experience with other formulations of ciprofloxacin has not identified differences in responses between the elderly and younger patients, but greater sensitivity of some older individuals cannot be ruled out. Ciprofloxacin is known to be substantially excreted by the kidney, and the risk of adverse reactions may be greater in patients with impaired renal function. No alteration of dosage is necessary for patients greater than 65 years of age with normal renal function. However, since some older individuals experience reduced renal function by virtue of their advanced age, care should be taken in dose selection for elderly patients, and renal function monitoring may be useful in these patients. (See **CLINICAL PHARMACOLOGY** and **DOSAGE AND ADMINISTRATION**.)

ADVERSE REACTIONS

Clinical trials in patients with urinary tract infections enrolled 961 patients treated with 500 mg or 1000 mg CIPRO XR. Most adverse events reported were described as mild to moderate in severity and required no treatment. The overall incidence, type and distribution of adverse events were similar in patients receiving both 500 mg and 1000 mg of CIPRO XR. Because clinical trials are conducted under widely varying conditions, adverse reaction rates observed in clinical trials of a drug cannot be directly compared to rates observed in clinical trials of another drug and may not reflect the rates observed in practice. The adverse reaction information from clinical studies does, however, provide a basis for identifying the adverse events that appear to be related to drug use and for approximating rates.

In the clinical trial of uncomplicated urinary tract infection, CIPRO XR (500 mg once daily) in 444 patients was compared to ciprofloxacin immediate-release tablets (250 mg twice daily) in 447 patients for 3 days. Discontinuations due to adverse reactions thought to be drug-related occurred in 0.2% (1/444) of patients in the CIPRO XR arm and in 0% (0/447) of patients in the control arm.

In the clinical trial of complicated urinary tract infection and acute uncomplicated pyelonephritis, CIPRO XR (1000 mg once daily) in 517 patients was compared to ciprofloxacin immediate-release tablets (500 mg twice daily) in 518 patients for 7 to 14 days. Discontinuations due to adverse reactions thought to be drug-related occurred in 3.1% (16/517) of patients in the CIPRO XR arm and in 2.3% (12/518) of patients in the control arm. The most common reasons for discontinuation in the CIPRO XR arm were nausea/vomiting (4 patients) and dizziness (3 patients). In the control arm the most common reason for discontinuation was nausea/vomiting (3 patients).

In these clinical trials, the following events occurred in ≥2% of all CIPRO XR patients, regardless of drug relationship: nausea (4%), headache (3%), dizziness (2%), diarrhea (2%), vomiting (2%) and vaginal moniliasis (2%).

Adverse events, judged by investigators to be at least possibly drug-related, occurring in greater than or equal to 1% of all CIPRO XR treated patients were: nausea (3%), diarrhea (2%), headache (1%), dyspepsia (1%), dizziness (1%), and vaginal moniliasis (1%). Vomiting (1%) occurred in the 1000 mg group.

Additional uncommon events, judged by investigators to be at least possibly drug-related, that occurred in less than 1% of CIPRO XR treated patients were:

BODY AS A WHOLE: abdominal pain, asthenia, malaise, photosensitivity reaction
CARDIOVASCULAR: bradycardia, migraine, syncope
DIGESTIVE: anorexia, constipation, dry mouth, flatulence, liver function tests abnormal, thirst
HEMIC/LYMPHATIC: prothrombin decrease
CENTRAL NERVOUS SYSTEM: abnormal dreams, depersonalization, depression, hypertonia, incoordination, insomnia, somnolence, tremor, vertigo
METABOLIC: hyperglycemia
SKIN/APPENDAGES: dry skin, maculopapular rash, pruritus, rash, skin disorder, urticaria, vesiculobullous rash
SPECIAL SENSES: diplopia, taste perversion
UROGENITAL: dysmenorrhea, hematuria, kidney function abnormal, vaginitis

The following additional adverse events, some of them life threatening, regardless of incidence or relationship to drug, have been reported during clinical trials and from worldwide post-marketing experience in patients given ciprofloxacin (includes all formulations, all dosages, all drug-therapy durations, and all indications). Because these reactions have been reported voluntarily from a population of uncertain size, it is not always possible to reliably estimate their frequency or a causal relationship to drug exposure. The events in alphabetical order are:

abnormal gait, achiness, acidosis, agitation, agranulocytosis, allergic reactions (ranging from urticaria to anaphylactic reactions and including life-threatening anaphylactic shock), amylase increase, anemia, angina pectoris, angioedema, anosmia, anxiety, arrhythmia, arthralgia, ataxia, atrial flutter, bleeding diathesis, blurred vision, bronchospasm, *C. difficile* associated diarrhea, candidiasis (cutaneous, oral), candiduria, cardiac murmur, cardiopulmonary arrest, cardiovascular collapse, cerebral thrombosis, chills, cholestatic jaundice, chromatopsia, confusion, convulsion, delirium, drowsiness, dysphagia, dysphasia, dyspnea, edema (conjunctivae, face, hands, laryngeal, lips, lower extremities, neck, pulmonary), epistaxis, erythema multiforme, erythema nodosum, exfoliative dermatitis, fever, fixed eruptions, flushing, gastrointestinal bleeding, gout (flare up), grand mal convulsion, gynecomastia, hallucinations, hearing loss, hemolytic anemia, hemoptysis, hemorrhagic cystitis, hepatic failure, hepatic necrosis, hepatitis, hiccup, hyperesthesia, hyperpigmentation, hypertension, hypertonia, hypesthesia, hypotension, ileus, interstitial nephritis, intestinal perforation, jaundice, joint stiffness, lethargy, lightheadedness, lipase increase, lymphadenopathy, manic reaction, marrow depression, migraine, moniliasis (oral, gastrointestinal, vaginal), myalgia, myasthenia, myasthenia gravis (possible exacerbation), myocardial infarction, myoclonus, nephritis, nightmares, nystagmus, oral ulceration, pain (arm, back, breast, chest, epigastric, eye, extremities, foot, jaw, neck, oral mucosa), palpitation, pancreatitis, pancytopenia, paranoia, paresthesia, peripheral neuropathy, perspiration (increased), petechia, phlebitis, phobia, pleural effusion, polyuria, postural hypotension, prothrombin time prolongation, pseudomembranous colitis (the onset of symptoms may occur during or after antimicrobial treatment), pulmonary embolism, purpura, renal calculi, renal failure, respiratory arrest, respiratory distress, restlessness, serum sickness-like reaction, Stevens-Johnson syndrome, sweating, tachycardia, taste loss, tendinitis, tendon rupture, tinnitus, torsade de pointes, toxic epidermal necrolysis (Lyell's syndrome), toxic psychosis, twitching, unresponsiveness, urethral bleeding, urinary retention, urination (frequent), vaginal pruritus, vasculitis, ventricular ectopy, vesicles, visual acuity (decreased), visual disturbances (flashing lights, change in color perception, overbrightness of lights).

Laboratory Changes:

The following adverse laboratory changes, in alphabetical order, regardless of incidence or relationship to drug, have been reported in patients given ciprofloxacin (includes all formulations, all dosages, all drug-therapy durations, and all indications):

Decreases in blood glucose, BUN, hematocrit, hemoglobin, leukocyte counts, platelet counts, prothrombin time, serum albumin, serum potassium, total serum protein, uric acid.

Increases in alkaline phosphatase, ALT (SGPT), AST (SGOT), atypical lymphocyte counts, blood glucose, blood monocytes, BUN, cholesterol, eosinophil counts, LDH, platelet counts, prothrombin time, sedimentation rate, serum amylase, serum bilirubin, serum calcium, serum cholesterol, serum creatine phosphokinase, serum creatinine, serum gamma-glutamyl transpeptidase (GGT), serum potassium, serum theophylline (in patients receiving theophylline concomitantly), serum triglycerides, uric acid.

Others: albuminuria, change in serum phenytoin, crystalluria, cylindruria, immature WBCs, leukocytosis, methemoglobinemia, pancytopenia.

OVERDOSAGE

In the event of acute excessive overdosage, reversible renal toxicity has been reported in some cases. The stomach should be emptied by inducing vomiting or by gastric lavage. The patient should be carefully observed and given supportive treatment, including monitoring of renal function and administration of magnesium or calcium containing antacids which can reduce the absorption of ciprofloxacin. Adequate hydration must be maintained. Only a small amount of ciprofloxacin (< 10%) is removed from the body after hemodialysis or peritoneal dialysis.

In mice, rats, rabbits and dogs, significant toxicity including tonic/clonic convulsions was observed at intravenous doses of ciprofloxacin between 125 and 300 mg/kg.

Single doses of ciprofloxacin were relatively non-toxic via the oral route of administration in mice, rats, and dogs. No deaths occurred within a 14-day post treatment observation period at the highest oral doses tested; up to 5000 mg/kg in either rodent species, or up to 2500 mg/kg in the dog. Clinical signs observed included hypoactivity and cyanosis in both rodent species and severe vomiting in dogs. In rabbits, significant mortality was seen at doses of ciprofloxacin > 2500 mg/kg. Mortality was delayed in these animals, occurring 10-14 days after dosing.

DOSAGE AND ADMINISTRATION

CIPRO XR and ciprofloxacin immediate-release tablets are not interchangeable. Cipro XR should be administered orally once daily as described in the following Dosage Guidelines table:

[See first table above]

Patients whose therapy is started with CIPRO I.V. for urinary tract infections may be switched to CIPRO XR when clinically indicated at the discretion of the physician.

DOSAGE GUIDELINES

Indication	Unit Dose	Frequency	Usual Duration
Uncomplicated Urinary Tract Infection (Acute Cystitis)	500 mg	Q24h	3 Days
Complicated Urinary Tract Infection	1000 mg	Q24h	7-14 Days
Acute Uncomplicated Pyelonephritis	1000 mg	Q24h	7-14 Days

	CIPRO XR 500 mg QD × 3 Days	CIPRO 250 mg BID × 3 Days
Randomized Patients	452	453
Per Protocol Patients[†]	199	223
Bacteriologic Eradication at TOC (n/N)*	188/199 (94.5%)	209/223 (93.7%)
	CI [-3.5%, 5.1%]	
Bacteriologic Eradication (by organism) at TOC (n/N)**		
E. coli	156/160 (97.5%)	176/181 (97.2%)
E. faecalis	10/11 (90.9%)	17/21 (81.0%)
P. mirabilis	11/12 (91.7%)	7/7 (100%)
S. saprophyticus	6/7 (85.7%)	9/9 (100%)
Clinical Response at TOC (n/N)***	189/199 (95.0%)	204/223 (91.5%)
	CI [-1.1%, 8.1%]	

* n/N = patients with baseline organism(s) eradicated and no new infections or superinfections/total number of patients
** n/N = patients with specified baseline organism eradicated/patients with specified baseline organism
*** n/N = patients with clinical success/total number of patients
[†] The presence of a pathogen at a level of $\geq 10^5$ CFU/mL was required for microbiological evaluability criteria, except for *S. saprophyticus* ($\geq 10^4$ CFU/mL).

CIPRO XR should be administered at least 2 hours before or 6 hours after antacids containing magnesium or aluminum, as well as sucralfate, VIDEX® (didanosine) chewable/buffered tablets or pediatric powder, other highly buffered drugs, metal cations such as iron, and multivitamin preparations with zinc. Although CIPRO XR may be taken with meals that include milk, concomitant administration with dairy products alone, or with calcium-fortified products should be avoided, since decreased absorption is possible. A 2-hour window between substantial calcium intake (> 800 mg) and dosing with CIPRO XR is recommended. CIPRO XR should be swallowed whole. **DO NOT SPLIT, CRUSH, OR CHEW THE TABLET.** (See **CLINICAL PHARMACOLOGY, Drug-drug Interactions, PRECAUTIONS, Drug Interactions** and **Information for Patients**.)

Impaired Renal Function:

Ciprofloxacin is eliminated primarily by renal excretion; however, the drug is also metabolized and partially cleared through the biliary system of the liver and through the intestine. These alternate pathways of drug elimination appear to compensate for the reduced renal excretion in patients with renal impairment. No dosage adjustment is required for patients with uncomplicated urinary tract infections receiving 500 mg CIPRO XR. In patients with complicated urinary tract infections and acute uncomplicated pyelonephritis, who have a creatinine clearance of < 30 mL/min, the dose of CIPRO XR should be reduced from 1000 mg to 500 mg daily. For patients on hemodialysis or peritoneal dialysis, administer CIPRO XR after the dialysis procedure is completed. (See **CLINICAL PHARMACOLOGY, Special Populations**, and **PRECAUTIONS, Geriatric Use**.)

Impaired Hepatic Function:

No dosage adjustment is required with CIPRO XR in patients with stable chronic cirrhosis. The kinetics of ciprofloxacin in patients with acute hepatic insufficiency, however, have not been fully elucidated. (See **CLINICAL PHARMACOLOGY, Special Populations**.)

HOW SUPPLIED

CIPRO XR is available as nearly white to slightly yellowish, film-coated, oblong-shaped tablets containing 500 mg or 1000 mg ciprofloxacin. The 500 mg tablet is coded with the word "BAYER" on one side and "C500 QD" on the reverse side. The 1000 mg tablet is coded with the word "BAYER" on one side and "C1000 QD" on the reverse side.

	Strength	NDC Code
Bottles of 50	500 mg	0085-1775-02
Bottles of 100	500 mg	0085-1775-01
Bottles of 50	1000 mg	0085-1778-03
Bottles of 100	1000 mg	0085-1778-01
Unit Dose Pack of 30	1000 mg	0085-1778-02

Store at 25°C (77°F); excursions permitted to 15-30°C (59-86°F) [see USP Controlled Room Temperature].

ANIMAL PHARMACOLOGY

Ciprofloxacin and other quinolones have been shown to cause arthropathy in immature animals of most species tested. (See **WARNINGS**.) Damage of weight bearing joints was observed in juvenile dogs and rats. In young beagles, 100 mg/kg ciprofloxacin, given daily for 4 weeks, caused degenerative articular changes of the knee joint. At 30 mg/kg, the effect on the joint was minimal. In a subsequent study in beagles, removal of weight bearing from the joint reduced the lesions but did not totally prevent them.

Crystalluria, sometimes associated with secondary nephropathy, occurs in laboratory animals dosed with ciprofloxacin. This is primarily related to the reduced solubility of ciprofloxacin under alkaline conditions, which predominate in the urine of test animals; in man, crystalluria is rare since human urine is typically acidic. In rhesus monkeys, crystalluria without nephropathy has been noted after single oral doses as low as 5 mg/kg. After 6 months of intravenous dosing at 10 mg/kg/day, no nephropathological changes were noted; however, nephropathy was observed after dosing at 20 mg/kg/day for the same duration.

In mice, concomitant administration of nonsteroidal anti-inflammatory drugs such as phenylbutazone and indomethacin with quinolones has been reported to enhance the CNS stimulatory effect of quinolones.

Ocular toxicity seen with some related drugs has not been observed in ciprofloxacin-treated animals.

CLINICAL STUDIES

Uncomplicated Urinary Tract Infections (acute cystitis)

CIPRO XR was evaluated for the treatment of uncomplicated urinary tract infections (acute cystitis) in a randomized, double-blind, controlled clinical trial conducted in the US. This study compared CIPRO XR (500 mg once daily for three days) with ciprofloxacin immediate-release tablets (CIPRO® 250 mg BID for three days). Of the 905 patients enrolled, 452 were randomly assigned to the CIPRO XR treatment group and 453 were randomly assigned to the control group. The primary efficacy variable was bacteriologic eradication of the baseline organism(s) with no new infection or superinfection at test-of-cure (Day 4–11 Post-therapy).

The bacteriologic eradication and clinical success rates were similar between CIPRO XR and the control group. The eradication and clinical success rates and their corresponding 95% confidence intervals for the differences between rates (CIPRO XR minus control group) are given in the following table:

[See second table above]

Complicated Urinary Tract Infections and Acute Uncomplicated Pyelonephritis

CIPRO XR was evaluated for the treatment of complicated urinary tract infections (cUTI) and acute uncomplicated pyelonephritis (AUP) in a randomized, double-blind, controlled clinical trial conducted in the US and Canada. The study enrolled 1,042 patients (521 patients per treatment arm) and compared CIPRO XR (1000 mg once daily for 7 to 14 days) with immediate-release ciprofloxacin (500 mg BID for 7 to 14 days). The primary efficacy endpoint for this trial was bacteriologic eradication of the baseline organism(s) with no new infection or superinfection at 5 to 11 days post-therapy (test-of-cure or TOC) for the Per Protocol and Modified Intent-To-Treat (MITT) populations.

The Per Protocol population was defined as patients with a diagnosis of cUTI or AUP, a causative organism(s) at baseline present at $\geq 10^5$ CFU/mL, no inclusion criteria violation, a valid test-of-cure urine culture within the TOC window, an organism susceptible to study drug, no premature discontinuation or loss to follow-up, and compliance with the dosage regimen (among other criteria). More patients in the CIPRO XR arm than in the control arm were excluded from the Per Protocol population and this should be considered in the interpretation of the study results. Reasons for

Continued on next page

Cipro XR—Cont.

exclusion with the greatest discrepancy between the two arms were no valid test-of-cure urine culture, an organism resistant to the study drug, and premature discontinuation due to adverse events.

An analysis of all patients with a causative organism(s) isolated at baseline and who received study medication, defined as the MITT population, included 342 patients in the CIPRO XR arm and 324 patients in the control arm. Patients with missing responses were counted as failures in this analysis. In the MITT analysis of cUTI patients, bacteriologic eradication was 160/271 (59.0%) versus 156/248 (62.9%) in CIPRO XR and control arm, respectively [97.5% CI* (-13.5%, 5.7%)]. Clinical cure was 184/271 (67.9%) for CIPRO XR and 182/248 (73.4%) for control arm, respectively [97.5% CI* (-14.4%, 3.5%)]. Bacterial eradication in the MITT analysis of patients with AUP at TOC was 47/71 (66.2%) and 58/76 (76.3%) for CIPRO XR and control arm, respectively [97.5% CI* (-26.8%, 6.5%)]. Clinical cure at TOC was 50/71 (70.4%) for CIPRO XR and 58/76 (76.3%) for the control arm [97.5% CI* (-22.0%, 10.4%)].

* confidence interval of the difference in rates (CIPRO XR minus control).

In the Per Protocol population, the differences between CIPRO XR and the control arm in bacteriologic eradication rates at the TOC visit were not consistent between AUP and cUTI patients. The bacteriologic eradication rate for cUTI patients was higher in the CIPRO XR arm than in the control arm. For AUP patients, the bacteriologic eradication rate was lower in the CIPRO XR arm than in the control arm. This inconsistency was not observed between the two treatment groups for clinical cure rates. Clinical cure rates were 96.1% (198/206) and 92.1% (211/229) for CIPRO XR and the control arm, respectively.

The bacterial eradication and clinical cure rates by infection type for CIPRO XR and the control arm at the TOC visit and their corresponding 97.5% confidence intervals for the differences between rates (CIPRO XR minus control arm) are given below for the Per Protocol population analysis:

[See table below]

Of the 166 cUTI patients treated with CIPRO XR, 148 (89%) had the causative organism(s) eradicated, 8 (5%) had persistence, 5 (3%) patients developed superinfections and 5 (3%) developed new infections. Of the 177 cUTI patients treated in the control arm, 144 (81%) had the causative organism(s) eradicated, 16 (9%) patients had persistence, 3 (2%) developed superinfections and 14 (8%) developed new infections. Of the 40 patients with AUP treated with CIPRO XR, 35 (87.5%) had the causative organism(s) eradicated, 2 (5%) patients had persistence and 3 (7.5%) developed new infections. Of the 5 CIPRO XR AUP patients without eradication at TOC, 4 were considered clinical cures and did not receive alternative antibiotic therapy. Of the 52 patients with AUP treated in the control arm, 51 (98%) had the causative organism(s) eradicated. One patient (2%) had persistence.

REFERENCES

1. NCCLS, Methods for Dilution Antimicrobial Susceptibility Tests for Bacteria That Grow Aerobically-Sixth Edition. Approved Standard NCCLS Document M7-A6, Vol. 23, No. 2, NCCLS, Wayne, PA, January, 2003.
2. NCCLS, Performance Standards for Antimicrobial Disk Susceptibility Tests-Eighth Edition. Approved Standard NCCLS Document M2-A8, Vol. 23, No. 1, NCCLS, Wayne, PA, January, 2003.

PATIENT INFORMATION ABOUT CIPRO® XR

(ciprofloxacin extended-release tablets)

This section contains important patient information about CIPRO XR and should be read completely before you begin treatment. This section does not take the place of discussion with your doctor or health care professional about your medical condition or your treatment. This section does not list all benefits and risks of CIPRO XR. CIPRO XR can be prescribed only by a licensed health care professional. Your doctor has prescribed CIPRO XR only for you.

CIPRO XR is intended only to treat urinary tract infections and acute uncomplicated pyelonephritis (also known as a kidney infection). It should not be used to treat other infections. Do not give it to other people even if they have a similar condition. Do not use it for a condition for which it was not prescribed. If you have any concerns about your condition or your medicine, ask your doctor. Only your doctor can determine if CIPRO XR is right for you.

What is CIPRO XR?

CIPRO XR is an antibiotic in the quinolone class that contains the active ingredient ciprofloxacin. CIPRO XR is specifically formulated to be taken just once daily to kill bacteria causing infection in the urinary tract. CIPRO XR has been shown in clinical trials to be effective in the treatment of urinary tract infections. You should contact your doctor if your condition is not improving while taking CIPRO XR.

CIPRO XR tablets are nearly white to slightly yellowish, film-coated, oblong-shaped tablets. CIPRO XR is available in 500 mg and 1000 mg tablet strengths.

How and when should I take CIPRO XR?

CIPRO XR should be taken once a day for three (3) to fourteen (14) days depending on your infection. Take CIPRO XR at approximately the same time each day with food or on an empty stomach. CIPRO XR should not be taken with dairy products (like milk or yogurt) or calcium-fortified juices alone; however, CIPRO XR may be taken with a meal that contains these products. Should you forget to take it at the usual time, you may take your dose later in the day. Do not take more than one CIPRO XR tablet per day even if you missed a dose. Swallow the CIPRO XR tablet whole. **DO NOT SPLIT, CRUSH, OR CHEW THE TABLET.**

You should take CIPRO XR for as long as your doctor prescribes it, even after you start to feel better. Stopping an antibiotic too early may result in failure to cure your infection.

Who should not take CIPRO XR?

You should not take CIPRO XR if you have ever had a severe reaction to any of the group of antibiotics known as "quinolones."

CIPRO XR is not recommended for use during pregnancy or nursing, as the effects on the unborn child or nursing infant are unknown. If you are pregnant or plan to become pregnant while taking CIPRO XR, talk to your doctor before taking this medication.

CIPRO XR is not recommended for persons less than 18 years of age.

What are the possible side effects of CIPRO XR?

CIPRO XR is generally well tolerated. The most common side effects, which are usually mild, include nausea, headache, dyspepsia, dizziness, vaginal yeast infection and diarrhea. If diarrhea persists, call your health care professional. Antibiotics of the quinolone class may also cause vomiting, rash, and abdominal pain/discomfort.

You should be careful about driving or operating machinery until you are sure CIPRO XR is not causing dizziness.

Rare cases of allergic reactions have been reported in patients receiving quinolones, including ciprofloxacin, even after just one dose. If you develop hives, difficulty breathing, or other symptoms of a severe allergic reaction, seek emergency treatment right away. If you develop a skin rash, you should stop taking CIPRO XR and call your health care professional.

Some patients taking quinolone antibiotics may become more sensitive to sunlight or ultraviolet light such as that used in tanning salons. You should avoid excessive exposure to sunlight or ultraviolet light while you are taking CIPRO XR.

Ciprofloxacin has been rarely associated with inflammation of tendons. If you experience pain, swelling or rupture of a tendon, you should stop taking CIPRO XR and call your health care professional.

Convulsions have been reported in patients receiving quinolone antibiotics including ciprofloxacin. If you have experienced convulsions in the past, be sure to let your physician know that you have a history of convulsions. Quinolones, including ciprofloxacin, have been rarely associated with other central nervous system events including confusion, tremors, hallucinations, and depression.

If you notice any side effects not mentioned in this section, or if you have any concerns about side effects you may be experiencing, please inform your health care professional.

What about other medications I am taking?

CIPRO XR can affect how other medicines work. Tell your doctor about all other prescriptions and nonprescription medicines or supplements you are taking. This is especially important if you are taking theophylline or VIDEX® (didanosine) chewable/buffered tablets or pediatric powder. Other medications including warfarin, glyburide, and phenytoin may also interact with CIPRO XR.

Many antacids, multivitamins, and other dietary supplements containing magnesium, calcium, aluminum, iron or zinc can interfere with the absorption of CIPRO XR and may prevent it from working. You should take CIPRO XR either 2 hours before or 6 hours after taking these products.

Remember:

Do not give CIPRO XR to anyone other than the person for whom it was prescribed.

Complete the course of CIPRO XR even if you are feeling better.

Keep CIPRO XR and all medications out of reach of children.

This information does not take the place of discussions with your doctor or health care professional about your medication or treatment.

℞ Only

Manufactured by
Bayer HealthCare
Bayer Pharmaceuticals Corporation
400 Morgan Lane
West Haven, CT 06516
Made in Germany
Distributed by
Schering-Plough
Schering Corporation
Kenilworth, NJ 07033
CIPRO is a registered trademark of Bayer Aktiengesellschaft and is used under license by Schering Corporation.
08918573, R.0   Bay o 9867/q 3939   10/04   12541
©2004 Bayer Pharmaceuticals Corporation

Printed in U.S.A.

	CIPRO XR 1000 mg QD	CIPRO 500 mg BID
Randomized Patients	521	521
Per Protocol Patient^	206	229
cUTI Patients		
Bacteriologic Eradication at TOC (n/N)*	148/166 (89.2%)	144/177 (81.4%)
CI [-0.7%, 16.3%]		
Bacteriologic Eradication (by organism) at TOC (n/N)**		
E. coli	91/94 (96.8%)	90/92 (97.8%)
K. pneumoniae	20/21 (95.2%)	19/23 (82.6%)
E. faecalis	17/17 (100%)	14/21 (66.7%)
P. mirabilis	11/12 (91.6%)	10/10 (100%)
P. aeruginosa	3/3 (100%)	3/3 (100%)
Clinical Cure at TOC (n/N)***	159/166 (95.8%)	161/177 (91.0%)
CI [-1.1%, 10.8%]		
AUP Patients		
Bacteriologic Eradication at TOC (n/N)*	35/40 (87.5%)	51/52 (98.1%)
CI [-34.8%, 6.2%]		
Bacteriologic Eradication of E. coli at TOC (n/N)**	35/36 (97.2%)	41/41 (100%)
Clinical Cure at TOC (n/N)***	39/40 (97.5%)	50/52 (96.2%)
CI [-15.3%, 21.1%]		

^Patients excluded from the Per Protocol population were primarily those with no causative organism(s) at baseline or no organism present at ≥ 10^5 CFU/mL at baseline, inclusion criteria violation, no valid test-of-cure urine culture within the TOC window, an organism resistant to study drug, premature discontinuation due to an adverse event, lost to follow-up, and non-compliance with dosage regimen (among other criteria).
* n/N = patients with baseline organism(s) eradicated and no new infections or superinfections/total number of patients
**n/N = patients with specified baseline organism eradicated/patients with specified baseline organism
***n/N = patients with clinical success/total number of patients

CLARINEX-D® 24-HOUR ℞

[klă-rĭ-nĕks D]

(desloratadine 5 mg and pseudoephedrine sulfate, USP 240 mg)
EXTENDED RELEASE TABLETS

DESCRIPTION

CLARINEX-D® 24 HOUR Extended Release Tablets are light blue oval shaped tablets containing 5 mg desloratadine in the tablet coating for immediate release and 240 mg pseudoephedrine sulfate, USP in the tablet core for extended release.

The inactive ingredients contained in CLARINEX-D® 24 HOUR Extended Release Tablets are hypromellose USP, ethylcellulose NF, dibasic calcium phosphate dihydrate USP, magnesium stearate NF, povidone USP, silicone dioxide NF, talc USP, polyacrylate dispersion, polyethylene glycol NF, simethicone USP, Blue Lake Blend 50726 (FD&C Blue No. 2 Lake, titanium dioxide USP and edetate disodium USP), and ink (Opacode® S-1-17746 or Opacode® S-1-4159).

Desloratadine, one of the two active ingredients of CLARINEX-D® 24 HOUR Extended Release Tablets, is a white to off-white powder that is slightly soluble in water, but very soluble in ethanol and propylene glycol. It has an empirical formula: $C_{19}H_{19}ClN_2$ and a molecular weight of 310.8. The chemical name is 8-chloro-6,11-dihydro-11-(4-piperdinylidene)-5*H*-benzo[5,6]cyclohepta[1,2-*b*]pyridine and has the following structure:

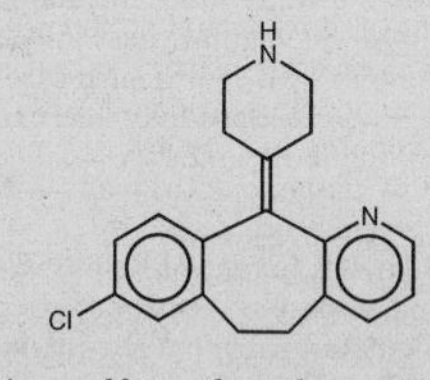

Pseudoephedrine sulfate, the other active ingredient of CLARINEX-D® 24 HOUR Extended Release Tablets, is the synthetic salt of one of the naturally occurring dextrorotatory diastereomers of ephedrine and is classified as an indirect sympathomimetic amine. Pseudoephedrine sulfate is a colorless hygroscopic crystal or white, hygroscopic crystalline powder, practically odorless, with a bitter taste. It is very soluble in water, freely soluble in alcohol, and sparingly soluble in ether. The empirical formula for pseudoephedrine sulfate is $(C_{10}H_{15}NO)_2 \bullet H_2SO_4$; the chemical name is benzenemethanol, α-[1-(methylamino) ethyl]-,[*S*-(*R**,*R**)]-, sulfate (2:1)(salt); and the chemical structure is:

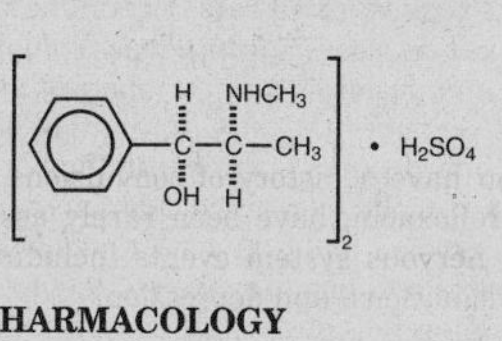

CLINICAL PHARMACOLOGY

Mechanism of Action: Desloratadine is a long-acting tricyclic histamine antagonist with selective H_1-receptor histamine antagonist activity. Receptor binding data indicate that at a concentration of 2-3 ng/mL (7 nanomolar), desloratadine shows significant interaction with the human histamine H_1-receptor. Desloratadine inhibited histamine release from human mast cells *in vitro*.

Results of a radiolabeled tissue distribution study in rats and a radioligand H_1-receptor binding study in guinea pigs showed that desloratadine did not readily cross the blood brain barrier.

Pseudoephedrine sulfate is an orally active sympathomimetic amine and exerts a decongestant action on the nasal mucosa. Pseudoephedrine sulfate is recognized as an effective agent for the relief of nasal congestion due to allergic rhinitis. Pseudoephedrine produces peripheral effects similar to those of ephedrine and central effects similar to, but less intense than, amphetamines. It has the potential for excitatory side effects.

Pharmacokinetics: Absorption: A bioequivalence study that compared CLARINEX-D® 24 HOUR Extended Release Tablets to the monotherapy (desloratadine 5 mg, and pseudoephedrine 240 mg) showed that CLARINEX-D® 24 HOUR Extended Release Tablets was not bioequivalent to the monotherapy (desloratadine 5 mg tablet). The systemic exposure to desloratadine and 3-hydroxydesloratadine was 15-20% lower from CLARINEX-D® 24 HOUR Extended Release Tablets than those from desloratadine 5 mg tablet. Clinical trials were therefore necessary to support efficacy of CLARINEX-D® 24 HOUR Extended Release Tablets (see **Clinical Trials** section).

In the above single dose pharmacokinetic study, the mean time to maximum plasma concentrations (T_{max}) for desloratadine occurred at approximately 6-7 hours post dose and mean peak plasma concentrations (C_{max}) and area under the concentration-time curve (AUC(tf)) of approximately 1.79 ng/mL and 61.1 ng•hr/mL, respectively, were observed. In another pharmacokinetic study, food and grapefruit juice had no effect on the bioavailability (C_{max}) and AUC) of desloratadine. For pseudoephedrine, the mean T_{max} occurred at 8-9 hours post dose and mean peak plasma concentrations (C_{max}) and AUC(tf) of 328 ng/mL and 6438 ng•hr/mL, respectively, were observed. The ingestion of food did not affect the absorption of pseudoephedrine from CLARINEX-D® 24 HOUR Extended Release Tablets.

Following oral administrations of CLARINEX-D® 24 HOUR Extended Release Tablets once daily for 14 days to healthy volunteers, steady-state conditions were reached on day 12 for desloratadine and day 10 for pseudoephedrine. For desloratadine, mean steady-state C_{max} and AUC (0-24 h) of approximately 2.44 ng/mL and 34.8 ng•hr/mL, respectively were observed. For pseudoephedrine, mean steady-state peak plasma concentrations (C_{max}) and AUC (0-24 h) of 523 ng/mL and 8795 ng•hr/mL, respectively were observed.

Distribution: Desloratadine and 3-hydroxydesloratadine are approximately 82% to 87% and 85% to 89%, bound to plasma proteins, respectively. Protein binding of desloratadine and 3-hydroxydesloratadine was unaltered in subjects with impaired renal function.

Table 1

Changes in Desloratadine and 3-hydroxydesloratadine Pharmacokinetics in Healthy Male and Female Subjects

	Desloratadine		3-hydroxy-desloratadine	
	C_{max}	AUC 0-24 hrs	C_{max}	AUC 0-24 hrs
Erythromycin (500 mg Q8h)	+24%	+14%	+43%	+40%
Ketoconazole (200 mg Q12h)	+45%	+39%	+43%	+72%
Azithromycin (500 mg day 1, 250 mg QD × 4 days)	+15%	+5%	+15%	+4%
Fluoxetine (20 mg QD)	+15%	+0%	+17%	+13%
Cimetidine (600 mg Q12h)	+12%	+19%	-11%	-3%

Metabolism: Desloratadine (a major metabolite of loratadine) is extensively metabolized to 3-hydroxydesloratadine, an active metabolite, which is subsequently glucuronidated. The enzyme(s) responsible for the formation of 3-hydroxydesloratadine have not been identified. Data from clinical trials with desloratadine indicate that a subset of the general population has a decreased ability to form 3-hydroxydesloratadine, and are poor metabolizers of desloratadine. In pharmacokinetic studies (n=3748), approximately 6% of subjects were poor metabolizers of desloratadine (defined as a subject with an AUC ratio of 3-hydroxydesloratadine to desloratadine less than 0.1, or a subject with a desloratadine half-life exceeding 50 hours). These pharmacokinetic studies included subjects between the ages of 2 and 70 years, including 977 subjects aged 2-5 years, 1575 subjects aged 6-11 years, and 1196 subjects aged 12-70 years. There was no difference in the prevalence of poor metabolizers across age groups. The frequency of poor metabolizers was higher in Blacks (17%, n=988) as compared to Caucasians (2%, n=1462) and Hispanics (2%, n=1063). The median exposure (AUC) to desloratadine in the poor metabolizers was approximately 6-fold greater than in the subjects who are not poor metabolizers. Subjects who are poor metabolizers of desloratadine cannot be prospectively identified and will be exposed to higher levels of desloratadine following dosing with the recommended dose of desloratadine. In multidose clinical safety studies, where metabolizer status was prospectively identified, a total of 94 poor metabolizers and 123 normal metabolizers were enrolled and treated with CLARINEX® Syrup for 15-35 days. In these studies, no overall differences in safety were observed between poor metabolizers and normal metabolizers. Although not seen in these studies, an increased risk of exposure-related adverse events in patients who are poor metabolizers cannot be ruled out.

Pseudoephedrine alone is incompletely metabolized (less than 1%) in the liver by N-demethylation to an inactive metabolite. The drug and its metabolite are excreted in the urine. About 55-96% of an administered dose of pseudoephedrine hydrochloride is excreted unchanged in the urine.

Elimination: Following single dose administration of CLARINEX-D® 24 HOUR Extended Release Tablets, the mean plasma elimination half-life of desloratadine was similar to the desloratadine 5 mg tablet, approximately 24 and 27 hours, respectively.

In another study, following administration of single oral doses of desloratadine 5 mg, C_{max} and AUC values increased in a dose proportional manner between 5 and 20 mg. The degree of accumulation after 14 days of dosing was consistent with the half-life and dosing frequency. A human mass balance study documented a recovery of approximately 87% of the ^{14}C-desloratadine dose, which was equally distributed in urine and feces as metabolic products. Analysis of plasma 3-hydroxydesloratadine showed similar T_{max} and half-life values compared to desloratadine.

The mean elimination half-life of pseudoephedrine is dependent on urinary pH. The elimination half-life is approximately 3-6 or 9-16 hours when the urinary pH is 5 or 8, respectively.

Special Populations: Geriatric: The number of patients (n=8)≥ 65 years old treated with CLARINEX-D® 24 HOUR Extended Release Tablets was too limited to make any clinically relevant judgment regarding the efficacy or safety of this drug product in this age group. Following multiple-dose administration of CLARINEX Tablets, the mean C_{max} and AUC values for desloratadine were 20% greater than in younger subjects (< 65 years old). The oral total body clearance (CL/F), when normalized for body weight, was similar between the two age groups. The mean plasma elimination half-life of desloratadine was 33.7 hr in subjects ≥ 65 years old. The pharmacokinetics for 3-hydroxydesloratadine appeared unchanged in older versus younger subjects. These age-related differences are unlikely to be clinically relevant and no dosage adjustment is recommended in elderly subjects.

Pediatric Subjects: CLARINEX-D® 24 HOUR Extended Release Tablets are not an appropriate dosage form for use in pediatric patients below 12 years of age.

Renally Impaired: No studies with CLARINEX-D® 24 HOUR Extended Release Tablets have been conducted in patients with renal insufficiency. Following a single dose of desloratadine 7.5 mg, pharmacokinetics were characterized in patients with mild (n=7; creatinine clearance 51-69 mL/min/1.73 m²), moderate (n=6; creatinine clearance 34-43 mL/min/1.73 m²), and severe (n=6; creatinine clearance 5-29 mL/min/1.73 m²) renal impairment or hemodialysis dependent (n=6) patients. In patients with mild and moderate renal impairment, median C_{max} and AUC values increased by approximately 1.2- and 1.9-fold, respectively, relative to subjects with normal renal function. In patients with severe renal impairment or who were hemodialysis dependent, C_{max} and AUC values increased by approximately 1.7- and 2.5-fold, respectively. Minimal changes in 3-hydroxydesloratadine concentrations were observed. Desloratadine and 3-hydroxydesloratadine were poorly removed by hemodialysis. Plasma protein binding of desloratadine and 3-hydroxydesloratadine was unaltered by renal impairment.

Pseudoephedrine is primarily excreted unchanged in the urine as unchanged drug, the remainder is apparently metabolized in the liver. Therefore, pseudoephedrine may accumulate in patients with renal insufficiency. Dosage adjustment for patients with renal impairment is recommended (see **PRECAUTIONS** and **DOSAGE AND ADMINISTRATION** section).

Hepatically Impaired: No studies with CLARINEX-D® 24 HOUR Extended Release Tablets or pseudoephedrine have been conducted in patients with hepatic impairment. Following a single oral dose of desloratadine, pharmacokinetics were characterized in patients with mild (n=4), moderate (n=4), and severe (n=4) hepatic impairment as defined by the Child-Pugh classification of hepatic function and 8 subjects with normal hepatic function. Patients with hepatic impairment, regardless of severity, had approximately a 2.4-fold increase in AUC as compared with normal subjects. The apparent oral clearance of desloratadine in patients with mild, moderate, and severe hepatic impairment was 37%, 36%, and 28% of that in normal subjects, respectively. An increase in the mean elimination half-life of desloratadine in patients with hepatic impairment was observed. For 3-hydroxydesloratadine, the mean C_{max} and AUC values for patients with hepatic impairment were not statistically significantly different from subjects with normal hepatic function. CLARINEX-D® 24 HOUR Extended Release Tablets should generally be avoided in patients with hepatic insufficiency (see **PRECAUTIONS** and **DOSAGE AND ADMINISTRATION**).

Gender: No clinically significant gender-related differences were observed in the pharmacokinetic parameters of desloratadine, 3-hydroxydesloratadine, or pseudoephedrine following administration of CLARINEX-D® 24 HOUR Extended Release Tablets. Female subjects treated for 14 days with CLARINEX Tablets had 10% and 3% higher desloratadine C_{max} and AUC values, respectively, compared with male subjects. The 3-hydroxydesloratadine C_{max} and AUC values were also increased by 45% and 48%, respectively, in females compared with males. However, these apparent differences are not likely to be clinically relevant and therefore no dosage adjustment is recommended.

Race: No studies have been conducted to evaluate the effect of race on the pharmacokinetics of CLARINEX-D® 24 HOUR Extended Release Tablets. Following 14 days of treatment with CLARINEX Tablets, the C_{max} and AUC values for desloratadine were 18% and 32% higher, respectively, in Blacks compared with Caucasians. For 3-hydroxydesloratadine there was a corresponding 10% reduction in C_{max} and AUC values in Blacks compared to Caucasians. These differences are not likely to be clinically relevant and therefore no dose adjustment is recommended.

Drug Interactions: No specific interaction studies have been conducted with CLARINEX-D 24 HOUR Extended Release Tablets. However, in two controlled crossover clinical pharmacology studies in healthy male (n=12 in each study) and female (n=12 in each study) subjects, desloratadine 7.5 mg (1.5 times the daily dose) once daily was coadministered with erythromycin 500 mg every 8 hours or ketoconazole 200 mg every 12 hours for 10 days. In 3 separate controlled, parallel group clinical pharmacology studies, desloratadine at the clinical dose of 5 mg has been coadministered with azithromycin 500 mg followed by 250 mg once daily for 4 days (n=18) or with fluoxetine 20 mg once daily for 7 days after a 23-day pretreatment period with fluoxetine (n=18) or with cimetidine 600 mg every 12 hours for 14 days (n=18) under steady state conditions to healthy male and female subjects. Although increased plasma concentrations (C_{max} and AUC 0-24 hrs) of desloratadine and 3-hydroxydesloratadine were observed (see Table 1), there were no clinically relevant changes in the safety profile of desloratadine, as assessed by electrocardiographic para-

Continued on next page

Clarinex-D—Cont.

meters (including the corrected QT interval), clinical laboratory tests, vital signs, and adverse events.
[See table 1 at top of previous page]
Due to the pseudoephedrine component, CLARINEX-D® 24 HOUR Extended Release Tablets should not be used by patients taking monoamine oxidase inhibitors or within 14 days after stopping such treatment. The antihypertensive effects of beta-adrenergic blocking agents, methyldopa, mecamylamine, reserpine, and veratrum alkaloids may be reduced by sympathomimetics. Increased ectopic pacemaker activity can occur when pseudoephedrine is used concomitantly with digitalis.

Pharmacodynamics: Wheal and Flare: Human histamine skin wheal studies following single and repeated 5 mg doses of desloratadine have shown that the drug exhibits an antihistaminic effect by 1 hour; this activity may persist for as long as 24 hours. There was no evidence of histamine-induced skin wheal tachyphylaxis within the desloratadine 5 mg group over the 28-day treatment period. The clinical relevance of histamine wheal skin testing is unknown.

Effects on QTc: In clinical trials for CLARINEX-D® 24 HOUR Extended Release Tablets, ECGs were recorded at baseline and after two weeks of treatment within 1 to 3 hours after dosing. No clinically meaningful changes were observed following treatment with CLARINEX-D® 24 HOUR Extended Release Tablets for any ECG parameter, including the QTc interval. An increase in the ventricular rate of 6.7 and 5.4 bpm was observed in the CLARINEX-D® 24 HOUR Extended Release Tablets and pseudoephedrine groups, respectively, compared to an increase of 2.8 bpm in patients receiving desloratadine. Single dose administration of desloratadine did not alter the corrected QT interval (QTc) in rats (up to 12 mg/kg, oral), or guinea pigs (25 mg/kg, intravenous). Repeated oral administration at doses up to 24 mg/kg for durations up to 3 months in monkeys did not alter the QTc at an estimated desloratadine exposure (AUC) that was approximately 955 times the mean AUC in humans at the recommended daily oral dose. See **OVERDOSAGE** section for information on human QTc experience.

CLINICAL TRIALS

The clinical efficacy and safety of CLARINEX-D® 24 HOUR Extended Release Tablets was evaluated in two 2-week, multicenter, randomized parallel group clinical trials involving 2852 patients 12 to 78 years of age with seasonal allergic rhinitis, 708 of whom received CLARINEX-D® 24 HOUR Extended Release Tablets. In the two trials patients were randomized to receive CLARINEX-D® 24 HOUR Extended Release Tablets, once daily, CLARINEX Tablets 5 mg once daily, and sustained-release pseudoephedrine tablet 240 mg once daily for two weeks. Primary efficacy variable was twice-daily reflective patient scoring of four nasal symptoms (rhinorrhea, nasal stuffiness/congestion, nasal itching, and sneezing) and four non-nasal symptoms (itching/burning eyes, tearing/watering eyes, redness of eyes, and itching of ears/palate) on a four point scale (0=none, 1=mild, 2=moderate, and 3=severe). In both trials, the antihistaminic efficacy of CLARINEX-D® 24 HOUR Extended Release Tablets, as measured by total symptom score excluding nasal congestion, was significantly greater than pseudoephedrine alone over the 2-week treatment period; and the decongestant efficacy of CLARINEX-D® 24 HOUR Extended Release Tablets, as measured by nasal stuffiness/congestion, was significantly greater than desloratadine alone over the 2-week treatment period. Primary efficacy variable results from one of two trials are shown in Table 2.
[See table 2 below]
There were no significant differences in the efficacy of CLARINEX-D® 24 HOUR Extended Release Tablets across subgroups of patients defined by gender, age, or race.

INDICATIONS AND USAGE

CLARINEX-D® 24 HOUR Extended Release Tablets is indicated for the relief of the nasal and non-nasal symptoms of seasonal allergic rhinitis including nasal congestion, in patients 12 years of age and older. CLARINEX-D® 24 HOUR Extended Release Tablets should be administered when the antihistaminic properties of desloratadine and the nasal decongestant properties of pseudoephedrine are desired (see **CLINICAL PHARMACOLOGY**).

CONTRAINDICATIONS

CLARINEX-D® 24 HOUR Extended Release Tablets is contraindicated in patients who are hypersensitive to this medication or to any of its ingredients, or to loratadine. Due to its pseudoephedrine component, it is contraindicated in patients with narrow-angle glaucoma or urinary retention, and in patients receiving monoamine oxidase (MAO) inhibitor therapy or within fourteen (14) days of stopping such treatment (see **Drug Interactions** section). It is also contraindicated in patients with severe hypertension, severe coronary artery disease, and in those who have shown hypersensitivity or idiosyncrasy to its components, to adrenergic agents, or to other drugs of similar chemical structures. Manifestations of patient idiosyncrasy to adrenergic agents include insomnia, dizziness, weakness, tremor, or arrhythmias.

WARNINGS

CLARINEX-D® 24 HOUR Extended Release Tablets should be used with caution in patients with hypertension, diabetes mellitus, ischemic heart disease, increased intraocular pressure, hyperthyroidism, renal impairment, or prostatic hypertrophy. Central nervous system stimulation with convulsions or cardiovascular collapse with accompanying hypotension may be produced by sympathomimetic amines.

PRECAUTIONS

General: Patients with decreased renal function should be dosed with CLARINEX-D® 24 HOUR Extended Release Tablets once every other day because they have reduced elimination of desloratadine and pseudoephedrine. CLARINEX-D® 24 HOUR Extended Release Tablets should generally be avoided in patients with hepatic insufficiency (see **CLINICAL PHARMACOLOGY**, and **DOSAGE AND ADMINISTRATION**).

Information for Patients: Patients should be instructed to use CLARINEX-D® 24 HOUR Extended Release Tablets as directed. As there are no food effects on bioavailability, patients can be instructed that CLARINEX-D® 24 HOUR Extended Release Tablets may be taken without regard to meals. Patients should be advised not to increase the dose or dosing frequency as studies have not demonstrated increased effectiveness and at higher doses, somnolence may occur. Patients should also be advised against the concurrent use of CLARINEX-D® 24 HOUR Extended Release Tablets with over-the-counter antihistamines and decongestants.
Patients should be instructed not to break or chew the tablet; swallow whole.
Patients who are hypersensitive to it or to any of its ingredients should not use this product. Due to its pseudoephedrine component, this product should not be used by patients with narrow-angle glaucoma, urinary retention, or by patients receiving a monoamine oxidase (MAO) inhibitor or within 14 days of stopping use of an MAO inhibitor. It also should not be used by patients with severe hypertension or severe coronary artery disease.
CLARINEX-D® 24 HOUR Extended Release Tablets should generally be avoided in patients with hepatic insufficiency. Patients who have renal impairment should modify the dosing to every other day.
Patients who are or may become pregnant should be told that this product should be used in pregnancy or during lactation only if the potential benefit justifies the potential risk to the fetus or nursing infant.

Carcinogenesis, Mutagenesis, Impairment of Fertility: There are no animal or laboratory studies on the combination product of desloratadine and pseudoephedrine sulfate to evaluate carcinogenesis, mutagenesis, or impairment of fertility.
The carcinogenic potential of desloratadine was assessed using a loratadine study in rats and a desloratadine study in mice. In a 2-year study in rats, loratadine was administered in the diet at doses up to 25 mg/kg/day (estimated desloratadine and desloratadine metabolite exposures were approximately 30 times the AUC in humans at the recommended daily oral dose). A significantly higher incidence of hepatocellular tumors (combined adenomas and carcinomas) was observed in males given 10 mg/kg/day of loratadine and in males and females given 25 mg/kg/day of loratadine. The estimated desloratadine and desloratadine metabolite exposures in rats given 10 mg/kg of loratadine were approximately 7 times the AUC in humans at the recommended daily oral dose. The clinical significance of these findings during long-term use of desloratadine is not known.
In a 2-year dietary study in mice, males and females given up to 16 mg/kg/day and 32 mg/kg/day desloratadine, respectively, did not show significant increases in the incidence of any tumors. The estimated desloratadine and metabolite exposures in mice at these doses were 12 and 27 times, respectively, the AUC in humans at the recommended daily oral dose.
In genotoxicity studies with desloratadine, there was no evidence of genotoxic potential in a reverse mutation assay (*Salmonella/E. coli* mammalian microsome bacterial mutagenicity assay) or in two assays for chromosomal aberrations (human peripheral blood lymphocyte clastogenicity assay and mouse bone marrow micronucleus assay).
There was no effect on female fertility in rats at desloratadine doses up to 24 mg/kg/day (estimated desloratadine and desloratadine metabolite exposures were approximately 130 times the AUC in humans at the recommended daily oral dose). A male specific decrease in fertility, demonstrated by reduced female conception rates, decreased sperm numbers and motility, and histopathologic testicular changes, occurred at an oral desloratadine dose of 12 mg/kg in rats (estimated desloratadine exposures were approximately 45 times the AUC in humans at the recommended daily oral dose). Desloratadine had no effect on fertility in rats at an oral dose of 3 mg/kg/day (estimated desloratadine and desloratadine metabolite exposures were approximately 8 times the AUC in humans at the recommended daily oral dose).

Pregnancy Category C: There have been no reproduction studies conducted with the combination of desloratadine and pseudoephedrine. Desloratadine was not teratogenic in rats at doses up to 48 mg/kg/day (estimated desloratadine and desloratadine metabolite exposures were approximately 210 times the AUC in humans at the recommended daily oral dose) or in rabbits at doses up to 60 mg/kg/day (estimated desloratadine exposures were approximately 230 times the AUC in humans at the recommended daily oral dose). In a separate study, an increase in pre-implantation loss and a decreased number of implantations and fetuses were noted in female rats at 24 mg/kg (estimated desloratadine and desloratadine metabolite exposures were approximately 120 times the AUC in humans at the recommended daily oral dose). Reduced body weight and slow righting reflex were reported in pups at doses of 9 mg/kg/day or greater (estimated desloratadine and desloratadine metabolite exposures were approximately 50 times or greater than the AUC in humans at the recommended daily oral dose). Desloratadine had no effect on pup development at an oral dose of 3 mg/kg/day (estimated desloratadine and desloratadine metabolite exposures were approximately 7 times the AUC in humans at the recommended daily oral dose). There are, however, no adequate and well-controlled studies in pregnant women. Because animal reproduction

Table 2
Changes in Symptoms in a 2-Week Clinical Trial
in Patients with Seasonal Allergic Rhinitis

Treatment Group (n)	Mean Baseline* (sem)	Change (% change) from Baseline** (sem)	CLARINEX-D® 24-HOUR Comparison to Components*** (*P*-value)
Total Symptom Score (Excluding Nasal Congestion)			
CLARINEX-D® 24 HOUR Extended Release Tablets (333)	14.84 (0.15)	-5.71 (-37.4) (0.22)	–
Pseudoephedrine tablet 240 mg (337)	15.03 (0.15)	-4.95 (-32.0) (0.22)	**P = 0.015**
CLARINEX 5 mg Tablets (337)	15.06 (0.15)	-4.78 (-30.8) (0.22)	P = 0.003
Nasal Stuffiness/Congestion			
CLARINEX-D® 24 HOUR Extended Release Tablets (333)	2.56 (0.020)	-0.85 (-32.3) (0.034)	–
Pseudoephedrine tablet 240 mg (337)	2.54 (0.020)	-0.70 (-27.1) (0.034)	P= 0.002
CLARINEX 5 mg Tablets (337)	2.57 (0.020)	-0.65 (-24.8) (0.034)	**P < 0.001**

*To qualify at Baseline, the sum of the twice-daily diary reflective scores for the three days prior to Baseline and the morning of the Baseline visit were to total ≥42 for total nasal symptom score (sum of 4 nasal symptoms of rhinorrhea, nasal stuffiness/congestion, nasal itching, and sneezing) and a total of ≥35 for total non-nasal symptoms score (sum of 4 non-nasal symptoms of itching/burning eyes, tearing/watering eyes, redness of eyes, and itching of ears/palate), and a score of ≥14 for each of the individual symptoms of nasal stuffiness/congestion and rhinorrhea. Each symptom was scored on a 4-point severity scale (0=none, 1=mild, 2=moderate, 3=severe).
**Mean reduction in score averaged over the 2-week treatment period.
***The comparison of interest is shown bolded.

Table 3
Incidence of Adverse Events Reported by ≥ 2% of Patients Receiving
CLARINEX-D® 24 HOUR Extended Release Tablets

Adverse Reaction	CLARINEX-D® 24 HOUR (N = 708)	Desloratadine 5 mg (N = 712)	Pseudoephedrine 240 mg (N = 719)
Mouth Dry	8%	2%	11%
Headache	6%	5%	7%
Insomnia	5%	1%	8%
Fatigue	3%	3%	2%
Pharyngitis	3%	2%	3%
Somnolence	3%	2%	3%
Nausea	2%	1%	3%
Dizziness	2%	1%	2%
Nervousness	2%	1%	1%
Hyperactivity	2%	0%	2%
Anorexia	2%	0%	2%

studies are not always predictive of human response, desloratadine should be used during pregnancy only if clearly needed.
Nursing Mothers: Desloratadine passes into breast milk, therefore a decision should be made whether to discontinue nursing or to discontinue CLARINEX-D® 24 HOUR Extended Release Tablets, taking into account the importance of the drug to the mother. Caution should be exercised when CLARINEX-D® 24 HOUR Extended Release Tablets are administered to a nursing woman.
Pediatric Use: CLARINEX-D® 24 HOUR Extended Release Tablets is not an appropriate formulation for use in pediatric patients under 12 years of age.
Geriatric Use: Clinical studies of CLARINEX-D® 24 HOUR Extended Release Tablets did not include sufficient numbers of subjects aged 65 and over to determine whether they respond differently from younger subjects. Other reported clinical experience has not identified differences between the elderly and younger patients, although the elderly are more likely to have adverse reactions to sympathomimetic amines. In general, dose selection for an elderly patient should be cautious, reflecting the greater frequency of decreased hepatic, renal, or cardiac function, and of concomitant disease or other drug therapy (see **CLINICAL PHARMACOLOGY–Special Populations**).
Pseudoephedrine, desloratadine, and their metabolites are known to be substantially excreted by the kidney, and the risk of adverse reactions may be greater in patients with impaired renal function. Because elderly patients are more likely to have decreased renal function, care should be taken in dose selection, and it may be useful to monitor the patient for adverse events (see **CLINICAL PHARMACOLOGY–Special Populations**).

ADVERSE REACTIONS
Adults and Adolescents: The clinical trials with CLARINEX-D® 24 HOUR Extended Release Tablets included 2852 patients, of which 708 patients received CLARINEX-D® 24 HOUR Extended Release Tablets daily for up to 15 days. The percentage of patients receiving CLARINEX-D® 24 HOUR Extended Release Tablets, and who discontinued from the study because of an adverse event was 3.4%. Adverse events that were reported by ≥ 2% of patients receiving CLARINEX-D® 24 HOUR Extended Release Tablets, regardless of relationship to study drugs, are shown in Table 3.
[See table 3 above]
There were no differences in adverse events for subgroups of patients as defined by gender, age, or race.
Observed During Clinical Practice: The following spontaneous adverse events have been reported during the marketing of desloratadine as a single ingredient product: headache, somnolence, dizziness, tachycardia, palpitations and rarely hypersensitivity reactions (such as rash, pruritus, urticaria, edema, dyspnea, and anaphylaxis), and elevated liver enzymes including bilirubin and very rarely hepatitis.

DRUG ABUSE AND DEPENDENCE
There is no information to indicate that abuse or dependency occurs with CLARINEX or the combination of the CLARINEX product with pseudoephedrine.

OVERDOSAGE
Information regarding acute overdosage with desloratadine is limited to experience from post-marketing adverse event reports and from clinical trials conducted during the development of the CLARINEX product. In the reported cases of overdose, there were no significant adverse events that were attributed to desloratadine. In a dose ranging trial, at doses of 10 mg and 20 mg/day somnolence was reported.
Single daily doses of desloratadine 45 mg were given to normal male and female subjects for 10 days. All ECGs obtained in this study were manually read in a blinded fashion by a cardiologist. In CLARINEX-treated subjects, there was an increase in mean heart rate of 9.2 bpm relative to placebo. The QT interval was corrected for heart rate (QTc) by both the Bazett and Fridericia methods. Using the QTc

(Bazett), there was a mean increase of 8.1 msec in CLARINEX-treated subjects relative to placebo. Using QTc (Fridericia) there was a mean increase of 0.4 msec in CLARINEX-treated subjects relative to placebo. No clinically relevant adverse events were reported.
In large doses, sympathomimetics may give rise to giddiness, headache, nausea, vomiting, sweating, thirst, tachycardia, precordial pain, palpitations, difficulty in micturition, muscular weakness and tenseness, anxiety, restlessness, and insomnia. Many patients can present a toxic psychosis with delusions and hallucinations. Some may develop cardiac arrhythmias, circulatory collapse, convulsions, coma, and respiratory failure.
In the event of overdose, consider standard measures to remove any unabsorbed drug. Symptomatic and supportive treatment is recommended. Desloratadine and 3-hydroxydesloratadine are not eliminated by hemodialysis.
Lethality occurred in rats at oral doses of 250 mg/kg or greater (estimated desloratadine and desloratadine metabolite exposures were approximately 120 times the AUC in humans at the recommended daily oral dose). The oral median lethal dose in mice was 353 mg/kg (estimated desloratadine exposures were approximately 290 times the human daily oral dose on a mg/m² basis). No deaths occurred at oral doses up to 250 mg/kg in monkeys (estimated desloratadine exposures were approximately 810 times the human daily oral dose on a mg/m² basis).

DOSAGE AND ADMINISTRATION
Adults and children 12 years of age and over: The recommended dose of CLARINEX-D® 24 HOUR Extended Release Tablets is one tablet once daily, administered with or without a meal. A dose of one tablet every other day is recommended in patients with renal impairment. CLARINEX-D® 24 HOUR Extended Release Tablets should generally be avoided in patients with hepatic insufficiency.
CAUTION: Do not break or crush the tablet; swallow whole.

HOW SUPPLIED
CLARINEX-D® 24 HOUR Extended Release Tablets contain 5 mg desloratadine in the tablet coating for immediate release and 240 mg pseudoephedrine sulfate, USP in an extended release core. CLARINEX-D® 24 HOUR Extended Release Tablets are light blue oval shaped coated tablets with "D 24" branded in black on one side; high-density polyethylene bottles of 100 (NDC 0085-1317-01).
Protect from excessive moisture.
Store at 25°C (77°F); excursions permitted to 15-30°C (59-86°F) [see USP Controlled Room Temperature]. Heat Sensitive. Avoid exposure at or above 30°C (86°F).
Schering®
Schering Corporation
Kenilworth, NJ 07033 USA
3/05   28226705T
U.S. Patent Nos. 4,659,716; 4,863,931; 5,595,997; and 6,100,274
Copyright © 2005, Schering Corporation. All rights reserved.

LEVITRA®   ℞
[lĕ-vē-trǎ]
(vardenafil HCl)
TABLETS

DESCRIPTION
LEVITRA® is an oral therapy for the treatment of erectile dysfunction. This monohydrochloride salt of vardenafil is a selective inhibitor of cyclic guanosine monophosphate (cGMP)-specific phosphodiesterase type 5 (PDE5).
Vardenafil HCl is designated chemically as piperazine, 1-[[3-(1,4-dihydro-5-methyl-4-oxo-7-propylimidazo[5,1-f][1,

2,4]triazin-2-yl)-4-ethoxyphenyl]sulfonyl]-4-ethyl-, monohydrochloride and has the following structural formula:

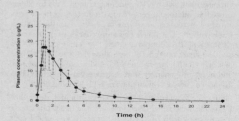

Vardenafil HCl is a nearly colorless, solid substance with a molecular weight of 579.1 g/mol and a solubility of 0.11 mg/mL in water. LEVITRA is formulated as orange, round, film-coated tablets with "BAYER" cross debossed on one side and "2.5", "5", "10", and "20" on the other side corresponding to 2.5 mg, 5 mg, 10 mg, and 20 mg of vardenafil, respectively. In addition to the active ingredient, vardenafil HCl, each tablet contains microcrystalline cellulose, crospovidone, colloidal silicon dioxide, magnesium stearate, hypromellose, polyethylene glycol, titanium dioxide, yellow ferric oxide, and red ferric oxide.

CLINICAL PHARMACOLOGY
Mechanism of Action
Penile erection is a hemodynamic process initiated by the relaxation of smooth muscle in the corpus cavernosum and its associated arterioles. During sexual stimulation, nitric oxide is released from nerve endings and endothelial cells in the corpus cavernosum. Nitric oxide activates the enzyme guanylate cyclase resulting in increased synthesis of cyclic guanosine monophosphate (cGMP) in the smooth muscle cells of the corpus cavernosum. The cGMP in turn triggers smooth muscle relaxation, allowing increased blood flow into the penis, resulting in erection. The tissue concentration of cGMP is regulated by both the rates of synthesis and degradation via phosphodiesterases (PDEs). The most abundant PDE in the human corpus cavernosum is the cGMP-specific phosphodiesterase type 5 (PDE5); therefore, the inhibition of PDE5 enhances erectile function by increasing the amount of cGMP. Because sexual stimulation is required to initiate the local release of nitric oxide, the inhibition of PDE5 has no effect in the absence of sexual stimulation.
In vitro studies have shown that vardenafil is a selective inhibitor of PDE5. The inhibitory effect of vardenafil is more selective on PDE5 than for other known phosphodiesterases (>15-fold relative to PDE6, >130-fold relative to PDE1, >300-fold relative to PDE11, and >1,000-fold relative to PDE2, 3, 4, 7, 8, 9, and 10).
Pharmacokinetics
The pharmacokinetics of vardenafil are approximately dose proportional over the recommended dose range. Vardenafil is eliminated predominantly by hepatic metabolism, mainly by CYP3A4 and to a minor extent, CYP2C isoforms. Concomitant use with strong CYP3A4 inhibitors such as ritonavir, indinavir, ketoconazole, itraconazole as well as moderate CYP3A inhibitors such as erythromycin results in significant increases of plasma levels of vardenafil (see **PRECAUTIONS, WARNINGS** and **DOSAGE AND ADMINISTRATION**). Mean vardenafil plasma concentrations measured after the administration of a single oral dose of 20 mg to healthy male volunteers are depicted in Figure 1.

Figure 1: Plasma Vardenafil Concentration (Mean ± SD) Curve for a Single 20 mg LEVITRA Dose

Absorption: Vardenafil is rapidly absorbed with absolute bioavailability of approximately 15%. Maximum observed plasma concentrations after a single 20 mg dose in healthy volunteers are usually reached between 30 minutes and 2 hours (median 60 minutes) after oral dosing in the fasted state. Two food-effect studies were conducted which showed that high-fat meals caused a reduction in C_{max} by 18%-50%.
Distribution: The mean steady-state volume of distribution (Vss) for vardenafil is 208 L, indicating extensive tissue distribution. Vardenafil and its major circulating metabolite, M1, are highly bound to plasma proteins (about 95% for parent drug and M1). This protein binding is reversible and independent of total drug concentrations.
Following a single oral dose of 20 mg vardenafil in healthy volunteers, a mean of 0.00018% of the administered dose was obtained in semen 1.5 hours after dosing.

Continued on next page

Levitra—Cont.

Metabolism: Vardenafil is metabolized predominantly by the hepatic enzyme CYP3A4, with contribution from the CYP3A5 and CYP2C isoforms. The major circulating metabolite, M1, results from desethylation at the piperazine moiety of vardenafil. M1 is subject to further metabolism. The plasma concentration of M1 is approximately 26% that of the parent compound. This metabolite shows a phosphodiesterase selectivity profile similar to that of vardenafil and an *in vitro* inhibitory potency for PDE5 28% of that of vardenafil. Therefore, M1 accounts for approximately 7% of total pharmacologic activity.
Excretion: The total body clearance of vardenafil is 56 L/h, and the terminal half-life of vardenafil and its primary metabolite (M1) is approximately 4-5 hours. After oral administration, vardenafil is excreted as metabolites predominantly in the feces (approximately 91-95% of administered oral dose) and to a lesser extent in the urine (approximately 2-6% of administered oral dose).
Pharmacokinetics in Special Populations
Pediatrics: Vardenafil trials were not conducted in the pediatric population.
Geriatrics: In a healthy volunteer study of elderly males (≥ 65 years) and younger males (18-45 years), mean C_{max} and AUC were 34% and 52% higher, respectively, in the elderly males (see **PRECAUTIONS, Geriatric Use** and **DOSAGE AND ADMINISTRATION**). Consequently, a lower starting dose of LEVITRA (5 mg) in patients ≥ 65 years of age should be considered.
Renal Insufficiency: In volunteers with mild renal impairment (CL_{cr} = 50-80 ml/min), the pharmacokinetics of vardenafil were similar to those observed in a control group with normal renal function. In the moderate (CL_{cr} = 30-50 ml/min) or severe (CL_{cr} <30 ml/min) renal impairment groups, the AUC of vardenafil was 20-30% higher compared to that observed in a control group with normal renal function (CL_{cr} >80 ml/min). Vardenafil pharmacokinetics have not been evaluated in patients requiring renal dialysis (see **PRECAUTIONS, Renal Insufficiency,** and **DOSAGE AND ADMINISTRATION**).
Hepatic Insufficiency: In volunteers with mild hepatic impairment (Child-Pugh A), the C_{max} and AUC following a 10 mg vardenafil dose were increased by 22% and 17%, respectively, compared to healthy control subjects. In volunteers with moderate hepatic impairment (Child-Pugh B), the C_{max} and AUC following a 10 mg vardenafil dose were increased by 130% and 160%, respectively, compared to healthy control subjects. Consequently, a starting dose of 5 mg is recommended for patients with moderate hepatic impairment, and the maximum dose should not exceed 10 mg (see **PRECAUTIONS** and **DOSAGE AND ADMINISTRATION**). Vardenafil has not been evaluated in patients with severe (Child-Pugh C) hepatic impairment.
Pharmacodynamics
Effects on Blood Pressure: In a clinical pharmacology study of patients with erectile dysfunction, single doses of vardenafil 20 mg caused a mean maximum decrease in supine blood pressure of 7 mm Hg systolic and 8 mm Hg diastolic (compared to placebo), accompanied by a mean maximum increase of heart rate of 4 beats per minute. The maximum decrease in blood pressure occurred between 1 and 4 hours after dosing. Following multiple dosing for 31 days, similar blood pressure responses were observed on Day 31 as on Day 1. Vardenafil may add to the blood pressure lowering effects of antihypertensive agents (see **CONTRAINDICATIONS, PRECAUTIONS, Drug Interactions**).
Effects on Blood Pressure and Heart Rate when LEVITRA is Combined with Nitrates: A study was conducted in which the blood pressure and heart rate response to 0.4 mg nitroglycerin (NTG) sublingually was evaluated in 18 healthy subjects following pretreatment with LEVITRA 20 mg at various times before NTG administration. LEVITRA 20 mg caused an additional time-related reduction in blood pressure and increase in heart rate in association with NTG administration. The blood pressure effects were observed when LEVITRA 20 mg was dosed 1 or 4 hours before NTG and the heart rate effects were observed when 20 mg was dosed 1, 4, or 8 hours before NTG. Additional blood pressure and heart rate changes were not detected when LEVITRA 20 mg was dosed 24 hours before NTG. (See Figure 2.)

Figure 2: Placebo-subtracted point estimates (with 90% CI) of mean maximal blood pressure and heart rate effects of pre-dosing with LEVITRA 20 mg at 24, 8, 4, and 1 hour before 0.4 mg NTG sublingually.

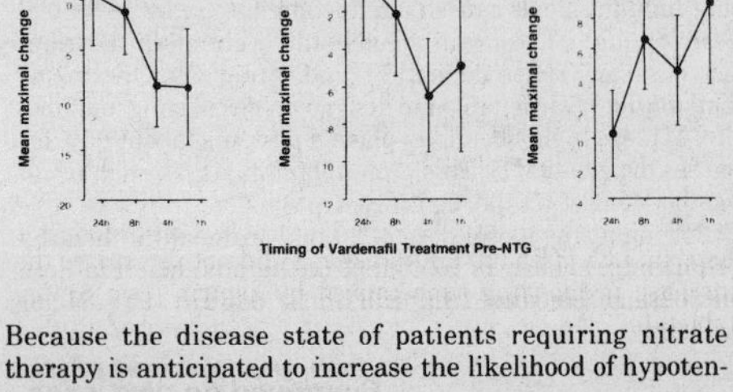

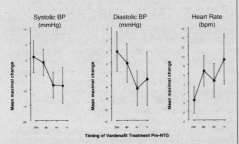

Because the disease state of patients requiring nitrate therapy is anticipated to increase the likelihood of hypotension, the use of vardenafil by patients on nitrate therapy or on nitric oxide donors is contraindicated (see **CONTRAINDICATIONS**).
Electrophysiology: The effect of 10 mg and 80 mg vardenafil on QT interval was evaluated in a single-dose, double-blind, randomized, placebo- and active-controlled (moxifloxacin 400 mg) crossover study in 59 healthy males (81% White, 12% Black, 7% Hispanic) aged 45-60 years. The QT interval was measured at one hour post dose because this time point approximates the average time of peak vardenafil concentration. The 80 mg dose of LEVITRA (four times the highest recommended dose) was chosen because this dose yields plasma concentrations covering those observed upon co-administration of a low-dose of LEVITRA (5 mg) and 600 mg BID of ritonavir. Of the CYP3A4 inhibitors that have been studied, ritonavir causes the most significant drug-drug interaction with vardenafil. Table 1 summarizes the effect on mean uncorrected QT and mean corrected QT interval (QT_c) with different methods of correction (Fridericia and a linear individual correction method) at one hour post-dose. No single correction method is known to be more valid than the other. In this study, the mean increase in heart rate associated with a 10 mg dose of LEVITRA compared to placebo was 5 beats/minute and with an 80 mg dose of LEVITRA the mean increase was 6 beats/minute.
[See table 1 above]

Table 1. Mean QT and QT_c changes in msec (90% CI) from baseline relative to placebo at 1 hour post-dose with different methodologies to correct for the effect of heart rate.

Drug/Dose	QT Uncorrected (msec)	Fridericia QT Correction (msec)	Individual QT Correction (msec)
Vardenafil 10 mg	-2 (-4, 0)	8 (6, 9)	4 (3, 6)
Vardenafil 80 mg	-2 (-4, 0)	10 (8, 11)	6 (4, 7)
Moxifloxacin* 400 mg	3 (1, 5)	8 (6, 9)	7 (5, 8)

*Active control (drug known to prolong QT)

Therapeutic and supratherapeutic doses of vardenafil and the active control moxifloxacin produced similar increases in QT_c interval. This study, however, was not designed to make direct statistical comparisons between the drug or the dose levels. The clinical impact of these QT_c changes is unknown (see **PRECAUTIONS**).
Effects on Exercise Treadmill Test in Patients with Coronary Artery Disease (CAD): In two independent trials that assessed 10 mg (n=41) and 20 mg (n=39) vardenafil, respectively, vardenafil did not alter the total treadmill exercise time compared to placebo. The patient population included men aged 40-80 years with stable exercise-induced angina documented by at least one of the following: 1) prior history of MI, CABG, PTCA, or stenting (not within 6 months); 2) positive coronary angiogram showing at least 60% narrowing of the diameter of at least one major coronary artery; or 3) a positive stress echocardiogram or stress nuclear perfusion study.
Results of these studies showed that LEVITRA did not alter the total treadmill exercise time compared to placebo (10 mg LEVITRA vs. placebo: 433±109 and 426±105 seconds, respectively; 20 mg LEVITRA vs. placebo: 414±114 and 411±124 seconds, respectively). The total time to angina was not altered by LEVITRA when compared to placebo (10 mg LEVITRA vs. placebo: 291±123 and 292±110 seconds; 20 mg LEVITRA vs. placebo: 354±137 and 347±143 seconds, respectively). The total time to 1 mm or greater ST-segment depression was similar to placebo in both the 10 mg and the 20 mg LEVITRA groups (10 mg LEVITRA vs. placebo: 380±108 and 334±108 seconds; 20 mg LEVITRA vs. placebo: 364±101 and 366±105 seconds, respectively).
Effects on Vision: Single oral doses of phosphodiesterase inhibitors have demonstrated transient dose-related impairment of color discrimination (blue/green) using the Farnsworth-Munsell 100-hue test and reductions in electroretinogram (ERG) b-wave amplitudes, with peak effects near the time of peak plasma levels. These findings are consistent with the inhibition of PDE6 in rods and cones, which is involved in phototransduction in the retina. The findings were most evident one hour after administration, diminishing but still present 6 hours after administration. In a single dose study in 25 normal males, LEVITRA 40 mg, twice the maximum daily recommended dose, did not alter visual acuity, intraocular pressure, fundoscopic and slit lamp findings.

CLINICAL STUDIES

LEVITRA was evaluated in four major double-blind, randomized, placebo-controlled, fixed-dose, parallel design, multicenter trials in 2431 men aged 20–83 (mean age 57 years; 78% White, 7% Black, 2% Asian, 3% Hispanic and 10% Other/Unknown). The doses of LEVITRA in these studies were 5 mg, 10 mg, and 20 mg. Two of these trials were conducted in the general ED population and two in special ED populations (one in patients with diabetes mellitus and one in post-prostatectomy patients). LEVITRA was dosed without regard to meals on an as needed basis in men with erectile dysfunction (ED), many of whom had multiple other medical conditions. The primary endpoints were assessed at 3 months.
Primary efficacy assessment in all four major trials was by means of the Erectile Function (EF) Domain score of the validated International Index of Erectile Function (IIEF) Questionnaire and two questions from the Sexual Encounter Profile (SEP) dealing with the ability to achieve vaginal penetration (SEP2), and the ability to maintain an erection long enough for successful intercourse (SEP3).
In all four fixed-dose efficacy trials, LEVITRA showed clinically meaningful and statistically significant improvement in the EF Domain, SEP2, and SEP3 scores compared to placebo. The mean baseline EF Domain score in these trials was 11.8 (scores range from 0–30 where lower scores represent more severe disease). LEVITRA (5 mg, 10 mg, and 20 mg) was effective in all age categories (<45, 45 to <65, and ≥65 years) and was also effective regardless of race (White, Black, Other).
Trials in a General Erectile Dysfunction Population: In the major North American fixed-dose trial, 762 patients (mean age 57, range 20-83 years; 79% White, 13% Black, 4% Hispanic, 2% Asian and 2% Other) were evaluated. The mean baseline EF Domain scores were 13, 13, 13, 14 for the LEVITRA 5 mg, 10 mg, 20 mg and placebo groups, respectively. There was significant improvement (p<0.0001) at 3 months with LEVITRA (EF Domain scores of 18, 21, 21, for the 5 mg, 10 mg, and 20 mg dose groups, respectively) compared to the placebo group (EF Domain score of 15). The European trial (total N=803) confirmed these results. The improvement in mean score was maintained at all doses at 6 months in the North American trial.
In the North American trial, LEVITRA significantly improved the rates of achieving an erection sufficient for penetration (SEP2) at doses of 5 mg, 10 mg, and 20 mg compared to placebo (65%, 75%, and 80%, respectively, compared to a 52% response in the placebo group at 3 months; p< 0.0001). The European trial confirmed these results.
LEVITRA demonstrated a clinically meaningful and statistically significant increase in the overall per-patient rate of maintenance of erection to successful intercourse (SEP3) (51% on 5 mg, 64% on 10 mg, and 65% on 20 mg, respectively, compared to 32% on placebo; p< 0.0001) at 3 months in the North American trial. The European trial showed comparable efficacy. This improvement in mean score was maintained at all doses at 6 months in the North American trial.
Trial in Patients with ED and Diabetes Mellitus: LEVITRA demonstrated clinically meaningful and statistically significant improvement in erectile function in a prospective, fixed-dose (10 and 20 mg LEVITRA), double-blind, placebo-controlled trial of patients with diabetes mellitus (n=439; mean age 57 years, range 33–81; 80% White, 9% Black, 8% Hispanic, and 3% Other).
Significant improvements in the EF Domain were shown in this study (EF Domain scores of 17 on 10 mg LEVITRA and 19 on 20 mg LEVITRA compared to 13 on placebo; p< 0.0001).
LEVITRA significantly improved the overall per-patient rate of achieving an erection sufficient for penetration (SEP2) (61% on 10 mg and 64% on 20 mg LEVITRA compared to 36% on placebo; p< 0.0001).
LEVITRA demonstrated a clinically meaningful and statistically significant increase in the overall per-patient rate of maintenance of erection to successful intercourse (SEP3) (49% on 10 mg, 54% on 20 mg LEVITRA compared to 23% on placebo; p< 0.0001).
Trial in Patients with ED after Radical Prostatectomy: LEVITRA demonstrated clinically meaningful and statistically significant improvement in erectile function in a prospective, fixed-dose (10 and 20 mg LEVITRA), double-blind, placebo-controlled trial in post-prostatectomy patients (n=427, mean age 60, range 44-77 years; 93% White, 5% Black, 2% Other).
Significant improvements in the EF Domain were shown in this study (EF Domain scores of 15 on 10 mg LEVITRA and 15 on 20 mg LEVITRA compared to 9 on placebo; p< 0.0001).
LEVITRA significantly improved the overall per-patient rate of achieving an erection sufficient for penetration (SEP2) (47% on 10 mg and 48% on 20 mg LEVITRA compared to 22% on placebo; p <0.0001).
LEVITRA demonstrated a clinically meaningful and statistically significant increase in the overall per-patient rate of maintenance of erection to successful intercourse (SEP3) (37% on 10 mg, 34% on 20 mg LEVITRA compared to 10% on placebo; p< 0.0001).

INDICATIONS AND USAGE

LEVITRA is indicated for the treatment of erectile dysfunction.

CONTRAINDICATIONS

Nitrates: Administration of LEVITRA with nitrates (either regularly and/or intermittently) and nitric oxide donors is contraindicated (see **CLINICAL PHARMACOLOGY, Pharmacodynamics, Effects on Blood Pressure and Heart Rate when LEVITRA is Combined with Nitrates**). Consistent with the effects of PDE5 inhibition on the nitric oxide/cyclic guanosine monophosphate pathway, PDE5 inhibitors may potentiate the hypotensive effects of nitrates. A suitable time interval following LEVITRA dosing for the safe administration of nitrates or nitric oxide donors has not been determined.

Alpha-Blockers: Because the co-administration of alpha-blockers and LEVITRA can produce hypotension, LEVITRA is contraindicated in patients taking alpha-blockers (see **PRECAUTIONS, Drug Interactions**).

Hypersensitivity: LEVITRA is contraindicated for patients with a known hypersensitivity to any component of the tablet.

WARNINGS

Cardiovascular effects

General: Physicians should consider the cardiovascular status of their patients, since there is a degree of cardiac risk associated with sexual activity. In men for whom sexual activity is not recommended because of their underlying cardiovascular status, any treatment for erectile dysfunction, including LEVITRA, generally should not be used.

Left Ventricular Outflow Obstruction: Patients with left ventricular outflow obstruction, e.g., aortic stenosis and idiopathic hypertrophic subaortic stenosis, can be sensitive to the action of vasodilators including Type 5 phosphodiesterase inhibitors.

Blood Pressure Effects: LEVITRA has systemic vasodilatory properties that resulted in transient decreases in supine blood pressure in healthy volunteers (mean maximum decrease of 7 mmHg systolic and 8 mmHg diastolic) (see **CLINICAL PHARMACOLOGY, Pharmacodynamics**). While this normally would be expected to be of little consequence in most patients, prior to prescribing LEVITRA, physicians should carefully consider whether their patients with underlying cardiovascular disease could be affected adversely by such vasodilatory effects.

Effect of Co-administration of Strong CYP3A4 Inhibitors

Long-term safety information is not available on the concomitant administration of vardenafil with HIV protease inhibitors. Concomitant administration with ritonavir or indinavir substantially increases plasma concentrations of vardenafil. To decrease the chance of adverse events in patients concomitantly taking ritonavir or indinavir, which are strong inhibitors of CYP3A4 metabolism, a maximum single dose of 2.5 mg LEVITRA should not be exceeded. Because ritonavir prolongs LEVITRA elimination half-life (5-6-fold), no more than a single 2.5 mg dose of LEVITRA should be taken in a 72-hour period by patients also taking ritonavir. Patients taking indinavir, ketoconazole 400 mg daily, or itraconazole 400 mg daily should not exceed LEVITRA 2.5 mg once daily. For patients taking ketoconazole or itraconazole 200 mg daily, a single dose of 5 mg LEVITRA should not be exceeded in a 24-hour period (see **PRECAUTIONS, Drug Interactions** and **DOSAGE AND ADMINISTRATION**).

Other Effects

There have been rare reports of prolonged erections greater than 4 hours and priapism (painful erections greater than 6 hours in duration) for this class of compounds, including vardenafil. In the event that an erection persists longer than 4 hours, the patient should seek immediate medical assistance. If priapism is not treated immediately, penile tissue damage and permanent loss of potency may result.

Patient Subgroups Not Studied in Clinical Trials

There is no controlled clinical data on the safety or efficacy of LEVITRA in the following patients; and therefore its use is not recommended until further information is available.

- unstable angina; hypotension (resting systolic blood pressure of <90 mm Hg); uncontrolled hypertension (>170/110 mm Hg); recent history of stroke, life-threatening arrhythmia, or myocardial infarction (within the last 6 months); severe cardiac failure
- severe hepatic impairment (Child-Pugh C)
- end stage renal disease requiring dialysis
- known hereditary degenerative retinal disorders, including retinitis pigmentosa

PRECAUTIONS

The evaluation of erectile dysfunction should include a determination of potential underlying causes, a medical assessment, and the identification of appropriate treatment.

Before prescribing LEVITRA, it is important to note the following:

Hepatic Insufficiency: In volunteers with moderate impairment (Child-Pugh B), the C_{max} and AUC following a 10 mg vardenafil dose were increased 130% and 160%, respectively, compared to healthy control subjects. Consequently, a starting dose of 5 mg is recommended for patients with moderate hepatic impairment and the maximum dose should not exceed 10 mg (see **CLINICAL PHARMACOLOGY, Pharmacokinetics in Special Populations**, and **DOSAGE AND ADMINISTRATION**). Vardenafil has not been evaluated in patients with severe hepatic impairment (Child-Pugh C).

Congenital or Acquired QT Prolongation: In a study of the effect of LEVITRA on QT interval in 59 healthy males (see **CLINICAL PHARMACOLOGY, Electrophysiology**), therapeutic (10 mg) and supratherapeutic (80 mg) doses of LEVITRA and the active control moxifloxacin (400 mg) produced similar increases in QT_c interval. This observation should be considered in clinical decisions when prescribing LEVITRA. Patients with congenital QT prolongation and those taking Class IA (e.g., quinidine, procainamide) or Class III (e.g., amiodarone, sotalol) antiarrhythmic medications should avoid using LEVITRA.

Renal Insufficiency: In patients with moderate (CL_{cr} = 30-50 ml/min) to severe (CL_{cr} <30 ml/min) renal impairment, the AUC of vardenafil was 20-30% higher compared to that observed in a control group with normal renal function (CL_{cr} >80 ml/min) (see **CLINICAL PHARMACOLOGY, Pharmacokinetics in Special Populations**). Vardenafil pharmacokinetics have not been evaluated in patients requiring renal dialysis.

General: In humans, vardenafil alone in doses up to 20 mg does not prolong the bleeding time. There is no clinical evidence of any additive prolongation of the bleeding time when vardenafil is administered with aspirin. Vardenafil has not been administered to patients with bleeding disorders or significant active peptic ulceration. Therefore LEVITRA should be administered to these patients after careful benefit-risk assessment.

Treatment for erectile dysfunction should generally be used with caution by patients with anatomical deformation of the penis (such as angulation, cavernosal fibrosis, or Peyronie's disease) or by patients who have conditions that may predispose them to priapism (such as sickle cell anemia, multiple myeloma, or leukemia).

The safety and efficacy of LEVITRA used in combination with other treatments for erectile dysfunction have not been studied. Therefore, the use of such combinations is not recommended.

Information for Patients

Physicians should discuss with patients the contraindication of LEVITRA with regular and/or intermittent use of organic nitrates. Patients should be counseled that concomitant use of LEVITRA with nitrates could cause blood pressure to suddenly drop to an unsafe level, resulting in dizziness, syncope, or even heart attack or stroke.

Physicians should inform their patients that concomitant use of LEVITRA with alpha-blockers is contraindicated because co-administration can produce hypotension.

Physicians should discuss with patients the appropriate use of LEVITRA and its anticipated benefits. It should be explained that sexual stimulation is required for an erection to occur after taking LEVITRA. LEVITRA should be taken approximately 60 minutes before sexual activity. Patients should be counseled regarding the dosing of LEVITRA. Patients should be advised to contact their healthcare provider for dose modification if they are not satisfied with the quality of their sexual performance with LEVITRA or in the case of an unwanted effect. Patients should be advised to contact the prescribing physician if new medications that may interact with LEVITRA are prescribed by another healthcare provider.

Physicians should discuss with patients the potential cardiac risk of sexual activity for patients with preexisting cardiovascular risk factors.

The use of LEVITRA offers no protection against sexually transmitted diseases. Counseling of patients about protective measures necessary to guard against sexually transmitted diseases, including the Human Immunodeficiency Virus (HIV), should be considered.

Physicians should inform patients that there have been rare reports of prolonged erections greater than 4 hours and priapism (painful erections greater than 6 hours in duration) for LEVITRA and this class of compounds. In the event that an erection persists longer than 4 hours, the patient should seek immediate medical assistance. If priapism is not treated immediately, penile tissue damage and permanent loss of potency may result.

Drug Interactions

Effect of other drugs on LEVITRA

In vitro studies: Studies in human liver microsomes showed that vardenafil is metabolized primarily by cytochrome P450 (CYP) isoforms 3A4/5, and to a lesser degree by CYP2C9. Therefore, inhibitors of these enzymes are expected to reduce vardenafil clearance (see **WARNINGS** and **DOSAGE AND ADMINISTRATION**).

In vivo studies: Cytochrome P450 Inhibitors

Cimetidine (400 mg b.i.d.) had no effect on vardenafil bioavailability (AUC) and maximum concentration (C_{max}) of vardenafil when co-administered with 20 mg LEVITRA in healthy volunteers.

Erythromycin (500 mg t.i.d) produced a 4-fold increase in vardenafil AUC and a 3-fold increase in C_{max} when co-administered with LEVITRA 5 mg in healthy volunteers (see **DOSAGE AND ADMINISTRATION**). It is recommended not to exceed a single 5 mg dose of LEVITRA in a 24-hour period when used in combination with erythromycin.

Ketoconazole (200 mg once daily) produced a 10-fold increase in vardenafil AUC and a 4-fold increase in C_{max} when co-administered with LEVITRA (5 mg) in healthy volunteers. A 5-mg LEVITRA dose should not be exceeded when used in combination with 200 mg once daily ketoconazole. Since higher doses of ketoconazole (400 mg daily) may result in higher increases in C_{max} and AUC, a single 2.5 mg dose of LEVITRA should not be exceeded in a 24-hour

period when used in combination with ketoconazole 400 mg daily (see **WARNINGS** and **DOSAGE AND ADMINISTRATION**).

HIV Protease Inhibitors:

Indinavir (800 mg t.i.d.) co-administered with LEVITRA 10 mg resulted in a 16-fold increase in vardenafil AUC, a 7-fold increase in vardenafil C_{max} and a 2-fold increase in vardenafil half-life. It is recommended not to exceed a single 2.5 mg LEVITRA dose in a 24-hour period when used in combination with indinavir (see **WARNINGS** and **DOSAGE AND ADMINISTRATION**).

Ritonavir (600 mg b.i.d.) co-administered with LEVITRA 5 mg resulted in a 49-fold increase in vardenafil AUC and a 13-fold increase in vardenafil C_{max}. The interaction is a consequence of blocking hepatic metabolism of vardenafil by ritonavir, a highly potent CYP3A4 inhibitor, which also inhibits CYP2C9. Ritonavir significantly prolonged the half-life of vardenafil to 26 hours. Consequently, it is recommended not to exceed a single 2.5 mg LEVITRA dose in a 72-hour period when used in combination with ritonavir (see **WARNINGS** and **DOSAGE AND ADMINISTRATION**).

Other Drug Interactions: No pharmacokinetic interactions were observed between vardenafil and the following drugs: glyburide, warfarin, digoxin, Maalox, and ranitidine. In the warfarin study, vardenafil had no effect on the prothrombin time or other pharmacodynamic parameters.

Effects of LEVITRA on other drugs

In vitro studies:

Vardenafil and its metabolites had no effect on CYP1A2, 2A6, and 2E1 (Ki > 100µM). Weak inhibitory effects toward other isoforms (CYP2C8, 2C9, 2C19, 2D6, 3A4) were found, but Ki values were in excess of plasma concentrations achieved following dosing. The most potent inhibitory activity was observed for vardenafil metabolite M1, which had a Ki of 1.4 µM toward CYP3A4, which is about 20 times higher than the M1 C_{max} values after an 80 mg LEVITRA dose.

In vivo studies:

Nitrates: The blood pressure lowering effects of sublingual nitrates (0.4 mg) taken 1 and 4 hours after vardenafil and increases in heart rate when taken at 1, 4 and 8 hours were potentiated by a 20 mg dose of LEVITRA in healthy middle-aged subjects. These effects were not observed when LEVITRA 20 mg was taken 24 hours before the NTG. Potentiation of the hypotensive effects of nitrates for patients with ischemic heart disease has not been evaluated, and concomitant use of LEVITRA and nitrates is contraindicated (see **CLINICAL PHARMACOLOGY, Pharmacodynamics, Effects on Blood Pressure and Heart Rate when LEVITRA is Combined with Nitrates; CONTRAINDICATIONS**).

Nifedipine: Vardenafil 20 mg, when co-administered with slow-release nifedipine 30 mg or 60 mg once daily, did not affect the relative bioavailability (AUC) or maximum concentration (C_{max}) of nifedipine, a drug that is metabolized via CYP3A4. Nifedipine did not alter the plasma levels of LEVITRA when taken in combination. In these patients whose hypertension was controlled with nifedipine, LEVITRA 20 mg produced mean additional supine systolic/diastolic blood pressure reductions of 6/5 mm Hg compared to placebo.

Alpha-blockers: When LEVITRA 10 or 20 mg was given to healthy volunteers either simultaneously or 6 hours after a 10 mg dose of terazosin, significant hypotension developed in a substantial number of subjects. With simultaneous dosing of LEVITRA 10 mg and terazosin 10 mg, 6 of 8 subjects experienced a standing systolic blood pressure of less than 85 mm Hg. With simultaneous dosing of LEVITRA 20 mg and terazosin 10 mg, 2 of 9 subjects experienced a standing systolic blood pressure of less than 85 mm Hg. When LEVITRA dosing was separated from terazosin 10 mg by 6 hours, 7 of 28 subjects who received 20 mg of LEVITRA experienced a decrease in standing systolic blood pressure below 85 mm Hg. In a similar study with tamsulosin in healthy volunteers, 1 of 24 subjects dosed with LEVITRA 20 mg and tamsulosin 0.4 mg separated by 6 hours experienced a standing systolic blood pressure below 85 mm Hg. Two of 16 subjects dosed simultaneously with LEVITRA 10 mg and tamsulosin 0.4 mg experienced a standing systolic blood pressure below 85 mm Hg. The administration of lower doses of LEVITRA with alpha-blockers has not been completely evaluated to determine if they can be safely administered together. Based on these data, LEVITRA should not be used in patients on alpha-blocker therapy (see **CONTRAINDICATIONS**).

Ritonavir and indinavir: Upon concomitant administration of 5 mg of LEVITRA with 600 mg BID ritonavir, the C_{max} and AUC of ritonavir were reduced by approximately 20%. Upon administration of 10 mg of LEVITRA with 800 mg TID indinavir, the C_{max} and AUC of indinavir were reduced by 40% and 30%, respectively.

Alcohol: Alcohol (0.5 g/kg body weight: approximately 40 mL of absolute alcohol in a 70 kg person) and vardenafil plasma levels were not altered when dosed simultaneously. LEVITRA (20 mg) did not potentiate the hypotensive effects of alcohol during the 4-hour observation period in healthy volunteers when administered with alcohol (0.5 g/kg body weight).

Aspirin: LEVITRA (10 mg and 20 mg) did not potentiate the increase in bleeding time caused by aspirin (two 81 mg tablets).

Continued on next page

Levitra—Cont.

Other interactions: LEVITRA had no effect on the pharmacodynamics of glyburide (glucose and insulin concentrations) and warfarin (prothrombin time or other pharmacodynamic parameters).

Carcinogenesis, Mutagenesis, Impairment of Fertility

Vardenafil was not carcinogenic in rats and mice when administered daily for 24 months. In these studies systemic drug exposures (AUCs) for unbound (free) vardenafil and its major metabolite were approximately 400- and 170-fold for male and female rats, respectively, and 21- and 37-fold for male and female mice, respectively, the exposures observed in human males given the Maximum Recommended Human Dose (MRHD) of 20 mg. Vardenafil was not mutagenic as assessed in either the *in vitro* bacterial Ames assay or the forward mutation assay in Chinese hamster V79 cells. Vardenafil was not clastogenic as assessed in either the *in vitro* chromosomal aberration test or the *in vivo* mouse micronucleus test. Vardenafil did not impair fertility in male and female rats administered doses up to 100 mg/kg/day for 28 days prior to mating in male, and for 14 days prior to mating and through day 7 of gestation in females. In a corresponding 1-month rat toxicity study, this dose produced an AUC value for unbound vardenafil 200 fold greater than AUC in humans at the MRHD of 20 mg.

There was no effect on sperm motility or morphology after single 20 mg oral doses of vardenafil in healthy volunteers.

Pregnancy, Nursing Mothers and Pediatric Use

LEVITRA is not indicated for use in women, newborns, or children. Vardenafil was secreted into the milk of lactating rats at concentrations approximately 10-fold greater than found in the plasma. Following a single oral dose of 3 mg/kg, 3.3% of the administered dose was excreted into the milk within 24 hours. It is not known if vardenafil is excreted in human breast milk.

Pregnancy Category B: No evidence of specific potential for teratogenicity, embryotoxicity or fetotoxicity was observed in rats and rabbits that received vardenafil at up to 18 mg/kg/day during organogenesis. This dose is approximately 100 fold (rat) and 29 fold (rabbit) greater than the AUC values for unbound vardenafil and its major metabolite in humans given the MRHD of 20 mg. In the rat pre- and postnatal development study, the NOAEL (no observed adverse effect level) for maternal toxicity was 8 mg/kg/day. Retarded physical development of pups in the absence of maternal effects was observed following maternal exposure to 1 and 8 mg/kg possibly due to vasodilatation and/or secretion of the drug into milk. The number of living pups born to rats exposed pre- and postnatally was reduced at 60 mg/kg/day. Based on the results of the pre- and postnatal study, the developmental NOAEL is less than 1 mg/kg/day. Based on plasma exposures in the rat developmental toxicity study, 1mg/kg/day in the pregnant rat is estimated to produce total AUC values for unbound vardenafil and its major metabolite comparable to the human AUC at the MRHD of 20 mg. There are no adequate and well-controlled trials of vardenafil in pregnant women.

Geriatric Use

Elderly males age 65 years and older have higher vardenafil plasma concentrations than younger males (18-45 years), mean C_{max} and AUC were 34% and 52% higher, respectively (see **CLINICAL PHARMACOLOGY, Pharmacokinetics in Special Populations**, and **DOSAGE AND ADMINISTRATION**). Phase 3 clinical trials included more than 834 elderly patients, and no differences in safety or effectiveness of LEVITRA 5, 10, or 20 mg were noted when these elderly patients were compared to younger patients. However, due to increased vardenafil concentrations in the elderly, a starting dose of 5 mg LEVITRA should be considered in patients ≥ 65 years of age.

ADVERSE REACTIONS

LEVITRA was administered to over 4430 men (mean age 56, range 18-89 years; 81% White, 6% Black, 2% Asian, 2% Hispanic and 9% Other) during controlled and uncontrolled clinical trials worldwide. Over 2200 patients were treated for 6 months or longer, and 880 patients were treated for at least 1 year.

In placebo-controlled clinical trials, the discontinuation rate due to adverse events was 3.4% for LEVITRA compared to 1.1% for placebo.

When LEVITRA was taken as recommended in placebo-controlled clinical trials, the following adverse events were reported (see Table 2).

Table 2: Adverse Events Reported By ≥ 2% of Patients Treated with LEVITRA and More Frequent on Drug than Placebo in Fixed and Flexible[γ] Dose Randomized, Controlled Trials of 5 mg, 10 mg, or 20 mg Vardenafil

Adverse Event	Percentage of Patients Reporting Event	
	Placebo N = 1199	LEVITRA N = 2203
Headache	4%	15%
Flushing	1%	11%
Rhinitis	3%	9%
Dyspepsia	1%	4%
Accidental Injury*	2%	3%
Sinusitis	1%	3%
Flu Syndrome	2%	3%
Dizziness	1%	2%
Increased Creatine Kinase	1%	2%
Nausea	1%	2%

*All the events listed in the above table were deemed to be adverse drug reactions with the exception of accidental injury.
[γ] Flexible dose studies started all patients at LEVITRA 10 mg and allowed decrease in dose to 5 mg or increase in dose to 20 mg based on side effects and efficacy.

Back pain was reported in 2.0% of patients treated with LEVITRA and 1.7% of patients on placebo.

Placebo-controlled trials suggested a dose effect in the incidence of some adverse events (headache, flushing, dyspepsia, nausea, rhinitis) over the 5 mg, 10 mg, and 20 mg doses of LEVITRA. The following section identifies additional, less frequent events (<2%) reported during the clinical development of LEVITRA. Excluded from this list are those events that are infrequent and minor, those events that may be commonly observed in the absence of drug therapy, and those events that are not reasonably associated with the drug.

BODY AS A WHOLE: anaphylactic reaction (including laryngeal edema), asthenia, face edema, pain
AUDITORY: tinnitus
CARDIOVASCULAR: angina pectoris, chest pain, hypertension, hypotension, myocardial ischemia, myocardial infarction, palpitation, postural hypotension, syncope, tachycardia
DIGESTIVE: abdominal pain, abnormal liver function tests, diarrhea, dry mouth, dysphagia, esophagitis, gastritis, gastroesophageal reflux, GGTP increased, vomiting
MUSCULOSKELETAL: arthralgia, back pain, myalgia, neck pain
NERVOUS: hypertonia, hypesthesia, insomnia, paresthesia, somnolence, vertigo
RESPIRATORY: dyspnea, epistaxis, pharyngitis
SKIN AND APPENDAGES: photosensitivity reaction, pruritus, rash, sweating
OPHTHALMOLOGIC: abnormal vision, blurred vision, chromatopsia, changes in color vision, conjunctivitis (increased redness of the eye), dim vision, eye pain, glaucoma, photophobia, watery eyes
UROGENITAL: abnormal ejaculation, priapism (including prolonged or painful erections)

OVERDOSAGE

The maximum dose of LEVITRA for which human data are available is a single 120 mg dose administered to eight healthy male volunteers. The majority of these subjects experienced reversible back pain/myalgia and/or "abnormal vision."

In cases of overdose, standard supportive measures should be taken as required. Renal dialysis is not expected to accelerate clearance because vardenafil is highly bound to plasma proteins and is not significantly eliminated in the urine.

DOSAGE AND ADMINISTRATION

For most patients, the recommended starting dose of LEVITRA is 10 mg, taken orally approximately 60 minutes before sexual activity. The dose may be increased to a maximum recommended dose of 20 mg or decreased to 5 mg based on efficacy and side effects. The maximum recommended dosing frequency is once per day. LEVITRA can be taken with or without food. Sexual stimulation is required for a response to treatment.

Geriatrics: A starting dose of 5 mg LEVITRA should be considered in patients ≥ 65 years of age (see **CLINICAL PHARMACOLOGY, Pharmacokinetics in Special Populations** and **PRECAUTIONS**).

Hepatic Impairment: For patients with mild hepatic impairment (Child-Pugh A), no dose adjustment of LEVITRA is required. Vardenafil clearance is reduced in patients with moderate hepatic impairment (Child-Pugh B), and a starting dose of 5 mg LEVITRA is recommended. The maximum dose in patients with moderate hepatic impairment should not exceed 10 mg. LEVITRA has not been evaluated in patients with severe hepatic impairment (Child-Pugh C) (see **CLINICAL PHARMACOLOGY, Metabolism and Excretion, WARNINGS** and **PRECAUTIONS**).

Renal Impairment: For patients with mild (CL_{cr} = 50-80 ml/min), moderate (CL_{cr} = 30-50 ml/min), or severe (CL_{cr} <30 ml/min) renal impairment, no dose adjustment is required. LEVITRA has not been evaluated in patients on renal dialysis (see **CLINICAL PHARMACOLOGY, Metabolism and Excretion** and **PRECAUTIONS**).

Concomitant Medications: The dosage of LEVITRA may require adjustment in patients receiving certain CYP3A4 inhibitors (e.g., ketoconazole, itraconazole, ritonavir, indinavir, and erythromycin) (see **WARNINGS, PRECAUTIONS, Drug Interactions**). For ritonavir, a single dose of 2.5 mg LEVITRA should not be exceeded in a 72-hour period. For indinavir, ketoconazole 400 mg daily, and itraconazole 400 mg daily, a single dose of 2.5 mg LEVITRA should not be exceeded in a 24-hour period. For ketoconazole 200 mg daily, itraconazole 200 mg daily, and erythromycin, a single dose of 5 mg LEVITRA should not be exceeded in a 24-hour period.

HOW SUPPLIED

LEVITRA (vardenafil HCl) is formulated as orange, film-coated round tablets with debossed "BAYER" cross on one side and "2.5", "5", "10", and "20" on the other side equivalent to 2.5 mg, 5 mg, 10 mg, and 20 mg of vardenafil, respectively.

Package	Strength	NDC Code
Bottles of 30	2.5 mg	0085-1923-01
	5 mg	0085-1945-01
	10 mg	0085-1901-01
	20 mg	0085-1934-01

Recommended Storage: Store at 25°C (77°F); excursions permitted to 15-30°C (59-86°F) [see USP Controlled Room Temperature].

Manufactured by:
Bayer HealthCare
Bayer Pharmaceuticals Corporation
400 Morgan Lane
West Haven, CT 06516
Made in Germany
Distributed by:
Schering-Plough
Schering Corporation
Kenilworth, NJ 07033
LEVITRA is a registered trademark of Bayer Aktiengesellschaft and is used under license by Schering Corporation.
℞ Only
08918646, R.0   10/04   12532
©2004 Bayer Pharmaceuticals Corporation
Printed in U.S.A.

Patient Information
LEVITRA® (Luh-VEE-Trah)
(vardenafil HCl) Tablets
Read the Patient Information about LEVITRA before you start taking it and again each time you get a refill. There may be new information. You may also find it helpful to share this information with your partner. This leaflet does not take the place of talking with your doctor. You and your doctor should talk about LEVITRA when you start taking it and at regular checkups. If you do not understand the information, or have questions, talk with your doctor or pharmacist.

WHAT IMPORTANT INFORMATION SHOULD YOU KNOW ABOUT LEVITRA?
LEVITRA can cause your blood pressure to drop suddenly to an unsafe level if it is taken with certain other medicines. With a sudden drop in blood pressure, you could get dizzy, faint, or have a heart attack or stroke.
Do not take LEVITRA if you:
• **take any medicines called "nitrates."**
• **use recreational drugs called "poppers" like amyl nitrate and butyl nitrate.**
• **take medicines called alpha-blockers.**
(See "Who Should Not Take LEVITRA?")
Tell all your healthcare providers that you take LEVITRA. If you need emergency medical care for a heart problem, it will be important for your healthcare provider to know when you last took LEVITRA.

WHAT IS LEVITRA?
LEVITRA is a prescription medicine taken by mouth for the treatment of erectile dysfunction (ED) in men.
ED is a condition where the penis does not harden and expand when a man is sexually excited, or when he cannot keep an erection. A man who has trouble getting or keeping an erection should see his doctor for help if the condition bothers him. LEVITRA may help a man with ED get and keep an erection when he is sexually excited.
LEVITRA does not:
• cure ED
• increase a man's sexual desire
• protect a man or his partner from sexually transmitted diseases, including HIV. Speak to your doctor about ways to guard against sexually transmitted diseases.
• serve as a male form of birth control
LEVITRA is only for men with ED. LEVITRA is not for women or children. LEVITRA must be used only under a doctor's care.

HOW DOES LEVITRA WORK?
When a man is sexually stimulated, his body's normal physical response is to increase blood flow to his penis. This results in an erection. LEVITRA helps increase blood flow to the penis and may help men with ED get and keep an erection satisfactory for sexual activity. Once a man has completed sexual activity, blood flow to his penis decreases, and his erection goes away.

WHO CAN TAKE LEVITRA?
Talk to your doctor to decide if LEVITRA is right for you. LEVITRA has been shown to be effective in men over the age of 18 years who have erectile dysfunction, including men with diabetes or who have undergone prostatectomy.

WHO SHOULD NOT TAKE LEVITRA?
Do not take LEVITRA if you:
• **take any medicines called "nitrates"** (See "What important information should you know about LEVITRA?"). Nitrates are commonly used to treat angina. Angina is a symptom of heart disease and can cause pain in your chest, jaw, or down your arm.
Medicines called nitrates include nitroglycerin that is found in tablets, sprays, ointments, pastes, or patches. Nitrates can also be found in other medicines such as isosorbide dinitrate or isosorbide mononitrate. Some recreational drugs called "poppers" also contain nitrates, such as amyl nitrate and butyl nitrate. Do not use LEVITRA if you are using these drugs. Ask your doctor or pharmacist if you are not sure if any of your medicines are nitrates.
• **take medicines called "alpha-blockers."** Alpha-blockers are sometimes prescribed for prostate problems or high blood pressure. If LEVITRA is taken with alpha-blockers, your blood pressure could suddenly drop to an unsafe level. You could get dizzy and faint.

- **you have been told by your healthcare provider to not have sexual activity because of health problems.** Sexual activity can put an extra strain on your heart, especially if your heart is already weak from a heart attack or heart disease.
- **are allergic to LEVITRA or any of its ingredients.** The active ingredient in LEVITRA is called vardenafil. See the end of this leaflet for a complete list of ingredients.

WHAT SHOULD YOU DISCUSS WITH YOUR DOCTOR BEFORE TAKING LEVITRA?

Before taking LEVITRA, tell your doctor about all your medical problems, including if you:

- **have heart problems** such as angina, heart failure, irregular heartbeats, or have had a heart attack. Ask your doctor if it is safe for you to have sexual activity.
- **have low blood pressure** or have high blood pressure that is not controlled
- **have had a stroke**
- **or any family members have a rare heart condition known as prolongation of the QT interval (long QT syndrome)**
- **have liver problems**
- **have kidney problems and require dialysis**
- **have retinitis pigmentosa,** a rare genetic (runs in families) eye disease
- **have stomach ulcers**
- **have a bleeding problem**
- **have a deformed penis shape** or Peyronie's disease
- **have had an erection that lasted more than 4 hours**
- **have blood cell problems** such as sickle cell anemia, multiple myeloma, or leukemia

CAN OTHER MEDICATIONS AFFECT LEVITRA?

Tell your doctor about all the medicines you take including prescription and non-prescription medicines, vitamins, and herbal supplements. LEVITRA and other medicines may affect each other. Always check with your doctor before starting or stopping any medicines. Especially tell your doctor if you take any of the following:

- medicines called nitrates (See "What important information should you know about LEVITRA?")
- medicines called alpha-blockers. These include Hytrin® (terazosin HCl), Flomax® (tamsulosin HCl), Cardura® (doxazosin mesylate), Minipress® (prazosin HCl) or Uroxatral® (alfuzosin HCl).
- medicines that treat abnormal heartbeat. These include quinidine, procainamide, amiodarone and sotalol.
- ritonavir (Norvir®) or indinavir sulfate (Crixivan®)
- ketoconazole or itraconazole (such as Nizoral® or Sporanox®)
- erythromycin
- other medicines or treatments for ED

HOW SHOULD YOU TAKE LEVITRA?

Take LEVITRA exactly as your doctor prescribes. LEVITRA comes in different doses (2.5 mg, 5 mg, 10 mg, and 20 mg). For most men, the recommended starting dose is 10 mg. **Take LEVITRA no more than once a day.** Doses should be taken at least 24 hours apart. Some men can only take a low dose of LEVITRA because of medical conditions or medicines they take. Your doctor will prescribe the dose that is right for you.

- If you are older than 65 or have liver problems, your doctor may start you on a lower dose of LEVITRA.
- If you are taking certain other medicines your doctor may prescribe a lower starting dose and limit you to one dose of LEVITRA in a 72-hour (3 days) period.

Take 1 LEVITRA tablet about 1 hour (60 minutes) before sexual activity. Some form of sexual stimulation is needed for an erection to happen with LEVITRA. LEVITRA may be taken with or without meals.

Do not change your dose of LEVITRA without talking to your doctor. Your doctor may lower your dose or raise your dose, depending on how your body reacts to LEVITRA.

If you take too much LEVITRA, call your doctor or emergency room right away.

WHAT ARE THE POSSIBLE SIDE EFFECTS OF LEVITRA?

The most common side effects with LEVITRA are headache, flushing, stuffy or runny nose, indigestion, upset stomach, or dizziness. These side effects usually go away after a few hours. Call your doctor if you get a side effect that bothers you or one that will not go away.

LEVITRA may uncommonly cause:

- **an erection that won't go away (priapism).** If you get an erection that lasts more than 4 hours, get medical help right away. Priapism must be treated as soon as possible or lasting damage can happen to your penis including the inability to have erections.
- **vision changes,** such as seeing a blue tinge to objects or having difficulty telling the difference between the colors blue and green.

These are not all the side effects of LEVITRA. For more information, ask your doctor or pharmacist.

HOW SHOULD LEVITRA BE STORED?

- Store LEVITRA at room temperature between 59° and 86° F (15° to 30° C).
- **Keep LEVITRA and all medicines out of the reach of children.**

GENERAL INFORMATION ABOUT LEVITRA.

Medicines are sometimes prescribed for conditions other than those described in patient information leaflets. Do not use LEVITRA for a condition for which it was not prescribed. Do not give LEVITRA to other people, even if they have the same symptoms that you have. It may harm them. This leaflet summarizes the most important information about LEVITRA. If you would like more information, talk with your healthcare provider. You can ask your doctor or pharmacist for information about LEVITRA that is written for health professionals.

For more information you can also visit www.LEVITRA.com, or call 1-866-LEVITRA.

WHAT ARE THE INGREDIENTS OF LEVITRA?

Active Ingredient: vardenafil hydrochloride

Inactive Ingredients: microcrystalline cellulose, crospovidone, colloidal silicon dioxide, magnesium stearate, hypromellose, polyethylene glycol, titanium dioxide, yellow ferric oxide, and red ferric oxide.

Norvir (ritonavir) is a trademark of Abbott Laboratories
Crixivan (indinavir sulfate) is a trademark of Merck & Co., Inc.
Nizoral (ketoconazole) is a trademark of Johnson & Johnson
Sporanox (itraconazole) is a trademark of Johnson & Johnson
Hytrin (terazosin HCl) is a trademark of Abbott Laboratories
Flomax (tamsulosin HCl) is a trademark of Yamanouchi Pharmaceutical Co., Ltd.
Cardura (doxazosin mesylate) is a trademark of Pfizer Inc.
Minipress (prazosin HCl) is a trademark of Pfizer Inc.
Uroxatral (alfuzosin HCl) is a trademark of Sanofi-Synthelabo

Manufactured by:
Bayer HealthCare
Bayer Pharmaceuticals Corporation
400 Morgan Lane
West Haven, CT 06516
Made in Germany
Distributed by:
Schering-Plough
Schering Corporation
Kenilworth, NJ 07033

LEVITRA is a registered trademark of Bayer Aktiengesellschaft and is used under license by Schering Corporation.

℞ Only

08918646IP, R.0 10/04 12532

Printed in U.S.A.

PROVENTIL® HFA ℞

[*prō-vĕn-tĭl*]

(albuterol sulfate)
Inhalation Aerosol
FOR ORAL INHALATION ONLY
Prescribing Information

DESCRIPTION

The active component of PROVENTIL HFA (albuterol sulfate) Inhalation Aerosol is albuterol sulfate, USP racemic α^1[(*tert*-Butylamino)methyl]-4-hydroxy-*m*-xylene-α,α′-diol sulfate (2:1)(salt), a relatively selective $beta_2$-adrenergic bronchodilator having the following chemical structure:

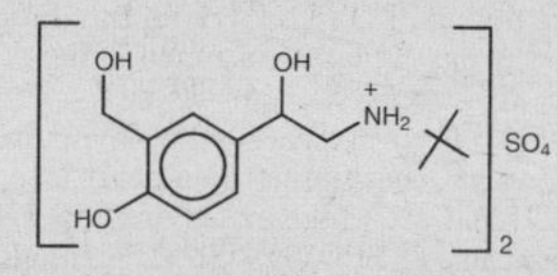

Albuterol sulfate is the official generic name in the United States. The World Health Organization recommended name for the drug is salbutamol sulfate. The molecular weight of albuterol sulfate is 576.7, and the empirical formula is $(C_{13}H_{21}NO_3)_2 \cdot H_2SO_4$. Albuterol sulfate is a white to off-white crystalline solid. It is soluble in water and slightly soluble in ethanol. PROVENTIL HFA Inhalation Aerosol is a pressurized metered-dose aerosol unit for oral inhalation. It contains a microcrystalline suspension of albuterol sulfate in propellant HFA-134a (1,1,1,2-tetrafluoroethane), ethanol, and oleic acid.

Each actuation delivers 120 mcg albuterol sulfate, USP from the valve and 108 mcg albuterol sulfate, USP from the mouthpiece (equivalent to 90 mcg of albuterol base from the mouthpiece). Each canister provides 200 inhalations. It is recommended to prime the inhaler before using for the first time and in cases where the inhaler has not been used for more than 2 weeks by releasing four "test sprays" into the air, away from the face.

This product does not contain chlorofluorocarbons (CFCs) as the propellant.

CLINICAL PHARMACOLOGY

Mechanism of Action *In vitro* studies and *in vivo* pharmacologic studies have demonstrated that albuterol has a preferential effect on $beta_2$-adrenergic receptors compared with isoproterenol. While it is recognized that $beta_2$-adrenergic receptors are the predominant receptors on bronchial smooth muscle, data indicate that there is a population of $beta_2$ receptors in the human heart existing in a concentration between 10% and 50% of cardiac beta-adrenergic receptors. The precise function of these receptors has not been established. (See **WARNINGS** for **Cardiovascular Effects.**)

Activation of $beta_2$-adrenergic receptors on airway smooth muscle leads to the activation of adenylcyclase and to an increase in the intracellular concentration of cyclic-3′,5′-adenosine monophosphate (cyclic AMP). This increase of cyclic AMP leads to the activation of protein kinase A, which inhibits the phosphorylation of myosin and lowers intracellular ionic calcium concentrations, resulting in relaxation. Albuterol relaxes the smooth muscles of all airways, from the trachea to the terminal bronchioles. Albuterol acts as a functional antagonist to relax the airway irrespective of the spasmogen involved, thus protecting against all bronchoconstrictor challenges. Increased cyclic AMP concentrations are also associated with the inhibition of release of mediators from mast cells in the airway.

Albuterol has been shown in most clinical trials to have more effect on the respiratory tract, in the form of bronchial smooth muscle relaxation, than isoproterenol at comparable doses while producing fewer cardiovascular effects. Controlled clinical studies and other clinical experience have shown that inhaled albuterol, like other beta-adrenergic agonist drugs, can produce a significant cardiovascular effect in some patients, as measured by pulse rate, blood pressure, symptoms, and/or electrocardiographic changes.

Preclinical Intravenous studies in rats with albuterol sulfate have demonstrated that albuterol crosses the blood-brain barrier and reaches brain concentrations amounting to approximately 5% of the plasma concentrations. In structures outside the blood-brain barrier (pineal and pituitary glands), albuterol concentrations were found to be 100 times those in the whole brain.

Studies in laboratory animals (minipigs, rodents, and dogs) have demonstrated the occurrence of cardiac arrhythmias and sudden death (with histologic evidence of myocardial necrosis) when β-agonists and methylxanthines were administered concurrently. The clinical significance of these findings is unknown.

Propellant HFA-134a is devoid of pharmacological activity except at very high doses in animals (380-1300 times the maximum human exposure based on comparisons of AUC values), primarily producing ataxia, tremors, dyspnea, or salivation. These are similar to effects produced by the structurally related chlorofluorocarbons (CFCs), which have been used extensively in metered dose inhalers.

In animals and humans, propellant HFA-134a was found to be rapidly absorbed and rapidly eliminated, with an elimination half-life of 3 to 27 minutes in animals and 5 to 7 minutes in humans. Time to maximum plasma concentration (T_{max}) and mean residence time are both extremely short leading to a transient appearance of HFA-134a in the blood with no evidence of accumulation.

Pharmacokinetics In a single-dose bioavailability study which enrolled six healthy, male volunteers, transient low albuterol levels (close to the lower limit of quantitation) were observed after administration of two puffs from both PROVENTIL HFA Inhalation Aerosol and a CFC 11/12 propelled albuterol inhaler. No formal pharmacokinetic analyses were possible for either treatment, but systemic albuterol levels appeared similar.

Clinical Trials In a 12-week, randomized, double-blind, double-dummy, active- and placebo-controlled trial, 565 patients with asthma were evaluated for the bronchodilator efficacy of PROVENTIL HFA Inhalation Aerosol (193 patients) in comparison to a CFC 11/12 propelled albuterol inhaler (186 patients) and an HFA-134a placebo inhaler (186 patients).

Serial FEV_1 measurements (shown below as percent change from test-day baseline) demonstrated that two inhalations of PROVENTIL HFA Inhalation Aerosol produced significantly greater improvement in pulmonary function than placebo and produced outcomes which were clinically comparable to a CFC 11/12 propelled albuterol inhaler.

The mean time to onset of a 15% increase in FEV_1 was 6 minutes and the mean time to peak effect was 50 to 55 minutes. The mean duration of effect as measured by a 15% increase in FEV_1 was 3 hours. In some patients, duration of effect was as long as 6 hours.

In another clinical study in adults, two inhalations of PROVENTIL HFA Inhalation Aerosol taken 30 minutes before exercise prevented exercise-induced bronchospasm as demonstrated by the maintenance of FEV_1 within 80% of baseline values in the majority of patients.

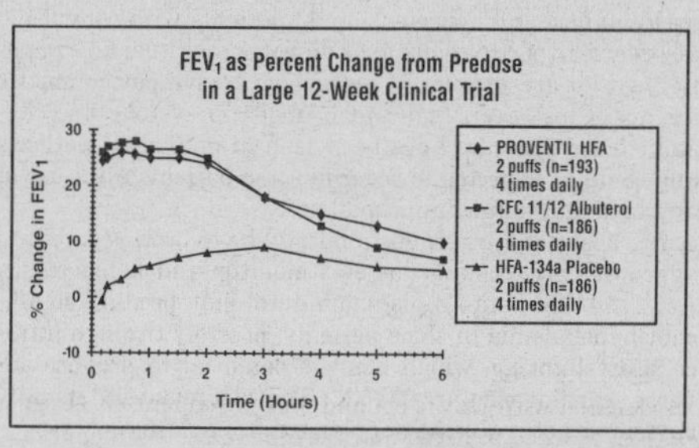

In a 4-week, randomized, open-label trial, 63 children, 4 to 11 years of age, with asthma were evaluated for the bronchodilator efficacy of PROVENTIL HFA Inhalation Aerosol (33 pediatric patients) in comparison to a CFC 11/12 propelled albuterol inhaler (30 pediatric patients).

Serial FEV_1 measurements as percent change from test-day baseline demonstrated that two inhalations of PROVENTIL HFA Inhalation Aerosol produced outcomes which were clinically comparable to a CFC 11/12 propelled albuterol inhaler.

The mean time to onset of a 12% increase in FEV_1 for PROVENTIL HFA Inhalation Aerosol was 7 minutes and the mean time to peak effect was approximately 50 minutes.

Continued on next page

Proventil HFA—Cont.

The mean duration of effect as measured by a 12% increase in FEV_1 was 2.3 hours. In some pediatric patients, duration of effect was as long as 6 hours.
In another clinical study in pediatric patients, two inhalations of PROVENTIL HFA Inhalation Aerosol taken 30 minutes before exercise provided comparable protection against exercise-induced bronchospasm as a CFC 11/12 propelled albuterol inhaler.

INDICATIONS AND USAGE

PROVENTIL HFA Inhalation Aerosol is indicated in adults and children 4 years of age and older for the treatment or prevention of bronchospasm with reversible obstructive airway disease and for the prevention of exercise-induced bronchospasm.

CONTRAINDICATIONS

PROVENTIL HFA Inhalation Aerosol is contraindicated in patients with a history of hypersensitivity to albuterol or any other PROVENTIL HFA components.

WARNINGS

1. Paradoxical Bronchospasm: Inhaled albuterol sulfate can produce paradoxical bronchospasm that may be life threatening. If paradoxical bronchospasm occurs, PROVENTIL HFA Inhalation Aerosol should be discontinued immediately and alternative therapy instituted. It should be recognized that paradoxical bronchospasm, when associated with inhaled formulations, frequently occurs with the first use of a new canister.
2. Deterioration of Asthma: Asthma may deteriorate acutely over a period of hours or chronically over several days or longer. If the patient needs more doses of PROVENTIL HFA Inhalation Aerosol than usual, this may be a marker of destabilization of asthma and requires reevaluation of the patient and treatment regimen, giving special consideration to the possible need for anti-inflammatory treatment, eg, corticosteroids.
3. Use of Anti-inflammatory Agents: The use of beta-adrenergic-agonist bronchodilators alone may not be adequate to control asthma in many patients. Early consideration should be given to adding anti-inflammatory agents, eg, corticosteroids, to the therapeutic regimen.
4. Cardiovascular Effects: PROVENTIL HFA Inhalation Aerosol, like other beta-adrenergic agonists, can produce clinically significant cardiovascular effects in some patients as measured by pulse rate, blood pressure, and/or symptoms. Although such effects are uncommon after administration of PROVENTIL HFA Inhalation Aerosol at recommended doses, if they occur, the drug may need to be discontinued. In addition, beta agonists have been reported to produce ECG changes, such as flattening of the T wave, prolongation of the QTc interval, and ST segment depression. The clinical significance of these findings is unknown. Therefore, PROVENTIL HFA Inhalation Aerosol, like all sympathomimetic amines, should be used with caution in patients with cardiovascular disorders, especially coronary insufficiency, cardiac arrhythmias, and hypertension.
5. Do Not Exceed Recommended Dose: Fatalities have been reported in association with excessive use of inhaled sympathomimetic drugs in patients with asthma. The exact cause of death is unknown, but cardiac arrest following an unexpected development of a severe acute asthmatic crisis and subsequent hypoxia is suspected.
6. Immediate Hypersensitivity Reactions: Immediate hypersensitivity reactions may occur after administration of albuterol sulfate, as demonstrated by rare cases of urticaria, angioedema, rash, bronchospasm, anaphylaxis, and oropharyngeal edema.

PRECAUTIONS

General Albuterol sulfate, as with all sympathomimetic amines should be used with caution in patients with cardiovascular disorders, especially coronary insufficiency, cardiac arrhythmias, and hypertension; in patients with convulsive disorders, hyperthyroidism, or diabetes mellitus; and in patients who are unusually responsive to sympathomimetic amines. Clinically significant changes in systolic and diastolic blood pressure have been seen in individual patients and could be expected to occur in some patients after use of any beta-adrenergic bronchodilator.
Large doses of intravenous albuterol have been reported to aggravate pre-existing diabetes mellitus and ketoacidosis. As with other beta-agonists, albuterol may produce significant hypokalemia in some patients, possibly through intracellular shunting, which has the potential to produce adverse cardiovascular effects. The decrease is usually transient, not requiring supplementation.
Information for Patients See illustrated **Patient's Instructions for Use.** SHAKE WELL BEFORE USING. Patients should be given the following information:
It is recommended to prime the inhaler before using for the first time and in cases where the inhaler has not been used for more than 2 weeks by releasing four "test sprays" into the air, away from the face.
KEEPING THE PLASTIC MOUTHPIECE CLEAN IS VERY IMPORTANT TO PREVENT MEDICATION BUILD-UP AND BLOCKAGE. THE MOUTHPIECE SHOULD BE WASHED, SHAKEN TO REMOVE EXCESS WATER AND AIR DRIED THOROUGHLY AT LEAST ONCE A WEEK. INHALER MAY CEASE TO DELIVER MEDICATION IF NOT PROPERLY CLEANED.
The mouthpiece should be cleaned (with the canister removed) by running warm water through the top and bottom for 30 seconds at least once a week. The mouthpiece must be shaken to remove excess water, then air dried thoroughly (such as overnight). Blockage from medication build-up or improper medication delivery may result from failure to thoroughly air dry the mouthpiece.
If the mouthpiece should become blocked (little or no medication coming out of the mouthpiece), the blockage may be removed by washing as described above.
If it is necessary to use the inhaler before it is completely dry, shake off excess water, replace canister, test spray twice away from face, and take the prescribed dose. After such use, the mouthpiece should be rewashed and allowed to air dry thoroughly.
The action of PROVENTIL HFA Inhalation Aerosol should last up to 4 to 6 hours. PROVENTIL HFA Inhalation Aerosol should not be used more frequently than recommended. Do not increase the dose or frequency of doses of PROVENTIL HFA Inhalation Aerosol without consulting your physician. If you find that treatment with PROVENTIL HFA Inhalation Aerosol becomes less effective for symptomatic relief, your symptoms become worse, and/or you need to use the product more frequently than usual, medical attention should be sought immediately. While you are taking PROVENTIL HFA Inhalation Aerosol, other inhaled drugs and asthma medications should be taken only as directed by your physician.
Common adverse effects of treatment with inhaled albuterol include palpitations, chest pain, rapid heart rate, tremor, or nervousness. If you are pregnant or nursing, contact your physician about use of PROVENTIL HFA Inhalation Aerosol. Effective and safe use of PROVENTIL HFA Inhalation Aerosol includes an understanding of the way that it should be administered. Use PROVENTIL HFA Inhalation Aerosol only with the actuator supplied with the product. Discard the canister after 200 sprays have been used.
In general, the technique for administering PROVENTIL HFA Inhalation Aerosol to children is similar to that for adults. Children should use PROVENTIL HFA Inhalation Aerosol under adult supervision, as instructed by the patient's physician. (See **Patient's Instructions for Use.**)

Drug Interactions
1. Beta Blockers: Beta-adrenergic-receptor blocking agents not only block the pulmonary effect of beta agonists, such as PROVENTIL HFA Inhalation Aerosol, but may produce severe bronchospasm in asthmatic patients. Therefore, patients with asthma should not normally be treated with beta blockers. However, under certain circumstances, eg, as prophylaxis after myocardial infarction, there may be no acceptable alternatives to the use of beta-adrenergic-blocking agents in patients with asthma. In this setting, cardioselective beta blockers should be considered, although they should be administered with caution.
2. Diuretics: The ECG changes and/or hypokalemia which may result from the administration of nonpotassium sparing diuretics (such as loop or thiazide diuretics) can be acutely worsened by beta agonists, especially when the recommended dose of the beta agonist is exceeded. Although the clinical significance of these effects is not known, caution is advised in the coadministration of beta agonists with nonpotassium sparing diuretics.
3. Albuterol-Digoxin: Mean decreases of 16% and 22% in serum digoxin levels were demonstrated after single-dose intravenous and oral administration of albuterol, respectively, to normal volunteers who had received digoxin for 10 days. The clinical significance of these findings for patients with obstructive airway disease who are receiving albuterol and digoxin on a chronic basis is unclear; nevertheless, it would be prudent to carefully evaluate the serum digoxin levels in patients who are currently receiving digoxin and albuterol.
4. Monoamine Oxidase Inhibitors or Tricyclic Antidepressants: PROVENTIL HFA Inhalation Aerosol should be administered with extreme caution to patients being treated with monoamine oxidase inhibitors or tricyclic antidepressants, or within 2 weeks of discontinuation of such agents, because the action of albuterol on the cardiovascular system may be potentiated.

Carcinogenesis, Mutagenesis, and Impairment of Fertility
In a 2-year study in Sprague-Dawley rats, albuterol sulfate caused a dose-related increase in the incidence of benign leiomyomas of the mesovarium at and above dietary doses of 2 mg/kg (approximately 15 times the maximum recommended daily inhalation dose for adults on a mg/m^2 basis and approximately 6 times the maximum recommended daily inhalation dose for children on a mg/m^2 basis). In another study this effect was blocked by the coadministration of propranolol, a nonselective beta-adrenergic antagonist. In an 18-month study in CD-1 mice, albuterol sulfate showed no evidence of tumorigenicity at dietary doses of up to 500 mg/kg (approximately 1700 times the maximum recommended daily inhalation dose for adults on a mg/m^2 basis and approximately 800 times the maximum recommended daily inhalation dose for children on a mg/m^2 basis). In a 22-month study in Golden Hamsters, albuterol sulfate showed no evidence of tumorigenicity at dietary doses of up to 50 mg/kg (approximately 225 times the maximum recommended daily inhalation dose for adults on a mg/m^2 basis and approximately 110 times the maximum recommended daily inhalation dose for children on a mg/m^2 basis).
Albuterol sulfate was not mutagenic in the Ames test or a mutation test in yeast. Albuterol sulfate was not clastogenic in a human peripheral lymphocyte assay or in an AH1 strain mouse micronucleus assay.
Reproduction studies in rats demonstrated no evidence of impaired fertility at oral doses up to 50 mg/kg (approximately 340 times the maximum recommended daily inhalation dose for adults on a mg/m^2 basis).

Pregnancy: ***Teratogenic Effects:*** **Pregnancy Category C**
Albuterol sulfate has been shown to be teratogenic in mice. A study in CD-1 mice given albuterol sulfate subcutaneously showed cleft palate formation in 5 of 111 (4.5%) fetuses at 0.25 mg/kg (less than the maximum recommended daily inhalation dose for adults on a mg/m^2 basis) and in 10 of 108 (9.3%) fetuses at 2.5 mg/kg (approximately 8 times the maximum recommended daily inhalation dose for adults on a mg/m^2 basis). The drug did not induce cleft palate formation at a dose of 0.025 mg/kg (less than the maximum recommended daily inhalation dose for adults on a mg/m^2 basis). Cleft palate also occurred in 22 of 72 (30.5%) fetuses from females treated subcutaneously with 2.5 mg/kg of isoproterenol (positive control).
A reproduction study in Stride Dutch rabbits revealed cranioschisis in 7 of 19 (37%) fetuses when albuterol sulfate was administered orally at 50 mg/kg dose (approximately 680 times the maximum recommended daily inhalation dose for adults on a mg/m^2 basis).
In an inhalation reproduction study in Sprague-Dawley rats, the albuterol sulfate/HFA-134a formulation did not exhibit any teratogenic effects at 10.5 mg/kg (approximately 70 times the maximum recommended daily inhalation dose for adults on a mg/m^2 basis).
A study in which pregnant rats were dosed with radiolabeled albuterol sulfate demonstrated that drug-related material is transferred from the maternal circulation to the fetus.
There are no adequate and well-controlled studies of PROVENTIL HFA Inhalation Aerosol or albuterol sulfate in pregnant women. PROVENTIL HFA Inhalation Aerosol should be used during pregnancy only if the potential benefit justifies the potential risk to the fetus.

Adverse Experience Incidences (% of patients) in a Large 12-week Clinical Trial*

Body System/	Adverse Event (Preferred Term)	PROVENTIL HFA Inhalation Aerosol (N = 193)	CFC 11/12 Propelled Albuterol Inhaler (N = 186)	HFA-134a Placebo Inhaler (N = 186)
Application Site Disorders	Inhalation Site Sensation	6	9	2
	Inhalation Taste Sensation	4	3	3
Body as a Whole	Allergic Reaction/Symptoms	6	4	<1
	Back Pain	4	2	3
	Fever	6	2	5
Central and Peripheral Nervous System	Tremor	7	8	2
Gastrointestinal System	Nausea	10	9	5
	Vomiting	7	2	3
Heart Rate and Rhythm Disorder	Tachycardia	7	2	<1
Psychiatric Disorders	Nervousness	7	9	3
Respiratory System Disorders	Respiratory Disorder (unspecified)	6	4	5
	Rhinitis	16	22	14
	Upper Resp Tract Infection	21	20	18
Urinary System Disorder	Urinary Tract Infection	3	4	2

*This table includes all adverse events (whether considered by the investigator drug related or unrelated to drug) which occurred at an incidence rate of at least 3.0% in the PROVENTIL HFA Inhalation Aerosol group and more frequently in the PROVENTIL HFA Inhalation Aerosol group than in the HFA-134a placebo inhaler group.

During worldwide marketing experience, various congenital anomalies, including cleft palate and limb defects, have been reported in the offspring of patients being treated with albuterol. Some of the mothers were taking multiple medications during their pregnancies. Because no consistent pattern of defects can be discerned, a relationship between albuterol use and congenital anomalies has not been established.

Use in Labor and Delivery

Because of the potential for beta-agonist interference with uterine contractility, use of PROVENTIL HFA Inhalation Aerosol for relief of bronchospasm during labor should be restricted to those patients in whom the benefits clearly outweigh the risk.

Tocolysis: Albuterol has not been approved for the management of preterm labor. The benefit:risk ratio when albuterol is administered for tocolysis has not been established. Serious adverse reactions, including pulmonary edema, have been reported during or following treatment of premature labor with $beta_2$-agonists, including albuterol.

Nursing Mothers

Plasma levels of albuterol sulfate and HFA-134a after inhaled therapeutic doses are very low in humans, but it is not known whether the components of PROVENTIL HFA Inhalation Aerosol are excreted in human milk.

Because of the potential for tumorigenicity shown for albuterol in animal studies and lack of experience with the use of PROVENTIL HFA Inhalation Aerosol by nursing mothers, a decision should be made whether to discontinue nursing or to discontinue the drug, taking into account the importance of the drug to the mother. Caution should be exercised when albuterol sulfate is administered to a nursing woman.

Pediatrics

The safety and effectiveness of PROVENTIL HFA Inhalation Aerosol in pediatric patients below the age of 4 years have not been established.

Geriatrics

PROVENTIL HFA Inhalation Aerosol has not been studied in a geriatric population. As with other $beta_2$-agonists, special caution should be observed when using PROVENTIL HFA Inhalation Aerosol in elderly patients who have concomitant cardiovascular disease that could be adversely affected by this class of drug.

ADVERSE REACTIONS

Adverse reaction information concerning PROVENTIL HFA Inhalation Aerosol is derived from a 12-week, double-blind, double-dummy study which compared PROVENTIL HFA Inhalation Aerosol, a CFC 11/12 propelled albuterol inhaler, and an HFA-134a placebo inhaler in 565 asthmatic patients. The following table lists the incidence of all adverse events (whether considered by the investigator drug related or unrelated to drug) from this study which occurred at a rate of 3% or greater in the PROVENTIL HFA Inhalation Aerosol treatment group and more frequently in the PROVENTIL HFA Inhalation Aerosol treatment group than in the placebo group. Overall, the incidence and nature of the adverse reactions reported for PROVENTIL HFA Inhalation Aerosol and a CFC 11/12 propelled albuterol inhaler were comparable.

[See table at top of previous page]

Adverse events reported by less than 3% of the patients receiving PROVENTIL HFA Inhalation Aerosol, and by a greater proportion of PROVENTIL HFA Inhalation Aerosol patients than placebo patients, which have the potential to be related to PROVENTIL HFA Inhalation Aerosol include: dysphonia, increased sweating, dry mouth, chest pain, edema, rigors, ataxia, leg cramps, hyperkinesia, eructation, flatulence, tinnitus, diabetes mellitus, anxiety, depression, somnolence, rash. Palpitation and dizziness have also been observed with PROVENTIL HFA Inhalation Aerosol.

Adverse events reported in a 4-week pediatric clinical trial comparing PROVENTIL HFA Inhalation Aerosol and a CFC 11/12 propelled albuterol inhaler occurred at a low incidence rate and were similar to those seen in the adult trials.

In small, cumulative dose studies, tremor, nervousness, and headache appeared to be dose related.

Rare cases of urticaria, angioedema, rash, bronchospasm, and oropharyngeal edema have been reported after the use of inhaled albuterol. In addition, albuterol, like other sympathomimetic agents, can cause adverse reactions such as hypertension, angina, vertigo, central nervous system stimulation, insomnia, headache, and drying or irritation of the oropharynx.

OVERDOSAGE

The expected symptoms with overdosage are those of excessive beta-adrenergic stimulation and/or occurrence or exaggeration of any of the symptoms listed under **ADVERSE REACTIONS**, eg, seizures, angina, hypertension or hypotension, tachycardia with rates up to 200 beats per minute, arrhythmias, nervousness, headache, tremor, dry mouth, palpitation, nausea, dizziness, fatigue, malaise, and insomnia.

Hypokalemia may also occur. As with all sympathomimetic medications, cardiac arrest and even death may be associated with abuse of PROVENTIL HFA Inhalation Aerosol. Treatment consists of discontinuation of PROVENTIL HFA Inhalation Aerosol together with appropriate symptomatic therapy. The judicious use of a cardioselective beta-receptor blocker may be considered, bearing in mind that such medication can produce bronchospasm. There is insufficient evidence to determine if dialysis is beneficial for overdosage of PROVENTIL HFA Inhalation Aerosol.

The oral median lethal dose of albuterol sulfate in mice is greater than 2000 mg/kg (approximately 6800 times the maximum recommended daily inhalation dose for adults on a mg/m^2 basis and approximately 3200 times the maximum recommended daily inhalation dose for children on a mg/m^2 basis.). In mature rats, the subcutaneous median lethal dose of albuterol sulfate is approximately 450 mg/kg (approximately 3000 times the maximum recommended daily inhalation dose for adults on a mg/m^2 basis and approximately 1400 times the maximum recommended daily inhalation dose for children on a mg/m^2 basis). In young rats, the subcutaneous median lethal dose is approximately 2000 mg/kg (approximately 14,000 times the maximum recommended daily inhalation dose for adults on a mg/m^2 basis and approximately 6400 times the maximum recommended daily inhalation dose for children on a mg/m^2 basis). The inhalation median lethal dose has not been determined in animals.

DOSAGE AND ADMINISTRATION

For treatment of acute episodes of bronchospasm or prevention of asthmatic symptoms, the usual dosage for adults and children 4 years of age and older is two inhalations repeated every 4 to 6 hours. More frequent administration or a larger number of inhalations is not recommended. In some patients, one inhalation every 4 hours may be sufficient. Each actuation of PROVENTIL HFA Inhalation Aerosol delivers 108 mcg of albuterol sulfate (equivalent to 90 mcg of albuterol base) from the mouthpiece. It is recommended to prime the inhaler before using for the first time and in cases where the inhaler has not been used for more than 2 weeks by releasing four "test sprays" into the air, away from the face.

Exercise Induced Bronchospasm Prevention: The usual dosage for adults and children 4 years of age and older is two inhalations 15 to 30 minutes before exercise.

To maintain proper use of this product, it is important that the mouthpiece be washed and dried thoroughly at least once a week. The inhaler may cease to deliver medication if not properly cleaned and dried thoroughly. See **Information for Patients**. Keeping the plastic mouthpiece clean is very important to prevent medication build-up and blockage. The inhaler may cease to deliver medication if not properly cleaned and air dried thoroughly. If the mouthpiece becomes blocked, washing the mouthpiece will remove the blockage.

If a previously effective dose regimen fails to provide the usual response, this may be a marker of destabilization of asthma and requires reevaluation of the patient and the treatment regimen, giving special consideration to the possible need for anti-inflammatory treatment, eg, corticosteroids.

HOW SUPPLIED

PROVENTIL HFA (albuterol sulfate) Inhalation Aerosol is supplied as a pressurized aluminum canister with a yellow plastic actuator and orange dust cap each in boxes of one. Each actuation delivers 120 mcg of albuterol sulfate from the valve and 108 mcg of albuterol sulfate from the mouthpiece (equivalent to 90 mcg of albuterol base). Canisters with a labeled net weight of 6.7 g contain 200 inhalations (NDC 0085-1132-01).

Rx only. Store between 15° and 25°C (59° and 77°F). For best results, canister should be at room temperature before use.

SHAKE WELL BEFORE USING.

The yellow actuator supplied with PROVENTIL HFA Inhalation Aerosol should not be used with any other product canisters, and actuator from other products should not be used with a PROVENTIL HFA Inhalation Aerosol canister. The correct amount of medication in each canister cannot be assured after 200 actuations, even though the canister is not completely empty. The canister should be discarded when the labeled number of actuations have been used.

WARNING: Avoid spraying in eyes. Contents under pressure. Do not puncture or incinerate. Exposure to temperatures above 120°F may cause bursting. Keep out of reach of children.

PROVENTIL HFA Inhalation Aerosol does not contain chlorofluorocarbons (CFCs) as the propellant.

Developed and Manufactured by
3M Health Care Limited
Loughborough UK
or
3M Pharmaceuticals,
Northridge, CA 91324
for
Key Pharmaceuticals, Inc.
Kenilworth, NJ 07033 USA

Copyright © 1996, 1999, Key Pharmaceuticals, Inc. All rights reserved.

Rev. 10/01 **23800110T**

To keep your **PDR** up to date
throughout the year, note these revisions
on the corresponding pages of the annual
volume. Simply write **"See Supplement A"**
next to the product heading.

Schwarz Pharma, Inc.

6140 W. EXECUTIVE DRIVE
MEQUON, WI 53092

For Medical Information Contact:
Schwarz Pharma, Inc.
Medical and Drug Information
(262) 238-9994
(800) 558-5114

NIRAVAM™ Ⓒ℞
[ni-ra-vam]
(alprazolam orally disintegrating tablets)
Rx Only

DESCRIPTION

NIRAVAM™ (alprazolam orally disintegrating tablets) contains alprazolam which is a triazolo analog of the 1,4 benzodiazepine class of central nervous system-active compounds. NIRAVAM™ is an orally administered formulation of alprazolam which rapidly disintegrates on the tongue and does not require water to aid dissolution or swallowing.

The chemical name of alprazolam is 8-Chloro-1-methyl-6-phenyl-4H-*s*-triazolo [4,3-α] [1,4] benzodiazepine. The empirical formula is $C_{17}H_{13}ClN_4$ and the molecular weight is 308.76. The structural formula is:

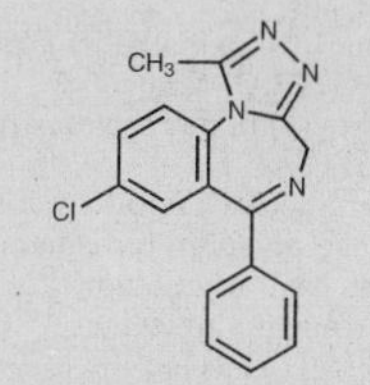

Alprazolam is a white crystalline powder, which is soluble in methanol or ethanol but which has no appreciable solubility in water at physiological pH.

Each orally disintegrating tablet contains either 0.25, 0.5, 1 or 2 mg of alprazolam and the following inactive ingredients: colloidal silicon dioxide, corn starch, crospovidone, magnesium stearate, mannitol, methacrylic acid copolymer, microcrystalline cellulose, natural and artificial orange flavor, sucralose and sucrose. In addition, the 0.25 mg and 0.5 mg tablets contain yellow iron oxide.

CLINICAL PHARMACOLOGY

Pharmacodynamics

CNS agents of the 1,4 benzodiazepine class presumably exert their effects by binding at stereo specific receptors at several sites within the central nervous system. Their exact mechanism of action is unknown. Clinically, all benzodiazepines cause a dose-related central nervous system depressant activity varying from mild impairment of task performance to hypnosis.

Pharmacokinetics

Absorption

Following oral administration, alprazolam is readily absorbed. The peak plasma concentration is reached about 1.5 to 2 hours after administration of NIRAVAM™ given with or without water. When taken with water, mean T_{max} occurs about 15 minutes earlier than when taken without water with no change in C_{max} or AUC. Plasma levels are proportional to the dose given; over the dose range of 0.5 to 3.0 mg, peak levels of 8.0 to 37 ng/mL are observed. The elimination half-life of alprazolam is approximately 12.5 hours (range 7.9-19.2 hours) after administration of NIRAVAM™ in healthy adults.

Food decreased the mean C_{max} by about 25% and increased the mean T_{max} by 2 hours from 2.2 hours to 4.4 hours after the ingestion of a high-fat meal. Food did not affect the extent of absorption (AUC) or the elimination half-life.

Distribution

In vitro, alprazolam is bound (80 percent) to human serum protein. Serum albumin accounts for the majority of the binding.

Metabolism/Elimination

Alprazolam is extensively metabolized in humans, primarily by cytochrome P450 3A4 (CYP3A4), to two major metabolites in the plasma: 4-hydroxyalprazolam and α-hydroxyalprazolam. A benzophenone derived from alprazolam is also found in humans. Their half-lives appear to be similar to that of alprazolam. The plasma concentrations of 4-hydroxyalprazolam and α-hydroxyalprazolam relative to unchanged alprazolam concentration were always less than 4%. The reported relative potencies in benzodiazepine receptor binding experiments and in animal models of induced seizure inhibition are 0.20 and 0.66, respectively, for 4-hydroxyalprazolam and α-hydroxyalprazolam. Such low concentrations and the lesser potencies of 4-hydroxyalprazolam and α-hydroxyalprazolam suggest that they are unlikely to contribute much to the pharmacological effects of alprazolam. The benzophenone metabolite is essentially inactive.

Alprazolam and its metabolites are excreted primarily in the urine.

Continued on next page

Niravam—Cont.

Special Populations
Changes in the absorption, distribution, metabolism and excretion of benzodiazepines have been reported in a variety of disease states including alcoholism, impaired hepatic function and impaired renal function. Changes have also been demonstrated in geriatric patients. A mean half-life of alprazolam of 16.3 hours has been observed in healthy elderly subjects (range: 9.0-26.9 hours, n=16) compared to 11.0 hours (range: 6.3-15.8 hours, n=16) in healthy adult subjects. In patients with alcoholic liver disease, the half-life of alprazolam ranged between 5.8 and 65.3 hours (mean: 19.7 hours, n=17) as compared to between 6.3 and 26.9 hours (mean=11.4 hours, n=17) in healthy subjects. In an obese group of subjects, the half-life of alprazolam ranged between 9.9 and 40.4 hours (mean=21.8 hours, n=12) as compared to between 6.3 and 15.8 hours (mean=10.6 hours, n=12) in healthy subjects.

Because of its similarity to other benzodiazepines, it is assumed that alprazolam undergoes transplacental passage and that it is excreted in human milk.

Race — Maximal concentrations and half-life of alprazolam are approximately 15% and 25% higher in Asians compared to Caucasians.

Pediatrics — The pharmacokinetics of alprazolam in pediatric patients have not been studied.

Gender — Gender has no effect on the pharmacokinetics of alprazolam.

Cigarette Smoking — Alprazolam concentrations may be reduced by up to 50% in smokers compared to non-smokers.

Drug-Drug Interactions
Alprazolam is primarily eliminated by metabolism via cytochrome P450 3A (CYP3A). Most of the interactions that have been documented with alprazolam are with drugs that inhibit or induce CYP3A4.

Compounds that are potent inhibitors of CYP3A would be expected to increase plasma alprazolam concentrations. Drug products that have been studied *in vivo*, along with their effect on increasing alprazolam AUC, are as follows: ketoconazole, 3.98 fold; itraconazole, 2.70 fold; nefazodone, 1.98 fold; fluvoxamine, 1.96 fold; and erythromycin, 1.61 fold (see CONTRAINDICATIONS, WARNINGS, and PRECAUTIONS—Drug Interactions).

CYP3A inducers would be expected to decrease alprazolam concentrations and this has been observed *in vivo*. The oral clearance of alprazolam (given in a 0.8 mg single dose) was increased from 0.90 ± 0.21 mL/min/kg to 2.13 ± 0.54 mL/min/kg and the elimination $t_{1/2}$ was shortened (from 17.1 ± 4.9 to 7.7 ± 1.7 h) following administration of 300 mg/day carbamazepine for 10 days (see PRECAUTIONS—Drug Interactions). However, the carbamazepine dose used in this study was fairly low compared to the recommended doses (1000-1200 mg/day); the effect at usual carbamazepine doses is unknown.

The ability of alprazolam to induce or inhibit human hepatic enzyme systems has not been determined. However, this is not a property of benzodiazepines in general. Further, alprazolam did not affect the prothrombin or plasma warfarin levels in male volunteers administered sodium warfarin orally.

CLINICAL STUDIES
Anxiety Disorders
Alprazolam was compared to placebo in double blind clinical studies (doses up to 4 mg/day) in patients with a diagnosis of anxiety or anxiety with associated depressive symptomatology. Alprazolam was significantly better than placebo at each of the evaluation periods of these 4-week studies as judged by the following psychometric instruments: Physician's Global Impressions, Hamilton Anxiety Rating Scale, Target Symptoms, Patient's Global Impressions and Self-Rating Symptom Scale.

Panic Disorder
Support for the effectiveness of alprazolam in the treatment of panic disorder came from three short-term, placebo-controlled studies (up to 10 weeks) in patients with diagnoses closely corresponding to DSM-III-R criteria for panic disorder.

The average dose of alprazolam was 5-6 mg/day in two of the studies, and the doses of alprazolam were fixed at 2 and 6 mg/day in the third study. In all three studies, alprazolam was superior to placebo on a variable defined as "the number of patients with zero panic attacks" (range, 37-83% met this criterion), as well as on a global improvement score. In two of the three studies, alprazolam was superior to placebo on a variable defined as "change from baseline on the number of panic attacks per week" (range, 3.3-5.2), and also on a phobia rating scale. A subgroup of patients who were improved on alprazolam during short-term treatment in one of these trials was continued on an open basis up to 8 months, without apparent loss of benefit.

INDICATIONS AND USAGE
Anxiety Disorders
NIRAVAM™ is indicated for the management of anxiety disorder (a condition corresponding most closely to the APA Diagnostic and Statistical Manual [DSM-III-R] diagnosis of generalized anxiety disorder) or the short-term relief of symptoms of anxiety. Anxiety or tension associated with the stress of everyday life usually does not require treatment with an anxiolytic.

Generalized anxiety disorder is characterized by unrealistic or excessive anxiety and worry (apprehensive expectation) about two or more life circumstances, for a period of 6 months or longer, during which the person has been bothered more days than not by these concerns. At least 6 of the following 18 symptoms are often present in these patients: *Motor Tension* (trembling, twitching, or feeling shaky; muscle tension, aches, or soreness; restlessness; easy fatigability); *Autonomic Hyperactivity* (shortness of breath or smothering sensations; palpitations or accelerated heart rate; sweating, or cold clammy hands; dry mouth; dizziness or lightheadedness; nausea, diarrhea, or other abdominal distress; flushes or chills; frequent urination; trouble swallowing or 'lump in throat'); *Vigilance and Scanning* (feeling keyed up or on edge; exaggerated startle response; difficulty concentrating or 'mind going blank' because of anxiety; trouble falling or staying asleep; irritability). These symptoms must not be secondary to another psychiatric disorder or caused by some organic factor.

Anxiety associated with depression is responsive to alprazolam.

Panic Disorder
NIRAVAM™ is also indicated for the treatment of panic disorder, with or without agoraphobia.

Studies supporting this claim were conducted in patients whose diagnoses corresponded closely to the DSM-III-R/IV criteria for panic disorder (see CLINICAL STUDIES).

Panic disorder (DSM-IV) is characterized by recurrent unexpected panic attacks, ie, a discrete period of intense fear or discomfort in which four (or more) of the following symptoms develop abruptly and reach a peak within 10 minutes: (1) palpitations, pounding heart, or accelerated heart rate; (2) sweating; (3) trembling or shaking; (4) sensations of shortness of breath or smothering; (5) feeling of choking; (6) chest pain or discomfort; (7) nausea or abdominal distress; (8) feeling dizzy, unsteady, lightheaded, or faint; (9) derealization (feelings of unreality) or depersonalization (being detached from oneself); (10) fear of losing control; (11) fear of dying; (12) paresthesias (numbness or tingling sensations); (13) chills or hot flushes.

Demonstrations of the effectiveness of alprazolam by systematic clinical study are limited to 4 months duration for anxiety disorder and 4 to 10 weeks duration for panic disorder; however, patients with panic disorder have been treated on an open basis for up to 8 months without apparent loss of benefit. The physician should periodically reassess the usefulness of the drug for the individual patient.

CONTRAINDICATIONS
NIRAVAM™ is contraindicated in patients with known sensitivity to this drug or other benzodiazepines. NIRAVAM™ may be used in patients with open angle glaucoma who are receiving appropriate therapy, but is contraindicated in patients with acute narrow angle glaucoma.

NIRAVAM™ is contraindicated with ketoconazole and itraconazole, since these medications significantly impair the oxidative metabolism mediated by cytochrome P450 3A (CYP3A) (see CLINICAL PHARMACOLOGY, WARNINGS and PRECAUTIONS—Drug Interactions).

WARNINGS
Dependence and Withdrawal Reactions, Including Seizures
Certain adverse clinical events, some life-threatening, are a direct consequence of physical dependence to alprazolam. These include a spectrum of withdrawal symptoms; the most important is seizure (see DRUG ABUSE AND DEPENDENCE). Even after relatively short-term use at the doses recommended for the treatment of transient anxiety and anxiety disorder (ie, 0.75 to 4.0 mg per day), there is some risk of dependence. Spontaneous reporting system data suggest that the risk of dependence and its severity appear to be greater in patients treated with doses greater than 4 mg/day and for long periods (more than 12 weeks). However, in a controlled postmarketing discontinuation study of panic disorder patients, the duration of treatment (3 months compared to 6 months) had no effect on the ability of patients to taper to zero dose. In contrast, patients treated with doses of alprazolam greater than 4 mg/day had more difficulty tapering to zero dose than those treated with less than 4 mg/day.

The importance of dose and the risks of alprazolam as a treatment for panic disorder
Because the management of panic disorder often requires the use of average daily doses of alprazolam above 4 mg, the risk of dependence among panic disorder patients may be higher than that among those treated for less severe anxiety. Experience in randomized placebo-controlled discontinuation studies of patients with panic disorder showed a high rate of rebound and withdrawal symptoms in patients treated with alprazolam compared to placebo-treated patients.

Relapse or return of illness was defined as a return of symptoms characteristic of panic disorder (primarily panic attacks) to levels approximately equal to those seen at baseline before active treatment was initiated. Rebound refers to a return of symptoms of panic disorder to a level substantially greater in frequency, or more severe in intensity than seen at baseline. Withdrawal symptoms were identified as those which were generally not characteristic of panic disorder and which occurred for the first time more frequently during discontinuation than at baseline.

In a controlled clinical trial in which 63 patients were randomized to alprazolam and where withdrawal symptoms were specifically sought, the following were identified as symptoms of withdrawal: heightened sensory perception, impaired concentration, dysosmia, clouded sensorium, paresthesias, muscle cramps, muscle twitch, diarrhea, blurred vision, appetite decrease, and weight loss. Other symptoms, such as anxiety and insomnia, were frequently seen during discontinuation, but it could not be determined if they were due to return of illness, rebound, or withdrawal.

In two controlled trials of 6 to 8 weeks duration where the ability of patients to discontinue medication was measured, 71%-93% of patients treated with alprazolam tapered completely off therapy compared to 89%-96% of placebo-treated patients. In a controlled postmarketing discontinuation study of panic disorder patients, the duration of treatment (3 months compared to 6 months) had no effect on the ability of patients to taper to zero dose.

Seizures attributable to alprazolam were seen after drug discontinuance or dose reduction in 8 of 1980 patients with panic disorder or in patients participating in clinical trials where doses of alprazolam greater than 4 mg/day for over 3 months were permitted. Five of these cases clearly occurred during abrupt dose reduction, or discontinuation from daily doses of 2 to 10 mg. Three cases occurred in situations where there was not a clear relationship to abrupt dose reduction or discontinuation. In one instance, seizure occurred after discontinuation from a single dose of 1 mg after tapering at a rate of 1 mg every 3 days from 6 mg daily. In two other instances, the relationship to taper is indeterminate; in both of these cases the patients had been receiving doses of 3 mg daily prior to seizure. The duration of use in the above 8 cases ranged from 4 to 22 weeks. There have been occasional voluntary reports of patients developing seizures while apparently tapering gradually from alprazolam. The risk of seizure seems to be greatest 24-72 hours after discontinuation (see DOSAGE AND ADMINISTRATION for recommended tapering and discontinuation schedule).

Status Epilepticus
The medical event voluntary reporting system shows that withdrawal seizures have been reported in association with the discontinuation of alprazolam. In most cases, only a single seizure was reported; however, multiple seizures and status epilepticus were reported as well.

Interdose Symptoms
Early morning anxiety and emergence of anxiety symptoms between doses of alprazolam have been reported in patients with panic disorder taking prescribed maintenance doses of alprazolam. These symptoms may reflect the development of tolerance or a time interval between doses which is longer than the duration of clinical action of the administered dose. In either case, it is presumed that the prescribed dose is not sufficient to maintain plasma levels above those needed to prevent relapse, rebound or withdrawal symptoms over the entire course of the interdosing interval. In these situations, it is recommended that the same total daily dose be given divided as more frequent administrations (see DOSAGE AND ADMINISTRATION).

Risk of Dose Reduction
Withdrawal reactions may occur when dosage reduction occurs for any reason. This includes purposeful tapering, but also inadvertent reduction of dose (eg, the patient forgets, the patient is admitted to a hospital). Therefore, the dosage of NIRAVAM™ should be reduced or discontinued gradually (see DOSAGE AND ADMINISTRATION).

CNS Depression and Impaired Performance
Because of its CNS depressant effects, patients receiving alprazolam should be cautioned against engaging in hazardous occupations or activities requiring complete mental alertness such as operating machinery or driving a motor vehicle. For the same reason, patients should be cautioned about the simultaneous ingestion of alcohol and other CNS depressant drugs during treatment with alprazolam.

Risk of Fetal Harm
Benzodiazepines can potentially cause fetal harm when administered to pregnant women. If alprazolam is used during pregnancy, or if the patient becomes pregnant while taking this drug, the patient should be apprised of the potential hazard to the fetus. Because of experience with other members of the benzodiazepine class, alprazolam is assumed to be capable of causing an increased risk of congenital abnormalities when administered to a pregnant woman during the first trimester. Because use of these drugs is rarely a matter of urgency, their use during the first trimester should almost always be avoided. The possibility that a woman of childbearing potential may be pregnant at the time of institution of therapy should be considered. Patients should be advised that if they become pregnant during therapy or intend to become pregnant they should communicate with their physicians about the desirability of discontinuing the drug.

Alprazolam Interaction with Drugs that Inhibit Metabolism via Cytochrome P450 3A
The initial step in alprazolam metabolism is hydroxylation catalyzed by cytochrome P450 3A (CYP3A). Drugs that inhibit this metabolic pathway may have a profound effect on the clearance of alprazolam. Consequently, alprazolam should be avoided in patients receiving very potent inhibitors of CYP3A. With drugs inhibiting CYP3A to a lesser but still significant degree, alprazolam should be used only with caution and consideration of appropriate dosage reduction. For some drugs, an interaction with alprazolam has been quantified with clinical data; for other drugs, interactions are predicted from *in vitro* data and/or experience with similar drugs in the same pharmacologic class.

The following are examples of drugs known to inhibit the metabolism of alprazolam and/or related benzodiazepines, presumably through inhibition of CYP3A.

Potent CYP3A Inhibitors
Azole antifungal agents — Ketoconazole and itraconazole are potent CYP3A inhibitors and have been shown *in vivo* to increase plasma alprazolam concentrations 3.98 fold and

2.70 fold, respectively. The coadministration of alprazolam with these agents is not recommended. Other azole-type antifungal agents should also be considered potent CYP3A inhibitors and the coadministration of alprazolam with them is not recommended (see CONTRAINDICATIONS).

Drugs demonstrated to be CYP3A inhibitors on the basis of clinical studies involving alprazolam (caution and consideration of appropriate alprazolam dose reduction are recommended during coadministration with the following drugs)

Nefazodone — Coadministration of nefazodone increased alprazolam concentration two-fold.

Fluvoxamine — Coadministration of fluvoxamine approximately doubled the maximum plasma concentration of alprazolam, decreased clearance by 49%, increased half-life by 71%, and decreased measured psychomotor performance.

Cimetidine — Coadministration of cimetidine increased the maximum plasma concentration of alprazolam by 86%, decreased clearance by 42%, and increased half-life by 16%.

Other drugs possibly affecting alprazolam metabolism

Other drugs possibly affecting alprazolam metabolism by inhibition of CYP3A are discussed in the PRECAUTIONS section (see PRECAUTIONS—Drug Interactions).

PRECAUTIONS

General

Suicide

As with other psychotropic medications, the usual precautions with respect to administration of the drug and size of the prescription are indicated for severely depressed patients or those in whom there is reason to expect concealed suicidal ideation or plans. Panic disorder has been associated with primary and secondary major depressive disorders and increased reports of suicide among untreated patients.

Mania

Episodes of hypomania and mania have been reported in association with the use of alprazolam in patients with depression.

Uricosuric Effect

Alprazolam has a weak uricosuric effect. Although other medications with weak uricosuric effect have been reported to cause acute renal failure, there have been no reported instances of acute renal failure attributable to therapy with alprazolam.

Use in Patients with Concomitant Illness

It is recommended that the dosage be limited to the smallest effective dose to preclude the development of ataxia or oversedation which may be a particular problem in elderly or debilitated patients. (See DOSAGE AND ADMINISTRATION.) The usual precautions in treating patients with impaired renal, hepatic or pulmonary function should be observed. There have been rare reports of death in patients with severe pulmonary disease shortly after the initiation of treatment with alprazolam. A decreased systemic alprazolam elimination rate (eg, increased plasma half-life) has been observed in both alcoholic liver disease patients and obese patients receiving alprazolam (see CLINICAL PHARMACOLOGY).

Information for Patients

For all users of NIRAVAM™

To assure safe and effective use of benzodiazepines, all patients prescribed NIRAVAM™ should be provided with the following guidance.

1. Do not remove NIRAVAM™ tablets from the bottle until just prior to dosing. With dry hands, open the bottle, remove the tablet, and immediately place on the tongue to dissolve and be swallowed with the saliva. The tablet may also be taken with water.
2. Discard any cotton that was included in the bottle and reseal the bottle tightly to prevent introducing moisture that might cause the tablets to disintegrate.
3. If only one-half of a scored tablet is used for dosing, the unused portion of the tablet should be discarded immediately because it may not remain stable.
4. Store away from moisture.
5. Inform your physician about any alcohol consumption and medicine you are taking now, including medication you may buy without a prescription. Alcohol should generally not be used during treatment with benzodiazepines.
6. Not recommended for use in pregnancy. Therefore, inform your physician if you are pregnant, if you are planning to have a child, or if you become pregnant while you are taking this medication.
7. Inform your physician if you are nursing.
8. Until you experience how this medication affects you, do not drive a car or operate potentially dangerous machinery, etc.
9. Do not increase the dose even if you think the medication "does not work anymore" without consulting your physician. Benzodiazepines, even when used as recommended, may produce emotional and/or physical dependence.
10. Do not stop taking this medication abruptly or decrease the dose without consulting your physician, since withdrawal symptoms can occur.

Additional advice for panic disorder patients

The use of alprazolam at doses greater than 4 mg/day, often necessary to treat panic disorder, is accompanied by risks that you need to carefully consider. When used at doses greater than 4 mg/day, which may or may not be required for your treatment, alprazolam has the potential to cause severe emotional and physical dependence in some patients and these patients may find it exceedingly difficult to terminate treatment. In two controlled trials of 6 to 8 weeks duration where the ability of patients to discontinue medication was measured, 7 to 29% of patients treated with alprazolam did not completely taper off therapy. In a controlled post-marketing discontinuation study of panic disorder patients, the patients treated with doses of alprazolam greater than 4 mg/day had more difficulty tapering to zero dose than patients treated with less than 4 mg/day. In all cases, it is important that your physician help you discontinue this medication in a careful and safe manner to avoid overly extended use of alprazolam.

In addition, the extended use at doses greater than 4 mg/day appears to increase the incidence and severity of withdrawal reactions when alprazolam is discontinued. These are generally minor but seizure can occur, especially if you reduce the dose too rapidly or discontinue the medication abruptly. Seizure can be life-threatening.

Treatment-Emergent Adverse Events Reported in Placebo-Controlled Trials of Anxiety Disorders

ANXIETY DISORDERS

	Treatment-Emergent Symptom Incidence† ALPRAZOLAM	PLACEBO	Incidence of Intervention Because of Symptom ALPRAZOLAM
Number of Patients	565	505	565
% of Patients Reporting:			
Central Nervous System			
Drowsiness	41.0	21.6	15.1
Lightheadedness	20.8	19.3	1.2
Depression	13.9	18.1	2.4
Headache	12.9	19.6	1.1
Confusion	9.9	10.0	0.9
Insomnia	8.9	18.4	1.3
Nervousness	4.1	10.3	1.1
Syncope	3.1	4.0	*
Dizziness	1.8	0.8	2.5
Akathisia	1.6	1.2	*
Tiredness/Sleepiness	*	*	1.8
Gastrointestinal			
Dry Mouth	14.7	13.3	0.7
Constipation	10.4	11.4	0.9
Diarrhea	10.1	10.3	1.2
Nausea/Vomiting	9.6	12.8	1.7
Increased Salivation	4.2	2.4	*
Cardiovascular			
Tachycardia/Palpitations	7.7	15.6	0.4
Hypotension	4.7	2.2	*
Sensory			
Blurred Vision	6.2	6.2	0.4
Musculoskeletal			
Rigidity	4.2	5.3	*
Tremor	4.0	8.8	0.4
Cutaneous			
Dermatitis/Allergy	3.8	3.1	0.6
Other			
Nasal Congestion	7.3	9.3	*
Weight Gain	2.7	2.7	*
Weight Loss	2.3	3.0	*

**None reported*

†Events reported by 1% or more of alprazolam patients are included.

Laboratory Tests

Laboratory tests are not ordinarily required in otherwise healthy patients. However, when treatment is protracted, periodic blood counts, urinalysis, and blood chemistry analyses are advisable in keeping with good medical practice.

Drug Interactions

Use with Other CNS Depressants

If NIRAVAM™ is to be combined with other psychotropic agents or anticonvulsant drugs, careful consideration should be given to the pharmacology of the agents to be employed, particularly with compounds which might potentiate the action of benzodiazepines. The benzodiazepines, including alprazolam, produce additive CNS depressant effects when co-administered with other psychotropic medications, anticonvulsants, antihistaminics, ethanol and other drugs which themselves produce CNS depression.

Drugs Effecting Salivary Flow and Stomach pH

Because NIRAVAM™ disintegrates in the presence of saliva and the formulation requires an acidic environment to dissolve, concomitant drugs or diseases that cause dry mouth or raise stomach pH might slow disintegration or dissolution, resulting in slowed or decreased absorption.

Use with Imipramine and Desipramine

The steady state plasma concentrations of imipramine and desipramine have been reported to be increased an average of 31% and 20%, respectively, by the concomitant administration of alprazolam in doses up to 4 mg/day. The clinical significance of these changes is unknown.

Drugs that inhibit alprazolam metabolism via cytochrome P450 3A

The initial step in alprazolam metabolism is hydroxylation catalyzed by cytochrome P450 3A (CYP3A). Drugs which inhibit this metabolic pathway may have a profound effect on the clearance of alprazolam (see CONTRAINDICATIONS and WARNINGS for additional drugs of this type).

Drugs demonstrated to be CYP3A inhibitors of possible clinical significance on the basis of clinical studies involving alprazolam (caution is recommended during coadministration with alprazolam)

Fluoxetine — Coadministration of fluoxetine with alprazolam increased the maximum plasma concentration of alprazolam by 46%, decreased clearance by 21%, increased half-life by 17%, and decreased measured psychomotor performance.

Propoxyphene — Coadministration of propoxyphene decreased the maximum plasma concentration of alprazolam by 6%, decreased clearance by 38%, and increased half-life by 58%.

Oral Contraceptives — Coadministration of oral contraceptives increased the maximum plasma concentration of alprazolam by 18%, decreased clearance by 22%, and increased half-life by 29%.

Drugs and other substances demonstrated to be CYP3A inhibitors on the basis of clinical studies involving benzodiazepines metabolized similarly to alprazolam or on the basis of *in vitro* studies with alprazolam or other benzodiazepines (caution is recommended during coadministration with alprazolam)

Available data from clinical studies of benzodiazepines other than alprazolam suggest a possible drug interaction with alprazolam for the following: diltiazem, isoniazid, macrolide antibiotics such as erythromycin and clarithromycin, and grapefruit juice. Data from *in vitro* studies of alprazolam suggest a possible drug interaction with alprazolam for the following: sertraline and paroxetine. However, data from an *in vivo* drug interaction study involving a single dose of alprazolam 1 mg and steady state doses of sertraline (50 to 150 mg/day) did not reveal any clinically significant changes in the pharmacokinetics of alprazolam. Data from *in vitro* studies of benzodiazepines other than alprazolam suggest a possible drug interaction for the following: ergotamine, cyclosporine, amiodarone, nicardipine, and nifedipine. Caution is recommended during the coadministration of any of these with alprazolam (see WARNINGS).

Drugs demonstrated to be inducers of CYP3A

Carbamazepine can increase alprazolam metabolism and therefore can decrease plasma levels of alprazolam.

Drug/Laboratory Test Interactions

Although interactions between benzodiazepines and commonly employed clinical laboratory tests have occasionally been reported, there is no consistent pattern for a specific drug or specific test.

Carcinogenesis, Mutagenesis, Impairment of Fertility

No evidence of carcinogenic potential was observed during 2-year bioassay studies of alprazolam in rats at doses up to 30 mg/kg/day (150 times the maximum recommended daily human dose of 10 mg/day) and in mice at doses up to 10 mg/kg/day (50 times the maximum recommended daily human dose).

Alprazolam was not mutagenic in the rat micronucleus test at doses up to 100 mg/kg, which is 500 times the maximum recommended daily human dose of 10 mg/day. Alprazolam also was not mutagenic *in vitro* in the DNA Damage/Alkaline Elution Assay or the Ames Assay.

Alprazolam produced no impairment of fertility in rats at doses up to 5 mg/kg/day, which is 25 times the maximum recommended daily human dose of 10 mg/day.

Pregnancy

Teratogenic Effects: Pregnancy Category D: (See WARNINGS section).

Continued on next page

Niravam—Cont.

Nonteratogenic Effects: It should be considered that the child born of a mother who is receiving benzodiazepines may be at some risk for withdrawal symptoms from the drug during the postnatal period. Also, neonatal flaccidity and respiratory problems have been reported in children born of mothers who have been receiving benzodiazepines.

Labor and Delivery

NIRAVAM™ has no established use in labor or delivery.

Nursing Mothers

Benzodiazepines are known to be excreted in human milk. It should be assumed that alprazolam is as well. Chronic administration of diazepam to nursing mothers has been reported to cause their infants to become lethargic and to lose weight. As a general rule, nursing should not be undertaken by mothers who must use NIRAVAM™.

Pediatric Use

Safety and effectiveness of NIRAVAM™ in individuals below 18 years of age have not been established.

Geriatric Use

The elderly may be more sensitive to the effects of benzodiazepines. They exhibit higher plasma alprazolam concentrations due to reduced clearance of the drug as compared with a younger population receiving the same doses. The smallest effective dose of NIRAVAM™ should be used in the elderly to preclude the development of ataxia and oversedation (see CLINICAL PHARMACOLOGY and DOSAGE AND ADMINISTRATION).

ADVERSE REACTIONS

Side effects to alprazolam, if they occur, are generally observed at the beginning of therapy and usually disappear upon continued medication. In the usual patient, the most frequent side effects are likely to be an extension of the pharmacological activity of alprazolam, eg, drowsiness or lightheadedness.

The data cited in the two tables below are estimates of untoward clinical event incidence among patients who participated under the following clinical conditions: relatively short duration (ie, four weeks) placebo-controlled clinical studies with dosages up to 4 mg/day of alprazolam (for the management of anxiety disorders or for the short-term relief of the symptoms of anxiety) and short-term (up to ten weeks) placebo-controlled clinical studies with dosages up to 10 mg/day of alprazolam in patients with panic disorder, with or without agoraphobia.

These data cannot be used to predict precisely the incidence of untoward events in the course of usual medical practice where patient characteristics, and other factors often differ from those in clinical trials. These figures cannot be compared with those obtained from other clinical studies involving related drug products and placebo as each group of drug trials are conducted under a different set of conditions.

Comparison of the cited figures, however, can provide the prescriber with some basis for estimating the relative contributions of drug and non-drug factors to the untoward event incidence in the population studied. Even this use must be approached cautiously, as a drug may relieve a symptom in one patient but induce it in others. (For example, an anxiolytic drug may relieve dry mouth [a symptom of anxiety] in some subjects but induce it [an untoward event] in others.)

Additionally, for anxiety disorders the cited figures can provide the prescriber with an indication as to the frequency with which physician intervention (eg, increased surveillance, decreased dosage or discontinuation of drug therapy) may be necessary because of the untoward clinical event.

[See table at top of previous page]

In addition to the relatively common (ie, greater than 1%) untoward events enumerated in the table above, the following adverse events have been reported in association with the use of benzodiazepines: dystonia, irritability, concentration difficulties, anorexia, transient amnesia or memory impairment, loss of coordination, fatigue, seizures, sedation, slurred speech, jaundice, musculoskeletal weakness, pruritus, diplopia, dysarthria, changes in libido, menstrual irregularities, incontinence and urinary retention.

Treatment-Emergent Adverse Events Reported in Placebo-Controlled Trials of Panic Disorder

PANIC DISORDER

	Treatment-Emergent Symptom Incidence*	
	ALPRAZOLAM	PLACEBO
Number of Patients	1388	1231
% of Patients Reporting:		
Central Nervous System		
Drowsiness	76.8	42.7
Fatigue and Tiredness	48.6	42.3
Impaired Coordination	40.1	17.9
Irritability	33.1	30.1
Memory Impairment	33.1	22.1
Lightheadedness/ Dizziness	29.8	36.9
Insomnia	29.4	41.8
Headache	29.2	35.6
Cognitive Disorder	28.8	20.5
Dysarthria	23.3	6.3
Anxiety	16.6	24.9
Abnormal Involuntary Movement	14.8	21.0
Decreased Libido	14.4	8.0
Depression	13.8	14.0
Confusional State	10.4	8.2
Muscular Twitching	7.9	11.8
Increased Libido	7.7	4.1
Change in Libido (Not Specified)	7.1	5.6
Weakness	7.1	8.4
Muscle Tone Disorders	6.3	7.5
Syncope	3.8	4.8
Akathisia	3.0	4.3
Agitation	2.9	2.6
Disinhibition	2.7	1.5
Paresthesia	2.4	3.2
Talkativeness	2.2	1.0
Vasomotor Disturbances	2.0	2.6
Derealization	1.9	1.2
Dream Abnormalities	1.8	1.5
Fear	1.4	1.0
Feeling Warm	1.3	0.5
Gastrointestinal		
Decreased Salivation	32.8	34.2
Constipation	26.2	15.4
Nausea/Vomiting	22.0	31.8
Diarrhea	20.6	22.8
Abdominal Distress	18.3	21.5
Increased Salivation	5.6	4.4
Cardio-Respiratory		
Nasal Congestion	17.4	16.5
Tachycardia	15.4	26.8
Chest Pain	10.6	18.1
Hyperventilation	9.7	14.5
Upper Respiratory Infection	4.3	3.7
Sensory		
Blurred Vision	21.0	21.4
Tinnitus	6.6	10.4
Musculoskeletal		
Muscular Cramps	2.4	2.4
Muscle Stiffness	2.3	3.3
Cutaneous		
Sweating	15.1	23.5
Rash	10.8	8.1
Other		
Increased Appetite	32.7	22.8
Decreased Appetite	27.8	24.1
Weight Gain	27.2	17.9
Weight Loss	22.6	16.5
Micturition Difficulties	12.2	8.6
Menstrual Disorders	10.4	8.7
Sexual Dysfunction	7.4	3.7
Edema	4.9	5.6
Incontinence	1.5	0.6
Infection	1.3	1.7

Events reported by 1% or more of alprazolam patients are included.

In addition to the relatively common (ie, greater than 1%) untoward events enumerated in the table above, the following adverse events have been reported in association with the use of alprazolam: seizures, hallucinations, depersonalization, taste alterations, diplopia, elevated bilirubin, elevated hepatic enzymes, and jaundice.

Panic disorder has been associated with primary and secondary major depressive disorders and increased reports of suicide among untreated patients (see PRECAUTIONS, General).

Adverse Events Reported as Reasons for Discontinuation in Treatment of Panic Disorder in Placebo-Controlled Trials

In a larger database comprised of both controlled and uncontrolled studies in which 641 patients received alprazolam, discontinuation-emergent symptoms which occurred at a rate of over 5% in patients treated with alprazolam and at a greater rate than the placebo-treated group were as follows:

[See table above]

DISCONTINUATION-EMERGENT SYMPTOM INCIDENCE

Percentage of 641 Alprazolam-Treated Panic Disorder Patients Reporting Events

Body System/Event		Body System/Event	
Neurologic		**Gastrointestinal**	
Insomnia	29.5	Nausea/Vomiting	16.5
Lightheadedness	19.3	Diarrhea	13.6
Abnormal involuntary movement	17.3	Decreased salivation	10.6
Headache	17.0	**Metabolic-Nutritional**	
Muscular twitching	6.9	Weight loss	13.3
Impaired coordination	6.6	Decreased appetite	12.8
Muscle tone disorders	5.9		
Weakness	5.8	**Dermatological**	
		Sweating	14.4
Psychiatric			
Anxiety	19.2	**Cardiovascular**	
Fatigue and Tiredness	18.4	Tachycardia	12.2
Irritability	10.5		
Cognitive Disorder	10.3	**Special Senses**	
Memory impairment	5.5	Blurred vision	10.0
Depression	5.1		
Confusional state	5.0		

From the studies cited, it has not been determined whether these symptoms are clearly related to the dose and duration of therapy with alprazolam in patients with panic disorder.

There have also been reports of withdrawal seizures upon rapid decrease or abrupt discontinuation of alprazolam (see WARNINGS).

To discontinue treatment in patients taking NIRAVAM™, the dosage should be reduced slowly in keeping with good medical practice. It is suggested that the daily dosage of NIRAVAM™ be decreased by no more than 0.5 mg every three days (see DOSAGE AND ADMINISTRATION). Some patients may benefit from an even slower dosage reduction. In a controlled postmarketing discontinuation study of panic disorder patients which compared this recommended taper schedule with a slower taper schedule, no difference was observed between the groups in the proportion of patients who tapered to zero dose; however, the slower schedule was associated with a reduction in symptoms associated with a withdrawal syndrome.

As with all benzodiazepines, paradoxical reactions such as stimulation, increased muscle spasticity, sleep disturbances, hallucinations and other adverse behavioral effects such as agitation, rage, irritability, and aggressive or hostile behavior have been reported rarely. In many of the spontaneous case reports of adverse behavioral effects, patients were receiving other CNS drugs concomitantly and/or were described as having underlying psychiatric conditions. Should any of the above events occur, alprazolam should be discontinued. Isolated published reports involving small numbers of patients have suggested that patients who have borderline personality disorder, a prior history of violent or aggressive behavior, or alcohol or substance abuse may be at risk for such events. Instances of irritability, hostility, and intrusive thoughts have been reported during discontinuation of alprazolam in patients with posttraumatic stress disorder.

Post Introduction Reports: Various adverse drug reactions have been reported in association with the use of alprazolam since market introduction. The majority of these reactions were reported through the medical event voluntary reporting system. Because of the spontaneous nature of the reporting of medical events and the lack of controls, a causal relationship to the use of alprazolam cannot be readily determined. Reported events include: liver enzyme elevations, hepatitis, hepatic failure, Stevens-Johnson syndrome, hyperprolactinemia, gynecomastia, and galactorrhea.

DRUG ABUSE AND DEPENDENCE

Physical and Psychological Dependence

Withdrawal symptoms similar in character to those noted with sedative/hypnotics and alcohol have occurred following discontinuance of benzodiazepines, including alprazolam. The symptoms can range from mild dysphoria and insomnia to a major syndrome that may include abdominal and muscle cramps, vomiting, sweating, tremors and convulsions. Distinguishing between withdrawal emergent signs and symptoms and the recurrence of illness is often difficult in patients undergoing dose reduction. The long term strategy for treatment of these phenomena will vary with their cause and the therapeutic goal. When necessary, immediate management of withdrawal symptoms requires re-institution of treatment at doses of alprazolam sufficient to suppress symptoms. There have been reports of failure of other benzodiazepines to fully suppress these withdrawal symptoms. These failures have been attributed to incomplete cross-tolerance but may also reflect the use of an inadequate dosing regimen of the substituted benzodiazepine or the effects of concomitant medications.

While it is difficult to distinguish withdrawal and recurrence for certain patients, the time course and the nature of the symptoms may be helpful. A withdrawal syndrome typically includes the occurrence of new symptoms, tends to appear toward the end of taper or shortly after discontinuation, and will decrease with time. In recurring panic disorder, symptoms similar to those observed before treatment may recur either early or late, and they will persist. While the severity and incidence of withdrawal phenomena appear to be related to dose and duration of treatment, withdrawal symptoms, including seizures, have been reported after only brief therapy with alprazolam at doses within the recommended range for the treatment of anxiety (eg, 0.75 to 4 mg/day). Signs and symptoms of withdrawal are often more prominent after rapid decrease of dosage or abrupt discontinuance. The risk of withdrawal seizures may be increased at doses above 4 mg/day (see WARNINGS).

Patients, especially individuals with a history of seizures or epilepsy, should not be abruptly discontinued from any CNS depressant agent, including alprazolam. It is recommended that all patients on NIRAVAM™ who require a dosage reduction be gradually tapered under close supervision (see WARNINGS and DOSAGE AND ADMINISTRATION).

Psychological dependence is a risk with all benzodiazepines, including NIRAVAM™. The risk of psychological dependence may also be increased at doses greater than 4 mg/day and with longer term use, and this risk is further increased in patients with a history of alcohol or drug abuse. Some patients have experienced considerable difficulty in tapering and discontinuing from alprazolam, especially those receiving higher doses for extended periods. Addiction-prone individuals should be under careful surveillance when receiving NIRAVAM™. As with all anxiolytics, repeat prescriptions should be limited to those who are under medical supervision.

Controlled Substance Class

Alprazolam is a controlled substance under the Controlled Substance Act by the Drug Enforcement Administration and NIRAVAM™ has been assigned to Schedule IV.

OVERDOSAGE

Clinical Experience

Manifestations of alprazolam overdosage include somnolence, confusion, impaired coordination, diminished reflexes and coma. Death has been reported in association with overdoses of alprazolam by itself, as it has with other benzodiazepines. In addition, fatalities have been reported in patients who have overdosed with a combination of a single benzodiazepine, including alprazolam, and alcohol; alcohol levels seen in some of these patients have been lower than those usually associated with alcohol-induced fatality.

The acute oral LD_{50} in rats is 331-2171 mg/kg. Other experiments in animals have indicated that cardiopulmonary collapse can occur following massive intravenous doses of alprazolam (over 195 mg/kg; 975 times the maximum recommended daily human dose of 10 mg/day). Animals could be resuscitated with positive mechanical ventilation and the intravenous infusion of norepinephrine bitartrate. Animal experiments have suggested that forced diuresis or hemodialysis are probably of little value in treating overdosage.

General Treatment of Overdose

Overdosage reports with alprazolam are limited. As in all cases of drug overdosage, respiration, pulse rate, and blood pressure should be monitored. General supportive measures should be employed, along with immediate gastric lavage. Intravenous fluids should be administered and an adequate airway maintained. If hypotension occurs, it may be combated by the use of vasopressors. Dialysis is of limited value. As with the management of intentional overdosing with any drug, it should be borne in mind that multiple agents may have been ingested.

Flumazenil, a specific benzodiazepine receptor antagonist, is indicated for the complete or partial reversal of the sedative effects of benzodiazepines and may be used in situations when an overdose with a benzodiazepine is known or suspected. Prior to the administration of flumazenil, necessary measures should be instituted to secure airway, ventilation and intravenous access. Flumazenil is intended as an adjunct to, not as a substitute for, proper management of benzodiazepine overdose. Patients treated with flumazenil should be monitored for re-sedation, respiratory depression, and other residual benzodiazepine effects for an appropriate period after treatment. **The prescriber should be aware of a risk of seizure in association with flumazenil treatment, particularly in long-term benzodiazepine users and in cyclic antidepressant overdose.** The complete flumazenil package insert including CONTRAINDICATIONS, WARNINGS and PRECAUTIONS should be consulted prior to use.

DOSAGE AND ADMINISTRATION

Dosage should be individualized for maximum beneficial effect. While the usual daily dosages given below will meet the needs of most patients, there will be some who require doses greater than 4 mg/day. In such cases, dosage should be increased cautiously to avoid adverse effects.

Anxiety Disorders and Transient Symptoms of Anxiety

Treatment for patients with anxiety should be initiated with a dose of 0.25 to 0.5 mg given three times daily. The dose may be increased to achieve a maximum therapeutic effect, at intervals of 3 to 4 days, to a maximum daily dose of 4 mg, given in divided doses. The lowest possible effective dose should be employed and the need for continued treatment reassessed frequently. The risk of dependence may increase with dose and duration of treatment.

In all patients, dosage should be reduced gradually when discontinuing therapy or when decreasing the daily dosage. Although there are no systematically collected data to support a specific discontinuation schedule, it is suggested that the daily dosage be decreased by no more than 0.5 mg every 3 days. Some patients may require an even slower dosage reduction.

Panic Disorder

The successful treatment of many panic disorder patients has required the use of alprazolam at doses greater than 4 mg daily. In controlled trials conducted to establish the efficacy of alprazolam in panic disorder, doses in the range of 1 to 10 mg daily were used. The mean dosage employed was approximately 5 to 6 mg daily. Among the approximately 1700 patients participating in the panic disorder development program, about 300 received alprazolam in dosages of greater than 7 mg/day, including approximately 100 patients who received maximum dosages of greater than 9 mg/day. Occasional patients required as much as 10 mg a day to achieve a successful response.

Dose Titration

Treatment may be initiated with a dose of 0.5 mg three times daily. Depending on the response, the dose may be increased at intervals of 3 to 4 days in increments of no more than 1 mg per day. Slower titration to the dose levels greater than 4 mg/day may be advisable to allow full expression of the pharmacodynamic effect of alprazolam. To lessen the possibility of interdose symptoms, the times of administration should be distributed as evenly as possible throughout the waking hours, that is, on a three or four times per day schedule.

Generally, therapy should be initiated at a low dose to minimize the risk of adverse responses in patients especially sensitive to the drug. Dose should be advanced until an acceptable therapeutic response (ie, a substantial reduction in or total elimination of panic attacks) is achieved, intolerance occurs, or the maximum recommended dose is attained.

Dose Maintenance

For patients receiving doses greater than 4 mg/day, periodic reassessment and consideration of dosage reduction is advised. In a controlled postmarketing dose-response study, patients treated with doses of alprazolam greater than 4 mg/day for 3 months were able to taper to 50% of their total maintenance dose without apparent loss of clinical benefit. Because of the danger of withdrawal, abrupt discontinuation of treatment should be avoided. (See WARNINGS, PRECAUTIONS, DRUG ABUSE AND DEPENDENCE.)

The necessary duration of treatment for panic disorder patients responding to alprazolam is unknown. After a period of extended freedom from attacks, a carefully supervised tapered discontinuation may be attempted, but there is evidence that this may often be difficult to accomplish without recurrence of symptoms and/or the manifestation of withdrawal phenomena.

Dose Reduction

Because of the danger of withdrawal, abrupt discontinuation of treatment should be avoided (see WARNINGS, PRECAUTIONS, DRUG ABUSE AND DEPENDENCE.)

In all patients, dosage should be reduced gradually when discontinuing therapy or when decreasing the daily dosage. Although there are no systematically collected data to support a specific discontinuation schedule, it is suggested that the daily dosage be decreased by no more than 0.5 mg every three days. Some patients may require an even slower dosage reduction.

In any case, reduction of dose must be undertaken under close supervision and must be gradual. If significant withdrawal symptoms develop, the previous dosing schedule should be reinstituted and, only after stabilization, should a less rapid schedule of discontinuation be attempted. In a controlled postmarketing discontinuation study of panic disorder patients which compared this recommended taper schedule with a slower taper schedule, no difference was observed between the groups in the proportion of patients who tapered to zero dose; however, the slower schedule was associated with a reduction in symptoms associated with a withdrawal syndrome. It is suggested that the dose be reduced by no more than 0.5 mg every 3 days, with the understanding that some patients may benefit from an even more gradual discontinuation. Some patients may prove resistant to all discontinuation regimens.

Dosing in Special Populations

In elderly patients, in patients with advanced liver disease or in patients with debilitating disease, the usual starting dose is 0.25 mg, given two or three times daily. This may be gradually increased if needed and tolerated. The elderly may be especially sensitive to the effects of benzodiazepines. If side effects occur at the recommended starting dose, the dose may be lowered.

Instructions to be Given to Patients for Use/Handling NIRAVAM™ Tablets

Just prior to administration, with dry hands, remove the tablet from the bottle. Immediately place the NIRAVAM™ tablet on top of the tongue where it will disintegrate, and be swallowed with saliva. Administration with liquid is not necessary.

If only one-half of a scored tablet is used for dosing, the unused portion of the tablet should be discarded immediately because it may not remain stable.

Discard any cotton that was included in the bottle and reseal the bottle tightly to prevent introducing moisture that might cause the tablets to disintegrate.

HOW SUPPLIED

NIRAVAM™ (alprazolam orally disintegrating tablets) 0.25 mg are yellow, round, orange-flavored, scored and engraved "SP 321" on the unscored side and "0.25" on the scored side. They are supplied as follows:

Bottles of 100 NDC 0091-3321-01

NIRAVAM™ (alprazolam orally disintegrating tablets) 0.5 mg are yellow, round, orange-flavored, scored and engraved "SP 322" on the unscored side and "0.5" on the scored side. They are supplied as follows:

Bottles of 100 NDC 0091-3322-01

NIRAVAM™ (alprazolam orally disintegrating tablets) 1 mg are white, round, orange-flavored, scored and engraved "SP 323" on the unscored side and "1" on the scored side. They are supplied as follows:

Bottles of 100 NDC 0091-3323-01

NIRAVAM™ (alprazolam orally disintegrating tablets) 2 mg are white, round, orange-flavored, scored and engraved "SP 324" on the unscored side and "2" on the scored side. They are supplied as follows:

Bottles of 100 NDC 0091-3324-01

Store at 20° to 25°C (68° to 77°F); excursions permitted between 15° to 30°C (59° to 86°F) [See USP Controlled Room Temperature]. Protect from moisture.

Dispense in a tight container as defined in the USP/NF.

ANIMAL STUDIES

When rats were treated with alprazolam at 3, 10, and 30 mg/kg/day (15 to 150 times the maximum recommended human dose) orally for 2 years, a tendency for a dose related increase in the number of cataracts was observed in females and a tendency for a dose related increase in corneal vascularization was observed in males. These lesions did not appear until after 11 months of treatment.

Manufactured for:

SCHWARZ
PHARMA
Milwaukee, WI 53201, USA

By: CIMA LABS INC.®
Eden Prairie, MN 55344, USA

NIRAVAM™ uses CIMA LABS INC.® U.S. Patent Nos. 6,024,981 and 6,221,392.

PC4714B
Rev. 1/05

Scios Inc.

6500 PASEO PADRE PARKWAY
FREMONT, CA 94555

Direct Inquiries to:
1-877-4 NATRECOR
(1-877-462-8732)
(510)-595-8183 (fax)

NATRECOR® ℞

[*nā-trĕ-kōr*]

(nesiritide)

for Injection

FOR INTRAVENOUS INFUSION ONLY

℞ Only

DESCRIPTION

Natrecor® (nesiritide) is a sterile, purified preparation of a new drug class, human B-type natriuretic peptide (hBNP), and is manufactured from *E.* coli using recombinant DNA technology. Nesiritide has a molecular weight of 3464 g/mol and an empirical formula of $C_{143}H_{244}N_{50}O_{42}S_4$. Nesiritide has the same 32 amino acid sequence as the endogenous peptide, which is produced by the ventricular myocardium.

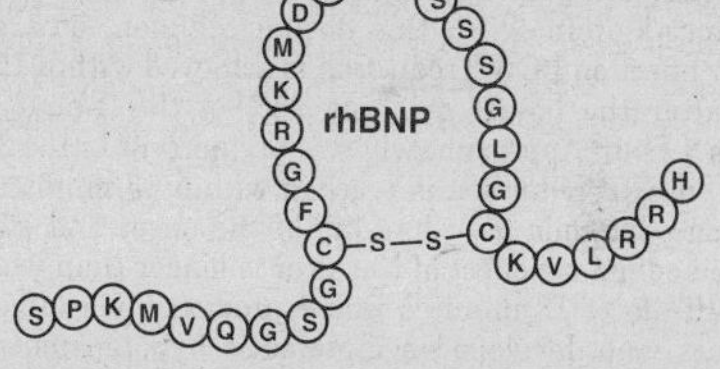

Natrecor is formulated as the citrate salt of rhBNP, and is provided in a sterile, single-use vial. Each 1.5 mg vial contains a white- to off-white lyophilized powder for intravenous (IV) administration after reconstitution. The quantitative composition of the lyophilized drug per vial is: nesiritide 1.58 mg, mannitol 20.0 mg, citric acid monohydrate 2.1 mg, and sodium citrate dihydrate 2.94 mg.

Mechanism of Action

Human BNP binds to the particulate guanylate cyclase receptor of vascular smooth muscle and endothelial cells, leading to increased intracellular concentrations of guanosine 3′5′-cyclic monophosphate (cGMP) and smooth muscle cell relaxation. Cyclic GMP serves as a second messenger to dilate veins and arteries. Nesiritide has been shown to relax isolated human arterial and venous tissue preparations that were precontracted with either endothelin-1 or the alpha-adrenergic agonist, phenylephrine.

In human studies, nesiritide produced dose-dependent reductions in pulmonary capillary wedge pressure (PCWP) and systemic arterial pressure in patients with heart failure.

In animals, nesiritide had no effects on cardiac contractility or on measures of cardiac electrophysiology such as atrial and ventricular effective refractory times or atrioventricular node conduction.

Naturally occurring atrial natriuretic peptide (ANP), a related peptide, increases vascular permeability in animals and humans and may reduce intravascular volume. The effect of nesiritide on vascular permeability has not been studied.

Pharmacokinetics

In patients with congestive heart failure (CHF), Natrecor administered intravenously by infusion or bolus exhibits biphasic disposition from the plasma. The mean terminal elimination half-life ($t_{½}$) of Natrecor is approximately 18 minutes and was associated with approximately 2/3 of the area-under-the-curve (AUC). The mean initial elimination

Continued on next page

Natrecor—Cont.

phase was estimated to be approximately 2 minutes. In these patients, the mean volume of distribution of the central compartment (Vc) of Natrecor was estimated to be 0.073 L/kg, the mean steady-state volume of distribution (Vss) was 0.19 L/kg, and the mean clearance (CL) was approximately 9.2 mL/min/kg. At steady state, plasma BNP levels increase from baseline endogenous levels by approximately 3-fold to 6-fold with Natrecor infusion doses ranging from 0.01 to 0.03 mcg/kg/min.

Elimination

Human BNP is cleared from the circulation via the following three independent mechanisms, in order of decreasing importance: 1) binding to cell surface clearance receptors with subsequent cellular internalization and lysosomal proteolysis; 2) proteolytic cleavage of the peptide by endopeptidases, such as neutral endopeptidase, which are present on the vascular lumenal surface; and 3) renal filtration.

Special Populations

Although Natrecor is eliminated, in part, through renal clearance, clinical data suggest that dose adjustment is not required in patients with renal insufficiency. The effects of Natrecor on PCWP, cardiac index (CI), and systolic blood pressure (SBP) were not significantly different in patients with chronic renal insufficiency (baseline serum creatinine ranging from 2 mg/dL to 4.3 mg/dL), and patients with normal renal function. The population pharmacokinetic (PK) analyses carried out to determine the effects of demographics and clinical variables on PK parameters showed that clearance of Natrecor is proportional to body weight, supporting the administration of weight-adjusted dosing of Natrecor (i.e., administration on a mcg/kg/min basis). Clearance was not influenced significantly by age, gender, race/ethnicity, baseline endogenous hBNP concentration, severity of CHF (as indicated by baseline PCWP, baseline Cl, or New York Heart Association [NYHA] classification), or concomitant administration of an ACE inhibitor.

Effects of Concomitant Medications

The co-administration of Natrecor with enalapril did not have significant effects on the PK of Natrecor. The PK effect of co-administration of Natrecor with other IV vasodilators such as nitroglycerin, nitroprusside, milrinone, or IV ACE inhibitors has not been evaluated. During clinical studies, Natrecor was administered concomitantly with other medications, including: diuretics, digoxin, oral ACE inhibitors, anticoagulants, oral nitrates, statins, class III antiarrhythmic agents, beta-blockers, dobutamine, calcium channel blockers, angiotensin II receptor antagonists, and dopamine. Although no PK interactions were specifically assessed, there did not appear to be evidence suggesting any clinically significant PK interaction.

Pharmacodynamics

The recommended dosing regimen of Natrecor is a 2 mcg/kg IV bolus followed by an intravenous infusion dose of 0.01 mcg/kg/min. With this dosing regimen, 60% of the 3-hour effect on PCWP reduction is achieved within 15 minutes after the bolus, reaching 95% of the 3-hour effect within 1 hour. Approximately seventy percent of the 3-hour effect on SBP reduction is reached within 15 minutes. The pharmacodynamic (PD) half-life of the onset and offset of the hemodynamic effect of Natrecor is longer than what the PK half-life of 18 minutes would predict. For example, in patients who developed symptomatic hypotension in the VMAC (Vasodilation in the Management of Acute Congestive Heart Failure) trial, half of the recovery of SBP toward the baseline value after discontinuation or reduction of the dose of Natrecor was observed in about 60 minutes. When higher doses of Natrecor were infused, the duration of hypotension was sometimes several hours.

Clinical Trials

Natrecor has been studied in 10 clinical trials including 941 patients with CHF (NYHA class II-III 61%, NYHA class IV 36%; mean age 60 years, women 28%). There were five randomized, multi-center, placebo- or active-controlled studies (comparative agents included nitroglycerin, dobutamine, milrinone, nitroprusside, or dopamine) in which 772 patients with decompensated CHF received continuous infusions of Natrecor at doses ranging from 0.01 to 0.03 mcg/kg/min. (See the ADVERSE REACTIONS section for relative frequency of adverse events at doses ranging from the recommended dose up to 0.03 mcg/kg/min). Of these patients, the majority (n = 541, 70%) received the Natrecor infusion for at least 24 hours; 371 (48%) received Natrecor for 24–48 hours, and 170 (22%) received Natrecor for greater than 48 hours.

In controlled trials, Natrecor has been used alone or in conjunction with other standard therapies, including diuretics (79%), digoxin (62%), oral ACE inhibitors (55%), anticoagulants (38%), oral nitrates (32%), statins (18%), class III antiarrhythmic agents (16%), beta-blockers (15%), dobutamine (15%), calcium channel blockers (11%), angiotensin II receptor antagonists (6%), and dopamine (4%). Natrecor has been studied in a broad range of patients, including the elderly (42% >65 years of age), women (30%), minorities (26% black), and patients with a history of significant morbidities such as hypertension (67%), previous myocardial infarction (50%), diabetes (44%), atrial fibrillation/flutter (34%), nonsustained ventricular tachycardia (25%), ventricular tachycardia/ fibrillation (12%), preserved systolic function (9%), and acute coronary syndromes less than 7 days before the start of Natrecor (4%).

The VMAC (Vasodilation in the Management of Acute Congestive Heart Failure) trial was a randomized, double-blind study of 489 patients (246 patients requiring a right heart catheter, 243 patients without a right heart catheter) who required hospitalization for management of shortness of breath at rest due to acutely decompensated CHF. The study compared the effects of Natrecor, placebo, and IV nitroglycerin when added to background therapy (IV and oral diuretics, non-IV cardiac medications, dobutamine, and dopamine). Patients with acute coronary syndrome, preserved systolic function, arrhythmia, and renal insufficiency were not excluded. The primary endpoints of the study were the change from baseline in PCWP and the change from baseline in patients' dyspnea, evaluated after three hours. Close attention was also paid to the occurrence and persistence of hypotension, given nesiritide's relatively long (compared to nitroglycerin) PK and PD half-life.

Natrecor was administered as a 2 mcg/kg bolus over approximately 60 seconds, followed by a continuous fixed dose infusion of 0.01 mcg/kg/min. After the 3-hour placebo-controlled period, patients receiving placebo crossed over to double-blinded active therapy with either Natrecor or nitroglycerin. The nitroglycerin dose was titrated at the physician's discretion. A subset of patients in the VMAC trial with central hemodynamic monitoring who were treated with Natrecor (62 of 124 patients) were allowed dose increases of Natrecor after the first 3 hours of treatment if the PCWP was ≥20 mm Hg and the SBP was ≥100 mm Hg. Dose increases of a 1 mcg/kg bolus followed by an increase of the infusion dose by 0.005 mcg/kg/min were allowed every 3 hours, up to a maximum dose of 0.03 mcg/kg/min. Overall, 23 patients in this subset had the dose of Natrecor increased in the VMAC trial.

In a second double-blind study, 127 patients requiring hospitalization for symptomatic CHF were randomized to placebo or to one of two doses of Natrecor (0.015 mcg/kg/min preceded by an IV bolus of 0.3 mcg/kg, and 0.03 mcg/kg/min preceded by an IV bolus of 0.6 mcg/kg). The primary endpoint of the trial was the change in PCWP from baseline to 6 hours, but the effect on symptoms also was examined.

Effects on Symptoms

In the VMAC study, patients receiving Natrecor reported greater improvement in their dyspnea at 3 hours than patients receiving placebo (p = 0.034).

In the dose-response study, patients receiving both doses of Natrecor reported greater improvement in dyspnea at 6 hours than patients receiving placebo.

Effects on Hemodynamics

The PCWP, right atrial pressure (RAP), CI, and other hemodynamic variables were monitored in 246 of the patients in the VMAC trial. There was a reduction in mean PCWP within 15 minutes of starting the Natrecor infusion, with most of the effect seen at 3 hours being achieved within the first 60 minutes of the infusion (see Pharmacodynamics).

In several studies, hemodynamic parameters were measured after Natrecor withdrawal. Following discontinuation of Natrecor, PCWP returns to within 10% of baseline within 2 hours, but no rebound increase to levels above baseline state was observed. There was also no evidence of tachyphylaxis to the hemodynamic effects of Natrecor in the clinical trials.

The following table and graph summarize the changes in the VMAC trial in PCWP and other measures during the first 3 hours.

[See table below]

PCWP through 3 Hours

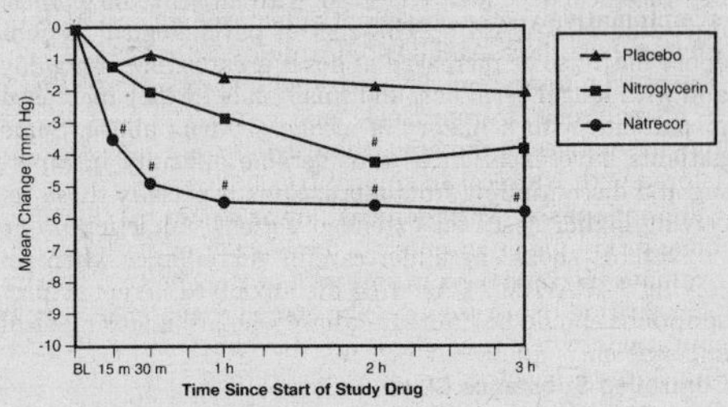

*p<0.05 compared to placebo

The VMAC study does not constitute an adequate effectiveness comparison with nitroglycerin. In this trial, the nitroglycerin group provides a rough landmark using a familiar therapy and regimen.

Effect on Urine Output

In the VMAC trial, in which the use of diuretics was not restricted, the mean change in volume status (output minus input) during the first 24 hours in the nitroglycerin and Natrecor groups was similar: 1279 ± 1455 mL and 1257 ± 1657 mL, respectively.

INDICATIONS AND USAGE

Natrecor (nesiritide) is indicated for the intravenous treatment of patients with acutely decompensated congestive heart failure who have dyspnea at rest or with minimal activity. In this population, the use of Natrecor reduced pulmonary capillary wedge pressure and improved dyspnea.

CONTRAINDICATIONS

Natrecor is contraindicated in patients who are hypersensitive to any of its components. Natrecor should not be used as primary therapy for patients with cardiogenic shock or in patients with a systolic blood pressure <90 mm Hg.

WARNINGS

Administration of Natrecor should be avoided in patients suspected of having, or known to have, low cardiac filling pressures.

PRECAUTIONS

General: Parenteral administration of protein pharmaceuticals or *E.* coli-derived products should be attended by appropriate precautions in case of an allergic or untoward reaction. No serious allergic or anaphylactic reactions have been reported with Natrecor.

Natrecor is not recommended for patients for whom vasodilating agents are not appropriate, such as patients with significant valvular stenosis, restrictive or obstructive cardiomyopathy, constrictive pericarditis, pericardial tamponade, or other conditions in which cardiac output is dependent upon venous return, or for patients suspected to have low cardiac filling pressures. (See CONTRAINDICATIONS.)

Renal: Natrecor may affect renal function in susceptible individuals. In patients with severe heart failure whose renal function may depend on the activity of the renin-angiotensin-aldosterone system, treatment with Natrecor may be associated with azotemia. When Natrecor was initiated at doses higher than 0.01 mcg/kg/min (0.015 and 0.03 mcg/kg/min), there was an increased rate of elevated serum creatinine over baseline compared with standard therapies, although the rate of acute renal failure and need for dialysis was not increased. In the 30-day follow-up period in the VMAC trial, 5 patients in the nitroglycerin group (2%) and 9 patients in the Natrecor group (3%) required first-time dialysis.

Cardiovascular: Natrecor may cause hypotension. In the VMAC trial, in patients given the recommended dose (2 mcg/kg bolus followed by a 0.01 mcg/kg/min infusion) or the adjustable dose, the incidence of symptomatic hypotension in the first 24 hours was similar for Natrecor (4%) and IV nitroglycerin (5%). When hypotension occurred, however, the duration of symptomatic hypotension was longer with Natrecor (mean duration was 2.2 hours) than with nitroglycerin (mean duration was 0.7 hours). In earlier trials, when Natrecor was initiated at doses higher than the 2 mcg/kg bolus followed by a 0.01 mcg/kg/min infusion (i.e., 0.015 and 0.03 mcg/kg/min preceded by a small bolus), there were more hypotensive episodes and these episodes were of greater intensity and duration. They were also more often symptomatic and/or more likely to require medical intervention (see ADVERSE REACTIONS). Natrecor should be administered only in settings where blood pressure can be monitored closely, and the dose of Natrecor should be reduced or the drug discontinued in patients who develop hypotension (see Dosing Instructions). The rate of symptomatic hypotension may be increased in patients with a blood pressure <100 mm Hg at baseline, and Natrecor should be used cautiously in these patients. The potential for hypotension may be increased by combining Natrecor with other drugs that may cause hypotension. For example, in the VMAC trial in patients treated with either Natrecor or nitroglycerin therapy, the frequency of symptomatic hypotension in patients who received an oral ACE inhibitor was 6%, compared to a frequency of symptomatic hypotension of 1% in patients who did not receive an oral ACE inhibitor.

Mean Hemodynamic Change from Baseline

Effects at 3 Hours	Placebo (n = 62)	Nitroglycerin (n = 60)	Natrecor (n = 124)
Pulmonary capillary wedge pressure (mm Hg)	−2.0	−3.8	−5.8‡
Right atrial pressure (mm Hg)	0.0	−2.6	−3.1‡
Cardiac index (L/min/M²)	0.0	0.2	0.1
Mean pulmonary artery pressure (mm Hg)	−1.1	−2.5	−5.4‡
Systemic vascular resistance (dynes*sec*cm⁻⁵)	−44	−105	−144
Systolic blood pressure† (mm Hg)	−2.5	−5.7‡	−5.6‡

† Based on all treated subjects: placebo n = 142, nitroglycerin n = 143, Natrecor n = 204
‡ p<0.05 compared to placebo

Drug Interactions: No trials specifically examining potential drug interactions with Natrecor were conducted, although many concomitant drugs were used in clinical trials. No drug interactions were detected except for an increase in symptomatic hypotension in patients receiving oral ACE inhibitors (see PRECAUTIONS, Cardiovascular).

The co-administration of Natrecor with IV vasodilators such as nitroglycerin, nitroprusside, milrinone, or IV ACE inhibitors has not been evaluated (these drugs were not co-administered with Natrecor in clinical trials).

Carcinogenesis, Mutagenesis, Impairment of Fertility: Long-term studies in animals have not been performed to evaluate the carcinogenic potential or the effect on fertility of nesiritide. Nesiritide did not increase the frequency of mutations when used in an in vitro bacterial cell assay (Ames test). No other genotoxicity studies were performed.

Pregnancy: Category C: Animal developmental and reproductive toxicity studies have not been conducted with nesiritide. It is also not known whether Natrecor can cause fetal harm when administered to pregnant women or can affect reproductive capacity. Natrecor should be used during pregnancy only if the potential benefit justifies any possible risk to the fetus.

Nursing Mothers: It is not known whether this drug is excreted in human milk. Therefore, caution should be exercised when Natrecor is administered to a nursing woman.

Pediatric Use: The safety and effectiveness of Natrecor in pediatric patients has not been established.

Geriatric Use: Of the total number of subjects in clinical trials treated with Natrecor (n = 941), 38% were 65 years or older and 16% were 75 years or older. No overall differences in effectiveness were observed between these subjects and younger subjects, and other reported clinical experience has not identified differences in responses between the elderly and younger patients. Some older individuals may be more sensitive to the effect of Natrecor than younger individuals.

ADVERSE REACTIONS

Adverse events that occurred with at least a 3% frequency during the first 24 hours of Natrecor infusion are shown in the following table.

[See table above]

Adverse events that are not listed in the above table that occurred in at least 1% of patients who received any of the above Natrecor doses included: Tachycardia, atrial fibrillation, AV node conduction abnormalities, catheter pain, fever, injection site reaction, confusion, paresthesia, somnolence, tremor, increased cough, hemoptysis, apnea, increased creatinine, sweating, pruritus, rash, leg cramps, amblyopia, anemia. All reported events (at least 1%) are included except those already listed, those too general to be informative, and those not reasonably associated with the use of the drug because they were associated with the condition being treated or are very common in the treated population.

In placebo and active-controlled clinical trials, Natrecor has not been associated with an increase in atrial or ventricular tachyarrhythmias. In placebo-controlled trials, the incidence of VT in both Natrecor and placebo patients was 2%. In the PRECEDENT (Prospective Randomized Evaluation of Cardiac Ectopy with Dobutamine or Natrecor Therapy) trial, the effects of Natrecor (n = 163) and dobutamine (n = 83) on the provocation or aggravation of existing ventricular arrhythmias in patients with decompensated CHF was compared using Holter monitoring. Treatment with Natrecor (0.015 and 0.03 mcg/kg/min without an initial bolus) for 24 hours did not aggravate pre-existing VT or the frequency of premature ventricular beats, compared to a baseline 24-hour Holter tape.

Clinical Laboratory

In the PRECEDENT trial, the incidence of elevations in serum creatinine to >0.5 mg/dL above baseline through day 14 was higher in the Natrecor 0.015 mcg/kg/min group (17%) and the Natrecor 0.03 mcg/kg/min group (19%) than with standard therapy (11%). In the VMAC trial, through day 30, the incidence of elevations in creatinine to >0.5 mg/dL above baseline was 28% and 21% in the Natrecor (2 mcg/kg bolus followed by 0.01 mcg/kg/min) and nitroglycerin groups, respectively.

Effect on Mortality

Data from all seven studies in which 30-day data were collected are presented in the chart below. The data depict hazard ratios and confidence intervals of mortality data for randomized and treated patients with Natrecor® relative to active controls through day 30 for each of the 7 individual studies (Studies 311, 325, 326, 329 [PRECEDENT], 339 [VMAC], 341 [PROACTION], and 348 [FUSION I]).

The figure (on logarithmic scale) also contains a plot for the six studies involving hospitalized or Emergency Department patients combined (n = 1507), and for all 7 studies combined (n = 1717). The percentage is the Kaplan-Meier estimate.

[See first figure at right]

The figure below represents 180-day mortality hazard ratios for randomized and treated patients from all four individual studies where 180-day data were collected, 16 week hazard ratios for Study 348 (180-day data were not collected), and the four studies with 180-day data pooled (n = 1167).

[See second figure at right]

There were few deaths in these studies, so the confidence limits around the hazard ratios for mortality are wide. The studies are also small, so some potentially important baseline imbalances exist among the treatment groups, the effects of which cannot be ascertained.

	VMAC Trial		Other Long Infusion Trials		
				Natrecor mcg/kg/min	
Adverse Events	Nitroglycerin (n = 216)	Natrecor Recommended Dose (n = 273)	Control* (n = 256)	0.015 (n = 253)	0.03 (n = 246)
Cardiovascular					
Hypotension	25 (12%)	31 (11%)	20 (8%)	56 (22%)	87 (35%)
Symptomatic Hypotension	10 (5%)	12 (4%)	8 (3%)	28 (11%)	42 (17%)
Asymptomatic Hypotension	17 (8%)	23 (8%)	13 (5%)	31 (12%)	49 (20%)
Ventricular Tachycardia (VT)	11 (5%)	9 (3%)	25 (10%)	25 (10%)	10 (4%)
Non–sustained VT	11 (5%)	9 (3%)	23 (9%)	24 (9%)	9 (4%)
Ventricular Extrasystoles	2 (1%)	7 (3%)	15 (6%)	10 (4%)	9 (4%)
Angina Pectoris	5 (2%)	5 (2%)	6 (2%)	14 (6%)	6 (2%)
Bradycardia	1 (<1%)	3 (1%)	1 (<1%)	8 (3%)	13 (5%)
Body as a Whole					
Headache	44 (20%)	21 (8%)	23 (9%)	23 (9%)	17 (7%)
Abdominal Pain	11 (5%)	4 (1%)	10 (4%)	6 (2%)	8 (3%)
Back Pain	7 (3%)	10 (4%)	4 (2%)	5 (2%)	3 (1%)
Nervous					
Insomnia	9 (4%)	6 (2%)	7 (3%)	15 (6%)	15 (6%)
Dizziness	4 (2%)	7 (3%)	7 (3%)	16 (6%)	12 (5%)
Anxiety	6 (3%)	8 (3%)	2 (1%)	8 (3%)	4 (2%)
Digestive					
Nausea	13 (6%)	10 (4%)	12 (5%)	24 (9%)	33 (13%)
Vomiting	4 (2%)	4 (1%)	2 (1%)	6 (2%)	10 (4%)

* Includes dobutamine, milrinone, nitroglycerin, placebo, dopamine, nitroprusside, or amrinone.

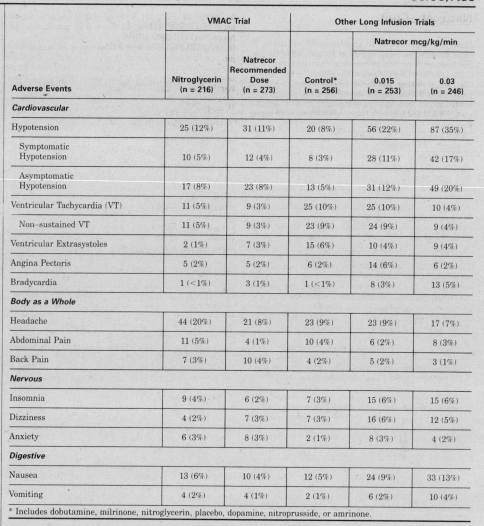

	Natrecor* N (Percentage)	Control N (Percentage)
704.311	2/74 (2.7%)	2/29 (7.5%)
704.325	5/85 (5.9%)	2/42 (4.8%)
704.326	14/203 (6.9%)	5/102 (4.9%)
704.329	6/163 (3.7%)	5/83 (6.1%)
704.339	22/273 (8.1%)	11/216 (5.1%)
704.341	5/120 (4.2%)	1/117 (0.9%)
704.348	2/141 (1.4%)	2/69 (2.9%)
Pooled (6 Studies)*	54/918 (5.9%)	26/589 (4.4%)
Pooled (7 Studies)†	56/1059 (5.3%)	28/658 (4.3%)

*Studies 704.311, 704.325, 704.326, 704.329, 704.339, and 704.341
†Studies 704.311, 704.325, 704.326, 704.329, 704.339, 704.341, and 704.348

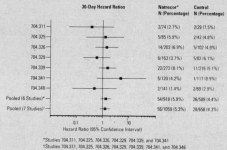

180-Day Hazard Ratios

	Natrecor* N (Percentage)	Control N (Percentage)
704.325	19/85 (23.1%)	8/42 (19.3%)
704.326	42/203 (20.8%)	24/102 (23.5%)
704.329	26/163 (16.3%)	18/83 (22.2%)
704.339	67/273 (25.1%)	44/216 (20.8%)
704.348*	13/141 (9.4%)	9/69 (13.5%)
Pooled (4 Studies)†	154/724 (21.7%)	94/443 (21.5%)

*Data collected through week 16
†Studies 704.325, 704.326, 704.329, and 704.339

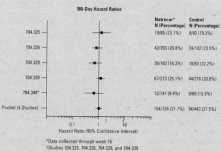

OVERDOSAGE

No data are available with respect to overdosage in humans. The expected reaction would be excessive hypotension, which should be treated with drug discontinuation or reduction (see PRECAUTIONS) and appropriate measures.

DOSAGE AND ADMINISTRATION

The Natrecor bolus must be drawn from the prepared infusion bag.

Natrecor (nesiritide) is for intravenous use only. There is limited experience with administering Natrecor for longer than 48 hours. Blood pressure should be monitored closely during Natrecor administration.

If hypotension occurs during the administration of Natrecor, the dose should be reduced or discontinued and other measures to support blood pressure should be started (IV fluids, changes in body position). In the VMAC trial, when symptomatic hypotension occurred, Natrecor was discontinued and subsequently could be restarted at a dose that was reduced by 30% (with no bolus administration) once the patient was stabilized. Because hypotension caused by Natrecor may be prolonged (up to hours), a period of observation may be necessary before restarting the drug.

Preparation

The Natrecor bolus must be drawn from the prepared infusion bag.

1. Reconstitute one 1.5 mg vial of Natrecor by adding 5 mL of diluent removed from a pre-filled 250 mL plastic IV bag containing the diluent of choice. After reconstitution of the vial, each mL contains 0.32 mg of nesiritide. The following preservative-free diluents are recommended for reconstitution: 5% Dextrose Injection (D5W), USP; 0.9% Sodium Chloride Injection, USP; 5% Dextrose and 0.45% Sodium Chloride Injection, USP, or 5% Dextrose and 0.2% Sodium Chloride Injection, USP.

2. Do not shake the vial. Rock the vial gently so that all surfaces, including the stopper, are in contact with the diluent to ensure complete reconstitution. Use only a clear, essentially colorless solution.

3. **Withdraw the entire contents of the reconstituted Natrecor vial** and add to the 250 mL plastic IV bag. This will yield a solution with a concentration of Natrecor of approximately 6 mcg/mL. The IV bag should be inverted several times to ensure complete mixing of the solution.

4. Use the reconstituted solution within 24 hours, as Natrecor contains no antimicrobial preservative. Parenteral drug products should be inspected visually for particulate matter and discoloration prior to administration, whenever solution and container permit. Reconstituted vials of Natrecor may be left at Controlled Room Temperature (20–25°C; 68–77°F) as per United States Pharmacopeia (USP) or may be refrigerated (2–8°C; 36–46°F) for up to 24 hours.

Dosing Instructions

The Natrecor bolus must be drawn from the prepared infusion bag.

The recommended dose of Natrecor is an IV bolus of 2 mcg/kg followed by a continuous infusion of 0.01 mcg/kg/min. Natrecor should not be initiated at a dose that is above the recommended dose.

Prime the IV tubing with 5 mL of the solution for infusion prior to connecting to the patient's vascular access port and prior to administering the bolus or starting the infusion.

The administration of the recommended dose of Natrecor is a two step process:

Step 1. Administration of the IV Bolus

After preparation of the infusion bag, as described previously, withdraw the bolus volume (see Weight-Adjusted Bolus Volume table) from the Natrecor infusion bag, and administer it over approximately 60 seconds through an IV port in the tubing.

Continued on next page

Natrecor—Cont.

Bolus Volume (mL) = Patient Weight (kg) / 3

Natrecor Weight-Adjusted Bolus Volume Administered Over 60 Seconds (Final Concentration = 6 mcg/mL)

Patient Weight (kg)	Volume of Bolus (mL = kg/3)
60	20.0
70	23.3
80	26.7
90	30.0
100	33.3
110	36.7

Step 2. Administration of the Continuous Infusion
Immediately following the administration of the bolus, infuse Natrecor at a flow rate of 0.1 mL/kg/hr. This will deliver a Natrecor infusion dose of 0.01 mcg/kg/min.
To calculate the infusion flow rate to deliver a 0.01 mcg/kg/min dose, use the following formula (see the following Weight-Adjusted Infusion Flow Rate for Dosing table):

Infusion Flow Rate (mL/hr) = Patient Weight (kg) × 0.1

Natrecor Weight-Adjusted Infusion Flow Rate for a 0.01 mcg/kg/min Dose following Bolus (Final Concentration = 6 mcg/mL)

Patient Weight (kg)	Infusion Flow Rate (mL/hr)
60	6
70	7
80	8
90	9
100	10
110	11

Dose Adjustments: The dose-limiting side effect of Natrecor is hypotension. Do not initiate Natrecor at a dose that is higher than the recommended dose of a 2 mcg/kg bolus followed by an infusion of 0.01 mcg/kg/min. In the VMAC trial there was limited experience with increasing the dose of Natrecor above the recommended dose (23 patients, all of whom had central hemodynamic monitoring). In those patients, the infusion dose of Natrecor was increased by 0.005 mcg/kg/min (preceded by a bolus of 1 mcg/kg), no more frequently than every 3 hours up to a maximum dose of 0.03 mcg/kg/min. Natrecor should not be titrated at frequent intervals as is done with other IV agents that have a shorter half-life (see Clinical Trials).

Chemical/Physical Interactions

Natrecor is physically and/or chemically incompatible with injectable formulations of heparin, insulin, ethacrynate sodium, bumetanide, enalaprilat, hydralazine, and furosemide. These drugs should not be co-administered as infusions with Natrecor through the same IV catheter. The preservative sodium metabisulfite is incompatible with Natrecor. Injectable drugs that contain sodium metabisulfite should not be administered in the same infusion line as Natrecor. The catheter must be flushed between administration of Natrecor and incompatible drugs.
Natrecor binds to heparin and therefore could bind to the heparin lining of a heparin-coated catheter, decreasing the amount of Natrecor delivered to the patient for some period of time. Therefore, Natrecor must not be administered through a central heparin-coated catheter. Concomitant administration of a heparin infusion through a separate catheter is acceptable.

Storage

Store Natrecor at controlled room temperature (20–25°C; 68–77°F); excursions permitted to 15–30°C (59–86°F; see USP Controlled Room Temperature), or refrigerated (2–8°C; 36–46°F). Keep in carton until time of use.

HOW SUPPLIED

Natrecor (nesiritide) is provided as a sterile lyophilized powder in 1.5 mg, single-use vials. Each carton contains one vial and is available in the following package:
1 vial/carton (NDC 65847-205-25)
US patent No. 5,114,923 and 5,674,710.
Distributed by Scios Inc.
6500 Paseo Padre Parkway
Fremont, CA 94555

20030302
Revised April 2005

Sepracor Inc.

84 WATERFORD DRIVE
MARLBOROUGH, MA 01752

For Medical Information for Healthcare Professionals Contact:
1-800-739-0565
For Direct Inquiries to the Customer Assistance Center (CAC) Contact:
1-888-394-7377
FAX 1-508-357-7589
E-mail CAC@sepracor.com
or write to Sepracor CAC at the address above.

LUNESTA™ Ⓒ℞
(eszopiclone) TABLETS
[lew-nĕs-tă]
1 mg, 2 mg, 3 mg
℞ only

PRESCRIBING INFORMATION

DESCRIPTION

LUNESTA (eszopiclone) is a nonbenzodiazepine hypnotic agent that is a pyrrolopyrazine derivative of the cyclopyrrolone class. The chemical name of eszopiclone is (+)-(5S)-6-(chloropyridin-2-yl)-7-oxo-6,7-dihydro-5H-pyrrolo[3,4-b] pyrazin-5-yl 4-methylpiperazine-1-carboxylate. Its molecular weight is 388.81, and its empirical formula is $C_{17}H_{17}ClN_6O_3$. Eszopiclone has a single chiral center with an (*S*)-configuration. It has the following chemical structure:

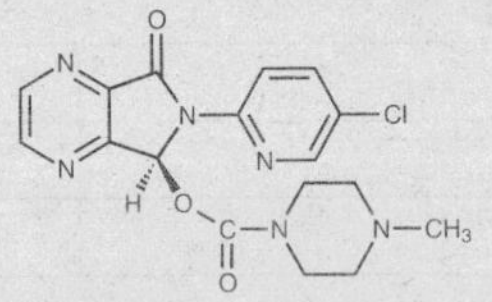

Eszopiclone is a white to light-yellow crystalline solid. Eszopiclone is very slightly soluble in water, slightly soluble in ethanol, and soluble in phosphate buffer (pH 3.2).
Eszopiclone is formulated as film-coated tablets for oral administration. LUNESTA tablets contain 1 mg, 2 mg, or 3 mg eszopiclone and the following inactive ingredients: calcium phosphate, colloidal silicon dioxide, croscarmellose sodium, hypromellose, lactose, magnesium stearate, microcrystalline cellulose, polyethylene glycol, titanium dioxide, and triacetin. In addition, both the 1 mg and 3 mg tablets contain FD&C Blue #2.

CLINICAL PHARMACOLOGY

Pharmacodynamics

The precise mechanism of action of eszopiclone as a hypnotic is unknown, but its effect is believed to result from its interaction with GABA-receptor complexes at binding domains located close to or allosterically coupled to benzodiazepine receptors. Eszopiclone is a nonbenzodiazepine hypnotic that is a pyrrolopyrazine derivative of the cyclopyrrolone class with a chemical structure unrelated to pyrazolopyrimidines, imidazopyridines, benzodiazepines, barbiturates, or other drugs with known hypnotic properties.

Pharmacokinetics

The pharmacokinetics of eszopiclone have been investigated in healthy subjects (adult and elderly) and in patients with hepatic disease or renal disease. In healthy subjects, the pharmacokinetic profile was examined after single doses of up to 7.5 mg and after once-daily administration of 1, 3, and 6 mg for 7 days. Eszopiclone is rapidly absorbed, with a time to peak concentration (t_{max}) of approximately 1 hour and a terminal-phase elimination half-life ($t_{1/2}$) of approximately 6 hours. In healthy adults, LUNESTA does not accumulate with once-daily administration, and its exposure is dose-proportional over the range of 1 to 6 mg.

Absorption And Distribution

Eszopiclone is rapidly absorbed following oral administration. Peak plasma concentrations are achieved within approximately 1 hour after oral administration. Eszopiclone is weakly bound to plasma protein (52-59%). The large free fraction suggests that eszopiclone disposition should not be affected by drug-drug interactions caused by protein binding. The blood-to-plasma ratio for eszopiclone is less than one, indicating no selective uptake by red blood cells.

Metabolism

Following oral administration, eszopiclone is extensively metabolized by oxidation and demethylation. The primary plasma metabolites are (*S*)-zopiclone-N-oxide and (*S*)-N-desmethyl zopiclone; the latter compound binds to GABA receptors with substantially lower potency than eszopiclone, and the former compound shows no significant binding to this receptor. *In vitro* studies have shown that CYP3A4 and CYP2E1 enzymes are involved in the metabolism of eszopiclone. Eszopiclone did not show any inhibitory potential on CYP450 1A2, 2A6, 2C9, 2C19, 2D6, 2E1, and 3A4 in cryopreserved human hepatocytes.

Elimination

After oral administration, eszopiclone is eliminated with a mean $t_{1/2}$ of approximately 6 hours. Up to 75% of an oral dose of racemic zopiclone is excreted in the urine, primarily as metabolites. A similar excretion profile would be expected for eszopiclone, the S-isomer of racemic zopiclone. Less than 10% of the orally administered eszopiclone dose is excreted in the urine as parent drug.

Effect Of Food

In healthy adults, administration of a 3 mg dose of eszopiclone after a high-fat meal resulted in no change in AUC, a reduction in mean C_{max} of 21%, and delayed t_{max} by approximately 1 hour. The half-life remained unchanged, approximately 6 hours. The effects of LUNESTA on sleep onset may be reduced if it is taken with or immediately after a high-fat/heavy meal.

Special Populations

Age

Compared with non-elderly adults, subjects 65 years and older had an increase of 41% in total exposure (AUC) and a slightly prolonged elimination of eszopiclone ($t_{1/2}$ approximately 9 hours). C_{max} was unchanged. Therefore, in elderly patients the starting dose of LUNESTA should be decreased to 1 mg and the dose should not exceed 2 mg.

Gender

The pharmacokinetics of eszopiclone in men and women are similar.

Race

In an analysis of data on all subjects participating in Phase 1 studies of eszopiclone, the pharmacokinetics for all races studied appeared similar.

Hepatic Impairment

Pharmacokinetics of a 2 mg eszopiclone dose were assessed in 16 healthy volunteers and in 8 subjects with mild, moderate, and severe liver disease. Exposure was increased 2-fold in severely impaired patients compared with the healthy volunteers. C_{max} and t_{max} were unchanged. The dose of LUNESTA should not be increased above 2 mg in patients with severe hepatic impairment. No dose adjustment is necessary for patients with mild-to-moderate hepatic impairment. LUNESTA should be used with caution in patients with hepatic impairment. (See **DOSAGE AND ADMINISTRATION.**)

Renal Impairment

The pharmacokinetics of eszopiclone were studied in 24 patients with mild, moderate, or severe renal impairment. AUC and C_{max} were similar in the patients compared with demographically matched healthy control subjects. No dose adjustment is necessary in patients with renal impairment, since less than 10% of the orally administered eszopiclone dose is excreted in the urine as parent drug.

Drug Interactions

Eszopiclone is metabolized by CYP3A4 and CYP2E1 via demethylation and oxidation. There were no pharmacokinetic or pharmacodynamic interactions between eszopiclone and paroxetine, digoxin, or warfarin. When eszopiclone was coadministered with olanzapine, no pharmacokinetic interaction was detected in levels of eszopiclone or olanzapine, but a pharmacodynamic interaction was seen on a measure of psychomotor function. Eszopiclone and lorazepam decreased each other's C_{max} by 22%. Coadministration of eszopiclone 3 mg to subjects receiving ketoconazole 400 mg, a potent inhibitor of CYP3A4, resulted in a 2.2-fold increase in exposure to eszopiclone. LUNESTA would not be expected to alter the clearance of drugs metabolized by common CYP450 enzymes. (See **PRECAUTIONS.**)

CLINICAL TRIALS

The effect of LUNESTA on reducing sleep latency and improving sleep maintenance was established in studies with 2100 subjects (ages 18-86) with chronic and transient insomnia in six placebo-controlled trials of up to 6 months' duration. Two of these trials were in elderly patients (n=523). Overall, at the recommended adult dose (2-3 mg) and elderly dose (1-2 mg), LUNESTA significantly decreased sleep latency and improved measures of sleep maintenance (objectively measured as wake time after sleep onset [WASO] and subjectively measured as total sleep time).

Transient Insomnia

Healthy adults were evaluated in a model of transient insomnia (n=436) in a sleep laboratory in a double-blind, parallel-group, single-night trial comparing two doses of eszopiclone and placebo. LUNESTA 3 mg was superior to placebo on measures of sleep latency and sleep maintenance, including polysomnographic (PSG) parameters of latency to persistent sleep (LPS) and WASO.

Chronic Insomnia (Adults And Elderly)

The effectiveness of LUNESTA was established in five controlled studies in chronic insomnia. Three controlled studies were in adult subjects, and two controlled studies were in elderly subjects with chronic insomnia.

Adults

In the first study, adults with chronic insomnia (n=308) were evaluated in a double-blind, parallel-group trial of 6 weeks' duration comparing LUNESTA 2 mg and 3 mg with placebo. Objective endpoints were measured for 4 weeks. Both 2 mg and 3 mg were superior to placebo on LPS at 4 weeks. The 3 mg dose was superior to placebo on WASO.
In the second study, adults with chronic insomnia (n=788) were evaluated using subjective measures in a double-blind, parallel-group trial comparing the safety and efficacy of LUNESTA 3 mg with placebo administered nightly for 6 months. LUNESTA was superior to placebo on subjective measures of sleep latency, total sleep time, and WASO.
In addition, a 6-period cross-over PSG study evaluating eszopiclone doses of 1 to 3 mg, each given over a 2-day period, demonstrated effectiveness of all doses on LPS, and of 3 mg on WASO. In this trial, the response was dose-related.

Elderly

Elderly subjects (ages 65-86) with chronic insomnia were evaluated in two double-blind, parallel-group trials of 2 weeks' duration. One study (n=231) compared the effects of LUNESTA with placebo on subjective outcome measures, and the other (n=292) on objective and subjective outcome measures. The first study compared 1 mg and 2 mg of LUNESTA with placebo, while the second study compared 2 mg of LUNESTA with placebo. All doses were superior to placebo on measures of sleep latency. In both studies, 2 mg of LUNESTA was superior to placebo on measures of sleep maintenance.

Studies Pertinent To Safety Concerns For Sedative/Hypnotic Drugs

Cognitive, Memory, Sedative, and Psychomotor Effects

In two double-blind, placebo-controlled, single-dose crossover studies of 12 patients each (one study in patients with insomnia; one in normal volunteers), the effects of LUNESTA 2 and 3 mg were assessed on 20 measures of cognitive function and memory at 9.5 and 12 hours after a nighttime dose. Although results suggested that patients receiving LUNESTA 3 mg performed more poorly than patients receiving placebo on a very small number of these measures at 9.5 hours post-dose, no consistent pattern of abnormalities was seen.

In a 6-month double-blind, placebo-controlled trial of nightly administered LUNESTA 3 mg, 8/593 subjects treated with LUNESTA 3 mg (1.3%) and 0/195 subjects treated with placebo (0%) spontaneously reported memory impairment. The majority of these events were mild in nature (5/8), and none were reported as severe. Four of these events occurred within the first 7 days of treatment and did not recur. The incidence of spontaneously reported confusion in this 6-month study was 0.5% in both treatment arms. In a 6-week adult study of nightly administered LUNESTA 2 mg or 3 mg or placebo, the spontaneous reporting rates for confusion were 0%, 3.0%, and 0%, respectively, and for memory impairment were 1%, 1%, and 0%, respectively.

In a 2-week study of 264 elderly insomniacs randomized to either nightly LUNESTA 2 mg or placebo, spontaneous reporting rates of confusion and memory impairment were 0% vs. 0.8% and 1.5% vs. 0%, respectively. In another 2-week study of 231 elderly insomniacs, the spontaneous reporting rates for the 1 mg, 2 mg, and placebo groups for confusion were 0%, 2.5%, and 0%, respectively, and for memory impairment were 1.4%, 0%, and 0%, respectively.

A study of normal subjects exposed to single fixed doses of LUNESTA from 1 to 7.5 mg using the DSST to assess sedation and psychomotor function at fixed times after dosing (hourly up to 16 hours) found the expected sedation and reduction in psychomotor function. This was maximal at 1 hour and present up to 4 hours, but was no longer present by 5 hours.

In another study, patients with insomnia were given 2 or 3 mg doses of LUNESTA nightly, with DSST assessed on the mornings following days 1, 15, and 29 of treatment. While both the placebo and LUNESTA 3 mg groups showed an improvement in DSST scores relative to baseline the following morning (presumably due to a learning effect), the improvement in the placebo group was greater and reached statistical significance on night 1, although not on nights 15 and 29. For the LUNESTA 2 mg group, DSST change scores were not significantly different from placebo at any time point.

Withdrawal-Emergent Anxiety And Insomnia

During nightly use for an extended period, pharmacodynamic tolerance or adaptation has been observed with other hypnotics. If a drug has a short elimination half-life, it is possible that a relative deficiency of the drug or its active metabolites (i.e., in relationship to the receptor site) may occur at some point in the interval between each night's use. This is believed to be responsible for two clinical findings reported to occur after several weeks of nightly use of other rapidly eliminated hypnotics: increased wakefulness during the last quarter of the night and the appearance of increased signs of daytime anxiety.

In a 6-month double-blind, placebo-controlled study of nightly administration of LUNESTA 3 mg, rates of anxiety reported as an adverse event were 2.1% in the placebo arm and 3.7% in the LUNESTA arm. In a 6-week adult study of nightly administration, anxiety was reported as an adverse event in 0%, 2.9%, and 1.0% of the placebo, 2 mg, and 3 mg treatment arms, respectively. In this study, single-blind placebo was administered on nights 45 and 46, the first and second days of withdrawal from study drug. New adverse events were recorded during the withdrawal period, beginning with day 45, up to 14 days after discontinuation. During this withdrawal period, 105 subjects previously taking nightly LUNESTA 3 mg for 44 nights spontaneously reported anxiety (1%), abnormal dreams (1.9%), hyperesthesia (1%), and neurosis (1%), while none of 99 subjects previously taking placebo reported any of these adverse events during the withdrawal period.

Rebound insomnia, defined as a dose-dependent temporary worsening in sleep parameters (latency, sleep efficiency, and number of awakenings) compared with baseline following discontinuation of treatment, is observed with short- and intermediate-acting hypnotics. Rebound insomnia following discontinuation of LUNESTA relative to placebo and baseline was examined objectively in a 6-week adult study on the first 2 nights of discontinuation (nights 45 and 46) following 44 nights of active treatment with 2 mg or 3 mg. In the LUNESTA 2 mg group, compared with baseline, there was a significant increase in WASO and a decrease in sleep

efficiency, both occurring only on the first night after discontinuation of treatment. No changes from baseline were noted in the LUNESTA 3 mg group on the first night after discontinuation, and there was a significant improvement in LPS and sleep efficiency compared with baseline following the second night of discontinuation. Comparisons of changes from baseline between LUNESTA and placebo were also performed. On the first night after discontinuation of LUNESTA 2 mg, LPS and WASO were significantly increased and sleep efficiency was reduced; there were no significant differences on the second night. On the first night following discontinuation of LUNESTA 3 mg, sleep efficiency was significantly reduced. No other differences from placebo were noted in any other sleep parameter on either the first or second night following discontinuation. For both doses, the discontinuation-emergent effect was mild, had the characteristics of the return of the symptoms of chronic insomnia, and appeared to resolve by the second night after LUNESTA discontinuation.

INDICATIONS AND USAGE

LUNESTA is indicated for the treatment of insomnia. In controlled outpatient and sleep laboratory studies, LUNESTA administered at bedtime decreased sleep latency and improved sleep maintenance.

CONTRAINDICATIONS

None known.

WARNINGS

Because sleep disturbances may be the presenting manifestation of a physical and/or psychiatric disorder, symptomatic treatment of insomnia should be initiated only after a careful evaluation of the patient. The failure of insomnia to remit after 7 to 10 days of treatment may indicate the presence of a primary psychiatric and/or medical illness that should be evaluated. Worsening of insomnia or the emergence of new thinking or behavior abnormalities may be the consequence of an unrecognized psychiatric or physical disorder. Such findings have emerged during the course of treatment with sedative/hypnotic drugs, including LUNESTA. Because some of the important adverse effects of LUNESTA appear to be dose-related, it is important to use the lowest possible effective dose, especially in the elderly (see **DOSAGE AND ADMINISTRATION**).

A variety of abnormal thinking and behavior changes have been reported to occur in association with the use of sedative/hypnotics. Some of these changes may be characterized by decreased inhibition (e.g., aggressiveness and extroversion that seem out of character), similar to effects produced by alcohol and other CNS depressants. Other reported behavioral changes have included bizarre behavior, agitation, hallucinations, and depersonalization. Amnesia and other neuropsychiatric symptoms may occur unpredictably. In primarily depressed patients, worsening of depression, including suicidal thinking, has been reported in association with the use of sedative/hypnotics.

It can rarely be determined with certainty whether a particular instance of the abnormal behaviors listed above are drug-induced, spontaneous in origin, or a result of an underlying psychiatric or physical disorder. Nonetheless, the emergence of any new behavioral sign or symptom of concern requires careful and immediate evaluation.

Following rapid dose decrease or abrupt discontinuation of the use of sedative/hypnotics, there have been reports of signs and symptoms similar to those associated with withdrawal from other CNS-depressant drugs (see **DRUG ABUSE AND DEPENDENCE**).

LUNESTA, like other hypnotics, has CNS-depressant effects. Because of the rapid onset of action, LUNESTA should only be ingested immediately prior to going to bed or after the patient has gone to bed and has experienced difficulty falling asleep. Patients receiving LUNESTA should be cautioned against engaging in hazardous occupations requiring complete mental alertness or motor coordination (e.g., operating machinery or driving a motor vehicle) after ingesting the drug, and be cautioned about potential impairment of the performance of such activities on the day following ingestion of LUNESTA. LUNESTA, like other hypnotics, may produce additive CNS-depressant effects when coadministered with other psychotropic medications, anticonvulsants, antihistamines, ethanol, and other drugs that themselves produce CNS depression. LUNESTA should not be taken with alcohol. Dose adjustment may be necessary when LUNESTA is administered with other CNS-depressant agents, because of the potentially additive effects.

PRECAUTIONS

General

Timing Of Drug Administration

LUNESTA should be taken immediately before bedtime. Taking a sedative/hypnotic while still up and about may result in short-term memory impairment, hallucinations, impaired coordination, dizziness, and lightheadedness.

Use In The Elderly And/Or Debilitated Patients

Impaired motor and/or cognitive performance after repeated exposure or unusual sensitivity to sedative/hypnotic drugs is a concern in the treatment of elderly and/or debilitated patients. The recommended starting dose of LUNESTA for these patients is 1 mg. (See **DOSAGE AND ADMINISTRATION**.)

Use In Patients With Concomitant Illness

Clinical experience with eszopiclone in patients with concomitant illness is limited. Eszopiclone should be used with caution in patients with diseases or conditions that could affect metabolism or hemodynamic responses.

A study in healthy volunteers did not reveal respiratory-depressant effects at doses 2.5-fold higher (7 mg) than the recommended dose of eszopiclone. Caution is advised, however, if LUNESTA is prescribed to patients with compromised respiratory function.

The dose of LUNESTA should be reduced to 1 mg in patients with severe hepatic impairment, because systemic exposure is doubled in such subjects. No dose adjustment appears necessary for subjects with mild or moderate hepatic impairment. No dose adjustment appears necessary in subjects with any degree of renal impairment, since less than 10% of eszopiclone is excreted unchanged in the urine.

The dose of LUNESTA should be reduced in patients who are administered potent inhibitors of CYP3A4, such as ketoconazole, while taking LUNESTA. Downward dose adjustment is also recommended when LUNESTA is administered with agents having known CNS-depressant effects.

Use In Patients With Depression

Sedative/hypnotic drugs should be administered with caution to patients exhibiting signs and symptoms of depression. Suicidal tendencies may be present in such patients, and protective measures may be required. Intentional overdose is more common in this group of patients; therefore, the least amount of drug that is feasible should be prescribed for the patient at any one time.

Information For Patients

Patient information is printed at the bottom of this insert. To assure safe and effective use of LUNESTA, this information and the instructions provided in the patient information section should be discussed with patients.

Laboratory Tests

There are no specific laboratory tests recommended.

Drug Interactions

CNS-Active Drugs

Ethanol: An additive effect on psychomotor performance was seen with coadministration of eszopiclone and ethanol 0.70 g/kg for up to 4 hours after ethanol administration.

Paroxetine: Coadministration of single doses of eszopiclone 3 mg and paroxetine 20 mg daily for 7 days produced no pharmacokinetic or pharmacodynamic interaction.

Lorazepam: Coadministration of single doses of eszopiclone 3 mg and lorazepam 2 mg did not have clinically relevant effects on the pharmacodynamics or pharmacokinetics of either drug.

Olanzapine: Coadministration of eszopiclone 3 mg and olanzapine 10 mg produced a decrease in DSST scores. The interaction was pharmacodynamic; there was no alteration in the pharmacokinetics of either drug.

Drugs That Inhibit CYP3A4 (Ketoconazole)

CYP3A4 is a major metabolic pathway for elimination of eszopiclone. The AUC of eszopiclone was increased 2.2-fold by coadministration of ketoconazole, a potent inhibitor of CYP3A4, 400 mg daily for 5 days. C_{max} and $t_{1/2}$ were increased 1.4-fold and 1.3-fold, respectively. Other strong inhibitors of CYP3A4 (e.g., itraconazole, clarithromycin, nefazodone, troleandomycin, ritonavir, nelfinavir) would be expected to behave similarly.

Drugs That Induce CYP3A4 (Rifampicin)

Racemic zopiclone exposure was decreased 80% by concomitant use of rifampicin, a potent inducer of CYP3A4. A similar effect would be expected with eszopiclone.

Drugs Highly Bound To Plasma Protein

Eszopiclone is not highly bound to plasma proteins (52-59% bound); therefore, the disposition of eszopiclone is not expected to be sensitive to alterations in protein binding. Administration of eszopiclone 3 mg to a patient taking another drug that is highly protein-bound would not be expected to cause an alteration in the free concentration of either drug.

Drugs With A Narrow Therapeutic Index

Digoxin: A single dose of eszopiclone 3 mg did not affect the pharmacokinetics of digoxin measured at steady state following dosing of 0.5 mg twice daily for one day and 0.25 mg daily for the next 6 days.

Warfarin: Eszopiclone 3 mg administered daily for 5 days did not affect the pharmacokinetics of (R)- or (S)-warfarin, nor were there any changes in the pharmacodynamic profile (prothrombin time) following a single 25 mg oral dose of warfarin.

Carcinogenesis, Mutagenesis, Impairment Of Fertility

Carcinogenesis

In a carcinogenicity study in Sprague-Dawley rats in which eszopiclone was given by oral gavage, no increases in tumors were seen; plasma levels (AUC) of eszopiclone at the highest dose used in this study (16 mg/kg/day) are estimated to be 80 (females) and 20 (males) times those in humans receiving the maximum recommended human dose (MRHD). However, in a carcinogenicity study in Sprague-Dawley rats in which racemic zopiclone was given in the diet, and in which plasma levels of eszopiclone were reached that were greater than those reached in the above study of eszopiclone, an increase in mammary gland adenocarcinomas in females and an increase in thyroid gland follicular cell adenomas and carcinomas in males were seen at the highest dose of 100 mg/kg/day. Plasma levels of eszopiclone at this dose are estimated to be 150 (females) and 70 (males) times those in humans receiving the MRHD. The mechanism for the increase in mammary adenocarcinomas is unknown. The increase in thyroid tumors is thought to be due to increased levels of TSH secondary to increased metabolism of circulating thyroid hormones, a mechanism that is not considered to be relevant to humans.

Continued on next page

Lunesta—Cont.

In a carcinogenicity study in B6C3F1 mice in which racemic zopiclone was given in the diet, an increase in pulmonary carcinomas and carcinomas plus adenomas in females and an increase in skin fibromas and sarcomas in males were seen at the highest dose of 100 mg/kg/day. Plasma levels of eszopiclone at this dose are estimated to be 8 (females) and 20 (males) times those in humans receiving the MRHD. The skin tumors were due to skin lesions induced by aggressive behavior, a mechanism that is not relevant to humans. A carcinogenicity study was also performed in which CD-1 mice were given eszopiclone at doses up to 100 mg/kg/day by oral gavage; although this study did not reach a maximum tolerated dose, and was thus inadequate for overall assessment of carcinogenic potential, no increases in either pulmonary or skin tumors were seen at doses producing plasma levels of eszopiclone estimated to be 90 times those in humans receiving the MRHD — i.e., 12 times the exposure in the racemate study.
Eszopiclone did not increase tumors in a p53 transgenic mouse bioassay at oral doses up to 300 mg/kg/day.

Mutagenesis
Eszopiclone was positive in the mouse lymphoma chromosomal aberration assay and produced an equivocal response in the Chinese hamster ovary cell chromosomal aberration assay. It was not mutagenic or clastogenic in the bacterial Ames gene mutation assay, in an unscheduled DNA synthesis assay, or in an *in vivo* mouse bone marrow micronucleus assay.
(S)-N-desmethyl zopiclone, a metabolite of eszopiclone, was positive in the Chinese hamster ovary cell and human lymphocyte chromosomal aberration assays. It was negative in the bacterial Ames mutation assay, in an *in vitro* ^{32}P-postlabeling DNA adduct assay, and in an *in vivo* mouse bone marrow chromosomal aberration and micronucleus assay.

Impairment Of Fertility
Eszopiclone was given by oral gavage to male rats at doses up to 45 mg/kg/day from 4 weeks premating through mating and to female rats at doses up to 180 mg/kg/day from 2 weeks premating through day 7 of pregnancy. An additional study was performed in which only females were treated, up to 180 mg/kg/day. Eszopiclone decreased fertility, probably

because of effects in both males and females, with no females becoming pregnant when both males and females were treated with the highest dose; the no-effect dose in both sexes was 5 mg/kg (16 times the MRHD on a mg/m² basis). Other effects included increased pre-implantation loss (no-effect dose 25 mg/kg), abnormal estrus cycles (no-effect dose 25 mg/kg), and decreases in sperm number and motility and increases in morphologically abnormal sperm (no-effect dose 5 mg/kg).

Pregnancy
Pregnancy Category C
Eszopiclone administered by oral gavage to pregnant rats and rabbits during the period of organogenesis showed no evidence of teratogenicity up to the highest doses tested (250 and 16 mg/kg/day in rats and rabbits, respectively; these doses are 800 and 100 times, respectively, the maximum recommended human dose [MRHD] on a mg/m² basis). In the rat, slight reductions in fetal weight and evidence of developmental delay were seen at maternally toxic doses of 125 and 150 mg/kg/day, but not at 62.5 mg/kg/day (200 times the MRHD on a mg/m² basis).
Eszopiclone was also administered by oral gavage to pregnant rats throughout the pregnancy and lactation periods at doses of up to 180 mg/kg/day. Increased post-implantation loss, decreased postnatal pup weights and survival, and increased pup startle response were seen at all doses; the lowest dose tested, 60 mg/kg/day, is 200 times the MRHD on a mg/m² basis. These doses did not produce significant maternal toxicity. Eszopiclone had no effects on other behavioral measures or reproductive function in the offspring.
There are no adequate and well-controlled studies of eszopiclone in pregnant women. Eszopiclone should be used during pregnancy only if the potential benefit justifies the potential risk to the fetus.

Labor And Delivery
LUNESTA has no established use in labor and delivery.

Nursing Mothers
It is not known whether LUNESTA is excreted in human milk. Because many drugs are excreted in human milk, caution should be exercised when LUNESTA is administered to a nursing woman.

Pediatric Use
Safety and effectiveness of eszopiclone in children below the age of 18 have not been established.

Geriatric Use
A total of 287 subjects in double-blind, parallel-group, placebo-controlled clinical trials who received eszopiclone were 65 to 86 years of age. The overall pattern of adverse events for elderly subjects (median age = 71 years) in 2-week studies with nighttime dosing of 2 mg eszopiclone was not different from that seen in younger adults (see AD-VERSE REACTIONS, Table 2). LUNESTA 2 mg exhibited significant reduction in sleep latency and improvement in sleep maintenance in the elderly population.

ADVERSE REACTIONS
The premarketing development program for LUNESTA included eszopiclone exposures in patients and/or normal subjects from two different groups of studies: approximately 400 normal subjects in clinical pharmacology/pharmacokinetic studies, and approximately 1550 patients in placebo-controlled clinical effectiveness studies, corresponding to approximately 263 patient-exposure years. The conditions and duration of treatment with LUNESTA varied greatly and included (in overlapping categories) open-label and double-blind phases of studies, inpatients and outpatients, and short-term and longer-term exposure. Adverse reactions were assessed by collecting adverse events, results of physical examinations, vital signs, weights, laboratory analyses, and ECGs.
Adverse events during exposure were obtained primarily by general inquiry and recorded by clinical investigators using terminology of their own choosing. Consequently, it is not possible to provide a meaningful estimate of the proportion of individuals experiencing adverse events without first grouping similar types of events into a smaller number of standardized event categories. In the tables and tabulations that follow, COSTART terminology has been used to classify reported adverse events.
The stated frequencies of adverse events represent the proportion of individuals who experienced, at least once, a treatment-emergent adverse event of the type listed. An event was considered treatment-emergent if it occurred for the first time or worsened while the patient was receiving therapy following baseline evaluation.

Adverse Findings Observed In Placebo-Controlled Trials
Adverse Events Resulting In Discontinuation Of Treatment
In placebo-controlled, parallel-group clinical trials in the elderly, 3.8% of 208 patients who received placebo, 2.3% of 215 patients who received 2 mg LUNESTA, and 1.4% of 72 patients who received 1 mg LUNESTA discontinued treatment due to an adverse event. In the 6-week parallel-group study in adults, no patients in the 3 mg arm discontinued because of an adverse event. In the long-term 6-month study in adult insomnia patients, 7.2% of 195 patients who received placebo and 12.8% of 593 patients who received 3 mg LUNESTA discontinued due to an adverse event. No event that resulted in discontinuation occurred at a rate of greater than 2%.
Adverse Events Observed At An Incidence Of ≥2% In Controlled Trials
Table 1 shows the incidence of treatment-emergent adverse events from a Phase 3 placebo-controlled study of LUNESTA at doses of 2 or 3 mg in non-elderly adults. Treatment duration in this trial was 44 days. The table includes only events that occurred in 2% or more of patients treated with LUNESTA 2 mg or 3 mg in which the incidence in patients treated with LUNESTA was greater than the incidence in placebo-treated patients.
[See table 1 at left]
Adverse events from Table 1 that suggest a dose-response relationship in adults include viral infection, dry mouth, dizziness, hallucinations, infection, rash, and unpleasant taste, with this relationship clearest for unpleasant taste.
Table 2 shows the incidence of treatment-emergent adverse events from combined Phase 3 placebo-controlled studies of LUNESTA at doses of 1 or 2 mg in elderly adults (ages 65-86). Treatment duration in these trials was 14 days. The table includes only events that occurred in 2% or more of patients treated with LUNESTA 1 mg or 2 mg in which the incidence in patients treated with LUNESTA was greater than the incidence in placebo-treated patients.
[See table 2 at top of next page]
Adverse events from Table 2 that suggest a dose-response relationship in elderly adults include pain, dry mouth, and unpleasant taste, with this relationship again clearest for unpleasant taste.
These figures cannot be used to predict the incidence of adverse events in the course of usual medical practice because patient characteristics and other factors may differ from those that prevailed in the clinical trials. Similarly, the cited frequencies cannot be compared with figures obtained from other clinical investigations involving different treatments, uses, and investigators. The cited figures, however, do provide the prescribing physician with some basis for estimating the relative contributions of drug and non-drug factors to the adverse event incidence rate in the population studied.

Other Events Observed During The Premarketing Evaluation Of LUNESTA
Following is a list of modified COSTART terms that reflect treatment-emergent adverse events as defined in the introduction to the ADVERSE REACTIONS section and reported by approximately 1550 subjects treated with LUNESTA at doses in the range of 1 to 3.5 mg/day during Phase 2 and 3 clinical trials throughout the United States and Canada. All reported events are included except those already listed in Tables 1 and 2 or elsewhere in labeling, minor events common in the general population, and events

Table 1: Incidence (%) of Treatment-Emergent Adverse Events in a 6-Week Placebo-Controlled Study in Non-Elderly Adults with LUNESTA[1]

Adverse Event	Placebo (n=99)	LUNESTA 2 mg (n=104)	LUNESTA 3 mg (n=105)
Body as a Whole			
Headache	13	21	17
Viral Infection	1	3	3
Digestive System			
Dry Mouth	3	5	7
Dyspepsia	4	4	5
Nausea	4	5	4
Vomiting	1	3	0
Nervous System			
Anxiety	0	3	1
Confusion	0	0	3
Depression	0	4	1
Dizziness	4	5	7
Hallucinations	0	1	3
Libido Decreased	0	0	3
Nervousness	3	5	0
Somnolence	3	10	8
Respiratory System			
Infection	3	5	10
Skin and Appendages			
Rash	1	3	4
Special Senses			
Unpleasant Taste	3	17	34
Urogenital System			
Dysmenorrhea*	0	3	0
Gynecomastia**	0	3	0

[1] Events for which the LUNESTA incidence was equal to or less than placebo are not listed on the table, but included the following: abnormal dreams, accidental injury, back pain, diarrhea, flu syndrome, myalgia, pain, pharyngitis, and rhinitis.
* Gender-specific adverse event in females
** Gender-specific adverse event in males

unlikely to be drug-related. Although the events reported occurred during treatment with LUNESTA, they were not necessarily caused by it.

Events are further categorized by body system and listed in order of decreasing frequency according to the following definitions: **frequent** adverse events are those that occurred on one or more occasions in at least 1/100 patients; **infrequent** adverse events are those that occurred in fewer than 1/100 patients but in at least 1/1,000 patients; **rare** adverse events are those that occurred in fewer than 1/1,000 patients. Gender-specific events are categorized based on their incidence for the appropriate gender.

Body as a Whole: **Frequent**: chest pain; **Infrequent**: allergic reaction, cellulitis, face edema, fever, halitosis, heat stroke, hernia, malaise, neck rigidity, photosensitivity.

Cardiovascular System: **Frequent**: migraine; **Infrequent**: hypertension; **Rare**: thrombophlebitis.

Digestive System: **Infrequent**: anorexia, cholelithiasis, increased appetite, melena, mouth ulceration, thirst, ulcerative stomatitis; **Rare**: colitis, dysphagia, gastritis, hepatitis, hepatomegaly, liver damage, stomach ulcer, stomatitis, tongue edema, rectal hemorrhage.

Hemic and Lymphatic System: **Infrequent**: anemia, lymphadenopathy.

Metabolic and Nutritional: **Frequent**: peripheral edema; **Infrequent**: hypercholesteremia, weight gain, weight loss; **Rare**: dehydration, gout, hyperlipemia, hypokalemia.

Musculoskeletal System: **Infrequent**: arthritis, bursitis, joint disorder (mainly swelling, stiffness, and pain), leg cramps, myasthenia, twitching; **Rare**: arthrosis, myopathy, ptosis.

Nervous System: **Infrequent**: agitation, apathy, ataxia, emotional lability, hostility, hypertonia, hypesthesia, incoordination, insomnia, memory impairment, neurosis, nystagmus, paresthesia, reflexes decreased, thinking abnormal (mainly difficulty concentrating), vertigo; **Rare**: abnormal gait, euphoria, hyperesthesia, hypokinesia, neuritis, neuropathy, stupor, tremor.

Respiratory System: **Infrequent**: asthma, bronchitis, dyspnea, epistaxis, hiccup, laryngitis.

Skin and Appendages: **Infrequent**: acne, alopecia, contact dermatitis, dry skin, eczema, skin discoloration, sweating, urticaria; **Rare**: erythema multiforme, furunculosis, herpes zoster, hirsutism, maculopapular rash, vesiculobullous rash.

Special Senses: **Infrequent**: conjunctivitis, dry eyes, ear pain, otitis externa, otitis media, tinnitus, vestibular disorder; **Rare**: hyperacusis, iritis, mydriasis, photophobia.

Urogenital System: **Infrequent**: amenorrhea, breast engorgement, breast enlargement, breast neoplasm, breast pain, cystitis, dysuria, female lactation, hematuria, kidney calculus, kidney pain, mastitis, menorrhagia, metrorrhagia, urinary frequency, urinary incontinence, uterine hemorrhage, vaginal hemorrhage, vaginitis; **Rare**: oliguria, pyelonephritis, urethritis.

DRUG ABUSE AND DEPENDENCE
Controlled Substance Class
LUNESTA is a Schedule IV controlled substance under the Controlled Substances Act. Other substances under the same classification are benzodiazepines and the nonbenzodiazepine hypnotics zaleplon and zolpidem. While eszopiclone is a hypnotic agent with a chemical structure unrelated to benzodiazepines, it shares some of the pharmacologic properties of the benzodiazepines.

Abuse, Dependence, And Tolerance
Abuse And Dependence
In a study of abuse liability conducted in individuals with known histories of benzodiazepine abuse, eszopiclone at doses of 6 and 12 mg produced euphoric effects similar to those of diazepam 20 mg. In this study, at doses 2-fold or greater than the maximum recommended doses, a dose-related increase in reports of amnesia and hallucinations was observed for both LUNESTA and diazepam.

The clinical trial experience with LUNESTA revealed no evidence of a serious withdrawal syndrome. Nevertheless, the following adverse events included in DSM-IV criteria for uncomplicated sedative/hypnotic withdrawal were reported during clinical trials following placebo substitution occurring within 48 hours following the last LUNESTA treatment: anxiety, abnormal dreams, nausea, and upset stomach. These reported adverse events occurred at an incidence of 2% or less. Use of benzodiazepines and similar agents may lead to physical and psychological dependence. The risk of abuse and dependence increases with the dose and duration of treatment and concomitant use of other psychoactive drugs. The risk is also greater for patients who have a history of alcohol or drug abuse or history of psychiatric disorders. These patients should be under careful surveillance when receiving LUNESTA or any other hypnotic.

Tolerance
Some loss of efficacy to the hypnotic effect of benzodiazepines and benzodiazepine-like agents may develop after repeated use of these drugs for a few weeks.

No development of tolerance to any parameter of sleep measurement was observed over six months. Tolerance to the efficacy of LUNESTA 3 mg was assessed by 4-week objective and 6-week subjective measurements of time to sleep onset and sleep maintenance for LUNESTA in a placebo-controlled 44-day study, and by subjective assessments of time to sleep onset and WASO in a placebo-controlled study for 6 months.

OVERDOSAGE
There is limited premarketing clinical experience with the effects of an overdosage of LUNESTA. In clinical trials with

Table 2: Incidence (%) of Treatment-Emergent Adverse Events in Elderly Adults (Ages 65-86) in 2-Week Placebo-Controlled Trials with LUNESTA[1]

Adverse Event	Placebo (n=208)	LUNESTA 1 mg (n=72)	LUNESTA 2 mg (n=215)
Body as a Whole			
Accidental Injury	1	0	3
Headache	14	15	13
Pain	2	4	5
Digestive System			
Diarrhea	2	4	2
Dry Mouth	2	3	7
Dyspepsia	2	6	2
Nervous System			
Abnormal Dreams	0	3	1
Dizziness	2	1	6
Nervousness	1	0	2
Neuralgia	0	3	0
Skin and Appendages			
Pruritus	1	4	1
Special Senses			
Unpleasant Taste	0	8	12
Urogenital System			
Urinary Tract Infection	0	3	0

[1] Events for which the LUNESTA incidence was equal to or less than placebo are not listed on the table, but included the following: abdominal pain, asthenia, nausea, rash, and somnolence.

eszopiclone, one case of overdose with up to 36 mg of eszopiclone was reported in which the subject fully recovered. Individuals have fully recovered from racemic zopiclone overdoses up to 340 mg (56 times the maximum recommended dose of eszopiclone).

Signs And Symptoms
Signs and symptoms of overdose effects of CNS depressants can be expected to present as exaggerations of the pharmacological effects noted in preclinical testing. Impairment of consciousness ranging from somnolence to coma has been described. Rare individual instances of fatal outcomes following overdose with racemic zopiclone have been reported in European postmarketing reports, most often associated with overdose with other CNS-depressant agents.

Recommended Treatment
General symptomatic and supportive measures should be used along with immediate gastric lavage where appropriate. Intravenous fluids should be administered as needed. Flumazenil may be useful. As in all cases of drug overdose, respiration, pulse, blood pressure, and other appropriate signs should be monitored and general supportive measures employed. Hypotension and CNS depression should be monitored and treated by appropriate medical intervention. The value of dialysis in the treatment of overdosage has not been determined.

Poison Control Center
As with the management of all overdosage, the possibility of multiple drug ingestion should be considered. The physician may wish to consider contacting a poison control center for up-to-date information on the management of hypnotic drug product overdosage.

DOSAGE AND ADMINISTRATION
The dose of LUNESTA should be individualized. The recommended starting dose for LUNESTA for most non-elderly adults is 2 mg immediately before bedtime. Dosing can be initiated at or raised to 3 mg if clinically indicated, since 3 mg is more effective for sleep maintenance (see **PRECAUTIONS**).

The recommended starting dose of LUNESTA for elderly patients whose primary complaint is difficulty falling asleep is 1 mg immediately before bedtime. In these patients, the dose may be increased to 2 mg if clinically indicated. For elderly patients whose primary complaint is difficulty staying asleep, the recommended dose is 2 mg immediately before bedtime (see **PRECAUTIONS**).

Taking LUNESTA with or immediately after a heavy, high-fat meal results in slower absorption and would be expected to reduce the effect of LUNESTA on sleep latency (see **Pharmacokinetics** under **CLINICAL PHARMACOLOGY**).

Special Populations
Hepatic
The starting dose of LUNESTA should be 1 mg in patients with severe hepatic impairment. LUNESTA should be used with caution in these patients.

Coadministration With CYP3A4 Inhibitors
The starting dose of LUNESTA should not exceed 1 mg in patients coadministered LUNESTA with potent CYP3A4 inhibitors. If needed, the dose can be raised to 2 mg.

HOW SUPPLIED
LUNESTA 3 mg tablets are round, dark blue, film-coated, and identified with debossed markings of S193 on one side, and are supplied as:

NDC 63402-193-10   bottle of 100 tablets
NDC 63402-193-09   carton of 90 tablets

LUNESTA 2 mg tablets are round, white, film-coated, and identified with debossed markings of S191 on one side, and are supplied as:

NDC 63402-191-10   bottle of 100 tablets
NDC 63402-191-09   carton of 90 tablets

LUNESTA 1 mg tablets are round, light blue, film-coated, and identified with debossed markings of S190 on one side, and are supplied as:

NDC 63402-190-10   bottle of 100 tablets

Store at 25°C (77°F); excursions permitted to 15°C to 30°C (59°F to 86°F) [see USP Controlled Room Temperature].

SEPRACOR
Manufactured for:
Sepracor Inc.
Marlborough, MA 01752 USA
by Patheon Inc., Mississauga, Ontario L5N 7K9 Canada
For customer service, call 1-888-394-7377.
To report adverse events, call 1-877-737-7226.
For medical information, call 1-800-739-0565.
February 2005
IN-5254/S

PHARMACIST — DETACH HERE AND GIVE INFORMATION TO PATIENT.

- -

Rx only   C-IV
LUNESTA™ (eszopiclone) TABLETS
1 mg, 2 mg, 3 mg
INFORMATION FOR PATIENTS TAKING LUNESTA
Your doctor has prescribed LUNESTA to help you sleep. The following information is intended to guide you in the safe use of this medicine. It is not meant to take the place of your doctor's instructions. If you have any questions about LUNESTA tablets, be sure to ask your doctor or pharmacist.

LUNESTA is used to treat different types of sleep problems, such as difficulty in falling asleep, difficulty in maintaining sleep during the night, and waking up too early in the morning. Most people with insomnia have more than one of these problems. You should take LUNESTA immediately before going to bed because of the risk of falling.

LUNESTA belongs to a group of medicines known as "hypnotics" or, simply, sleep medicines. There are many different sleep medicines available to help people sleep better. Insomnia is often transient and intermittent. It usually requires treatment for only a short time, usually 7 to 10 days up to 2 weeks. Some people have chronic sleep problems that may require more prolonged use of sleep medicine. However, you should not use these medicines for long periods without talking with your doctor about the risks and benefits of prolonged use.

Continued on next page

Lunesta—Cont.

Side Effects
All medicines have side effects. The most common side effects of sleep medicines are:
- Drowsiness
- Dizziness
- Lightheadedness
- Difficulty with coordination

Sleep medicines can make you sleepy during the day. How drowsy you feel depends upon how your body reacts to the medicine, which sleep medicine you are taking, and how large a dose your doctor has prescribed. Daytime drowsiness is best avoided by taking the lowest dose possible that will still help you sleep at night. Your doctor will work with you to find the dose of LUNESTA that is best for you. Some patients taking LUNESTA have reported next-day sleepiness.
To manage these side effects while you are taking this medicine:
- When you first start taking LUNESTA or any other sleep medicine, until you know whether the medicine will still have some effect on you the next day, use extreme care while doing anything that requires complete alertness, such as driving a car, operating machinery, or piloting an aircraft.
- Do not drink alcohol when you are taking LUNESTA or any sleep medicine. Alcohol can increase the side effects of LUNESTA or any other sleep medicine.
- Do not take any other medicines without asking your doctor first. This includes medicines you can buy without a prescription. Some medicines can cause drowsiness and are best avoided while taking LUNESTA.
- Always take the exact dose of LUNESTA prescribed by your doctor. Never change your dose without talking to your doctor first.

Special Concerns
There are some special problems that may occur while taking sleep medicines.
Memory Problems
Sleep medicines may cause a special type of memory loss or "amnesia." When this occurs, a person may not remember what has happened for several hours after taking the medicine. This is usually not a problem since most people fall asleep after taking the medicine. Memory loss can be a problem, however, when sleep medicines are taken while traveling, such as during an airplane flight and the person wakes up before the effect of the medicine is gone. This has been called "traveler's amnesia." Memory problems have been reported rarely by patients taking LUNESTA in clinical studies. In most cases, memory problems can be avoided if you take LUNESTA only when you are able to get a full night of sleep before you need to be active again. Be sure to talk to your doctor if you think you are having memory problems.
Tolerance
When sleep medicines are used every night for more than a few weeks, they may lose their effectiveness in helping you sleep. This is known as "tolerance." Development of tolerance to LUNESTA was not observed in a clinical study of 6 months' duration. Insomnia is often transient and intermittent, and prolonged use of sleep medicines is generally not necessary. Some people, though, have chronic sleep problems that may require more prolonged use of sleep medicine. If your sleep problems continue, consult your doctor, who will determine whether other measures are needed to overcome your sleep problems.
Dependence
Sleep medicines can cause dependence in some people, especially when these medicines are used regularly for longer than a few weeks or at high doses. Dependence is the need to continue taking a medicine because stopping it is unpleasant.
When people develop dependence, stopping the medicine suddenly may cause unpleasant symptoms (see *Withdrawal* below). They may find they have to keep taking the medicine either at the prescribed dose or at increasing doses just to avoid withdrawal symptoms.
All people taking sleep medicines have some risk of becoming dependent on the medicine. However, people who have been dependent on alcohol or other drugs in the past may have a higher chance of becoming addicted to sleep medicines. This possibility must be considered before using these medicines for more than a few weeks. If you have been addicted to alcohol or drugs in the past, it is important to tell your doctor before starting LUNESTA or any sleep medicine.
Withdrawal
Withdrawal symptoms may occur when sleep medicines are stopped suddenly after being used daily for a long time. In some cases, these symptoms can occur even if the medicine has been used for only a week or two. In mild cases, withdrawal symptoms may include unpleasant feelings. In more severe cases, abdominal and muscle cramps, vomiting, sweating, shakiness, and, rarely, seizures may occur. These more severe withdrawal symptoms are very uncommon. Although withdrawal symptoms have not been observed in the relatively limited controlled trials experience with LUNESTA, there is, nevertheless, the risk of such events in association with the use of any sleep medicine.
Another problem that may occur when sleep medicines are stopped is known as "rebound insomnia." This means that a person may have more trouble sleeping the first few nights after the medicine is stopped than before starting the medicine. If you should experience rebound insomnia, do not get discouraged. This problem usually goes away on its own after 1 or 2 nights. If you have been taking LUNESTA or any other sleep medicine for more than 1 or 2 weeks, do not stop taking it on your own. Always follow your doctor's directions.
Changes In Behavior And Thinking
Some people using sleep medicines have experienced unusual changes in their thinking and/or behavior. These effects are not common. However, they have included:
- More outgoing or aggressive behavior than normal
- Confusion
- Strange behavior
- Agitation
- Hallucinations
- Worsening of depression
- Suicidal thoughts

How often these effects occur depends on several factors, such as a person's general health, the use of other medicines, and which sleep medicine is being used. Clinical experience with LUNESTA suggests that it is rarely associated with these behavior changes.
It is also important to realize that it is rarely clear whether these behavior changes are caused by the medicine, are caused by an illness, or have occurred on their own. In fact, sleep problems that do not improve may be due to illnesses that were present before the medicine was used. If you or your family notice any changes in your behavior, or if you have any unusual or disturbing thoughts, call your doctor immediately.
Pregnancy And Breastfeeding
Sleep medicines may cause sedation or other potential effects in the unborn baby when used during the last weeks of pregnancy. Be sure to tell your doctor if you are pregnant, if you are planning to become pregnant, or if you become pregnant while taking LUNESTA.
In addition, a very small amount of LUNESTA may be present in breast milk after use of the medication. The effects of very small amounts of LUNESTA on an infant are not known; therefore, as with all other prescription sleep medicines, it is recommended that you not take LUNESTA if you are breastfeeding a baby.
Safe Use Of Sleep Medicines
To ensure the safe and effective use of LUNESTA or any other sleep medicine, you should observe the following cautions:
1. LUNESTA is a prescription medicine and should be used ONLY as directed by your doctor. Follow your doctor's instructions about how to take, when to take, and how long to take LUNESTA.
2. Never use LUNESTA or any other sleep medicine for longer than directed by your doctor.
3. If you notice any unusual and/or disturbing thoughts or behavior during treatment with LUNESTA or any other sleep medicine, contact your doctor.
4. Tell your doctor about any medicines you may be taking, including medicines you may buy without a prescription and herbal preparations. You should also tell your doctor if you drink alcohol. DO NOT use alcohol while taking LUNESTA or any other sleep medicine.
5. Do not take LUNESTA unless you are able to get 8 or more hours of sleep before you must be active again.
6. Do not increase the prescribed dose of LUNESTA or any other sleep medicine unless instructed by your doctor.
7. When you first start taking LUNESTA or any other sleep medicine, until you know whether the medicine will still have some effect on you the next day, use extreme care while doing anything that requires complete alertness, such as driving a car, operating machinery, or piloting an aircraft.
8. Be aware that you may have more sleeping problems the first night or two after stopping any sleep medicine.
9. Be sure to tell your doctor if you are pregnant, if you are planning to become pregnant, if you become pregnant, or if you are breastfeeding a baby while taking LUNESTA.
10. As with all prescription medicines, never share LUNESTA or any other sleep medicine with anyone else. Always store LUNESTA or any other sleep medicine in the original container and out of reach of children.
11. Be sure to tell your doctor if you suffer from depression.
12. LUNESTA works very quickly. You should only take LUNESTA immediately before going to bed.
13. For LUNESTA to work best, you should not take it with or immediately after a high-fat, heavy meal.
14. Some people, such as older adults (i.e., ages 65 and over) and people with liver disease, should start with the lower dose (1 mg) of LUNESTA. Your doctor may choose to start therapy at 2 mg. In general, adults under age 65 should be treated with 2 or 3 mg.
15. Each tablet is a single dose; do not crush or break the tablet.

SEPRACOR
Manufactured for:
Sepracor Inc.
Marlborough, MA 01752 USA
by Patheon Inc., Mississauga, Ontario L5N 7K9 Canada
For customer service, call 1-888-394-7377.
To report adverse events, call 1-877-737-7226.
For medical information, call 1-800-739-0565.
February 2005
IN-5254/S

Shire US Inc.
725 CHESTERBROOK BLVD.
WAYNE, PA 19087

Direct Inquiries to:
Customer Service
(800) 828-2088

For Medical Information Contact:
(800) 828-2088

EQUETRO™ ℞
[ē-kwĕ-trō]
(carbamazepine) Extended-Release Capsules
Rx only

WARNING
APLASTIC ANEMIA AND AGRANULOCYTOSIS HAVE BEEN REPORTED IN ASSOCIATION WITH THE USE OF CARBAMAZEPINE. DATA FROM A POPULATION-BASED CASE-CONTROL STUDY DEMONSTRATE THAT THE RISK OF DEVELOPING THESE REACTIONS IS 5-8 TIMES GREATER THAN IN THE GENERAL POPULATION. HOWEVER, THE OVERALL RISK OF THESE REACTIONS IN THE UNTREATED GENERAL POPULATION IS LOW. APPROXIMATELY SIX PATIENTS PER ONE MILLION POPULATION PER YEAR FOR AGRANULOCYTOSIS AND TWO PATIENTS PER ONE MILLION POPULATION PER YEAR FOR APLASTIC ANEMIA.
ALTHOUGH REPORTS OF TRANSIENT OR PERSISTENT DECREASED PLATELET OR WHITE BLOOD CELL COUNTS ARE NOT UNCOMMON IN ASSOCIATION WITH THE USE OF CARBAMAZEPINE, DATA ARE NOT AVAILABLE TO ESTIMATE ACCURATELY THEIR INCIDENCE OR OUTCOME. HOWEVER, THE VAST MAJORITY OF THE CASES OF LEUKOPENIA HAVE NOT PROGRESSED TO THE MORE SERIOUS CONDITIONS OF APLASTIC ANEMIA OR AGRANULOCYTOSIS.
BECAUSE OF THE VERY LOW INCIDENCE OF AGRANULOCYTOSIS AND APLASTIC ANEMIA, THE VAST MAJORITY OF MINOR HEMATOLOGIC CHANGES OBSERVED IN MONITORING OF PATIENTS ON CARBAMAZEPINE ARE UNLIKELY TO SIGNAL THE OCCURRENCE OF EITHER ABNORMALITY. NONETHELESS, COMPLETE PRETREATMENT HEMATOLOGICAL TESTING SHOULD BE OBTAINED AS A BASELINE. IF A PATIENT IN THE COURSE OF TREATMENT EXHIBITS LOW OR DECREASED WHITE BLOOD CELL OR PLATELET COUNTS, THE PATIENT SHOULD BE MONITORED CLOSELY. DISCONTINUATION OF THE DRUG SHOULD BE CONSIDERED IF ANY EVIDENCE OF SIGNIFICANT BONE MARROW DEPRESSION DEVELOPS.

Before prescribing EQUETRO™, the physician should be thoroughly familiar with the details of this prescribing information, particularly regarding use with other drugs, especially those which accentuate toxicity potential.

DESCRIPTION
EQUETRO™ is available for oral administration as 100 mg, 200 mg and 300 mg extended-release capsules of carbamazepine, USP. Carbamazepine is a white to off-white powder, practically insoluble in water and soluble in alcohol and in acetone. Its molecular weight is 236.27. Its chemical name is 5H-dibenz[b,f]azepine-5-carboxamide, and its structural formula is:

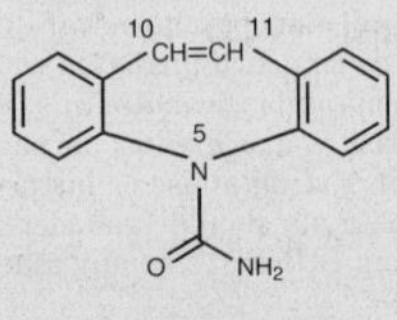

CARBAMAZEPINE

EQUETRO™ is a multi-component capsule formulation consisting of three different types of beads: immediate-release beads, extended-release beads, and enteric-release beads. The three bead types are combined in a specific ratio to provide twice daily dosing of Equetro™.
Inactive ingredients: citric acid, colloidal silicon dioxide, lactose monohydrate, microcrystalline cellulose, polyethylene glycol, povidone, sodium lauryl sulfate, talc, triethyl citrate and other ingredients.
The 100 mg capsule shells contain gelatin-NF, FD&C Blue #2, Yellow Iron Oxide, Titanium Dioxide and are imprinted with white ink; the 200 mg capsule shells contain gelatin-NF, Yellow Iron Oxide, FD&C Blue #2, and Titanium Diox-

ide, and are imprinted with white ink; and the 300 mg capsule shells contain gelatin-NF, FD&C Blue #2, Yellow Iron Oxide, and Titanium Dioxide, and are imprinted with white ink.

CLINICAL PHARMACOLOGY

In controlled clinical trials, carbamazepine has been shown to be effective in the treatment of Bipolar I Disorder.

Mechanism of Action

The mechanism(s) of action of carbamazepine in the treatment of bipolar disorder has not been elucidated. Although numerous pharmacological effects of carbamazepine have been described in the published literature (e.g., modulation of ion channels [sodium and calcium], receptor-mediated neurotransmission [GABAergic, glutamatergic, and monoaminergic], and intracellular signaling pathways in experimental preparations), the contribution of these effects to the efficacy of carbamazepine in bipolar disorder is unknown.

Pharmacokinetics

Carbamazepine (CBZ): Following a single 200 mg oral extended-release dose of carbamazepine, peak plasma concentration was 1.9 ± 0.3 µg/mL and the time to reach the peak was 19 ± 7 hours. Following repeat dose administration (800 mg every 12 hours), the peak levels were 11.0 ± 2.5 µg/mL and the time to reach the peak was 5.9 ± 1.8 hours. The pharmacokinetics of extended-release carbamazepine is linear over the single dose range of 200-800 mg.

Carbamazepine is 76% bound to plasma proteins. Carbamazepine is primarily metabolized in the liver. Cytochrome P450 3A4 was identified as the major isoform responsible for the formation of carbamazepine-10,11-epoxide. Since carbamazepine induces its own metabolism, the half-life is also variable. Following a single extended-release dose of carbamazepine, the average half-life ranged from 35-40 hours and 12-17 hours following repeated dosing. The apparent oral clearance following a single dose was 25 ± 5 mL/min and following multiple dosing was 80 ± 30 mL/min.

After oral administration of ^{14}C-carbamazepine, 72% of the administered radioactivity was found in the urine and 28% in the feces. This urinary radioactivity was composed largely of hydroxylated and conjugated metabolites, with only 3% of unchanged carbamazepine.

Carbamazepine-10,11-epoxide (CBZ-E): Carbamazepine-10,11-epoxide is considered to be an active metabolite of carbamazepine. Following a single 200 mg oral extended-release dose of carbamazepine, the peak plasma concentration of carbamazepine-10,11-epoxide was 0.11 ± 0.012 µg/mL and the time to reach the peak was 36 ± 6 hours. Following chronic administration of an extended-release dose of carbamazepine (800 mg every 12 hours), the peak levels of carbamazepine-10,11-epoxide were 2.2 ± 0.9 µg/mL and the time to reach the peak was 14 ± 8 hours. The plasma half-life of carbamazepine-10,11-epoxide following administration of carbamazepine is 34 ± 9 hours. Following a single oral dose of extended-release carbamazepine (200-800 mg) the AUC and C_{max} of carbamazepine-10,11-epoxide were less than 10% of carbamazepine. Following multiple dosing of extended-release carbamazepine (800-1600 mg daily for 14 days), the AUC and C_{max} of carbamazepine-10,11-epoxide were dose related, ranging from 15.7 µg.hr/mL and 1.5 µg/mL at 800 mg/day to 32.6 µg.hr/mL and 3.2 µg/mL at 1600 mg/day, respectively, and were less than 30% of carbamazepine. Carbamazepine-10,11-epoxide is 50% bound to plasma proteins.

Food Effect: A high fat meal diet increased the rate of absorption of a single 400 mg dose (mean T_{max} was reduced from 24 hours, in the fasting state, to 14 hours and C_{max} increased from 3.2 to 4.3 µg/mL) but not the extent (AUC) of absorption. The elimination half-life remained unchanged between fed and fasting state. The multiple dose study conducted in the fed state showed that the steady-state C_{max} values were within the therapeutic concentration range. The pharmacokinetic profile of extended-release carbamazepine was similar when given by sprinkling the beads over applesauce compared to the intact capsule administered in the fasted state.

Special Populations

Hepatic Dysfunction: The effect of hepatic impairment on the pharmacokinetics of carbamazepine is not known. However, given that carbamazepine is primarily metabolized in the liver, it is prudent to proceed with caution in patients with hepatic dysfunction.

Renal Dysfunction: The effect of renal impairment on the pharmacokinetics of carbamazepine is not known.

Gender: No difference in the mean AUC and C_{max} of carbamazepine and carbamazepine-10,11-epoxide was found between males and females.

Age: Carbamazepine is more rapidly metabolized to carbamazepine-10,11-epoxide in young children than adults. In children below the age of 15, there is an inverse relationship between CBZ-E/CBZ ratio and increasing age. The safety and effectiveness of EQUETRO™ in pediatric and adolescent patients have not been established.

Race: No information is available on the effect of race on the pharmacokinetics of carbamazepine.

CLINICAL STUDIES

The effectiveness of EQUETRO™ in the acute treatment of manic and mixed symptoms in patients with Bipolar I Disorder was established in 2 (3 week) multicenter, randomized, double-blind, flexible dose, placebo controlled studies in adult patients who met the DSM-IV criteria for Bipolar I Disorder with manic or mixed episode. In both studies, pa-

tients were titrated to a dose range from 400 mg/day to 1600 mg/day, given in divided doses, twice daily. The mean carbamazepine ER dose during the last week was 952 mg/day in the first study, and 726 mg/day in the second.

The primary rating instrument used for assessing manic symptoms in these trials was the Young Mania Rating Scale (YMRS), an 11-item clinician-rated scale traditionally used to assess the degree of manic symptomatology in a range from 0 (no manic features) to 60 (maximum score). The primary outcome in these trials was change from baseline in the YMRS total score.

EQUETRO™ was significantly more effective than placebo in reduction of the YMRS total score for both studies.

INDICATIONS AND USAGE

EQUETRO™ is indicated for the treatment of acute manic and mixed episodes associated with Bipolar I Disorder.

A manic episode is a distinct period of abnormally and persistently elevated, expansive, or irritable mood. A mixed episode is characterized by the criteria for a manic episode in conjunction with those for a major depressive episode (depressed mood, loss of interest or pleasure in nearly all activities).

The efficacy of EQUETRO™ in acute mania was established in 2 placebo-controlled, double-blind, 3-week studies in patients meeting DSM-IV criteria for Bipolar I Disorder who currently displayed an acute manic or mixed episode (see CLINICAL PHARMACOLOGY).

The effectiveness of EQUETRO™ for longer-term use and for prophylactic use in mania has not been systematically evaluated in controlled clinical trials. Therefore, physicians who elect to use EQUETRO™ for extended periods should periodically re-evaluate the long-term risks and benefits of the drug for the individual patient (see DOSAGE AND ADMINISTRATION).

CONTRAINDICATIONS

Carbamazepine should not be used in patients with a history of previous bone marrow depression, hypersensitivity to the drug, or known sensitivity to any of the tricyclic compounds, such as amitriptyline, desipramine, imipramine, protriptyline and nortriptyline. Likewise, on theoretical grounds its use with monoamine oxidase inhibitors is not recommended. Before administration of carbamazepine, MAO inhibitors should be discontinued for a minimum of 14 days, or longer if the clinical situation permits.

WARNINGS

Patients should be made aware that EQUETRO™ contains carbamazepine and should not be used in combination with any other medications containing carbamazepine.

Usage in Pregnancy

Carbamazepine can cause fetal harm when administered to a pregnant woman.

Epidemiological data suggest that there may be an association between the use of carbamazepine during pregnancy and congenital malformations, including spina bifida. The prescribing physician will wish to weigh the benefits of therapy against the risks in treating or counseling women of childbearing potential. If this drug is used during pregnancy, or if the patient becomes pregnant while taking this drug, the patient should be apprised of the potential hazard to the fetus.

Retrospective case reviews suggest that, compared with monotherapy, there may be a higher prevalence of teratogenic effects associated with the use of anticonvulsants in combination therapy.

In humans, transplacental passage of carbamazepine is rapid (30-60 minutes), and the drug is accumulated in the fetal tissues, with higher levels found in liver and kidney than in brain and lung.

Carbamazepine has been shown to have adverse effects in reproduction studies in rats when given orally in dosages 10-25 times a human daily dosage of 1200 mg on a mg/kg basis or 1.5-4 times the human daily dosage on a mg/m² basis. In rat teratology studies, 2 of 135 offspring showed kinked ribs at 250 mg/kg and 4 of 119 offspring at 650 mg/kg showed other anomalies (cleft palate, 1; talipes, 1; anophthalmos, 2). In reproduction studies in rats, nursing offspring demonstrated a lack of weight gain and an unkempt appearance at a maternal dosage level of 200 mg/kg.

Tests to detect defects using current accepted procedures should be considered a part of routine prenatal care in childbearing women receiving carbamazepine.

General

Patients with a history of adverse hematologic reaction to any drug may be particularly at risk.

Severe dermatologic reactions, including toxic epidermal necrolysis (Lyell's syndrome) and Stevens-Johnson syndrome have been reported with carbamazepine. These reactions have been extremely rare. However, a few fatalities have been reported.

In patients with seizure disorder, carbamazepine should not be discontinued abruptly because of the strong possibility of precipitating status epilepticus with attendant hypoxia and threat to life.

Carbamazepine has shown mild anticholinergic activity; therefore, patients with increased intraocular pressure should be closely observed during therapy.

Because of the relationship of the drug to other tricyclic compounds, the possibility of activation of a latent psychosis and, in elderly patients, of confusion or agitation should be considered.

Co-administration of carbamazepine and delavirdine may lead to loss of virologic response and possible resistance to RESCRIPTOR or to the class of non-nucleoside reverse transcriptase inhibitors.

PRECAUTIONS

General

Before initiating therapy, a detailed history and physical examination should be made.

Therapy should be prescribed only after critical benefit-to-risk appraisal in patients with a history of cardiac, hepatic, or renal damage; adverse hematologic reaction to other drugs; or interrupted courses of therapy with carbamazepine.

Suicide: The possibility of suicide attempt is inherent in Bipolar Disorder and close supervision of high risk patients should accompany drug therapy. Prescriptions for EQUETRO™ should be written for the smallest quantity consistent with good patient management in order to reduce the risk of overdose.

Information for Patients

Patients should be made aware of the early toxic signs and symptoms of a potential hematologic problem, such as fever, sore throat, rash, ulcers in the mouth, easy bruising, petechial or purpuric hemorrhage, and should be advised to report to the physician immediately if any such signs or symptoms appear.

Since dizziness and drowsiness may occur, patients should be cautioned about the hazards of operating machinery or automobiles or engaging in other potentially dangerous tasks.

If necessary, the EQUETRO™ capsules can be opened and the contents sprinkled over food, such as a teaspoon of applesauce or other similar food products. EQUETRO™ capsules or their contents should not be crushed or chewed. EQUETRO™ may interact with some drugs. Therefore, patients should be advised to report to their doctors the use of any other prescription or non-prescription medication or herbal products.

Laboratory Tests

Complete pretreatment blood counts, including platelets and possibly reticulocytes and serum iron, should be obtained as a baseline. If a patient in the course of treatment exhibits low or decreased white blood cell or platelet counts, the patient should be monitored closely. Discontinuation of the drug should be considered if any evidence of significant bone marrow depression develops.

Baseline and periodic evaluations of liver function, particularly in patients with a history of liver disease, must be performed during treatment with this drug since liver damage may occur. The drug should be discontinued immediately in cases of aggravated liver dysfunction or active liver disease.

Baseline and periodic eye examinations, including slit-lamp, funduscopy, and tonometry, are recommended since many phenothiazines and related drugs have been shown to cause eye changes.

Baseline and periodic complete urinalysis and BUN determinations are recommended for patients treated with this agent because of observed renal dysfunction.

Increases in total cholesterol, LDL and HDL have been observed in some patients taking anticonvulsants. Therefore, periodic evaluation of these parameters is also recommended.

Monitoring of blood levels (see CLINICAL PHARMACOLOGY) may be useful for verification of drug compliance, assessing safety and determining the cause of toxicity including when more than one medication is being used.

Thyroid function tests have been reported to show decreased values with carbamazepine administered alone.

Hyponatremia has been reported in association with carbamazepine use, either alone or in combination with other drugs.

Interference with some pregnancy tests has been reported.

Drug Interactions

Clinically meaningful drug interactions have occurred with concomitant medications and include, but are not limited to the following:

Agents Highly Bound to Plasma Protein:

Carbamazepine is not highly bound to plasma proteins; therefore, administration of EQUETRO™ to a patient taking another drug that is highly protein bound should not cause increased free concentrations of the other drug.

Agents that Inhibit Cytochrome P450 Isoenzymes and/or Epoxide Hydrolase:

Carbamazepine is metabolized mainly by cytochrome P450 (CYP) 3A4 to the active carbamazepine 10,11-epoxide, which is further metabolized to the trans-diol by epoxide hydrolase. Therefore, the potential exists for interaction between carbamazepine and any agent that inhibits CYP3A4 and/or epoxide hydrolase. Agents that are CYP3A4 inhibitors that have been found, or are expected, to increase plasma levels of EQUETRO™ are the following:

Acetazolamide, azole antifungals, cimetidine, clarithromycin[1], dalfopristin, danazol, delavirdine, diltiazem, erythromycin[1], fluoxetine, fluvoxamine, grapefruit juice, isoniazid, itraconazole, ketoconazole, loratadine, nefazodone, niacinamide, nicotinamide, protease inhibitors, propoxyphene, quinine, quinupristin, troleandomycin, valproate[1], verapamil, zileuton.

[1]also inhibits epoxide hydrolase resulting in increased levels of the active metabolite carbamazepine 10, 11-epoxide

Continued on next page

Equetro—Cont.

Thus, if a patient has been titrated to a stable dosage of EQUETRO™, and then begins a course of treatment with one of these CYP3A4 or epoxide hydrolase inhibitors, it is reasonable to expect that a dose reduction for EQUETRO™ may be necessary.

Agents that Induce Cytochrome P450 Isoenzymes:
Carbamazepine is metabolized by CYP3A4. Therefore, the potential exists for interaction between carbamazepine and any agent that induces CYP3A4. Agents that are CYP inducers that have been found, or are expected, to decrease plasma levels of EQUETRO™ are the following:

Cisplatin, doxorubicin HCL, felbamate, rifampin, phenobarbital, Phenytoin(2)*, primidone, methsuximide, and theophylline*

(2)Phenytoin plasma levels have also been reported to increase and decrease in the presence of carbamazepine, see below.

Thus, if a patient has been titrated to a stable dosage on EQUETRO™, and then begins a course of treatment with one of these CYP3A4 inducers, it is reasonable to expect that a dose increase for EQUETRO™may be necessary.

Agents with Decreased Levels in the Presence of Carbamazepine due to Induction of Cytochrome P450 Enzymes:
Carbamazepine is known to induce CYP1A2 and CYP3A4. Therefore, the potential exists for interaction between carbamazepine and any agent metabolized by one (or more) of these enzymes. Agents that have been found, or are expected to have decreased plasma levels in the presence of EQUETRO™ due to induction of CYP enzymes are the following:

Acetaminophen, alprazolam, amitriptyline, bupropion, buspirone, citalopram, clobazam, clonazepam, clozapine, cyclosporin, delavirdine, desipramine, diazepam, dicumarol, doxycycline, ethosuximide, felbamate, felodipine, glucocorticoids, haloperidol, itraconazole, lamotrigine, levothyroxine, lorazepam, methadone, midazolam, mirtazapine, nortriptyline, olanzapine, oral contraceptives(3)*, oxcarbazepine, Phenytoin*(4)*, praziquantel, protease inhibitors, quetiapine, risperidone, theophylline, topiramate, tiagabine, tramadol, triazolam, valproate, warfarin*(5)*, ziprasidone, and zonisamide.*

(3)Break through bleeding has been reported among patients receiving concomitant oral contraceptives and their reliability may be adversely affected.

(4)Phenytoin has also been reported to increase in the presence of carbamazepine. Careful monitoring of phenytoin plasma levels following co-medication with carbamazepine is advised.

(5)Warfarin's anticoagulant effect can be reduced in the presence of carbamazepine.

Thus, if a patient has been titrated to a stable dosage on one of the agents in this category, and then begins a course of treatment with EQUETRO™, it is reasonable to expect that a dose increase for the concomitant agent may be necessary.

Agents with Increased Levels in the Presence of Carbamazepine:
EQUETRO™ increases the plasma levels of the following agents:

Clomipramine HCl, Phenytoin(6)*, and primidone*

(6)Phenytoin has also been reported to decrease in the presence of carbamazepine. Careful monitoring of phenytoin plasma levels following co-medication with carbamazepine is advised.

Thus, if a patient has been titrated to a stable dosage on one of the agents in this category, and then begins a course of the treatment with EQUETRO™, it is reasonable to expect that a dose decrease for the concomitant agent may be necessary.

Pharmacological/Pharmacodynamic Interactions with Carbamazepine:
Concomitant administration of carbamazepine and lithium may increase the risk of neurotoxic side effects.
Given the anticonvulsant properties of carbamazepine, EQUETRO™ may reduce the thyroid function as has been reported with other anticonvulsants. Additionally, antimalarial drugs, such as chloroquine and mefloquine, may antagonize the activity of carbamazepine.
Thus if a patient has been titrated to a stable dosage on one of the agents in this category, and then begins a course of treatment with EQUETRO™, it is reasonable to expect that a dose adjustment may be necessary.
Because of its primary CNS effect, caution should be used when EQUETRO™ is taken with other centrally acting drugs and alcohol.

Carcinogenesis, Mutagenesis, Impairment of Fertility:
Administration of carbamazepine to Sprague-Dawley rats for two years in the diet at doses of 25, 75, and 250 mg/kg/day (low dose approximately 0.2 times the human daily dose of 1200 mg on a mg/m^2 basis), resulted in a dose-related increase in the incidence of hepatocellular tumors in females and of benign interstitial cell adenomas in the testes of males.
Carbamazepine must, therefore, be considered to be carcinogenic in Sprague-Dawley rats. Bacterial and mammalian mutagenicity studies using carbamazepine produced negative results. The significance of these findings relative to the use of carbamazepine in humans is, at present, unknown.

Usage in Pregnancy: Pregnancy Category D (See WARNINGS)

Labor and Delivery: The effect of carbamazepine on human labor and delivery is unknown.

Nursing Mothers: Carbamazepine and its epoxide metabolite are transferred to breast milk and during lactation. Because of the potential for serious adverse reactions in nursing infants from carbamazepine, a decision should be made whether to discontinue nursing or to discontinue the drug, taking into account the importance of the drug to the mother.

Pediatric Use: The safety and effectiveness of EQUETRO in pediatric and adolescent patients have not been established.

Geriatric Use: No systematic studies in geriatric patients have been conducted.

ADVERSE REACTIONS

General: The most severe adverse reactions previously observed with carbamazepine were reported in the hemopoietic system (see BOX WARNING), the skin, and the cardiovascular system.
The most frequently observed adverse reactions, particularly during the initial phases of therapy, are dizziness, drowsiness, unsteadiness, nausea, and vomiting. To minimize the possibility of such reactions, therapy should be initiated at the lowest dosage recommended.
The most commonly observed adverse experiences (5% and at least twice placebo) seen in association with the use of EQUETRO™ (400 to 1600 mg/day, dose adjusted in 200mg daily increments in week 1 in Bipolar I Disorder in the double-blind, placebo-controlled trials of 3 weeks' duration are included in Table 3 below:

Table 3. Most Common Adverse Events Reported in Double-Blind, Placebo Controlled Trials (Incidence >=5% and at least twice Placebo)

Adverse Events	EQUETRO™ (N = 251)	Placebo (N = 248)
DIZZINESS	44%	12%
SOMNOLENCE	32%	13%
NAUSEA	29%	10%
VOMITING	18%	3%
ATAXIA	15%	0%
PRURITUS	8%	2%
DRY MOUTH	8%	3%
AMBLYOPIA*	6%	2%
SPEECH DISORDER	6%	0%

* reported as blurred vision

EQUETRO™ and placebo-treated patients from the two double-blind, placebo-controlled studies were enrolled in a 6-month open-label study. The table below summarizes the most common adverse events with an incidence of 5% or more.
[See table 4 below]
Other significant adverse events seen in less than 5% of patients include:

Suicide Attempt, Manic Reaction, Insomnia, Nervousness, Depersonalization and Extrapyramidal Symptoms, Infections (Fungal, Viral, Bacterial), Pharyngitis, Rhinitis, Sinusitis, Bronchitis, Urinary Tract Infection, Leukopenia and Lymphadenopathy, Liver Function Tests Abnormal, Edema, Peripheral Edema, Allergic Reaction, Photosensitivity Reaction, Alopecia, Diplopia and Ear Pain.

The following additional adverse reactions were previously reported with carbamazepine:

Hemopoietic System: Aplastic anemia, agranulocytosis, pancytopenia, bone marrow depression, thrombocytopenia, leukopenia, leukocytosis, eosinophilia, acute intermittent porphyria

Skin: Pruritic and erythematous rashes, urticaria, toxic epidermal necrolysis (Lyell's syndrome) (see WARNINGS), Stevens-Johnson syndrome (see WARNINGS), photosensitivity reactions, alterations in skin pigmentation, exfoliative dermatitis, erythema multiforme and nodosum, purpura, aggravation of disseminated lupus erythematosus, alopecia, and diaphoresis. In certain cases, discontinuation of therapy may be necessary. Isolated cases of hirsutism have been reported, but a causal relationship is not clear.

Cardiovascular System: Congestive heart failure, edema, aggravation of hypertension, hypotension, syncope and collapse, aggravation of coronary artery disease, arrhythmias and AV block, thrombophlebitis, thromboembolism, and adenopathy or lymphadenopathy. Some of these cardiovascular complications have resulted in fatalities. Myocardial infarction has been associated with other tricyclic compounds.

Liver: Abnormalities in liver function tests, cholestatic and hepatocellular jaundice, hepatitis.

Respiratory System: Pulmonary hypersensitivity characterized by fever, dyspnea, pneumonitis, or pneumonia.

Genitourinary System: Urinary frequency, acute urinary retention, oliguria with elevated blood pressure, azotemia, renal failure, and impotence. Albuminuria, glycosuria, elevated BUN, and microscopic deposits in the urine have also been reported.
Testicular atrophy occurred in rats receiving carbamazepine orally from 4-52 weeks at dosage levels of 50-400 mg/kg/day. Additionally, rats receiving carbamazepine in the diet for 2 years at dosage levels of 25, 75, and 250 mg/kg/day had a dose-related incidence of testicular atrophy and aspermatogenesis. In dogs, it produced a brownish discoloration, presumably a metabolite, in the urinary bladder at dosage levels of 50 mg/kg/day and higher. Relevance of these findings to humans is unknown.

Nervous System: Dizziness, drowsiness, disturbances of coordination, confusion, headache, fatigue, blurred vision, visual hallucinations, transient diplopia, oculomotor disturbances, nystagmus, speech disturbances, abnormal involuntary movements, peripheral neuritis and paresthesias, depression with agitation, talkativeness, tinnitus, and hyperacusis.
There have been reports of associated paralysis and other symptoms of cerebral arterial insufficiency, but the exact relationship of these reactions to the drug has not been established.
Isolated cases of neuroleptic malignant syndrome have been reported with concomitant use of psychotropic drugs.

Digestive System: Nausea, vomiting, gastric distress and abdominal pain, diarrhea, constipation, anorexia, and dryness of the mouth and pharynx, including glossitis and stomatitis.

Eyes: Scattered punctate cortical lens opacities, as well as conjunctivitis, have been reported. Although a direct causal relationship has not been established, many phenothiazines and related drugs have been shown to cause eye changes.

Musculoskeletal System: Aching joints and muscles, and leg cramps.

Metabolism: Fever and chills, inappropriate antidiuretic hormone (ADH) secretion syndrome has been reported. Cases of frank water intoxication, with decreased serum sodium (hyponatremia) and confusion have been reported in association with carbamazepine use (see PRECAUTIONS, Laboratory Tests). Decreased levels of plasma calcium have been reported.

Other: Isolated cases of a lupus erythematosus-like syndrome have been reported. There have been occasional reports of elevated levels of cholesterol, HDL cholesterol, and triglycerides in patients taking anticonvulsants.

Table 4. Most Common Adverse Events Reported in Open Label (Incidence >=5%)

Body As A Whole	**% events reported**	**Nervous System**	**% events reported**
Headache	22%	Dizziness	16%
Infection	12%	Somnolence	12%
Pain	12%	Amnesia^	8%
Asthenia	8%	Anxiety	7%
Accidental Injury	7%	Depression*	7%
Chest Pain	5%	Manic Depressive Reaction	7%
Back Pain	5%	Ataxia	5%
Digestive		**Skin Appendages**	
Diarrhea	10%	Rash	13%
Dyspepsia	10%	Pruritis	5%
Nausea	10%		
Constipation	5%		

^Amnesia includes poor memory, forgetful and memory disturbance
*Depression includes suicidal ideation

A case of aseptic meningitis, accompanied by myoclonus and peripheral eosinophilia, has been reported in a patient taking carbamazepine in combination with other medications. The patient was successfully dechallenged, and the meningitis reappeared upon rechallenge with carbamazepine.

DRUG ABUSE AND DEPENDENCE

No evidence of abuse potential has been associated with carbamazepine, nor is there evidence of psychological or physical dependence in humans.

OVERDOSAGE

Acute Toxicity

Lowest known lethal dose: adults, >60 g (39-year-old man). Highest known doses survived: adults, 30 g (31-year-old woman); children, 10 g (6-year-old boy); small children, 5 g (3-year-old girl).

Oral LD_{50} in animals (mg/kg): mice, 1100-3750; rats, 3850-4025; rabbits, 1500-2680; guinea pigs, 920.

Signs and Symptoms

The first signs and symptoms appear after 1-3 hours. Neuromuscular disturbances are the most prominent. Cardiovascular disorders are generally milder, and severe cardiac complications occur only when very high doses (>60 g) have been ingested.

Respiration: Irregular breathing, respiratory depression.
Cardiovascular System: Tachycardia, hypotension or hypertension, shock, conduction disorders.
Nervous System and Muscles: Impairment of consciousness ranging in severity to deep coma. Convulsions, especially in small children. Motor restlessness, muscular twitching, tremor, athetoid movements, opisthotonos, ataxia, drowsiness, dizziness, mydriasis, nystagmus, adiadochokinesia, ballism, psychomotor disturbances, dysmetria. Initial hyperreflexia, followed by hyporeflexia.
Gastrointestinal Tract: Nausea, vomiting.
Kidneys and Bladder: Anuria or oliguria, urinary retention.
Laboratory Findings: Isolated instances of overdosage have included leukocytosis, reduced leukocyte count, glycosuria, and acetonuria. EEG may show dysrhythmias.
Combined Poisoning: When alcohol, tricyclic antidepressants, barbiturates, or hydantoins are taken at the same time, the signs and symptoms of acute poisoning with carbamazepine may be aggravated or modified.

Treatment

For the most up to date information on management of carbamazepine overdose, please contact the poison center for your area by calling 1-800-222-1222. The prognosis in cases of carbamazepine poisoning is generally favorable. Of 5,645 cases of carbamazepine exposures reported to US poison centers in 2002, a total of 8 deaths (0.14% mortality rate) occurred. Over 39% of the cases reported to these poison centers were managed safely at home with conservative care. Successful management of large or intentional carbamazepine exposures requires implementation of supportive care, frequent monitoring of serum drug concentrations, as well as aggressive but appropriate gastric decontamination.

Elimination of the Drug: The primary method for gastric decontamination of carbamazepine overdose is use of activated charcoal. For substantial recent ingestions, gastric lavage may also be considered. Administration of activated charcoal prior to hospital assessment has the potential to significantly reduce drug absorption. There is no specific antidote. In overdose, absorption of carbamazepine may be prolonged and delayed. More than one dose of activated charcoal may be beneficial in patients that have evidence of continued absorption (e.g., rising serum carbamazepine levels).

Measures to Accelerate Elimination: The data on use of dialysis to enhance elimination in carbamazepine is scarce. Dialysis, particularly high flux or high efficiency hemodialysis, may be considered in patients with severe carbamazepine poisoning associated with renal failure or in cases of status epilepticus, or where there are rising serum drug levels and worsening clinical status despite appropriate supportive care and gastric decontamination. For severe cases of carbamazepine overdose unresponsive to other measures, charcoal hemoperfusion may be used to enhance drug clearance.

Respiratory Depression: Keep the airways free; resort, if necessary, to endotracheal intubation, artificial respiration, and administration of oxygen.

Hypotension, Shock: Keep the patient's legs raised and administer a plasma expander. If blood pressure fails to rise despite measures taken to increase plasma volume, use of vasoactive substances should be considered.

Convulsions: Diazepam or barbiturates.

Warning: Diazepam or barbiturates may aggravate respiratory depression (especially in children), hypotension, and coma. However, barbiturates should not be used if drugs that inhibit monoamine oxidase have also been taken by the patient either in overdosage or in recent therapy (within 1 week).

Surveillance: Respiration, cardiac function (ECG monitoring), blood pressure, body temperature, pupillary reflexes, and kidney and bladder function should be monitored for several days.

Treatment of Blood Count Abnormalities: If evidence of significant bone marrow depression develops, the following recommendations are suggested: (1) stop the drug, (2) perform daily CBC, platelet, and reticulocyte counts, (3) do a bone marrow aspiration and trephine biopsy immediately and repeat with sufficient frequency to monitor recovery.

Special periodic studies might be helpful as follows: (1) white cell and platelet antibodies, (2) ^{59}Fe-ferrokinetic studies, (3) peripheral blood cell typing, (4) cytogenetic studies on marrow and peripheral blood, (5) bone marrow culture studies for colony-forming units, (6) hemoglobin electrophoresis for A_2 and F hemoglobin, and (7) serum folic acid and B_{12} levels.

A fully developed aplastic anemia will require appropriate, intensive monitoring and therapy, for which specialized consultation should be sought.

DOSAGE AND ADMINISTRATION

The recommended initial dose of EQUETRO™ is 400 mg/day given in divided doses, twice daily. The dose should be adjusted in 200 mg daily increments to achieve optimal clinical response. Doses higher than 1600mg/day have not been studied.

Monitoring of blood levels (see PRECAUTIONS), Laboratory Tests may be useful for verification of drug compliance, assessing safety and determining the cause of toxicity including when more than one medication is being used.

The EQUETRO™ capsules may be opened and the beads sprinkled over food, such as a teaspoon of applesauce or other similar food products if this method of administration is preferred. EQUETRO™ capsules or their contents should not be crushed or chewed. EQUETRO™ can be taken with or without meals.

HOW SUPPLIED

EQUETRO™ (carbamazepine) extended-release capsules is supplied in three dosage strengths.

100 mg-Two-piece hard gelatin capsule yellow opaque cap with bluish green opaque body printed with the SPD 417 on one end, SPD417 and 100 mg on the other in white ink: Supplied in bottles of 120 NDC 54092-419-12

200 mg-Two-piece hard gelatin capsule yellow opaque cap with blue opaque body printed with the SPD 417 on one end and SPD417 and 200 mg on the other in white ink: Supplied in bottles of 120 NDC 54092-421-12

300 mg-Two-piece hard gelatin capsule yellow opaque cap with blue body printed with the SPD 417 on one end and SPD417 and 300 mg on the other in white ink: Supplied in bottles of 120 .... NDC 54092-423-12

Store at 25° C (77° F); excursions permitted to 15-30° C (59-86° F) [see USP controlled room temperature]. PROTECT FROM LIGHT.

Manufactured for: **Shire US Inc.,** 725 Chesterbrook Blvd., Wayne, PA 19087
1-800-828-2088, Made in U.S.A.
© 2004 Shire US Inc.
001212
419 1207 001
(Rev 12/2004)
EQU-PI   Shire

FOSRENOL®   ℞
[fos-wren-all]
(lanthanum carbonate) 250 mg and 500 mg
Chewable Tablets

DESCRIPTION

FOSRENOL® contains lanthanum carbonate (2:3) hydrate with molecular formula $La_2(CO_3)_3 \cdot xH_2O$ (on average x=4-5 moles of water) and molecular weight 457.8 (anhydrous mass). Lanthanum (La) is a naturally occurring rare earth element. Lanthanum carbonate is practically insoluble in water.

Each FOSRENOL®, white to off-white, chewable tablet contains lanthanum carbonate hydrate equivalent to 250 or 500 mg of elemental lanthanum and the following inactive ingredients: dextrates (hydrated) NF, colloidal silicon dioxide NF, magnesium stearate NF, and talc USP.

CLINICAL PHARMACOLOGY

Patients with end stage renal disease (ESRD) can develop hyperphosphatemia that may be associated with secondary hyperparathyroidism and elevated calcium phosphate product. Elevated calcium phosphate product increases the risk of ectopic calcification. Treatment of hyperphosphatemia usually includes all of the following: reduction in dietary intake of phosphate, removal of phosphate by dialysis and inhibition of intestinal phosphate absorption with phosphate binders. FOSRENOL® does not contain calcium or aluminum.

Pharmacodynamics:
Lanthanum carbonate dissociates in the acid environment of the upper GI tract to release lanthanum ions that bind dietary phosphate released from food during digestion. FOSRENOL® inhibits absorption of phosphate by forming highly insoluble lanthanum phosphate complexes, consequently reducing both serum phosphate and calcium phosphate product.

In vitro studies have shown that in the physiologically relevant pH range of 3 to 5 in gastric fluid, lanthanum binds approximately 97% of the available phosphate when lanthanum is present in a two-fold molar excess to phosphate. In order to bind dietary phosphate efficiently, lanthanum should be administered with or immediately after a meal.

Pharmacokinetics:
Absorption/Distribution:
Following single or multiple dose oral administration of FOSRENOL® to healthy subjects, the concentration of lanthanum in plasma was very low (bioavailability <0.002%).

Following oral administration in ESRD patients, the mean lanthanum C_{max} was 1.0 ng/mL. During long-term administration (52 weeks) in ESRD patients, the mean lanthanum concentration in plasma was approximately 0.6 ng/mL. There was minimal increase in plasma lanthanum concentrations with increasing doses within the therapeutic dose range. The effect of food on the bioavailability of FOSRENOL® has not been evaluated, but the timing of food intake relative to lanthanum administration (during and 30 minutes after food intake) has a negligible effect on the systemic level of lanthanum.

In vitro, lanthanum is highly bound (>99%) to human plasma proteins, including human serum albumin, α1-acid glycoprotein, and transferrin. Binding to erythrocytes in vivo is negligible in rats.

In 105 bone biopsies from patients treated with FOSRENOL® for up to 4.5 years, rising levels of lanthanum were noted over time. Estimates of elimination half-life from bone ranged from 2.0 to 3.6 years. Steady state bone concentrations were not reached during the period studied. In studies in mice, rats and dogs, lanthanum concentrations in many tissues increased over time and were several orders of magnitude higher than plasma concentrations (particularly in the GI tract, bone and liver). Steady state tissue concentrations in bone and liver were achieved in dogs between 4 and 26 weeks. Relatively high levels of lanthanum remained in these tissues for longer than 6 months after cessation of dosing in dogs. There is no evidence from animal studies that lanthanum crosses the blood-brain barrier.

Metabolism/Elimination:
Lanthanum is not metabolized and is not a substrate of CYP450. In vitro metabolic inhibition studies showed that lanthanum at concentrations of 10 and 40 µg/ml does not have relevant inhibitory effects on any of the CYP450 isoenzymes tested (1A2, 2C9/10, 2C19, 2D6, and 3A4/5). Lanthanum was cleared from plasma following discontinuation of therapy with an elimination half-life 53 hours.

No information is available regarding the mass balance of lanthanum in humans after oral administration. In rats and dogs, the mean recovery of lanthanum after an oral dose was about 99% and 94% respectively and was essentially all from feces. Biliary excretion is the predominant route of elimination for circulating lanthanum in rats. In healthy volunteers administered intravenous lanthanum as the soluble chloride salt (120 µg), renal clearance was less than 2% of total plasma clearance. Quantifiable amounts of lanthanum were not measured in the dialysate of treated ESRD patients.

In Vitro- Drug Interactions:
Gastric Fluid: The potential for a physico-chemical interaction (precipitation) between lanthanum and six commonly used medications (warfarin, digoxin, furosemide, phenytoin, metoprolol, and enalapril) was investigated in simulated gastric fluid. The results suggest that precipitation in the stomach of insoluble complexes of these drugs with lanthanum is unlikely.

In Vivo- Drug Interactions:
Lanthanum carbonate is neither a substrate nor an inhibitor of CYP450 enzymes.

The absorption of a single dose of 1000 mg of FOSRENOL® is unaffected by co-administration of citrate. No effects of lanthanum were found on the absorption of digoxin (0.5-mg), metoprolol (100-mg), or warfarin (10-mg) in healthy subjects co-administered lanthanum carbonate (three doses of 1000 mg on the day prior to exposure and one dose of 1000 mg on the day of co-administration). Potential pharmacodynamic interactions between lanthanum and these drugs (e.g., bleeding time or prothrombin time) were not evaluated. None of the drug interaction studies was done with the maximum recommended therapeutic dose of lanthanum carbonate. No drug interaction studies assessed the effects of drugs on phosphate binding by lanthanum carbonate.

Clinical Trials:
The effectiveness of FOSRENOL® in reducing serum phosphorus in ESRD patients was demonstrated in one short-term, placebo-controlled, double-blind dose-ranging study, two placebo-controlled randomized withdrawal studies and two long-term, active-controlled, open-label studies in both hemodialysis and peritoneal dialysis (PD) patients.

Double-Blind Placebo-Controlled Studies:
One hundred forty-four patients with chronic renal failure undergoing hemodialysis and with elevated phosphate levels were randomized to double-blind treatment at a fixed dose of lanthanum carbonate of 225 mg (n=27), 675 mg (n=29), 1350 mg (n=30) or 2250 mg (n=26) or placebo (n=32) in divided doses with meals. Fifty-five percent of subjects were male, 71% black, 25% white and 4% of other races. The mean age was 56 years and the duration of dialysis ranged from 0.5 to 15.3 years. Steady-state effects were achieved after two weeks. The effect after six weeks of treatment is shown in Figure 1.

[See figure 1 at top of next column]

One-hundred eighty five patients with end-stage renal disease undergoing either hemodialysis (n=146) or peritoneal dialysis (n=39) were enrolled in two placebo-controlled, randomized withdrawal studies. Sixty-four percent of subjects were male, 28% black, 62% white and 10% of other races. The mean age was 58.4 years and the duration of dialysis ranged from 0.2 to 21.4 years. After titration of lanthanum carbonate to achieve a phosphate level between 4.2 and 5.6 mg/dl in one study (doses up to 2250 mg/day) or

Continued on next page

Fosrenol—Cont.

Figure 1. Difference in Phosphate Reduction in the FOSRENOL® and Placebo Group in a 6-Week, Dose-Ranging, Double-Blind Study in ESRD Patients (with 95% Confidence Intervals)

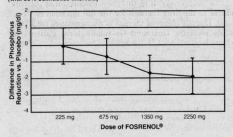

≤5.9 mg/dl in the second study (doses up to 3000 mg/day) and maintenance through 6 weeks, patients were randomized to lanthanum or placebo. During the placebo-controlled, randomized withdrawal phase (four weeks), the phosphorus concentration rose in the placebo group by 1.9 mg/dl in both studies relative to patients who remained on lanthanum carbonate therapy.

Open-Label Active-Controlled Studies:

Two long-term open-label studies were conducted, involving a total of 2028 patients with ESRD undergoing hemodialysis. Patients were randomized to receive FOSRENOL® or alternative phosphate binders for up to six months in one study and two years in the other. The daily FOSRENOL® doses, divided and taken with meals, ranged from 375 mg to 3000 mg. Doses were titrated to reduce serum phosphate levels to a target level. The daily doses of the alternative therapy were based on current prescribing information or those commonly utilized. Both treatment groups had similar reductions in serum phosphate of about 1.8 mg/dL. Maintenance of reduction was observed for up to three years in patients treated with FOSRENOL® in long-term, open label extensions.

No effects of FOSRENOL® on serum levels of 25-dihydroxy vitamin D3, vitamin A, vitamin B12, vitamin E and vitamin K were observed in patients who were monitored for 6 months.

Paired bone biopsies (at baseline and at one or two years) in 69 patients randomized to either FOSRENOL® or calcium carbonate in one study and 71 patients randomized to either FOSRENOL® or alternative therapy in a second study showed no differences in the development of mineralization defects between the groups.

Vital Status was known for over 2000 patients, 97% of those participating in the clinical program during and after receiving treatment. The adjusted yearly mortality rate (rate/years of observation) for patients treated with FOSRENOL® or alternative therapy was 6.6%.

INDICATIONS AND USAGE

FOSRENOL® is indicated to reduce serum phosphate in patients with end-stage renal disease.

CONTRAINDICATIONS

None known.

PRECAUTIONS

General:

Patients with acute peptic ulcer, ulcerative colitis, Crohn's disease or bowel obstruction were not included in FOSRENOL® clinical studies. Caution should be used in patients with these conditions.

Long-term Effects:

There were no differences in the rates of fracture or mortality in patients treated with FOSRENOL® compared to alternative therapy for up to 3 years. The duration of treatment exposure and time of observation in the clinical program are too short to conclude that FOSRENOL® does not affect the risk of fracture or mortality beyond 3 years.

Information for the Patient:

FOSRENOL® tablets should be taken with or immediately after meals. Tablets should be chewed completely before swallowing. Intact tablets should not be swallowed.

Drug Interactions:

FOSRENOL® is not metabolized.

Studies in healthy subjects have shown that FOSRENOL® does not adversely affect the pharmacokinetics of warfarin, digoxin or metoprolol. The absorption and pharmacokinetics of FOSRENOL® are unaffected by co-administration with citrate-containing compounds (see **CLINICAL PHARMACOLOGY: In Vitro/In Vivo Drug Interactions**).

An *in vitro* study showed no evidence that FOSRENOL® forms insoluble complexes with warfarin, digoxin, furosemide, phenytoin, metoprolol and enalapril in simulated gastric fluid. However, it is recommended that compounds known to interact with antacids should not be taken within 2 hours of dosing with FOSRENOL®.

Carcinogenesis, Mutagenesis, Impairment of Fertility:

Oral administration of lanthanum carbonate to rats for up to 104 weeks, at doses up to 1500 mg of the salt per kg/day [2.5 times the maximum recommended daily human dose (MRHD) of 5725 mg, on a mg/m² basis, assuming a 60-kg patient] revealed no evidence of carcinogenic potential. In the mouse, oral administration of lanthanum carbonate for up to 99 weeks, at a dose of 1500 mg/kg/day (1.3 times the MRHD) was associated with an increased incidence of glandular stomach adenomas in male mice.

Lanthanum carbonate tested negative for mutagenic activity in an *in vitro* Ames assay using *Salmonella typhimurium* and *Escherichia coli* strains and *in vitro* HGPRT gene mutation and chromosomal aberration assays in Chinese hamster ovary cells. Lanthanum carbonate also tested negative in an oral mouse micronucleus assay at doses up to 2000 mg/kg (1.7 times the MRHD), and in micronucleus and unscheduled DNA synthesis assays in rats given IV lanthanum chloride at doses up to 0.1 mg/kg, a dose that produced plasma lanthanum concentrations >2000 times the peak human plasma concentration.

Lanthanum carbonate, at doses up to 2000 mg/kg/day (3.4 times the MRHD), did not affect fertility or mating performance of male or female rats.

Pregnancy:

Pregnancy Category C. No adequate and well-controlled studies have been conducted in pregnant women. The effect of FOSRENOL® on the absorption of vitamins and other nutrients has not been studied in pregnant women. FOSRENOL® is not recommended for use during pregnancy.

In pregnant rats, oral administration of lanthanum carbonate at doses as high as 2000 mg/kg/day (3.4 times the MRHD) resulted in no evidence of harm to the fetus. In pregnant rabbits, oral administration of lanthanum carbonate at 1500 mg/kg/day (5 times the MRHD) was associated with a reduction in maternal body weight gain and food consumption, increased post-implantation loss, reduced fetal weights, and delayed fetal ossification. Lanthanum carbonate administered to rats from implantation through lactation at 2000 mg/kg/day (3.4 times the MRHD) caused delayed eye opening, reduction in body weight gain, and delayed sexual development (preputial separation and vaginal opening) of the offspring.

Labor and Delivery

No lanthanum carbonate treatment-related effects on labor and delivery were seen in animal studies. The effects of lanthanum carbonate on labor and delivery in humans is unknown.

Nursing Mothers:

It is not known whether lanthanum carbonate is excreted in human milk. Because many drugs are excreted in human milk, caution should be exercised when FOSRENOL® is administered to a nursing woman.

Geriatric Use:

Of the total number of patients in clinical studies of FOSRENOL®, 32% (538) were ≥ 65, while 9.3% (159) were ≥ 75. No overall differences in safety or effectiveness were observed between patients ≥65 years of age and younger patients.

Pediatric Use:

While growth abnormalities were not identified in long-term animal studies, lanthanum was deposited into developing bone including growth plate. The consequences of such deposition in developing bone in pediatric patients are unknown. Therefore, the use of FOSRENOL® in this population is not recommended.

ADVERSE REACTIONS

The most common adverse events for FOSRENOL® were gastrointestinal events, such as nausea and vomiting and they generally abated over time with continued dosing.

In double-blind, placebo-controlled studies where a total of 180 and 95 ESRD patients were randomized to FOSRENOL® and placebo, respectively, for 4-6 weeks of treatment, the most common events that were more frequent (≥5% difference) in the FOSRENOL® group were nausea, vomiting, dialysis graft occlusion, and abdominal pain (Table 1).

Table 1. Adverse Events That Were More Common on FOSRENOL® in Placebo-Controlled, Double-Blind Studies with Treatment Periods of 4-6 Weeks.

	FOSRENOL® % (N=180)	Placebo % (N=95)
Nausea	11	5
Vomiting	9	4
Dialysis graft occlusion	8	1
Abdominal pain	5	0

The safety of FOSRENOL® was studied in two long-term clinical trials that included 1215 patients treated with FOSRENOL® and 943 with alternative therapy. Fourteen percent (14%) of patients in these comparative, open-label studies discontinued in the FOSRENOL®-treated group due to adverse events. Gastrointestinal adverse events, such as nausea, diarrhea and vomiting, were the most common type of event leading to discontinuation.

The most common adverse events (≥5% in either treatment group) in both the long-term (2 year), open-label, active controlled, study of FOSRENOL® vs. alternative therapy (Study A) and the 6-month, comparative study of FOSRENOL® vs. calcium carbonate (Study B) are shown in Table 2. In Table 2, Study A events have been adjusted for mean exposure differences between treatment groups (with a mean exposure of 0.9 years on lanthanum and 1.3 years on alternative therapy). The adjustment for mean exposure was achieved by multiplying the observed adverse event rates in the alternative therapy group by 0.71.

[See table 2 below]

OVERDOSAGE

There is no experience with FOSRENOL® overdosage. Lanthanum carbonate was not acutely toxic in animals by the oral route. No deaths and no adverse effects occurred in mice, rats or dogs after single oral doses of 2000 mg/kg. In clinical trials, daily doses up to 4718 mg/day of lanthanum were well tolerated in healthy adults when administered with food, with the exception of GI symptoms. Given the topical activity of lanthanum in the gut, and the excretion in feces of the majority of the dose, supportive therapy is recommended for overdosage.

DOSAGE AND ADMINISTRATION

The total daily dose of FOSRENOL® should be divided and taken with meals. The recommended initial total daily dose of FOSRENOL® is 750-1500 mg. The dose should be titrated every 2-3 weeks until an acceptable serum phosphate level is reached. Serum phosphate levels should be monitored as needed during dose titration and on a regular basis thereafter.

In clinical studies of ESRD patients, FOSRENOL® doses up to 3750 mg were evaluated. Most patients required a total daily dose between 1500 mg and 3000 mg to reduce plasma phosphate levels to less than 6.0 mg/dL. Doses were generally titrated in increments of 750 mg/day.

Tablets should be chewed completely before swallowing. Intact tablets should not be swallowed.

HOW SUPPLIED

FOSRENOL® is supplied as a chewable tablet in two dosage strengths for oral administration: 250 mg tablets and 500 mg tablets. Each chewable tablet is white to off-white and embossed on one side with 'S405' and the dosage

Table 2. Incidence of Treatment-Emergent Adverse Events that Occurred in ≥5% of Patients (in Either Treatment Group) and in Both Comparative Studies A and B

	Study A %		Study B %	
	FOSRENOL® (N = 682)	Alternative Therapy Adjusted Rates (N=676)	FOSRENOL® (N=533)	Calcium Carbonate (N=267)
Nausea	36	28	16	13
Vomiting	26	21	18	11
Dialysis graft complication	26	25	3	5
Diarrhea	23	22	13	10
Headache	21	20	5	5
Dialysis graft occlusion	21	20	4	6
Abdominal pain	17	17	5	3
Hypotension	16	17	8	9
Constipation	14	13	6	7
Bronchitis	5	6	5	6
Rhinitis	5	7	7	6
Hypercalcemia	4	8	0	20

strength corresponding to the content of elemental lanthanum. The 250 mg tablets are round/convex and the 500 mg tablets are flat with a beveled edge.

250 mg supplied in bottles of 100 .... NDC 54092-247-01
500 mg supplied in bottles of 100 .... NDC 54092-249-01

Storage

Store at 25°C (77°F): excursions permitted to 15-30°C (59-86°F)
[See USP controlled room temperature]
Protect from moisture

Rx only

Manufactured for Shire US Inc.
Wayne, PA 19087-2088, USA
1-800-828-2088
Rev: 10/2004
247 0107 001 **Shire**

Wyeth Pharmaceuticals

Division of Wyeth
P.O. BOX 8299
PHILADELPHIA, PA 19101

For Product Information Contact:
(800) 934-5556
For Product Quality Contact:
(800) 999-9384
For Sales Representative Information Contact:
(800) 395-9938
For Customer Service and Ordering Information Contact:
Pharmaceuticals and Vaccines: (800) 666-7248
For Patient Assistance Program Contact:
(800) 568-9938
For All Other Inquiries:
(610) 688-4400
www.wyeth.com

TRECATOR® ℞

[*trĕk"ă'tōr*]
(ethionamide tablets, USP)
Tablets
Rx only

This product's label may have been revised after this insert was used in production. For further product information and current package insert, please visit www.wyeth.com or call our medical communications department toll-free at 1-800-934-5556.

Complete Prescribing Information for Trecator® (ethionamide Tablets, USP), appears below. Trecator®-SC (ethionamide Tablets, USP), as listed on pages 3406–3407 of the 2005 PDR, has been discontinued.

DESCRIPTION

Trecator® (ethionamide tablets, USP) is used in the treatment of tuberculosis. The chemical name for ethionamide is 2-ethylthioisonicotinamide with the following structural formula:

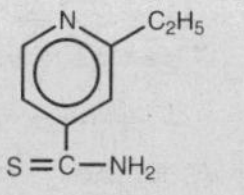

$C_8H_{10}N_2S$ M.W. 166.24

Ethionamide is a yellow crystalline, nonhygroscopic compound with a faint to moderate sulfide odor and a melting point of 162°C. It is practically insoluble in water and ether, but soluble in methanol and ethanol. It has a partition coefficient (octanol/water) Log P value of 0.3699. Trecator tablets contain 250 mg of ethionamide. The inactive ingredients present are croscarmellose sodium, FD&C Yellow #6, magnesium stearate, microcrystalline cellulose, polyethylene glycol, polyvinyl alcohol, povidone, silicon dioxide, talc, and titanium dioxide.

CLINICAL PHARMACOLOGY

Absorption

Ethionamide is essentially completely absorbed following oral administration and is not subjected to any appreciable first pass metabolism. Ethionamide tablets may be administered without regard to the timing of meals.

The pharmacokinetic parameters of ethionamide following single oral-dose administration of 250 mg of Trecator film-coated tablets under fasted conditions to 40 healthy adult volunteers are provided in Table 1.

Table 1: Mean (SD) Pharmacokinetic Parameters for Ethionamide Following Single-dose Administration of 250 mg Trecator Film-Coated Tablets to Healthy Adult Volunteers

	C_{max} (µg/mL)	T_{max} (hrs)	AUC (µg•hr/mL)
Film-Coated Tablet	2.16	1.02	7.67
	(0.61)	(0.55)	(1.69)

Trecator tablets have been reformulated from a sugar-coated tablet to a film-coated tablet. The C_{max} for the film-coated tablets (2.16 µg/mL) was significantly higher than that of sugar-coated tablets (1.48 µg/mL) (see **DOSAGE AND ADMINISTRATION**).

Distribution

Ethionamide is rapidly and widely distributed into body tissues and fluids following administration of a sugar-coated tablet, with concentrations in plasma and various organs being approximately equal. Significant concentrations are also present in cerebrospinal fluid following administration of a sugar-coated tablet. Distribution of ethionamide into the same body tissues and fluids, including cerebrospinal fluid following administration of the film-coated tablet, has not been studied, but is not expected to differ significantly from that of the sugar-coated tablet. The drug is approximately 30% bound to proteins. The mean (SD) apparent oral volume of distribution observed in 40 healthy volunteers following a 250 mg oral dose of film-coated tablets was 93.5 (19.2) L.

Metabolism

Ethionamide is extensively metabolized to active and inactive metabolites. Metabolism is presumed to occur in the liver and thus far 6 metabolites have been isolated: 2-ethylisonicotinamide, carbonyl-dihydropyridine, thiocarbonyl-dihydropyridine, S-oxocarbamoyl dihydropyridine, 2-ethylthioiso-nicotinamide, and ethionamide sulphoxide. The sulphoxide metabolite has been demonstrated to have antimicrobial activity against *Mycobacterium tuberculosis*.

Elimination

The mean (SD) half-life observed in 40 healthy volunteers following a 250 mg oral dose of film-coated tablets was 1.92 (0.27) hours. Less than 1% of the oral dose is excreted as ethionamide in urine.

Mechanism of Action

Ethionamide may be bacteriostatic or bactericidal in action, depending on the concentration of the drug attained at the site of infection and the susceptibility of the infecting organism. The exact mechanism of action of ethionamide has not been fully elucidated, but the drug appears to inhibit peptide synthesis in susceptible organisms.

Microbiology

In Vitro Activity

Ethionamide exhibits bacteriostatic activity against extracellular and intracellular *Mycobacterium tuberculosis* organisms. The development of ethionamide resistant *M. tuberculosis* isolates can be obtained by repeated subculturing in liquid or on solid media containing increasing concentrations of ethionamide. Multi-drug resistant strains of *M. tuberculosis* may have acquired resistance to both isoniazid and ethionamide. However, the majority of *M. tuberculosis* isolates that are resistant to one are usually susceptible to the other. There is no evidence of cross-resistance between ethionamide and para-aminosalicylic acid (PAS), streptomycin, or cycloserine. However, limited data suggest that cross-resistance may exist between ethionamide and thiosemicarbazones (i.e., thiacetazone) as well as isoniazid.

In Vivo Activity

Ethionamide administered orally initially decreased the number of culturable *Mycobacterium tuberculosis* organisms from the lungs of H37Rv infected mice. Drug resistance developed with continued ethionamide monotherapy, but did not occur when mice received ethionamide in combination with streptomycin or isoniazid.

SUSCEPTIBILITY TESTING

Ethionamide susceptibility testing should only be performed by qualified or reference laboratories.

Two standardized *in vitro* susceptibility methods are available for testing ethionamide against *M. tuberculosis* organisms. The modified proportion method (CDC or NCCLS M24-P) utilizes Middlebrook and Cohn 7H10 agar medium impregnated with ethionamide at a final concentration of 5.0 µg/mL. After 2 to 3 weeks of incubation, MIC_{99} values are calculated by comparing the quantity of organisms growing in the medium containing drug to the control cultures. Mycobacterial growth in the presence of drug, of at least 1% of the growth in the control culture, indicates resistance.

The radiometric broth method employs the BACTEC 460 machine to compare the growth index from untreated control cultures to cultures grown in the presence of 5.0 µg/mL of ethionamide. Strict adherence to the manufacturer's instructions for sample processing and data interpretation is required for this assay.

Susceptibility test results obtained by these two different methods cannot be compared unless equivalent drug concentrations are evaluated.

The clinical relevance of *in vitro* susceptibility test results for mycobacterial species other than *M. tuberculosis* using either the radiometric or the proportion method has not been determined.

INDICATIONS AND USAGE

Trecator is primarily indicated for the treatment of active tuberculosis in patients with *M. tuberculosis* resistant to isoniazid or rifampin, or when there is intolerance on the part of the patient to other drugs. Its use alone in the treatment of tuberculosis results in the rapid development of resistance. It is essential, therefore, to give a suitable companion drug or drugs, the choice being based on the results of susceptibility tests. If the susceptibility tests indicate that the patient's organism is resistant to one of the first-line antituberculosis drugs (i.e., isoniazid or rifampin) yet susceptible to ethionamide, ethionamide should be accompanied by at least one drug to which the *M. tuberculosis* isolate is known to be susceptible.[3] If the tuberculosis is resistant to both isoniazid and rifampin, yet susceptible to ethionamide, ethionamide should be accompanied by at least two other drugs to which the *M. tuberculosis* isolate is known to be susceptible.[3]

Patient nonadherence to prescribed treatment can result in treatment failure and in the development of drug-resistant tuberculosis, which can be life-threatening and lead to other serious health risks. It is, therefore, essential that patients adhere to the drug regimen for the full duration of treatment. Directly observed therapy is recommended for all patients receiving treatment for tuberculosis. Patients in whom drug-resistant *M. tuberculosis* organisms are isolated should be managed in consultation with an expert in the treatment of drug-resistant tuberculosis.

CONTRAINDICATIONS

Ethionamide is contraindicated in patients with severe hepatic impairment and in patients who are hypersensitive to the drug.

WARNINGS

The use of Trecator alone in the treatment of tuberculosis results in rapid development of resistance. It is essential, therefore, to give a suitable companion drug or drugs, the choice being based on the results of susceptibility testing. However, therapy may be initiated prior to receiving the results of susceptibility tests as deemed appropriate by the physician. Ethionamide should be administered with at least one, sometimes two, other drugs to which the organism is known to be susceptible (see **INDICATIONS AND USAGE**). Drugs which have been used as companion agents are rifampin, ethambutol, pyrazinamide, cycloserine, kanamycin, streptomycin, and isoniazid. The usual warnings, precautions, and dosage regimens for these companion drugs should be observed.

Patient compliance is essential to the success of the antituberculosis therapy and to prevent the emergence of drug-resistant organisms. Therefore, patients should adhere to the drug regimen for the full duration of treatment. It is recommended that directly observed therapy be practiced when patients are receiving antituberculous medication. Additional consultation from experts in the treatment of drug-resistant tuberculosis is recommended when patients develop drug-resistant organisms.

PRECAUTIONS

General

Ethionamide may potentiate the adverse effects of the other antituberculous drugs administered concomitantly (see **Drug Interactions**). Ophthalmologic examinations (including ophthalmoscopy) should be performed before and periodically during therapy with Trecator.

Information For Patients

Patients should be advised to consult their physician should blurred vision or any loss of vision, with or without eye pain, occur during treatment.

Excessive ethanol ingestion should be avoided because a psychotic reaction has been reported.

Laboratory Tests

Determination of serum transaminases (SGOT, SGPT) should be made prior to initiation of therapy and should be monitored monthly. If serum transaminases become elevated during therapy, ethionamide and the companion antituberculosis drug or drugs may be discontinued temporarily until the laboratory abnormalities have resolved. Ethionamide and the companion antituberculosis medication(s) then should be reintroduced sequentially to determine which drug (or drugs) is (are) responsible for the hepatotoxicity.

Blood glucose determinations should be made prior to and periodically throughout therapy with Trecator. Diabetic patients should be particularly alert for episodes of hypoglycemia.

Periodic monitoring of thyroid function tests is recommended as hypothyroidism, with or without goiter, has been reported with ethionamide therapy.

Drug Interactions

Trecator has been found to temporarily raise serum concentrations of isoniazid. Trecator may potentiate the adverse effects of other antituberculous drugs administered concomitantly. In particular, convulsions have been reported when ethionamide is administered with cycloserine and special care should be taken when the treatment regimen includes both of these drugs. Excessive ethanol ingestion should be avoided because a psychotic reaction has been reported.

Carcinogenesis, Mutagenesis, Impairment of Fertility

Teratogenic Effects: Pregnancy Category C

Animal studies conducted with Trecator indicate that the drug has teratogenic potential in rabbits and rats. The doses used in these studies on a mg/kg basis were considerably in excess of those recommended in humans. There are no adequate and well-controlled studies in pregnant women. Because of these animal studies, however, it must be recommended that Trecator be withheld from women who are pregnant, or who are likely to become pregnant while under therapy, unless the prescribing physician considers it to be an essential part of the treatment.

Labor and Delivery

The effect of Trecator on labor and delivery in pregnant women is unknown.

Nursing Mothers

Because no information is available on the excretion of ethionamide in human milk, Trecator should be adminis-

Continued on next page

Trecator—Cont.

tered to nursing mothers only if the benefits outweigh the risks. Newborns who are breast-fed by mothers who are taking Trecator should be monitored for adverse effects.

Pediatric Use

Due to the fact that pulmonary tuberculosis resistant to primary therapy is rarely found in neonates, infants, and children, investigations have been limited in these age groups. At present, the drug should not be used in pediatric patients under 12 years of age except when the organisms are definitely resistant to primary therapy and systemic dissemination of the disease, or other life-threatening complications of tuberculosis, is judged to be imminent.

ADVERSE REACTIONS

Gastrointestinal: The most common side effects of ethionamide are gastrointestinal disturbances including nausea, vomiting, diarrhea, abdominal pain, excessive salivation, metallic taste, stomatitis, anorexia and weight loss. Adverse gastrointestinal effects appear to be dose related, with approximately 50% of patients unable to tolerate 1 gm as a single dose. Gastrointestinal effects may be minimized by decreasing dosage, by changing the time of drug administration, or by the concurrent administration of an antiemetic agent.

Nervous System: Psychotic disturbances (including mental depression), drowsiness, dizziness, restlessness, headache, and postural hypotension have been reported with ethionamide. Rare reports of peripheral neuritis, optic neuritis, diplopia, blurred vision, and a pellagra-like syndrome also have been reported. Concurrent administration of pyridoxine has been recommended to prevent or relieve neurotoxic effects.

Hepatic: Transient increases in serum bilirubin, SGOT, SGPT; Hepatitis (with or without jaundice).

Other: Hypersensitivity reactions including rash, photosensitivity, thrombocytopenia and purpura have been reported rarely. Hypoglycemia, gynecomastia, impotence, and acne also have occurred. The management of patients with diabetes mellitus may become more difficult in those receiving ethionamide.

OVERDOSAGE

No specific information is available on the treatment of overdosage with Trecator. If it should occur, standard procedures to evacuate gastric contents and to support vital functions should be employed.

DOSAGE AND ADMINISTRATION

In the treatment of tuberculosis, a major cause of the emergence of drug-resistant organisms, and thus treatment failure, is patient nonadherence to prescribed treatment. Treatment failure and drug-resistant organisms can be life-threatening and may result in other serious health risks. It is, therefore, important that patients adhere to the drug regimen for the full duration of treatment. Directly observed therapy is recommended when patients are receiving treatment for tuberculosis. Consultation with an expert in the treatment of drug-resistant tuberculosis is advised for patients in whom drug-resistant tuberculosis is suspected or likely. Ethionamide should be administered with at least one, sometimes two, other drugs to which the organism is known to be susceptible (see **INDICATIONS AND USAGE**).

Trecator is administered orally. The usual adult dose is 15 to 20 mg/kg/day, administered once daily or, if patient exhibits poor gastrointestinal tolerance, in divided doses, with a maximum daily dosage of 1 gram.

Trecator tablets have been reformulated from a sugarcoated tablet to a film-coated tablet. Patients should be monitored and have their dosage retitrated when switching from the sugar-coated tablet to the film-coated tablet (see **CLINICAL PHARMACOLOGY**).

Therapy should be initiated at a dose of 250 mg daily, with gradual titration to optimal doses as tolerated by the patient. A regimen of 250 mg daily for 1 or 2 days, followed by 250 mg twice daily for 1 or 2 days with a subsequent increase to 1 gm in 3 or 4 divided doses has been reported.[4,5] Thus far, there is insufficient evidence to indicate the lowest effective dosage levels. Therefore, in order to minimize the risk of resistance developing to the drug or to the companion drug, the principle of giving the highest tolerated dose (based on gastrointestinal intolerance) has been followed. In the adult this would seem to be between 0.5 and 1.0 gm daily, with an average of 0.75 gm daily.

The optimum dosage for pediatric patients has not been established. However, pediatric dosages of 10 to 20 mg/kg p.o. daily in 2 or 3 divided doses given after meals or 15 mg/kg/24 hrs as a single daily dose have been recommended.[1,2] As with adults, ethionamide may be administered to pediatric patients once daily. It should be noted that in patients with concomitant tuberculosis and HIV infection, malabsorption syndrome may be present. Drug malabsorption should be suspected in patients who adhere to therapy, but who fail to respond appropriately. In such cases, consideration should be given to therapeutic drug monitoring (see **CLINICAL PHARMACOLOGY**).

The best times of administration are those which the individual patient finds most suitable in order to avoid or minimize gastrointestinal intolerance, which is usually at mealtimes. Every effort should be made to encourage patients to persevere with treatment when gastrointestinal side effects appear, since they may diminish in severity as treatment proceeds.

Concomitant administration of pyridoxine is recommended. Duration of treatment should be based on individual clinical response. In general, continue therapy until bacteriological conversion has become permanent and maximal clinical improvement has occurred.

HOW SUPPLIED

Trecator® (ethionamide tablets, USP) are supplied in bottles of 100 tablets as follows:

250 mg, orange film-coated tablet marked "W" on one side and "4117" on reverse side, NDC 0008-4117-01.

Store at controlled room temperature 20° to 25°C (68° to 77°F). Dispense in a tight container.

REFERENCES

1) Feigin, R.D., and Cherry, J.D.: Textbook of Pediatric Infectious Diseases, 2nd Edition. Philadelphia, W.B. Saunders Co., 1987, pp. 1371-1372.

2) Nelson, W.E., Behrman, R.E., Vaughan, V.C. (eds.): Nelson Textbook of Pediatrics, 13th edition. Philadelphia, W.B. Saunders Co., 1987, p.636.

3) Treatment of Tuberculosis and Tuberculosis Infection in Adults and Children, Am J Respiratory and Critical Care Medicine, 149:1359-1374, 1994.

4) Peloquin, CA: Pharmacology of the Antimycobacterial Drugs, Med Clin North Am 77(6): 1230-1262, 1993.

5) American Thoracic Society. Am J Respir Crit Care Med 1997;156:S1-S25.

Wyeth®
Manufactured for
Wyeth Pharmaceuticals Inc.   W10479C003
Philadelphia, PA 19101   ET01
By OSG Norwich Pharmaceuticals Inc.   Rev 02/05
Norwich, New York 13815

REVISED INFORMATION

As new research data and clinical findings become available, the product information in *PDR* is revised accordingly. Revisions submitted since the 2005 edition went to press can be found below. To remind yourself of a revision, write "See Supplement A" next to the product's heading in the book.

Abbott Laboratories
Pharmaceutical Products Division
NORTH CHICAGO, IL 60064, U.S.A.

Pharmaceutical Products Division—
Direct Inquiries to:
Customer Service:
(800) 255-5162
Technical Services:
(800) 441-4987
For Medical Information Contact:
Generally:
(800) 633-9110
Adverse experiences or side effects
(for all Abbott drug products):
(800) 633-9110
Sales and Ordering:
(800) 255-5162

TRICOR® 48 mg and 145 mg
[tri cŏr]
(fenofibrate tablets)
℞ only

Ŗ

Prescribing information for this product, which appears on pages 523–526 of the 2005 PDR, has been completely revised as follows. Please write "See Supplement A" next to the product heading.

DESCRIPTION
TRICOR (fenofibrate tablets), is a lipid regulating agent available as tablets for oral administration. Each tablet contains 48 mg or 145 mg of fenofibrate. The chemical name for fenofibrate is 2-[4-(4-chlorobenzoyl) phenoxy]-2-methyl-propanoic acid, 1-methylethyl ester with the following structural formula:

The empirical formula is $C_{20}H_{21}O_4Cl$ and the molecular weight is 360.83; fenofibrate is insoluble in water. The melting point is 79-82°C. Fenofibrate is a white solid which is stable under ordinary conditions.
Inactive Ingredients: Each tablet contains hypromellose 2910 (3cps), docusate sodium, sucrose, sodium lauryl sulfate, lactose monohydrate, silicified microcrystalline cellulose, crospovidone, and magnesium stearate.
In addition, individual tablets contain:
48 mg tablets: polyvinyl alcohol, titanium dioxide, talc, soybean lecithin, xanthan gum, D&C Yellow #10 aluminum lake, FD&C Yellow #6/sunset yellow FCF aluminum lake, FD&C Blue #2/indigo carmine aluminum lake. 145 mg tablets: polyvinyl alcohol, titanium dioxide, talc, soybean lecithin, xanthan gum.

CLINICAL PHARMACOLOGY
A variety of clinical studies have demonstrated that elevated levels of total cholesterol (total-C), low density lipoprotein cholesterol (LDL-C), and apolipoprotein B (apo B), an LDL membrane complex, are associated with human atherosclerosis. Similarly, decreased levels of high density lipoprotein cholesterol (HDL-C) and its transport complex, apolipoprotein A (apo AI and apo AII) are associated with the development of atherosclerosis. Epidemiologic investigations have established that cardiovascular morbidity and mortality vary directly with the level of total-C, LDL-C, and triglycerides, and inversely with the level of HDL-C. The independent effect of raising HDL-C or lowering triglycerides (TG) on the risk of cardiovascular morbidity and mortality has not been determined.
Fenofibric acid, the active metabolite of fenofibrate, produces reductions in total cholesterol, LDL cholesterol, apo-

lipoprotein B, total triglycerides and triglyceride rich lipoprotein (VLDL) in treated patients. In addition, treatment with fenofibrate results in increases in high density lipoprotein (HDL) and apoproteins apoAI and apoAII.
The effects of fenofibric acid seen in clinical practice have been explained *in vivo* in transgenic mice and *in vitro* in human hepatocyte cultures by the activation of peroxisome proliferator activated receptor α (PPARα). Through this mechanism, fenofibrate increases lipolysis and elimination of triglyceride-rich particles from plasma by activating lipoprotein lipase and reducing production of apoprotein C-III (an inhibitor of lipoprotein lipase activity).
The resulting fall in triglycerides produces an alteration in the size and composition of LDL from small, dense particles (which are thought to be atherogenic due to their susceptibility to oxidation), to large buoyant particles. These larger particles have a greater affinity for cholesterol receptors and are catabolized rapidly. Activation of PPARα also induces an increase in the synthesis of apoproteins A-I, A-II and HDL-cholesterol.
Fenofibrate also reduces serum uric acid levels in hyperuricemic and normal individuals by increasing the urinary excretion of uric acid.

Pharmacokinetics/Metabolism
Plasma concentrations of fenofibric acid after administration of three 48 mg or one 145 mg tablets are equivalent under fed conditions to one 200 mg capsule.

Absorption
The absolute bioavailability of fenofibrate cannot be determined as the compound is virtually insoluble in aqueous media suitable for injection. However, fenofibrate is well absorbed from the gastrointestinal tract. Following oral administration in healthy volunteers, approximately 60% of a single dose of radiolabelled fenofibrate appeared in urine, primarily as fenofibric acid and its glucuronate conjugate, and 25% was excreted in the feces. Peak plasma levels of fenofibric acid occur within 6 to 8 hours after administration.
Exposure to fenofibric acid in plasma, as measured by C_{max} and AUC, is not significantly different when a single 145 mg dose of fenofibrate is administered under fasting or nonfasting conditions.

Distribution
In healthy volunteers, steady-state plasma levels of fenofibric acid were shown to be achieved within 5 days of dosing and did not demonstrate accumulation across time following multiple dose administration. Serum protein binding was approximately 99% in normal and hyperlipidemic subjects.

Metabolism
Following oral administration, fenofibrate is rapidly hydrolyzed by esterases to the active metabolite, fenofibric acid; no unchanged fenofibrate is detected in plasma.
Fenofibric acid is primarily conjugated with glucuronic acid and then excreted in urine. A small amount of fenofibric acid is reduced at the carbonyl moiety to a benzhydrol metabolite which is, in turn, conjugated with glucuronic acid and excreted in urine.
In vivo metabolism data indicate that neither fenofibrate nor fenofibric acid undergo oxidative metabolism (e.g., cytochrome P450) to a significant extent.

Excretion
After absorption, fenofibrate is mainly excreted in the urine in the form of metabolites, primarily fenofibric acid and fenofibric acid glucuronide. After administration of radiolabelled fenofibrate, approximately 60% of the dose appeared in the urine and 25% was excreted in the feces.
Fenofibric acid is eliminated with a half-life of 20 hours, allowing once daily administration in a clinical setting.

Special Populations
Geriatrics
In elderly volunteers 77-87 years of age, the oral clearance of fenofibric acid following a single oral dose of fenofibrate was 1.2 L/h, which compares to 1.1 L/h in young adults. This

indicates that a similar dosage regimen can be used in the elderly, without increasing accumulation of the drug or metabolites.
Pediatrics
TRICOR has not been investigated in adequate and well-controlled trials in pediatric patients.
Gender
No pharmacokinetic difference between males and females has been observed for fenofibrate.
Race
The influence of race on the pharmacokinetics of fenofibrate has not been studied, however fenofibrate is not metabolized by enzymes known for exhibiting inter-ethnic variability. Therefore, inter-ethnic pharmacokinetic differences are very unlikely.
Renal insufficiency
In a study in patients with severe renal impairment (creatinine clearance < 50 mL/min), the rate of clearance of fenofibric acid was greatly reduced, and the compound accumulated during chronic dosage. However, in patients having moderate renal impairment (creatinine clearance of 50 to 90 mL/min), the oral clearance and the oral volume of distribution of fenofibric acid are increased compared to healthy adults (2.1 L/h and 95 L versus 1.1 L/h and 30 L, respectively). Therefore, the dosage of TRICOR should be minimized in patients who have severe renal impairment, while no modification of dosage is required in patients having moderate renal impairment.
Hepatic insufficiency
No pharmacokinetic studies have been conducted in patients having hepatic insufficiency.
Drug-drug interactions
In vitro studies using human liver microsomes indicate that fenofibrate and fenofibric acid are not inhibitors of cytochrome (CYP) P450 isoforms CYP3A4, CYP2D6, CYP2E1, or CYP1A2. They are weak inhibitors of CYP2C19 and CYP2A6, and mild-to-moderate inhibitors of CYP2C9 at therapeutic concentrations.
Potentiation of coumarin-type anticoagulants has been observed with prolongation of the prothrombin time/INR.
Bile acid sequestrants have been shown to bind other drugs given concurrently. Therefore, fenofibrate should be taken at least 1 hour before or 4-6 hours after a bile acid binding resin to avoid impeding its absorption. (See WARNINGS and PRECAUTIONS).
Concomitant administration of fenofibrate (equivalent to 145 mg TRICOR) with pravastatin (40 mg) once daily for 10 days has been shown to increase the mean C_{max} and AUC values for pravastatin by 36% (range from 69% decrease to 321% increase) and 28% (range from 54% decrease to 128% increase), respectively, and for 3α-hydroxy-iso-pravastatin by 55% (range from 32% decrease to 314% increase) and 39% (range from 24% decrease to 261% increase), respectively in 23 healthy adults.
A single dose of pravastatin had no clinically important effect on the pharmacokinetics of fenofibric acid.
Concomitant administration of fenofibrate (equivalent to 145 mg TRICOR) with atorvastatin (20 mg) once daily for 10 days resulted in approximately 17% decrease (range from 67% decrease to 44% increase) in atorvastatin AUC values in 22 healthy males. The atorvastatin C_{max} values were not significantly affected by fenofibrate. The pharmacokinetics of fenofibric acid were not significantly affected by atorvastatin.

Clinical Trials

Hypercholesterolemia (Heterozygous Familial and Nonfamilial) and Mixed Dyslipidemia (Fredrickson Types IIa and IIb)
The effects of fenofibrate at a dose equivalent to 145 mg TRICOR (fenofibrate tablets) per day were assessed from four randomized, placebo-controlled, double-blind, parallel-group studies including patients with the following mean

Continued on next page

Tricor—Cont.

baseline lipid values: total-C 306.9 mg/dL; LDL-C 213.8 mg/dL; HDL-C 52.3 mg/dL; and triglycerides 191.0 mg/dL. TRICOR therapy lowered LDL-C, Total-C, and the LDL-C/HDL-C ratio. TRICOR therapy also lowered triglycerides and raised HDL-C (see Table 1).
[See table 1 at right]

In a subset of the subjects, measurements of apo B were conducted. TRICOR treatment significantly reduced apo B from baseline to endpoint as compared with placebo (-25.1% vs. 2.4%, p<0.0001, n=213 and 143 respectively).

Hypertriglyceridemia (Fredrickson Type IV and V)

The effects of fenofibrate on serum triglycerides were studied in two randomized, double-blind, placebo-controlled clinical trials[1] of 147 hypertriglyceridemic patients (Fredrickson Types IV and V). Patients were treated for eight weeks under protocols that differed only in that one entered patients with baseline triglyceride (TG) levels of 500 to 1500 mg/dL, and the other TG levels of 350 to 500 mg/dL. In patients with hypertriglyceridemia and normal cholesterolemia with or without hyperchylomicronemia (Type IV/V hyperlipidemia), treatment with fenofibrate at dosages equivalent to 145 mg TRICOR per day decreased primarily very low density lipoprotein (VLDL) triglycerides and VLDL cholesterol. Treatment of patients with Type IV hyperlipoproteinemia and elevated triglycerides often results in an increase of low density lipoprotein (LDL) cholesterol (see Table 2).
[See table 2 at right]

The effect of TRICOR on cardiovascular morbidity and mortality has not been determined.

INDICATIONS AND USAGE

Treatment of Hypercholesterolemia

TRICOR is indicated as adjunctive therapy to diet to reduce elevated LDL-C, Total-C, Triglycerides and Apo B, and to increase HDL-C in adult patients with primary hypercholesterolemia or mixed dyslipidemia (Fredrickson Types IIa and IIb). Lipid-altering agents should be used in addition to a diet restricted in saturated fat and cholesterol when response to diet and non-pharmacological interventions alone has been inadequate (see National Cholesterol Education Program [NCEP] Treatment Guidelines, below).

Treatment of Hypertriglyceridemia

TRICOR is also indicated as adjunctive therapy to diet for treatment of adult patients with hypertriglyceridemia (Fredrickson Types IV and V hyperlipidemia). Improving glycemic control in diabetic patients showing fasting chylomicronemia will usually reduce fasting triglycerides and eliminate chylomicronemia thereby obviating the need for pharmacologic intervention.

Markedly elevated levels of serum triglycerides (e.g. > 2,000 mg/dL) may increase the risk of developing pancreatitis. The effect of TRICOR therapy on reducing this risk has not been adequately studied.

Drug therapy is not indicated for patients with Type I hyperlipoproteinemia, who have elevations of chylomicrons and plasma triglycerides, but who have normal levels of very low density lipoprotein (VLDL). Inspection of plasma refrigerated for 14 hours is helpful in distinguishing Types I, IV and V hyperlipoproteinemia[2].

The initial treatment for dyslipidemia is dietary therapy specific for the type of lipoprotein abnormality. Excess body weight and excess alcoholic intake may be important factors in hypertriglyceridemia and should be addressed prior to any drug therapy. Physical exercise can be an important ancillary measure. Diseases contributory to hyperlipidemia, such as hypothyroidism or diabetes mellitus should be looked for and adequately treated. Estrogen therapy, thiazide diuretics and beta-blockers, are sometimes associated with massive rises in plasma triglycerides, especially in subjects with familial hypertriglyceridemia. In such cases, discontinuation of the specific etiologic agent may obviate the need for specific drug therapy of hypertriglyceridemia. The use of drugs should be considered only when reasonable attempts have been made to obtain satisfactory results with non-drug methods. If the decision is made to use drugs, the patient should be instructed that this does not reduce the importance of adhering to diet. (See WARNINGS and PRECAUTIONS).

Fredrickson Classification of Hyperlipoproteinemias

Type	Lipoprotein Elevated	Lipid Elevation Major	Lipid Elevation Minor
I (rare)	chylomicrons	TG	↑↔C
IIa	LDL	C	–
IIb	LDL, VLDL	C	TG
III (rare)	IDL	C, TG	–
IV	VLDL	TG	↑↔C
V (rare)	chylomicrons, VLDL	TG	↑↔C

C = cholesterol
TG = triglycerides
LDL = low density lipoprotein
VLDL = very low density lipoprotein
IDL = intermediate density lipoprotein

[See third table at right]

After the LDL-C goal has been achieved, if the TG is still >200 mg/dL, non HDL-C (total-C minus HDL-C) becomes a secondary target of therapy. Non-HDL-C goals are set 30 mg/dL higher than LDL-C goals for each risk category.

CONTRAINDICATIONS

TRICOR is contraindicated in patients who exhibit hypersensitivity to fenofibrate.

TRICOR is contraindicated in patients with hepatic or severe renal dysfunction, including primary biliary cirrhosis, and patients with unexplained persistent liver function abnormality.

TRICOR is contraindicated in patients with preexisting gallbladder disease (see WARNINGS).

WARNINGS

Liver Function: Fenofibrate at doses equivalent to 96 mg to 145 mg TRICOR per day has been associated with increases in serum transaminases [AST (SGOT) or ALT (SGPT)]. In a pooled analysis of 10 placebo-controlled trials, increases to > 3 times the upper limit of normal occurred in 5.3% of patients taking fenofibrate versus 1.1% of patients treated with placebo.

When transaminase determinations were followed either after discontinuation of treatment or during continued treatment, a return to normal limits was usually observed. The incidence of increases in transaminases related to fenofibrate therapy appear to be dose related. In an 8-week dose-ranging study, the incidence of ALT or AST elevations to at least three times the upper limit of normal was 13% in patients receiving dosages equivalent to 96 mg to 145 mg TRICOR per day and was 0% in those receiving dosages equivalent to 48 mg or less TRICOR per day, or placebo. Hepatocellular, chronic active and cholestatic hepatitis associated with fenofibrate therapy have been reported after exposures of weeks to several years. In extremely rare cases, cirrhosis has been reported in association with chronic active hepatitis.

Regular periodic monitoring of liver function, including serum ALT (SGPT) should be performed for the duration of therapy with TRICOR, and therapy discontinued if enzyme levels persist above three times the normal limit.

Table 1
Mean Percent Change in Lipid Parameters at End of Treatment[†]

Treatment Group	Total-C	LDL-C	HDL-C	TG
Pooled Cohort				
Mean baseline lipid values (n=646)	306.9 mg/dL	213.8 mg/dL	52.3 mg/dL	191.0 mg/dL
All FEN (n=361)	-18.7%*	-20.6%*	+11.0%*	-28.9%*
Placebo (n=285)	-0.4%	-2.2%	+0.7%	+7.7%
Baseline LDL-C > 160 mg/dL and TG < 150 mg/dL (Type IIa)				
Mean baseline lipid values (n=334)	307.7 mg/dL	227.7 mg/dL	58.1 mg/dL	101.7 mg/dL
All FEN (n=193)	-22.4%*	-31.4%*	+9.8%*	-23.5%*
Placebo (n=141)	+0.2%	-2.2%	+2.6%	+11.7%
Baseline LDL-C > 160 mg/dL and TG ≥ 150 mg/dL (Type IIb)				
Mean baseline lipid values (n=242)	312.8 mg/dL	219.8 mg/dL	46.7 mg/dL	231.9 mg/dL
All FEN (n=126)	-16.8%*	-20.1%*	+14.6%*	-35.9%*
Placebo (n=116)	-3.0%	-6.6%	+2.3%	+0.9%

[†]Duration of study treatment was 3 to 6 months.
*p= <0.05 vs. Placebo

Table 2
Effects of TRICOR in Patients With Fredrickson Type IV/V Hyperlipidemia

Study 1	Placebo				TRICOR			
Baseline TG levels 350 to 499 mg/dL	N	Baseline (Mean)	Endpoint (Mean)	% Change (Mean)	N	Baseline (Mean)	Endpoint (Mean)	% Change (Mean)
Triglycerides	28	449	450	-0.5	27	432	223	-46.2*
VLDL Triglycerides	19	367	350	2.7	19	350	178	-44.1*
Total Cholesterol	28	255	261	2.8	27	252	227	-9.1*
HDL Cholesterol	28	35	36	4	27	34	40	19.6*
LDL Cholesterol	28	120	129	12	27	128	137	14.5
VLDL Cholesterol	27	99	99	5.8	27	92	46	-44.7*

Study 2	Placebo				TRICOR			
Baseline TG levels 500 to 1500 mg/dL	N	Baseline (Mean)	Endpoint (Mean)	% Change (Mean)	N	Baseline (Mean)	Endpoint (Mean)	% Change (Mean)
Triglycerides	44	710	750	7.2	48	726	308	-54.5*
VLDL Triglycerides	29	537	571	18.7	33	543	205	-50.6*
Total Cholesterol	44	272	271	0.4	48	261	223	-13.8*
HDL Cholesterol	44	27	28	5.0	48	30	36	22.9*
LDL Cholesterol	42	100	90	-4.2	45	103	131	45.0*
VLDL Cholesterol	42	137	142	11.0	45	126	54	-49.4*

* = p<0.05 vs. Placebo

NCEP Treatment Guidelines: LDL-C Goals and Cutpoints for Therapeutic Lifestyle Changes and Drug Therapy in Different Risk Categories

Risk Category	LDL Goal (mg/dL)	LDL Level at Which to Initiate Therapeutic Lifestyle Changes (mg/dL)	LDL Level at which to Consider Drug Therapy (mg/dL)
CHD[†] or CHD risk equivalents (10-years risk >20%)	<100	≥100	≥130 (100-129:drug optional)[††]
2+ Risk Factors (10-years risk ≤20%)	<130	≥130	10-year risk 10%-20%:≥130 10-Year risk <10%: ≥160
0-1 Risk Factor[†††]	<160	≥160	≥190 (160-189: LDL-lowering drug optional)

[†] CHD = coronary heart disease
[††] Some authorities recommend use of LDL-lowering drugs in this category if an LDL-C level of <100 mg/dL cannot be achieved by therapeutic lifestyle changes. Others prefer use of drugs that primarily modify triglycerides and HDL-C, e.g., nicotinic acid or fibrate. Clinical judgement also may call for deferring drug therapy in this subcategory.
[†††] Almost all people with 0-1 risk factor have 10-year risk <10%; thus, 10-year risk assessment in people with 0-1 risk factor is not necessary.

Cholelithiasis: Fenofibrate, like clofibrate and gemfibrozil, may increase cholesterol excretion into the bile, leading to cholelithiasis. If cholelithiasis is suspected, gallbladder studies are indicated. TRICOR therapy should be discontinued if gallstones are found.

Concomitant Oral Anticoagulants: Caution should be exercised when anticoagulants are given in conjunction with TRICOR because of the potentiation of coumarin-type anticoagulants in prolonging the prothrombin time/INR. The dosage of the anticoagulant should be reduced to maintain the prothrombin time/INR at the desired level to prevent bleeding complications. Frequent prothrombin time/INR determinations are advisable until it has been definitely determined that the prothrombin time/INR has stabilized.

Concomitant HMG-CoA Reductase Inhibitors: The combined use of TRICOR and HMG-CoA reductase inhibitors should be avoided unless the benefit of further alterations in lipid levels is likely to outweigh the increased risk of this drug combination.

Concomitant administration of fenofibrate (equivalent to 145 mg TRICOR) and pravastatin (40 mg) once daily for 10 days increased the mean C_{max} and AUC values for pravastatin by 36% (range from 69% decrease to 321% increase) and 28% (range from 54% decrease to 128% increase), respectively, and for 3α-hydroxy-iso-pravastatin by 55% (range from 32% decrease to 314% increase) and 39% (range from 24% decrease to 261% increase), respectively. (See also **CLINICAL PHARMACOLOGY**, Drug-drug interactions).

The combined use of fibric acid derivatives and HMG-CoA reductase inhibitors has been associated, in the absence of a marked pharmacokinetic interaction, in numerous case reports, with rhabdomyolysis, markedly elevated creatine kinase (CK) levels and myoglobinuria, leading in a high proportion of cases to acute renal failure.

The use of fibrates alone, including TRICOR, may occasionally be associated with myositis, myopathy, or rhabdomyolysis. Patients receiving TRICOR and complaining of muscle pain, tenderness, or weakness should have prompt medical evaluation for myopathy, including serum creatine kinase level determination. If myopathy/myositis is suspected or diagnosed, TRICOR therapy should be stopped.

Mortality: The effect of TRICOR on coronary heart disease morbidity and mortality and non-cardiovascular mortality has not been established.

Other Considerations: In the Coronary Drug Project, a large study of post myocardial infarction of patients treated for 5 years with clofibrate, there was no difference in mortality seen between the clofibrate group and the placebo group. There was however, a difference in the rate of cholelithiasis and cholecystitis requiring surgery between the two groups (3.0% vs. 1.8%).

Because of chemical, pharmacological, and clinical similarities between TRICOR (fenofibrate tablets), Atromid-S (clofibrate), and Lopid (gemfibrozil), the adverse findings in 4 large randomized, placebo-controlled clinical studies with these other fibrate drugs may also apply to TRICOR.

In a study conducted by the World Health Organization (WHO), 5000 subjects without known coronary artery disease were treated with placebo or clofibrate for 5 years and followed for an additional one year. There was a statistically significant, higher age-adjusted all-cause mortality in the clofibrate group compared with the placebo group (5.70% vs. 3.96%, p=<0.01). Excess mortality was due to a 33% increase in non-cardiovascular causes, including malignancy, post-cholecystectomy complications, and pancreatitis. This appeared to confirm the higher risk of gallbladder disease seen in clofibrate-treated patients studied in the Coronary Drug Project.

The Helsinki Heart Study was a large (n=4081) study of middle-aged men without a history of coronary artery disease. Subjects received either placebo or gemfibrozil for 5 years, with a 3.5 year open extension afterward. Total mortality was numerically higher in the gemfibrozil randomization group but did not achieve statistical significance (p=0.19, 95% confidence interval for relative risk G:P=.91-1.64). Although cancer deaths trended higher in the gemfibrozil group (p=0.11), cancers (excluding basal cell carcinoma) were diagnosed with equal frequency in both study groups. Due to the limited size of the study, the relative risk of death from any cause was not shown to be different than that seen in the 9 year follow-up data from World Health Organization study (RR=1.29). Similarly, the numerical excess of gallbladder surgeries in the gemfibrozil group did not differ statistically from that observed in the WHO study.

A secondary prevention component of the Helsinki Heart Study enrolled middle-aged men excluded from the primary prevention study because of known or suspected coronary heart disease. Subjects received gemfibrozil or placebo for 5 years. Although cardiac deaths trended higher in the gemfibrozil group, this was not statistically significant (hazard ratio 2.2, 95% confidence interval: 0.94-5.05). The rate of gallbladder surgery was not statistically significant between study groups, but did trend higher in the gemfibrozil group, (1.9% vs. 0.3%, p=0.07). There was a statistically significant difference in the number of appendectomies in the gemfibrozil group (6/311 vs. 0/317, p=0.029).

PRECAUTIONS

Initial therapy: Laboratory studies should be done to ascertain that the lipid levels are consistently abnormal before instituting TRICOR therapy. Every attempt should be made to control serum lipids with appropriate diet, exercise, weight loss in obese patients, and control of any medical problems such as diabetes mellitus and hypothyroidism that are contributing to the lipid abnormalities. Medications known to exacerbate hypertriglyceridemia (beta-blockers, thiazides, estrogens) should be discontinued or changed if possible prior to consideration of triglyceride-lowering drug therapy.

BODY SYSTEM Adverse Event	Fenofibrate* (N=439)	Placebo (N=365)
BODY AS A WHOLE		
Abdominal Pain	4.6%	4.4%
Back Pain	3.4%	2.5%
Headache	3.2%	2.7%
Asthenia	2.1%	3.0%
Flu Syndrome	2.1%	2.7%
DIGESTIVE		
Liver Function Tests Abnormal	7.5%**	1.4%
Diarrhea	2.3%	4.1%
Nausea	2.3%	1.9%
Constipation	2.1%	1.4%
METABOLIC AND NUTRITIONAL DISORDERS		
SGPT Increased	3.0%	1.6%
Creatine Phosphokinase Increased	3.0%	1.4%
SGOT Increased	3.4%**	0.5%
RESPIRATORY		
Respiratory Disorder	6.2%	5.5%
Rhinitis	2.3%	1.1%

* Dosage equivalent to 145 mg TRICOR
** Significantly different from Placebo

Continued therapy: Periodic determination of serum lipids should be obtained during initial therapy in order to establish the lowest effective dose of TRICOR. Therapy should be withdrawn in patients who do not have an adequate response after two months of treatment with the maximum recommended dose of 145 mg per day.

Pancreatitis: Pancreatitis has been reported in patients taking fenofibrate, gemfibrozil, and clofibrate. This occurrence may represent a failure of efficacy in patients with severe hypertriglyceridemia, a direct drug effect, or a secondary phenomenon mediated through biliary tract stone or sludge formation with obstruction of the common bile duct.

Hypersensitivity Reactions: Acute hypersensitivity reactions including severe skin rashes requiring patient hospitalization and treatment with steroids have occurred very rarely during treatment with fenofibrate, including rare spontaneous reports of Stevens-Johnson syndrome, and toxic epidermal necrolysis. Urticaria was seen in 1.1 vs. 0%, and rash in 1.4 vs. 0.8% of fenofibrate and placebo patients respectively in controlled trials.

Hematologic Changes: Mild to moderate hemoglobin, hematocrit, and white blood cell decreases have been observed in patients following initiation of fenofibrate therapy. However, these levels stabilize during long-term administration. Extremely rare spontaneous reports of thrombocytopenia and agranulocytosis have been received during post-marketing surveillance outside of the U.S. Periodic blood counts are recommended during the first 12 months of TRICOR administration.

Skeletal muscle: The use of fibrates alone, including TRICOR, may occasionally be associated with myopathy. Treatment with drugs of the fibrate class has been associated on rare occasions with rhabdomyolysis, usually in patients with impaired renal function. Myopathy should be considered in any patient with diffuse myalgias, muscle tenderness or weakness, and/or marked elevations of creatine phosphokinase levels.

Patients should be advised to report promptly unexplained muscle pain, tenderness or weakness, particularly if accompanied by malaise or fever. CPK levels should be assessed in patients reporting these symptoms, and fenofibrate therapy should be discontinued if markedly elevated CPK levels occur or myopathy is diagnosed.

Drug Interactions

Oral Anticoagulants: CAUTION SHOULD BE EXERCISED WHEN COUMARIN ANTICOAGULANTS ARE GIVEN IN CONJUNCTION WITH TRICOR. THE DOSAGE OF THE ANTICOAGULANTS SHOULD BE REDUCED TO MAINTAIN THE PROTHROMBIN TIME/INR AT THE DESIRED LEVEL TO PREVENT BLEEDING COMPLICATIONS. FREQUENT PROTHROMBIN TIME/INR DETERMINATIONS ARE ADVISABLE UNTIL IT HAS BEEN DEFINITELY DETERMINED THAT THE PROTHROMBIN TIME/INR HAS STABILIZED.

HMG-CoA reductase inhibitors: The combined use of TRICOR and HMG-CoA reductase inhibitors should be avoided unless the benefit of further alterations in lipid levels is likely to outweigh the increased risk of this drug combination (see WARNINGS).

Resins: Since bile acid sequestrants may bind other drugs given concurrently, patients should take TRICOR at least 1 hour before or 4-6 hours after a bile acid binding resin to avoid impeding its absorption.

Cyclosporine: Because cyclosporine can produce nephrotoxicity with decreases in creatinine clearance and rises in serum creatinine, and because renal excretion is the primary elimination route of fibrate drugs including TRICOR, there is a risk that an interaction will lead to deterioration. The benefits and risks of using TRICOR (fenofibrate tablets) with immunosuppressants and other potentially nephrotoxic agents should be carefully considered, and the lowest effective dose employed.

Carcinogenesis, Mutagenesis, Impairment of Fertility: Two dietary carcinogenicity studies have been conducted in rats with fenofibrate. In the first 24-month study, rats were dosed with fenofibrate at 10, 45, and 200 mg/kg/day, approximately 0.3, 1, and 6 times the maximum recommended human dose (MRHD) of 145 mg/day, based on mg/meter^2 of surface area). At a dose of 200 mg/kg/day (at 6 times the MRHD), the incidence of liver carcinomas was significantly increased in both sexes. A statistically significant increase in pancreatic carcinomas was observed in males at 1 and 6 times the MRHD; an increase in pancreatic adenomas and benign testicular interstitial cell tumors was observed at 6 times the MRHD in males. In a second 24-month study in a different strain of rats, doses of 10 and 60 mg/kg/day (0.3 and 2 times the MRHD based on mg/meter^2 surface area) produced significant increases in the incidence of pancreatic acinar adenomas in both sexes and increases in testicular interstitial cell tumors in males at 2 times the MRHD (200 mg/kg/day).

A 117-week carcinogenicity study was conducted in rats comparing three drugs: fenofibrate 10 and 60 mg/kg/day (0.3 and 2 times the MRHD), clofibrate (400 mg/kg/day; 2 times the human dose), and Gemfibrozil (250 mg/kg/day; 2 times the human dose) (multiples based on mg/meter^2 surface area). Fenofibrate increased pancreatic acinar adenomas in both sexes. Clofibrate increased hepatocellular carcinoma and pancreatic acinar adenomas in males and hepatic neoplastic nodules in females. Gemfibrozil increased hepatic neoplastic nodules in males and females, while all three drugs increased testicular interstitial cell tumors in males.

In a 21-month study in mice, fenofibrate 10, 45, and 200 mg/kg/day (approximately 0.2, 0.7, and 3 times the MRHD on the basis of mg/meter^2 surface area) significantly increased the liver carcinomas in both sexes at 3 times the MRHD. In a second 18-month study at the same doses, fenofibrate significantly increased the liver carcinomas in male mice and liver adenomas in female mice at 3 times the MRHD.

Electron microscopy studies have demonstrated peroxisomal proliferation following fenofibrate administration to the rat. An adequate study to test for peroxisome proliferation in humans has not been done, but changes in peroxisome morphology and numbers have been observed in humans after treatment with other members of the fibrate class when liver biopsies were compared before and after treatment in the same individual.

Fenofibrate has been demonstrated to be devoid of mutagenic potential in the following tests: Ames, mouse lymphoma, chromosomal aberration and unscheduled DNA synthesis.

Pregnancy Category C: Safety in pregnant women has not been established. Fenofibrate has been shown to be embryocidal and teratogenic in rats when given in doses 7 to 10 times the maximum recommended human dose (MRHD) and embryocidal in rabbits when given at 9 times the MRHD (on the basis of mg/meter^2 surface area). There are no adequate and well-controlled studies in pregnant women. Fenofibrate should be used during pregnancy only if the potential benefit justifies the potential risk to the fetus.

Administration of approximately 9 times the MRHD of 145mg/day of fenofibrate to female rats before and throughout gestation caused 100% of dams to delay delivery and resulted in a 60% increase in post-implantation loss, a decrease in litter size, a decrease in birth weight, a 40% survival of pups at birth, a 4% survival of pups as neonates, and a 0% survival of pups to weaning, and an increase in spina bifida.

Administration of approximately 10 times the MRHD to female rats on days 6-15 of gestation caused an increase in gross, visceral and skeletal findings in fetuses (domed head/hunched shoulders/rounded body/abnormal chest, kyphosis, stunted fetuses, elongated sternal ribs, malformed sternebrae, extra foramen in palatine, misshapen vertebrae, supernumerary ribs).

Administration of approximately 7 times the MRHD to female rats from day 15 of gestation through weaning caused a delay in delivery, a 40% decrease in live births, a 75% decrease in neonatal survival, and decreases in pup weight, at birth as well as on days 4 and 21 post-partum.

Administration of fenofibrate at 9 to 18 times the MRHD to female rabbits caused abortions in 10% to 25% of dams and death in 7% of fetuses at 18 times the MRHD.

Nursing mothers: Fenofibrate should not be used in nursing mothers. Because of the potential for tumorigenicity

Continued on next page

Tricor—Cont.

seen in animal studies, a decision should be made whether to discontinue nursing or to discontinue the drug.

Pediatric Use: Safety and efficacy in pediatric patients have not been established.

Geriatric Use: Fenofibric acid is known to be substantially excreted by the kidney, and the risk of adverse reactions to this drug may be greater in patients with impaired renal function. Because elderly patients are more likely to have decreased renal function, care should be taken in dose selection.

ADVERSE REACTIONS

CLINICAL: Adverse events reported by 2% or more of patients treated with fenofibrate during the double-blind, placebo-controlled trials, regardless of causality, are listed in the table below. Adverse events led to discontinuation of treatment in 5.0% of patients treated with fenofibrate and in 3.0% treated with placebo. Increases in liver function tests were the most frequent events, causing discontinuation of fenofibrate treatment in 1.6% of patients in double-blind trials.

[See table at top of previous page]

Additional adverse events reported by three or more patients in placebo-controlled trials or reported in other controlled or open trials, regardless of causality are listed below.

BODY AS A WHOLE: Chest pain, pain (unspecified), infection, malaise, allergic reaction, cyst, hernia, fever, photosensitivity reaction, and accidental injury.

CARDIOVASCULAR SYSTEM: Angina pectoris, hypertension, vasodilatation, coronary artery disorder, electrocardiogram abnormal, ventricular extrasystoles, myocardial infarct, peripheral vascular disorder, migraine, varicose vein, cardiovascular disorder, hypotension, palpitation, vascular disorder, arrhythmia, phlebitis, tachycardia, extrasystoles, and atrial fibrillation.

DIGESTIVE SYSTEM: Dyspepsia, flatulence, nausea, increased appetite, gastroenteritis, cholelithiasis, rectal disorder, esophagitis, gastritis, colitis, tooth disorder, vomiting, anorexia, gastrointestinal disorder, duodenal ulcer, nausea and vomiting, peptic ulcer, rectal hemorrhage, liver fatty deposit, cholecystitis, eructation, gamma glutamyl transpeptidase, and diarrhea.

ENDOCRINE SYSTEM: Diabetes mellitus.

HEMIC AND LYMPHATIC SYSTEM: Anemia, leukopenia, ecchymosis, eosinophilia, lymphadenopathy, and thrombocytopenia.

METABOLIC AND NUTRITIONAL DISORDERS: Creatinine increased, weight gain, hypoglycemia, gout, weight loss, edema, hyperuricemia, and peripheral edema.

MUSCULOSKELETAL SYSTEM: Myositis, myalgia, arthralgia, arthritis, tenosynovitis, joint disorder, arthrosis, leg cramps, bursitis, and myasthenia.

NERVOUS SYSTEM: Dizziness, insomnia, depression, vertigo, libido decreased, anxiety, paresthesia, dry mouth, hypertonia, nervousness, neuralgia, and somnolence.

RESPIRATORY SYSTEM: Pharyngitis, bronchitis, cough increased, dyspnea, asthma, allergic pulmonary alveolitis, pneumonia, laryngitis, and sinusitis.

SKIN AND APPENDAGES: Rash, pruritus, eczema, herpes zoster, urticaria, acne, sweating, fungal dermatitis, skin disorder, alopecia, contact dermatitis, herpes simplex, maculopapular rash, nail disorder, and skin ulcer.

SPECIAL SENSES: Conjunctivitis, eye disorder, amblyopia, ear pain, otitis media, abnormal vision, cataract specified, and refraction disorder.

UROGENITAL SYSTEM: Urinary frequency, prostatic disorder, dysuria, abnormal kidney function, urolithiasis, gynecomastia, unintended pregnancy, vaginal moniliasis, and cystitis.

OVERDOSAGE

There is no specific treatment for overdose with TRICOR. General supportive care of the patient is indicated, including monitoring of vital signs and observation of clinical status, should an overdose occur. If indicated, elimination of unabsorbed drug should be achieved by emesis or gastric lavage; usual precautions should be observed to maintain the airway. Because fenofibrate is highly bound to plasma proteins, hemodialysis should not be considered.

DOSAGE AND ADMINISTRATION

Patients should be placed on an appropriate lipid-lowering diet before receiving TRICOR, and should continue this diet during treatment with TRICOR. TRICOR tablets can be given without regard to meals.

For the treatment of adult patients with primary hypercholesterolemia or mixed hyperlipidemia, the initial dose of TRICOR is 145 mg per day.

For adult patients with hypertriglyceridemia, the initial dose is 48 to 145 mg per day. Dosage should be individualized according to patient response, and should be adjusted if necessary following repeat lipid determinations at 4 to 8 week intervals. The maximum dose is 145 mg per day.

Treatment with TRICOR should be initiated at a dose of 48 mg/day in patients having impaired renal function, and increased only after evaluation of the effects on renal function and lipid levels at this dose. In the elderly, the initial dose should likewise be limited to 48 mg/day.

Lipid levels should be monitored periodically and consideration should be given to reducing the dosage of TRICOR if lipid levels fall significantly below the targeted range.

HOW SUPPLIED

TRICOR® (fenofibrate tablets) is available in two strengths:
48 mg yellow tablets, imprinted with a and Abbo-Code identification letters "FI", available in bottles of 90 (NDC 0074-6122-90).
145 mg white tablets, imprinted with a and Abbo-Code identification letters "FO", available in bottles of 90 (NDC 0074-6123-90).

Storage

Store at 25°C (77°F); excursions permitted to 15-30°C (59-86°F) [see USP Controlled Room Temperature]. Keep out of the reach of children. Protect from moisture.

Manufactured for Abbott Laboratories, North Chicago, IL 60064, U.S.A. by Fournier Laboratories Ireland Limited, Anngrove, Carrigtwohill Co. Cork, Ireland

REFERENCES

1. GOLDBERG AC, *et al.* Fenofibrate for the Treatment of Type IV and V Hyperlipoproteinemias: A Double-Blind, Placebo-Controlled Multicenter US Study. *Clinical Therapeutics*, 11, pp. 69-83, 1989.
2. NIKKILA EA. Familial Lipoprotein Lipase Deficiency and Related Disorders of Chylomicron Metabolism. In Stanbury J.B., *et al.* (eds.): *The Metabolic Basis of Inherited Disease*, 5th edition, McGraw-Hill, 1983, Chap. 30, pp. 622-642.
3. BROWN WV, *et al.* Effects of Fenofibrate on Plasma Lipids: Double-Blind, Multicenter Study In Patients with Type IIA or IIB Hyperlipidemia. *Arteriosclerosis*. 6, pp. 670-678, 1986.

Ref.: 03-5344-R1
Revised: November, 2004
ABBOTT LABORATORIES
NORTH CHICAGO, IL 60064, U.S.A.
PRINTED IN U.S.A.

AstraZeneca LP

WILMINGTON, DE 19850-5437

For Product Full Prescribing Information, Business Information, Medical Information, Adverse Drug Experiences, and Customer Service:

Information Center
1-800-236-9933

For Product Ordering:

Trade Customer Service
1-800-842-9920

For Product Full Prescribing Information:

Internet: www.astrazeneca-us.com

ATACAND® ℞

[ăt'-ă-kănd]
(candesartan cilexetil)
TABLETS

Prescribing information for this product, which appears on pages 610–612 of the 2005 PDR, has been completely revised as follows. Please write "See Supplement A" next to the product heading.

USE IN PREGNANCY
When used in pregnancy during the second and third trimesters, drugs that act directly on the renin-angiotensin system can cause injury and even death to the developing fetus. When pregnancy is detected, ATACAND should be discontinued as soon as possible. See WARNINGS, Fetal/Neonatal Morbidity and Mortality.

DESCRIPTION

ATACAND (candesartan cilexetil), a prodrug, is hydrolyzed to candesartan during absorption from the gastrointestinal tract. Candesartan is a selective AT_1 subtype angiotensin II receptor antagonist.

Candesartan cilexetil, a nonpeptide, is chemically described as (±)-1-Hydroxyethyl 2-ethoxy-1-[*p*-(o-1*H*-tetrazol-5-ylphenyl)benzyl]-7-benzimidazolecarboxylate, cyclohexyl carbonate (ester).

Its empirical formula is $C_{33}H_{34}N_6O_6$, and its structural formula is

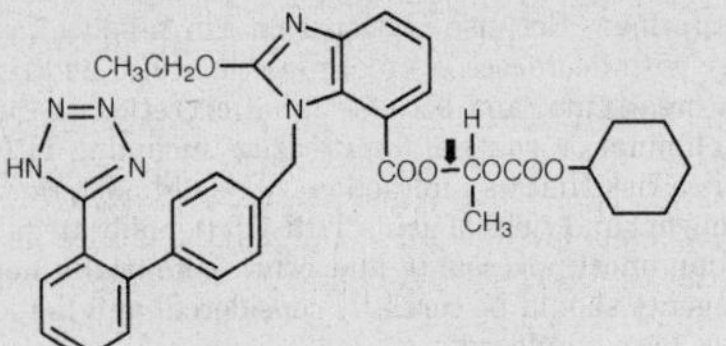

Candesartan cilexetil is a white to off-white powder with a molecular weight of 610.67. It is practically insoluble in water and sparingly soluble in methanol. Candesartan cilexetil is a racemic mixture containing one chiral center at the cyclohexyloxycarbonyloxy ethyl ester group. Following oral administration, candesartan cilexetil undergoes hydrolysis at the ester link to form the active drug, candesartan, which is achiral.

ATACAND is available for oral use as tablets containing either 4 mg, 8 mg, 16 mg, or 32 mg of candesartan cilexetil and the following inactive ingredients: hydroxypropyl cellulose, polyethylene glycol, lactose, corn starch, carboxymethylcellulose calcium, and magnesium stearate. Ferric oxide (reddish brown) is added to the 8-mg, 16-mg, and 32-mg tablets as a colorant.

CLINICAL PHARMACOLOGY

Mechanism of Action

Angiotensin II is formed from angiotensin I in a reaction catalyzed by angiotensin-converting enzyme (ACE, kininase II). Angiotensin II is the principal pressor agent of the renin-angiotensin system, with effects that include vasoconstriction, stimulation of synthesis and release of aldosterone, cardiac stimulation, and renal reabsorption of sodium. Candesartan blocks the vasoconstrictor and aldosterone-secreting effects of angiotensin II by selectively blocking the binding of angiotensin II to the AT_1 receptor in many tissues, such as vascular smooth muscle and the adrenal gland. Its action is, therefore, independent of the pathways for angiotensin II synthesis.

There is also an AT_2 receptor found in many tissues, but AT_2 is not known to be associated with cardiovascular homeostasis. Candesartan has much greater affinity (>10,000-fold) for the AT_1 receptor than for the AT_2 receptor.

Blockade of the renin-angiotensin system with ACE inhibitors, which inhibit the biosynthesis of angiotensin II from angiotensin I, is widely used in the treatment of hypertension. ACE inhibitors also inhibit the degradation of bradykinin, a reaction also catalyzed by ACE. Because candesartan does not inhibit ACE (kininase II), it does not affect the response to bradykinin. Whether this difference has clinical relevance is not known. Candesartan does not bind to or block other hormone receptors or ion channels known to be important in cardiovascular regulation.

Blockade of the angiotensin II receptor inhibits the negative regulatory feedback of angiotensin II on renin secretion, but the resulting increased plasma renin activity and angiotensin II circulating levels do not overcome the effect of candesartan on blood pressure.

Pharmacokinetics

General

Candesartan cilexetil is rapidly and completely bioactivated by ester hydrolysis during absorption from the gastrointestinal tract to candesartan, a selective AT_1 subtype angiotensin II receptor antagonist. Candesartan is mainly excreted unchanged in urine and feces (via bile). It undergoes minor hepatic metabolism by O-deethylation to an inactive metabolite. The elimination half-life of candesartan is approximately 9 hours. After single and repeated administration, the pharmacokinetics of candesartan are linear for oral doses up to 32 mg of candesartan cilexetil. Candesartan and its inactive metabolite do not accumulate in serum upon repeated once-daily dosing.

Following administration of candesartan cilexetil, the absolute bioavailability of candesartan was estimated to be 15%. After tablet ingestion, the peak serum concentration (C_{max}) is reached after 3 to 4 hours. Food with a high fat content does not affect the bioavailability of candesartan after candesartan cilexetil administration.

Metabolism and Excretion

Total plasma clearance of candesartan is 0.37 mL/min/kg, with a renal clearance of 0.19 mL/min/kg. When candesartan is administered orally, about 26% of the dose is excreted unchanged in urine. Following an oral dose of C-labeled candesartan cilexetil, approximately 33% of radioactivity is recovered in urine and approximately 67% in feces. Following an intravenous dose of ^{14}C-labeled candesartan, approximately 59% of radioactivity is recovered in urine and approximately 36% in feces. Biliary excretion contributes to the elimination of candesartan.

Distribution

The volume of distribution of candesartan is 0.13 L/kg. Candesartan is highly bound to plasma proteins (>99%) and does not penetrate red blood cells. The protein binding is constant at candesartan plasma concentrations well above the range achieved with recommended doses. In rats, it has been demonstrated that candesartan crosses the blood-brain barrier poorly, if at all. It has also been demonstrated in rats that candesartan passes across the placental barrier and is distributed in the fetus.

Special Populations

Pediatric—The pharmacokinetics of candesartan cilexetil have not been investigated in patients <18 years of age.

Geriatric and Gender—The pharmacokinetics of candesartan have been studied in the elderly (≥65 years) and in both sexes. The plasma concentration of candesartan was higher in the elderly (C_{max} was approximately 50% higher, and AUC was approximately 80% higher) compared with younger subjects administered the same dose. The pharmacokinetics of candesartan were linear in the elderly, and candesartan and its inactive metabolite did not accumulate in the serum of these subjects upon repeated, once-daily administration. No initial dosage adjustment is necessary. (See DOSAGE AND ADMINISTRATION.) There is no difference in the pharmacokinetics of candesartan between male and female subjects.

Renal Insufficiency—In hypertensive patients with renal insufficiency, serum concentrations of candesartan were elevated. After repeated dosing, the AUC and C_{max} were approximately doubled in patients with severe renal

impairment (creatinine clearance <30 mL/min/1.73m²) compared with patients with normal kidney function. The pharmacokinetics of candesartan in hypertensive patients undergoing hemodialysis are similar to those in hypertensive patients with severe renal impairment. Candesartan cannot be removed by hemodialysis. No initial dosage adjustment is necessary in patients with renal insufficiency. (See DOSAGE AND ADMINISTRATION.)
In heart failure patients with renal impairment, AUC_{0-72} was 36% and 65% higher in mild and moderate renal impairment, respectively. C_{max} was 15% and 55% higher in mild and moderate renal impairment, respectively.
Hepatic Insufficiency—The pharmacokinetics of candesartan were compared in patients with mild and moderate hepatic impairment to matched healthy volunteers following a single oral dose of 16 mg candesartan cilexetil. The increase in AUC for candesartan was 30% in patients with mild hepatic impairment (Child-Pugh A) and 145% in patients with moderate hepatic impairment (Child-Pugh B). The increase in C_{max} for candesartan was 56% in patients with mild hepatic impairment and 73% in patients with moderate hepatic impairment. The pharmacokinetics after candesartan cilexetil administration have not been investigated in patients with severe hepatic impairment. No initial dosage adjustment is necessary in patients with mild hepatic impairment. In hypertensive patients with moderate hepatic impairment, consideration should be given to initiation of ATACAND at a lower dose. (See DOSAGE AND ADMINISTRATION.)
Heart Failure—The pharmacokinetics of candesartan were linear in patients with heart failure (NYHA Class II and III) after candesartan cilexetil doses of 4, 8, and 16 mg. After repeated dosing, the AUC was approximately doubled in these patients compared with healthy, younger patients. The pharmacokinetics in heart failure patients is similar to that in healthy elderly volunteers. (See DOSAGE AND ADMINISTRATION, Heart Failure.)

Drug Interactions

See PRECAUTIONS, Drug Interactions.

Pharmacodynamics

Candesartan inhibits the pressor effects of angiotensin II infusion in a dose-dependent manner. After 1 week of once daily dosing with 8 mg of candesartan cilexetil, the pressor effect was inhibited by approximately 90% at peak with approximately 50% inhibition persisting for 24 hours.
Plasma concentrations of angiotensin I and angiotensin II, and plasma renin activity (PRA), increased in a dose-dependent manner after single and repeated administration of candesartan cilexetil to healthy subjects, hypertensive, and heart failure patients. ACE activity was not altered in healthy subjects after repeated candesartan cilexetil administration. The once-daily administration of up to 16 mg of candesartan cilexetil to healthy subjects did not influence plasma aldosterone concentrations, but a decrease in the plasma concentration of aldosterone was observed when 32 mg of candesartan cilexetil was administered to hypertensive patients. In spite of the effect of candesartan cilexetil on aldosterone secretion, very little effect on serum potassium was observed.
Hypertension
In multiple-dose studies with hypertensive patients, there were no clinically significant changes in metabolic function, including serum levels of total cholesterol, triglycerides, glucose, or uric acid. In a 12-week study of 161 patients with non-insulin-dependent (type 2) diabetes mellitus and hypertension, there was no change in the level of HbA_{1c}.

Clinical Trials

Hypertension
The antihypertensive effects of ATACAND were examined in 14 placebo-controlled trials of 4- to 12-weeks duration, primarily at daily doses of 2 to 32 mg per day in patients with baseline diastolic blood pressures of 95 to 114 mm Hg. Most of the trials were of candesartan cilexetil as a single agent, but it was also studied as add-on to hydrochlorothiazide and amlodipine. These studies included a total of 2350 patients randomized to one of several doses of candesartan cilexetil and 1027 to placebo. Except for a study in diabetics, all studies showed significant effects, generally dose related, of 2 to 32 mg on trough (24 hour) systolic and diastolic pressures compared to placebo, with doses of 8 to 32 mg giving effects of about 8-12/4-8 mm Hg. There were no exaggerated first-dose effects in these patients. Most of the antihypertensive effect was seen within 2 weeks of initial dosing, and the full effect in 4 weeks. With once-daily dosing, blood pressure effect was maintained over 24 hours, with trough to peak ratios of blood pressure effect generally over 80%. Candesartan cilexetil had an additional blood pressure lowering effect when added to hydrochlorothiazide.
The antihypertensive effects of candesartan cilexetil and losartan potassium at their highest recommended doses administered once-daily were compared in two randomized, double-blind trials. In a total of 1268 patients with mild to moderate hypertension who were not receiving other antihypertensive therapy, candesartan cilexetil 32 mg lowered systolic and diastolic blood pressure by 2 to 3 mm Hg on average more than losartan potassium 100 mg, when measured at the time of either peak or trough effect. The antihypertensive effects of twice daily dosing of either candesartan cilexetil or losartan potassium were not studied.
The antihypertensive effect was similar in men and women and in patients older and younger than 65. Candesartan was effective in reducing blood pressure regardless of race, although the effect was somewhat less in blacks (usually a low-renin population). This has been generally true for angiotensin II antagonists and ACE inhibitors.

Table 1
CHARM – Alternative: Primary Endpoint and its Components

Endpoint (time to first event)	ATACAND (n=1013)	Placebo (n=1015)	Hazard Ratio (95% CI)	p-value (logrank)
CV death or CHF hospitalization	334	406	.077 (0.67–0.89)	<0.001
CV death	219	252	0.85 (0.71–1.02)	0.072
CHF hospitalization	207	286	0.68 (0.57–0.81)	<0.001

In long-term studies of up to 1 year, the antihypertensive effectiveness of candesartan cilexetil was maintained, and there was no rebound after abrupt withdrawal.
There were no changes in the heart rate of patients treated with candesartan cilexetil in controlled trials.
Heart Failure
CHARM-Alternative was an international, double-blind, placebo-controlled, parallel study in which 2028 subjects with NYHA Class II-IV heart failure, ejection fraction ≤40%, and intolerance to ACE inhibitors were randomized to placebo or ATACAND (initially 4-8 mg daily, titrated as tolerated to 32 mg daily) and followed for up to 4 years. Patients with serum creatinine >3 mg/dL, serum potassium >5.5 mg/dL, symptomatic hypotension or known bilateral renal artery stenosis were to be excluded. The primary end point was time to either cardiovascular mortality or hospitalization for heart failure. The mean age was 67 years, 47.6% were NYHA II, 48.8% were NYHA III, 3.6% were NYHA IV, the mean ejection fraction was 30%, and 32% were female. Sixty-two percent had a history of myocardial infarction, 50% had a history of hypertension, and 27% had diabetes. Common drugs at baseline were diuretics (85%), digoxin (46%), beta-blockers (55%), and spironolactone (24%).
After a median follow-up of 34 months, there was a 23% reduction in the risk of cardiovascular death or heart failure hospitalization on ATACAND (p<0.001), with both components contributing to the overall effect (Table 1).
[See table 1 above]
This finding was supported by a second study (CHARM – Added) of 2548 subjects with NYHA Class II-IV heart failure and ejection fraction ≤40% in which subjects were mostly on submaximal doses of ACE inhibitors. Together, in these studies, subjects on ATACAND had a 15% lower risk of cardiovascular mortality (p=0.005). In these studies, symptoms of heart failure as assessed by NYHA functional class were also improved (p<0.001).

INDICATIONS AND USAGE

Hypertension
ATACAND is indicated for the treatment of hypertension. It may be used alone or in combination with other antihypertensive agents.
Heart Failure
ATACAND is indicated for the treatment of heart failure (NYHA Class II-IV and ejection fraction ≤40%) to reduce the risk of death from cardiovascular causes and reduce hospitalizations for heart failure (see Clinical Trials).

CONTRAINDICATIONS

ATACAND is contraindicated in patients who are hypersensitive to any component of this product.

WARNINGS

Fetal/Neonatal Morbidity and Mortality

Drugs that act directly on the renin-angiotensin system can cause fetal and neonatal morbidity and death when administered to pregnant women. Several dozen cases have been reported in the world literature in patients who were taking angiotensin-converting enzyme inhibitors. Post-marketing experience has identified reports of fetal and neonatal toxicity in babies born to women treated with ATACAND during pregnancy. When pregnancy is detected, ATACAND should be discontinued as soon as possible.
The use of drugs that act directly on the renin-angiotensin system during the second and third trimesters of pregnancy has been associated with fetal and neonatal injury, including hypotension, neonatal skull hypoplasia, anuria, reversible or irreversible renal failure, and death. Oligohydramnios has also been reported, presumably resulting from decreased fetal renal function; oligohydramnios in this setting has been associated with fetal limb contractures, craniofacial deformation, and hypoplastic lung development. Prematurity, intrauterine growth retardation, and patent ductus arteriosus have also been reported, although it is not clear whether these occurrences were due to exposure to the drug.
These adverse effects do not appear to have resulted from intrauterine drug exposure that has been limited to the first trimester. Mothers whose embryos and fetuses are exposed to an angiotensin II receptor antagonist only during the first trimester should be so informed. Nonetheless, when patients become pregnant, physicians should have the patient discontinue the use of ATACAND as soon as possible.
Rarely (probably less often than once in every thousand pregnancies), no alternative to a drug acting on the renin-angiotensin system will be found. In these rare cases, the mothers should be apprised of the potential hazards to their fetuses, and serial ultrasound examinations should be performed to assess the intra-amniotic environment.
If oligohydramnios is observed, ATACAND should be discontinued unless it is considered life saving for the mother. Contraction stress testing (CST), a nonstress test (NST), or biophysical profiling (BPP) may be appropriate, depending upon the week of pregnancy. Patients and physicians should be aware, however, that oligohydramnios may not appear until after the fetus has sustained irreversible injury.
Infants with histories of *in utero* exposure to an angiotensin II receptor antagonist should be closely observed for hypotension, oliguria, and hyperkalemia. If oliguria occurs, attention should be directed toward support of blood pressure and renal perfusion. Exchange transfusion or dialysis may be required as means of reversing hypotension and/or substituting for disordered renal function.
Oral doses ≥10 mg of candesartan cilexetil/kg/day administered to pregnant rats during late gestation and continued through lactation were associated with reduced survival and an increased incidence of hydronephrosis in the offspring. The 10-mg/kg/day dose in rats is approximately 2.8 times the maximum recommended daily human dose (MRHD) of 32 mg on a mg/m² basis (comparison assumes human body weight of 50 kg). Candesartan cilexetil given to pregnant rabbits at an oral dose of 3 mg/kg/day (approximately 1.7 times the MRHD on a mg/m² basis) caused maternal toxicity (decreased body weight and death) but, in surviving dams, had no adverse effects on fetal survival, fetal weight, or external, visceral, or skeletal development. No maternal toxicity or adverse effects on fetal development were observed when oral doses up to 1000 mg of candesartan cilexetil/kg/day (approximately 138 times the MRHD on a mg/m² basis) were administered to pregnant mice.

Hypotension in Volume- and Salt-Depleted Patients

In patients with an activated renin-angiotensin system, such as volume- and/or salt-depleted patients (eg, those being treated with diuretics), symptomatic hypotension may occur. These conditions should be corrected prior to administration of ATACAND, or the treatment should start under close medical supervision (see DOSAGE AND ADMINISTRATION).
If hypotension occurs, the patients should be placed in the supine position and, if necessary, given an intravenous infusion of normal saline. A transient hypotensive response is not a contraindication to further treatment which usually can be continued without difficulty once the blood pressure has stabilized.

Hypotension in Heart Failure Patients

Caution should be observed when initiating therapy in patients with heart failure. Patients with heart failure given ATACAND commonly have some reduction in blood pressure. In patients with symptomatic hypotension this may require temporarily reducing the dose of ATACAND, or diuretic, or both, and volume repletion. In the CHARM program, hypotension was reported in 18.8% of patients on candesartan versus 9.8% of patients on placebo; the incidence of hypotension leading to drug discontinuation in candesartan-treated patients was 4.1% compared with 2.0% in placebo-treated patients. Monitoring of blood pressure is recommended during dose escalation and periodically thereafter.

PRECAUTIONS

General

Impaired Hepatic Function—Based on pharmacokinetic data that demonstrate significant increases in candesartan AUC and C_{max} in patients with moderate hepatic impairment, a lower initiating dose should be considered for patients with moderate hepatic impairment. (See DOSAGE AND ADMINISTRATION, and CLINICAL PHARMACOLOGY, Special Populations.)
Impaired Renal Function—As a consequence of inhibiting the renin-angiotensin-aldosterone system, changes in renal function may be anticipated in susceptible individuals treated with ATACAND. In patients whose renal function may depend upon the activity of the renin-angiotensin-aldosterone system (eg, patients with severe congestive heart failure), treatment with angiotensin-converting enzyme inhibitors and angiotensin receptor antagonists has been associated with oliguria and/or progressive azotemia and (rarely) with acute renal failure and/or death. Similar results may be anticipated in patients treated with ATACAND. (See CLINICAL PHARMACOLOGY, Special Populations.)
In studies of ACE inhibitors in patients with unilateral or bilateral renal artery stenosis, increases in serum creatinine or blood urea nitrogen (BUN) have been reported. There has been no long-term use of ATACAND in patients with unilateral or bilateral renal artery stenosis, but similar results may be expected.

Continued on next page

Atacand—Cont.

In heart failure patients treated with ATACAND, increases in serum creatinine may occur. Dosage reduction or discontinuation of the diuretic or ATACAND, and volume repletion may be required. In the CHARM program, the incidence of abnormal renal function (e.g., creatinine increase) was 12.5% in patients treated with candesartan versus 6.3% in patients treated with placebo. In the CHARM program, the incidence of abnormal renal function (eg, creatinine increase) leading to drug discontinuation in candesartan-treated patients was 6.3% compared with 2.9% in placebo-treated patients. Evaluation of patients with heart failure should always include assessment of renal function and volume status. Monitoring of serum creatinine is recommended during dose escalation and periodically thereafter.

Hyperkalemia
In heart failure patients treated with ATACAND, hyperkalemia may occur, especially when taken concomitantly with ACE inhibitors and potassium-sparing diuretics such as spironolactone. In the CHARM program, the incidence of hyperkalemia was 6.3% in patients treated with candesartan versus 2.1% in patients treated with placebo. The incidence of hyperkalemia leading to drug discontinuation in candesartan-treated patients was 2.4% compared with 0.6% in placebo-treated patients. During treatment with ATACAND in patients with heart failure, monitoring of serum potassium is recommended during dose escalation and periodically thereafter.

Information for Patients
Pregnancy—Female patients of childbearing age should be told about the consequences of second- and third-trimester exposure to drugs that act on the renin-angiotensin system, and they should also be told that these consequences do not appear to have resulted from intrauterine drug exposure that has been limited to the first trimester. These patients should be asked to report pregnancies to their physicians as soon as possible.

Drug Interactions
No significant drug interactions have been reported in studies of candesartan cilexetil given with other drugs such as glyburide, nifedipine, digoxin, warfarin, hydrochlorothiazide, and oral contraceptives in healthy volunteers, or given with enalapril to patients with heart failure (NYHA Class II and III). Because candesartan is not significantly metabolized by the cytochrome P450 system and at therapeutic concentrations has no effects on P450 enzymes, interactions with drugs that inhibit or are metabolized by those enzymes would not be expected.
Lithium—Reversible increases in serum lithium concentrations and toxicity have been reported during concomitant administration of lithium with ACE inhibitors, and with some angiotensin II receptor antagonists. An increase in serum lithium concentration has been reported during concomitant administration of lithium with ATACAND, so careful monitoring of serum lithium levels is recommended during concomitant use.

Carcinogenesis, Mutagenesis, Impairment of Fertility
There was no evidence of carcinogenicity when candesartan cilexetil was orally administered to mice and rats for up to 104 weeks at doses up to 100 and 1000 mg/kg/day, respectively. Rats received the drug by gavage, whereas mice received the drug by dietary administration. These (maximally-tolerated) doses of candesartan cilexetil provided systemic exposures to candesartan (AUCs) that were, in mice, approximately 7 times and, in rats, more than 70 times the exposure in man at the maximum recommended daily human dose (32 mg).
Candesartan and its O-deethyl metabolite tested positive for genotoxicity in the *in vitro* Chinese hamster lung (CHL) chromosomal aberration assay. Neither compound tested positive in the Ames microbial mutagenesis assay or the *in vitro* mouse lymphoma cell assay. Candesartan (but not its O-deethyl metabolite) was also evaluated *in vivo* in the mouse micronucleus test and *in vitro* in the Chinese hamster ovary (CHO) gene mutation assay, in both cases with negative results. Candesartan cilexetil was evaluated in the Ames test, the *in vitro* mouse lymphoma cell and rat hepatocyte unscheduled DNA synthesis assays and the *in vivo* mouse micronucleus test, in each case with negative results. Candesartan cilexetil was not evaluated in the CHL chromosomal aberration or CHO gene mutation assay.
Fertility and reproductive performance were not affected in studies with male and female rats given oral doses of up to 300 mg/kg/day (83 times the maximum daily human dose of 32 mg on a body surface area basis).

Pregnancy
Pregnancy Categories C (first trimester) *and D* (second and third trimesters)—See WARNINGS, Fetal/Neonatal Morbidity and Mortality.

Nursing Mothers
It is not known whether candesartan is excreted in human milk, but candesartan has been shown to be present in rat milk. Because of the potential for adverse effects on the nursing infant, a decision should be made whether to discontinue nursing or discontinue the drug, taking into account the importance of the drug to the mother.

Pediatric Use
Safety and effectiveness in pediatric patients have not been established.

Geriatric Use
Hypertension
Of the total number of subjects in clinical studies of ATACAND, 21% (683/3260) were 65 and over, while 3% (87/

3260) were 75 and over. No overall differences in safety or effectiveness were observed between these subjects and younger subjects, and other reported clinical experience has not identified differences in responses between the elderly and younger patients, but greater sensitivity of some older individuals cannot be ruled out. In a placebo-controlled trial of about 200 elderly hypertensive patients (ages 65 to 87 years), administration of candesartan cilexetil was well tolerated and lowered blood pressure by about 12/6 mm Hg more than placebo.
Heart Failure
Of the 7599 patients with heart failure in the CHARM program, 4343 (57%) were age 65 years or older and 1736 (23%) were 75 years or older. In patients ≥75 years of age, the incidence of drug discontinuations due to adverse events was higher for those treated with ATACAND or placebo compared with patients <75 years of age. In these patients, the most common adverse events leading to drug discontinuation at an incidence of at least 3%, and more frequent with ATACAND than placebo, were abnormal renal function (7.9% vs. 4.0%), hypotension (5.2% vs. 3.2%) and hyperkalemia (4.2% vs. 0.9%). In addition to monitoring of serum creatinine, potassium, and blood pressure during dose escalation and periodically thereafter, greater sensitivity of some older individuals with heart failure must be considered.

ADVERSE REACTIONS
Hypertension
ATACAND has been evaluated for safety in more than 3600 patients/subjects, including more than 3200 patients treated for hypertension. About 600 of these patients were studied for at least 6 months and about 200 for at least 1 year. In general, treatment with ATACAND was well tolerated. The overall incidence of adverse events reported with ATACAND was similar to placebo.
The rate of withdrawals due to adverse events in all trials in patients (7510 total) was 3.3% (ie, 108 of 3260) of patients treated with candesartan cilexetil as monotherapy and 3.5% (ie, 39 of 1106) of patients treated with placebo. In placebo-controlled trials, discontinuation of therapy due to clinical adverse events occurred in 2.4% (ie, 57 of 2350) of patients treated with ATACAND and 3.4% (ie, 35 of 1027) of patients treated with placebo.
The most common reasons for discontinuation of therapy with ATACAND were headache (0.6%) and dizziness (0.3%).
The adverse events that occurred in placebo-controlled clinical trials in at least 1% of patients treated with ATACAND and at a higher incidence in candesartan cilexetil (n=2350) than placebo (n=1027) patients included back pain (3% vs 2%), dizziness (4% vs 3%), upper respiratory tract infection (6% vs 4%), pharyngitis (2% vs 1%), and rhinitis (2% vs 1%). The following adverse events occurred in placebo-controlled clinical trials at a more than 1% rate but at about the same or greater incidence in patients receiving placebo compared to candesartan cilexetil: fatigue, peripheral edema, chest pain, headache, bronchitis, coughing, sinusitis, nausea, abdominal pain, diarrhea, vomiting, arthralgia, albuminuria.
Other potentially important adverse events that have been reported, whether or not attributed to treatment, with an incidence of 0.5% or greater from the 3260 patients worldwide treated in clinical trials with ATACAND are listed below. It cannot be determined whether these events were causally related to ATACAND. **Body as a Whole:** asthenia, fever; **Central and Peripheral Nervous System:** paresthesia, vertigo; **Gastrointestinal System Disorder:** dyspepsia, gastroenteritis; **Heart Rate and Rhythm Disorders:** tachycardia, palpitation; **Metabolic and Nutritional Disorders:** creatine phosphokinase increased, hyperglycemia, hypertriglyceridemia, hyperuricemia; **Musculoskeletal System Disorders:** myalgia; **Platelet/Bleeding-Clotting Disorders:** epistaxis; **Psychiatric Disorders:** anxiety, depression, somnolence; **Respiratory System Disorders:** dyspnea; **Skin and Appendages Disorders:** rash, sweating increased; **Urinary System Disorders:** hematuria.
Other reported events seen less frequently included angina pectoris, myocardial infarction, and angioedema.
Adverse events occurred at about the same rates in men and women, older and younger patients, and black and non-black patients.

Heart Failure
The adverse event profile of ATACAND in heart failure patients was consistent with the pharmacology of the drug and the health status of the patients. In the CHARM program, comparing ATACAND in total daily doses up to 32 mg once daily (n=3803) with placebo (n=3796), 21.0% of ATACAND patients discontinued for adverse events vs. 16.1% of placebo patients.

Post-Marketing Experience:
The following have been very rarely reported in post-marketing experience:
Digestive: Abnormal hepatic function and hepatitis.
Hematologic: Neutropenia, leukopenia, and agranulocytosis.
Metabolic and Nutritional Disorders: hyperkalemia, hyponatremia.
Renal: renal impairment, renal failure.
Skin and Appendages Disorders: Pruritus and urticaria.
Rare reports of rhabdomyolysis have been reported in patients receiving angiotensin II receptor blockers.

Laboratory Test Findings
Hypertension
In controlled clinical trials, clinically important changes in standard laboratory parameters were rarely associated with the administration of ATACAND.

Creatinine, Blood Urea Nitrogen—Minor increases in blood urea nitrogen (BUN) and serum creatinine were observed infrequently.
Hyperuricemia—Hyperuricemia was rarely found (19 or 0.6% of 3260 patients treated with candesartan cilexetil and 5 or 0.5% of 1106 patients treated with placebo).
Hemoglobin and Hematocrit—Small decreases in hemoglobin and hematocrit (mean decreases of approximately 0.2 grams/dL and 0.5 volume percent, respectively) were observed in patients treated with ATACAND alone but were rarely of clinical importance. Anemia, leukopenia, and thrombocytopenia were associated with withdrawal of one patient each from clinical trials.
Potassium—A small increase (mean increase of 0.1 mEq/L) was observed in patients treated with ATACAND alone but was rarely of clinical importance. One patient from a congestive heart failure trial was withdrawn for hyperkalemia (serum potassium = 7.5 mEq/L). This patient was also receiving spironolactone.
Liver Function Tests—Elevations of liver enzymes and/or serum bilirubin were observed infrequently. Five patients assigned to candesartan cilexetil in clinical trials were withdrawn because of abnormal liver chemistries. All had elevated transaminases. Two had mildly elevated total bilirubin, but one of these patients was diagnosed with Hepatitis A.
Heart Failure
In the CHARM program, small increases in serum creatinine (mean increase 0.2 mg/dL in candesartan-treated patients and 0.1 mg/dL in placebo-treated patients) and serum potassium (mean increase 0.15 mEq/L in candesartan-treated patients and 0.02 mEq/L in placebo-treated patients), and small decreases in hemoglobin (mean decrease 0.5 gm/dL in candesartan-treated patients and 0.3 gm/dL in placebo-treated patients) and hematocrit (mean decrease 1.6% in candesartan-treated patients and 0.9% in placebo-treated patients) were observed.

OVERDOSAGE
No lethality was observed in acute toxicity studies in mice, rats, and dogs given single oral doses of up to 2000 mg/kg of candesartan cilexetil. In mice given single oral doses of the primary metabolite, candesartan, the minimum lethal dose was greater than 1000 mg/kg but less than 2000 mg/kg.
The most likely manifestation of overdosage with ATACAND would be hypotension, dizziness, and tachycardia; bradycardia could occur from parasympathetic (vagal) stimulation. If symptomatic hypotension should occur, supportive treatment should be instituted.
Candesartan cannot be removed by hemodialysis.
Treatment: To obtain up-to-date information about the treatment of overdose, consult your Regional Poison Control Center. Telephone numbers of certified poison control centers are listed in the *Physicians' Desk Reference (PDR)*. In managing overdose, consider the possibilities of multiple-drug overdoses, drug-drug interactions, and altered pharmacokinetics in your patient.

DOSAGE AND ADMINISTRATION
Hypertension
Dosage must be individualized. Blood pressure response is dose related over the range of 2 to 32 mg. The usual recommended starting dose of ATACAND is 16 mg once daily when it is used as monotherapy in patients who are not volume depleted. ATACAND can be administered once or twice daily with total daily doses ranging from 8 mg to 32 mg. Larger doses do not appear to have a greater effect, and there is relatively little experience with such doses. Most of the antihypertensive effect is present within 2 weeks, and maximal blood pressure reduction is generally obtained within 4 to 6 weeks of treatment with ATACAND.
No initial dosage adjustment is necessary for elderly patients, for patients with mildly impaired renal function, or for patients with mildly impaired hepatic function (see CLINICAL PHARMACOLOGY, Special Populations). In patients with moderate hepatic impairment, consideration should be given to initiation of ATACAND at a lower dose (See CLINICAL PHARMACOLOGY, Special Populations). For patients with possible depletion of intravascular volume (eg, patients treated with diuretics, particularly those with impaired renal function), ATACAND should be initiated under close medical supervision and consideration should be given to administration of a lower dose (see WARNINGS, Hypotension in Volume- and Salt-Depleted Patients).
ATACAND may be administered with or without food.
If blood pressure is not controlled by ATACAND alone, a diuretic may be added. ATACAND may be administered with other antihypertensive agents.

Heart Failure
The recommended initial dose for treating heart failure is 4 mg once daily. The target dose is 32 mg once daily, which is achieved by doubling the dose at approximately 2-week intervals, as tolerated by the patient.

HOW SUPPLIED
No. 3782—Tablets ATACAND, 4 mg, are white to off-white, circular/biconvex-shaped, non-film-coated tablets, coded ACF on one side and 004 on the other. They are supplied as follows:
NDC 0186-0004-31 unit of use bottles of 30.
No. 3780—Tablets ATACAND, 8 mg, are light pink, circular/biconvex-shaped, non-film-coated tablets, coded ACG on one side and 008 on the other. They are supplied as follows:
NDC 0186-0008-31 unit of use bottles of 30.

No. 3781—Tablets ATACAND, 16 mg, are pink, circular/ biconvex-shaped, non-film-coated tablets, coded ACH on one side and 016 on the other. They are supplied as follows:
NDC 0186-0016-31 unit of use bottles of 30
NDC 0186-0016-54 unit of use bottles of 90
NDC 0186-0016-28 unit dose packages of 100.
No. 3791—Tablets ATACAND, 32 mg, are pink, circular/ biconvex-shaped, non-film-coated tablets, coded ACL on one side and 032 on the other. They are supplied as follows:
NDC 0186-0032-31 unit of use bottles of 30
NDC 0186-0032-54 unit of use bottles of 90
NDC 0186-0032-28 unit dose packages of 100.

Storage
Store at 25°C (77°F); excursions permitted to 15–30°C (59–86°F) [see USP Controlled Room Temperature]. Keep container tightly closed.

ATACAND is a trademark of the AstraZeneca group of companies
© AstraZeneca 2005
Manufactured under the license from
Takeda Chemical Industries, Ltd.
by: AstraZeneca AB, S-151 85 Södertälje, Sweden
for: AstraZeneca LP, Wilmington, DE 19850
Made in Sweden
9174311
3102700 Rev. 02/05 **AstraZeneca**

ATACAND HCT® 16-12.5 ℞
[ăt ă-kănd]
(candesartan cilexetil – hydrochlorothiazide)

ATACAND HCT® 32-12.5 ℞
(candesartan cilexetil – hydrochlorothiazide)
TABLETS

Prescribing information for this product, which appears on pages 612–615 of the 2005 PDR, has been completely revised as follows. Please write "See Supplement A" next to the product heading.

USE IN PREGNANCY
When used in pregnancy during the second and third trimesters, drugs that act directly on the renin-angiotensin system can cause injury and even death to the developing fetus. When pregnancy is detected, ATACAND HCT should be discontinued as soon as possible. See WARNINGS, Fetal/Neonatal Morbidity and Mortality.

DESCRIPTION
ATACAND HCT (candesartan cilexetil-hydrochlorothiazide) combines an angiotensin II receptor (type AT_1) antagonist and a diuretic, hydrochlorothiazide.
Candesartan cilexetil, a nonpeptide, is chemically described as (±)-1-Hydroxyethyl 2-ethoxy-1-[*p*-(*o*-1*H*-tetrazol-5-ylphenyl)benzyl]-7-benzimidazolecarboxylate, cyclohexyl carbonate (ester).
Its empirical formula is $C_{33}H_{34}N_6O_6$, and its structural formula is

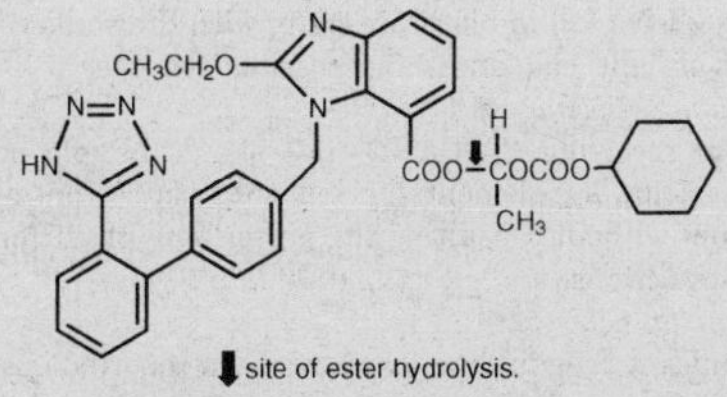

Candesartan cilexetil is a white to off-white powder with a molecular weight of 610.67. It is practically insoluble in water and sparingly soluble in methanol. Candesartan cilexetil is a racemic mixture containing one chiral center at the cyclohexyloxycarbonyloxy ethyl ester group. Following oral administration, candesartan cilexetil undergoes hydrolysis at the ester link to form the active drug, candesartan, which is achiral.
Hydrochlorothiazide is 6-chloro-3,4-dihydro-2*H*-1,2,4-benzothiadiazine-7-sulfonamide 1,1-dioxide. Its empirical formula is $C_7H_8ClN_3O_4S_2$ and its structural formula is

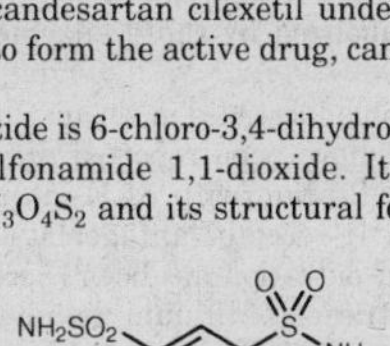

Hydrochlorothiazide is a white, or practically white, crystalline powder with a molecular weight of 297.72, which is slightly soluble in water, but freely soluble in sodium hydroxide solution.
ATACAND HCT is available for oral administration in two tablet strengths of candesartan cilexetil and hydrochlorothiazide.
ATACAND HCT 16-12.5 contains 16 mg of candesartan cilexetil and 12.5 mg of hydrochlorothiazide. ATACAND HCT 32-12.5 contains 32 mg of candesartan cilexetil and 12.5 mg of hydrochlorothiazide. The inactive ingredients of the tablets are calcium carboxymethylcellulose, hydroxypropyl cellulose, lactose monohydrate, magnesium stearate, corn starch, polyethylene glycol 8000, and ferric oxide (yellow). Ferric oxide (reddish brown) is also added to the 16-12.5 mg tablet as colorant.

CLINICAL PHARMACOLOGY
Mechanism of Action
Angiotensin II is formed from angiotensin I in a reaction catalyzed by angiotensin-converting enzyme (ACE, kininase II). Angiotensin II is the principal pressor agent of the renin-angiotensin system, with effects that include vasoconstriction, stimulation of synthesis and release of aldosterone, cardiac stimulation, and renal reabsorption of sodium. Candesartan blocks the vasoconstrictor and aldosterone-secreting effects of angiotensin II by selectively blocking the binding of angiotensin II to the AT_1 receptor in many tissues, such as vascular smooth muscle and the adrenal gland. Its action is, therefore, independent of the pathways for angiotensin II synthesis.
There is also an AT_2 receptor found in many tissues, but AT_2 is not known to be associated with cardiovascular homeostasis. Candesartan has much greater affinity (>10,000-fold) for the AT_1 receptor than for the AT_2 receptor.
Blockade of the renin-angiotensin system with ACE inhibitors, which inhibit the biosynthesis of angiotensin II from angiotensin I, is widely used in the treatment of hypertension. ACE inhibitors also inhibit the degradation of bradykinin, a reaction also catalyzed by ACE. Because candesartan does not inhibit ACE (kininase II), it does not affect the response to bradykinin. Whether this difference has clinical relevance is not yet known. Candesartan does not bind to or block other hormone receptors or ion channels known to be important in cardiovascular regulation.
Blockade of the angiotensin II receptor inhibits the negative regulatory feedback of angiotensin II on renin secretion, but the resulting increased plasma renin activity and angiotensin II circulating levels do not overcome the effect of candesartan on blood pressure.
Hydrochlorothiazide is a thiazide diuretic. Thiazides affect the renal tubular mechanisms of electrolyte reabsorption, directly increasing excretion of sodium and chloride in approximately equivalent amounts. Indirectly, the diuretic action of hydrochlorothiazide reduces plasma volume, with consequent increases in plasma renin activity, increases in aldosterone secretion, increases in urinary potassium loss, and decreases in serum potassium. The renin-aldosterone link is mediated by angiotensin II, so coadministration of an angiotensin II receptor antagonist tends to reverse the potassium loss associated with these diuretics.
The mechanism of the antihypertensive effect of thiazides is unknown.

Pharmacokinetics
General
Candesartan Cilexetil
Candesartan cilexetil is rapidly and completely bioactivated by ester hydrolysis during absorption from the gastrointestinal tract to candesartan, a selective AT_1 subtype angiotensin II receptor antagonist. Candesartan is mainly excreted unchanged in urine and feces (via bile). It undergoes minor hepatic metabolism by O-deethylation to an inactive metabolite. The elimination half-life of candesartan is approximately 9 hours. After single and repeated administration, the pharmacokinetics of candesartan are linear for oral doses up to 32 mg of candesartan cilexetil. Candesartan and its inactive metabolite do not accumulate in serum upon repeated once-daily dosing.
Following administration of candesartan cilexetil, the absolute bioavailability of candesartan was estimated to be 15%. After tablet ingestion, the peak serum concentration (C_{max}) is reached after 3 to 4 hours. Food with a high fat content does not affect the bioavailability of candesartan after candesartan cilexetil administration.
Hydrochlorothiazide
When plasma levels have been followed for at least 24 hours, the plasma half-life has been observed to vary between 5.6 and 14.8 hours.

Metabolism and Excretion
Candesartan Cilexetil
Total plasma clearance of candesartan is 0.37 mL/min/kg, with a renal clearance of 0.19 mL/min/kg. When candesartan is administered orally, about 26% of the dose is excreted unchanged in urine. Following an oral dose of ^{14}C-labeled candesartan cilexetil, approximately 33% of radioactivity is recovered in urine and approximately 67% in feces. Following an intravenous dose of ^{14}C-labeled candesartan, approximately 59% of radioactivity is recovered in urine and approximately 36% in feces. Biliary excretion contributes to the elimination of candesartan.
Hydrochlorothiazide
Hydrochlorothiazide is not metabolized but is eliminated rapidly by the kidney. At least 61% of the oral dose is eliminated unchanged within 24 hours.

Distribution
Candesartan Cilexetil
The volume of distribution of candesartan is 0.13 L/kg. Candesartan is highly bound to plasma proteins (>99%) and does not penetrate red blood cells. The protein binding is constant at candesartan plasma concentrations well above the range achieved with recommended doses. In rats, it has been demonstrated that candesartan crosses the blood-brain barrier poorly, if at all. It has also been demonstrated in rats that candesartan passes across the placental barrier and is distributed in the fetus.
Hydrochlorothiazide
Hydrochlorothiazide crosses the placental but not the blood-brain barrier and is excreted in breast milk.

Special Populations
Pediatric
The pharmacokinetics of candesartan cilexetil have not been investigated in patients <18 years of age.
Geriatric
The pharmacokinetics of candesartan have been studied in the elderly (≥65 years). The plasma concentration of candesartan was higher in the elderly (C_{max} was approximately 50% higher, and AUC was approximately 80% higher) compared to younger subjects administered the same dose. The pharmacokinetics of candesartan were linear in the elderly, and candesartan and its inactive metabolite did not accumulate in the serum of these subjects upon repeated, once-daily administration. No initial dosage adjustment is necessary. (See DOSAGE AND ADMINISTRATION.)
Gender
There is no difference in the pharmacokinetics of candesartan between male and female subjects.
Renal Insufficiency
In hypertensive patients with renal insufficiency, serum concentrations of candesartan were elevated. After repeated dosing, the AUC and C_{max} were approximately doubled in patients with severe renal impairment (creatinine clearance <30 mL/min/1.73m^2) compared to patients with normal kidney function. The pharmacokinetics of candesartan in hypertensive patients undergoing hemodialysis are similar to those in hypertensive patients with severe renal impairment. Candesartan cannot be removed by hemodialysis. No initial dosage adjustment is necessary in patients with renal insufficiency.
Thiazide diuretics are eliminated by the kidney, with a terminal half-life of 5-15 hours. In a study of patients with impaired renal function (mean creatinine clearance of 19 mL/ min), the half-life of hydrochlorothiazide elimination was lengthened to 21 hours. (See DOSAGE AND ADMINISTRATION.)
Hepatic Insufficiency
The pharmacokinetics of candesartan were compared in patients with mild (Child-Pugh A) or moderate (Child-Pugh B) hepatic impairment to matched healthy volunteers following a single dose of 16 mg candesartan cilexetil. The AUC for candesartan in patients with mild and moderate hepatic impairment was increased 30% and 145% respectively. The C_{max} for candesartan was increased 56% and 73% respectively. The pharmacokinetics of candesartan in severe hepatic impairment have not been studied. No dose adjustment is recommended for patients with mild hepatic impairment. In patients with moderate hepatic impairment, consideration should be given to initiation of ATACAND at a lower dose, such as 8 mg. If a lower starting dose is selected for candesartan cilexetil, ATACAND HCT is not recommended for initial titration because the appropriate initial starting dose of candesartan cilexetil cannot be given. (See DOSAGE AND ADMINISTRATION.)
Thiazide diuretics should be used with caution in patients with hepatic impairment. (See DOSAGE AND ADMINISTRATION.)

Pharmacodynamics
Candesartan Cilexetil
Candesartan inhibits the pressor effects of angiotensin II infusion in a dose-dependent manner. After 1 week of once-daily dosing with 8 mg of candesartan cilexetil, the pressor effect was inhibited by approximately 90% at peak with approximately 50% inhibition persisting for 24 hours.
Plasma concentrations of angiotensin I and angiotensin II, and plasma renin activity (PRA), increased in a dose-dependent manner after single and repeated administration of candesartan cilexetil to healthy subjects and hypertensive patients. ACE activity was not altered in healthy subjects after repeated candesartan cilexetil administration. The once-daily administration of up to 16 mg of candesartan cilexetil to healthy subjects did not influence plasma aldosterone concentrations, but a decrease in the plasma concentration of aldosterone was observed when 32 mg of candesartan cilexetil was administered to hypertensive patients. In spite of the effect of candesartan cilexetil on aldosterone secretion, very little effect on serum potassium was observed.
In multiple-dose studies with hypertensive patients, there were no clinically significant changes in metabolic function including serum levels of total cholesterol, triglycerides, glucose, or uric acid. In a 12-week study of 161 patients with non-insulin-dependent (type 2) diabetes mellitus and hypertension, there was no change in the level of HbA_{1c}.
Hydrochlorothiazide
After oral administration of hydrochlorothiazide, diuresis begins within 2 hours, peaks in about 4 hours and lasts about 6 to 12 hours.

Clinical Trials
Candesartan Cilexetil–Hydrochlorothiazide
Of 12 controlled clinical trials involving 4588 patients, 5 were double-blind, placebo controlled and evaluated the antihypertensive effects of single entities vs the combination. These 5 trials, of 8 to 12 weeks duration, randomized 3037 hypertensive patients. Doses ranged from 2 to 32 mg candesartan cilexetil and from 6.25 to 25 mg hydrochlorothiazide administered once daily in various combinations.
The combination of candesartan cilexetil-hydrochlorothiazide resulted in placebo-adjusted decreases in sitting systolic and diastolic blood pressures of 14-18/8-11 mm Hg at doses of 16-12.5 mg and 32-12.5 mg. The combination of candesartan cilexetil and hydrochlorothiazide 32-25 mg re-

Continued on next page

Atacand HCT—Cont.

sulted in placebo-adjusted decreases in sitting systolic and diastolic blood pressures of 16-19/9-11 mm Hg. The placebo corrected trough to peak ratio was evaluated in a study of candesartan cilexetil-hydrochlorothiazide 32-12.5 mg and was 88%.

Most of the antihypertensive effect of the combination of candesartan cilexetil and hydrochlorothiazide was seen in 1 to 2 weeks with the full effect observed within 4 weeks. In long-term studies of up to 1 year, the blood pressure lowering effect of the combination was maintained. The antihypertensive effect was similar regardless of age or gender, and overall response to the combination was similar in black and non-black patients. No appreciable changes in heart rate were observed with combination therapy in controlled trials.

INDICATIONS AND USAGE

ATACAND HCT is indicated for the treatment of hypertension. This fixed dose combination is not indicated for initial therapy (see DOSAGE AND ADMINISTRATION).

CONTRAINDICATIONS

ATACAND HCT is contraindicated in patients who are hypersensitive to any component of this product.

Because of the hydrochlorothiazide component, this product is contraindicated in patients with anuria or hypersensitivity to other sulfonamide-derived drugs.

WARNINGS

Fetal/Neonatal Morbidity and Mortality

Drugs that act directly on the renin-angiotensin system can cause fetal and neonatal morbidity and death when administered to pregnant women. Several dozen cases have been reported in the world literature in patients who were taking angiotensin-converting enzyme inhibitors. Post-marketing experience has identified reports of fetal and neonatal toxicity in babies born to women treated with candesartan cilexetil during pregnancy. Because candesartan cilexetil is a component of ATACAND HCT, when pregnancy is detected, ATACAND HCT should be discontinued as soon as possible.

The use of drugs that act directly on the renin-angiotensin system during the second and third trimesters of pregnancy has been associated with fetal and neonatal injury, including hypotension, neonatal skull hypoplasia, anuria, reversible or irreversible renal failure, and death. Oligohydramnios has also been reported, presumably resulting from decreased fetal renal function; oligohydramnios in this setting has been associated with fetal limb contractures, craniofacial deformation, and hypoplastic lung development. Prematurity, intrauterine growth retardation, and patent ductus arteriosus have also been reported, although it is not clear whether these occurrences were due to exposure to the drug.

These adverse effects do not appear to have resulted from intrauterine drug exposure that has been limited to the first trimester. Mothers whose embryos and fetuses are exposed to an angiotensin II receptor antagonist only during the first trimester should be so informed. Nonetheless, when patients become pregnant, physicians should have the patient discontinue the use of ATACAND HCT as soon as possible.

Rarely (probably less often than once in every thousand pregnancies), no alternative to a drug acting on the renin-angiotensin system will be found. In these rare cases, the mothers should be apprised of the potential hazards to their fetuses, and serial ultrasound examinations should be performed to assess the intra-amniotic environment.

If oligohydramnios is observed, ATACAND HCT should be discontinued unless it is considered life saving for the mother. Contraction stress testing (CST), a nonstress test (NST), or biophysical profiling (BPP) may be appropriate, depending upon the week of pregnancy. Patients and physicians should be aware, however, that oligohydramnios may not appear until after the fetus has sustained irreversible injury.

Infants with histories of *in utero* exposure to an angiotensin II receptor antagonist should be closely observed for hypotension, oliguria, and hyperkalemia. If oliguria occurs, attention should be directed toward support of blood pressure and renal perfusion. Exchange transfusion or dialysis may be required as means of reversing hypotension and/or substituting for disordered renal function.

Candesartan Cilexetil-Hydrochlorothiazide

There was no evidence of teratogenicity or other adverse effects on embryo-fetal development when pregnant mice, rats or rabbits were treated orally with candesartan cilexetil alone or in combination with hydrochlorothiazide. For mice, the maximum dose of candesartan cilexetil was 1000 mg/kg/day (about 150 times the maximum recommended daily human dose [MRHD]*). For rats, the maximum dose of candesartan cilexetil was 100 mg/kg/day (about 31 times the MRHD*). For rabbits, the maximum dose of candesartan cilexetil was 1 mg/kg/day (a maternally toxic dose that is about half the MRHD*). In each of these studies, hydrochlorothiazide was tested at the same dose level (10 mg/kg/day, about 4, 8, and 15 times the MRHD* in mouse, rats, and rabbit, respectively). There was no evidence of harm to the rat or mouse fetus or embryo in studies in which hydrochlorothiazide was administered alone to the pregnant rat or mouse at doses of up to 1000 and 3000 mg/kg/day, respectively.

* Doses compared on the basis of body surface area. MRHD considered to be 32 mg for candesartan cilexetil and 12.5 mg for hydrochlorothiazide.

Thiazides cross the placental barrier and appear in cord blood. There is a risk of fetal or neonatal jaundice, thrombocytopenia, and possibly other adverse reactions that have occurred in adults.

Hypotension in Volume- and Salt-Depleted Patients

Based on adverse events reported from all clinical trials of ATACAND HCT, excessive reduction of blood pressure was rarely seen in patients with uncomplicated hypertension treated with candesartan cilexetil and hydrochlorothiazide (0.4%). Initiation of antihypertensive therapy may cause symptomatic hypotension in patients with intravascular volume- or sodium-depletion, eg, in patients treated vigorously with diuretics or in patients on dialysis. These conditions should be corrected prior to administration of ATACAND HCT, or the treatment should start under close medical supervision (see DOSAGE AND ADMINISTRATION).

If hypotension occurs, the patients should be placed in the supine position and, if necessary, given an intravenous infusion of normal saline. A transient hypotensive response is not a contraindication to further treatment which usually can be continued without difficulty once the blood pressure has stabilized.

Hydrochlorothiazide

Impaired Hepatic Function

Thiazide diuretics should be used with caution in patients with impaired hepatic function or progressive liver disease, since minor alterations of fluid and electrolyte balance may precipitate hepatic coma.

Hypersensitivity Reaction

Hypersensitivity reactions to hydrochlorothiazide may occur in patients with or without a history of allergy or bronchial asthma, but are more likely in patients with such a history.

Systemic Lupus Erythematosus

Thiazide diuretics have been reported to cause exacerbation or activation of systemic lupus erythematosus.

Lithium Interaction

Lithium generally should not be given with thiazides (see PRECAUTIONS, Drug Interactions, Hydrochlorothiazide, Lithium).

PRECAUTIONS

General

Candesartan Cilexetil–Hydrochlorothiazide

In clinical trials of various doses of candesartan cilexetil and hydrochlorothiazide, the incidence of hypertensive patients who developed hypokalemia (serum potassium <3.5 mEq/L) was 2.5% versus 2.1% for placebo; the incidence of hyperkalemia (serum potassium >5.7 mEq/L) was 0.4% versus 1.0% for placebo. No patient receiving ATACAND HCT 16-12.5 mg or 32-12.5 mg was discontinued due to increases or decreases in serum potassium. Overall, the combination of candesartan cilexetil and hydrochlorothiazide had no clinically significant effect on serum potassium.

Hydrochlorothiazide

Periodic determination of serum electrolytes to detect possible electrolyte imbalance should be performed at appropriate intervals.

All patients receiving thiazide therapy should be observed for clinical signs of fluid or electrolyte imbalance: namely, hyponatremia, hypochloremic alkalosis, and hypokalemia. Serum and urine electrolyte determinations are particularly important when the patient is vomiting excessively or receiving parenteral fluids. Warning signs or symptoms of fluid and electrolyte imbalance, irrespective of cause, include dryness of mouth, thirst, weakness, lethargy, drowsiness, restlessness, confusion, seizures, muscle pains or cramps, muscular fatigue, hypotension, oliguria, tachycardia, and gastrointestinal disturbances such as nausea and vomiting.

Hypokalemia may develop, especially with brisk diuresis, when severe cirrhosis is present, or after prolonged therapy. Interference with adequate oral electrolyte intake will also contribute to hypokalemia. Hypokalemia may cause cardiac arrhythmia and may also sensitize or exaggerate the response of the heart to the toxic effects of digitalis (eg, increased ventricular irritability).

Although any chloride deficit is generally mild and usually does not require specific treatment, except under extraordinary circumstances (as in liver disease or renal disease), chloride replacement may be required in the treatment of metabolic alkalosis.

Dilutional hyponatremia may occur in edematous patients in hot weather; appropriate therapy is water restriction, rather than administration of salt, except in rare instances when the hyponatremia is life-threatening. In actual salt depletion, appropriate replacement is the therapy of choice.

Hyperuricemia may occur or acute gout may be precipitated in certain patients receiving thiazide therapy.

In diabetic patients dosage adjustments of insulin or oral hypoglycemic agents may be required. Hyperglycemia may occur with thiazide diuretics. Thus latent diabetes mellitus may become manifest during thiazide therapy.

The antihypertensive effects of the drug may be enhanced in the post-sympathectomy patient.

If progressive renal impairment becomes evident consider withholding or discontinuing diuretic therapy.

Thiazides have been shown to increase the urinary excretion of magnesium; this may result in hypomagnesemia.

Thiazides may decrease urinary calcium excretion. Thiazides may cause intermittent and slight elevation of serum calcium in the absence of known disorders of calcium metabolism. Marked hypercalcemia may be evidence of hidden hyperparathyroidism. Thiazides should be discontinued before carrying out tests for parathyroid function.

Increases in cholesterol and triglyceride levels may be associated with thiazide diuretic therapy.

Impaired Renal Function

Candesartan Cilexetil

As a consequence of inhibiting the renin-angiotensin-aldosterone system, changes in renal function may be anticipated in susceptible individuals treated with candesartan cilexetil. In patients whose renal function may depend upon the activity of the renin-angiotensin-aldosterone system (eg, patients with severe congestive heart failure), treatment with angiotensin-converting enzyme inhibitors and angiotensin receptor antagonists has been associated with oliguria and/or progressive azotemia and (rarely) with acute renal failure and/or death. Similar results may be anticipated in patients treated with candesartan cilexetil. (See CLINICAL PHARMACOLOGY, Special Populations.)

In studies of ACE inhibitors in patients with unilateral or bilateral renal artery stenosis, increases in serum creatinine or blood urea nitrogen (BUN) have been reported. There has been no long-term use of candesartan cilexetil in patients with unilateral or bilateral renal artery stenosis, but similar results may be expected.

Hydrochlorothiazide

Thiazides should be used with caution in severe renal disease. In patients with renal disease, thiazides may precipitate azotemia. Cumulative effects of the drug may develop in patients with impaired renal function.

Impaired Hepatic Function

Candesartan Cilexetil

Based on pharmacokinetic data significant increases in candesartan AUC and C_{max} in patients with moderate hepatic impairment have been demonstrated. (See CLINICAL PHARMACOLOGY, Special Populations.)

Information for Patients

Pregnancy

Female patients of childbearing age should be told about the consequences of second- and third-trimester exposure to drugs that act on the renin-angiotensin system, and they should also be told that these consequences do not appear to have resulted from intrauterine drug exposure that has been limited to the first trimester. These patients should be asked to report pregnancies to their physicians as soon as possible.

Symptomatic Hypotension

A patient receiving ATACAND HCT should be cautioned that lightheadedness can occur, especially during the first days of therapy, and that it should be reported to the prescribing physician. The patients should be told that if syncope occurs, ATACAND HCT should be discontinued until the physician has been consulted.

All patients should be cautioned that inadequate fluid intake, excessive perspiration, diarrhea, or vomiting can lead to an excessive fall in blood pressure, with the same consequences of lightheadedness and possible syncope.

Potassium Supplements

A patient receiving ATACAND HCT should be told not to use potassium supplements or salt substitutes containing potassium without consulting the prescribing physician.

Drug Interactions

Candesartan Cilexetil

No significant drug interactions have been reported in studies of candesartan cilexetil given with other drugs such as glyburide, nifedipine, digoxin, warfarin, hydrochlorothiazide, and oral contraceptives in healthy volunteers. Because candesartan is not significantly metabolized by the cytochrome P450 system and at therapeutic concentrations has no effects on P450 enzymes, interactions with drugs that inhibit or are metabolized by those enzymes would not be expected.

Lithium – Reversible increases in serum lithium concentrations and toxicity have been reported during concomitant administration of lithium with ACE inhibitors, and with some angiotensin II receptor antagonists. An increase in serum lithium concentration has been reported during concomitant administration of lithium with candesartan cilexetil, so careful monitoring of serum lithium levels is recommended during concomitant use.

Hydrochlorothiazide

When administered concurrently the following drugs may interact with thiazide diuretics:

Alcohol, barbiturates, or narcotics – Potentiation of orthostatic hypotension may occur.

Antidiabetic drugs (oral agents and insulin) – Dosage adjustment of the antidiabetic drug may be required.

Other antihypertensive drugs – Additive effect or potentiation.

Cholestyramine and colestipol resins – Absorption of hydrochlorothiazide is impaired in the presence of anionic exchange resins. Single doses of either cholestyramine or colestipol resins bind the hydrochlorothiazide and reduce its absorption from the gastrointestinal tract by up to 85 and 43 percent, respectively.

Corticosteroids, ACTH – Intensified electrolyte depletion, particularly hypokalemia.
Pressor amines (eg, norepinephrine) – Possible decreased response to pressor amines but not sufficient to preclude their use.
Skeletal muscle relaxants, nondepolarizing (eg, tubocurarine) – Possible increased responsiveness to the muscle relaxant.
Lithium – Generally should not be given with diuretics. Diuretic agents reduce the renal clearance of lithium and add a high risk of lithium toxicity. Refer to the package insert for lithium preparations before use of such preparations with ATACAND HCT.
Non-steroidal Anti-inflammatory Drugs – In some patients, the administration of a non-steroidal anti-inflammatory agent can reduce the diuretic, natriuretic, and antihypertensive effects of loop, potassium-sparing and thiazide diuretics. Therefore, when ATACAND HCT and non-steroidal anti-inflammatory agents are used concomitantly, the patient should be observed closely to determine if the desired effect of the diuretic is obtained.

Carcinogenesis, Mutagenesis, Impairment of Fertility
No carcinogenicity studies have been conducted with the combination of candesartan cilexetil and hydrochlorothiazide. There was no evidence of carcinogenicity when candesartan cilexetil was orally administered to mice and rats for up to 104 weeks at doses up to 100 and 1000 mg/kg/day, respectively. Rats received the drug by gavage whereas mice received the drug by dietary administration. These (maximally-tolerated) doses of candesartan cilexetil provided systemic exposures to candesartan (AUCs) that were, in mice, approximately 7 times and, in rats, more than 70 times the exposure in man at the maximum recommended daily human dose (32 mg). Two-year feeding studies in mice and rats conducted under the auspices of the National Toxicology Program (NTP) uncovered no evidence of a carcinogenic potential of hydrochlorothiazide in female mice (at doses of up to approximately 600 mg/kg/day) or in male and female rats (at doses of up to approximately 100 mg/kg/day). The NTP, however, found equivocal evidence for hepatocarcinogenicity in male mice.
Candesartan cilexetil or candesartan (the active metabolite), in combination with hydrochlorothiazide, tested positive *in vitro* in the Chinese hamster lung (CHL) chromosomal aberration assay and mouse lymphoma mutagenicity assay. The candesartan cilexetil/hydrochlorothiazide combination tested negative for mutagenicity in bacteria (Ames test), for unscheduled DNA synthesis in rat liver, for chromosomal aberrations in rat bone marrow and for micronuclei in mouse bone marrow.
Both candesartan and its O-deethyl metabolite tested positive for genotoxicity in the *in vitro* CHL chromosomal aberration assay. Neither compound tested positive in the Ames microbial mutagenesis assay or in the *in vitro* mouse lymphoma cell assay. Candesartan (but not its O-deethyl metabolite) was also evaluated *in vivo* in the mouse micronucleus test and *in vitro* in the Chinese hamster ovary (CHO) gene mutation assay, in both cases with negative results. Candesartan cilexetil was evaluated in the Ames test, the *in vitro* mouse lymphoma cell assay, the *in vivo* rat hepatocyte unscheduled DNA synthesis assay and the *in vivo* mouse micronucleus test, in each case with negative results. Candesartan cilexetil was not evaluated in the CHL chromosomal aberration or CHO gene mutation assays.
When hydrochlorothiazide was tested alone, positive results were obtained *in vitro* in the CHO sister chromatid exchange (clastogenicity) and mouse lymphoma cell (mutagenicity) assays and in the *Aspergillus nidulans* nondisjunciton assay.
Hydrochlorothiazide was not genotoxic *in vitro* in the Ames test for point mutations and the CHO test for chromosomal aberrations, or *in vivo* in assays using mouse germinal cell chromosomes, Chinese hamster bone marrow chromosomes, and the Drosophila sex-linked recessive lethal trait gene.
No fertility studies have been conducted with the combination of candesartan cilexetil and hydrochlorothiazide. Fertility and reproductive performance were not affected in studies with male and female rats given oral doses of up to 300 mg candesartan cilexetil/kg/day (83 times the maximum daily human dose of 32 mg on a body surface area basis). Hydrochlorothiazide had no adverse effects on the fertility of mice and rats of either sex in studies wherein these species were exposed, via their diet, to doses of up to 100 and 4 mg/kg, respectively, prior to conception and throughout gestation.

Pregnancy
Pregnancy Categories C (first trimester) *and D* (second and third trimesters). See WARNINGS, Fetal/Neonatal Morbidity and Mortality.

Nursing Mothers
It is not known whether candesartan is excreted in human milk, but candesartan has been shown to be present in rat milk. Thiazides appear in human milk. Because of the potential for adverse effects on the nursing infant, a decision should be made whether to discontinue nursing or discontinue the drug, taking into account the importance of the drug to the mother.

Pediatric Use
Safety and effectiveness in pediatric patients have not been established.

Geriatric Use
Of the total number of subjects in all clinical studies of ATACAND HCT (2831), 611 (22%) were 65 and over, while 94 (3%) were 75 and over. No overall differences in safety or effectiveness were observed between these subjects and younger subjects. Other reported clinical experience has not identified differences in responses between the elderly and younger patients, but greater sensitivity of some older individuals cannot be ruled out.
Hydrochlorothiazide is known to be substantially excreted by the kidney, and the risk of toxic reactions to this drug may be greater in patients with impaired renal function.

ADVERSE REACTIONS

Candesartan Cilexetil-Hydrochlorothiazide
ATACAND HCT has been evaluated for safety in more than 2800 patients treated for hypertension. More than 750 of these patients were studied for at least six months and more than 500 patients were treated for at least one year. Adverse experiences have generally been mild and transient in nature and have only infrequently required discontinuation of therapy. The overall incidence of adverse events reported with ATACAND HCT was comparable to placebo. The overall frequency of adverse experiences was not related to dose, age, gender, or race.
In placebo-controlled trials that included 1089 patients treated with various combinations of candesartan cilexetil (doses of 2-32 mg) and hydrochlorothiazide (doses of 6.25-25 mg) and 592 patients treated with placebo, adverse events, whether or not attributed to treatment, occurring in greater than 2% of patients treated with ATACAND HCT and that were more frequent for ATACAND HCT than placebo were: ***Respiratory System Disorder:*** upper respiratory tract infection (3.6% vs 3.0%); ***Body as a Whole:*** back pain (3.3% vs 2.4%); influenza-like symptoms (2.5% vs 1.9%); ***Central/Peripheral Nervous System:*** dizziness (2.9% vs 1.2%).
The frequency of headache was greater than 2% (2.9%) in patients treated with ATACAND HCT but was less frequent than the rate in patients treated with placebo (5.2%).
Other adverse events that have been reported, whether or not attributed to treatment, with an incidence of 0.5% or greater from the more than 2800 patients worldwide treated with ATACAND HCT included: ***Body as a Whole:*** inflicted injury, fatigue, pain, chest pain, peripheral edema, asthenia; ***Central and Peripheral Nervous System:*** vertigo, paresthesia, hypesthesia; ***Respiratory System Disorders:*** bronchitis, sinusitis, pharyngitis, coughing, rhinitis, dyspnea; ***Musculoskeletal System Disorders:*** arthralgia, myalgia, arthrosis, arthritis, leg cramps, sciatica; ***Gastrointestinal System Disorders:*** nausea, abdominal pain, diarrhea, dyspepsia, gastritis, gastroenteritis, vomiting; ***Metabolic and Nutritional Disorders:*** hyperuricemia, hyperglycemia, hypokalemia, increased BUN, creatine phosphokinase increased; ***Urinary System Disorders:*** urinary tract infection, hematuria, cystitis; ***Liver/Biliary System Disorders:*** hepatic function abnormal, increased transaminase levels; ***Heart Rate and Rhythm Disorders:*** tachycardia, palpitation, extrasystoles, bradycardia; ***Psychiatric Disorders:*** depression, insomnia, anxiety; ***Cardiovascular Disorders:*** ECG abnormal; ***Skin and Appendages Disorders:*** eczema, sweating increased, pruritus, dermatitis, rash; ***Platelet/Bleeding-Clotting Disorders:*** epistaxis; ***Resistance Mechanism Disorders:*** infection, viral infection; ***Vision Disorders:*** conjunctivitis; ***Hearing and Vestibular Disorders:*** tinnitus.
Reported events seen less frequently than 0.5% included angina pectoris, myocardial infarction and angioedema.
Candesartan Cilexetil
Other adverse experiences that have been reported with candesartan cilexetil, without regard to causality, were: ***Body as a Whole:*** fever; ***Metabolic and Nutritional Disorders:*** hypertriglyceridemia; ***Psychiatric Disorders:*** somnolence; ***Urinary System Disorders:*** albuminuria.
Post-Marketing Experience
The following have been very rarely reported in post-marketing experience with candesartan cilexetil:
Digestive: Abnormal hepatic function and hepatitis.
Hematologic: Neutropenia, leukopenia, and agranulocytosis.
Metabolic and Nutritional Disorders: hyperkalemia, hyponatremia.
Renal: renal impairment, renal failure.
Skin and Appendages Disorders: Pruritus and urticaria.
Rare reports of rhabdomyolysis have been reported in patients receiving angiotensin II receptor blockers.
Hydrochlorothiazide
Other adverse experiences that have been reported with hydrochlorothiazide, without regard to causality, are listed below:
Body As A Whole: weakness; ***Cardiovascular:*** hypotension including orthostatic hypotension (may be aggravated by alcohol, barbiturates, narcotics or antihypertensive drugs); ***Digestive:*** pancreatitis, jaundice (intrahepatic cholestatic jaundice), sialadenitis, cramping, constipation, gastric irritation, anorexia; ***Hematologic:*** aplastic anemia, agranulocytosis, leukopenia, hemolytic anemia, thrombocytopenia; ***Hypersensitivity:*** anaphylactic reactions, necrotizing angiitis (vasculitis and cutaneous vasculitis), respiratory distress including pneumonitis and pulmonary edema, photosensitivity, urticaria, purpura; ***Metabolic:*** electrolyte imbalance, glycosuria; ***Musculoskeletal:*** muscle spasm; ***Nervous System/Psychiatric:*** restlessness; ***Renal:*** renal failure, renal dysfunction, interstitial nephritis; ***Skin:*** erythema multiforme including Stevens-Johnson syndrome, exfoliative dermatitis including toxic epidermal necrolysis, alopecia; ***Special Senses:*** transient blurred vision, xanthopsia; ***Urogenital:*** impotence.

Laboratory Test Findings
In controlled clinical trials, clinically important changes in standard laboratory parameters were rarely associated with the administration of ATACAND HCT.
Creatinine, Blood Urea Nitrogen—Minor increases in blood urea nitrogen (BUN) and serum creatinine were observed infrequently. One patient was discontinued from ATACAND HCT due to increased BUN. No patient was discontinued due to an increase in serum creatinine.
Hemoglobin and Hematocrit—Small decreases in hemoglobin and hematocrit (mean decreases of approximately 0.2 g/dL and 0.4 volume percent, respectively) were observed in patients treated with ATACAND HCT, but were rarely of clinical importance.
Potassium— A small decrease (mean decrease of 0.1 mEq/L) was observed in patients treated with ATACAND HCT. In placebo-controlled trials, hypokalemia was reported in 0.4% of patients treated with ATACAND HCT as compared to 1.0% of patients treated with hydrochlorothiazide or 0.2% of patients treated with placebo.
Liver Function Tests—Occasional elevations of liver enzymes and/or serum bilirubin have occurred.

OVERDOSAGE

Candesartan Cilexetil-Hydrochlorothiazide
No lethality was observed in acute toxicity studies in mice, rats and dogs given single oral doses of up to 2000 mg/kg of candesartan cilexetil or in rats given single oral doses of up to 2000 mg/kg of candesartan cilexetil in combination with 1000 mg/kg of hydrochlorothiazide. In mice given single oral doses of the primary metabolite, candesartan, the minimum lethal dose was greater than 1000 mg/kg but less than 2000 mg/kg.
Limited data are available in regard to overdosage with candesartan cilexetil in humans. The most likely manifestations of overdosage with candesartan cilexetil would be hypotension, dizziness, and tachycardia; bradycardia could occur from parasympathetic (vagal) stimulation. If symptomatic hypotension should occur, supportive treatment should be initiated. For hydrochlorothiazide, the most common signs and symptoms observed are those caused by electrolyte depletion (hypokalemia, hypochloremia, hyponatremia) and dehydration resulting from excessive diuresis. If digitalis has also been administered, hypokalemia may accentuate cardiac arrhythmias.
Candesartan cannot be removed by hemodialysis. The degree to which hydrochlorothiazide is removed by hemodialysis has not been established.
Treatment
To obtain up-to-date information about the treatment of overdose, consult your Regional Poison Control Center. Telephone numbers of certified poison control centers are listed in the *Physicians' Desk Reference (PDR)*. In managing overdose, consider the possibilities of multiple-drug overdoses, drug-drug interactions, and altered pharmacokinetics in your patient.

DOSAGE AND ADMINISTRATION

The usual recommended starting dose of candesartan cilexetil is 16 mg once daily when it is used as monotherapy in patients who are not volume depleted. ATACAND can be administered once or twice daily with total daily doses ranging from 8 mg to 32 mg. Patients requiring further reduction in blood pressure should be titrated to 32 mg. Doses larger than 32 mg do not appear to have a greater blood pressure lowering effect.
Hydrochlorothiazide is effective in doses of 12.5 to 50 mg once daily.
To minimize dose-independent side effects, it is usually appropriate to begin combination therapy only after a patient has failed to achieve the desired effect with monotherapy.
The side effects (See WARNINGS) of candesartan cilexetil are generally rare and apparently independent of dose; those of hydrochlorothiazide are a mixture of dose-dependent phenomena (primarily hypokalemia) and dose-independent phenomena (eg, pancreatitis), the former much more common than the latter.
Therapy with any combination of candesartan cilexetil and hydrochlorothiazide will be associated with both sets of dose-independent side effects.
Replacement Therapy: The combination may be substituted for the titrated components.
Dose Titration by Clinical Effect: A patient whose blood pressure is not controlled on 25 mg of hydrochlorothiazide once daily can expect an incremental effect from ATACAND HCT 16-12.5 mg. A patient whose blood pressure is controlled on 25 mg of hydrochlorothiazide but is experiencing decreases in serum potassium can expect the same or incremental blood pressure effects from ATACAND HCT 16-12.5 mg and serum potassium may improve.
A patient whose blood pressure is not controlled on 32 mg of ATACAND can expect incremental blood pressure effects from ATACAND HCT 32-12.5 mg and then 32-25 mg. The maximal antihypertensive effect of any dose of ATACAND HCT can be expected within 4 weeks of initiating that dose.
Patients with Renal Impairment: The usual regimens of therapy with ATACAND HCT may be followed as long as the patient's creatinine clearance is > 30 mL/min. In patients with more severe renal impairment, loop diuretics are preferred to thiazides, so ATACAND HCT is not recommended.
Patients with Hepatic Impairment: The usual regimens of therapy with ATACAND HCT may be followed in patients with mild hepatic impairment. In patients with moderate hepatic impairment, consideration should be given to initiation of ATACAND at a lower dose, such as 8 mg. If a lower starting dose is selected for candesartan cilexetil, ATACAND HCT is not recommended for initial titration be-

Continued on next page

Atacand HCT—Cont.

cause the appropriate initial starting dose of candesartan cilexetil cannot be given. (See CLINICAL PHARMACOLOGY, Special Populations, *Hepatic Insufficiency*).

Thiazide diuretics should be used with caution in patients with hepatic impairment; therefore, care should be exercised with dosing of ATACAND HCT.

ATACAND HCT may be administered with other antihypertensive agents.

ATACAND HCT may be administered with or without food.

HOW SUPPLIED

No. 3825—Tablets ATACAND HCT 16-12.5, are peach, oval, biconvex, non-film-coated tablets, coded ACS on one side and 162 on the other. They are supplied as follows:

NDC 0186-0162-28 unit dose packages of 100.

NDC 0186-0162-54 unit of use bottles of 90.

No. 3826—Tablets ATACAND HCT 32-12.5, are yellow, oval, biconvex, non-film-coated tablets, coded ACJ on one side and 322 on the other. They are supplied as follows:

NDC 0186-0322-28 unit dose packages of 100.

NDC 0186-0322-54 unit of use bottles of 90.

Storage

Store at 25°C (77°F); excursions permitted to 15-30°C (59-86°F) [see USP Controlled Room Temperature]. Keep container tightly closed.

ATACAND HCT is a trademark of the AstraZeneca group of companies.
©AstraZeneca 2003, 2004

Manufactured under the license
from Takeda Chemical Industries, Ltd.
by: AstraZeneca AB, S-151 85 Södertälje, Sweden
for: AstraZeneca LP, Wilmington, DE 19850
Made in Sweden
9329103
610517-03 Rev. 05/04
AstraZeneca

NEXIUM® ℞

(esomeprazole magnesium)
DELAYED-RELEASE CAPSULES

Rx only

Prescribing information for this product, which appears on pages 621–625 of the 2005 PDR, has been completely revised as follows. Please write "See Supplement A" next to the product heading.

DESCRIPTION

The active ingredient in NEXIUM® (esomeprazole magnesium) Delayed-Release Capsules is bis(5-methoxy-2-[(S)-[(4-methoxy-3,5-dimethyl-2-pyridinyl)methyl]sulfinyl]-1*H*-benzimidazole-1-yl) magnesium trihydrate, a compound that inhibits gastric acid secretion. Esomeprazole is the S-isomer of omeprazole, which is a mixture of the S- and R-isomers. Its empirical formula is $(C_{17}H_{18}N_3O_3S)_2Mg \times 3\ H_2O$ with molecular weight of 767.2 as a trihydrate and 713.1 on an anhydrous basis. The structural formula is:

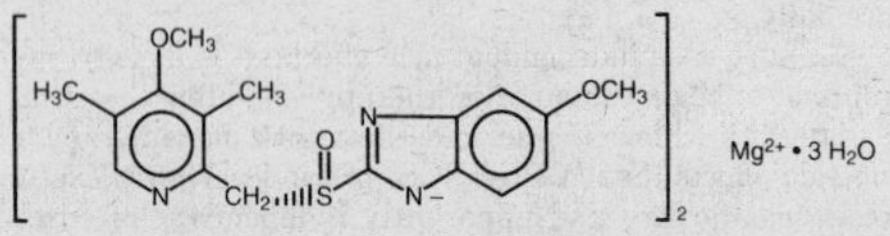

The magnesium salt is a white to slightly colored crystalline powder. It contains 3 moles of water of solvation and is slightly soluble in water.

The stability of esomeprazole magnesium is a function of pH; it rapidly degrades in acidic media, but it has acceptable stability under alkaline conditions. At pH 6.8 (buffer), the half-life of the magnesium salt is about 19 hours at 25°C and about 8 hours at 37°C.

NEXIUM is supplied as Delayed-Release Capsules for oral administration. Each delayed-release capsule contains 20 mg or 40 mg of esomeprazole (present as 22.3 mg or 44.5 mg esomeprazole magnesium trihydrate) in the form of enteric-coated pellets with the following inactive ingredients: glyceryl monostearate 40-50, hydroxypropyl cellulose, hypromellose, magnesium stearate, methacrylic acid copolymer type C, polysorbate 80, sugar spheres, talc, and triethyl citrate. The capsule shells have the following inactive ingredients: gelatin, FD&C Blue #1, FD&C Red #40, D&C Red #28, titanium dioxide, shellac, ethyl alcohol, isopropyl alcohol, n-butyl alcohol, propylene glycol, sodium hydroxide, polyvinyl pyrrolidone, and D&C Yellow #10.

CLINICAL PHARMACOLOGY

Pharmacokinetics

Absorption

NEXIUM Delayed-Release Capsules contain an enteric-coated pellet formulation of esomeprazole magnesium. After oral administration peak plasma levels (C_{max}) occur at approximately 1.5 hours (T_{max}). The C_{max} increases proportionally when the dose is increased, and there is a three-fold increase in the area under the plasma concentration-time curve (AUC) from 20 to 40 mg. At repeated once-daily dosing with 40 mg, the systemic bioavailability is approximately 90% compared to 64% after a single dose of 40 mg. The mean exposure (AUC) to esomeprazole increases from 4.32 μmol*hr/L on day 1 to 11.2 μmol*hr/L on day 5 after 40 mg once daily dosing.

The AUC after administration of a single 40 mg dose of esomeprazole is decreased by 43-53% after food intake compared to fasting conditions. Esomeprazole should be taken at least one hour before meals.

The pharmacokinetic profile of esomeprazole was determined in 36 patients with symptomatic gastroesophageal reflux disease following repeated once daily administration of 20 mg and 40 mg capsules of NEXIUM over a period of five days. The results are shown in the following table:

Pharmacokinetic Parameters of NEXIUM Following Oral Dosing for 5 days

Parameter	NEXIUM 40 mg	NEXIUM 20 mg
AUC (μmol*h/L)	12.6	4.2
Coefficient of variation	42%	59%
C_{max} (μmol/L)	4.7	2.1
T_{max} (h)	1.6	1.6
$t_{1/2}$ (h)	1.5	1.2

Values represent the geometric mean, except the T_{max}, which is the arithmetic mean.

Distribution

Esomeprazole is 97% bound to plasma proteins. Plasma protein binding is constant over the concentration range of 2-20 μmol/L. The apparent volume of distribution at steady state in healthy volunteers is approximately 16 L.

Metabolism

Esomeprazole is extensively metabolized in the liver by the cytochrome P450 (CYP) enzyme system. The metabolites of esomeprazole lack antisecretory activity. The major part of esomeprazole's metabolism is dependent upon the CYP2C19 isoenzyme, which forms the hydroxy and desmethyl metabolites. The remaining amount is dependent on CYP3A4 which forms the sulphone metabolite. CYP2C19 isoenzyme exhibits polymorphism in the metabolism of esomeprazole, since some 3% of Caucasians and 15-20% of Asians lack CYP2C19 and are termed Poor metabolizers. At steady state, the ratio of AUC in Poor metabolizers to AUC in the rest of the population (Extensive metabolizers) is approximately 2.

Following administration of equimolar doses, the S- and R-isomers are metabolized differently by the liver, resulting in higher plasma levels of the S- than of the R-isomer.

Excretion

The plasma elimination half-life of esomeprazole is approximately 1–1.5 hours. Less than 1% of parent drug is excreted in the urine. Approximately 80% of an oral dose of esomeprazole is excreted as inactive metabolites in the urine, and the remainder is found as inactive metabolites in the feces.

Special Populations

Geriatric

The AUC and C_{max} values were slightly higher (25% and 18%, respectively) in the elderly as compared to younger subjects at steady state. Dosage adjustment based on age is not necessary.

Pediatric

The pharmacokinetics of esomeprazole have not been studied in patients <18 years of age.

Gender

The AUC and C_{max} values were slightly higher (13%) in females than in males at steady state. Dosage adjustment based on gender is not necessary.

Hepatic Insufficiency

The steady state pharmacokinetics of esomeprazole obtained after administration of 40 mg once daily to 4 patients each with mild (Child Pugh A), moderate (Child Pugh Class B), and severe (Child Pugh Class C) liver insufficiency were compared to those obtained in 36 male and female GERD patients with normal liver function. In patients with mild and moderate hepatic insufficiency, the AUCs were within the range that could be expected in patients with normal liver function. In patients with severe hepatic insufficiency the AUCs were 2 to 3 times higher than in the patients with normal liver function. No dosage adjustment is recommended for patients with mild to moderate hepatic insufficiency (Child Pugh Classes A and B). However, in patients with severe hepatic insufficiency (Child Pugh Class C) a dose of 20 mg once daily should not be exceeded (See **DOSAGE AND ADMINISTRATION**).

Renal Insufficiency

The pharmacokinetics of esomeprazole in patients with renal impairment are not expected to be altered relative to healthy volunteers as less than 1% of esomeprazole is excreted unchanged in urine.

Pharmacokinetics: Combination Therapy with Antimicrobials

Esomeprazole magnesium 40 mg once daily was given in combination with clarithromycin 500 mg twice daily and amoxicillin 1000 mg twice daily for 7 days to 17 healthy male and female subjects. The mean steady state AUC and C_{max} of esomeprazole increased by 70% and 18%, respectively, during triple combination therapy compared to treatment with esomeprazole alone. The observed increase in esomeprazole exposure during co-administration with clarithromycin and amoxicillin is not expected to produce significant safety concerns.

The pharmacokinetic parameters for clarithromycin and amoxicillin were similar during triple combination therapy and administration of each drug alone. However, the mean AUC and C_{max} for 14-hydroxyclarithromycin increased by 19% and 22%, respectively, during triple combination therapy compared to treatment with clarithromycin alone. This increase in exposure to 14-hydroxyclarithromycin is not considered to be clinically significant.

Pharmacodynamics

Mechanism of Action

Esomeprazole is a proton pump inhibitor that suppresses gastric acid secretion by specific inhibition of the H^+/K^+-ATPase in the gastric parietal cell. The S- and R-isomers of omeprazole are protonated and converted in the acidic compartment of the parietal cell forming the active inhibitor, the achiral sulphenamide. By acting specifically on the proton pump, esomeprazole blocks the final step in acid production, thus reducing gastric acidity. This effect is dose-related up to a daily dose of 20 to 40 mg and leads to inhibition of gastric acid secretion.

Antisecretory Activity

The effect of esomeprazole on intragastric pH was determined in patients with symptomatic gastroesophageal reflux disease in two separate studies. In the first study of 36 patients, NEXIUM 40 mg and 20 mg capsules were administered over 5 days. The results are shown in the following table:

Effect on Intragastric pH on Day 5 (N=36)

Parameter	NEXIUM 40 mg	NEXIUM 20 mg
% Time Gastric pH >4† (Hours)	70%* (16.8 h)	53% (12.7 h)
Coefficient of variation	26%	37%
Median 24 Hour pH	4.9*	4.1
Coefficient of variation	16%	27%

† Gastric pH was measured over a 24-hour period
* p<0.01 NEXIUM 40 mg vs NEXIUM 20 mg

In a second study, the effect on intragastric pH of NEXIUM 40 mg administered once daily over a five day period was similar to the first study, (% time with pH>4 was 68% or 16.3 hours).

Serum Gastrin Effects

The effect of NEXIUM on serum gastrin concentrations was evaluated in approximately 2,700 patients in clinical trials up to 8 weeks and in over 1,300 patients for up to 6-12 months. The mean fasting gastrin level increased in a dose-related manner. This increase reached a plateau within two to three months of therapy and returned to baseline levels within four weeks after discontinuation of therapy.

Enterochromaffin-like (ECL) Cell Effects

In 24-month carcinogenicity studies of omeprazole in rats, a dose-related significant occurrence of gastric ECL cell carcinoid tumors and ECL cell hyperplasia was observed in both male and female animals (see **PRECAUTIONS**, Carcinogenesis, Mutagenesis, Impairment of Fertility). Carcinoid tumors have also been observed in rats subjected to fundectomy or long-term treatment with other proton pump inhibitors or high doses of H_2-receptor antagonists.

Human gastric biopsy specimens have been obtained from more than 3,000 patients treated with omeprazole in long-term clinical trials. The incidence of ECL cell hyperplasia in these studies increased with time; however, no case of ECL cell carcinoids, dysplasia, or neoplasia has been found in these patients.

In over 1,000 patients treated with NEXIUM (10, 20 or 40 mg/day) up to 6-12 months, the prevalence of ECL cell hyperplasia increased with time and dose. No patient developed ECL cell carcinoids, dysplasia, or neoplasia in the gastric mucosa.

Endocrine Effects

NEXIUM had no effect on thyroid function when given in oral doses of 20 or 40 mg for 4 weeks. Other effects of NEXIUM on the endocrine system were assessed using omeprazole studies. Omeprazole given in oral doses of 30 or 40 mg for 2 to 4 weeks had no effect on carbohydrate metabolism, circulating levels of parathyroid hormone, cortisol, estradiol, testosterone, prolactin, cholecystokinin or secretin.

Microbiology

Esomeprazole magnesium, amoxicillin and clarithromycin triple therapy has been shown to be active against most strains of *Helicobacter pylori (H. pylori) in vitro* and in clinical infections as described in the **Clinical Studies** and **INDICATIONS AND USAGE** sections.

Helicobacter

Helicobacter pylori: Susceptibility testing of *H. pylori* isolates was performed for amoxicillin and clarithromycin using agar dilution methodology, and minimum inhibitory concentrations (MICs) were determined.

Pretreatment Resistance: Clarithromycin pretreatment resistance rate (MIC ≥1 μg/mL) to *H. pylori* was 15% (66/445) at baseline in all treatment groups combined. A total of >99% (394/395) of patients had *H. pylori* isolates which were considered to be susceptible (MIC ≤0.25 μg/mL) to amoxicillin at baseline. One patient had a baseline *H. pylori* isolate with an amoxicillin MIC=0.5 μg/mL.

Clarithromycin Susceptibility Test Results and Clinical/Bacteriologic Outcomes: The baseline *H. pylori* clarithromycin susceptibility results and the *H. pylori* eradication results at the Day 38 visit are shown in the table below:

Clarithromycin Susceptibility Test Results and Clinical/Bacteriological Outcomes[a] for Triple Therapy – (Esomeprazole magnesium 40 mg once daily/amoxicillin 1000 mg twice daily/clarithromycin 500 mg twice daily for 10 days)

Clarithromycin Pretreatment Results	H. pylori negative (Eradicated)	H. pylori positive (Not Eradicated) Post-treatment susceptibility results			
		S[b]	I[b]	R[b]	No MIC
Susceptible[b] 182	162	4	0	2	14
Intermediate[b] 1	1	0	0	0	0
Resistant[b] 29	13	1	0	13	2

[a] Includes only patients with pretreatment and post-treatment clarithromycin susceptibility test results
[b] Susceptible (S) MIC ≤0.25 μg/mL, Intermediate (I) MIC=0.5 μg/mL, Resistant (R) MIC ≥1.0 μg/mL

Patients not eradicated of *H. pylori* following esomeprazole magnesium/amoxicillin/clarithromycin triple therapy will likely have clarithromycin resistant *H. pylori* isolates. Therefore, clarithromycin susceptibility testing should be done, when possible. Patients with clarithromycin resistant *H. pylori* should not be re-treated with a clarithromycin-containing regimen.

Amoxicillin Susceptibility Test Results and Clinical/Bacteriological Outcomes: In the esomeprazole magnesium/amoxicillin/clarithromycin clinical trials, 83% (176/212) of the patients in the esomeprazole magnesium/amoxicillin/clarithromycin treatment group who had pretreatment amoxicillin susceptible MICs (≤0.25 μg/mL) were eradicated of *H. pylori*, and 17% (36/212) were not eradicated of *H. pylori*. Of the 36 patients who were not eradicated of *H. pylori* on triple therapy, 16 had no post-treatment susceptibility test results and 20 had post-treatment *H. pylori* isolates with amoxicillin susceptible MICs. Fifteen of the patients who were not eradicated of *H. pylori* on triple therapy also had post-treatment *H. pylori* isolates with clarithromycin resistant MICs. There were no patients with *H. pylori* isolates who developed treatment emergent resistance to amoxicillin.

Susceptibility Test for Helicobacter pylori: The reference methodology for susceptibility testing of *H. pylori* is agar dilution MICs. One to three microliters of an inoculum equivalent to a No.2 McFarland standard (1×10^7 – 1×10^8 CFU/mL for *H. pylori*) are inoculated directly onto freshly prepared antimicrobial containing Mueller-Hinton agar plates with 5% aged defibrinated sheep blood (≥2 weeks old). The agar dilution plates are incubated at 35°C in a microaerobic environment produced by a gas generating system suitable for *Campylobacter*. After 3 days of incubation, the MICs are recorded as the lowest concentration of antimicrobial agent required to inhibit growth of the organism. The clarithromycin and amoxicillin MIC values should be interpreted according to the following criteria:

Clarithromycin MIC (μg/mL)[a]	Interpretation	
≤0.25	Susceptible	(S)
0.5	Intermediate	(I)
≥1.0	Resistant	(R)
Amoxicillin MIC (μg/mL)[a,b]	Interpretation	
≤0.25	Susceptible	(S)

[a] These are breakpoints for the agar dilution methodology and they should not be used to interpret results obtained using alternative methods.
[b] There were not enough organisms with MICs >0.25 μg/mL to determine a resistance breakpoint.

Standardized susceptibility test procedures require the use of laboratory control microorganisms to control the technical aspects of the laboratory procedures. Standard clarithromycin and amoxicillin powders should provide the following MIC values:

Microorganism	Antimicrobial Agent	MIC (μg/mL)[a]
H. pylori ATCC 43504	Clarithromycin	0.016 – 0.12 (μg/mL)
H. pylori ATCC 43504	Amoxicillin	0.016 – 0.12 (μg/mL)

[a] These are quality control ranges for the agar dilution methodology and they should not be used to control test results obtained using alternative methods.

Clinical Studies
Healing of Erosive Esophagitis
The healing rates of NEXIUM 40 mg, NEXIUM 20 mg, and omeprazole 20 mg (the approved dose for this indication) were evaluated in patients with endoscopically diagnosed erosive esophagitis in four multicenter, double-blind, randomized studies. The healing rates at weeks 4 and 8 were evaluated and are shown in the table below:
[See first table above]

Erosive Esophagitis Healing Rate (Life-Table Analysis)

Study	No. of Patients	Treatment Groups	Week 4	Week 8	Significance Level*
1	588 588	NEXIUM 20 mg Omeprazole 20 mg	68.7% 69.5%	90.6% 88.3%	N.S.
2	654 656 650	NEXIUM 40 mg NEXIUM 20 mg Omeprazole 20 mg	75.9% 70.5% 64.7%	94.1% 89.9% 86.9%	p <0.001 p <0.05
3	576 572	NEXIUM 40 mg Omeprazole 20 mg	71.5% 68.6%	92.2% 89.8%	N.S.
4	1216 1209	NEXIUM 40 mg Omeprazole 20 mg	81.7% 68.7%	93.7% 84.2%	p <0.001

*log-rank test vs omeprazole 20 mg
N.S. = not significant (p > 0.05).

Sustained Resolution[‡] of Heartburn (Erosive Esophagitis Patients)

Study	No. of Patients	Treatment Groups	Cumulative Percent[#] with Sustained Resolution		Significance Level*
			Day 14	Day 28	
1	573 555	NEXIUM 20 mg Omeprazole 20 mg	64.3% 64.1%	72.7% 70.9%	N.S.
2	621 620 626	NEXIUM 40 mg NEXIUM 20 mg Omeprazole 20 mg	64.8% 62.9% 56.5%	74.2% 70.1% 66.6%	p <0.001 N.S.
3	568 551	NEXIUM 40 mg Omeprazole 20 mg	65.4% 65.5%	73.9% 73.1%	N.S.
4	1187 1188	NEXIUM 40 mg Omeprazole 20 mg	67.6% 62.5%	75.1% 70.8%	p <0.001

[‡] Defined as 7 consecutive days with no heartburn reported in daily patient diary.
[#] Defined as the cumulative proportion of patients who have reached the start of sustained resolution
*log-rank test vs omeprazole 20 mg
N.S. = not significant (p > 0.05).

In these same studies of patients with erosive esophagitis, sustained heartburn resolution and time to sustained heartburn resolution were evaluated and are shown in the table below:
[See second table above]
In these four studies, the range of median days to the start of sustained resolution (defined as 7 consecutive days with no heartburn) was 5 days for NEXIUM 40 mg, 7–8 days for NEXIUM 20 mg and 7–9 days for omeprazole 20 mg.
There are no comparisons of 40 mg of NEXIUM with 40 mg of omeprazole in clinical trials assessing either healing or symptomatic relief of erosive esophagitis.
Long-Term Maintenance of Healing of Erosive Esophagitis
Two multicenter, randomized, double-blind placebo-controlled 4-arm trials were conducted in patients with endoscopically confirmed, healed erosive esophagitis to evaluate NEXIUM 40 mg (n=174), 20 mg (n=180), 10 mg (n=168) or placebo (n=171) once daily over six months of treatment. No additional clinical benefit was seen with NEXIUM 40 mg over NEXIUM 20 mg.
The percentage of patients that maintained healing of erosive esophagitis at the various time points are shown in the figure below:

Maintenance of Healing Rates by Month (Study 177)

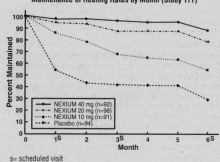

s= scheduled visit

[See figure at top of next column]
Patients remained in remission significantly longer and the number of recurrences of erosive esophagitis was significantly less in patients treated with NEXIUM compared to placebo.
In both studies, the proportion of patients on NEXIUM who remained in remission and were free of heartburn and other GERD symptoms was well differentiated from placebo.
In a third multicenter open label study of 808 patients treated for 12 months with NEXIUM 40 mg, the percentage of patients that maintained healing of erosive esophagitis was 93.7% for six months and 89.4% for one year.
Symptomatic Gastroesophageal Reflux Disease (GERD)
Two multicenter, randomized, double-blind, placebo-controlled studies were conducted in a total of 717 patients comparing four weeks of treatment with NEXIUM 20 mg or 40 mg once daily versus placebo for resolution of GERD

Maintenance of Healing Rates by Month (Study 178)

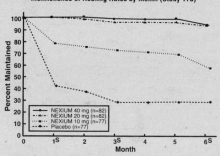

s= scheduled visit

symptoms. Patients had ≥6-month history of heartburn episodes, no erosive esophagitis by endoscopy, and heartburn on at least four of the seven days immediately preceding randomization.
The percentage of patients that were symptom-free of heartburn was significantly higher in the NEXIUM groups compared to placebo at all follow-up visits (Weeks 1, 2, and 4). No additional clinical benefit was seen with NEXIUM 40 mg over NEXIUM 20 mg.
The percent of patients symptom-free of heartburn by day are shown in the figures below:

Percent of Patients Symptom-Free of Heartburn by Day (Study 225)

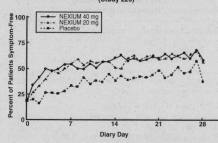

[See figure at top of next column]
In three European symptomatic GERD trials, NEXIUM 20 mg and 40 mg and omeprazole 20 mg were evaluated. No significant treatment related differences were seen.
Risk Reduction of NSAID-Associated Gastric Ulcer
Two multicenter, double-blind, placebo-controlled studies were conducted in patients at risk of developing gastric and/or duodenal ulcers associated with continuous use of

Continued on next page

Nexium—Cont.

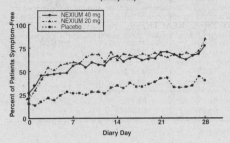

Percent of Patients Symptom-Free of Heartburn by Day (Study 226)

non-selective and COX-2 selective NSAIDs. A total of 1429 patients were randomized across the 2 studies. Patients ranged in age from 19 to 89 (median age 66.0 years) with 70.7% female, 29.3% male, 82.9% Caucasian, 5.5% Black, 3.7% Asian, and 8.0% Others. At baseline, the patients in these studies were endoscopically confirmed not to have ulcers but were determined to be at risk for ulcer occurrence due to their age (≥60 years) and/or history of a documented gastric or duodenal ulcer within the past 5 years. Patients receiving NSAIDs and treated with NEXIUM 20 mg or 40 mg once-a-day experienced significant reduction in gastric ulcer occurrences relative to placebo treatment at 26 weeks. No additional benefit was seen with NEXIUM 40 mg over NEXIUM 20 mg. These studies did not demonstrate significant reduction in the development of NSAID-associated duodenal ulcer due to the low incidence.

Cumulative percentage of patients without gastric ulcers at 26 weeks:

Study	No. of Patients	Treatment Group	% of Patients Remaining Gastric Ulcer Free[1]
1	191	NEXIUM 20 mg	95.4
	194	NEXIUM 40 mg	96.7
	184	Placebo	88.2
2	267	NEXIUM 20 mg	94.7
	271	NEXIUM 40 mg	95.3
	257	Placebo	83.3

[1]%= Life Table Estimate. Significant difference from placebo ($p<0.01$).

Helicobacter pylori (H. pylori) Eradication in Patients with Duodenal Ulcer Disease
Triple Therapy (NEXIUM / amoxicillin / clarithromycin): Two multicenter, randomized, double-blind studies were conducted using a 10 day treatment regimen. The first study (191) compared NEXIUM 40 mg once daily in combination with amoxicillin 1000 mg twice daily and clarithromycin 500 mg twice daily to NEXIUM 40 mg once daily plus clarithromycin 500 mg twice daily. The second study (193) compared NEXIUM 40 mg once daily in combination with amoxicillin 1000 mg twice daily and clarithromycin 500 mg twice daily to NEXIUM 40 mg once daily. *H. pylori* eradication rates, defined as at least two negative tests and no positive tests from CLOtest®, histology and/or culture, at 4 weeks post-therapy were significantly higher in the NEXIUM plus amoxicillin and clarithromycin group than in the NEXIUM plus clarithromycin or NEXIUM alone group. The results are shown in the following table:

H. pylori Eradication Rates at 4 Weeks after 10 Day Treatment Regimen
% of Patients Cured
[95% Confidence Interval]
(Number of patients)

Study	Treatment Group	Per-Protocol[†]	Intent-to-Treat[‡]
191	NEXIUM plus amoxicillin and clarithromycin	84%* [78, 89] (n=196)	77%* [71, 82] (n=233)
	NEXIUM plus clarithromycin	55% [48, 62] (n=187)	52% [45, 59] (n=215)
193	NEXIUM plus amoxicillin and clarithromycin	85%** [74, 93] (n=67)	78%** [67, 87] (n=74)
	NEXIUM	5% [0, 23] (n=22)	4% [0, 21] (n=24)

[†] Patients were included in the analysis if they had *H. pylori* infection documented at baseline, had at least one endoscopically verified duodenal ulcer ≥0.5 cm in diameter at baseline or had a documented history of duodenal ulcer disease within the past 5 years, and were not protocol vio-

lators. Patients who dropped out of the study due to an adverse event related to the study drug were included in the analysis as not *H. pylori* eradicated.
[‡] Patients were included in the analysis if they had documented *H. pylori* infection at baseline, had at least one documented duodenal ulcer at baseline, or had a documented history of duodenal ulcer disease, and took at least one dose of study medication. All dropouts were included as not *H. pylori* eradicated.
*p <0.05 compared to NEXIUM plus clarithromycin
**p <0.05 compared to NEXIUM alone

The percentage of patients with a healed baseline duodenal ulcer by 4 weeks after the 10 day treatment regimen in the NEXIUM plus amoxicillin and clarithromycin group was 75% (n=156) and 57% (n=60) respectively, in the 191 and 193 studies (per-protocol analysis).

INDICATIONS AND USAGE
Treatment of Gastroesophageal Reflux Disease (GERD)
Healing of Erosive Esophagitis
NEXIUM is indicated for the short-term treatment (4 to 8 weeks) in the healing and symptomatic resolution of diagnostically confirmed erosive esophagitis. For those patients who have not healed after 4–8 weeks of treatment, an additional 4–8-week course of NEXIUM may be considered.
Maintenance of Healing of Erosive Esophagitis
NEXIUM is indicated to maintain symptom resolution and healing of erosive esophagitis. Controlled studies do not extend beyond 6 months.
Symptomatic Gastroesophageal Reflux Disease
NEXIUM is indicated for treatment of heartburn and other symptoms associated with GERD.
Risk Reduction of NSAID-Associated Gastric Ulcer
NEXIUM is indicated for the reduction in the occurrence of gastric ulcers associated with continuous NSAID therapy in patients at risk for developing gastric ulcers. Patients are considered to be at risk due to their age (≥60) and/or documented history of gastric ulcers. Controlled studies do not extend beyond 6 months.
H. pylori Eradication to Reduce the Risk of Duodenal Ulcer Recurrence
Triple Therapy (NEXIUM plus amoxicillin and clarithromycin): NEXIUM, in combination with amoxicillin and clarithromycin, is indicated for the treatment of patients with *H. pylori* infection and duodenal ulcer disease (active or history of within the past 5 years) to eradicate *H. pylori*. Eradication of *H. pylori* has been shown to reduce the risk of duodenal ulcer recurrence. (See **Clinical Studies** and **DOSAGE AND ADMINISTRATION**.)
In patients who fail therapy, susceptibility testing should be done. If resistance to clarithromycin is demonstrated or susceptibility testing is not possible, alternative antimicrobial therapy should be instituted. (See **CLINICAL PHARMACOLOGY, Microbiology** and the clarithromycin package insert, **CLINICAL PHARMACOLOGY, Microbiology**.)

CONTRAINDICATIONS
NEXIUM is contraindicated in patients with known hypersensitivity to any component of the formulation or to substituted benzimidazoles.
Clarithromycin is contraindicated in patients with a known hypersensitivity to any macrolide antibiotic.
Concomitant administration of clarithromycin with pimozide is contraindicated. There have been post-marketing reports of drug interactions when clarithromycin and/or erythromycin are co-administered with pimozide resulting in cardiac arrhythmias (QT prolongation, ventricular tachycardia, ventricular fibrillation, and torsade de pointes) most likely due to inhibition of hepatic metabolism of pimozide by erythromycin and clarithromycin. Fatalities have been reported. (Please refer to full prescribing information for clarithromycin.)
Amoxicillin is contraindicated in patients with a known hypersensitivity to any penicillin. (Please refer to full prescribing information for amoxicillin.)

WARNINGS
CLARITHROMYCIN SHOULD NOT BE USED IN PREGNANT WOMEN EXCEPT IN CLINICAL CIRCUMSTANCES WHERE NO ALTERNATIVE THERAPY IS APPROPRIATE. IF PREGNANCY OCCURS WHILE TAKING CLARITHROMYCIN, THE PATIENT SHOULD BE APPRISED OF THE POTENTIAL HAZARD TO THE FETUS. (See WARNINGS in prescribing information for clarithromycin.)
Amoxicillin: Serious and occasionally fatal hypersensitivity (anaphylactic) reactions have been reported in patients on penicillin therapy. These reactions are more apt to occur in individuals with a history of penicillin hypersensitivity and/or a history of sensitivity to multiple allergens. There have been well documented reports of individuals with a history of penicillin hypersensitivity reactions who have experienced severe hypersensitivity reactions when treated with a cephalosporin. Before initiating therapy with any penicillin, careful inquiry should be made concerning previous hypersensitivity reactions to penicillins, cephalosporins, and other allergens. If an allergic reaction occurs, amoxicillin should be discontinued and the appropriate therapy instituted.
SERIOUS ANAPHYLACTIC REACTIONS REQUIRE IMMEDIATE EMERGENCY TREATMENT WITH EPINEPHRINE. OXYGEN, INTRAVENOUS STEROIDS, AND AIRWAY MANAGEMENT, INCLUDING INTUBATION, SHOULD ALSO BE ADMINISTERED AS INDICATED.
Pseudomembranous colitis has been reported with nearly all antibacterial agents, including clarithromycin and amoxicillin, and may range in severity from mild to life threaten-

ing. Therefore, it is important to consider this diagnosis in patients who present with diarrhea subsequent to the administration of antibacterial agents.
Treatment with antibacterial agents alters the normal flora of the colon and may permit overgrowth of clostridia. Studies indicate that a toxin produced by *Clostridium difficile* is a primary cause of "antibiotic-associated colitis."
After the diagnosis of pseudomembranous colitis has been established, therapeutic measures should be initiated. Mild cases of pseudomembranous colitis usually respond to discontinuation of the drug alone. In moderate to severe cases, consideration should be given to management with fluids and electrolytes, protein supplementation, and treatment with an antibacterial drug clinically effective against *Clostridium difficile* colitis.

PRECAUTIONS
General
Symptomatic response to therapy with NEXIUM does not preclude the presence of gastric malignancy.
Atrophic gastritis has been noted occasionally in gastric corpus biopsies from patients treated long-term with omeprazole, of which NEXIUM is an enantiomer.
Information for Patients
Patients should be informed of the following:
NEXIUM Delayed-Release Capsules should be taken at least one hour before meals.
For patients who have difficulty swallowing capsules, one tablespoon of applesauce can be added to an empty bowl and the NEXIUM Delayed-Release Capsule can be opened, and the pellets inside the capsule carefully emptied onto the applesauce. The pellets should be mixed with the applesauce and then swallowed immediately. The applesauce used should not be hot and should be soft enough to be swallowed without chewing. The pellets should not be chewed or crushed. The pellet/applesauce mixture should not be stored for future use.
Antacids may be used while taking NEXIUM.
Drug Interactions
Esomeprazole is extensively metabolized in the liver by CYP2C19 and CYP3A4.
In vitro and *in vivo* studies have shown that esomeprazole is not likely to inhibit CYPs 1A2, 2A6, 2C9, 2D6, 2E1 and 3A4. No clinically relevant interactions with drugs metabolized by these CYP enzymes would be expected. Drug interaction studies have shown that esomeprazole does not have any clinically significant interactions with phenytoin, warfarin, quinidine, clarithromycin or amoxicillin. Post-marketing reports of changes in prothrombin measures have been received among patients on concomitant warfarin and esomeprazole therapy. Increases in INR and prothrombin time may lead to abnormal bleeding and even death. Patients treated with proton pump inhibitors and warfarin concomitantly may need to be monitored for increases in INR and prothrombin time.
Esomeprazole may potentially interfere with CYP2C19, the major esomeprazole metabolizing enzyme. Coadministration of esomeprazole 30 mg and diazepam, a CYP2C19 substrate, resulted in a 45% decrease in clearance of diazepam. Increased plasma levels of diazepam were observed 12 hours after dosing and onwards. However, at that time, the plasma levels of diazepam were below the therapeutic interval, and thus this interaction is unlikely to be of clinical relevance.
Coadministration of oral contraceptives, diazepam, phenytoin, or quinidine did not seem to change the pharmacokinetic profile of esomeprazole.
Studies evaluating concomitant administration of esomeprazole and either naproxen (non-selective NSAID) or rofecoxib (COX-2 selective NSAID) did not identify any clinically relevant changes in the pharmacokinetic profiles of esomeprazole or these NSAIDs.
Esomeprazole inhibits gastric acid secretion. Therefore, esomeprazole may interfere with the absorption of drugs where gastric pH is an important determinant of bioavailability (eg, ketoconazole, iron salts and digoxin).
Combination Therapy with Clarithromycin
Co-administration of esomeprazole, clarithromycin, and amoxicillin has resulted in increases in the plasma levels of esomeprazole and 14-hydroxyclarithromycin. (See **CLINICAL PHARMACOLOGY, Pharmacokinetics: Combination Therapy with Antimicrobials**.)
Concomitant administration of clarithromycin with pimozide is contraindicated. (See clarithromycin package insert.)
Carcinogenesis, Mutagenesis, Impairment of Fertility
The carcinogenic potential of esomeprazole was assessed using omeprazole studies. In two 24-month oral carcinogenicity studies in rats, omeprazole at daily doses of 1.7, 3.4, 13.8, 44.0 and 140.8 mg/kg/day (about 0.7 to 57 times the human dose of 20 mg/day expressed on a body surface area basis) produced gastric ECL cell carcinoids in a dose-related manner in both male and female rats; the incidence of this effect was markedly higher in female rats, which had higher blood levels of omeprazole. Gastric carcinoids seldom occur in the untreated rat. In addition, ECL cell hyperplasia was present in all treated groups of both sexes. In one of these studies, female rats were treated with 13.8 mg omeprazole/kg/day (about 5.6 times the human dose on a body surface area basis) for 1 year, then followed for an additional year without the drug. No carcinoids were seen in these rats. An increased incidence of treatment-related ECL cell hyperplasia was observed at the end of 1 year (94% treated vs 10% controls). By the second year the difference between treated and control rats was much smaller (46% vs 26%) but still

showed more hyperplasia in the treated group. Gastric adenocarcinoma was seen in one rat (2%). No similar tumor was seen in male or female rats treated for 2 years. For this strain of rat no similar tumor has been noted historically, but a finding involving only one tumor is difficult to interpret. A 78-week mouse carcinogenicity study of omeprazole did not show increased tumor occurrence, but the study was not conclusive.

Esomeprazole was negative in the Ames mutation test, in the *in vivo* rat bone marrow cell chromosome aberration test, and the *in vivo* mouse micronucleus test. Esomeprazole, however, was positive in the *in vitro* human lymphocyte chromosome aberration test. Omeprazole was positive in the *in vitro* human lymphocyte chromosome aberration test, the *in vivo* mouse bone marrow cell chromosome aberration test, and the *in vivo* mouse micronucleus test.

The potential effects of esomeprazole on fertility and reproductive performance were assessed using omeprazole studies. Omeprazole at oral doses up to 138 mg/kg/day in rats (about 56 times the human dose on a body surface area basis) was found to have no effect on reproductive performance of parental animals.

Pregnancy

Teratogenic Effects. Pregnancy Category B
Teratology studies have been performed in rats at oral doses up to 280 mg/kg/day (about 57 times the human dose on a body surface area basis) and in rabbits at oral doses up to 86 mg/kg/day (about 35 times the human dose on a body surface area basis) and have revealed no evidence of impaired fertility or harm to the fetus due to esomeprazole. There are, however, no adequate and well-controlled studies in pregnant women. Because animal reproduction studies are not always predictive of human response, this drug should be used during pregnancy only if clearly needed.
Teratology studies conducted with omeprazole in rats at oral doses up to 138 mg/kg/day (about 56 times the human dose on a body surface area basis) and in rabbits at doses up to 69 mg/kg/day (about 56 times the human dose on a body surface area basis) did not disclose any evidence for a teratogenic potential of omeprazole. In rabbits, omeprazole in a dose range of 6.9 to 69.1 mg/kg/day (about 5.5 to 56 times the human dose on a body surface area basis) produced dose-related increases in embryo-lethality, fetal resorptions, and pregnancy disruptions. In rats, dose-related embryo/fetal toxicity and postnatal developmental toxicity were observed in offspring resulting from parents treated with omeprazole at 13.8 to 138.0 mg/kg/day (about 5.6 to 56 times the human doses on a body surface area basis). There are no adequate and well-controlled studies in pregnant women. Sporadic reports have been received of congenital abnormalities occurring in infants born to women who have received omeprazole during pregnancy.

Amoxicillin
Pregnancy Category B. See full prescribing information for amoxicillin before using in pregnant women.

Clarithromycin
Pregnancy Category C. See **WARNINGS** (above) and full prescribing information for clarithromycin before using in pregnant women.

Nursing Mothers
The excretion of esomeprazole in milk has not been studied. However, omeprazole concentrations have been measured in breast milk of a woman following oral administration of 20 mg. Because esomeprazole is likely to be excreted in human milk, because of the potential for serious adverse reactions in nursing infants from esomeprazole, and because of the potential for tumorigenicity shown for omeprazole in rat carcinogenicity studies, a decision should be made whether to discontinue nursing or to discontinue the drug, taking into account the importance of the drug to the mother.

Pediatric Use
Safety and effectiveness in pediatric patients have not been established.

Geriatric Use
Of the total number of patients who received NEXIUM in clinical trials, 1459 were 65 to 74 years of age and 354 patients were ≥75 years of age.
No overall differences in safety and efficacy were observed between the elderly and younger individuals, and other reported clinical experience has not identified differences in responses between the elderly and younger patients, but greater sensitivity of some older individuals cannot be ruled out.

ADVERSE REACTIONS

The safety of NEXIUM was evaluated in over 15,000 patients (aged 18-84 years) in clinical trials worldwide including over 8,500 patients in the United States and over 6,500 patients in Europe and Canada. Over 2,900 patients were treated in long-term studies for up to 6-12 months. In general, NEXIUM was well tolerated in both short- and long-term clinical trials.

The safety in the treatment of healing of erosive esophagitis was assessed in four randomized comparative clinical trials, which included 1,240 patients on NEXIUM 20 mg, 2,434 patients on NEXIUM 40 mg, and 3,008 patients on omeprazole 20 mg daily. The most frequently occurring adverse events (≥1%) in all three groups was headache (5.5, 5.0, and 3.8, respectively) and diarrhea (no difference among the three groups). Nausea, flatulence, abdominal pain, constipation, and dry mouth occurred at similar rates among patients taking NEXIUM or omeprazole.

Additional adverse events that were reported as possibly or probably related to NEXIUM with an incidence <1% are listed below by body system:

Body as a Whole: abdomen enlarged, allergic reaction, asthenia, back pain, chest pain, chest pain substernal, facial edema, peripheral edema, hot flushes, fatigue, fever, flu-like disorder, generalized edema, leg edema, malaise, pain, rigors; *Cardiovascular:* flushing, hypertension, tachycardia; *Endocrine:* goiter; *Gastrointestinal:* bowel irregularity, constipation aggravated, dyspepsia, dysphagia, dysplasia GI, epigastric pain, eructation, esophageal disorder, frequent stools, gastroenteritis, GI hemorrhage, GI symptoms not otherwise specified, hiccup, melena, mouth disorder, pharynx disorder, rectal disorder, serum gastrin increased, tongue disorder, tongue edema, ulcerative stomatitis, vomiting; *Hearing:* earache, tinnitus; *Hematologic:* anemia, anemia hypochromic, cervical lymphoadenopathy, epistaxis, leukocytosis, leukopenia, thrombocytopenia; *Hepatic:* bilirubinemia, hepatic function abnormal, SGOT increased, SGPT increased; *Metabolic/Nutritional:* glycosuria, hyperuricemia, hyponatremia, increased alkaline phosphatase, thirst, vitamin B12 deficiency, weight increase, weight decrease; *Musculoskeletal:* arthralgia, arthritis aggravated, arthropathy, cramps, fibromyalgia syndrome, hernia, polymyalgia rheumatica; *Nervous System/Psychiatric:* anorexia, apathy, appetite increased, confusion, depression aggravated, dizziness, hypertonia, nervousness, hypoesthesia, impotence, insomnia, migraine, migraine aggravated, paresthesia, sleep disorder, somnolence, tremor, vertigo, visual field defect; *Reproductive:* dysmenorrhea, menstrual disorder, vaginitis; *Respiratory:* asthma aggravated, coughing, dyspnea, larynx edema, pharyngitis, rhinitis, sinusitis; *Skin and Appendages:* acne, angioedema, dermatitis, pruritus, pruritus ani, rash, rash erythematous, rash maculopapular, skin inflammation, sweating increased, urticaria; *Special Senses:* otitis media, parosmia, taste loss, taste perversion; *Urogenital:* abnormal urine, albuminuria, cystitis, dysuria, fungal infection, hematuria, micturition frequency, moniliasis, genital moniliasis, polyuria; *Visual:* conjunctivitis, vision abnormal.

Endoscopic findings that were reported as adverse events include: duodenitis, esophagitis, esophageal stricture, esophageal ulceration, esophageal varices, gastric ulcer, gastritis, hernia, benign polyps or nodules, Barrett's esophagus, and mucosal discoloration.

The incidence of treatment-related adverse events during 6-month maintenance treatment was similar to placebo. There were no differences in types of related adverse events seen during maintenance treatment up to 12 months compared to short-term treatment.

Two placebo-controlled studies were conducted in 710 patients for the treatment of symptomatic gastroesophageal reflux disease. The most common adverse events that were reported as possibly or probably related to NEXIUM were diarrhea (4.3%), headache (3.8%), and abdominal pain (3.8%).

Postmarketing Reports – There have been spontaneous reports of adverse events with postmarketing use of esomeprazole. These reports have included rare cases of anaphylactic reaction and myalgia, severe dermatologic reactions, including toxic epidermal necrolysis (TEN, some fatal), Stevens-Johnson syndrome, and erythema multiforme, and pancreatitis. Very rarely, hepatitis with or without jaundice has been reported.

Other adverse events not observed with NEXIUM, but occurring with omeprazole can be found in the omeprazole package insert, **ADVERSE REACTIONS** section.

Combination Treatment with Amoxicillin and Clarithromycin
In clinical trials using combination therapy with NEXIUM plus amoxicillin and clarithromycin, no adverse events peculiar to these drug combinations were observed. Adverse events that occurred have been limited to those that had been observed with NEXIUM, amoxicillin, or clarithromycin alone.

The most frequently reported drug-related adverse events for patients who received triple therapy for 10 days were diarrhea (9.2%), taste perversion (6.6%), and abdominal pain (3.7%). No treatment-emergent adverse events were observed at higher rates with triple therapy than were observed with NEXIUM alone.

For more information on adverse events with amoxicillin or clarithromycin, refer to their package inserts, **ADVERSE REACTIONS** sections.

Laboratory Events
The following potentially clinically significant laboratory changes in clinical trials, irrespective of relationship to NEXIUM, were reported in ≤1% of patients: increased creatinine, uric acid, total bilirubin, alkaline phosphatase, ALT, AST, hemoglobin, white blood cell count, platelets, serum gastrin, potassium, sodium, thyroxine and thyroid stimulating hormone (see **CLINICAL PHARMACOLOGY,** *Endocrine Effects* for further information on thyroid effects). Decreases were seen in hemoglobin, white blood cell count, platelets, potassium, sodium, and thyroxine.

In clinical trials using combination therapy with NEXIUM plus amoxicillin and clarithromycin, no additional increased laboratory abnormalities particular to these drug combinations were observed.

For more information on laboratory changes with amoxicillin or clarithromycin, refer to their package inserts, **ADVERSE REACTIONS** section.

OVERDOSAGE

A single oral dose of esomeprazole at 510 mg/kg (about 103 times the human dose on a body surface area basis), was lethal to rats. The major signs of acute toxicity were reduced motor activity, changes in respiratory frequency, tremor, ataxia, and intermittent clonic convulsions.

There have been some reports of overdosage with esomeprazole. Reports have been received of overdosage with omeprazole in humans. Doses ranged up to 2,400 mg (120 times the usual recommended clinical dose). Manifestations were variable, but included confusion, drowsiness, blurred vision, tachycardia, nausea, diaphoresis, flushing, headache, dry mouth, and other adverse reactions similar to those seen in normal clinical experience (see omeprazole package insert – **ADVERSE REACTIONS**). No specific antidote for esomeprazole is known. Since esomeprazole is extensively protein bound, it is not expected to be removed by dialysis. In the event of overdosage, treatment should be symptomatic and supportive.

As with the management of any overdose, the possibility of multiple drug ingestion should be considered. For current information on treatment of any drug overdose, a certified Regional Poison Control Center should be contacted. Telephone numbers are listed in the Physicians' Desk Reference (PDR) or local telephone book.

DOSAGE AND ADMINISTRATION

The recommended adult dosages are outlined in the table below. NEXIUM Delayed-Release Capsules should be swallowed whole and taken at least one hour before eating.
For patients who have difficulty swallowing capsules, one tablespoon of applesauce can be added to an empty bowl and the NEXIUM Delayed-Release Capsule can be opened, and the pellets inside the capsule carefully emptied onto the applesauce. The pellets should be mixed with the applesauce and then swallowed immediately. The applesauce used should not be hot and should be soft enough to be swallowed without chewing. The pellets should not be chewed or crushed. The pellet/applesauce mixture should not be stored for future use.
For patients who have a nasogastric tube in place, NEXIUM Delayed-Release Capsules can be opened and the intact granules emptied into a 60 mL syringe and mixed with 50 mL of water. Replace the plunger and shake the syringe vigorously for 15 seconds. Hold the syringe with the tip up and check for granules remaining in the tip. Attach the syringe to a nasogastric tube and deliver the contents of the syringe through the nasogastric tube into the stomach. After administering the granules, the nasogastric tube should be flushed with additional water. Do not administer the pellets if they have dissolved or disintegrated.
The suspension must be used immediately after preparation.

Recommended Adult Dosage Schedule of NEXIUM

Indication	Dose	Frequency
Gastroesophageal Reflux Disease (GERD)		
Healing of Erosive Esophagitis	20 mg or 40 mg	Once Daily for 4 to 8 Weeks*
Maintenance of Healing of Erosive Esophagitis	20 mg	Once Daily**
Symptomatic Gastroesophageal Reflux Disease	20 mg	Once Daily for 4 Weeks***
Risk Reduction of NSAID-Associated Gastric Ulcer	20 mg or 40 mg	Once Daily for up to 6 months**
H. pylori Eradication to Reduce the Risk of Duodenal Ulcer Recurrence		
Triple Therapy:		
NEXIUM	40 mg	Once Daily for 10 Days
Amoxicillin	1000 mg	Twice Daily for 10 Days
Clarithromycin	500 mg	Twice Daily for 10 Days

* (see **CLINICAL STUDIES**). The majority of patients are healed within 4 to 8 weeks. For patients who do not heal after 4–8 weeks, an additional 4–8 weeks of treatment may be considered.

** Controlled studies did not extend beyond six months.

*** If symptoms do not resolve completely after 4 weeks, an additional 4 weeks of treatment may be considered.

Please refer to amoxicillin and clarithromycin full prescribing information for **CONTRAINDICATIONS, WARNINGS** and dosing in elderly and renally-impaired patients.

Special Populations
Geriatric: No dosage adjustment is necessary. (See **CLINICAL PHARMACOLOGY, Pharmacokinetics**.)
Renal Insufficiency: No dosage adjustment is necessary. (See **CLINICAL PHARMACOLOGY, Pharmacokinetics**.)
Hepatic Insufficiency: No dosage adjustment is necessary in patients with mild to moderate liver impairment (Child Pugh Classes A and B). For patients with severe liver impairment (Child Pugh Class C), a dose of 20 mg of NEXIUM should not be exceeded (See **CLINICAL PHARMACOLOGY, Pharmacokinetics**.)
Gender: No dosage adjustment is necessary. (See **CLINICAL PHARMACOLOGY, Pharmacokinetics**.)

HOW SUPPLIED

NEXIUM Delayed-Release Capsules, 20 mg, are opaque, hard gelatin, amethyst colored capsules with two radial bars in yellow on the cap and NEXIUM 20 mg in yellow on the body. They are supplied as follows:

Continued on next page

Nexium—Cont.

NDC 0186-5020-31 unit of use bottles of 30
NDC 0186-5022-28 unit dose packages of 100
NDC 0186-5020-54 bottles of 90
NDC 0186-5020-82 bottles of 1000
NEXIUM Delayed-Release Capsules, 40 mg, are opaque, hard gelatin, amethyst colored capsules with three radial bars in yellow on the cap and NEXIUM 40 mg in yellow on the body. They are supplied as follows:
NDC 0186-5040-31 unit of use bottles of 30
NDC 0186-5042-28 unit dose packages of 100
NDC 0186-5040-54 bottles of 90
NDC 0186-5040-82 bottles of 1000

Storage

Store at 25°C (77°F); excursions permitted to 15–30°C (59–86°F). [See USP Controlled Room Temperature]. Keep container tightly closed. Dispense in a tight container if the product package is subdivided.

REFERENCES

1. National Committee for Clinical Laboratory Standards. Methods for Dilution Antimicrobial Susceptibility Tests for Bacteria That Grow Aerobically. Fifth Edition: Approved Standard NCCLS Document M7-A5, Vol. 20, no. 2, NCCLS, Wayne, PA, January 2000.

NEXIUM and the color purple as applied to the capsule are registered trademarks of the AstraZeneca group of companies
© AstraZeneca 2004

Distributed by:
AstraZeneca LP
Wilmington, DE 19850
Product of France
9346609
620514-09
Rev. 12/04 AstraZeneca

RHINOCORT AQUA® ℞

[rī-nə-kort ăquă]
(budesonide)
Nasal Spray 32 mcg
For Intranasal Use Only.
℞ only

Prescribing information for this product, which appears on pages 630–632 of the 2005 PDR, has been completely revised as follows. Please write "See Supplement A" next to the product heading.

DESCRIPTION

Budesonide, the active ingredient of RHINOCORT AQUA® Nasal Spray, is an anti-inflammatory synthetic corticosteroid.

It is designated chemically as (RS)-11-beta, 16-alpha, 17, 21-tetrahydroxypregna-1,4-diene-3,20-dione cyclic 16, 17-acetal with butyraldehyde.

Budesonide is provided as the mixture of two epimers (22R and 22S).

The empirical formula of budesonide is $C_{25}H_{34}O_6$ and its molecular weight is 430.5.

Its structural formula is:

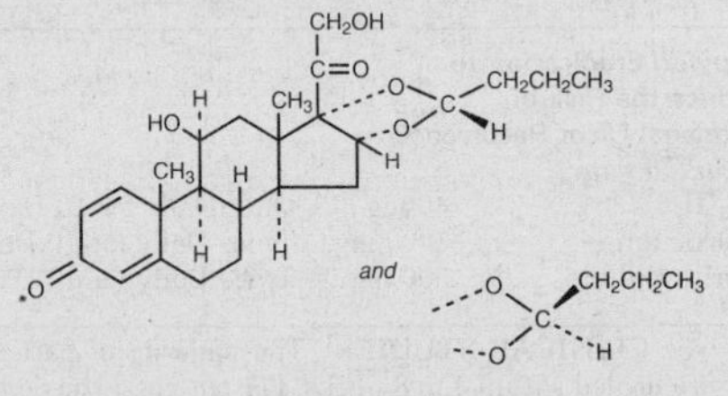

Budesonide is a white to off-white, odorless powder that is practically insoluble in water and in heptane, sparingly soluble in ethanol, and freely soluble in chloroform.

Its partition coefficient between octanol and water at pH 5 is 1.6×10^3.

RHINOCORT AQUA is an unscented, metered-dose, manual-pump spray formulation containing a micronized suspension of budesonide in an aqueous medium. Microcrystalline cellulose and carboxymethyl cellulose sodium, dextrose anhydrous, polysorbate 80, disodium edetate, potassium sorbate, and purified water are contained in this medium; hydrochloric acid is added to adjust the pH to a target of 4.5.

RHINOCORT AQUA Nasal Spray delivers 32 mcg of budesonide per spray.

Each bottle of RHINOCORT AQUA Nasal Spray 32 mcg contains 120 metered sprays after initial priming.

Prior to initial use, the container must be shaken gently and the pump must be primed by actuating eight times. If used daily, the pump does not need to be reprimed. If not used for two consecutive days, reprime with one spray or until a fine spray appears. If not used for more than 14 days, rinse the applicator and reprime with two sprays or until a fine spray appears.

CLINICAL PHARMACOLOGY

Budesonide is a synthetic corticosteroid having potent glucocorticoid activity and weak mineralocorticoid activity. In standard *in vitro* and animal models, budesonide has approximately a 200-fold higher affinity for the glucocorticoid receptor and a 1000-fold higher topical anti-inflammatory potency than cortisol (rat croton oil ear edema assay). As a measure of systemic activity, budesonide is 40 times more potent than cortisol when administered subcutaneously and 25 times more potent when administered orally in the rat thymus involution assay. In glucocorticoid receptor affinity studies, the 22R form was twice as active as the 22S epimer. The precise mechanism of corticosteroid actions in seasonal and perennial allergic rhinitis is not known. Corticosteroids have been shown to have a wide range of inhibitory activities against multiple cell types (eg, mast cells, eosinophils, neutrophils, macrophages, and lymphocytes) and mediators (eg, histamine, eicosanoids, leukotrienes, and cytokines) involved in allergic mediated inflammation.

Corticosteroids affect the delayed (6 hour) response to an allergen challenge more than the histamine-associated immediate response (20 minute). The clinical significance of these findings is unknown.

Pharmacokinetics

The pharmacokinetics of budesonide have been studied following nasal, oral, and intravenous administration. Budesonide is relatively well absorbed after both inhalation and oral administration, and is rapidly metabolized into metabolites with low corticosteroid potency. The clinical activity of RHINOCORT AQUA Nasal Spray is therefore believed to be due to the parent drug, budesonide. *In vitro* studies indicate that the two epimeric forms of budesonide do not interconvert.

Absorption

Following intranasal administration of RHINOCORT AQUA, the mean peak plasma concentration occurs at approximately 0.7 hours. Compared to an intravenous dose, approximately 34% of the delivered intranasal dose reaches the systemic circulation, most of which is absorbed through the nasal mucosa. While budesonide is well absorbed from the GI tract, the oral bioavailability of budesonide is low (~10%) primarily due to extensive first pass metabolism in the liver.

Distribution

Budesonide has a volume of distribution of approximately 2-3 L/kg. The volume of distribution for the 22R epimer is almost twice that of the 22S epimer. Protein binding of budesonide *in vitro* is constant (85-90%) over a concentration range (1-100 nmol/L) which exceeded that achieved after administration of recommended doses. Budesonide shows little to no binding to glucocorticosteroid binding globulin. It rapidly equilibrates with red blood cells in a concentration independent manner with a blood/plasma ratio of about 0.8.

Metabolism

Budesonide is rapidly and extensively metabolized in humans by the liver. Two major metabolites (16α-hydroxyprednisolone and 6β-hydroxybudesonide) are formed via cytochrome P450 (CYP) isoenzyme 3A4 (CYP3A4)-catalyzed biotransformation. Known metabolic inhibitors of CYP3A4 (eg, ketoconazole), or significant hepatic impairment, may increase the systemic exposure of unmetabolized budesonide (see WARNINGS and PRECAUTIONS). *In vitro* studies on the binding of the two primary metabolites to the glucocorticoid receptor indicate that they have less than 1% of the affinity for the receptor as the parent compound budesonide. *In vitro* studies have evaluated sites of metabolism and showed negligible metabolism in skin, lung, and serum. No qualitative difference between the *in vitro* and *in vivo* metabolic patterns could be detected.

Elimination

Budesonide is excreted in the urine and feces in the form of metabolites. After intranasal administration of a radiolabeled dose, 2/3 of the radioactivity was found in the urine and the remainder in the feces. The main metabolites of budesonide in the 0-24 hour urine sample following IV administration are 16α-hydroxyprednisolone (24%) and 6β-hydroxybudesonide (5%). An additional 34% of the radioactivity recovered in the urine was identified as conjugates. The 22R form was preferentially cleared with clearance value of 1.4 L/min vs. 1.0 L/min for the 22S form. The terminal half-life, 2 to 3 hours, was similar for both epimers and it appeared to be independent of dose.

Special Populations

Geriatric: No specific pharmacokinetic study has been undertaken in subjects >65 years of age.

Pediatric: After administration of RHINOCORT AQUA Nasal Spray, the time to reach peak drug concentrations and plasma half-life were similar in children and in adults. Children had plasma concentrations approximately twice those observed in adults due primarily to differences in weight between children and adults.

Gender: No specific pharmacokinetic study has been conducted to evaluate the effect of gender on budesonide pharmacokinetics. However, following administration of 400 mcg of RHINOCORT AQUA Nasal Spray to 7 male and 8 female volunteers in a pharmacokinetic study, no major gender differences in the pharmacokinetic parameters were found.

Race: No specific study has been undertaken to evaluate the effect of race on budesonide pharmacokinetics.

Renal Insufficiency: The pharmacokinetics of budesonide have not been investigated in patients with renal insufficiency.

Hepatic Insufficiency: Reduced liver function may affect the elimination of corticosteroids. The pharmacokinetics of orally administered budesonide were affected by compromised liver function as evidenced by a doubled systemic availability. The relevance of this finding to intranasally administered budesonide has not been established.

Pharmacodynamics

A 3-week clinical study in seasonal rhinitis, comparing RHINOCORT Nasal Inhaler, orally ingested budesonide, and placebo in 98 patients with allergic rhinitis due to birch pollen, demonstrated that the therapeutic effect of RHINOCORT Nasal Inhaler can be attributed to the topical effects of budesonide.

The effects of RHINOCORT AQUA Nasal Spray on adrenal function have been evaluated in several clinical trials. In a four-week clinical trial, 61 adult patients who received 256 mcg daily of RHINOCORT AQUA Nasal Spray demonstrated no significant differences from patients receiving placebo in plasma cortisol levels measured before and 60 minutes after 0.25 mg intramuscular cosyntropin. There were no consistent differences in 24-hour urinary cortisol measurements in patients receiving up to 400 mcg daily. Similar results were seen in a study of 150 children and adolescents aged 6 to 17 with perennial rhinitis who were treated with 256 mcg daily for up to 12 months.

After treatment with the recommended maximal daily dose of RHINOCORT AQUA (256 mcg) for seven days, there was a small, but statistically significant decrease in the area under the plasma cortisol-time curve over 24 hours (AUC_{0-24h}) in healthy adult volunteers.

A dose-related suppression of 24-hour urinary cortisol excretion was observed after administration of RHINOCORT AQUA doses ranging from 100–800 mcg daily for up to four days in 78 healthy adult volunteers. The clinical relevance of these results is unknown.

Clinical Trials

The therapeutic efficacy of RHINOCORT AQUA Nasal Spray has been evaluated in placebo-controlled clinical trials of seasonal and perennial allergic rhinitis of 3–6 weeks duration.

The number of patients treated with budesonide in these studies was 90 males and 51 females aged 6–12 years and 691 males and 694 females 12 years and above. The patients were predominantly Caucasian.

Overall, the results of these clinical trials showed that RHINOCORT AQUA Nasal Spray administered once daily provides statistically significant reduction in the severity of nasal symptoms of seasonal and perennial allergic rhinitis including runny nose, sneezing, and nasal congestion.

An improvement in nasal symptoms may be noted in patients within 10 hours of first using RHINOCORT AQUA Nasal Spray. This time to onset is supported by an environmental exposure unit study in seasonal allergic rhinitis patients which demonstrated that RHINOCORT AQUA Nasal Spray led to a statistically significant improvement in nasal symptoms compared to placebo by 10 hours. Further support comes from a clinical study of patients with perennial allergic rhinitis which demonstrated a statistically significant improvement in nasal symptoms for both RHINOCORT AQUA Nasal Spray and for the active comparator (mometasone furoate) compared to placebo by 8 hours. Onset was also assessed in this study with peak nasal inspiratory flow rate and this endpoint failed to show efficacy for either active treatment. Although statistically significant improvements in nasal symptoms compared to placebo were noted within 8–10 hours in these studies, about one half to two thirds of the ultimate clinical improvement with RHINOCORT AQUA Nasal Spray occurs over the first 1–2 days, and maximum benefit may not be achieved until approximately 2 weeks after initiation of treatment.

INDICATIONS AND USAGE

RHINOCORT AQUA Nasal Spray is indicated for the management of nasal symptoms of seasonal or perennial allergic rhinitis in adults and children six years of age and older.

CONTRAINDICATIONS

Hypersensitivity to any of the ingredients in this preparation contraindicates the use of RHINOCORT AQUA Nasal Spray.

WARNINGS

The replacement of a systemic corticosteroid with a topical corticosteroid can be accompanied by signs of adrenal insufficiency, and in addition some patients may experience symptoms of corticosteroid withdrawal, eg, joint and/or muscular pain, lassitude, and depression. Patients previously treated for prolonged periods with systemic corticosteroids and transferred to topical corticosteroids should be carefully monitored for acute adrenal insufficiency in response to stress. In those patients who have asthma or other clinical conditions requiring long-term systemic corticosteroid treatment, too rapid a decrease in systemic corticosteroids may cause a severe exacerbation of their symptoms.

Patients who are on drugs which suppress the immune system are more susceptible to infections than healthy individuals. Chicken pox and measles, for example, can have a more serious or even fatal course in non-immune children or adults on immunosuppressant doses of corticosteroids. In such children or adults who have not had these diseases, particular care should be taken to avoid exposure. How the dose, route, and duration of corticosteroid administration affects the risk of developing a disseminated infection is not known. The contribution of the underlying disease and/or prior corticosteroid treatment to the risk is also not known. If exposed to chicken pox, prophylaxis with varicella zoster immune globulin (VZIG) may be indicated. If exposed to measles, prophylaxis with pooled intramuscular immunoglobulin (IG) may be indicated. (See the respective package inserts for complete VZIG and IG prescribing information). If chicken pox develops, treatment with antiviral agents may be considered.

PRECAUTIONS

General

Intranasal corticosteroids may cause a reduction in growth velocity when administered to pediatric patients (see PRECAUTIONS, Pediatric Use).

Rarely, immediate and/or delayed hypersensitivity reactions may occur after the intranasal administration of budesonide. Rare instances of wheezing, nasal septum perforation, and increased intraocular pressure have been reported following the intranasal application of corticosteroids, including budesonide.

Although systemic effects have been minimal with recommended doses of RHINOCORT AQUA Nasal Spray, any such effect is dose dependent. Therefore, larger than recommended doses of RHINOCORT AQUA Nasal Spray should be avoided and the minimal effective dose for the patient should be used (see DOSAGE AND ADMINISTRATION).

When used at larger doses, systemic corticosteroid effects such as hypercorticism and adrenal suppression may appear. If such changes occur, the dosage of RHINOCORT AQUA Nasal Spray should be discontinued slowly, consistent with accepted procedures for discontinuing oral corticosteroid therapy.

In clinical studies with budesonide administered intranasally, the development of localized infections of the nose and pharynx with *Candida albicans* has occurred only rarely. When such an infection develops, it may require treatment with appropriate local or systemic therapy and discontinuation of treatment with RHINOCORT AQUA Nasal Spray. Patients using RHINOCORT AQUA Nasal Spray over several months or longer should be examined periodically for evidence of *Candida* infection or other signs of adverse effects on the nasal mucosa.

RHINOCORT AQUA Nasal Spray should be used with caution, if at all, in patients with active or quiescent tuberculous infection, untreated fungal, bacterial, or systemic viral infections, or ocular herpes simplex.

Because of the inhibitory effect of corticosteroids on wound healing, patients who have experienced recent nasal septal ulcers, nasal surgery, or nasal trauma should not use a nasal corticosteroid until healing has occurred.

Hepatic dysfunction influences the pharmacokinetics of budesonide, similar to the effect on other corticosteroids, with a reduced elimination rate and increased systemic availability (see CLINICAL PHARMACOLOGY, Special Populations).

Information for Patients

Patients being treated with RHINOCORT AQUA Nasal Spray should receive the following information and instructions. Patients who are on immunosuppressant doses of corticosteroids should be warned to avoid exposure to chicken pox or measles and, if exposed, to obtain medical advice.

Patients should use RHINOCORT AQUA Nasal Spray at regular intervals since its effectiveness depends on its regular use (see DOSAGE AND ADMINISTRATION).

An improvement in nasal symptoms may be noted in patients within 10 hours of first using RHINOCORT AQUA Nasal Spray. This time to onset is supported by an environmental exposure unit study in seasonal allergic rhinitis patients which demonstrated that RHINOCORT AQUA Nasal Spray led to a statistically significant improvement in nasal symptoms compared to placebo by 10 hours. Further support comes from a clinical study of patients with perennial allergic rhinitis which demonstrated a statistically significant improvement in nasal symptoms for both RHINOCORT AQUA Nasal Spray and for the active comparator (mometasone furoate) compared to placebo by 8 hours. Onset was also assessed in this study with peak nasal inspiratory flow rate and this endpoint failed to show efficacy for either active treatment. Although statistically significant improvements in nasal symptoms compared to placebo were noted within 8–10 hours in these studies, about one half to two thirds of the ultimate clinical improvement with RHINOCORT AQUA Nasal Spray occurs over the first 1–2 days, and maximum benefit may not be achieved until approximately 2 weeks after initiation of treatment. Initial assessment for response should be made during this time frame and periodically until the patient's symptoms are stabilized.

The patient should take the medication as directed and should not exceed the prescribed dosage. The patient should contact the physician if symptoms do not improve after two weeks, or if the condition worsens. Patients who experience recurrent episodes of epistaxis (nosebleeds) or nasal septum discomfort while taking this medication should contact their physician. For proper use of this unit and to attain maximum improvement, the patient should read and follow the accompanying patient instructions carefully.

It is important to shake the bottle well before each use. The RHINOCORT AQUA Nasal Spray 32 mcg bottle has been filled with an excess to accommodate the priming activity. The bottle should be discarded after 120 sprays following initial priming, since the amount of budesonide delivered per spray thereafter may be substantially less than the labeled dose. Do not transfer any remaining suspension to another bottle.

Drug Interactions

The main route of metabolism of budesonide, as well as other corticosteroids, is via cytochrome P450 (CYP) isoenzyme 3A4 (CYP3A4). After oral administration of ketoconazole, a potent inhibitor of CYP3A4, the mean plasma concentration of orally administered budesonide increased by more than seven-fold. Concomitant administration of other known inhibitors of CYP3A4 (eg, itraconazole, clarithromycin, erythromycin, etc.) may inhibit the metabolism of, and increase the systemic exposure to, budesonide (see WARNINGS and PRECAUTIONS, General). Care should be exercised when budesonide is coadministered with long-term ketoconazole and other known CYP3A4 inhibitors.

Omeprazole, an inhibitor of CYP2C19, did not have effects on the pharmacokinetics of oral budesonide, while cimetidine, primarily an inhibitor of CYP1A2, caused a slight decrease in budesonide clearance and corresponding increase in its oral bioavailability.

Carcinogenesis, Mutagenesis, Impairment of Fertility

In a two-year study in Sprague-Dawley rats, budesonide caused a statistically significant increase in the incidence of gliomas in the male rats receiving an oral dose of 50 mcg/kg (approximately twice the maximum recommended daily intranasal dose in adults and children on a mcg/m² basis). No tumorigenicity was seen in male and female rats at respective oral doses up to 25 and 50 mcg/kg (approximately equal to and two times the maximum recommended daily intranasal dose in adults and children on a mcg/m² basis, respectively). In two additional two-year studies in male Fischer and Sprague-Dawley rats, budesonide caused no gliomas at an oral dose of 50 mcg/kg (approximately twice the maximum recommended daily intranasal dose in adults and children on a mcg/m² basis). However, in male Sprague-Dawley rats, budesonide caused a statistically significant increase in the incidence of hepatocellular tumors at an oral dose of 50 mcg/kg (approximately twice the maximum recommended daily intranasal dose in adults and children on a mcg/m² basis). The concurrent reference corticosteroids (prednisolone and triamcinolone acetonide) in these two studies showed similar findings.

In a 91-week study in mice, budesonide caused no treatment-related carcinogenicity at oral doses up to 200 mcg/kg (approximately 3 times the maximum recommended daily intranasal dose in adults and children on a mcg/m² basis).

Budesonide was not mutagenic or clastogenic in six different test systems: Ames *Salmonella*/microsome plate test, mouse micronucleus test, mouse lymphoma test, chromosome aberration test in human lymphocytes, sex-linked recessive lethal test in *Drosophila melanogaster*, and DNA repair analysis in rat hematocyte culture.

In rats, budesonide caused a decrease in prenatal viability and viability of the pups at birth and during lactation, along with a decrease in maternal body-weight gain, at subcutaneous doses of 20 mcg/kg and above (less than the maximum recommended daily intranasal dose in adults on a mcg/m² basis). No such effects were noted at 5 mcg/kg (less than the maximum recommended daily intranasal dose in adults on a mcg/m² basis).

Pregnancy

Teratogenic Effects: Pregnancy Category B: The impact of budesonide on human pregnancy outcomes has been evaluated through assessments of birth registries linked with maternal usage of inhaled budesonide (ie, PULMICORT TURBUHALER) and intranasally administered budesonide (ie, RHINOCORT AQUA Nasal Spray). The results from population-based prospective cohort epidemiological studies reviewing data from three Swedish registries covering approximately 99% of the pregnancies from 1995–2001 (ie, Swedish Medical Birth Registry; Registry of Congenital Malformations; Child Cardiology Registry) indicate no increased risk for overall congenital malformations from the use of inhaled or intranasal budesonide during early pregnancy.

Congenital malformations were studied in 2,014 infants born to mothers reporting the use of inhaled budesonide for asthma in early pregnancy (usually 10–12 weeks after the last menstrual period), the period when most major organ malformations occur.[1] The rate of overall congenital malformations was similar compared to the general population rate (3.8 % vs. 3.5%, respectively). The number of infants born with orofacial clefts and cardiac defects was similar to the expected number in the general population (4 children vs. 3.3 and 18 children vs. 17–18, respectively). In a follow-on study bringing the total number of infants to 2,534, the rate of overall congenital malformations among infants whose mothers were exposed to inhaled budesonide during early pregnancy was not different from the rate for all newborn babies during the same period (3.6%).[2] A third study from the Swedish Medical Birth Registry of 2,968 pregnancies exposed to inhaled budesonide, the majority of which were first trimester exposures, reported gestational birth weight, birth length, stillbirths, and multiple births similar for exposed infants compared to nonexposed infants.[3]

Congenital malformations were studied in 2,113 infants born to mothers reporting the use intranasal budesonide in early pregnancy. The rate of overall congenital malformations was similar compared to the general population rate (4.5% vs. 3.5%, respectively). The adjusted odds ratio (OR) was 1.06 (95% CI 0.86–1.31). The number of infants born with orofacial clefts was similar to the expected number in the general population (3 children vs. 3, respectively).The number of infants born with cardiac defects exceeded that expected in the general population (28 children vs. 17.8 respectively). The systemic exposure from intranasal budesonide is 6-fold less than from inhaled budesonide and an association of cardiac defects was not seen with higher exposures of budesonide.

As with other corticosteroids, budesonide was teratogenic and embryocidal in rabbits and rats. Budesonide produced fetal loss, decreased pup weights, and skeletal abnormalities at subcutaneous doses of 25 mcg/kg in rabbits and 500 mcg/kg in rats (approximately 2 and 16 times the maximum recommended daily intranasal dose in adults on a mcg/m² basis). In another study in rats, no teratogenic or embryocidal effects were seen at inhalation doses up to 250 mcg/kg (approximately 8 times the maximum recommended daily intranasal dose in adults on a mcg/m² basis).

Experience with oral corticosteroids since their introduction in pharmacologic, as opposed to physiologic doses suggests that rodents are more prone to teratogenic effects from corticosteroids than humans. In addition, because there is an increase in corticosteroid production during pregnancy, most women will require a lower exogenous corticosteroid dose and many will not need corticosteroid treatment during pregnancy.

Despite the animal findings, it would appear that the possibility of fetal harm remote if the drug is used during pregnancy. Nevertheless, because the studies in humans cannot rule out the possibility of harm, RHINOCORT AQUA should be used during pregnancy only if clearly needed.

Nonteratogenic Effects: Hypoadrenalism may occur in infants born of mothers receiving corticosteroids during pregnancy. Such infants should be carefully observed.

Nursing Mothers

It is not known whether budesonide is excreted in human milk. Because other corticosteroids are excreted in human milk, caution should be exercised when RHINOCORT AQUA Nasal Spray is administered to nursing women.

Pediatric Use

Safety and effectiveness in pediatric patients below 6 years of age have not been established.

Controlled clinical studies have shown that intranasal corticosteroids may cause a reduction in growth velocity in pediatric patients. This effect has been observed in the absence of laboratory evidence of hypothalamic-pituitary-adrenal (HPA)-axis suppression, suggesting that growth velocity is a more sensitive indicator of systemic corticosteroid exposure in pediatric patients than some commonly used tests of HPA-axis function. The long-term effects of this reduction in growth velocity associated with intranasal corticosteroids, including the impact on final adult height, are unknown. The potential for "catch-up" growth following discontinuation of treatment with intranasal corticosteroids has not been adequately studied. The growth of pediatric patients receiving intranasal corticosteroids, including RHINOCORT AQUA Nasal Spray, should be monitored routinely (eg, via stadiometry). The potential growth effects of prolonged treatment should be weighed against clinical benefits obtained and the availability of safe and effective noncorticosteroid treatment alternatives. To minimize the systemic effects of intranasal corticosteroids, including RHINOCORT AQUA Nasal Spray, each patient should be titrated to the lowest dose that effectively controls his/her symptoms.

A one-year placebo-controlled clinical growth study was conducted in 229 pediatric patients (ages 4 through 8 years of age) to assess the effect of RHINOCORT AQUA (single-daily dose of 64 mcg, the recommended starting dose for children ages 6 years and above) on growth velocity. From a population of 141 patients receiving RHINOCORT AQUA Nasal Spray and 67 receiving placebo, the point estimate for growth velocity with RHINOCORT AQUA Nasal Spray was 0.25 cm/year lower than that noted with placebo (95% confidence interval ranging from 0.59 cm/year lower than placebo to 0.08 cm/year higher than placebo).

The potential RHINOCORT AQUA to cause growth suppression in susceptible patients or when given at doses above 64 mcg daily cannot ruled out. The recommended dosage range in patients 6 to 11 years of age is 64 to 128 mcg per day (see **DOSAGE AND ADMINISTRATION**).

Geriatric Use

Of the 2,461 patients in clinical studies of RHINOCORT AQUA Nasal Spray, 5% were 60 years of age and over. No overall differences in safety or effectiveness were observed between these subjects and younger subjects, except for an adverse event reporting frequency of epistaxis which increased with age. Further, other reported clinical experience has not identified any other differences in responses between elderly and younger patients, but greater sensitivity of some older individuals cannot be ruled out.

ADVERSE REACTIONS

The incidence of common adverse reactions is based upon two U.S. and five non-U.S. controlled clinical trials in 1,526 patients [110 females and 239 males less than 18 years of age, and 635 females and 542 males 18 years of age and older] treated with RHINOCORT AQUA Nasal Spray at doses up to 400 mcg once daily for 3–6 weeks. The table below describes adverse events occurring at an incidence of 2% or greater and more common among RHINOCORT AQUA Nasal Spray-treated patients than in placebo-treated patients in controlled clinical trials. The overall incidence of adverse events was similar between RHINOCORT AQUA and placebo.

Adverse Event	RHINOCORT AQUA	Placebo Vehicle
Epistaxis	8%	5%
Pharyngitis	4%	3%
Bronchospasm	2%	1%

Continued on next page

Rhinocort Aqua—Cont.

Coughing	2%	<1%
Nasal Irritation	2%	<1%

A similar adverse event profile was observed in the subgroup of pediatric patients 6 to 12 years of age.
Two to three percent (2–3%) of patients in clinical trials discontinued because of adverse events. Systemic corticosteroid side effects were not reported during controlled clinical studies with RHINOCORT AQUA Nasal Spray.
If recommended doses are exceeded, however, or if individuals are particularly sensitive, symptoms of hypercorticism, ie, Cushing's Syndrome, could occur.
Rare adverse events reported from post-marketing experience include: nasal septum perforation, pharynx disorders (throat irritation, throat pain, swollen throat, burning throat, and itchy throat), angioedema, anosmia, and palpitations.
Cases of growth suppression have been reported for intranasal corticosteroids including RHINOCORT AQUA Nasal Spray (see PRECAUTIONS Pediatric Use).

OVERDOSAGE

Acute overdosage with this dosage form is unlikely since one 120 spray bottle of RHINOCORT AQUA Nasal Spray 32 mcg only contains approximately 5.4 mg of budesonide. Chronic overdosage may result in signs/symptoms of hypercorticism (see WARNINGS and PRECAUTIONS).

DOSAGE AND ADMINISTRATION

The recommended starting dose for adults and children 6 years of age and older is 64 mcg per day administered as one spray per nostril of RHINOCORT AQUA Nasal Spray 32 mcg once daily. The maximum recommended dose for adults (12 years of age and older) is 256 mcg per day administered as four sprays per nostril once daily of RHINOCORT AQUA Nasal Spray 32 mcg and the maximum recommended dose for pediatric patients (<12 years of age) is 128 mcg per day administered as two sprays per nostril once daily of RHINOCORT AQUA Nasal Spray 32 mcg (see HOW SUPPLIED).
Prior to initial use, the container must be shaken gently and the pump must be primed by actuating eight times. If used daily, the pump does not need to be reprimed. If not used for two consecutive days, reprime with one spray or until a fine spray appears. If not used for more than 14 days, rinse the applicator and reprime with two sprays or until a fine spray appears.

Individualization of Dosage

It is always desirable to titrate an individual patient to the minimum effective dose to reduce the possibility of side effects. In adults and children 6 years of age and older, the recommended starting dose is 64 mcg daily administered as one spray per nostril of RHINOCORT AQUA Nasal Spray 32 mcg, once daily. Some patients who do not achieve symptom control at the recommended starting dose may benefit from an increased dose. The maximum daily dose is 256 mcg for adults and 128 mcg for pediatric patients (<12 years of age). When the maximum benefit has been achieved and symptoms have been controlled, reducing the dose may be effective in maintaining control of the allergic rhinitis symptoms in patients who were initially controlled on higher doses.
An improvement in nasal symptoms may be noted in patients within 10 hours of first using RHINOCORT AQUA Nasal Spray. This time to onset is supported by an environmental exposure unit study in seasonal allergic rhinitis patients which demonstrated that RHINOCORT AQUA Nasal Spray led to a statistically significant improvement in nasal symptoms compared to placebo by 10 hours. Further support comes from a clinical study of patients with perennial allergic rhinitis which demonstrated a statistically significant improvement in nasal symptoms for both RHINOCORT AQUA Nasal Spray and for the active comparator (mometasone furoate) compared to placebo by 8 hours. Onset was also assessed in this study with peak nasal inspiratory flow rate and this endpoint failed to show efficacy for either active treatment. Although statistically significant improvements in nasal symptoms compared to placebo were noted within 8–10 hours in these studies, about one half to two thirds of the ultimate clinical improvement with RHINOCORT AQUA Nasal Spray occurs over the first 1–2 days, and maximum benefit may not be achieved until approximately 2 weeks after initiation of treatment. Initial assessment for response should be made during this time frame and periodically until the patient's symptoms are stabilized.

Directions for Use

Illustrated *Patient's Instructions for Use* accompany each package of RHINOCORT AQUA Nasal Spray 32 mcg.

HOW SUPPLIED

RHINOCORT AQUA Nasal Spray 32 mcg is available in an amber glass bottle with a metered-dose pump spray and a green protection cap. RHINOCORT AQUA Nasal Spray 32 mcg provides 120 metered sprays after initial priming; net fill weight 8.6 g. The RHINOCORT AQUA Nasal Spray 32 mcg bottle has been filled with an excess to accommodate the priming activity. The bottle should be discarded after 120 sprays following initial priming, since the amount of budesonide delivered per spray thereafter may be substantially less than the labeled dose. Each spray delivers 32 mcg of budesonide to the patient.
NDC 0186-1070-08
RHINOCORT AQUA Nasal Spray
32 mcg, 120 metered sprays; net fill weight 8.6 g
RHINOCORT AQUA Nasal Spray should be stored at controlled room temperature, 20 to 25°C (68 to 77°F) with the valve up. Do not freeze. Protect from light. **Shake gently before use.** Do not spray in eyes.

REFERENCES

1. Kallen B, Rydhstroem H, Aberg A. Congenital malformations after the use of inhaled budesonide in early pregnancy. Obstet Gynecol 1999;93:392-395.
2. Ericson A, Kallen B. Use of drugs during pregnancy: unique Swedish registration method that can be improved. Swedish Medical Products Agency 1999;1:8-11.
3. Norjavaara E, Gerhardsson de Verdier M. Normal pregnancy outcomes in a population-based study including 2968 pregnant women exposed to budesonide. J Allergy Clin Immunol 2003;111:736-742.

All trademarks are the property of the AstraZeneca group
© AstraZeneca 2001, 2004
Distributed by:
AstraZeneca LP, Wilmington, DE 19850
Rev. 1/05 30516-00
AstraZeneca

TOPROL-XL® ℞

[*tō'prōl*]
(metoprolol succinate)
EXTENDED-RELEASE TABLETS
TABLETS: 25 mg, 50 mg, 100 mg, and 200 mg

Prescribing information for this product, which appears on pages 632–635 of the 2005 PDR, has been completely revised as follows. Please write "See Supplement A" next to the product heading.

DESCRIPTION

TOPROL-XL, metoprolol succinate, is a $beta_1$-selective (cardioselective) adrenoceptor blocking agent, for oral administration, available as extended release tablets. TOPROL-XL has been formulated to provide a controlled and predictable release of metoprolol for once-daily administration. The tablets comprise a multiple unit system containing metoprolol succinate in a multitude of controlled release pellets. Each pellet acts as a separate drug delivery unit and is designed to deliver metoprolol continuously over the dosage interval. The tablets contain 23.75, 47.5, 95 and 190 mg of metoprolol succinate equivalent to 25, 50, 100 and 200 mg of metoprolol tartrate, USP, respectively. Its chemical name is (±)1-(isopropylamino)-3-[p-(2-methoxyethyl) phenoxy]-2-propanol succinate (2:1) (salt). Its structural formula is:

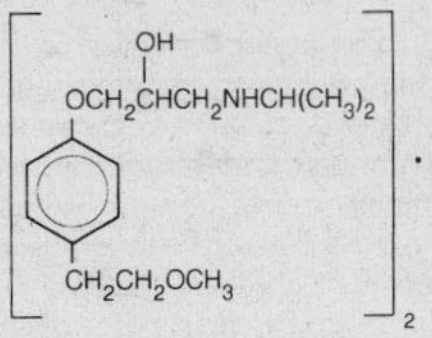

Metoprolol succinate is a white crystalline powder with a molecular weight of 652.8. It is freely soluble in water; soluble in methanol; sparingly soluble in ethanol; slightly soluble in dichloromethane and 2-propanol; practically insoluble in ethyl-acetate, acetone, diethylether and heptane. Inactive ingredients: silicon dioxide, cellulose compounds, sodium stearyl fumarate, polyethylene glycol, titanium dioxide, paraffin.

CLINICAL PHARMACOLOGY

General

Metoprolol is a $beta_1$-selective (cardioselective) adrenergic receptor blocking agent. This preferential effect is not absolute, however, and at higher plasma concentrations, metoprolol also inhibits $beta_2$-adrenoreceptors, chiefly located in the bronchial and vascular musculature. Metoprolol has no intrinsic sympathomimetic activity, and membrane-stabilizing activity is detectable only at plasma concentrations much greater than required for beta-blockade. Animal and human experiments indicate that metoprolol slows the sinus rate and decreases AV nodal conduction.
Clinical pharmacology studies have confirmed the beta-blocking activity of metoprolol in man, as shown by (1) reduction in heart rate and cardiac output at rest and upon exercise, (2) reduction of systolic blood pressure upon exercise, (3) inhibition of isoproterenol-induced tachycardia, and (4) reduction of reflex orthostatic tachycardia.
The relative $beta_1$-selectivity of metoprolol has been confirmed by the following: (1) In normal subjects, metoprolol is unable to reverse the $beta_2$-mediated vasodilating effects of epinephrine. This contrasts with the effect of nonselective beta-blockers, which completely reverse the vasodilating effects of epinephrine. (2) In asthmatic patients, metoprolol reduces FEV_1 and FVC significantly less than a nonselective beta-blocker, propranolol, at equivalent $beta_1$-receptor blocking doses.
In five controlled studies in normal healthy subjects, the same daily doses of TOPROL-XL and immediate release metoprolol were compared in terms of the extent and duration of $beta_1$-blockade produced. Both formulations were given in a dose range equivalent to 100-400 mg of immediate release metoprolol per day. In these studies, TOPROL-XL was administered once a day and immediate release metoprolol was administered once to four times a day. A sixth controlled study compared the $beta_1$-blocking effects of a 50 mg daily dose of the two formulations. In each study, $beta_1$-blockade was expressed as the percent change from baseline in exercise heart rate following standardized submaximal exercise tolerance tests at steady state. TOPROL-XL administered once a day, and immediate release metoprolol administered once to four times a day, provided comparable total $beta_1$-blockade over 24 hours (area under the $beta_1$-blockade versus time curve) in the dose range 100-400 mg. At a dosage of 50 mg once daily, TOPROL-XL produced significantly higher total $beta_1$-blockade over 24 hours than immediate release metoprolol. For TOPROL-XL, the percent reduction in exercise heart rate was relatively stable throughout the entire dosage interval and the level of $beta_1$-blockade increased with increasing doses from 50 to 300 mg daily. The effects at peak/trough (ie, at 24-hours post-dosing) were: 14/9, 16/10, 24/14, 27/22 and 27/20% reduction in exercise heart rate for doses of 50, 100, 200, 300 and 400 mg TOPROL-XL once a day, respectively. In contrast to TOPROL-XL, immediate release metoprolol given at a dose of 50-100 mg once a day produced a significantly larger peak effect on exercise tachycardia, but the effect was not evident at 24 hours. To match the peak to trough ratio obtained with TOPROL-XL over the dosing range of 200 to 400 mg, a t.i.d. to q.i.d. divided dosing regimen was required for immediate release metoprolol. A controlled cross-over study in heart failure patients compared the plasma concentrations and $beta_1$-blocking effects of 50 mg immediate release metoprolol administered t.i.d., 100 mg and 200 mg TOPROL-XL once daily. A 50 mg dose of immediate release metoprolol t.i.d. produced a peak plasma level of metoprolol similar to the peak level observed with 200 mg of TOPROL-XL. A 200 mg dose of TOPROL-XL produced a larger effect on suppression of exercise-induced and Holter-monitored heart rate over 24 hours compared to 50 mg t.i.d. of immediate release metoprolol.
The relationship between plasma metoprolol levels and reduction in exercise heart rate is independent of the pharmaceutical formulation. Using an E_{max} model, the maximum effect is a 30% reduction in exercise heart rate, is attributed to $beta_1$-blockade. $Beta_1$-blocking effects in the range of 30-80% of the maximal effect (approximately 8-23% reduction in exercise heart rate) correspond to metoprolol plasma concentrations from 30-540 nmol/L. The relative $beta_1$-selectivity of metoprolol diminishes and blockade of $beta_2$-adrenoceptors increases at plasma concentrations above 300 nmol/L.
Although beta-adrenergic receptor blockade is useful in the treatment of angina, hypertension, and heart failure there are situations in which sympathetic stimulation is vital. In patients with severely damaged hearts, adequate ventricular function may depend on sympathetic drive. In the presence of AV block, beta-blockade may prevent the necessary facilitating effect of sympathetic activity on conduction. $Beta_2$-adrenergic blockade results in passive bronchial constriction by interfering with endogenous adrenergic bronchodilator activity in patients subject to bronchospasm and may also interfere with exogenous bronchodilators in such patients.
In other studies, treatment with TOPROL-XL produced an improvement in left ventricular ejection fraction. TOPROL-XL was also shown to delay the increase in left ventricular end-systolic and end-diastolic volumes after 6 months of treatment.

Pharmacokinetics

In man, absorption of metoprolol is rapid and complete. Plasma levels following oral administration of conventional metoprolol tablets, however, approximate 50% of levels following intravenous administration, indicating about 50% first-pass metabolism. Metoprolol crosses the blood-brain barrier and has been reported in the CSF in a concentration 78% of the simultaneous plasma concentration.
Plasma levels achieved are highly variable after oral administration. Only a small fraction of the drug (about 12%) is bound to human serum albumin. Metoprolol is a racemic mixture of R- and S-enantiomers, and is primarily metabolized by CYP2D6. When administered orally, it exhibits stereoselective metabolism that is dependent on oxidation phenotype. Elimination is mainly by biotransformation in the liver, and the plasma half-life ranges from approximately 3 to 7 hours. Less than 5% of an oral dose of metoprolol is recovered unchanged in the urine; the rest is excreted by the kidneys as metabolites that appear to have no beta-blocking activity. Following intravenous administration of metoprolol, the urinary recovery of unchanged drug is approximately 10%. The systemic availability and half-life of metoprolol in patients with renal failure do not differ to a clinically significant degree from those in normal subjects. Consequently, no reduction in dosage is usually needed in patients with chronic renal failure.
Metoprolol is metabolized predominantly by CYP2D6, an enzyme that is absent in about 8% of Caucasians (poor metabolizers) and about 2% of most other populations. CYP2D6 can be inhibited by a number of drugs. Concomitant use of inhibiting drugs in poor metabolizers will increase blood levels of metoprolol several-fold, decreasing metoprolol's cardioselectivity. (See PRECAUTIONS, Drug Interactions.)
In comparison to conventional metoprolol, the plasma metoprolol levels following administration of TOPROL-XL are characterized by lower peaks, longer time to peak and significantly lower peak to trough variation. The peak plasma levels following once-daily administration of TOPROL-XL

average one-fourth to one-half the peak plasma levels obtained following a corresponding dose of conventional metoprolol, administered once daily or in divided doses. At steady state the average bioavailability of metoprolol following administration of TOPROL-XL, across the dosage range of 50 to 400 mg once daily, was 77% relative to the corresponding single or divided doses of conventional metoprolol. Nevertheless, over the 24-hour dosing interval, β_1-blockade is comparable and dose-related (see CLINICAL PHARMACOLOGY). The bioavailability of metoprolol shows a dose-related, although not directly proportional, increase with dose and is not significantly affected by food following TOPROL-XL administration.

Hypertension

The mechanism of the antihypertensive effects of beta-blocking agents has not been elucidated. However, several possible mechanisms have been proposed: (1) competitive antagonism of catecholamines at peripheral (especially cardiac) adrenergic neuron sites, leading to decreased cardiac output; (2) a central effect leading to reduced sympathetic outflow to the periphery; and (3) suppression of renin activity.

Clinical Trials

In a double-blind study, 1092 patients with mild-to-moderate hypertension were randomized to once daily TOPROL-XL (25, 100, or 400 mg), PLENDIL® (felodipine extended release tablets), the combination, or placebo. After 9 weeks, TOPROL-XL alone decreased sitting blood pressure by 6-8/4-7 mmHg (placebo-corrected change from baseline) at 24 hours post-dose. The combination of TOPROL-XL with PLENDIL has greater effects on blood pressure.

In controlled clinical studies, an immediate release dosage form of metoprolol was an effective antihypertensive agent when used alone or as concomitant therapy with thiazide-type diuretics at dosages of 100-450 mg daily. TOPROL-XL, in dosages of 100 to 400 mg once daily, produces similar β_1-blockade as conventional metoprolol tablets administered two to four times daily. In addition, TOPROL-XL administered at a dose of 50 mg once daily lowered blood pressure 24-hours post-dosing in placebo-controlled studies. In controlled, comparative, clinical studies, immediate release metoprolol appeared comparable as an antihypertensive agent to propranolol, methyldopa, and thiazide-type diuretics, and affected both supine and standing blood pressure. Because of variable plasma levels attained with a given dose and lack of a consistent relationship of antihypertensive activity to drug plasma concentration, selection of proper dosage requires individual titration.

Angina Pectoris

By blocking catecholamine-induced increases in heart rate, in velocity and extent of myocardial contraction, and in blood pressure, metoprolol reduces the oxygen requirements of the heart at any given level of effort, thus making it useful in the long-term management of angina pectoris.

Clinical Trials

In controlled clinical trials, an immediate release formulation of metoprolol has been shown to be an effective antianginal agent, reducing the number of angina attacks and increasing exercise tolerance. The dosage used in these studies ranged from 100 to 400 mg daily. TOPROL-XL, in dosages of 100 to 400 mg once daily, has been shown to possess beta-blockade similar to conventional metoprolol tablets administered two to four times daily.

Heart Failure

The precise mechanism for the beneficial effects of beta-blockers in heart failure has not been elucidated.

Clinical Trials

MERIT-HF was a double-blind, placebo-controlled study of TOPROL-XL conducted in 14 countries including the US. It randomized 3991 patients (1990 to TOPROL-XL) with ejection fraction ≤ 0.40 and NYHA Class II-IV heart failure attributable to ischemia, hypertension, or cardiomyopathy. The protocol excluded patients with contraindications to beta-blocker use, those expected to undergo heart surgery, and those within 28 days of myocardial infarction or unstable angina. The primary endpoints of the trial were (1) all-cause mortality plus all-cause hospitalization (time to first event) and (2) all-cause mortality. Patients were stabilized on optimal concomitant therapy for heart failure, including diuretics, ACE inhibitors, cardiac glycosides, and nitrates. At randomization, 41% of patients were NYHA Class II, 55% NYHA Class III; 65% of patients had heart failure attributed to ischemic heart disease; 44% had a history of hypertension; 25% had diabetes mellitus; 48% had a history of myocardial infarction. Among patients in the trial, 90% were on diuretics, 89% were on ACE inhibitors, 64% were on digitalis, 27% were on a lipid-lowering agent, 37% were on an oral anticoagulant, and the mean ejection fraction was 0.28. The mean duration of follow-up was one year. At the end of the study, the mean daily dose of TOPROL-XL was 159 mg.

The trial was terminated early for a statistically significant reduction in all-cause mortality (34%, nominal p=0.00009). The risk of all-cause mortality plus all-cause hospitalization was reduced by 19% (p=0.00012). The trial also showed improvements in heart failure-related mortality and heart failure-related hospitalizations, and NYHA functional class. The table below shows the principal results for the overall study population. The figure below illustrates principal results for a wide variety of subgroup comparisons, including US vs. non-US populations (the latter of which was not prespecified). The combined endpoints of all-cause mortality plus all-cause hospitalization and of mortality plus heart failure hospitalization showed consistent effects in the overall study population and the subgroups, including women

Clinical Endpoints in the MERIT-HF Study

Clinical Endpoint	Number of Patients		Relative Risk (95% CI)	Risk Reduction w/TOPROL-XL	Nominal P-value
	Placebo n=2001	TOPROL-XL n=1990			
All-cause mortality plus all-cause hospitalization†	767	641	0.81 (0.73-0.90)	19%	0.00012
All-cause mortality	217	145	0.66 (0.53-0.81)	34%	0.00009
All-cause mortality plus heart failure hospitalization†	439	311	0.69 (0.60-0.80)	31%	0.0000008
Cardiovascular mortality	203	128	0.62 (0.50-0.78)	38%	0.000022
Sudden death	132	79	0.59 (0.45-0.78)	41%	0.0002
Death due to worsening heart failure	58	30	0.51 (0.33-0.79)	49%	0.0023
Hospitalizations due to worsening heart failure‡	451	317	N/A	N/A	0.0000076
Cardiovascular hospitalization‡	773	649	N/A	N/A	0.00028

† Time to first event
‡ Comparison of treatment groups examines the number of hospitalizations (Wilcoxon test); relative risk and risk reduction are not applicable.

Results for Subgroups in MERIT-HF

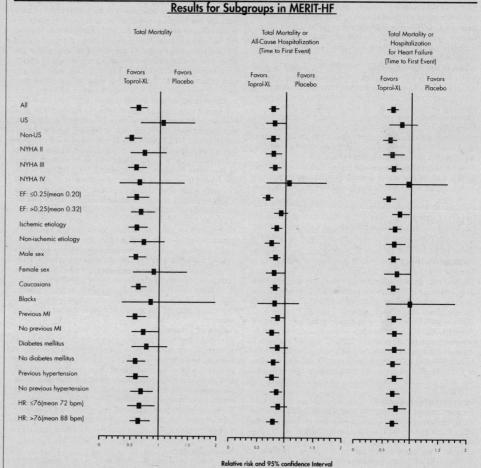

US = United States; NYHA = New York Heart Association; EF = ejection fraction; MI = myocardial infarction; HR = heart rate.

and the US population. However, in the US subgroup (n=1071) and women (n=898), overall mortality and cardiovascular mortality appeared less affected. Analyses of female and US patients were carried out because they each represented about 25% of the overall population. Nonetheless, subgroup analyses can be difficult to interpret and it is not known whether these represent true differences or chance effects.

[See table above]
[See figure above]

INDICATIONS AND USAGE

Hypertension

TOPROL-XL is indicated for the treatment of hypertension. It may be used alone or in combination with other antihypertensive agents.

Angina Pectoris

TOPROL-XL is indicated in the long-term treatment of angina pectoris.

Heart Failure

TOPROL-XL is indicated for the treatment of stable, symptomatic (NYHA Class II or III) heart failure of ischemic, hypertensive, or cardiomyopathic origin. It was studied in patients already receiving ACE inhibitors, diuretics, and, in the majority of cases, digitalis. In this population, TOPROL-XL decreased the rate of mortality plus hospitalization, largely through a reduction in cardiovascular mortality and hospitalizations for heart failure.

CONTRAINDICATIONS

TOPROL-XL is contraindicated in severe bradycardia, heart block greater than first degree, cardiogenic shock, decompensated cardiac failure, sick sinus syndrome (unless a permanent pacemaker is in place) (see WARNINGS) and in patients who are hypersensitive to any component of this product.

WARNINGS

Ischemic Heart Disease: Following abrupt cessation of therapy with certain beta-blocking agents, exacerbations of angina pectoris and, in some cases, myocardial infarction have occurred. When discontinuing chronically administered TOPROL-XL, particularly in patients with ischemic heart disease, the dosage should be gradually reduced over a period of 1-2 weeks and the patient should be carefully monitored. If angina markedly worsens or acute coronary insufficiency develops,

Continued on next page

Toprol-XL—Cont.

TOPROL-XL administration should be reinstated promptly, at least temporarily, and other measures appropriate for the management of unstable angina should be taken. Patients should be warned against interruption or discontinuation of therapy without the physician's advice. Because coronary artery disease is common and may be unrecognized, it may be prudent not to discontinue TOPROL-XL therapy abruptly even in patients treated only for hypertension.

Bronchospastic Diseases: PATIENTS WITH BRONCHOSPASTIC DISEASES SHOULD, IN GENERAL, NOT RECEIVE BETA-BLOCKERS. Because of its relative $beta_1$-selectivity, however, TOPROL-XL may be used with caution in patients with bronchospastic disease who do not respond to, or cannot tolerate, other antihypertensive treatment. Since $beta_1$-selectivity is not absolute, a $beta_2$-stimulating agent should be administered concomitantly, and the lowest possible dose of TOPROL-XL should be used (see DOSAGE AND ADMINISTRATION).

Major Surgery: The necessity or desirability of withdrawing beta-blocking therapy prior to major surgery is controversial; the impaired ability of the heart to respond to reflex adrenergic stimuli may augment the risks of general anesthesia and surgical procedures.

TOPROL-XL, like other beta-blockers, is a competitive inhibitor of beta-receptor agonists, and its effects can be reversed by administration of such agents, eg, dobutamine or isoproterenol. However, such patients may be subject to protracted severe hypotension. Difficulty in restarting and maintaining the heart beat has also been reported with beta-blockers.

Diabetes and Hypoglycemia: TOPROL-XL should be used with caution in diabetic patients if a beta-blocking agent is required. Beta-blockers may mask tachycardia occurring with hypoglycemia, but other manifestations such as dizziness and sweating may not be significantly affected.

Thyrotoxicosis: Beta-adrenergic blockade may mask certain clinical signs (eg, tachycardia) of hyperthyroidism. Patients suspected of developing thyrotoxicosis should be managed carefully to avoid abrupt withdrawal of beta-blockade, which might precipitate a thyroid storm.

Peripheral Vascular Disease: Beta-blockers can precipitate or aggravate symptoms of arterial insufficiency in patients with peripheral vascular disease. Caution should be exercised in such individuals.

Calcium Channel Blockers: Because of significant inotropic and chronotropic effects in patients treated with beta-blockers and calcium channel blockers of the verapamil and diltiazem type, caution should be exercised in patients treated with these agents concomitantly.

PRECAUTIONS

General

TOPROL-XL should be used with caution in patients with impaired hepatic function. In patients with pheochromocytoma, an alpha-blocking agent should be initiated prior to the use of any beta-blocking agent.

Worsening cardiac failure may occur during up-titration of TOPROL-XL. If such symptoms occur, diuretics should be increased and the dose of TOPROL-XL should not be advanced until clinical stability is restored (see DOSAGE AND ADMINISTRATION). It may be necessary to lower the dose of TOPROL-XL or temporarily discontinue it. Such episodes do not preclude subsequent successful titration of TOPROL-XL.

Information for Patients

Patients should be advised to take TOPROL-XL regularly and continuously, as directed, preferably with or immediately following meals. If a dose should be missed, the patient should take only the next scheduled dose (without doubling it). Patients should not interrupt or discontinue TOPROL-XL without consulting the physician.

Patients should be advised (1) to avoid operating automobiles and machinery or engaging in other tasks requiring alertness until the patient's response to therapy with TOPROL-XL has been determined; (2) to contact the physician if any difficulty in breathing occurs; (3) to inform the physician or dentist before any type of surgery that he or she is taking TOPROL-XL.

Heart failure patients should be advised to consult their physician if they experience signs or symptoms of worsening heart failure such as weight gain or increasing shortness of breath.

Laboratory Tests

Clinical laboratory findings may include elevated levels of serum transaminase, alkaline phosphatase, and lactate dehydrogenase.

Drug Interactions

Catecholamine-depleting drugs (eg, reserpine, mono amine oxidase (MAO) inhibitors) may have an additive effect when given with beta-blocking agents. Patients treated with TOPROL-XL plus a catecholamine depletor should therefore be closely observed for evidence of hypotension or marked bradycardia, which may produce vertigo, syncope, or postural hypotension.

Drugs that inhibit CYP2D6 such as quinidine, fluoxetine, paroxetine, and propafenone are likely to increase metoprolol concentration. In healthy subjects with CYP2D6 extensive metabolizer phenotype, coadministration of quinidine 100 mg and immediate release metoprolol 200 mg tripled the concentration of S-metoprolol and doubled the metoprolol elimination half-life. In four patients with cardiovascular disease, coadministration of propafenone 150 mg t.i.d. with immediate release metoprolol 50 mg t.i.d. resulted in two- to five-fold increases in the steady-state concentration of metoprolol. These increases in plasma concentration would decrease the cardioselectivity of metoprolol.

Tablet	Shape	Engraving	Bottle of 100 NDC 0186-	Unit Dose Packages of 100 NDC 0186-
25 mg*	Oval	A β	1088-05	1088-39
50 mg	Round	A mo	1090-05	1090-39
100 mg	Round	A ms	1092-05	1092-39
200 mg	Oval	A my	1094-05	N/A

* The 25-mg tablet is scored on both sides.

Beta-blockers may exacerbate the rebound hypertension which can follow the withdrawal of clonidine. If the two drugs are coadministered, the beta blocker should be withdrawn several days before the gradual withdrawal of clonidine. If replacing clonidine by beta-blocker therapy, the introduction of beta-blockers should be delayed for several days after clonidine administration has stopped.

Carcinogenesis, Mutagenesis, Impairment of Fertility

Long-term studies in animals have been conducted to evaluate the carcinogenic potential of metoprolol tartrate. In 2-year studies in rats at three oral dosage levels of up to 800 mg/kg/day (41 times, on a mg/m^2 basis, the daily dose of 200 mg for a 60-kg patient), there was no increase in the development of spontaneously occurring benign or malignant neoplasms of any type. The only histologic changes that appeared to be drug related were an increased incidence of generally mild focal accumulation of foamy macrophages in pulmonary alveoli and a slight increase in biliary hyperplasia. In a 21-month study in Swiss albino mice at three oral dosage levels of up to 750 mg/kg/day (18 times, on a mg/m^2 basis, the daily dose of 200 mg for a 60-kg patient), benign lung tumors (small adenomas) occurred more frequently in female mice receiving the highest dose than in untreated control animals. There was no increase in malignant or total (benign plus malignant) lung tumors, nor in the overall incidence of tumors or malignant tumors. This 21-month study was repeated in CD-1 mice, and no statistically or biologically significant differences were observed between treated and control mice of either sex for any type of tumor.

All genotoxicity tests performed on metoprolol tartrate (a dominant lethal study in mice, chromosome studies in somatic cells, a *Salmonella*/mammalian-microsome mutagenicity test, and a nucleus anomaly test in somatic interphase nuclei) and metoprolol succinate (a *Salmonella*/mammalian-microsome mutagenicity test) were negative.

No evidence of impaired fertility due to metoprolol tartrate was observed in a study performed in rats at doses up to 22 times, on a mg/m^2 basis, the daily dose of 200 mg in a 60-kg patient.

Pregnancy Category C

Metoprolol tartrate has been shown to increase post-implantation loss and decrease neonatal survival in rats at doses up to 22 times, on a mg/m^2 basis, the daily dose of 200 mg in a 60-kg patient. Distribution studies in mice confirm exposure of the fetus when metoprolol tartrate is administered to the pregnant animal. These studies have revealed no evidence of impaired fertility or teratogenicity. There are no adequate and well-controlled studies in pregnant women. Because animal reproduction studies are not always predictive of human response, this drug should be used during pregnancy only if clearly needed.

Nursing Mothers

Metoprolol is excreted in breast milk in very small quantities. An infant consuming 1 liter of breast milk daily would receive a dose of less than 1 mg of the drug. Caution should be exercised when TOPROL-XL is administered to a nursing woman.

Pediatric Use

Safety and effectiveness in pediatric patients have not been established.

Geriatric Use

Clinical studies of TOPROL-XL in hypertension did not include sufficient numbers of subjects aged 65 and over to determine whether they respond differently from younger subjects. Other reported clinical experience in hypertensive patients has not identified differences in responses between elderly and younger patients.

Of the 1,990 patients with heart failure randomized to TOPROL-XL in the MERIT-HF trial, 50% (990) were 65 years of age and older and 12% (238) were 75 years of age and older. There were no notable differences in efficacy or the rate of adverse events between older and younger patients.

In general, dose selection for an elderly patient should be cautious, usually starting at the low end of the dosing range, reflecting greater frequency of decreased hepatic, renal, or cardiac function, and of concomitant disease or other drug therapy.

Risk of Anaphylactic Reactions

While taking beta-blockers, patients with a history of severe anaphylactic reactions to a variety of allergens may be more reactive to repeated challenge, either accidental, diagnostic, or therapeutic. Such patients may be unresponsive to the usual doses of epinephrine used to treat allergic reaction.

ADVERSE REACTIONS

Hypertension and Angina

Most adverse effects have been mild and transient. The following adverse reactions have been reported for immediate release metoprolol tartrate.

Central Nervous System: Tiredness and dizziness have occurred in about 10 of 100 patients. Depression has been reported in about 5 of 100 patients. Mental confusion and short-term memory loss have been reported. Headache, somnolence, nightmares, and insomnia have also been reported.

Cardiovascular: Shortness of breath and bradycardia have occurred in approximately 3 of 100 patients. Cold extremities; arterial insufficiency, usually of the Raynaud type; palpitations; congestive heart failure; peripheral edema; syncope; chest pain; and hypotension have been reported in about 1 of 100 patients (see CONTRAINDICATIONS, WARNINGS, and PRECAUTIONS).

Respiratory: Wheezing (bronchospasm) and dyspnea have been reported in about 1 of 100 patients (see WARNINGS).

Gastrointestinal: Diarrhea has occurred in about 5 of 100 patients. Nausea, dry mouth, gastric pain, constipation, flatulence, digestive tract disorders, and heartburn have been reported in about 1 of 100 patients.

Hypersensitive Reactions: Pruritus or rash have occurred in about 5 of 100 patients. Worsening of psoriasis has also been reported.

Miscellaneous: Peyronie's disease has been reported in fewer than 1 of 100,000 patients. Musculoskeletal pain, blurred vision, decreased libido, and tinnitus have also been reported.

There have been rare reports of reversible alopecia, agranulocytosis, and dry eyes. Discontinuation of the drug should be considered if any such reaction is not otherwise explicable. The oculomucocutaneous syndrome associated with the beta-blocker practolol has not been reported with metoprolol.

Potential Adverse Reactions

In addition, there are a variety of adverse reactions not listed above, which have been reported with other beta-adrenergic blocking agents and should be considered potential adverse reactions to TOPROL-XL.

Central Nervous System: Reversible mental depression progressing to catatonia; an acute reversible syndrome characterized by disorientation for time and place, short-term memory loss, emotional lability, slightly clouded sensorium, and decreased performance on neuropsychometrics.

Cardiovascular: Intensification of AV block (see CONTRAINDICATIONS).

Hematologic: Agranulocytosis, nonthrombocytopenic purpura, thrombocytopenic purpura.

Hypersensitive Reactions: Fever combined with aching and sore throat, laryngospasm, and respiratory distress.

Heart Failure

In the MERIT-HF study, serious adverse events and adverse events leading to discontinuation of study medication were systematically collected. In the MERIT-HF study comparing TOPROL-XL in daily doses up to 200 mg (mean dose 159 mg once-daily) (n=1990) to placebo (n=2001), 10.3% of TOPROL-XL patients discontinued for adverse events vs. 12.2% of placebo patients.

The table below lists adverse events in the MERIT-HF study that occurred at an incidence of equal to or greater than 1% in the TOPROL-XL group and greater than placebo by more than 0.5%, regardless of the assessment of causality.

Adverse Events Occurring in the MERIT-HF Study at an Incidence ≥ 1% in the TOPROL-XL Group and Greater Than Placebo by More Than 0.5%

	TOPROL-XL N=1990 % of patients	Placebo N=2001 % of patients
Dizziness/vertigo	1.8	1.0
Bradycardia	1.5	0.4
Accident and/or injury	1.4	0.8

Other adverse events with an incidence of > 1% on TOPROL-XL and as common on placebo (within 0.5%) included myocardial infarction, pneumonia, cerebrovascular disorder, chest pain, dyspnea/dyspnea aggravated, syncope, coronary artery disorder, ventricular tachycardia/arrhythmia aggravated, hypotension, diabetes mellitus/diabetes mellitus aggravated, abdominal pain, and fatigue.

Post-Marketing Experience

The following adverse reactions have been reported with TOPROL-XL in worldwide post-marketing use, regardless of causality:

Cardiovascular: 2nd and 3rd degree heart block.
Gastrointestinal: hepatitis, vomiting.
Hematologic: thrombocytopenia.
Musculoskeletal: arthralgia.
Nervous System/Psychiatric: anxiety/nervousness, hallucinations, paresthesia.
Reproductive, male: impotence.
Skin: increased sweating, photosensitivity, urticaria.
Special Sense Organs: taste disturbances.

OVERDOSAGE

Acute Toxicity

There have been a few reports of overdosage with TOPROL-XL and no specific overdosage information was obtained with this drug, with the exception of animal toxicology data. However, since TOPROL-XL (metoprolol succinate salt) contains the same active moiety, metoprolol, as conventional metoprolol tablets (metoprolol tartrate salt), the recommendations on overdosage for metoprolol conventional tablets are applicable to TOPROL-XL.

Signs and Symptoms

Overdosage of TOPROL-XL may lead to severe hypotension, sinus bradycardia, atrioventricular block, heart failure, cardiogenic shock, cardiac arrest, bronchospasm, impairment of consciousness/coma, nausea, vomiting, and cyanosis.

Treatment

In general, patients with acute or recent myocardial infarction or congestive heart failure may be more hemodynamically unstable than other patients and should be treated accordingly. When possible the patient should be treated under intensive care conditions. On the basis of the pharmacologic actions of metoprolol, the following general measures should be employed:

Elimination of the Drug: Gastric lavage should be performed.

Bradycardia: Atropine should be administered. If there is no response to vagal blockade, isoproterenol should be administered cautiously.

Hypotension: A vasopressor should be administered, eg, levarterenol or dopamine.

Bronchospasm: A $beta_2$-stimulating agent and/or a theophylline derivative should be administered.

Cardiac Failure: A digitalis glycoside and diuretics should be administered. In shock resulting from inadequate cardiac contractility, administration of dobutamine, isoproterenol, or glucagon may be considered.

DOSAGE AND ADMINISTRATION

TOPROL-XL is an extended release tablet intended for once daily administration. For treatment of hypertension and angina, when switching from immediate release metoprolol to TOPROL-XL, the same total daily dose of TOPROL-XL should be used. Dosages of TOPROL-XL should be individualized and titration may be needed in some patients.

TOPROL-XL tablets are scored and can be divided; however, the whole or half tablet should be swallowed whole and not chewed or crushed.

Hypertension

The usual initial dosage is 25 to 100 mg daily in a single dose, whether used alone or added to a diuretic. The dosage may be increased at weekly (or longer) intervals until optimum blood pressure reduction is achieved. In general, the maximum effect of any given dosage level will be apparent after 1 week of therapy. Dosages above 400 mg per day have not been studied.

Angina Pectoris

The dosage of TOPROL-XL should be individualized. The usual initial dosage is 100 mg daily, given in a single dose. The dosage may be gradually increased at weekly intervals until optimum clinical response has been obtained or there is a pronounced slowing of the heart rate. Dosages above 400 mg per day have not been studied. If treatment is to be discontinued, the dosage should be reduced gradually over a period of 1-2 weeks (see WARNINGS).

Heart Failure

Dosage must be individualized and closely monitored during up-titration. Prior to initiation of TOPROL-XL, the dosing of diuretics, ACE inhibitors, and digitalis (if used) should be stabilized. The recommended starting dose of TOPROL-XL is 25 mg once daily for two weeks in patients with NYHA Class II heart failure and 12.5 mg once daily in patients with more severe heart failure. The dose should then be doubled every two weeks to the highest dosage level tolerated by the patient or up to 200 mg of TOPROL-XL. If transient worsening of heart failure occurs, it may be treated with increased doses of diuretics, and it may also be necessary to lower the dose of TOPROL-XL or temporarily discontinue it. The dose of TOPROL-XL should not be increased until symptoms of worsening heart failure have been stabilized. Initial difficulty with titration should not preclude later attempts to introduce TOPROL-XL. If heart failure patients experience symptomatic bradycardia, the dose of TOPROL-XL should be reduced.

HOW SUPPLIED

Tablets containing metoprolol succinate equivalent to the indicated weight of metoprolol tartrate, USP, are white, biconvex, film-coated, and scored.

[See table at top of previous page]

Store at 25°C (77°F). Excursions permitted to 15-30°C (59-86°F). (See USP Controlled Room Temperature.)

Manufactured for: AstraZeneca LP
Wilmington, DE 19850
By: AstraZeneca AB
S-151 85 Södertälje, Sweden
Made in Sweden
30015-01
Rev 02/05

AstraZeneca

AstraZeneca Pharmaceuticals LP

1800 CONCORD PIKE
WILMINGTON, DE 19850-5437 USA

For Product Full Prescribing Information, Business Information, Medical Information, Adverse Drug Experiences, and Customer Service:

Information Center
1-800-236-9933

For Product Ordering:

Trade Customer Service
1-800-842-9920

For Product Full Prescribing Information:

Internet: www.astrazeneca-us.com

ACCOLATE ℞

[*ac-cō'late*]
(zafirlukast) TABLETS

Prescribing information for this product, which appears on pages 635–637 of the 2005 PDR, has been revised as follows. Please write "See Supplement A" next to the product heading.

Change appears under the ADVERSE REACTION section. The seventh paragraph has been revised to include insomnia, malaise, and pruritus.

The paragraph now reads:

"Hypersensitivity reactions, including urticaria, angioedema and rashes, with or without blistering, have been reported in association with ACCOLATE therapy. Additionally, there have been reports of patients experiencing agranulocytosis, bleeding, bruising, or edema, arthralgia, myalgia, insomnia, malaise, and pruritus in association with ACCOLATE therapy."

-Also, 2004 has been added to the copyright.

-The revision date is now Rev. 07/04

ARIMIDEX® ℞

[*ă-rĭ-mĭ-dĕx*]
(anastrozole) TABLETS

Prescribing information for this product, which appears on page 637–642 of the 2005 PDR, has been completely revised as follows. Please write "See Supplement A" next to the product heading.

DESCRIPTION

ARIMIDEX® (anastrozole) tablets for oral administration contain 1 mg of anastrozole, a non-steroidal aromatase inhibitor. It is chemically described as 1,3-Benzenediacetonitrile, a, a, a', a'-tetramethyl-5-(1H-1,2,4-triazol-1-ylmethyl). Its molecular formula is $C_{17}H_{19}N_5$ and its structural formula is:

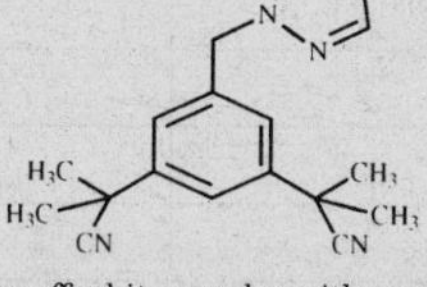

Anastrozole is an off-white powder with a molecular weight of 293.4. Anastrozole has moderate aqueous solubility (0.5 mg/mL at 25°C); solubility is independent of pH in the physiological range. Anastrozole is freely soluble in methanol, acetone, ethanol, and tetrahydrofuran, and very soluble in acetonitrile.

Each tablet contains as inactive ingredients: lactose, magnesium stearate, hydroxypropylmethylcellulose, polyethylene glycol, povidone, sodium starch glycolate, and titanium dioxide.

CLINICAL PHARMACOLOGY

Mechanism of Action

Many breast cancers have estrogen receptors and growth of these tumors can be stimulated by estrogen. In postmenopausal women, the principal source of circulating estrogen (primarily estradiol) is conversion of adrenally-generated androstenedione to estrone by aromatase in peripheral tissues, such as adipose tissue, with further conversion of estrone to estradiol. Many breast cancers also contain aromatase; the importance of tumor-generated estrogens is uncertain.

Treatment of breast cancer has included efforts to decrease estrogen levels, by ovariectomy premenopausally and by use of anti-estrogens and progestational agents both pre- and post-menopausally; and these interventions lead to decreased tumor mass or delayed progression of tumor growth in some women.

Anastrozole is a potent and selective non-steroidal aromatase inhibitor. It significantly lowers serum estradiol concentrations and has no detectable effect on formation of adrenal corticosteroids or aldosterone.

Pharmacokinetics

Inhibition of aromatase activity is primarily due to anastrozole, the parent drug. Studies with radiolabeled drug have demonstrated that orally administered anastrozole is well absorbed into the systemic circulation with 83 to 85% of the radiolabel recovered in urine and feces. Food does not affect the extent of absorption. Elimination of anastrozole is primarily via hepatic metabolism (approximately 85%) and to a lesser extent, renal excretion (approximately 11%), and anastrozole has a mean terminal elimination half-life of approximately 50 hours in postmenopausal women. The major circulating metabolite of anastrozole, triazole, lacks pharmacologic activity. The pharmacokinetic parameters are similar in patients and in healthy postmenopausal volunteers. The pharmacokinetics of anastrozole are linear over the dose range of 1 to 20 mg and do not change with repeated dosing. Consistent with the approximately 2-day terminal elimination half-life, plasma concentrations approach steady-state levels at about 7 days of once daily dosing and steady-state levels are approximately three- to four-fold higher than levels observed after a single dose of ARIMIDEX. Anastrozole is 40% bound to plasma proteins in the therapeutic range.

Metabolism and Excretion

Studies in postmenopausal women demonstrated that anastrozole is extensively metabolized with about 10% of the dose excreted in the urine as unchanged drug within 72 hours of dosing, and the remainder (about 60% of the dose) is excreted in urine as metabolites. Metabolism of anastrozole occurs by N-dealkylation, hydroxylation and glucuronidation. Three metabolites of anastrozole have been identified in human plasma and urine. The known metabolites are triazole, a glucuronide conjugate of hydroxy-anastrozole, and a glucuronide of anastrozole itself. Several minor (less than 5% of the radioactive dose) metabolites have not been identified.

Because renal elimination is not a significant pathway of elimination, total body clearance of anastrozole is unchanged even in severe (creatinine clearance less than 30 mL/min/1.73m²) renal impairment, dosing adjustment in patients with renal dysfunction is not necessary (see **Special Populations** and **DOSAGE AND ADMINISTRATION** sections). Dosage adjustment is also unnecessary in patients with stable hepatic cirrhosis (see **Special Populations** and **DOSAGE AND ADMINISTRATION** sections).

Special Populations

Geriatric

Anastrozole pharmacokinetics have been investigated in postmenopausal female volunteers and patients with breast cancer. No age related effects were seen over the range <50 to >80 years.

Race

Estradiol and estrone sulfate levels were similar between Japanese and Caucasian postmenopausal women who received 1 mg of anastrozole daily for 16 days. Anastrozole mean steady-state minimum plasma concentrations in Caucasian and Japanese postmenopausal women were 25.7 and 30.4 ng/mL, respectively.

Renal Insufficiency

Anastrozole pharmacokinetics have been investigated in subjects with renal insufficiency. Anastrozole renal clearance decreased proportionally with creatinine clearance and was approximately 50% lower in volunteers with severe renal impairment (creatinine clearance < 30 mL/min/1.73m²) compared to controls. Since only about 10% of anastrozole is excreted unchanged in the urine, the reduction in renal clearance did not influence the total body clearance (See **DOSAGE AND ADMINISTRATION**).

Hepatic Insufficiency

Hepatic metabolism accounts for approximately 85% of anastrozole elimination. Anastrozole pharmacokinetics have been investigated in subjects with hepatic cirrhosis related to alcohol abuse. The apparent oral clearance (CL/F) of anastrozole was approximately 30% lower in subjects with stable hepatic cirrhosis than in control subjects with normal liver function. However, plasma anastrozole concentrations in the subjects with hepatic cirrhosis were within the range of concentrations seen in normal subjects across all clinical trials (see **DOSAGE AND ADMINISTRATION**), so that no dosage adjustment is needed.

Drug-Drug Interactions

Anastrozole inhibited reactions catalyzed by cytochrome P450 1A2, 2C8/9, and 3A4 *in vitro* with Ki values which were approximately 30 times higher than the mean steady-state C_{max} values observed following a 1 mg daily dose. Anastrozole had no inhibitory effect on reactions catalyzed by cytochrome P450 2A6 or 2D6 *in vitro*. Administration of a single 30 mg/kg or multiple 10 mg/kg doses of anastrozole to healthy subjects had no effect on the clearance of antipyrine or urinary recovery of antipyrine metabolites. Based on these *in vitro* and *in vivo* results, it is unlikely that co-administration of ARIMIDEX 1 mg with other drugs will result in clinically significant inhibition of cytochrome P450 mediated metabolism.

Continued on next page

Arimidex—Cont.

In a study conducted in 16 male volunteers, anastrozole did not alter the pharmacokinetics as measured by C_{max} and AUC, and anticoagulant activity as measured by prothrombin time, activated partial thromboplastine time, and thrombin time of both R- and S-warfarin.

Co-administration of anastrozole and tamoxifen in breast cancer patients reduced anastrozole plasma concentration by 27% compared to those achieved with anastrozole alone; however, the coadministration did not affect the pharmacokinetics of tamoxifen or N-desmethyltamoxifen (see **PRE-CAUTIONS-Drug Interactions**).

Pharmacodynamics

Effect on Estradiol: Mean serum concentrations of estradiol were evaluated in multiple daily dosing trials with 0.5, 1, 3, 5, and 10 mg of ARIMIDEX in postmenopausal women with advanced breast cancer. Clinically significant suppression of serum estradiol was seen with all doses. Doses of 1 mg and higher resulted in suppression of mean serum concentrations of estradiol to the lower limit of detection (3.7 pmol/L). The recommended daily dose, ARIMIDEX 1 mg, reduced estradiol by approximately 70% within 24 hours and by approximately 80% after 14 days of daily dosing. Suppression of serum estradiol was maintained for up to 6 days after cessation of daily dosing with ARIMIDEX 1 mg.

The effect of ARIMIDEX on estradiol levels in premenopausal women has not been studied. Because aromatization of adrenal androgens is not a significant source of estradiol in premenopausal women (women with functioning ovaries as evidenced by menstruation and/or premenopausal LH, FSH and estradiol levels), ARIMIDEX would not be expected to lower estradiol levels in premenopausal women.

Effect on Corticosteroids

In multiple daily dosing trials with 3, 5, and 10 mg, the selectivity of anastrozole was assessed by examining effects on corticosteroid synthesis. For all doses, anastrozole did not affect cortisol or aldosterone secretion at baseline or in response to ACTH. No glucocorticoid or mineralocorticoid replacement therapy is necessary with anastrozole.

Other Endocrine Effects

In multiple daily dosing trials with 5 and 10 mg, thyroid stimulating hormone (TSH) was measured; there was no increase in TSH during the administration of ARIMIDEX. ARIMIDEX does not possess direct progestogenic, androgenic, or estrogenic activity in animals, but does perturb the circulating levels of progesterone, androgens, and estrogens.

Clinical Studies

Adjuvant Treatment of Breast Cancer in Postmenopausal Women: A multicenter, double-blind trial (ATAC) randomized 9,366 postmenopausal women with operable breast cancer to adjuvant treatment with ARIMIDEX 1 mg daily, tamoxifen 20 mg daily, or a combination of the two treatments for five years or until recurrence of the disease. At the time of the efficacy analysis, women had received a median of 31 months of treatment and had been followed for recurrence-free survival for a median of 33 months.

The primary endpoint of the trial is recurrence-free survival, ie, time to occurrence of a distant or local recurrence, or contralateral breast primary or death from any cause. Time to distant recurrence and the incidence of contralateral breast primaries were analyzed.

Demographic and other baseline characteristics were similar among the three treatment groups (see Table 1).
[See table 1 below]

The recommended duration of tamoxifen therapy is five years; continued benefit of tamoxifen after 3 years has been documented. The results of the ATAC trial in a patient population treated for a median of 31 months, thus allow only a preliminary comparison of ARIMIDEX and tamoxifen therapy. At this time, recurrence-free survival was improved in the ARIMIDEX arm compared to the tamoxifen arm: Hazard Ratio (HR) = 0.83, 95% CI 0.71-0.96, p=0.0144. Results were essentially the same in the hormone receptor positive patients (about 84% of the patients): HR=0.78, 95% CI 0.65-0.93.

Recurrence-free survival in the combination treatment arm was similar to that in the tamoxifen group.

Duration of follow-up in this ongoing trial is too short to permit a mature survival analysis. The duration of therapy on the study arms and frequency of individual events comprising recurrence are described in Table 2.
[See table 2 at top of next page]

First Line Therapy in Postmenopausal Women with Advanced Breast Cancer: Two double-blind, well-controlled clinical studies of similar design (0030, a North American study and 0027, a predominately European study) were conducted to assess the efficacy of ARIMIDEX compared with tamoxifen as first-line therapy for hormone receptor positive or hormone receptor unknown locally advanced or metastatic breast cancer in postmenopausal women. A total of 1021 patients between the ages of 30 and 92 years old were randomized to receive trial treatment. Patients were randomized to receive 1 mg of ARIMIDEX once daily or 20 mg of tamoxifen once daily. The primary end points for both trials were time to tumor progression, objective tumor response rate, and safety.

Demographics and other baseline characteristics, including patients who had measurable and no measurable disease, patients who were given previous adjuvant therapy, the site of metastatic disease and ethnic origin were similar for the two treatment groups for both trials. The following table summarizes the hormone receptor status at entry for all randomized patients in trials 0030 and 0027.
[See table 3 on next page]

For the primary endpoints, trial 0030 showed ARIMIDEX was at least as effective as tamoxifen for objective tumor response rate. ARIMIDEX had a statistically significant advantage over tamoxifen (p=0.006) for time to tumor progression (see Table 4 and Figure 1). Trial 0027 showed ARIMIDEX was at least as effective as tamoxifen for objective tumor response rate and time to tumor progression (See Table 4 and Figure 2).

Table 4 below summarizes the results of trial 0030 and trial 0027 for the primary efficacy endpoints.
[See table 4 on next page]

Table 1 - Demographic and Baseline Characteristics for ATAC Trial

Demographic Characteristic	ARIMIDEX 1 mg (*N=3125)	Tamoxifen 20 mg (*N=3116)	ARIMIDEX 1 mg plus Tamoxifen 20 mg (*N=3125)
Mean Age (yrs.)	64.1	64.1	64.3
Age Range (yrs.)	38.1–92.8	32.8–94.9	37.0–92.2
Age Distribution (%)			
<45 yrs.	0.7	0.4	0.5
45-60 yrs.	34.6	35.0	34.5
>60 <70 yrs.	38.0	37.1	37.7
>70 yrs.	26.7	27.4	27.3
Mean Weight (kg)	70.8	71.1	71.3
Receptor Status (%)			
Positive[1]	83.5	83.1	83.8
Negative[2]	7.4	8.0	7.0
Other[3]	8.8	8.6	9.1
Other Treatment (%) prior to Randomization			
Mastectomy	47.8	47.3	48.1
Breast conservation[4]	52.3	52.8	52
Axillary surgery	95.5	95.7	95.2
Radiotherapy	63.3	62.5	62.0
Chemotherapy	22.3	20.8	20.8
Neoadjuvant Tamoxifen	1.6	1.6	1.7
Primary Tumor Size (%)			
T1 (≤2 cm)	63.9	62.9	64.1
T2 (>2 cm and ≤5 cm)	32.6	34.2	32.9
T3 (>5 cm)	2.7	2.2	2.3
Nodal Status (%)			
Node positive	34.9	33.6	33.5
1-3 (# of nodes)	24.4	24.4	24.3
4-9	7.5	6.4	6.8
>9	2.9	2.7	2.3
Tumor Grade (%)			
Well-differentiated	20.8	20.5	21.2
Moderately differentiated	46.8	47.8	46.6
Poorly/undifferentiated	23.7	23.3	23.7
Not assessed/recorded	8.7	8.4	8.5

[1] Includes patients who were estrogen receptor (ER) positive or progesterone receptor (PgR) positive, or both positive
[2] Includes patients with both ER negative and PgR negative receptor status
[3] Includes all other combinations of ER and PgR receptor status unknown
[4] Among the patients who had breast conservation, radiotherapy was administered to 95.0% of patients in the ARIMIDEX arm, 94.1% in the tamoxifen arm and 94.5% in the ARIMIDEX plus tamoxifen arm.
* N=Number of patients randomized to the treatment

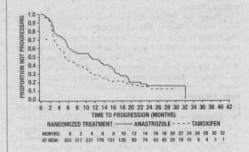

Figure 1 - Kaplan-Meier probability of time to disease progression for all randomized patients (intent-to-treat) in Trial 0030

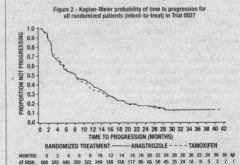

Figure 2 - Kaplan-Meier probability of time to progression for all randomized patients (intent-to-treat) in Trial 0027

Results from the secondary endpoints of time to treatment failure, duration of tumor response, and duration of clinical benefit were supportive of the results of the primary efficacy endpoints. There were too few deaths occurring across treatment groups of both trials to draw conclusions on overall survival differences.

Second Line Therapy in Postmenopausal Women with Advanced Breast Cancer who had Disease Progression following Tamoxifen Therapy: Anastrozole was studied in two well-controlled clinical trials (0004, a North American study; 0005, a predominately European study) in postmenopausal women with advanced breast cancer who had disease progression following tamoxifen therapy for either advanced or early breast cancer. Some of the patients had also received previous cytotoxic treatment. Most patients were ER-positive; a smaller fraction were ER-unknown or ER-negative; the ER-negative patients were eligible only if they had had a positive response to tamoxifen. Eligible patients with measurable and non-measurable disease were randomized to receive either a single daily dose of 1 mg or 10 mg of ARIMIDEX or megestrol acetate 40 mg four times a day. The studies were double-blinded with respect to ARIMIDEX. Time to progression and objective response (only patients with measurable disease could be considered partial responders) rates were the primary efficacy variables. Objective response rates were calculated based on the Union Internationale Contre le Cancer (UICC) criteria. The rate of prolonged (more than 24 weeks) stable disease, the rate of progression, and survival were also calculated.

Both trials included over 375 patients; demographics and other baseline characteristics were similar for the three treatment groups in each trial. Patients in the 0005 trial had responded better to prior tamoxifen treatment. Of the patients entered who had prior tamoxifen therapy for advanced disease (58% in Trial 0004; 57% in Trial 0005), 18% of these patients in Trial 0004 and 42% in Trial 0005 were reported by the primary investigator to have responded. In Trial 0004, 81% of patients were ER-positive, 13% were ER-unknown, and 6% were ER-negative. In Trial 0005, 58% of patients were ER-positive, 37% were ER-unknown, and 5% were ER-negative. In Trial 0004, 62% of patients had measurable disease compared to 79% in Trial 0005. The sites of metastatic disease were similar among treatment groups for each trial. On average, 40% of the patients had soft tissue metastases; 60% had bone metastases; and 40% had visceral (15% liver) metastases.

As shown in the table below, similar results were observed among treatment groups and between the two trials. None of the within-trial differences were statistically significant. [See table 5 at top of next page]

More than 1/3 of the patients in each treatment group in both studies had either an objective response or stabilization of their disease for greater than 24 weeks. Among the 263 patients who received ARIMIDEX 1 mg, there were 11 complete responders and 22 partial responders. In patients who had an objective response, more than 80% were still responding at 6 months from randomization and more than 45% were still responding at 12 months from randomization.

When data from the two controlled trials are pooled, the objective response rates and median times to progression and death were similar for patients randomized to ARIMIDEX 1 mg and megestrol acetate. There is, in this data, no indication that ARIMIDEX 10 mg is superior to ARIMIDEX 1 mg.

[See table 6 at top of next page]

Objective response rates and median times to progression and death for ARIMIDEX 1 mg were similar to megestrol acetate for women over or under 65. There were too few nonwhite patients studied to draw conclusions about racial differences in response.

INDICATIONS AND USAGE

ARIMIDEX is indicated for adjuvant treatment of postmenopausal women with hormone receptor positive early breast cancer.

The effectiveness of ARIMIDEX in early breast cancer is based on an analysis of recurrence-free survival in patients treated for a median of 31 months (see **CLINICAL PHARMACOLOGY-Clinical Studies** subsection). Further follow-up of study patients will be required to determine long-term outcomes.

ARIMIDEX is indicated for the first-line treatment of postmenopausal women with hormone receptor positive or hormone receptor unknown locally advanced or metastatic breast cancer.

ARIMIDEX is indicated for the treatment of advanced breast cancer in postmenopausal women with disease progression following tamoxifen therapy. Patients with ER-negative disease and patients who did not respond to previous tamoxifen therapy rarely responded to ARIMIDEX.

CONTRAINDICATIONS

ARIMIDEX is contraindicated in any patient who has shown a hypersensitivity reaction to the drug or to any of the excipients.

WARNINGS

ARIMIDEX can cause fetal harm when administered to a pregnant woman. Anastrozole has been found to cross the placenta following oral administration of 0.1 mg/kg in rats and rabbits (about 1 and 1.9 times the recommended human dose, respectively, on a mg/m^2 basis). Studies in both rats and rabbits at doses equal to or greater than 0.1 and 0.02 mg/kg/day, respectively (about 1 and 1/3, respectively, the recommended human dose on a mg/m^2 basis), adminis-

Table 2 – ATAC Endpoint Summary

	ARIMIDEX 1 mg (N=3125)	Tamoxifen 20 mg (N=3116)	ARIMIDEX 1 mg plus Tamoxifen 20 mg (N=3125)
Median Duration of Therapy (mo.)[1]	30.9	30.7	30.4
Range Duration of Therapy (mo.)	<1 to 55.3	<1 to 55.7	<1 to 54.5
Median Efficacy Follow-UP (mo.)	33.6	33.2	32.9
Range Follow-Up (mo.)	<1 to 55.2	<1 to 55.7	<1 to 54.4
Recurrence-Free Survival			
First Event (n,%)	318 (10.2)	379 (12.2)	383 (12.3)
Locoregional[2]	67 (2.1)	83 (2.7)	81 (2.6)
Distant	157 (5.0)	181 (5.8)	202 (6.5)
New Contralateral Primaries	14 (0.4)	33 (1.1)	28 (0.9)
Invasive	9 (0.3)	30 (1.0)	23 (0.7)
Ductal carcinoma in situ	5 (0.2)	3 (<0.1)	5 (0.2)
Deaths[3]			
Death – breast cancer	4 (0.12)	1 (0.03)	0 (0.00)
Death – other reason	76 (2.4)	81 (2.6)	72 (2.3)

[1]Based on treatment received
[2]Includes new primary ipsilateral breast cancer (including DCIS), and recurrences at the chest wall, axillary and other regional lymph nodes
[3]Includes only deaths that were first events

Table 3
Number (%) of subjects

	Trial 0030		Trial 0027	
Receptor status	ARIMIDEX 1 mg (n=171)	Tamoxifen 20 mg (n=182)	ARIMIDEX 1 mg (n=340)	Tamoxifen 20 mg (n=328)
ER+ and/or PgR+	151 (88.3)	162 (89.0)	154 (45.3)	144 (43.9)
ER unknown, PgR Unknown	19 (11.1)	20 (11.0)	185 (54.4)	183 (55.8)

ER = Estrogen receptor
PgR = Progesterone receptor

Table 4
Number (%) of subjects

	Trial 0030		Trial 0027	
End point	ARIMIDEX 1 mg (n=171)	Tamoxifen 20 mg (n=182)	ARIMIDEX 1 mg (n=340)	Tamoxifen 20 mg (n=328)
Time to progression (TTP)				
Median TTP (months)	11.1	5.6	8.2	8.3
Number (%) of subjects who progressed	114 (67%)	138 (76%)	249 (73%)	247 (75%)
Hazard ratio (LCL)[1]	1.42 (1.15)		1.01 (0.87)	
2-sided 95% CI	(1.11, 1.82)		(0.85, 1.20)	
p-value[2]	0.006		0.920	
Best objective response rate				
Number (%) of subjects With CR + PR[3]	36 (21.1%)	31 (17.0%)	112 (32.9%)	107 (32.6%)
Odds Ratio (LCL)[3]	1.30 (0.83)		1.01 (0.77)	

CR = Complete Response
PR = Partial Response
CI = Confidence Interval
LCL = Lower Confidence Limit
[1] Tamoxifen:ARIMIDEX
[2] Two-sided Log Rank
[3] ARIMIDEX:Tamoxifen

tered during the period of organogenesis showed that anastrozole increased pregnancy loss (increased pre- and/or post-implantation loss, increased resorption, and decreased numbers of live fetuses); effects were dose related in rats. Placental weights were significantly increased in rats at doses of 0.1 mg/kg/day or more.

Evidence of fetotoxicity, including delayed fetal development (i.e., incomplete ossification and depressed fetal body weights), was observed in rats administered doses of 1 mg/kg/day (which produced plasma anastrozole C_{ssmax} and $AUC_{0-24\ hr}$ that were 19 times and 9 times higher than the respective values found in postmenopausal volunteers at the recommended dose). There was no evidence of teratogenicity in rats administered doses up to 1.0 mg/kg/day. In rabbits, anastrozole caused pregnancy failure at doses equal to or greater than 1.0 mg/kg/day (about 16 times the recommended human dose on a mg/m^2 basis); there was no evidence of teratogenicity in rabbits administered 0.2 mg/kg/day (about 3 times the recommended human dose on a mg/m^2 basis).

There are no adequate and well-controlled studies in pregnant women using ARIMIDEX. If ARIMIDEX is used during pregnancy, or if the patient becomes pregnant while receiving this drug, the patient should be apprised of the potential hazard to the fetus or potential risk for loss of the pregnancy.

PRECAUTIONS

General

ARIMIDEX is not recommended for use in premenopausal women as safety and efficacy has not been established (see **CLINICAL PHARMACOLOGY, Pharmacodynamics, Effect on Estradiol** section).

Before starting treatment with ARIMIDEX, pregnancy must be excluded (see **WARNINGS**). ARIMIDEX should be administered under the supervision of a qualified physician experienced in the use of anticancer agents.

Laboratory Tests

Results from the ATAC trial bone substudy, at 12 and 24 months demonstrated that patients receiving ARIMIDEX had a mean decrease in both lumbar spine and total hip

Continued on next page

Arimidex—Cont.

bone mineral density (BMD) compared to baseline. Patients receiving tamoxifen had a mean increase in both lumbar spine and total hip BMD compared to baseline.

Because ARIMIDEX lowers circulating estrogen levels it may cause a reduction in bone mineral density.

During the ATAC trial, more patients receiving ARIMIDEX were reported to have an elevated serum cholesterol compared to patients receiving tamoxifen (7% versus 3%, respectively).

Drug Interactions

(See **CLINICAL PHARMACOLOGY**) Anastrozole inhibited *in vitro* metabolic reactions catalyzed by cytochromes P450 1A2, 2C8/9, and 3A4 but only at relatively high concentrations. Anastrozole did not inhibit P450 2A6 or the polymorphic P450 2D6 in human liver microsomes. Anastrozole did not alter the pharmacokinetics of antipyrine. Although there have been no formal interaction studies other than with antipyrine, based on these *in vivo* and *in vitro* studies, it is unlikely that co-administration of a 1 mg dose of ARIMIDEX with other drugs will result in clinically significant drug inhibition of cytochrome P450-mediated metabolism of the other drugs.

An interaction study with warfarin showed no clinically significant effect of anastrozole on warfarin pharmacokinetics or anticoagulant activity.

Clinical and pharmacokinetic results from the ATAC trial suggest that tamoxifen should not be administered with anastrozole (see **CLINICAL PHARMACOLOGY – Drug Interactions and Clinical Studies** subsections). Co-administration of anastrozole and tamoxifen resulted in a reduction of anastrozole plasma levels by 27% compared with those achieved with anastrozole alone.

Estrogen-containing therapies should not be used with ARIMIDEX as they may diminish its pharmacologic action.

Drug/Laboratory Test Interactions

No clinically significant changes in the results of clinical laboratory tests have been observed.

Carcinogenesis

A conventional carcinogenesis study in rats at doses of 1.0 to 25 mg/kg/day (about 10 to 243 times the daily maximum recommended human dose on a mg/m^2 basis) administered by oral gavage for up to 2 years revealed an increase in the incidence of hepatocellular adenoma and carcinoma and uterine stromal polyps in females and thyroid adenoma in males at the high dose. A dose related increase was observed in the incidence of ovarian and uterine hyperplasia in females. At 25 mg/kg/day, plasma $AUC_{0-24\ hr}$ levels in rats were 110 to 125 times higher than the level exhibited in postmenopausal volunteers at the recommended dose. A separate carcinogenicity study in mice at oral doses of 5 to 50 mg/kg/day (about 24 to 243 times the daily maximum recommended human dose on a mg/m^2 basis) for up to 2 years produced an increase in the incidence of benign ovarian stromal, epithelial and granulosa cell tumors at all dose levels. A dose related increase in the incidence of ovarian hyperplasia was also observed in female mice. These ovarian changes are considered to be rodent-specific effects of aromatase inhibition and are of questionable significance to humans. The incidence of lymphosarcoma was increased in males and females at the high dose. At 50 mg/kg/day, plasma AUC levels in mice were 35 to 40 times higher than the level exhibited in postmenopausal volunteers at the recommended dose.

Mutagenesis

ARIMIDEX has not been shown to be mutagenic in *in vitro* tests (Ames and E. coli bacterial tests, CHO-K1 gene mutation assay) or clastogenic either *in vitro* (chromosome aberrations in human lymphocytes) or *in vivo* (micronucleus test in rats).

Impairment of Fertility

Oral administration of anastrozole to female rats (from 2 weeks before mating to pregnancy day 7) produced significant incidence of infertility and reduced numbers of viable pregnancies at 1 mg/kg/day (about 10 times the recommended human dose on a mg/m^2 basis and 9 times higher than the $AUC_{0-24\ hr}$ found in postmenopausal volunteers at the recommended dose). Pre-implantation loss of ova or fetus was increased at doses equal to or greater than 0.02 mg/kg/day (about one-fifth the recommended human dose on a mg/m^2 basis). Recovery of fertility was observed following a 5-week non-dosing period which followed 3 weeks of dosing. It is not known whether these effects observed in female rats are indicative of impaired fertility in humans.

Multiple-dose studies in rats administered anastrozole for 6 months at doses equal to or greater than 1 mg/kg/day (which produced plasma anastrozole C_{ssmax} and $AUC_{0-24\ hr}$ that were 19 and 9 times higher than the respective values found in postmenopausal volunteers at the recommended dose) resulted in hypertrophy of the ovaries and the presence of follicular cysts. In addition, hyperplastic uteri were observed in 6-month studies in female dogs administered doses equal to or greater than 1 mg/kg/day (which produced plasma anastrozole C_{ssmax} and $AUC_{0-24\ hr}$ that were 22 times and 16 times higher than the respective values found in postmenopausal women at the recommended dose). It is not known whether these effects on the reproductive organs of

animals are associated with impaired fertility in premenopausal women.

Pregnancy

Pregnancy Category D
(See **WARNINGS**)

Table 5

Trial 0004	ARIMIDEX 1 mg	ARIMIDEX 10 mg	Megestrol Acetate 160 mg
(N. America)	(n=128)	(n=130)	(n=128)
Median Follow-up (months)*	31.3	30.9	32.9
Median Time to Death (months)	29.6	25.7	26.7
2 Year Survival Probability (%)	62.0	58.0	53.1
Median Time to Progression (months)	5.7	5.3	5.1
Objective Response (all patients) (%)	12.5	10.0	10.2
Stable Disease for >24 weeks (%)	35.2	29.2	32.8
Progression (%)	86.7	85.4	90.6
Trial 0005			
(Europe, Australia, S. Africa)	(n=135)	(n=118)	(n=125)
Median Follow-up (months)*	31.0	30.9	31.5
Median Time to Death (months)	24.3	24.8	19.8
2 Year Survival Probability (%)	50.5	50.9	39.1
Median Time to Progression (months)	4.4	5.3	3.9
Objective Response (all patients) (%)	12.6	15.3	14.4
Stable Disease for >24 weeks (%)	24.4	25.4	23.2
Progression (%)	91.9	89.8	92.0

*Surviving Patients

Table 6

Trials 0004 & 0005 (Pooled Data)	ARIMIDEX 1 mg N=263	ARIMIDEX 10 mg N=248	Megestrol Acetate 160 mg N=253
Median Time to Death (months)	26.7	25.5	22.5
2 Year Survival Probability (%)	56.1	54.6	46.3
Median Time to Progression	4.8	5.3	4.6
Objective Response (all patients) (%)	12.5	12.5	12.3

Table 7 – Adverse events occurring with an incidence of at least 5% in any treatment group during treatment, or within 14 days of the end of treatment

Body system and adverse event by COSTART-preferred term*	Number (%) of patients		
	ARIMIDEX 1 mg (N = 3092)	Tamoxifen 20 mg (N = 3093)	ARIMIDEX 1 mg plus Tamoxifen 20 mg (N = 3098)
Body as a whole			
Asthenia	512 (17)	491 (16)	468 (15)
Pain	461 (15)	435 (14)	407 (13)
Back pain	256 (8)	255 (8)	258 (8)
Headache	277 (9)	216 (7)	214 (7)
Abdominal pain	227 (7)	228 (7)	219 (7)
Infection	223 (7)	225 (7)	211 (7)
Accidental injury	221 (7)	221 (7)	226 (7)
Flu syndrome	154 (5)	170 (5)	170 (5)
Chest pain	164 (5)	122 (4)	152 (5)
Cardiovascular			
Vasodilatation	1082 (35)	1246 (40)	1261 (41)
Hypertension	292 (9)	252 (8)	270 (9)
Digestive			
Nausea	307 (10)	298 (10)	324 (10)
Constipation	201 (7)	214 (7)	232 (7)
Diarrhea	227 (7)	186 (6)	193 (6)
Dyspepsia	166 (5)	137 (4)	156 (5)
Gastrointestinal disorder	155 (5)	122 (4)	127 (4)
Hemic and lymphatic			
Lymphoedema	267 (9)	299 (10)	296 (10)
Metabolic and nutritional			
Peripheral edema	255 (8)	275 (9)	281 (9)
Weight gain	253 (8)	250 (8)	264 (9)
Hypercholesteremia	210 (7)	79 (3)	72 (2)
Musculoskeletal			
Arthritis	431 (14)	344 (11)	364 (12)
Arthralgia	390 (13)	251 (8)	265 (9)
Osteoporosis	229 (7)	161 (5)	174 (6)
Fracture	219 (7)	137 (4)	178 (6)
Bone pain	165 (5)	149 (5)	143 (5)
Arthrosis	179 (6)	136 (4)	119 (4)
Nervous system			
Depression	348 (11)	341 (11)	342 (11)
Insomnia	266 (9)	245 (8)	227 (7)
Dizziness	198 (6)	207 (7)	190 (6)
Anxiety	168 (5)	157 (5)	140 (5)
Paraesthesia	195 (6)	116 (4)	120 (4)
Respiratory			
Pharyngitis	376 (12)	359 (12)	350 (11)
Cough increased	212 (7)	237 (8)	203 (7)
Dyspnea	186 (6)	185 (6)	175 (6)
Skin and appendages			
Rash	300 (10)	331 (11)	326 (11)
Sweating	121 (4)	165 (5)	142 (5)
Urogenital			
Leukorrhea	75 (2)	265 (9)	277 (9)
Urinary tract infection	192 (6)	252 (8)	228 (7)
Breast pain	205 (7)	136 (4)	182 (6)
Vulvovaginitis	180 (6)	134 (4)	134 (4)

COSTART Coding Symbols for Thesaurus of Adverse Reaction Terms.
N = Number of patients receiving the treatment.
*A patient may have had more than 1 adverse event, including more than 1 adverse event in the same body system.

Nursing Mothers

It is not known if anastrozole is excreted in human milk. Because many drugs are excreted in human milk, caution should be exercised when ARIMIDEX is administered to a nursing woman (See **WARNINGS** and **PRECAUTIONS**).

Pediatric Use

The safety and efficacy of ARIMIDEX in pediatric patients have not been established.

Geriatric Use

In studies 0030 and 0027 about 50% of patients were 65 or older. Patients ≥ 65 years of age had moderately better tumor response and time to tumor progression than patients < 65 years of age regardless of randomized treatment. In studies 0004 and 0005 50% of patients were 65 or older. Response rates and time to progression were similar for the over 65 and younger patients. In the ATAC adjuvant study, 35% of patients were <60 years of age; 38% were ≥ 60 to ≤ 70 years of age; and 27% were > 70 years of age. The number of events by age group was insufficient to perform a subset efficacy analysis.

ADVERSE REACTIONS

Adjuvant Therapy

The median duration of adjuvant treatment for safety evaluation was 37.3 months, 36.9 months, and 36.5 months for patients receiving ARIMIDEX 1 mg, tamoxifen 20 mg, and the combination of ARIMIDEX 1 mg plus tamoxifen 20 mg, respectively.

Adverse events occurring with an incidence of at least 5% in any treatment group during treatment or within 14 days of the end of treatment are presented in Table 7.

[See table 7 on previous page]

Non-pathologic fractures were reported more frequently in the ARIMIDEX-treated patients (219 [7%]) than in the tamoxifen-treated patients (137 [4%]).

Certain adverse events and combinations of adverse events were prospectively specified for analysis, based on the known pharmacologic properties and side effect profiles of the two drugs (See table 8). Patients receiving ARIMIDEX had an increase in musculoskeletal events and fractures (including fractures of spine, hip and wrist) compared with patients receiving tamoxifen. Patients receiving ARIMIDEX had a decrease in hot flashes, vaginal bleeding, vaginal discharge, endometrial cancer, venous thromboembolic events (including deep venous thrombosis) and ischemic cerebrovascular events compared with patients receiving tamoxifen.

[See table 8 at right]

Angina pectoris was reported more frequently in the ARIMIDEX-treated patients (52 [1.7%]) than in the tamoxifen-treated patients (30 [1.0%]); the incidence of myocardial infarction was comparable (ARIMIDEX 24 patients [0.8%]; tamoxifen 25 patients [0.8%]).

Results from the ATAC trial bone substudy, at 12 and 24 months demonstrated that patients receiving ARIMIDEX had a mean decrease in both lumbar spine and total hip bone mineral density (BMD) compared to baseline. Patients receiving tamoxifen had a mean increase in both lumbar spine and total hip BMD compared to baseline.

First Line Therapy

ARIMIDEX was generally well tolerated in two well-controlled clinical trials (ie, Trials 0030 and 0027). Adverse events occurring with an incidence of at least 5% in either treatment group of trials 0030 and 0027 during or within 2 weeks of the end of treatment are shown in Table 9.

Table 9

Body system Adverse event[a]	ARIMIDEX (n=506)	Tamoxifen (n=511)
Whole body		
Asthenia	83 (16)	81 (16)
Pain	70 (14)	73 (14)
Back pain	60 (12)	68 (13)
Headache	47 (9)	40 (8)
Abdominal pain	40 (8)	38 (7)
Chest pain	37 (7)	37 (7)
Flu syndrome	35 (7)	30 (6)
Pelvic pain	23 (5)	30 (6)
Cardiovascular		
Vasodilation	128 (25)	106 (21)
Hypertension	25 (5)	36 (7)
Digestive		
Nausea	94 (19)	106 (21)
Constipation	47 (9)	66 (13)
Diarrhea	40 (8)	33 (6)
Vomiting	38 (8)	36 (7)
Anorexia	26 (5)	46 (9)
Metabolic and nutritional		
Peripheral edema	51 (10)	41 (8)
Musculoskeletal		
Bone pain	54 (11)	52 (10)
Nervous		
Dizziness	30 (6)	22 (4)
Insomnia	30 (6)	38 (7)
Depression	23 (5)	32 (6)
Hypertonia	16 (3)	26 (5)
Respiratory		
Cough increased	55 (11)	52 (10)
Dyspnea	51 (10)	47 (9)
Pharyngitis	49 (10)	68 (13)
Skin and appendages		
Rash	38 (8)	34 (8)
Urogenital		
Leukorrhea	9 (2)	31 (6)

[a] A patient may have had more than 1 adverse event.

Table 8 – Number (%) of patients with Pre-Specified Adverse Event in ATAC Trial

	ARIMIDEX N=3092 (%)	Tamoxifen N=3093 (%)	Odds-ratio	95% CI
All Fractures	224 (7)	145 (5)	1.59	1.28 – 1.97
Fractures of Spine, Hip, Wrist	89 (3)	62 (2)	1.45	1.04 – 2.04
Musculo-skeletal disorders[1]	940 (30)	737 (24)	1.41	1.28 – 1.55
Ischemic Cardiovascular Disease	92 (3)	74 (2)	1.25	0.91 – 1.72
Asthenia	513 (17)	491 (16)	1.05	0.93 – 1.20
Nausea and Vomiting	348 (11)	342 (11)	1.02	0.88 – 1.19
Mood Disturbances	521 (17)	511 (17)	1.02	0.90 – 1.16
Cataracts	128 (4)	140 (5)	0.91	0.71 – 1.17
Hot Flashes	1082 (35)	1246 (40)	0.80	0.73 – 0.87
Venous Thromboembolic events	73 (2)	120 (4)	0.60	0.44 – 0.81
Deep Venous Thromboembolic Events	40 (1)	60 (2)	0.66	0.43 – 1.00
Ischemic Cerebrovascular Event	40 (1)	74 (2)	0.53	0.35 – 0.80
Vaginal Bleeding	147 (5)	270 (9)	0.52	0.42 – 0.64
Vaginal Discharge	94 (3)	378 (12)	0.23	0.18 – 0.28
Endometrial Cancer	3 (0.1)	15 (0.5)	0.20	0.04 – 0.70

[1] Refers to joint symptoms, including arthritis, arthrosis and arthralgia.

Less frequent adverse experiences reported in patients receiving ARIMIDEX 1 mg in either Trial 0030 or Trial 0027 were similar to those reported for second-line therapy. Based on results from second-line therapy and the established safety profile of tamoxifen, the incidences of 9 pre-specified adverse event categories potentially causally related to one or both of the therapies because of their pharmacology were statistically analyzed. No significant differences were seen between treatment groups.

Table 10 Number (n) and Percentage of Patients

	ARIMIDEX 1 mg (n = 506)	NOLVADEX 20 mg (n = 511)
Adverse Event Group[a]	n (%)	n (%)
Depression	23 (5)	32 (6)
Tumor Flare	15 (3)	18 (4)
Thromboembolic Disease[a]	18 (4)	33 (6)
Venous[b]	5	15
Coronary and Cerebral[c]	13	19
Gastrointestinal Disturbance	170 (34)	196 (38)
Hot Flushes	134 (26)	118 (23)
Vaginal Dryness	9 (2)	3 (1)
Lethargy	6 (1)	15 (3)
Vaginal Bleeding	5 (1)	11 (2)
Weight Gain	11(2)	8 (2)

[a] A patient may have had more than 1 adverse event
[b] Includes pulmonary embolus, thrombophlebitis, retinal vein thrombosis
[c] Includes myocardial infarction, myocardial ischemia, angina pectoris, cerebrovascular accident, cerebral ischemia and cerebral infarct

Despite the lack of estrogenic activity for ARIMIDEX, there was no increase in myocardial infarction or fracture when compared with tamoxifen.

Second Line Therapy

ARIMIDEX was generally well tolerated in two well-controlled clinical trials (ie, Trials 0004 and 0005), with less than 3.3% of the ARIMIDEX-treated patients and 4.0% of the megestrol acetate-treated patients withdrawing due to an adverse event.

The principal adverse event more common with ARIMIDEX than megestrol acetate was diarrhea. Adverse events reported in greater than 5% of the patients in any of the treatment groups in these two well-controlled clinical trials, regardless of causality, are presented below:

Table 11 – Number (n) and Percentage of Patients with Adverse Event[†]

	ARIMIDEX 1 mg (n = 262)	ARIMIDEX 10 mg (n = 246)	Megestrol Acetate 160 mg (n = 253)
Adverse Event	n (%)	n (%)	n (%)
Asthenia	42 (16)	33 (13)	47 (19)
Nausea	41 (16)	48 (20)	28 (11)
Headache	34 (13)	44 (18)	24 (9)
Hot Flashes	32 (12)	29 (11)	21 (8)
Pain	28 (11)	38 (15)	29 (11)
Back Pain	28 (11)	26 (11)	19 (8)
Dyspnea	24 (9)	27 (11)	53 (21)
Vomiting	24 (9)	26 (11)	16 (6)
Cough Increased	22 (8)	18 (7)	19 (8)
Diarrhea	22 (8)	18 (7)	7 (3)
Constipation	18 (7)	18 (7)	21 (8)
Abdominal Pain	18 (7)	14 (6)	18 (7)
Anorexia	18 (7)	19 (8)	11 (4)
Bone Pain	17 (6)	26 (12)	19 (8)
Pharyngitis	16 (6)	23 (9)	15 (6)
Dizziness	16 (6)	12 (5)	15 (6)
Rash	15 (6)	15 (6)	19 (8)
Dry Mouth	15 (6)	11 (4)	13 (5)
Peripheral Edema	14 (5)	21 (9)	28 (11)
Pelvic Pain	14 (5)	17 (7)	13 (5)
Depression	14 (5)	6 (2)	5 (2)
Chest Pain	13 (2)	18 (7)	13 (5)
Paresthesia	12 (5)	15 (6)	9 (4)
Vaginal Hemorrhage	6 (2)	4 (2)	13 (5)
Weight Gain	4 (2)	9 (4)	30 (12)
Sweating	4 (2)	3 (1)	16 (6)
Increased Appetite	0 (0)	1 (0)	13 (5)

[†] A patient may have more than one adverse event.

Other less frequent (2% to 5%) adverse experiences reported in patients receiving ARIMIDEX 1 mg in either Trial 0004 or Trial 0005 are listed below. These adverse experiences are listed by body system and are in order of decreasing frequency within each body system regardless of assessed causality.

Body as a Whole: Flu syndrome; fever; neck pain; malaise; accidental injury; infection

Cardiovascular: Hypertension; thrombophlebitis

Hepatic: Gamma GT increased; SGOT increased; SGPT increased

Hematologic: Anemia; leukopenia

Metabolic and Nutritional: Alkaline phosphatase increased; weight loss

Mean serum total cholesterol levels increased by 0.5 mmol/L among patients receiving ARIMIDEX. Increases in LDL cholesterol have been shown to contribute to these changes.

Musculoskeletal: Myalgia; arthralgia; pathological fracture

Nervous: Somnolence; confusion; insomnia; anxiety; nervousness

Respiratory: Sinusitis; bronchitis; rhinitis

Skin and Appendages: Hair thinning; pruritus

Urogenital: Urinary tract infection; breast pain

The incidences of the following adverse event groups potentially causally related to one or both of the therapies because of their pharmacology, were statistically analyzed: weight gain, edema, thromboembolic disease, gastrointestinal disturbance, hot flushes, and vaginal dryness. These six groups, and the adverse events captured in the groups, were prospectively defined. The results are shown in the table below.

Continued on next page

Arimidex—Cont.

Table 12 – Number (n) and Percentage of Patients

Adverse Event Group	ARIMIDEX 1 mg (n = 262) n (%)	ARIMIDEX 10 mg (n = 246) n (%)	Megestrol Acetate 160 mg (n = 253) n (%)
Gastrointestinal Disturbance	77 (29)	81 (33)	54 (21)
Hot Flushes	33 (13)	29 (12)	35 (14)
Edema	19 (7)	28 (11)	35 (14)
Thromboembolic Disease	9 (3)	4 (2)	12 (5)
Vaginal Dryness	5 (2)	3 (1)	2 (1)
Weight Gain	4 (2)	10 (4)	30 (12)

More patients treated with megestrol acetate reported weight gain as an adverse event compared to patients treated with ARIMIDEX 1 mg ($p<0.0001$). Other differences were not statistically significant.

An examination of the magnitude of change in weight in all patients was also conducted. Thirty-four percent (87/253) of the patients treated with megestrol acetate experienced weight gain of 5% or more and 11% (27/253) of the patients treated with megestrol acetate experienced weight gain of 10% or more. Among patients treated with ARIMIDEX 1 mg, 13% [33/262] experienced weight gain of 5% or more and 3% [6/262] experienced weight gain of 10% or more. On average, this 5 to 10% weight gain represented between 6 and 12 pounds.

No patients receiving ARIMIDEX or megestrol acetate discontinued treatment due to drug-related weight gain.

Vaginal bleeding has been reported infrequently, mainly in patients during the first few weeks after changing from existing hormonal therapy to treatment with ARIMIDEX. If bleeding persists, further evaluation should be considered.

During clinical trials and postmarketing experience joint pain/stiffness has been reported in association with the use of ARIMIDEX.

ARIMIDEX may also be associated with rash including very rare cases of mucocutaneous disorders such as erythema multiforme and Stevens-Johnson syndrome. Very rare cases of allergic reactions including angioedema, urticaria and anaphylaxis have been reported in patients receiving ARIMIDEX.

OVERDOSAGE

Clinical trials have been conducted with ARIMIDEX, up to 60 mg in a single dose given to healthy male volunteers and up to 10 mg daily given to postmenopausal women with advanced breast cancer; these dosages were well tolerated. A single dose of ARIMIDEX that results in life-threatening symptoms has not been established. In rats, lethality was observed after single oral doses that were greater than 100 mg/kg (about 800 times the recommended human dose on a mg/m^2 basis) and was associated with severe irritation to the stomach (necrosis, gastritis, ulceration, and hemorrhage).

In an oral acute toxicity study in the dog the median lethal dose was greater than 45 mg/kg/day.

There is no specific antidote to overdosage and treatment must be symptomatic. In the management of an overdose, consider that multiple agents may have been taken. Vomiting may be induced if the patient is alert. Dialysis may be helpful because ARIMIDEX is not highly protein bound. General supportive care, including frequent monitoring of vital signs and close observation of the patient, is indicated.

DOSAGE AND ADMINISTRATION

The dose of ARIMIDEX is one 1 mg tablet taken once a day. For patients with advanced breast cancer, ARIMIDEX should be continued until tumor progression.

For adjuvant treatment of early breast cancer in postmenopausal women, the optimal duration of therapy is unknown. The median duration of therapy at the time of data analysis was 31 months; the ongoing ATAC trial is planned for five years of treatment.

Patients with Hepatic Impairment

(See **CLINICAL PHARMACOLOGY**) Hepatic metabolism accounts for approximately 85% of anastrozole elimination. Although clearance of anastrozole was decreased in patients with cirrhosis due to alcohol abuse, plasma anastrozole concentrations stayed in the usual range seen in patients without liver disease. Therefore, no changes in dose are recommended for patients with mild-to-moderate hepatic impairment, although patients should be monitored for side effects. ARIMIDEX has not been studied in patients with severe hepatic impairment.

Patients with Renal Impairment

No changes in dose are necessary for patients with renal impairment.

Use in the Elderly

No dosage adjustment is necessary.

HOW SUPPLIED

White, biconvex, film-coated tablets containing 1 mg of anastrozole. The tablets are impressed on one side with a logo consisting of a letter "A" (upper case) with an arrowhead attached to the foot of the extended right leg of the "A" and on the reverse with the tablet strength marking "Adx 1". These tablets are supplied in bottles of 30 tablets (NDC 0310-0201-30).

Storage

Store at controlled room temperature, 20-25°C (68-77°F) [see USP].

AstraZeneca Pharmaceuticals LP
Wilmington, Delaware 19850
Made in USA

ARIMIDEX is a trademark of the AstraZeneca group of companies.

Rev 08-04 SIC No. XXXXX-XX

CRESTOR® ℞

[krĕs-tōr]

(rosuvastatin calcium)

Prescribing information for this product, which appears on pages 644–647 of the 2005 PDR, has been completely revised as follows. Please write "See Supplement A" next to the product heading.

DESCRIPTION

CRESTOR® (rosuvastatin calcium) is a synthetic lipid-lowering agent. Rosuvastatin is an inhibitor of 3-hydroxy-3-methylglutaryl-coenzyme A (HMG-CoA) reductase. This enzyme catalyzes the conversion of HMG-CoA to mevalonate, an early and rate-limiting step in cholesterol biosynthesis.

Rosuvastatin calcium is bis[(E)-7-[4-(4-fluorophenyl)-6-isopropyl-2-[methyl(methylsulfonyl)amino] pyrimidin-5-yl](3R,5S)-3,5-dihydroxyhept-6-enoic acid] calcium salt. The empirical formula for rosuvastatin calcium is $(C_{22}H_{27}FN_3O_6S)_2Ca$. Its molecular weight is 1001.14. Its structural formula is:

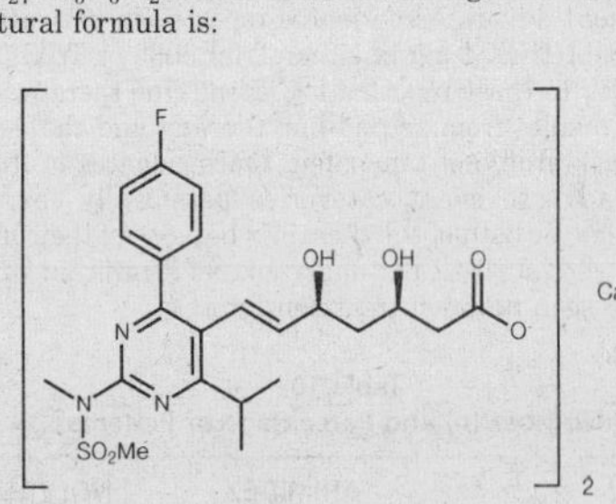

Rosuvastatin calcium is a white amorphous powder that is sparingly soluble in water and methanol, and slightly soluble in ethanol. Rosuvastatin is a hydrophilic compound with a partition coefficient (octanol/water) of 0.13 at pH of 7.0.

CRESTOR Tablets for oral administration contain 5, 10, 20, or 40 mg of rosuvastatin and the following inactive ingredients: microcrystalline cellulose NF, lactose monohydrate NF, tribasic calcium phosphate NF, crospovidone NF, magnesium stearate NF, hypromellose NF, triacetin NF, titanium dioxide USP, yellow ferric oxide, and red ferric oxide NF.

CLINICAL PHARMACOLOGY

General: In the bloodstream, cholesterol and triglycerides (TG) circulate as part of lipoprotein complexes. With ultracentrifugation, these complexes separate into very-low-density lipoprotein (VLDL), intermediate-density lipoprotein (IDL), and low-density lipoprotein (LDL) fractions that contain apolipoprotein B-100 (ApoB-100) and high-density lipoprotein (HDL) fractions.

Cholesterol and TG synthesized in the liver are incorporated into VLDL and secreted into the circulation for delivery to peripheral tissues. TG are removed by the action of lipases, and in a series of steps, the modified VLDL is transformed first into IDL and then into cholesterol-rich LDL. IDL and LDL are removed from the circulation mainly by high affinity ApoB/E receptors, which are expressed to the greatest extent on liver cells. HDL is hypothesized to participate in the reverse transport of cholesterol from tissues back to the liver.

Epidemiologic, experimental, and clinical studies have established that high LDL cholesterol (LDL-C), low HDL cholesterol (HDL-C), and high plasma TG promote human atherosclerosis and are risk factors for developing cardiovascular disease. In contrast, higher levels of HDL-C are associated with decreased cardiovascular risk.

Like LDL, cholesterol-enriched triglyceride-rich lipoproteins, including VLDL, IDL, and remnants, can also promote atherosclerosis. Elevated plasma triglycerides are frequently found with low HDL-C levels and small LDL particles, as well as in association with non-lipid metabolic risk factors for coronary heart disease (CHD). As such, total plasma TG has not consistently been shown to be an independent risk factor for CHD. Furthermore, the independent effect of raising HDL or lowering TG on the risk of coronary and cardiovascular morbidity and mortality has not been determined.

Mechanism of Action: Rosuvastatin is a selective and competitive inhibitor of HMG-CoA reductase, the rate-limiting enzyme that converts 3-hydroxy-3-methylglutaryl coenzyme A to mevalonate, a precursor of cholesterol. *In vivo* studies in animals, and *in vitro* studies in cultured animal and human cells have shown rosuvastatin to have a high uptake into, and selectivity for, action in the liver, the target organ for cholesterol lowering. In *in vivo* and *in vitro* studies, rosuvastatin produces its lipid-modifying effects in two ways. First, it increases the number of hepatic LDL receptors on the cell-surface to enhance uptake and catabolism of LDL. Second, rosuvastatin inhibits hepatic synthesis of VLDL, which reduces the total number of VLDL and LDL particles.

Rosuvastatin reduces total cholesterol (total-C), LDL-C, ApoB, and nonHDL-C (total cholesterol minus HDL-C) in patients with homozygous and heterozygous familial hypercholesterolemia (FH), nonfamilial forms of hypercholesterolemia, and mixed dyslipidemia. Rosuvastatin also reduces TG and produces increases in HDL-C. Rosuvastatin reduces total-C, LDL-C, VLDL-cholesterol (VLDL-C), ApoB, non-HDL-C, and TG, and increases HDL-C in patients with isolated hypertriglyceridemia. The effect of rosuvastatin on cardiovascular morbidity and mortality has not been determined.

Pharmacokinetics and Drug Metabolism

Absorption: In clinical pharmacology studies in man, peak plasma concentrations of rosuvastatin were reached 3 to 5 hours following oral dosing. Both peak concentration (C_{max}) and area under the plasma concentration-time curve (AUC) increased in approximate proportion to rosuvastatin dose. The absolute bioavailability of rosuvastatin is approximately 20%.

Administration of rosuvastatin with food decreased the rate of drug absorption by 20% as assessed by C_{max}, but there was no effect on the extent of absorption as assessed by AUC.

Plasma concentrations of rosuvastatin do not differ following evening or morning drug administration.

Significant LDL-C reductions are seen when rosuvastatin is given with or without food, and regardless of the time of day of drug administration.

Distribution: Mean volume of distribution at steady-state of rosuvastatin is approximately 134 liters. Rosuvastatin is 88% bound to plasma proteins, mostly albumin. This binding is reversible and independent of plasma concentrations.

Metabolism: Rosuvastatin is not extensively metabolized; approximately 10% of a radiolabeled dose is recovered as metabolite. The major metabolite is N-desmethyl rosuvastatin, which is formed principally by cytochrome P450 2C9, and *in vitro* studies have demonstrated that N-desmethyl rosuvastatin has approximately one-sixth to one-half the HMG-CoA reductase inhibitory activity of rosuvastatin. Overall, greater than 90% of active plasma HMG-CoA reductase inhibitory activity is accounted for by rosuvastatin.

Excretion: Following oral administration, rosuvastatin and its metabolites are primarily excreted in the feces (90%). The elimination half-life ($t_{1/2}$) of rosuvastatin is approximately 19 hours.

After an intravenous dose, approximately 28% of total body clearance was via the renal route, and 72% by the hepatic route.

Special Populations

Race: A population pharmacokinetic analysis revealed no clinically relevant differences in pharmacokinetics among Caucasian, Hispanic, and Black or Afro-Caribbean groups. However, pharmacokinetic studies, including one conducted in the US, have demonstrated an approximate 2-fold elevation in median exposure (AUC and C_{max}) in Asian subjects when compared with a Caucasian control group (see WARNINGS, Myopathy/Rhabdomyolysis, PRECAUTIONS, General and DOSAGE AND ADMINISTRATION).

Gender: There were no differences in plasma concentrations of rosuvastatin between men and women.

Geriatric: There were no differences in plasma concentrations of rosuvastatin between the nonelderly and elderly populations (age ≥65 years).

Pediatric: In a pharmacokinetic study, 18 patients (9 boys and 9 girls) 10 to 17 years of age with heterozygous FH received single and multiple oral doses of rosuvastatin. Both C_{max} and AUC of rosuvastatin were similar to values observed in adult subjects administered the same doses.

Renal Insufficiency: Mild to moderate renal impairment (creatinine clearance ≥ 30 mL/min/1.73m^2) had no influence on plasma concentrations of rosuvastatin when oral doses of 20 mg rosuvastatin were administered for 14 days. However, plasma concentrations of rosuvastatin increased to a clinically significant extent (about 3-fold) in patients with severe renal impairment (CL_{cr} < 30 mL/min/1.73m^2) compared with healthy subjects (CL_{cr} > 80 mL/min/1.73m^2) (see PRECAUTIONS, General).

Hemodialysis: Steady-state plasma concentrations of rosuvastatin in patients on chronic hemodialysis were approximately 50% greater compared with healthy volunteer subjects with normal renal function.

Hepatic Insufficiency: In patients with chronic alcohol liver disease, plasma concentrations of rosuvastatin were modestly increased. In patients with Child-Pugh A disease, C_{max} and AUC were increased by 60% and 5%, respectively, as compared with patients with normal liver function. In patients with Child-Pugh B disease, C_{max} and AUC were increased 100% and 21%, respectively, compared with patients with normal liver function (see CONTRAINDICATIONS and WARNINGS, Liver Enzymes).

Drug-Drug Interactions

Cytochrome P450 3A4: *In vitro* and *in vivo* data indicate that rosuvastatin clearance is not dependent on metabolism by cytochrome P450 3A4 to a clinically significant extent. This has been confirmed in studies with known cytochrome P450 3A4 inhibitors (ketoconazole, erythromycin, itraconazole).

Ketoconazole: Coadministration of ketoconazole (200 mg twice daily for 7 days) with rosuvastatin (80 mg) resulted in no change in plasma concentrations of rosuvastatin.

Erythromycin: Coadministration of erythromycin (500 mg four times daily for 7 days) with rosuvastatin (80 mg) decreased AUC and C_{max} of rosuvastatin by 20% and 31%, respectively. These reductions are not considered clinically significant.

Itraconazole: Itraconazole (200 mg once daily for 5 days) resulted in a 39% and 28% increase in AUC of rosuvastatin after 10 mg and 80 mg dosing, respectively. These increases are not considered clinically significant.

Fluconazole: Coadministration of fluconazole (200 mg once daily for 11 days) with rosuvastatin (80 mg) resulted in a 14% increase in AUC of rosuvastatin. This increase is not considered clinically significant.

Cyclosporine: Coadministration of cyclosporine with rosuvastatin resulted in no significant changes in cyclosporine plasma concentrations. However, C_{max} and AUC of rosuvastatin increased 11- and 7-fold, respectively, compared with historical data in healthy subjects. These increases are considered to be clinically significant (see PRECAUTIONS Drug Interactions, WARNINGS, Myopathy/Rhabdomyolysis, and DOSAGE AND ADMINISTRATION).

Warfarin: Coadministration of warfarin (25 mg) with rosuvastatin (40 mg) did not change warfarin plasma concentrations but increased the International Normalized Ratio (INR) (see PRECAUTIONS, Drug Interactions).

Digoxin: Coadministration of digoxin (0.5 mg) with rosuvastatin (40 mg) resulted in no change to digoxin plasma concentrations.

Fenofibrate: Coadministration of fenofibrate (67 mg three times daily) with rosuvastatin (10 mg) resulted in no significant changes in plasma concentrations of rosuvastatin or fenofibrate (see PRECAUTIONS, Drug Interactions, and WARNINGS, Myopathy/Rhabdomyolysis).

Gemfibrozil: Coadministration of gemfibrozil (600 mg twice daily for 7 days) with rosuvastatin (80 mg) resulted in a 90% and 120% increase for AUC and C_{max} of rosuvastatin, respectively. This increase is considered to be clinically significant (see PRECAUTIONS, Drug Interactions, WARNINGS, Myopathy/Rhabdomyolysis, DOSAGE AND ADMINISTRATION).

Antacid: Coadministration of an antacid (aluminum and magnesium hydroxide combination) with rosuvastatin (40 mg) resulted in a decrease in plasma concentrations of rosuvastatin by 54%. However, when the antacid was given 2 hours after rosuvastatin, there were no clinically significant changes in plasma concentrations of rosuvastatin (see PRECAUTIONS, Information for Patients).

Oral contraceptives: Coadministration of oral contraceptives (ethinyl estradiol and norgestrel) with rosuvastatin resulted in an increase in plasma concentrations of ethinyl estradiol and norgestrel by 26% and 34%, respectively.

Clinical Studies

Hypercholesterolemia (Heterozygous Familial and Nonfamilial) and Mixed Dyslipidemia (Fredrickson Type IIa and IIb)

CRESTOR reduces total-C, LDL-C, ApoB, nonHDL-C, and TG, and increases HDL-C, in patients with hypercholesterolemia and mixed dyslipidemia. Therapeutic response is seen within 1 week, and maximum response is usually achieved within 4 weeks and maintained during long-term therapy.

CRESTOR is effective in a wide variety of adult patient populations with hypercholesterolemia, with and without hypertriglyceridemia, regardless of race, gender, or age and in special populations such as diabetics or patients with heterozygous FH. Experience in pediatric patients has been limited to patients with homozygous FH.

Dose-Ranging Study: In a multicenter, double-blind, placebo-controlled, dose-ranging study in patients with hypercholesterolemia, CRESTOR given as a single daily dose for 6 weeks significantly reduced total-C, LDL-C, nonHDL-C, and ApoB, across the dose range (Table 1).

Table 1.
Dose-Response in Patients With Primary Hypercholesterolemia (Adjusted Mean % Change From Baseline at Week 6)

Dose	N	Total-C	LDL-C	HDL-C	ApoB	TG	Non HDL-C
Placebo	13	-5	-7	-7	-3	-3	3
5	17	-33	-45	-44	-38	-35	13
10	17	-36	-52	-48	-42	-10	14
20	17	-40	-55	-51	-46	-23	8
40	18	-46	-63	-60	-54	-28	10

Active-Controlled Study: CRESTOR was compared with the HMG-CoA reductase inhibitors atorvastatin, simvastatin, and pravastatin in a multicenter, open-label, dose-ranging study of 2,240 patients with Type IIa and IIb hypercholesterolemia. After randomization, patients were treated for 6 weeks with a single daily dose of either CRESTOR, atorvastatin, simvastatin, or pravastatin (Figure 1 and Table 2).

Table 3.
Mean LDL-C Percentage Change from Baseline

		CRESTOR (n=435) LS Mean* (95% CI)	Atorvastatin (n=187) LS Mean (95% CI)
Week 6	20 mg	-47% (-49%, -46%)	-38% (-40%, -36%)
Week 12	40 mg	-55% (-57%, -54%)	-47% (-49%, -45%)
Week 18	80 mg	NA	-52% (-54%, -50%)

*LS Means are least square means adjusted for baseline LDL.

Table 4.
Dose-Response in Patients With Primary Hypertriglyceridemia Over 6 Weeks
Dosing Median (Min, Max) Percent Change From Baseline

Dose	Placebo N=26	CRESTOR 5 mg N=25	CRESTOR 10 mg N=23	CRESTOR 20 mg N=27	CRESTOR 40 mg N=25
Triglycerides	1 (-40, 72)	-21 (-58, 38)	-37 (-65, 5)	-37 (-72, 11)	-43 (-80, -7)
NonHDL-C	2 (-13, 19)	-29 (-43, -8)	-49 (-59, -20)	-43 (-74, 12)	-51 (-62, -6)
VLDL-C	2 (-36, 53)	-25 (-62, 49)	-48 (-72, 14)	-49 (-83, 20)	-56 (-83, 10)
Total-C	1 (-13, 17)	-24 (-40, -4)	-40 (-51, -14)	-34 (-61, -11)	-40 (-51, -4)
LDL-C	5 (-30, 52)	-28 (-71, 2)	-45 (-59, 7)	-31 (-66, 34)	-43 (-61, -3)
HDL-C	-3 (-25, 18)	3 (-38, 33)	8 (-8, 24)	22 (-5, 50)	17 (-14, 63)

Table 5.
NCEP Treatment Guidelines: LDL-C Goals and Cutpoints for Therapeutic Lifestyle Changes and Drug Therapy in Different Risk Categories

Risk Category	LDL Goal	LDL level at which to initiate TLC	LDL level at which to consider drug therapy
CHD[a] or CHD Risk Equivalent (10-year risk > 20%)	<100 mg/dL	≥100 mg/dL	≥130 mg/dL (100-129 mg/dL: drug optional)[b]
2+ Risk Factors (10-year risk ≤ 20%)	<130 mg/dL	≥130 mg/dL	≥130 mg/dL 10-year risk 10-20% ≥160 mg/dL 10-year risk <10%
0-1 Risk Factor[c]	<160 mg/dL	≥160 mg/dL	≥190 mg/dL (160-189 mg/dL (LDL-lowering drug optional)

[a] CHD = coronary heart disease.
[b] Some authorities recommend use of LDL-lowering drugs in this category if an LDL-C <100 mg/dL cannot be achieved by TLC. Others prefer use of drugs that primarily modify triglycerides and HDL-C, e.g., nicotinic acid or fibrate. Clinical judgment also may call for deferring drug therapy in this subcategory.
[c] Almost all people with 0-1 risk factor have 10-year risk <10%; thus, 10-year risk assessment in people with 0-1 risk factor is not necessary.

Figure 1.
Percent LDL-C Change by Dose of CRESTOR, Atorvastatin, Simvastatin, and Pravastatin at Week 6 in Patients With Type IIa/IIb Dyslipidemia

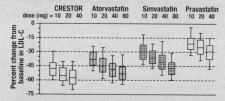

Box plots are a representation of the 25th, 50th, and 75th percentile values, with whiskers representing the 10th and 90th percentile values.
Mean baseline LDL-C: 189 mg/dL.

Table 2.
Percent Change in LDL-C From Baseline to Week 6 (LS means[§]) by Treatment Group (sample sizes ranging from 156–157 patients per group)

Treatment	Treatment Daily Dose 10 mg	20 mg	40 mg	80 mg
CRESTOR	-46*	-52[†]	-55[‡]	—
Atorvastatin	-37	-43	-48	-51
Pravastatin	-20	-24	-30	—
Simvastatin	-28	-35	-39	-46

*CRESTOR 10 mg reduced LDL-C significantly more than atorvastatin 10 mg; pravastatin 10 mg, 20 mg, and 40 mg; simvastatin 10 mg, 20 mg, and 40 mg. (p<0.002)
[†] CRESTOR 20 mg reduced LDL-C significantly more than atorvastatin 20 mg and 40 mg; pravastatin 20 mg and 40 mg; simvastatin 20 mg, 40 mg, and 80 mg. (p<0.002)
[‡] CRESTOR 40 mg reduced LDL-C significantly more than atorvastatin 40 mg; pravastatin 40 mg; simvastatin 40 mg and 80 mg. (p<0.002)
[§] Corresponding standard errors are approximately 1.00

Heterozygous Familial Hypercholesterolemia

In a study of patients with heterozygous FH (baseline mean LDL of 291), patients were randomized to CRESTOR 20 mg or atorvastatin 20 mg. The dose was increased by 6-week intervals. Significant LDL-C reductions from baseline were seen at each dose in both treatment groups (Table 3).
[See table 3 above]

Hypertriglyceridemia (Fredrickson Type IIb & IV)

In a double-blind, placebo-controlled dose-response study in patients with baseline TG levels from 273 to 817 mg/dL, CRESTOR given as a single daily dose (5 to 40 mg) over 6 weeks significantly reduced serum TG levels (Table 4).
[See table 4 above]

Homozygous Familial Hypercholesterolemia

In an open-label, forced-titration study, homozygous FH patients (n=40, 8-63 years) were evaluated for their response to CRESTOR 20 to 40 mg titrated at a 6-week interval. In the overall population, the mean LDL-C reduction from baseline was 22%. About one-third of the patients benefited from increasing their dose from 20 mg to 40 mg with further LDL lowering of greater than 6%. In the 27 patients with at least a 15% reduction in LDL-C, the mean LDL-C reduction was 30% (median 28% reduction). Among 13 patients with an LDL-C reduction of <15%, 3 had no change or an increase in LDL-C. Reductions in LDL-C of 15% or greater were observed in 3 of 5 patients with known receptor negative status.

INDICATIONS AND USAGE

CRESTOR is indicated:
1. as an adjunct to diet to reduce elevated total-C, LDL-C, ApoB, nonHDL-C, and TG levels and to increase HDL-C in patients with primary hypercholesterolemia (heterozygous familial and nonfamilial) and mixed dyslipidemia (Fredrickson Type IIa and IIb);
2. as an adjunct to diet for the treatment of patients with elevated serum TG levels (Fredrickson Type IV);
3. to reduce LDL-C, total-C, and ApoB in patients with homozygous familial hypercholesterolemia as an adjunct to other lipid-lowering treatments (e.g., LDL apheresis) or if such treatments are unavailable.

According to NCEP-ATPIII guidelines, therapy with lipid-altering agents should be a component of multiple-risk-factor intervention in individuals at increased risk for coronary heart disease due to hypercholesterolemia. The two major modalities of LDL-lowering therapy are therapeutic lifestyle changes (TLC) and drug therapy. The TLC Diet stresses reductions in saturated fat and cholesterol intake. Table 5 defines LDL-C goals and cutpoints for initiation of TLC and for drug consideration.
[See table 5 above]

After the LDL-C goal has been achieved, if the TG is still ≥ 200 mg/dL, nonHDL-C (total-C minus HDL-C) becomes a secondary target of therapy. NonHDL-C goals are set 30 mg/dL higher than LDL-C goals for each risk category. At the time of hospitalization for a coronary event, consideration can be given to initiating drug therapy at discharge if the LDL-C is ≥ 130 mg/dL (see NCEP Treatment Guidelines, above).

Continued on next page

Crestor—Cont.

Patients >20 years of age should be screened for elevated cholesterol levels every 5 years.

Prior to initiating therapy with CRESTOR, secondary causes for hypercholesterolemia (e.g., poorly-controlled diabetes mellitus, hypothyroidism, nephrotic syndrome, dyslipoproteinemias, obstructive liver disease, other drug therapy, and alcoholism) should be excluded, and a lipid profile performed to measure total-C, LDL-C, HDL-C, and TG. For patients with TG <400 mg/dL (<4.5 mmol/L), LDL-C can be estimated using the following equation: LDL-C = total-C - (0.20 × [TG] + HDL-C). For TG levels >400 mg/dL (>4.5 mmol/L), this equation is less accurate and LDL-C concentrations should be determined by ultracentrifugation.

CRESTOR has not been studied in Fredrickson Type I, III, and V dyslipidemias.

CONTRAINDICATIONS

CRESTOR is contraindicated in patients with a known hypersensitivity to any component of this product.

Rosuvastatin is contraindicated in patients with active liver disease or with unexplained persistent elevations of serum transaminases (see WARNINGS, Liver Enzymes).

Pregnancy and Lactation

Atherosclerosis is a chronic process and discontinuation of lipid-lowering drugs during pregnancy should have little impact on the outcome of long-term therapy of primary hypercholesterolemia. Cholesterol and other products of cholesterol biosynthesis are essential components for fetal development (including synthesis of steroids and cell membranes). Since HMG-CoA reductase inhibitors decrease cholesterol synthesis and possibly the synthesis of other biologically active substances derived from cholesterol, they may cause fetal harm when administered to pregnant women. Therefore, HMG-CoA reductase inhibitors are contraindicated during pregnancy and in nursing mothers. ROSUVASTATIN SHOULD BE ADMINISTERED TO WOMEN OF CHILDBEARING AGE ONLY WHEN SUCH PATIENTS ARE HIGHLY UNLIKELY TO CONCEIVE AND HAVE BEEN INFORMED OF THE POTENTIAL HAZARDS. If the patient becomes pregnant while taking this drug, therapy should be discontinued immediately and the patient apprised of the potential hazard to the fetus.

WARNINGS

Liver Enzymes

HMG-CoA reductase inhibitors, like some other lipid-lowering therapies, have been associated with biochemical abnormalities of liver function. The incidence of persistent elevations (>3 times the upper limit of normal [ULN] occurring on 2 or more consecutive occasions) in serum transaminases in fixed dose studies was 0.4, 0, 0, and 0.1% in patients who received rosuvastatin 5, 10, 20, and 40 mg, respectively. In most cases, the elevations were transient and resolved or improved on continued therapy or after a brief interruption in therapy. There were two cases of jaundice, for which a relationship to rosuvastatin therapy could not be determined, which resolved after discontinuation of therapy. There were no cases of liver failure or irreversible liver disease in these trials.

It is recommended that liver function tests be performed before and at 12 weeks following both the initiation of therapy and any elevation of dose, and periodically (e.g., semiannually) thereafter. Liver enzyme changes generally occur in the first 3 months of treatment with rosuvastatin. Patients who develop increased transaminase levels should be monitored until the abnormalities have resolved. Should an increase in ALT or AST of >3 times ULN persist, reduction of dose or withdrawal of rosuvastatin is recommended. Rosuvastatin should be used with caution in patients who consume substantial quantities of alcohol and/or have a history of liver disease (see CLINICAL PHARMACOLOGY, Special Populations, Hepatic Insufficiency). Active liver disease or unexplained persistent transaminase elevations are contraindications to the use of rosuvastatin (see CONTRAINDICATIONS).

Myopathy/Rhabdomyolysis

Rare cases of rhabdomyolysis with acute renal failure secondary to myoglobinuria have been reported with rosuvastatin and with other drugs in this class.

Uncomplicated myalgia has been reported in rosuvastatin-treated patients (see ADVERSE REACTIONS). Creatine kinase (CK) elevations (>10 times upper limit of normal) occurred in 0.2% to 0.4% of patients taking rosuvastatin at doses up to 40 mg in clinical studies. Treatment-related myopathy, defined as muscle aches or muscle weakness in conjunction with increases in CK values >10 times upper limit of normal, was reported in up to 0.1% of patients taking rosuvastatin doses of up to 40 mg in clinical studies. In clinical trials, the incidence of myopathy and rhabdomyolysis increased at doses of rosuvastatin above the recommended dosage range (5 to 40 mg). In postmarketing experience, effects on skeletal muscle, e.g. uncomplicated myalgia, myopathy and, rarely, rhabdomyolysis have been reported in patients treated with HMG-CoA reductase inhibitors including rosuvastatin. As with other HMG-CoA reductase inhibitors, reports of rhabdomyolysis with rosuvastatin are rare, but higher at the highest marketed dose (40 mg). Factors that may predispose patients to myopathy with HMG-CoA reductase inhibitors include advanced age (≥65 years), hypothyroidism, and renal insufficiency.

Consequently:

1. Rosuvastatin should be prescribed with caution in patients with predisposing factors for myopathy, such as, re-

nal impairment (see DOSAGE AND ADMINISTRATION), advanced age, and inadequately treated hypothyroidism.

2. Patients should be advised to promptly report unexplained muscle pain, tenderness, or weakness, particularly if accompanied by malaise or fever. Rosuvastatin therapy should be discontinued if markedly elevated CK levels occur or myopathy is diagnosed or suspected.

3. The 40 mg dose of rosuvastatin is reserved only for those patients who have not achieved their LDL-C goal utilizing the 20 mg dose of rosuvastatin once daily (see DOSAGE AND ADMINISTRATION).

4. The risk of myopathy during treatment with rosuvastatin may be increased with concurrent administration of other lipid-lowering therapies or cyclosporine, (see CLINICAL PHARMACOLOGY, Drug Interactions, PRECAUTIONS, Drug Interactions, and DOSAGE AND ADMINISTRATION). **The benefit of further alterations in lipid levels by the combined use of rosuvastatin with fibrates or niacin should be carefully weighed against the potential risks of this combination. Combination therapy with rosuvastatin and gemfibrozil should generally be avoided. (See DOSAGE AND ADMINISTRATION and PRECAUTIONS, Drug Interactions).**

5. **The risk of myopathy during treatment with rosuvastatin may be increased in circumstances which increase rosuvastatin drug levels (see CLINICAL PHARMACOLOGY, Special Populations, Race and Renal Insufficiency, and PRECAUTIONS, General).**

6. **Rosuvastatin therapy should also be temporarily withheld in any patient with an acute, serious condition suggestive of myopathy or predisposing to the development of renal failure secondary to rhabdomyolysis (e.g., sepsis, hypotension, major surgery, trauma, severe metabolic, endocrine, and electrolyte disorders, or uncontrolled seizures).**

PRECAUTIONS

General

Before instituting therapy with rosuvastatin, an attempt should be made to control hypercholesterolemia with appropriate diet and exercise, weight reduction in obese patients, and treatment of underlying medical problems (see INDICATIONS AND USAGE).

Administration of rosuvastatin 20 mg to patients with severe renal impairment (CL_{cr} <30 mL/min/1.73 m^2) resulted in a 3-fold increase in plasma concentrations of rosuvastatin compared with healthy volunteers (see WARNINGS, Myopathy/Rhabdomyolysis and DOSAGE AND ADMINISTRATION).

The result of a large pharmacokinetic study conducted in the US demonstrated an approximate 2-fold elevation in median exposure in Asian subjects (having either Filipino, Chinese, Japanese, Korean, Vietnamese or Asian-Indian origin) compared with a Caucasian control group. This increase should be considered when making rosuvastatin dosing decisions for Asian patients (see WARNINGS Myopathy/Rhabdomyolysis; CLINICAL PHARMACOLOGY, Special Populations, Race, and DOSAGE AND ADMINISTRATION).

Information for Patients

Patients should be advised to report promptly unexplained muscle pain, tenderness, or weakness, particularly if accompanied by malaise or fever.

When taking rosuvastatin with an aluminum and magnesium hydroxide combination antacid, the antacid should be taken at least 2 hours after rosuvastatin administration (see CLINICAL PHARMACOLOGY, Drug Interactions).

Laboratory Tests

In the rosuvastatin clinical trial program, dipstick-positive proteinuria and microscopic hematuria were observed among rosuvastatin treated patients, predominantly in patients dosed above the recommended dose range (i.e., 80 mg). However, this finding was more frequent in patients taking rosuvastatin 40 mg, when compared to lower doses of rosuvastatin or comparator statins, though it was generally transient and was not associated with worsening renal function. Although the clinical significance of this finding is unknown, a dose reduction should be considered for patients on rosuvastatin 40 mg therapy with unexplained persistent proteinuria during routine urinalysis testing.

Drug Interactions

Cyclosporine: When rosuvastatin 10 mg was coadministered with cyclosporine in cardiac transplant patients, rosuvastatin mean C_{max} and mean AUC were increased 11-fold and 7-fold, respectively, compared with healthy volunteers. These increases are considered to be clinically significant and require special consideration in the dosing of rosuvastatin to patients taking concomitant cyclosporine (see WARNINGS, Myopathy/Rhabdomyolysis, and DOSAGE AND ADMINISTRATION).

Warfarin: Coadministration of rosuvastatin to patients on stable warfarin therapy resulted in clinically significant rises in INR (>4, baseline 2-3). In patients taking coumarin anticoagulants and rosuvastatin concomitantly, INR should be determined before starting rosuvastatin and frequently enough during early therapy to ensure that no significant alteration of INR occurs. Once a stable INR time has been documented, INR can be monitored at the intervals usually recommended for patients on coumarin anticoagulants. If the dose of rosuvastatin is changed, the same procedure should be repeated. Rosuvastatin therapy has not been associated with bleeding or with changes in INR in patients not taking anticoagulants.

Gemfibrozil: Coadministration of a single rosuvastatin dose to healthy volunteers on gemfibrozil (600 mg twice daily) resulted in 2.2- and 1.9-fold, respectively, increase in mean C_{max} and mean AUC of rosuvastatin (see DOSAGE AND ADMINISTRATION).

Endocrine Function

Although clinical studies have shown that rosuvastatin alone does not reduce basal plasma cortisol concentration or impair adrenal reserve, caution should be exercised if any HMG-CoA reductase inhibitor or other agent used to lower cholesterol levels is administered concomitantly with drugs that may decrease the levels or activity of endogenous steroid hormones such as ketoconazole, spironolactone, and cimetidine.

CNS Toxicity

CNS vascular lesions, characterized by perivascular hemorrhages, edema, and mononuclear cell infiltration of perivascular spaces, have been observed in dogs treated with several other members of this drug class. A chemically similar drug in this class produced dose-dependent optic nerve degeneration (Wallerian degeneration of retinogeniculate fibers) in dogs, at a dose that produced plasma drug levels about 30 times higher than the mean drug level in humans taking the highest recommended dose. Edema, hemorrhage, and partial necrosis in the interstitium of the choroid plexus was observed in a female dog sacrificed moribund at day 24 at 90 mg/kg/day by oral gavage (systemic exposures 100 times the human exposure at 40 mg/day based on AUC comparisons). Corneal opacity was seen in dogs treated for 52 weeks at 6 mg/kg/day by oral gavage (systemic exposures 20 times the human exposure at 40 mg/day based on AUC comparisons). Cataracts were seen in dogs treated for 12 weeks by oral gavage at 30 mg/kg/day (systemic exposures 60 times the human exposure at 40 mg/day based on AUC comparisons). Retinal dysplasia and retinal loss were seen in dogs treated for 4 weeks by oral gavage at 90 mg/kg/day (systemic exposures 100 times the human exposure at 40 mg/day based on AUC). Doses ≤30 mg/kg/day (systemic exposures ≤60 times the human exposure at 40 mg/day based on AUC comparisons) following treatment up to one year, did not reveal retinal findings.

Carcinogenesis, Mutagenesis, Impairment of Fertility

In a 104-week carcinogenicity study in rats at dose levels of 2, 20, 60, or 80 mg/kg/day by oral gavage, the incidence of uterine stromal polyps was significantly increased in females at 80 mg/kg/day at systemic exposure 20 times the human exposure at 40 mg/day based on AUC. Increased incidence of polyps was not seen at lower doses.

In a 107-week carcinogenicity study in mice given 10, 60, 200 mg/kg/day by oral gavage, an increased incidence of hepatocellular adenoma/carcinoma was observed at 200 mg/kg/day at systemic exposures 20 times human exposure at 40 mg/day based on AUC. An increased incidence of hepatocellular tumors was not seen at lower doses.

Rosuvastatin was not mutagenic or clastogenic with or without metabolic activation in the Ames test with *Salmonella typhimurium* and *Escherichia coli*, the mouse lymphoma assay, and the chromosomal aberration assay in Chinese hamster lung cells. Rosuvastatin was negative in the *in vivo* mouse micronucleus test.

In rat fertility studies with oral gavage doses of 5, 15, 50 mg/kg/day, males were treated for 9 weeks prior to and throughout mating and females were treated 2 weeks prior to mating and throughout mating until gestation day 7. No adverse effect on fertility was observed at 50 mg/kg/day (systemic exposures up to 10 times human exposure at 40 mg/day based on AUC comparisons). In testicles of dogs treated with rosuvastatin at 30 mg/kg/day for one month, spermatidic giant cells were seen. Spermatidic giant cells were observed in monkeys after 6-month treatment at 30 mg/kg/day in addition to vacuolation of seminiferous tubular epithelium. Exposures in the dog were 20 times and in the monkey 10 times human exposure at 40 mg/day based on body surface area comparisons. Similar findings have been seen with other drugs in this class.

Pregnancy

Pregnancy Category X

See CONTRAINDICATIONS.

Rosuvastatin may cause fetal harm when administered to a pregnant woman. Rosuvastatin is contraindicated in women who are or may become pregnant. Safety in pregnant women has not been established. There are no adequate and well-controlled studies of rosuvastatin in pregnant women. Rosuvastatin crosses the placenta and is found in fetal tissue and amniotic fluid at 3% and 20%, respectively, of the maternal plasma concentration following a single 25 mg/kg oral gavage dose on gestation day 16 in rats. A higher fetal tissue distribution (25% maternal plasma concentration) was observed in rabbits after a single oral gavage dose of 1 mg/kg on gestation day 18. If this drug is administered to a woman with reproductive potential, the patient should be apprised of the potential hazard to a fetus.

In female rats given oral gavage doses of 5, 15, 50 mg/kg/day rosuvastatin before mating and continuing through day 7 postcoitus results in decreased fetal body weight (female pups) and delayed ossification at the high dose (systemic exposures 10 times human exposure at 40 mg/day based on AUC comparisons).

In pregnant rats given oral gavage doses of 2, 10, 50 mg/kg/day from gestation day 7 through lactation day 21 (weaning), decreased pup survival occurred in groups given 50 mg/kg/day, systemic exposures ≥12 times human exposure at 40 mg/day based on body surface area comparisons.

In pregnant rabbits given oral gavage doses of 0.3, 1, 3 mg/kg/day from gestation day 6 to lactation day 18 (weaning),

exposures equivalent to human exposure at 40 mg/day based on body surface area comparisons, decreased fetal viability and maternal mortality was observed.
Rosuvastatin was not teratogenic in rats at ≤25 mg/kg/day or in rabbits ≤3 mg/kg/day (systemic exposures equivalent to human exposure at 40 mg/day based on AUC or body surface comparison, respectively).

Nursing Mothers
It is not known whether rosuvastatin is excreted in human milk. Studies in lactating rats have demonstrated that rosuvastatin is secreted into breast milk at levels 3 times higher than that obtained in the plasma following oral gavage dosing. Because many drugs are excreted in human milk and because of the potential for serious adverse reactions in nursing infants from rosuvastatin, a decision should be made whether to discontinue nursing or administration of rosuvastatin taking into account the importance of the drug to the lactating woman.

Pediatric Use
The safety and effectiveness in pediatric patients have not been established. Treatment experience with rosuvastatin in a pediatric population is limited to 8 patients with homozygous FH. None of these patients was below 8 years of age.

Geriatric Use
Of the 10,275 patients in clinical studies with rosuvastatin, 3,159 (31%) were 65 years and older, and 698 (6.8%) were 75 years and older. The overall frequency of adverse events and types of adverse events were similar in patients above and below 65 years of age. (See WARNINGS, Myopathy/Rhabdomyolysis.)
The efficacy of rosuvastatin in the geriatric population (≥65 years of age) was comparable to the efficacy observed in the non-elderly.

ADVERSE REACTIONS

Rosuvastatin is generally well tolerated. Adverse reactions have usually been mild and transient. In clinical studies of 10,275 patients, 3.7% were discontinued due to adverse experiences attributable to rosuvastatin. The most frequent adverse events thought to be related to rosuvastatin were myalgia, constipation, asthenia, abdominal pain, and nausea.

Clinical Adverse Experiences
Adverse experiences, regardless of causality assessment, reported in ≥2% of patients in placebo-controlled clinical studies of rosuvastatin are shown in Table 6; discontinuations due to adverse events in these studies of up to 12 weeks duration occurred in 3% of patients on rosuvastatin and 5% on placebo.

Table 6. Adverse Events in Placebo-Controlled Studies

Adverse Event	Rosuvastatin N=744	Placebo N=382
Pharyngitis	9.0	7.6
Headache	5.5	5.0
Diarrhea	3.4	2.9
Dyspepsia	3.4	3.1
Nausea	3.4	3.1
Myalgia	2.8	1.3
Asthenia	2.7	2.6
Back Pain	2.6	2.4
Flu syndrome	2.3	1.8
Urinary tract infection	2.3	1.6
Rhinitis	2.2	2.1
Sinusitis	2.0	1.8

In addition, the following adverse events were reported, regardless of causality assessment, in ≥1% of 10,275 patients treated with rosuvastatin in clinical studies. The events in *italics* occurred in ≥2% of these patients.
Body as a Whole: *Abdominal pain, accidental injury, chest pain, infection, pain*, pelvic pain, and neck pain.
Cardiovascular System: *Hypertension*, angina pectoris, vasodilatation, and palpitation.
Digestive System: *Constipation, gastroenteritis*, vomiting, flatulence, periodontal abscess, and gastritis.
Endocrine: Diabetes mellitus.
Hemic and Lymphatic System: Anemia and ecchymosis.
Metabolic and Nutritional Disorders: *Peripheral edema*.
Musculoskeletal System: *Arthritis, arthralgia*, and pathological fracture.
Nervous System: *Dizziness, insomnia, hypertonia, paresthesia, depression*, anxiety, vertigo and neuralgia.
Respiratory System: *Bronchitis, cough increased*, dyspnea, pneumonia, and asthma.
Skin and Appendages: *Rash* and pruritus.
Laboratory Abnormalities: In the rosuvastatin clinical trial program, dipstick-positive proteinuria and microscopic hematuria were observed among rosuvastatin-treated patients, predominantly in patients dosed above the recommended dose range (i.e., 80 mg). However, this finding was more frequent in patients taking rosuvastatin 40 mg, when compared to lower doses of rosuvastatin or comparator statins, though it was generally transient and was not associated with worsening renal function. (See PRECAUTIONS, Laboratory Tests.)
Other abnormal laboratory values reported were elevated creatine phosphokinase, transaminases, hyperglycemia, glutamyl transpeptidase, alkaline phosphatase, bilirubin, and thyroid function abnormalities.
Other adverse events reported less frequently than 1% in the rosuvastatin clinical study program, regardless of causality assessment, included arrhythmia, hepatitis, hypersensitivity reactions (i.e., face edema, thrombocytopenia, leukopenia, vesiculobullous rash, urticaria, and angioedema), kidney failure, syncope, myasthenia, myositis, pancreatitis, photosensitivity reaction, myopathy, and rhabdomyolysis.

Postmarketing Experience
In addition to the events reported above, as with other drugs in this class, the following event has been reported during postmarketing experience with CRESTOR, regardless of causality assessment: very rare cases of jaundice.

OVERDOSAGE

There is no specific treatment in the event of overdose. In the event of overdose, the patient should be treated symptomatically and supportive measures instituted as required. Hemodialysis does not significantly enhance clearance of rosuvastatin.

DOSAGE AND ADMINISTRATION

The patient should be placed on a standard cholesterol-lowering diet before receiving CRESTOR and should continue on this diet during treatment. CRESTOR can be administered as a single dose at any time of day, with or without food.

Hypercholesterolemia (Heterozygous Familial and Nonfamilial) and Mixed Dyslipidemia (Fredrickson Type IIa and IIb)
The dose range for CRESTOR is 5 to 40 mg once daily. Therapy with CRESTOR should be individualized according to goal of therapy and response. The usual recommended starting dose of CRESTOR is 10 mg once daily. However, initiation of therapy with 5 mg once daily should be considered for patients requiring less aggressive LDL-C reductions, who have predisposing factors for myopathy, and as noted below for special populations such as patients taking cyclosporine, Asian patients, and patients with severe renal insufficiency (see CLINICAL PHARMACOLOGY, Race, and Renal Insufficiency, and Drug Interactions). For patients with marked hypercholesterolemia (LDL-C > 190 mg/dL) and aggressive lipid targets, a 20-mg starting dose may be considered. After initiation and/or upon titration of CRESTOR, lipid levels should be analyzed within 2 to 4 weeks and dosage adjusted accordingly.
The 40-mg dose of CRESTOR is reserved only for those patients who have not achieved their LDL-C goal utilizing the 20 mg dose of CRESTOR once daily (see WARNINGS, Myopathy/Rhabdomyolysis). When initiating statin therapy or switching from another statin therapy, the appropriate CRESTOR starting dose should first be utilized, and only then titrated according to the patient's individualized goal of therapy.

Homozygous Familial Hypercholesterolemia
The recommended starting dose of CRESTOR is 20 mg once daily in patients with homozygous FH. The maximum recommended daily dose is 40 mg. CRESTOR should be used in these patients as an adjunct to other lipid-lowering treatments (e.g., LDL apheresis) or if such treatments are unavailable. Response to therapy should be estimated from pre-apheresis LDL-C levels.

Dosage in Asian Patients
Initiation of CRESTOR therapy with 5 mg once daily should be considered for Asian patients. The potential for increased systemic exposures relative to Caucasians is relevant when considering escalation of dose in cases where hypercholesterolemia is not adequately controlled at doses of 5, 10, or 20 mg once daily (see WARNINGS, Myopathy/Rhabdomyolysis, CLINICAL PHARMACOLOGY, Special Populations, Race, and PRECAUTIONS, General).

Dosage in Patients Taking Cyclosporine
In patients taking cyclosporine, therapy should be limited to CRESTOR 5 mg once daily (see WARNINGS Myopathy/Rhabdomyolysis, and PRECAUTIONS, Drug Interactions).

Concomitant Lipid-Lowering Therapy
The effect of CRESTOR on LDL-C and total-C may be enhanced when used in combination with a bile acid binding resin. If CRESTOR is used in combination with gemfibrozil, the dose of CRESTOR should be limited to 10 mg once daily (see WARNINGS, Myopathy/Rhabdomyolysis, and PRECAUTIONS, Drug Interactions).

Dosage in Patients With Renal Insufficiency
No modification of dosage is necessary for patients with mild to moderate renal insufficiency. For patients with severe renal impairment (CL_{cr} <30 mL/min/1.73 m^2) not on hemodialysis, dosing of CRESTOR should be started at 5 mg once daily and not to exceed 10 mg once daily (see PRECAUTIONS, General, and CLINICAL PHARMACOLOGY, Special Populations, Renal Insufficiency).

HOW SUPPLIED

CRESTOR® (rosuvastatin calcium) Tablets are supplied as:
5 mg tablets: Yellow, round, biconvex, coated tablets identified as "CRESTOR" and "5" debossed on one side and plain on the other side of the tablet.
(NDC 0310-0755-90) bottles of 90
10 mg tablets: Pink, round, biconvex, coated tablets identified as "CRESTOR" and "10" debossed on one side and plain on the other side of the tablet.
(NDC 0310-0751-90) bottles of 90
(NDC 0310-0751-39) unit dose packages of 100
20 mg tablets: Pink, round, biconvex, coated tablets identified as "CRESTOR" and "20" debossed on one side and plain on the other side of the tablet.
(NDC 0310-0752-90) bottles of 90
(NDC 0310-0752-39) unit dose packages of 100
40 mg tablets: Pink, oval, biconvex, coated tablets identified as "CRESTOR" debossed on one side and "40" debossed on the other side of the tablet.
(NDC 0310-0754-30) bottles of 30
(NDC 0310-0754-39) unit dose packages of 100

Storage
Store at controlled room temperature, 20–25°C (68–77°F) [see USP]. Protect from moisture.

Rx only
CRESTOR is a trademark of the AstraZeneca group of companies.
© AstraZeneca 2003, 2005
Licensed from SHIONOGI & CO., LTD., Osaka, Japan
Manufactured for:
AstraZeneca Pharmaceuticals LP
Wilmington, DE 19850
By: IPR Pharmaceuticals, Inc.
Carolina, PR 00984
630301
Rev. 03/05 **AstraZeneca**

DIPRIVAN® ℞
[*dĭ′prĭ-văn*]
(propofol) INJECTABLE EMULSION

Prescribing information for this product, which appears on pages 647–653 of the 2004 PDR, has been revised as follows. Please write "See Supplement A" next to the product heading.

Delete the following paragraph from the PRECAUTIONS, Intensive Care Unit Sedation, Adult Patients section of the PI and replace with a new paragraph.
Delete: "There have been very rare reports of rhabdomyolysis associated with the administration of DIPRIVAN Injectable Emulsion for ICU sedation."
Replace with: "Very rare reports of metabolic acidosis, rhabdomyolysis, hyperklalemia, and/or cardiac failure, in some cases with a fatal outcome, have been received concerning seriously ill patients receiving DIPRIVAN for ICU sedation. These reports demonstrated that a failure of oxygen delivery to the tissues was likely to have occurred. A causal relationship between these reported events and DIPRIVAN has not been established. All sedative and therapeutic agents used in the ICU (including DIPRIVAN) should be titrated to maintain optimal oxygen delivery and hemodynamic parameters."
SIC 64180-03
Rev 07/04

FASLODEX® ℞
[*făs′lō-dĕks*]
(fulvestrant) INJECTION

Prescribing information for this product, which appears on pages 653–658 of the 2005 PDR, has been completely revised as follows. Please write "See Supplement A" next to the product heading.

DESCRIPTION

FASLODEX® (fulvestrant) Injection for intramuscular administration is an estrogen receptor antagonist without known agonist effects. The chemical name is 7-alpha-[9-(4,4,5,5,5-penta fluoropentylsulphinyl) nonyl]estra-1,3,5-(10)- triene-3,17-beta-diol. The molecular formula is $C_{32}H_{47}F_5O_3S$ and its structural formula is:

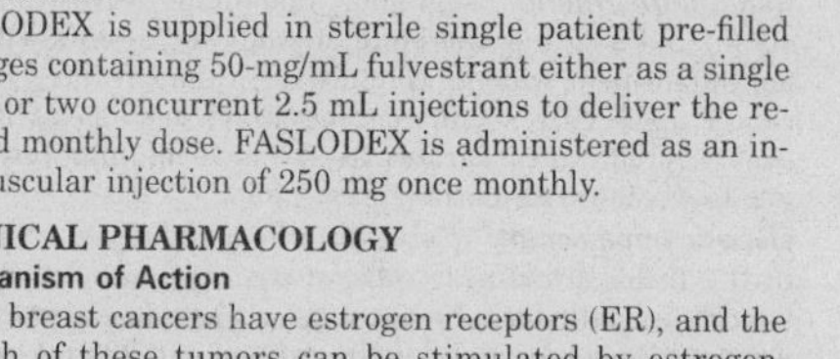

Fulvestrant is a white powder with a molecular weight of 606.77. The solution for injection is a clear, colorless to yellow, viscous liquid.
Each injection contains as inactive ingredients: Alcohol, USP, Benzyl Alcohol, NF, and Benzyl Benzoate, USP, as co-solvents, and Castor Oil, USP as a co-solvent and release rate modifier.
FASLODEX is supplied in sterile single patient pre-filled syringes containing 50-mg/mL fulvestrant either as a single 5 mL or two concurrent 2.5 mL injections to deliver the required monthly dose. FASLODEX is administered as an intramuscular injection of 250 mg once monthly.

CLINICAL PHARMACOLOGY

Mechanism of Action
Many breast cancers have estrogen receptors (ER), and the growth of these tumors can be stimulated by estrogen. Fulvestrant is an estrogen receptor antagonist that binds to the estrogen receptor in a competitive manner with affinity comparable to that of estradiol. Fulvestrant downregulates the ER protein in human breast cancer cells.
In a clinical study in postmenopausal women with primary breast cancer treated with single doses of FASLODEX 15-22 days prior to surgery, there was evidence of increasing down regulation of ER with increasing dose. This was associated with a dose-related decrease in the expression of the progesterone receptor, an estrogen-regulated protein. These effects on the ER pathway were also associated with a decrease in Ki67 labeling index, a marker of cell proliferation.
In vitro studies demonstrated that fulvestrant is a reversible inhibitor of the growth of tamoxifen-resistant, as well

Continued on next page

Faslodex—Cont.

as estrogen-sensitive human breast cancer (MCF-7) cell lines. In *in vivo* tumor studies, fulvestrant delayed the establishment of tumors from xenografts of human breast cancer MCF-7 cells in nude mice. Fulvestrant inhibited the growth of established MCF-7 xenografts and of tamoxifen-resistant breast tumor xenografts. Fulvestrant resistant breast tumor xenografts may also be cross-resistant to tamoxifen.

Fulvestrant showed no agonist-type effects in *in vivo* uterotropic assays in immature or ovariectomized mice and rats. In *in vivo* studies in immature rats and ovariectomized monkeys, fulvestrant blocked the uterotrophic action of estradiol. In postmenopausal women, the absence of changes in plasma concentrations of FSH and LH in response to fulvestrant treatment (250 mg monthly) suggests no peripheral steroidal effects.

Pharmacokinetics

Following intravenous administration, fulvestrant is rapidly cleared at a rate approximating hepatic blood flow (about 10.5 mL plasma/min/Kg). After an intramuscular injection plasma concentrations are maximal at about 7 days and are maintained over a period of at least one month, with trough concentration about one-third of C_{max}. The apparent half-life was about 40 days. After administration of 250 mg of fulvestrant intramuscularly every month, plasma levels approach steady-state after 3 to 6 doses, with an average 2.5 fold increase in plasma AUC, compared to single dose AUC and trough levels about equal to the single dose C_{max} (see **Table 1**).

[See table 1 at right]

Table 1: Summary of fulvestrant pharmacokinetic parameters in postmenopausal advanced breast cancer patients after intramuscular administration of a 250 mg dose (Mean ± SD)

	C_{max} ng/mL	C_{min} ng/mL	AUC ng.d/mL	t½ days	CL mL/min
Single dose	8.5 ± 5.4	2.6 ± 1.1	131 ± 62	40 ± 11	690 ± 226
Multiple dose steady state	15.8 ± 2.4	7.4 ± 1.7	328 ± 48		

Fulvestrant was subject to extensive and rapid distribution. The apparent volume of distribution at steady state was approximately 3 to 5 L/kg. This suggests that distribution is largely extravascular. Fulvestrant was highly (99%) bound to plasma proteins; VLDL, LDL and HDL lipoprotein fractions appear to be the major binding components. The role of sex hormone-binding globulin, if any, could not be determined.

Metabolism and Excretion:

Biotransformation and disposition of fulvestrant in humans have been determined following intramuscular and intravenous administration of ^{14}C-labeled fulvestrant. Metabolism of fulvestrant appears to involve combinations of a number of possible biotransformation pathways analogous to those of endogenous steroids, including oxidation, aromatic hydroxylation, conjugation with glucuronic acid and/or sulphate at the 2, 3 and 17 positions of the steroid nucleus, and oxidation of the side chain sulphoxide. Identified metabolites are either less active or exhibit similar activity to fulvestrant in antiestrogen models. Studies using human liver preparations and recombinant human enzymes indicate that cytochrome P-450 3A4 (CYP 3A4) is the only P-450 isoenzyme involved in the oxidation of fulvestrant; however, the relative contribution of P-450 and non-P-450 routes *in vivo* is unknown.

Fulvestrant was rapidly cleared by the hepatobiliary route, with excretion primarily via the feces (approximately 90%). Renal elimination was negligible (less than 1%).

Special Populations:

Geriatric: In patients with breast cancer, there was no difference in fulvestrant pharmacokinetic profile related to age (range 33 to 89 years).

Gender: Following administration of a single intravenous dose, there were no pharmacokinetic differences between men and women or between premenopausal and postmenopausal women. Similarly, there were no differences between men and postmenopausal women after intramuscular administration.

Race: In the advanced breast cancer treatment trials, the potential for pharmacokinetic differences due to race have been evaluated in 294 women including 87.4% Caucasian, 7.8% Black, and 4.4% Hispanic. No differences in fulvestrant plasma pharmacokinetics were observed among these groups. In a separate trial, pharmacokinetic data from postmenopausal ethnic Japanese women were similar to those obtained in non-Japanese patients.

Renal Impairment: Negligible amounts of fulvestrant are eliminated in urine; therefore, a study in patients with renal impairment was not conducted. In the advanced breast cancer trials, fulvestrant concentrations in women with estimated creatinine clearance as low as 30 mL/min were similar to women with normal creatinine.

Hepatic Impairment: Fulvestrant is metabolized primarily in the liver. In clinical trials in patients with locally advanced or metastatic breast cancer, pharmacokinetic data were obtained following administration of a 250 mg dose of FASLODEX to 261 patients classified as having normal liver function and to 24 patients with mild impairment. Mild impairment was defined as an alanine aminotransferase concentration (at any visit) greater than the upper limit of the normal (ULN) reference range, but less than 2 times the ULN; or if any 2 of the following 3 parameters were between 1- and 2-times the ULN: aspartate aminotransferase, alkaline phosphatase, or total bilirubin.

There was no clear relationship between fulvestrant clearance and hepatic impairment and the safety profile in patients with mild hepatic impairment was similar to that seen in patients with no hepatic impairment. Safety and efficacy have not been evaluated in patients with moderate to severe hepatic impairment (see **PRECAUTIONS-Hepatic Impairment** and **DOSAGE AND ADMINISTRATION-Hepatic Impairment** sections).

Table 2: Study Population Demographics

Parameter	North American Trial FASLODEX 250 mg	North American Trial Anastrozole 1 mg	European Trial FASLODEX 250 mg	European Trial Anastrozole 1 mg
No. of Participants	206	194	222	229
Median Age (yrs)	64	61	64	65
Age Range (yrs)	33–89	36–94	35–86	33–89
Receptor Status # (%)				
ER Positive	170 (83%)	156 (80%)	156 (70%)	173 (76%)
ER/PgR Positive	179 (87%)	169 (87%)	163 (73%)	183 (80%)
ER/PgR Unknown	13 (6%)	15 (8%)	51 (23%)	37 (16%)
Previous Therapy				
Tamoxifen	196 (95%)	187 (96%)	215 (97%)	225 (98%)
Adjuvant antiestrogen only	94 (46%)	94 (48%)	95 (43%)	100 (44%)
Antiestrogen for advanced disease +/- adjuvant use	110 (53%)	97 (50%)	126 (57%)	129 (56%)
Cytotoxic Chemotherapy	129 (63%)	122 (63%)	94 (42%)	98 (43%)
Site of Metastases				
Visceral only*	39 (19%)	45 (23%)	30 (14%)	41 (18%)
Visceral Liver involvement	47 (23%)	45 (23%)	48 (22%)	56 (24%)
Visceral Lung involvement	63 (31%)	60 (31%)	56 (25%)	60 (26%)
Bone only	47 (23%)	43 (22%)	38 (17%)	40 (17%)
Soft Tissue only	12 (6%)	13 (7%)	11 (5%)	8 (3%)
Skin and soft tissue	43 (21%)	41 (21%)	40 (18%)	35 (15%)

*Defined as liver or lung metastatic, or recurrent, disease
ER/PgR Positive defined as ER positive or PgR positive
ER/PgR Unknown defined as ER unknown and PgR unknown

Table 3: Efficacy Results

Endpoint	North American Trial FASLODEX 250 mg (n=206)	North American Trial Anastrozole 1 mg (n=194)	European Trial FASLODEX 250 mg (n=222)	European Trial Anastrozole 1 mg (n=229)
Objective tumor response				
Number (%) of subjects with CR + PR	35 (17.0)	33 (17.0)	45 (20.3)	34 (14.9)
% Difference in Tumor Response Rate (FAS-ANA)	0.0		5.4	
2-sided 95.4% CI	(-6.3, 8.9)		(-1.4, 14.8)	
Time to progression (TTP)				
Median TTP (days)	165	103	166	156
Hazard ratio (FAS/ANA)	0.9		1.0	
2-sided 95.4% CI	(0.7, 1.1)		(0.8, 1.2)	
Stable Disease for ≥24 weeks (%)	26.7	19.1	24.3	30.1
Survival Time				
Died n (%)	152 (73.8%)	149 (76.8%)	167 (75.2%)	173 (75.5%)
Median Survival (days)	844	913	803	736
Hazard ratio	0.98		0.97	
2-sided 95% CI	(0.78, 1.24)		(0.78, 1.21)	

CR = Complete Response; PR = Partial Response; CI = Confidence Interval; FAS = FASLODEX; ANA = anastrazole

Pediatric: The pharmacokinetics of fulvestrant have not been evaluated in pediatric patients.

Drug-Drug Interactions

There are no known drug-drug interactions. Fulvestrant does not significantly inhibit any of the major CYP isoenzymes, including CYP 1A2, 2C9, 2C19, 2D6, and 3A4 *in vitro*, and studies of co-administration of fulvestrant with midazolam indicate that therapeutic doses of fulvestrant have no inhibitory effects on CYP 3A4 or alter blood levels of drug metabolized by that enzyme. Although fulvestrant is partly metabolized by CYP 3A4, a clinical study with rifampin, an inducer of CYP 3A4, showed no effect on the pharmacokinetics of fulvestrant. Also results from a healthy volunteer study with ketoconazole, a potent inhibitor of CYP 3A4, indicated that ketoconazole had no effect on the pharmacokinetics of fulvestrant and dosage adjustment is not necessary in patients co-prescribed CYP 3A4 inhibitors or inducers.

Clinical Studies

Efficacy of FASLODEX was established by comparison to the selective aromatase inhibitor anastrozole in two randomized, controlled clinical trials (one conducted in North America, the other in predominately Europe) in postmenopausal women with locally advanced or metastatic breast cancer. All patients had progressed after previous therapy with an antiestrogen or progestin for breast cancer in the adjuvant or advanced disease setting. The majority of patients in these trials had ER+ and/or PgR+ tumors. Patients who had ER-/PgR- or unknown disease must have shown prior response to endocrine therapy.

In both trials, eligible patients with measurable and/or evaluable disease were randomized to receive either FASLODEX 250 mg intramuscularly once a month (28 days ± 3 days) or anastrozole 1 mg orally once a day. All patients were assessed monthly for the first three months and every three months thereafter. The North American trial was a double-blind, randomized trial in 400 postmenopausal women. The European trial was an open, randomized trial conducted in 451 patients. Patients on the FASLODEX arm of the North American trial received two separate injections (2 x 2.5 mL), whereas FASLODEX patients received a single injection (1 x 5 mL) in the European trial. In both trials, patients were initially randomized to a 125 mg per month dose as well, but interim analysis showed a very low response rate and low dose groups were dropped.

The effectiveness endpoints were response rates (RR), based on the Union Internationale Contre le Cancer (UICC) criteria, and time to progression (TTP). Survival time was also determined. Confidence intervals (95.4%) were calculated for the difference in RR between the FASLODEX and anastrozole groups. The hazard ratio for an unfavorable event, (such as disease progression or death) between FASLODEX and anastrozole groups was also determined.

Table 2 provides the demographics and baseline characteristics of the postmenopausal women randomized to FASLODEX 250 mg or anastrozole 1 mg.

[See table 2 above]

Results of the trials, after a minimum follow-up duration of 14.6 months, are summarized in Table 3. The effectiveness of FASLODEX 250 mg was determined by comparing RR and TTP results to anastrozole 1 mg, the active control. With respect to response rate, the two studies ruled out (by one-sided 97.7% confidence limit) inferiority of FASLODEX to anastrozole of 6.3% and 1.4%. There was no statistically significant difference in the survival time between the two treatment groups.

[See table 3 above]

There no efficacy data for the use of FASLODEX in premenopausal women with advanced breast cancer (women with functioning ovaries as evidenced by menstruation and/or premenopausal LH, FSH and estradiol levels).

INDICATIONS AND USAGE

FASLODEX is indicated for the treatment of hormone receptor positive metastatic breast cancer in postmenopausal women with disease progression following antiestrogen therapy.

CONTRAINDICATIONS

FASLODEX is contraindicated in pregnant women, and in patients with a known hypersensitivity to the drug or to any of its components.

WARNINGS

Women of childbearing potential should be advised not to become pregnant while receiving FASLODEX. FASLODEX can cause fetal harm when administered to a pregnant woman and has been shown to cross the placenta following single intramuscular doses in rats and in rabbits. In studies in the pregnant rat, intramuscular doses of fulvestrant 100 times lower than the maximum recommended human dose (based on body surface area [BSA]), caused an increased incidence of fetal abnormalities and death. Similarly, rabbits failed to maintain pregnancy and the fetuses showed an increased incidence of skeletal variations when fulvestrant was administered at one-half the recommended human dose (based on BSA).

There are no studies in pregnant women using FASLODEX. If FASLODEX is used during pregnancy or if the patient becomes pregnant while receiving this drug, the patient should be apprised of the potential hazard to the fetus, or potential risk for loss of the pregnancy. See **Pregnancy** section of **PRECAUTIONS**.

Because FASLODEX is administered intramuscularly, it should not be used in patients with bleeding diatheses, thrombocytopenia or in patients on anticoagulants.

PRECAUTIONS

General

Before starting treatment with FASLODEX, pregnancy must be excluded (see **WARNINGS**).

Hepatic Impairment

Safety and efficacy have not been evaluated in patients with moderate to severe hepatic impairment (see **CLINICAL PHARMACOLOGY-Hepatic Impairment** and **DOSAGE AND ADMINISTRATION-Hepatic Impairment** sections).

Drug Interactions

There are no known drug-drug interactions. Although, fulvestrant is metabolized by CYP 3A4 *in vitro*, drug interactions studies with ketoconazole or rifampin did not alter fulvestrant pharmacokinetics. Dose adjustment is not needed in patients co-prescribed CYP3A4 inhibitors or inducers (see **CLINICAL PHARMACOLOGY-Drug-Drug Interactions**).

Carcinogenesis, Mutagenesis and Impairment of Fertility

A two-year carcinogenesis study was conducted in female and male rats, at intramuscular doses of 15 mg/kg/30 days, 10 mg/rat/30 days and 10 mg/rat/15 days. These doses correspond to approximately 1-, 3-, and 5-fold (in females) and 1.3-, 1.3-, and 1.6-fold (in males) the systemic exposure [$AUC_{0-30\ days}$] achieved in women receiving the recommended dose of 250 mg/month. An increased incidence of benign ovarian granulosa cell tumors and testicular Leydig cell tumors was evident, in females dosed at 10 mg/rat/15 days and males dosed at 15 mg/rat/30 days, respectively. Induction of such tumors is consistent with the pharmacology-related endocrine feedback alterations in gonadotropin levels caused by an antiestrogen.

Fulvestrant was not mutagenic or clastogenic in multiple *in vitro* tests with and without the addition of a mammalian liver metabolic activation factor (bacterial mutation assay in strains of Salmonella typhimurium and Escherichia coli, in vitro cytogenetics study in human lymphocytes, mammalian cell mutation assay in mouse lymphoma cells and *in vivo* micronucleus test in rat.

In female rats, fulvestrant administered at doses ≥ 0.01 mg/kg/day (approximately one-hundredth of the human recommended dose based on body surface area [BSA], for 2 weeks prior to and for 1 week following mating, caused a reduction in fertility and embryonic survival. No adverse effects on female fertility and embryonic survival were evident in female animals dosed at 0.001 mg/kg/day (approximately one-thousandth of the human dose based on BSA). Restoration of female fertility to values similar to controls was evident following a 29-day withdrawal period after dosing at 2 mg/kg/day (twice the human dose based on BSA). The effects of fulvestrant on the fertility of female rats appear to be consistent with its antiestrogenic activity. The potential effects of fulvestrant on the fertility of male animals were not studied but, in a 6-month toxicology study, male rats treated with intramuscular doses of 15 mg/kg/30 days, 10 mg/rat/30 days, or 10 mg/rat/15 days fulvestrant showed a loss of spermatozoa from the seminiferous tubules, seminiferous tubular atrophy, and degenerative changes in the epididymides. Changes in the testes and epididymides had not recovered 20 weeks after cessation of dosing. These fulvestrant doses correspond to approximately 2-, 3-, and 3-fold the systemic exposure [$AUC_{0-30\ days}$] achieved in women.

Pregnancy

Pregnancy Category D: (See **WARNINGS**).

In studies in female rats at doses ≥ 0.01 mg/kg/day (IM; approximately one-hundredth of the human recommended dose based on body surface area [BSA]), fulvestrant caused a reversible reduction in female fertility, as well as effects on embryo/fetal development consistent with its antiestrogenic activity. Fulvestrant caused an increased incidence of fetal abnormalities in rats (tarsal flexure of the hind paw at 2 mg/kg/day IM; twice the human dose on BSA) and non-ossification of the odontoid and ventral tubercle of the first cervical vertebra at doses ≥ 0.1 mg/kg/day IM (approximately one-tenth of the human dose on BSA) when administered during the period of organogenesis. Rabbits failed to maintain pregnancy when dosed with 1 mg/kg/day fulvestrant IM (twice the human dose on BSA) during the period of organogenesis. Further, in rabbits dosed at 0.25 mg/kg/day (about one-half the human dose on BSA), increases in placental weight and post-implantation loss were observed but, there were no observed effects on fetal development. Fulvestrant was associated with an increased incidence of fetal variations in rabbits (backwards displacement of the pelvic girdle, and 27 pre-sacral vertebrae at 0.25 mg/kg/day IM; one-half the human dose on BSA) when administered during the period of organogenesis. Because pregnancy could not be maintained in the rabbit following doses of fulvestrant of 1 mg/kg/day and above, this study was inadequate to fully define the possible adverse effects on fetal development at clinically relevant exposures.

Nursing Mothers

Fulvestrant is found in rat milk at levels significantly higher (approximately 12-fold) than plasma after administration of 2 mg/kg. Drug exposure in rodent pups from fulvestrant-treated lactating dams was estimated as 10% of the administered dose. It is not known if fulvestrant is excreted in human milk. Because many drugs are excreted in human milk, and because of the potential for serious adverse reactions from FASLODEX in nursing infants, a decision should be made whether to discontinue nursing or to discontinue the drug taking into account the importance of the drug to the mother.

Pediatric Use

The safety and efficacy of FASLODEX in pediatric patients have not been established.

Geriatric Use

When tumor response was considered by age, objective responses were seen in 24% and 22% of patients under 65 years of age and in 16% and 11% of patients 65 years of age and older, who were treated with FASLODEX in the European and North American trials, respectively.

ADVERSE REACTIONS

The most commonly reported adverse experiences in the FASLODEX and anastrozole treatment groups, regardless of the investigator's assessment of causality, were gastrointestinal symptoms (including nausea, vomiting, constipation, diarrhea and abdominal pain), headache, back pain, vasodilatation (hot flushes), and pharyngitis.

Injection site reactions with mild transient pain and inflammation were seen with FASLODEX and occurred in 7% of patients (1% of treatments) given the single 5 mL injection (predominately European Trial) and in 27% of patients (4.6% of treatments) given the 2 x 2.5 mL injections (North American Trial).

Table 4 lists adverse experiences reported with an incidence of 5% or greater, regardless of assessed causality, from the two controlled clinical trials comparing the administration of FASLODEX 250 mg intramuscularly once a month with anastrozole 1 mg orally once a day.

Table 4: Combined Trials Adverse Events ≥ 5%

Body system and adverse event[a]	FASLODEX 250 mg N=423 (%)	Anastrozole 1 mg N=423 (%)
Body as a whole	68.3	67.6
Asthenia	22.7	27.0
Pain	18.9	20.3
Headache	15.4	16.8
Back pain	14.4	13.2
Abdominal pain	11.8	11.6
Injection site pain*	10.9	6.6
Pelvic pain	9.9	9.0
Chest pain	7.1	5.0
Flu syndrome	7.1	6.4
Fever	6.4	6.4
Accidental injury	4.5	5.7
Cardiovascular system	30.3	27.9
Vasodilatation	17.7	17.3
Digestive system	51.5	48.0
Nausea	26.0	25.3
Vomiting	13.0	11.8
Constipation	12.5	10.6
Diarrhea	12.3	12.8
Anorexia	9.0	10.9
Hemic and lymphatic systems	13.7	13.5
Anemia	4.5	5.0
Metabolic and Nutritional disorders	18.2	17.7
Peripheral edema	9.0	10.2
Musculoskeletal system	25.5	27.9
Bone pain	15.8	13.7
Arthritis	2.8	6.1
Nervous system	34.3	33.8
Dizziness	6.9	6.6
Insomnia	6.9	8.5
Paresthesia	6.4	7.6
Depression	5.7	6.9
Anxiety	5.0	3.8
Respiratory system	38.5	33.6
Pharyngitis	16.1	11.6
Dyspnea	14.9	12.3
Cough increased	10.4	10.4
Skin and appendages	22.2	23.4
Rash	7.3	8.0
Sweating	5.0	5.2
Urogenital system	18.2	14.9
Urinary tract infection	6.1	3.5

[a] A patient may have more than one adverse event.
* All patients on FASLODEX received injections, but only those anastrozole patients who were in the North American study received placebo injections.

Other adverse events reported as drug-related and seen infrequently (<1%) include thromboembolic phenomena, myalgia, vertigo, leukopenia and hypersensitivity reactions including angioedema and urticaria.

Vaginal bleeding has been reported infrequently (<1%), mainly in patients during the first 6 weeks after changing from existing hormonal therapy to treatment with FASLODEX. If bleeding persists, further evaluation should be considered.

OVERDOSAGE

Animal studies have shown no effects other than those related directly or indirectly to antiestrogen activity with intramuscular doses of fulvestrant higher than the recommended human dose. There is no clinical experience with overdosage in humans. No adverse effects were seen in healthy male and female volunteers who received intravenous fulvestrant, which resulted in peak plasma concentrations at the end of the infusion, that were approximately 10 to 15 times those seen after intramuscular injection.

DOSAGE AND ADMINISTRATION

Adults (including the elderly): The recommended dose is 250 mg to be administered intramuscularly into the buttock at intervals of one month as either a single 5 mL injection or two concurrent 2.5 mL injections (see **HOW SUPPLIED**). The injection should be administered slowly.

Patients with Hepatic Impairment

FASLODEX has not been studied in patients with moderate or severe hepatic compromise. No dosage adjustment is recommended in patients with mild hepatic impairment (see **CLINICAL PHARMACOLOGY-Hepatic Impairment** and **PRECAUTIONS-Hepatic Impairment** sections).

Instructions for Intramuscular use, handling and disposal

1. Remove glass syringe barrel from tray and check that it is not damaged.
2. Remove perforated patient record label from syringe.
3. Peel open the safety needle (SafetyGlide™) outer packaging. For complete SafetyGlide™ instructions refer below to the "Directions for Use of SafetyGlide™."
4. Break the seal of the white plastic cover on the syringe luer connector to remove the cover with the attached rubber tip cap (see Figure 1).
5. Twist to lock the needle to the luer connector.
6. Remove needle sheath.
7. Remove excess gas from the syringe (a small gas bubble may remain).
8. Administer intramuscularly slowly in the buttock.
9. Immediately activate needle protection device upon withdrawal from patient by pushing lever arm completely forward until needle tip is fully covered (see Figure 2).
10. Visually confirm that the lever arm has fully advanced and the needle tip is covered. If unable to activate, discard immediately into an approved sharps collector.
11. Repeat steps 1 through 10 for second syringe.

For the 2 x 2.5 mL syringe package only, both syringes must be administered to receive the 250 mg recommended monthly dose.

SAFETYGLIDE™ INSTRUCTIONS FROM BECTON DICKINSON

SafetyGlide™ is a trademark of Becton Dickinson and Company

Reorder number 305917

CAUTION CONCERNING SAFETYGLIDE™

Federal (USA) law restricts this device to sale by or on the order of a physician. To help avoid HIV (AIDS), HBV (Hepatitis), and other infectious diseases due to accidental needlesticks, contaminated needles should not be recapped or removed, unless there is no alternative or that such action is required by a specific medical procedure.

WARNING CONCERNING SAFETYGLIDE™

Do not autoclave SafetyGlide™ Needle before use. Hands must remain behind the needle at all times during use and disposal.

DIRECTIONS FOR USE OF SAFETYGLIDE™

Peel apart packaging of the SafetyGlide™, break the seal of the white plastic cover on the syringe Luer connector and attach the SafetyGlide™ needle to the Luer Lock of the syringe by twisting.

Transport filled syringe to point of administration.

Pull shield straight off needle to avoid damaging needle point.

Administer injection following package instruction.

For user convenience, the needle 'bevel up' position is orientated to the lever arm, as shown in Figure 3.

Immediately activate needle protection device upon withdrawal from patient by pushing lever arm completely forward until needle tip is fully covered (Figure 2).

Visually confirm that the lever arm has fully advanced and the needle tip is covered. If unable to activate, discard immediately into an approved sharps collector.

Activation of the protective mechanism may cause minimal splatter of fluid that may remain on the needle after injection.

For greatest safety, use a one-handed technique and activate away from self and others.

After single use, discard in an approved sharps collector in accordance with applicable regulations and institutional policy.

Continued on next page

Faslodex—Cont.

Becton Dickinson guarantees the contents of their un-opened or undamaged packages to be sterile, non-toxic and non-pyrogenic.

HOW SUPPLIED

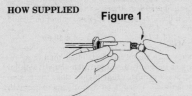

Figure 1

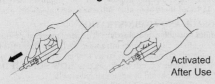

Figure 2

Activated
After Use

Figure 3

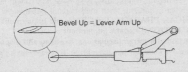

Bevel Up = Lever Arm Up

FASLODEX is supplied in two different packaging configurations:

1. FASLODEX is supplied as one clear neutral glass (Type 1) barrel containing 250 mg/5mL (50 mg/mL) FASLODEX Injection for intramuscular injection and fitted with a tamper evident closure.
NDC 0310-0720-50

2. FASLODEX is also supplied as two clear neutral glass (Type 1) barrels each containing 125 mg/2.5 mL (50 mg/mL) FASLODEX Injection for intramuscular injection and fitted with a tamper-evident closure. **PLEASE NOTE: THE SYRINGES ARE SUPPLIED HALF FULL. BOTH SYRINGES MUST BE ADMINISTERED TO RECEIVE THE 250 MG RECOMMENDED MONTHLY DOSE.**
NDC 0310-0720-25

The syringes are presented in a tray with polystyrene plunger rod and safety needles (SafetyGlide™) for connection to the barrel.

Storage

REFRIGERATE, 2°-8°C (36°-46°F). TO PROTECT FROM LIGHT, STORE IN THE ORIGINAL CARTON UNTIL TIME OF USE.

SafetyGlide™ is a trademark of Becton Dickinson and Company

FASLODEX is a trademark of the AstraZeneca group of companies.

© AstraZeneca 2002, 2004
Distributed by:
AstraZeneca Pharmaceuticals LP
Wilmington, DE 19850
Manufactured for:
AstraZeneca UK Ltd.
Macclesfield, England
By: Vetter Pharma-Fertigung GmbH & Co. KG
Ravensburg, Germany
Made in Germany
31003-00
Rev 08/04
AstraZeneca

IRESSA®

[ēr′ əs-sə]
(gefitinib) TABLETS
250 mg
FOR ONCOLOGY USE ONLY

℞

Prescribing information for this product, which appears on pages 656–658 of the 2005 PDR, has been completely revised as follows. Please write "See Supplement A" next to the product heading.

DESCRIPTION

IRESSA® (gefitinib tablets) contain 250 mg of gefitinib and are available as brown film-coated tablets for daily oral administration.

Gefitinib is an anilinoquinazoline with the chemical name 4-Quinazolinamine, N-(3-chloro-4-fluorophenyl)-7-methoxy-6-[3-4-morpholin) propoxy] and the following structural formula:

[See chemical structure at top of next column]

It has the molecular formula $C_{22}H_{24}ClFN_4O_3$, a relative molecular mass of 446.9 and is a white-colored powder. Gefitinib is a free base. The molecule has pK_as of 5.4 and 7.2 and therefore ionizes progressively in solution as the pH falls. Gefitinib can be defined as sparingly soluble at pH 1, but is practically insoluble above pH 7, with the solubility

dropping sharply between pH 4 and pH 6. In non-aqueous solvents, gefitinib is freely soluble in glacial acetic acid and dimethylsulphoxide, soluble in pyridine, sparingly soluble in tetrahydrofuran, and slightly soluble in methanol, ethanol (99.5%), ethyl acetate, propan-2-ol and acetonitrile.

The inactive ingredients of IRESSA tablets are: **Tablet core:** Lactose monohydrate, microcrystalline cellulose, croscarmellose sodium, povidone, sodium lauryl sulfate and magnesium stearate. **Coating:** Hypromellose, polyethylene glycol 300, titanium dioxide, red ferric oxide and yellow ferric oxide.

CLINICAL PHARMACOLOGY

Mechanism of Action

The mechanism of the clinical antitumor action of gefitinib is not fully characterized. Gefitinib inhibits the intracellular phosphorylation of numerous tyrosine kinases associated with transmembrane cell surface receptors, including the tyrosine kinases associated with the epidermal growth factor receptor (EGFR-TK). EGFR is expressed on the cell surface of many normal cells and cancer cells. No clinical studies have been performed that demonstrate a correlation between EGFR receptor expression and response to gefitinib.

Pharmacokinetics

Gefitinib is absorbed slowly after oral administration with mean bioavailability of 60%. Elimination is by metabolism (primarily CYP3A4) and excretion in feces. The elimination half-life is about 48 hours. Daily oral administration of gefitinib to cancer patients resulted in a 2-fold accumulation compared to single dose administration. Steady state plasma concentrations are achieved within 10 days.

Absorption and Distribution:

Gefitinib is slowly absorbed, with peak plasma levels occurring 3-7 hours after dosing and mean oral bioavailability of 60%. Bioavailability is not significantly altered by food. Gefitinib is extensively distributed throughout the body with a mean steady state volume of distribution of 1400 L following intravenous administration. *In vitro* binding of gefitinib to human plasma proteins (serum albumin and α1-acid glycoprotein) is 90% and is independent of drug concentrations.

Metabolism and Elimination:

Gefitinib undergoes extensive hepatic metabolism in humans, predominantly by CYP3A4. Three sites of biotransformation have been identified: metabolism of the N-propoxymorpholino-group, demethylation of the methoxy-substituent on the quinazoline, and oxidative defluorination of the halogenated phenyl group.

Five metabolites were identified in human plasma. Only O-desmethyl gefitinib has exposure comparable to gefitinib. Although this metabolite has similar EGFR-TK activity to gefitinib in the isolated enzyme assay, it had only 1/14 of the potency of gefitinib in one of the cell-based assays.

Gefitinib is cleared primarily by the liver, with total plasma clearance and elimination half-life values of 595 mL/min and 48 hours, respectively, after intravenous administration. Excretion is predominantly via the feces (86%), with renal elimination of drug and metabolites accounting for less than 4% of the administered dose.

Table 1: Demographic and Disease Characteristics

Characteristic	IRESSA Dose	
	250 mg/day N = 66 (%)	500 mg/day N = (76%)
Age Group		
18-64 years	43 (65)	43 (57)
64-74 years	19 (29)	30 (39)
75 years and above	4 (6)	3 (4)
Sex		
Male	38 (58)	41 (54)
Female	28 (42)	35 (46)
Race		
White	61 (92)	68 (89)
Black	1 (2)	2 (3)
Asian/Oriental	1 (2)	2 (3)
Hispanic	0 (0)	3 (4)
Other	3 (5)	1 (1)
Smoking History		
Yes (Previous or current smoker)	45 (68)	62 (82)
No (Never smoked)	21 (32)	14 (18)
Baseline WHO Performance Status		
0	14 (21)	9 (12)
1	36 (55)	53 (70)
2	15 (23)	14 (18)
Not recorded	1 (2)	0 (0)
Tumor Histology		
Squamous	9 (14)	11 (14)
Adenocarcinoma	47 (71)	50 (66)
Undifferentiated	6 (9)	4 (5)
Large Cell	1 (2)	2 (3)
Squamous & Adenocarcinoma	3 (5)	7 (9)
Not Recorded	0 (0)	2 (3)
Current Disease Status		
Locally advanced	11 (17)	5 (7)
Metastatic	55 (83)	71 (93)

Special Populations:

In population based data analyses, no relationships were identified between predicted steady state trough concentration and patient age, body weight, gender, ethnicity or creatinine clearance.

Pediatric:

There are no pharmacokinetic data in pediatric patients.

Hepatic Impairment:

The influence of hepatic metastases with elevation of serum aspartate aminotransferase (AST/SGOT), alkaline phosphatase, and bilirubin has been evaluated in patients with normal (14 patients), moderately elevated (13 patients) and severely elevated (4 patients) levels of one or more of these biochemical parameters. Patients with moderately and severely elevated biochemical liver abnormalities had gefitinib pharmacokinetics similar to individuals without liver abnormalities (see **PRECAUTIONS** section).

Renal Impairment:

No clinical studies were conducted with IRESSA in patients with severely compromised renal function (see **PRECAUTIONS** section). Gefitinib and its metabolites are not significantly excreted via the kidney (<4%).

Drug-Drug Interactions:

In human liver microsome studies, gefitinib had no inhibitory effect on CYP1A2, CYP2C9, and CYP3A4 activities at concentrations ranging from 2–5000 ng/mL. At the highest concentration studied (5000 ng/mL), gefitinib inhibited CYP2C19 by 24% and CYP2D6 by 43%. Exposure to metoprolol, a substrate of CYP2D6, was increased by 30% when it was given in combination with gefitinib (500 mg daily for 28 days) in patients with solid tumors.

Rifampicin, an inducer of CYP3A4, reduced mean AUC of gefitinib by 85% in healthy male volunteers (see **PRECAUTIONS—Drug Interactions** and **DOSAGE AND ADMINISTRATION—Dosage Adjustment** sections).

Concomitant administration of itraconazole (200 mg QD for 12 days), an inhibitor of CYP3A4, with gefitinib (250 mg single dose) to healthy male volunteers, increased mean gefitinib AUC by 88% (see **PRECAUTIONS—Drug Interactions** section).

Co-administration of high doses of ranitidine with sodium bicarbonate (to maintain the gastric pH above pH 5.0) reduced mean gefitinib AUC by 44% (see **PRECAUTIONS—Drug Interactions** section).

International Normalized Ratio (INR) elevations and/or bleeding events have been reported in some patients taking warfarin while on IRESSA therapy. Patients taking warfarin should be monitored regularly for changes in prothrombin time or INR (see **PRECAUTIONS—Drug Interactions** and **ADVERSE REACTIONS** sections).

Clinical Studies

Non-Small Cell Lung Cancer (NSCLC)—A multicenter clinical trial in the United States evaluated the tumor response rate of IRESSA 250 and 500 mg/day in patients with advanced non-small cell lung cancer whose disease had progressed after at least two prior chemotherapy regimens including a platinum drug and docetaxel. IRESSA was taken once daily at approximately the same time each day.

Two hundred and sixteen patients received IRESSA, 102 (47%) and 114 (53%) receiving 250 mg and 500 mg daily doses, respectively. Study patient demographics and disease characteristics are summarized in Table 1. Forty-one percent of the patients had received two prior treatment regimens, 33% three prior treatment regimens, and 25% four or more prior treatment regimens. Effectiveness of IRESSA as third line therapy was determined in the 142 evaluable patients with documented disease progression on platinum and docetaxel therapies or who had had unacceptable toxicity on these agents.

[See table 1 at top of previous page]

Table 2 shows tumor response rates and response duration. The overall response rate for the 250 and 500 mg doses combined was 10.6% (95% CI: 6%, 16.8%). Response rates appeared to be highly variable in subgroups of the treated population: 5.1% (4/79) in males, 17.5% (11/63) in females, 4.6% (5/108) in previous or current smokers, 29.4% (10/34) in nonsmokers, 12.4% (12/97) with adenocarcinoma histology, and 6.7% (3/45) with other NSCLC histologies. Similar differences in response were seen in a multinational study in patients who had received 1 or 2 prior chemotherapy regimens, at least 1 of which was platinum-based. In responders, the median time from diagnosis to study randomization was 16.7 months (range 8 to 34 months).

[See table 2 at right]

Table 2 - Efficacy Results

	Evaluable Patients		
	250 mg (N=66)	500 mg (N=76)	Combined (N=142)
Objective Tumor Response Rate (%)	13.6	7.9	10.6
95% CI (%)	6.4-24.3	3.0-16.4	6.0-16.8
Median Duration of Objective Response (months)	8.9	4.5	7.0
Range (months)	4.6-18.6+	4.4-7.6	4.4-18.6+

+=data are ongoing

Non-Small Cell Lung Cancer (NSCLC); Studies of First-line Treatment in Combination with Chemotherapy—Two large trials were conducted in chemotherapy-naïve patients with stage III and IV non-small cell lung cancer. Two thousand one hundred thirty patients were randomized to receive IRESSA 250 mg daily, IRESSA 500 mg daily, or placebo in combination with platinum-based chemotherapy regimens. The chemotherapies given in these first-line trials were gemcitabine and cis-platinum (N=1093) or carboplatin and paclitaxel (N=1037). The addition of IRESSA did not demonstrate any increase, or trend toward such an increase, in tumor response rates, time to progression, or overall survival.

INDICATIONS AND USAGE

IRESSA is indicated as monotherapy for the treatment of patients with locally advanced or metastatic non-small cell lung cancer after failure of both platinum-based and docetaxel chemotherapies.

The effectiveness of IRESSA is based on objective response rates (see **CLINICAL PHARMACOLOGY—Clinical Studies** section). There are no controlled trials demonstrating a clinical benefit, such as improvement in disease-related symptoms or increased survival.

Results from two large, controlled, randomized trials in first-line treatment of non-small cell lung cancer showed no benefit from adding IRESSA to doublet, platinum-based chemotherapy. Therefore, IRESSA is not indicated for use in this setting.

CONTRAINDICATIONS

IRESSA is contraindicated in patients with severe hypersensitivity to gefitinib or to any other component of IRESSA.

WARNINGS

Pulmonary Toxicity

Cases of interstitial lung disease (ILD) have been observed in patients receiving IRESSA at an overall incidence of about 1%. Approximately 1/3 of the cases have been fatal. The reported incidence of ILD was about 2% in the Japanese post-marketing experience, about 0.3% in approximately 23,000 patients treated with IRESSA in a US expanded access program and about 1% in the studies of first-line use in NSCLC (but with similar rates in both treatment and placebo groups). Reports have described the adverse event as interstitial pneumonia, pneumonitis and alveolitis. Patients often present with the acute onset of dyspnea, sometimes associated with cough or low-grade fever, often becoming severe within a short time and requiring hospitalization. ILD has occurred in patients who have received prior radiation therapy (31% of reported cases), prior chemotherapy (57% of reported patients), and no previous therapy (12% of reported cases). Patients with concurrent idiopathic pulmonary fibrosis whose condition worsens while receiving IRESSA have been observed to have an increased mortality compared to those without concurrent idiopathic pulmonary fibrosis.

In the event of acute onset or worsening of pulmonary symptoms (dyspnea, cough, fever), IRESSA therapy should be interrupted and a prompt investigation of these symptoms should occur. If interstitial lung disease is confirmed, IRESSA should be discontinued and the patient treated appropriately (see **PRECAUTIONS—Information for Patients, ADVERSE REACTIONS** and **DOSAGE AND ADMINISTRATION—Dosage Adjustment** sections).

Pregnancy Category D

IRESSA may cause fetal harm when administered to a pregnant woman. A single dose study in rats showed that gefitinib crosses the placenta after an oral dose of 5 mg/kg (30 mg/m^2, about 1/5 the recommended human dose on a mg/m^2 basis). When pregnant rats were treated with 5 mg/kg from the beginning of organogenesis to the end of weaning gave birth, there was a reduction in the number of offspring born alive. This effect was more severe at 20 mg/kg and was accompanied by high neonatal mortality soon after parturition. In this study a dose of 1 mg/kg caused no adverse effects.

In rabbits, a dose of 20 mg/kg/day (240 mg/m^2, about twice the recommended dose in humans on a mg/m^2 basis) caused reduced fetal weight.

There are no adequate and well-controlled studies in pregnant women using IRESSA. If IRESSA is used during pregnancy or if the patient becomes pregnant while receiving this drug, she should be apprised of the potential hazard to the fetus or potential risk for loss of the pregnancy.

PRECAUTIONS

Hepatotoxicity

Asymptomatic increases in liver transaminases have been observed in IRESSA-treated patients; therefore, periodic liver function (transaminases, bilirubin, and alkaline phosphatase) testing should be considered. Discontinuation of IRESSA should be considered if changes are severe.

Patients with Hepatic Impairment

In vitro and *in vivo* evidence suggest that gefitinib is cleared primarily by the liver. Therefore, gefitinib exposure may be increased in patients with hepatic dysfunction. In patients with liver metastases and moderately to severely elevated biochemical liver abnormalities, however, gefitinib pharmacokinetics were similar to the pharmacokinetics of individuals without liver abnormalities (see **CLINICAL PHARMACOLOGY—Pharmacokinetics—Special Populations** section). The influence of non-cancer related hepatic impairment on the pharmacokinetics of gefitinib has not been evaluated.

Information for Patients

Patients should be advised to seek medical advice promptly if they develop 1) severe or persistent diarrhea, nausea, anorexia, or vomiting, as these have sometimes been associated with dehydration; 2) an onset or worsening of pulmonary symptoms, ie, shortness of breath or cough; 3) an eye irritation; or, 4) any other new symptom (see **WARNINGS—Pulmonary Toxicity, ADVERSE REACTIONS** and **DOSAGE AND ADMINISTRATION—Dosage Adjustment** sections).

Women of childbearing potential must be advised to avoid becoming pregnant (see **WARNINGS—Pregnancy Category D**).

Drug Interactions

Substances that are inducers of CYP3A4 activity increase the metabolism of gefitinib and decrease its plasma concentrations. In patients receiving a potent CYP3A4 inducer such as rifampicin or phenytoin, a dose increase to 500 mg daily should be considered in the absence of severe adverse drug reaction, and clinical response and adverse events should be carefully monitored (see **CLINICAL PHARMACOLOGY—Pharmacokinetics—Drug-Drug Interactions** and **DOSAGE AND ADMINISTRATION—Dosage Adjustment** sections).

International Normalized Ratio (INR) elevations and/or bleeding events have been reported in some patients taking warfarin while on IRESSA therapy. Patients taking warfarin should be monitored regularly for changes in prothrombin time or INR (see **CLINICAL PHARMACOLOGY—Pharmacokinetics—Drug-Drug Interactions** and **ADVERSE REACTIONS** sections).

Substances that are potent inhibitors of CYP3A4 activity (eg, ketoconazole and itraconazole) decrease gefitinib metabolism and increase gefitinib plasma concentrations. This increase may be clinically relevant as adverse experiences are related to dose and exposure; therefore, caution should be used when administering CYP3A4 inhibitors with IRESSA (see **CLINICAL PHARMACOLOGY—Pharmacokinetics—Drug-Drug Interactions** and **ADVERSE REACTIONS** sections).

Drugs that cause significant sustained elevation in gastric pH (histamine H_2-receptor antagonists such as ranitidine or cimetidine) may reduce plasma concentrations of IRESSA and therefore potentially may reduce efficacy (see **CLINICAL PHARMACOLOGY—Drug-Drug Interactions** section).

Phase II clinical trial data, where IRESSA and vinorelbine have been used concomitantly, indicate that IRESSA may exacerbate the neutropenic effect of vinorelbine.

Carcinogenesis, Mutagenesis, Impairment of Fertility

Gefitinib has been tested for genotoxicity in a series of *in vitro* (bacterial mutation, mouse lymphoma, and human lymphocyte) assays and an *in vivo* rat micronucleus test. Under the conditions of these assays, gefitinib did not cause genetic damage.

Carcinogenicity studies have not been conducted with gefitinib.

Pregnancy

Pregnancy Category D (see **WARNINGS** and **PRECAUTIONS—Information for Patients** sections).

Nursing Mothers

It is not known whether IRESSA is excreted in human milk. Following oral administration of carbon-14 labeled gefitinib to rats 14 days postpartum, concentrations of radioactivity in milk were higher than in blood. Levels of gefitinib and its metabolites were 11-to-19-fold higher in milk than in blood, after oral exposure of lactating rats to a dose of 5 mg/kg. Because many drugs are excreted in human milk and because of the potential for serious adverse reactions in nursing infants, women should be advised against breast-feeding while receiving IRESSA therapy.

Pediatric Use

IRESSA is not indicated for use in pediatric patients, as safety and effectiveness have not been established. In clinical trials of IRESSA alone or with radiation in pediatric patients with primary Central Nervous System (CNS) tumors, cases of CNS hemorrhage and death have been reported. There are insufficient data in pediatric patients to establish a causal relationship. There is no evidence to suggest increased risk of cerebral hemorrhage in adult patients with NSCLC receiving IRESSA.

Geriatric Use

Of the total number of patients participating in trials of second- and third-line IRESSA treatment of NSCLC, 65% were aged 64 years or less, 30.5% were aged 65 to 74 years, and 5% of patients were aged 75 years or older. No differences in safety or efficacy were observed between younger and older patients.

Patients with Severe Renal Impairment

The effect of severe renal impairment on the pharmacokinetics of gefitinib is not known. Patients with severe renal impairment should be treated with caution when given IRESSA.

ADVERSE REACTIONS

The safety database includes 941 patients from clinical trials and approximately 23,000 patients in the Expanded Access Program.

Table 3 includes drug-related adverse events with an incidence of ≥5% for the 216 patients who received either 250 mg or 500 mg of IRESSA monotherapy for treatment of NSCLC. The most common adverse events reported at the recommended 250 mg daily dose were diarrhea, rash, acne, dry skin, nausea, and vomiting (see **PRECAUTIONS—Information for Patients** and **DOSAGE AND ADMINISTRATION—Dosage Adjustment** sections). The 500 mg dose showed a higher rate for most of these adverse events.

Table 4 provides drug-related adverse events with an incidence of ≥5% by CTC grade for the patients who received the 250 mg/day dose of IRESSA monotherapy for treatment of NSCLC. Only 2% of patients stopped therapy due to an adverse drug reaction (ADR). The onset of these ADRs occurred within the first month of therapy.

Table 3 - Drug-Related Adverse Events with an Incidence of ≥5% in either 250 mg or 500 mg Dose Group

	Number (%) of Patients	
Drug-related adverse event[a]	250 mg/day (N=102) %	500 mg/day (N=114) %
Diarrhea	49 (48)	76 (67)
Rash	44 (43)	61 (54)
Acne	25 (25)	37 (33)
Dry skin	13 (13)	30 (26)
Nausea	13 (13)	20 (18)
Vomiting	12 (12)	10 (9)
Pruritus	8 (8)	10 (9)
Anorexia	7 (7)	11 (10)
Asthenia	6 (6)	5 (4)
Weight loss	3 (3)	6 (5)

[a]A patient may have had more than 1 drug-related adverse event.

Table 4 - Drug Related Adverse Events ≥5% at 250 mg dose by Worst CTC Grade (n=102)

	% of Patients				
Adverse event	All Grades	CTC Grade 1	CTC Grade 2	CTC Grade 3	CTC Grade 4
Diarrhea	48	41	6	1	0
Rash	43	39	4	0	0
Acne	25	19	6	0	0
Dry Skin	13	12	1	0	0
Nausea	13	7	5	1	0
Vomiting	12	9	2	1	0
Pruritus	8	7	1	0	0
Anorexia	7	3	4	0	0
Asthenia	6	2	2	1	1

Other adverse events reported at an incidence of <5% in patients who received either 250 mg or 500 mg as monotherapy for treatment of NSCLC (along with their frequency at the 250 mg recommended dose) include the following: peripheral edema (2%), amblyopia (2%), dyspnea (2%), conjunctivitis (1%), vesiculobullous rash (1%), and mouth ulceration (1%).

Interstitial Lung Disease

Cases of interstitial lung disease (ILD) have been observed in patients receiving IRESSA at an overall incidence of

Continued on next page

Iressa—Cont:

about 1%. Approximately 1/3 of the cases have been fatal. The reported incidence of ILD was about 2% in the Japanese post-marketing experience, about 0.3% in approximately 23,000 patients treated with IRESSA in a US expanded access program and about 1% in the studies of first-line use in NSCLC (but with similar rates in both treatment and placebo groups). Reports have described the adverse event as interstitial pneumonia, pneumonitis and alveolitis. Patients often present with the acute onset of dyspnea, sometimes associated with cough or low-grade fever, often becoming severe within a short time and requiring hospitalization. ILD has occurred in patients who have received prior radiation therapy (31% of reported cases), prior chemotherapy (57% of reported patients), and no previous therapy (12% of reported cases). Patients with concurrent idiopathic pulmonary fibrosis whose condition worsens while receiving IRESSA have been observed to have an increased mortality compared to those without concurrent idiopathic pulmonary fibrosis.

In the event of acute onset or worsening of pulmonary symptoms (dyspnea, cough, fever), IRESSA therapy should be interrupted and a prompt investigation of these symptoms should occur. If interstitial lung disease is confirmed, IRESSA should be discontinued and the patient treated appropriately (see **WARNINGS—Pulmonary Toxicity**, **PRECAUTIONS—Information for Patients** and **DOSAGE AND ADMINISTRATION—Dosage Adjustment** sections).

In patients receiving IRESSA therapy, there were reports of eye pain and corneal erosion/ulcer, sometimes in association with aberrant eyelash growth (see **PRECAUTIONS—Information for Patients** section). Hemorrhage, such as epistaxis and hematuria have been reported in patients receiving IRESSA. There were also rare reports of pancreatitis and very rare reports of corneal membrane sloughing, ocular ischemia/hemorrhage, toxic epidermal necrolysis, erythema multiforme, and allergic reactions, including angioedema and urticaria.

International Normalized Ratio (INR) elevations and/or bleeding events have been reported in some patients taking warfarin while on IRESSA therapy. Patients taking warfarin should be monitored regularly for changes in prothrombin time or INR (see **CLINICAL PHARMACOLOGY—Drug-Drug Interactions** and **PRECAUTIONS—Drug Interactions** sections).

Data from non-clinical (*in vitro and in vivo*) studies indicate that gefitinib has the potential to inhibit the cardiac action potential repolarization process (eg, QT interval). The clinical relevance of these findings is unknown.

OVERDOSAGE

The acute toxicity of gefitinib up to 500 mg in clinical studies has been low. In non-clinical studies, a single dose of 12,000 mg/m^2 (about 80 times the recommended clinical dose on a mg/m^2 basis) was lethal to rats. Half this dose caused no mortality in mice.

There is no specific treatment for an IRESSA overdose and possible symptoms of overdose are not established. However, in phase 1 clinical trials, a limited number of patients were treated with daily doses of up to 1000 mg. An increase in frequency and severity of some adverse reactions was observed, mainly diarrhea and skin rash. Adverse reactions associated with overdose should be treated symptomatically; in particular, severe diarrhea should be managed appropriately.

DOSAGE AND ADMINISTRATION

The recommended daily dose of IRESSA is one 250 mg tablet with or without food. Higher doses do not give a better response and cause increased toxicity.

For Patient who have Difficulty Swallowing Solids

IRESSA tablets can also be dispersed in half a glass of drinking water (noncarbonated). No other liquids should be used. Drop the tablet in the water, without crushing it, stir until the tablet is dispersed (approximately 10 minutes) and drink liquid immediately. Rinse the glass with half a glass of water and drink. The liquid can also be administered through a naso-gastric tube.

Dosage Adjustment

Patients with poorly tolerated diarrhea (sometimes associated with dehydration) or skin adverse drug reactions may be successfully managed by providing a brief (up to 14 days) therapy interruption followed by reinstatement of the 250 mg daily dose.

In the event of acute onset or worsening of pulmonary symptoms (dyspnea, cough, fever), IRESSA therapy should be interrupted and a prompt investigation of these symptoms should occur and appropriate treatment initiated. If interstitial lung disease is confirmed, IRESSA should be discontinued and the patient treated appropriately (see **WARNINGS—Pulmonary Toxicity**, **PRECAUTIONS—Information for Patients** and **ADVERSE REACTIONS** sections).

Patients who develop onset of new eye symptoms such as pain should be medically evaluated and managed appropriately, including IRESSA therapy interruption and removal of an aberrant eyelash if present. After symptoms and eye changes have resolved, the decision should be made concerning reinstatement of the 250 mg daily dose (see **PRECAUTIONS—Information for Patients** and **ADVERSE REACTIONS** sections).

In patients receiving a potent CYP3A4 inducer such as rifampicin or phenytoin, a dose increase to 500 mg daily should be considered in the absence of severe adverse drug reaction, and clinical response and adverse events should be carefully monitored (see **CLINICAL PHARMACOLOGY—Pharmacokinetics—Drug-Drug Interactions** and **PRECAUTIONS—Drug Interactions** sections).

No dosage adjustment is required on the basis of patient age, body weight, gender, ethnicity, or renal function; or in patients with moderate to severe hepatic impairment due to liver metastases (see **CLINICAL PHARMACOLOGY—Pharmacokinetics—Special Populations** section).

HOW SUPPLIED

IRESSA tablets are supplied as round, biconvex, brown film-coated tablets intagliated with "IRESSA 250" on one side and plain on the other side, each containing 250 mg of gefitinib.

Bottles of 30 Tablets (NDC 0310-0482-30)

Storage

Store at controlled room temperature 20-25°C (68-77°F) [see USP].

IRESSA is a trademark of the AstraZeneca group of companies.

Manufactured for:
AstraZeneca Pharmaceuticals LP
Wilmington, DE 19850
By: AstraZeneca UK Limited
Macclesfield, Cheshire, England
Made in the United Kingdom
30020-00
Rev 11/04
AstraZeneca

SEROQUEL® ℞

[sē-rō-kwĕl]
(quetiapine fumarate)

Prescribing information for this product, which appears on pages 662–667 of the 2005 PDR, has been completely revised as follows. Please write "See Supplement A" next to the product heading.

DESCRIPTION

SEROQUEL (quetiapine fumarate) is a psychotropic agent belonging to a chemical class, the dibenzothiazepine derivatives. The chemical designation is 2-[2-(4-dibenzo [*b,f*] [1,4]thiazepin-11-yl-1-piperazinyl)ethoxy]-ethanol fumarate (2:1) (salt). It is present in tablets as the fumarate salt. All doses and tablet strengths are expressed as milligrams of base, not as fumarate salt. Its molecular formula is $C_{42}H_{50}N_6O_4S_2 \cdot C_4H_4O_4$ and it has a molecular weight of 883.11 (fumarate salt). The structural formula is:

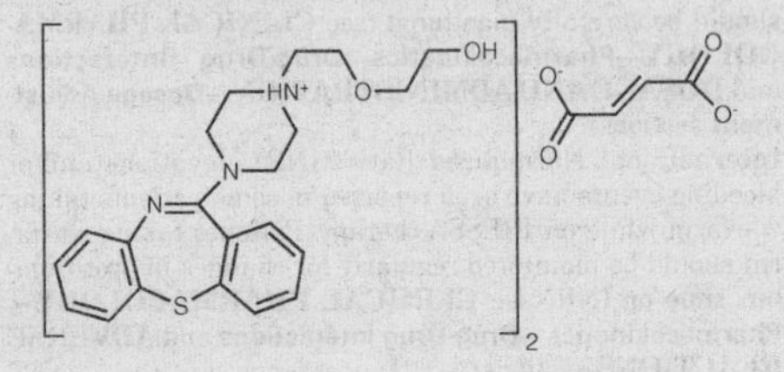

Quetiapine fumarate is a white to off-white crystalline powder which is moderately soluble in water.

SEROQUEL is supplied for oral administration as 25 mg (round, peach), 100 mg (round, yellow), 200 mg (round, white), and 300 mg (capsule-shaped, white) tablets.

Inactive ingredients are povidone, dibasic dicalcium phosphate dihydrate, microcrystalline cellulose, sodium starch glycolate, lactose monohydrate, magnesium stearate, hypromellose, polyethylene glycol and titanium dioxide.

The 25 mg tablets contain red ferric oxide and yellow ferric oxide and the 100 mg tablets contain only yellow ferric oxide.

CLINICAL PHARMACOLOGY

Pharmacodynamics

SEROQUEL is an antagonist at multiple neurotransmitter receptors in the brain: serotonin $5HT_{1A}$ and $5HT_2$ (IC_{50s}=717 & 148nM respectively), dopamine D_1 and D_2 (IC_{50s}=1268 & 329nM respectively), histamine H_1 (IC_{50}=30nM), and adrenergic α_1 and α_2 receptors (IC_{50s}=94 & 271nM, respectively). SEROQUEL has no appreciable affinity at cholinergic muscarinic and benzodiazepine receptors (IC_{50s}>5000 nM).

The mechanism of action of SEROQUEL, as with other drugs having efficacy in the treatment of schizophrenia and acute manic episodes associated with bipolar disorder, is unknown. However, it has been proposed that this drug's efficacy in schizophrenia is mediated through a combination of dopamine type 2 (D_2) and serotonin type 2 ($5HT_2$) antagonism. Antagonism at receptors other than dopamine and $5HT_2$ with similar receptor affinities may explain some of the other effects of SEROQUEL.

SEROQUEL's antagonism of histamine H_1 receptors may explain the somnolence observed with this drug.

SEROQUEL's antagonism of adrenergic α_1 receptors may explain the orthostatic hypotension observed with this drug.

Pharmacokinetics

Quetiapine fumarate activity is primarily due to the parent drug. The multiple-dose pharmacokinetics of quetiapine are dose-proportional within the proposed clinical dose range, and quetiapine accumulation is predictable upon multiple dosing. Elimination of quetiapine is mainly via hepatic metabolism with a mean terminal half-life of about 6 hours within the proposed clinical dose range. Steady-state concentrations are expected to be achieved within two days of dosing. Quetiapine is unlikely to interfere with the metabolism of drugs metabolized by cytochrome P450 enzymes.

Absorption: Quetiapine fumarate is rapidly absorbed after oral administration, reaching peak plasma concentrations in 1.5 hours. The tablet formulation is 100% bioavailable relative to solution. The bioavailability of quetiapine is marginally affected by administration with food, with C_{max} and AUC values increased by 25% and 15%, respectively.

Distribution: Quetiapine is widely distributed throughout the body with an apparent volume of distribution of 10±4 L/kg. It is 83% bound to plasma proteins at therapeutic concentrations. *In vitro*, quetiapine did not affect the binding of warfarin or diazepam to human serum albumin. In turn, neither warfarin nor diazepam altered the binding of
quetiapine.

Metabolism and Elimination: Following a single oral dose of ^{14}C-quetiapine, less than 1% of the administered dose was excreted as unchanged drug, indicating that quetiapine is highly metabolized. Approximately 73% and 20% of the dose was recovered in the urine and feces, respectively.

Quetiapine is extensively metabolized by the liver. The major metabolic pathways are sulfoxidation to the sulfoxide metabolite and oxidation to the parent acid metabolite; both metabolites are pharmacologically inactive. *In vitro* studies using human liver microsomes revealed that the cytochrome P450 3A4 isoenzyme is involved in the metabolism of quetiapine to its major, but inactive, sulfoxide metabolite.

Population Subgroups:

Age: Oral clearance of quetiapine was reduced by 40% in elderly patients (≥ 65 years, n=9) compared to young patients (n=12), and dosing adjustment may be necessary (See **DOSAGE AND ADMINISTRATION**).

Gender: There is no gender effect on the pharmacokinetics of quetiapine.

Race: There is no race effect on the pharmacokinetics of quetiapine.

Smoking: Smoking has no effect on the oral clearance of quetiapine.

Renal Insufficiency: Patients with severe renal impairment (Clcr=10-30 mL/min/1.73 m^2, n=8) had a 25% lower mean oral clearance than normal subjects (Clcr > 80 mL/min/1.73 m^2, n=8), but plasma quetiapine concentrations in the subjects with renal insufficiency were within the range of concentrations seen in normal subjects receiving the same dose. Dosage adjustment is therefore not needed in these patients.

Hepatic Insufficiency: Hepatically impaired patients (n=8) had a 30% lower mean oral clearance of quetiapine than normal subjects. In two of the 8 hepatically impaired patients, AUC and C_{max} were 3-times higher than those observed typically in healthy subjects. Since quetiapine is extensively metabolized by the liver, higher plasma levels are expected in the hepatically impaired population, and dosage adjustment may be needed (See **DOSAGE AND ADMINISTRATION**).

Drug-Drug Interactions: *In vitro* enzyme inhibition data suggest that quetiapine and 9 of its metabolites would have little inhibitory effect on *in vivo* metabolism mediated by cytochromes P450 1A2, 2C9, 2C19, 2D6 and 3A4.

Quetiapine oral clearance is increased by the prototype cytochrome P450 3A4 inducer, phenytoin, and decreased by the prototype cytochrome P450 3A4 inhibitor, ketoconazole. Dose adjustment of quetiapine will be necessary if it is coadministered with phenytoin or ketoconazole (See **Drug Interactions** under **PRECAUTIONS** and **DOSAGE AND ADMINISTRATION**).

Quetiapine oral clearance is not inhibited by the nonspecific enzyme inhibitor, cimetidine.

Quetiapine at doses of 750 mg/day did not affect the single dose pharmacokinetics of antipyrine, lithium or lorazepam (See **Drug Interactions** under **PRECAUTIONS**).

Clinical Efficacy Data

Bipolar Mania

The efficacy of SEROQUEL in the treatment of acute manic episodes was established in 3 placebo-controlled trials in patients who met DSM-IV criteria for bipolar I disorder with manic episodes. These trials included patients with or without psychotic features and excluded patients with rapid cycling and mixed episodes. Of these trials, 2 were monotherapy (12 weeks) and 1 was adjunct therapy (3 weeks) to either lithium or divalproex. Key outcomes in these trials were change from baseline in the Young Mania Rating Scale (YMRS) score at 3 and 12 weeks for monotherapy and at 3 weeks for adjunct therapy. Adjunct therapy is defined as the simultaneous initiation or subsequent administration of SEROQUEL with lithium or divalproex.

The primary rating instrument used for assessing manic symptoms in these trials was the YMRS, an 11-item clinician-rated scale traditionally used to assess the degree of manic symptomatology (irritability, disruptive/aggressive behavior, sleep, elevated mood, speech, increased activity, sexual interest, language/thought disorder, thought content, appearance, and insight) in a range from 0 (no manic features) to 60 (maximum score).

The results of the trials follow:

Monotherapy

In two 12-week trials (n=300, n=299) comparing SEROQUEL to placebo, SEROQUEL was superior to placebo in the reduction of the YMRS total score at weeks 3 and 12. The majority of patients in these trials taking SEROQUEL were dosed in a range between 400 and 800 mg per day.

Adjunct Therapy

In this 3-week placebo-controlled trial, 170 patients with acute bipolar mania (YMRS ≥ 20) were randomized to receive SEROQUEL or placebo as adjunct treatment to lithium or divalproex. Patients may or may not have received an adequate treatment course of lithium or divalproex prior to randomization. SEROQUEL was superior to placebo when added to lithium or divalproex alone in the reduction of YMRS total score.

The majority of patients in this trial taking SEROQUEL were dosed in a range between 400 and 800 mg per day. In a similarly designed trial (n=200), SEROQUEL was associated with an improvement in YMRS scores but did not demonstrate superiority to placebo, possibly due to a higher placebo effect.

Schizophrenia

The efficacy of SEROQUEL in the treatment of schizophrenia was established in 3 short-term (6-week) controlled trials of inpatients with schizophrenia who met DSM III-R criteria for schizophrenia. Although a single fixed dose haloperidol arm was included as a comparative treatment in one of the three trials, this single haloperidol dose group was inadequate to provide a reliable and valid comparison of SEROQUEL and haloperidol.

Several instruments were used for assessing psychiatric signs and symptoms in these studies, among them the Brief Psychiatric Rating Scale (BPRS), a multi-item inventory of general psychopathology traditionally used to evaluate the effects of drug treatment in schizophrenia. The BPRS psychosis cluster (conceptual disorganization, hallucinatory behavior, suspiciousness, and unusual thought content) is considered a particularly useful subset for assessing actively psychotic schizophrenic patients. A second traditional assessment, the Clinical Global Impression (CGI), reflects the impression of a skilled observer, fully familiar with the manifestations of schizophrenia, about the overall clinical state of the patient. In addition, the Scale for Assessing Negative Symptoms (SANS), a more recently developed but less well evaluated scale, was employed for assessing negative symptoms.

The results of the trials follow:

(1) In a 6-week, placebo-controlled trial (n=361) involving 5 fixed doses of SEROQUEL (75, 150, 300, 600 and 750 mg/day on a tid schedule), the 4 highest doses of SEROQUEL were generally superior to placebo on the BPRS total score, the BPRS psychosis cluster and the CGI severity score, with the maximal effect seen at 300 mg/day, and the effects of doses of 150 to 750 mg/day were generally indistinguishable. SEROQUEL, at a dose of 300 mg/day, was superior to placebo on the SANS.

(2) In a 6-week, placebo-controlled trial (n=286) involving titration of SEROQUEL in high (up to 750 mg/day on a tid schedule) and low (up to 250 mg/day on a tid schedule) doses, only the high dose SEROQUEL group (mean dose, 500 mg/day) was generally superior to placebo on the BPRS total score, the BPRS psychosis cluster, the CGI severity score, and the SANS.

(3) In a 6-week dose and dose regimen comparison trial (n=618) involving two fixed doses of SEROQUEL (450 mg/day on both bid and tid schedules and 50 mg/day on a bid schedule), only the 450 mg/day (225 mg bid schedule) dose group was generally superior to the 50 mg/day (25 mg bid) SEROQUEL dose group on the BPRS total score, the BPRS psychosis cluster, the CGI severity score, and on the SANS.

Examination of population subsets (race, gender, and age) did not reveal any differential responsiveness on the basis of race or gender, with an apparently greater effect in patients under the age of 40 compared to those older than 40. The clinical significance of this finding is unknown.

INDICATIONS AND USAGE

Bipolar Mania

SEROQUEL is indicated for the treatment of acute manic episodes associated with bipolar I disorder, as either monotherapy or adjunct therapy to lithium or divalproex.

The efficacy of SEROQUEL in acute bipolar mania was established in two 12-week monotherapy trials and one 3-week adjunct therapy trial of bipolar I patients initially hospitalized for up to 7 days for acute mania (See **CLINICAL PHARMACOLOGY**). Effectiveness has not been systematically evaluated in clinical trials for more than 12 weeks in monotherapy and 3 weeks in adjunct therapy. Therefore, the physician who elects to use SEROQUEL for extended periods should periodically reevaluate the long-term risks and benefits of the drug for the individual patient (See **DOSAGE AND ADMINISTRATION**).

Schizophrenia

SEROQUEL is indicated for the treatment of schizophrenia. The efficacy of SEROQUEL in schizophrenia was established in short-term (6-week) controlled trials of schizophrenic inpatients (See **CLINICAL PHARMACOLOGY**). The effectiveness of SEROQUEL in long-term use, that is, for more than 6 weeks, has not been systematically evaluated in controlled trials. Therefore, the physician who elects to use SEROQUEL for extended periods should periodically reevaluate the long-term usefulness of the drug for the individual patient (See **DOSAGE AND ADMINISTRATION**).

CONTRAINDICATIONS

SEROQUEL is contraindicated in individuals with a known hypersensitivity to this medication or any of its ingredients.

WARNINGS

Neuroleptic Malignant Syndrome (NMS)

A potentially fatal symptom complex sometimes referred to as Neuroleptic Malignant Syndrome (NMS) has been reported in association with administration of antipsychotic drugs, including SEROQUEL. Rare cases of NMS have been reported with SEROQUEL. Clinical manifestations of NMS are hyperpyrexia, muscle rigidity, altered mental status, and evidence of autonomic instability (irregular pulse or blood pressure, tachycardia, diaphoresis, and cardiac dysrhythmia). Additional signs may include elevated creatine phosphokinase, myoglobinuria (rhabdomyolysis) and acute renal failure.

The diagnostic evaluation of patients with this syndrome is complicated. In arriving at a diagnosis, it is important to exclude cases where the clinical presentation includes both serious medical illness (e.g., pneumonia, systemic infection, etc.) and untreated or inadequately treated extrapyramidal signs and symptoms (EPS). Other important considerations in the differential diagnosis include central anticholinergic toxicity, heat stroke, drug fever and primary central nervous system (CNS) pathology.

The management of NMS should include: 1) immediate discontinuation of antipsychotic drugs and other drugs not essential to concurrent therapy; 2) intensive symptomatic treatment and medical monitoring; and 3) treatment of any concomitant serious medical problems for which specific treatments are available. There is no general agreement about specific pharmacological treatment regimens for NMS.

If a patient requires antipsychotic drug treatment after recovery from NMS, the potential reintroduction of drug therapy should be carefully considered. The patient should be carefully monitored since recurrences of NMS have been reported.

Tardive Dyskinesia

A syndrome of potentially irreversible, involuntary, dyskinetic movements may develop in patients treated with antipsychotic drugs. Although the prevalence of the syndrome appears to be highest among the elderly, especially elderly women, it is impossible to rely upon prevalence estimates to predict, at the inception of antipsychotic treatment, which patients are likely to develop the syndrome. Whether antipsychotic drug products differ in their potential to cause tardive dyskinesia is unknown.

The risk of developing tardive dyskinesia and the likelihood that it will become irreversible are believed to increase as the duration of treatment and the total cumulative dose of antipsychotic drugs administered to the patient increase. However, the syndrome can develop, although much less commonly, after relatively brief treatment periods at low doses.

There is no known treatment for established cases of tardive dyskinesia, although the syndrome may remit, partially or completely, if antipsychotic treatment is withdrawn. Antipsychotic treatment, itself, however, may suppress (or partially suppress) the signs and symptoms of the syndrome and thereby may possibly mask the underlying process. The effect that symptomatic suppression has upon the long-term course of the syndrome is unknown.

Given these considerations, SEROQUEL should be prescribed in a manner that is most likely to minimize the occurrence of tardive dyskinesia. Chronic antipsychotic treatment should generally be reserved for patients who appear to suffer from a chronic illness that (1) is known to respond to antipsychotic drugs, and (2) for whom alternative, equally effective, but potentially less harmful treatments are not available or appropriate. In patients who do require chronic treatment, the smallest dose and the shortest duration of treatment producing a satisfactory clinical response should be sought. The need for continued treatment should be reassessed periodically.

If signs and symptoms of tardive dyskinesia appear in a patient on SEROQUEL, drug discontinuation should be considered. However, some patients may require treatment with SEROQUEL despite the presence of the syndrome.

Hyperglycemia and Diabetes Mellitus

Hyperglycemia, in some cases extreme and associated with ketoacidosis or hyperosmolar coma or death, has been reported in patients treated with atypical antipsychotics, including SEROQUEL. Assessment of the relationship between atypical antipsychotic use and glucose abnormalities is complicated by the possibility of an increased background risk of diabetes mellitus in patients with schizophrenia and the increasing incidence of diabetes mellitus in the general population. Given these confounders, the relationship between atypical antipsychotic use and hyperglycemia-related adverse events is not completely understood. However, epidemiological studies suggest an increased risk of treatment-emergent hyperglycemia-related adverse events in patients treated with the atypical antipsychotics. Precise risk estimates for hyperglycemia-related adverse events in patients treated with atypical antipsychotics are not available.

Patients with an established diagnosis of diabetes mellitus who are started on atypical antipsychotics should be monitored regularly for worsening of glucose control. Patients with risk factors for diabetes mellitus (eg, obesity, family history of diabetes) who are starting treatment with atypical antipsychotics should undergo fasting blood glucose testing at the beginning of treatment and periodically during treatment. Any patient treated with atypical antipsychotics should be monitored for symptoms of hyperglycemia including polydipsia, polyuria, polyphagia, and weakness. Patients who develop symptoms of hyperglycemia during treatment with atypical antipsychotics should undergo fasting blood glucose testing. In some cases, hyperglycemia has resolved when the atypical antipsychotic was discontinued; however, some patients required continuation of anti-diabetic treatment despite discontinuation of the suspect drug.

PRECAUTIONS

General:

Orthostatic Hypotension: SEROQUEL may induce orthostatic hypotension associated with dizziness, tachycardia and, in some patients, syncope, especially during the initial dose-titration period, probably reflecting its α_1-adrenergic antagonist properties. Syncope was reported in 1% (23/2567) of the patients treated with SEROQUEL, compared with 0% (0/607) on placebo and about 0.4% (2/527) on active control drugs.

SEROQUEL should be used with particular caution in patients with known cardiovascular disease (history of myocardial infarction or ischemic heart disease, heart failure or conduction abnormalities), cerebrovascular disease or conditions which would predispose patients to hypotension (dehydration, hypovolemia and treatment with antihypertensive medications). The risk of orthostatic hypotension and syncope may be minimized by limiting the initial dose to 25 mg bid (See **DOSAGE AND ADMINISTRATION**). If hypotension occurs during titration to the target dose, a return to the previous dose in the titration schedule is appropriate.

Cataracts: The development of cataracts was observed in association with quetiapine treatment in chronic dog studies (see Animal Toxicology). Lens changes have also been observed in patients during long-term SEROQUEL treatment, but a causal relationship to SEROQUEL use has not been established. Nevertheless, the possibility of lenticular changes cannot be excluded at this time. Therefore, examination of the lens by methods adequate to detect cataract formation, such as slit lamp exam or other appropriately sensitive methods, is recommended at initiation of treatment or shortly thereafter, and at 6 month intervals during chronic treatment.

Seizures: During clinical trials, seizures occurred in 0.6% (18/2792) of patients treated with SEROQUEL compared to 0.2% (1/607) on placebo and 0.7% (4/527) on active control drugs. As with other antipsychotics SEROQUEL should be used cautiously in patients with a history of seizures or with conditions that potentially lower the seizure threshold, e.g., Alzheimer's dementia. Conditions that lower the seizure threshold may be more prevalent in a population of 65 years or older.

Hypothyroidism: Clinical trials with SEROQUEL demonstrated a dose-related decrease in total and free thyroxine (T4) of approximately 20% at the higher end of the therapeutic dose range and was maximal in the first two to four weeks of treatment and maintained without adaptation or progression during more chronic therapy. Generally, these changes were of no clinical significance and TSH was unchanged in most patients, and levels of TBG were unchanged. In nearly all cases, cessation of SEROQUEL treatment was associated with a reversal of the effects on total and free T4, irrespective of the duration of treatment. About 0.4% (12/2791) of SEROQUEL patients did experience TSH increases in monotherapy studies. Six of the patients with TSH increases needed replacement thyroid treatment. In the mania adjunct studies, where SEROQUEL was added to lithium or divalproate, 12% (24/196) of SEROQUEL treated patients compared to 7% (15/203) of placebo treated patients had elevated TSH levels. Of the SEROQUEL treated patients with elevated TSH levels, 3 had simultaneous low free T4 levels.

Cholesterol and Triglyceride Elevations: In schizophrenia trials, SEROQUEL treated patients had increases from baseline in cholesterol and triglyceride of 11% and 17%, respectively, compared to slight decreases for placebo patients. These changes were only weakly related to the increases in weight observed in SEROQUEL treated patients.

Hyperprolactinemia: Although an elevation of prolactin levels was not demonstrated in clinical trials with SEROQUEL, increased prolactin levels were observed in rat studies with this compound, and were associated with an increase in mammary gland neoplasia in rats (see **Carcinogenesis**). Tissue culture experiments indicate that approximately one-third of human breast cancers are prolactin dependent *in vitro*, a factor of potential importance if the prescription of these drugs is contemplated in a patient with previously detected breast cancer. Although disturbances such as galactorrhea, amenorrhea, gynecomastia, and impotence have been reported with prolactin-elevating compounds, the clinical significance of elevated serum prolactin levels is unknown for most patients. Neither clinical studies nor epidemiologic studies conducted to date have shown an association between chronic administration of this class of drugs and tumorigenesis in humans; the available evidence is considered too limited to be conclusive at this time.

Transaminase Elevations: Asymptomatic, transient and reversible elevations in serum transaminases (primarily ALT) have been reported. In schizophrenia trials, the proportions of patients with transaminase elevations of > 3 times the upper limits of the normal reference range in a pool of 3- to 6-week placebo-controlled trials were approximately 6% for SEROQUEL compared to 1% for placebo. In acute bipolar mania trials, the proportions of patients with transaminase elevations of > 3 times the upper limits of the normal reference range in a pool of 3- to 12-week placebo-controlled trials were approximately 1% for both SEROQUEL and placebo. These hepatic enzyme elevations usually occurred within the first 3 weeks of drug treatment and promptly returned to pre-study levels with ongoing treatment with SEROQUEL.

Continued on next page

Seroquel—Cont.

Potential for Cognitive and Motor Impairment: Somnolence was a commonly reported adverse event reported in patients treated with SEROQUEL especially during the 3-5 day period of initial dose-titration. In schizophrenia trials, somnolence was reported in 18% of patients on SEROQUEL compared to 11% of placebo patients. In acute bipolar mania trials using SEROQUEL as monotherapy, somnolence was reported in 16% of patients on SEROQUEL compared to 4% of placebo patients. In acute bipolar mania trials using SEROQUEL as adjunct therapy, somnolence was reported in 34% of patients on SEROQUEL compared to 9% of placebo patients. Since SEROQUEL has the potential to impair judgment, thinking, or motor skills, patients should be cautioned about performing activities requiring mental alertness, such as operating a motor vehicle (including automobiles) or operating hazardous machinery until they are reasonably certain that SEROQUEL therapy does not affect them adversely.

Priapism: One case of priapism in a patient receiving SEROQUEL has been reported prior to market introduction. While a causal relationship to use of SEROQUEL has not been established, other drugs with alpha-adrenergic blocking effects have been reported to induce priapism, and it is possible that SEROQUEL may share this capacity. Severe priapism may require surgical intervention.

Body Temperature Regulation: Although not reported with SEROQUEL, disruption of the body's ability to reduce core body temperature has been attributed to antipsychotic agents. Appropriate care is advised when prescribing SEROQUEL for patients who will be experiencing conditions which may contribute to an elevation in core body temperature, e.g., exercising strenuously, exposure to extreme heat, receiving concomitant medication with anticholinergic activity, or being subject to dehydration.

Dysphagia: Esophageal dysmotility and aspiration have been associated with antipsychotic drug use. Aspiration pneumonia is a common cause of morbidity and mortality in elderly patients, in particular those with advanced Alzheimer's dementia. SEROQUEL and other antipsychotic drugs should be used cautiously in patients at risk for aspiration pneumonia.

Suicide: The possibility of a suicide attempt is inherent in bipolar disorder and schizophrenia: close supervision of high risk patients should accompany drug therapy. Prescriptions for SEROQUEL should be written for the smallest quantity of tablets consistent with good patient management in order to reduce the risk of overdose.

Use in Patients with Concomitant Illness: Clinical experience with SEROQUEL in patients with certain concomitant systemic illnesses (see Renal Impairment and Hepatic Impairment under **CLINICAL PHARMACOLOGY**, Special Populations) is limited.

SEROQUEL has not been evaluated or used to any appreciable extent in patients with a recent history of myocardial infarction or unstable heart disease. Patients with these diagnoses were excluded from premarketing clinical studies. Because of the risk of orthostatic hypotension with SEROQUEL, caution should be observed in cardiac patients (see **Orthostatic Hypotension**).

Information for Patients

Physicians are advised to discuss the following issues with patients for whom they prescribe SEROQUEL.

Orthostatic Hypotension: Patients should be advised of the risk of orthostatic hypotension, especially during the 3-5 day period of initial dose titration, and also at times of re-initiating treatment or increases in dose.

Interference with Cognitive and Motor Performance: Since somnolence was a commonly reported adverse event associated with SEROQUEL treatment, patients should be advised of the risk of somnolence, especially during the 3-5 day period of initial dose titration. Patients should be cautioned about performing any activity requiring mental alertness, such as operating a motor vehicle (including automobiles) or operating hazardous machinery, until they are reasonably certain that SEROQUEL therapy does not affect them adversely.

Pregnancy: Patients should be advised to notify their physician if they become pregnant or intend to become pregnant during therapy.

Nursing: Patients should be advised not to breast feed if they are taking SEROQUEL.

Concomitant Medication: As with other medications, patients should be advised to notify their physicians if they are taking, or plan to take, any prescription or over-the-counter drugs.

Alcohol: Patients should be advised to avoid consuming alcoholic beverages while taking SEROQUEL.

Heat Exposure and Dehydration: Patients should be advised regarding appropriate care in avoiding overheating and dehydration.

Laboratory Tests

No specific laboratory tests are recommended.

Drug Interactions

The risks of using SEROQUEL in combination with other drugs have not been extensively evaluated in systematic studies. Given the primary CNS effects of SEROQUEL, caution should be used when it is taken in combination with other centrally acting drugs. SEROQUEL potentiated the cognitive and motor effects of alcohol in a clinical trial in subjects with selected psychotic disorders, and alcoholic beverages should be avoided while taking SEROQUEL.

Because of its potential for inducing hypotension, SEROQUEL may enhance the effects of certain antihypertensive agents.

SEROQUEL may antagonize the effects of levodopa and dopamine agonists.

The Effect of Other Drugs on Quetiapine

Phenytoin: Coadministration of quetiapine (250 mg tid) and phenytoin (100 mg tid) increased the mean oral clearance of quetiapine by 5-fold. Increased doses of SEROQUEL may be required to maintain control of symptoms of schizophrenia in patients receiving quetiapine and phenytoin, or other hepatic enzyme inducers (e.g., carbamazepine, barbiturates, rifampin, glucocorticoids). Caution should be taken if phenytoin is withdrawn and replaced with a non-inducer (e.g., valproate) (see **DOSAGE AND ADMINISTRATION**).

Divalproex: Coadministration of quetiapine (150 mg bid) and divalproex (500 mg bid) increased the mean maximum plasma concentration of quetiapine at steady state by 17% without affecting the extent of absorption or mean oral clearance.

Thioridazine: Thioridazine (200 mg bid) increased the oral clearance of quetiapine (300 mg bid) by 65%.

Cimetidine: Administration of multiple daily doses of cimetidine (400 mg tid for 4 days) resulted in a 20% decrease in the mean oral clearance of quetiapine (150 mg tid). Dosage adjustment for quetiapine is not required when it is given with cimetidine.

P450 3A Inhibitors: Coadministration of ketoconazole (200 mg once daily for 4 days), a potent inhibitor of cytochrome P450 3A, reduced oral clearance of quetiapine by 84%, resulting in a 335% increase in maximum plasma concentration of quetiapine. Caution is indicated when SEROQUEL is administered with ketoconazole and other inhibitors of cytochrome P450 3A (e.g., itraconazole, fluconazole, and erythromycin).

Fluoxetine, Imipramine, Haloperidol, and Risperidone: Coadministration of fluoxetine (60 mg once daily); imipramine (75 mg bid), haloperidol (7.5 mg bid), or risperidone (3 mg bid) with quetiapine (300 mg bid) did not alter the steady-state pharmacokinetics of quetiapine.

Effect of Quetiapine on Other Drugs

Lorazepam: The mean oral clearance of lorazepam (2 mg, single dose) was reduced by 20% in the presence of quetiapine administered as 250 mg tid dosing.

Divalproex: The mean maximum concentration and extent of absorption of total and free valproic acid at steady state were decreased by 10 to 12% when divalproex (500 mg bid) was administered with quetiapine (150 mg bid). The mean oral clearance of total valproic acid (administered as divalproex 500 mg bid) was increased by 11% in the presence of quetiapine (150 mg bid). The changes were not significant.

Lithium: Concomitant administration of quetiapine (250 mg tid) with lithium had no effect on any of the steady-state pharmacokinetic parameters of lithium.

Antipyrine: Administration of multiple daily doses up to 750 mg/day (on a tid schedule) of quetiapine to subjects with selected psychotic disorders had no clinically relevant effect on the clearance of antipyrine or urinary recovery of antipyrine metabolites. These results indicate that quetiapine does not significantly induce hepatic enzymes responsible for cytochrome P450 mediated metabolism of antipyrine.

Carcinogenesis, Mutagenesis, Impairment of Fertility

Carcinogenesis: Carcinogenicity studies were conducted in C57BL mice and Wistar rats. Quetiapine was administered in the diet to mice at doses of 20, 75, 250, and 750 mg/kg and to rats by gavage at doses of 25, 75, and 250 mg/kg for two years. These doses are equivalent to 0.1, 0.5, 1.5, and 4.5 times the maximum human dose (800 mg/day) on a mg/m^2 basis (mice) or 0.3, 0.9, and 3.0 times the maximum human dose on a mg/m^2 basis (rats). There were statistically significant increases in thyroid gland follicular adenomas in male mice at doses of 250 and 750 mg/kg or 1.5 and 4.5 times the maximum human dose on a mg/m^2 basis and in male rats at a dose of 250 mg/kg or 3.0 times the maximum human dose on a mg/m^2 basis. Mammary gland adenocarcinomas were statistically significantly increased in female rats at all doses tested (25, 75, and 250 mg/kg or 0.3, 0.9, and 3.0 times the maximum recommended human dose on a mg/m^2 basis).

Thyroid follicular cell adenomas may have resulted from chronic stimulation of the thyroid gland by thyroid stimulating hormone (TSH) resulting from enhanced metabolism and clearance of thyroxine by rodent liver. Changes in TSH, thyroxine, and thyroxine clearance consistent with this mechanism were observed in subchronic toxicity studies in rat and mouse and in a 1-year toxicity study in rat; however, the results of these studies were not definitive. The relevance of the increases in thyroid follicular cell adenomas to human risk, through whatever mechanism, is unknown.

Antipsychotic drugs have been shown to chronically elevate prolactin levels in rodents. Serum measurements in a 1-yr toxicity study showed that quetiapine increased median serum prolactin levels a maximum of 32- and 13-fold in male and female rats, respectively. Increases in mammary neoplasms have been found in rodents after chronic administration of other antipsychotic drugs and are considered to be prolactin-mediated. The relevance of this increased incidence of prolactin-mediated mammary gland tumors in rats to human risk is unknown (see Hyperprolactinemia in **PRECAUTIONS, General**).

Mutagenesis: The mutagenic potential of quetiapine was tested in six *in vitro* bacterial gene mutation assays and in an *in vitro* mammalian gene mutation assay in Chinese Hamster Ovary cells. However, sufficiently high concentrations of quetiapine may not have been used for all tester strains. Quetiapine did produce a reproducible increase in mutations in one *Salmonella typhimurium* tester strain in the presence of metabolic activation. No evidence of clastogenic potential was obtained in an *in vitro* chromosomal aberration assay in cultured human lymphocytes or in the *in vivo* micronucleus assay in rats.

Impairment of Fertility: Quetiapine decreased mating and fertility in male Sprague-Dawley rats at oral doses of 50 and 150 mg/kg or 0.6 and 1.8 times the maximum human dose on a mg/m^2 basis. Drug-related effects included increases in interval to mate and in the number of matings required for successful impregnation. These effects continued to be observed at 150 mg/kg even after a two-week period without treatment. The no-effect dose for impaired mating and fertility in male rats was 25 mg/kg, or 0.3 times the maximum human dose on a mg/m^2 basis. Quetiapine adversely affected mating and fertility in female Sprague-Dawley rats at an oral dose of 50 mg/kg, or 0.6 times the maximum human dose on a mg/m^2 basis. Drug-related effects included decreases in matings and in matings resulting in pregnancy, and an increase in the interval to mate. An increase in irregular estrus cycles was observed at doses of 10 and 50 mg/kg, or 0.1 and 0.6 times the maximum human dose on a mg/m^2 basis. The no-effect dose in female rats was 1 mg/kg, or 0.01 times the maximum human dose on a mg/m^2 basis.

Pregnancy

Pregnancy Category C:

The teratogenic potential of quetiapine was studied in Wistar rats and Dutch Belted rabbits dosed during the period of organogenesis. No evidence of a teratogenic effect was detected in rats at doses of 25 to 200 mg/kg or 0.3 to 2.4 times the maximum human dose on a mg/m^2 basis or in rabbits at 25 to 100 mg/kg or 0.6 to 2.4 times the maximum human dose on a mg/m^2 basis. There was, however, evidence of embryo/fetal toxicity. Delays in skeletal ossification were detected in rat fetuses at doses of 50 and 200 mg/kg (0.6 and 2.4 times the maximum human dose on a mg/m^2 basis) and in rabbits at 50 and 100 mg/kg (1.2 and 2.4 times the maximum human dose on a mg/m^2 basis). Fetal body weight was reduced in rat fetuses at 200 mg/kg and rabbit fetuses at 100 mg/kg (2.4 times the maximum human dose on a mg/m^2 basis for both species). There was an increased incidence of a minor soft tissue anomaly (carpal/tarsal flexure) in rabbit fetuses at a dose of 100 mg/kg (2.4 times the maximum human dose on a mg/m^2 basis). Evidence of maternal toxicity (i.e., decreases in body weight gain and/or death) was observed at the high dose in the rat study and at all doses in the rabbit study. In a peri/postnatal reproductive study in rats, no drug-related effects were observed at doses of 1, 10, and 20 mg/kg or 0.01, 0.12, and 0.24 times the maximum human dose on a mg/m^2 basis. However, in a preliminary peri/postnatal study, there were increases in fetal and pup death, and decreases in mean litter weight at 150 mg/kg, or 3.0 times the maximum human dose on a mg/m^2 basis.

There are no adequate and well-controlled studies in pregnant women and quetiapine should be used during pregnancy only if the potential benefit justifies the potential risk to the fetus.

Labor and Delivery: The effect of SEROQUEL on labor and delivery in humans is unknown.

Nursing Mothers: SEROQUEL was excreted in milk of treated animals during lactation. It is not known if SEROQUEL is excreted in human milk. It is recommended that women receiving SEROQUEL should not breast feed.

Pediatric Use: The safety and effectiveness of SEROQUEL in pediatric patients have not been established.

Geriatric Use: Of the approximately 3400 patients in clinical studies with SEROQUEL, 7% (232) were 65 years of age or over. In general, there was no indication of any different tolerability of SEROQUEL in the elderly compared to younger adults. Nevertheless, the presence of factors that might decrease pharmacokinetic clearance, increase the pharmacodynamic response to SEROQUEL, or cause poorer tolerance or orthostasis, should lead to consideration of a lower starting dose, slower titration, and careful monitoring during the initial dosing period in the elderly. The mean plasma clearance of SEROQUEL was reduced by 30% to 50% in elderly patients when compared to younger patients (see Pharmacokinetics under **CLINICAL PHARMACOLOGY** and **DOSAGE AND ADMINISTRATION**).

ADVERSE REACTIONS

The information below is derived from a clinical trial database for SEROQUEL consisting of over 3000 patients. This database includes 405 patients exposed to SEROQUEL for the treatment of acute bipolar mania (monotherapy and adjunct therapy) and approximately 2600 patients and/or normal subjects exposed to 1 or more doses of SEROQUEL for the treatment of schizophrenia.

Of these approximately 3000 subjects, approximately 2700 (2300 in schizophrenia and 405 in acute bipolar mania) were patients who participated in multiple dose effectiveness trials, and their experience corresponded to approximately 914.3 patient-years. The conditions and duration of treatment with SEROQUEL varied greatly and included (in overlapping categories) open-label and double-blind phases of studies, inpatients and outpatients, fixed-dose and dose-titration studies, and short-term or longer-term exposure. Adverse reactions were assessed by collecting adverse events, results of physical examinations, vital signs, weights, laboratory analyses, ECGs, and results of ophthalmologic examinations.

Adverse events during exposure were obtained by general inquiry and recorded by clinical investigators using terminology of their own choosing. Consequently, it is not possible to provide a meaningful estimate of the proportion of individuals experiencing adverse events without first grouping similar types of events into a smaller number of standardized event categories. In the tables and tabulations that follow, standard COSTART terminology has been used to classify reported adverse events.

The stated frequencies of adverse events represent the proportion of individuals who experienced, at least once, a treatment-emergent adverse event of the type listed. An event was considered treatment emergent if it occurred for the first time or worsened while receiving therapy following baseline evaluation.

Adverse Findings Observed in Short-Term, Controlled Trials

Adverse Events Associated with Discontinuation of Treatment in Short-Term, Placebo-Controlled Trials

Bipolar Mania: Overall, discontinuations due to adverse events were 5.7% for SEROQUEL vs. 5.1% for placebo in monotherapy and 3.6% for SEROQUEL vs. 5.9% for placebo in adjunct therapy.

Schizophrenia: Overall, there was little difference in the incidence of discontinuation due to adverse events (4% for SEROQUEL vs. 3% for placebo) in a pool of controlled trials. However, discontinuations due to somnolence and hypotension were considered to be drug related (see **PRECAUTIONS**):

Adverse Event	SEROQUEL	Placebo
Somnolence	0.8%	0%
Hypotension	0.4%	0%

Adverse Events Occurring at an Incidence of 1% or More Among SEROQUEL Treated Patients in Short-Term, Placebo-Controlled Trials: The prescriber should be aware that the figures in the tables and tabulations cannot be used to predict the incidence of side effects in the course of usual medical practice where patient characteristics and other factors differ from those that prevailed in the clinical trials. Similarly, the cited frequencies cannot be compared with figures obtained from other clinical investigations involving different treatments, uses, and investigators. The cited figures, however, do provide the prescribing physician with some basis for estimating the relative contribution of drug and nondrug factors to the side effect incidence in the population studied.

Table 1 enumerates the incidence, rounded to the nearest percent, of treatment-emergent adverse events that occurred during acute therapy of schizophrenia (up to 6 weeks) and bipolar mania (up to 12 weeks) in 1% or more of patients treated with SEROQUEL (doses ranging from 75 to 800 mg/day) where the incidence in patients treated with SEROQUEL was greater than the incidence in placebo-treated patients.

Table 1. Treatment-Emergent Adverse Experience Incidence in 3- to 12-Week Placebo-Controlled Clinical Trials[1] for the Treatment of Schizophrenia and Bipolar Mania (monotherapy)

Body System/ Preferred Term	SEROQUEL (n=719)	Placebo (n=404)
Body as a Whole		
Headache	21%	14%
Pain	7%	5%
Asthenia	5%	3%
Abdominal Pain	4%	1%
Back Pain	3%	1%
Fever	2%	1%
Cardiovascular		
Tachycardia	6%	4%
Postural Hypotension	4%	1%
Digestive		
Dry Mouth	9%	3%
Constipation	8%	3%
Vomiting	6%	5%
Dyspepsia	5%	1%
Gastroenteritis	2%	0%
Gamma Glutamyl Transpeptidase Increased	1%	0%
Metabolic and Nutritional		
Weight Gain	5%	1%
SGPT Increased	5%	1%
SGOT Increased	3%	1%
Nervous		
Agitation	20%	17%
Somnolence	18%	8%
Dizziness	11%	5%
Anxiety	4%	3%
Respiratory System		
Pharyngitis	4%	3%
Rhinitis	3%	1%
Skin and Appendages		
Rash	4%	2%
Special Senses		
Amblyopia	2%	1%

[1] Events for which the SEROQUEL incidence was equal to or less than placebo are not listed in the table, but included the following: accidental injury, akathisia, chest pain, cough increased, depression, diarrhea, extrapyramidal syndrome, hostility, hypertension, hypertonia, hypotension, increased appetite, infection, insomnia, leukopenia, malaise, nausea, nervousness, paresthesia, peripheral edema, sweating, tremor, and weight loss.

In these studies, the most commonly observed adverse events associated with the use of SEROQUEL (incidence of 5% or greater) and observed at a rate on SEROQUEL at least twice that of placebo were somnolence (18%), dizziness (11%), dry mouth (9%), constipation (8%), SGPT increased (5%), weight gain (5%), and dyspepsia (5%).

Table 2 enumerates the incidence, rounded to the nearest percent, of treatment-emergent adverse events that occurred during therapy (up to 3-weeks) of acute mania in 5% or more of patients treated with SEROQUEL (doses ranging from 100 to 800 mg/day) used as adjunct therapy to lithium and divalproex where the incidence in patients treated with SEROQUEL was greater than the incidence in placebo-treated patients.

Table 2. Treatment-Emergent Adverse Experience Incidence in 3-Week Placebo-Controlled Clinical Trials[1] for the Treatment of Bipolar Mania (Adjunct Therapy)

Body System/ Preferred Term	SEROQUEL (n=196)	Placebo (n=203)
Body as a Whole		
Headache	17%	13%
Asthenia	10%	4%
Abdominal Pain	7%	3%
Back Pain	5%	3%
Cardiovascular		
Postural Hypotension	7%	2%
Digestive		
Dry Mouth	19%	3%
Constipation	10%	5%
Metabolic and Nutritional		
Weight Gain	6%	3%
Nervous		
Somnolence	34%	9%
Dizziness	9%	6%
Tremor	8%	7%
Agitation	6%	4%
Respiratory		
Pharyngitis	6%	3%

[1] Events for which the SEROQUEL incidence was equal to or less than placebo are not listed in the table, but included the following: akathisia, diarrhea, insomnia, and nausea.

In these studies, the most commonly observed adverse events associated with the use of SEROQUEL (incidence of 5% or greater) and observed at a rate on SEROQUEL at least twice that of placebo were somnolence (34%), dry mouth (19%), asthenia (10%), constipation (10%), abdominal pain (7%), postural hypotension (7%), pharyngitis (6%), and weight gain (6%).

Explorations for interactions on the basis of gender, age, and race did not reveal any clinically meaningful differences in the adverse event occurrence on the basis of these demographic factors.

Dose Dependency of Adverse Events in Short-Term, Placebo-Controlled Trials

Dose-related Adverse Events: Spontaneously elicited adverse event data from a study of schizophrenia comparing five fixed doses of SEROQUEL (75 mg, 150 mg, 300 mg, 600 mg, and 750 mg/day) to placebo were explored for dose-relatedness of adverse events. Logistic regression analyses revealed a positive dose response ($p<0.05$) for the following adverse events: dyspepsia, abdominal pain, and weight gain.

Extrapyramidal Symptoms: Data from one 6-week clinical trial of schizophrenia comparing five fixed doses of SEROQUEL (75, 150, 300, 600, 750 mg/day) provided evidence for the lack of treatment-emergent extrapyramidal symptoms (EPS) and dose-relatedness for EPS associated with SEROQUEL treatment. Three methods were used to measure EPS: (1) Simpson-Angus total score (mean change from baseline) which evaluates parkinsonism and akathisia, (2) incidence of spontaneous complaints of EPS (akathisia, akinesia, cogwheel rigidity, extrapyramidal syndrome, hypertonia, hypokinesia, neck rigidity, and tremor), and (3) use of anticholinergic medications to treat emergent EPS.

		SEROQUEL				
Dose Groups	Placebo	75 mg	150 mg	300 mg	600 mg	750 mg
Parkinsonism	0.6	-1.0	-1.2	-1.6	-1.8	-1.8
EPS incidence	16%	6%	6%	4%	8%	6%
Anticholinergic Medications	14%	11%	10%	8%	12%	11%

In six additional placebo-controlled clinical trials trials (3 in acute mania and 3 in schizophrenia) using variable doses of SEROQUEL, there were no differences between the SEROQUEL and placebo treatment groups in the incidence of EPS, as assessed by Simpson-Angus total scores, spontaneous complaints of EPS and the use of concomitant anticholinergic medications to treat EPS.

Vital Signs and Laboratory Studies

Vital Sign Changes: SEROQUEL is associated with orthostatic hypotension (see **PRECAUTIONS**).

Weight Gain: In schizophrenia trials the proportions of patients meeting a weight gain criterion of ≥7% of body weight were compared in a pool of four 3- to 6-week placebo-controlled clinical trials, revealing a statistically significantly greater incidence of weight gain for SEROQUEL (23%) compared to placebo (6%). In mania monotherapy trials the proportions of patients meeting the same weight gain criterion were 21% compared to 7% for placebo and in mania adjunct therapy trials the proportion of patients meeting the same weight criterion were 13% compared to 4% for placebo.

Laboratory Changes: An assessment of the premarketing experience for SEROQUEL suggested that it is associated with asymptomatic increases in SGPT and increases in both total cholesterol and triglycerides (see **PRECAUTIONS**).

An assessment of hematological parameters in short-term, placebo-controlled trials revealed no clinically important differences between SEROQUEL and placebo.

ECG Changes: Between group comparisons for pooled placebo-controlled trials revealed no statistically significant SEROQUEL/placebo differences in the proportions of patients experiencing potentially important changes in ECG parameters, including QT, QTc, and PR intervals. However, the proportions of patients meeting the criteria for tachycardia were compared in four 3- to 6-week placebo-controlled clinical trials for the treatment of schizophrenia revealing a 1% (4/399) incidence for SEROQUEL compared to 0.6% (1/156) incidence for placebo. In acute (monotherapy) bipolar mania trials the proportions of patients meeting the criteria for tachycardia was 0.5% (1/192) for SEROQUEL compared to 0% (0/178) incidence for placebo. In acute bipolar mania (adjunct) trials the proportions of patients meeting the same criteria was 0.6% (1/166) for SEROQUEL compared to 0% (0/171) incidence for placebo. SEROQUEL use was associated with a mean increase in heart rate, assessed by ECG, of 7 beats per minute compared to a mean increase of 1 beat per minute among placebo patients. This slight tendency to tachycardia may be related to SEROQUEL's potential for inducing orthostatic changes (see **PRECAUTIONS**).

Other Adverse Events Observed During the Pre-Marketing Evaluation of SEROQUEL

Following is a list of COSTART terms that reflect treatment-emergent adverse events as defined in the introduction to the ADVERSE REACTIONS section reported by patients treated with SEROQUEL at multiple doses ≥ 75 mg/day during any phase of a trial within the premarketing database of approximately 2200 patients treated for schizophrenia. All reported events are included except those already listed in Table 1 or elsewhere in labeling, those events for which a drug cause was remote, and those event terms which were so general as to be uninformative. It is important to emphasize that, although the events reported occurred during treatment with SEROQUEL, they were not necessarily caused by it.

Events are further categorized by body system and listed in order of decreasing frequency according to the following definitions: frequent adverse events are those occurring in at least 1/100 patients (only those not already listed in the tabulated results from placebo-controlled trials appear in this listing); infrequent adverse events are those occurring in 1/100 to 1/1000 patients; rare events are those occurring in fewer than 1/1000 patients.

Nervous System: ***Frequent:*** hypertonia, dysarthria; ***Infrequent:*** abnormal dreams, dyskinesia, thinking abnormal, tardive dyskinesia, vertigo, involuntary movements, confusion, amnesia, psychosis, hallucinations, hyperkinesia, libido increased*, urinary retention, incoordination, paranoid reaction, abnormal gait, myoclonus, delusions, manic reaction, apathy, ataxia, depersonalization, stupor, bruxism, catatonic reaction, hemiplegia; ***Rare:*** aphasia, buccoglossal syndrome, choreoathetosis, delirium, emotional lability, euphoria, libido decreased*, neuralgia, stuttering, subdural hematoma.

Body as a Whole: ***Frequent:*** flu syndrome; ***Infrequent:*** neck pain, pelvic pain*, suicide attempt, malaise, photosensitivity reaction, chills, face edema, moniliasis; ***Rare:*** abdomen enlarged.

Digestive System: ***Frequent:*** anorexia; ***Infrequent:*** increased salivation, increased appetite, gamma glutamyl transpeptidase increased, gingivitis, dysphagia, flatulence, gastroenteritis, gastritis, hemorrhoids, stomatitis, thirst, tooth caries, fecal incontinence, gastroesophageal reflux, gum hemorrhage, mouth ulceration, rectal hemorrhage, tongue edema; ***Rare:*** glossitis, hematemesis, intestinal obstruction, melena, pancreatitis.

Cardiovascular System: ***Frequent:*** palpitation; ***Infrequent:*** vasodilatation, QT interval prolonged, migraine, bradycardia, cerebral ischemia, irregular pulse, T wave abnormality, bundle branch block, cerebrovascular accident, deep thrombophlebitis, T wave inversion; ***Rare:*** angina pectoris, atrial fibrillation, AV block first degree, congestive heart failure, ST elevated, thrombophlebitis, T wave flattening, ST abnormality, increased QRS duration.

Respiratory System: ***Frequent:*** pharyngitis, rhinitis, cough increased, dyspnea; ***Infrequent:*** pneumonia, epistaxis, asthma; ***Rare:*** hiccup, hyperventilation.

Metabolic and Nutritional System: ***Frequent:*** peripheral edema; ***Infrequent:*** weight loss, alkaline phosphatase increased, hyperlipemia, alcohol intolerance, dehydration, hyperglycemia, creatinine increased, hypoglycemia; ***Rare:*** glycosuria, gout, hand edema, hypokalemia, water intoxication.

Skin and Appendages System: ***Frequent:*** sweating; ***Infrequent:*** pruritis, acne, eczema, contact dermatitis, maculopapular rash, seborrhea, skin ulcer; ***Rare:*** exfoliative dermatitis, psoriasis, skin discoloration.

Continued on next page

Seroquel—Cont.

Urogenital System: ***Infrequent:*** dysmenorrhea*, vaginitis*, urinary incontinence, metrorrhagia*, impotence*, dysuria, vaginal moniliasis*, abnormal ejaculation*, cystitis, urinary frequency, amenorrhea*, female lactation*, leukorrhea*, vaginal hemorrhage*, vulvovaginitis* orchitis*; ***Rare:*** gynecomastia*, nocturia, polyuria, acute kidney failure.

Special Senses: ***Infrequent:*** conjunctivitis, abnormal vision, dry eyes, tinnitus, taste perversion, blepharitis, eye pain; ***Rare:*** abnormality of accommodation, deafness, glaucoma.

Musculoskeletal System: ***Infrequent:*** pathological fracture, myasthenia, twitching, arthralgia, arthritis, leg cramps, bone pain.

Hemic and Lymphatic System: ***Frequent:*** leukopenia; ***Infrequent:*** leukocytosis, anemia, ecchymosis, eosinophilia, hypochromic anemia; lymphadenopathy, cyanosis; ***Rare:*** hemolysis, thrombocytopenia.

Endocrine System: ***Infrequent:*** hypothyroidism, diabetes mellitus; ***Rare:*** hyperthyroidism.

---

*adjusted for gender

Post Marketing Experience: Adverse events reported since market introduction which were temporally related to SEROQUEL therapy include: leukopenia/neutropenia. If a patient develops a low white cell count consider discontinuation of therapy. Possible risk factors for leukopenia/neutropenia include pre-existing low white cell count and history of drug induced leukopenia/neutropenia.

Other adverse events reported since market introduction, which were temporally related to SEROQUEL therapy, but not necessarily causally related, include the following: agranulocytosis, anaphylaxis, hyponatremia, rhabdomyolysis, syndrome of inappropriate antidiuretic hormone secretion (SIADH), and Steven Johnson syndrome (SJS).

DRUG ABUSE AND DEPENDENCE

Controlled Substance Class: SEROQUEL is not a controlled substance.

Physical and Psychologic dependence: SEROQUEL has not been systematically studied, in animals or humans, for its potential for abuse, tolerance or physical dependence. While the clinical trials did not reveal any tendency for any drug-seeking behavior, these observations were not systematic and it is not possible to predict on the basis of this limited experience the extent to which a CNS-active drug will be misused, diverted, and/or abused once marketed. Consequently, patients should be evaluated carefully for a history of drug abuse, and such patients should be observed closely for signs of misuse or abuse of SEROQUEL, e.g., development of tolerance, increases in dose, drug-seeking behavior.

OVERDOSAGE

Human experience: Experience with SEROQUEL (quetiapine fumarate) in acute overdosage was limited in the clinical trial database (6 reports) with estimated doses ranging from 1200 mg to 9600 mg and no fatalities. In general, reported signs and symptoms were those resulting from an exaggeration of the drug's known pharmacological effects, i.e., drowsiness and sedation, tachycardia and hypotension. One case, involving an estimated overdose of 9600 mg, was associated with hypokalemia and first degree heart block. In post-marketing experience, there have been very rare reports of overdose of SEROQUEL alone resulting in death, coma or QTc prolongation.

Management of Overdosage: In case of acute overdosage, establish and maintain an airway and ensure adequate oxygenation and ventilation. Gastric lavage (after intubation, if patient is unconscious) and administration of activated charcoal together with a laxative should be considered. The possibility of obtundation, seizure or dystonic reaction of the head and neck following overdose may create a risk of aspiration with induced emesis. Cardiovascular monitoring should commence immediately and should include continuous electrocardiographic monitoring to detect possible arrhythmias. If antiarrhythmic therapy is administered, disopyramide, procainamide and quinidine carry a theoretical hazard of additive QT-prolonging effects when administered in patients with acute overdosage of SEROQUEL. Similarly it is reasonable to expect that the alpha-adrenergic-blocking properties of bretylium might be additive to those of quetiapine, resulting in problematic hypotension.

There is no specific antidote to SEROQUEL. Therefore appropriate supportive measures should be instituted. The possibility of multiple drug involvement should be considered. Hypotension and circulatory collapse should be treated with appropriate measures such as intravenous fluids and/or sympathomimetic agents (epinephrine and dopamine should not be used, since beta stimulation may worsen hypotension in the setting of quetiapine-induced alpha blockade). In cases of severe extrapyramidal symptoms, anticholinergic medication should be administered. Close medical supervision and monitoring should continue until the patient recovers.

DOSAGE AND ADMINISTRATION

Bipolar Mania

Usual Dose: When used as monotherapy or adjunct therapy (with lithium or divalproex), SEROQUEL should be initiated in BID doses totaling 100 mg/day on Day 1, increased to 400 mg/day on Day 4 in increments of up to 100 mg/day in BID divided doses. Further dosage adjustments up to 800 mg/day by Day 6 should be in increments of no greater than 200 mg/day. Data indicates that the majority of patients responded between 400 to 800 mg/day. The safety of doses above 800 mg/day has not been evaluated in clinical trials.

Schizophrenia

Usual Dose: SEROQUEL should generally be administered with an initial dose of 25 mg bid, with increases in increments of 25-50 mg bid or tid on the second and third day, as tolerated, to a target dose range of 300 to 400 mg daily by the fourth day, given bid or tid. Further dosage adjustments, if indicated, should generally occur at intervals of not less than 2 days, as steady state for SEROQUEL would not be achieved for approximately 1-2 days in the typical patient. When dosage adjustments are necessary, dose increments/decrements of 25-50 mg bid are recommended. Most efficacy data with SEROQUEL were obtained using tid regimens, but in one controlled trial 225 mg bid was also effective.

Efficacy in schizophrenia was demonstrated in a dose range of 150 to 750 mg/day in the clinical trials supporting the effectiveness of SEROQUEL. In a dose response study, doses above 300 mg/day were not demonstrated to be more efficacious than the 300 mg/day dose. In other studies, however, doses in the range of 400-500 mg/day appeared to be needed. The safety of doses above 800 mg/day has not been evaluated in clinical trials.

Dosing in Special Populations

Consideration should be given to a slower rate of dose titration and a lower target dose in the elderly and in patients who are debilitated or who have a predisposition to hypotensive reactions (see **CLINICAL PHARMACOLOGY**). When indicated, dose escalation should be performed with caution in these patients.

Patients with hepatic impairment should be started on 25 mg/day. The dose should be increased daily in increments of 25-50 mg/day to an effective dose, depending on the clinical response and tolerability of the patient.

The elimination of quetiapine was enhanced in the presence of phenytoin. Higher maintenance doses of quetiapine may be required when it is coadministered with phenytoin and other enzyme inducers such as carbamazepine and phenobarbital (See Drug Interactions under **PRECAUTIONS**).

Maintenance Treatment: While there is no body of evidence available to answer the question of how long the patient treated with SEROQUEL should remain on it, the effectiveness of maintenance treatment is well established for many other drugs used to treat schizophrenia. It is recommended that responding patients be continued on SEROQUEL, but at the lowest dose needed to maintain remission. Patients should be periodically reassessed to determine the need for maintenance treatment.

Reinitiation of Treatment in Patients Previously Discontinued: Although there are no data to specifically address reinitiation of treatment, it is recommended that when restarting patients who have had an interval of less than one week off SEROQUEL, titration of SEROQUEL is not required and the maintenance dose may be reinitiated. When restarting therapy of patients who have been off SEROQUEL for more than one week, the initial titration schedule should be followed.

Switching from Antipsychotics: There are no systematically collected data to specifically address switching patients with schizophrenia from antipsychotics to SEROQUEL, or concerning concomitant administration with antipsychotics. While immediate discontinuation of the previous antipsychotic treatment may be acceptable for some patients with schizophrenia, more gradual discontinuation may be most appropriate for others. In all cases, the period of overlapping antipsychotic administration should be minimized. When switching patients with schizophrenia from depot antipsychotics, if medically appropriate, initiate SEROQUEL therapy in place of the next scheduled injection. The need for continuing existing EPS medication should be reevaluated periodically.

HOW SUPPLIED

25 mg Tablets (NDC 0310-0275) peach, round, biconvex, film coated tablets, identified with 'SEROQUEL' and '25' on one side and plain on the other side, are supplied in bottles of 100 tablets and 1000 tablets, and hospital unit dose packages of 100 tablets.

100 mg Tablets (NDC 0310-0271) yellow, round, biconvex film coated tablets, identified with 'SEROQUEL' and '100' on one side and plain on the other side, are supplied in bottles of 100 tablets and hospital unit dose packages of 100 tablets.

200 mg Tablets (NDC 0310-0272) white, round, biconvex, film coated tablets, identified with 'SEROQUEL' and '200' on one side and plain on the other side, are supplied in bottles of 100 tablets and hospital unit dose packages of 100 tablets.

300 mg Tablets (NDC 0310-0274) white, capsule-shaped, biconvex, film coated tablets, intagliated with 'SEROQUEL' on one side and '300' on the other side, are supplied in bottles of 60 tablets and hospital unit dose packages of 100 tablets.

Store at 25°C (77°F); excursions permitted to 15-30°C (59-86°F) [See USP].

ANIMAL TOXICOLOGY

Quetiapine caused a dose-related increase in pigment deposition in thyroid gland in rat toxicity studies which were 4 weeks in duration or longer and in a mouse 2 year carcinogenicity study. Doses were 10-250 mg/kg in rats, 75-750 mg/kg in mice; these doses are 0.1-3.0, and 0.1-4.5 times the maximum recommended human dose (on a mg/m^2 basis), respectively. Pigment deposition was shown to be irreversible in rats. The identity of the pigment could not be determined, but was found to be co-localized with quetiapine in thyroid gland follicular epithelial cells. The functional effects and the relevance of this finding to human risk are unknown.

In dogs receiving quetiapine for 6 or 12 months, but not for 1 month, focal triangular cataracts occurred at the junction of posterior sutures in the outer cortex of the lens at a dose of 100 mg/kg, or 4 times the maximum recommended human dose on a mg/m^2 basis. This finding may be due to inhibition of cholesterol biosynthesis by quetiapine. Quetiapine caused a dose related reduction in plasma cholesterol levels in repeat-dose dog and monkey studies; however, there was no correlation between plasma cholesterol and the presence of cataracts in individual dogs. The appearance of delta-8-cholestanol in plasma is consistent with inhibition of a late stage in cholesterol biosynthesis in these species. There also was a 25% reduction in cholesterol content of the outer cortex of the lens observed in a special study in quetiapine treated female dogs. Drug-related cataracts have not been seen in any other species; however, in a 1-year study in monkeys, a striated appearance of the anterior lens surface was detected in 2/7 females at a dose of 225 mg/kg or 5.5 times the maximum recommended human dose on a mg/m^2 basis.

SEROQUEL is a trademark of the AstraZeneca group of companies.

AstraZeneca Pharmaceuticals LP
Wilmington, DE 19850
Made in USA
64251-00
Rev 07/04
AstraZeneca

Axcan Scandipharm Inc.

22 INVERNESS CENTER PARKWAY
BIRMINGHAM, AL 35242

Direct Inquiries to:
Customer Service
(800) 950-8085
Fax: (205) 991-8426

For Medical Information Contact:
(800) 565-3255
Fax: (450) 467-5857

CANASA® ℞

[*kă-nă-să*]
(Mesalamine, USP)
Rectal Suppositories 500 mg and 1000 mg
NDC 58914-500-56 and NDC 58914-501-56
Rx Only

Prescribing information for this product, which appears on pages 765–767 of the 2005 PDR, has been completely revised as follows. Please write "See Supplement A" next to the product heading.

DESCRIPTION

The active ingredient in **CANASA®** 500 mg and 1000 mg suppositories is mesalamine, also known as mesalazine or 5-aminosalicylic acid (5-ASA). Chemically, mesalamine is 5-amino-2-hydroxybenzoic acid, and is classified as an anti-inflammatory drug.

The empirical formula is $C_7H_7NO_3$, representing a molecular weight of 153.14. The structural formula is:

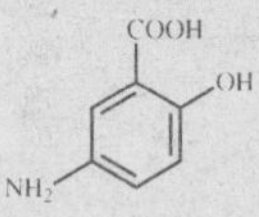

Each **CANASA®** rectal suppository contains 500 mg or 1000 mg of mesalamine (USP) in a base of Hard Fat NF.

CLINICAL PHARMACOLOGY

Sulfasalazine has been used in the treatment of ulcerative colitis for over 55 years. It is split by bacterial action in the colon into sulfapyridine (SP) and mesalamine (5-ASA). It is thought that the mesalamine component only is therapeutically active in ulcerative colitis.

Mechanism of Action

The mechanism of action of mesalamine (and sulfasalazine) is not fully understood, but appears to be topical rather than systemic. Although the pathology of inflammatory bowel disease is uncertain, both prostaglandins and leukotrienes have been implicated as mediators of mucosal injury and inflammation. Recently, however, the role of mesalamine as a free radical scavenger or inhibitor of tumor necrosis factor (TNF) has also been postulated.

Pharmacokinetics

Absorption: Mesalamine (5-ASA) administered as a rectal suppository is variably absorbed. In patients with ulcerative colitis treated with mesalamine 500 mg rectal suppositories, administered once every eight hours for six days, the mean mesalamine peak plasma concentration (C_{max}) was 353 ng/mL (CV=55 %) following the initial dose and 361 ng/mL (CV=67 %) at steady state. The mean minimum steady state plasma concentration (C_{min}) was 89 ng/mL (CV=89 %). Absorbed mesalamine does not accumulate in the plasma.

Distribution: Mesalamine administered as rectal suppositories distributes in rectal tissue to some extent. In patients with ulcerative proctitis treated with **CANASA®** (mesalamine, USP) 500 mg or 1000 mg rectal suppositories, rectal tissue concentrations for 5-ASA and N-acetyl 5-ASA have not been rigorously quantified.

Metabolism: Mesalamine is extensively metabolized, mainly to N-acetyl-5-ASA. The site of metabolism has not been elucidated. In patients with ulcerative colitis treated with one 500 mg mesalamine rectal suppository every eight hours for six days, peak concentration (C_{max}) of N-acetyl-5-ASA ranged from 467 ng/mL to 1399 ng/mL following the initial dose and from 193 ng/mL to 1304 ng/mL at steady state.

Elimination: Mesalamine is eliminated from plasma mainly by urinary excretion, predominantly as N-acetyl-5-ASA. In patients with ulcerative proctitis treated with one mesalamine 500 mg rectal suppository every eight hours for six days, ≤12% of the dose was eliminated in urine as unchanged 5-ASA and 8-77% as N-acetyl-5-ASA following the initial dose. At steady state, ≤ 11% of the dose was eliminated as unchanged 5-ASA and 3-35% as N-acetyl-5-ASA. The mean elimination half-life was five hours (CV=73%) for 5-ASA and six hours (CV=63%) for N-acetyl-5-ASA following the initial dose. At steady state, the mean elimination half-life was seven hours for both 5-ASA and N-acetyl-5-ASA (CV=102% for 5-ASA and 82% for N-acetyl-5-ASA).

Drug-Drug Interactions: The potential for interactions between mesalamine, administered as 500 mg or 1000 mg rectal suppositories, and other drugs has not been studied.

Special Populations (Patients with Renal or Hepatic Impairment): The effect of renal or hepatic impairment on elimination of mesalamine in ulcerative proctitis patients treated with mesalamine 500 mg or 1000 mg suppositories has not been studied.

Preclinical Toxicology

Preclinical studies of mesalamine were conducted in rats, mice, rabbits and dogs and kidney was the main target organ of toxicity. In rats, adverse renal effects were observed at a single oral dose of 600 mg/kg (about 3.2 times the recommended human intra-rectal dose, based on body surface area) and at IV doses of >214 mg/kg (about 1.2 times the recommended human intra-rectal dose, based on body surface area). In a 13-week oral gavage toxicity study in rats, papillary necrosis and/or multifocal tubular injury were observed in males receiving 160 mg/kg (about 0.86 times the recommended human intra-rectal dose, based on body surface area) and in both males and females at 640 mg/kg (about 3.5 times the recommended human intra-rectal dose, based on body surface area). In a combined 52-week toxicity and 127-week carcinogenicity study in rats, degeneration of the kidneys and hyalinization of basement membranes and Bowman's capsule were observed at oral doses of 100 mg/kg/day (about 0.54 times the recommended human intra-rectal dose, based on body surface area) and above. In a 14-day rectal toxicity study of mesalamine suppositories in rabbits, intra-rectal doses up to 800 mg/kg (about 8.6 times the recommended human intra-rectal dose, based on body surface area) was not associated with any adverse effects. In a six-month oral toxicity study in dogs, doses of 80 mg/kg (about 1.4 times the recommended human intra-rectal dose, based on body surface area) and higher caused renal pathology similar to that described for the rat. In a rectal toxicity study of mesalamine suppositories in dogs, a dose of 166.6 mg/kg (about 3.0 times the recommended human intra-rectal dose, based on body surface area) produced chronic nephritis and pyelitis. In the 12-month eye toxicity study in dogs, Keratoconjunctivitis sicca (KCS) occurred at oral doses of 40 mg/kg (about 0.72 times the recommended human intra-rectal dose, based on body surface area) and above.

CLINICAL STUDIES

Two double-blind placebo-controlled multicenter studies were conducted in North America in patients with mild to moderate active ulcerative proctitis. The primary measures of efficacy were the same in all trials (clinical disease activity index, sigmoidoscopic and histologic evaluations). The main difference between the studies was dosage regimen: 500 mg three times daily (1.5 g/d) in Study 1; and 500 mg twice daily (1.0 g/d) in Study 2. A total of 173 patients were studied (Study 1, N=79; Study 2, N=94). Eighty-nine (89) patients received mesalamine suppositories, and eighty-four (84) patients received placebo suppositories. Patients were evaluated clinically and sigmoidoscopically after three and six weeks of suppository treatment. In Study No. 1 patients were 17 to 73 years of age (mean = 39 yrs), 57% were female, and 97% were white. Patients had an average extent of proctitis (upper disease boundary) of 10.8 cm. Eighty-four percent (84%) of the study patients had multiple prior episodes of proctitis. In Study No. 2, patients were 21 to 72 years of age (mean = 39 yrs), 62% were female, and 96% were white. Patients had an average extent of proctitis (upper disease boundary) of 10.3 cm. Seventy-eight percent (78%) of the study patients had multiple prior episodes of proctitis.

Compared to placebo, mesalamine suppository treatment was statistically (p<0.01) superior to placebo in all trials with respect to improvement in stool frequency, rectal bleeding, mucosal appearance, disease severity, and overall disease activity after three and six weeks of treatment. Daily diary records indicated significant improvement in rectal bleeding in the first week of therapy while tenesmus and diarrhea improved significantly within two weeks. Investigators rated patients receiving mesalamine much improved compared to patients receiving placebo (p<0.001).

The effectiveness of mesalamine suppositories was statistically significant irrespective of sex, extent of proctitis, duration of current episode or duration of disease.

A multicenter, open-label, randomized, parallel group study in ninety-nine (99) patients diagnosed with mild to moderate ulcerative proctitis compared the clinical efficacy of the **CANASA®** 1000 mg suppository to that of the **CANASA®** 500 mg suppository. The primary measures of efficacy included clinical disease activity index, sigmoidoscopic and histologic evaluations. Patients were randomized to one of two treatment groups, with a dosage regimen of one 500 mg mesalamine suppository BID, morning and HS, or one 1000 mg mesalamine suppository HS for 6 weeks. Patients were evaluated clinically and sigmoidoscopically after three and six weeks of suppository treatment. Of the 81 patients in the Per Protocol population, forty-six (46) patients received mesalamine 500 mg suppositories BID, and thirty-five (35) patients received mesalamine 1000 mg suppositories HS.

The efficacy of the 1000 mg HS treatment was not statistically or clinically different after 6 weeks from the 500 mg BID treatment, and both were effective in the treatment of ulcerative proctitis. Both treatments resulted in a significant decrease between Baseline and 6 weeks in the Disease Activity Index (DAI), a composite index reflecting rectal bleeding, stool frequency, mucosal appearance at endoscopy, and a global assessment of disease. In the 500 mg BID group, the mean DAI value decreased from 6.6 to 1.6, and in the 1000 mg HS group, the mean DAI value decreased from 6.2 to 1.3 over 6 weeks of treatment, representing a decrease of greater than 75% in both groups. Seventy-eight percent (78%; 36/46) of patients in the 500 mg BID group and 86% (30/35) of the patients in the 1000 mg HS group achieved a substantial improvement in symptoms (defined as a DAI score of less than 3) after 6 weeks of treatment. These patients regained normal daily stools, lost their rectal bleeding, and lost signs of inflammation at endoscopic visualization. The time to onset of response to the study drug was within 3 weeks of initiation of therapy in each treatment group, but further improvement was observed between 3 and 6 weeks of treatment.

INDICATIONS AND USAGE

CANASA® 500 mg and 1000 mg Suppositories are indicated for the treatment of active ulcerative proctitis.

CONTRAINDICATIONS

CANASA® 500 mg and 1000 mg Suppositories are contraindicated in patients who have demonstrated hypersensitivity to mesalamine (5-aminosalicylic acid) or to the suppository vehicle [saturated vegetable fatty acid esters (Hard Fat, NF)], or to salicylates (including aspirin).

PRECAUTIONS

Mesalamine has been implicated in the production of an acute intolerance syndrome characterized by cramping, acute abdominal pain and bloody diarrhea, sometimes fever, headache and a rash; in such cases prompt withdrawal is required. The patient's history of sulfasalazine intolerance, if any, should be re-evaluated. If a rechallenge is performed later in order to validate the hypersensitivity it should be carried out under close supervision and only if clearly needed, giving consideration to reduced dosage. In the literature one patient previously sensitive to sulfasalazine was rechallenged with 400 mg oral mesalamine; within eight hours she experienced headache, fever, intensive abdominal colic, profuse diarrhea and was readmitted as an emergency. She responded poorly to steroid therapy and two weeks later a pancolectomy was required. The possibility of increased absorption of mesalamine and concomitant renal tubular damage as noted in the preclinical studies must be kept in mind. Patients on **CANASA®** 500 mg or 1000 mg, especially those on concurrent oral products which contain or release mesalamine and those with pre-existing renal disease, should be carefully monitored with urinalysis, BUN and creatinine testing.

In a clinical trial most patients who were hypersensitive to sulfasalazine were able to take mesalamine enemas without evidence of any allergic reaction. Nevertheless, caution should be exercised when mesalamine is initially used in patients known to be allergic to sulfasalazine. These patients should be instructed to discontinue therapy if signs of rash or fever become apparent.

A small proportion of patients have developed pancolitis while using mesalamine. However, extension of upper disease boundary and/or flare-ups occurred less often in the mesalamine-treated group than in the placebo-treated group.

Rare instances of pericarditis have been reported with mesalamine containing products including sulfasalazine. Cases of pericarditis have also been reported as manifestations of inflammatory bowel disease. In the cases reported there have been positive rechallenges with mesalamine or mesalamine containing products. In one of these cases, however, a second rechallenge with sulfasalazine was negative throughout a 2 month follow-up. Chest pain or dyspnea in patients treated with mesalamine should be investigated with this information in mind. Discontinuation of **CANASA®** suppositories may be warranted in some cases, but rechallenge with mesalamine can be performed under careful clinical observation should the continued therapeutic need for mesalamine be present.

There have been two reports in the literature of additional serious adverse events: one patient who developed leukopenia and thrombocytopenia after seven months of treatment with one 500 mg suppository nightly, and one patient with rash and fever which was a similar reaction to sulfasalazine.

Information for Patients: See patient information printed at the end of this insert.

Carcinogenesis, Mutagenesis, Impairment of Fertility

Mesalamine caused no increase in the incidence of neoplastic lesions over controls in a two-year study of Wistar rats fed up to 320 mg/kg/day of mesalamine admixed with diet (about 1.7 times the recommended human intra-rectal dose, based on body surface area).

Mesalamine was not mutagenic in the Ames test, the mouse lymphoma cell ($TK^{+/-}$) forward mutation test, or the mouse micronucleus test.

No effects on fertility or reproductive performance of the male and female rats were observed at oral mesalamine doses up to 320 mg/kg/day (about 1.7 times the recommended human intra-rectal dose, based on body surface area). The oligospermia and infertility in men associated with sulfasalazine have not been reported with mesalamine.

Pregnancy, Teratogenic Effects, Pregnancy Category B

Teratology studies have been performed in rats at oral doses up to 320 mg/kg/day (about 1.7 times the recommended human intra-rectal dose, based on body surface area) and in rabbits at oral doses up to 495 mg/kg/day (about 5.4 times the recommended human intra-rectal dose, based on body surface area) and have revealed no evidence of impaired fertility or harm to the fetus due to mesalamine. There are, however, no adequate and well controlled studies in pregnant women. Because animal reproduction studies are not always predictive of human response, this drug should be used in pregnancy only if clearly needed.

Nursing Mothers

It is not known whether mesalamine or its metabolite(s) are excreted in human milk. Because many drugs are excreted in human milk, caution should be exercised when **CANASA®** 500 mg or 1000 mg suppositories are administered to a nursing woman.

Pediatric Use

Safety and effectiveness in pediatric patients have not been established.

Geriatric Use

Clinical studies of **CANASA®** did not include sufficient numbers of subjects aged 65 and over to determine whether they respond differently from younger subjects. Other reported clinical experience has not identified differences in responses between the elderly and younger patients. In general, dose selection for an elderly patient should be cautious, reflecting the greater frequency of decreased hepatic, renal, or cardiac function, and of concomitant disease or other drug therapy.

Mesalamine is known to be substantially excreted by the kidney, and the risk of toxic reactions to this drug may be greater in patients with impaired renal function. Because elderly patients are more likely to have decreased renal function, it may be useful to monitor renal function.

ADVERSE REACTIONS

Clinical Adverse Experience

The most frequent adverse reactions observed in the double-blind, placebo-controlled trials are summarized in the Table below.

ADVERSE REACTIONS OCCURRING IN MORE THAN 1% OF MESALAMINE SUPPOSITORY TREATED PATIENTS (COMPARISON TO PLACEBO)

Symptom	Mesalamine (n=177)		Placebo (n=84)	
	N	%	N	%
Dizziness	5	3.0	2	2.4
Rectal Pain	3	1.8	0	0.0
Fever	2	1.2	0	0.0
Rash	2	1.2	0	0.0
Acne	2	1.2	0	0.0
Colitis	2	1.2	0	0.0

In the multicenter, open-label, randomized, parallel group study comparing the **CANASA®** 1000 mg suppository (HS) to that of the **CANASA®** 500 mg suppository (BID), there were no differences between the two treatment groups in the adverse event profile. The most frequent AEs were headache (14.4%), flatulence (5.2%), abdominal pain (5.2%), diarrhea (3.1%), and nausea (3.1%). Three (3) patients had to discontinue medication because of a treatment emergent AE; one of these AEs (headache) was deemed possibly related to study medication.

In addition to the events observed in the clinical trials, the following adverse events have been associated with mesalamine containing products: nephrotoxicity, pancreatitis, fibrosing alveolitis and elevated liver enzymes. Cases of pancreatitis and fibrosing alveolitis have been reported as manifestations of inflammatory bowel disease as well.

Continued on next page

Canasa—Cont.

Hair Loss

Mild hair loss characterized by "more hair in the comb" but no withdrawal from clinical trials has been observed in seven of 815 mesalamine patients but none of the placebo-treated patients. In the literature there are at least six additional patients with mild hair loss who received either mesalamine or sulfasalazine. Retreatment is not always associated with repeated hair loss.

OVERDOSAGE

There have been no documented reports of serious toxicity in man resulting from massive overdosing with mesalamine. Under ordinary circumstances, mesalamine absorption from the colon is limited.

DOSAGE AND ADMINISTRATION

The usual dosage of **CANASA®** (mesalamine, USP) 500 mg Suppositories is one 500 mg rectal suppository 2 times daily with possible increase to 3 times daily if inadequate response at two weeks. The usual dosage of **CANASA®** (mesalamine, USP) 1000 mg Suppositories is one rectal suppository 1 time daily at bedtime.

The suppository should be retained for one to three hours or longer, if possible, to achieve the maximum benefit. While the effect of **CANASA®** Suppositories may be seen within three to twenty-one days, the usual course of therapy would be from three to six weeks depending on symptoms and sigmoidoscopic findings. Studies have suggested that **CANASA®** Suppositories will delay relapse after the six-week short-term treatment.

Patient Instructions:
NOTE: CANASA® Suppositories will cause staining of direct contact surfaces, including but not limited to fabrics, flooring, painted surfaces, marble, granite, vinyl, and enamel.
I. Detach one suppository from strip of suppositories.
II. Hold suppository upright and carefully remove the plastic wrapper.
III. Avoid excessive handling of suppository, which is designed to melt at body temperature.
IV. Insert suppository completely into rectum with gentle pressure, pointed end first.
V. A small amount of lubricating gel may be used on the tip of the suppository to assist insertion.

HOW SUPPLIED

CANASA® (Mesalamine, USP) 500 mg Suppositories:
CANASA® 500 mg Suppositories for rectal administration are available as bullet shaped, light tan suppositories containing 500 mg mesalamine supplied in boxes of 30 individually plastic wrapped suppositories (NDC 58914-500-56).

CANASA® (Mesalamine, USP) 1000 mg Suppositories:
CANASA® 1000 mg Suppositories for rectal administration are available as bullet shaped, light tan suppositories containing 1000 mg mesalamine supplied in boxes of 30 individually plastic wrapped suppositories (NDC 58914-501-56). Store below 25°C, (77°F), do not freeze. Keep away from direct heat, light or humidity.
Rx only
Axcan Scandipharm, Inc.
Birmingham, AL 35242
Date: September 23, 2004

Patient Information

CANASA® Rectal Suppositories
(Mesalamine, USP) 500 and 1000 mg
Read this information carefully before you begin treatment. Also, read the information you get whenever you get more medicine. There may be new information. This information does not take the place of talking with your doctor about your medical condition or your treatment. If you have any questions about this medicine, ask your doctor or pharmacist.

What is CANASA®?

CANASA® (can-AH-sah) is a medicine used to treat ulcerative proctitis (ulcerative rectal colitis). CANASA® works inside your rectum (lower intestine) to help reduce bleeding, mucous and bloody diarrhea caused by inflammation (swelling and soreness) of the rectal area. You use CANASA® by inserting it into your rectum.

Who should not use CANASA®?

Do not use CANASA® if you are allergic to the active ingredient mesalamine (also found in drugs such as Rowasa, Asacol, Pentasa, Azulfidine, and Dipentum), if you are allergic to the inactive ingredients, or if you have had any unusual reaction to the ingredients.
Tell your doctor if you:
• Have kidney problems. Using CANASA® may make them worse.
• Have had inflamed pancreas (pancreatitis).
• Are pregnant. You and your doctor will decide if you should use CANASA®.
• Have ever had pericarditis (inflamed sac around your heart).
• Are allergic to sulfasalazine. You may need to watch for signs of an allergic reaction to CANASA®.
• Are allergic to aspirin.
• Are allergic to other things, such as foods, preservatives, or dyes.

How should I use CANASA®?

Follow your doctor's instructions about how often to use CANASA® and how long to use it. For the 500 mg suppository, the usual dose is one suppository 2 times a day for 3-6 weeks. For the 1000 mg suppository, the usual dose is one suppository at bedtime for 3-6 weeks. We do not know if CANASA® will work for children or is safe for them.
Follow these steps to use CANASA®:
1. For best results, empty your rectum (have a bowel movement) just before using CANASA®.
2. Detach one CANASA® suppository from the strip of suppositories.
3. Hold the suppository upright and carefully peel open the plastic at the pre-cut line to take out the suppository.
4. Insert the suppository with the pointed end first completely into your rectum, using gentle pressure.
5. For best results, keep the suppository in your rectum for 3 hours or longer, if possible.
If you have trouble inserting CANASA®, you may put a little bit of lubricating gel on the suppository.
Do not handle the suppository too much, since it may begin to melt from the heat from your hands and body.
If you miss a dose of CANASA®, use it as soon as possible, unless it is almost time for next dose. Do not use two CANASA® suppositories at the same time to make up for a missed dose.
Keep using CANASA® as long as your doctor tells you to use it, even if you feel better.
CANASA® can cause stains on things it touches. Therefore keep it away from clothing and other fabrics, flooring, painted surfaces, marble, granite, plastics, and enamel. Be careful since CANASA® may stain clothing.

What should I avoid while taking CANASA®?

Do not breast feed while using CANASA®. We do not know if CANASA® can pass through the milk and harm the baby. Tell your doctor if you become pregnant while using CANASA®.

What are the possible side effects of CANASA®?

• The most common side effects of CANASA® are: headache, gas or flatulence, and diarrhea. These events also occurred when patients were given an inactive suppository.
• Less common, but possibly serious side effects include a reaction to the medicine (acute intolerance syndrome) that includes cramps, sharp abdominal (stomach area) pain, bloody diarrhea, and sometimes fever, headache and rash. Stop use and tell your doctor right away if you get any of these symptoms.
• In rare cases, the sac around the heart may become inflamed (pericarditis). Tell your doctor right away if you develop chest pain or shortness of breath, which are signs of this problem.
• In rare cases, patients using CANASA® develop worsening colitis (pancolitis).
• A very few patients using CANASA® may have mild hair loss.
• Other side effects not listed above may also occur in some patients.
If you notice any other side effects, check with your doctor or pharmacist.

How should I store CANASA®?

Store CANASA® below 25°C, (77° F), do not freeze it. Keep it away from direct heat, light, or humidity. Keep it out of the reach of children.

General advice about prescription medicines

Medicines are sometimes prescribed for conditions that are not mentioned in patient information leaflets. Do not use CANASA® for a condition for which it was not prescribed. Do not give CANASA® to other people, even if they have the same symptoms you have.
This leaflet summarizes the most important information about CANASA®. If you would like more information, talk with your doctor. You can ask your pharmacist or doctor for information about CANASA® that is written for health professionals.

Bayer Pharmaceuticals Corporation

400 MORGAN LANE
WEST HAVEN, CT 06516

For Medical Information Contact:
Director, Medical Services
(800) 468-0894
(203) 812-2000

AVELOX®

[ā´ vē-lŏks]
(moxifloxacin hydrochloride) Tablets

AVELOX® I.V.

(moxifloxacin hydrochloride in sodium chloride injection)

This product is now marketed and distributed by Schering Corporation, 2000 Galloping Hill Road, Kenilworth NJ 07033.

CIPRO® I.V.

[sĭprō]
(ciprofloxacin)
For Intravenous Infusion

This product is now marketed and distributed by Schering Corporation, 2000 Galloping Hill Road, Kenilworth NJ 07033.

CIPRO® XR

[sĭ´prō]
(ciprofloxacin* extended-release tablets)

This product is now marketed and distributed by Schering Corporation, 2000 Galloping Hill Road, Kenilworth NJ 07033.

LEVITRA

[lĕ-vē-tră]
vardenafil HCl

This product is now marketed and distributed by Schering Corporation, 2000 Galloping Hill Road, Kenilworth NJ 07033.

Biogen Idec

14 CAMBRIDGE CENTER
CAMBRIDGE, MA 02142

Direct Inquiries to:
AMEVIVE Customer Service:
Tel: 866-263-8483
Fax: 866-420-8888
AVONEX Customer Service:
Tel: 800-456-2255
Fax: 617-679-8100
RITUXAN Customer Service:
Tel: 800-821-8590
ZEVALIN Customer Service:
Tel: 877-433-4332

AMEVIVE®

[ă´ mĕ-vēv]
(alefacept)

Prescribing information for this product, which appears on pages 949–951 of the 2005 PDR, has been completely revised as follows. Please write "See Supplement A" next to the product heading.

DESCRIPTION

AMEVIVE® (alefacept) is an immunosuppressive dimeric fusion protein that consists of the extracellular CD2-binding portion of the human leukocyte function antigen-3 (LFA-3) linked to the Fc (hinge, C_H2 and C_H3 domains) portion of human IgG1. Alefacept is produced by recombinant DNA technology in a Chinese Hamster Ovary (CHO) mammalian cell expression system. The molecular weight of alefacept is 91.4 kilodaltons.
AMEVIVE® is supplied as a sterile, white-to-off-white, preservative-free, lyophilized powder for parenteral administration. After reconstitution with 0.6 mL of the supplied Sterile Water for Injection, USP, the solution of AMEVIVE® is clear, with a pH of approximately 6.9.
AMEVIVE® is available in two formulations. AMEVIVE® for intramuscular injection contains 15 mg alefacept per 0.5 mL of reconstituted solution. AMEVIVE® for intravenous injection contains 7.5 mg alefacept per 0.5 mL of reconstituted solution. Both formulations also contain 12.5 mg sucrose, 5.0 mg glycine, 3.6 mg sodium citrate dihydrate, and 0.06 mg citric acid monohydrate per 0.5 mL.

CLINICAL PHARMACOLOGY

AMEVIVE® interferes with lymphocyte activation by specifically binding to the lymphocyte antigen, CD2, and inhibiting LFA-3/CD2 interaction. Activation of T lymphocytes involving the interaction between LFA-3 on antigen-presenting cells and CD2 on T lymphocytes plays a role in the pathophysiology of chronic plaque psoriasis. The majority of T lymphocytes in psoriatic lesions are of the memory effector phenotype characterized by the presence of the CD45RO marker[1], express activation markers (e.g., CD25, CD69) and release inflammatory cytokines, such as interferon γ.
AMEVIVE® also causes a reduction in subsets of CD2+ T lymphocytes (primarily CD45RO+), presumably by bridging between CD2 on target lymphocytes and immunoglobulin Fc receptors on cytotoxic cells, such as natural killer cells. Treatment with AMEVIVE® results in a reduction in circulating total CD4+ and CD8+ T lymphocyte counts. CD2 is also expressed at low levels on the surface of natural killer cells and certain bone marrow B lymphocytes. Therefore, the potential exists for AMEVIVE® to affect the activation and numbers of cells other than T lymphocytes. In clinical studies of AMEVIVE®, minor changes in the numbers of circulating cells other than T lymphocytes have been observed.

Pharmacokinetics

In patients with moderate to severe plaque psoriasis, following a 7.5 mg intravenous (IV) administration, the mean volume of distribution of alefacept was 94 mL/kg, the mean clearance was 0.25 mL/h/kg, and the mean elimination half-life was approximately 270 hours. Following an intramuscular (IM) injection, bioavailability was 63%.

The pharmacokinetics of alefacept in pediatric patients have not been studied. The effects of renal or hepatic impairment on the pharmacokinetics of alefacept have not been studied.

Pharmacodynamics

At doses tested in clinical trials, AMEVIVE® therapy resulted in a dose-dependent decrease in circulating total lymphocytes[2]. This reduction predominantly affected the memory effector subset of the CD4+ and CD8+ T lymphocyte compartments (CD4+CD45RO+ and CD8+CD45RO+), the predominant phenotype in psoriatic lesions. Circulating naive T lymphocyte and natural killer cell counts appeared to be only minimally susceptible to AMEVIVE® treatment, while circulating B lymphocyte counts appeared not to be affected by AMEVIVE® (see **ADVERSE REACTIONS, Effect on Lymphocyte Counts**).

CLINICAL STUDIES

AMEVIVE® was evaluated in two randomized, double-blind, placebo-controlled studies in adults with chronic (≥1 year) plaque psoriasis and a minimum body surface area involvement of 10% who were candidates for or had previously received systemic therapy or phototherapy. Each course consisted of once-weekly administration for 12 weeks (IV for Study 1, IM for Study 2) of placebo or AMEVIVE®. Patients could receive concomitant low potency topical steroids. Concomitant phototherapy or systemic therapy was not allowed.

In Study 1, patients were randomized to receive one or two courses of AMEVIVE® 7.5 mg administered by IV bolus. The first and second courses in the two-course cohort were separated by at least a 12-week post-dosing interval. A total of 553 patients were randomized into three cohorts (Table 1).

Table 1. Treatment Group and Number of Patients Dosed in Study 1

	Course 1 (No. of patients)	Course 2 (No. of patients)
Cohort 1	AMEVIVE® (183)	AMEVIVE® (154)
Cohort 2	AMEVIVE® (184)	Placebo (142)
Cohort 3	Placebo (186)	AMEVIVE® (153)

Study 2 provided a basis for comparison of patients treated with either 10 mg or 15 mg AMEVIVE® IM. One hundred seventy-three patients were randomized to receive 10 mg of AMEVIVE® IM, 166 to receive 15 mg of AMEVIVE® IM, and 168 to receive placebo.

In Studies 1 and 2, 77% of patients had previously received systemic therapy and/or phototherapy for psoriasis. Of these, 23% and 19%, respectively, had failed to respond to at least one of these previous therapies.

Table 2 shows the treatment response in the first course of Study 1 and Study 2. Response to treatment in both studies was defined as the proportion of patients with a reduction in score on the Psoriasis Area and Severity Index (PASI)[3] of at least 75% from baseline at two weeks following the 12-week treatment period.

Other treatment responses included the proportion of patients who achieved a scoring of "almost clear" or "clear" by Physician Global Assessment (PGA) and the proportion of patients with a reduction in PASI of at least 50% from baseline two weeks after the 12-week treatment period.

[See table 2 above]

In Study 2, the proportion of responders to the 10 mg IM dose was higher than placebo, but the difference was not statistically significant.

In both studies, onset of response to AMEVIVE® treatment (at least a 50% reduction of baseline PASI) began 60 days after the start of therapy.

With one course of therapy in Study 1 (IV route), the median duration of response (defined as maintenance of a 75% or greater reduction in PASI) was 3.5 months for AMEVIVE®-treated patients and 1 month for placebo-treated patients. In Study 2 (IM route), the median duration of response was approximately 2 months for both AMEVIVE®-treated patients and placebo-treated patients.

Most patients who had responded to either AMEVIVE® or placebo maintained a 50% or greater reduction in PASI through the 3-month observation period.

Among responders in study 1 who received AMEVIVE® 7.5 mg IV or in study 2 who received AMEVIVE® 15 mg IM and were followed off active treatment before AMEVIVE® retreatment, a 50% or greater reduction in PASI was maintained for a median of 7 months.

Some patients achieved their maximal response beyond 2 weeks post-dosing. In Studies 1 and 2, an additional 11% (42/367) and 7% (12/166) of patients treated with AMEVIVE®, respectively, achieved a 75% reduction from baseline PASI score at one or more visits after the first 2 weeks of the follow-up period.

Retreatment

Patients in Study 1 who had completed the first IV treatment course were eligible to receive a second treatment course if their psoriasis was less than "clear" by PGA and

Table 2. Percentage of Patients Responding to the First Course of Treatment in Study 1 (the Intravenous Study) and Study 2 (the Intramuscular Study) Two Weeks Post Dosing

Treatment response: (reduction in disease activity from baseline)	Study 1			Study 2		
	Placebo (N=186)	AMEVIVE® 7.5 mg IV (N=367)[1]	Difference (95% CI)	Placebo (N=168)	AMEVIVE® 15 mg IM (N=166)	Difference (95% CI)
≥75% reduction PASI	4%	14%	10* (6, 15)	5%	21%	16* (9, 23)
≥50% reduction PASI	10%	38%	28* (22, 35)	18%	42%	24* (14, 33)
PGA "almost clear" or "clear"	4%	11%	7+ (3, 12)	5%	14%	9§ (3, 15)

[1]Cohorts 1 and 2 are combined.
*p values <0.001
+p value 0.004
§p value 0.006

Figure 1. Median PASI Score Over Time

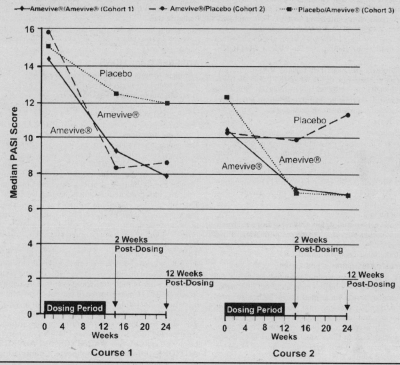

their CD4+ T lymphocyte count was above the lower limit of normal. The level of response (decrease in median PASI score) over the two courses of IV treatment is shown in Figure 1. The median reduction in PASI score was greater in patients who received a second course of AMEVIVE® treatment (see Cohort 1) compared to patients who received placebo (see Cohort 2).

[See figure 1 above]

Data on the safety and efficacy of AMEVIVE® treatment beyond two courses are limited.

INDICATIONS AND USAGE

AMEVIVE® is indicated for the treatment of adult patients with moderate to severe chronic plaque psoriasis who are candidates for systemic therapy or phototherapy.

CONTRAINDICATIONS

AMEVIVE® should not be administered to patients with known hypersensitivity to AMEVIVE® or any of its components.

WARNINGS

LYMPHOPENIA

AMEVIVE® INDUCES DOSE-DEPENDENT REDUCTIONS IN CIRCULATING CD4+ AND CD8+ T LYMPHOCYTE COUNTS. A COURSE OF AMEVIVE® THERAPY SHOULD NOT BE INITIATED IN PATIENTS WITH A CD4+ T LYMPHOCYTE COUNT BELOW NORMAL. THE CD4+ T LYMPHOCYTE COUNTS OF PATIENTS RECEIVING AMEVIVE® SHOULD BE MONITORED WEEKLY THROUGHOUT THE COURSE OF THE 12-WEEK DOSING REGIMEN. DOSING SHOULD BE WITHHELD IF CD4+ T LYMPHOCYTE COUNTS ARE BELOW 250 CELLS/μL. THE DRUG SHOULD BE DISCONTINUED IF THE COUNTS REMAIN BELOW 250 CELLS/μL FOR ONE MONTH (SEE DOSAGE AND ADMINISTRATION).

Malignancies

AMEVIVE® may increase the risk of malignancies. Some patients who received AMEVIVE® in clinical studies developed malignancies (**see ADVERSE REACTIONS, Malignancies**). In preclinical studies, animals developed B cell hyperplasia, and one animal developed a lymphoma (**see PRECAUTIONS, Carcinogenesis, Mutagenesis, and Fertility**). AMEVIVE® should not be administered to patients

with a history of systemic malignancy. Caution should be exercised when considering the use of AMEVIVE® in patients at high risk for malignancy. If a patient develops a malignancy, AMEVIVE® should be discontinued.

Serious Infections

AMEVIVE® is an immunosuppressive agent and, therefore, has the potential to increase the risk of infection and reactivate latent, chronic infections. AMEVIVE® should not be administered to patients with a clinically important infection. Caution should be exercised when considering the use of AMEVIVE® in patients with chronic infections or a history of recurrent infection. Patients should be monitored for signs and symptoms of infection during or after a course of AMEVIVE®. New infections should be closely monitored. If a patient develops a serious infection, AMEVIVE® should be discontinued (see **ADVERSE REACTIONS, Infections**).

PRECAUTIONS

Effects on the Immune System

Patients receiving other immunosuppressive agents or phototherapy should not receive concurrent therapy with AMEVIVE® because of the possibility of excessive immunosuppression. The duration of the period following treatment with AMEVIVE® before one should consider starting other immunosuppressive therapy has not been evaluated.

The safety and efficacy of vaccines, specifically live or live-attenuated vaccines, administered to patients being treated with AMEVIVE® have not been studied. In a study of 46 patients with chronic plaque psoriasis, the ability to mount immunity to tetanus toxoid (recall antigen) and an experimental neo-antigen was preserved in those patients undergoing AMEVIVE® therapy.

Allergic Reactions

Hypersensitivity reactions (urticaria, angioedema) were associated with the administration of AMEVIVE®. If an anaphylactic reaction or other serious allergic reaction occurs, administration of AMEVIVE® should be discontinued immediately and appropriate therapy initiated.

Hepatic Injury

In post-marketing experience there have been reports of liver injury, including asymptomatic transaminase eleva-

Continued on next page

Amevive—Cont.

tion, fatty infiltration of the liver, hepatitis, decompensation of cirrhosis with liver failure, and acute failure. Two cases of liver failure were reported with concomitant alcohol use (see **ADVERSE REACTIONS, Hepatic Injury**). While the exact relationship of these occurrences with the use of AMEVIVE® has not been established, patients with signs or symptoms of liver injury should be fully evaluated. AMEVIVE® should be discontinued in patients who develop significant clinical signs of liver injury. In clinical trials, AMEVIVE®-treated patients experienced rare cases (9) of transaminase elevations to 5 to 10 times the upper limit of normal.

Information Patients

Patients should be informed of the need for regular monitoring of white blood cell (lymphocyte) counts during therapy and that AMEVIVE® must be administered under the supervision of a physician. Patients should also be informed that AMEVIVE® reduces lymphocyte counts, which could increase their chances of developing an infection or a malignancy. Patients should be advised to inform their physician promptly if they develop any signs of an infection or malignancy while undergoing a course of treatment with AMEVIVE®.

Female patients should also be advised to notify their physicians if they become pregnant while taking AMEVIVE® (or within 8 weeks of discontinuing AMEVIVE®) and be advised of the existence of and encouraged to enroll in the Pregnancy Registry. Call 1-866-AMEVIVE (1-866-263-8483) to enroll into the Registry (see **PRECAUTIONS, Pregnancy**).

Patients should be advised that serious liver injury has been reported in patients receiving AMEVIVE®. Patients should be advised to report to their physician persistent nausea, anorexia, fatigue, vomiting, abdominal pain, jaundice, easy bruising, dark urine or pale stools.

Laboratory Tests

CD4+ T lymphocyte counts should be monitored weekly during the 12-week dosing period and used to guide dosing. Patients should have normal CD4+ T lymphocyte counts prior to an initial or a subsequent course of treatment with AMEVIVE®. Dosing should be withheld if CD4+ T lymphocyte counts are below 250 cells/μL. AMEVIVE® should be discontinued if CD4+ T lymphocyte counts remain below 250 cells/μL for one month.

Drug Interactions

No formal interaction studies have been performed. The duration of the period following treatment with AMEVIVE® before one should consider starting other immunosuppressive therapy has not been evaluated.

Carcinogenesis, Mutagenesis, and Fertility

In a chronic toxicity study, cynomolgus monkeys were dosed weekly for 52 weeks with intravenous alefacept at 1 mg/kg/dose or 20 mg/kg/dose. One animal in the high dose group developed a B-cell lymphoma that was detected after 28 weeks of dosing. Additional animals in both dose groups developed B-cell hyperplasia of the spleen and lymph nodes. One-year post-treatment there was no evidence of alefacept-related lymphoma or B-cell hyperplasia in any of the remaining treated monkeys.

All animals in the study were positive for an endemic primate gammaherpes virus also known as lymphocryptovirus (LCV). Latent LCV infection is generally asymptomatic, but can lead to B-cell lymphomas when animals are immune suppressed.

In a separate study, baboons given 3 doses of alefacept at 1 mg/kg every 8 weeks were found to have centroblast proliferation in B-cell dependent areas in the germinal centers of the spleen following a 116-day washout period.

The role of AMEVIVE® in the development of the lymphoid malignancy and the hyperplasia observed in non-human primates and the relevance to humans is unknown. Immunodeficiency-associated lymphocyte disorders (plasmacytic hyperplasia, polymorphic proliferation, and B-cell lymphomas) occur in patients who have congenital or acquired immunodeficiencies including those resulting from immunosuppressive therapy.

No formal carcinogenicity or fertility studies were conducted.

Mutagenicity studies were conducted *in vitro* and *in vivo;* no evidence of mutagenicity was observed.

Pregnancy (Category B)

Women of childbearing potential make up a considerable segment of the patient population affected by psoriasis. Since the effect of AMEVIVE® on pregnancy and fetal development, including immune system development, is not known, health care providers are encouraged to enroll patients currently taking AMEVIVE® who become pregnant into the Biogen Idec Pregnancy Registry by calling 1-866-AMEVIVE (1-866-263-8483).

Reproductive toxicology studies have been performed in cynomolgus monkeys at doses up to 5 mg/kg/week (about 62 times the human dose based on body weight) and have revealed no evidence of impaired fertility or harm to the fetus due to AMEVIVE®. No abortifacient or teratogenic effects were observed in cynomolgus monkeys following intravenous bolus injections of AMEVIVE® administered weekly during the period of organogenesis to gestation. AMEVIVE® underwent trans-placental passage and produced *in utero* exposure in the developing monkeys. *In utero*, serum levels of exposure in these monkeys were 23%

of maternal serum levels. No evidence of fetal toxicity including adverse effects on immune system development was observed in any of these animals.

Animal reproduction studies, however, are not always predictive of human response and there are no adequate and well-controlled studies in pregnant women. Because the risk to the development of the fetal immune system and postnatal immune function in humans is unknown, AMEVIVE® should be used during pregnancy only if clearly needed. If pregnancy occurs while taking AMEVIVE®, continued use of the drug should be assessed.

Nursing Mothers

It is not known whether AMEVIVE® is excreted in human milk. Because many drugs are excreted in human milk, and because there exists the potential for serious adverse reactions in nursing infants from AMEVIVE®, a decision should be made whether to discontinue nursing while taking the drug or to discontinue the use of the drug, taking into account the importance of the drug to the mother.

Geriatric Use

Of the 1357 patients who received AMEVIVE® in clinical trials, a total of 100 patients were ≥ 65 years of age and 13 patients were ≥ 75 years of age. No differences in safety or efficacy were observed between older and younger patients, but there were not sufficient data to exclude important differences. Because the incidence of infections and certain malignancies is higher in the elderly population, in general, caution should be used in treating the elderly.

Pediatric Use

The safety and efficacy of AMEVIVE® in pediatric patients have not been studied. AMEVIVE® is not indicated for pediatric patients.

ADVERSE REACTIONS

The most serious adverse reactions were:
- Lymphopenia (see **WARNINGS**)
- Malignancies (see **WARNINGS**)
- Serious Infections requiring hospitalization (see **WARNINGS**)
- Hypersensitivity Reactions (see **PRECAUTIONS, Allergic Reactions**)

Commonly observed adverse events seen in the first course of placebo-controlled clinical trials with at least a 2% higher incidence in the AMEVIVE®-treated patients compared to placebo-treated patients were: pharyngitis, dizziness, increased cough, nausea, pruritus, myalgia, chills, injection site pain, injection site inflammation, and accidental injury. The only adverse event that occurred at a 5% or higher incidence among AMEVIVE®-treated patients compared to placebo-treated patients was chills (1% placebo *vs.* 6% AMEVIVE®), which occurred predominantly with intravenous administration.

The adverse reactions which most commonly resulted in clinical intervention were cardiovascular events including coronary artery disorder in <1% of patients and myocardial infarct in <1% of patients. These events were not observed in any of the 413 placebo-treated patients. The total number of patients hospitalized for cardiovascular events in the AMEVIVE®-treated group was 1.2% (11/876).

The most common events resulting in discontinuation of treatment with AMEVIVE® were CD4+ T lymphocyte levels below 250 cells/μL (see **WARNINGS**, and **ADVERSE REACTIONS, Effect on Lymphocyte Counts**), headache (0.2%), and nausea (0.2%).

Because clinical trials are conducted under widely varying conditions, adverse event rates observed in the clinical trials of a drug cannot be directly compared to rates in the clinical trials of another drug and may not reflect the rates observed in practice. The adverse reaction information does, however, provide a basis for identifying the adverse events that appear to be related to drug use and a basis for approximating rates.

The data described below reflect exposure to AMEVIVE® in a total of 1357 psoriasis patients, 85% of whom received 1 to 2 courses of therapy and the rest received 3 to 6 courses and were followed for up to three years. Of the 1357 total patients, 876 received their first course in placebo-controlled studies. The population studied ranged in age from 16 to 84 years, and included 69% men and 31% women. The patients were mostly Caucasian (89%), reflecting the general psoriatic population. Disease severity at baseline was moderate to severe psoriasis.

Effect on Lymphocyte Counts

In the intramuscular study (Study 2), 4% of patients temporarily discontinued treatment and no patients permanently discontinued treatment due to CD4+ T lymphocyte counts below the specified threshold of 250 cells/μL. In Study 2, 10%, 28%, and 42% of patients had total lymphocyte, CD4+, and CD8+ T lymphocyte counts below normal, respectively. Twelve weeks after a course of therapy (12 weekly doses), 2%, 8%, and 21% of patients had total lymphocyte, CD4+, and CD8+ T cell counts below normal.

In the first course of the intravenous study (Study 1), 10% of patients temporarily discontinued treatment and 2% permanently discontinued treatment due to CD4+ T lymphocyte counts below the specified threshold of 250 cells/μL. During the first course of Study 1, 22% of patients had total lymphocyte counts below normal, 48% had CD4+ T lymphocyte counts below normal and 59% had CD8+ T lymphocyte counts below normal. The maximal effect on lymphocytes was observed within 6 to 8 weeks of initiation of treatment. Twelve weeks after a course of therapy (12 weekly doses), 4% of patients had total lymphocyte counts below normal, 19% had CD4+ T lymphocyte counts below normal, and 36% had CD8+ T lymphocyte counts below normal.

For patients receiving a second course of AMEVIVE® in Study 1, 17% of patients had total lymphocyte counts below normal, 44% had CD4+ T lymphocyte counts below normal, and 56% had CD8+ T lymphocyte counts below normal. Twelve weeks after completing dosing, 3% of patients had total lymphocyte counts below normal, 17% had CD4+ T lymphocyte counts below normal, and 35% had CD8+ T lymphocyte counts below normal (see **WARNINGS**, and **PRECAUTIONS, Laboratory Tests**).

Malignancies

In the 24-week period constituting the first course of placebo-controlled studies, 13 malignancies were diagnosed in 11 AMEVIVE®-treated patients. The incidence of malignancies was 1.3% (11/876) for AMEVIVE®-treated patients compared to 0.5% (2/413) in the placebo group.

Among 1357 patients who received AMEVIVE®, 25 patients were diagnosed with 35 treatment-emergent malignancies. The majority of these malignancies (23 cases) were basal (6) or squamous cell cancers (17) of the skin. Three cases of lymphoma were observed; one was classified as non-Hodgkin's follicle-center cell lymphoma and two were classified as Hodgkin's disease.

Infections

In the 24-week period constituting the first course of placebo-controlled studies, serious infections (infections requiring hospitalization) were seen at a rate of 0.9% (8/876) in AMEVIVE®-treated patients and 0.2% (1/413) in the placebo group. In patients receiving repeated courses of AMEVIVE® therapy, the rates of serious infections were 0.7% (5/756) and 1.5% (3/199) in the second and third course of therapy, respectively. Serious infections among 1357 AMEVIVE®-treated patients included necrotizing cellulitis, peritonsillar abscess, post-operative and burn wound infection, toxic shock, pneumonia, appendicitis, pre-septal cellulitis, cholecystitis, gastroenteritis and herpes simplex infection.

Hypersensitivity Reactions

In clinical studies two patients were reported to experience angioedema, one of whom was hospitalized. In the 24-week period constituting the first course of placebo-controlled studies, urticaria was reported in 6 (<1%) AMEVIVE®-treated patients *vs.* 1 patient in the control group. Urticaria resulted in discontinuation of therapy in one of the AMEVIVE®-treated patients.

Hepatic Injury

In post-marketing experience there have been reports of asymptomatic transaminase elevation, fatty infiltration of the liver, hepatitis, and severe liver failure (see **PRECAUTIONS, Hepatic Injury**).

Injection Site Reactions

In the intramuscular study (Study 2), 16% of AMEVIVE®-treated patients and 8% of placebo-treated patients reported injection site reactions. Reactions at the site of injection were generally mild, typically occurred on single occasions, and included either pain (7%), inflammation (4%), bleeding (4%), edema (2%), non-specific reaction (2%), mass (1%), or skin hypersensitivity (<1%). In the clinical trials, a single case of injection site reaction led to the discontinuation of AMEVIVE®.

Immunogenicity

Approximately 3% (35/1306) of patients receiving AMEVIVE® developed low-titer antibodies to alefacept. No apparent correlation of antibody development and clinical response or adverse events was observed. The long-term immunogenicity of AMEVIVE® is unknown.

The data reflect the percentage of patients whose test results were considered positive for antibodies to alefacept in an ELISA assay, and are highly dependent on the sensitivity and specificity of the assay. Additionally, the observed incidence of antibody positivity in an assay may be influenced by several factors including sample handling, timing of sample collection, concomitant medications, and underlying disease. For these reasons, comparison of the incidence of antibodies to alefacept with the incidence of antibodies to other products may be misleading.

OVERDOSAGE

The highest dose tested in humans (0.75 mg/kg IV) was associated with chills, headache, arthralgia, and sinusitis within one day of dosing. Patients who have been inadvertently administered an excess of the recommended dose should be closely monitored for effects on total lymphocyte count and CD4+ T lymphocyte count.

DOSAGE AND ADMINISTRATION

AMEVIVE® should only be used under the guidance and supervision of a physician.

The recommended dose of AMEVIVE® is 7.5 mg given once weekly as an IV bolus or 15 mg given once weekly as an IM injection. The recommended regimen is a course of 12 weekly injections. Retreatment with an additional 12-week course may be initiated provided that CD4+ T lymphocyte counts are within the normal range, and a minimum of a 12-week interval has passed since the previous course of treatment. Data on retreatment beyond two cycles are limited.

The CD4+ T lymphocyte counts of patients receiving AMEVIVE® should be monitored weekly before initiating dosing and throughout the course of the 12-week dosing regimen. Dosing should be withheld if CD4+ T lymphocyte counts are below 250 cells/μL. The drug should be discontinued if the counts remain below 250 cells/μL for one month (see **PRECAUTIONS, Laboratory Tests**).

Preparation Instructions

AMEVIVE® should be reconstituted by a health care professional using aseptic technique. Each vial is intended for single patient use only.

Do not use AMEVIVE® beyond the date stamped on the carton, dose pack lid (IV), drug/diluent pack (IM), AMEVIVE® vial label, or diluent container label.

AMEVIVE® 15 mg lyophilized powder for IM administration should be reconstituted with 0.6 mL of the supplied diluent (Sterile Water for Injection, USP). 0.5 mL of the reconstituted solution contains 15 mg of alefacept.

AMEVIVE® 7.5 mg lyophilized powder for IV administration should be reconstituted with 0.6 mL of the supplied diluent. 0.5 mL of the reconstituted solution contains 7.5 mg of alefacept.

Do not add other medications to solutions containing AMEVIVE®. Do not reconstitute AMEVIVE® with other diluents. Do not filter reconstituted solution during preparation or administration.

All procedures require the use of aseptic technique. Using the supplied syringe and one of the supplied needles, withdraw **only 0.6 mL** of the supplied diluent, (Sterile Water for Injection, USP). Keeping the needle pointed at the sidewall of the vial, slowly inject the diluent into the vial of AMEVIVE®. Some foaming will occur, which is normal. To avoid excessive foaming, do not shake or vigorously agitate. The contents should be swirled gently during dissolution. Generally, dissolution of AMEVIVE® takes less than two minutes. The solution should be used as soon as possible after reconstitution.

The reconstituted solution should be clear and colorless to slightly yellow. Visually inspect the solution for particulate matter and discoloration prior to administration. The solution should not be used if discolored or cloudy, or if undissolved material remains.

Following reconstitution, the product should be used immediately or within 4 hours if stored in the vial at 2-8°C (36-46°F). AMEVIVE® NOT USED WITHIN 4 HOURS OF RECONSTITUTION SHOULD BE DISCARDED.

Remove the needle used for reconstitution and attach the other supplied needle. Withdraw 0.5 mL of the AMEVIVE® solution into the syringe. Some foam or bubbles may remain in the vial.

Administration Instructions

For intramuscular use, inject the full 0.5 mL of solution. Rotate injection sites so that a different site is used for each new injection. New injections should be given at least 1 inch from an old site and never into areas where the skin is tender, bruised, red, or hard.

For intravenous use,

- Prepare 2 syringes with 3.0 mL Normal Saline, USP for pre- and post-administration flush.
- Prime the winged infusion set with 3.0 mL saline and insert the set into the vein.
- Attach the AMEVIVE®-filled syringe to the infusion set and administer the solution over no more than 5 seconds.
- Flush the infusion set with 3.0 mL saline, USP.

HOW SUPPLIED

AMEVIVE® for IV administration is supplied in either a carton containing four administration dose packs, or in a carton containing one administration dose pack. Each dose pack contains one 7.5-mg single-use vial of AMEVIVE®, one 10 mL single-use diluent vial (Sterile Water for Injection, USP), one syringe, one 23 gauge, ¾ inch winged infusion set, and two 23 gauge, 1 ¼ inch needles. The NDC number for the four administration dose pack carton is 59627-020-01. The NDC number for the one administration dose pack carton is 59627-020-02.

AMEVIVE® for IM administration is supplied in either a carton containing four doses, or in a carton containing one dose. Each four-dose carton contains one removable drug/diluent pack for refrigeration, four 1 mL syringes, and eight 23 gauge, 1 ¼ inch needles. Each four-dose drug/diluent pack for refrigeration contains: four 15-mg single-use vials of AMEVIVE® and four 10 mL single-use diluent vials of Sterile Water for Injection, USP. Each single-dose carton contains one removable drug/diluent pack for refrigeration, one syringe and two 23 gauge, 1 ¼ inch needles. Each single-dose drug/diluent pack for refrigeration contains: one 15-mg single-use vial of AMEVIVE® and one 10 mL single-use diluent vial of Sterile Water for Injection, USP. The NDC number for the four-dose carton is 59627-021-03. The NDC number for the single-dose carton is 59627-021-04.

AMEVIVE® is reconstituted with 0.6 mL of the 10 mL single-use diluent.

Storage

The dose pack (IV) and drug/diluent pack (IM) containing AMEVIVE® (lyophilized powder) should be stored in a refrigerator between 2-8°C/36-46°F. PROTECT FROM LIGHT. Retain in carton (IV) or drug/diluent pack (IM) until time of use.

Rx only

REFERENCES

1. Bos JD, Hagenaars C, Das PK, et al. Predominance of "memory" T cells (CD4+, CDw29+) over "naïve" T cells (CD4+, CD45R+) in both normal and diseased human skin. Arch Dermatol Res 1989; 281:24–30.
2. Ellis C, Krueger GG. Treatment of chronic plaque psoriasis by selective targeting of memory effector T lymphocytes. N Engl J Med 2001; 345:248–255.
3. Fredriksson T, Pettersson U. Severe psoriasis–oral therapy with a new retinoid. Dermatologica 1978; 157:238–244.

Issued: January/2005
AMEVIVE® (alefacept)
Manufactured by:
BIOGEN IDEC INC.
14 Cambridge Center
Cambridge, MA 02142 USA

©2005 Biogen Idec Inc. All rights reserved.

1-866-263-8483
U.S. Patents:
4,956,281
5,547,853
5,728,677
5,914,111
5,928,643
6,162,432
Additional U.S. Patents Pending
I63007-4

AVONEX® ℞

[a-vuh-necks]

(Interferon beta-1a)

IM Injection

Prescribing information for this product, which appears on pages 951–957 of the 2005 PDR, has been completely revised as follows. Please write "See Supplement A" next to the product heading.

DESCRIPTION

AVONEX® (Interferon beta-1a) is a 166 amino acid glycoprotein with a predicted molecular weight of approximately 22,500 daltons. It is produced by recombinant DNA technology using genetically engineered Chinese Hamster Ovary cells into which the human interferon beta gene has been introduced. The amino acid sequence of AVONEX® is identical to that of natural human interferon beta.

Using the World Health Organization (WHO) natural interferon beta standard, Second International Standard for Interferon, Human Fibroblast (Gb-23-902-531), AVONEX® has a specific activity of approximately 200 million international units (IU) of antiviral activity per mg of Interferon beta-1a determined specifically by an *in vitro* cytopathic effect bioassay using lung carcinoma cells (A549) and Encephalomyocarditis virus (ECM). AVONEX® 30 mcg contains approximately 6 million IU of antiviral activity using this method. The activity against other standards is not known. Comparison of the activity of AVONEX® with other Interferon betas is not appropriate, because of differences in the reference standards and assays used to measure activity.

30 mcg Lyophilized Powder Vial

A vial of AVONEX® is formulated as a sterile, white to off-white lyophilized powder for intramuscular injection after reconstitution with supplied diluent (Sterile Water for Injection, USP). Each vial of reconstituted AVONEX® contains 30 mcg of Interferon beta-1a; 15 mg Albumin (Human), USP; 5.8 mg Sodium Chloride, USP; 5.7 mg Dibasic Sodium Phosphate, USP; and 1.2 mg Monobasic Sodium Phosphate, USP, in 1.0 mL at a pH of approximately 7.3.

30 mcg Prefilled Syringe

A prefilled syringe of AVONEX® is formulated as a sterile liquid for intramuscular injection. Each 0.5 mL (30 mcg dose) of AVONEX® in a prefilled glass syringe contains 30 mcg of Interferon beta-1a, 0.79 mg Sodium Acetate Trihydrate, USP; 0.25 mg Glacial Acetic Acid, USP; 15.8 mg Arginine Hydrochloride, USP; and 0.025 mg Polysorbate 20 in Water for Injection, USP at a pH of approximately 4.8.

CLINICAL PHARMACOLOGY

General

Interferons are a family of naturally occurring proteins and glycoproteins that are produced by eukaryotic cells in response to viral infection and other biological inducers. Interferon beta, one member of this family, is produced by various cell types including fibroblasts and macrophages. Natural interferon beta and Interferon beta-1a are glycosylated, with each containing a single N-linked complex carbohydrate moiety. Glycosylation of other proteins is known to affect their stability, activity, aggregation, biodistribution, and half-life in blood. However, the effects of glycosylation of interferon beta on these properties have not been fully defined.

Biologic Activities

Interferons are cytokines that mediate antiviral, antiproliferative and immunomodulatory activities in response to viral infection and other biological inducers. Three major interferons have been distinguished: alpha, beta, and gamma. Interferons alpha and beta form the Type I class of interferons, and interferon gamma is a Type II interferon. These interferons have overlapping but clearly distinct biological activities.

Interferon beta exerts its biological effects by binding to specific receptors on the surface of human cells. This binding initiates a complex cascade of intracellular events that leads to the expression of numerous interferon-induced gene products and markers. These include 2′, 5′-oligoadenylate synthetase, β_2-microglobulin, and neopterin. These products have been measured in the serum and cellular fractions of blood collected from patients treated with AVONEX®.

The specific interferon-induced proteins and mechanisms by which AVONEX® exerts its effects in multiple sclerosis have not been fully defined. Clinical studies conducted in multiple sclerosis patients showed that interleukin 10 (IL-10) levels in cerebrospinal fluid were increased in patients treated with AVONEX® compared to placebo. Serum IL-10 levels were increased 48 hours after intramuscular (IM) injection of AVONEX® and remained elevated for 1 week. However, no relationship has been established between absolute levels of IL-10 and clinical outcome in multiple sclerosis.

Pharmacokinetics

Pharmacokinetics of AVONEX® in multiple sclerosis patients have not been evaluated. The pharmacokinetic and pharmacodynamic profiles of AVONEX® in healthy subjects following doses of 30 mcg through 75 mcg have been investigated. Serum levels of AVONEX® as measured by antiviral activity are slightly above detectable limits following a 30 mcg IM dose, and increase with higher doses.

After an IM dose, serum levels of AVONEX® typically peak between 3 and 15 hours and then decline at a rate consistent with a 10 hour elimination half-life. Serum levels of AVONEX® may be sustained after IM administration due to prolonged absorption from the IM site. Systemic exposure, as determined by AUC and C_{max} values, is greater following IM than subcutaneous (SC) administration.

Subcutaneous administration of AVONEX® should not be substituted for intramuscular administration. Subcutaneous and intramuscular administration have been observed to have non-equivalent pharmacokinetic and pharmacodynamic parameters following administration to healthy volunteers.

Biological response markers (e.g., neopterin and β_2-microglobulin) are induced by AVONEX® following parenteral doses of 15 mcg through 75 mcg in healthy subjects and treated patients. Biological response marker levels increase within 12 hours of dosing and remain elevated for at least 4 days. Peak biological response marker levels are typically observed 48 hours after dosing. The relationship of serum AVONEX® levels or levels of these induced biological response markers to the mechanisms by which AVONEX® exerts its effects in multiple sclerosis is unknown.

Clinical Studies

The clinical effects of AVONEX® in multiple sclerosis were studied in two randomized, multicenter, double-blind, placebo-controlled studies in patients with multiple sclerosis.[1,2] Safety and efficacy of treatment with AVONEX® beyond 3 years is not known.

In Study 1, 301 patients received either 30 mcg of AVONEX® (n=158) or placebo (n=143) by IM injection once weekly. Patients were entered into the trial over a 2½ year period, received injections for up to 2 years, and continued to be followed until study completion. Two hundred eighty-two patients completed 1 year on study, and 172 patients completed 2 years on study. There were 144 patients treated with AVONEX® for more than 1 year, 115 patients for more than 18 months and 82 patients for 2 years.

All patients had a definite diagnosis of multiple sclerosis of at least 1 year duration and had at least 2 exacerbations in the 3 years prior to study entry (or 1 per year if the duration of disease was less than 3 years). At entry, study participants were without exacerbation during the prior 2 months and had Kurtzke Expanded Disability Status Scale (EDSS[3]) scores ranging from 1.0 to 3.5. Patients with chronic progressive multiple sclerosis were excluded from this study.

The primary outcome assessment was time to progression in disability, measured as an increase in the EDSS score of at least 1.0 point that was sustained for at least 6 months. An increase in EDSS score reflects accumulation of disability. This endpoint was used to ensure that progression reflected permanent increase in disability rather than a transient effect due to an exacerbation.

Secondary outcomes included exacerbation frequency and results of magnetic resonance imaging (MRI) scans including gadolinium (Gd)-enhanced lesion number and volume and T2-weighted (proton density) lesion volume. Additional secondary endpoints included 2 upper limb (tested in both arms) and 3 lower limb function tests.

Twenty-three of the 301 patients (8%) discontinued treatment prematurely. Of these, 1 patient treated with placebo (1%) and 6 patients treated with AVONEX® (4%) discontinued treatment due to adverse events. Thirteen of these 23 patients remained on study and were evaluated for clinical endpoints.

Figure 1

Onset of Sustained Disability Progression by Time on Study (Kaplan-Meier Methodology)

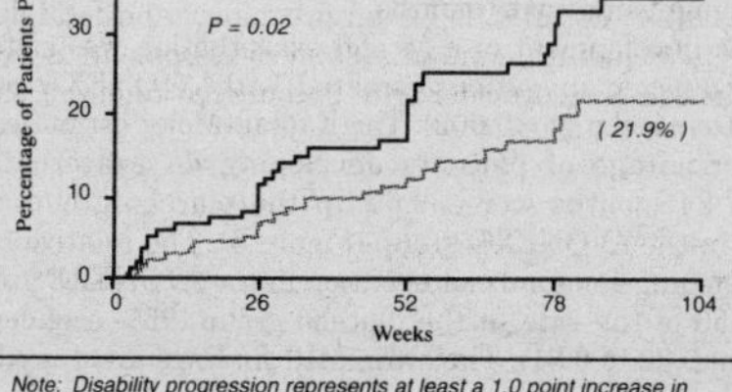

Note: Disability progression represents at least a 1.0 point increase in EDSS score sustained for at least 6 months.

Time to onset of sustained progression in disability was significantly longer in patients treated with AVONEX® than in patients receiving placebo (p = 0.02). The Kaplan-Meier plots of these data are presented in Figure 1. The Kaplan-Meier estimate of the percentage of patients progressing by

Continued on next page

Avonex—Cont.

the end of 2 years was 34.9% for placebo-treated patients and 21.9% for AVONEX®-treated patients, indicating a slowing of the disease process. This represents a 37% relative reduction in the risk of accumulating disability in the AVONEX®-treated group compared to the placebo-treated group.

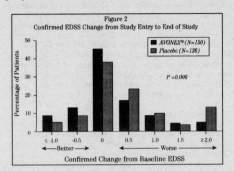

Figure 2
Confirmed EDSS Change from Study Entry to End of Study

The distribution of confirmed EDSS change from study entry (baseline) to the end of the study is shown in Figure 2. There was a statistically significant difference between treatment groups in confirmed change for patients with at least 2 scheduled visits (136 placebo-treated and 150 AVONEX®-treated patients; p = 0.006; see Table 1).

The rate and frequency of exacerbations were determined as secondary outcomes. For all patients included in the study, irrespective of time on study, the annual exacerbation rate was 0.67 per year in the AVONEX®-treated group and 0.82 per year in the placebo-treated group (p = 0.04).

AVONEX® treatment significantly decreased the frequency of exacerbations in the subset of patients who were enrolled in the study for at least 2 years (87 placebo-treated patients and 85 AVONEX®-treated patients; p = 0.03; see Table 1). Gd-enhanced and T2-weighted (proton density) MRI scans of the brain were obtained in most patients at baseline and at the end of 1 and 2 years of treatment. Gd-enhancing lesions seen on brain MRI scans represent areas of breakdown of the blood brain barrier thought to be secondary to inflammation. Patients treated with AVONEX® demonstrated significantly lower Gd-enhanced lesion number after 1 and 2 years of treatment (p ≤ 0.05; see Table 1). The volume of Gd-enhanced lesions was also analyzed, and showed similar treatment effects (p ≤ 0.03). Percentage change in T2-weighted lesion volume from study entry to Year 1 was significantly lower in AVONEX®-treated than placebo-treated patients (p = 0.02). A significant difference in T2-weighted lesion volume change was not seen between study entry and Year 2.

The exact relationship between MRI findings and the clinical status of patients is unknown. The prognostic significance of MRI findings in these studies has not been evaluated.

Of the limb function tests, only 1 demonstrated a statistically significant difference between treatment groups (favoring AVONEX®). A summary of the effects of AVONEX® on the clinical and MRI endpoints of this study is presented in Table 1.

[See table 1 above]

In Study 2, 383 patients who had recently experienced an isolated demyelinating event involving the optic nerve, spinal cord, or brainstem/cerebellum, and who had lesions typical of multiple sclerosis on brain MRI, received either 30 mcg AVONEX® (n = 193) or placebo (n = 190) by IM injection once weekly. All patients received intravenous steroid treatment for the initiating clinical exacerbation. Patients were enrolled into the study over a two-year period and followed for up to three years or until they developed a second clinical exacerbation in an anatomically distinct region of the central nervous system. Sixteen percent of subjects on AVONEX® and 14% of subjects on placebo withdrew from the study for a reason other than the development of a second exacerbation[2].

The primary outcome measure was time to development of a second exacerbation in an anatomically distinct region of the central nervous system. Secondary outcomes were brain MRI measures, including the cumulative increase in the number of new or enlarging T2 lesions, T2 lesion volume compared to baseline at 18 months, and the number of Gd-enhancing lesions at 6 months.

Time to development of a second exacerbation was significantly delayed in patients treated with AVONEX® compared to placebo (p = 0.002). The Kaplan-Meier estimates of the percentage of patients developing an exacerbation within 24 months were 38.6% in the placebo group and 21.1% in the AVONEX® group (Figure 3). The relative rate of developing a second exacerbation in the AVONEX® group was 0.56 of the rate in the placebo group (95% confidence interval 0.38 to 0.81). The brain MRI findings are described in Table 2.

[See figure 3 above]

[See table 2 at top of next page]

INDICATIONS AND USAGE

AVONEX® (Interferon beta-1a) is indicated for the treatment of patients with relapsing forms of multiple sclerosis to slow the accumulation of physical disability and decrease the frequency of clinical exacerbations. Patients with mul-

Table 1
Clinical and MRI Endpoints in Study 1

Endpoint	Placebo	AVONEX®	P-Value
PRIMARY ENDPOINT:			
Time to sustained progression in disability (N: 143, 158)[1]	–See Figure 1–		0.02[2]
Percentage of patients progressing in disability at 2 years (Kaplan-Meier estimate)[1]	34.9%	21.9%	
SECONDARY ENDPOINTS:			
DISABILITY			
Mean confirmed change in EDSS from study entry to end of study (N: 136, 150)[1]	0.50	0.20	0.006[3]
EXACERBATIONS			
Number of exacerbations in subset completing 2 years (N: 87, 85)			
0	26%	38%	0.03[3]
1	30%	31%	
2	11%	18%	
3	14%	7%	
≥4	18%	7%	
Percentage of patients exacerbation-free in subset completing 2 years (N: 87, 85)	26%	38%	0.10[4]
Annual exacerbation rate (N: 143, 158)[1]	0.82	0.67	0.04[5]
MRI			
Number of Gd-enhanced lesions:			
At study entry (N: 132, 141)			
Mean (Median)	2.3 (1.0)	3.2 (1.0)	
Range	0-23	0-56	
Year 1 (N: 123, 134)			
Mean (Median)	1.6 (0)	1.0 (0)	0.02[3]
Range	0-22	0-28	
Year 2 (N: 82, 83)			
Mean (Median)	1.6 (0)	0.8 (0)	0.05[3]
Range	0-34	0-13	
T2 lesion volume:			
Percentage change from study entry to Year 1 (N: 116, 123)			
Median	-3.3%	-13.1%	0.02[3]
Percentage change from study entry to Year 2 (N: 83, 81)			
Median	-6.5%	-13.2%	0.36[3]

Note: (N: ,) denotes the number of evaluable placebo and AVONEX® patients, respectively.
[1] Patient data included in this analysis represent variable periods of time on study.
[2] Analyzed by Mantel-Cox (logrank) test.
[3] Analyzed by Mann-Whitney rank-sum test.
[4] Analyzed by Cochran-Mantel-Haenszel test.
[5] Analyzed by likelihood ratio test.

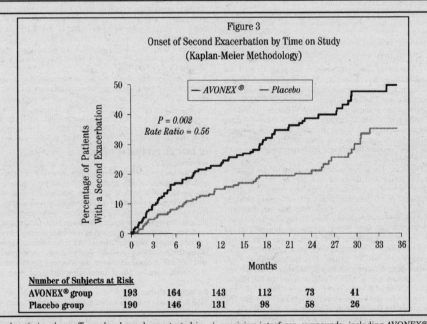

Figure 3
Onset of Second Exacerbation by Time on Study
(Kaplan-Meier Methodology)

P = 0.002
Rate Ratio = 0.56

Number of Subjects at Risk

AVONEX® group	193	164	143	112	73	41
Placebo group	190	146	131	98	58	26

tiple sclerosis in whom efficacy has been demonstrated include patients who have experienced a first clinical episode and have MRI features consistent with multiple sclerosis. Safety and efficacy in patients with chronic progressive multiple sclerosis have not been established.

CONTRAINDICATIONS

AVONEX® is contraindicated in patients with a history of hypersensitivity to natural or recombinant interferon beta, or any other component of the formulation.

The lyophilized vial formulation of AVONEX® is contraindicated in patients with a history of hypersensitivity to albumin (human).

WARNINGS

Depression and Suicide

AVONEX® should be used with caution in patients with depression or other mood disorders, conditions that are common with multiple sclerosis. Depression and suicide have been reported to occur with increased frequency in patients receiving interferon compounds, including AVONEX®. Patients treated with AVONEX® should be advised to report immediately any symptoms of depression and/or suicidal ideation to their prescribing physicians. If a patient develops depression or other severe psychiatric symptoms, cessation of AVONEX® therapy should be considered. In Study 2, AVONEX®-treated patients were more likely to experience depression than placebo-treated patients. An equal incidence of depression was seen in the placebo-treated and AVONEX®-treated patients in Study 1. Additionally, there have been post-marketing reports of depression, suicidal ideation and/or development of new or worsening of pre-existing other psychiatric disorders, including psychosis. Some of these patients improved upon cessation of AVONEX® dosing.

Anaphylaxis

Anaphylaxis has been reported as a rare complication of AVONEX® use. Other allergic reactions have included dyspnea, orolingual edema, skin rash and urticaria (see ADVERSE REACTIONS).

Decreased Peripheral Blood Counts
Decreased peripheral blood counts in all cell lines, including rare pancytopenia and thrombocytopenia, have been reported from post-marketing experience (see ADVERSE REACTIONS). Some cases of thrombocytopenia have had nadirs below 10,000/μL. Some cases reoccur with rechallenge (see ADVERSE REACTIONS). Patients should be monitored for signs of these disorders (see Precautions: Laboratory Tests).

Hepatic Injury
Severe hepatic injury, including cases of hepatic failure, has been reported rarely in patients taking AVONEX®. Asymptomatic elevation of hepatic transaminases has also been reported, and in some patients has recurred upon rechallenge with AVONEX®. In some cases, these events have occurred in the presence of other drugs that have been associated with hepatic injury. The potential risk of AVONEX® used in combination with known hepatotoxic drugs or other products (e.g. alcohol) should be considered prior to AVONEX® administration, or when adding new agents to the regimen of patients already on AVONEX®. Patients should be monitored for signs of hepatic injury (see Precautions: Laboratory Tests).

Albumin (Human)
The lyophilized vial of AVONEX® contains albumin, a derivative of human blood. Based on effective donor screening and product manufacturing processes, it carries an extremely remote risk for transmission of viral diseases. A theoretical risk for transmission of Creutzfeldt-Jakob disease (CJD) also is considered extremely remote. No cases of transmission of viral diseases or CJD have been identified for albumin. The prefilled syringe of AVONEX® does not contain albumin.

PRECAUTIONS

Seizures
Caution should be exercised when administering AVONEX® to patients with pre-existing seizure disorders. In the two placebo-controlled studies in multiple sclerosis, 4 patients receiving AVONEX® experienced seizures, while no seizures occurred in the placebo group. Three of these 4 patients had no prior history of seizure (see ADVERSE REACTIONS). It is not known whether these events were related to the effects of multiple sclerosis alone, to AVONEX®, or to a combination of both. The effect of AVONEX® administration on the medical management of patients with seizure disorder is unknown.

Cardiomyopathy and Congestive Heart Failure
Patients with cardiac disease, such as angina, congestive heart failure, or arrhythmia, should be closely monitored for worsening of their clinical condition during initiation and continued treatment with AVONEX®. While AVONEX® does not have any known direct-acting cardiac toxicity, during the post-marketing period infrequent cases of congestive heart failure, cardiomyopathy, and cardiomyopathy with congestive heart failure have been reported in patients without known predisposition to these events, and without other known etiologies being established. In rare cases, these events have been temporally related to the administration of AVONEX®. In some of these instances recurrence upon rechallenge was observed.

Autoimmune Disorders
Autoimmune disorders of multiple target organs have been reported post-marketing including idiopathic thrombocytopenia, hyper- and hypothyroidism, and rare cases of autoimmune hepatitis have also been reported. Patients should be monitored for signs of these disorders (see Precautions: Laboratory Tests) and appropriate treatment implemented when observed.

Information to Patients
All patients should be instructed to read the AVONEX® Medication Guide supplied to them. Patients should be cautioned not to change the dosage or the schedule of administration without medical consultation.

Patients should be informed of the most serious (see WARNINGS) and the most common adverse events associated with AVONEX® administration, including symptoms associated with flu syndrome (see ADVERSE REACTIONS). Symptoms of flu syndrome are most prominent at the initiation of therapy and decrease in frequency with continued treatment. Concurrent use of analgesics and/or antipyretics may help ameliorate flu-like symptoms on treatment days.

Patients should be cautioned to report depression or suicidal ideation (see WARNINGS).

Patients should be advised about the abortifacient potential of AVONEX® (see Precautions: Pregnancy—Teratogenic Effects). If a woman becomes pregnant while taking AVONEX®, she should be advised to consider enrolling in the AVONEX® Pregnancy Registry by calling 1-800-456-2255.

The prefilled syringe cap contains dry natural rubber.

When a physician determines that AVONEX® can be used outside of the physician's office, persons who will be administering AVONEX® should receive instruction in reconstitution and injection, including the review of the injection procedures. If a patient is to self-administer, the physical ability of that patient to self-inject intramuscularly should be assessed. The first injection should be performed under the supervision of a qualified health care professional. A puncture-resistant container for disposal of needles and syringes should be used. Patients should be instructed in the technique and importance of proper syringe and needle disposal and be cautioned against reuse of these items.

Table 2
Brain MRI Data According to Treatment Group

	AVONEX®	Placebo
CHANGE IN T2 VOLUME @ 18 MONTHS:	N = 119	N = 109
Actual Change (mm^3)[1]*		
Median (25th%, 75th%)	28 (-576, 397)	313 (5, 1140)
Percentage Change[1]*		
Median (25th%, 75th%)	1 (-24, 29)	16 (0, 53)
NUMBER OF NEW OR ENLARGING T2 LESIONS @ 18 MONTHS[1]*:	N = 132	N = 119
	N (%)	N (%)
0	62 (47)	22 (18)
1–3	41 (31)	47 (40)
≥4	29 (22)	50 (42)
Mean (SD)	2.13 (3.19)	4.97 (7.71)
NUMBER OF GD-ENHANCING LESIONS @ 6 MONTHS[2]*:	N = 165	N = 152
	N (%)	N (%)
0	115 (70)	93 (61)
1	27 (16)	16 (11)
>1	23 (14)	43 (28)
Mean (SD)	0.87 (2.28)	1.49 (3.14)

[1]P value <0.001
[2]P value <0.03
*P value from a Mann-Whitney rank-sum test

Laboratory Tests
In addition to those laboratory tests normally required for monitoring patients with multiple sclerosis, complete blood and differential white blood cell counts, platelet counts, and blood chemistries, including liver function tests, are recommended during AVONEX® therapy (see WARNINGS: Decreased Peripheral Blood Counts and PRECAUTIONS: Cardiomyopathy and Congestive Heart Failure, and Autoimmune Disorders). During the placebo-controlled studies in multiple sclerosis, these tests were performed at least every 6 months. There were no significant differences between the placebo and AVONEX® groups in the incidence of liver enzyme elevation, leukopenia, or thrombocytopenia. However, these are known to be dose-related laboratory abnormalities associated with the use of interferons. Patients with myelosuppression may require more intensive monitoring of complete blood cell counts, with differential and platelet counts. Thyroid function should be monitored periodically. If patients have or develop symptoms of thyroid dysfunction (hypo- or hyperthyroidism), thyroid function tests should be performed according to standard medical practice.

Drug Interactions
No formal drug interaction studies have been conducted with AVONEX®. In the placebo-controlled studies in multiple sclerosis, corticosteroids or ACTH were administered for treatment of exacerbations in some patients concurrently receiving AVONEX®. In addition, some patients receiving AVONEX® were also treated with anti-depressant therapy and/or oral contraceptive therapy. No unexpected adverse events were associated with these concomitant therapies. However, the potential for hepatic injury should be considered when AVONEX® is used in combination with other products associated with hepatic injury, or when new agents are added to the regimen of patients already on AVONEX® (see WARNINGS: Hepatic Injury).

Carcinogenesis, Mutagenesis, and Impairment of Fertility
Carcinogenesis: No carcinogenicity data for AVONEX® are available in animals or humans.
Mutagenesis: AVONEX® was not mutagenic when tested in the Ames bacterial test and in an *in vitro* cytogenetic assay in human lymphocytes in the presence and absence of metabolic activation. These assays are designed to detect agents that interact directly with and cause damage to cellular DNA. AVONEX® is a glycosylated protein that does not directly bind to DNA.
Impairment of Fertility: No studies were conducted to evaluate the effects of AVONEX® on fertility in normal women or women with multiple sclerosis. It is not known whether AVONEX® can affect human reproductive capacity. Menstrual irregularities were observed in monkeys administered AVONEX® at a dose 100 times the recommended weekly human dose (based upon a body surface area comparison). Anovulation and decreased serum progesterone levels were also noted transiently in some animals. These effects were reversible after discontinuation of drug.
Treatment of monkeys with AVONEX® at 2 times the recommended weekly human dose (based upon a body surface area comparison) had no effects on cycle duration or ovulation.
The accuracy of extrapolating animal doses to human doses is not known. In the placebo-controlled studies in multiple sclerosis, 5% of patients receiving placebo and 6% of patients receiving AVONEX® experienced menstrual disorder. If menstrual irregularities occur in humans, it is not known how long they will persist following treatment.

Pregnancy—Teratogenic Effects
Pregnancy Category C: The reproductive toxicity of AVONEX® has not been studied in animals or humans. In pregnant monkeys given AVONEX® at 100 times the recommended weekly human dose (based upon a body surface area comparison), no teratogenic or other adverse effects on fetal development were observed. Abortifacient activity was evident following 3 to 5 doses at this level. No abortifacient effects were observed in monkeys treated at 2 times the recommended weekly human dose (based upon a body surface area comparison). Although no teratogenic effects were seen in these studies, it is not known if teratogenic effects would be observed in humans. There are no adequate and well-controlled studies with interferons in pregnant women. If a woman becomes pregnant or plans to become pregnant while taking AVONEX®, she should be informed of the potential hazards to the fetus, and discontinuation of AVONEX® therapy should be considered.
If a woman becomes pregnant while taking AVONEX®, consider enrolling her in the AVONEX® Pregnancy Registry by calling 1-800-456-2255.

Nursing Mothers
It is not known whether AVONEX® is excreted in human milk. Because of the potential of serious adverse reactions in nursing infants, a decision should be made to either discontinue nursing or to discontinue AVONEX®.

Pediatric Use
Safety and effectiveness of AVONEX® in pediatric patients below the age of 18 years have not been evaluated.

Geriatric Use
Clinical studies of AVONEX® did not include sufficient numbers of patients aged 65 and over to determine whether they respond differently than younger patients.

ADVERSE REACTIONS

Depression, suicidal ideation, and new or worsening other psychiatric disorders have been observed to be increased in patients using interferon compounds including AVONEX® (see WARNINGS: Depression and Suicide). Anaphylaxis and other allergic reactions have been reported in patients using AVONEX® (see WARNINGS: Anaphylaxis). Decreased peripheral blood counts have been reported in patients using AVONEX® (see WARNINGS: Decreased Peripheral Blood Counts). Hepatic injury, including hepatic failure, hepatitis, and elevated serum hepatic enzyme levels, has been reported in post-marketing experience (see WARNINGS: Hepatic Injury). Seizures, cardiovascular adverse events, and autoimmune disorders also have been reported in association with the use of AVONEX® (see Precautions).
The adverse reactions most commonly reported in patients associated with the use of AVONEX® were flu-like and other symptoms occurring within hours to days following an injection. Symptoms can include myalgia, fever, fatigue, headaches, chills, nausea, and vomiting. Some patients have experienced paresthesias, hypertonia and myasthenia. The most frequently reported adverse reactions resulting in clinical intervention (e.g., discontinuation of AVONEX®, or the need for concomitant medication to treat an adverse reaction symptom) were flu-like symptoms and depression.
Because clinical trials are conducted under widely varying conditions, adverse reaction rates observed in the clinical trials of AVONEX® cannot be directly compared to rates in clinical trials of other drugs and may not reflect the rates observed in practice.
The data described below reflect exposure to AVONEX® in 351 patients, including 319 patients exposed for 6 months, and 288 patients exposed for greater than one year in placebo-controlled trials. The mean age of patients receiving AVONEX® was 35 years, 74% were women and 89% were Caucasian. Patients received either 30 mcg AVONEX® or placebo.
Table 3 enumerates adverse events and selected laboratory abnormalities that occurred at an incidence of at least 2% higher frequency in AVONEX®-treated subjects than was observed in the placebo group. Reported adverse events have been classified using standard COSTART terms.
[See table 3 at top of next page]
No AVONEX®-treated patients attempted suicide in the two placebo-controlled studies. In Study 2, AVONEX®-treated patients were more likely to experience depression than placebo-treated patients (20% in AVONEX® group vs. 13% in placebo group). The incidences of depression in the placebo-treated and AVONEX®-treated patients in Study 1 were similar. In Study 1, suicidal tendency was seen more frequently in AVONEX®-treated patients (4% in AVONEX® group vs. 1% in placebo group) (see WARNINGS).

Continued on next page

Avonex—Cont.

Seizures

Seizures have been reported in 4 of 351 AVONEX®-treated patients in the placebo-controlled studies, compared to none in the placebo-treated patients (see Precautions: Seizures).

Post-Marketing Experience

The following adverse events have been identified and reported during post-approval use of AVONEX®: New or worsening other psychiatric disorders, and anaphylaxis (see WARNINGS). Autoimmune disorders including autoimmune hepatitis, idiopathic thrombocytopenia, hyper- and hypothyroidism, and seizures in patients without prior history (see Precautions).

Infrequent reports of congestive heart failure, cardiomyopathy, and cardiomyopathy with congestive heart failure with rare cases being temporally related to the administration of AVONEX® (see Precautions: Cardiomyopathy and Congestive Heart Failure).

Decreased peripheral blood counts in all cell lines, including rare pancytopenia and thrombocytopenia (see WARNINGS: Decreased Peripheral Blood Counts). Some cases of thrombocytopenia have had nadirs below 10,000/μL. Some of these cases reoccur upon rechallenge.

Hepatic injury, including hepatic failure and elevated serum hepatic enzyme levels, some of which have been severe, has been reported post-marketing (see WARNINGS: Hepatic Injury).

Meno- and metrorrhagia, rash (including vesicular rash), and rare cases of injection site abscess or cellulitis that may require surgical intervention have also been reported in post-marketing experience.

Because reports of these reactions are voluntary and the population is of an uncertain size, it is not always possible to reliably estimate the frequency of the event or establish a causal relationship to drug exposure.

Adverse Reactions Associated with Subcutaneous Use

AVONEX® has also been evaluated in 290 patients with diseases other than multiple sclerosis, primarily chronic viral hepatitis B and C, in which the doses studied ranged from 15 mcg to 75 mcg, given SC, 3 times a week, for up to 6 months. Inflammation at the site of the subcutaneous injection was observed in 52% of treated patients in these studies. Subcutaneous injections were also associated with the following local reactions: injection site necrosis, injection site atrophy, injection site edema and injection site hemorrhage. None of the above was observed in the multiple sclerosis patients participating in Study 1. Injection site edema and injection site hemorrhage were observed in multiple sclerosis patients participating in Study 2.

Immunogenicity

As with all therapeutic proteins, there is a potential for immunogenicity. In recent studies assessing immunogenicity in multiple sclerosis patients administered AVONEX® for at least 1 year, 5% (21 of 390 patients) showed the presence of neutralizing antibodies at one or more times. The clinical significance of neutralizing antibodies to AVONEX® is unknown.

These data reflect the percentage of patients whose test results were considered positive for antibodies to AVONEX® using a two-tiered assay (ELISA binding assay followed by an antiviral cytopathic effect assay), and are highly dependent on the sensitivity and specificity of the assay. Additionally, the observed incidence of neutralizing activity in an assay may be influenced by several factors including sample handling, timing of sample collection, concomitant medications, and underlying disease. For these reasons, comparison of the incidence of antibodies to AVONEX® with the incidence of antibodies to other products may be misleading.

Anaphylaxis has been reported as a rare complication of AVONEX® use. Other allergic reactions have included dyspnea, orolingual edema, skin rash and urticaria (see WARNINGS: Anaphylaxis).

DRUG ABUSE AND DEPENDENCE

There is no evidence that abuse or dependence occurs with AVONEX® therapy. However, the risk of dependence has not been systematically evaluated.

OVERDOSAGE

Safety of doses higher than 60 mcg once a week have not been adequately evaluated. The maximum amount of AVONEX® that can be safely administered has not been determined.

DOSAGE AND ADMINISTRATION

The recommended dosage of AVONEX® (Interferon beta-1a) is 30 mcg injected intramuscularly once a week.

AVONEX® is intended for use under the guidance and supervision of a physician. Patients may self-inject only if their physician determines that it is appropriate and with medical follow-up, as necessary, after proper training in intramuscular injection technique. Sites for injection include the thigh or upper arm (see Medication Guide).

Reconstitution of AVONEX® Vials

Use appropriate aseptic technique during the preparation of AVONEX®. To reconstitute lyophilized AVONEX®, use a sterile syringe and MICRO PIN® to inject 1.1 mL of the supplied diluent, Sterile Water for Injection, USP, into the AVONEX® vial. Gently swirl the vial of AVONEX® to dissolve the drug completely. **DO NOT SHAKE.** The reconstituted solution should be clear to slightly yellow without particles. Inspect the reconstituted product visually prior to

use. Discard the product if it contains particulate matter or is discolored. Each vial of reconstituted solution contains 30 mcg/1.0 mL Interferon beta-1a.

Withdraw 1.0 mL of reconstituted solution from the vial into a sterile syringe. Replace the cover on the MICRO PIN® and attach the sterile 23 gauge, 1¼ inch needle and inject the solution intramuscularly. The AVONEX® and diluent vials are for single-use only; unused portions should be discarded.

Using Avonex® Prefilled Syringes

The AVONEX® prefilled syringe should be held upright (rubber cap faces up). Remove the protective cover by turning and gently pulling the rubber cap in a clockwise motion. Attach the 23 gauge, 1¼ inch needle and inject the solution intramuscularly. The AVONEX® prefilled syringe is for single-use only.

HOW SUPPLIED

30 mcg Lyophilized Powder Vial

A vial of AVONEX® is supplied as a lyophilized powder in a single-use vial containing 33 mcg (6.6 million IU) of Interferon beta-1a; 16.5 mg Albumin (Human), USP; 6.4 mg Sodium Chloride, USP; 6.3 mg Dibasic Sodium Phosphate, USP; and 1.3 mg Monobasic Sodium Phosphate, USP, and is preservative-free. Diluent is supplied in a single-use vial (Sterile Water for Injection, USP).

AVONEX® lyophilized vials are available in the following package configuration (NDC 59627-001-03): A package containing four Administration Dose Packs (each containing one vial of AVONEX®, one 10 mL diluent vial, two alcohol wipes, one gauze pad, one 3 mL syringe, one MICRO PIN®* vial access pin, one 23 gauge, 1¼ inch needle, and one adhesive bandage).

30 mcg Prefilled Syringe

A prefilled syringe of AVONEX® is supplied as a sterile liquid albumin-free formulation containing 30 mcg of Interferon beta-1a, 0.79 mg Sodium Acetate Trihydrate, USP; 0.25 mg Glacial Acetic Acid, USP; 15.8 mg Arginine Hydrochloride, USP; and 0.025 mg Polysorbate 20 in Water for Injection, USP. Each prefilled glass syringe contains 0.5 mL for IM injection.

AVONEX® prefilled syringes are available in the following package configuration (NDC 59627-002-05): A package containing four Administration Dose Packs (each containing one single-use syringe of AVONEX® and one 23 gauge, 1¼ inch needle), and a recloseable accessory pouch containing 4 alcohol wipes, 4 gauze pads, and 4 adhesive bandages.

Stability and Storage

30 mcg Lyophilized Powder Vial

Vials of AVONEX® must be stored in a 2-8°C (36-46°F) refrigerator. Should refrigeration be unavailable, vials of AVONEX® can be stored at 25°C (77°F) for a period of up to 30 days. DO NOT EXPOSE TO HIGH TEMPERATURES. DO NOT FREEZE. Protect from light. Do not use beyond the expiration date stamped on the vial. Following reconstitution, it is recommended the product be used as soon as possible within 6 hours stored at 2-8°C (36-46°F). DO NOT FREEZE RECONSTITUTED AVONEX®.

30 mcg Prefilled Syringe

AVONEX® in prefilled syringes must be stored in a 2-8°C (36-46°F) refrigerator. Once removed from the refrigerator, AVONEX® in a prefilled syringe should be allowed to warm to room temperature (about 30 minutes) and used within 12 hours. Do not use external heat sources such as hot water to warm AVONEX® in a prefilled syringe. DO NOT EXPOSE TO HIGH TEMPERATURES. DO NOT FREEZE. Protect from light. Do not use beyond the expiration date stamped on the syringe.

REFERENCES

1. Jacobs LD, et al. Intramuscular interferon beta-1a for disease progression in relapsing multiple sclerosis. Ann Neurol 1996;39(3):285-294.
2. Jacobs LD, et al. Intramuscular interferon beta-1a initiated during a first demyelinating event in multiple sclerosis. NEJM 2000;343:898-904.
3. Kurtzke JF. Rating neurologic impairment in multiple sclerosis: an expanded disability status scale (EDSS). Neurology 1983;33:1444-1452.

AVONEX® (Interferon beta-1a)
Manufactured by:
BIOGEN IDEC INC.
14 Cambridge Center
Cambridge, MA 02142 USA
©2005 Biogen Idec Inc. All rights reserved.
1-800-456-2255
U.S. Patent Pending
(Issue Date 03/2005)
Rx only
*Micro Pin® is the trademark of B. Braun Medical Inc.

MEDICATION GUIDE

AVONEX®
Interferon beta-1a
(Including appendix with instructions for using AVONEX® Prefilled Syringe or the AVONEX® vials)

Please read this guide carefully before you start to use AVONEX® (a-vuh-necks) and each time your prescription is refilled since there may be new information. The information in this guide does not take the place of talking with your doctor or healthcare professional.

What is the most important information I should know about AVONEX®?

AVONEX® will not cure multiple sclerosis (MS) but it has been shown to decrease the number of flare-ups and slow the occurrence of some of the physical disability that is common in people with MS. AVONEX® can cause serious side effects, so before you start taking AVONEX®, you should talk with your doctor about the possible benefits of AVONEX® and its possible side effects to decide if AVONEX® is right for you. Potential serious side effects include:

• **Depression**—Some people treated with interferons, including AVONEX®, have become depressed (feeling sad, feeling low or feeling bad about oneself). Some people have thought about killing themselves and a few have committed suicide. Depression is common in people with

Table 3
Adverse Events and Selected Laboratory Abnormalities in the Placebo-Controlled Studies

Adverse Event	Placebo (N = 333)	AVONEX® (N = 351)
Body as a Whole		
Headache	55%	58%
Flu-like symptoms (otherwise unspecified)	29%	49%
Pain	21%	23%
Asthenia	18%	24%
Fever	9%	20%
Chills	5%	19%
Abdominal pain	6%	8%
Injection site pain	6%	8%
Infection	4%	7%
Injection site inflammation	2%	6%
Chest pain	2%	5%
Injection site reaction	1%	3%
Toothache	1%	3%
Nervous System		
Depression	14%	18%
Dizziness	12%	14%
Respiratory System		
Upper respiratory tract infection	12%	14%
Sinusitis	12%	14%
Bronchitis	5%	8%
Digestive System		
Nausea	19%	23%
Musculoskeletal System		
Myalgia	22%	29%
Arthralgia	6%	9%
Urogenital		
Urinary tract infection	15%	17%
Urine constituents abnormal	0%	3%
Skin and Appendages		
Alopecia	2%	4%
Special Senses		
Eye disorder	2%	4%
Hemic and Lymphatic System		
Injection site ecchymosis	4%	6%
Anemia	1%	4%
Cardiovascular System		
Migraine	3%	5%
Vasodilation	0%	2%

MS. If you are noticeably sadder or feeling more hopeless, you should tell a family member or friend right away and call your doctor as soon as possible. You should tell the doctor if you have ever had any mental illness, including depression, and if you take any medicines for depression.

- **Liver problems**—Your liver may be affected by taking AVONEX® and a few patients have developed severe liver injury. Your healthcare provider may ask you to have regular blood tests to make sure that your liver is working properly. If your skin or the whites of your eyes become yellow or if you are bruising easily you should call your doctor immediately.

- **Risk to pregnancy**—If you become pregnant while taking AVONEX®, you should stop using AVONEX® immediately and call your doctor. AVONEX® may cause you to lose your baby (miscarry) or may cause harm to your unborn child. You and your doctor will need to decide whether the potential benefit of taking AVONEX® is greater than the risks are to your unborn child.

- **Allergic reactions**—Some patients taking AVONEX® have had severe allergic reactions leading to difficulty breathing. Allergic reactions can happen after your first dose or may not happen until after you have taken AVONEX® many times. Less severe allergic reactions such as rash, itching, skin bumps or swelling of the mouth and tongue can also happen. If you think you are having an allergic reaction, stop using AVONEX® immediately and call your doctor.

- **Blood problems**—You may have a drop in the levels of infection-fighting blood cells, red blood cells or cells that help to form blood clots. If the drop in levels are severe, they can lessen your ability to fight infections, make you feel tired or sluggish or cause you to bruise or bleed easily.

- **Seizures**—Some patients have had seizures while taking AVONEX®, including some patients who have never had seizures before. It is not known whether the seizures were related to the effects of their MS, to AVONEX®, or to a combination of both. If you have a seizure while taking AVONEX®, you should stop taking AVONEX® and call your doctor right away.

- **Heart problems**—While AVONEX® is not known to have direct effects on the heart, a few patients who did not have a history of heart problems developed heart muscle problems or congestive heart failure after taking AVONEX®. Some of the symptoms of heart problems are swollen ankles, shortness of breath, decreased ability to exercise, fast heartbeat, tightness in chest, increased need to urinate at night, and not being able to lay flat in bed. If you develop these symptoms or any heart problems while taking AVONEX®, you should call your doctor right away.

For more information on possible side effects with AVONEX®, please read the section on **"What are the possible side effects of AVONEX®?"** in this Medication Guide.

What is AVONEX®?

AVONEX® is a form of a protein called beta interferon that occurs naturally in the body. It is used to treat relapsing forms of multiple sclerosis. It will not cure your MS but may decrease the number of flare-ups of the disease and slow the occurrence of some of the physical disability that is common in people with MS. MS is a life-long disease that affects your nervous system by destroying the protective covering (myelin) that surrounds your nerve fibers. The way AVONEX® works in MS is not known.

Who should not take AVONEX®?

Do not take AVONEX® if you have had an allergic reaction (difficulty breathing, itching, flushing or skin bumps spread widely over the body) to interferon beta.

Do not take the vial formulation of AVONEX® if you have a history of hypersensitivity to albumin (human).

If you have ever had any of the following conditions or serious medical problems, you should tell your doctor before taking AVONEX®:

- Depression (sinking feeling or sadness), anxiety (feeling uneasy or fearful for no reason), or trouble sleeping
- Problems with your thyroid gland
- Blood problems such as bleeding or bruising easily and anemia (low red blood cells) or low white blood cells
- Seizures (for example, epilepsy)
- Heart problems
- Liver disease
- Are planning to become pregnant

You should tell your doctor if you are taking any other prescription or nonprescription medicines. This includes any vitamin or mineral supplements, or herbal products.

You should tell your doctor if you have had a natural rubber sensitivity since the AVONEX® prefilled syringe cap contains dry natural rubber, which may cause allergic reactions.

How should I take AVONEX®?

To get the most benefit from this medicine, it is important that you take AVONEX® exactly as your doctor tells you. AVONEX® is given by injection into the muscle (intramuscular injection) once a week, on the same day (for example, every Monday right before bedtime). If you miss a dose, you should take your next dose as soon as you remember. You should continue your regular schedule the following week. **Do not take AVONEX® on two consecutive days.** Take only the dose your doctor has prescribed for you. Do not change your dose unless you are told to by your doctor. If you take more than your prescribed dose, call your healthcare provider right away. Your doctor may want to monitor you more closely.

You should always follow your doctor's instructions and advice about how to take this medication. If your doctor feels that you, or a family member or friend, may give you the

injections, then you and/or the other person should be instructed by your doctor or other healthcare provider in how to prepare and inject your dose of AVONEX®. Do not try to give yourself injections at home until you are sure that you (or the person who will be giving you the injections) fully understands and is comfortable with how to prepare and inject the product. At the end of this guide there are detailed instructions on how to prepare and give yourself an injection of AVONEX® that will help remind you of the instructions from your doctor or healthcare provider.

Always use a new, unopened AVONEX® vial or prefilled syringe for each injection. Never reuse the vials or syringes. It is important to keep your work area, your hands, and your injection site clean to minimize risk of infection. You should wash your hands prior to handling the syringe.

It is important that you change your injection site each week.

Do not inject into an area of the body where the skin is irritated, reddened, bruised, infected or scarred in any way. Use the alcohol wipe to **thoroughly** clean the skin at the injection site you have chosen. Using a circular motion, and starting at the injection site and moving outward, clean the injection site with an alcohol wipe. Let the skin area dry before you inject the AVONEX®.

AVONEX® comes in two different forms (a powder in a single-use vial and a liquid in a prefilled syringe). **See the attached appendix for detailed instructions for preparing and giving a dose of AVONEX®. These instructions are specific to the form of AVONEX® chosen for you by your healthcare provider.**

What should I avoid while taking AVONEX®?

- **Pregnancy**—You should avoid becoming pregnant while taking AVONEX® until you have talked with your doctor. AVONEX® can cause you to lose your baby (miscarry). If you become pregnant while taking AVONEX® you should stop using AVONEX® immediately and tell your doctor. You and your doctor will need to decide whether the potential benefit of taking AVONEX® is greater than the risk to your unborn child. If you become pregnant while taking AVONEX®, consider enrolling in the AVONEX® Pregnancy Registry by calling 1-800-456-2255.

- **Breast-feeding**—You should talk to your doctor if you are breast-feeding an infant. It is not known if the interferon in AVONEX® gets into the breast milk, or if it could harm your nursing baby.

What are the possible side effects of AVONEX®?

- **Flu-like symptoms**—Most people who take AVONEX® have flu-like symptoms (fever, chills, sweating, muscle aches, and tiredness) early during the course of therapy. Usually, these symptoms last for a day after the injection. You may be able to manage these flu-like symptoms by injecting your AVONEX® dose at bedtime and taking over-the-counter pain and fever reducers. For many people, these symptoms lessen or go away over time. Talk to your doctor if these symptoms continue longer than the first few months of therapy, or if they are difficult to manage.

- **Depression**—Some patients taking interferons have become severely depressed and/or anxious. If you feel sad or hopeless you should tell a friend or family member right away and call your doctor immediately. Your doctor or healthcare provider may ask that you stop taking AVONEX®, and/or may recommend that you take a medication to treat your depression. (See **"What is the most important information I should know about AVONEX®?"**)

- **Liver problems**—Your liver function may be affected. If you develop symptoms of changes in your liver, including yellowing of the skin and whites of the eyes and easy bruising, call your doctor immediately. (See **"What is the most important information I should know about AVONEX®?"**)

- **Blood problems**—A drop in the levels of white (infection-fighting) blood cells, red blood cells, or a part of your blood that helps to form blood clots (platelets) can happen. If this drop in blood levels is severe, it can lessen your ability to fight infections, make you feel very tired or sluggish, or cause you to bruise or bleed easily. Your doctor may ask you to have periodic blood tests. (See **"What is the most important information I should know about AVONEX®?"**)

- **Thyroid problems**—Some people taking AVONEX® develop changes in the function of their thyroid. Symptoms of these changes include feeling cold or hot all the time, a change in your weight (gain or loss) without a change in your diet or amount of exercise you get, or feeling emotional.

- **Seizures**—Some patients have had seizures while taking AVONEX®, including patients who have never had seizures before. It is not known whether the seizures were related to the effects of their MS, to AVONEX®, or to a combination of both. If you have a seizure while taking AVONEX®, you should call your doctor right away. (See **"What is the most important information I should know about AVONEX®?"**)

- **Heart problems**—While AVONEX® is not known to have any direct effects on the heart, a few patients who did not have a history of heart problems developed heart muscle problems or congestive heart failure after taking AVONEX®. Some of the symptoms of heart problems are swollen ankles, shortness of breath, decreased ability to exercise, fast heartbeat, tightness in chest, increased need to urinate at night, and not being able to lay flat in bed. If you develop these symptoms or any heart problems while

taking AVONEX®, you should call your doctor right away. (See **"What is the most important information I should know about AVONEX®?"**)

If you get any of the symptoms listed in this section or any listed in the section **"What is the most important information I should know about AVONEX®?"**, you should call your doctor right away. Whether you experience any side effects or not, you and your doctor should periodically discuss your general health. Your doctor may want to monitor you more closely or may ask you to have blood tests more frequently.

General advice about prescription medicines

Medicines are sometimes prescribed for purposes other than those listed in a Medication Guide. This medication has been prescribed for your particular condition. Do not use it for another condition or give this drug to anyone else. If you have questions you should speak with your doctor or healthcare professional. You may also ask your doctor or pharmacist for a copy of the information provided to them with the product.

Keep this and all drugs out of the reach of children.

This Medication Guide has been approved by the U.S. Food and Drug Administration.

Manufactured by:
Biogen Idec Inc.
14 Cambridge Center
Cambridge, MA 02142 USA
©2005 Biogen Idec Inc. All rights reserved.
1-800-456-2255
(Issue date 03/2005)

Medication Guide Appendix: Instructions for Preparing and Giving a Dose with an AVONEX® Prefilled Syringe

Storing AVONEX® Prefilled Syringes

AVONEX® in prefilled syringes should be refrigerated (36-46°F or 2-8°C). Once removed from the refrigerator, AVONEX® in a prefilled syringe should be allowed to warm to room temperature (about 30 minutes) and used within 12 hours. Do not use external heat sources such as hot water to warm AVONEX® in a prefilled syringe. Do not expose to high temperatures. Do not freeze. Protect from light.

How do I prepare and inject a dose of AVONEX®?

Find a well lit, clean, flat work surface like a table and collect all the supplies you will need to give yourself or receive an injection. Take one AVONEX® Administration Dose Pack out of the refrigerator about 30 minutes before you plan on injecting your dose to allow it to reach room temperature. A room temperature solution is more comfortable to inject. You will need the following supplies:

- single-use prefilled syringe
- sterile needle
- alcohol wipe
- gauze pad
- adhesive bandage
- a puncture resistant container for disposal of used syringes and needles

Preparing AVONEX® prefilled syringe

It is important to keep your work area, your hands, and your injection site clean to minimize risk of infection. You should wash your hands prior to handling the syringe.

1. Check the expiration date. The expiration date is printed on the AVONEX® prefilled syringe, syringe package, and the carton. Do not use if the medication is expired.

2. Check the contents of the syringe. The solution in the syringe should be clear and colorless. If the solution is colored or cloudy, do not use the syringe. Get a new syringe.

3. Hold the syringe so the rubber cap is facing down and the 0.5 mL mark is at eye level. Check to make sure the amount of liquid in the syringe is the same or very close to the 0.5 mL mark. If the syringe does not have the correct amount of liquid, DO NOT USE THAT SYRINGE. Call your pharmacist.

4. Hold the AVONEX® prefilled syringe upright (rubber cap facing up).

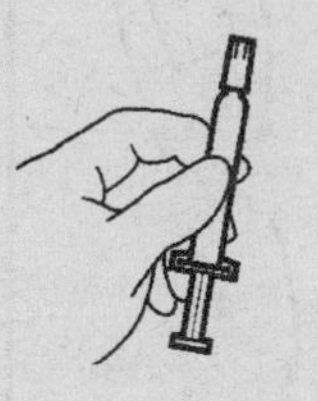

5. Remove the protective rubber cap by turning and gently pulling the cap in a clockwise motion.

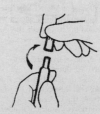

6. Open the package with the 23 gauge 1¼ inch needle. Attach the needle by firmly pressing it onto the syringe and turning it a half turn clockwise.

Continued on next page

Avonex—Cont.

NOTE: If you do not firmly attach the needle to the syringe, it may leak so you may not get your full dose of AVONEX®.

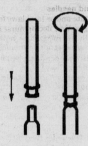

Selecting an injection site

You should use a different site each time you inject. This can be as simple as switching between thighs (if you are always injecting yourself), or if another person is helping you, you can rotate between your upper arms and your thighs. Keeping a record of the date and location of each injection will help you.

Do not inject into an area of the body where the skin is irritated, reddened, bruised, infected or scarred in any way. The best sites for intramuscular injection are the thigh and upper arm:
• thigh

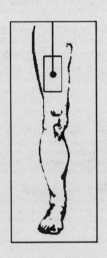

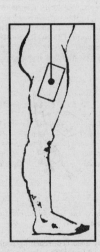

• upper arm
  [See first figure at top of next column]

Injecting the AVONEX® dose

1. Use the alcohol wipe to clean the skin at the injection site you choose. Then, pull the protective cover **straight** off the needle; do not twist the cover off.
2. With one hand, stretch the skin out around the injection site. Hold the syringe like a pencil with the other hand, and using a quick motion insert the needle at a 90° angle, through the skin and into the muscle.
3. Once the needle is in, let go of the skin and slowly push the plunger down until the syringe is empty.
   [See second figure at top of next column]

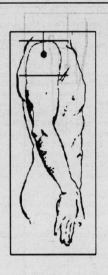

4. Take the gauze pad and hold it near the needle at the injection site and pull the needle straight out. Use the gauze pad to apply pressure to the site for a few seconds or rub gently in a circular motion.

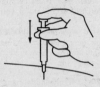

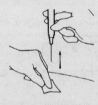

5. If there is bleeding at the site, wipe it off and, if necessary, apply an adhesive bandage.
6. After 2 hours, check the injection site for redness, swelling or tenderness. If you have a skin reaction and it does not clear up in a few days, contact your doctor or nurse.
7. Dispose of the used syringe and needle in your puncture resistant container. This is a single-use syringe. DO NOT USE a syringe or needle more than once.

Disposal of syringes and needles

There may be special state and/or local laws for disposing of used needles and syringes. Your doctor, nurse or pharmacist should provide you with instructions on how to dispose of your used needles and syringes.
• **Always keep your disposal container out of the reach of children.**
• DO NOT throw used needles and syringes into the household trash and DO NOT RECYCLE.

Appendix Revision Date: 03/2005

Medication Guide Appendix: Instructions for Preparing and Giving a Dose with an AVONEX® Vial

Storing AVONEX® Vials

Prior to use, AVONEX® should be refrigerated (36-46°F or 2-8°C) but can be kept for up to 30 days at room temperature (77°F or 25°C). You should avoid exposing AVONEX® to high temperatures and freezing. After mixing, AVONEX® solution should be used immediately, within 6 hours when stored refrigerated at 36-46°F or 2-8°C. Do not freeze the AVONEX® solution.

How do I prepare and inject a dose of AVONEX®?

Find a well-lit, clean, flat work surface like a table and collect all the supplies you will need to give yourself or receive an injection. You may want to take one AVONEX® Administration Dose Pack out of the refrigerator about 30 minutes before you plan on injecting your dose to allow it to reach room temperature. A room temperature solution is more comfortable to inject.

You will need the following supplies:
• vial of AVONEX® (white to off-white powder or cake)
• vial of diluent, single-use (Sterile Water for Injection, USP)
• 3 mL syringe
• blue MICRO PIN® (vial access pin)
• sterile needle
• alcohol wipes
• gauze pad
• adhesive bandage
• a puncture resistant container for disposal of used syringes, needles, and MICRO PINS.

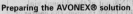

Preparing the AVONEX® solution

It is important to keep your work area, your hands, and your injection site clean to minimize risk of infection. You should wash your hands prior to preparing the medication.

1. Check the expiration date on the AVONEX® vial and the vial of diluent; do not use if the medication or diluent is expired.
2. Remove the caps from the vial of AVONEX® and the vial of diluent, and clean the rubber stopper on the top of each vial with an alcohol wipe.

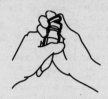

3. Attach the blue MICRO PIN® to the syringe by turning clockwise until secure. *NOTE: Over-tightening can make the MICRO PIN® difficult to remove.*

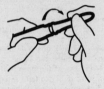

4. Pull the MICRO PIN® cover straight off; do not twist. Save the cover for later use.

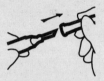

5. Pull back the syringe plunger to the 1.1 mL mark.

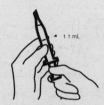

6. Firmly push the MICRO PIN® down through the **center** of the rubber stopper of the diluent vial.

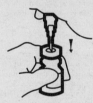

7. Inject the air in the syringe into the diluent vial by pushing down on the plunger until it cannot be pushed any further.
8. Keeping the MICRO PIN® in the vial, turn the diluent vial and syringe upside down.
9. While keeping the MICRO PIN® in the fluid, slowly pull back on the plunger to withdraw 1.1 mL of diluent into the syringe.

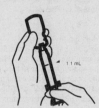

10. Gently tap the syringe with your finger to make any air bubbles rise to the top. If bubbles are present, slowly press the plunger in (to push just the bubbles out through the needle). Make sure there is still 1.1 mL of diluent in the syringe.

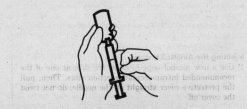

11. Slowly pull the MICRO PIN® out of the diluent vial.
12. Carefully insert the MICRO PIN® through the **center** of the rubber stopper of the vial of AVONEX®. *NOTE: Off-center punctures can push the stopper into the vial. If the stopper falls into the vial, do not use.*
13. **Slowly** inject the diluent into the vial of AVONEX®. DO NOT aim the stream of diluent directly on the AVONEX® powder. Too direct or forceful a stream of diluent onto the powder may cause foaming, and make it difficult to withdraw AVONEX®.

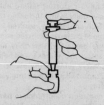

14. Without removing the syringe, **gently** swirl the vial until the AVONEX® is dissolved. ***DO NOT SHAKE.***

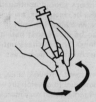

15. Check to see that all of the AVONEX® is dissolved. Check the solution in the vial of AVONEX®. It should be clear to slightly yellow in color and should not have any particles. Do not use the vial if the solution is cloudy, has particles in it or is a color other than clear to slightly yellow.
16. Turn the vial and syringe upside down. Slowly pull back on the plunger to withdraw 1.0 mL of AVONEX®. If bubbles appear, push solution slowly back into the vial and withdraw the solution again.

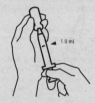

17. With the vial still upside down, tap the syringe **gently** to make any air bubbles rise to the top. Then press the plunger in until the AVONEX® is at the top of the syringe. Check the volume (should be 1.0 mL) and withdraw more medication if necessary. Withdraw the MICRO PIN® and syringe from the vial.
18. Replace the cover on the MICRO PIN® and remove from the syringe with a counterclockwise turn.
19. Attach the sterile needle for injection to the syringe turning clockwise until the needle is secure. A secure attachment will prevent leakage during the injection.

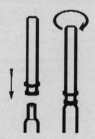

Selecting an injection site
You should use a different site each time you inject. This can be as simple as switching between thighs (if you are always injecting yourself), or if another person is helping you, you can rotate between your upper arms and your thighs. Keeping a record of the date and location of each injection will help you.

Do not inject into an area of the body where the skin is irritated, reddened, bruised, infected or scarred in any way. The best sites for intramuscular injection are the thigh and upper arm:
* thigh
  [See first figure at top of next column]
  [See second figure at top of next column]
* upper arm
  [See third figure in next column]

Injecting the AVONEX® dose
1. Use a new alcohol wipe to clean the skin at one of the recommended intramuscular injection sites. Then, pull the protective cover **straight** off the needle; do not twist the cover off.

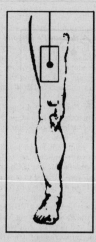

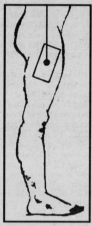

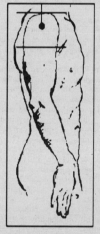

2. With one hand, stretch the skin out around the injection site. Hold the syringe like a pencil with the other hand, and using a quick motion insert the needle at a 90° angle, through the skin and into the muscle.
3. Once the needle is in, let go of the skin and use that hand to gently pull back slightly on the plunger. If you see blood come into the syringe, withdraw the needle from the injection site and put pressure the site with a gauze pad. You will need to replace the needle and choose clean a new site for injection.
4. If no blood came into the syringe, slowly push the plunger in the syringe is empty.

5. Hold a gauze pad near the needle at the injection site and pull the needle straight out. Use the pad to apply pressure to the site for a few seconds or rub gently in a circular motion.

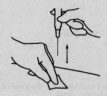

6. If there is bleeding at the site, wipe it off and, if necessary, apply an adhesive bandage.
7. Dispose of the used syringe, needle and blue MICRO PIN® in your puncture resistant container. DO NOT USE a syringe, MICRO PIN®, or needle more than once. The AVONEX® and diluent vials should be put in the trash.

Disposal of syringes and needles
There may be special state and/or local laws for disposing of used needles and syringes. Your doctor, nurse or pharmacist should provide you with instructions on how to dispose of your used needles and syringes.
* **Always keep your disposal container out of the reach of children.**
* DO NOT throw used needles and syringes into the household trash and DO NOT RECYCLE.

Appendix Revision Date: 11/2004

Boehringer Ingelheim Pharmaceuticals, Inc.
A subsidiary of Boehringer Ingelheim Corporation
900 RIDGEBURY ROAD
POST OFFICE BOX 368
RIDGEFIELD, CT 06877-0368

For Medical Information Contact:
1–800–542–6257
or email:
druginfo@rdg.boehringer-ingelheim.com

MIRAPEX® ℞
[mĭ-ră·pĕks]
(pramipexole dihydrochloride)
0.125 mg, 0.25 mg, 0.5 mg, 1 mg, and 1.5 mg Tablets

Prescribing information for this product, which appears on pages 1002–1006 of the 2005 PDR, has been completely revised as follows. Please write "See Supplement A" next to the product heading.

DESCRIPTION
MIRAPEX® (pramipexole dihydrochloride) Tablets contain pramipexole, a dopamine agonist indicated for the treatment of the signs and symptoms of idiopathic Parkinson's disease. The chemical name of pramipexole dihydrochloride is (S)-2-amino-4,5,6,7-tetrahydro-6-(propylamino)benzothiazole dihydrochloride monohydrate. Its empirical formula is $C_{10}H_{17}N_3S \cdot 2\,HCl \cdot H_2O$, and its molecular weight is 302.27. The structural formula is:

$$H_2N \quad \cdots \quad \cdot 2\,HCl \cdot H_2O$$

Pramipexole dihydrochloride is a white to off-white powder substance. Melting occurs in the range of 296°C to 301°C, with decomposition. Pramipexole dihydrochloride is more than 20% soluble in water, about 8% in methanol, about 0.5% in ethanol, and practically insoluble in dichloromethane.

MIRAPEX Tablets, for oral administration, contain 0.125 mg, 0.25 mg, 0.5 mg, 1.0 mg, or 1.5 mg of pramipexole dihydrochloride monohydrate. Inactive ingredients consist of mannitol, corn starch, colloidal silicon dioxide, povidone, and magnesium stearate.

CLINICAL PHARMACOLOGY
Pramipexole is a nonergot dopamine agonist with high relative in vitro specificity and full intrinsic activity at the D_2 subfamily of dopamine receptors, binding with higher affinity to D_3 than to D_2 or D_4 receptor subtypes. The relevance of D_3 receptor binding in Parkinson's disease is unknown.

The precise mechanism of action of pramipexole as a treatment for Parkinson's disease is unknown, although it is believed to be related to its ability to stimulate dopamine receptors in the striatum. This conclusion is supported by electrophysiologic studies in animals that have demonstrated that pramipexole influences striatal neuronal firing rates via activation of dopamine receptors in the striatum and the substantia nigra, the site of neurons that send projections to the striatum.

Pharmacokinetics
Pramipexole is rapidly absorbed, reaching peak concentrations in approximately 2 hours. The absolute bioavailability of pramipexole is greater than 90%, indicating that it is well absorbed and undergoes little presystemic metabolism. Food does not affect the extent of pramipexole absorption, although the time of maximum plasma concentration (T_{max}) is increased by about 1 hour when the drug is taken with a meal.

Pramipexole is extensively distributed, having a volume of distribution of about 500 L (coefficient of variation [CV]=20%). It is about 15% bound to plasma proteins. Pramipexole distributes into red blood cells as indicated by an erythrocyte-to-plasma ratio of approximately 2.

Continued on next page

Mirapex—Cont.

Pramipexole displays linear pharmacokinetics over the clinical dosage range. Its terminal half-life is about 8 hours in young healthy volunteers and about 12 hours in elderly volunteers (see **CLINICAL PHARMACOLOGY**, *Pharmacokinetics in Special Populations*). Steady-state concentrations are achieved within 2 days of dosing.

Metabolism and elimination: Urinary excretion is the major route of pramipexole elimination, with 90% of a pramipexole dose recovered in urine, almost all as unchanged drug. Nonrenal routes may contribute to a small extent to pramipexole elimination, although no metabolites have been identified in plasma or urine. The renal clearance of pramipexole is approximately 400 mL/min (CV=25%), approximately three times higher than the glomerular filtration rate. Thus, pramipexole is secreted by the renal tubules, probably by the organic cation transport system.

Pharmacokinetics in Special Populations
Because therapy with pramipexole is initiated at a subtherapeutic dosage and gradually titrated upward according to clinical tolerability to obtain the optimum therapeutic effect, adjustment of the initial dose based on gender, weight, or age is not necessary. However, renal insufficiency, which can cause a large decrease in the ability to eliminate pramipexole, may necessitate dosage adjustment (see **CLINICAL PHARMACOLOGY**, *Renal Insufficiency*).

Gender: Pramipexole clearance is about 30% lower in women than in men, but most of this difference can be accounted for by differences in body weight. There is no difference in half-life between males and females.

Age: Pramipexole clearance decreases with age as the half-life and clearance are about 40% longer and 30% lower, respectively, in elderly (aged 65 years or older) compared with young healthy volunteers (aged less than 40 years). This difference is most likely due to the well-known reduction in renal function with age, since pramipexole clearance is correlated with renal function, as measured by creatinine clearance (see **CLINICAL PHARMACOLOGY**, *Renal Insufficiency*).

Parkinson's disease patients: A cross-study comparison of data suggests that the clearance of pramipexole may be reduced by about 30% in Parkinson's disease patients compared with healthy elderly volunteers. The reason for this difference appears to be reduced renal function in Parkinson's disease patients, which may be related to their poorer general health. The pharmacokinetics of pramipexole were comparable between early and advanced Parkinson's disease patients.

Pediatric: The pharmacokinetics of pramipexole in the pediatric population have not been evaluated.

Hepatic insufficiency: The influence of hepatic insufficiency on pramipexole pharmacokinetics has not been evaluated. Because approximately 90% of the recovered dose is excreted in the urine as unchanged drug, hepatic impairment would not be expected to have a significant effect on pramipexole elimination.

Renal insufficiency: The clearance of pramipexole was about 75% lower in patients with severe renal impairment (creatinine clearance approximately 20 mL/min) and about 60% lower in patients with moderate impairment (creatinine clearance approximately 40 mL/min) compared with healthy volunteers. A lower starting and maintenance dose is recommended in these patients (see **PRECAUTIONS** and **DOSAGE AND ADMINISTRATION**). In patients with varying degrees of renal impairment, pramipexole clearance correlates well with creatinine clearance. Therefore, creatinine clearance can be used as a predictor of the extent of decrease in pramipexole clearance. Pramipexole clearance is extremely low in dialysis patients, as a negligible amount of pramipexole is removed by dialysis. Caution should be exercised when administering pramipexole to patients with renal disease.

CLINICAL STUDIES
The effectiveness of MIRAPEX (pramipexole dihydrochloride) Tablets in the treatment of Parkinson's disease was evaluated in a multinational drug development program consisting of seven randomized, controlled trials. Three were conducted in patients with early Parkinson's disease who were not receiving concomitant levodopa, and four were conducted in patients with advanced Parkinson's disease who were receiving concomitant levodopa. Among these seven studies, three studies provide the most persuasive evidence of pramipexole's effectiveness in the management of patients with Parkinson's disease who were and were not receiving concomitant levodopa. Two of these three trials enrolled patients with early Parkinson's disease (not receiving levodopa), and one enrolled patients with advanced Parkinson's disease who were receiving maximally tolerated doses of levodopa.

In all studies, the Unified Parkinson's Disease Rating Scale (UPDRS), or one or more of its subparts, served as the primary outcome assessment measure. The UPDRS is a four-part multi-item rating scale intended to evaluate mentation (part I), activities of daily living (part II), motor performance (part III), and complications of therapy (part IV). Part II of the UPDRS contains 13 questions relating to activities of daily living (ADL), which are scored from 0 (normal) to 4 (maximal severity) for a maximum (worst) score of 52. Part III of the UPDRS contains 27 questions (for 14 items) and is scored as described for part II. It is designed to assess the severity of the cardinal motor findings in patients

with Parkinson's disease (e.g., tremor, rigidity, bradykinesia, postural instability, etc), scored for different body regions, and has a maximum (worst) score of 108.

Studies in Patients With Early Parkinson's Disease
Patients (N=599) in the two studies of early Parkinson's disease had a mean disease duration of 2 years, limited or no prior exposure to levodopa (generally none in the preceding 6 months), and were not experiencing the "on-off" phenomenon and dyskinesia characteristic of later stages of the disease.

One of the two early Parkinson's disease studies (N=335) was a double-blind, placebo-controlled, parallel trial consisting of a 7-week dose-escalation period and a 6-month maintenance period. Patients could be on selegiline, anticholinergics, or both, but could not be on levodopa products or amantadine. Patients were randomized to MIRAPEX or placebo. Patients treated with MIRAPEX had a starting daily dose of 0.375 mg and were titrated to a maximally tolerated dose, but no higher than 4.5 mg/day in three divided doses. At the end of the 6-month maintenance period, the mean improvement from baseline on the UPDRS part II (ADL) total score was 1.9 in the group receiving MIRAPEX and –0.4 in the placebo group, a difference that was statistically significant. The mean improvement from baseline on the UPDRS part III total score was 5.0 in the group receiving MIRAPEX and –0.8 in the placebo group, a difference that was also statistically significant. A statistically significant difference between groups in favor of MIRAPEX was seen beginning at week 2 of the UPDRS part II (maximum dose 0.75 mg/day) and at week 3 of the UPDRS part III (maximum dose 1.5 mg/day).

The second early Parkinson's disease study (N=264) was a double-blind, placebo-controlled, parallel trial consisting of a 6-week dose-escalation period and a 4-week maintenance period. Patients could be on selegiline, anticholinergics, amantadine, or any combination of these, but could not be on levodopa products. Patients were randomized to 1 of 4 fixed doses of MIRAPEX (1.5 mg, 3.0 mg, 4.5 mg, or 6.0 mg per day) or placebo. At the end of the 4-week maintenance period, the mean improvement from baseline on the UPDRS part II total score was 1.8 in the patients treated with MIRAPEX, regardless of assigned dose group, and 0.3 in placebo-treated patients. The mean improvement from baseline on the UPDRS part III total score was 4.2 in patients treated with MIRAPEX and 0.6 in placebo-treated patients. No dose-response relationship was demonstrated. The between-treatment differences on both parts of the UPDRS were statistically significant in favor of MIRAPEX for all doses.

No differences in effectiveness based on age or gender were detected. There were too few non-Caucasian patients to evaluate the effect of race. Patients receiving selegiline or anticholinergics had responses similar to patients not receiving these drugs.

Studies in Patients With Advanced Parkinson's Disease
In the advanced Parkinson's disease study, the primary assessments were the UPDRS and daily diaries that quantified amounts of "on" and "off" time.

Patients in the advanced Parkinson's disease study (N=360) had a mean disease duration of 9 years, had been exposed to levodopa for long periods of time (mean 8 years), used concomitant levodopa during the trial, and had "on-off" periods. The advanced Parkinson's disease study was a double-blind, placebo-controlled, parallel trial consisting of a 7-week dose-escalation period and a 6-month maintenance period. Patients were all treated with concomitant levodopa products and could additionally be on concomitant selegiline, anticholinergics, amantadine, or any combination. Patients treated with MIRAPEX had a starting dose of 0.375 mg/day and were titrated to a maximally tolerated dose, but no higher than 4.5 mg/day in three divided doses. At selected times during the 6-month maintenance period, patients were asked to record the amount of "off," "on," or "on with dyskinesia" time per day for several sequential days. At the end of the 6-month maintenance period, the mean improvement from baseline on the UPDRS part II total score was 2.7 in the group treated with MIRAPEX and 0.5 in the placebo group, a difference that was statistically significant. The mean improvement from baseline on the UPDRS part III total score was 5.6 in the group treated with MIRAPEX and 2.8 in the placebo group, a difference that was statistically significant. A statistically significant difference between groups in favor of MIRAPEX was seen at week 3 of the UPDRS part II (maximum dose 1.5 mg/day) and at week 2 of the UPDRS part III (maximum dose 0.75 mg/day). Dosage reduction of levodopa was allowed during this study if dyskinesia (or hallucinations) developed; levodopa dosage reduction occurred in 76% of patients treated with MIRAPEX versus 54% of placebo patients. On average, the levodopa dose was reduced 27%.

The mean number of "off" hours per day during baseline was 6 hours for both treatment groups. Throughout the trial, patients treated with MIRAPEX had a mean of 4 "off" hours per day, while placebo-treated patients continued to experience 6 "off" hours per day.

No differences in effectiveness based on age or gender were detected. There were too few non-Caucasian patients to evaluate the effect of race.

INDICATIONS AND USAGE
MIRAPEX (pramipexole dihydrochloride) Tablets are indicated for the treatment of the signs and symptoms of idiopathic Parkinson's disease.

The effectiveness of MIRAPEX was demonstrated in randomized, controlled trials in patients with early Parkinson's

disease who were not receiving concomitant levodopa therapy as well as in patients with advanced disease on concomitant levodopa (see **CLINICAL STUDIES**).

CONTRAINDICATIONS
MIRAPEX (pramipexole dihydrochloride) Tablets are contraindicated in patients who have demonstrated hypersensitivity to the drug or its ingredients.

WARNINGS
Falling Asleep During Activities of Daily Living:
Patients treated with MIRAPEX (pramipexole dihydrochloride) have reported falling asleep while engaged in activities of daily living, including the operation of motor vehicles which sometimes resulted in accidents. Although many of these patients reported somnolence while on MIRAPEX, some perceived that they had no warning signs such as excessive drowsiness, and believed that they were alert immediately prior to the event. Some of these events have been reported as late as one year after the initiation of treatment.

Somnolence is a common occurrence in patients receiving MIRAPEX at doses above 1.5 mg/day. Many clinical experts believe that falling asleep while engaged in activities of daily living always occurs in a setting of pre-existing somnolence, although patients may not give such a history. For this reason, prescribers should continually reassess patients for drowsiness or sleepiness, especially since some of the events occur well after the start of treatment. Prescribers should also be aware that patients may not acknowledge drowsiness or sleepiness until directly questioned about drowsiness or sleepiness during specific activities.

Before initiating treatment with MIRAPEX, patients should be advised of the potential to develop drowsiness and specifically asked about factors that may increase the risk with MIRAPEX such as concomitant sedating medications, the presence of sleep disorders, and concomitant medications that increase pramipexole plasma levels (e.g., cimetidine — see PRECAUTIONS, Drug Interactions). If a patient develops significant daytime sleepiness or episodes of falling asleep during activities that require active participation (e.g., conversations, eating, etc.), MIRAPEX should ordinarily be discontinued. If a decision is made to continue MIRAPEX, patients should be advised to not drive and to avoid other potentially dangerous activities. While dose reduction clearly reduces the degree of somnolence, there is insufficient information to establish that dose reduction will eliminate episodes of falling asleep while engaged in activities of daily living.

Symptomatic Hypotension: Dopamine agonists, in clinical studies and clinical experience, appear to impair the systemic regulation of blood pressure, with resulting orthostatic hypotension, especially during dose escalation. Parkinson's disease patients, in addition, appear to have an impaired capacity to respond to an orthostatic challenge. For these reasons, Parkinson's disease patients being treated with dopaminergic agonists ordinarily require careful monitoring for signs and symptoms of orthostatic hypotension, especially during dose escalation, and should be informed of this risk (see **PRECAUTIONS**, *Information for Patients*).

In clinical trials of pramipexole, however, and despite clear orthostatic effects in normal volunteers, the reported incidence of clinically significant orthostatic hypotension was not greater among those assigned to MIRAPEX Tablets than among those assigned to placebo. This result is clearly unexpected in light of the previous experience with the risks of dopamine agonist therapy.

While this finding could reflect a unique property of pramipexole, it might also be explained by the conditions of the study and the nature of the population enrolled in the clinical trials. Patients were very carefully titrated, and patients with active cardiovascular disease or significant orthostatic hypotension at baseline were excluded.

Hallucinations: In the three double-blind, placebo-controlled trials in early Parkinson's disease, hallucinations were observed in 9% (35 of 388) of patients receiving MIRAPEX, compared with 2.6% (6 of 235) of patients receiving placebo. In the four double-blind, placebo-controlled trials in advanced Parkinson's disease, where patients received MIRAPEX and concomitant levodopa, hallucinations were observed in 16.5% (43 of 260) of patients receiving MIRAPEX compared with 3.8% (10 of 264) of patients receiving placebo. Hallucinations were of sufficient severity to cause discontinuation of treatment in 3.1% of the early Parkinson's disease patients and 2.7% of the advanced Parkinson's disease patients compared with about 0.4% of placebo patients in both populations.

Age appears to increase the risk of hallucinations attributable to pramipexole. In the early Parkinson's disease patients, the risk of hallucinations was 1.9 times greater than placebo in patients younger than 65 years and 6.8 times greater than placebo in patients older than 65 years. In the advanced Parkinson's disease patients, the risk of hallucinations was 3.5 times greater than placebo in patients younger than 65 years and 5.2 times greater than placebo in patients older than 65 years.

PRECAUTIONS
Rhabdomyolysis: A single case of rhabdomyolysis occurred in a 49-year-old male with advanced Parkinson's disease treated with MIRAPEX (pramipexole dihydrochloride) Tablets. The patient was hospitalized with an elevated CPK (10,631 IU/L). The symptoms resolved with discontinuation of the medication.

Renal: Since pramipexole is eliminated through the kidneys, caution should be exercised when prescribing MIRAPEX to patients with renal insufficiency (see **DOSAGE AND ADMINISTRATION**).

Dyskinesia: MIRAPEX may potentiate the dopaminergic side effects of levodopa and may cause or exacerbate pre-existing dyskinesia. Decreasing the dose of levodopa may ameliorate this side effect.

Retinal pathology in albino rats: Pathologic changes (degeneration and loss of photoreceptor cells) were observed in the retina of albino rats in the 2-year carcinogenicity study. While retinal degeneration was not diagnosed in pigmented rats treated for 2 years, a thinning in the outer nuclear layer of the retina was slightly greater in rats given drug compared with controls. Evaluation of the retinas of albino mice, monkeys, and minipigs did not reveal similar changes. The potential significance of this effect in humans has not been established, but cannot be disregarded because disruption of a mechanism that is universally present in vertebrates (i.e., disk shedding) may be involved (see **ANIMAL TOXICOLOGY**).

Events Reported With Dopaminergic Therapy

Although the events enumerated below have not been reported in association with the use of pramipexole in its development program, they are associated with the use of other dopaminergic drugs. The expected incidence of these events, however, is so low that even if pramipexole caused these events at rates similar to those attributable to other dopaminergic therapies, it would be unlikely that even a single case would have occurred in a cohort of the size exposed to pramipexole in studies to date.

Withdrawal-emergent hyperpyrexia and confusion: Although not reported with pramipexole in the clinical development program, a symptom complex resembling the neuroleptic malignant syndrome (characterized by elevated temperature, muscular rigidity, altered consciousness, and autonomic instability), with no other obvious etiology, has been reported in association with rapid dose reduction, withdrawal of, or changes in antiparkinsonian therapy.

Fibrotic complications: Although not reported with pramipexole in the clinical development program, cases of retroperitoneal fibrosis, pulmonary infiltrates, pleural effusion, and pleural thickening have been reported in some patients treated with ergot-derived dopaminergic agents. While these complications may resolve when the drug is discontinued, complete resolution does not always occur.

Although these adverse events are believed to be related to the ergoline structure of these compounds, whether other, nonergot derived dopamine agonists can cause them is unknown.

Information for Patients: Patients should be instructed to take MIRAPEX only as prescribed.

Patients should be alerted to the potential sedating effects associated with MIRAPEX, including somnolence and the possibility of falling asleep while engaged in activities of daily living. Since somnolence is a frequent adverse event with potentially serious consequences, patients should neither drive a car nor engage in other potentially dangerous activities until they have gained sufficient experience with MIRAPEX to gauge whether or not it affects their mental and/or motor performance adversely. Patients should be advised that if increased somnolence or new episodes of falling asleep during activities of daily living (e.g., watching television, passenger in a car, etc.) are experienced at any time during treatment, they should not drive or participate in potentially dangerous activities until they have contacted their physician. Because of possible additive effects, caution should be advised when patients are taking other sedating medications or alcohol in combination with MIRAPEX and when taking concomitant medications that increase plasma levels of pramipexole (e.g., cimetidine).

Patients should be informed that hallucinations can occur and that the elderly are at a higher risk than younger patients with Parkinson's disease.

Patients may develop postural (orthostatic) hypotension, with or without symptoms such as dizziness, nausea, fainting or blackouts, and sometimes, sweating. Hypotension may occur more frequently during initial therapy. Accordingly, patients should be cautioned against rising rapidly after sitting or lying down, especially if they have been doing so for prolonged periods and especially at the initiation of treatment with MIRAPEX.

Because the teratogenic potential of pramipexole has not been completely established in laboratory animals, and because experience in humans is limited, patients should be advised to notify their physicians if they become pregnant or intend to become pregnant during therapy (see **PRECAUTIONS**, *Pregnancy*).

Because of the possibility that pramipexole may be excreted in breast milk, patients should be advised to notify their physicians if they intend to breast-feed or are breast-feeding an infant.

If patients develop nausea, they should be advised that taking MIRAPEX with food may reduce the occurrence of nausea.

Laboratory Tests: During the development of MIRAPEX, no systematic abnormalities on routine laboratory testing were noted. Therefore, no specific guidance is offered regarding routine monitoring; the practitioner retains responsibility for determining how best to monitor the patient in his or her care.

Drug Interactions

Carbidopa/levodopa: Carbidopa/levodopa did not influence the pharmacokinetics of pramipexole in healthy volunteers (N=10). Pramipexole did not alter the extent of absorption (AUC) or the elimination of carbidopa/levodopa, although it caused an increase in levodopa C_{max} by about 40% and a decrease in T_{max} from 2.5 to 0.5 hours.

Selegiline: In healthy volunteers (N=11), selegiline did not influence the pharmacokinetics of pramipexole.

Amantadine: Population pharmacokinetic analysis suggests that amantadine is unlikely to alter the oral clearance of pramipexole (N=54).

Cimetidine: Cimetidine, a known inhibitor of renal tubular secretion of organic bases via the cationic transport system, caused a 50% increase in pramipexole AUC and a 40% increase in half-life (N=12).

Probenecid: Probenecid, a known inhibitor of renal tubular secretion of organic acids via the anionic transporter, did not noticeably influence pramipexole pharmacokinetics (N=12).

Other drugs eliminated via renal secretion: Population pharmacokinetic analysis suggests that coadministration of drugs that are secreted by the cationic transport system (e.g., cimetidine, ranitidine, diltiazem, triamterene, verapamil, quinidine, and quinine) decreases the oral clearance of pramipexole by about 20%, while those secreted by the anionic transport system (e.g., cephalosporins, penicillins, indomethacin, hydrochlorothiazide, and chlorpropamide) are likely to have little effect on the oral clearance of pramipexole.

CYP interactions: Inhibitors of cytochrome P450 enzymes would not be expected to affect pramipexole elimination because pramipexole is not appreciably metabolized by these enzymes in vivo or in vitro. Pramipexole does not inhibit CYP enzymes CYP1A2, CYP2C9, CYP2C19, CYP2E1, and CYP3A4. Inhibition of CYP2D6 was observed with an apparent Ki of 30 μM, indicating that pramipexole will not inhibit CYP enzymes at plasma concentrations observed following the highest recommended clinical dose (1.5 mg tid).

Dopamine antagonists: Since pramipexole is a dopamine agonist, it is possible that dopamine antagonists, such as the neuroleptics (phenothiazines, butyrophenones, thioxanthenes) or metoclopramide, may diminish the effectiveness of MIRAPEX.

Drug/Laboratory Test Interactions: There are no known interactions between MIRAPEX and laboratory tests.

Carcinogenesis, Mutagenesis, Impairment of Fertility: Two-year carcinogenicity studies with pramipexole have been conducted in mice and rats. Pramipexole was administered in the diet to Chbb:NMRI mice at doses of 0.3, 2, and 10 mg/kg/day (0.3, 2.2, and 11 times the highest recommended clinical dose [1.5 mg tid] on a mg/m² basis). Pramipexole was administered in the diet to Wistar rats at 0.3, 2, and 8 mg/kg/day (plasma AUCs equal to 0.3, 2.5, and 12.5 times the AUC in humans receiving 1.5 mg tid). No significant increases in tumors occurred in either species.

Pramipexole was not mutagenic or clastogenic in a battery of assays, including the in vitro Ames assay, V79 gene mutation assay for HGPRT mutants, chromosomal aberration assay in Chinese hamster ovary cells, and in vivo mouse micronucleus assay.

In rat fertility studies, pramipexole at a dose of 2.5 mg/kg/day (5.4 times the highest clinical dose on a mg/m² basis) prolonged estrus cycles and inhibited implantation. These effects were associated with reductions in serum levels of prolactin, a hormone necessary for implantation and maintenance of early pregnancy in rats.

Pregnancy: Pregnancy Category C. When pramipexole was given to female rats throughout pregnancy, implantation was inhibited at a dose of 2.5 mg/kg/day (5.4 times the highest clinical dose on a mg/m² basis). Administration of 1.5 mg/kg/day of pramipexole to pregnant rats during the period of organogenesis (gestation days 7 through 16) resulted in a high incidence of total resorption of embryos. The plasma AUC in rats dosed at this level was 4.3 times the AUC in humans receiving 1.5 mg tid. These findings are thought to be due to the prolactin-lowering effect of pramipexole, since prolactin is necessary for implantation and maintenance of early pregnancy in rats (but not rabbits or humans). Because of pregnancy disruption and early embryonic loss in these studies, the teratogenic potential of pramipexole could not be adequately evaluated. There was no evidence of adverse effects on embryo-fetal development following administration of up to 10 mg/kg/day to pregnant rabbits during organogenesis (plasma AUC was 71 times that in humans receiving 1.5 mg tid). Postnatal growth was inhibited in the offspring of rats treated with 0.5 mg/kg/day (approximately equivalent to the highest clinical dose on a mg/m² basis) or greater during the latter part of pregnancy and throughout lactation.

There are no studies of pramipexole in human pregnancy. Because animal reproduction studies are not always predictive of human response, pramipexole should be used during pregnancy only if the potential benefit outweighs the potential risk to the fetus.

Nursing Mothers: A single-dose, radio-labeled study showed that drug-related materials were excreted into the breast milk of lactating rats. Concentrations of radioactivity in milk were three to six times higher than concentrations in plasma at equivalent time points.

Other studies have shown that pramipexole treatment resulted in an inhibition of prolactin secretion in humans and rats.

It is not known whether this drug is excreted in human milk. Because many drugs are excreted in human milk and because of the potential for serious adverse reactions in nursing infants from pramipexole, a decision should be made as to whether to discontinue nursing or to discontinue the drug, taking into account the importance of the drug to the mother.

Pediatric Use: The safety and efficacy of MIRAPEX® in pediatric patients has not been established.

Geriatric Use: Pramipexole total oral clearance was approximately 30% lower in subjects older than 65 years compared with younger subjects, because of a decline in pramipexole renal clearance due to an age-related reduction in renal function. This resulted in an increase in elimination half-life from approximately 8.5 hours to 12 hours. In clinical studies, 38.7% of patients were older than 65 years. There were no apparent differences in efficacy or safety between older and younger patients, except that the relative risk of hallucination associated with the use of MIRAPEX was increased in the elderly.

ADVERSE EVENTS

During the premarketing development of pramipexole, patients with either early or advanced Parkinson's disease were enrolled in clinical trials. Apart from the severity and duration of their disease, the two populations differed in their use of concomitant levodopa therapy. Patients with early disease did not receive concomitant levodopa therapy during treatment with pramipexole; those with advanced Parkinson's disease all received concomitant levodopa treatment. Because these two populations may have differential risks for various adverse events, this section will, in general, present adverse-event data for these two populations separately.

Because the controlled trials performed during premarketing development all used a titration design, with a resultant confounding of time and dose, it was impossible to adequately evaluate the effects of dose on the incidence of adverse events.

Early Parkinson's Disease

In the three double-blind, placebo-controlled trials of patients with early Parkinson's disease, the most commonly observed adverse events (>5%) that were numerically more frequent in the group treated with MIRAPEX (pramipexole dihydrochloride) Tablets were nausea, dizziness, somnolence, insomnia, constipation, asthenia, and hallucinations. Approximately 12% of 388 patients with early Parkinson's disease and treated with MIRAPEX who participated in the double-blind, placebo-controlled trials discontinued treatment due to adverse events compared with 11% of 235 patients who received placebo. The adverse events most commonly causing discontinuation of treatment were related to the nervous system (hallucinations [3.1% on MIRAPEX vs 0.4% on placebo]; dizziness [2.1% on MIRAPEX vs 1% on placebo]; somnolence [1.6% on MIRAPEX vs 0% on placebo]; extrapyramidal syndrome [1.6% on MIRAPEX vs 6.4% on placebo]; headache and confusion [1.3% and 1.0%, respectively, on MIRAPEX vs 0% on placebo]); and gastrointestinal system (nausea [2.1% on MIRAPEX vs 0.4% on placebo]).

Adverse-event incidence in controlled clinical studies in early Parkinson's disease: Table 1 lists treatment-emergent adverse events that occurred in the double-blind, placebo-controlled studies in early Parkinson's disease that were reported by ≥1% of patients treated with MIRAPEX and were numerically more frequent than in the placebo group. In these studies, patients did not receive concomitant levodopa. Adverse events were usually mild or moderate in intensity.

The prescriber should be aware that these figures cannot be used to predict the incidence of adverse events in the course of usual medical practice where patient characteristics and other factors differ from those that prevailed in the clinical studies. Similarly, the cited frequencies cannot be compared with figures obtained from other clinical investigations involving different treatments, uses, and investigators. However, the cited figures do provide the prescribing physician with some basis for estimating the relative contribution of drug and nondrug factors to the adverse-event incidence rate in the population studied.

Table 1: Treatment-Emergent Adverse-Event* Incidence in Double-Blind, Placebo-Controlled Trials in Early Parkinson's Disease (Events ≥ 1% of Patients Treated With MIRAPEX and Numerically More Frequent Than in the Placebo Group)

Body System/ Adverse Event	MIRAPEX N=388	Placebo N=235
Body as a Whole		
Asthenia	14	12
General edema	5	3
Malaise	2	1
Reaction unevaluable	2	1
Fever	1	0
Digestive System		
Nausea	28	18
Constipation	14	6

Continued on next page

Mirapex—Cont.

Anorexia	4	2
Dysphagia	2	0

Metabolic & Nutritional System

Peripheral edema	5	4
Decreased weight	2	0

Nervous System

Dizziness	25	24
Somnolence	22	9
Insomnia	17	12
Hallucinations	9	3
Confusion	4	1
Amnesia	4	2
Hypesthesia	3	1
Dystonia	2	1
Akathisia	2	0
Thinking abnormalities	2	0
Decreased libido	1	0
Myoclonus	1	0

Special Senses

Vision abnormalities	3	0

Urogenital System

Impotence	2	1

*Patients may have reported multiple adverse experiences during the study or at discontinuation; thus, patients may be included in more than one category.

Other events reported by 1% or more of patients with early Parkinson's disease and treated with MIRAPEX but reported equally or more frequently in the placebo group were infection, accidental injury, headache, pain, tremor, back pain, syncope, postural hypotension, hypertonia, depression, abdominal pain, anxiety, dyspepsia, flatulence, diarrhea, rash, ataxia, dry mouth, extrapyramidal syndrome, leg cramps, twitching, pharyngitis, sinusitis, sweating, rhinitis, urinary tract infection, vasodilation, flu syndrome, increased saliva, tooth disease, dyspnea, increased cough, gait abnormalities, urinary frequency, vomiting, allergic reaction, hypertension, pruritus, hypokinesia, increased creatine PK, nervousness, dream abnormalities, chest pain, neck pain, paresthesia, tachycardia, vertigo, voice alteration, conjunctivitis, paralysis, accommodation abnormalities, tinnitus, diplopia, and taste perversions.

In a fixed-dose study in early Parkinson's disease, occurrence of the following events increased in frequency as the dose increased over the range from 1.5 mg/day to 6 mg/day: postural hypotension, nausea, constipation, somnolence, and amnesia. The frequency of these events was generally 2-fold greater than placebo for pramipexole doses greater than 3 mg/day. The incidence of somnolence with pramipexole at a dose of 1.5 mg/day was comparable to that reported for placebo.

Advanced Parkinson's Disease

In the four double-blind, placebo-controlled trials of patients with advanced Parkinson's disease, the most commonly observed adverse events (>5%) that were numerically more frequent in the group treated with MIRAPEX and concomitant levodopa were postural (orthostatic) hypotension, dyskinesia, extrapyramidal syndrome, insomnia, dizziness, hallucinations, accidental injury, dream abnormalities, confusion, constipation, asthenia, somnolence, dystonia, gait abnormality, hypertonia, dry mouth, amnesia, and urinary frequency.

Approximately 12% of 260 patients with advanced Parkinson's disease who received MIRAPEX and concomitant levodopa in the double-blind, placebo-controlled trials discontinued treatment due to adverse events compared with 16% of 264 patients who received placebo and concomitant levodopa. The events most commonly causing discontinuation of treatment were related to the nervous system (hallucinations [2.7% on MIRAPEX vs 0.4% on placebo]; dyskinesia [1.9% on MIRAPEX vs 0.8% on placebo]; extrapyramidal syndrome [1.5% on MIRAPEX vs 4.9% on placebo]; dizziness [1.2% on MIRAPEX vs 1.5% on placebo]; confusion [1.2% on MIRAPEX vs 2.3% on placebo]; and cardiovascular system (postural [orthostatic] hypotension [2.3% on MIRAPEX vs 1.1% on placebo]).

Adverse-event incidence in controlled clinical studies in advanced Parkinson's disease: Table 2 lists treatment-emergent adverse events that occurred in the double-blind, placebo-controlled studies in advanced Parkinson's disease that were reported by ≥1% of patients treated with

MIRAPEX and were numerically more frequent than in the placebo group. In these studies, MIRAPEX or placebo was administered to patients who were also receiving concomitant levodopa. Adverse events were usually mild or moderate in intensity.

The prescriber should be aware that these figures cannot be used to predict the incidence of adverse events in the course of usual medical practice where patient characteristics and other factors differ from those that prevailed in the clinical studies. Similarly, the cited frequencies cannot be compared with figures obtained from other clinical investigations involving different treatments, uses, and investigators. However, the cited figures do provide the prescribing physician with some basis for estimating the relative contribution of drug and nondrug factors to the adverse-events incidence rate in the population studied.

Table 2:   Treatment-Emergent Adverse-Event* Incidence in Double-Blind, Placebo-Controlled Trials in Advanced Parkinson's Disease (Events ≥ 1% of Patients Treated With MIRAPEX and Numerically More Frequent Than in the Placebo Group)

Body System/ Adverse Event	MIRAPEX[†] (pramipexole (dihydrochloride) N=260	Placebo[†] N=264
Body as a Whole		
Accidental injury	17	15
Asthenia	10	8
General edema	4	3
Chest pain	3	2
Malaise	3	2
Cardiovascular System		
Postural hypotension	53	48
Digestive System		
Constipation	10	9
Dry mouth	7	3
Metabolic & Nutritional System		
Peripheral edema	2	1
Increased creatine PK	1	0
Musculoskeletal System		
Arthritis	3	1
Twitching	2	0
Bursitis	2	0
Myasthenia	1	0
Nervous System		
Dyskinesia	47	31
Extrapyramidal syndrome	28	26
Insomnia	27	22
Dizziness	26	25
Hallucinations	17	4
Dream abnormalities	11	10
Confusion	10	7
Somnolence	9	6
Dystonia	8	7
Gait abnormalities	7	5
Hypertonia	7	6
Amnesia	6	4
Akathisia	3	2
Thinking abnormalities	3	2
Paranoid reaction	2	0
Delusions	1	0
Sleep disorders	1	0
Respiratory System		
Dyspnea	4	3
Rhinitis	3	1
Pneumonia	2	0
Skin & Appendages		
Skin disorders	2	1
Special Senses		
Accommodation abnormalities	4	2
Vision abnormalities	3	1
Diplopia	1	0
Urogenital System		
Urinary frequency	6	3
Urinary tract infection	4	3
Urinary incontinence	2	1

*Patients may have reported multiple adverse experiences during the study or at discontinuation; thus, patients may be included in more than one category.
[†] Patients received concomitant levodopa.

Other events reported by 1% or more of patients with advanced Parkinson's disease and treated with MIRAPEX but reported equally or more frequently in the placebo group were nausea, pain, infection, headache, depression, tremor, hypokinesia, anorexia, back pain, dyspepsia, flatulence, ataxia, flu syndrome, sinusitis, diarrhea, myalgia, abdominal pain, anxiety, rash, paresthesia, hypertension, increased saliva, tooth disorder, apathy, hypotension, sweating, vasodilation, vomiting, increased cough, nervousness, pruritus, hypesthesia, neck pain, syncope, arthralgia, dysphagia, palpitations, pharyngitis, vertigo, leg cramps, conjunctivitis, and lacrimation disorders.

Adverse Events; Relationship to Age, Gender, and Race: Among the treatment-emergent adverse events in patients treated with MIRAPEX, hallucination appeared to exhibit a positive relationship to age. No gender-related differences were observed. Only a small percentage (4%) of patients enrolled were non-Caucasian, therefore, an evaluation of adverse events related to race is not possible.

Other Adverse Events Observed During All Phase 2 and 3 Clinical Trials: MIRAPEX has been administered to 1,408 individuals during all clinical trials (Parkinson's disease and other patient populations), 648 of whom were in seven double-blind, placebo-controlled Parkinson's disease trials. During these trials, all adverse events were recorded by the clinical investigators using terminology of their own choosing. To provide a meaningful estimate of the proportion of individuals having adverse events, similar types of events were grouped into a smaller number of standardized categories using modified COSTART dictionary terminology. These categories are used in the listing below. The events listed below occurred in less than 1% of the 1,408 individuals exposed to MIRAPEX and occurred on at least two occasions (on one occasion if the event was serious). All reported events, except those already listed above, are included, without regard to determination of a causal relationship to MIRAPEX.

Events are listed within body-system categories in order of decreasing frequency.

Body as a whole: enlarged abdomen, death, fever, suicide attempt.

Cardiovascular system: peripheral vascular disease, myocardial infarction, angina pectoris, atrial fibrillation, heart failure, arrhythmia, atrial arrhythmia, pulmonary embolism.

Digestive system: thirst.

Musculoskeletal system: joint disorder, myasthenia.

Nervous system: agitation, CNS stimulation, hyperkinesia, psychosis, convulsions.

Respiratory system: pneumonia.

Special senses: cataract, eye disorder, glaucoma.

Urogenital system: dysuria, abnormal ejaculation, prostate cancer, hematuria, prostate disorder.

Falling Asleep During Activities of Daily Living: Patients treated with MIRAPEX have reported falling asleep while engaged in activities of daily living, including operation of a motor vehicle which sometimes resulted in accidents (see bolded WARNING).

Post-Marketing Experience: In addition to the adverse events reported during clinical trials, the following adverse reactions have been identified during post-approval use of MIRAPEX Tablets. Because these reactions are reported voluntarily from a population of uncertain size, it is not always possible to reliably estimate their frequency or establish a causal relationship to drug exposure. Decisions to include these reactions in labeling are typically based on one or more of the following factors: (1) seriousness of the reaction, (2) frequency of reporting, or (3) strength of causal connection to MIRAPEX Tablets. Similar types of events were grouped into a smaller number of standardized categories using the MedDRA dictionary: accidents (including fall), compulsive behaviors (including sexual and pathological gambling), fatigue, hallucinations (all kind), headache, hypotension (including postural hypotension), libido disorders, syncope, and blackouts.

DRUG ABUSE AND DEPENDENCE

Pramipexole is not a controlled substance. Pramipexole has not been systematically studied in animals or humans for its potential for abuse, tolerance, or physical dependence. However, in a rat model on cocaine self-administration, pramipexole had little or no effect.

OVERDOSAGE

There is no clinical experience with massive overdosage. One patient, with a 10-year history of schizophrenia, took 11 mg/day of pramipexole for 2 days; this is two to three times the protocol recommended daily dose. No adverse events were reported related to the increased dose. Blood pressure remained stable although pulse rate increased to between 100 and 120 beats/minute. The patient withdrew from the study at the end of week 2 due to lack of efficacy. There is no known antidote for overdosage of a dopamine agonist. If signs of central nervous system stimulation are present, a phenothiazine or other butyrophenone neuroleptic agent may be indicated; the efficacy of such drugs in reversing the effects of overdosage has not been assessed. Management of overdose may require general supportive measures along with gastric lavage, intravenous fluids, and electrocardiogram monitoring.

DOSAGE AND ADMINISTRATION

In all clinical studies, dosage was initiated at a subtherapeutic level to avoid intolerable adverse effects and orthostatic hypotension. MIRAPEX (pramipexole dihydrochloride) should be titrated gradually in all patients. The dosage should be increased to achieve a maximum therapeutic effect, balanced against the principal side effects of dyskinesia, hallucinations, somnolence, and dry mouth.

Dosing in Patients With Normal Renal Function

Initial Treatment: Dosages should be increased gradually from a starting dose of 0.375 mg/day given in three divided doses and should not be increased more frequently than every 5 to 7 days. A suggested ascending dosage schedule that was used in clinical studies is shown in the following table:

Table 3: Ascending Dosage Schedule of MIRAPEX

Week	Dosage (mg)	Total Daily Dose (mg)
1	0.125 tid	0.375
2	0.25 tid	0.75
3	0.5 tid	1.50
4	0.75 tid	2.25
5	1.0 tid	3.0
6	1.25 tid	3.75
7	1.5 tid	4.50

Maintenance Treatment: MIRAPEX Tablets were effective and well tolerated over a dosage range of 1.5 to 4.5 mg/day administered in equally divided doses three times per day with or without concomitant levodopa (approximately 800 mg/day).

In a fixed-dose study in early Parkinson's disease patients, doses of 3 mg, 4.5 mg, and 6 mg per day of MIRAPEX were not shown to provide any significant benefit beyond that achieved at a daily dose of 1.5 mg/day. However, in the same fixed-dose study, the following adverse events were dose related: postural hypotension, nausea, constipation, somnolence, and amnesia. The frequency of these events was generally 2-fold greater than placebo for pramipexole doses greater than 3 mg/day. The incidence of somnolence reported with pramipexole at a dose of 1.5 mg/day was comparable to placebo.

When MIRAPEX is used in combination with levodopa, a reduction of the levodopa dosage should be considered. In a controlled study in advanced Parkinson's disease, the dosage of levodopa was reduced by an average of 27% from baseline.

Table 4: Patients with Renal Impairment Pramipexole Dosage in the Renally Impaired

Renal Status	Starting Dose (mg)	Maximum Dose (mg)
Normal to mild impairment (creatinine Cl > 60 mL/min)	0.125 tid	1.5 tid
Moderate impairment (creatinine Cl = 35 to 59 mL/min)	0.125 bid	1.5 bid
Severe impairment (creatinine Cl = 15 to 34 mL/min)	0.125 qd	1.5 qd
Very severe impairment (creatinine Cl < 15 mL/min and hemodialysis patients)	The use of MIRAPEX (pramipexole dihydrochloride) has not been adequately studied in this group of patients.	

Discontinuation of Treatment: It is recommended that MIRAPEX be discontinued over a period of 1 week; in some studies, however, abrupt discontinuation was uneventful.

HOW SUPPLIED

MIRAPEX (pramipexole dihydrochloride) Tablets are available as follows:

0.125 mg: white, round tablet with "U" on one side and "2" on the reverse side.

Bottles of 63 NDC 0597-0083-53

0.25 mg: white, oval, scored tablet with "U" twice on one side and "4" twice on the reverse side.

Bottles of 90 NDC 0597-0084-90
Unit dose packages of 100 NDC 0597-0084-61

0.5 mg: white, oval, scored tablet with "U" twice on one side and "8" twice on the reverse side.

Bottles of 90 NDC 0597-0085-90
Unit dose packages of 100 NDC 0597-0085-61

1 mg: white, round, scored tablet with "U" twice on one side and "6" twice on the reverse side.

Bottles of 90 NDC 0597-0090-90
Unit dose packages of 100 NDC 0597-0090-61

1.5 mg: white, round, scored tablet with "U" twice on one side and "37" twice on the reverse side.

Bottles of 90 NDC 0597-0091-90
Unit dose packages of 100 NDC 0597-0091-61

Store at 25°C (77°F); excursions permitted to 15°-30°C (59°-86°F) [see USP Controlled Room Temperature]. Protect from light.

Store in a safe place out of the reach of children.

℞ only

ANIMAL TOXICOLOGY

Retinal Pathology in Albino Rats

Pathologic changes (degeneration and loss of photoreceptor cells) were observed in the retina of albino rats in the 2-year carcinogenicity study with pramipexole. These findings were first observed during week 76 and were dose dependent in animals receiving 2 or 8 mg/kg/day (plasma AUCs equal to 2.5 and 12.5 times the AUC in humans that received 1.5 mg tid). In a similar study of pigmented rats with 2 years exposure to pramipexole at 2 or 8 mg/kg/day, retinal degeneration was not diagnosed. Animals given drug had thinning in the outer nuclear layer of the retina that was only slightly greater than that seen in control rats utilizing morphometry.

Investigative studies demonstrated that pramipexole reduced the rate of disk shedding from the photoreceptor rod cells of the retina in albino rats, which was associated with enhanced sensitivity to the damaging effects of light. In a comparative study, degeneration and loss of photoreceptor cells occurred in albino rats after 13 weeks of treatment with 25 mg/kg/day of pramipexole (54 times the highest clinical dose on a mg/m^2 basis) and constant light (100 lux) but not in pigmented rats exposed to the same dose and higher light intensities (500 lux). Thus, the retina of albino rats is considered to be uniquely sensitive to the damaging effects of pramipexole and light. Similar changes in the retina did not occur in a 2-year carcinogenicity study in albino mice treated with 0.3, 2, or 10 mg/kg/day (0.3, 2.2 and 11 times the highest clinical dose on a mg/m^2 basis). Evaluation of the retinas of monkeys given 0.1, 0.5, or 2.0 mg/kg/day of pramipexole (0.4, 2.2, and 8.6 times the highest clinical dose on a mg/m^2 basis) for 12 months and minipigs given 0.3, 1, or 5 mg/kg/day of pramipexole for 13 weeks also detected no changes.

The potential significance of this effect in humans has not been established, but cannot be disregarded because disruption of a mechanism that is universally present in vertebrates (i.e., disk shedding) may be involved.

Fibro-osseous Proliferative Lesions in Mice

An increased incidence of fibro-osseous proliferative lesions occurred in the femurs of female mice treated for 2 years with 0.3, 2.0, or 10 mg/kg/day (0.3, 2.2, and 11 times the highest clinical dose on a mg/m^2 basis). Lesions occurred at a lower rate in control animals. Similar lesions were not observed in male mice or rats and monkeys of either sex that were treated chronically with pramipexole. The significance of this lesion to humans is not known.

Distributed by: Boehringer Ingelheim Pharmaceuticals, Inc. Ridgefield, CT 06877 USA

Licensed from: Boehringer Ingelheim International GmbH

Trademark under license from:
Boehringer Ingelheim International GmbH
U.S. Patent Nos. 4,886,812 and 4,843,086
©2005, Boehringer Ingelheim International GmbH
ALL RIGHTS RESERVED
Revised March 3, 2005
OT10017
MP-10552

To keep your **PDR** up to date throughout the year, note these revisions on the corresponding pages of the annual volume. Simply write **"See Supplement A"** next to the product heading.

Centocor, Inc.
200 GREAT VALLEY PARKWAY
MALVERN, PA 19355
USA

Direct General Inquiries to:
Ph: (610) 651-6000
(888) 874-3083
Fax: (610) 651-6100

Medical Emergency Contact:
Ph: (800)-457-6399

For Medical Information/Adverse Experience Reporting Contact:
Medical Information
Ph: (800) 457-6399

REMICADE® ℞

[*rĕm-ĭ-kād*]
(infliximab)
for IV Injection

Prescribing information for this product, which appears on pages 1117-1122 of the 2005 PDR, has been completely revised as follows. Please write "See Supplement A" next to the product heading.

> **WARNING**
> **RISK OF INFECTIONS**
> **TUBERCULOSIS (FREQUENTLY DISSEMINATED OR EXTRAPULMONARY AT CLINICAL PRESENTATION), INVASIVE FUNGAL INFECTIONS, AND OTHER OPPORTUNISTIC INFECTIONS, HAVE BEEN OBSERVED IN PATIENTS RECEIVING REMICADE. SOME OF THESE INFECTIONS HAVE BEEN FATAL (SEE WARNINGS).**
> **PATIENTS SHOULD BE EVALUATED FOR LATENT TUBERCULOSIS INFECTION WITH A TUBERCULIN SKIN TEST.[1] TREATMENT OF LATENT TUBERCULOSIS INFECTION SHOULD BE INITIATED PRIOR TO THERAPY WITH REMICADE.**

DESCRIPTION

REMICADE is a chimeric IgG1κ monoclonal antibody with an approximate molecular weight of 149,100 daltons. It is composed of human constant and murine variable regions. Infliximab binds specifically to human tumor necrosis factor alpha (TNFα) with an association constant of 10^{10} M^{-1}. Infliximab is produced by a recombinant cell line cultured by continuous perfusion and is purified by a series of steps that includes measures to inactivate and remove viruses.

REMICADE is supplied as a sterile, white, lyophilized powder for intravenous infusion. Following reconstitution with 10 mL of Sterile Water for Injection, USP, the resulting pH is approximately 7.2. Each single-use vial contains 100 mg infliximab, 500 mg sucrose, 0.5 mg polysorbate 80, 2.2 mg monobasic sodium phosphate, monohydrate, and 6.1 mg dibasic sodium phosphate, dihydrate. No preservatives are present.

CLINICAL PHARMACOLOGY

General

Infliximab neutralizes the biological activity of TNFα by binding with high affinity to the soluble and transmembrane forms of TNFα and inhibits binding of TNFα with its receptors.[2,3] Infliximab does not neutralize TNFβ (lymphotoxin α), a related cytokine that utilizes the same receptors as TNFα. Biological activities attributed to TNFα include: induction of pro-inflammatory cytokines such as interleukins (IL) 1 and 6, enhancement of leukocyte migration by increasing endothelial layer permeability and expression of adhesion molecules by endothelial cells and leukocytes, activation of neutrophil and eosinophil functional activity, induction of acute phase reactants and other liver proteins, as well as tissue degrading enzymes produced by synoviocytes and/or chondrocytes. Cells expressing transmembrane TNFα bound by infliximab can be lysed *in vitro*[3] or *in vivo*.[4] Infliximab inhibits the functional activity of TNFα in a wide variety of *in vitro* bioassays utilizing human fibroblasts, endothelial cells, neutrophils, B and T lymphocytes and epithelial cells. Anti-TNFα antibodies reduce disease activity in the cotton-top tamarin colitis model, and decrease synovitis and joint erosions in a murine model of collagen-induced arthritis. Infliximab prevents disease in transgenic mice that develop polyarthritis as a result of constitutive expression of human TNFα, and when administered after disease onset, allows eroded joints to heal.

Pharmacodynamics

Elevated concentrations of TNFα have been found in involved tissues and fluids of patients with rheumatoid arthritis, Crohn's disease and ankylosing spondylitis. In rheumatoid arthritis, treatment with REMICADE reduced infiltration of inflammatory cells into inflamed areas of the joint as well as expression of molecules mediating cellular adhesion [E-selectin, intercellular adhesion molecule-1 (ICAM-1) and vascular cell adhesion molecule-1 (VCAM-1)], chemoattraction [IL-8 and monocyte chemotactic protein (MCP-1)] and tissue degradation [matrix metalloproteinase (MMP) 1 and 3]. In Crohn's disease, treatment with

Continued on next page

Remicade—Cont.

REMICADE reduced infiltration of inflammatory cells and TNFα production in inflamed areas of the intestine, and reduced the proportion of mononuclear cells from the lamina propria able to express TNFα and interferon. After treatment with REMICADE, patients with rheumatoid arthritis or Crohn's disease exhibited decreased levels of serum IL-6 and C-reactive protein (CRP) compared to baseline. Peripheral blood lymphocytes from REMICADE-treated patients showed no significant decrease in number or in proliferative responses to *in vitro* mitogenic stimulation when compared to cells from untreated patients.

Pharmacokinetics

Single intravenous (IV) infusions of 3 mg/kg to 20 mg/kg showed a linear relationship between the dose administered and the maximum serum concentration. The volume of distribution at steady state was independent of dose and indicated that infliximab was distributed primarily within the vascular compartment. Median pharmacokinetic results for doses of 3 mg/kg to 10 mg/kg in rheumatoid arthritis and 5 mg/kg in Crohn's disease indicate that the terminal half-life of infliximab is 8.0 to 9.5 days.

Following an initial dose of REMICADE, repeated infusions at 2 and 6 weeks resulted in predictable concentration-time profiles following each treatment. No systemic accumulation of infliximab occurred upon continued repeated treatment with 3 mg/kg or 10 mg/kg at 4- or 8-week intervals. Development of antibodies to infliximab increased infliximab clearance. At 8 weeks after a maintenance dose of 3 to 10 mg/kg of REMICADE, median infliximab serum concentrations ranged from approximately 0.5 to 6 mcg/mL; however, infliximab concentrations were not detectable (<0.1 mcg/mL) in patients who became positive for antibodies to infliximab. No major differences in clearance or volume of distribution were observed in patient subgroups defined by age, weight, or gender. It is not known if there are differences in clearance or volume of distribution in patients with marked impairment of hepatic or renal function.

A pediatric Crohn's disease pharmacokinetic study was conducted in 21 patients aged 11 to 17 years old. No notable differences in single-dose pharmacokinetic parameters were observed between pediatric and adult Crohn's disease patients (see PRECAUTIONS, Pediatric Use).

CLINICAL STUDIES

Rheumatoid Arthritis

The safety and efficacy of infliximab were assessed in two multicenter, randomized, double-blind, pivotal trials: ATTRACT (Study RA I) and ASPIRE (Study RA II). Concurrent use of stable doses of folic acid, oral corticosteroids (≤10 mg/day) and/or non-steroidal anti-inflammatory drugs was permitted.

Study RA I was a placebo-controlled study of 428 patients with active rheumatoid arthritis despite treatment with MTX. Patients enrolled had a median age of 54 years, median disease duration of 8.4 years, median swollen and tender joint count of 20 and 31 respectively, and were on a median dose of 15 mg/wk of MTX. Patients received either placebo + MTX or one of 4 doses/schedules of REMICADE + MTX: 3 mg/kg or 10 mg/kg of REMICADE by IV infusion at weeks 0, 2 and 6 followed by additional infusions every 4 or 8 weeks in combination with MTX.

Study RA II was a placebo-controlled study of three active treatment arms in 1004 MTX naive patients of 3 or fewer years duration active rheumatoid arthritis. Patients enrolled had a median age of 51 years with a median disease duration of 0.6 years, median swollen and tender joint count of 19 and 31, respectively, and >80% of patients had baseline joint erosions. At randomization, all patients received MTX (optimized to 20 mg/wk by week 8) and either placebo, 3mg/kg or 6 mg/kg REMICADE at weeks 0, 2, and 6 and every 8 weeks thereafter.

Data on use of REMICADE without concurrent MTX are limited (see ADVERSE REACTIONS, Immunogenicity).[5,6]

Clinical response

In Study RA I, all doses/schedules of REMICADE + MTX resulted in improvement in signs and symptoms as measured by the American College of Rheumatology response criteria (ACR 20) with a higher percentage of patients achieving an ACR 20, 50 and 70 compared to placebo + MTX (Table 1). This improvement was observed at week 2 and maintained through week 102. Greater effects on each component of the ACR 20 were observed in all patients treated with REMICADE + MTX compared to placebo + MTX (Table 2). More patients treated with REMICADE reached a major clinical response than placebo-treated patients (Table 1).

In Study RA II, after 54 weeks of treatment, both doses of REMICADE + MTX resulted in statistically significantly greater response in signs and symtoms compared to MTX alone as measured by the production of patients achieving ACR 20, 50 and 70 responses (Table 1). More patients treated with REMICADE reached a major clinical response than placebo-treated patients (Table 1).

[See table 1 above]
[See table 2 above]

Radiographic response

Structural damage in both hands and feet was assessed radiographically at week 54 by the change from baseline in the van der Heijde-modified Sharp (vdH-S) score, a composite score of structural damage that measures the number and size of joint erosions and the degree of joint space narrowing in hands/wrists and feet.[7]

In Study RA I, approximately 80% of patients had paired x-ray data at 54 weeks and approximately 70% at 102 weeks. The inhibition of progression of structural damage was observed at 54 weeks (Table 3) and maintained through 102 weeks.

In Study RA II, >90% of patients had at least two evaluable x-rays. Inhibition of progression of structural damage was observed at weeks 30 and 54 (Table 3) in the REMICADE + MTX groups compared to MTX alone. In an exploratory analysis of Study RA II, patients treated with REMICADE + MTX demonstrated less progression of structural damage compared to MTX alone, whether baseline acute phase reactants (ESR and CRP) were normal or elevated: patients with elevated baseline acute phase reactants treated with MTX alone demonstrated a mean progression in vdH-S score of 4.2 units compared to patients treated with REMICADE + MTX who demonstrated 0.5 units of progression; patients with normal baseline acute phase reactants

Table 1
ACR RESPONSE (PERCENT OF PATIENTS)

Response	Study RA I					Study RA II		
		REMICADE + MTX					REMICADE + MTX	
		3 mg/kg		10 mg/kg			3 mg/kg	6 mg/kg
	Placebo + MTX (n=88)	q 8 wks (n=86)	q 4 wks (n=86)	q 8 wks (n=87)	q 4 wks (n=81)	Placebo + MTX (n=274)	q 8 wks (n=351)	q 8 wks (n=355)
ACR 20								
Week 30	20%	50%[a]	50%[a]	52%[a]	58%[a]	N/A	N/A	N/A
Week 54	17%	42%[a]	48%[a]	59%[a]	59%[a]	54%	62%[c]	66%[a]
ACR 50								
Week 30	5%	27%[a]	29%[a]	31%[a]	26%[a]	N/A	N/A	N/A
Week 54	9%	21%[c]	34%[a]	40%[a]	38%[a]	32%	46%[a]	50%[a]
ACR 70								
Week 30	0%	8%[b]	11%[b]	18%[a]	11%[a]	N/A	N/A	N/A
Week 54	2%	11%[c]	18%[a]	26%[a]	19%[a]	21%	33%[b]	37%[a]
Major clinical response[#]	0%	7%[c]	8%[b]	15%[a]	6%[c]	8%	12%	17%[a]

A major clinical response was defined as a 70% ACR response for 6 consecutive months (consecutive visits spanning at least 26 weeks) through week 102 for Study RA I and week 54 for Study RA II.
[a] $p \leq 0.001$
[b] $p < 0.01$
[c] $p < 0.05$

Table 2
COMPONENTS OF ACR 20 AT BASELINE AND 54 WEEKS (Study RA I)

Parameter (medians)	Placebo + MTX		REMICADE + MTX[a]	
	(n=88)		(n=340)	
	Baseline	Week 54	Baseline	Week 54
No. of Tender Joints	24	16	32	8
No. of Swollen Joints	19	13	20	7
Pain[b]	6.7	6.1	6.8	3.3
Physician's Global Assessment[b]	6.5	5.2	6.2	2.1
Patient's Global Assessment[b]	6.2	6.2	6.3	3.2
Disability Index (HAQ)[c]	1.8	1.5	1.8	1.3
CRP (mg/dL)	3.0	2.3	2.4	0.6

[a] All doses/schedules of REMICADE + MTX
[b] Visual Analog Scale (0=best, 10=worst)
[c] Health Assessment Questionnaire, measurement of 8 categories: dressing and grooming, arising, eating, walking, hygiene, reach, grip, and activities (0=best, 3=worst)

Table 3
RADIOGRAPHIC CHANGE FROM BASELINE TO WEEK 54

	Study RA I			Study RA II		
		REMICADE + MTX			REMICADE + MTX	
		3 mg/kg	10 mg/kg		3 mg/kg	6 mg/kg
	Placebo + MTX (n=64)	q 8 wks (n=71)	q 8 wks (n=77)	Placebo + MTX (n=282)	q 8 wks (n=359)	q 8 wks (n=363)
Total Score						
Baseline						
Mean	79	78	65	11.3	11.6	11.2
Median	55	57	56	5.1	5.2	5.3
Change from baseline						
Mean	6.9	1.3[a]	0.2[a]	3.7	0.4[a]	0.5[a]
Median	4.0	0.5	0.5	0.4	0.0	0.0
Erosion Score						
Baseline						
Mean	44	44	33	8.3	8.8	8.3
Median	25	29	22	3.0	3.8	3.8
Change from baseline						
Mean	4.1	0.2[a]	0.2[a]	3.0	0.3[a]	0.1[a]
Median	2.0	0.0	0.5	0.3	0.0	0.0
JSN Score						
Baseline						
Mean	36	34	31	3.0	2.9	2.9
Median	26	29	24	1.0	1.0	1.0
Change from baseline						
Mean	2.9	1.1[a]	0.0[a]	0.6	0.1[a]	0.2
Median	1.5	0.0	0.0	0.0	0.0	0.0

[a] $P < 0.001$ for each outcome against placebo.

Table 4
CLINICAL REMISSION AND STEROID WITHDRAWAL

	Single 5 mg/kg Dose[a] Placebo Maintenance	Three Dose Induction[b] Infliximab Maintenance q 8 wks 5 mg/kg	10 mg/kg
Week 30			
Clinical remission	25/102 25%	41/104 39%	48/105 46%
p-value[c]		0.022	0.001
Week 54			
Patients in remission able to discontinue corticosteroid use[d]	6/54 11%	14/56 25%	18/53 34%
p-value[c]		0.059	0.005

[a] REMICADE at week 0
[b] REMICADE 5 mg/kg administered at weeks 0, 2 and 6
[c] p-values represent pairwise comparisons to placebo
[d] Of those receiving corticosteroids at baseline

treated with MTX alone demonstrated a mean progression in vdH-S score of 1.8 units compared to REMICADE + MTX who demonstrated 0.2 units of progression. Of patients receiving REMICADE + MTX, 59% had no progression (vdH-S) ≤ 0 unit) of structural damage compared to 45% patients receiving MTX alone. In a subset of patients who began the study without erosions, REMICADE + MTX maintained an erosion free state at 1 year in a greater proportion of patients than MTX alone, 79% (77/98) vs. 58% (23/40), respectively (p<0.01). Fewer patients in the REMICADE + MTX groups (47%) developed erosions in uninvolved joints compared to MTX alone (59%).

[See table 3 on previous page]

Physical function response

Physical function and disability were assessed using the Health Assessment Questionnaire (HAQ) and the general health-related quality of life questionnaire SF-36.

In Study RA I, all doses/schedules of REMICADE + MTX showed significantly greater improvement from baseline in HAQ and SF-36 physical component summary score averaged over time through week 54 compared to placebo + MTX, and no worsening in the SF-36 mental component summary score. The median (interquartile range) improvement from baseline to week 54 in HAQ was 0.1 (-0.1, 0.5) for the placebo + MTX group and 0.4 (0.1, 0.9) for REMICADE + MTX (p<0.001). Both HAQ and SF-36 effects were maintained through week 102. Approximately 80% of patients in all doses/schedules of REMICADE + MTX remained in the trial through 102 weeks.

In Study RA II, both REMICADE treatment groups showed greater improvement in HAQ from baseline averaged over time through week 54 compared to MTX alone; 0.7 for REMICADE + MTX vs. 0.6 for MTX alone (p≤0.001). No worsening in the SF-36 mental component summary score was observed.

Active Crohn's Disease

The safety and efficacy of single and multiple doses of REMICADE were assessed in two randomized, double-blind, placebo-controlled clinical studies in 653 patients with moderate to severely active Crohn's disease [Crohn's Disease Activity Index (CDAI) ≥220 and ≤400] with an inadequate response to prior conventional therapies. Concomitant stable doses of aminosalicylates, corticosteroids and/or immunomodulatory agents were permitted and 92% of patients continued to receive at least one of these medications.

In the single-dose trial[8] of 108 patients, 16% (4/25) of placebo patients achieved a clinical response (decrease in CDAI ≥70 points) at week 4 vs. 81% (22/27) of patients receiving 5 mg/kg REMICADE (p<0.001, two-sided, Fisher's Exact test). Additionally, 4% (1/25) of placebo patients and 48% (13/27) of patients receiving 5 mg/kg REMICADE achieved clinical remission (CDAI<150) at week 4.

In a multidose trial (ACCENT I [Study Crohn's I])[9], 545 patients received 5 mg/kg at week 0 and were then randomized to one of three treatment groups; the placebo maintenance group received placebo at weeks 2 and 6, and then every 8 weeks; the 5 mg/kg maintenance group received 5 mg/kg at weeks 2 and 6, and then every 8 weeks; and the 10 mg/kg maintenance group received 5 mg/kg at weeks 2 and 6, and then 10 mg/kg every 8 weeks. Patients in response at week 2 were randomized and analyzed separately from those not in response at week 2. Corticosteroid taper was permitted after week 6.

At week 2, 57% (311/545) of patients were in clinical response. At week 30, a significantly greater proportion of these patients in the 5 mg/kg and 10 mg/kg maintenance groups achieved clinical remission compared to patients in the placebo maintenance group (Table 4).

Additionally, a significantly greater proportion of patients in the 5 mg/kg and 10 mg/kg infliximab maintenance groups were in clinical remission and were able to discontinue corticosteroid use compared to patients in the placebo maintenance group at week 54 (Table 4).

[See table 4 above]

Patients in the infliximab maintenance groups (5 mg/kg and 10 mg/kg) had a longer time to loss of response than patients in the placebo maintenance group (Figure 1). At weeks 30 and 54, significant improvement from baseline was seen among the 5 mg/kg and 10 mg/kg infliximab-treated groups compared to the placebo group in the disease specific inflammatory bowel disease questionnaire (IBDQ), particularly the bowel and systemic components, and in the physical component summary score of the general health-related quality of life questionnaire SF-36.

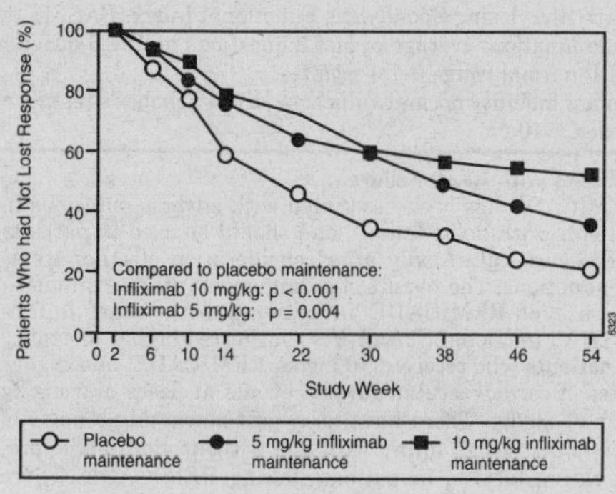

Figure 1
Kaplan-Meier estimate of the proportion of patients who had not lost response through week 54

In a subset of 78 patients who had mucosal ulceration at baseline and who participated in an endoscopic substudy, 13 of 43 patients in the infliximab maintenance group had endoscopic evidence of mucosal healing compared to 1 of 28 patients in the placebo group at week 10. Of the infliximab-treated patients showing mucosal healing at week 10, 9 of 12 patients also showed mucosal healing at week 54.

Patients who achieved a response and subsequently lost response were eligible to receive infliximab on an episodic basis at a dose that was 5 mg/kg higher than the dose to which they were randomized. The majority of such patients responded to the higher dose. Among patients who were not in response at week 2, 59% (92/157) of infliximab maintenance patients responded by week 14 compared to 51% (39/77) of placebo maintenance patients. Among patients who did not respond by week 14, additional therapy did not result in significantly more responses (see DOSAGE AND ADMINISTRATION).

Fistulizing Crohn's Disease

The safety and efficacy of REMICADE were assessed in 2 randomized, double-blind, placebo-controlled studies in patients with fistulizing Crohn's disease with fistula(s) that were of at least 3 months duration. Concurrent use of stable doses of corticosteroids, 5-aminosalicylates, antibiotics, MTX, 6-mercaptopurine (6-MP) and/or azathioprine (AZA) was permitted.

In the first trial,[10] 94 patients received three doses of either placebo or REMICADE at weeks 0, 2 and 6. Fistula response (≥50% reduction in number of enterocutaneous fistulas draining upon gentle compression on at least two consecutive visits without an increase in medication or surgery for Crohn's disease) was seen in 68% (21/31) of patients in the 5 mg/kg REMICADE group (p=0.002) and 56% (18/32) of patients in the 10 mg/kg REMICADE group (p=0.021) vs. 26% (8/31) of patients in the placebo arm. The median time to onset of response and median duration of response in REMICADE-treated patients was 2 and 12 weeks, respectively. Closure of all fistula was achieved in 52% of REMICADE-treated patients compared with 13% of placebo-treated patients (p<0.001).

In the second trial (ACCENT II [Study Crohn's II]), patients who were enrolled had to have at least one draining enterocutaneous (perianal,abdominal) fistula. All patients received 5 mg/kg REMICADE at weeks 0, 2 and 6. Patients were randomized to placebo or 5 mg/kg REMICADE maintenance at week 14. Patients received maintenance doses at week 14 and then every eight weeks through week 46. Patients who were in fistula response (fistula response was defined the same as in the first trial) at both weeks 10 and 14 were randomized separately from those not in response. The primary endpoint was time from randomization to loss of response among those patients who were in fistula response.

Among the randomized patients (273 of the 296 initially enrolled), 87% had perianal fistulas and 14% had abdominal fistulas. Eight percent also had rectovaginal fistulas. Greater than 90% of the patients had received previous immunosuppressive and antibiotic therapy.

At week 14, 65% (177/273) of patients were in fistula response. Patients randomized to REMICADE maintenance had a longer time to loss of fistula response compared to the placebo maintenance group (Figure 2). At week 54, 38% (33/87) of REMICADE-treated patients had no draining fistulas compared with 22% (20/90) of placebo-treated patients (p=0.02). Compared to placebo maintenance, patients on REMICADE maintenance had a trend toward fewer hospitalizations.

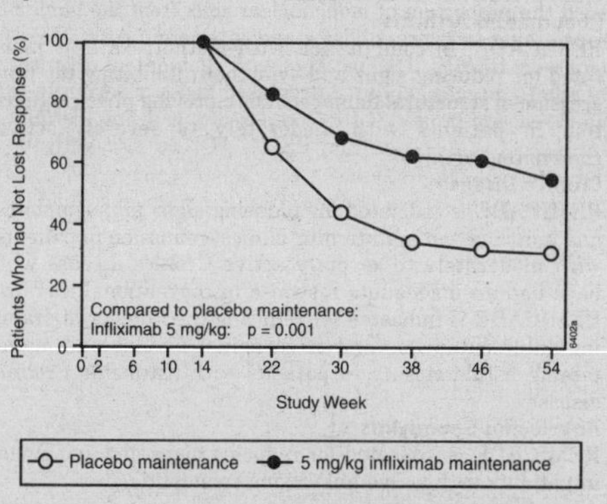

Figure 2
Life table estimates of the proportion of patients who had not lost fistula response through week 54

Patients who achieved a fistula response and subsequently lost response were eligible to receive REMICADE maintenance therapy at a dose that was 5 mg/kg higher than the dose to which they were randomized. Of the placebo maintenance patients, 66% (25/38) responded to 5 mg/kg REMICADE, and 57% (12/21) of REMICADE maintenance patients responded to 10 mg/kg.

Patients who had not achieved a response by week 14 were unlikely to respond to additional doses of REMICADE.

Similar proportions of patients in either group developed new fistulas (17% overall) and similar numbers developed abscesses (15% overall).

Ankylosing Spondylitis

The safety and efficacy of REMICADE were assessed in a randomized, multicenter, double-blind, placebo-controlled study in 279 patients with active ankylosing spondylitis. Patients were between 18 and 74 years of age, and had ankylosing spondylitis as defined by the modified New York criteria for Ankylosing Spondylitis.[11] Patients were to have had active disease as evidenced by both a Bath Ankylosing Spondylitis Disease Activity Index (BASDAI) score >4 (possible range 0-10) and spinal pain >4 (on Visual Analog Scale [VAS] of 0-10). Patients with complete ankylosis of the spine were excluded from study participation, and the use of Disease Modifying Anti-Rheumatic Drugs (DMARDs) and systemic corticosteroids were prohibited. Doses of REMICADE 5 mg/kg or placebo were administered intravenously at Weeks 0, 2, 6, 12 and 18.

At 24 weeks, improvement in the signs and symptoms of ankylosing spondylitis, as measured by the proportion of patients achieving a 20% improvement in ASAS response criteria (ASAS 20), was seen in 60% of patients in the REMICADE-treated group vs. 18% of patients in the placebo group (p<0.001). Improvement was observed at week 2 and maintained through week 24 (Figure 3 and Table 5).

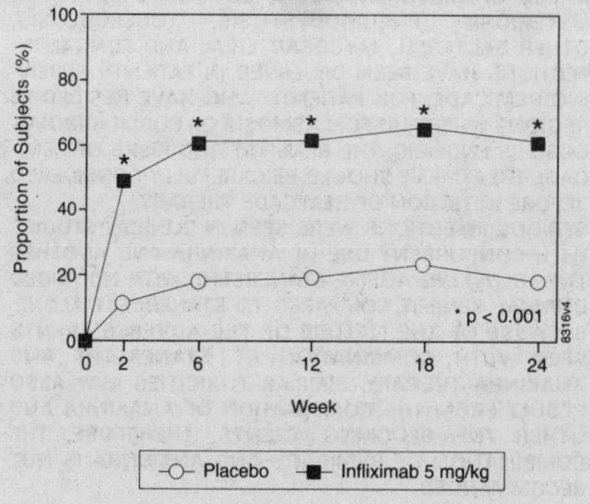

Figure 3
Proportion of patients achieving ASAS 20 response

At 24 weeks, the proportions of patients achieving a 50% and a 70% improvement in the signs and symptoms of ankylosing spondylitis, as measured by ASAS response criteria (ASAS 50 and ASAS 70, respectively), were 44% and 28%, respectively, for patients receiving REMICADE, compared to 9% and 4%, respectively, for patients receiving placebo (p<0.001, REMICADE vs. placebo). A low level of disease activity (defined as a value <20 [on a scale of 0-100 mm] in each of the four ASAS response parameters) was achieved in 22% of REMICADE-treated patients vs. 1% in placebo-treated patients (p<0.001).

[See table 5 at top of next page]

The median improvement from baseline in the general health-related quality of life questionnaire SF-36 physical component summary score at week 24 was 10.2 for the REMICADE group vs. 0.8 for the placebo group (p<0.001). There was no change in the SF-36 mental component summary score in either the REMICADE group or the placebo group.

Results of this study were similar to those seen in a multicenter double-blind, placebo-controlled study of 70 patients with ankylosing spondylitis.

Continued on next page

Remicade—Cont.

INDICATIONS AND USAGE

Rheumatoid Arthritis

REMICADE, in combination with methotrexate, is indicated for reducing signs and symptoms, inhibiting the progression of structural damage, and improving physical function in patients with moderately to severely active rheumatoid arthritis.

Crohn's Disease

REMICADE is indicated for reducing signs and symptoms and inducing and maintaining clinical remission in patients with moderately to severely active Crohn's disease who have had an inadequate response to conventional therapy. REMICADE is indicated for reducing the number of draining enterocutaneous and rectovaginal fistulas and maintaining fistula closure in patients with fistulizing Crohn's disease.

Ankylosing Spondylitis

REMICADE is indicated for reducing signs and symptoms in patients with active ankylosing spondylitis.

CONTRAINDICATIONS

REMICADE at doses >5 mg/kg should not be administered to patients with moderate to severe heart failure. In a randomized study evaluating REMICADE in patients with moderate to severe heart failure (New York Heart Association [NYHA] Functional Class III/IV), REMICADE treatment at 10 mg/kg was associated with an increased incidence of death and hospitalization due to worsening heart failure (see WARNINGS and ADVERSE REACTIONS, Patients with Heart Failure).

REMICADE should not be administered to patients with known hypersensitivity to any murine proteins or other component of the product.

WARNINGS

RISK OF INFECTIONS

(See boxed WARNING)

SERIOUS INFECTIONS, INCLUDING SEPSIS AND PNEUMONIA, HAVE BEEN REPORTED IN PATIENTS RECEIVING TNF-BLOCKING AGENTS. SOME OF THESE INFECTIONS HAVE BEEN FATAL. MANY OF THE SERIOUS INFECTIONS IN PATIENTS TREATED WITH REMICADE HAVE OCCURRED IN PATIENTS ON CONCOMITANT IMMUNOSUPPRESSIVE THERAPY THAT, IN ADDITION TO THEIR CROHN'S DISEASE OR RHEUMATOID ARTHRITIS, COULD PREDISPOSE THEM TO INFECTIONS.

REMICADE SHOULD NOT BE GIVEN TO PATIENTS WITH A CLINICALLY IMPORTANT, ACTIVE INFECTION. CAUTION SHOULD BE EXERCISED WHEN CONSIDERING THE USE OF REMICADE IN PATIENTS WITH A CHRONIC INFECTION OR A HISTORY OF RECURRENT INFECTION. PATIENTS SHOULD BE MONITORED FOR SIGNS AND SYMPTOMS OF INFECTION WHILE ON OR AFTER TREATMENT WITH REMICADE. NEW INFECTIONS SHOULD BE CLOSELY MONITORED. IF A PATIENT DEVELOPS A SERIOUS INFECTION, REMICADE THERAPY SHOULD BE DISCONTINUED (see ADVERSE REACTIONS, Infections).

CASES OF HISTOPLASMOSIS, COCCIDIOIDOMYCOSIS, LISTERIOSIS, PNEUMOCYSTOSIS, TUBERCULOSIS, OTHER BACTERIAL, MYCOBACTERIAL AND FUNGAL INFECTIONS HAVE BEEN OBSERVED IN PATIENTS RECEIVING REMICADE. FOR PATIENTS WHO HAVE RESIDED IN REGIONS WHERE HISTOPLASMOSIS OR COCCIDIOIDOMYCOSIS IS ENDEMIC, THE BENEFITS AND RISKS OF REMICADE TREATMENT SHOULD BE CAREFULLY CONSIDERED BEFORE INITIATION OF REMICADE THERAPY.

SERIOUS INFECTIONS WERE SEEN IN CLINICAL STUDIES WITH CONCURRENT USE OF ANAKINRA AND ANOTHER TNFα-BLOCKING AGENT, ETANERCEPT, WITH NO ADDED CLINICAL BENEFIT COMPARED TO ETANERCEPT ALONE. BECAUSE OF THE NATURE OF THE ADVERSE EVENTS SEEN WITH COMBINATION OF ETANERCEPT AND ANAKINRA THERAPY, SIMILAR TOXICITIES MAY ALSO RESULT FROM THE COMBINATION OF ANAKINRA AND OTHER TNFα-BLOCKING AGENTS. THEREFORE, THE COMBINATION OF REMICADE AND ANAKINRA IS NOT RECOMMENDED.

Hepatotoxicity

Severe hepatic reactions, including acute liver failure, jaundice, hepatitis and cholestasis have been reported rarely in postmarketing data in patients receiving REMICADE. Autoimmune hepatitis has been diagnosed in some of these cases. Severe hepatic reactions occurred between two weeks to more than a year after initiation of REMICADE; elevations in hepatic aminotransferase levels were not noted prior to discovery of the liver injury in many of these cases. Some of these cases were fatal or necessitated liver transplantation. Patients with symptoms or signs of liver dysfunction should be evaluated for evidence of liver injury. If jaundice and/or marked liver enzyme elevations (e.g., ≥5 times the upper limit of normal) develops, REMICADE should be discontinued, and a thorough investigation of the abnormality should be undertaken. As with other immunosuppressive drugs, use of REMICADE has been associated with reactivation of hepatitis B in patients who are chronic carriers of this virus (i.e., surface antigen positive). Chronic carriers of hepatitis B should be appropriately evaluated and monitored prior to the initiation of and during treatment with REMICADE. In clinical trials, mild or moderate elevations of ALT and AST have been observed in patients receiving REMICADE without progression to severe hepatic injury (see ADVERSE REACTIONS, Hepatotoxicity).

Table 5
Components of Ankylosing Spondylitis Disease Activity

	Placebo (n=78)		REMICADE 5mg/kg (n=201)		
	Baseline	24 Weeks	Baseline	24 Weeks	p-value
ASAS 20 response Criteria (Mean)					
Patient global assessment[a]	6.6	6.0	6.8	3.8	<0.001
Spinal pain[a]	7.3	6.5	7.6	4.0	<0.001
BASFI[b]	5.8	5.6	5.7	3.6	<0.001
Inflammation[c]	6.9	5.8	6.9	3.4	<0.001
Acute Phase Reactants					
Median CRP[d] (mg/dL)	1.7	1.5	1.5	0.4	<0.001
Spinal Mobility (cm, Mean)					
Modified Schober's test[e]	4.0	5.0	4.3	4.4	0.75
Chest expansion[e]	3.6	3.7	3.3	3.9	0.04
Tragus to wall[e]	17.3	17.4	16.9	15.7	0.02
Lateral spinal flexion	10.6	11.0	11.4	12.9	0.03

[a]measured on a VAS with 0= "none" and 10= "severe"
[b]Bath Ankylosing Spondylitis Functional Index (BASFI), average of 10 questions
[c]Inflammation, average of last 2 questions on the 6 question BASDAI
[d]CRP normal range 0-1.0 mg/dL
[e]Spinal mobility normal values: modified Schober's test:>4 cm; chest expansion:>6 cm; tragus to wall: <15 cm; lateral spinal flexion: >10 cm

Patients with Heart Failure

REMICADE has been associated with adverse outcomes in patients with heart failure, and should be used in patients with heart failure only after consideration of other treatment options. The results of a randomized study evaluating the use of REMICADE in patients with heart failure (NYHA Functional Class III/IV) suggested higher mortality in patients who received 10 mg/kg REMICADE, and higher rates of cardiovascular adverse events at doses of 5 mg/kg and 10 mg/kg. There have been post-marketing reports of worsening heart failure, with and without identifiable precipitating factors, in patients taking REMICADE. There have also been rare post-marketing reports of new onset heart failure, including heart failure in patients without known pre-existing cardiovascular disease. Some of these patients have been under 50 years of age. If a decision is made to administer REMICADE to patients with heart failure, they should be closely monitored during therapy, and REMICADE should be discontinued if new or worsening symptoms of heart failure appear. (See CONTRAINDICATIONS and ADVERSE REACTIONS, Patients with Heart Failure.)

Hematologic Events

Cases of leukopenia, neutropenia, thrombocytopenia, and pancytopenia, some with a fatal outcome, have been reported in patients receiving REMICADE. The causal relationship to REMICADE therapy remains unclear. Although no high-risk group(s) has been identified, caution should be exercised in patients being treated with REMICADE who have ongoing or a history of significant hematologic abnormalities. All patients should be advised to seek immediate medical attention if they develop signs and symptoms suggestive of blood dyscrasias or infection (e.g., persistent fever) while on REMICADE. Discontinuation of REMICADE therapy should be considered in patients who develop significant hematologic abnormalities.

Hypersensitivity

REMICADE has been associated with hypersensitivity reactions that vary in their time of onset and required hospitalization in some cases. Most hypersensitivity reactions, which include urticaria, dyspnea, and/or hypotension, have occurred during or within 2 hours of REMICADE infusion. However, in some cases, serum sickness-like reactions have been observed in Crohn's disease patients 3 to 12 days after REMICADE therapy was reinstituted following an extended period without REMICADE treatment. Symptoms associated with these reactions include fever, rash, headache, sore throat, myalgias, polyarthralgias, hand and facial edema and/or dysphagia. These reactions were associated with marked increase in antibodies to infliximab, loss of detectable serum concentrations of infliximab, and possible loss of drug efficacy. REMICADE should be discontinued for severe reactions. Medications for the treatment of hypersensitivity reactions (e.g., acetaminophen, antihistamines, corticosteroids and/or epinephrine) should be available for immediate use in the event of a reaction (see ADVERSE REACTIONS, Infusion-related Reactions).

Neurologic Events

Infliximab and other agents that inhibit TNF have been associated in rare cases with optic neuritis, seizure and new onset or exacerbation of clinical symptoms and/or radiographic evidence of central nervous system demyelinating disorders, including multiple sclerosis, and CNS manifestation of systemic vasculitis. Prescribers should exercise caution in considering the use of REMICADE in patients with pre-existing or recent onset of central nervous system demyelinating or seizure disorders. Discontinuation of REMICADE should be considered in patients who develop significant central nervous system adverse reactions.

Malignancies

In the controlled portions of clinical trials of all the TNFα-blocking agents, more cases of lymphoma have been observed among patients receiving a TNF blocker compared with control patients. During the controlled portions of REMICADE trials in patients with moderately to severely active rheumatoid arthritis and Crohn's disease, 1 patient developed lymphoma among 1389 REMICADE-treated patients versus 0 among 483 control patients (median duration of follow-up 1.1 years). In the controlled and open-label portions of these clinical trials of REMICADE, 3 patients developed lymphomas (1 patient with rheumatoid arthritis and 2 patients with Crohn's disease) among 2410 patients (median duration of follow-up 1.1 years). In rheumatoid arthritis patients, this is approximately 3-fold higher than expected in the general population. In the combined clinical trial population for rheumatoid arthritis and Crohn's disease, this is approximately 6-fold higher than expected in the general population. Rates in clinical trials for REMICADE cannot be compared to rates of clinical trials of other TNF blockers and may not predict rates observed in a broader patient population. Patients with Crohn's disease or rheumatoid arthritis, particularly patients with highly active disease and/or chronic exposure to immunosuppressant therapies, may be at a higher risk (up to several fold) than the general population for the development of lymphoma. The potential role of TNFα-blocking therapy in the development of malignancies is not known (see ADVERSE REACTIONS, Malignancies). No studies have been conducted that include patients with a history of malignancy or that continue treatment in patients who develop malignancy while receiving REMICADE; thus additional caution should be exercised in considering REMICADE treatment of these patients.

PRECAUTIONS

Autoimmunity

Treatment with REMICADE may result in the formation of autoantibodies and, rarely, in the development of a lupus-like syndrome. If a patient develops symptoms suggestive of a lupus-like syndrome following treatment with REMICADE, treatment should be discontinued (see ADVERSE REACTIONS, Autoantibodies/Lupus-like Syndrome).

Vaccinations

No data are available on the response to vaccination with live vaccines or on the secondary transmission of infection by live vaccines in patients receiving anti-TNF therapy. It is recommended that live vaccines not be given concurrently.

Information for Patients

Patients should be provided the REMICADE Patient Information Sheet and provided an opportunity to read it prior to each treatment infusion session. Because caution should be exercised in administering REMICADE to patients with clinically important active infections, it is important that the patient's overall health be assessed at each treatment visit and any questions resulting from the patient's reading of the Patient Information Sheet be discussed.

Drug Interactions

Concurrent administration of etanercept (another TNFα-blocking agent) and anakinra (an interleukin-1 antagonist) has been associated with an increased risk of serious infections, and increased risk of neutropenia and no additional benefit compared to these medicinal products alone. Other TNFα-blocking agents (including REMICADE) used in combination with anakinra may also result in similar toxicities (see WARNINGS, RISK OF INFECTIONS).

Specific drug interaction studies, including interactions with MTX, have not been conducted. The majority of patients in rheumatoid arthritis or Crohn's disease clinical studies received one or more concomitant medications. In rheumatoid arthritis, concomitant medications besides MTX were nonsteroidal anti-inflammatory agents, folic acid, corticosteroids and/or narcotics. Concomitant Crohn's disease medications were antibiotics, antivirals, corticosteroids, 6-MP/AZA and aminosalicylates. Patients with Crohn's disease who received immunosuppressants tended to experience fewer infusion reactions compared to patients on no immunosuppressants (see ADVERSE REACTIONS, Immunogenicity and Infusion-related Reactions).

Serum infliximab concentrations appeared to be unaffected by baseline use of medications for the treatment of Crohn's disease including corticosteroids, antibiotics (metronidazole or ciprofloxacin) and aminosalicylates.

Carcinogenesis, Mutagenesis and Impairment of Fertility

A repeat dose toxicity study was conducted with mice given cV1q anti-mouse TNFα to evaluate tumorigenicity. CV1q is an analogous antibody that inhibits the function of TNFα in mice. Animals were assigned to 1 of 3 dose groups: control,

10 mg/kg or 40 mg/kg cV1q given weekly for 6 months. The weekly doses of 10 mg/kg and 40 mg/kg are 2 and 8 times, respectively, the human dose of 5 mg/kg for Crohn's disease. Results indicated that cV1q did not cause tumorigenicity in mice. No clastogenic or mutagenic effects of infliximab were observed in the *in vivo* mouse micronucleus test or the *Salmonella-Escherichia coli* (Ames) assay, respectively. Chromosomal aberrations were not observed in an assay performed using human lymphocytes. The significance of these findings for human risk is unknown. It is not known whether infliximab can impair fertility in humans. No impairment of fertility was observed in a fertility and general reproduction toxicity study with the analogous mouse antibody used in the 6-month chronic toxicity study.

Pregnancy Category B

Since infliximab does not cross-react with TNFα in species other than humans and chimpanzees, animal reproduction studies have not been conducted with REMICADE. No evidence of maternal toxicity, embryotoxicity or teratogenicity was observed in a developmental toxicity study conducted in mice using an analogous antibody that selectively inhibits the functional activity of mouse TNFα. Doses of 10 to 15 mg/kg in pharmacodynamic animal models with the anti-TNF analogous antibody produced maximal pharmacologic effectiveness. Doses up to 40 mg/kg were shown to produce no adverse effects in animal reproduction studies. It is not known whether REMICADE can cause fetal harm when administered to a pregnant woman or can affect reproduction capacity. REMICADE should be given to a pregnant woman only if clearly needed.

Nursing Mothers

It is not known whether infliximab is excreted in human milk or absorbed systemically after ingestion. Because many drugs and immunoglobulins are excreted in human milk, and because of the potential for adverse reactions in nursing infants from REMICADE, a decision should be made whether to discontinue nursing or to discontinue the drug, taking into account the importance of the drug to the mother.

Pediatric Use

Safety and effectiveness of REMICADE in patients with juvenile rheumatoid arthritis and in pediatric patients with Crohn's disease have not been established.

Geriatric Use

In rheumatoid arthritis clinical trials, no overall differences were observed in effectiveness or safety in 181 patients aged 65 or older compared to younger patients although the incidence of serious adverse events in patients aged 65 or older was higher in both infliximab and control groups compared to younger patients. In Crohn's disease and ankylosing spondylitis studies, there were insufficient numbers of patients aged 65 and over to determine whether they respond differently from patients aged 18 to 65. Because there is a higher incidence of infections in the elderly population in general, caution should be used in treating the elderly (see ADVERSE REACTIONS, Infections).

ADVERSE REACTIONS

The data described herein reflect exposure to REMICADE in 2629 patients, including 1484 patients exposed beyond 30 weeks and 296 exposed beyond one year. The most common reason for discontinuation of treatment was infusion-related reactions (e.g. dyspnea, flushing, headache and rash). Adverse events have been reported in a higher proportion of rheumatoid arthritis patients receiving the 10 mg/kg dose than the 3 mg/kg dose, however, no differences were observed in the frequency of adverse events between the 5 mg/kg dose and 10 mg/kg dose in patients with Crohn's disease.

Infusion-related Reactions

Acute infusion reactions

An infusion reaction was defined in clinical trials as any adverse event occurring during an infusion or within 1 to 2 hours after an infusion. Approximately 20% of REMICADE-treated patients in all clinical studies experienced an infusion reaction compared to approximately 10% of placebo-treated patients. Among all REMICADE infusions, 3% were accompanied by nonspecific symptoms such as fever or chills, 1% were accompanied by cardiopulmonary reactions (primarily chest pain, hypotension, hypertension or dyspnea), and <1% were accompanied by pruritus, urticaria, or the combined symptoms of pruritus/urticaria and cardiopulmonary reactions. Serious infusion reactions occurred in <1% of patients and included anaphylaxis, convulsions, erythematous rash and hypotension. Approximately 3% of patients discontinued REMICADE because of infusion reactions, and all patients recovered with treatment and/or discontinuation of the infusion. REMICADE infusions beyond the initial infusion were not associated with a higher incidence of reactions.

Patients who became positive for antibodies to infliximab were more likely (approximately 2- to 3-fold) to have an infusion reaction than were those who were negative. Use of concomitant immunosuppressant agents appeared to reduce the frequency of antibodies to infliximab and infusion reactions (see ADVERSE REACTIONS, Immunogenicity and PRECAUTIONS, Drug Interactions).

In post-marketing experience, cases of anaphylactic-like reactions, including laryngeal/pharyngeal edema and severe bronchospasm, and seizure have been associated with REMICADE administration.

Reactions following readministration

In a study where 37 of 41 patients with Crohn's disease were retreated with infliximab following a 2 to 4 year period without infliximab treatment, 10 patients experienced adverse events manifesting 3 to 12 days following infusion of which 6 were considered serious. Signs and symptoms included myalgia and/or arthralgia with fever and/or rash, with some patients also experiencing pruritus, facial, hand or lip edema, dysphagia, urticaria, sore throat, and headache. Patients experiencing these adverse events had not experienced infusion-related adverse events associated with their initial infliximab therapy. These adverse events occurred in 39% (9/23) of patients who had received liquid formulation which is no longer in use and 7% (1/14) of patients who received lyophilized formulation. The clinical data are not adequate to determine if occurrence of these reactions is due to differences in formulation. Patients' signs and symptoms improved substantially or resolved with treatment in all cases. There are insufficient data on the incidence of these events after drug-free intervals of 1 to 2 years. These events have been observed only infrequently in clinical studies and post-marketing surveillance with retreatment intervals up to 1 year.

Infections

In REMICADE clinical studies, treated infections were reported in 36% of REMICADE-treated patients (average of 53 weeks of follow-up) and in 28% of placebo-treated patients (average of 47 weeks of follow-up). The infections most frequently reported were respiratory tract infections (including sinusitis, pharyngitis, and bronchitis) and urinary tract infections. Among REMICADE-treated patients, serious infections included pneumonia, cellulitis, abscess, skin ulceration, sepsis, and bacterial infection. In all clinical trials, three opportunistic infections were reported; coccidioidomycosis (which resulted in death), nocardiosis and cytomegalovirus. Tuberculosis was reported in six patients, one of whom died due to miliary tuberculosis. Other cases of tuberculosis, including disseminated tuberculosis, also have been reported post-marketing. Most of these cases of tuberculosis occurred within the first two months after initiation of therapy with infliximab and may reflect recrudescence of latent disease (see WARNINGS, RISK OF INFECTIONS). In the RA trials at 1 year, 5.3% of patients receiving infliximab and MTX every 8 weeks developed serious infections as compared to 3.4% of placebo patients receiving MTX. Of 924 patients receiving infliximab, 1.7% developed pneumonia and 0.4% developed TB, when compared to 0.3% and 0.0% in the placebo arm respectively. During the 54 weeks Crohn's II Study, 15% of patients with fistulizing Crohn's disease developed a new fistula-related abscess.

In post-marketing experience, infections have been observed with various pathogens including viral, bacterial, fungal, and protozoal organisms. Infections have been noted in all organ systems and have been reported in patients receiving REMICADE alone or in combination with immunosuppressive agents.

Autoantibodies/Lupus-like Syndrome

Approximately half of infliximab-treated patients in clinical trials who were antinuclear antibody (ANA) negative at baseline developed a positive ANA during the trial compared with approximately one-fifth of placebo-treated patients. Anti-dsDNA antibodies were newly detected in approximately one-fifth of infliximab-treated patients compared with 0% of placebo-treated patients. Reports of lupus and lupus-like syndromes, however, remain uncommon.

Malignancies

Among 2410 patients with moderately to severely active rheumatoid arthritis and Crohn's disease treated with REMICADE in clinical trials with a median of 1.1 years of follow-up, 3 patients developed lymphomas, for a rate of 0.07 cases per 100 patient-years of follow-up in patients with rheumatoid arthritis and 0.12 cases per 100 patient-years of follow up in the combined clinical trial data for rheumatoid arthritis and Crohn's disease patients. This is approximately 3-fold higher in the RA clinical trial population and 6-fold higher in the overall clinical trial population than expected in an age-, gender-, and race-matched general population based on the Surveillance, Epidemiology and End Results Database. Rates in clinical trials for REMICADE cannot be compared to rates of clinical trials of other TNF blockers and may not predict rates observed in a broader patient population. An increased rate of lymphoma up to several fold has reported in the Crohn's disease and rheumatoid arthritis patient populations, and may be further increased in patients with more severe disease activity. Other than lymphoma, 13 patients developed malignancies, which was similar in number to what would be expected the general population. Of these, the most common malignancies were breast, colorectal, and melanoma. (See WARNINGS, Malignancies.)

Malignancies, including non-Hodgkin's lymphoma and Hodgkin's disease, have also been reported in patients receiving REMICADE during post-approval use.

Patients with Heart Failure

In a randomized study evaluating REMICADE in moderate to severe heart failure (NYHA Class III/IV; left ventricular ejection fraction ≤35%), 150 patients were randomized to receive treatment with 3 infusions of REMICADE 10 mg/kg, 5 mg/kg, or placebo, at 0, 2, and 6 weeks. Higher incidences of mortality and hospitalization due to worsening heart failure were observed in patients receiving the 10 mg/kg REMICADE dose. At 1 year, 8 patients in the 10 mg/kg REMICADE group had died compared with 4 deaths each in the 5 mg/kg REMICADE and the placebo groups. There were trends towards increased dyspnea, hypotension, angina, and dizziness in both the 10 mg/kg and 5 mg/kg REMICADE treatment groups, versus placebo. REMICADE has not been studied in patients with mild heart failure (NYHA Class I/II). (See CONTRAINDICATIONS and WARNINGS, Patients with Heart Failure.)

Immunogenicity

Treatment with REMICADE can be associated with the development of antibodies to infliximab. The incidence of antibodies to infliximab in patients given a 3-dose induction regimen followed by maintenance dosing was approximately 10% as assessed through one to two years of REMICADE treatment. A higher incidence of antibodies to infliximab was observed in Crohn's disease patients receiving REMICADE after drug free intervals >16 weeks. The majority of antibody-positive patients had low titers. Patients who were antibody-positive were more likely to have higher rates of clearance, reduced efficacy and to experience an infusion reaction (see ADVERSE REACTIONS, Infusion-related Reactions) than were patients who were antibody negative. Antibody development was lower among rheumatoid arthritis and Crohn's disease patients receiving immunosuppressant therapies such as 6-MP/AZA or MTX.

The data reflect the percentage of patients whose test results were positive for antibodies to infliximab in an ELISA assay, and are highly dependent on the sensitivity and specificity of the assay. Additionally, the observed incidence of antibody positivity in an assay may be influenced by several factors including sample handling, timing of sample collection, concomitant medication, and underlying disease. For these reasons, comparison of the incidence of antibodies to infliximab with the incidence of antibodies to other products may be misleading.

Hepatotoxicity

Severe liver injury, including acute liver failure and autoimmune hepatitis, has been reported rarely in patients receiving REMICADE (see WARNINGS, Hepatotoxicity). Reactivation of hepatitis B has occurred in patients receiving REMICADE who are chronic carriers of this virus (i.e., surface antigen positive) (see WARNINGS, Hepatotoxicity).

In clinical trials in RA, Crohn's disease and ankylosing spondylitis, elevations of aminotransferases were observed (ALT more common than AST) in a greater proportion of patients receiving REMICADE than in controls, both when REMICADE was given as monotherapy and when it was used in combination with other immunosuppressive agents. In general, patients who developed ALT and AST elevations were asymptomatic, and the abnormalities decreased or resolved with either continuation or discontinuation of REMICADE, or modification of concomitant medications. ALT elevations ≥5 times the upper limit of normal were observed in 1% of patients receiving REMICADE.

In rheumatoid arthritis clinical trials, 34% of patients who received REMICADE + MTX experienced transient mild (<2 times the upper limit of normal) or moderate (≥2 but <3 times the upper limit of normal) elevations in ALT compared to 24% of patients treated with placebo + MTX. ALT elevations ≥3 times the upper limit of normal were observed in 3.9% of patients who received REMICADE + MTX compared with 3.2% of patients who received MTX alone (median follow up approximately 1 year).

In Crohn's disease clinical trials (median follow up 54 weeks), 39% of patients receiving REMICADE-maintenance experienced mild to moderate elevations in ALT, compared to 34% of patients treated with placebo-maintenance. ALT elevations ≥3 times the upper limit of normal were observed in 5.0% of patients who received REMICADE-maintenance compared with 4.0% of patients who received placebo-maintenance.

In an ankylosing spondylitis clinical trial in which patients were not receiving MTX, 40% of patients who received REMICADE experienced mild to moderate elevations in ALT compared to 13% of patients treated with placebo. ALT elevations ≥3 times the upper limit of normal were observed in 12 (6%) REMICADE-treated patients compared to none in placebo-treated patients.

Other Adverse Reactions

Safety data are available from 2629 REMICADE-treated patients, including 1304 with rheumatoid arthritis, and 1106 with Crohn's disease, 202 with ankylosing spondylitis and 17 with other conditions. Adverse events reported in ≥5% of all patients with rheumatoid arthritis receiving 4 or more infusions are in Table 6. The types and frequencies of adverse reactions observed were similar in REMICADE-treated rheumatoid arthritis, ankylosing spondylitis and Crohn's disease patients except for abdominal pain, which occurred in 26% of REMICADE-treated patients with Crohn's disease. In the Crohn's disease studies, there were insufficient numbers and duration of follow-up for patients who never received REMICADE to provide meaningful comparisons.

Table 6

ADVERSE EVENTS OCCURRING IN 5% OR MORE OF PATIENTS RECEIVING 4 OR MORE INFUSIONS FOR RHEUMATOID ARTHRITIS

	Placebo (n=350)	REMICADE (n=1129)
Average weeks of follow-up	59	66
Gastrointestinal		
Nausea	20%	21%
Abdominal Pain	8%	12%
Diarrhea	12%	12%
Dyspepsia	7%	10%

Continued on next page

Remicade—Cont.

Respiratory

Upper respiratory tract infection	25%	32%
Sinusitis	8%	14%
Pharyngitis	8%	12%
Coughing	8%	12%
Bronchitis	9%	10%
Rhinitis	5%	8%
Skin and appendages disorders		
Rash	5%	10%
Pruritis	2%	7%
Body as a whole–general disorders		
Fatigue	7%	9%
Pain	7%	8%
Resistance mechanism disorders		
Fever	4%	7%
Moniliasis	3%	5%
Central and peripheral nervous system disorders		
Headache	14%	18%
Musculoskeletal system disorders		
Back pain	5%	8%
Arthralgia	7%	8%
Urinary system disorders		
Urinary tract infection	6%	8%
Cardiovascular disorders, general		
Hypertension	5%	7%

Because clinical trials are conducted under widely varying conditions, adverse reaction rates observed in clinical trials of a drug cannot be directly compared to rates in clinical trials of another drug and may not predict the rates observed in broader patient populations in clinical practice. The most common serious adverse events observed in clinical trials were infections (see ADVERSE REACTIONS, Infections). Other serious, medically relevant adverse events ≥0.2% or clinically significant adverse events by body system were as follows:
Body as a whole: allergic reaction, diaphragmatic hernia, edema, surgical/procedural sequela
Blood: pancytopenia
Cardiovascular: circulatory failure, hypotension, syncope
Gastrointestinal: constipation, gastrointestinal hemorrhage, ileus, intestinal obstruction, intestinal perforation, intestinal stenosis, pancreatitis, peritonitis, proctalgia
Central & Peripheral Nervous: meningitis, neuritis, peripheral neuropathy, dizziness
Heart Rate and Rhythm: arrhythmia, bradycardia, cardiac arrest, tachycardia
Liver and Biliary: biliary pain, cholecystitis, cholelithiasis, hepatitis
Metabolic and Nutritional: dehydration
Musculoskeletal: intervertebral disk herniation, tendon disorder
Myo-, Endo-, Pericardial and Coronary Valve: myocardial infarction
Platelet, Bleeding and Clotting: thrombocytopenia
Neoplasms: basal cell, breast, lymphoma
Psychiatric: confusion, suicide attempt
Red Blood Cell: anemia, hemolytic anemia
Reproductive: menstrual irregularity
Resistance Mechanism: cellulitis, sepsis, serum sickness
Respiratory: adult respiratory distress syndrome, lower respiratory tract infection (including pneumonia), pleural effusion, pleurisy, pulmonary edema, respiratory insufficiency
Skin and Appendages: increased sweating, ulceration
Urinary: renal calculus, renal failure
Vascular (Extracardiac): brain infarction, pulmonary embolism, thrombophlebitis
White Cell and Reticuloendothelial: leukopenia, lymphadenopathy
The following adverse events have been reported during post-approval use of REMICADE: neutropenia (see WARNINGS, Hematologic Events), interstitial pneumonitis/fibrosis, idiopathic thrombocytopenic purpura, thrombotic thrombocytopenic purpura, pericardial effusion, systemic and cutaneous vasculitis, Guillain-Barré syndrome, transverse myelitis, and neuropathies (additional neurologic events have also been observed, see WARNINGS, Neurologic Events). Because these events are reported voluntarily from a population of uncertain size, it is not always possible to reliably estimate their frequency or establish a causal relationship to REMICADE exposure.

OVERDOSAGE

Single doses up to 20 mg/kg have been administered without any direct toxic effect. In case of overdosage, it is recommended that the patient be monitored for any signs or symptoms of adverse reactions or effects and appropriate symptomatic treatment instituted immediately.

DOSAGE AND ADMINISTRATION

Rheumatoid Arthritis
The recommended dose of REMICADE is 3 mg/kg given as an intravenous infusion followed with additional similar doses at 2 and 6 weeks after the first infusion then every 8 weeks thereafter. REMICADE should be given in combination with methotrexate. For patients who have an incomplete response, consideration may be given to adjusting the dose up to 10 mg/kg or treating as often as every 4 weeks.

Crohn's Disease or Fistulizing Crohn's Disease
The recommended dose of REMICADE is 5 mg/kg given as an induction regimen at 0, 2 and 6 weeks followed by a maintenance regimen of 5 mg/kg every 8 weeks thereafter for the treatment of moderately to severely active Crohn's disease or fistulizing disease. For patients who respond and then lose their response, consideration may be given to treatment with 10 mg/kg. Patients who do not respond by week 14 are unlikely to respond with continued dosing and consideration should be given to discontinue REMICADE in these patients.

Ankylosing Spondylitis
The recommended dose of REMICADE is 5 mg/kg given as an intravenous infusion followed with additional similar doses at 2 and 6 weeks after the first infusion, then every 6 weeks thereafter.

Preparation and Administration Instructions
Use aseptic technique.
REMICADE vials do not contain antibacterial preservatives. Therefore, the vials after reconstitution should be used immediately, not re-entered or stored. The diluent to be used for reconstitution is 10 mL of Sterile Water for Injection, USP. The total dose of the reconstituted product must be further diluted to 250 mL with 0.9% Sodium Chloride Injection, USP. The infusion concentration should range between 0.4 mg/mL and 4 mg/mL. The REMICADE infusion should begin within 3 hours of preparation.

1. Calculate the dose and the number of REMICADE vials needed. Each REMICADE vial contains 100 mg of infliximab. Calculate the total volume of reconstituted REMICADE solution required.
2. Reconstitute each REMICADE vial with 10 mL of Sterile Water for Injection, USP, using a syringe equipped with a 21-gauge or smaller needle. Remove the flip-top from the vial and wipe the top with an alcohol swab. Insert the syringe needle into the vial through the center of the rubber stopper and direct the stream of Sterile Water for Injection, USP, to the glass wall of the vial. Do not use the vial if the vacuum is not present. Gently swirl the solution by rotating the vial to dissolve the lyophilized powder. Avoid prolonged or vigorous agitation. DO NOT SHAKE. Foaming of the solution on reconstitution is not unusual. Allow the reconstituted solution to stand for 5 minutes. The solution should be colorless to light yellow and opalescent, and the solution may develop a few translucent particles as infliximab is a protein. Do not use if opaque particles, discoloration, or other foreign particles are present.
3. Dilute the total volume of the reconstituted REMICADE solution dose to 250 mL with 0.9% Sodium Chloride Injection, USP, by withdrawing a volume of 0.9% Sodium Chloride Injection, USP, equal to the volume of reconstituted REMICADE from the 0.9% Sodium Chloride Injection, USP, 250 mL bottle or bag. Slowly add the total volume of reconstituted REMICADE solution to the 250 mL infusion bottle or bag. Gently mix.
4. The infusion solution must be administered over a period of not less than 2 hours and must use an infusion set with an in-line, sterile, non-pyrogenic, low-protein-binding filter (pore size of 1.2 μm or less). Any unused portion of the infusion solution should not be stored for reuse.
5. No physical biochemical compatibility studies have been conducted to evaluate the co-administration of REMICADE with other agents. REMICADE should not be infused concomitantly in the same intravenous line with other agents.
6. Parenteral drug products should be inspected visually for particulate matter and discoloration prior to administration, whenever solution and container permit. If visibly opaque particles, discoloration or other foreign particulates are observed, the solution should not be used.

Storage
Store the lyophilized product under refrigeration at 2°C to 8°C (36°F to 46°F). Do not freeze. Do not use beyond the expiration date. This product contains no preservative.

HOW SUPPLIED

REMICADE lyophilized concentrate for IV injection is supplied in individually-boxed single-use vials in the following strength:
NDC 57894-030-01   100 mg infliximab in a 20 mL vial

REFERENCES

1. American Thoracic Society, Centers for Disease Control and Prevention. Targeted tuberculin testing and treatment of latent tuberculosis infection. *Am J Respir Crit Care Med* 2000;161:S221-S247.
2. Knight DM, Trinh H, Le J, et al. Construction and initial characterization of a mouse-human chimeric anti-TNF antibody. *Molec Immunol* 1993;30:1443-1453.
3. Scallon BJ, Moore MA, Trinh H, et al. Chimeric anti-TNFα monoclonal antibody cA2 binds recombinant transmembrane TNFα and activates immune effector functions. *Cytokine* 1995;7:251-259.
4. ten Hove T, van Montfrans C, Peppelenbosch MP, et al. Infliximab treatment induces apoptosis of lamina propria T lymphocytes in Crohn's disease. *Gut* 2002;50:206-211.
5. Maini RN, Breedveld FC, Kalden JR, et al. Therapeutic efficacy of multiple intravenous infusions of anti-tumor necrosis factor α monoclonal antibody combined with low-dose weekly methotrexate in rheumatoid arthritis. *Arthritis Rheum* 1998;41(9):1552-1563.
6. Elliott MJ, Maini RN, Feldmann M, et al. Randomised double-blind comparison of chimeric monoclonal antibody to tumour necrosis factor alpha (cA2) vs. placebo in rheumatoid arthritis. *Lancet* 1994;344(8930):1105-1110.
7. Van der Heijde DM, van Leeuwen MA, van Riel PL, et al. Biannual radiographic assessments of hands and feet in a three-year prospective follow-up of patients with early rheumatoid arthritis. *Arthritis Rheum* 1992;35(1):26-34.
8. Targan SR, Hanauer SR, van Deventer SJH, et al. A short-term study of chimeric monoclonal antibody cA2 to tumor necrosis factor α for Crohn's disease. *N Engl J Med* 1997;337(15):1029-1035.
9. Hanauer SB, Feagan BG, Lichtenstein GR, et al. Maintenance infliximab for Crohn's disease: the ACCENT I randomized trial. *Lancet* 2002; 359:1541-1549.
10. Present DH, Rutgeerts P, Targan S, et al. Infliximab for the treatment of fistulas in patients with Crohn's disease. *N Engl J Med* 1999;340:1398-1405.
11. van der Linden S, Valkenburg Cats A. Evaluation of diagnostic criteria for ankylosing spondylitis. A proposal for modification of the New York criteria. *Arthritis Rheum.* 1984;27(4):361-368.

©Centocor, Inc. 2004
Malvern, PA 19355, USA   License #1242
1-800-457-6399   Revised December 2004
Rx Only

REMICADE® (infliximab)
Patient Information Sheet

You should read this information sheet before you start using REMICADE® (pronounced rem-eh-kaid) and before each time you are scheduled to receive REMICADE. This information sheet does not take the place of talking with your doctor. You and your doctor should talk about your health and how you are feeling before you start taking REMICADE, while you are taking it and at regular checkups. If you do not understand any of the information in this sheet, you should ask your doctor to explain what it means.

What is REMICADE?
REMICADE is a medicine that is used to treat adults with moderately to severely active rheumatoid arthritis, Crohn's disease and ankylosing spondylitis. In Crohn's disease, REMICADE is for people who have not responded well enough to other medicines.

How does REMICADE work?
The medicine REMICADE is a type of protein that recognizes, attaches to and blocks the action of a substance in your body called tumor necrosis factor. Tumor necrosis factor (TNF) is made by certain blood cells in your body. REMICADE will not cure rheumatoid arthritis, Crohn's disease or ankylosing spondylitis, but blocking TNF with REMICADE may reduce the inflammation caused by too much TNF in your body. You should also know that REMICADE may help you feel better but can also cause serious side effects and can reduce your body's ability to fight infections (see below).

What should I know about the immune system, and taking REMICADE for Rheumatoid Arthritis, Crohn's Disease or Ankylosing Spondylitis?
The immune system protects the body by responding to "invaders" like bacteria, viruses and other foreign matter that enter your body by producing antibodies and putting them into action to fight off the "invaders." In diseases like rheumatoid arthritis, Crohn's disease and ankylosing spondylitis, your body's immune system produces too much TNF. Too much TNF can cause your immune system to attack healthy tissues in your body and cause inflammation. If this condition is left untreated, it can cause permanent damage to the body's bones, cartilage and tissue.
While taking REMICADE can block the TNF that causes inflammation, it can also lower your body's ability to fight infections. So, taking REMICADE can make you more prone to getting infections or it can make an infection that you already have worse. You should call your doctor right away if you think you have an infection.

What important information should I know about treatment with REMICADE?
REMICADE, like other medicines that affect your immune system, is a strong medicine that can cause serious side effects. Possible serious side effects include:
Serious Infections:
• Some patients have had serious infections while receiving REMICADE. Some of the patients have died from these infections. Serious infections include TB (tuberculosis), and infections caused by viruses, fungi or bacteria that have spread throughout the body. If you develop a fever, feel very tired, have a cough, or have flu-like symptoms, these could be signs that you may be getting an infection. If you have any of these symptoms while you are taking or after you have taken REMICADE, you should tell your doctor right away.
Heart Failure:
• If you have been told that you have a heart problem called congestive heart failure and you are currently being treated with REMICADE, you will need to be closely monitored by your doctor. If you develop new or worse symptoms that are related to your heart condition, such as shortness of breath or swelling of your ankles or feet, you must contact your doctor immediately.
Blood Problems:
• In some patients the body may fail to produce enough of the blood cells that help your body fight infections or help you stop bleeding. Some of the patients have died from this failure to produce blood cells. If you develop a fever that doesn't go away, bruise or bleed very easily or look

very pale, call your doctor right away. Your doctor may decide to stop your treatment.

Allergic Reactions:

- Some patients have had severe allergic reactions to REMICADE. These reactions can happen while you are getting your REMICADE infusion or shortly afterwards. The symptoms of an allergic reaction may include hives (red, raised, itchy patches of skin), difficulty breathing, chest pain and high or low blood pressure. Your doctor may decide to stop REMICADE treatment and give you medicines to treat the allergic reaction.
- Some patients who have been taking REMICADE for Crohn's disease have had allergic reactions 3 to 12 days after receiving their REMICADE treatment. The symptoms of this type of delayed reaction may include fever, rash, headache and muscle or joint pain. Call your doctor right away if you develop any of these symptoms or any other unusual symptoms such as difficulty swallowing.

Nervous System Disorders:

- There have been rare cases where people taking REMICADE or other TNF blockers have developed disorders that affected their nervous system. Signs that you could be having a problem include: changes in your vision, weakness in your arms and/or legs, and numbness or tingling in any part of your body.

Malignancy

- Reports of a type of blood cancer called lymphoma in patients on REMICADE or other TNF blockers are rare but occur more often than expected for people in general. People who have been treated for rheumatoid arthritis, Crohn's disease or ankylosing spondylitis for a long time, particularly those with highly active disease may be more prone to develop lymphoma. If you take REMICADE or other TNF blockers, your risk for developing lymphoma may increase. You should also tell your doctor if you have had or develop lymphoma or other cancers while you are taking REMICADE.

Liver Injury

- There have been rare cases where people taking REMICADE have developed liver problems. Signs that you could be having problem include: jaundice (skin and eyes turning yellow), dark brown-colored urine, right sided abdominal pain, fever, and severe fatigue (tiredness). You should contact your doctor immediately if you develop any of these symptoms.

Other Important Information

Some patients have developed symptoms that can resemble disease called lupus. Lupus-like symptoms may include chest discomfort or pain that doesn't go away, shortness of breath, joint pain, or a rash on the cheeks or arms that gets worse in the sun. If you develop any of these symptoms your doctor may decide to stop your treatment with REMICADE.

What are the more common side effects of REMICADE?

The more common side effects with REMICADE are respiratory infections (that may include sinus infections and sore throat), coughing and stomach pain.

Who should not take REMICADE?

YOU SHOULD NOT take REMICADE if you have:

- Heart failure, unless your doctor has talked to you and decided that you are able to take REMICADE.
- Had an allergic reaction to REMICADE or any other product that was made with murine (mouse) proteins.

What health concerns should I talk to my doctor about?

Before receiving your first treatment with REMICADE you should tell your doctor if you:

- Have or think you may have any kind of infection. The infection could be in only one place in your body (such as an open cut or sore), or an infection that affects your whole body (such as the flu). Having an infection could put you at risk for serious side effects from REMICADE.
- Have an infection that won't go away or a history of infection that keeps coming back.
- Have had TB (tuberculosis), or if you have recently been with anyone who might have TB. Your doctor will examine you for TB and perform a skin test. If your doctor feels that you are at risk for TB, he or she may start treating you for TB before you begin REMICADE therapy.
- Have lived in or visited an area of the country where an infection called histoplasmosis or coccidioidomycosis (an infection caused by a fungus that affects the lungs) is common. If you don't know if the area you live in is one where histoplasmosis or coccidioidomycosis is common, ask your doctor.
- Have or have previously had heart failure or other heart conditions.
- Have or have had a condition that affects your nervous system, like multiple sclerosis, or Guillain-Barré syndrome, or if you experience any numbness, or tingling, or have had a seizure.
- Are pregnant or nursing.
- Have recently received or are scheduled to receive a vaccine.

Can I take REMICADE while I am on other medicines?

Tell your doctor if you are taking any other medicines including over the counter medicines, supplements or herbal products before you are treated with REMICADE. If you start taking or plan to start taking any new medicine while you are taking REMICADE, tell your doctor.

REMICADE and KINERET should not be taken together.

How will REMICADE be given to me?

REMICADE will be given to you by a healthcare professional. REMICADE will be given to you by an IV. This means that the medicine will be given to you through a needle placed in a vein in your arm. It will take about 2 hours to give you the full dose of medicine. During that time and for a period after you receive REMICADE, you will be monitored by a healthcare professional. Your doctor may ask you to take other medicines along with REMICADE.

Only a health care professional should prepare the medicine and administer it to you.

How often will I receive REMICADE?

Rheumatoid Arthritis

If you are receiving REMICADE for rheumatoid arthritis you will receive your first dose followed by additional doses at 2 and 6 weeks after the first dose. You will then receive a dose every 8 weeks. Your doctor will monitor your response to REMICADE and may change your dose or treat you more frequently (as often as every 4 weeks).

Crohn's Disease or Fistulizing Crohn's Disease

If you are receiving REMICADE for active Crohn's disease or fistulizing Crohn's disease, you will receive your first dose followed by additional doses at 2 and 6 weeks after the first dose. You will then receive a dose every 8 weeks. Your doctor will monitor your response to REMICADE and may change your dose.

Ankylosing Spondylitis

If you are receiving REMICADE for ankylosing spondylitis you will receive your first dose followed by additional doses at 2 and 6 weeks after the first dose. You will then receive a dose every 6 weeks.

What if I still have questions?

If you have any questions, or problems, always talk first with your doctor. You can also visit the REMICADE internet site at www.remicade.com.

Product developed and manufactured by:

Centocor, Inc.
200 Great Valley Parkway
Malvern, PA 19355
Revised December 2004
IN04810

Cephalon, Inc.

41 MOORES ROAD
PO BOX 4011
FRAZER, PA 19355

For Medical Information and Adverse Drug Experience/Product Complaint Reporting Contact:
(800) 896-5855
Fax 610-738-6669

GABITRIL® ℞

[*găb-ĭ-trĭl*]
(tiagabine hydrochloride)
Tablets
Rx only

Prescribing information for this product, which appears on pages 1126–1131 of the 2005 PDR, has been completely revised as follows. Please write "See Supplement A" next to the product heading.

DESCRIPTION

GABITRIL (tiagabine HCl) is an antiepilepsy drug available as 2 mg, 4 mg, 12 mg, and 16 mg tablets for oral administration. Its chemical name is (-)-(R)-1-[4,4-Bis(3-methyl-2-thienyl)-3-butenyl]nipecotic acid hydrochloride, its molecular formula is $C_{20}H_{25}NO_2S_2$ HCl, and its molecular weight is 412.0. Tiagabine HCl is a white to off-white, odorless, crystalline powder. It is insoluble in heptane, sparingly soluble in water, and soluble in aqueous base. The structural formula is:

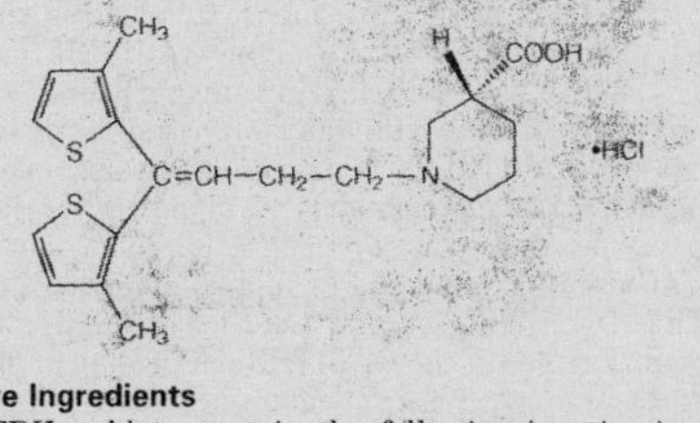

Inactive Ingredients

GABITRIL tablets contain the following inactive ingredients: Ascorbic acid, colloidal silicon dioxide, crospovidone, hydrogenated vegetable oil wax, hydroxypropyl cellulose, hypromellose, lactose, magnesium stearate, microcrystalline cellulose, pregelatinized starch, stearic acid, and titanium dioxide.

In addition, individual tablets contain:

2 mg tablets: FD&C Yellow No. 6.
4 mg tablets: D&C Yellow No. 10.
12 mg tablets: D&C Yellow No. 10 and FD&C Blue No. 1.
16 mg tablets: FD&C Blue No. 2.

CLINICAL PHARMACOLOGY

Mechanism of Action

The precise mechanism by which tiagabine exerts its antiseizure effect is unknown, although it is believed to be related to its ability, documented in *in vitro* experiments, to enhance the activity of gamma aminobutyric acid (GABA), the major inhibitory neurotransmitter in the central nervous system. These experiments have shown that tiagabine binds to recognition sites associated with the GABA uptake carrier. It is thought that, by this action, tiagabine blocks GABA uptake into presynaptic neurons, permitting more GABA to be available for receptor binding on the surfaces of post-synaptic cells. Inhibition of GABA uptake has been shown for synaptosomes, neuronal cell cultures, and glial cell cultures. In rat-derived hippocampal slices, tiagabine has been shown to prolong GABA-mediated inhibitory postsynaptic potentials. Tiagabine increases the amount of GABA available in the extracellular space of the globus pallidus, ventral palladum, and substantia nigra in rats at the ED_{50} and ED_{85} doses for inhibition of pentylenetetrazol (PTZ)-induced tonic seizures. This suggests that tiagabine prevents the propagation of neural impulses that contribute to seizures by a GABA-ergic action.

Tiagabine has shown efficacy in several animal models of seizures. It is effective against the tonic phase of subcutaneous PTZ-induced seizures in mice and rats, seizures induced by the proconvulsant DMCM in mice, audiogenic seizures in genetically epilepsy-prone rats (GEPR), and amygdala-kindled seizures in rats. Tiagabine has little efficacy against maximal electroshock seizures in rats and is only partially effective against subcutaneous PTZ-induced clonic seizures in mice, picrotoxin-induced tonic seizures in the mouse, bicuculline-induced seizures in the rat, and photic seizures in photosensitive baboons. Tiagabine produces a biphasic dose-response curve against PTZ- and DMCM-induced convulsions, with attenuated effectiveness at higher doses.

Based on *in vitro* binding studies, tiagabine does not significantly inhibit the uptake of dopamine, norepinephrine, serotonin, glutamate, or choline and shows little or no binding to dopamine D1 and D2, muscarinic, serotonin $5HT_{1A}$, $5HT_2$, and $5HT_3$, beta-1 and 2 adrenergic, alpha-1 and alpha-2 adrenergic, histamine H2 and H3, adenosine A_1 and A_2, opiate µ and K_1, NMDA glutamate, and $GABA_A$ receptors at 100 µM. It also lacks significant affinity for sodium or calcium channels. Tiagabine binds to histamine H1, serotonin $5HT_{1B}$, benzodiazepine, and chloride channel receptors at concentrations 20 to 400 times those inhibiting the uptake of GABA.

PHARMACOKINETICS

Tiagabine is well absorbed, with food slowing absorption rate but not altering the extent of absorption. The elimination half-life of tiagabine is 7 to 9 hours in normal volunteers. In epilepsy clinical trials, most patients were receiving hepatic enzyme-inducing agents (e.g., carbamazepine, phenytoin, primidone, and phenobarbital). The pharmacokinetic profile in induced patients is significantly different from the non-induced population (see **PRECAUTIONS - Use in Non-Induced Patients**). The systemic clearance of tiagabine in induced patients is approximately 60% greater resulting in considerably lower plasma concentrations and an elimination half-life of 2 to 5 hours. Given this difference in clearance, the systemic exposure after a dose of 32 mg/day in an induced population is expected to be comparable to the systemic exposure after a dose of 12 mg/day in a non-induced population. Similarly, the systemic exposure after a dose of 56 mg/day in an induced population is expected to be comparable to the systemic exposure after a dose of 22 mg/day in a non-induced population.

Absorption and Distribution: Absorption of tiagabine is rapid, with peak plasma concentrations occurring at approximately 45 minutes following an oral dose in the fasting state. Tiagabine is nearly completely absorbed (>95%), with an absolute oral bioavailability of about 90%. A high fat meal decreases the rate (mean T_{max} was prolonged to 2.5 hours, and mean C_{max} was reduced by about 40%) but not the extent (AUC) of tiagabine absorption. In all clinical trials, tiagabine was given with meals.

The pharmacokinetics of tiagabine are linear over the single dose range of 2 to 24 mg. Following multiple dosing, steady state is achieved within 2 days.

Tiagabine is 96% bound to human plasma proteins, mainly to serum albumin and α1-acid glycoprotein over the concentration range of 10 ng/mL to 10,000 ng/mL. While the relationship between tiagabine plasma concentrations and clinical response is not currently understood, trough plasma concentrations observed in controlled clinical trials at doses from 30 to 56 mg/day ranged from <1 ng/mL to 234 ng/mL.

Metabolism and Elimination: Although the metabolism of tiagabine has not been fully elucidated, *in vivo* and *in vitro* studies suggest that at least two metabolic pathways for tiagabine have been identified in humans: 1) thiophene ring oxidation leading to the formation of 5-oxo-tiagabine; and 2) glucuronidation. The 5-oxo-tiagabine metabolite does not contribute to the pharmacologic activity of tiagabine.

Based on *in vitro* data, tiagabine is likely to be metabolized primarily by the 3A isoform subfamily of hepatic cytochrome P450 (CYP 3A), although contributions to the metabolism of tiagabine from CYP 1A2, CYP 2D6 or CYP 2C19 have not been excluded.

Approximately 2% of an oral dose of tiagabine is excreted unchanged, with 25% and 63% of the remaining dose excreted into the urine and feces, respectively, primarily as metabolites, at least 2 of which have not been identified. The mean systemic plasma clearance is 109 mL/min (CV = 23%) and the average elimination half-life for tiagabine in healthy subjects ranged from 7 to 9 hours. The elimination half-life decreased by 50 to 65% in hepatic enzyme-induced patients with epilepsy compared to uninduced patients with epilepsy.

A diurnal effect on the pharmacokinetics of tiagabine was observed. Mean steady-state C_{min} values were 40% lower in the evening than in the morning. Tiagabine steady-state AUC values were also found to be 15% lower following the evening tiagabine dose compared to the AUC following the morning dose.

Continued on next page

Gabitril—Cont.

SPECIAL POPULATIONS

Renal Insufficiency: The pharmacokinetics of total and unbound tiagabine were similar in subjects with normal renal function (creatinine clearance >80 mL/min) and in subjects with mild (creatinine clearance 40 to 80 mL/min), moderate (creatinine clearance 20 to 39 mL/min), or severe (creatinine clearance 5 to 19 mL/min) renal impairment. The pharmacokinetics of total and unbound tiagabine were also unaffected in subjects with renal failure requiring hemodialysis.

Hepatic Insufficiency: In patients with moderate hepatic impairment (Child-Pugh Class B), clearance of unbound tiagabine was reduced by about 60%. Patients with impaired liver function may require reduced initial and maintenance doses of tiagabine and/or longer dosing intervals compared to patients with normal hepatic function (see **PRECAUTIONS**).

Geriatric: The pharmacokinetic profile of tiagabine was similar in healthy elderly and healthy young adults.

Pediatric: Tiagabine has not been investigated in adequate and well-controlled clinical trials in patients below the age of 12. The apparent clearance and volume of distribution of tiagabine per unit body surface area or per kg were fairly similar in 25 children (age: 3 to 10 years) and in adults taking enzyme-inducing antiepilepsy drugs ([AEDs] e.g., carbamazepine or phenytoin). In children who were taking a non-inducing AED (e.g., valproate), the clearance of tiagabine based upon body weight and body surface area was 2 and 1.5-fold higher, respectively, than in non-induced adults with epilepsy.

Gender, Race and Cigarette Smoking: No specific pharmacokinetic studies were conducted to investigate the effect of gender, race and cigarette smoking on the disposition of tiagabine. Retrospective pharmacokinetic analyses, however, suggest that there is no clinically important difference between the clearance of tiagabine in males and females, when adjusted for body weight. Population pharmacokinetic analyses indicated that tiagabine clearance values were not significantly different in Caucasian (N=463), Black (N=23), or Hispanic (N=17) patients with epilepsy, and that tiagabine clearance values were not significantly affected by tobacco use.

Interactions with other Antiepilepsy Drugs: The clearance of tiagabine is affected by the co-administration of hepatic enzyme-inducing antiepilepsy drugs. Tiagabine is eliminated more rapidly in patients who have been taking hepatic enzyme-inducing drugs, e.g., carbamazepine, phenytoin, primidone and phenobarbital than in patients not receiving such treatment (see **PRECAUTIONS, Drug Interactions**).

Interactions with Other Drugs: See **PRECAUTIONS, Drug Interactions.**

CLINICAL STUDIES

The effectiveness of GABITRIL as adjunctive therapy (added to other antiepilepsy drugs) was examined in three multi-center, double-blind, placebo-controlled, parallel-group, clinical trials in 769 patients with refractory partial seizures who were taking at least one hepatic enzyme-inducing antiepilepsy drug (AED), and two placebo-controlled cross-over studies in 90 patients. In the parallel-group trials, patients had a history of at least six complex partial seizures (Study 1 and Study 2, U.S. studies), or six partial seizures of any type (Study 3, European study), occurring alone or in combination with any other seizure type within the 8-week period preceding the first study visit in spite of receiving one or more AEDs at therapeutic concentrations.

In the first two studies, the primary protocol-specified outcome measure was the median reduction from baseline in the 4-week complex partial seizure (CPS) rates during treatment. In the third study, the protocol-specified primary outcome measure was the proportion of patients achieving a 50% or greater reduction from baseline in the 4-week seizure rate of all partial seizures during treatment. The results given below include data for complex partial seizures and all partial seizures for the intent-to-treat population (all patients who received at least one dose of treatment and at least one seizure evaluation) in each study.

Study 1 was a double-blind, placebo-controlled, parallel-group trial comparing GABITRIL 16 mg/day, GABITRIL 32 mg/day, GABITRIL 56 mg/day, and placebo. Study drug was given as a four times a day regimen. After a prospective Baseline Phase of 12 weeks, patients were randomized to one of the four treatment groups described above. The 16-week Treatment Phase consisted of a 4-week Titration Period, followed by a 12-week Fixed-Dose Period, during which concomitant AED doses were held constant. The primary outcome was assessed for the combined 32 and 56 mg/day groups compared to placebo.

Study 2 was a double-blind, placebo-controlled, parallel-group trial consisting of an 8-week Baseline Phase and a 12-week Treatment Phase, the first 4 weeks of which constituted a Titration Period and the last 8 weeks a Fixed-Dose Period. This study compared GABITRIL 16 mg BID and 8 mg QID to placebo. The protocol-specified primary outcome measure was assessed separately for each group treated with GABITRIL.

The following tables display the results of the analyses of these two trials.

[See table 1 above]

[See table 2 above]

Continued on next page

Table 1
Median Reduction and Median Percent Reduction
from Baseline in 4-Week Seizure Rates in Study 1

		Placebo (N=91)	GABITRIL 16 mg/day (N=61)	GABITRIL 32 mg/day (N=87)	GABITRIL 56 mg/day (N=56)	Combined 32 + 56 mg/day (N=143)
Complex Partial	Median Reduction	0.6	0.8	2.2*	2.9*	2.6*
	Median % Reduction[†]	9%	13%	25%	32%	29%
All Partial	Median Reduction	0.2	1.2	2.7*	3.5*	2.9*
	Median % Reduction[†]	3%	12%	24%	36%	27%

* p<0.05
[†] Statistical significance was not assessed for median % reduction.

Table 2
Median Reduction and Median Percent Reduction
from Baseline in 4-Week Seizure Rates in Study 2

		Placebo (N=107)	GABITRIL 16 mg BID (N=106)	GABITRIL 8 mg QID (N=104)
Complex Partial	Median Reduction	0.3	1.6	1.3*
	Median % Reduction[†]	4%	22%	15%
All Partial	Median Reduction	0.5	1.6	1.3
	Median % Reduction[†]	5%	19%	13%

* p < 0.027, necessary for statistical significance due to multiple comparisons.
[†] Statistical significance was not assessed for median % reduction.

Figures 1 to 4 present the proportion of patients (X-axis) whose percent reduction from baseline in the all partial seizure rate was at least as great as that indicated on the Y axis in the three placebo-controlled adjunctive studies (Studies 1, 2, and 3). A positive value on the Y axis indicates an improvement from baseline (i.e., a decrease in seizure rate), while a negative value indicates a worsening from baseline (i.e., an increase in seizure rate). Thus, in a display of this type, the curve for an effective treatment is shifted to the left of the curve for placebo.

Figure 1 indicates that the proportion of patients achieving any particular level of reduction in seizure rate was consistently higher for the combined GABITRIL 32 mg and 56 mg groups compared to the placebo group in Study 1. For example, Figure 1 indicates that approximately 24% of patients treated with GABITRIL experienced a 50% or greater reduction, compared to 4% in the placebo group.

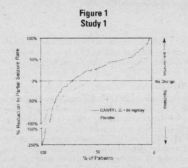
Figure 1
Study 1

Figure 2 also displays the results for Study 1, which was a dose-response study, by treatment group. Figure 2 indicates a dose-response relationship across the three GABITRIL groups. The proportion of patients achieving any particular level of reduction in all partial seizure rates was consistently higher as the dose of GABITRIL was increased. For example, Figure 2 indicates that approximately 4% of patients in the placebo group experienced a 50% or greater reduction in all partial seizure rate, compared to approximately 10% of the GABITRIL 16 mg/day group, 21% of the GABITRIL 32 mg/day group, and 30% of the GABITRIL 56 mg/day group.

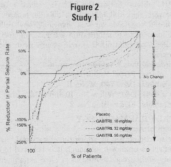
Figure 2
Study 1

Figure 3 indicates that the proportion of patients achieving any particular level of reduction in partial seizure rate was consistently greater in patients taking GABITRIL than in those taking placebo in Study 2. (Study 2 compared placebo to GABITRIL 32 mg/day; one of the GABITRIL groups re-

ceived 8 mg QID, while the other GABITRIL group received 16 mg BID). For example, Figure 3 indicates that approximately 7% of patients in the placebo group experienced a 50% or greater reduction in their partial seizure rate, compared to approximately 23% of patients in the GABITRIL 8 mg QID group and 28% of patients in the GABITRIL 16 mg BID group.

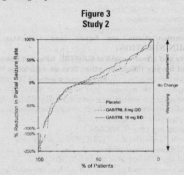
Figure 3
Study 2

Study 3 was a double-blind, placebo-controlled, parallel-group trial that compared GABITRIL 10 mg TID (N=77) with placebo (N=77). In this trial, patients were followed prospectively during a 12-week Baseline Phase and then randomized to receive study drug during an 18-week Treatment Phase. During the first 6 weeks of treatment (Titration Period), patients were titrated to 30 mg/day, after which they were maintained on this dose during the 12-week Fixed-Dose Period. The protocol-specified primary outcome measure (proportion of patients who achieved at least a 50% reduction from baseline in partial seizure rate) did not reach statistical significance. However, analyses of the median reduction from baseline in 4-week partial seizure rate (the analyses presented above for Study 1 and Study 2) were performed and showed a statistically significant improvement compared to placebo in all partial and complex partial seizure rates (Table 3):

[See table 3 at bottom of next page]

Figure 4 indicates that the proportion of patients achieving any particular level of reduction in seizure activity was consistently higher in those taking GABITRIL than those taking placebo in Study 3. For example, Figure 4 indicates that approximately 5% of patients in the placebo group experienced a 50% or greater reduction in their partial seizure rate compared to approximately 10% of patients in the GABITRIL group.

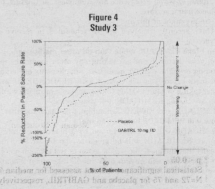
Figure 4
Study 3

The two other placebo-controlled trials that examined the effectiveness of GABITRIL were small cross-over trials (N=46 and 44). Both trials included an open Screening Phase during which patients were titrated to an optimal dose and then treated with this dose for an additional 4 weeks. After this Open Phase, patients were randomized to one of two blinded treatment sequences (GABITRIL followed by placebo or placebo followed by GABITRIL). The Double-Blind Phase consisted of two Treatment Periods, each lasting 7 weeks (with a 3 week washout between periods). The outcome measures were median with-in patient differences between placebo and GABITRIL Treatment Periods in 4-week complex partial and all partial seizure rates. The reductions in seizure rates were statistically significant in both studies.

INDICATIONS AND USAGE

GABITRIL (tiagabine hydrochloride) is indicated as adjunctive therapy in adults and children 12 years and older in the treatment of partial seizures.

CONTRAINDICATIONS

GABITRIL is contraindicated in patients who have demonstrated hypersensitivity to the drug or its ingredients.

WARNINGS

Seizures in Patients Without Epilepsy: Post-marketing reports have shown that GABITRIL use has been associated with new onset seizures and status epilepticus in patients without epilepsy. Dose may be an important predisposing factor in the development of seizures, although seizures have been reported in patients taking daily doses of GABITRIL as low as 4 mg/day. In most cases, patients were using concomitant medications (antidepressants, antipsychotics, stimulants, narcotics) that are thought to lower the seizure threshold. Some seizures occurred near the time of a dose increase, even after periods of prior stable dosing.

The GABITRIL dosing recommendations in current labeling for treatment of epilepsy were based on use in patients with partial seizures 12 years of age and older, most of whom were taking enzyme-inducing antiepileptic drugs (AEDs; e.g., carbamazepine, phenytoin, primidone and phenobarbital) which lower plasma levels of GABITRIL by inducing its metabolism. Use of GABITRIL without enzyme-inducing antiepileptic drugs results in blood levels about twice those attained in the studies on which current dosing recommendations are based (see DOSAGE AND ADMINISTRATION).

Safety and effectiveness of GABITRIL have not been established for any indication other than as adjunctive therapy for partial seizures in adults and children 12 years and older.

In nonepileptic patients who develop seizures while on GABITRIL treatment, GABITRIL should be discontinued and patients should be evaluated for an underlying seizure disorder.

Seizures and status epilepticus are known to occur with GABITRIL overdosage (see OVERDOSAGE).

Withdrawal Seizures: As a rule, antiepilepsy drugs should not be abruptly discontinued because of the possibility of increasing seizure frequency. In a placebo-controlled, double-blind, dose-response study (Study 1 described in CLINICAL STUDIES) designed, in part, to investigate the capacity of GABITRIL to induce withdrawal seizures, study drug was tapered over a 4-week period after 16 weeks of treatment. Patients' seizure frequency during this 4-week withdrawal period was compared to their baseline seizure frequency (before study drug). For each partial seizure type, for all partial seizure types combined, and for secondarily generalized tonic-clonic seizures, more patients experienced increases in their seizure frequencies during the withdrawal period in the three GABITRIL groups than in the placebo group. The increase in seizure frequency was not affected by dose. GABITRIL should be withdrawn gradually to minimize the potential of increased seizure frequency, unless safety concerns require a more rapid withdrawal.

Cognitive/Neuropsychiatric Adverse Events: Adverse events most often associated with the use of GABITRIL were related to the central nervous system. The most significant of these can be classified into 2 general categories: 1) impaired concentration, speech or language problems, and confusion (effects on thought processes); and 2) somnolence and fatigue (effects on level of consciousness). The majority of these events were mild to moderate. In controlled clinical trials, these events led to discontinuation of treatment with GABITRIL in 6% (31 of 494) of patients compared to 2% (5 of 275) of the placebo-treated patients. A total

of 1.6% (8 of 494) of the GABITRIL treated patients in the controlled trials were hospitalized secondary to the occurrence of these events compared to 0% of the placebo treated patients. Some of these events were dose related and usually began during initial titration.

Patients with a history of spike and wave discharges on EEG have been reported to have exacerbations of their EEG abnormalities associated with these cognitive/neuropsychiatric events. This raises the possibility that these clinical events may, in some cases, be a manifestation of underlying seizure activity (see PRECAUTIONS, EEG). In the documented cases of spike and wave discharges on EEG with cognitive/neuropsychiatric events, patients usually continued tiagabine, but required dosage adjustment.

Additionally, there have been postmarketing reports of patients who have experienced cognitive/neuropsychiatric symptoms, some accompanied by EEG abnormalities such as generalized spike and wave activity, that have been reported as nonconvulsant status epilepticus. Some reports describe recovery following reduction of dose or discontinuation of GABITRIL.

Status Epilepticus: In the three double-blind, placebo-controlled, parallel-group studies (Studies 1, 2, and 3), the incidence of any type of status epilepticus (simple, complex, or generalized tonic-clonic) in patients receiving GABITRIL was 0.8% (4 of 494 patients) versus 0.7% (2 of 275 patients) receiving placebo. Among the patients treated with GABITRIL across all epilepsy studies (controlled and uncontrolled), 5% had some form of status epilepticus. Of the 5%, 57% of patients experienced complex partial status epilepticus. A critical risk factor for status epilepticus was the presence of a previous history; 33% of patients with a history of status epilepticus had recurrence during GABITRIL treatment. Because adequate information about the incidence of status epilepticus in a similar population of patients with epilepsy who have not received treatment with GABITRIL is not available, it is impossible to state whether or not treatment with GABITRIL is associated with a higher or lower rate of status epilepticus than would be expected to occur in a similar population not treated with GABITRIL.

Sudden Unexpected Death In Epilepsy (SUDEP): There have been as many as 10 cases of sudden unexpected deaths during the clinical development of tiagabine among 2531 patients with epilepsy (3831 patient-years of exposure). This represents an estimated incidence of 0.0026 deaths per patient-year. This rate is within the range of estimates for the incidence of sudden and unexpected deaths in patients with epilepsy not receiving GABITRIL (ranging from 0.0005 for the general population with epilepsy, 0.003 to 0.004 for clinical trial populations similar to that in the clinical development program for GABITRIL, to 0.005 for patients with refractory epilepsy). The estimated SUDEP rates in patients receiving GABITRIL are also similar to those observed in patients receiving other antiepilepsy drugs, chemically unrelated to GABITRIL, that underwent clinical testing in similar populations at about the same time. This evidence suggests that the SUDEP rates reflect population rates, not a drug effect.

PRECAUTIONS

General

Use in Non-Induced Patients: Virtually all experience with GABITRIL has been obtained in patients with epilepsy receiving at least one concomitant enzyme-inducing antiepilepsy drug (AED), which lowers the plasma levels of tiagabine. Use in non-induced patients requires lower doses of GABITRIL. These patients may also require a slower titration of GABITRIL compared to that of induced patients (see DOSAGE AND ADMINISTRATION). Patients taking a combination of inducing and non-inducing agents (e.g., carbamazepine and valproate) should be considered to be induced. Patients not receiving hepatic enzyme-inducing agents are referred to as non-induced patients.

Generalized Weakness: Moderately severe to incapacitating generalized weakness has been reported following administration of GABITRIL in 28 of 2531 (approximately 1%) patients with epilepsy. The weakness resolved in all cases after a reduction in dose or discontinuation of GABITRIL.

Binding in the Eye and Other Melanin-Containing Tissues: When dogs received a single dose of radiolabeled tiagabine, there was evidence of residual binding in the retina and uvea after 3 weeks (the latest time point measured). Although not directly measured, melanin binding is suggested. The ability of available tests to detect potentially adverse consequences, if any, of the binding of tiagabine to melanin-containing tissue is unknown and there was no systematic monitoring for relevant ophthalmological

changes during the clinical development of GABITRIL. However, long term (up to one year) toxicological studies of tiagabine in dogs showed no treatment-related ophthalmoscopic changes and macro- and microscopic examinations of the eye were unremarkable. Accordingly, although there are no specific recommendations for periodic ophthalmologic monitoring, prescribers should be aware of the possibility of long-term ophthalmologic effects.

Use in Hepatically-Impaired Patients: Because the clearance of tiagabine is reduced in patients with liver disease, dosage reduction may be necessary in these patients.

Serious Rash: Four patients treated with tiagabine during the product's premarketing clinical testing developed what were considered to be serious rashes. In two patients, the rash was described as maculopapular; in one it was described as vesiculobullous; and in the 4th case, a diagnosis of Stevens Johnson Syndrome was made. In none of the 4 cases is it certain that tiagabine was the primary, or even a contributory, cause of the rash. Nevertheless, drug associated rash can, if extensive and serious, cause irreversible morbidity, even death.

Information for Patients: Patients should be instructed to take GABITRIL only as prescribed.

Patients should be advised that GABITRIL may cause dizziness, somnolence, and other symptoms and signs of CNS depression. Accordingly, patients should be advised neither to drive nor to operate other complex machinery until they have gained sufficient experience on GABITRIL to gauge whether or not it affects their mental and/or motor performance adversely. Because of the possible additive depressive effects, caution should also be used when patients are taking other CNS depressants in combination with GABITRIL.

Because teratogenic effects were seen in the offspring of rats exposed to maternally toxic doses of tiagabine and because experience in humans is limited, patients should be advised to notify their physicians if they become pregnant or intend to become pregnant during therapy.

Because of the possibility that tiagabine may be excreted in breast milk, patients should be advised to notify those providing care to themselves and their children if they intend to breast-feed or are breast-feeding an infant.

Laboratory Tests

Therapeutic Monitoring of Plasma Concentrations of Tiagabine: A therapeutic range for tiagabine plasma concentrations has not been established. In controlled trials, trough plasma concentrations observed among patients randomized to doses of tiagabine that were statistically significantly more effective than placebo ranged from <1 ng/mL to 234 ng/mL (median, 10th and 90th percentiles are 23.7 ng/mL, 5.4 ng/mL, and 69.8 ng/mL, respectively). Because of the potential for pharmacokinetic interactions between GABITRIL and drugs that induce or inhibit hepatic metabolizing enzymes, it may be useful to obtain plasma levels of tiagabine before and after changes are made in the therapeutic regimen.

Clinical Chemistry and Hematology: During the development of GABITRIL, no systematic abnormalities on routine laboratory testing were noted. Therefore, no specific guidance is offered regarding routine monitoring; the practitioner retains responsibility for determining how best to monitor the patient in his/her care.

EEG: Patients with a history of spike and wave discharges on EEG have been reported to have exacerbations of their EEG abnormalities associated with cognitive/neuropsychiatric events. This raises the possibility that these clinical events may, in some cases, be a manifestation of underlying seizure activity (see WARNINGS, Cognitive/Neuropsychiatric Adverse Events). In the documented cases of spike and wave discharges on EEG with cognitive/neuropsychiatric events, patients usually continued tiagabine, but required dosage adjustment.

Drug Interactions

In evaluating the potential for interactions among co-administered antiepilepsy drugs (AEDs), whether or not an AED induces or does not induce metabolic enzymes is an important consideration. Carbamazepine, phenytoin, primidone, and phenobarbitalare generally classified as enzyme inducers; valproate and gabapentin are not. GABITRIL is considered to be a non-enzyme inducing AED (see PRECAUTIONS, Use in Non-Induced Patients).

The drug interaction data described in this section were obtained from studies involving either healthy subjects or patients with epilepsy.

Effects of GABITRIL on other Antiepilepsy Drugs (AEDs):

Phenytoin: Tiagabine had no effect on the steady-state plasma concentrations of phenytoin in patients with epilepsy.

Carbamazepine: Tiagabine had no effect on the steady-state plasma concentrations of carbamazepine or its epoxide metabolite in patients with epilepsy.

Valproate: Tiagabine causes a slight decrease (about 10%) in steady-state valproate concentrations.

Phenobarbital or Primidone: No formal pharmacokinetic studies have been performed examining the addition of tiagabine to regimens containing phenobarbital or primidone. The addition of tiagabine in a limited number of patients in three well-controlled studies caused no systematic changes in phenobarbital or primidone concentrations when compared to placebo.

Effects of other Antiepilepsy Drugs (AEDs) on GABITRIL:

Carbamazepine: Population pharmacokinetic analyses indicate that tiagabine clearance is 60% greater in patients taking carbamazepine with or without other enzyme-inducing AEDs.

Table 3
Median Reduction and Median Percent Reduction
from Baseline in 4-Week Seizure Rates in Study 3

		Placebo (N=77)	GABITRIL 30 mg/day (N=77)
Complex Partial[‡]	Median Reduction	−0.1	1.3*
	Median % Reduction[†]	−1%	14%
All Partial	Median Reduction	−0.5	1.1*
	Median % Reduction[†]	−7%	11%

---

* p <0.05
[†] Statistical significance was not assessed for median % reduction.
[‡] N=72 and 75 for placebo and GABITRIL, respectively.

Continued on next page

Gabitril—Cont.

Phenytoin: Population pharmacokinetic analyses indicate that tiagabine clearance is 60% greater in patients taking phenytoin with or without other enzyme-inducing AEDs.
Phenobarbital (Primidone): Population pharmacokinetic analyses indicate that tiagabine clearance is 60% greater in patients taking phenobarbital (primidone) with or without other enzyme-inducing AEDs.
Valproate: The addition of tiagabine to patients taking valproate chronically had no effect on tiagabine pharmacokinetics, but valproate significantly decreased tiagabine binding *in vitro* from 96.3 to 94.8%, which resulted in an increase of approximately 40% in the free tiagabine concentration. The clinical relevance of this *in vitro* finding is unknown.

Interaction of GABITRIL with Other Drugs:
Cimetidine: Co-administration of cimetidine (800 mg/day) to patients taking tiagabine chronically had no effect on tiagabine pharmacokinetics.
Theophylline: A single 10 mg dose of tiagabine did not affect the pharmacokinetics of theophylline at steady state.
Warfarin: No significant differences were observed in the steady-state pharmacokinetics of R-warfarin or S-warfarin with the addition of tiagabine given as a single dose. Prothrombin times were not affected by tiagabine.
Digoxin: Concomitant administration of tiagabine did not affect the steady-state pharmacokinetics of digoxin or the mean daily trough serum level of digoxin.
Ethanol or Triazolam: No significant differences were observed in the pharmacokinetics of triazolam (0.125 mg) and tiagabine (10 mg) when given together as a single dose. The pharmacokinetics of ethanol were not affected by multiple-dose administration of tiagabine. Tiagabine has shown no clinically important potentiation of the pharmacodynamic effects of triazolam or alcohol. Because of the possible additive effects of drugs that may depress the nervous system, ethanol or triazolam should be used cautiously in combination with tiagabine.
Oral Contraceptives: Multiple dose administration of tiagabine (8 mg/day monotherapy) did not alter the pharmacokinetics of oral contraceptives in healthy women of child-bearing age.
Antipyrine: Antipyrine pharmacokinetics were not significantly different before and after tiagabine multiple-dose regimens. This indicates that tiagabine does not cause induction or inhibition of the hepatic microsomal enzyme systems responsible for the metabolism of antipyrine.

Interaction of GABITRIL with Highly Protein Bound Drugs: *In vitro* data showed that tiagabine is 96% bound to human plasma protein and therefore has the potential to interact with other highly protein bound compounds. Such an interaction can potentially lead to higher free fractions of either tiagabine or the competing drug.

Carcinogenesis: In rats, a study of the potential carcinogenicity associated with tiagabine HCl administration showed that 200 mg/kg/day (plasma exposure [AUC] 36 to 100 times that at the maximum recommended human dosage [MRHD] of 56 mg/day) for 2 years resulted in small, but statistically significant increases in the incidences of hepatocellular adenomas in females and Leydig cell tumors of the testis in males. The significance of these findings relative to the use of GABITRIL in humans is unknown. The no effect dosage for induction of tumors in this study was 100 mg/kg/day (17 to 50 times the exposure at the MRHD). No statistically significant increases in tumor formation were noted in mice at dosages up to 250 mg/kg/day (20 times the MRHD on a mg/m^2 basis).

Mutagenesis: Tiagabine produced an increase in structural chromosome aberration frequency in human lymphocytes *in vitro* in the absence of metabolic activation. No increase in chromosomal aberration frequencies was demonstrated in this assay in the presence of metabolic activation. No evidence of genetic toxicity was found in the *in vitro* bacterial gene mutation assays, the *in vitro* HGPRT forward mutation assay in Chinese hamster lung cells, the *in vivo* mouse micronucleus test, or an unscheduled DNA synthesis assay.

Impairment of Fertility: Studies of male and female rats administered dosages of tiagabine HCl prior to and during mating, gestation, and lactation have shown no impairment of fertility at doses up to 100 mg/kg/day. This dose represents approximately 16 times the maximum recommended human dose (MRHD) of 56 mg/day, based on body surface area (mg/m^2). Lowered maternal weight gain and decreased viability and growth in the rat pups were found at 100 mg/kg, but not at 20 mg/kg/day (3 times the MRHD on a mg/m^2 basis).

Pregnancy: Pregnancy Category C: Tiagabine has been shown to have adverse effects on embryo-fetal development, including teratogenic effects, when administered to pregnant rats and rabbits at doses greater than the human therapeutic dose.
An increased incidence of malformed fetuses (various craniofacial, appendicular, and visceral defects) and decreased fetal weights were observed following oral administration of 100 mg/kg/day to pregnant rats during the period of organogenesis. This dose is approximately 16 times the maximum recommended human dose (MRHD) of 56 mg/day, based on body surface area (mg/m^2). Maternal toxicity (transient weight loss/reduced maternal weight gain during gestation) was associated with this dose, but there is no evidence to suggest that the teratogenic effects were secondary to the maternal effects. No adverse maternal or embryo-fetal effects were seen at a dose of 20 mg/kg/day (3 times the MRHD on a mg/m^2 basis).
Decreased maternal weight gain, increased resorption of embryos and increased incidences of fetal variations, but not malformations, were observed when pregnant rabbits were given 25 mg/kg/day (8 times the MRHD on a mg/m^2 basis) during organogenesis. The no effect level for maternal and embryo-fetal toxicity in rabbits was 5 mg/kg/day (equivalent to the MRHD on a mg/m^2 basis).
When female rats were given tiagabine 100 mg/kg/day during late gestation and throughout parturition and lactation, decreased maternal weight gain during gestation, an increase in stillbirths, and decreased postnatal offspring viability and growth were found. There are no adequate and well-controlled studies in pregnant women. Tiagabine should be used during pregnancy only if clearly needed.

Use in Nursing Mothers: Studies in rats have shown that tiagabine HCl and/or its metabolites are excreted in the milk of that species. Levels of excretion of tiagabine and/or its metabolites in human milk have not been determined and effects on the nursing infant are unknown. GABITRIL should be used in women who are nursing only if the benefits clearly outweigh the risks.

Pediatric Use: Safety and effectiveness in pediatric patients below the age of 12 have not been established. The pharmacokinetics of tiagabine were evaluated in pediatric patients age 3 to 10 years (see **CLINICAL PHARMACOLOGY—Pediatric**).

Geriatric Use: Because few patients over the age of 65 (approximately 20) were exposed to GABITRIL during its clinical evaluation, no specific statements about the safety or effectiveness of GABITRIL in this age group could be made.

ADVERSE REACTIONS

The most commonly observed adverse events in placebo-controlled, parallel-group, add-on epilepsy trials associated with the use of GABITRIL in combination with other antiepilepsy drugs not seen at an equivalent frequency among placebo-treated patients were dizziness/light-headedness, asthenia/lack of energy, somnolence, nausea, nervousness/irritability, tremor, abdominal pain, and thinking abnormal/difficulty with concentration or attention.
Approximately 21% of the 2531 patients who received GABITRIL in clinical trials of epilepsy discontinued treatment because of an adverse event. The adverse events most commonly associated with discontinuation were dizziness (1.7%), somnolence (1.6%), depression (1.3%), confusion (1.1%), and asthenia (1.1%).
In Studies 1 and 2 (U.S. studies), the double-blind, placebo-controlled, parallel-group, add-on studies, the proportion of patients who discontinued treatment because of adverse events was 11% for the group treated with GABITRIL and 6% for the placebo group. The most common adverse events considered the primary reason for discontinuation were confusion (1.2%), somnolence (1.0%), and ataxia (1.0%).

Adverse Event Incidence in Controlled Clinical Trials: Table 4 lists treatment-emergent signs and symptoms that occurred in at least 1% of patients treated with GABITRIL for epilepsy participating in parallel-group, placebo-controlled trials and were numerically more common in the GABITRIL group. In these studies, either GABITRIL or placebo was added to the patient's current antiepilepsy drug therapy. Adverse events were usually mild or moderate in intensity.
The prescriber should be aware that these figures, obtained when GABITRIL was added to concurrent antiepilepsy drug therapy, cannot be used to predict the frequency of adverse events in the course of usual medical practice when patient characteristics and other factors may differ from those prevailing during clinical studies. Similarly, the cited frequencies cannot be directly compared with figures obtained from other clinical investigations involving different treatments, uses, or investigators. An inspection of these frequencies, however, does provide the prescribing physician with one basis to estimate the relative contribution of drug and non-drug factors to the adverse event incidences in the population studied.
[See table 4 at left]

Table 4
Treatment-Emergent Adverse Event[1] Incidence in Parallel-Group, Placebo-Controlled, Add-On Trials (events in at least 1% of patients treated with GABITRIL and numerically more frequent than in the placebo group)

Body System/ COSTART	GABITRIL N=494 %	Placebo N=275 %
Body as a Whole		
Abdominal Pain	7	3
Pain (unspecified)	5	3
Cardiovascular		
Vasodilation	2	1
Digestive		
Nausea	11	9
Diarrhea	7	3
Vomiting	7	4
Increased Appetite	2	0
Mouth Ulceration	1	0
Musculoskeletal		
Myasthenia	1	0
Nervous System		
Dizziness	27	15
Asthenia	20	14
Somnolence	18	15
Nervousness	10	3
Tremor	9	3
Difficulty With Concentration/Attention*	6	2
Insomnia	6	4
Ataxia	5	3
Confusion	5	3
Speech Disorder	4	2
Difficulty With Memory*	4	3
Paresthesia	4	2
Depression	3	1
Emotional Lability	3	2
Abnormal Gait	3	2
Hostility	2	1
Nystagmus	2	1
Language Problems*	2	0
Agitation	1	0
Respiratory System		
Pharyngitis	7	4
Cough Increased	4	3
Skin and Appendages		
Rash	5	4
Pruritus	2	0

[1]Patients in these add-on studies were receiving one to three concomitant enzyme-inducing antiepilepsy drugs in addition to GABITRIL or placebo. Patients may have reported multiple adverse experiences; thus, patients may be included in more than one category.
* COSTART term substituted with a more clinically descriptive term.

Other events reported by 1% or more of patients treated with GABITRIL but equally or more frequent in the placebo group were: accidental injury, chest pain, constipation, flu syndrome, rhinitis, anorexia, back pain, dry mouth, flatulence, ecchymosis, twitching, fever, amblyopia, conjunctivitis, urinary tract infection, urinary frequency, infection, dyspepsia, gastroenteritis, nausea and vomiting, myalgia, diplopia, headache, anxiety, acne, sinusitis, and incoordination.
Study 1 was a dose-response study including doses of 32 mg and 56 mg. Table 5 shows adverse events reported at a rate of ≥ 5% in at least one GABITRIL group and more frequent than in the placebo group. Among these events, depression, tremor, nervousness, difficulty with concentration/attention, and perhaps asthenia exhibited a positive relationship to dose.
[See table 5 at top of next page]
The effects of GABITRIL in relation to those of placebo on the incidence of adverse events and the types of adverse events reported were independent of age, weight, and gen-

der. Because only 10% of patients were non-Caucasian in parallel-group, placebo-controlled trials, there is insufficient data to support a statement regarding the distribution of adverse experience reports by race.

Other Adverse Events Observed During All Clinical Trials: GABITRIL has been administered to 2531 patients during all phase 2/3 clinical trials, only some of which were placebo-controlled. During these trials, all adverse events were recorded by the clinical investigators using terminology of their own choosing. To provide a meaningful estimate of the proportion of individuals having adverse events, similar types of events were grouped into a smaller number of standardized categories using modified COSTART dictionary terminology. These categories are used in the listing below. The frequencies presented represent the proportion of the 2531 patients exposed to GABITRIL who experienced events of the type cited on at least one occasion while receiving GABITRIL. All reported events are included except those already listed above, events seen only three times or fewer (unless potentially important), events very unlikely to be drug-related, and those too general to be informative. Events are included without regard to determination of a causal relationship to tiagabine.

Events are further classified within body system categories and enumerated in order of decreasing frequency using the following definitions: frequent adverse events are defined as those occurring in at least 1/100 patients; infrequent adverse events are those occurring in 1/100 to 1/1000 patients; rare events are those occurring in fewer than 1/1000 patients.

Body as a Whole: *Frequent:* Allergic reaction, chest pain, chills, cyst, neck pain, and malaise. *Infrequent:* Abscess, cellulitis, facial edema, halitosis, hernia, neck rigidity, neoplasm, pelvic pain, photosensitivity reaction, sepsis, sudden death, and suicide attempt.

Cardiovascular System: *Frequent:* Hypertension, palpitation, syncope, and tachycardia. *Infrequent:* Angina pectoris, cerebral ischemia, electrocardiogram abnormal, hemorrhage, hypotension, myocardial infarct, pallor, peripheral vascular disorder, phlebitis, postural hypotension, and thrombophlebitis.

Digestive System: *Frequent:* Gingivitis and stomatitis. *Infrequent:* Abnormal stools, cholecystitis, cholelithiasis, dysphagia, eructation, esophagitis, fecal incontinence, gastritis, gastrointestinal hemorrhage, glossitis, gum hyperplasia, hepatomegaly, increased salivation, liver function tests abnormal, melena, periodontal abscess, rectal hemorrhage, thirst, tooth caries, and ulcerative stomatitis.

Endocrine System: *Infrequent:* Goiter and hypothyroidism.

Hemic and Lymphatic System: *Frequent:* Lymphadenopathy. *Infrequent:* Anemia, erythrocytes abnormal, leukopenia, petechia, and thrombocytopenia.

Metabolic and Nutritional: *Frequent:* Edema, peripheral edema, weight gain, and weight loss. *Infrequent:* Dehydration, hypercholesteremia, hyperglycemia, hyperlipemia, hypoglycemia, hypokalemia, and hyponatremia.

Musculoskeletal System: *Frequent:* Arthralgia. *Infrequent:* Arthritis, arthrosis, bursitis, generalized spasm, and tendinous contracture.

Nervous System: *Frequent:* Depersonalization, dysarthria, euphoria, hallucination, hyperkinesia, hypertonia, hypesthesia, hypokinesia, hypotonia, migraine, myoclonus, paranoid reaction, personality disorder, reflexes decreased, stupor, twitching, and vertigo. *Infrequent:* Abnormal dreams, apathy, choreoathetosis, circumoral paresthesia, CNS neoplasm, coma, delusions, dry mouth, dystonia, encephalopathy, hemiplegia, leg cramps, libido increased, libido decreased, movement disorder, neuritis, neurosis, paralysis, peripheral neuritis, psychosis, reflexes increased, and urinary retention.

Respiratory System: *Frequent:* Bronchitis, dyspnea, epistaxis, and pneumonia. *Infrequent:* Apnea, asthma, hemoptysis, hiccups, hyperventilation, laryngitis, respiratory disorder, and voice alteration.

Skin and Appendages: *Frequent:* Alopecia, dry skin, and sweating. *Infrequent:* Contact dermatitis, eczema, exfoliative dermatitis, furunculosis, herpes simplex, herpes zoster, hirsutism, maculopapular rash, psoriasis, skin benign neoplasm, skin carcinoma, skin discolorations, skin nodules, skin ulcer, subcutaneous nodule, urticaria, and vesiculobullous rash.

Special Senses: *Frequent:* Abnormal vision, ear pain, otitis media, and tinnitus. *Infrequent:* Blepharitis, blindness, deafness, eye pain, hyperacusis, keratoconjunctivitis, otitis externa, parosmia, photophobia, taste loss, taste perversion, and visual field defect.

Urogenital System: *Frequent:* Dysmenorrhea, dysuria, metrorrhagia, urinary incontinence, and vaginitis. *Infrequent:* Abortion, amenorrhea, breast enlargement, breast pain, cystitis, fibrocystic breast, hematuria, impotence, kidney failure, menorrhagia, nocturia, papanicolaou smear suspicious, polyuria, pyelonephritis, salpingitis, urethritis, urinary urgency, and vaginal hemorrhage.

DRUG ABUSE AND DEPENDENCE

The abuse and dependence potential of GABITRIL have not been evaluated in human studies.

OVERDOSAGE

Human Overdose Experience: Human experience of acute overdose with GABITRIL is limited. Eleven patients in clinical trials took single doses of GABITRIL up to 800 mg. All patients fully recovered, usually within one day. The most common symptoms reported after overdose included somnolence, impaired consciousness, agitation, confusion, speech difficulty, hostility, depression, weakness, and myoclonus. One patient who ingested a single dose of 400 mg experienced generalized tonic-clonic status epilepticus, which responded to intravenous phenobarbital.

From post-marketing experience, there have been no reports of fatal overdoses involving GABITRIL alone (doses up to 720 mg), although a number of patients required intubation and ventilatory support as part of the management of their status epilepticus. Overdoses involving multiple drugs, including GABITRIL, have resulted in fatal outcomes. Symptoms most often accompanying GABITRIL overdose, alone or in combination with other drugs, have included: seizures including status epilepticus in patients with and without underlying seizure disorders, nonconvulsive status epilepticus, coma, ataxia, confusion, somnolence, drowsiness, impaired speech, agitation, lethargy, myoclonus, spike wave stupor, tremors, disorientation, vomiting, hostility, and temporary paralysis. Respiratory depression was seen in a number of patients, including children, in the context of seizures.

Management of Overdose: There is no specific antidote for overdose with GABITRIL. If indicated, elimination of unabsorbed drug should be achieved by emesis or gastric lavage; usual precautions should be observed to maintain the airway. General supportive care of the patient is indicated including monitoring of vital signs and observation of clinical status of the patient. Since tiagabine is mostly metabolized by the liver and is highly protein bound, dialysis is unlikely to be beneficial. A Certified Poison Control Center should be consulted for up to date information on the management of overdose with GABITRIL.

DOSAGE AND ADMINISTRATION

General:

The blood level of tiagabine obtained after a given dose depends on whether the patient also is receiving a drug that induces the metabolism of tiagabine. The presence of an inducer means that the attained blood level will be substantially reduced. Dosing should take the presence of concomitant medications into account.

GABITRIL (tiagabine HCl) is recommended as adjunctive therapy for the treatment of partial seizures in patients 12 years and older.

The following dosing recommendations apply to all patients taking GABITRIL:

- GABITRIL is given orally and should be taken with food.
- Do not use a loading dose of GABITRIL.
- Dose titration: Rapid escalation and/or large dose increments of GABITRIL should not be used.
- Missed dose(s): If the patient forgets to take the prescribed dose of GABITRIL at the scheduled time, the patient should not attempt to make up for the missed dose by increasing the next dose. If a patient has missed multiple doses, patient should refer back to his or her physician for possible re-titration as clinically indicated.
- Dosage adjustment of GABITRIL should be considered whenever a change in patient's enzyme-inducing status occurs as a result of the addition, discontinuation, or dose change of the enzyme-inducing agent.

Induced Adults and Adolescents 12 Years or Older: The dosing recommendations apply to patients who are already taking enzyme-inducing antiepilepsy drugs (AEDs) (e.g., carbamazepine, phenytoin, primidone, and phenobarbital). Such patients are considered induced patients when administering GABITRIL.

In adolescents 12 to 18 years old, GABITRIL should be initiated at 4 mg once daily. Modification of concomitant antiepilepsy drugs is not necessary, unless clinically indicated. The total daily dose of GABITRIL may be increased by 4 mg at the beginning of Week 2. Thereafter, the total daily dose may be increased by 4 to 8 mg at weekly intervals until clinical response is achieved or up to 32 mg/day. The total daily dose should be given in divided doses two to four times daily. Doses above 32 mg/day have been tolerated in a small number of adolescent patients for a relatively short duration.

In adults, GABITRIL should be initiated at 4 mg once daily. Modification of concomitant antiepilepsy drugs is not necessary, unless clinically indicated. The total daily dose of GABITRIL may be increased by 4 to 8 mg at weekly inter-

Continued on next page

Table 5
Treatment-Emergent Adverse Event Incidence in Study 1[†]
(events in at least 5% of patients treated with GABITRIL 32 or 56 mg and numerically more frequent than in the placebo group)

Body System/ COSTART Term	GABITRIL 56 mg (N=57) %	GABITRIL 32 mg (N=88) %	Placebo (N=91) %
Body as a Whole			
Accidental Injury	21	15	20
Infection	19	10	12
Flu Syndrome	9	6	3
Pain	7	2	3
Abdominal Pain	5	7	4
Digestive System			
Diarrhea	2	10	6
Hemic and Lymphatic System			
Ecchymosis	0	6	1
Musculoskeletal System			
Myalgia	5	2	3
Nervous System			
Dizziness	28	31	12
Asthenia	23	18	15
Tremor	21	14	1
Somnolence	19	21	17
Nervousness	14	11	6
Difficulty With Concentration/Attention*	14	7	3
Ataxia	9	6	6
Depression	7	1	0
Insomnia	5	6	3
Abnormal Gait	5	5	3
Hostility	5	5	2
Respiratory System			
Pharyngitis	7	8	6
Special Senses			
Amblyopia	4	9	8
Urogenital System			
Urinary Tract Infection	5	0	2

[†]Patients in this study were receiving one to three concomitant enzyme-inducing antiepilepsy drugs in addition to GABITRIL or placebo. Patients may have reported multiple adverse experiences; thus, patients may be included in more than one category.

* COSTART term substituted with a more clinically descriptive term.

Table 6
Typical Dosing Titration Regimen for Patients Taking Enzyme-Inducing AEDs

	Initiation and Titration Schedule	Total Daily Dose
Week 1	Initiate at 4 mg once daily	4 mg/day
Week 2	Increase total daily dose by 4 mg	8 mg/day (in two divided doses)
Week 3	Increase total daily dose by 4 mg	12 mg/day (in three divided doses)
Week 4	Increase total daily dose by 4 mg	16 mg/day (in two to four divided doses)
Week 5	Increase total daily dose by 4 to 8 mg	20 to 24 mg/day (in two to four divided doses)
Week 6	Increase total daily dose by 4 to 8 mg	24 to 32 mg/day (in two to four divided doses)
Usual Adult Maintenance Dose in Induced Patients:	32 to 56 mg/day in two to four divided doses	

Gabitril—Cont.

vals until clinical response is achieved or, up to 56 mg/day. The total daily dose should be given in divided doses two to four times daily. Doses above 56 mg/day have not been systematically evaluated in adequate and well-controlled clinical trials.

Experience is limited in patients taking total daily doses above 32 mg/day using twice daily dosing. A typical dosing titration regimen for patients taking enzyme-inducing AEDs (induced patients) is provided in Table 6.

[See table 6 on previous page]

Non-Induced Adults and Adolescents 12 Years or Older: The following dosing recommendations apply to patients who are taking only non-enzyme-inducing AEDs. Such patients are considered non-induced patients:

Following a given dose of GABITRIL, the estimated plasma concentration in the non-induced patients is more than twice that in patients receiving enzyme-inducing agents. Use in non-induced patients requires lower doses of GABITRIL. These patients may also require a slower titration of GABITRIL compared to that of induced patients (see **PHARMACOKINETICS** and **PRECAUTIONS, Use in Non-Induced Patients**).

HOW SUPPLIED

GABITRIL tablets are available in four dosage strengths. 2 mg orange-peach, round tablets, debossed with [C] on one side and 402 on the opposite side, are available in bottles of 100 (**NDC** 63459-402-01).

4 mg yellow, round tablets, debossed with [C] on one side and 404 on the opposite side, are available in bottles of 100 (**NDC** 63459-404-01).

12 mg green, ovaloid tablets, debossed with [C] on one side and 412 on the opposite side, are available in bottles of 100 (**NDC** 63459-412-01).

16 mg blue, ovaloid tablets, debossed with [C] on one side and 416 on the opposite side, are available in bottles of 100 (**NDC** 63459-416-01).

Recommended Storage: Store tablets at controlled room temperature, between 20–25°C (68–77°F). See USP. Protect from light and moisture.

ANIMAL TOXICOLOGY

In repeat dose toxicology studies, dogs receiving daily oral doses of 5 mg/kg/day or greater experienced unexpected CNS effects throughout the study. These effects occurred acutely and included marked sedation and apparent visual impairment which was characterized by a lack of awareness of objects, failure to fix on and follow moving objects, and absence of a blink reaction. Plasma exposures (AUCs) at 5 mg/kg/day were equal to those in humans receiving the maximum recommended daily human dose of 56 mg/day. The effects were reversible upon cessation of treatment and were not associated with any observed structural abnormality. The implications of these findings for humans are unknown.

Manufactured for:
Cephalon, Inc.
West Chester, PA 19380
Revised: February, 2005
©1997-2005 Cephalon, Inc.
All rights reserved.
PRINTED IN U.S.A.

C. B. Fleet Co., Inc.
4615 MURRAY PLACE
LYNCHBURG, VA 24502

Direct Inquiries to:
Sherrie Scott RN. M.S.N.
Director of Medical Affairs
(434) 528-4000

FLEET® PHOSPHO-SODA®   OTC
AN ORAL SALINE LAXATIVE

Prescribing information for this product, which appears on page 1264 of the 2005 PDR, has been completely revised as follows. Please write "See Supplement A" next to the product heading.

COMPOSITION

Each Tablespoon (15 mL) of Unflavored or Natural Ginger-lemon flavor FLEET® Phospho-soda® contains 7.2 g mono-basic sodium phosphate monohydrate and 2.7 g dibasic sodium phosphate heptahydrate in a stable, buffered aqueous solution.

ELEMENTAL AND ELECTROLYTIC CONTENT

mEq Phosphate (PO_4) per mL	12.45
mEq Sodium (Na) per mL	4.82
mg Sodium (Na) per mL	111
mmole Phosphorus (P) per mL	4.15

INDICATIONS

As a laxative, for the relief of occasional constipation. For use as part of a bowel cleansing regimen in preparing the colon for colonoscopy, other endoscopic and radiologic examinations and surgery.

ACTION AND USES

Versatile in action as a laxative or purgative, according to dosage. This product produces a bowel movement in $1/2$ to 6 hours, depending on dosage.

PROFESSIONAL USE WARNINGS AND PRECAUTIONS. **Do not use** in patients with megacolon, gastrointestinal obstruction, ascites, congestive heart failure, kidney disease or in children under 5 years of age. **Use with caution** in patients with impaired renal function, heart disease, acute myocardial infarction, unstable angina, pre-existing electrolyte disturbances, increased risk for electrolyte disturbances (e.g., dehydration, gastric retention, bowel perforation, colitis, ileus, inability to take adequate oral fluid, concomitant use of diuretics or other medications that affect electrolytes), with debilitated or elderly patients or with patients who are taking medications known to prolong the QT interval. **In at-risk patients, including elderly patients, consider obtaining baseline and post-treatment sodium, potassium, calcium, chloride, bicarbonate, phosphate, blood urea nitrogen and creatinine values, and consider using the lower end of the dosage range.** There is a risk of elevated serum levels of sodium and phosphate and decreased levels of calcium and potassium; consequently, hypernatremia, hyperphosphatemia, hypocalcemia, hypokalemia, and acidosis may occur. Nephrocalcinosis associated with transient renal insufficiency and renal failure has been very rarely reported in patients using sodium phosphates for bowel cleansing. Care should be taken to prescribe Fleet® Phospho-soda® as a bowel cleanser by volumes, not "by the bottle" (see WARNINGS), per recommendations with a particular attention to known contraindications and adequate hydration (See DOSAGE AND ADMINISTRATION and INFORMATION FOR PATIENT). **Additional fluids by mouth are recommended with all bowel cleansing dosages.** Encourage patients to drink large amounts of clear liquids to prevent dehydration. Drinking large amounts of clear liquids also helps ensure that the patient's bowel will be clean for the procedure. No other sodium phosphate preparations should be given concomitantly.

OVERDOSAGE

Overdosage or retention may lead to severe electrolyte disturbances, including hyperphosphatemia, hypernatremia, hypocalcemia, and hypokalemia, as well as dehydration and hypovolemia, with attendant signs and symptoms of these disturbances (such as metabolic acidosis, renal failure, and tetany). Certain severe electrolyte disturbances may lead to cardiac arrhythmia and death. The patient who has taken an overdose should be monitored carefully. **Treatment of electrolyte imbalance may require immediate medical intervention with appropriate electrolyte and fluid replacement.**

WARNINGS

TAKING MORE THAN THE RECOMMENDED DOSE IN 24 HOURS CAN BE HARMFUL. IF THERE IS NO BOWEL MOVEMENT AFTER MAXIMUM DOSAGE, CONTACT A PHYSICIAN, AS DEHYDRATION COULD OCCUR.
SINCE FLEET® PHOSPHO-SODA® IS AVAILABLE IN TWO SIZES, PRESCRIBE BY VOLUME. DO NOT PRESCRIBE "BY THE BOTTLE," AS SERIOUS SIDE EFFECTS FROM OVERDOSAGE MAY OCCUR.

INFORMATION FOR PATIENT

DO NOT USE if you have megacolon, gastrointestinal obstruction, ascites, congestive heart failure, kidney disease or in children under 5 years of age. Ask a doctor before using this product if you are on a sodium-restricted diet, or are pregnant or nursing a baby. Ask a doctor before using any laxative if you have nausea, vomiting or abdominal pain; have a sudden change in bowel habits lasting more than 2 weeks; or have already used a laxative for more than 1 week. Stop using this product and consult a doctor if you have rectal bleeding or have no bowel movement after use, as dehydration may occur. These symptoms may indicate a serious condition.
Keep this and all drugs out of the reach of children. In case of overdose or accidental ingestion, seek professional assistance or contact a Poison Control Center immediately.

DOSAGE AND ADMINISTRATION

For laxative use: Dilute dose in the table below with one-half glass (4 fl. oz.) cool water. Drink, then follow with at least one additional glass (8 fl. oz.) cool water. For bowel cleansing prior to medical procedures only when prescribed by a doctor: Dilute dose in the table below with one glass (8 fl. oz.) clear liquid. Drink, then follow with at least three glasses (24 fl. oz.) clear liquids.
DOSAGE: DO NOT EXCEED RECOMMENDED DOSAGE, AS SERIOUS SIDE EFFECTS MAY OCCUR. **NEVER TAKE MORE THAN 3 TABLESPOONS AT ONE TIME.** SINGLE DAILY DOSAGE: DO NOT TAKE MORE UNLESS DIRECTED BY A DOCTOR. SEE WARNINGS.

Ages (years)	Laxative Use	Medical Procedure
12 & older	1 Tablespoon	2 or 3 Tablespoons
10 & 11	1 Tablespoon	Ask Your Doctor
5 to 9	½ Tablespoon	Ask Your Doctor
under 5	DO NOT USE	DO NOT USE

* DO NOT TAKE MORE THAN THIS AMOUNT IN A 24-HOUR PERIOD.

HYDRATION AND DIET:

Clear liquid beverages may be consumed throughout the day and should be encouraged.

During bowel preparation you will lose significant amounts of fluid. THIS IS NORMAL. It is very important that you replace this fluid to prevent dehydration. Drink large amounts of clear liquids. Drinking large amounts of clear liquids also helps ensure that your bowel will be clean for the examination. (See "Clear Liquids Diet List" below).

Day before the exam – eat a regular breakfast.
DO NOT DRINK OR EAT ANYTHING COLORED RED OR PURPLE.

Low residue lunch (must be eaten before 2 PM). Do not eat anything that is not on this diet. Do not eat more than the allowed portions. Lunch may include any of the following items:
- Main entrée – choose one of the following:
  - 3 oz. of skinless chicken, turkey, fish or seafood
  - 1 large or 2 medium eggs
  - 1 can of chicken noodle soup without vegetables
- Vegetable / Fruit – choose one of the following:
  - ½ cup applesauce
  - ½ cup of cooked or canned vegetables without seeds. *No corn.*
- Bread – choose one of the following:
  - 1 white potato roll
  - 2 slices of white bread
  - 1 cup of cooked white rice or 1 cup of cooked pasta
  - 1 small skinless potato
- Condiments – choose one of the following:
  - 2 tsp. of soft tub margarine
  - 1 tsp. mustard or mayonnaise
- Dessert – choose one of the following:
  - 4 vanilla wafers
  - ¼ cup pretzels
  - ½ cup sherbet
- Any items from the "Clear Liquids Diet List" below:

CLEAR LIQUIDS DIET LIST:
BEVERAGES:
- Water, tea or coffee (no milk or non-dairy creamer); sweetners are okay to use
- Soft drinks (orange, ginger ale, cola, Sprite®, 7-Up®, etc.), Gatorade®, Kool-Aid®
- Strained fruit juices without pulp (apple, white grape, orange, lemonade, etc.)

Dosing: Each of the two doses consists of 2 or 3 tablespoons of Fleet® Phospho-soda®, according to the doctor's prescription. The doctor should also prescribe the timing of the two doses of diluted Fleet® Phospho-soda® so the doses are separated by 10–12 hours. See References.

Dilution Alternatives:
1) Mix 2 or 3 Tablespoons (use measuring Tablespoon, not tableware) Fleet® Phospho-soda® with 8 fl.oz. of cold, clear liquid. Then follow with at least 24 fl.oz. of clear liquid.

OR

2) Mix 2 or 3 Tablespoons Fleet® Phospho-soda® with two or three 8 fl. oz. glasses cold, clear liquid (one Tablespoon of Fleet® Phospho-soda® per glass). Drink two glasses within 20 minutes or three glasses within 30 minutes.

The taste of Fleet® Phospho-soda® is improved by mixing it with ginger ale, apple juice, or lemon-lime type drinks.

HOW SUPPLIED

Unflavored or Natural Ginger-lemon flavor, in bottles of 1.5 fl. oz. and 3 fl. oz. FLEET® Phospho-soda® should not be confused with FLEET® Enema, a sodium phosphates disposable ready-to-use enema. FLEET® Enema and Fleet® Enema for Children ARE NOT INTENDED FOR ORAL CONSUMPTION in any dosage size.

IS THIS PRODUCT OTC?

Yes.

REFERENCES

1. Balaban, D.H. et al. Low Volume Bowel Preparation for Colonoscopy: Randomized, Endoscopist-Blinded Trial of Liquid Sodium Phosphate versus Tablet Sodium Phosphate. The American Journal of Gastroenterology, 2003; 98(4):827
2. Cohen, S.M. et al. Prospective, Randomized, Endoscopic-Blinded Trial Comparing Precolonoscopy Bowel Cleansing Methods. Diseases of the Colon & Rectum. 1994; 37(7):689.
3. Hookey, L.C. et al. The Safety Profile of Oral Sodium Phosphate for Colonic Cleansing before Colonoscopy in Adults. Gastrointestinal Endoscopy, 2002; 56(6):895
4. Barclay, R.L. et al. Carbohydrate-electrolyte Rehydration Protects against Intravascular Volume Contraction during Colonic Cleansing with Orally Administered Sodium Phosphate. Gastrointestinal Endoscopy, 2002. 56(5):633
5. Allaire, J. et al. A Quality Improvement Project Comparing Two Regimens of Medication for Colonoscopy Preparation. Gastroenterology Nursing, 2003. 27(1):3
6. Oliveira, L. et al. Mechanical Bowel Preparation for Elective Colorectal Surgery. Diseases of the Colon & Rectum. 1997; 40(5):585.
7. Vanner, S. J. et al. A Randomized Prospective Trial Comparing Oral Sodium Phosphate with Standard Polyethylene Glycol-Based Lavage Solution (Golytely) in the Preparation of Patients for Colonoscopy. The American Journal of Gastroenterology. 1990; 85(4):422.

FLEET® PHOSPHO-SODA® ACCU-PREP® OTC

Prescribing information for this product, which appears on pages 1264–1265 of the 2005 PDR, has been completely revised as follows. Please write "See Supplement A" next to the product heading.

DESCRIPTION

COMPOSITION OF FLEET® PHOSPHO-SODA® ACCU-PREP® BOWEL CLEANSING SYSTEM

Fleet® Phospho-soda® ACCU-PREP® contains:

1. Six 15-mL (1/2 fl. oz.) units of Fleet® Phospho-soda®, net contents 3 fl. oz. (90 mL).
   Active Ingredients: Each Unit (15-mL) contains monobasic sodium phosphate monohydrate 7.2g/dibasic sodium phosphate heptahydrate 2.7g.
2. Four Fleet® Relief™ Pre-Moistened Anorectal Wipes.
   Active Ingredients: Each wipe is moistened with Pramoxine hydrochloride 1% and Glycerin 12%.
3. Patient mixing instructions.

Fleet® Phospho-soda®

COMPOSITION

Each 15-mL of Natural Ginger-lemon flavor Fleet® Phospho-soda® contains 7.2 g monobasic sodium phosphate monohydrate and 2.7 g dibasic sodium phosphate heptahydrate in a stable, aqueous solution.

ELEMENTAL AND ELECTROLYTIC CONTENT:

mEq Phosphate (PO_4) per 15 mL	186.75
mEq Sodium (Na) per 15 mL	72.30
mg Sodium (Na) per 15 mL	1668
mmole Phosphorus (P) per 15 mL	62.25

ACTIONS

Fleet® Phospho-soda® is an oral saline laxative.

INDICATIONS AND USES

For use as part of a bowel cleansing regimen in preparing the colon for colonoscopy, other endoscopic and radiologic examinations and surgery. See DOSAGE AND ADMINISTRATION. This product generally produces a bowel movement in ½ to 6 hours.

PROFESSIONAL USE WARNINGS

Do not use in patients with megacolon, gastrointestinal obstruction, ascites, congestive heart failure, kidney disease or in children under 5 years of age. **Use with caution** in patients with impaired renal function, heart disease, acute myocardial infarction, unstable angina, pre-existing electrolyte disturbances, increased risk for electrolyte disturbances (e.g., dehydration, gastric retention, bowel perforation, colitis, ileus, inability to take adequate oral fluid, concomitant use of diuretics or other medications that affect electrolytes), with debilitated or elderly patients or with patients who are taking medications known to prolong the QT interval. **In at-risk patients, including elderly patients, consider obtaining baseline and post-treatment sodium, potassium, calcium, chloride, bicarbonate, phosphate, blood urea nitrogen and creatinine values, and consider using the lower end of the dosage range.** There is a risk of elevated serum levels of sodium and phosphate and decreased levels of calcium and potassium; consequently, hypernatremia, hyperphosphatemia, hypocalcemia, hypokalemia, and acidosis may occur. Nephrocalcinosis associated with transient renal insufficiency and renal failure has been very rarely reported in patients using sodium phosphates for bowel cleansing. Care should be taken to prescribe Fleet® Phospho-soda® as a bowel cleanser by volumes, not "by the bottle" (see WARNINGS), per recommendations with a particular attention to known contraindications and adequate hydration (see DOSAGE AND ADMINISTRATION and INFORMATION FOR PATIENT). **Additional fluids by mouth are recommended with all bowel cleansing dosages.** Encourage patients to drink large amounts of clear liquids to prevent dehydration. Drinking large amounts of clear liquids also helps ensure that the patient's bowel will be clean for the procedure. No other sodium phosphate preparations should be given concomitantly.

OVERDOSAGE

Overdosage or retention may lead to severe electrolyte disturbances, including hypernatremia, hyperphosphatemia, hypocalcemia and hypokalemia, as well as dehydration and hypovolemia, with attendant signs and symptoms of these disturbances (such as metabolic acidosis, renal failure, and tetany). Certain severe electrolyte disturbances may lead to cardiac arrhythmia and death. The patient who has taken an overdose should be monitored carefully. **Treatment of electrolyte imbalance may require immediate medical intervention with appropriate electrolyte and fluid replacement.**

PRECAUTIONS

GENERAL

Taking more than the recommended dose in 24 hours can be harmful.

The patient should be instructed to open and read directions at least two days in advance of the examination.

Instruct the patient to contact a physician if there is no bowel movement after maximum dosage as dehydration can occur.

INFORMATION FOR PATIENT

DO NOT USE if you have megacolon, gastrointestinal obstruction, ascites, congestive heart failure, kidney disease or in children under 5 years of age.

Patients should ask a doctor before using this product if they are on a sodium-restricted diet, or are pregnant or nursing a baby. Patients should contact a doctor before using any laxative if they have nausea, vomiting or abdominal pain; have a sudden change in bowel habits lasting more than 2 weeks or have already used a laxative for more than 1 week. Patients should stop using the product and call a doctor if they have rectal bleeding, or have no bowel movement with use, as dehydration may occur. These symptoms may indicate a serious condition.

Keep this and all drugs out of the reach of children. In case of overdose or accidental ingestion, seek professional assistance or contact a Poison Control Center immediately.

DOSAGE AND ADMINISTRATION

Each of the two doses consists of 2–3 pre-measured 15-mL (1/2 fl. oz.) units of Phospho-soda. Dilute each pre-measured 15-mL (1/2 fl. oz.) unit in an 8 fl. oz. glass of clear liquid. Repeat for each pre-measured unit (2–3 units according to the doctor's instructions) at the prescribed times. The doses should be separated by 10–12 hours. Drink at least 3 additional 8 fl. oz. glasses of clear liquid after the first dose.

adults and children 12 years & over	2–3 15-mL pre-measured units*
children 5 to 11 years	ask a doctor
children under 5 years	**DO NOT USE**

***DO NOT TAKE MORE THAN 3 PRE-MEASURED UNITS IN EACH DOSE.**

HYDRATION AND DIET

Clear liquid beverages may be consumed throughout the day and should be encouraged. (See "Clear Liquids Diet List" below).

During bowel preparation you will lose significant amounts of fluid. THIS IS NORMAL. It is very important that you replace this fluid to prevent dehydration. Drink large amounts of clear liquids. Drinking large amounts of clear liquids also helps ensure that your bowel will be clean for the examination.

Day before the exam – eat a regular breakfast.

DO NOT DRINK OR EAT ANYTHING COLORED RED OR PURPLE.

Low residue lunch (must be eaten before 2 PM). Do not eat anything that is not on this diet. Do not eat more than the allowed portions. Lunch may include any of the following items:

- Main entrée – choose one of the following:
  - 3 oz. of skinless chicken, turkey, fish or seafood
  - 1 large or 2 medium eggs
  - 1 can of chicken noodle soup without vegetables
- Vegetable/Fruit – choose one of the following
  - ½ cup applesauce
  - ½ cup of cooked or canned vegetables without seeds. ***No corn.***
- Bread – choose one of the following:
  - 1 white potato roll
  - 2 slices of white bread
  - 1 cup of cooked white rice or 1 cup of cooked pasta
  - 1 small skinless potato
- Condiments – choose one of the following:
  - 2 tsp. of soft tub margarine
  - 1 tsp. mustard or mayonnaise
- Dessert – choose one of the following:
  - 4 vanilla wafers
  - ¼ cup pretzels
  - ½ cup sherbet
- Any items from the "Clear Liquids Diet List" below:

CLEAR LIQUIDS DIET LIST:

BEVERAGES:

- Water, tea or coffee (no milk or non-dairy creamer); sweeteners are okay to use
- Soft drinks (orange, ginger ale, cola, Sprite®, 7-Up®, etc.), Gatorade®, Kool-Aid®
- Strained fruit juices without pulp (apple, white grape, orange, lemonade, etc.)

Fleet® Relief™ Pre-Moistened Anorectal Wipes

COMPOSITION

Each wipe is moistened with Pramoxine hydrochloride 1%; Glycerin 12%.

ACTIONS

Fleet® Relief™ Pre-Moistened Anorectal Wipes act as a local anesthetic and protectant for temporary relief of pain, soreness or burning.

INDICATIONS AND USES

For the temporary relief of local itching and discomfort associated with hemorrhoids. Temporarily forms a protective coating over inflamed tissues to help prevent drying of tissues and temporarily provides a coating for relief of anorectal discomfort.

WARNINGS

FOR EXTERNAL USE ONLY

INFORMATION FOR THE PATIENT

Do not exceed the recommended daily dosage. Consult a doctor promptly in case of bleeding. Do not put the product into the rectum by using fingers or any mechanical device or applicator.

Stop use and ask a doctor if the condition worsens or does not improve within 7 days; or if redness, irritation, swelling, pain or other symptoms develop or increase. Certain persons can develop allergic reactions to ingredients in this product.

DIRECTIONS

Adults & children 12 years & over: When practical, cleanse the affected area with mild soap and warm water and rinse thoroughly. Gently dry by patting or blotting with toilet tissue or a soft cloth. Open the sealed pouch and remove one Fleet® Relief™ Wipe and gently apply to the affected area. Apply after each bowel movement, up to 5 times daily. Discard the wipe after use. There are four Fleet® Relief™ Wipes. They can be used after a bowel movement or whenever anorectal discomfort is felt.

HOW SUPPLIED

This complete, simple, convenient bowel cleansing kit includes six 15-mL units of Phospho-soda® (Natural ginger-lemon flavor) and four Fleet® Relief™ Pre-Moistened Anorectal Wipes. Fleet® Phospho-soda® ACCU-PREP® is available in 12 units per case.

Fleet® Phospho-soda® ACCU-PREP® should not be confused with Fleet® Enema, a sodium phosphates disposable ready-to-use enema. Fleet® Enemas, Adult and Children size, ARE NOT INTENDED FOR ORAL CONSUMPTION in any dosage size.

IS THIS PRODUCT OTC?

Yes. Fleet® Phospho-soda® ACCU-PREP® is an OTC product, but it may be stocked behind the pharmacy counter. Patients should be directed to ask their pharmacists for Fleet® Phospho-soda® ACCU-PREP®.

Forest Pharmaceuticals, Inc.

(Subsidiary of Forest Laboratories, Inc.)
13600 SHORELINE DRIVE
ST. LOUIS, MO 63045

Direct Inquiries to:
Professional Affairs Department
13600 Shoreline Drive
St. Louis, MO 63045
(800) 678-1605

CELEXA® ℞
[sĕ-lĕk-să]
(citalopram hydrobromide)
Tablets/Oral Solution
Rx Only

Prescribing information for this product, which appears on pages 1269–1273 of the 2005 PDR, has been completely revised as follows. Please write "See Supplement A" next to the product heading.

Suicidality in Children and Adolescents
Antidepressants increased the risk of suicidal thinking and behavior (suicidality) in short-term studies in children and adolescents with Major Depressive Disorder (MDD) and other psychiatric disorders. Anyone considering the use of Celexa or any other antidepressant in a child or adolescent must balance this risk with the clinical need. Patients who are started on therapy should be observed closely for clinical worsening, suicidality, or unusual changes in behavior. Families and caregivers should be advised of the need for close observation and communication with the prescriber. Celexa is not approved for use in pediatric patients. (See Warnings and Precautions: Pediatric Use)
Pooled analyses of short-term (4 to 16 weeks) placebo-controlled trials of 9 antidepressant drugs (SSRIs and others) in children and adolescents with major depressive disorder (MDD), obsessive compulsive disorder (OCD), or other psychiatric disorders (a total of 24 trials involving over 4400 patients) have revealed a greater risk of adverse events representing suicidal thinking or behavior (suicidality) during the first few months of treatment in those receiving antidepressants. The average risk of such events in patients receiving antidepressants was 4%, twice the placebo risk of 2%. No suicides occurred in these trials.

DESCRIPTION

Celexa® (citalopram HBr) is an orally administered selective serotonin reuptake inhibitor (SSRI) with a chemical structure unrelated to that of other SSRIs or of tricyclic, tetracyclic, or other available antidepressant agents. Citalopram HBr is a racemic bicyclic phthalane derivative desig-

Continued on next page

Celexa—Cont.

nated (±)-1-(3-dimethylaminopropyl)-1-(4-fluorophenyl)-1,3-dihydroisobenzofuran-5-carbonitrile, HBr with the following structural formula:

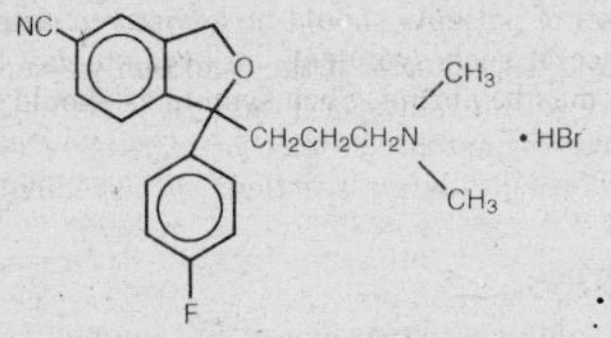

The molecular formula is $C_{20}H_{22}BrFN_2O$ and its molecular weight is 405.35.
Citalopram HBr occurs as a fine, white to off-white powder. Citalopram HBr is sparingly soluble in water and soluble in ethanol.
Celexa (citalopram hydrobromide) is available as tablets or as an oral solution.
Celexa 10 mg tablets are film-coated, oval tablets containing citalopram HBr in strengths equivalent to 10 mg citalopram base. Celexa 20 mg and 40 mg tablets are film-coated, oval, scored tablets containing citalopram HBr in strengths equivalent to 20 mg or 40 mg citalopram base. The tablets also contain the following inactive ingredients: copolyvidone, corn starch, crosscarmellose sodium, glycerin, lactose monohydrate, magnesium stearate, hypromellose, microcrystalline cellulose, polyethylene glycol, and titanium dioxide. Iron oxides are used as coloring agents in the beige (10 mg) and pink (20 mg) tablets.
Celexa oral solution contains citalopram HBr equivalent to 2 mg/mL citalopram base. It also contains the following inactive ingredients: sorbitol, purified water, propylene glycol, methylparaben, natural peppermint flavor, and propylparaben.

CLINICAL PHARMACOLOGY

Pharmacodynamics

The mechanism of action of citalopram HBr as an antidepressant is presumed to be linked to potentiation of serotonergic activity in the central nervous system (CNS) resulting from its inhibition of CNS neuronal reuptake of serotonin (5-HT). *In vitro* and *in vivo* studies in animals suggest that citalopram is a highly selective serotonin reuptake inhibitor (SSRI) with minimal effects on norepinephrine (NE) and dopamine (DA) neuronal reuptake. Tolerance to the inhibition of 5-HT uptake is not induced by long-term (14-day) treatment of rats with citalopram. Citalopram is a racemic mixture (50/50), and the inhibition of 5-HT reuptake by citalopram is primarily due to the (S)-enantiomer.
Citalopram has no or very low affinity for 5-HT_{1A}, 5-HT_{2A}, dopamine D_1 and D_2 α_1-, α_2-, and β-adrenergic, histamine H_1, gamma aminobutyric acid (GABA), muscarinic cholinergic, and benzodiazepine receptors. Antagonism of muscarinic, histaminergic, and adrenergic receptors has been hypothesized to be associated with various anticholinergic, sedative, and cardiovascular effects of other psychotropic drugs.

Pharmacokinetics

The single- and multiple-dose pharmacokinetics of citalopram are linear and dose-proportional in a dose range of 10–60 mg/day. Biotransformation of citalopram is mainly hepatic, with a mean terminal half-life of about 35 hours. With once daily dosing, steady state plasma concentrations are achieved within approximately one week. At steady state, the extent of accumulation of citalopram in plasma, based on the half-life, is expected to be 2.5 times the plasma concentrations observed after a single dose. The tablet and oral solution dosage forms of citalopram HBr are bioequivalent.

Absorption and Distribution

Following a single oral dose (40 mg tablet) of citalopram, peak blood levels occur at about 4 hours. The absolute bioavailability of citalopram was about 80% relative to an intravenous dose, and absorption is not affected by food. The volume of distribution of citalopram is about 12 L/kg and the binding of citalopram (CT), demethylcitalopram (DCT) and didemethylcitalopram (DDCT) to human plasma proteins is about 80%.

Metabolism and Elimination

Following intravenous administrations of citalopram, the fraction of drug recovered in the urine as citalopram and DCT was about 10% and 5%, respectively. The systemic clearance of citalopram was 330 mL/min, with approximately 20% of that due to renal clearance.
Citalopram is metabolized to demethylcitalopram (DCT), didemethylcitalopram (DDCT), citalopram-N-oxide, and a deaminated propionic acid derivative. In humans, unchanged citalopram is the predominant compound in plasma. At steady state, the concentrations of citalopram's metabolites, DCT and DDCT, in plasma are approximately one-half and one-tenth, respectively, that of the parent drug. *In vitro* studies show that citalopram is at least 8 times more potent than its metabolites in the inhibition of serotonin reuptake, suggesting that the metabolites evaluated do not likely contribute significantly to the antidepressant actions of citalopram.
In vitro studies using human liver microsomes indicated that CYP3A4 and CYP2C19 are the primary isozymes involved in the N-demethylation of citalopram.

Population Subgroups

Age - Citalopram pharmacokinetics in subjects ≥ 60 years of age were compared to younger subjects in two normal volunteer studies. In a single-dose study, citalopram AUC and half-life were increased in the elderly subjects by 30% and 50%, respectively, whereas in a multiple-dose study they were increased by 23% and 30%, respectively. 20 mg is the recommended dose for most elderly patients (see **DOSAGE AND ADMINISTRATION**).
Gender - In three pharmacokinetic studies (total N=32), citalopram AUC in women was one and a half to two times that in men. This difference was not observed in five other pharmacokinetic studies (total N=114). In clinical studies, no differences in steady state serum citalopram levels were seen between men (N=237) and women (N=388). There were no gender differences in the pharmacokinetics of DCT and DDCT. No adjustment of dosage on the basis of gender is recommended.
Reduced hepatic function - Citalopram oral clearance was reduced by 37% and half-life was doubled in patients with reduced hepatic function compared to normal subjects. 20 mg is the recommended dose for most hepatically impaired patients (see **DOSAGE AND ADMINISTRATION**).
Reduced renal function - In patients with mild to moderate renal function impairment, oral clearance of citalopram was reduced by 17% compared to normal subjects. No adjustment of dosage for such patients is recommended. No information is available about the pharmacokinetics of citalopram in patients with severely reduced renal function (creatinine clearance < 20 mL/min).

Drug-Drug Interactions

In vitro enzyme inhibition data did not reveal an inhibitory effect of citalopram on CYP3A4, -2C9, or -2E1, but did suggest that it is a weak inhibitor of CYP1A2, -2D6, and -2C19. Citalopram would be expected to have little inhibitory effect on *in vivo* metabolism mediated by these cytochromes. However, *in vivo* data to address this question are limited.
Since CYP3A4 and 2C19 are the primary enzymes involved in the metabolism of citalopram, it is expected that potent inhibitors of 3A4 (e.g., ketoconazole, itraconazole, and macrolide antibiotics) and potent inhibitors of CYP2C19 (e.g., omeprazole) might decrease the clearance of citalopram. However, coadministration of citalopram and the potent 3A4 inhibitor ketoconazole did not significantly affect the pharmacokinetics of citalopram. Because citalopram is metabolized by multiple enzyme systems, inhibition of a single enzyme may not appreciably decrease citalopram clearance. Citalopram steady state levels were not significantly different in poor metabolizers and extensive 2D6 metabolizers after multiple-dose administration of Celexa, suggesting that coadministration, with Celexa, of a drug that inhibits CYP2D6, is unlikely to have clinically significant effects on citalopram metabolism. See **Drug Interactions** under **PRECAUTIONS** for more detailed information on available drug interaction data.

Clinical Efficacy Trials

The efficacy of Celexa as a treatment for depression was established in two placebo-controlled studies (of 4 to 6 weeks in duration) in adult outpatients (ages 18-66) meeting DSM-III or DSM-III-R criteria for major depression. Study 1, a 6-week trial in which patients received fixed Celexa doses of 10, 20, 40, and 60 mg/day, showed that Celexa at doses of 40 and 60 mg/day was effective as measured by the Hamilton Depression Rating Scale (HAMD) total score, the HAMD depressed mood item (Item 1), the Montgomery Asberg Depression Rating Scale, and the Clinical Global Impression (CGI) Severity scale. This study showed no clear effect of the 10 and 20 mg/day doses, and the 60 mg/day dose was not more effective than the 40 mg/day dose. In study 2, a 4-week, placebo-controlled trial in depressed patients, of whom 85% met criteria for melancholia, the initial dose was 20 mg/day, followed by titration to the maximum tolerated dose or a maximum dose of 80 mg/day. Patients treated with Celexa showed significantly greater improvement than placebo patients on the HAMD total score, HAMD item 1, and the CGI Severity score. In three additional placebo-controlled depression trials, the difference in response to treatment between patients receiving Celexa and patients receiving placebo was not statistically significant, possibly due to high spontaneous response rate, smaller sample size, or, in the case of one study, too low a dose.
In two long-term studies, depressed patients who had responded to Celexa during an initial 6 or 8 weeks of acute treatment (fixed doses of 20 or 40 mg/day in one study and flexible doses of 20-60 mg/day in the second study) were randomized to continuation of Celexa or to placebo. In both studies, patients receiving continued Celexa treatment experienced significantly lower relapse rates over the subsequent 6 months compared to those receiving placebo. In the fixed-dose study, the decreased rate of depression relapse was similar in patients receiving 20 or 40 mg/day of Celexa.
Analyses of the relationship between treatment outcome and age, gender, and race did not suggest any differential responsiveness on the basis of these patient characteristics.

Comparison of Clinical Trial Results

Highly variable results have been seen in the clinical development of all antidepressant drugs. Furthermore, in those circumstances when the drugs have not been studied in the same controlled clinical trial(s), comparisons among the results of studies evaluating the effectiveness of different antidepressant drug products are inherently unreliable. Because conditions of testing (e.g., patient samples, investigators, doses of the treatments administered and compared, outcome measures, etc.) vary among trials, it is virtually impossible to distinguish a difference in drug effect from a difference due to one of the confounding factors just enumerated.

INDICATIONS AND USAGE

Celexa (citalopram HBr) is indicated for the treatment of depression.
The efficacy of Celexa in the treatment of depression was established in 4-6 week, controlled trials of outpatients whose diagnosis corresponded most closely to the DSM-III and DSM-III-R category of major depressive disorder (see **CLINICAL PHARMACOLOGY**).
A major depressive episode (DSM-IV) implies a prominent and relatively persistent (nearly every day for at least 2 weeks) depressed or dysphoric mood that usually interferes with daily functioning, and includes at least five of the following nine symptoms: depressed mood, loss of interest in usual activities, significant change in weight and/or appetite, insomnia or hypersomnia, psychomotor agitation or retardation, increased fatigue, feelings of guilt or worthlessness, slowed thinking or impaired concentration, a suicide attempt or suicidal ideation.
The antidepressant action of Celexa in hospitalized depressed patients has not been adequately studied.
The efficacy of Celexa in maintaining an antidepressant response for up to 24 weeks following 6 to 8 weeks of acute treatment was demonstrated in two placebo-controlled trials (see **CLINICAL PHARMACOLOGY**). Nevertheless, the physician who elects to use Celexa for extended periods should periodically re-evaluate the long-term usefulness of the drug for the individual patient.

CONTRAINDICATIONS

Concomitant use in patients taking monoamine oxidase inhibitors (MAOIs) is contraindicated (see **WARNINGS**).
Concomitant use in patients taking pimozide is contraindicated (see **PRECAUTIONS**).
Celexa is contraindicated in patients with a hypersensitivity to citalopram or any of the inactive ingredients in Celexa.

WARNINGS

WARNINGS—Clinical Worsening and Suicide Risk

Clinical Worsening and Suicide Risk

Patients with major depressive disorder (MDD), both adult and pediatric, may experience worsening of their depression and/or the emergence of suicidal ideation and behavior (suicidality) or unusual changes in behavior, whether or not they are taking antidepressant medications, and this risk may persist until significant remission occurs. There has been a long-standing concern that antidepressants may have a role in inducing worsening of depression and the emergence of suicidality in certain patients. Antidepressants increased the risk of suicidal thinking and behavior (suicidality) in short-term studies in children and adolescents with Major Depressive Disorder (MDD) and other psychiatric disorders.
Pooled analyses of short-term placebo-controlled trials of 9 antidepressant drugs (SSRIs and others) in children and adolescents with MDD, OCD, or other psychiatric disorders (a total of 24 trials involving over 4400 patients) have revealed a greater risk of adverse events representing suicidal behavior or thinking (suicidality) during the first few months of treatment in those receiving antidepressants. The average risk of such events in patients receiving antidepressants was 4%, twice the placebo risk of 2%. There was considerable variation in risk among drugs, but a tendency toward an increase for almost all drugs studied. The risk of suicidality was most consistently observed in the MDD trials, but there were signals of risk arising from some trials in other psychiatric indications (obsessive compulsive disorder and social anxiety disorder) as well. **No suicides occurred in any of these trials.** It is unknown whether the suicidality risk in pediatric patients extends to longer-term use, i.e., beyond several months. It is also unknown whether the suicidality risk extends to adults.
All pediatric patients being treated with antidepressants for any indication should be observed closely for clinical worsenng, suicidality, and unusual changes in behavior, especially during the initial few months of a course of drug therapy, or at times of dose changes, either increases or decreases. Such observation would generally include at least weekly face-to-face contact with patients or their family members or caregivers during the first 4 weeks of treatment, then every other week visits for the next 4 weeks, then at 12 weeks, and as clinically indicated beyond 12 weeks. Additional contact by telephone may be appropriate between face-to-face visits.
Adults with MDD or co-morbid depression in the setting of other psychiatric illness being treated with antidepressants should be observed similarly for clinical worsening and suicidality, especially during the initial few months of a course of drug therapy, or at times of dose changes, either increases or decreases.
The following symptoms, anxiety, agitation, panic attacks, insomnia, irritability, hostility, aggressiveness, impulsivity, akathisia (psychomotor restlessness), hypomania, and mania, have been reported in adult and pediatric patients being treated with antidepressants for major depressive disorder as well as for other indications, both psychiatric and nonpsychiatric. Although a causal link between the emergence of such symptoms and either the worsening of depression and/or the emergence of suicidal impulses has not been established, there is concern that such symptoms may represent precursors to emerging suicidality.
Consideration should be given to changing the therapeutic regimen, including possibly discontinuing the medication, in patients whose depression is persistently worse, or who are experiencing emergent suicidality or symptoms that

might be precursors to worsening depression or suicidality, especially if these symptoms are severe, abrupt in onset, or were not part of the patient's presenting symptoms.

If the decision has been made to discontinue treatment, medication should be tapered, as rapidly as is feasible, but with recognition that abrupt discontinuation can be associated with certain symptoms (see PRECAUTIONS and DOSAGE AND ADMINISTRATION—Discontinuation of Treatment with Celexa, for a description of the risks of discontinuation of Celexa).

Families and caregivers of pediatric patients being treated with antidepressants for major depressive disorder or other indications, both psychiatric and nonpsychiatric, should be alerted about the need to monitor patients for the emergence of agitation, irritability, unusual changes in behavior, and the other symptoms described above, as well as the emergence of suicidality, and to report such symptoms immediately to health care providers. Such monitoring should include daily observation by families and caregivers. Prescriptions for Celexa should be written for the smallest quantity of tablets consistent with good patient management, in order to reduce the risk of overdose. Families and caregivers of adults being treated for depression should be similarly advised.

Screening Patients for Bipolar Disorder: A major depressive episode may be the initial presentation of bipolar disorder. It is generally believed (though not established in controlled trials) that treating such an episode with an antidepressant alone may increase the likelihood of precipitation of a mixed/manic episode in patients at risk for bipolar disorder. Whether any of the sympoms described above represent such a conversion is unknown. However, prior to initiating treatment with an antidepressant, patients with depressive symptoms should be adequately screened to determine if they are at risk for bipolar disorder; such screening should include a detailed psychiatric history, including a family history of suicide, bipolar disorder, and depression. It should be noted that Celexa is not approved for use in treating bipolar depression.

Potential for Interaction with Monoamine Oxidase Inhibitors

In patients receiving serotonin reuptake inhibitor drugs in combination with monoamine oxidase inhibitor (MAOI), there have been reports of serious, sometimes fatal, reactions including hyperthermia, rigidity, myoclonus, autonomic instability with possible rapid fluctuations of vital signs, and mental status changes that include extreme agitation progressing to delirium and coma. These reactions have also been reported in patients who have recently discontinued SSRI treatment and have been started on an MAOI. Some cases presented with features resembling neuroleptic malignant syndrome. Furthermore, limited animal data on the effects of combined use of SSRIs and MAOIs suggest that these drugs may act synergistically to elevate blood pressure and evoke behavioral excitation. Therefore, it is recommended that Celexa should not be used in combination with an MAOI, or within 14 days of discontinuing treatment with an MAOI. Similarly, at least 14 days should be allowed after stopping Celexa before starting an MAOI.

PRECAUTIONS

General

Discontinuation of Treatment with Celexa

During marketing of Celexa and other SSRIs and SNRIs (serotonin and norepinephrine reuptake inhibitors), there have been spontaneous reports of adverse events occurring upon discontinuation of these drugs, particularly when abrupt, including the following: dysphoric mood, irritability, agitation, dizziness, sensory disturbances (e.g., paresthesias such as electric shock sensations), anxiety, confusion, headache, lethargy, emotional lability, insomnia, and hypomania. While these events are generally self-limiting, there have been reports of serious discontinuation symptoms.

Patients should be monitored for these symptoms when discontinuing treatment with Celexa. A gradual reduction in the dose rather than abrupt cessation is recommended whenever possible. If intolerable symptoms occur following a decrease in the dose or upon discontinuation of treatment, then resuming the previously prescribed dose may be considered. Subsequently, the physician may continue decreasing the dose but at a more gradual rate (see **DOSAGE AND ADMINISTRATION**).

Abnormal Bleeding

Published case reports have documented the occurrence of bleeding episodes in patients treated with psychotropic drugs that interfere with serotonin reuptake. Subsequent epidemiological studies, both of the case-control and cohort design, have demonstrated an association between use of psychotropic drugs that interfere with serotonin reuptake and the occurrence of upper gastrointestinal bleeding. In two studies, concurrent use of a nonsteroidal anti-inflammatory drug (NSAID) or aspirin potentiated the risk of bleeding (see **Drug Interactions**). Although these studies focused on upper gastrointestinal bleeding, there is reason to believe that bleeding at other sites may be similarly potentiated. Patients should be cautioned regarding the risk of bleeding associated with the concomitant use of Celexa with NSAIDs, aspirin, or other drugs that affect coagulation.

Hyponatremia

Cases of hyponatremia and SIADH (syndrome of inappropriate antidiuretic hormone secretion) have been reported in association with Celexa treatment. All patients with these events have recovered with discontinuation of Celexa and/or medical intervention. Hyponatremia and SIADH have also been reported in association with other marketed drugs effective in the treatment of major depressive disorder.

Activation of Mania/Hypomania

In placebo-controlled trials of Celexa, some of which included patients with bipolar disorder, activation of mania/hypomania was reported in 0.2% of 1063 patients treated with Celexa and in none of the 446 patients treated with placebo. Activation of mania/hypomania has also been reported in a small proportion of patients with major affective disorders treated with other marketed antidepressants. As with all antidepressants, Celexa should be used cautiously in patients with a history of mania.

Seizures

Although anticonvulsant effects of citalopram have been observed in animal studies, Celexa has not been systematically evaluated in patients with a seizure disorder. These patients were excluded from clinical studies during the product's premarketing testing. In clinical trials of Celexa, seizures occurred in 0.3% of patients treated with Celexa (a rate of one patient per 98 years of exposure) and 0.5% of patients treated with placebo (a rate of one patient per 50 years of exposure). Like other antidepressants, Celexa should be introduced with care in patients with a history of seizure disorder.

Interference with Cognitive and Motor Performance

In studies in normal volunteers, Celexa in doses of 40 mg/day did not produce impairment of intellectual function or psychomotor performance. Because any psychoactive drug may impair judgment, thinking, or motor skills, however, patients should be cautioned about operating hazardous machinery, including automobiles, until they are reasonably certain that Celexa therapy does not affect their ability to engage in such activities.

Use in Patients with Concomitant Illness

Clinical experience with Celexa in patients with certain concomitant systemic illnesses is limited. Caution is advisable in using Celexa in patients with diseases or conditions that produce altered metabolism or hemodynamic responses.

Celexa has not been systematically evaluated in patients with a recent history of myocardial infarction or unstable heart disease. Patients with these diagnoses were generally excluded from clinical studies during the product's premarketing testing. However, the electrocardiograms of 1116 patients who received Celexa in clinical trials were evaluated and the data indicate that Celexa is not associated with the development of clinically significant ECG abnormalities.

In subjects with hepatic impairment, citalopram clearance was decreased and plasma concentrations were increased. The use of Celexa in hepatically impaired patients should be approached with caution and a lower maximum dosage is recommended (see **DOSAGE AND ADMINISTRATION**).

Because citalopram is extensively metabolized, excretion of unchanged drug in urine is a minor route of elimination. Until adequate numbers of patients with severe renal impairment have been evaluated during chronic treatment with Celexa, however, it should be used with caution in such patients (see **DOSAGE AND ADMINISTRATION**).

Information for Patients

Physicians are advised to discuss the following issues with patients for whom they prescribe Celexa.

Although in controlled studies Celexa has not been shown to impair psychomotor performance, any psychoactive drug may impair judgment, thinking, or motor skills, so patients should be cautioned about operating hazardous machinery, including automobiles, until they are reasonably certain that Celexa therapy does not affect their ability to engage in such activities.

Patients should be told that, although Celexa has not been shown in experiments with normal subjects to increase the mental and motor skill impairments caused by alcohol, the concomitant use of Celexa and alcohol in depressed patients is not advised.

Patients should be advised to inform their physician if they are taking, or plan to take, any prescription or over-the-counter drugs, as there is a potential for interactions.

Patients should be cautioned about the concomitant use of Celexa and NSAIDs, aspirin, or other drugs that affect coagulation since the combined use of psychotropic drugs that interfere with serotonin reuptake and these agents has been associated with an increased risk of bleeding.

Patients should be advised to notify their physician if they become pregnant or intend to become pregnant during therapy.

Patients should be advised to notify their physician if they are breastfeeding an infant.

While patients may notice improvement with Celexa therapy in 1 to 4 weeks, they should be advised to continue therapy as directed.

Prescribers or other health professionals should inform patients, their families, and their caregivers about the benefits and risks associated with treatment with Celexa and should counsel them in its appropriate use. A patient Medication Guide About Using Antidepressants in Children and Teenagers is available for Celexa. The prescriber or health professional should instruct patients, their families, and their caregivers to read the Medication Guide and should assist them in understanding its contents. Patients should be given the opportunity to discuss the contents of the Medication Guide and to obtain answers to any questions they may have. The complete text of the Medication Guide is reprinted at the end of this document.

Patients should be advised of the following issues and asked to alert their prescriber these occur while taking Celexa.

Clinical Worsening and Suicide Risk: Patients, their families, and their caregivers should be encouraged to be alert to the emergence of anxiety, agitation, panic attacks, insomnia, irritability, hostility, aggressiveness, impulsivity, akathisia (psychomotor restlessness), hypomania, mania, other unusual changes in behavior, worsening of depression, and suicidal ideation, especially early during antidepressant treatment and when the dose is adjusted up down. Families caregivers of patients should be advised to observe for the emergence of such symptoms on a day-to-day basis, since changes may be abrupt. Such symptoms should be reported to the patient's prescriber or health professional, especially if they are severe, abrupt in onset, or were not part of the patient's presenting symptoms. Symptoms such as these may be associated with an increased risk for suicidal thinking and behavior and indicate a need for very close monitoring and possibly changes in the medication.

Laboratory Tests

There are no specific laboratory tests recommended.

Drug Interactions

CNS Drugs - Given the primary CNS effects of citalopram, caution should be used when it is taken in combination with other centrally acting drugs.

Alcohol - Although citalopram did not potentiate the cognitive and motor effects of alcohol in a clinical trial, as with other psychotropic medications, the use of alcohol by depressed patients taking Celexa is not recommended.

Monoamine Oxidase Inhibitors (MAOIs) - See **CONTRAINDICATIONS** and **WARNINGS**.

Drugs That Interfere With Hemostasis (NSAIDs, Aspirin, Warfarin, etc.)- Serotonin release by platelets plays an important role in hemostasis. Epidemiological studies of the case-control and cohort design that have demonstrated an association between use of psychotropic drugs that interfere with serotonin reuptake and the occurrence of upper gastrointestinal bleeding have also shown that concurrent use of an NSAID or aspirin potentiated the risk of bleeding. Thus, patients should be cautioned about the use of such drugs concurrently with Celexa.

Cimetidine - In subjects who had received 21 days of 40 mg/day Celexa, combined administration of 400 mg/day cimetidine for 8 days resulted in an increase in citalopram AUC and C_{max} of 43% and 39%, respectively. The clinical significance of these findings is unknown.

Digoxin - In subjects who had received 21 days of 40 mg/day Celexa, combined administration of Celexa and digoxin (single dose of 1 mg) did not significantly affect the pharmacokinetics of either citalopram or digoxin.

Lithium - Coadministration of Celexa (40 mg/day for 10 days) and lithium (30 mmol/day for 5 days) had no significant effect on the pharmacokinetics of citalopram or lithium. Nevertheless, plasma lithium levels should be monitored with appropriate adjustment to the lithium dose in accordance with standard clinical practice. Because lithium may enhance the serotonergic effects of citalopram, caution should be exercised when Celexa and lithium are coadministered.

Pimozide - In a controlled study, a single dose of pimozide 2 mg co-administered with citalopram 40 mg given once daily for 11 days was associated with a mean increase in QTc values of approximately 10 msec compared to pimozide given alone. Citalopram did not alter the mean AUC or Cmax of pimozide. The mechanism of this pharmacodynamic interaction is not known.

Theophylline - Combined administration of Celexa (40 mg/day for 21 days) and the CYP1A2 substrate theophylline (single dose of 300 mg) did not affect the pharmacokinetics of theophylline. The effect of theophylline on the pharmacokinetics of citalopram was not evaluated.

Sumatriptan - There have been rare postmarketing reports describing patients with weakness, hyperreflexia, and incoordination following the use of a SSRI and sumatriptan. If concomitant treatment with sumatriptan and an SSRI (e.g., fluoxetine, fluvoxamine, paroxetine, sertraline, citalopram) is clinically warranted, appropriate observation of the patient is advised.

Warfarin - Administration of 40 mg/day Celexa for 21 days did not affect the pharmacokinetics of warfarin, a CYP3A4 substrate. Prothrombin time was increased by 5%, the clinical significance of which is unknown.

Carbamazepine - Combined administration of Celexa (40 mg/day for 14 days) and carbamazepine (titrated to 400 mg/day for 35 days) did not significantly affect the pharmacokinetics of carbamazepine, a CYP3A4 substrate. Although trough citalopram plasma levels were unaffected, given the enzyme-inducing properties of carbamazepine, the possibility that carbamazepine might increase the clearance of citalopram should be considered if the two drugs are coadministered.

Triazolam - Combined administration of Celexa (titrated to 40 mg/day for 28 days) and the CYP3A4 substrate triazolam (single dose of 0.25 mg) did not significantly affect the pharmacokinetics of either citalopram or triazolam.

Ketoconazole - Combined administration of Celexa (40 mg) and ketoconazole (200 mg) decreased the C_{max} and AUC of ketoconazole by 21% and 10%, respectively, and did not significantly affect the pharmacokinetics of citalopram.

CYP3A4 and 2C19 Inhibitors - *In vitro* studies indicated that CYP3A4 and 2C19 are the primary enzymes involved in the metabolism of citalopram. However, coadministration of citalopram (40 mg) and ketoconazole (200 mg), a potent inhibitor of CYP3A4, did not significantly affect the phar-

Continued on next page

Celexa—Cont.

macokinetics of citalopram. Because citalopram is metabolized by multiple enzyme systems, inhibition of a single enzyme may not appreciably decrease citalopram clearance.

Metoprolol - Administration of 40 mg/day Celexa for 22 days resulted in a two-fold increase in the plasma levels of the beta-adrenergic blocker metoprolol. Increased metoprolol plasma levels have been associated with decreased cardioselectivity. Coadministration of Celexa and metoprolol had no clinically significant effects on blood pressure or heart rate.

Imipramine and Other Tricyclic Antidepressants (TCAs) - *In vitro* studies suggest that citalopram is a relatively weak inhibitor of CYP2D6. Coadministration of Celexa (40 mg/day for 10 days) with the TCA imipramine (single dose of 100 mg), a substrate for CYP2D6, did not significantly affect the plasma concentrations of imipramine or citalopram. However, the concentration of the imipramine metabolite desipramine was increased by approximately 50%. The clinical significance of the desipramine change is unknown. Nevertheless, caution is indicated in the coadministration of TCAs with Celexa.

Electroconvulsive Therapy (ECT) - There are no clinical studies of the combined use of electroconvulsive therapy (ECT) and Celexa.

Carcinogenesis, Mutagenesis, Impairment of Fertility

Carcinogenesis

Citalopram was administered in the diet to NMRI/BOM strain mice and COBS WI strain rats for 18 and 24 months, respectively. There was no evidence for carcinogenicity of citalopram in mice receiving up to 240 mg/kg/day, which is equivalent to 20 times the maximum recommended human daily dose (MRHD) of 60 mg on a surface area (mg/m^2) basis. There was an increased incidence of small intestine carcinoma in rats receiving 8 or 24 mg/kg/day, doses which are approximately 1.3 and 4 times the MRHD, respectively, on a mg/m^2 basis. A no-effect dose for this finding was not established. The relevance of these findings to humans is unknown.

Mutagenesis

Citalopram was mutagenic in the *in vitro* bacterial reverse mutation assay (Ames test) in 2 of 5 bacterial strains (Salmonella TA98 and TA1537) in the absence of metabolic activation. It was clastogenic in the *in vitro* Chinese hamster lung cell assay for chromosomal aberrations in the presence and absence of metabolic activation. Citalopram was not mutagenic in the *in vitro* mammalian forward gene mutation assay (HPRT) in mouse lymphoma cells or in a coupled *in vitro/in vivo* unscheduled DNA synthesis (UDS) assay in rat liver. It was not clastogenic in the *in vitro* chromosomal aberration assay in human lymphocytes or in two *in vivo* mouse micronucleus assays.

Impairment of Fertility

When citalopram was administered orally to 16 male and 24 female rats prior to and throughout mating and gestation at doses of 32, 48, and 72 mg/kg/day, mating was decreased at all doses, and fertility was decreased at doses ≥ 32 mg/kg/day, approximately 5 times the MRHD of 60 mg/day on a body surface area (mg/m^2) basis. Gestation duration was increased at 48 mg/kg/day, approximately 8 times the MRHD.

Pregnancy

Pregnancy Category C

In animal reproduction studies, citalopram has been shown to have adverse effects on embryo/fetal and postnatal development, including teratogenic effects, when administered at doses greater than human therapeutic doses.

In two rat embryo/fetal development studies, oral administration of citalopram (32, 56, or 112 mg/kg/day) to pregnant animals during the period of organogenesis resulted in decreased embryo/fetal growth and survival and an increased incidence of fetal abnormalities (including cardiovascular and skeletal defects) at the high dose, which is approximately 18 times the MRHD of 60 mg/day on a body surface area (mg/m^2) basis. This dose was also associated with maternal toxicity (clinical signs, decreased body weight gain). The developmental, no-effect dose of 56 mg/kg/day is approximately 9 times the MRHD on a mg/m^2 basis. In a rabbit study, no adverse effects on embryo/fetal development were observed at doses of up to 16 mg/kg/day, or approximately 5 times the MRHD on a mg/m^2 basis. Thus, teratogenic effects were observed at a maternally toxic dose in the rat and were not observed in the rabbit.

When female rats were treated with citalopram (4.8, 12.8, or 32 mg/kg/day) from late gestation through weaning, increased offspring mortality during the first 4 days after birth and persistent offspring growth retardation were observed at the highest dose, which is approximately 5 times the MRHD on a mg/m^2 basis. The no-effect dose of 12.8 mg/kg/day is approximately 2 times the MRHD on a mg/m^2 basis. Similar effects on offspring mortality and growth were seen when dams were treated throughout gestation and early lactation at doses ≥ 24 mg/kg/day, approximately 4 times the MRHD on a mg/m^2 basis. A no-effect dose was not determined in that study.

There are no adequate and well-controlled studies in pregnant women; therefore, citalopram should be used during pregnancy only if the potential benefit justifies the potential risk to the fetus.

Pregnancy-Nonteratogenic Effects

Neonates exposed to Celexa and other SSRIs or SNRIs, late in the third trimester, have developed complications requiring prolonged hospitalization, respiratory support, and tube feeding. Such complications can arise immediately upon delivery. Reported clinical findings have included respiratory distress, cyanosis, apnea, seizures, temperature instability, feeding difficulty, vomiting, hypoglycemia, hypotonia, hypertonia, hyperreflexia, tremor, jitteriness, irritability, and constant crying. These features are consistent with either a direct toxic effect of SSRIs and SNRIs or, possibly, a drug discontinuation syndrome. It should be noted that, in some cases, the clinical picture is consistent with serotonin syndrome (see **WARNINGS**).

When treating a pregnant woman with Celexa during the third trimester, the physician should carefully consider the potential risks and benefits of treatment (see **DOSAGE AND ADMINISTRATION**).

Labor and Delivery

The effect of Celexa on labor and delivery in humans is unknown.

Nursing Mothers

As has been found to occur with many other drugs, citalopram is excreted in human breast milk. There have been two reports of infants experiencing excessive somnolence, decreased feeding, and weight loss in association with breastfeeding from a citalopram-treated mother; in one case, the infant was reported to recover completely upon discontinuation of citalopram by its mother and in the second case, no follow-up information was available. The decision whether to continue or discontinue either nursing or Celexa therapy should take into account the risks of citalopram exposure for the infant and the benefits of Celexa treatment for the mother.

Pediatric Use

Safety and effectiveness in the pediatric population have not been established (see BOX WARNING and WARNINGS—Clinical Worsening and Suicide Risk). Two placebo-controlled trials in 407 pediatric patients with MDD hae been conducted with Celexa, and the data were not sufficient to report a claim for use in pediatric patients. Anyone considering the use of Celexa in a child or adolescent must balance the potential risks with the clinical need.

Geriatric Use

Of 4422 patients in clinical studies of Celexa, 1357 were 60 and over, 1034 were 65 and over, and 457 were 75 and over. No overall differences in safety or effectiveness were observed between these subjects and younger subjects, and other reported clinical experience has not identified differences in responses between the elderly and younger patients, but greater sensitivity of some older individuals cannot be ruled out. Most elderly patients treated with Celexa in clinical trials received daily doses between 20 and 40 mg (see **DOSAGE AND ADMINISTRATION**).

In two pharmacokinetic studies, citalopram AUC was increased by 23% and 30%, respectively, in elderly subjects as compared to younger subjects, and its half-life was increased by 30% and 50%, respectively (see **CLINICAL PHARMACOLOGY**).

20 mg/day is the recommended dose for most elderly patients (see **DOSAGE AND ADMINISTRATION**).

ADVERSE REACTIONS

The premarketing development program for Celexa included citalopram exposures in patients and/or normal subjects from 3 different groups of studies: 429 normal subjects in clinical pharmacology/pharmacokinetic studies; 4422 exposures from patients in controlled and uncontrolled clinical trials, corresponding to approximately 1370 patient-exposure years. There were, in addition, over 19,000 exposures from mostly open-label, European postmarketing studies. The conditions and duration of treatment with Celexa varied greatly and included (in overlapping categories) open-label and double-blind studies, inpatient and outpatient studies, fixed-dose and dose-titration studies, and short-term and long-term exposure. Adverse reactions were assessed by collecting adverse events, results of physical examinations, vital signs, weights, laboratory analyses, ECGs, and results of ophthalmologic examinations.

Adverse events during exposure were obtained primarily by general inquiry and recorded by clinical investigators using terminology of their own choosing. Consequently, it is not possible to provide a meaningful estimate of the proportion of individuals experiencing adverse events without first grouping similar types of events into a smaller number of standardized event categories. In the tables and tabulations that follow, standard World Health Organization (WHO) terminology has been used to classify reported adverse events.

The stated frequencies of adverse events represent the proportion of individuals who experienced, at least once, a treatment-emergent adverse event of the type listed. An event was considered treatment-emergent if it occurred for the first time or worsened while receiving therapy following baseline evaluation.

Adverse Findings Observed in Short-Term, Placebo-Controlled Trials

Adverse Events Associated with Discontinuation of Treatment

Among 1063 depressed patients who received Celexa at doses ranging from 10 to 80 mg/day in placebo-controlled trials of up to 6 weeks in duration, 16% discontinued treatment due to an adverse event, as compared to 8% of 446 patients receiving placebo. The adverse events associated with discontinuation and considered drug-related (i.e., associated with discontinuation in at least 1% of Celexa-treated patients at a rate at least twice that of placebo) are shown in **TABLE 1**. It should be noted that one patient can report more than one reason for discontinuation and be counted more than once in this table.

TABLE 1
Adverse Events Associated with Discontinuation of Treatment in Short-Term, Placebo-Controlled, Depression Trials

	Percentage of Patients Discontinuing Due to Adverse Event	
	Citalopram (N=1063)	Placebo (N=446)
Body System/Adverse Event		
General		
Asthenia	1%	<1%
Gastrointestinal Disorders		
Nausea	4%	0%
Dry Mouth	1%	<1%
Vomiting	1%	0%
Central and Peripheral Nervous System Disorders		
Dizziness	2%	<1%
Psychiatric Disorders		
Insomnia	3%	1%
Somnolence	2%	1%
Agitation	1%	<1%

Adverse Events Occurring at an Incidence of 2% or More Among Celexa-Treated Patients

Table 2 enumerates the incidence, rounded to the nearest percent, of treatment-emergent adverse events that occurred among 1063 depressed patients who received Celexa at doses ranging from 10 to 80 mg/day in placebo-controlled trials of up to 6 weeks in duration. Events included are those occurring in 2% or more of patients treated with Celexa and for which the incidence in patients treated with Celexa was greater than the incidence in placebo-treated patients.

The prescriber should be aware that these figures cannot be used to predict the incidence of adverse events in the course of usual medical practice where patient characteristics and other factors differ from those which prevailed in the clinical trials. Similarly, the cited frequencies cannot be compared with figures obtained from other clinical investigations involving different treatments, uses, and investigators. The cited figures, however, do provide the prescribing physician with some basis for estimating the relative contribution of drug and non-drug factors to the adverse event incidence rate in the population studied.

The only commonly observed adverse event that occurred in Celexa patients with an incidence of 5% or greater and at least twice the incidence in placebo patients was ejaculation disorder (primarily ejaculatory delay) in male patients (see **TABLE 2**).

TABLE 2
Treatment-Emergent Adverse Events: Incidence in Placebo-Controlled Clinical Trials*

	(Percentage of Patients Reporting Event)	
Body System/Adverse Event	Celexa (N=1063)	Placebo (N=446)
Autonomic Nervous System Disorders		
Dry Mouth	20%	14%
Sweating Increased	11%	9%
Central & Peripheral Nervous System Disorders		
Tremor	8%	6%
Gastrointestinal Disorders		
Nausea	21%	14%
Diarrhea	8%	5%
Dyspepsia	5%	4%
Vomiting	4%	3%
Abdominal Pain	3%	2%
General		
Fatigue	5%	3%
Fever	2%	<1%
Musculoskeletal System Disorders		
Arthralgia	2%	1%
Myalgia	2%	1%
Psychiatric Disorders		
Somnolence	18%	10%
Insomnia	15%	14%
Anxiety	4%	3%
Anorexia	4%	2%
Agitation	3%	1%
Dysmenorrhea[1]	3%	2%
Libido Decreased	2%	<1%
Yawning	2%	<1%
Respiratory System Disorders		
Upper Respiratory Tract Infection	5%	4%
Rhinitis	5%	3%
Sinusitis	3%	<1%
Urogenital		
Ejaculation Disorder[2,3]	6%	1%
Impotence[3]	3%	<1%

*Events reported by at least 2% of patients treated with Celexa are reported, except for the following events which had an incidence on placebo ≥ Celexa: headache, asthenia, dizziness, constipation, palpitation, vision abnormal, sleep disorder, nervousness, pharyngitis, micturition disorder, back pain.

[1] Denominator used was for females only (N=638 Celexa; N=252 placebo).
[2] Primarily ejaculatory delay.
[3] Denominator used was for males only (N=425 Celexa; N=194 placebo).

Dose Dependency of Adverse Events
The potential relationship between the dose of Celexa administered and the incidence of adverse events was examined in a fixed-dose study in depressed patients receiving placebo or Celexa 10, 20, 40, and 60 mg. Jonckheere's trend test revealed a positive dose response ($p<0.05$) for the following adverse events: fatigue, impotence, insomnia, sweating increased, somnolence, and yawning.

Male and Female Sexual Dysfunction with SSRIs
Although changes in sexual desire, sexual performance, and sexual satisfaction often occur as manifestations of a psychiatric disorder, they may also be a consequence of pharmacologic treatment. In particular, some evidence suggests that SSRIs can cause such untoward sexual experiences.
Reliable estimates of the incidence and severity of untoward experiences involving sexual desire, performance, and satisfaction are difficult to obtain, however, in part because patients and physicians may be reluctant to discuss them. Accordingly, estimates of the incidence of untoward sexual experience and performance cited in product labeling, are likely to underestimate their actual incidence.
The table below displays the incidence of sexual side effects reported by at least 2% of patients taking Celexa in a pool of placebo-controlled clinical trials in patients with depression.

Treatment	Celexa (425 males)	Placebo (194 males)
Abnormal Ejaculation (mostly ejaculatory delay)	6.1% (males only)	1% (males only)
Libido Decreased	3.8% (males only)	<1% (males only)
Impotence	2.8% (males only)	<1% (males only)

In female depressed patients receiving Celexa, the reported incidence of decreased libido and anorgasmia was 1.3% (n=638 females) and 1.1% (n=252 females), respectively.
There are no adequately designed studies examining sexual dysfunction with citalopram treatment.
Priapism has been reported with all SSRIs.
While it is difficult to know the precise risk of sexual dysfunction associated with the use of SSRIs, physicians should routinely inquire about such possible side effects.

Vital Sign Changes
Celexa and placebo groups were compared with respect to (1) mean change from baseline in vital signs (pulse, systolic blood pressure, and diastolic blood pressure) and (2) the incidence of patients meeting criteria for potentially clinically significant changes from baseline in these variables. These analyses did not reveal any clinically important changes in vital signs associated with Celexa treatment. In addition, a comparison of supine and standing vital sign measures for Celexa and placebo treatments indicated that Celexa treatment is not associated with orthostatic changes.

Weight Changes
Patients treated with Celexa in controlled trials experienced a weight loss of about 0.5 kg compared to no change for placebo patients.

Laboratory Changes
Celexa and placebo groups were compared with respect to (1) mean change from baseline in various serum chemistry, hematology, and urinalysis variables, and (2) the incidence of patients meeting criteria for potentially clinically significant changes from baseline in these variables. These analyses revealed no clinically important changes in laboratory test parameters associated with Celexa treatment.

ECG Changes
Electrocardiograms from Celexa (N=802) and placebo (N=241) groups were compared with respect to (1) mean change from baseline in various ECG parameters, and (2) the incidence of patients meeting criteria for potentially clinically significant changes from baseline in these variables. The only statistically significant drug-placebo difference observed was a decrease in heart rate for Celexa of 1.7 bpm compared to no change in heart rate for placebo. There were no observed differences in QT or other ECG intervals.

Other Events Observed During the Premarketing Evaluation of Celexa (citalopram HBr)
Following is a list of WHO terms that reflect treatment-emergent adverse events, as defined in the introduction to the **ADVERSE REACTIONS** section, reported by patients treated with Celexa at multiple doses in a range of 10 to 80 mg/day during any phase of a trial within the premarketing database of 4422 patients. All reported events are included except those already listed in Table 2 or elsewhere in labeling, those events for which a drug cause was remote, those event terms which were so general as to be uninformative, and those occurring in only one patient. It is important to emphasize that, although the events reported occurred during treatment with Celexa, they were not necessarily caused by it.
Events are further categorized by body system and listed in order of decreasing frequency according to the following definitions: frequent adverse events are those occurring on one or more occasions in at least 1/100 patients; infrequent adverse events are those occurring in less than 1/100 patients but at least 1/1000 patients; rare events are those occurring in fewer than 1/1000 patients.

Cardiovascular - *Frequent*: tachycardia, postural hypotension, hypotension. *Infrequent* hypertension, bradycardia, edema (extremities), angina pectoris, extrasystoles, cardiac failure, flushing, myocardial infarction, cerebrovascular accident, myocardial ischemia. *Rare*: transient ischemic attack, phlebitis, atrial fibrillation, cardiac arrest, bundle branch block.

Central and Peripheral Nervous System Disorders - *Frequent*: paresthesia, migraine. *Infrequent*: hyperkinesia, vertigo, hypertonia, extrapyramidal disorder, leg cramps, involuntary muscle contractions, hypokinesia, neuralgia, dystonia, abnormal gait, hypesthesia, ataxia. *Rare*: abnormal coordination, hyperesthesia, ptosis, stupor.

Endocrine Disorders - *Rare*: hypothyroidism, goiter, gynecomastia.

Gastrointestinal Disorders - *Frequent*: saliva increased, flatulence. *Infrequent*: gastritis, gastroenteritis, stomatitis, eructation, hemorrhoids, dysphagia, teeth grinding, gingivitis, esophagitis. *Rare*: colitis, gastric ulcer, cholecystitis, cholelithiasis, duodenal ulcer, gastroesophageal reflux, glossitis, jaundice, diverticulitis, rectal hemorrhage, hiccups.

General - *Infrequent*: hot flushes, rigors, alcohol intolerance, syncope, influenza-like symptoms. *Rare*: hayfever.

Hemic and Lymphatic Disorders - *Infrequent*: purpura, anemia, epistaxis, leukocytosis, leucopenia, lymphadenopathy. *Rare*: pulmonary embolism, granulocytopenia, lymphocytosis, lymphopenia, hypochromic anemia, coagulation disorder, gingival bleeding.

Metabolic and Nutritional Disorders - *Frequent*: decreased weight, increased weight. *Infrequent*: increased hepatic enzymes, thirst, dry eyes, increased alkaline phosphatase, abnormal glucose tolerance. *Rare*: bilirubinemia, hypokalemia, obesity, hypoglycemia, hepatitis, dehydration.

Musculoskeletal System Disorders - *Infrequent*: arthritis, muscle weakness, skeletal pain. *Rare*: bursitis, osteoporosis.

Psychiatric Disorders - *Frequent*: impaired concentration, amnesia, apathy, depression, increased appetite, aggravated depression, suicide attempt, confusion. *Infrequent*: increased libido, aggressive reaction, paroniria, drug dependence, depersonalization, hallucination, euphoria, psychotic depression, delusion, paranoid reaction, emotional lability, panic reaction, psychosis. *Rare*: catatonic reaction, melancholia.

Reproductive Disorders/Female* - *Frequent*: amenorrhea. *Infrequent*: galactorrhea, breast pain, breast enlargement, vaginal hemorrhage.

*% based on female subjects only: 2955

Respiratory System Disorders - *Frequent*: coughing. *Infrequent*: bronchitis, dyspnea, pneumonia. *Rare*: asthma, laryngitis, bronchospasm, pneumonitis, sputum increased.

Skin and Appendages Disorders - *Frequent*: rash, pruritus. *Infrequent*: photosensitivity reaction, urticaria, acne, skin discoloration, eczema, alopecia, dermatitis, skin dry, psoriasis. *Rare*: hypertrichosis, decreased sweating, melanosis, keratitis, cellulitis, pruritus ani.

Special Senses - *Frequent*: accommodation abnormal, taste perversion. *Infrequent*: tinnitus, conjunctivitis, eye pain. *Rare* mydriasis, photophobia, diplopia, abnormal lacrimation, cataract, taste loss.

Urinary System Disorders - *Frequent* polyuria. *Infrequent*: micturition frequency, urinary incontinence, urinary retention, dysuria. *Rare*: facial edema, hematuria, oliguria, pyelonephritis, renal calculus, renal pain.

Other Events Observed During the Postmarketing Evaluation of Celexa (citalopram HBr)
It is estimated that over 30 million patients have been treated with Celexa since market introduction. Although no causal relationship to Celexa treatment has been found, the following adverse events have been reported to be temporally associated with Celexa treatment, and have not been described elsewhere in labeling: acute renal failure, akathisia, allergic reaction, anaphylaxis, angioedema, choreoathetosis, chest pain, delirium, dyskinesia, ecchymosis, epidermal necrolysis, erythema multiforme, gastrointestinal hemorrhage, grand mal convulsions, hemolytic anemia, hepatic necrosis, myoclonus, neuroleptic malignant syndrome, nystagmus, pancreatitis, priapism, prolactinemia, prothrombin decreased, QT prolonged, rhabdomyolysis, serotonin syndrome, spontaneous abortion, thrombocytopenia, thrombosis, ventricular arrhythmia, torsades de pointes, and withdrawal syndrome.

DRUG ABUSE AND DEPENDENCE

Controlled Substance Class
Celexa (citalopram HBr) is not a controlled substance.

Physical and Psychological Dependence
Animal studies suggest that the abuse liability of Celexa is low. Celexa has not been systematically studied in humans for its potential for abuse, tolerance, or physical dependence. The premarketing clinical experience with Celexa did not reveal any drug-seeking behavior. However, these observations were not systematic and it is not possible to predict, on the basis of this limited experience, the extent to which a CNS-active drug will be misused, diverted, and/or abused once marketed. Consequently, physicians should carefully evaluate Celexa patients for history of drug abuse and follow such patients closely, observing them for signs of misuse or abuse (e.g., development of tolerance, incrementations of dose, drug-seeking behavior).

OVERDOSAGE

Human Experience
In clinical trials of citalopram, there were reports of citalopram overdose, including overdoses of up to 2000 mg, with no associated fatalities. During the postmarketing evaluation of citalopram, Celexa overdoses, including overdoses of up to 6000 mg, have been reported. As with other SSRI's, a fatal outcome in a patient who has taken an overdose of citalopram has been rarely reported.
Symptoms most often accompanying citalopram overdose, alone or in combination with other drugs and/or alcohol, included dizziness, sweating, nausea, vomiting, tremor, somnolence, and sinus tachycardia. In more rare cases, observed symptoms included amnesia, confusion, coma, convulsions, hyperventilation, cyanosis, rhabdomyolysis, and ECG changes (including QTc prolongation, nodal rhythm, ventricular arrhythmia, and one possible case of torsades de pointes).

Management of Overdose
Establish and maintain an airway to ensure adequate ventilation and oxygenation. Gastric evacuation by lavage and use of activated charcoal should be considered. Careful observation and cardiac and vital sign monitoring are recommended, along with general symptomatic and supportive care. Due to the large volume of distribution of citalopram, forced diuresis, dialysis, hemoperfusion, and exchange transfusion are unlikely to be of benefit. There are no specific antidotes for Celexa.
In managing overdosage, consider the possibility of multiple-drug involvement. The physician should consider contacting a poison control center for additional information on the treatment of any overdose.

DOSAGE AND ADMINISTRATION

Initial Treatment
Celexa (citalopram HBr) should be administered at an initial dose of 20 mg once daily, generally with an increase to a dose of 40 mg/day. Dose increases should usually occur in increments of 20 mg at intervals of no less than one week. Although certain patients may require a dose of 60 mg/day, the only study pertinent to dose response for effectiveness did not demonstrate an advantage for the 60 mg/day dose over the 40 mg/day dose; doses above 40 mg are therefore not ordinarily recommended.
Celexa should be administered once daily, in the morning or evening, with or without food.

Special Populations
20 mg/day is the recommended dose for most elderly patients and patients with hepatic impairment, with titration to 40 mg/day only for nonresponding patients.
No dosage adjustment is necessary for patients with mild or moderate renal impairment. Celexa should be used with caution in patients with severe renal impairment.

Treatment of Pregnant Women During the Third Trimester
Neonates exposed to Celexa and other SSRIs or SNRIs, late in the third trimester, have developed complications requiring prolonged hospitalization, respiratory support, and tube feeding (see **PRECAUTIONS**). When treating pregnant women with Celexa during the third trimester, the physician should carefully consider the potential risks and benefits of treatment. The physician may consider tapering Celexa in the third trimester.

Maintenance Treatment
It is generally agreed that acute episodes of depression require several months or longer of sustained pharmacologic therapy. Systematic evaluation of Celexa in two studies has shown that its antidepressant efficacy is maintained for periods of up to 24 weeks following 6 or 8 weeks of initial treatment (32 weeks total). In one study, patients were assigned randomly to placebo or to the same dose of Celexa (20-60 mg/day) during maintenance treatment as they had received during the acute stabilization phase, while in the other study, patients were assigned randomly to continuation of Celexa 20 or 40 mg/day, or placebo, for maintenance treatment. In the latter study, the rates of relapse to depression were similar for the two dose groups (see **Clinical Trials** under **CLINICAL PHARMACOLOGY**). Based on these limited data, it is not known whether the dose of citalopram needed to maintain euthymia is identical to the dose needed to induce remission. If adverse reactions are bothersome, a decrease in dose to 20 mg/day can be considered.

Discontinuation of Treatment with Celexa
Symptoms associated with discontinuation of Celexa and other SSRIs and SNRIs have been reported (see **PRECAUTIONS**). Patients should be monitored for these symptoms when discontinuing treatment. A gradual reduction in the dose rather than abrupt cessation is recommended whenever possible. If intolerable symptoms occur following a decrease in the dose or upon discontinuation of treatment, then resuming the previously prescribed dose may be considered. Subsequently, the physician may continue decreasing the dose but at a more gradual rate.

Switching Patients To or From a Monoamine Oxidase Inhibitor
At least 14 days should elapse between discontinuation of an MAOI and initiation of Celexa therapy. Similarly, at least 14 days should be allowed after stopping Celexa before starting an MAOI (see **CONTRAINDICATIONS** and **WARNINGS**).

Continued on next page

Celexa—Cont.

HOW SUPPLIED

Tablets:

10 mg	Bottle of 100	NDC # 0456-4010-01

Beige, oval, film-coated.
Imprint on one side with "FP". Imprint on the other side with "10 mg".

20 mg	Bottle of 100	NDC # 0456-4020-01
	10 × 10 Unit Dose	NDC # 0456-4020-63

Pink, oval, scored, film-coated.
Imprint on scored side with "F" on the left side and "P" on the right side.
Imprint on the non-scored side with "20 mg".

40 mg	Bottle of 100	NDC # 0456-4040-01
	10 × 10 Unit Dose	NDC # 0456-4040-63

White, oval, scored, film-coated.
Imprint on scored side with "F" on the left side and "P" on the right side.
Imprint on the non-scored side with "40 mg".
Oral Solution:
10 mg/5 mL, peppermint flavor (240 mL) NDC 0456-4130-08
Store at 25°C (77°F); excursions permitted to 15-30°C (59-86°F).

ANIMAL TOXICOLOGY

Retinal Changes in Rats

Pathologic changes (degeneration/atrophy) were observed in the retinas of albino rats in the 2-year carcinogenicity study with citalopram. There was an increase in both incidence and severity of retinal pathology in both male and female rats receiving 80 mg/kg/day (13 times the maximum recommended daily human dose of 60 mg on a mg/m^2 basis). Similar findings were not present in rats receiving 24 mg/kg/day for two years, in mice treated for 18 months at doses up to 240 mg/kg/day, or in dogs treated for one year at doses up to 20 mg/kg/day (4, 20, and 10 times, respectively, the maximum recommended daily human dose on a mg/m^2 basis).

Additional studies to investigate the mechanism for this pathology have not been performed, and the potential significance of this effect in humans has not been established.

Cardiovascular Changes in Dogs

In a one-year toxicology study, 5 of 10 beagle dogs receiving oral doses of 8 mg/kg/day (4 times the maximum recommended daily human dose of 60 mg on a mg/m^2 basis) died suddenly between weeks 17 and 31 following initiation of treatment. Although appropriate data from that study are not available to directly compare plasma levels of citalopram (CT) and its metabolites, demethylcitalopram (DCT) and didemethylcitalopram (DDCT), to levels that have been achieved in humans, pharmacokinetic data indicate that the relative dog-to-human exposure was greater for the metabolites than for citalopram. Sudden deaths were not observed in rats at doses up to 120 mg/kg/day, which produced plasma levels of CT, DCT, and DDCT similar to those observed in dogs at doses of 8 mg/kg/day. A subsequent intravenous dosing study demonstrated that in beagle dogs, DDCT caused QT prolongation, a known risk factor for the observed outcome in dogs. This effect occurred in dogs at doses producing peak DDCT plasma levels of 810 to 3250 nM (39–155 times the mean steady state DDCT plasma level measured at the maximum recommended human daily dose of 60 mg). In dogs, peak DDCT plasma concentrations are approximately equal to peak CT plasma concentrations, whereas in humans, steady state DDCT plasma concentrations are less than 10% of steady state CT plasma concentrations. Assays of DDCT plasma concentrations in 2020 citalopram-treated individuals demonstrated that DDCT levels rarely exceeded 70 nM; the highest measured level of DDCT in human overdose was 138 nM. While DDCT is ordinarily present in humans at lower levels than in dogs, it is unknown whether there are individuals who may achieve higher DDCT levels. The possibility that DCT, a principal metabolite in humans, may prolong the QT interval in dogs has not been directly examined because DCT is rapidly converted to DDCT in that species.

Forest Pharmaceuticals, Inc.
Subsidiary of Forest Laboratories, Inc.
St. Louis, MO 63045 USA
Licensed from H. Lundbeck A/S
Rev. 02/05

MG #13940(20)

Medication Guide

About Using Antidepressants in Children and Teenagers

What is the most important information I should know if my child is being prescribed an antidepressant?

Parents or guardians need to think about 4 important things when their child is prescribed an antidepressant:

1. There is a risk of suicidal thoughts or actions
2. How to try to prevent suicidal thoughts or actions in your child
3. You should watch for certain signs if your child is taking an antidepressant
4. There are benefits and risks when using antidepressants

1. There is a Risk of Suicidal Thoughts or Actions

Children and teenagers sometimes think about suicide, and many report trying to kill themselves.

Antidepressants increase suicidal thoughts and actions in some children and teenagers. But suicidal thoughts and actions can also be caused by depression, a serious medical condition that is commonly treated with antidepressants. Thinking about killing yourself or trying to kill yourself is called *suicidality or being suicidal*.

A large study combined the results of 24 different studies of children and teenagers with depression or other illnesses. In these studies, patients took either a placebo (sugar pill) or an antidepressant for 1 to 4 months. ***No one committed suicide in these studies,*** but some patients became suicidal. On sugar pills, 2 out of every 100 became suicidal. On the antidepressants, 4 out of every 100 patients became suicidal.

For some children and teenagers, the risks of suicidal actions may be especially high. These include patients with

- Bipolar illness (sometimes called manic-depressive illness)
- A family history of bipolar illness
- A personal or family history of attempting suicide

If any of these are present, make sure you tell your healthcare provider before your child takes an antidepressant.

2. How to Try to Prevent Suicidal Thoughts and Actions

To try to prevent suicidal thoughts and actions in your child, pay close attention to changes in her or his moods or actions, especially if the changes occur suddenly. Other important people in your child's life can help by paying attention as well (e.g., your child, brothers and sisters, teachers, and other important people). The changes to look out for are listed in Section 3, on what to watch for.

Whenever an antidepressant is started or its dose is changed, pay close attention to your child.

After starting an antidepressant, your child should generally see his or her healthcare provider:

- Once a week for the first 4 weeks
- Every 2 weeks for the next 4 weeks
- After taking the antidepressant for 12 weeks
- After 12 weeks, follow your healthcare provider's advice about how often to come back
- More often if problems or questions arise (see Section 3)

You should call your child's healthcare provider between visits if needed.

3. You Should Watch for Certain Signs If Your Child is Taking an Antidepressant

Contact your child's healthcare provider ***right away*** if your child exhibits any of the following signs for the first time, or if they seem worse, or worry you, your child, or your child's teacher:

- Thoughts about suicide or dying
- Attempts to commit suicide
- New or worse depression
- New or worse anxiety
- Feeling very agitated or restless
- Panic attacks
- Difficulty sleeping (insomnia)
- New or worse irritability
- Acting aggressive, being angry, or violent
- Acting on dangerous impulses
- An extreme increase in activity and talking
- Other unusual changes in behavior or mood

Never let your child stop taking an antidepressant without first talking to his or her healthcare provider. Stopping an antidepressant suddenly can cause other symptoms.

4. There are Benefits and Risks When Using Antidepressants

Antidepressants are used to treat depression and other illnesses. Depression and other illnesses can lead to suicide. In some children and teenagers, treatment with an antidepressant increases suicidal thinking or actions. It is important to discuss all the risks of treating depression and also the risks of not treating it. You and your child should discuss all treatment choices with your healthcare provider, not just the use of antidepressants.

Other side effects can occur with antidepressants (see section below).

Of all the antidepressants, only fluoxetine (Prozac™) has been FDA approved to treat pediatric depression.

For obsessive compulsive disorder in children and teenagers, FDA has approved only fluoxetine (Prozac™), sertraline (Zoloft™), fluvoxamine, and clomipramine (Anafranil™).

Your healthcare provider may suggest other antidepressants based on the past experience of your child or other family members.

Is this all I need to know if my child is being prescribed an antidepressant?

No. This is a warning about the risk for suicidality. Other side effects can occur with antidepressants. Be sure to ask your healthcare provider to explain all the side effects of the particular drug he or she is prescribing. Also ask about drugs to avoid when taking an antidepressant. Ask your healthcare provider or pharmacist where to find more information.

*Prozac® is a registered trademark of Eli Lilly and Company
*Zoloft® is a registered trademark of Pfizer Pharmaceuticals
*Anafranil® is a registered trademark of Mallinckrodt Inc.

This Medication Guide has been approved by the U.S. Food and Drug Administration for all antidepressants.

LEVOTHROID® ℞

[lēv′o-throid″]
(levothyroxine sodium tablets, USP)
Rx Only

Prescribing information for this product, which appears on pages 1278–1282 of the 2005 PDR, has been completely revised as follows. Please write "See Supplement A" next to the product heading.

DESCRIPTION

LEVOTHROID® (levothyroxine sodium tablets, USP) contains synthetic crystalline L-3,3′,5,5′-tetraiodothyronine sodium salt [levothyroxine (T_4) sodium]. Synthetic T_4 is identical to that produced in the human thyroid gland. Levothyroxine (T_4) sodium has an empirical formula of $C_{15}H_{10}I_4N\ NaO_4 \times H_2O$, molecular weight of 798.86 g/mol (anhydrous), and structural formula as shown:

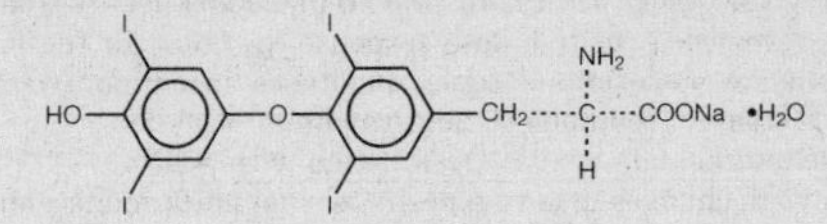

I
I
NH2
HO
O
CH2
C
COONa
•H2O
H
I
I

Inactive Ingredients: Microcrystalline cellulose, calcium phosphate dibasic, povidone and magnesium stearate. The following are the coloring additives per tablet strength.

Strength (mcg)	Color additive(s)
25	FD&C Yellow No. 6 Aluminum Lake
50	None
75	FD&C Blue No. 2 Aluminum Lake, FD&C Red No. 40 Aluminum Lake
88	FD&C Yellow No. 6 Aluminum Lake, FD&C Blue No. 1 Aluminum Lake, D&C Yellow No. 10 Aluminum Lake
100	FD&C Yellow No. 6 Aluminum Lake, D&C Yellow No. 10 Aluminum Lake
112	D&C Red No. 27 Aluminum Lake, D&C Red No. 30 Aluminum Lake
125	FD&C Blue No. 1 Aluminum Lake, FD&C Red No. 40 Aluminum Lake, FD&C Yellow No. 6 Aluminum Lake
137	FD&C Blue No. 1 Aluminum Lake
150	FD&C Blue No. 2 Aluminum Lake
175	FD&C Blue No. 1 Aluminum Lake, D&C Red No. 30 Aluminum Lake, D&C Red No. 27 Aluminum Lake
200	FD&C Red No. 40 Aluminum Lake
300	FD&C Yellow No. 6 Aluminum Lake, FD&C Blue No.1 Aluminum Lake, D&C Yellow No. 10 Aluminum Lake

CLINICAL PHARMACOLOGY

Thyroid hormone synthesis and secretion is regulated by the hypothalamic-pituitary-thyroid axis. Thyrotropin-releasing hormone (TRH) released from the hypothalamus stimulates secretion of thyrotropin-stimulating hormone, TSH, from the anterior pituitary. TSH, in turn, is the physiologic stimulus for the synthesis and secretion of thyroid hormones, L-thyroxine (T_4) and L-triiodothyronine (T_3), by the thyroid gland. Circulating serum T_3 and T_4 levels exert a feedback effect on both TRH and TSH secretion. When serum T_3 and T_4 levels increase, TRH and TSH secretion decrease. When thyroid hormone levels decrease, TRH and TSH secretion increase.

The mechanisms by which thyroid hormones exert their physiologic actions are not completely understood, but it is thought that their principal effects are exerted through control of DNA transcription and protein synthesis. T_3 and T_4 diffuse into the cell nucleus and bind to thyroid receptor proteins attached to DNA. This hormone nuclear receptor complex activates gene transcription and synthesis of messenger RNA and cytoplasmic proteins.

Thyroid hormones regulate multiple metabolic processes and play an essential role in normal growth and development, and normal maturation of the central nervous system and bone. The metabolic actions of thyroid hormones include augmentation of cellular respiration and thermogenesis, as well as metabolism of proteins, carbohydrates and lipids. The protein anabolic effects of thyroid hormones are essential to normal growth and development.

The physiological actions of thyroid hormones are produced predominantly by T_3, the majority of which (approximately 80%) is derived from T_4 by deiodination in peripheral tissues.

Levothyroxine, at doses individualized according to patient response, is effective as replacement or supplemental therapy in hypothyroidism of any etiology, except transient hypothyroidism during the recovery phase of subacute thyroiditis.

Levothyroxine is also effective in the suppression of pituitary TSH secretion in the treatment or prevention of various types of euthyroid goiters, including thyroid nodules, Hashimoto's thyroiditis, multinodular goiter and, as adjunctive therapy in the management of thyrotropin-dependent well-differentiated thyroid cancer (see **INDICATIONS AND USAGE, PRECAUTIONS, DOSAGE AND ADMINISTRATION**).

PHARMACOKINETICS

Absorption - Absorption of orally administered T_4 from the gastrointestinal (GI) tract ranges from 40% to 80%. The majority of the levothyroxine dose is absorbed from the jejunum and upper ileum. The relative bioavailability of LEVOTHROID® tablets, compared to an equal nominal dose of oral levothyroxine sodium solution, is approximately 94%. T_4 absorption is increased by fasting, and decreased in malabsorption syndromes and by certain foods such as soybean infant formula. Dietary fiber decreases bioavailability of T_4. Absorption may also decrease with age. In addition, many drugs and foods affect T_4 absorption (see **PRECAUTIONS, Drug Interactions** and **Drug-Food Interactions**).

Distribution - Circulating thyroid hormones are greater than 99% bound to plasma proteins, including thyroxine-binding globulin (TBG), thyroxine-binding prealbumin (TBPA), and albumin (TBA), whose capacities and affinities vary for each hormone. The higher affinity of both TBG and TBPA for T_4 partially explains the higher serum levels, slower metabolic clearance, and longer half-life of T_4 compared to T_3. Protein-bound thyroid hormones exist in reverse equilibrium with small amounts of free hormone. Only unbound hormone is metabolically active. Many drugs and physiologic conditions affect the binding of thyroid hormones to serum proteins (see **PRECAUTIONS, Drug Interactions** and **Drug-Laboratory Test Interactions**). Thyroid hormones do not readily cross the placental barrier (see **PRECAUTIONS, Pregnancy**).

Metabolism - T_4 is slowly eliminated (see **Table 1**). The major pathway of thyroid hormone metabolism is through sequential deiodination. Approximately eighty-percent of circulating T_3 is derived from peripheral T_4 by monodeiodination. The liver is the major site of degradation for both T_4 and T_3, with T_4 deiodination also occurring at a number of additional sites, including the kidney and other tissues. Approximately 80% of the daily dose of T_4 is deiodinated to yield equal amounts of T_3 and reverse T_3 (rT_3). T_3 and rT_3 are further deiodinated to diiodothyronine. Thyroid hormones are also metabolized via conjugation with glucuronides and sulfates and excreted directly into the bile and gut where they undergo enterohepatic recirculation.

Elimination - Thyroid hormones are primarily eliminated by the kidneys. A portion of the conjugated hormone reaches the colon unchanged and is eliminated in the feces. Approximately 20% of T_4 is eliminated in the stool. Urinary excretion of T_4 decreases with age.

Table 1: Pharmacokinetic Parameters of Thyroid Hormones in Euthyroid Patients

Hormone	Ratio in Thyro-globulin	Biologic Potency	$t_{1/2}$ (days)	Protein Binding (%)[2]
Levothyroxine (T_4)	10–20	1	6–7[1]	99.96
Liothyronine (T_3)	1	4	≤2	99.5

[1] 3 to 4 days in hyperthyroidism, 9 to 10 days in hypothyroidism; [2] Includes TBG, TBPA, and TBA

INDICATIONS AND USAGE

Levothyroxine sodium is used for the following indications:

Hypothyroidism - As replacement or supplemental therapy in congenital or acquired hypothyroidism of any etiology, except transient hypothyroidism during the recovery phase of subacute thyroiditis. Specific indications include: primary (thyroidal), secondary (pituitary), and tertiary (hypothalamic) hypothyroidism and subclinical hypothyroidism. Primary hypothyroidism may result from functional deficiency, primary atrophy, partial or total congenital absence of the thyroid gland, or from the effects of surgery, radiation, or drugs, with or without the presence of goiter.

Pituitary TSH Suppression - In the treatment or prevention of various types of euthyroid goiters (see **WARNINGS** and **PRECAUTIONS**), including thyroid nodules (see **WARNINGS** and **PRECAUTIONS**), subacute or chronic lymphocytic thyroiditis (Hashimoto's thyroiditis), multinodular goiter (see **WARNINGS** and **PRECAUTIONS**) and, as an adjunct to surgery and radioiodine therapy in the management of thyrotropin-dependent well-differentiated thyroid cancer.

CONTRAINDICATIONS

Levothyroxine is contraindicated in patients with untreated subclinical (suppressed serum TSH level with normal T_3 and T_4 levels) or overt thyrotoxicosis of any etiology and in patients with acute myocardial infarction. Levothyroxine is contraindicated in patients with uncorrected adrenal insufficiency since thyroid hormones may precipitate an acute adrenal crisis by increasing the metabolic clearance of glucocorticoids (see **PRECAUTIONS**). LEVOTHROID® is contraindicated in patients with hypersensitivity to any of the inactive ingredients in LEVOTHROID® tablets (see **DESCRIPTION, Inactive Ingredients**).

WARNINGS

> **WARNING: Thyroid hormones, including LEVOTHROID®, either alone or with other therapeutic agents, should not be used for the treatment of obesity or for weight loss. In euthyroid patients, doses within the range of daily hormonal requirements are ineffective for weight reduction. Larger doses may produce serious or even life threatening manifestations of toxicity, particularly when given in association with sympathomimetic amines such as those used for their anorectic effects.**

Levothyroxine sodium should not be used in the treatment of male or female infertility unless this condition is associated with hypothyroidism.

In patients with nontoxic diffuse goiter or nodular thyroid disease, particularly the elderly or those with underlying cardiovascular disease, levothyroxine sodium therapy is contraindicated if the serum TSH level is already suppressed due to the risk of precipitating overt thyrotoxicosis (see **CONTRAINDICATIONS**). If the serum TSH level is not suppressed, LEVOTHROID® should be used with caution in conjunction with careful monitoring of thyroid function for evidence of hyperthyroidism and clinical monitoring for potential associated adverse cardiovascular signs and symptoms of hyperthyroidism.

PRECAUTIONS

General

Levothyroxine has a narrow therapeutic index. Regardless of the indication for use, careful dosage titration is necessary to avoid the consequences of over- or under-treatment. These consequences include, among others, effects on growth and development, cardiovascular function, bone metabolism, reproductive function, cognitive function, emotional state, gastrointestinal function, and on glucose and lipid metabolism. Many drugs interact with levothyroxine sodium, necessitating adjustments in dosing to maintain therapeutic response (see **Drug Interactions**).

Effects on bone mineral density - In women, long-term levothyroxine sodium therapy has been associated with increased bone resorption, thereby decreasing bone mineral density, especially in post-menopausal women on greater than replacement doses or in women who are receiving suppressive doses of levothyroxine sodium. The increased bone resorption may be associated with increased serum levels and urinary excretion of calcium and phosphorous, elevations in bone alkaline phosphatase and suppressed serum parathyroid hormone levels. Therefore, it is recommended that patients receiving levothyroxine sodium be given the minimum dose necessary to achieve the desired clinical and biochemical response.

Patients with underlying cardiovascular disease - Exercise caution when administering levothyroxine to patients with cardiovascular disorders and to the elderly in whom there is an increased risk of occult cardiac disease. In these patients, levothyroxine therapy should be initiated at lower doses than those recommended in younger individuals or in patients without cardiac disease (see **WARNINGS; PRECAUTIONS, Geriatric Use; and DOSAGE AND ADMINISTRATION**). If cardiac symptoms develop or worsen, the levothyroxine dose should be reduced or withheld for one week and then cautiously restarted at a lower dose. Overtreatment with levothyroxine sodium may have adverse cardiovascular effects such as an increase in heart rate, cardiac wall thickness, and cardiac contractility and may precipitate angina or arrhythmias. Patients with coronary artery disease who are receiving levothyroxine therapy should be monitored closely during surgical procedures, since the possibility of precipitating cardiac arrhythmias may be greater in those treated with levothyroxine. Concomitant administration of levothyroxine and sympathomimetic agents to patients with coronary artery disease may precipitate coronary insufficiency.

Patients with nontoxic diffuse goiter or nodular thyroid disease - Exercise caution when administering levothyroxine to patients with nontoxic diffuse goiter or nodular thyroid disease in order to prevent precipitation of thyrotoxicosis (see **WARNINGS**). If the serum TSH is already suppressed, levothyroxine sodium should not be administered (see **CONTRAINDICATIONS**).

Associated endocrine disorders

Hypothalamic/pituitary hormone deficiencies - In patients with secondary or tertiary hypothyroidism, additional hypothalamic/pituitary hormone deficiencies should be considered, and, if diagnosed, treated (see **PRECAUTIONS, Autoimmune polyglandular syndrome** for adrenal insufficiency).

Autoimmune polyglandular syndrome - Occasionally, chronic autoimmune thyroiditis may occur in association with other autoimmune disorders such as adrenal insufficiency, pernicious anemia, and insulin-dependent diabetes mellitus. Patients with concomitant adrenal insufficiency should be treated with replacement glucocorticoids prior to initiation of treatment with levothyroxine sodium. Failure to do so may precipitate an acute adrenal crisis when thyroid hormone therapy is initiated, due to increased metabolic clearance of glucocorticoids by thyroid hormone. Patients with diabetes mellitus may require upward adjustments of their antidiabetic therapeutic regimens when treated with levothyroxine (see **PRECAUTIONS, Drug Interactions**).

Other associated medical conditions

Infants with congenital hypothyroidism appear to be at increased risk for other congenital anomalies, with cardiovascular anomalies (pulmonary stenosis, atrial septal defect, and ventricular septal defect) being the most common association.

Information for Patients

Patients should be informed of the following information to aid in the safe and effective use of LEVOTHROID®:

1. Notify your physician if you are allergic to any foods or medicines, are pregnant or intend to become pregnant, are breast-feeding or are taking any other medications, including prescription and over-the-counter preparations.

2. Notify your physician of any other medical conditions you may have, particularly heart disease, diabetes, clotting disorders, and adrenal or pituitary gland problems. Your dose of medications used to control these other conditions may need to be adjusted while you are taking LEVOTHROID®. If you have diabetes, monitor your blood and/or urinary glucose levels as directed by your physician and immediately report any changes to your physician. If you are taking anticoagulants (blood thinners), your clotting status should be checked frequently.

3. Use LEVOTHROID® only as prescribed by your physician. Do not discontinue or change the amount you take or how often you take it, unless directed to do so by your physician.

4. The levothyroxine in LEVOTHROID® is intended to replace a hormone that is normally produced by your thyroid gland. Generally, replacement therapy is to be taken for life, except in cases of transient hypothyroidism, which is usually associated with an inflammation of the thyroid gland (thyroiditis).

5. Take LEVOTHROID® as a single dose, preferably on an empty stomach, one-half to one hour before breakfast. Levothyroxine absorption is increased on an empty stomach.

6. It may take several weeks before you notice an improvement in your symptoms.

7. Notify your physician if you experience any of the following symptoms: rapid or irregular heartbeat, chest pain, shortness of breath, leg cramps, headache, nervousness, irritability, sleeplessness, tremors, change in appetite, weight gain or loss, vomiting, diarrhea, excessive sweating, heat intolerance, fever, changes in menstrual periods, hives or skin rash, or any other unusual medical event.

8. Notify your physician if you become pregnant while taking LEVOTHROID®. It is likely that your dose of LEVOTHROID® will need to be increased while you are pregnant.

9. Notify your physician or dentist that you are taking LEVOTHROID® prior to any surgery.

10. Partial hair loss may occur rarely during the first few months of LEVOTHROID® therapy, but this is usually temporary.

11. LEVOTHROID® should not be used as a primary or adjunctive therapy in a weight control program.

12. Keep LEVOTHROID® out of the reach of children. Store LEVOTHROID® away from heat, moisture, and light.

Laboratory Tests

General

The diagnosis of hypothyroidism is confirmed by measuring TSH levels using a sensitive assay (second generation assay sensitivity ≤0.1 mIU/L or third generation assay sensitivity ≤0.01 mIU/L) and measurement of free-T_4.

The adequacy of therapy is determined by periodic assessment of appropriate laboratory tests and clinical evaluation. The choice of laboratory tests depends on various factors including the etiology of the underlying thyroid disease, the presence of concomitant medical conditions, including pregnancy, and the use of concomitant medications (see **PRECAUTIONS, Drug Interactions** and **Drug-Laboratory Test Interactions**). Persistent clinical and laboratory evidence of hypothyroidism despite an apparent adequate replacement dose of LEVOTHROID® may be evidence of inadequate absorption, poor compliance, drug interactions, or decreased T_4 potency of the drug product.

Adults

In adult patients with primary (thyroidal) hypothyroidism, serum TSH levels (using a sensitive assay) alone may be used to monitor therapy. The frequency of TSH monitoring during levothyroxine dose titration depends on the clinical situation but it is generally recommended at 6-8 week intervals until normalization. For patients who have recently initiated levothyroxine therapy and whose serum TSH has normalized or in patients who have had their dosage or brand of levothyroxine changed, the serum TSH concentration should be measured after 8-12 weeks. When the optimum replacement dose has been attained, clinical (physical examination) and biochemical monitoring may be performed every 6-12 months, depending on the clinical situation, and whenever there is a change in the patient's status. It is recommended that a physical examination and a serum TSH measurement be performed at least annually in patients receiving LEVOTHROID® (see **WARNINGS, PRECAUTIONS, and DOSAGE AND ADMINISTRATION**).

Pediatrics

In patients with congenital hypothyroidism, the adequacy of replacement therapy should be assessed by measuring both serum TSH (using a sensitive assay) and total- or free-T_4. During the first three years of life, the serum total- or free-T_4 should be maintained at all times in the upper half of the normal range. While the aim of therapy is to also normalize the serum TSH level, this is not always possible in a small percentage of patients, particularly in the first few months of therapy. TSH may not normalize due to a resetting of the pituitary-thyroid feedback threshold as a result of in utero hypothyroidism. Failure of the serum T_4 to increase into the upper half of the normal range within 2

Continued on next page

Levothroid—Cont.

weeks of initiation of LEVOTHROID® therapy and/or of the serum TSH to decrease below 20mU/L within 4 weeks should alert the physician to the possibility that the child is not receiving adequate therapy. Careful inquiry should then be made regarding compliance, dose of medication administered, and method of administration prior to raising the dose of LEVOTHROID®.

The recommended frequency of monitoring of TSH and total- or free-T_4 in children is as follows: at 2 and 4 weeks after the initiation of treatment; every 1-2 months during the first year of life; every 2-3 months between 1 and 3 years of age; and every 3 to 12 months thereafter until growth is completed. More frequent intervals of monitoring may be necessary if poor compliance is suspected or abnormal values are obtained. It is recommended that TSH and T_4 levels, and a physical examination, if indicated, be performed 2 weeks after any change in LEVOTHROID® dosage. Routine clinical examination, including assessment of mental and physical growth and development, and bone maturation, should be performed at regular intervals (see **PRECAUTIONS, Pediatric Use** and **DOSAGE AND ADMINISTRATION**).

Secondary (pituitary) and tertiary (hypothalamic) hypothyroidism

Adequacy of therapy should be assessed by measuring serum free-T_4 levels, which should be maintained in the upper half of the normal range in these patients.

Drug Interactions

Many drugs affect thyroid hormone pharmacokinetics and metabolism (e.g., absorption, synthesis, secretion, catabolism, protein binding, and target tissue response) and may alter the therapeutic response to LEVOTHROID®. In addition, thyroid hormones and thyroid status have varied effects on the pharmacokinetics and actions of other drugs. A listing of drug-thyroidal axis interactions is contained in Table 2.

The list of drug-thyroidal axis interactions in Table 2 may not be comprehensive due to the introduction of new drugs that interact with the thyroidal axis or the discovery of previously unknown interactions. The prescriber should be aware of this fact and should consult appropriate reference sources (e.g., package inserts of newly approved drugs, medical literature) for additional information if a drug-drug interaction with levothyroxine is suspected.

[See table 2 at right and on next page]

Oral anticoagulants - Levothyroxine increases the response to oral anticoagulant therapy. Therefore, a decrease in the dose of anticoagulant may be warranted with correction of the hypothyroid state or when the LEVOTHROID® dose is increased. Prothrombin time should be closely monitored to permit appropriate and timely dosage adjustments (see **Table 2**).

Digitalis glycosides - The therapeutic effects of digitalis glycosides may be reduced by levothyroxine. Serum digitalis glycoside levels may be decreased when a hypothyroid patient becomes euthyroid, necessitating an increase in the dose of digitalis glycosides (see **Table 2**).

Drug-Food Interactions - Consumption of certain foods may affect levothyroxine absorption thereby necessitating adjustments in dosing. Soybean flour (infant formula), cotton seed meal, walnuts, and dietary fiber may bind and decrease the absorption of levothyroxine sodium from the GI tract.

Drug-Laboratory Test Interactions - Changes in TBG concentration must be considered when interpreting T_4 and T_3 values, which necessitates measurement and evaluation of unbound (free) hormone and/or determination of the free-T_4 index (FT_4I). Pregnancy, infectious hepatitis, estrogens, estrogen-containing oral contraceptives, and acute intermittent porphyria increase TBG concentrations. Decreases in TBG concentrations are observed in nephrosis, severe hypoproteinemia, severe liver disease, acromegaly, and after androgen or corticosteroid therapy (see also **Table 2**). Familial hyper- or hypo-thyroxine binding globulinemias have been described, with the incidence of TBG deficiency approximating 1 in 9000.

Carcinogenesis, Mutagenesis, and Impairment of Fertility - Animal studies have not been performed to evaluate the carcinogenic potential, mutagenic potential or effects on fertility of levothyroxine. The synthetic T_4 in LEVOTHROID® is identical to that produced naturally by the human thyroid gland. Although there has been a reported association between prolonged thyroid hormone therapy and breast cancer, this has not been confirmed. Patients receiving LEVOTHROID® for appropriate clinical indications should be titrated to the lowest effective replacement dose.

Pregnancy - Category A - Studies in women taking levothyroxine sodium during pregnancy have not shown an increased risk of congenital abnormalities. Therefore, the possibility of fetal harm appears remote. LEVOTHROID® should not be discontinued during pregnancy and hypothyroidism diagnosed during pregnancy should be promptly treated.

Hypothyroidism during pregnancy is associated with a higher rate of complications, including spontaneous abortion, pre-eclampsia, stillbirth and premature delivery. Maternal hypothyroidism may have an adverse effect on fetal and childhood growth and development. During pregnancy, serum T_4 levels may decrease and serum TSH levels increase to values outside the normal range. Since elevations in serum TSH may occur as early as 4 weeks gestation, pregnant women taking LEVOTHROID® should have their

Table 2: Drug-Thyroidal Axis Interactions

Drugs that may reduce TSH secretion - the reduction is not sustained; therefore, hypothyroidism does not occur

Drug or Drug Class		
Dopamine / Dopamine Agonists	Glucocorticoids	Octreotide

Effect - Use of these agents may result in a transient reduction in TSH secretion when administered at the following doses: Dopamine (≥1 μg/kg/min); Glucocorticoids (hydrocortisone ≥100 mg/day or equivalent); Octreotide (>100 μg/day).

Drugs that alter thyroid hormone secretion

Drugs that may decrease thyroid hormone secretion, which may result in hypothyroidism

Drug or Drug Class		
Aminoglutethimide	Iodide	Methimazole
Amiodarone	(including iodine-containing	Propylthiouracil (PTU)
	Radiographic contrast agents)	Sulfonamides
	Lithium	Tolbutamide

Effect - Long-term lithium therapy can result in goiter in up to 50% of patients, and either subclinical or overt hypothyroidism, each in up to 20% of patients. The fetus, neonate, elderly and euthyroid patients with underlying thyroid disease (e.g., Hashimoto's thyroiditis or with Grave's disease previously treated with radioiodine or surgery) are among those individuals who are particularly susceptible to iodine-induced hypothyroidism. Oral cholecystographic agents and amiodarone are slowly excreted, producing more prolonged hypothyroidism than parenterally administered iodinated contrast agents. Long-term aminoglutethimide therapy may minimally decrease T_4 and T_3 levels and increase TSH, although all values remain within normal limits in most patients.

Drugs that may increase thyroid hormone secretion, which may result in hyperthyroidism

Drug or Drug Class
Amiodarone
Iodide (including iodine-containing Radiographic contrast agents)

Effect - Iodide and drugs that contain pharmacological amounts of iodide may cause hyperthyroidism in euthyroid patients with Grave's disease previously treated with antithyroid drugs or in euthyroid patients with thyroid autonomy (e.g., multinodular goiter or hyperfunctioning thyroid adenoma). Hyperthyroidism may develop over several weeks and may persist for several months after therapy discontinuation. Amiodarone may induce hyperthyroidism by causing thyroiditis.

Drugs that may decrease T_4 absorption, which may result in hypothyroidism

Drug or Drug Class		
Antacids	Bile Acid Sequestrants	Cation Exchange Resins
- Aluminum & Magnesium	- Cholestyramine	- Kayexalate
Hydroxides	- Colestipol	Ferrous Sulfate
- Simethicone	Calcium Carbonate	Sucralfate

Effect - Concurrent use may reduce the efficacy of levothyroxine by binding and delaying or preventing absorption, potentially resulting in hypothyroidism. Calcium carbonate may form an insoluble chelate with levothyroxine, and ferrous sulfate likely forms a ferric-thyroxine complex. Administer levothyroxine at least 4 hours apart from these agents.

Drugs that may alter T_4 and T_3 serum transport - but FT_4 concentration remains normal; and, therefore, the patient remains euthyroid

Drugs that may increase serum TBG concentration

Clofibrate	Estrogens (oral)	Mitotane
Estrogen-containing	Heroin / Methadone	Tamoxifen
oral contraceptives	5-Flourouracil	

Drugs that may decrease serum TBG concentration

Androgens / Anabolic Steroids	Glucocorticoids
Asparaginase	Slow-Release Nicotinic Acid

Drugs that may cause protein-binding site displacement

Drug or Drug Class	
Furosemide (> 80 mg IV)	Non Steroidal Anti-Inflammatory Drugs
Heparin	- Fenamates
Hydantoins	- Phenylbutazone
	Salicylates (> 2 g/day)

Effect - Administration of these agents with levothyroxine results in an initial transient increase in FT_4. Continued administration results in a decrease in serum T_4 and normal FT_4 and TSH concentrations and, therefore, patients are clinically euthyroid. Salicylates inhibit binding of T_4 and T_3 to TBG and transthyretin. An initial increase in serum FT_4 is followed by return of FT_4 to normal levels with sustained therapeutic serum salicylate concentrations, although total-T_4 levels may decrease by as much as 30%.

Drugs that may alter T_4 and T_3 metabolism

Drugs that may increase hepatic metabolism, which may result in hypothyroidism

Drug or Drug Class			
Carbamazepine	Hydantoins	Phenobarbital	Rifampin

Effect - Stimulation of hepatic microsomal drug-metabolizing enzyme activity may cause increased hepatic degradation of levothyroxine, resulting in increased levothyroxine requirements. Phenytoin and carbamazepine reduce serum protein binding of levothyroxine, and total- and free-T_4 may be reduced by 20% to 40%, but most patients have normal serum TSH levels and are clinically euthyroid.

(Table continued on next page)

TSH measured during each trimester. An elevated serum TSH level should be corrected by an increase in the dose of LEVOTHROID®. Since postpartum TSH levels are similar to preconception values, the LEVOTHROID® dosage should return to the pre-pregnancy dose immediately after delivery. A serum TSH level should be obtained 6-8 weeks postpartum.

Thyroid hormones cross the placental barrier to some extent as evidenced by levels in cord blood of athyreotic fetuses being approximately one-third maternal levels. Transfer of thyroid hormone from the mother to the fetus, however, may not be adequate to prevent *in utero* hypothyroidism.

Nursing Mothers - Although thyroid hormones are excreted only minimally in human milk, caution should be exercised when LEVOTHROID® is administered to a nursing woman. However, adequate replacement doses of levothyroxine are generally needed to maintain normal lactation.

Pediatric Use

General

The goal of treatment in pediatric patients with hypothyroidism is to achieve and maintain normal intellectual and physical growth and development.

The initial dose of levothyroxine varies with age and body weight (see **DOSAGE AND ADMINISTRATION, Table 3**). Dosing adjustments are based on an assessment of the individual patient's clinical and laboratory parameters (see **PRECAUTIONS, Laboratory Tests**).

In children in whom a diagnosis of permanent hypothyroidism has not been established, it is recommended that levothyroxine administration be discontinued for a 30-day trial period, but only after the child is at least 3 years of age. Serum T_4 and TSH levels should then be obtained. If the T_4 is low and the TSH high, the diagnosis of permanent hypothyroidism is established, and levothyroxine therapy should be reinstituted. If the T_4 and TSH levels are normal, euthyroidism may be assumed and, therefore, the hypothyroidism can be considered to have been transient. In this instance, however, the physician should carefully monitor the child and repeat the thyroid function tests if any signs or symptoms of hypothyroidism develop. In this setting, the clinician should have a high index of suspicion of relapse. If the results of the levothyroxine withdrawal test are inconclusive, careful follow-up and subsequent testing will be necessary.

Since some more severely affected children may become clinically hypothyroid when treatment is discontinued for 30 days, an alternate approach is to reduce the replacement dose of levothyroxine by half during the 30-day trial period. If, after 30 days, the serum TSH is elevated above 20 mU/L, the diagnosis of permanent hypothyroidism is confirmed, and full replacement therapy should be resumed. However, if the serum TSH has not risen to greater than 20 mU/L, levothyroxine treatment should be discontinued for another 30-day trial period followed by repeat serum T_4 and TSH testing.

The presence of concomitant medical conditions should be considered in certain clinical circumstances and, if present, appropriately treated (see **PRECAUTIONS**).

Congenital Hypothyroidism (see **PRECAUTIONS, Laboratory Tests** and **DOSAGE AND ADMINISTRATION**)

Rapid restoration of normal serum T_4 concentrations is essential for preventing the adverse effects of congenital hypothyroidism on intellectual development as well as on overall physical growth and maturation. Therefore, LEVOTHROID® therapy should be initiated immediately upon diagnosis and is generally continued for life.

During the first 2 weeks of LEVOTHROID® therapy, infants should be closely monitored for cardiac overload, arrhythmias, and aspiration from avid suckling.

The patient should be monitored closely to avoid undertreatment or overtreatment. Undertreatment may have deleterious effects on intellectual development and linear growth. Overtreatment has been associated with craniosynostosis in infants, and may adversely affect the tempo of brain maturation and accelerate the bone age with resultant premature closure of the epiphyses and compromised adult stature.

Acquired Hypothyroidism in Pediatric Patients

The patient should be monitored closely to avoid undertreatment and overtreatment. Undertreatment may result in poor school performance due to impaired concentration and slowed mentation and in reduced adult height. Overtreatment may accelerate the bone age and result in premature epiphyseal closure and compromised adult stature.

Treated children may manifest a period of catch-up growth, which may be adequate in some cases to normalize adult height. In children with severe or prolonged hypothyroidism, catch-up growth may not be adequate to normalize adult height.

Geriatric Use

Because of the increased prevalence of cardiovascular disease among the elderly, levothyroxine therapy should not be initiated at the full replacement dose (see **WARNINGS, PRECAUTIONS,** and **DOSAGE AND ADMINISTRATION**).

ADVERSE REACTIONS

Adverse reactions associated with levothyroxine therapy are primarily those of hyperthyroidism due to therapeutic overdosage (see **PRECAUTIONS** and **OVERDOSAGE**). They include the following:

General: fatigue, increased appetite, weight loss, heat intolerance, fever, excessive sweating;

Central nervous system: headache, hyperactivity, nervousness, anxiety, irritability, emotional lability, insomnia;

Musculoskeletal: tremors, muscle weakness;

Cardiovascular: palpitations, tachycardia, arrhythmias, increased pulse and blood pressure, heart failure, angina, myocardial infarction, cardiac arrest;

Respiratory: dyspnea;

Gastrointestinal: diarrhea, vomiting, abdominal cramps and elevations in liver function tests;

Dermatologic: hair loss, flushing;

Endocrine: decreased bone mineral density;

Reproductive: menstrual irregularities, impaired fertility.

Pseudotumor cerebri and slipped capital femoral epiphysis have been reported in children receiving levothyroxine therapy. Overtreatment may result in craniosynostosis in infants and premature closure of the epiphyses in children with resultant compromised adult height.

Seizures have been reported rarely with the institution of levothyroxine therapy.

Inadequate levothyroxine dosage will produce or fail to ameliorate the signs and symptoms of hypothyroidism.

Hypersensitivity reactions to inactive ingredients have occurred in patients treated with thyroid hormone products. These include urticaria, pruritus, skin rash, flushing, angioedema, various GI symptoms (abdominal pain, nausea, vomiting and diarrhea), fever, arthralgia, serum sickness and wheezing. Hypersensitivity to levothyroxine itself is not known to occur.

OVERDOSAGE

The signs and symptoms of overdosage are those of hyperthyroidism (see **PRECAUTIONS** and **ADVERSE REACTIONS**). In addition, confusion and disorientation may occur. Cerebral embolism, shock, coma, and death have been reported. Seizures have occurred in a child ingesting 18 mg

---

Table 2 (cont.): Drug-Thyroidal Axis Interactions

Drugs that may decrease T_4 5'-deiodinase activity

Drug or Drug Class

Amiodarone	Glucocorticoids
Beta-adrenergic antagonists	- (e.g., Dexamethasone ≥4 mg/day)
- (e.g., Propranolol > 160 mg/day)	Propylthiouracil (PTU)

Effect - Administration of these enzyme inhibitors decreases the peripheral conversion of T_4 to T_3, leading to decreased T_3 levels. However, serum T_4 levels are usually normal but may occasionally be slightly increased. In patients treated with large doses of propranolol (> 160 mg/day), T_3 and T_4 levels change slightly, TSH levels remain normal, and patients are clinically euthyroid. It should be noted that actions of particular beta-adrenergic antagonists may be impaired when the hypothyroid patient is converted to the euthyroid state. Short-term administration of large doses of glucocorticoids may decrease serum T_3 concentrations by 30% with minimal change in serum T_4 levels. However, long-term glucocorticoid therapy may result in slightly decreased T_3 and T_4 levels due to decreased TBG production (see above).

Miscellaneous

Drug or Drug Class

Anticoagulants (oral)

- Coumarin Derivatives	- Indandione Derivatives

Effect - Thyroid hormones appear to increase the catabolism of vitamin K-dependent clotting factors, thereby increasing the anticoagulant activity of oral anticoagulants. Concomitant use of these agents impairs the compensatory increases in clotting factor synthesis. Prothrombin time should be carefully monitored in patients taking levothyroxine and oral anticoagulants and the dose of anticoagulant therapy adjusted accordingly.

Drug or Drug Class

Antidepressants

- Tricyclics (e.g., Amitriptyline)	- Selective Serotonin Reuptake Inhibitors
- Tetracyclics (e.g., Maprotiline)	(SSRIs; e.g., Sertraline)

Effect - Concurrent use of tri/tetracyclic antidepressants and levothyroxine may increase the therapeutic and toxic effects of both drugs, possibly due to increased receptor sensitivity to catecholamines. Toxic effects may include increased risk of cardiac arrhythmias and CNS stimulation; onset of action of tricyclics may be accelerated. Administration of sertraline in patients stabilized on levothyroxine may result in increased levothyroxine requirements.

Drug or Drug Class

Antidiabetic Agents	- Meglitinides	- Sulfonylureas
- Biguanides	- Thiazolidinediones	- Insulin

Effect - Addition of levothyroxine to antidiabetic or insulin therapy may result in increased antidiabetic agent or insulin requirements. Careful monitoring of diabetic control is recommended, especially when thyroid therapy is started, changed, or discontinued.

Drug or Drug Class

Cardiac Glycosides

Effect - Serum digitalis glycoside levels may be reduced in hyperthyroidism or when the hypothyroid patient is converted to the euthyroid state. Therapeutic effect of digitalis glycosides may be reduced.

Drug or Drug Class

Cytokines	- Interferon-α	- Interleukin-2

Effect - Therapy with interferon-α has been associated with the development of antithyroid microsomal antibodies in 20% of patients and some have transient hypothyroidism, hyperthyroidism, or both. Patients who have antithyroid antibodies before treatment are at higher risk for thyroid dysfunction during treatment. Interleukin-2 has been associated with transient painless thyroiditis in 20% of patients. Interferon-β and -γ have not been reported to cause thyroid dysfunction.

Drug or Drug Class

Growth Hormones	- Somatrem	- Somatropin

Effect - Excessive use of thyroid hormones with growth hormones may accelerate epiphyseal closure. However, untreated hypothyroidism may interfere with growth response to growth hormone.

Drug or Drug Class

Ketamine

Effect - Concurrent use may produce marked hypertension and tachycardia; cautious administration to patients receiving thyroid hormone therapy is recommended.

Drug or Drug Class

Methylxanthine Bronchodilators	- (e.g., Theophylline)

Effect - Decreased theophylline clearance may occur in hypothyroid patients; clearance returns to normal when the euthyroid state is achieved.

Drug or Drug Class

Radiographic Agents

Effect - Thyroid hormones may reduce the uptake of ^{123}I, ^{131}I, and ^{99m}Tc.

Drug or Drug Class

Sympathomimetics

Effect - Concurrent use may increase the effects of sympathomimetics or thyroid hormone. Thyroid hormones may increase the risk of coronary insufficiency when sympathomimetic agents are administered to patients with coronary artery disease.

Drug or Drug Class

Chloral Hydrate	Metoclopramide	Perphenazine
Diazepam	6-Mercaptopurine	Resorcinol
Ethionamide	Nitroprusside	(excessive topical use)
Lovastatin	Para-aminosalicylate sodium	Thiazide Diuretics

Effect - These agents have been associated with thyroid hormone and / or TSH level alterations by various mechanisms.

---

of levothyroxine. Symptoms may not necessarily be evident or may not appear until several days after ingestion of levothyroxine sodium.

Treatment of Overdosage

Levothyroxine sodium should be reduced in dose or temporarily discontinued if signs or symptoms of overdosage occur.

Acute Massive Overdosage - This may be a life-threatening emergency, therefore, symptomatic and supportive therapy should be instituted immediately. If not contraindicated (e.g., by seizures, coma, or loss of the gag reflex), the stomach should be emptied by emesis or gastric lavage to decrease gastrointestinal absorption. Activated charcoal or cholestyramine may also be used to decrease absorption. Central and peripheral increased sympathetic activity may be treated by administering β-receptor antagonists, e.g., propranolol, provided there are no medical contraindications to their use. Provide respiratory support as needed; control congestive heart failure and arrhythmia; control fever, hypoglycemia, and fluid loss as necessary. Large doses of antithyroid drugs (e.g., methimazole or propylthiouracil) followed in one to two hours by large doses of iodine may be given to inhibit synthesis and release of thyroid hormones. Glucocorticoids may be given to inhibit the conversion of T_4 to T_3. Plasmapheresis, charcoal hemoperfusion and exchange transfusion have been reserved for cases in which continued clinical deterioration occurs despite conventional therapy. Because T_4 is highly protein bound, very little drug will be removed by dialysis.

DOSAGE AND ADMINISTRATION

General Principles

The goal of replacement therapy is to achieve and maintain a clinical and biochemical euthyroid state. The goal of suppressive therapy is to inhibit growth and/or function of abnormal thyroid tissue. The dose of LEVOTHROID® that is

Continued on next page

Levothroid—Cont.

adequate to achieve these goals depends on a variety of factors including the patient's age, body weight, cardiovascular status, concomitant medical conditions, including pregnancy, concomitant medications, and the specific nature of the condition being treated (see **WARNINGS** and **PRECAUTIONS**). Hence, the following recommendations serve only as dosing guidelines. Dosing must be individualized and adjustments made based on periodic assessment of the patient's clinical response and laboratory parameters (see **PRECAUTIONS, Laboratory Tests**).

LEVOTHROID® is administered as a single daily dose, preferably one-half to one hour before breakfast. LEVOTHROID® should be taken at least 4 hours apart from drugs that are known to interfere with its absorption (see **PRECAUTIONS, Drug Interactions**).

Due to the long half-life of levothyroxine, the peak therapeutic effect at a given dose of levothyroxine sodium may not be attained for 4-6 weeks.

Caution should be exercised when administering LEVOTHROID® to patients with underlying cardiovascular disease, to the elderly, and to those with concomitant adrenal insufficiency (see **PRECAUTIONS**).

Specific Patient Populations

Hypothyroidism in Adults and in Children in Whom Growth and Puberty are Complete (see **WARNINGS and PRECAUTIONS, Laboratory Tests**)

Therapy may begin at full replacement doses in otherwise healthy individuals less than 50 years old and in those older than 50 years who have been recently treated for hyperthyroidism or who have been hypothyroid for only a short time (such as a few months). The average full replacement dose of levothyroxine sodium is approximately 1.7 mcg/kg/day (e.g., **100-125 mcg/day** for a 70 kg adult). Older patients may require less than 1 mcg/kg/day. Levothyroxine sodium doses greater than 200 mcg/day are seldom required. An inadequate response to daily doses ≥300 mcg/day is rare and may indicate poor compliance, malabsorption, and/or drug interactions.

For most patients older than 50 years or for patients under 50 years of age with underlying cardiac disease, an initial starting dose of **25-50 mcg/day** of levothyroxine sodium is recommended, with gradual increments in dose at 6-8 week intervals, as needed. The recommended starting dose of levothyroxine sodium in elderly patients with cardiac disease is **12.5-25 mcg/day**, with gradual dose increments at 4-6 week intervals. The levothyroxine sodium dose is generally adjusted in 12.5-25 mcg increments until the patient with primary hypothyroidism is clinically euthyroid and the serum TSH has normalized.

In patients with severe hypothyroidism, the recommended initial levothyroxine sodium dose is **12.5-25 mcg/day** with increases of 25 mcg/day every 2-4 weeks, accompanied by clinical and laboratory assessment, until the TSH level is normalized.

In patients with secondary (pituitary) or tertiary (hypothalamic) hypothyroidism, the levothyroxine sodium dose should be titrated until the patient is clinically euthyroid and the serum free-T_4 level is restored to the upper half of the normal range.

Pediatric Dosage - Congenital or Acquired Hypothyroidism (see **PRECAUTIONS, Laboratory Tests**)

General Principles

In general, levothyroxine therapy should be instituted at full replacement doses as soon as possible. Delays in diagnosis and institution of therapy may have deleterious effects on the child's intellectual and physical growth and development.

Undertreatment and overtreatment should be avoided (see **PRECAUTIONS, Pediatric Use**).

LEVOTHROID® may be administered to infants and children who cannot swallow intact tablets by crushing the tablet and suspending the freshly crushed tablet in a small amount (5-10 mL or 1-2 teaspoons) of water. This suspension can be administered by spoon or dropper. **DO NOT STORE THE SUSPENSION.** Foods that decrease absorption of levothyroxine, such as soybean infant formula, should not be used for administering levothyroxine sodium tablets (see **PRECAUTIONS, Drug-Food Interactions**).

Newborns

The recommended starting dose of levothyroxine sodium in newborn infants is **10-15 mcg/kg/day.** A lower starting dose (e.g., 25 mcg/day) should be considered in infants at risk for cardiac failure, and the dose should be increased in 4–6 weeks as needed based on clinical and laboratory response to treatment. In infants with very low (<5 mcg/dL) or undetectable serum T_4 concentrations, the recommended initial starting dose is **50 mcg/day** of levothyroxine sodium.

Infants and Children

Levothyroxine therapy is usually initiated at full replacement doses, with the recommended dose per body weight decreasing with age (see **Table 3**). However, in children with chronic or severe hypothyroidism, an initial dose of **25 mcg/day** of levothyroxine sodium is recommended with increments of 25 mcg every 2-4 weeks until the desired effect is achieved.

Hyperactivity in an older child can be minimized if the starting dose is one-fourth of the recommended full replacement dose, and the dose is then increased on a weekly basis by an amount equal to one-fourth the full-recommended replacement dose until the full recommended replacement dose is reached.

Table 3: Levothyroxine Sodium Dosing Guidelines for Pediatric Hypothyroidism

AGE	Daily Dose Per Kg Body Weight[a]
0–3 months	10–15 mcg/kg/day
3–6 months	8–10 mcg/kg/day
6–12 months	6–8 mcg/kg/day
1–5 years	5–6 mcg/kg/day
6–12 years	4–5 mcg/kg/day
>12 years but growth and puberty incomplete	2–3 mcg/kg/day
Growth and puberty complete	1.7 mcg/kg/day

[a] The dose should be adjusted based on clinical response and laboratory parameters (see **PRECAUTIONS, Laboratory Tests** and **Pediatric Use**).

Pregnancy - Pregnancy may increase levothyroxine requirements (see **Pregnancy**).

Subclinical Hypothyroidism - If this condition is treated, a lower levothyroxine sodium dose (e.g., **1 mcg/kg/day**) than that used for full replacement may be adequate to normalize the serum TSH level. Patients who are not treated should be monitored yearly for changes in clinical status and thyroid laboratory parameters.

TSH Suppression in Well-differentiated Thyroid Cancer and Thyroid Nodules - The target level for TSH suppression in these conditions has not been established with controlled studies. In addition, the efficacy of TSH suppression for benign nodular disease is controversial. Therefore, the dose of LEVOTHROID® used for TSH suppression should be individualized based on the specific disease and the patient being treated.

In the treatment of well-differentiated (papillary and follicular) thyroid cancer, levothyroxine is used as an adjunct to surgery and radioiodine therapy. Generally, TSH is suppressed to <0.1 mU/L, and this usually requires a levothyroxine sodium dose of **greater than 2 mcg/kg/day**. However, in patients with high-risk tumors, the target level for TSH suppression may be <0.01 mU/L.

In the treatment of benign nodules and nontoxic multinodular goiter, TSH is generally suppressed to a higher target (e.g., 0.1 to either 0.5 or 1.0 mU/L) than that used for the treatment of thyroid cancer. Levothyroxine sodium is contraindicated if the serum TSH is already suppressed due to the risk of precipitating overt thyrotoxicosis (see **CONTRAINDICATIONS, WARNINGS** and **PRECAUTIONS**).

Myxedema Coma - Myxedema coma is a life-threatening emergency characterized by poor circulation and hypometabolism, and may result in unpredictable absorption of levothyroxine sodium from the gastrointestinal tract. Therefore, oral thyroid hormone drug products are not recommended to treat this condition. Thyroid hormone drug products formulated for intravenous administration should be administered.

HOW SUPPLIED

LEVOTHROID® (levothyroxine sodium tablets, USP) are caplet-shaped, color-coded, potency marked tablets and are supplied as follows:

Strength (mcg)	Color	NDC # for bottles of 100	NDC # for bottles of 1000
25	Orange	NDC 0456-1320-01	NDC 0456-1320-00
50	White	NDC 0456-1321-01	NDC 0456-1321-00
75	Violet	NDC 0456-1322-01	NDC 0456-1322-00
88	Mint Green	NDC 0456-1329-01	NDC 0456-1329-00
100	Yellow	NDC 0456-1323-01	NDC 0456-1323-00
112	Rose	NDC 0456-1330-01	NDC 0456-1330-00
125	Brown	NDC 0456-1324-01	NDC 0456-1324-00
137	Deep Blue	NDC 0456-1331-01	NDC 0456-1331-00
150	Blue	NDC 0456-1325-01	NDC 0456-1325-00
175	Lilac	NDC 0456-1326-01	NDC 0456-1326-00
200	Pink	NDC 0456-1327-01	NDC 0456-1327-00
300	Green	NDC 0456-1328-01	NDC 0456-1328-00

STORAGE CONDITIONS

Store at 25°C (77°F) with excursions permitted to 15-30°C (59-86°F).

Protect from moisture and light.

Manufactured for:
FOREST PHARMACEUTICALS, INC.
Subsidiary of Forest Laboratories, Inc.
St. Louis, Missouri, 63045
by:
Lloyd Pharmaceutical
Division of Lloyd, Inc.
Shenandoah, IA 51601

Rev. 07/04
RMC 8950

LEXAPRO® ℞

[lĕks'ă-prō]
(escitalopram oxalate)
TABLETS/ORAL SOLUTION
Rx Only

Prescribing information for this product, which appears on pages 1282–1286 of the 2005 PDR, has been completely revised as follows. Please write "See Supplement A" next to the product heading.

Suicidality in Children and Adolescents

Antidepressants increased the risk of suicidal thinking and behavior (suicidality) in short-term studies in children and adolescents with Major Depressive Disorder (MDD) and other psychiatric disorders. Anyone considering the use of Lexapro or any other antidepressant in a child or adolescent must balance this risk with the clinical need. Patients who are started on therapy should be observed closely for clinical worsening, suicidality, or unusual changes in behavior. Families and caregivers should be advised of the need for close observation and communication with the prescriber. Lexapro is not approved for use in pediatric patients. (See Warnings and Precautions: Pediatric Use)

Pooled analyses of short-term (4 to 16 weeks) placebo-controlled trials of 9 antidepressant drugs (SSRIs and others) in children and adolescents with major depressive disorder (MDD), obsessive compulsive disorder (OCD), or other psychiatric disorders (a total of 24 trials involving over 4400 patients) have revealed a greater risk of adverse events representing suicidal thinking or behavior (suicidality) during the first few months of treatment in those receiving antidepressants. The average risk of such events in patients receiving antidepressants was 4%, twice the placebo risk of 2%. No suicides occurred in these trials.

DESCRIPTION

Lexapro® (escitalopram oxalate) is an orally administered selective serotonin reuptake inhibitor (SSRI). Escitalopram is the pure S-enantiomer (single isomer) of the racemic bicyclic phthalane derivative citalopram. Escitalopram oxalate is designated S-(+)-1-[3-(dimethyl-amino)propyl]-1-(*p*-fluorophenyl)-5-phthalancarbonitrile oxalate with the following structural formula:

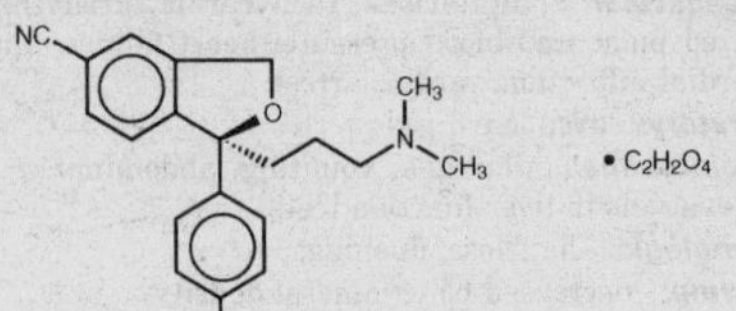

The molecular formula is $C_{20}H_{21}FN_2O \bullet C_2H_2O_4$ and the molecular weight is 414.40.

Escitalopram oxalate occurs as a fine, white to slightly-yellow powder and is freely soluble in methanol and dimethyl sulfoxide (DMSO), soluble in isotonic saline solution, sparingly soluble in water and ethanol, slightly soluble in ethyl acetate, and insoluble in heptane.

Lexapro (escitalopram oxalate) is available as tablets or as an oral solution.

Lexapro tablets are film-coated, round tablets containing escitalopram oxalate in strengths equivalent to 5 mg, 10 mg, and 20 mg escitalopram base. The 10 and 20 mg tablets are scored. The tablets also contain the following inactive ingredients: talc, croscarmellose sodium, microcrystalline cellulose/colloidal silicon dioxide, and magnesium stearate. The film coating contains hypromellose, titanium dioxide, and polyethylene glycol.

Lexapro oral solution contains escitalopram oxalate equivalent to 1 mg/mL escitalopram base. It also contains the following inactive ingredients: sorbitol, purified water, citric acid, sodium citrate, malic acid, glycerin, propylene glycol, methylparaben, propylparaben, and natural peppermint flavor.

CLINICAL PHARMACOLOGY
Pharmacodynamics

The mechanism of antidepressant action of escitalopram, the S-enantiomer of racemic citalopram, is presumed to be linked to potentiation of serotonergic activity in the central nervous system (CNS) resulting from its inhibition of CNS neuronal reuptake of serotonin (5-HT). In vitro and in vivo studies in animals suggest that escitalopram is a highly selective serotonin reuptake inhibitor (SSRI) with minimal effects on norepinephrine and dopamine neuronal reuptake. Escitalopram is at least 100-fold more potent than the R-enantiomer with respect to inhibition of 5-HT reuptake and inhibition of 5-HT neuronal firing rate. Tolerance to a model of antidepressant effect in rats was not induced by long-term (up to 5 weeks) treatment with escitalopram. Escitalopram has no or very low affinity for serotonergic $(5-HT_{1-7})$ or other receptors including alpha- and beta-adrenergic, dopamine (D_{1-5}), histamine (H_{1-3}), muscarinic (M_{1-5}), and benzodiazepine receptors. Escitalopram also does not bind to, or has low affinity for, various ion channels including Na^+, K^+, Cl^-, and Ca^{++} channels. Antagonism of muscarinic, histaminergic, and adrenergic receptors has been hypothesized to be associated with various anticholinergic, sedative, and cardiovascular side effects of other psychotropic drugs.

Pharmacokinetics

The single- and multiple-dose pharmacokinetics of escitalopram are linear and dose-proportional in a dose range of 10 to 30 mg/day. Biotransformation of escitalopram is mainly hepatic, with a mean terminal half-life of about 27-32 hours. With once-daily dosing, steady state plasma concentrations are achieved within approximately one week. At steady state, the extent of accumulation of escitalopram in plasma in young healthy subjects was 2.2-2.5 times the plasma concentrations observed after a single dose. The tablet and the oral solution dosage forms of escitalopram oxalate are bioequivalent.

Absorption and Distribution

Following a single oral dose (20 mg tablet or solution) of escitalopram, peak blood levels occur at about 5 hours. Absorption of escitalopram is not affected by food.

The absolute bioavailability of citalopram is about 80% relative to an intravenous dose, and the volume of distribution of citalopram is about 12 L/kg. Data specific on escitalopram are unavailable.

The binding of escitalopram to human plasma proteins is approximately 56%.

Metabolism and Elimination

Following oral administrations of escitalopram, the fraction of drug recovered in the urine as escitalopram and S-demethylcitalopram (S-DCT) is about 8% and 10%, respectively. The oral clearance of escitalopram is 600 mL/min, with approximately 7% of that due to renal clearance.

Escitalopram is metabolized to S-DCT and S-didemethylcitalopram (S-DDCT). In humans, unchanged escitalopram is the predominant compound in plasma. At steady state, the concentration of the escitalopram metabolite S-DCT in plasma is approximately one-third that of escitalopram. The level of S-DDCT was not detectable in most subjects. In vitro studies show that escitalopram is at least 7 and 27 times more potent than S-DCT and S-DDCT, respectively, in the inhibition of serotonin reuptake, suggesting that the metabolites of escitalopram do not contribute significantly to the antidepressant actions of escitalopram. S-DCT and S-DDCT also have no or very low affinity for serotonergic $(5-HT_{1-7})$ or other receptors including alpha- and beta-adrenergic, dopamine (D_{1-5}), histamine (H_{1-3}), muscarinic (M_{1-5}), and benzodiazepine receptors. S-DCT and S-DDCT also do not bind to various ion channels including Na^+, K^+, Cl^-, and Ca^{++} channels.

In vitro studies using human liver microsomes indicated that CYP3A4 and CYP2C19 are the primary isozymes involved in the N-demethylation of escitalopram.

Population Subgroups

Age—Escitalopram pharmacokinetics in subjects ≥ 65 years of age were compared to younger subjects in a single-dose and a multiple-dose study. Escitalopram AUC and half-life were increased by approximately 50% in elderly subjects, and C_{max} was unchanged. 10 mg is the recommended dose for elderly patients (see **DOSAGE AND ADMINISTRATION**).

Gender—In a multiple-dose study of escitalopram (10 mg/day for 3 weeks) in 18 male (9 elderly and 9 young) and 18 female (9 elderly and 9 young) subjects, there were no differences in AUC, C_{max}, and half-life between the male and female subjects. No adjustment of dosage on the basis of gender is needed.

Reduced hepatic function—Citalopram oral clearance was reduced by 37% and half-life was doubled in patients with reduced hepatic function compared to normal subjects. 10 mg is the recommended dose of escitalopram for most hepatically impaired patients (see **DOSAGE AND ADMINISTRATION**).

Reduced renal function—In patients with mild to moderate renal function impairment, oral clearance of citalopram was reduced by 17% compared to normal subjects. No adjustment of dosage for such patients is recommended. No information is available about the pharmacokinetics of escitalopram in patients with severely reduced renal function (creatinine clearance < 20 mL/min).

Drug-Drug Interactions

In vitro enzyme inhibition data did not reveal an inhibitory effect of escitalopram on CYP3A4, -1A2, -2C9, -2C19, and -2E1. Based on in vitro data, escitalopram would be expected to have little inhibitory effect on in vivo metabolism mediated by these cytochromes. While in vivo data to address this question are limited, results from drug interaction studies suggest that escitalopram, at a dose of 20 mg, has no 3A4 inhibitory effect and a modest 2D6 inhibitory effect. See **Drug Interactions** under **PRECAUTIONS** for more detailed information on available drug interaction data.

Clinical Efficacy Trials
Major Depressive Disorder

The efficacy of Lexapro as a treatment for major depressive disorder was established in three, 8-week, placebo-controlled studies conducted in outpatients between 18 and 65 years of age who met DSM-IV criteria for major depressive disorder. The primary outcome in all three studies was change from baseline to endpoint in the Montgomery Asberg Depression Rating Scale (MADRS).

A fixed-dose study compared 10 mg/day Lexapro and 20 mg/day Lexapro to placebo and 40 mg/day citalopram. The 10 mg/day and 20 mg/day Lexapro treatment groups showed significantly greater mean improvement compared to placebo on the MADRS. The 10 mg and 20 mg Lexapro groups were similar on this outcome measure.

In a second fixed-dose study of 10 mg/day Lexapro and placebo, the 10 mg/day Lexapro treatment group showed significantly greater mean improvement compared to placebo on the MADRS.

In a flexible-dose study, comparing Lexapro, titrated between 10 and 20 mg/day, to placebo and citalopram, titrated between 20 and 40 mg/day, the Lexapro treatment group showed significantly greater mean improvement compared to placebo on the MADRS.

Analyses of the relationship between treatment outcome and age, gender, and race did not suggest any differential responsiveness on the basis of these patient characteristics. In a longer-term trial, 274 patients meeting (DSM-IV) criteria for major depressive disorder, who had responded during an initial 8-week, open-label treatment phase with Lexapro 10 or 20 mg/day, were randomized to continuation of Lexapro at their same dose, or to placebo, for up to 36 weeks of observation for relapse. Response during the open-label phase was defined by having a decrease of the MADRS total score to ≤ 12. Relapse during the double-blind phase was defined as an increase of the MADRS total score to ≥ 22, or discontinuation due to insufficient clinical response. Patients receiving continued Lexapro experienced a significantly longer time to relapse over the subsequent 36 weeks compared to those receiving placebo.

Generalized Anxiety Disorder

The efficacy of Lexapro in the treatment of Generalized Anxiety Disorder (GAD) was demonstrated in three, 8-week, multicenter, flexible-dose, placebo-controlled studies that compared Lexapro 10–20 mg/day to placebo in outpatients between 18 and 80 years of age who met DSM-IV criteria for GAD. In all three studies, Lexapro showed significantly greater mean improvement compared to placebo on the Hamilton Anxiety Scale (HAM-A).

There were too few patients in differing ethnic and age groups to adequately assess whether or not Lexapro has differential effects in these groups. There was no difference in response to Lexapro between men and women.

INDICATIONS AND USAGE
Major Depressive Disorder

Lexapro (escitalopram) is indicated for the treatment of major depressive disorder.

The efficacy of Lexapro in the treatment of major depressive disorder was established in three, 8-week, placebo-controlled trials of outpatients whose diagnoses corresponded most closely to the DSM-IV category of major depressive disorder (see **CLINICAL PHARMACOLOGY**).

A major depressive episode (DSM-IV) implies a prominent and relatively persistent (nearly every day for at least 2 weeks) depressed or dysphoric mood that usually interferes with daily functioning, and includes at least five of the following nine symptoms: depressed mood, loss of interest in usual activities, significant change in weight and/or appetite, insomnia or hypersomnia, psychomotor agitation or retardation, increased fatigue, feelings of guilt or worthlessness, slowed thinking or impaired concentration, a suicide attempt or suicidal ideation.

The efficacy of Lexapro in hospitalized patients with major depressive disorders has not been adequately studied.

The efficacy of Lexapro in maintaining a response, in patients with major depressive disorder who responded during an 8-week, acute-treatment phase while taking Lexapro and were then observed for relapse during a period of up to 36 weeks, was demonstrated in a placebo-controlled trial (see **Clinical Efficacy Trials** under **CLINICAL PHARMACOLOGY**). Nevertheless, the physician who elects to use Lexapro for extended periods should periodically re-evaluate the long-term usefulness of the drug for the individual patient (see **DOSAGE AND ADMINISTRATION**).

Generalized Anxiety Disorder

Lexapro is indicated for the treatment of Generalized Anxiety Disorder (GAD). The efficacy of Lexapro was established in three, 8-week, placebo-controlled trials in patients with GAD (see **CLINICAL PHARMACOLOGY**).

Generalized Anxiety Disorder (DSM-IV) is characterized by excessive anxiety and worry (apprehensive expectation) that is persistent for at least 6 months and which the person finds difficult to control. It must be associated with at least 3 of the following symptoms: restlessness or feeling keyed up or on edge, being easily fatigued, difficulty concentrating or mind going blank, irritability, muscle tension, and sleep disturbance.

The efficacy of Lexapro in the long-term treatment of GAD, that is, for more than 8 weeks, has not been systematically evaluated in controlled trials. The physician who elects to use Lexapro for extended periods should periodically re-evaluate the long-term usefulness of the drug for the individual patient.

CONTRAINDICATIONS

Concomitant use in patients taking monoamine oxidase inhibitors (MAOIs) is contraindicated (see **WARNINGS**).

Concomitant use in patients taking pimozide is contraindicated (see **Drug Interactions** – Pimozide and Celexa).

Lexapro is contraindicated in patients with a hypersensitivity to escitalopram or citalopram or any of the inactive ingredients in Lexapro.

WARNINGS
WARNINGS—Clinical Worsening and Suicide Risk
Clinical Worsening and Suicide Risk

Patients with major depressive disorder (MDD), both adult and pediatric, may experience worsening of their depression and/or the emergence of suicidal ideation and behavior (suicidality) or unusual changes in behavior, whether or not they are taking antidepressant medications, and this risk may persist until significant remission occurs. There has been a long-standing concern that antidepressants may have a role in inducing worsening of depression and the emergence of suicidality in certain patients. Antidepressants increased the risk of suicidal thinking and behavior (suicidality) in short-term studies in children and adolescents with Major Depressive Disorder (MDD) and other psychiatric disorders.

Pooled analyses of short-term placebo-controlled trials of 9 antidepressant drugs (SSRIs and others) in children and adolescents with MDD, OCD, or other psychiatric disorders (a total of 24 trials involving over 4400 patients) have revealed a greater risk of adverse events representing suicidal behavior or thinking (suicidality) during the first few months of treatment in those receiving antidepressants. The average risk of such events in patients receiving antidepressants was 4%, twice the placebo risk of 2%. There was considerable variation in risk among drugs, but a tendency toward an increase for almost all drugs studied. The risk of suicidality was most consistently observed in the MDD trials, but there were signals of risk arising from some trials in other psychiatric indications (obsessive compulsive disorder and social anxiety disorder) as well. **No suicides occurred in any of these trials.** It is unknown whether the suicidality risk in pediatric patients extends to longer-term use, i.e., beyond several months. It is also unknown whether the suicidality risk extends to adults. **All pediatric patients being treated with antidepressants for any indication should be observed closely for clinical worsening, suicidality, and unusual changes in behavior, especially during the initial few months of a course of drug therapy, or at times of dose changes, either increases or decreases. Such observation would generally include at least weekly face-to-face contact with patients or their family members or caregivers during the first 4 weeks of treatment, then every other week visits for the next 4 weeks, then at 12 weeks, and as clinically indicated beyond 12 weeks. Additional contact by telephone may be appropriate between face-to-face visits. Adults with MDD or co-morbid depression in the setting of other psychiatric illness being treated with antidepressants should be observed similarly for clinical worsening and suicidality, especially during the initial few months of a course of drug therapy, or at times of dose changes, either increases or decreases.**

The following symptoms, anxiety, agitation, panic attacks, insomnia, irritability, hostility, aggressiveness, impulsivity, akathisia (psychomotor restlessness), hypomania, and mania, have been reported in adult and pediatric patients being treated with antidepressants for major depressive disorder as well as for other indications, both psychiatric and nonpsychiatric. Although a causal link between the emergence of such symptoms and either the worsening of depression and/or the emergence of suicidal impulses has not been established, there is concern that such symptoms may represent precursors to emerging suicidality.

Consideration should be given to changing the therapeutic regimen, including possibly discontinuing the medication, in patients whose depression is persistently worse, or who are experiencing emergent suicidality or symptoms that might be precursors to worsening depression or suicidality, especially if these symptoms are severe, abrupt in onset, or were not part of the patient's presenting symptoms.

If the decision has been made to discontinue treatment, medication should be tapered, as rapidly as is feasible, but with recognition that abrupt discontinuation can be associated with certain symptoms (see PRECAUTIONS and DOSAGE AND ADMINISTRATION—Discontinuation of Treatment with Lexapro, for a description of the risks of discontinuation of Lexapro).

Families and caregivers of pediatric patients being treated with antidepressants for major depressive disorder or other indications, both psychiatric and nonpsychiatric, should be alerted about the need to monitor patients for the emergence of agitation, irritability, unusual changes in behavior, and the other symptoms described above, as well as the emergence of suicidality, and to report such symptoms immediately to health care providers. Such monitoring should include daily observation by families and caregivers. Prescriptions for Lexapro should be written for the smallest quantity of tablets consistent with good pa-

Continued on next page

Lexapro—Cont.

tient management, in order to reduce the risk of overdose. Families and caregivers of adults being treated for depression should be similarly advised.

Screening Patients for Bipolar Disorder: A major depressive episode may be the initial presentation of bipolar disorder. It is generally believed (though not established in controlled trials) that treating such an episode with an antidepressant alone may increase the likelihood of precipitation of a mixed/manic episode in patients at risk for bipolar disorder. Whether any of the symptoms described above represent such a conversion is unknown. However, prior to initiating treatment with an antidepressant, patients with depressive symptoms should be adequately screened to determine if they are at risk for bipolar disorder; such screening should include a detailed psychiatric history, including a family history of suicide, bipolar disorder, and depression. It should be noted that Lexapro is not approved for use in treating bipolar depression.

Potential for Interaction with Monoamine Oxidase Inhibitors

In patients receiving serotonin reuptake inhibitor drugs in combination with a monoamine oxidase inhibitor (MAOI), there have been reports of serious, sometimes fatal, reactions including hyperthermia, rigidity, myoclonus, autonomic instability with possible rapid fluctuations of vital signs, and mental status changes that include extreme agitation progressing to delirium and coma. These reactions have also been reported in patients who have recently discontinued SSRI treatment and have been started on an MAOI. Some cases presented with features resembling neuroleptic malignant syndrome. Furthermore, limited animal data on the effects of combined use of SSRIs and MAOIs suggest that these drugs may act synergistically to elevate blood pressure and evoke behavioral excitation. Therefore, it is recommended that Lexapro should not be used in combination with an MAOI, or within 14 days of discontinuing treatment with an MAOI. Similarly, at least 14 days should be allowed after stopping Lexapro before starting an MAOI.

Serotonin syndrome has been reported in two patients who were concomitantly receiving linezolid, an antibiotic which is a reversible non-selective MAOI.

PRECAUTIONS

General

Discontinuation of Treatment with Lexapro

During marketing of Lexapro and other SSRIs and SNRIs (serotonin and norepinephrine reuptake inhibitors), there have been spontaneous reports of adverse events occurring upon discontinuation of these drugs, particularly when abrupt, including the following: dysphoric mood, irritability, agitation, dizziness, sensory disturbances (e.g., paresthesias such as electric shock sensations), anxiety, confusion, headache, lethargy, emotional lability, insomnia, and hypomania. While these events are generally self-limiting, there have been reports of serious discontinuation symptoms.

Patients should be monitored for these symptoms when discontinuing treatment with Lexapro. A gradual reduction in the dose rather than abrupt cessation is recommended whenever possible. If intolerable symptoms occur following a decrease in the dose or upon discontinuation of treatment, then resuming the previously prescribed dose may be considered. Subsequently, the physician may continue decreasing the dose but at a more gradual rate (see **DOSAGE AND ADMINISTRATION**).

Abnormal Bleeding

Published case reports have documented the occurrence of bleeding episodes in patients treated with psychotropic drugs that interfere with serotonin reuptake. Subsequent epidemiological studies, both of the case-control and cohort design, have demonstrated an association between use of psychotropic drugs that interfere with serotonin reuptake and the occurrence of upper gastrointestinal bleeding. In two studies, concurrent use of a nonsteroidal anti-inflammatory drug (NSAID) or aspirin potentiated the risk of bleeding (see **Drug Interactions**). Although these studies focused on upper gastrointestinal bleeding, there is reason to believe that bleeding at other sites may be similarly potentiated. Patients should be cautioned regarding the risk of bleeding associated with the concomitant use of Lexapro with NSAIDs, aspirin, or other drugs that affect coagulation.

Hyponatremia

Cases of hyponatremia and SIADH (syndrome of inappropriate antidiuretic hormone secretion) have been reported in association with Lexapro treatment. All patients with these events have recovered with discontinuation of escitalopram and/or medical intervention. Hyponatremia and SIADH have also been reported in association with other marketed drugs effective in the treatment of major depressive disorder.

Activation of Mania/Hypomania

In placebo-controlled trials of Lexapro in major depressive disorder, activation of mania/hypomania was reported in one (0.1%) of 715 patients treated with Lexapro and in none of the 592 patients treated with placebo. One additional case of hypomania has been reported in association with Lexapro treatment. Activation of mania/hypomania has also been reported in a small proportion of patients with major affective disorders treated with racemic citalopram and other marketed drugs effective in the treatment of major de-

pressive disorder. As with all drugs effective in the treatment of major depressive disorder, Lexapro should be used cautiously in patients with a history of mania.

Seizures

Although anticonvulsant effects of racemic citalopram have been observed in animal studies, Lexapro has not been systematically evaluated in patients with a seizure disorder. These patients were excluded from clinical studies during the product's premarketing testing. In clinical trials of Lexapro, cases of convulsion have been reported in association with Lexapro treatment. Like other drugs effective in the treatment of major depressive disorder, Lexapro should be introduced with care in patients with a history of seizure disorder.

Interference with Cognitive and Motor Performance

In a study in normal volunteers, Lexapro 10 mg/day did not produce impairment of intellectual function or psychomotor performance. Because any psychoactive drug may impair judgment, thinking, or motor skills, however, patients should be cautioned about operating hazardous machinery, including automobiles, until they are reasonably certain that Lexapro therapy does not affect their ability to engage in such activities.

Use in Patients with Concomitant Illness

Clinical experience with Lexapro in patients with certain concomitant systemic illnesses is limited. Caution is advisable in using Lexapro in patients with diseases or conditions that produce altered metabolism or hemodynamic responses.

Lexapro has not been systematically evaluated in patients with a recent history of myocardial infarction or unstable heart disease. Patients with these diagnoses were generally excluded from clinical studies during the product's premarketing testing.

In subjects with hepatic impairment, clearance of racemic citalopram was decreased and plasma concentrations were increased. The recommended dose of Lexapro in hepatically impaired patients is 10 mg/day (see **DOSAGE AND ADMINISTRATION**).

Because escitalopram is extensively metabolized, excretion of unchanged drug in urine is a minor route of elimination. Until adequate numbers of patients with severe renal impairment have been evaluated during chronic treatment with Lexapro, however, it should be used with caution in such patients (see **DOSAGE AND ADMINISTRATION**).

Information for Patients

Physicians are advised to discuss the following issues with patients for whom they prescribe Lexapro.

In a study in normal volunteers, Lexapro 10 mg/day did not impair psychomotor performance. The effect of Lexapro on psychomotor coordination, judgment, or thinking has not been systematically examined in controlled studies. Because psychoactive drugs may impair judgment, thinking, or motor skills, patients should be cautioned about operating hazardous machinery, including automobiles, until they are reasonably certain that Lexapro therapy does not affect their ability to engage in such activities.

Patients should be told that, although Lexapro has not been shown in experiments with normal subjects to increase the mental and motor skill impairments caused by alcohol, the concomitant use of Lexapro and alcohol in depressed patients is not advised.

Patients should be made aware that escitalopram is the active isomer of Celexa (citalopram hydrobromide) and that the two medications should not be taken concomitantly.

Patients should be advised to inform their physician if they are taking, or plan to take, any prescription or over-the-counter drugs, as there is a potential for interactions.

Patients should be cautioned about the concomitant use of Lexapro and NSAIDs, aspirin, or other drugs that affect coagulation since the combined use of psychotropic drugs that interfere with serotonin reuptake and these agents has been associated with an increased risk of bleeding.

Patients should be advised to notify their physician if they become pregnant or intend to become pregnant during therapy.

Patients should be advised to notify their physician if they are breastfeeding an infant.

While patients may notice improvement with Lexapro therapy in 1 to 4 weeks, they should be advised to continue therapy as directed.

Prescribers or other health professionals should inform patients, their families, and their caregivers about the benefits and risks associated with treatment with Lexapro and should counsel them in its appropriate use. A patient Medication Guide About Using Antidepressants in Children and Teenagers is available for Lexapro. The prescriber or health professional should instruct patients, their families, and their caregivers to read the Medication Guide and should assist them in understanding its contents. Patients should be given the opportunity to discuss the contents of the Medication Guide and to obtain answers to any questions they may have. The complete text of the Medication Guide is reprinted at the end of this document.

Patients should be advised of the following issues and asked to alert their prescriber if these occur while taking Lexapro.

Clinical Worsening and Suicide Risk: Patients, their families, and their caregivers should be encouraged to be alert to the emergence of anxiety, agitation, panic attacks, insomnia, irritability, hostility, aggressiveness, impulsivity, akathisia (psychomotor restlessness), hypomania, mania, other unusual changes in behavior, worsening of depression, and suicidal ideation, especially early during antidepressant treatment and when the dose is adjusted up or down. Families and caregivers of patients should be advised to observe

for the emergence of such symptoms on a day-to-day basis, since changes may be abrupt. Such symptoms should be reported to the patient's prescriber or health professional, especially if they are severe, abrupt in onset, or were not part of the patient's presenting symptoms. Symptoms such as these may be associated with an increased risk for suicidal thinking and behavior and indicate a need for very close monitoring and possibly changes in the medication.

Laboratory Tests

There are no specific laboratory tests recommended.

Concomitant Administration with Racemic Citalopram

Citalopram—Since escitalopram is the active isomer of racemic citalopram (Celexa), the two agents should not be coadministered.

Drug Interactions

CNS Drugs—Given the primary CNS effects of escitalopram, caution should be used when it is taken in combination with other centrally acting drugs.

Alcohol—Although Lexapro did not potentiate the cognitive and motor effects of alcohol in a clinical trial, as with other psychotropic medications, the use of alcohol by patients taking Lexapro is not recommended.

Monoamine Oxidase Inhibitors (MAOIs)—See **CONTRAINDICATIONS** and **WARNINGS**.

Drugs That Interfere With Hemostasis (NSAIDs, Aspirin, Warfarin, etc.)

Serotonin release by platelets plays an important role in hemostasis. Epidemiological studies of the case-control and cohort design that have demonstrated an association between use of psychotropic drugs that interfere with serotonin reuptake and the occurrence of upper gastrointestinal bleeding have also shown that concurrent use of an NSAID or aspirin potentiated the risk of bleeding. Thus, patients should be cautioned about the use of such drugs concurrently with Lexapro.

Cimetidine—In subjects who had received 21 days of 40 mg/day racemic citalopram, combined administration of 400 mg/day cimetidine for 8 days resulted in an increase in citalopram AUC and C_{max} of 43% and 39%, respectively. The clinical significance of these findings is unknown.

Digoxin—In subjects who had received 21 days of 40 mg/day racemic citalopram, combined administration of citalopram and digoxin (single dose of 1 mg) did not significantly affect the pharmacokinetics of either citalopram or digoxin.

Lithium—Coadministration of racemic citalopram (40 mg/day for 10 days) and lithium (30 mmol/day for 5 days) had no significant effect on the pharmacokinetics of citalopram or lithium. Nevertheless, plasma lithium levels should be monitored with appropriate adjustment to the lithium dose in accordance with standard clinical practice. Because lithium may enhance the serotonergic effects of escitalopram, caution should be exercised when Lexapro and lithium are coadministered.

Pimozide and Celexa—In a controlled study, a single dose of pimozide 2 mg co-administered with racemic citalopram 40 mg given once daily for 11 days was associated with a mean increase in QTc values of approximately 10 msec compared to pimozide given alone. Racemic citalopram did not alter the mean AUC or C_{max} of pimozide. The mechanism of this pharmacodynamic interaction is not known.

Sumatriptan—There have been rare postmarketing reports describing patients with weakness, hyperreflexia, and incoordination following the use of an SSRI and sumatriptan. If concomitant treatment with sumatriptan and an SSRI (e.g., fluoxetine, fluvoxamine, paroxetine, sertraline, citalopram, escitalopram) is clinically warranted, appropriate observation of the patient is advised.

Theophylline—Combined administration of racemic citalopram (40 mg/day for 21 days) and the CYP1A2 substrate theophylline (single dose of 300 mg) did not affect the pharmacokinetics of theophylline. The effect of theophylline on the pharmacokinetics of citalopram was not evaluated.

Warfarin—Administration of 40 mg/day racemic citalopram for 21 days did not affect the pharmacokinetics of warfarin, a CYP3A4 substrate. Prothrombin time was increased by 5%, the clinical significance of which is unknown.

Carbamazepine—Combined administration of racemic citalopram (40 mg/day for 14 days) and carbamazepine (titrated to 400 mg/day for 35 days) did not significantly affect the pharmacokinetics of carbamazepine, a CYP3A4 substrate. Although trough citalopram plasma levels were unaffected, given the enzyme-inducing properties of carbamazepine, the possibility that carbamazepine might increase the clearance of escitalopram should be considered if the two drugs are coadministered.

Triazolam—Combined administration of racemic citalopram (titrated to 40 mg/day for 28 days) and the CYP3A4 substrate triazolam (single dose of 0.25 mg) did not significantly affect the pharmacokinetics of either citalopram or triazolam.

Ketoconazole—Combined administration of racemic citalopram (40 mg) and ketoconazole (200 mg), a potent CYP3A4 inhibitor, decreased the C_{max} and AUC of ketoconazole by 21% and 10%, respectively, and did not significantly affect the pharmacokinetics of citalopram.

Ritonavir—Combined administration of a single dose of ritonavir (600 mg), both a CYP3A4 substrate and a potent inhibitor of CYP3A4, and escitalopram (20 mg) did not affect the pharmacokinetics of either ritonavir or escitalopram.

CYP3A4 and -2C19 Inhibitors—In vitro studies indicated that CYP3A4 and -2C19 are the primary enzymes involved in the metabolism of escitalopram. However, coadministration of escitalopram (20 mg) and ritonavir (600 mg), a potent inhibitor of CYP3A4, did not significantly affect the pharmacokinetics of escitalopram. Because escitalopram is metabolized by multiple enzyme systems, inhibition of a single enzyme may not appreciably decrease escitalopram clearance.

Drugs Metabolized by Cytochrome P4502D6—*In vitro* studies did not reveal an inhibitory effect of escitalopram on CYP2D6. In addition, steady state levels of racemic citalopram were not significantly different in poor metabolizers and extensive CYP2D6 metabolizers after multiple-dose administration of citalopram, suggesting that coadministration, with escitalopram, of a drug that inhibits CYP2D6, is unlikely to have clinically significant effects on escitalopram metabolism. However, there are limited *in vivo* data suggesting a modest CYP2D6 inhibitory effect for escitalopram, i.e., coadministration of escitalopram (20 mg/day for 21 days) with the tricyclic antidepressant desipramine (single dose of 50 mg), a substrate for CYP2D6, resulted in a 40% increase in C_{max} and a 100% increase in AUC of desipramine. The clinical significance of this finding is unknown. Nevertheless, caution is indicated in the coadministration of escitalopram and drugs metabolized by CYP2D6.

Metoprolol—Administration of 20 mg/day Lexapro for 21 days in healthy volunteers resulted in a 50% increase in C_{max} and 82% increase in AUC of the beta-adrenergic blocker metoprolol (given in a single dose of 100 mg). Increased metoprolol plasma levels have been associated with decreased cardioselectivity. Coadministration of Lexapro and metoprolol had no clinically significant effects on blood pressure or heart rate.

Electroconvulsive Therapy (ECT)—There are no clinical studies of the combined use of ECT and escitalopram.

Carcinogenesis, Mutagenesis, Impairment of Fertility

Carcinogenesis
Racemic citalopram was administered in the diet to NMRI/BOM strain mice and COBS WI strain rats for 18 and 24 months, respectively. There was no evidence for carcinogenicity of racemic citalopram in mice receiving up to 240 mg/kg/day. There was an increased incidence of small intestine carcinoma in rats receiving 8 or 24 mg/kg/day racemic citalopram. A no-effect dose for this finding was not established. The relevance of these findings to humans is unknown.

Mutagenesis
Racemic citalopram was mutagenic in the *in vitro* bacterial reverse mutation assay (Ames test) in 2 of 5 bacterial strains (Salmonella TA98 and TA1537) in the absence of metabolic activation. It was clastogenic in the *in vitro* Chinese hamster lung cell assay for chromosomal aberrations in the presence and absence of metabolic activation. Racemic citalopram was not mutagenic in the *in vitro* mammalian forward gene mutation assay (HPRT) in mouse lymphoma cells or in a coupled *in vitro/in vivo* unscheduled DNA synthesis (UDS) assay in rat liver. It was not clastogenic in the *in vitro* chromosomal aberration assay in human lymphocytes or in two *in vivo* mouse micronucleus assays.

Impairment of Fertility
When racemic citalopram was administered orally to 16 male and 24 female rats prior to and throughout mating and gestation at doses of 32, 48, and 72 mg/kg/day, mating was decreased at all doses, and fertility was decreased at doses ≥ 32 mg/kg/day. Gestation duration was increased at 48 mg/kg/day.

Pregnancy

Pregnancy Category C
In a rat embryo/fetal development study, oral administration of escitalopram (56, 112, or 150 mg/kg/day) to pregnant animals during the period of organogenesis resulted in decreased fetal body weight and associated delays in ossification at the two higher doses (approximately ≥ 56 times the maximum recommended human dose [MRHD] of 20 mg/day on a body surface area [mg/m^2] basis). Maternal toxicity (clinical signs and decreased body weight gain and food consumption), mild at 56 mg/kg/day, was present at all dose levels. The developmental no-effect dose of 56 mg/kg/day is approximately 28 times the MRHD on a mg/m^2 basis. No teratogenicity was observed at any of the doses tested (as high as 75 times the MRHD on a mg/m^2 basis).

When female rats were treated with escitalopram (6, 12, 24, or 48 mg/kg/day) during pregnancy and through weaning, slightly increased offspring mortality and growth retardation were noted at 48 mg/kg/day which is approximately 24 times the MRHD on a mg/m^2 basis. Slight maternal toxicity (clinical signs and decreased body weight gain and food consumption) was seen at this dose. Slightly increased offspring mortality was seen at 24 mg/kg/day. The no-effect dose was 12 mg/kg/day which is approximately 6 times the MRHD on a mg/m^2 basis.

In animal reproduction studies, racemic citalopram has been shown to have adverse effects on embryo/fetal and postnatal development, including teratogenic effects, when administered at doses greater than human therapeutic doses.

In two rat embryo/fetal development studies, oral administration of racemic citalopram (32, 56, or 112 mg/kg/day) to pregnant animals during the period of organogenesis resulted in decreased embryo/fetal growth and survival and an increased incidence of fetal abnormalities (including cardiovascular and skeletal defects) at the high dose. This dose was also associated with maternal toxicity (clinical signs, decreased body weight gain). The developmental no-effect dose was 56 mg/kg/day. In a rabbit study, no adverse effects on embryo/fetal development were observed at doses of racemic citalopram of up to 16 mg/kg/day. Thus, teratogenic

effects of racemic citalopram were observed at a maternally toxic dose in the rat and were not observed in the rabbit. When female rats were treated with racemic citalopram (4.8, 12.8, or 32 mg/kg/day) from late gestation through weaning, increased offspring mortality during the first 4 days after birth and persistent offspring growth retardation were observed at the highest dose. The no-effect dose was 12.8 mg/kg/day. Similar effects on offspring mortality and growth were seen when dams were treated throughout gestation and early lactation at doses ≥ 24 mg/kg/day. A no-effect dose was not determined in that study.

There are no adequate and well-controlled studies in pregnant women; therefore, escitalopram should be used during pregnancy only if the potential benefit justifies the potential risk to the fetus.

Pregnancy-Nonteratogenic Effects
Neonates exposed to Lexapro and other SSRIs or SNRIs, late in the third trimester, have developed complications requiring prolonged hospitalization, respiratory support, and tube feeding. Such complications can arise immediately upon delivery. Reported clinical findings have included respiratory distress, cyanosis, apnea, seizures, temperature instability, feeding difficulty, vomiting, hypoglycemia, hypotonia, hypertonia, hyperreflexia, tremor, jitteriness, irritability, and constant crying. These features are consistent with either a direct toxic effect of SSRIs and SNRIs or, possibly, a drug discontinuation syndrome. It should be noted that, in some cases, the clinical picture is consistent with serotonin syndrome (see **WARNINGS**).

When treating a pregnant woman with Lexapro during the third trimester, the physician should carefully consider the potential risks and benefits of treatment (see **DOSAGE AND ADMINISTRATION**).

Labor and Delivery
The effect of Lexapro on labor and delivery in humans is unknown.

Nursing Mothers
Racemic citalopram, like many other drugs, is excreted in human breast milk. There have been two reports of infants experiencing excessive somnolence, decreased feeding, and weight loss in association with breastfeeding from a citalopram-treated mother; in one case, the infant was reported to recover completely upon discontinuation of citalopram by its mother and, in the second case, no follow-up information was available. The decision whether to continue or discontinue either nursing or Lexapro therapy should take into account the risks of citalopram exposure for the infant and the benefits of Lexapro treatment for the mother.

Pediatric Use
Safety and effectiveness in the pediatric population have not been established (see BOX WARNING and WARNINGS—Clinical Worsening and Suicide Risk). One placebo-controlled trial in 264 pediatric patients with MDD has been conducted with Lexapro, and the data were not sufficient to support a claim for use in pediatric patients. Anyone considering the use of Lexapro in a child or adolescent must balance the potential risks with the clinical need.

Geriatric Use
Approximately 6% of the 1144 patients receiving escitalopram in controlled trials of Lexapro in major depressive disorder and GAD were 60 years of age or older; elderly patients in these trials received daily doses of Lexapro between 10 and 20 mg. The number of elderly patients in these trials was insufficient to adequately assess for possible differential efficacy and safety measures on the basis of age. Nevertheless, greater sensitivity of some elderly individuals to effects of Lexapro cannot be ruled out.

In two pharmacokinetic studies, escitalopram half-life was increased by approximately 50% in elderly subjects as compared to young subjects and C_{max} was unchanged (see **CLINICAL PHARMACOLOGY**). 10 mg/day is the recommended dose for elderly patients (see **DOSAGE AND ADMINISTRATION**).

Of 4422 patients in clinical studies of racemic citalopram, 1357 were 60 and over, 1034 were 65 and over, and 457 were 75 and over. No overall differences in safety or effectiveness were observed between these subjects and younger subjects, and other reported clinical experience has not identified differences in responses between the elderly and younger patients, but again, greater sensitivity of some elderly individuals cannot be ruled out.

ADVERSE REACTIONS

Adverse event information for Lexapro was collected from 715 patients with major depressive disorder who were exposed to escitalopram and from 592 patients who were exposed to placebo in double-blind, placebo-controlled trials. An additional 284 patients with major depressive disorder were newly exposed to escitalopram in open-label trials. The adverse event information for Lexapro in patients with GAD was collected from 429 patients exposed to escitalopram and from 427 patients exposed to placebo in double-blind, placebo-controlled trials.

Adverse events during exposure were obtained primarily by general inquiry and recorded by clinical investigators using terminology of their own choosing. Consequently, it is not possible to provide a meaningful estimate of the proportion of individuals experiencing adverse events without first grouping similar types of events into a smaller number of standardized event categories. In the tables and tabulations that follow, standard World Health Organization (WHO) terminology has been used to classify reported adverse events.

The stated frequencies of adverse events represent the proportion of individuals who experienced, at least once, a

treatment-emergent adverse event of the type listed. An event was considered treatment-emergent if it occurred for the first time or worsened while receiving therapy following baseline evaluation.

Adverse Events Associated with Discontinuation of Treatment

Major Depressive Disorder
Among the 715 depressed patients who received Lexapro in placebo-controlled trials, 6% discontinued treatment due to an adverse event, as compared to 2% of 592 patients receiving placebo. In two fixed-dose studies, the rate of discontinuation for adverse events in patients receiving 10 mg/day Lexapro was not significantly different from the rate of discontinuation for adverse events in patients receiving placebo. The rate of discontinuation for adverse events in patients assigned to a fixed dose of 20 mg/day Lexapro was 10%, which was significantly different from the rate of discontinuation for adverse events in patients receiving 10 mg/day Lexapro (4%) and placebo (3%). Adverse events that were associated with the discontinuation of at least 1% of patients treated with Lexapro, and for which the rate was at least twice that of placebo, were nausea (2%) and ejaculation disorder (2% of male patients).

Generalized Anxiety Disorder
Among the 429 GAD patients who received Lexapro 10–20 mg/day in placebo-controlled trials, 8% discontinued treatment due to an adverse event, as compared to 4% of 427 patients receiving placebo. Adverse events that were associated with the discontinuation of at least 1% of patients treated with Lexapro, and for which the rate was at least twice the placebo rate, were nausea (2%), insomnia (1%), and fatigue (1%).

Incidence of Adverse Events in Placebo-Controlled Clinical Trials

Major Depressive Disorder
Table 1 enumerates the incidence, rounded to the nearest percent, of treatment-emergent adverse events that occurred among 715 depressed patients who received Lexapro at doses ranging from 10 to 20 mg/day in placebo-controlled trials. Events included are those occurring in 2% or more of patients treated with Lexapro and for which the incidence in patients treated with Lexapro was greater than the incidence in placebo-treated patients.

The prescriber should be aware that these figures can not be used to predict the incidence of adverse events in the course of usual medical practice where patient characteristics and other factors differ from those which prevailed in the clinical trials. Similarly, the cited frequencies cannot be compared with figures obtained from other clinical investigations involving different treatments, uses, and investigators. The cited figures, however, do provide the prescribing physician with some basis for estimating the relative contribution of drug and non-drug factors to the adverse event incidence rate in the population studied.

The most commonly observed adverse events in Lexapro patients (incidence of approximately 5% or greater and approximately twice the incidence in placebo patients) were insomnia, ejaculation disorder (primarily ejaculatory delay), nausea, sweating increased, fatigue, and somnolence (see **TABLE 1**).

TABLE 1
Treatment-Emergent Adverse Events:
Incidence in Placebo-Controlled Clinical Trials for
Major Depressive Disorder*

Body System/ Adverse Event	(Percentage of Patients Reporting Event)	
	Lexapro (N=715)	Placebo (N=592)
Autonomic Nervous System Disorders		
Dry Mouth	6%	5%
Sweating Increased	5%	2%
Central & Peripheral Nervous System Disorders		
Dizziness	5%	3%
Gastrointestinal Disorders		
Nausea	15%	7%
Diarrhea	8%	5%
Constipation	3%	1%
Indigestion	3%	1%
Abdominal Pain	2%	1%
General		
Influenza-like Symptoms	5%	4%
Fatigue	5%	2%
Psychiatric Disorders		
Insomnia	9%	4%
Somnolence	6%	2%
Appetite Decreased	3%	1%
Libido Decreased	3%	1%
Respiratory System Disorders		
Rhinitis	5%	4%
Sinusitis	3%	2%
Urogenital		
Ejaculation Disorder[1,2]	9%*	<1%
Impotence[2]	3%	<1%
Anorgasmia[3]	2%	<1%

*Events reported by at least 2% of patients treated with Lexapro are reported, except for the following events which had an incidence on placebo ≥ Lexapro: headache, upper

Continued on next page

Lexapro—Cont.

respiratory tract infection, back pain, pharyngitis, inflicted injury, anxiety.
[1] Primarily ejaculatory delay.
[2] Denominator used was for males only (N=225 Lexapro; N=188 placebo).
[3] Denominator used was for females only (N=490 Lexapro; N=404 placebo).

Generalized Anxiety Disorder

Table 2 enumerates the incidence, rounded to the nearest percent of treatment-emergent adverse events that occurred among 429 GAD patients who received Lexapro 10 to 20 mg/day in placebo-controlled trials. Events included are those occurring in 2% or more of patients treated with Lexapro and for which the incidence in patients treated with Lexapro was greater than the incidence in placebo-treated patients.

The most commonly observed adverse events in Lexapro patients (incidence of approximately 5% or greater and approximately twice the incidence in placebo patients) were nausea, ejaculation disorder (primarily ejaculatory delay), insomnia, fatigue, decreased libido, and anorgasmia (see TABLE 2).

TABLE 2
Treatment-Emergent Adverse Events:
Incidence in Placebo-Controlled Clinical Trials for
Generalized Anxiety Disorder*

Body System/ Adverse Event	(Percentage of Patients Reporting Event)	
	Lexapro (N=429)	Placebo (N=427)
Autonomic Nervous System Disorders		
Dry Mouth	9%	5%
Sweating Increased	4%	1%
Central & Peripheral Nervous System Disorders		
Headache	24%	17%
Paresthesia	2%	1%
Gastrointestinal Disorders		
Nausea	18%	8%
Diarrhea	8%	6%
Constipation	5%	4%
Indigestion	3%	2%
Vomiting	3%	1%
Abdominal Pain	2%	1%
Flatulence	2%	1%
Toothache	2%	0%
General		
Fatigue	8%	2%
Influenza-like Symptoms	5%	4%
Musculoskeletal		
Neck/Shoulder Pain	3%	1%
Psychiatric Disorders		
Somnolence	13%	7%
Insomnia	12%	6%
Libido Decreased	7%	2%
Dreaming Abnormal	3%	2%
Appetite Decreased	3%	1%
Lethargy	3%	1%
Yawning	2%	1%
Urogenital		
Ejaculation Disorder[1,2]	14%	2%
Anorgasmia[3]	6%	<1%
Menstrual Disorder	2%	1%

*Events reported by at least 2% of patients treated with Lexapro are reported, except for the following events which had an incidence on placebo ≥ Lexapro: inflicted injury, dizziness, back pain, upper respiratory tract infection, rhinitis, pharyngitis.
[1] Primarily ejaculatory delay.
[2] Denominator used was for males only (N=182 Lexapro; N=195 placebo).
[3] Denominator used was for females only (N=247 Lexapro; N=232 placebo).

Dose Dependency of Adverse Events

The potential dose dependency of common adverse events (defined as an incidence rate of ≥5% in either the 10 mg or 20 mg Lexapro groups) was examined on the basis of the combined incidence of adverse events in two fixed-dose trials. The overall incidence rates of adverse events in 10 mg Lexapro-treated patients (66%) was similar to that of the placebo-treated patients (61%), while the incidence rate in 20 mg/day Lexapro-treated patients was greater (86%). Table 3 shows common adverse events that occurred in the 20 mg/day Lexapro group with an incidence that was approximately twice that of the 10 mg/day Lexapro group and approximately twice that of the placebo group.

TABLE 3
Incidence of Common Adverse Events* in Patients with
Major Depressive Disorder Receiving Placebo,
10 mg/day Lexapro, or 20 mg/day Lexapro

Adverse Event	Placebo (N=311)	10 mg/day Lexapro (N=310)	20 mg/day Lexapro (N=125)
Insomnia	4%	7%	14%
Diarrhea	5%	6%	14%
Dry Mouth	3%	4%	9%
Somnolence	1%	4%	9%
Dizziness	2%	4%	7%
Sweating Increased	<1%	3%	8%
Constipation	1%	3%	6%
Fatigue	2%	2%	6%
Indigestion	1%	2%	6%

*Adverse events with an incidence rate of at least 5% in either of the Lexapro groups and with an incidence rate in the 20 mg/day Lexapro group that was approximately twice that of the 10 mg/day Lexapro group and the placebo group.

Male and Female Sexual Dysfunction with SSRIs

Although changes in sexual desire, sexual performance, and sexual satisfaction often occur as manifestations of a psychiatric disorder, they may also be a consequence of pharmacologic treatment. In particular, some evidence suggests that SSRIs can cause such untoward sexual experiences.

Reliable estimates of the incidence and severity of untoward experiences involving sexual desire, performance, and satisfaction are difficult to obtain, however, in part because patients and physicians may be reluctant to discuss them. Accordingly, estimates of the incidence of untoward sexual experience and performance cited in product labeling are likely to underestimate their actual incidence.

Table 4 shows the incidence rates of sexual side effects in patients with major depressive disorder and GAD in placebo-controlled trials.

TABLE 4
Incidence of Sexual Side Effects in
Placebo-Controlled Clinical Trials

Adverse Event	Lexapro	Placebo
	In Males Only	
	(N=407)	(N=383)
Ejaculation Disorder (primarily ejaculatory delay)	12%	1%
Libido Decreased	6%	2%
Impotence	2%	<1%
	In Females Only	
	(N=737)	(N=636)
Libido Decreased	3%	1%
Anorgasmia	3%	<1%

There are no adequately designed studies examining sexual dysfunction with escitalopram treatment.

Priapism has been reported with all SSRIs.

While it is difficult to know the precise risk of sexual dysfunction associated with the use of SSRIs, physicians should routinely inquire about such possible side effects.

Vital Sign Changes

Lexapro and placebo groups were compared with respect to (1) mean change from baseline in vital signs (pulse, systolic blood pressure, and diastolic blood pressure) and (2) the incidence of patients meeting criteria for potentially clinically significant changes from baseline in these variables. These analyses did not reveal any clinically important changes in vital signs associated with Lexapro treatment. In addition, a comparison of supine and standing vital sign measures in subjects receiving Lexapro indicated that Lexapro treatment is not associated with orthostatic changes.

Weight Changes

Patients treated with Lexapro in controlled trials did not differ from placebo-treated patients with regard to clinically important change in body weight.

Laboratory Changes

Lexapro and placebo groups were compared with respect to (1) mean change from baseline in various serum chemistry, hematology, and urinalysis variables, and (2) the incidence of patients meeting criteria for potentially clinically significant changes from baseline in these variables. These analyses revealed no clinically important changes in laboratory test parameters associated with Lexapro treatment.

ECG Changes

Electrocardiograms from Lexapro (N=625), racemic citalopram (N=351), and placebo (N=527) groups were compared with respect to (1) mean change from baseline in various ECG parameters and (2) the incidence of patients meeting criteria for potentially clinically significant changes from baseline in these variables. These analyses revealed (1) a decrease in heart rate of 2.2 bpm for Lexapro and 2.7 bpm for racemic citalopram, compared to an increase of 0.3 bpm for placebo and (2) an increase in QTc interval of 3.9 msec for Lexapro and 3.7 msec for racemic citalopram, compared to 0.5 msec for placebo. Neither Lexapro nor racemic citalopram were associated with the development of clinically significant ECG abnormalities.

Other Events Observed During the Premarketing Evaluation of Lexapro.

Following is a list of WHO terms that reflect treatment-emergent adverse events, as defined in the introduction to the ADVERSE REACTIONS section, reported by the 1428 patients treated with Lexapro for periods of up to one year in double-blind or open-label clinical trials during its premarketing evaluation. All reported events are included except those already listed in Tables 1 & 2, those occurring in only one patient, event terms that are so general as to be uninformative, and those that are unlikely to be drug related. It is important to emphasize that, although the events reported occurred during treatment with Lexapro, they were not necessarily caused by it.

Events are further categorized by body system and listed in order of decreasing frequency according to the following definitions: frequent adverse events are those occurring on one or more occasions in at least 1/100 patients; infrequent adverse events are those occurring in less than 1/100 patients but at least 1/1000 patients.

Cardiovascular—*Frequent*: palpitation, hypertension. *Infrequent*: bradycardia, tachycardia, ECG abnormal, flushing, varicose vein.

Central and Peripheral Nervous System Disorders—*Frequent*: light-headed feeling, migraine. *Infrequent*: tremor, vertigo, restless legs, shaking, twitching, dysequilibrium, tics, carpal tunnel syndrome, muscle contractions involuntary, sluggishness, coordination abnormal, faintness, hyperreflexia, muscular tone increased.

Gastrointestinal Disorders—*Frequent*: heartburn, abdominal cramp, gastroenteritis. *Infrequent*: gastroesophageal reflux, bloating, abdominal discomfort, dyspepsia, increased stool frequency, belching, gastritis, hemorrhoids, gagging, polyposis gastric, swallowing difficult.

General—*Frequent*: allergy, pain in limb, fever, hot flushes, chest pain. *Infrequent*: edema of extremities, chills, tightness of chest, leg pain, asthenia, syncope, malaise, anaphylaxis, fall.

Hemic and Lymphatic Disorders—*Infrequent*: bruise, anemia, nosebleed, hematoma, lymphadenopathy cervical.

Metabolic and Nutritional Disorders—*Frequent*: increased weight. *Infrequent*: decreased weight, hyperglycemia, thirst, bilirubin increased, hepatic enzymes increased, gout, hypercholesterolemia.

Musculoskeletal System Disorders—*Frequent*: arthralgia, myalgia. *Infrequent*: jaw stiffness, muscle cramp, muscle stiffness, arthritis, muscle weakness, back discomfort, arthropathy, jaw pain, joint stiffness.

Psychiatric Disorders—*Frequent*: appetite increased, lethargy, irritability, concentration impaired. *Infrequent*: jitteriness, panic reaction, agitation, apathy, forgetfulness, depression aggravated, nervousness, restlessness aggravated, suicide attempt, amnesia, anxiety attack, bruxism, carbohydrate craving, confusion, depersonalization, disorientation, emotional lability, feeling unreal, tremulousness nervous, crying abnormal, depression, excitability, auditory hallucination, suicidal tendency.

Reproductive Disorders/Female*—*Frequent*: menstrual cramps, menstrual disorder. *Infrequent*: menorrhagia, breast neoplasm, pelvic inflammation, premenstrual syndrome, spotting between menses.

*% based on female subjects only: N= 905

Respiratory System Disorders—*Frequent*: bronchitis, sinus congestion, coughing, nasal congestion, sinus headache. *Infrequent*: asthma, breath shortness, laryngitis, pneumonia, tracheitis.

Skin and Appendages Disorders—*Frequent*: rash. *Infrequent*: pruritus, acne, alopecia, eczema, dermatitis, dry skin, folliculitis, lipoma, furunculosis, dry lips, skin nodule.

Special Senses—*Frequent*: vision blurred, tinnitus. *Infrequent*: taste alteration, earache, conjunctivitis, vision abnormal, dry eyes, eye irritation, visual disturbance, eye infection, pupils dilated, metallic taste.

Urinary System Disorders—*Frequent*: urinary frequency, urinary tract infection. *Infrequent*: urinary urgency, kidney stone, dysuria, blood in urine.

Events Reported Subsequent to the Marketing of Escitalopram

Although no causal relationship to escitalopram treatment has been found, the following adverse events have been reported to have occurred in patients and to be temporally associated with escitalopram treatment during postmarketing experience and were not observed during the premarketing evaluation of escitalopram: abnormal gait, acute renal failure, aggression, angioedema, atrial fibrillation, diplopia, dystonia, extrapyramidal disorders, gastrointestinal hemorrhage, grand mal seizures (or convulsions), hepatitis, hypotension, myocardial infarction, neuroleptic malignant syndrome, orthostatic hypotension, pancreatitis, pulmonary embolism, QT prolongation, rhabdomyolysis, seizures, serotonin syndrome, SIADH, thrombocytopenia, torsades de pointes, toxic epidermal necrolysis, ventricular tachycardia and visual hallucinations.

Events Reported Subsequent to the Marketing of Racemic Citalopram

Although no causal relationship to racemic citalopram treatment has been found, the following adverse events have been reported to have occurred in patients and to be temporally associated with racemic citalopram treatment and were not observed during the premarketing evaluation of citalopram: acute renal failure, akathisia, allergic reaction, anaphylaxis, angioedema, choreoathetosis, delirium, dyskinesia, ecchymosis, erythema multiforme, gastrointestinal hemorrhage, grand mal seizures (or convulsions), hemolytic anemia, hepatic necrosis, myoclonus, neuroleptic malignant syndrome, nystagmus, pancreatitis, priapism, prolactinemia, prothrombin decreased, QT prolongation, rhabdomyolysis, serotonin syndrome, spontaneous abortion, thrombocytopenia, thrombosis, torsades de pointes, toxic epidermal necrolysis and ventricular arrhythmia.

DRUG ABUSE AND DEPENDENCE

Controlled Substance Class

Lexapro is not a controlled substance.

Physical and Psychological Dependence

Animal studies suggest that the abuse liability of racemic citalopram is low. Lexapro has not been systematically studied in humans for its potential for abuse, tolerance, or physical dependence. The premarketing clinical experience with Lexapro did not reveal any drug-seeking behavior. However, these observations were not systematic and it is not possible to predict on the basis of this limited experience the extent to which a CNS-active drug will be misused, diverted, and/or abused once marketed. Consequently, physicians should carefully evaluate Lexapro patients for history of drug abuse and follow such patients closely, observing them for signs of misuse or abuse (e.g., development of tolerance, incrementations of dose, drug-seeking behavior).

OVERDOSAGE

Human Experience

In clinical trials of escitalopram, there were reports of escitalopram overdose, including overdoses of up to 600 mg, with no associated fatalities. During the postmarketing evaluation of escitalopram, Lexapro overdoses involving overdoses of over 1000 mg have been reported. As with other SSRI's, a fatal outcome in a patient who has taken an overdose of escitalopram has been rarely reported. Symptoms most often accompanying escitalopram overdose, alone or in combination with other drugs and/or alcohol, included convulsions, coma, dizziness, hypotension, insomnia, nausea, vomiting, sinus tachycardia, somnolence, and ECG changes (including QT prolongation).

Management of Overdose

Establish and maintain an airway to ensure adequate ventilation and oxygenation. Gastric evacuation by lavage and use of activated charcoal should be considered. Careful observation and cardiac and vital sign monitoring are recommended, along with general symptomatic and supportive care. Due to the large volume of distribution of escitalopram, forced diuresis, dialysis, hemoperfusion, and exchange transfusion are unlikely to be of benefit. There are no specific antidotes for Lexapro.

In managing overdosage, consider the possibility of multiple-drug involvement. The physician should consider contacting a poison control center for additional information on the treatment of any overdose.

DOSAGE AND ADMINISTRATION

Major Depressive Disorder

Initial Treatment

The recommended dose of Lexapro is 10 mg once daily. A fixed-dose trial of Lexapro demonstrated the effectiveness of both 10 mg and 20 mg of Lexapro, but failed to demonstrate a greater benefit of 20 mg over 10 mg (see **Clinical Efficacy Trials** under **CLINICAL PHARMACOLOGY**). If the dose is increased to 20 mg, this should occur after a minimum of one week.

Lexapro should be administered once daily, in the morning or evening, with or without food.

Special Populations

10 mg/day is the recommended dose for most elderly patients and patients with hepatic impairment.

No dosage adjustment is necessary for patients with mild or moderate renal impairment. Lexapro should be used with caution in patients with severe renal impairment.

Treatment of Pregnant Women During the Third Trimester

Neonates exposed to Lexapro and other SSRIs or SNRIs, late in the third trimester, have developed complications requiring prolonged hospitalization, respiratory support, and tube feeding (see **PRECAUTIONS**). When treating pregnant women with Lexapro during the third trimester, the physician should carefully consider the potential risks and benefits of treatment. The physician may consider tapering Lexapro in the third trimester.

Maintenance Treatment

It is generally agreed that acute episodes of major depressive disorder require several months or longer of sustained pharmacological therapy beyond response to the acute episode. Systematic evaluation of continuing Lexapro 10 or 20 mg/day for periods of up to 36 weeks in patients with major depressive disorder who responded while taking Lexapro during an 8-week, acute-treatment phase demonstrated a benefit of such maintenance treatment (see **Clinical Efficacy Trials** under **CLINICAL PHARMACOLOGY**). Nevertheless, patients should be periodically reassessed to determine the need for maintenance treatment.

Generalized Anxiety Disorder

Initial Treatment

The recommended starting dose of Lexapro is 10 mg once daily. If the dose is increased to 20 mg, this should occur after a minimum of one week.

Lexapro should be administered once daily, in the morning or evening, with or without food.

Maintenance Treatment

Generalized anxiety disorder is recognized as a chronic condition. The efficacy of Lexapro in the treatment of GAD beyond 8 weeks has not been systematically studied. The physician who elects to use Lexapro for extended periods should periodically re-evaluate the long-term usefulness of the drug for the individual patient.

Discontinuation of Treatment with Lexapro

Symptoms associated with discontinuation of Lexapro and other SSRIs and SNRIs have been reported (see **PRECAUTIONS**). Patients should be monitored for these symptoms when discontinuing treatment. A gradual reduction in the dose rather than abrupt cessation is recommended whenever possible. If intolerable symptoms occur following a decrease in the dose or upon discontinuation of treatment, then resuming the previously prescribed dose may be considered. Subsequently, the physician may continue decreasing the dose but at a more gradual rate.

Switching Patients To or From a Monoamine Oxidase Inhibitor

At least 14 days should elapse between discontinuation of an MAOI and initiation of Lexapro therapy. Similarly, at least 14 days should be allowed after stopping Lexapro before starting an MAOI (see **CONTRAINDICATIONS** and **WARNINGS**).

HOW SUPPLIED

5 mg Tablets:

Bottle of 100	NDC # 0456-2005-01

White to off-white, round, non-scored, film-coated. Imprint "FL" on one side of the tablet and "5" on the other side.

10 mg Tablets:

Bottle of 100	NDC # 0456-2010-01
10 × 10 Unit Dose	NDC # 0456-2010-63

White to off-white, round, scored, film-coated. Imprint on scored side with "F" on the left side and "L" on the right side.

Imprint on the non-scored side with "10".

20 mg Tablets:

Bottle of 100	NDC # 0456-2020-01
10 × 10 Unit Dose	NDC # 0456-2020-63

White to off-white, round, scored, film-coated. Imprint on scored side with "F" on the left side and "L" on the right side.

Imprint on the non-scored side with "20".

Oral Solution:

5 mg/5 mL, peppermint flavor (240 mL)	NDC # 0456-2101-08

Store at 25°C (77°F); excursions permitted to 15-30°C (59-86°F).

ANIMAL TOXICOLOGY

Retinal Changes in Rats

Pathologic changes (degeneration/atrophy) were observed in the retinas of albino rats in the 2-year carcinogenicity study with racemic citalopram. There was an increase in both incidence and severity of retinal pathology in both male and female rats receiving 80 mg/kg/day. Similar findings were not present in rats receiving 24 mg/kg/day of racemic citalopram for two years, in mice receiving up to 240 mg/kg/day of racemic citalopram for 18 months, or in dogs receiving up to 20 mg/kg/day of racemic citalopram for one year.

Additional studies to investigate the mechanism for this pathology have not been performed, and the potential significance of this effect in humans has not been established.

Cardiovascular Changes in Dogs

In a one-year toxicology study, 5 of 10 beagle dogs receiving oral racemic citalopram doses of 8 mg/kg/day died suddenly between weeks 17 and 31 following initiation of treatment. Sudden deaths were not observed in rats at doses of racemic citalopram up to 120 mg/kg/day, which produced plasma levels of citalopram and its metabolites demethylcitalopram and didemethylcitalopram (DDCT) similar to those observed in dogs at 8 mg/kg/day. A subsequent intravenous dosing study demonstrated that in beagle dogs, racemic DDCT caused QT prolongation, a known risk factor for the observed outcome in dogs.

Forest Pharmaceuticals, Inc.
Subsidiary of Forest Laboratories, Inc.
St. Louis, MO 63045 USA
Licensed from H. Lundbeck A/S
Rev. 02/05

MG #17541(10)

Medication Guide

About Using Antidepressants in Children and Teenagers

What is the most important information I should know if my child is being prescribed an antidepressant?

Parents or guardians need to think about 4 important things when their child is prescribed an antidepressant:

1. There is a risk of suicidal thoughts or actions
2. How to try to prevent suicidal thoughts or actions in your child
3. You should watch for certain signs if your child is taking an antidepressant
4. There are benefits and risks when using antidepressants

1. There is a Risk of Suicidal Thoughts or Actions

Children and teenagers sometimes think about suicide, and many report trying to kill themselves.

Antidepressants increase suicidal thoughts and actions in some children and teenagers. But suicidal thoughts and actions can also be caused by depression, a serious medical condition that is commonly treated with antidepressants. Thinking about killing yourself or trying to kill yourself is called *suicidality* or *being suicidal*.

A large study combined the results of 24 different studies of children and teenagers with depression or other illnesses. In these studies, patients took either a placebo (sugar pill) or an antidepressant for 1 to 4 months. ***No one committed suicide in these studies***, but some patients became suicidal. On sugar pills, 2 out of every 100 became suicidal. On the antidepressants, 4 out of every 100 patients became suicidal.

For some children and teenagers, the risks of suicidal actions may be especially high. These include patients with

- Bipolar illness (sometimes called manic-depressive illness)
- A family history of bipolar illness
- A personal or family history of attempting suicide

If any of these are present, make sure you tell your healthcare provider before your child takes an antidepressant.

2. How to Try to Prevent Suicidal Thoughts and Actions

To try to prevent suicidal thoughts and actions in your child, pay close attention to changes in her or his moods or actions, especially if the changes occur suddenly. Other important people in your child's life can help by paying attention as well (e.g., your child, brothers and sisters, teachers, and other important people). The changes to look out for are listed in Section 3, on what to watch for.

Whenever an antidepressant is started or its dose is changed, pay close attention to your child.

After starting an antidepressant, your child should generally see his or her healthcare provider:

- Once a week for the first 4 weeks
- Every 2 weeks for the next 4 weeks
- After taking the antidepressant for 12 weeks
- After 12 weeks, follow your healthcare provider's advice about how often to come back
- More often if problems or questions arise (see Section 3)

You should call your child's healthcare provider between visits if needed.

3. You Should Watch for Certain Signs If Your Child is Taking an Antidepressant

Contact your child's healthcare provider ***right away*** if your child exhibits any of the following signs for the first time, or if they seem worse, or worry you, your child, or your child's teacher:

- Thoughts about suicide or dying
- Attempts to commit suicide
- New or worse depression
- New or worse anxiety
- Feeling very agitated or restless
- Panic attacks
- Difficulty sleeping (insomnia)
- New or worse irritability
- Acting aggressive, being angry, or violent
- Acting on dangerous impulses
- An extreme increase in activity and talking
- Other unusual changes in behavior or mood

Never let your child stop taking an antidepressant without first talking to his or her healthcare provider.

Stopping an antidepressant suddenly can cause other symptoms.

4. There are Benefits and Risks When Using Antidepressants

Antidepressants are used to treat depression and other illnesses. Depression and other illnesses can lead to suicide. In some children and teenagers, treatment with an antidepressant increases suicidal thinking or actions. It is important to discuss all the risks of treating depression and also the risks of not treating it. You and your child should discuss all treatment choices with your healthcare provider, not just the use of antidepressants.

Other side effects can occur with antidepressants (see section below).

Of all the antidepressants, only fluoxetine (Prozac™) has been FDA approved to treat pediatric depression.

For obsessive compulsive disorder in children and teenagers, FDA has approved only fluoxetine (Prozac™), sertraline (Zoloft™), fluvoxamine, and clomipramine (Anafranil™).

Your healthcare provider may suggest other antidepressants based on the past experience of your child or other family members.

Is this all I need to know if my child is being prescribed an antidepressant?

No. This is a warning about the risk for suicidality. Other side effects can occur with antidepressants. Be sure to ask your healthcare provider to explain all the side effects of the particular drug he or she is prescribing. Also ask about drugs to avoid when taking an antidepressant. Ask your healthcare provider or pharmacist where to find more information.

*Prozac® is a registered trademark of Eli Lilly and Company
*Zoloft® is a registered trademark of Pfizer Pharmaceuticals
*Anafranil® is a registered trademark of Mallinckrodt Inc.

This Medication Guide has been approved by the U.S. Food and Drug Administration for all antidepressants.

NAMENDA® TABLETS ℞

[*nă-mĕn-dă*]

(memantine hydrochloride)

Rx Only

Prescribing information for this product, which appears on pages 1288–1291 of the 2005 PDR, has been completely revised as follows. Please write "See Supplement A" next to the product heading.

DESCRIPTION

Namenda® (memantine hydrochloride) is an orally active NMDA receptor antagonist. The chemical name for memantine hydrochloride is 1-amino-3,5-dimethyladamantane hydrochloride with the following structural formula:

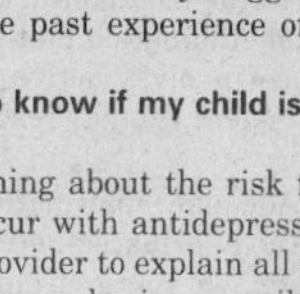

The molecular formula is $C_{12}H_{21}N \cdot HCl$ and the molecular weight is 215.76.

Memantine HCl occurs as a fine white to off-white powder and is soluble in water.

Namenda is available for oral administration as capsule-shaped, film-coated tablets containing 5 mg and 10 mg of

Continued on next page

Namenda—Cont.

memantine hydrochloride. The tablets also contain the following inactive ingredients: microcrystalline cellulose, lactose monohydrate, colloidal silicon dioxide, talc and magnesium stearate. In addition the following inactive ingredients are also present as components of the film coat: hypromellose, triacetin, titanium dioxide, FD&C yellow #6 and FD&C blue #2 (5 mg tablets), iron oxide black (10 mg tablets).

CLINICAL PHARMACOLOGY

Mechanism of Action and Pharmacodynamics

Persistent activation of central nervous system N-methyl-D-aspartate (NMDA) receptors by the excitatory amino acid glutamate has been hypothesized to contribute to the symptomatology of Alzheimer's disease. Memantine is postulated to exert its therapeutic effect through its action as a low to moderate affinity uncompetitive (open-channel) NMDA receptor antagonist which binds preferentially to the NMDA receptor-operated cation channels. There is no evidence that memantine prevents or slows neurodegeneration in patients with Alzheimer's disease.

Memantine showed low to negligible affinity for GABA, benzodiazepine, dopamine, adrenergic, histamine and glycine receptors and for voltage-dependent Ca^{2+}, Na^{+} or K^{+} channels. Memantine also showed antagonistic effects at the $5HT_3$ receptor with a potency similar to that for the NMDA receptor and blocked nicotinic acetylcholine receptors with one-sixth to one-tenth the potency.

In vitro studies have shown that memantine does not affect the reversible inhibition of acetylcholinesterase by donepezil, galantamine, or tacrine.

Pharmacokinetics

Memantine is well absorbed after oral administration and has linear pharmacokinetics over the therapeutic dose range. It is excreted predominantly in the urine, unchanged, and has a terminal elimination half life of about 60–80 hours.

Absorption and Distribution

Following oral administration memantine is highly absorbed with peak concentrations reached in about 3–7 hours. Food has no effect on the absorption of memantine. The mean volume of distribution of memantine is 9–11 L/kg and the plasma protein binding is low (45%).

Metabolism and Elimination

Memantine undergoes little metabolism, with the majority (57–82%) of an administered dose excreted unchanged in urine; the remainder is converted primarily to three polar metabolites: the N-gludantan conjugate, 6-hydroxy memantine, and 1-nitroso-deaminated memantine. These metabolites possess minimal NMDA receptor antagonist activity. The hepatic microsomal CYP450 enzyme system does not play a significant role in the metabolism of memantine. Memantine has a terminal elimination half-life of about 60–80 hours. Renal clearance involves active tubular secretion moderated by pH dependent tubular reabsorption.

Special Populations

Renal Impairment: Adequate information on the effect of renal impairment on the pharmacokinetics of memantine is not available. As the major route of elimination is renal, however, it is very likely that subjects with moderate and severe renal impairment will have significantly higher exposure than normal subjects.

Elderly: The pharmacokinetics of Namenda in young and elderly subjects are similar.

Gender: Following multiple dose administration of Namenda 20 mg b.i.d., females had about 45% higher exposure than males, but there was no difference in exposure when body weight was taken into account.

Drug-Drug Interactions

Substrates of Microsomal Enzymes: *In vitro* studies have shown that memantine produces minimal inhibition of CYP450 enzymes CYP1A2, CYP2A6, CYP2C9, CYP2D6, CYP2E1, and CYP3A4. These data indicate that no pharmacokinetic interactions with drugs metabolized by these enzymes are expected.

Inhibitors of Microsomal Enzymes: Since memantine undergoes minimal metabolism, with the majority of the dose excreted unchanged in urine, an interaction between memantine and drugs that are inhibitors of CYP450 enzymes is unlikely. Coadministration of Namenda with the AChE inhibitor donepezil HCl does not affect the pharmacokinetics of either compound.

Drugs Eliminated via Renal Mechanisms: Memantine is eliminated in part by tubular secretion. *In vivo* studies have shown that multiple doses of the diuretic hydrochlorothiazide/triamterene (HCTZ/TA) did not affect the AUC of memantine at steady state. Memantine did not affect the bioavailability of TA, and decreased AUC and C_{max} of HCTZ by about 20%.

Drugs that make the urine alkaline: The clearance of memantine was reduced by about 80% under alkaline urine conditions at pH 8. Therefore, alterations of urine pH towards the alkaline state may lead to an accumulation of the drug with a possible increase in adverse effects. Drugs that alkalinize the urine (e.g. carbonic anhydrase inhibitors, sodium bicarbonate) would be expected to reduce renal elimination of memantine.

Drugs highly bound to plasma proteins: Because the plasma protein binding of memantine is low (45%), an interaction with drugs that are highly bound to plasma proteins, such as warfarin and digoxin, is unlikely.

CLINICAL TRIALS

The effectiveness of Namenda (memantine hydrochloride) as a treatment for patients with moderate to severe Alzheimer's disease was demonstrated in 2 randomized, double-blind, placebo-controlled clinical studies (Studies 1 and 2) conducted in the United States that assessed both cognitive function and day to day function. The mean age of patients participating in these two trials was 76 with a range of 50–93 years. Approximately 66% of patients were female and 91% of patients were Caucasian.

A third study (Study 3), carried out in Latvia, enrolled patients with severe dementia, but did not assess cognitive function as a planned endpoint.

Study Outcome Measures: In each U.S. study, the effectiveness of Namenda was determined using both an instrument designed to evaluate overall function through caregiver-related assessment, and an instrument that measures cognition. Both studies showed that patients on Namenda experienced significant improvement on both measures compared to placebo.

Day-to-day function was assessed in both studies using the modified Alzheimer's disease Cooperative Study – Activities of Daily Living inventory (ADCS-ADL). The ADCS-ADL consists of a comprehensive battery of ADL questions used to measure the functional capabilities of patients. Each ADL item is rated from the highest level of independent performance to complete loss. The investigator performs the inventory by interviewing a caregiver familiar with the behavior of the patient. A subset of 19 items, including ratings of the patient's ability to eat, dress, bathe, telephone, travel, shop, and perform other household chores has been validated for the assessment of patients with moderate to severe dementia. This is the modified ADCS-ADL, which has a scoring range of 0 to 54, with the lower scores indicating greater functional impairment.

The ability of Namenda to improve cognitive performance was assessed in both studies with the Severe Impairment Battery (SIB), a multi-item instrument that has been validated for the evaluation of cognitive function in patients with moderate to severe dementia. The SIB examines selected aspects of cognitive performance, including elements of attention, orientation, language, memory, visuospatial ability, construction, praxis, and social interaction. The SIB scoring range is from 0 to 100, with lower scores indicating greater cognitive impairment.

Study 1 (Twenty-Eight-Week Study)

In a study of 28 weeks duration, 252 patients with moderate to severe probable Alzheimer's disease (diagnosed by DSM-IV and NINCDS-ADRDA criteria, with Mini-Mental State Examination scores ≥3 and ≤14 and Global Deterioration Scale Stages 5–6) were randomized to Namenda or placebo. For patients randomized to Namenda, treatment was initiated at 5 mg once daily and increased weekly by 5 mg/day in divided doses to a dose of 20 mg/day (10 mg twice a day).

Effects on the ADCS-ADL:

Figure 1 shows the time course for the change from baseline in the ADCS-ADL score for patients in the two treatment groups completing the 28 weeks of the study. At 28 weeks of treatment, the mean difference in the ADCS-ADL change scores for the Namenda-treated patients compared to the patients on placebo was 3.4 units. Using an analysis based on all patients and carrying their last study observation forward (LOCF analysis), Namenda treatment was statistically significantly superior to placebo.

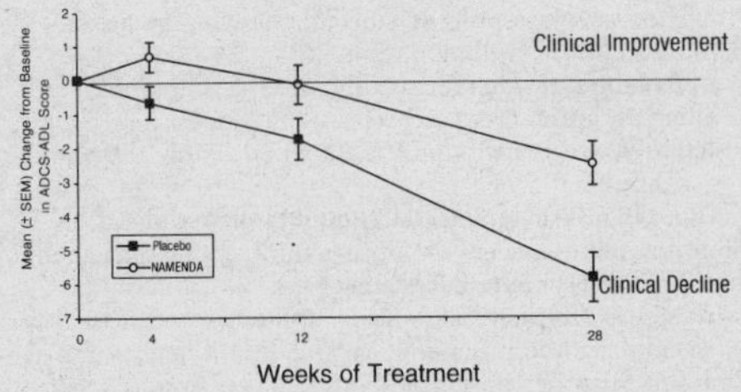

Figure 1: Time course of the change from baseline in ADCS-ADL score for patients completing 28 weeks of treatment.

Figure 2 shows the cumulative percentages of patients from each of the treatment groups who had attained at least the change in the ADCS-ADL shown on the X axis.

The curves show that both patients assigned to Namenda and placebo have a wide range of responses and generally show deterioration (a negative change in ADCS-ADL compared to baseline), but that the Namenda group is more likely to show a smaller decline or an improvement. (In a cumulative distribution display, a curve for an effective treatment would be shifted to the left of the curve for placebo, while an ineffective or deleterious treatment would be superimposed upon or shifted to the right of the curve for placebo.)

[See figure at top of next column]

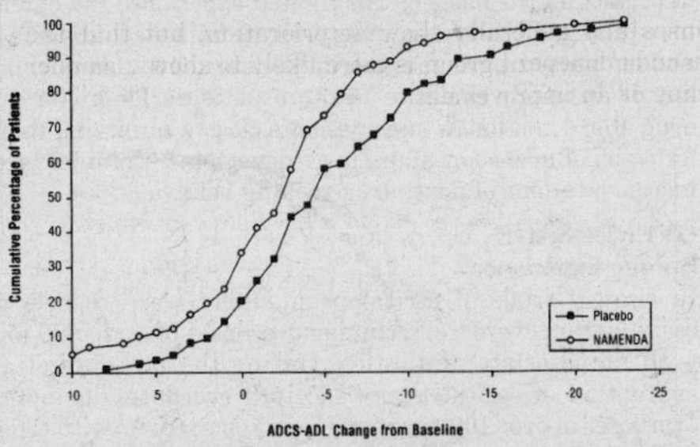

Figure 2: Cumulative percentage of patients completing 28 weeks of double-blind treatment with specified changes from baseline in ADCS-ADL scores.

Effects on the SIB:

Figure 3 shows the time course for the change from baseline in SIB score for the two treatment groups over the 28 weeks of the study. At 28 weeks of treatment, the mean difference in the SIB change scores for the Namenda-treated patients compared to the patients on placebo was 5.7 units. Using an LOCF analysis, Namenda treatment was statistically significantly superior to placebo.

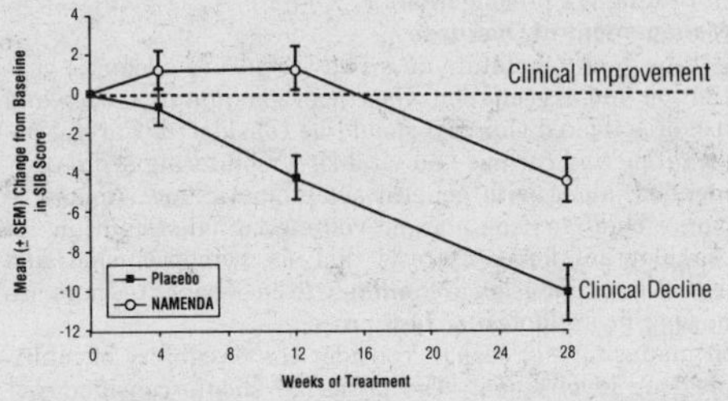

Figure 3: Time course of the change from baseline in SIB score for patients completing 28 weeks of treatment.

Figure 4 shows the cumulative percentages of patients from each treatment group who had attained at least the measure of change in SIB score shown on the X axis.

The curves show that both patients assigned to Namenda and placebo have a wide range of responses and generally show deterioration, but that the Namenda group is more likely to show a smaller decline or an improvement.

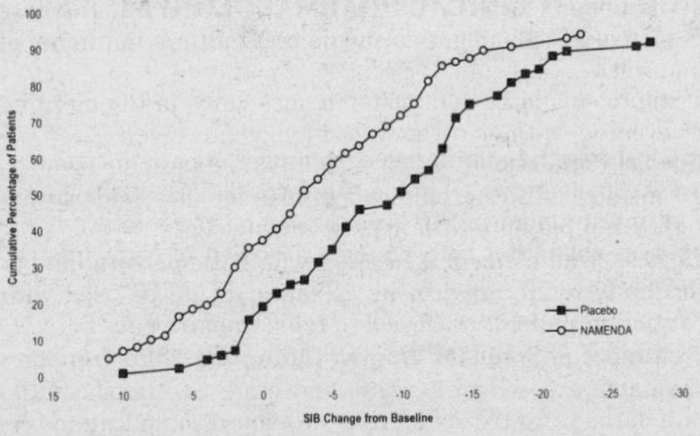

Figure 4: Cumulative percentage of patients completing 28 weeks of double-blind treatment with specified changes from baseline in SIB scores.

Study 2 (Twenty-Four-Week Study)

In a study of 24 weeks duration, 404 patients with moderate to severe probable Alzheimer's disease (diagnosed by NINCDS-ADRDA criteria, with Mini-Mental State Examination scores ≥5 and ≤14) who had been treated with donepezil for at least 6 months and who had been on a stable dose of donepezil for the last 3 months were randomized to Namenda or placebo while still receiving donepezil. For patients randomized to Namenda, treatment was initiated at 5 mg once daily and increased weekly by 5 mg/day in divided doses to a dose of 20 mg/day (10 mg twice a day).

Effects on the ADCS-ADL:

Figure 5 shows the time course for the change from baseline in the ADCS-ADL score for the two treatment groups over the 24 weeks of the study. At 24 weeks of treatment, the mean difference in the ADCS-ADL change scores for the Namenda/donepezil treated patients (combination therapy) compared to the patients on placebo/donepezil (monotherapy) was 1.6 units. Using an LOCF analysis, Namenda/donepezil treatment was statistically significantly superior to placebo/donepezil.

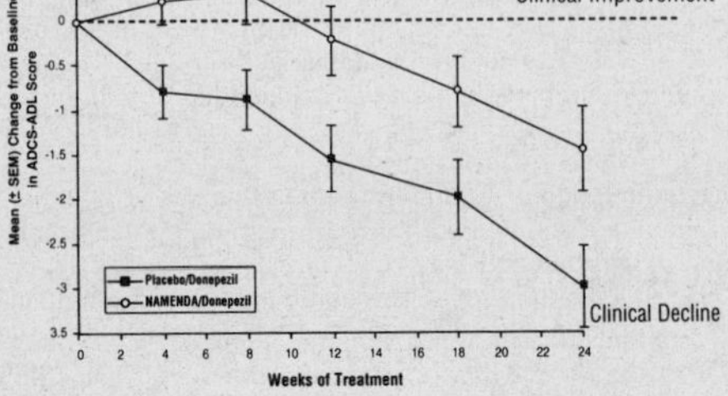

Figure 5: Time course of the change from baseline in ADCS-ADL score for patients completing 24 weeks of treatment.

Figure 6 shows the cumulative percentages of patients from each of the treatment groups who had attained at least the measure of improvement in the ADCS-ADL shown on the X axis.

The curves show that both patients assigned to Namenda/donepezil and placebo/donepezil have a wide range of responses and generally show deterioration, but that the Namenda/donepezil group is more likely to show a smaller decline or an improvement.

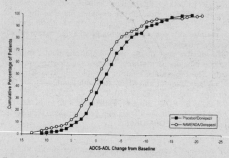

Figure 6: Cumulative percentage of patients completing 24 weeks of double-blind treatment with specified changes from baseline in ADCS-ADL scores.

Effects on the SIB:

Figure 7 shows the time course for the change from baseline in SIB score for the two treatment groups over the 24 weeks of the study. At 24 weeks of treatment, the mean difference in the SIB change scores for the Namenda/donepezil-treated patients compared to the patients on placebo/donepezil was 3.3 units. Using an LOCF analysis, Namenda/donepezil treatment was statistically significantly superior to placebo/donepezil.

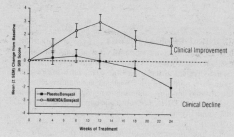

Figure 7: Time course of the change from baseline in SIB score for patients completing 24 weeks of treatment.

Figure 8 shows the cumulative percentages of patients from each treatment group who had attained at least the measure of improvement in SIB score shown on the X axis. The curves show that both patients assigned to Namenda/donepezil and placebo/donepezil have a wide range of responses, but that the Namenda/donepezil group is more likely to show an improvement or a smaller decline.

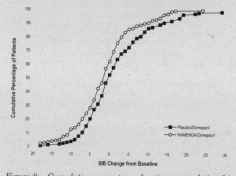

Figure 8: Cumulative percentage of patients completing 24 weeks of double-blind treatment with specified changes from baseline in SIB scores.

Study 3 (Twelve-Week Study)

In a double-blind study of 12 weeks duration, conducted in nursing homes in Latvia, 166 patients with dementia according to DSM-III-R, a Mini-Mental Status Examination score of <10, and Global Deterioration Scale staging of 5 to 7 were randomized to either Namenda or placebo. For patients randomized to Namenda, treatment was initiated at 5 mg once daily and increased to 10 mg once daily after 1 week. The primary efficacy measures were the care dependency subscale of the Behavioral Rating Scale for Geriatric Patients (BGP), a measure of day-to-day function, and a Clinical Global Impression of Change (CGI-C), a measure of overall clinical effect. No valid measure of cognitive function was used in this study. A statistically significant treatment difference at 12 weeks that favored Namenda over placebo was seen on both primary efficacy measures. Because the patients entered were a mixture of Alzheimer's disease and vascular dementia, an attempt was made to distinguish the two groups and all patients were later designated as having either vascular dementia or Alzheimer's disease, based on their scores on the Hachinski Ischemic Scale at study entry. Only about 50% of the patients had computerized tomography of the brain. For the subset designated as having Alzheimer's disease, a statistically significant treatment effect favoring Namenda over placebo at 12 weeks was seen on both the BGP and CGI-C.

INDICATIONS AND USAGE

Namenda (memantine hydrochloride) is indicated for the treatment of moderate to severe dementia of the Alzheimer's type.

CONTRAINDICATIONS

Namenda (memantine hydrochloride) is contraindicated in patients with known hypersensitivity to memantine hydrochloride or to any excipients used in the formulation.

PRECAUTIONS

Information for Patients and Caregivers: Caregivers should be instructed in the recommended administration (twice per day for doses above 5 mg) and dose escalation (minimum interval of one week between dose increases).

Neurological Conditions

Seizures: Namenda has not been systematically evaluated in patients with a seizure disorder. In clinical trials of Namenda, seizures occurred in 0.2% of patients treated with Namenda and 0.5% of patients treated with placebo.

Genitourinary Conditions

Conditions that raise urine pH may decrease the urinary elimination of memantine resulting in increased plasma levels of memantine.

Special Populations

Hepatic Impairment

Namenda undergoes partial hepatic metabolism, but the major fraction of a dose (57–82%) is excreted unchanged in urine. The pharmacokinetics of memantine in patients with hepatic impairment have not been investigated, but would be expected to be only modestly affected.

Renal Impairment

There are inadequate data available in patients with mild, moderate, and severe renal impairment but it is likely that patients with moderate renal impairment will have higher exposure than normal subjects. Dose reduction in these patients should be considered. The use of Namenda in patients with severe renal impairment is not recommended.

Drug-Drug Interactions

N-methyl-D-aspartate (NMDA) antagonists: The combined use of Namenda with other NMDA antagonists (amantadine, ketamine, and dextromethorphan) has not been systematically evaluated and such use should be approached with caution.

Effects of Namenda on substrates of microsomal enzymes: In vitro studies conducted with marker substrates of CYP450 enzymes (CYP1A2, −2A6, −2C9, −2D6, −2E1, −3A4) showed minimal inhibition of these enzymes by memantine. No pharmacokinetic interactions with drugs metabolized by these enzymes are expected.

Effects of inhibitors and/or substrates of microsomal enzymes on Namenda: Memantine is predominantly renally eliminated, and drugs that are substrates and/or inhibitors of the CYP450 system are not expected to alter the metabolism of memantine.

Acetylcholinesterase (AChE) inhibitors: Coadministration of Namenda with the AChE inhibitor donepezil HCl did not affect the pharmacokinetics of either compound. In a 24-week controlled clinical study in patients with moderate to severe Alzheimer's disease, the adverse event profile observed with a combination of memantine and donepezil was similar to that of donepezil alone.

Drugs eliminated via renal mechanisms: Because memantine is eliminated in part by tubular secretion, coadministration of drugs that use the same renal cationic system, including hydrochlorothiazide (HCTZ), triamterene (TA), cimetidine, ranitidine, quinidine, and nicotine, could potentially result in altered plasma levels of both agents. However, coadministration of Namenda and HCTZ/TA did not affect the bioavailability of either memantine or TA, and the bioavailability of HCTZ decreased by 20%.

Drugs that make the urine alkaline: The clearance of memantine was reduced by about 80% under alkaline urine conditions at pH 8. Therefore, alterations of urine pH towards the alkaline condition may lead to an accumulation of the drug with a possible increase in adverse effects. Urine pH is altered by diet, drugs (e.g. carbonic anhydrase inhibitors, sodium bicarbonate) and clinical state of the patient (e.g. renal tubular acidosis or severe infections of the urinary tract). Hence, memantine should be used with caution under these conditions.

Carcinogenesis, Mutagenesis and Impairment of Fertility

There was no evidence of carcinogenicity in a 113-week oral study in mice at doses up to 40 mg/kg/day (10 times the maximum recommended human dose [MRHD] on a mg/m² basis). There was also no evidence of carcinogenicity in rats orally dosed at up to 40 mg/kg/day for 71 weeks followed by 20 mg/kg/day (20 and 10 times the MRHD on a mg/m² basis, respectively) through 128 weeks.

Memantine produced no evidence of genotoxic potential when evaluated in the *in vitro S. typhimurium* or *E. coli* reverse mutation assay, an *in vitro* chromosomal aberration test in human lymphocytes, an *in vivo* cytogenetics assay for chromosome damage in rats, and the *in vivo* mouse micronucleus assay. The results were equivocal in an *in vitro* gene mutation assay using Chinese hamster V79 cells.

No impairment of fertility or reproductive performance was seen in rats administered up to 18 mg/kg/day (9 times the MRHD on a mg/m² basis) orally from 14 days prior to mating through gestation and lactation in females, or for 60 days prior to mating in males.

Pregnancy

Pregnancy Category B: Memantine given orally to pregnant rats and pregnant rabbits during the period of organogenesis was not teratogenic up to the highest doses tested (18 mg/kg/day in rats and 30 mg/kg/day in rabbits, which are 9 and 30 times, respectively, the maximum recommended human dose [MRHD] on a mg/m² basis).

Slight maternal toxicity, decreased pup weights and an increased incidence of non-ossified cervical vertebrae were

seen at an oral dose of 18 mg/kg/day in a study in which rats were given oral memantine beginning pre-mating and continuing through the postpartum period. Slight maternal toxicity and decreased pup weights were also seen at this dose in a study in which rats were treated from day 15 of gestation through the post-partum period. The no-effect dose for these effects was 6 mg/kg, which is 3 times the MRHD on a mg/m² basis.

There are no adequate and well-controlled studies of memantine in pregnant women. Memantine should be used during pregnancy only if the potential benefit justifies the potential risk to the fetus.

Nursing Mothers

It is not known whether memantine is excreted in human breast milk. Because many drugs are excreted in human milk, caution should be exercised when memantine is administered to a nursing mother.

Pediatric Use

There are no adequate and well-controlled trials documenting the safety and efficacy of memantine in any illness occurring in children.

ADVERSE REACTIONS

The experience described in this section derives from studies in patients with Alzheimer's disease and vascular dementia.

Adverse Events Leading to Discontinuation: In placebo-controlled trials in which dementia patients received doses of Namenda up to 20 mg/day, the likelihood of discontinuation because of an adverse event was the same in the Namenda group as in the placebo group. No individual adverse event was associated with the discontinuation of treatment in 1% or more of Namenda-treated patients and at a rate greater than placebo.

Adverse Events Reported in Controlled Trials: The reported adverse events in Namenda (memantine hydrochloride) trials reflect experience gained under closely monitored conditions in a highly selected patient population. In actual practice or in other clinical trials, these frequency estimates may not apply, as the conditions of use, reporting behavior and the types of patients treated may differ. Table 1 lists treatment-emergent signs and symptoms that were reported in at least 2% of patients in placebo-controlled dementia trials and for which the rate of occurrence was greater for patients treated with Namenda than for those treated with placebo. No adverse event occurred at a frequency of at least 5% and twice the placebo rate.

Table 1: Adverse Events Reported in Controlled Clinical Trials in at Least 2% of Patients Receiving Namenda and at a Higher Frequency than Placebo-treated Patients.

Body System Adverse Event	Placebo (N = 922) %	Namenda (N = 940) %
Body as a Whole		
Fatigue	1	2
Pain	1	3
Cardiovascular System		
Hypertension	2	4
Central and Peripheral Nervous System		
Dizziness	5	7
Headache	3	6
Gastrointestinal System		
Constipation	3	5
Vomiting	2	3
Musculoskeletal System		
Back pain	2	3
Psychiatric Disorders		
Confusion	5	6
Somnolence	2	3
Hallucination	2	3
Respiratory System		
Coughing	3	4
Dyspnea	1	2

Other adverse events occurring with an incidence of at least 2% in Namenda-treated patients but at a greater or equal rate on placebo were agitation, fall, inflicted injury, urinary incontinence, diarrhea, bronchitis, insomnia, urinary tract infection, influenza-like symptoms, abnormal gait, depression, upper respiratory tract infection, anxiety, peripheral edema, nausea, anorexia, and arthralgia.

Continued on next page

Namenda—Cont.

The overall profile of adverse events and the incidence rates for individual adverse events in the subpopulation of patients with moderate to severe Alzheimer's disease were not different from the profile and incidence rates described above for the overall dementia population.

Vital Sign Changes: Namenda and placebo groups were compared with respect to (1) mean change from baseline in vital signs (pulse, systolic blood pressure, diastolic blood pressure, and weight) and (2) the incidence of patients meeting criteria for potentially clinically significant changes from baseline in these variables. There were no clinically important changes in vital signs in patients treated with Namenda. A comparison of supine and standing vital sign measures for Namenda and placebo in elderly normal subjects indicated that Namenda treatment is not associated with orthostatic changes.

Laboratory Changes: Namenda and placebo groups were compared with respect to (1) mean change from baseline in various serum chemistry, hematology, and urinalysis variables and (2) the incidence of patients meeting criteria for potentially clinically significant changes from baseline in these variables. These analyses revealed no clinically important changes in laboratory test parameters associated with Namenda treatment.

ECG Changes: Namenda and placebo groups were compared with respect to (1) mean change from baseline in various ECG parameters and (2) the incidence of patients meeting criteria for potentially clinically significant changes from baseline in these variables. These analyses revealed no clinically important changes in ECG parameters associated with Namenda treatment.

Other Adverse Events Observed During Clinical Trials

Namenda has been administered to approximately 1350 patients with dementia, of whom more than 1200 received the maximum recommended dose of 20 mg/day. Patients received Namenda treatment for periods of up to 884 days, with 862 patients receiving at least 24 weeks of treatment and 387 patients receiving 48 weeks or more of treatment.

Treatment emergent signs and symptoms that occurred during 8 controlled clinical trials and 4 open-label trials were recorded as adverse events by the clinical investigators using terminology of their own choosing. To provide an overall estimate of the proportion of individuals having similar types of events, the events were grouped into a smaller number of standardized categories using WHO terminology, and event frequencies were calculated across all studies.

All adverse events occurring in at least two patients are included, except for those already listed in Table 1, WHO terms too general to be informative, minor symptoms or events unlikely to be drug-caused, e.g., because they are common in the study population. Events are classified by body system and listed using the following definitions: frequent adverse events – those occurring in at least 1/100 patients; infrequent adverse events – those occurring in 1/100 to 1/1000 patients. These adverse events are not necessarily related to Namenda treatment and in most cases were observed at a similar frequency in placebo-treated patients in the controlled studies.

Body as a Whole: *Frequent:* syncope. *Infrequent:* hypothermia, allergic reaction.

Cardiovascular System: *Frequent:* cardiac failure. *Infrequent:* angina pectoris, bradycardia, myocardial infarction, thrombophlebitis, atrial fibrillation, hypotension, cardiac arrest, postural hypotension, pulmonary embolism, pulmonary edema.

Central and Peripheral Nervous System: *Frequent:* transient ischemic attack, cerebrovascular accident, vertigo, ataxia, hypokinesia. *Infrequent:* paresthesia, convulsions, extrapyramidal disorder, hypertonia, tremor, aphasia, hypoesthesia, abnormal coordination, hemiplegia, hyperkinesia, involuntary muscle contractions, stupor, cerebral hemorrhage, neuralgia, ptosis, neuropathy.

Gastrointestinal System: *Infrequent:* gastroenteritis, diverticulitis, gastrointestinal hemorrhage, melena, esophageal ulceration.

Hemic and Lymphatic Disorders: *Frequent:* anemia. *Infrequent:* leukopenia.

Metabolic and Nutritional Disorders: *Frequent:* increased alkaline phosphatase, decreased weight. *Infrequent:* dehydration, hyponatremia, aggravated diabetes mellitus.

Psychiatric Disorders: *Frequent:* aggressive reaction. *Infrequent:* delusion, personality disorder, emotional lability, nervousness, sleep disorder, libido increased, psychosis, amnesia, apathy, paranoid reaction, thinking abnormal, crying abnormal, appetite increased, paroniria, delirium, depersonalization, neurosis, suicide attempt.

Respiratory System: *Frequent:* pneumonia. *Infrequent:* apnea, asthma, hemoptysis.

Skin and Appendages: *Frequent:* rash. *Infrequent:* skin ulceration, pruritus, cellulitis, eczema, dermatitis, erythematous rash, alopecia, urticaria

Special Senses: *Frequent:* cataract, conjunctivitis. *Infrequent:* macula lutea degeneration, decreased visual acuity, decreased hearing, tinnitus, blepharitis, blurred vision, corneal opacity, glaucoma, conjunctival hemorrhage, eye pain, retinal hemorrhage, xerophthalmia, diplopia, abnormal lacrimation, myopia, retinal detachment.

Urinary System: *Frequent:* frequent micturition. *Infrequent:* dysuria, hematuria, urinary retention

Events Reported Subsequent to the Marketing of Namenda, both US and Ex-US

Although no causal relationship to memantine treatment has been found, the following adverse events have been reported to be temporally associated with memantine treatment and are not described elsewhere in labeling: atrioventricular block, bone fracture, carpal tunnel syndrome, cerebral infarction, chest pain, claudication, colitis, dyskinesia, dysphagia, gastritis, gastroesophageal reflux, grand mal convulsions, intracranial hemorrhage, hepatic failure, hyperlipidemia, hypoglycemia, ileus, impotence, malaise, neuroleptic malignant syndrome, acute pancreatitis, aspiration pneumonia, acute renal failure, prolonged QT interval, restlessness, Stevens-Johnson syndrome, sudden death, supraventricular tachycardia, tachycardia, tardive dyskinesia, and thrombocytopenia.

ANIMAL TOXICOLOGY

Memantine induced neuronal lesions (vacuolation and necrosis) in the multipolar and pyramidal cells in cortical layers III and IV of the posterior cingulate and retrosplenial neocortices in rats, similar to those which are known to occur in rodents administered other NMDA receptor antagonists. Lesions were seen after a single dose of memantine. In a study in which rats were given daily oral doses of memantine for 14 days, the no-effect dose for neuronal necrosis was 6 times the maximum recommended human dose on a mg/m^2 basis. The potential for induction of central neuronal vacuolation and necrosis by NMDA receptor antagonists in humans is unknown.

DRUG ABUSE AND DEPENDENCE

Controlled Substance Class: Memantine HCl is not a controlled substance.

Physical and Psychological Dependence: Memantine HCl is a low to moderate affinity uncompetitive NMDA antagonist that did not produce any evidence of drug-seeking behavior or withdrawal symptoms upon discontinuation in 2,504 patients who participated in clinical trials at therapeutic doses. Post marketing data, outside the U.S., retrospectively collected, has provided no evidence of drug abuse or dependence.

OVERDOSAGE

Because strategies for the management of overdose are continually evolving, it is advisable to contact a poison control center to determine the latest recommendations for the management of an overdose of any drug.

As in any cases of overdose, general supportive measures should be utilized, and treatment should be symptomatic. Elimination of memantine can be enhanced by acidification of urine. In a documented case of an overdosage with up to 400 mg of memantine, the patient experienced restlessness, psychosis, visual hallucinations, somnolence, stupor and loss of consciousness. The patient recovered without permanent sequelae.

DOSAGE AND ADMINISTRATION

The dosage of Namenda (memantine hydrochloride) shown to be effective in controlled clinical trials is 20 mg/day.

The recommended starting dose of Namenda is 5 mg once daily. The recommended target dose is 20 mg/day. The dose should be increased in 5 mg increments to 10 mg/day (5 mg twice a day), 15 mg/day (5 mg and 10 mg as separate doses), and 20 mg/day (10 mg twice a day). The minimum recommended interval between dose increases is one week. Namenda can be taken with or without food.

Doses in Special Populations

Dose reduction in patients with moderate renal impairment should be considered. In patients with severe renal impairment the use of Namenda has not been systematically evaluated and is not recommended. (See Clinical Pharmacology—Pharmacokinetics).

HOW SUPPLIED

5 mg Tablet:

Bottle of 60 NDC #0456-3205-60
10 × 10 Unit Dose NDC #0456-3205-63

The capsule-shaped, film-coated tablets are tan, with the strength (5) debossed on one side and FL on the other.

10 mg Tablet:

Bottle of 60 NDC #0456-3210-60
10 × 10 Unit Dose NDC #0456-3210-63

The capsule-shaped, film-coated tablets are gray, with the strength (10) debossed on one side and FL on the other.

Titration Pak:

PVC/Aluminum Blister package containing 49 tablets. 28 × 5 mg and 21 × 10 mg tablets.
NDC #0456-3200-14

The 5 mg capsule-shaped, film-coated tablets are tan, with the strength (5) debossed on one side and FL on the other. The 10 mg capsule-shaped, film-coated tablets are gray, with the strength (10) debossed on one side and FL on the other.

Store at 25°C (77°F); excursions permitted to 15–30°C (59–86°F) [see USP Controlled Room Temperature].

Forest Pharmaceuticals, Inc.
Subsidiary of Forest Laboratories, Inc.
St. Louis, MO 63045
Licensed from Merz Pharmaceuticals GmbH
Rev. 05/05

MG #19109(03)

THYROLAR® Tablets ℞

[thī-rō-lär]
(Liotrix Tablets, USP)
Rx only

Prescribing information for this product, which appears on page 1292 of the 2005 PDR, has been completely revised as follows. Please write "See Supplement A" next to the product heading.

DESCRIPTION

Thyrolar Tablets (Liotrix Tablets, USP) contain triiodothyronine (T3 liothyronine) sodium and tetraiodothyronine (T4 levothyroxine) sodium in the amounts listed in the "How Supplied" section. (T3 liothyronine sodium is approximately four times as potent as T4 thyroxine on a microgram for microgram basis.)

The inactive ingredients are calcium phosphate, colloidal silicon dioxide, corn starch, lactose, and magnesium stearate. The tablets also contain the following dyes: Thyrolar $^1/_4$ - FD&C Blue #1 and FD&C Red #40; Thyrolar $^1/_2$ - FD&C Red #40 and D&C Yellow #10; Thyrolar 1 - FD&C Red #40; Thyrolar 2 - FD&C Blue #1, FD&C Red #40, and D&C Yellow #10; Thyrolar 3 - FD&C Red #40 and D&C Yellow #10.

STRUCTURAL FORMULAS

Liothyronine (T_3) Sodium

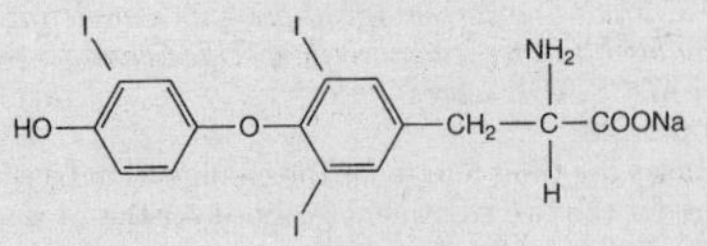

Levothyroxine (T_4) Sodium

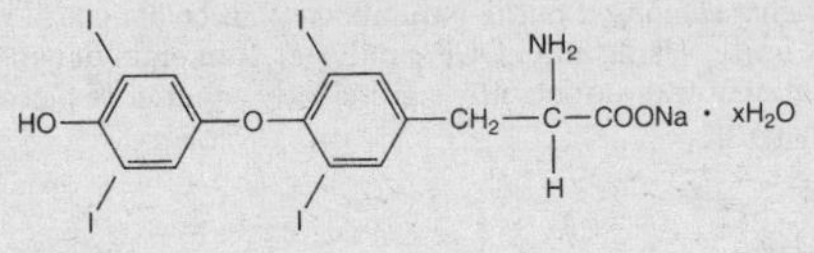

CLINICAL PHARMACOLOGY

The steps in the synthesis of the thyroid hormones are controlled by thyrotropin (Thyroid Stimulating Hormone, TSH) secreted by the anterior pituitary. This hormone's secretion is in turn controlled by a feedback mechanism effected by the thyroid hormones themselves and by thyrotropin releasing hormone (TRH), a tripeptide of hypothalamic origin. Endogenous thyroid hormone secretion is suppressed when exogenous thyroid hormones are administered to euthyroid individuals in excess of the normal gland's secretion.

The mechanisms by which thyroid hormones exert their physiologic action are not well understood. These hormones enhance oxygen consumption by most tissues of the body, increase the basal metabolic rate, and the metabolism of carbohydrates, lipids, and proteins. Thus, they exert a profound influence on every organ system in the body and are of particular importance in the development of the central nervous system.

The normal thyroid gland contains approximately 200 mcg of levothyroxine (T4) per gram of gland, and 15 mcg of triiodothyronine (T3) per gram. The ratio of these two hormones in the circulation does not represent the ratio in the thyroid gland, since about 80 percent of peripheral triiodothyronine comes from monodeiodination of levothyroxine. Peripheral monodeiodination of levothyroxine at the 5 position (inner ring) also results in the formation of reverse triiodothyronine (T3), which is calorigenically inactive.

Triiodothyronine (T3) levels are low in the fetus and newborn, in old age, in chronic caloric deprivation, hepatic cirrhosis, renal failure, surgical stress, and chronic illnesses representing what has been called the "low triiodothyronine syndrome."

Pharmacokinetics—Animal studies have shown that T4 is only partially absorbed from the gastrointestinal tract. The degree of absorption is dependent on the vehicle used for its administration and by the character of the intestinal contents, the intestinal flora, including plasma protein, soluble dietary factors, all of which bind thyroid and thereby make it unavailable for diffusion. Only 41 percent is absorbed when given in a gelatin capsule as opposed to a 74 percent absorption when given with an albumin carrier.

Depending on other factors, absorption has varied from 48 to 79 percent of the administered dose. Fasting increases absorption. Malabsorption syndromes, as well as dietary factors (children's soybean formula, concomitant use of anionic exchange resins such as cholestyramine) cause excessive fecal loss. T3 is almost totally absorbed, 95 percent in 4 hours. The hormones contained in the natural preparations are absorbed in a manner similar to the synthetic hormones.

More than 99 percent of circulating hormones are bound to serum proteins, including thyroid-binding globulin (TBg), thyroid-binding prealbumin (TBPA), and albumin (TBa), whose capacities and affinities vary for the hormones. The higher affinity of levothyroxine (T4) for both TBg and TBPA as compared to triiodothyronine (T3) partially explains the higher serum levels and longer half-life of the former hormone. Both protein-bound hormones exist in reverse equilibrium with minute amounts of free hormone, the latter accounting for the metabolic activity.

Deiodination of levothyroxine (T4) occurs at a number of sites, including liver, kidney, and other tissues. The conjugated hormone, in the form of glucuronide or sulfate, is found in the bile and gut where it may complete an enterohepatic circulation. Eighty-five percent of levothyroxine (T4) metabolized daily is deiodinated.

INDICATIONS AND USAGE

Thyrolar Tablets are indicated:

1. As replacement or supplemental therapy in patients with hypothyroidism of any etiology, except transient hypothy-

roidism during the recovery phase of subacute thyroiditis. This category includes cretinism, myxedema, and ordinary hypothyroidism in patients of any age (children, adults, the elderly), or state (including pregnancy); primary hypothyroidism resulting from functional deficiency, primary atrophy, partial or total absence of thyroid gland, or the effects of surgery, radiation, or drugs, with or without the presence of goiter; and secondary (pituitary), or tertiary (hypothalamic) hypothyroidism (See **WARNINGS**).
2. As pituitary TSH suppressants, in the treatment or prevention of various types of euthyroid goiters, including thyroid nodules, sub-acute or chronic lymphocytic thyroiditis (Hashimoto's), multinodular goiter, and in the management of thyroid cancer.
3. As diagnostic agents in suppression tests to differentiate suspected mild hyperthyroidism or thyroid gland autonomy.

CONTRAINDICATIONS

Thyroid hormone preparations are generally contraindicated in patients with diagnosed but as yet uncorrected adrenal cortical insufficiency, untreated thyrotoxicosis, and apparent hypersensitivity to any of their active or extraneous constituents. There is no well documented evidence from the literature, however, of true allergic or idiosyncratic reactions to thyroid hormone.

WARNINGS

Drugs with thyroid hormone activity, alone or together with other therapeutic agents, have been used for the treatment of obesity. In euthyroid patients, doses within the range of daily hormonal requirements are ineffective for weight reduction. Larger doses may produce serious or even lifethreatening manifestations of toxicity, particularly when given in association with sympathomimetic amines such as those used for their anorectic effects.
The use of thyroid hormones in the therapy of obesity, alone or combined with other drugs, is unjustified and has been shown to be ineffective. Neither is their use justified for the treatment of male or female infertility unless this condition is accompanied by hypothyroidism.

PRECAUTIONS

General—Thyroid hormones should be used with great caution in a number of circumstances where the integrity of the cardiovascular system, particularly the coronary arteries, is suspected.
These include patients with angina pectoris or the elderly, in whom there is a greater likelihood of occult cardiac disease. In these patients therapy should be initiated with low doses, i.e., one tablet of Thyrolar $^1/_4$ or Thyrolar $^1/_2$. When, in such patients, a euthyroid state can only be reached at the expense of an aggravation of the cardiovascular disease, thyroid hormone dosage should be reduced.
Thyroid hormone therapy in patients with concomitant diabetes mellitus or diabetes insipidus or adrenal cortical insufficiency aggravates the intensity of their symptoms. Appropriate adjustments of the various therapeutic measures directed at these concomitant endocrine diseases are required. The therapy of myxedema coma requires simultaneous administration of glucocorticoids (See **DOSAGE AND ADMINISTRATION**).
Hypothyroidism decreases and hyperthyroidism increases the sensitivity to oral anticoagulants. Prothrombin time should be closely monitored in thyroid treated patients on oral anticoagulants and dosage of the latter agents adjusted on the basis of frequent prothrombin time determinations.
In infants, excessive doses of thyroid hormone preparations may produce craniosynostosis.
Information for the Patient—Patients on thyroid hormone preparations and parents of children on thyroid therapy should be informed that:
1. Replacement therapy is to be taken essentially for life, with the exception of cases of transient hypothyroidism, usually associated with thyroiditis, and in those patients receiving a therapeutic trial of the drug.
2. They should immediately report during the course of therapy any signs or symptoms of thyroid hormone toxicity, e.g., chest pain, increased pulse rate, palpitations, excessive sweating, heat intolerance, nervousness, or any other unusual event.
3. In case of concomitant diabetes mellitus, the daily dosage of antidiabetic medication may need readjustment as thyroid hormone replacement is achieved. If thyroid medication is stopped, a downward readjustment of the dosage of insulin or oral hypoglycemic agent may be necessary to avoid hypoglycemia. At all times, close monitoring of urinary glucose levels is mandatory in such patients.
4. In case of concomitant oral anticoagulant therapy, the prothrombin time should be measured frequently to determine if the dosage of oral anticoagulants is to be readjusted.
5. Partial loss of hair may be experienced by children in the first few months of thyroid therapy, but this is usually a transient phenomenon and later recovery is usually the rule.
6. Tablets should be stored at cold temperature, between 36°F and 46°F (2°C and 8°C) in a tight, light-resistant container.
Laboratory Tests—Treatment of patients with thyroid hormones requires the periodic assessment of thyroid status by means of appropriate laboratory tests besides the full clinical evaluation. The TSH suppression test can be used to test the effectiveness of any thyroid preparation bearing in mind the relative insensitivity of the infant pituitary to the negative feedback effect of thyroid hormones. Serum T4 levels can be used to test the effectiveness of all thyroid medications except T3. When the total serum T4 is low but TSH is normal, a test specific to assess unbound (free) T4 levels is warranted. Specific measurements of T4 and T3 by competitive protein binding or radioimmunoassay are not influenced by blood levels of organic or inorganic iodine.

Name	Composition (T3/T4 per tablet)	Color	Armacode®	NDC
Thyrolar—$^1/_4$	3.1 mcg/12.5 mcg	Violet/White	YC	0456–0040–01
Thyrolar—$^1/_2$	6.25 mcg/25 mcg	Peach/White	YD	0456–0045–01
Thyrolar—1	12.5 mcg/50 mcg	Pink/White	YE	0456–0050–01
Thyrolar—2	25 mcg/100 mcg	Green/White	YF	0456–0055–01
Thyrolar—3	37.5 mcg/150 mcg	Yellow/White	YH	0456–0060–01

Drug Interactions—Oral Anticoagulants—Thyroid hormones appear to increase catabolism of vitamin K-dependent clotting factors. If oral anticoagulants are also being given, compensatory increases in clotting factor synthesis are impaired. Patients stabilized on oral anticoagulants who are found to require thyroid replacement therapy should be watched very closely when thyroid is started. If a patient is truly hypothyroid, it is likely that a reduction in anticoagulant dosage will be required. No special precautions appear to be necessary when oral anticoagulant therapy is begun in a patient already stabilized on maintenance thyroid replacement therapy.
Insulin or Oral Hypoglycemics—Initiating thyroid replacement therapy may cause increases in insulin or oral hypoglycemic requirements. The effects seen are poorly understood and depend upon a variety of factors such as dose and type of thyroid preparations and endocrine status of the patient. Patients receiving insulin or oral hypoglycemics should be closely watched during initiation of thyroid replacement therapy.
Cholestyramine or Colestipol—Cholestyramine or colestipol binds both T4 and T3 in the intestine thus impairing absorption of these thyroid hormones. In vitro studies indicate that the binding is not easily removed. Therefore, four to five hours should elapse between administration of cholestyramine or colestipol and thyroid hormones.
Estrogen, Oral Contraceptives—Estrogens tend to increase serum thyroxine-binding globulin (TBg). In a patient with a nonfunctioning thyroid gland who is receiving thyroid replacement therapy, free levothyroxine may be decreased when estrogens are started, thus increasing thyroid requirements. However, if the patient's thyroid gland has sufficient function, the decreased free thyroxine will result in a compensatory increase in thyroxine output by the thyroid. Therefore, patients without a functioning thyroid gland who are on thyroid replacement therapy may need to increase their thyroid dose if estrogens or estrogen-containing oral contraceptives are given.
Drug/Laboratory Test Interactions—The following drugs or moieties are known to interfere with laboratory tests performed in patients on thyroid hormone therapy: androgens, corticosteroids, estrogens, oral contraceptives containing estrogens, iodine-containing preparations, and the numerous preparations containing salicylates.
1. Changes in TBg concentration should be taken into consideration in the interpretation of T4 and T3 values. In such cases, the unbound (free) hormone should be measured. Pregnancy, estrogens, and estrogen-containing oral contraceptives increase TBg concentrations. TBg may also be increased during infectious hepatitis. Decreases in TBg concentrations are observed in nephrosis, acromegaly, and after androgen or corticosteroid therapy. Familial hyper- or hypothyroxine-binding-globulinemias have been described. The incidence of TBg deficiency approximates 1 in 9,000. The binding of thyroxine by TBPA is inhibited by salicylates.
2. Medicinal or dietary iodine interferes with all in vivo tests of radio-iodine uptake, producing low uptakes which may not be relative of a true decrease in hormone synthesis.
3. The persistence of clinical and laboratory evidence of hypothyroidism in spite of adequate dosage replacement indicates either poor patient compliance, poor absorption, excessive fecal loss, or inactivity of the preparation. Intracellular resistance to thyroid hormone is quite rare.
Carcinogenesis, Mutagenesis, and Impairment of Fertility—A reportedly apparent association between prolonged thyroid therapy and breast cancer has not been confirmed and patients on thyroid for established indications should not discontinue therapy. No confirmatory long-term studies in animals have been performed to evaluate carcinogenic potential, mutagenicity, or impairment of fertility in either males or females.
Pregnancy-Category A—Thyroid hormones do not readily cross the placental barrier. The clinical experience to date does not indicate any adverse effect on fetuses when thyroid hormones are administered to pregnant women. On the basis of current knowledge, thyroid replacement therapy to hypothyroid women should not be discontinued during pregnancy.
Nursing Mothers—Minimal amounts of thyroid hormones are excreted in human milk. Thyroid is not associated with serious adverse reactions and does not have a known tumorigenic potential. However, caution should be exercised when thyroid is administered to a nursing woman.
Pediatric Use—Pregnant mothers provide little or no thyroid hormone to the fetus. The incidence of congenital hypothyroidism is relatively high (1:4000) and the hypothyroid fetus would not derive any benefit from the small amounts of hormone crossing the placental barrier. Routine determinations of serum (T4) and/or TSH is strongly advised in neonates in view of the deleterious effects of thyroid deficiency on growth and development.
Treatment should be initiated immediately upon diagnosis, and maintained for life, unless transient hypothyroidism is suspected; in which case, therapy may be interrupted for 2 to 8 weeks after the age of 3 years to reassess the condition. Cessation of therapy is justified in patients who have maintained a normal TSH during those 2 to 8 weeks.

ADVERSE REACTIONS

During postmarketing surveillance, the following events have been observed to have occured in patients administered Thyrolar: fatigue, sluggishness, increase in weight, alopecia, palpitations, dry skin, urticaria, headache, hyperhidrosis, pruritus, asthenia, increased blood pressure, arthralgia, myalgia, tremor, hypothyroidism, increase in TSH, decrease in TSH, nausea, chest pain, hypersensitivity, keratoconjunctivitis sicca, increased heart rate, irregular heart rate, anxiety, depression, and insomnia. Adverse reactions other than those indicative of hyperthyroidism because of therapeutic overdosage, either initially or during the maintenance period, are rare (See **OVERDOSAGE**).

OVERDOSAGE

Signs and Symptoms—Excessive doses of thyroid result in a hypermetabolic state resembling in every respect the condition of endogenous origin. The condition may be self-induced.
Treatment of Overdosage—Dosage should be reduced or therapy temporarily discontinued if signs and symptoms of overdosage appear. Treatment may be reinstituted at a lower dosage. In normal individuals, normal hypothalamic-pituitary-thyroid axis function is restored in 6 to 8 weeks after thyroid suppression.
Treatment of acute massive thyroid hormone overdosage is aimed at reducing gastrointestinal absorption of the drugs and counteracting central and peripheral effects, mainly those of increased sympathetic activity. Vomiting may be induced initially if further gastrointestinal absorption can reasonably be prevented and barring contraindications such as coma, convulsions, or loss of the gagging reflex. Treatment is symptomatic and supportive. Oxygen may be administered and ventilation maintained. Cardiac glycosides may be indicated if congestive heart failure develops. Measures to control fever, hypoglycemia, or fluid loss should be instituted if needed. Antiadrenergic agents, particularly propranolol, have been used advantageously in the treatment of increased sympathetic activity. Propranolol may be administered intravenously at a dosage of 1 to 3 mg over a 10 minute period or orally, 80 to 160 mg/day, initially, especially when no contraindications exist for its use.

DOSAGE AND ADMINISTRATION

The dosage of Thyrolar Tablets (Liotrix Tablets, USP) is determined by the indication and must in every case be individualized according to patient response and laboratory findings.
Thyroid hormones are given orally. In acute, emergency conditions, injectable sodium levothyroxine may be given intravenously when oral administration is not feasible or desirable, as in the treatment of myxedema coma, or during total parenteral nutrition. Intramuscular administration is not advisable because of reported poor absorption.
Hypothyroidism—Therapy is usually instituted using low doses with increments which depend on the cardiovascular status of the patient. The usual starting dose is one tablet of Thyrolar $^1/_2$ with increments of one tablet of Thyrolar $^1/_4$ every 2 to 3 weeks. A lower starting dosage, one tablet of Thyrolar $^1/_4$/day, is recommended in patients with long-standing myxedema, particularly if cardiovascular impairment is suspected, in which case extreme caution is recommended. The appearance of angina is an indication for a reduction in dosage. Most patients require one tablet of Thyrolar 1 to one tablet of Thyrolar 2 per day. Failure to respond to doses of one tablet of Thyrolar 3 suggests lack of compliance or malabsorption. Maintenance dosages of one tablet of Thyrolar 1 to one tablet of Thyrolar 2 per day usually result in normal serum levothyroxine (T4) and triiodothyronine (T3) levels. Adequate therapy usually results in normal TSH and T4 levels after 2 to 3 weeks of therapy.
Readjustment of thyroid hormone dosage should be made within the first four weeks of therapy, after proper clinical and laboratory evaluations, including serum levels of T4, bound and free, and TSH. T3 may be used in preference to levothyroxine (T4) during radio-isotope scanning procedures, since induction of hypothyroidism in those cases is more abrupt and can be of shorter duration. It may also be preferred when impairment of peripheral conversion of T4 and T3 is suspected.
Myxedema Coma—Myxedema coma is usually precipitated in the hypothyroid patient of long-standing by intercurrent illness or drugs such as sedatives and anesthetics and should be considered a medical emergency. Therapy should be directed at the correction of electrolyte disturbances and possible infection besides the administration of thyroid hormones. Corticosteroids should be administered routinely. T4 and T3 may be administered via a nasogastric tube but the

Continued on next page

Thyrolar—Cont.

preferred route of administration of both hormones is intravenous. Sodium levothyroxine (T4) is given at a starting dose of 400 mcg (100 mcg/mL) given rapidly, and is usually well tolerated, even in the elderly. This initial dose is followed by daily supplements of 100 to 200 mcg given IV. Normal T4 levels are achieved in 24 hours followed in 3 days by threefold elevation of T3. Oral therapy with thyroid hormone would be resumed as soon as the clinical situation has been stabilized and the patient is able to take oral medication.

Thyroid Cancer—Exogenous thyroid hormone may produce regression of metastases from follicular and papillary carcinoma of the thyroid and is used as ancillary therapy of these conditions with radioactive iodine. TSH should be suppressed to low or undetectable levels. Therefore, larger amounts of thyroid hormone than those used for replacement therapy are required. Medullary carcinoma of the thyroid is usually unresponsive to this therapy.

Thyroid Suppression Therapy—Administration of thyroid hormone in doses higher than those produced physiologically by the gland results in suppression of the production of endogenous hormone. This is the basis for the thyroid suppression test and is used as an aid in the diagnosis of patients with signs of mild hyperthyroidism in whom baseline laboratory tests appear normal, or to demonstrate thyroid gland autonomy in patients with Grave's ophthalmopathy. 131I uptake is determined before and after the administration of the exogenous hormone. A fifty percent or greater suppression of uptake indicates a normal thyroid-pituitary axis and thus rules out thyroid gland autonomy.

For adults, the usual suppressive dose of levothyroxine (T4) is 1.56 mcg/kg of body weight per day given for 7 to 10 days. These doses usually yield normal serum T4 and T3 levels and lack of response to TSH.

Thyroid hormones should be administered cautiously to patients in whom there is strong suspicion of thyroid gland autonomy, in view of the fact that the exogenous hormone effects will be additive to the endogenous source.

Pediatric Dosage—Pediatric dosage should follow the recommendations summarized in Table 1. In infants with congenital hypothyroidism, therapy with full doses should be instituted as soon as the diagnosis has been made.

Recommended Pediatric Dosage for Congenital Hypothyroidism Table 1

Age	Dose per day in mcg T3/T4 to T3/T4
0-6 mos	3.1/12.5 to 6.25/25
6-12 mos	6.25/25 to 9.35/37.5
1-5 yrs	9.35/37.5 to 12.5/50
6-12 yrs	12.5/50 to 18.75/75
Over 12 yrs	over 18.75/75

HOW SUPPLIED

Thyrolar Tablets (Liotrix Tablets, USP) are available in five potencies coded as follows:

[See table at top of previous page]

Supplied in bottles of 100, two-layered compressed tablets. Tablets should be stored at cold temperature, between 36°F and 46°F (2°C and 8°C) in a tight, light-resistant container. Note: (T3 liothyronine sodium is approximately four times as potent as T4 thyroxine on a microgram for microgram basis.)

FOREST PHARMACEUTICALS, INC.
A Subsidiary of Forest Laboratories, Inc.
St. Louis, MO 63045
Rev. 07/04
RMC #1436
©2004 Forest Laboratories, Inc.

To keep your **PDR** up to date throughout the year, note these revisions on the corresponding pages of the annual volume. Simply write **"See Supplement A"** next to the product heading.

GlaxoSmithKline
FIVE MOORE DRIVE
RESEARCH TRIANGLE PARK, NC 27709

For Medical Information for Healthcare Professionals and Consumers, Contact:
1-888-825-5249
www.us.gsk.com

ADVAIR DISKUS® 100/50 ℞
[ad'vair disk'us]
(fluticasone propionate 100 mcg and salmeterol* 50 mcg inhalation powder)

ADVAIR DISKUS® 250/50 ℞
(fluticasone propionate 250 mcg and salmeterol* 50 mcg inhalation powder)

ADVAIR DISKUS® 500/50 ℞
(fluticasone propionate 500 mcg and salmeterol* 50 mcg inhalation powder)

***As salmeterol xinafoate salt 72.5 mcg, equivalent to salmeterol base 50 mcg**
FOR ORAL INHALATION ONLY

Prescribing information for this product, which appears on pages 1387–1396 of the 2005 PDR, has been revised as follows. Please write "See Supplement A" next to the product heading.
The boxed warning at the beginning of the package insert has been revised as follows.

> **WARNING:** Data from a large placebo-controlled US study that compared the safety of salmeterol (SEREVENT® Inhalation Aerosol) or placebo added to usual asthma therapy showed a small but significant increase in asthma-related deaths in patients receiving salmeterol (13 deaths out of 13,176 patients treated for 28 weeks) versus those on placebo (3 of 13,179) (see WARNINGS).

The first 4 paragraphs of the WARNINGS *section have been revised as follows.*

DATA FROM A LARGE PLACEBO-CONTROLLED SAFETY STUDY THAT WAS STOPPED EARLY SUGGEST THAT SALMETEROL, A COMPONENT OF ADVAIR DISKUS, MAY BE ASSOCIATED WITH RARE SERIOUS ASTHMA EPISODES OR ASTHMA-RELATED DEATHS. Data from this study further suggest that the risk might be greater in African American patients. The Salmeterol Multicenter Asthma Research Trial (SMART) was a randomized, double-blind study that enrolled long-acting beta$_2$-agonist-naive patients with asthma to assess the safety of salmeterol (SEREVENT Inhalation Aerosol) 42 mcg twice daily over 28 weeks compared to placebo when added to usual asthma therapy. The primary endpoint was the combined number of respiratory-related deaths or respiratory-related life-threatening experiences (intubation and mechanical ventilation). Secondary endpoints included combined asthma-related deaths or life-threatening experiences and asthma-related deaths.

A planned interim analysis was conducted when approximately half of the intended number of patients had been enrolled (N = 26,355). Due to the low rate of primary events in the study, the findings of the planned interim analysis were not conclusive. However, analyses of secondary endpoints suggested that patients receiving salmeterol may be at increased risk for some of these events compared to patients receiving placebo. The analysis for the total population showed a relative risk of 1.40 (95% CI 0.91, 2.14) for the primary endpoint in the salmeterol group relative to the placebo group (50 out of 13,176 vs. 36 out of 13,179, respectively). In the total population, a higher number of asthma-related deaths (13 vs. 3, RR 4.37, 95% CI 1.25, 15.34) and combined asthma-related deaths or life-threatening experiences (37 vs. 22, RR 1.71, 95% CI 1.01, 2.89) occurred in patients treated with salmeterol than those treated with placebo. The analysis of the African American subgroup showed a relative risk of 4.10 (95% CI 1.54, 10.90) for the primary endpoint in patients treated with salmeterol relative to those treated with placebo (20 out of 2,366 vs. 5 out of 2,319, respectively). In African Americans, a higher number of asthma-related deaths (7 vs. 1, RR 7.26, 95% CI 0.89, 58.94) and combined asthma-related deaths or life-threatening experiences (19 vs. 4, RR 4.92, 95% CI 1.68, 14.45) occurred in patients treated with salmeterol than those treated with placebo. Analysis of the Caucasian population showed a relative risk of 1.05 (95% CI 0.62, 1.76) for the primary endpoint for those treated with salmeterol relative to those treated with placebo (29 out of 9,281 vs. 28 out of 9,361, respectively). In Caucasians, a higher number of asthma-related deaths (6 vs. 1, RR 5.82, 95% CI 0.70, 48.37) occurred in patients treated with salmeterol than in patients treated with placebo. In Caucasians, the relative risk was 1.08 (17 vs. 16, 95% CI 0.55, 2.14) for combined asthma-related deaths or life-threatening experiences in patients treated with salmeterol relative to placebo. The numbers of patients from other ethnic groups were too small to draw any conclusions in these populations. Even though SMART did not reach predetermined stopping criteria for the total population, the study was stopped due to the findings in African American patients and difficulties in enrollment. The data from the SMART study are not adequate to determine whether concurrent use of inhaled corticosteroids, such as fluticasone propionate, a component of ADVAIR DISKUS, provides protection from this risk. Therefore, it is not known whether the findings seen with SEREVENT Inhalation Aerosol would apply to ADVAIR DISKUS. Given the similar basic mechanisms of action of beta$_2$-agonists, it is possible that the findings seen in the SMART study may be consistent with a class effect.

Findings similar to the SMART study findings were reported in a prior 16-week clinical study performed in the United Kingdom, the Salmeterol Nationwide Surveillance (SNS) study. In the SNS study, the incidence of asthma-related death was numerically, though not statistically, greater in patients with asthma treated with salmeterol (42 mcg twice daily) versus albuterol (180 mcg 4 times daily) added to usual asthma therapy.

GlaxoSmithKline, Research Triangle Park, NC 27709
©2004, GlaxoSmithKline. All rights reserved.
September 2004/RL-2128

ANCEF® ℞
[an' sef]
cefazolin for injection

Prescribing information for this product, which appears on pages 1415–1416 of the 2005 PDR, has been revised as follows. Please write "See Supplement A" next to the product heading.
The following PRECAUTIONS: Geriatric Use *section has been added.*

Of the 920 subjects who received ANCEF in clinical studies, 313 (34%) were 65 years and over, while 138 (15%) were 75 years and over. No overall differences in safety or effectiveness were observed between these subjects and younger subjects. Other reported clinical experience has not identified differences in responses between the elderly and younger patients, but greater sensitivity of some older individuals cannot be ruled out.

This drug is known to be substantially excreted by the kidney, and the risk of toxic reactions to this drug may be greater in patients with impaired renal function. Because elderly patients are more likely to have decreased renal function, care should be taken in dose selection, and it may be useful to monitor renal function (see PRECAUTIONS, General and DOSAGE AND ADMINISTRATION).

The following pack was added to the HOW SUPPLIED *section.*

Each vial contains cefazolin sodium equivalent to 10 grams of cefazolin. NDC 0007-3135-05 (package of 10 pharmacy bulk vials)

GlaxoSmithKline, Research Triangle Park, NC 27709
©2004, GlaxoSmithKline. All rights reserved.
September 2004/AF:L58, AF:L59

AVANDAMET® ℞
[ə-van' də-met]
(rosiglitazone maleate and metformin hydrochloride) Tablets

Prescribing information for this product, which appears on pages 1433-1438 of the 2005 PDR, has been revised as follows. Please write "See Supplement A" next to the product heading.
The following has been added to the end of the CLINICAL PHARMACOLOGY *section.*

Drug Interactions:

***Rosiglitazone maleate:* Drugs that Inhibit, Induce, or are Metabolized by Cytochrome P450:** In vitro drug metabolism studies suggest that rosiglitazone does not inhibit any of the major P450 enzymes at clinically relevant concentrations. In vitro data demonstrate that rosiglitazone is predominantly metabolized by CYP2C8, and to a lesser extent, 2C9.

Gemfibrozil: Concomitant administration of gemfibrozil (600 mg twice daily), an inhibitor of CYP2C8, and rosiglitazone (4 mg once daily) for 7 days increased rosiglitazone AUC by 127%, compared to the administration of rosiglitazone (4 mg once daily) alone. Given the potential for dose-related adverse events with rosiglitazone, a decrease in the dose of rosiglitazone may be needed when gemfibrozil is introduced.

Rifampin: Rifampin administration (600 mg once a day), an inducer of CYP2C8, for 6 days is reported to decrease rosiglitazone AUC by 66%, compared to the administration of rosiglitazone (8 mg) alone (see PRECAUTIONS).[1]

Rosiglitazone (4 mg twice daily) was shown to have no clinically relevant effect on the pharmacokinetics of nifedipine and oral contraceptives (ethinyl estradiol and norethindrone), which are predominantly metabolized by CYP3A4.

***Metformin hydrochloride:* Furosemide:** A single-dose, metformin-furosemide drug interaction study in healthy subjects demonstrated that pharmacokinetic parameters of both compounds were affected by coadministration. Furosemide increased the metformin plasma and blood C_{max} by 22% and blood AUC by 15%, without any significant change in metformin renal clearance. When administered with metformin, the C_{max} and AUC of furosemide were 31% and 12% smaller, respectively, than when administered alone, and the terminal half-life was decreased by 32%, without any significant change in furosemide renal clearance. No information is available about the interaction of metformin and furosemide when coadministered chronically.

Nifedipine: A single-dose, metformin-nifedipine drug interaction study in normal healthy volunteers demonstrated that coadministration of nifedipine increased plasma metformin C_{max} and AUC by 20% and 9%, respectively, and increased the amount excreted in the urine. T_{max} and half-life were unaffected. Nifedipine appears to enhance the absorption of metformin. Metformin had minimal effects on nifedipine.

Cationic Drugs: Cationic drugs (e.g., amiloride, digoxin, morphine, procainamide, quinidine, quinine, ranitidine, triamterene, trimethoprim, and vancomycin) that are eliminated by renal tubular secretion theoretically have the potential for interaction with metformin by competing for common renal tubular transport systems. Such interaction between metformin and oral cimetidine has been observed in normal healthy volunteers in both single- and multiple-dose, metformin-cimetidine drug interaction studies, with a 60% increase in peak metformin plasma and whole blood concentrations and a 40% increase in plasma and whole blood metformin AUC. There was no change in elimination half-life in the single-dose study. Metformin had no effect on cimetidine pharmacokinetics.

Other: Certain drugs tend to produce hyperglycemia and may lead to loss of glycemic control. These drugs include thiazides and other diuretics, corticosteroids, phenothiazines, thyroid products, estrogens, oral contraceptives, phenytoin, nicotinic acid, sympathomimetics, calcium channel blocking drugs, and isoniazid.

In healthy volunteers, the pharmacokinetics of metformin and propranolol and metformin and ibuprofen were not affected when coadministered in single-dose interaction studies.

Metformin is negligibly bound to plasma proteins and is therefore, less likely to interact with highly protein-bound drugs such as salicylates, sulfonamides, chloramphenicol, and probenecid.

The following PRECAUTIONS subsection has been revised.

Drug Interactions: An inhibitor of CYP2C8 (such as gemfibrozil) may increase the AUC of rosiglitazone and an inducer of CYP2C8 (such as rifampin) may decrease the AUC of rosiglitazone. Therefore, if an inhibitor or an inducer of CYP2C8 is started or stopped during treatment with rosiglitazone, changes in diabetes treatment may be needed based upon clinical response.

Although drug interactions with cationic drugs (e.g., amiloride, digoxin, morphine, procainamide, quinidine, quinine, ranitidine, triamterene, trimethoprim, and vancomycin) remain theoretical (except for cimetidine), careful patient monitoring and dose adjustment of AVANDAMET and/or the interfering drug is recommended in patients who are taking cationic medications that are excreted via the proximal renal tubular secretory system.

When drugs that produce hyperglycemia which may lead to loss of glycemic control are administered to a patient receiving AVANDAMET, the patient should be closely observed to maintain adequate glycemic control. (See CLINICAL PHARMACOLOGY, Drug Interactions.)

The following has been added to the end of the package insert.

REFERENCE

1. Park JY, Kim KA, Kang MH, et al. Effect of rifampin on the pharmacokinetics of rosiglitazone in healthy subjects. *Clin Pharmacol Ther* 2004;75:157–162.

GlaxoSmithKline, Research Triangle Park, NC 27709
©2005, GlaxoSmithKline. All rights reserved.
January 2005/AT:L7

AVANDIA®   ℞
[ə-van'dē-ə]
(rosiglitazone maleate)
Tablets

Prescribing information for this product, which appears on pages 1438–1443 of the 2005 PDR, has been completely revised as follows. Please write "See Supplement A" next to the product heading.

DESCRIPTION

AVANDIA (rosiglitazone maleate) is an oral antidiabetic agent which acts primarily by increasing insulin sensitivity. AVANDIA is used in the management of type 2 diabetes mellitus (also known as non-insulin-dependent diabetes mellitus [NIDDM] or adult-onset diabetes). AVANDIA improves glycemic control while reducing circulating insulin levels.

Pharmacological studies in animal models indicate that rosiglitazone improves sensitivity to insulin in muscle and adipose tissue and inhibits hepatic gluconeogenesis. Rosiglitazone maleate is not chemically or functionally related to the sulfonylureas, the biguanides, or the alpha-glucosidase inhibitors.

Chemically, rosiglitazone maleate is (±)-5-[[4-[2-(methyl-2-pyridinylamino)ethoxy]phenyl]methyl]-2,4-thiazolidinedione, (Z)-2-butenedioate (1:1) with a molecular weight of 473.52 (357.44 free base). The molecule has a single chiral center and is present as a racemate. Due to rapid interconversion, the enantiomers are functionally indistinguishable. The molecular formula is $C_{18}H_{19}N_3O_3S \cdot C_4H_4O_4$. Rosiglitazone maleate is a white to off-white solid with a melting point range of 122° to 123°C. The pKa values of rosiglitazone maleate are 6.8 and 6.1. It is readily soluble in ethanol and a buffered aqueous solution with pH of 2.3; solubility decreases with increasing pH in the physiological range. Each pentagonal film-coated TILTAB® tablet contains rosiglitazone maleate equivalent to rosiglitazone, 2 mg, 4 mg, or 8 mg, for oral administration. Inactive ingredients are: Hypromellose 2910, lactose monohydrate, magnesium stearate, microcrystalline cellulose, polyethylene glycol 3000, sodium starch glycolate, titanium dioxide, triacetin, and 1 or more of the following: Synthetic red and yellow iron oxides and talc.

CLINICAL PHARMACOLOGY

Mechanism of Action: Rosiglitazone, a member of the thiazolidinedione class of antidiabetic agents, improves glycemic control by improving insulin sensitivity. Rosiglitazone is a highly selective and potent agonist for the peroxisome proliferator-activated receptor-gamma (PPARγ). In humans, PPAR receptors are found in key target tissues for insulin action such as adipose tissue, skeletal muscle, and liver. Activation of PPARγ nuclear receptors regulates the transcription of insulin-responsive genes involved in the control of glucose production, transport, and utilization. In addition, PPARγ-responsive genes also participate in the regulation of fatty acid metabolism.

Insulin resistance is a common feature characterizing the pathogenesis of type 2 diabetes. The antidiabetic activity of rosiglitazone has been demonstrated in animal models of type 2 diabetes in which hyperglycemia and/or impaired glucose tolerance is a consequence of insulin resistance in target tissues. Rosiglitazone reduces blood glucose concentrations and reduces hyperinsulinemia in the ob/ob obese mouse, db/db diabetic mouse, and fa/fa fatty Zucker rat.

In animal models, rosiglitazone's antidiabetic activity was shown to be mediated by increased sensitivity to insulin's action in the liver, muscle, and adipose tissues. The expression of the insulin-regulated glucose transporter GLUT-4 was increased in adipose tissue. Rosiglitazone did not induce hypoglycemia in animal models of type 2 diabetes and/or impaired glucose tolerance.

Pharmacokinetics and Drug Metabolism: Maximum plasma concentration (C_{max}) and the area under the curve (AUC) of rosiglitazone increase in a dose-proportional manner over the therapeutic dose range (see Table 1). The elimination half-life is 3 to 4 hours and is independent of dose.

Table 1. Mean (SD) Pharmacokinetic Parameters for Rosiglitazone Following Single Oral Doses (N = 32)

Parameter	1 mg Fasting	2 mg Fasting	8 mg Fasting	8 mg Fed
AUC$_{0-inf}$ [ng.hr./mL]	358 (112)	733 (184)	2,971 (730)	2,890 (795)
C_{max} [ng/mL]	76 (13)	156 (42)	598 (117)	432 (92)
Half-life [hr.]	3.16 (0.72)	3.15 (0.39)	3.37 (0.63)	3.59 (0.70)
CL/F* [L/hr.]	3.03 (0.87)	2.89 (0.71)	2.85 (0.69)	2.97 (0.81)

*CL/F = Oral clearance.

Absorption: The absolute bioavailability of rosiglitazone is 99%. Peak plasma concentrations are observed about 1 hour after dosing. Administration of rosiglitazone with food resulted in no change in overall exposure (AUC), but there was an approximately 28% decrease in C_{max} and a delay in T_{max} (1.75 hours). These changes are not likely to be clinically significant; therefore, AVANDIA may be administered with or without food.

Distribution: The mean (CV%) oral volume of distribution (Vss/F) of rosiglitazone is approximately 17.6 (30%) liters, based on a population pharmacokinetic analysis. Rosiglitazone is approximately 99.8% bound to plasma proteins, primarily albumin.

Metabolism: Rosiglitazone is extensively metabolized with no unchanged drug excreted in the urine. The major routes of metabolism were N-demethylation and hydroxylation, followed by conjugation with sulfate and glucuronic acid. All the circulating metabolites are considerably less potent than parent and, therefore, are not expected to contribute to the insulin-sensitizing activity of rosiglitazone. In vitro data demonstrate that rosiglitazone is predominantly metabolized by Cytochrome P_{450} (CYP) isoenzyme 2C8, with CYP2C9 contributing as a minor pathway.

Excretion: Following oral or intravenous administration of [¹⁴C]rosiglitazone maleate, approximately 64% and 23% of the dose was eliminated in the urine and in the feces, respectively. The plasma half-life of [¹⁴C]related material ranged from 103 to 158 hours.

Population Pharmacokinetics in Patients with Type 2 Diabetes: Population pharmacokinetic analyses from 3 large clinical trials including 642 men and 405 women with type 2 diabetes (aged 35 to 80 years) showed that the pharmacokinetics of rosiglitazone are not influenced by age, race, smoking, or alcohol consumption. Both oral clearance (CL/F) and oral steady-state volume of distribution (Vss/F) were shown to increase with increases in body weight. Over the weight range observed in these analyses (50 to 150 kg), the range of predicted CL/F and Vss/F values varied by <1.7-fold and <2.3-fold, respectively. Additionally, rosiglitazone CL/F was shown to be influenced by both weight and gender, being lower (about 15%) in female patients.

Special Populations: Geriatric: Results of the population pharmacokinetic analysis (n = 716 <65 years; n = 331 ≥65 years) showed that age does not significantly affect the pharmacokinetics of rosiglitazone.

Gender: Results of the population pharmacokinetics analysis showed that the mean oral clearance of rosiglitazone in female patients (n = 405) was approximately 6% lower compared to male patients of the same body weight (n = 642). As monotherapy and in combination with metformin, AVANDIA improved glycemic control in both males and females. In metformin combination studies, efficacy was demonstrated with no gender differences in glycemic response. In monotherapy studies, a greater therapeutic response was observed in females; however, in more obese patients, gender differences were less evident. For a given body mass index (BMI), females tend to have a greater fat mass than males. Since the molecular target PPARγ is expressed in adipose tissues, this differentiating characteristic may account, at least in part, for the greater response to AVANDIA in females. Since therapy should be individualized, no dose adjustments are necessary based on gender alone.

Hepatic Impairment: Unbound oral clearance of rosiglitazone was significantly lower in patients with moderate to severe liver disease (Child-Pugh Class B/C) compared to healthy subjects. As a result, unbound C_{max} and AUC$_{0-inf}$ were increased 2- and 3-fold, respectively. Elimination half-life for rosiglitazone was about 2 hours longer in patients with liver disease, compared to healthy subjects.

Therapy with AVANDIA should not be initiated if the patient exhibits clinical evidence of active liver disease or increased serum transaminase levels (ALT >2.5× upper limit of normal) at baseline (see PRECAUTIONS, General, Hepatic Effects).

Renal Impairment: There are no clinically relevant differences in the pharmacokinetics of rosiglitazone in patients with mild to severe renal impairment or in hemodialysis-dependent patients compared to subjects with normal renal function. No dosage adjustment is therefore required in such patients receiving AVANDIA. Since metformin is contraindicated in patients with renal impairment, co-administration of metformin with AVANDIA is contraindicated in these patients.

Race: Results of a population pharmacokinetic analysis including subjects of Caucasian, black, and other ethnic origins indicate that race has no influence on the pharmacokinetics of rosiglitazone.

Drug Interactions:

Drugs that Inhibit, Induce, or are Metabolized by Cytochrome P_{450}: In vitro drug metabolism studies suggest that rosiglitazone does not inhibit any of the major P_{450} enzymes at clinically relevant concentrations. In vitro data demonstrate that rosiglitazone is predominantly metabolized by CYP2C8, and to a lesser extent, 2C9.

Gemfibrozil: Concomitant administration of gemfibrozil (600 mg twice daily), an inhibitor of CYP2C8, and rosiglitazone (4 mg once daily) for 7 days increased rosiglitazone AUC by 127%, compared to the administration of rosiglitazone (4 mg once daily) alone. Given the potential for dose-related adverse events with rosiglitazone, a decrease in the dose of rosiglitazone may be needed when gemfibrozil is introduced (see PRECAUTIONS).

Rifampin: Rifampin administration (600 mg once a day), an inducer of CYP2C8, for 6 days is reported to decrease rosiglitazone AUC by 66%, compared to the administration of rosiglitazone (8 mg) alone (see PRECAUTIONS).[1]

AVANDIA (4 mg twice daily) was shown to have no clinically relevant effect on the pharmacokinetics of nifedipine and oral contraceptives (ethinyl estradiol and norethindrone), which are predominantly metabolized by CYP3A4.

Glyburide: AVANDIA (2 mg twice daily) taken concomitantly with glyburide (3.75 to 10 mg/day) for 7 days did not alter the mean steady-state 24-hour plasma glucose concentrations in diabetic patients stabilized on glyburide therapy. Repeat doses of AVANDIA (8 mg once daily) for 8 days in healthy adult Caucasian subjects caused a decrease in glyburide AUC (32%) and C_{max} (35%). In Japanese subjects, glyburide AUC (14%) and C_{max} (31%) slightly increased following coadministration of AVANDIA.

Glimepiride: Single oral doses of glimepiride in 14 healthy adult subjects had no clinically significant effect on the steady-state pharmacokinetics of AVANDIA. No clinically significant reductions in glimepiride AUC and C_{max} were observed after repeat doses of AVANDIA (8 mg once daily) for 8 days in healthy adult subjects.

Metformin: Concurrent administration of AVANDIA (2 mg twice daily) and metformin (500 mg twice daily) in healthy volunteers for 4 days had no effect on the steady-state pharmacokinetics of either metformin or rosiglitazone.

Acarbose: Coadministration of acarbose (100 mg three times daily) for 7 days in healthy volunteers had no clinically relevant effect on the pharmacokinetics of a single oral dose of AVANDIA.

Digoxin: Repeat oral dosing of AVANDIA (8 mg once daily) for 14 days did not alter the steady-state pharmacokinetics of digoxin (0.375 mg once daily) in healthy volunteers.

Warfarin: Repeat dosing with AVANDIA had no clinically relevant effect on the steady-state pharmacokinetics of warfarin enantiomers.

Ethanol: A single administration of a moderate amount of alcohol did not increase the risk of acute hypoglycemia in type 2 diabetes mellitus patients treated with AVANDIA.

Continued on next page

Avandia—Cont.

Ranitidine: Pretreatment with ranitidine (150 mg twice daily for 4 days) did not alter the pharmacokinetics of either single oral or intravenous doses of rosiglitazone in healthy volunteers. These results suggest that the absorption of oral rosiglitazone is not altered in conditions accompanied by increases in gastrointestinal pH.

CLINICAL STUDIES

In clinical studies, treatment with AVANDIA resulted in an improvement in glycemic control, as measured by fasting plasma glucose (FPG) and hemoglobin A1c (HbA1c), with a concurrent reduction in insulin and C-peptide. Postprandial glucose and insulin were also reduced. This is consistent with the mechanism of action of AVANDIA as an insulin sensitizer. The improvement in glycemic control was durable, with maintenance of effect for 52 weeks. The maximum recommended daily dose is 8 mg. Dose-ranging studies suggested that no additional benefit was obtained with a total daily dose of 12 mg.

The addition of AVANDIA to either metformin, a sulfonylurea, or insulin resulted in significant reductions in hyperglycemia compared to any of these agents alone. These results are consistent with an additive effect on glycemic control when AVANDIA is used as combination therapy.

Patients with lipid abnormalities were not excluded from clinical trials of AVANDIA. In all 26-week controlled trials, across the recommended dose range, AVANDIA as monotherapy was associated with increases in total cholesterol, LDL, and HDL and decreases in free fatty acids. These changes were statistically significantly different from placebo or glyburide controls (see Table 2).

Increases in LDL occurred primarily during the first 1 to 2 months of therapy with AVANDIA and LDL levels remained elevated above baseline throughout the trials. In contrast, HDL continued to rise over time. As a result, the LDL/HDL ratio peaked after 2 months of therapy and then appeared to decrease over time. Because of the temporal nature of lipid changes, the 52-week glyburide-controlled study is most pertinent to assess long-term effects on lipids. At baseline, week 26, and week 52, mean LDL/HDL ratios were 3.1, 3.2, and 3.0, respectively, for AVANDIA 4 mg twice daily. The corresponding values for glyburide were 3.2, 3.1, and 2.9. The differences in change from baseline between AVANDIA and glyburide at week 52 were statistically significant.

The pattern of LDL and HDL changes following therapy with AVANDIA in combination with other hypoglycemic agents were generally similar to those seen with AVANDIA in monotherapy.

The changes in triglycerides during therapy with AVANDIA were variable and were generally not statistically different from placebo or glyburide controls.
[See table 2 above]

Monotherapy: A total of 2,315 patients with type 2 diabetes, previously treated with diet alone or antidiabetic medication(s), were treated with AVANDIA as monotherapy in 6 double-blind studies, which included two 26-week placebo-controlled studies, one 52-week glyburide-controlled study, and 3 placebo-controlled dose-ranging studies of 8 to 12 weeks duration. Previous antidiabetic medication(s) were withdrawn and patients entered a 2 to 4 week placebo run-in period prior to randomization.

Two 26-week, double-blind, placebo-controlled trials, in patients with type 2 diabetes (n = 1,401) with inadequate glycemic control (mean baseline FPG approximately 228 mg/dL [101 to 425 mg/dL] and mean baseline HbA1c 8.9% [5.2% to 16.2%]), were conducted. Treatment with AVANDIA produced statistically significant improvements in FPG and HbA1c compared to baseline and relative to placebo. Data from one of these studies are summarized in Table 3.
[See table 3 above]

When administered at the same total daily dose, AVANDIA was generally more effective in reducing FPG and HbA1c when administered in divided doses twice daily compared to once daily doses. However, for HbA1c, the difference between the 4 mg once daily and 2 mg twice daily doses was not statistically significant.

Long-term maintenance of effect was evaluated in a 52-week, double-blind, glyburide-controlled trial in patients with type 2 diabetes. Patients were randomized to treatment with AVANDIA 2 mg twice daily (N = 195) or AVANDIA 4 mg twice daily (N = 189) or glyburide (N = 202) for 52 weeks. Patients receiving glyburide were given an initial dosage of either 2.5 mg/day or 5.0 mg/day. The dosage was then titrated in 2.5 mg/day increments over the next 12 weeks, to a maximum dosage of 15.0 mg/day in order to optimize glycemic control. Thereafter the glyburide dose was kept constant.

The median titrated dose of glyburide was 7.5 mg. All treatments resulted in a statistically significant improvement in glycemic control from baseline (see Figure 1 and Figure 2). At the end of week 52, the reduction from baseline in FPG and HbA1c was -40.8 mg/dL and -0.53% with AVANDIA 4 mg twice daily; -25.4 mg/dL and -0.27% with AVANDIA 2 mg twice daily; and -30.0 mg/dL and -0.72% with glyburide. For HbA1c, the difference between AVANDIA 4 mg twice daily and glyburide was not statistically significant at week 52. The initial fall in FPG with glyburide was greater than with AVANDIA; however, this effect was less durable over time. The improvement in glycemic control seen with

Table 2. Summary of Mean Lipid Changes in 26-Week Placebo-Controlled and 52-Week Glyburide-Controlled Monotherapy Studies

| | Placebo-controlled Studies Week 26 | | | Glyburide-controlled Study Week 26 and Week 52 | | | |
| | Placebo | AVANDIA | | Glyburide Titration | | AVANDIA 8 mg | |
		4 mg daily*	8 mg daily*	Wk 26	Wk 52	Wk 26	Wk 52
Free Fatty Acids							
N	207	428	436	181	168	166	145
Baseline (mean)	18.1	17.5	17.9	26.4	26.4	26.9	26.6
% Change from baseline (mean)	+0.2%	-7.8%	-14.7%	-2.4%	-4.7%	-20.8%	-21.5%
LDL							
N	190	400	374	175	160	161	133
Baseline (mean)	123.7	126.8	125.3	142.7	141.9	142.1	142.1
% Change from baseline (mean)	+4.8%	+14.1%	+18.6%	-0.9%	-0.5%	+11.9%	+12.1%
HDL							
N	208	429	436	184	170	170	145
Baseline (mean)	44.1	44.4	43.0	47.2	47.7	48.4	48.3
% Change from baseline (mean)	+8.0%	+11.4%	+14.2%	+4.3%	+8.7%	+14.0%	+18.5%

*Once daily and twice daily dosing groups were combined.

Table 3. Glycemic Parameters in a 26-Week Placebo-Controlled Trial

| | | AVANDIA | | AVANDIA | |
	Placebo	4 mg once daily	2 mg twice daily	8 mg once daily	4 mg twice daily
N	173	180	186	181	187
FPG (mg/dL)					
Baseline (mean)	225	229	225	228	228
Change from baseline (mean)	8	-25	-35	-42	-55
Difference from placebo (adjusted mean)	-	-31*	-43*	-49*	-62*
% of patients with ≥30 mg/dL decrease from baseline	19%	45%	54%	58%	70%
HbA1c (%)					
Baseline (mean)	8.9	8.9	8.9	8.9	9.0
Change from baseline (mean)	0.8	0.0	-0.1	-0.3	-0.7
Difference from placebo (adjusted mean)	-	-0.8*	-0.9*	-1.1*	-1.5*
% of patients with ≥0.7% decrease from baseline	9%	28%	29%	39%	54%

*<0.0001 compared to placebo.

AVANDIA 4 mg twice daily at week 26 was maintained through week 52 of the study.

Figure 1. Mean FPG Over Time in a 52-Week Glyburide-Controlled Study

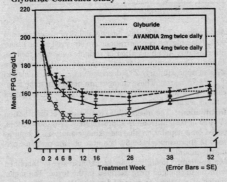

Legend: Glyburide; AVANDIA 2mg twice daily; AVANDIA 4mg twice daily. Mean FPG (mg/dL) vs Treatment Week (Error Bars = SE)

Figure 2. Mean HbA1c Over Time in a 52-Week Glyburide-Controlled Study

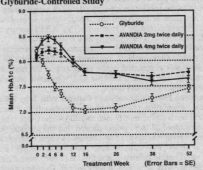

Legend: Glyburide; AVANDIA 2mg twice daily; AVANDIA 4mg twice daily. Mean HbA1c (%) vs Treatment Week (Error Bars = SE)

Hypoglycemia was reported in 12.1% of glyburide-treated patients versus 0.5% (2 mg twice daily) and 1.6% (4 mg twice daily) of patients treated with AVANDIA. The improvements in glycemic control were associated with a

mean weight gain of 1.75 kg and 2.95 kg for patients treated with 2 mg and 4 mg twice daily of AVANDIA, respectively, versus 1.9 kg in glyburide-treated patients. In patients treated with AVANDIA, C-peptide, insulin, pro-insulin, and pro-insulin split products were significantly reduced in a dose-ordered fashion, compared to an increase in the glyburide-treated patients.

Combination With Metformin: A total of 670 patients with type 2 diabetes participated in two 26-week, randomized, double-blind, placebo/active-controlled studies designed to assess the efficacy of AVANDIA in combination with metformin. AVANDIA, administered in either once daily or twice daily dosing regimens, was added to the therapy of patients who were inadequately controlled on a maximum dose (2.5 grams/day) of metformin.

In one study, patients inadequately controlled on 2.5 grams/day of metformin (mean baseline FPG 216 mg/dL and mean baseline HbA1c 8.8%) were randomized to receive 4 mg of AVANDIA once daily, 8 mg of AVANDIA once daily, or placebo in addition to metformin. A statistically significant improvement in FPG and HbA1c was observed in patients treated with the combinations of metformin and 4 mg of AVANDIA once daily and 8 mg of AVANDIA once daily, versus patients continued on metformin alone (see Table 4).
[See table 4 at top of next page]

In a second 26-week study, patients with type 2 diabetes inadequately controlled on 2.5 grams/day of metformin who were randomized to receive the combination of AVANDIA 4 mg twice daily and metformin (N = 105) showed a statistically significant improvement in glycemic control with a mean treatment effect for FPG of -56 mg/dL and a mean treatment effect for HbA1c of -0.8% over metformin alone. The combination of metformin and AVANDIA resulted in lower levels of FPG and HbA1c than either agent alone.

Patients who were inadequately controlled on a maximum dose (2.5 grams/day) of metformin and who were switched to monotherapy with AVANDIA demonstrated loss of glycemic control, as evidenced by increases in FPG and HbA1c. In this group, increases in LDL and VLDL were also seen.

Combination With a Sulfonylurea: A total of 3,457 patients with type 2 diabetes participated in ten 24- to 26-week randomized, double-blind, placebo/active-controlled studies and one 2-year double-blind, active-controlled study in elderly patients designed to assess the efficacy and safety of AVANDIA in combination with a sulfonylurea. AVANDIA 2 mg, 4 mg, or 8 mg daily, was administered either once daily (3 studies) or in divided doses twice daily (7 studies), to patients inadequately controlled on a submaximal or maximal dose of sulfonylurea.

In these studies, the combination of AVANDIA 4 mg or 8 mg daily (administered as single or twice daily divided doses) and a sulfonylurea significantly reduced FPG and HbA1c compared to placebo plus sulfonylurea or further up-titration of the sulfonylurea. Table 5 shows pooled data for 8 studies in which AVANDIA added to sulfonylurea was compared to placebo plus sulfonylurea.

[See table 5 at right]

One of the 24- to 26-week studies included patients who were inadequately controlled on maximal doses of glyburide and switched to 4 mg of AVANDIA daily as monotherapy; in this group, loss of glycemic control was demonstrated, as evidenced by increases in FPG and HbA1c.

In a 2-year double-blind study, elderly patients (aged 59 to 89 years) on half-maximal sulfonylurea (glipizide 10 mg twice daily) were randomized to the addition of AVANDIA (n = 115, 4 mg once daily to 8 mg as needed) or to continued up-titration of glipizide (n = 110), to a maximum of 20 mg twice daily. Mean baseline FPG and HbA1c were 157 mg/dL and 7.72%, respectively, for the AVANDIA plus glipizide arm and 159 mg/dL and 7.65%, respectively, for the glipizide up-titration arm. Loss of glycemic control (FPG ≥180 mg/dL) occurred in a significantly lower proportion of patients (2%) on AVANDIA plus glipizide compared to patients in the glipizide up-titration arm (28.7%). About 78% of the patients on combination therapy completed the 2 years of therapy while only 51% completed on glipizide monotherapy. The effect of combination therapy on FPG and HbA1c was durable over the 2-year study period, with patients achieving a mean of 132 mg/dL for FPG and a mean of 6.98% for HbA1c compared to no change on the glipizide arm.

Combination With Insulin: In two 26-week randomized, double-blind, fixed-dose studies designed to assess the efficacy and safety of AVANDIA in combination with insulin, patients inadequately controlled on insulin (65 to 76 units/day, mean range at baseline) were randomized to receive AVANDIA 4 mg plus insulin (n = 206) or placebo plus insulin (n = 203). The mean duration of disease in these patients was 12 to 13 years.

Compared to insulin plus placebo, single or divided doses of AVANDIA 4 mg daily plus insulin significantly reduced FPG (mean reduction of 32 to 40 mg/dL) and HbA1c (mean reduction of 0.6% to 0.7%). Approximately 40% of all patients treated with AVANDIA reduced their insulin dose.

Combination With Sulfonylurea and Metformin: In two 24- to 26-week, double-blind, placebo-controlled, studies designed to assess the efficacy and safety of AVANDIA in combination with sulfonylurea plus metformin, AVANDIA 4 mg or 8 mg daily, was administered in divided doses twice daily, to patients inadequately controlled on submaximal (10 mg) and maximal (20 mg) doses of glyburide and maximal dose of metformin (2 g/day). A statistically significant improvement in FPG and HbA1c was observed in patients treated with the combinations of sulfonylurea plus metformin and 4 mg of AVANDIA and 8 mg of AVANDIA versus patients continued on sulfonylurea plus metformin, as shown in Table 6.

[See table 6 at top of next page]

INDICATIONS AND USAGE

AVANDIA is indicated as an adjunct to diet and exercise to improve glycemic control in patients with type 2 diabetes mellitus.

- AVANDIA is indicated as monotherapy.
- AVANDIA is also indicated for use in combination with a sulfonylurea, metformin, or insulin when diet, exercise, and a single agent do not result in adequate glycemic control. For patients inadequately controlled with a maximum dose of a sulfonylurea or metformin, AVANDIA should be added to, rather than substituted for, a sulfonylurea or metformin.
- AVANDIA is also indicated for use in combination with a sulfonylurea plus metformin when diet, exercise, and both agents do not result in adequate glycemic control.

Management of type 2 diabetes should include diet control. Caloric restriction, weight loss, and exercise are essential for the proper treatment of the diabetic patient because they help improve insulin sensitivity. This is important not only in the primary treatment of type 2 diabetes, but also in maintaining the efficacy of drug therapy. Prior to initiation of therapy with AVANDIA, secondary causes of poor glycemic control, e.g., infection, should be investigated and treated.

CONTRAINDICATIONS

AVANDIA is contraindicated in patients with known hypersensitivity to this product or any of its components.

WARNINGS

Cardiac Failure and Other Cardiac Effects: AVANDIA, like other thiazolidinediones, alone or in combination with other antidiabetic agents, can cause fluid retention, which may exacerbate or lead to heart failure. Patients should be observed for signs and symptoms of heart failure. In combination with insulin, thiazolidinediones may also increase the risk of other cardiovascular adverse events. AVANDIA should be discontinued if any deterioration in cardiac status occurs.

Patients with New York Heart Association (NYHA) Class 3 and 4 cardiac status were not studied during the clinical trials. AVANDIA is not recommended in patients with NYHA Class 3 and 4 cardiac status.

In three 26-week trials in patients with type 2 diabetes, 216 received 4 mg of AVANDIA plus insulin, 322 received 8 mg of AVANDIA plus insulin, and 338 received insulin alone. These trials included patients with long-standing diabetes

Table 4. Glycemic Parameters in a 26-Week Combination Study of AVANDIA Plus Metformin

	Metformin	AVANDIA 4 mg once daily + metformin	AVANDIA 8 mg once daily + metformin
N	113	116	110
FPG (mg/dL)			
Baseline (mean)	214	215	220
Change from baseline (mean)	6	-33	-48
Difference from metformin alone (adjusted mean)	–	-40*	-53*
% of patients with ≥30 mg/dL decrease from baseline	20%	45%	61%
HbA1c (%)			
Baseline (mean)	8.6	8.9	8.9
Change from baseline (mean)	0.5	-0.6	-0.8
Difference from metformin alone (adjusted mean)	–	-1.0*	-1.2*
% of patients with ≥0.7% decrease from baseline	11%	45%	52%

*<0.0001 compared to metformin.

Table 5. Glycemic Parameters in 24- to 26-Week Combination Studies of AVANDIA Plus Sulfonylurea

Twice Daily Divided Dosing (5 Studies)	Sulfonylurea	AVANDIA 2 mg twice daily + sulfonylurea	Sulfonylurea	AVANDIA 4 mg twice daily + sulfonylurea
N	397	497	248	346
FPG (mg/dL)				
Baseline (mean)	204	198	188	187
Change from baseline (mean)	11	-29	8	-43
Difference from sulfonylurea alone (adjusted mean)	–	-42*	–	-53*
% of patients with ≥30 mg/dL decrease from baseline	17%	49%	15%	61%
HbA1c (%)				
Baseline (mean)	9.4	9.5	9.3	9.6
Change from baseline (mean)	0.2	-1.0	0.0	-1.6
Difference from sulfonylurea alone (adjusted mean)	–	-1.1*	–	-1.4*
% of patients with ≥0.7% decrease from baseline	21%	60%	23%	75%

Once Daily Dosing (3 Studies)	Sulfonylurea	AVANDIA 4 mg once daily + sulfonylurea	Sulfonylurea	AVANDIA 8 mg once daily + sulfonylurea
N	172	172	173	176
FPG (mg/dL)				
Baseline (mean)	198	206	188	192
Change from baseline (mean)	17	-25	17	-43
Difference from sulfonylurea alone (adjusted mean)	–	-47*	–	-66*
% of patients with ≥30 mg/dL decrease from baseline	17%	48%	19%	55%
HbA1c (%)				
Baseline (mean)	8.6	8.8	8.9	8.9
Change from baseline (mean)	0.4	-0.5	0.1	-1.2
Difference from sulfonylurea alone (adjusted mean)	–	-0.9*	–	-1.4*
% of patients with ≥0.7% decrease from baseline	11%	36%	20%	68%

*<0.0001 compared to sulfonylurea alone.

and a high prevalence of pre-existing medical conditions, including peripheral neuropathy, retinopathy, ischemic heart disease, vascular disease, and congestive heart failure. In these clinical studies an increased incidence of edema, cardiac failure, and other cardiovascular adverse events was seen in patients on AVANDIA and insulin combination therapy compared to insulin and placebo. Patients who experienced cardiovascular events were on average older and had a longer duration of diabetes. These cardiovascular events were noted at both the 4 mg and 8 mg daily doses of AVANDIA. In this population, however, it was not possible to determine specific risk factors that could be used to identify all patients at risk of heart failure and other cardiovascular events on combination therapy. Three of 10 patients who developed cardiac failure on combination therapy during the double-blind part of the fixed-dose studies had no known prior evidence of congestive heart failure, or pre-existing cardiac condition.

In a double-blind study in type 2 diabetes patients with chronic renal failure (112 received 4 mg or 8 mg of AVANDIA plus insulin and 108 received insulin control), there was no difference in cardiovascular adverse events with AVANDIA in combination with insulin compared to insulin control.

Patients treated with combination AVANDIA and insulin should be monitored for cardiovascular adverse events. This combination therapy should be discontinued in patients who do not respond as manifested by a reduction in HbA1c or insulin dose after 4 to 5 months of therapy or who develop any significant adverse events. (See ADVERSE REACTIONS).

PRECAUTIONS

General: Due to its mechanism of action, AVANDIA is active only in the presence of endogenous insulin. Therefore, AVANDIA should not be used in patients with type 1 diabetes or for the treatment of diabetic ketoacidosis.

Hypoglycemia: Patients receiving AVANDIA in combination with other hypoglycemic agents may be at risk for hypoglycemia, and a reduction in the dose of the concomitant agent may be necessary.

Edema: AVANDIA should be used with caution in patients with edema. In a clinical study in healthy volunteers who received 8 mg of AVANDIA once daily for 8 weeks, there was a statistically significant increase in median plasma volume compared to placebo.

Continued on next page

Avandia—Cont.

Since thiazolidinediones, including rosiglitazone, can cause fluid retention, which can exacerbate or lead to congestive heart failure, AVANDIA should be used with caution in patients at risk for heart failure. Patients should be monitored for signs and symptoms of heart failure (see WARNINGS, Cardiac Failure and Other Cardiac Effects and PRECAUTIONS, Information for Patients).

In controlled clinical trials of patients with type 2 diabetes, mild to moderate edema was reported in patients treated with AVANDIA, and may be dose related. Patients with ongoing edema are more likely to have adverse events associated with edema if started on combination therapy with insulin and AVANDIA (see ADVERSE REACTIONS).

Weight Gain: Dose-related weight gain was seen with AVANDIA alone and in combination with other hypoglycemic agents (see Table 7). The mechanism of weight gain is unclear but probably involves a combination of fluid retention and fat accumulation.

In postmarketing experience, there have been reports of unusually rapid increases in weight and increases in excess of that generally observed in clinical trials. Patients who experience such increases should be assessed for fluid accumulation and volume-related events such as excessive edema and congestive heart failure.

[See table 7 at right]

Hematologic: Across all controlled clinical studies, decreases in hemoglobin and hematocrit (mean decreases in individual studies ≤1.0 gram/dL and ≤3.3%, respectively) were observed for AVANDIA alone and in combination with other hypoglycemic agents. The changes occurred primarily during the first 3 months following initiation of therapy with AVANDIA or following a dose increase in AVANDIA. White blood cell counts also decreased slightly in patients treated with AVANDIA. The observed changes may be related to the increased plasma volume observed with treatment with AVANDIA and may be dose related (see ADVERSE REACTIONS, Laboratory Abnormalities, *Hematologic*).

Ovulation: Therapy with AVANDIA, like other thiazolidinediones, may result in ovulation in some premenopausal anovulatory women. As a result, these patients may be at an increased risk for pregnancy while taking AVANDIA (see PRECAUTIONS, Pregnancy, *Pregnancy Category C*). Thus, adequate contraception in premenopausal women should be recommended. This possible effect has not been specifically investigated in clinical studies so the frequency of this occurrence is not known.

Although hormonal imbalance has been seen in preclinical studies (see PRECAUTIONS, Carcinogenesis, Mutagenesis, Impairment of Fertility), the clinical significance of this finding is not known. If unexpected menstrual dysfunction occurs, the benefits of continued therapy with AVANDIA should be reviewed.

Hepatic Effects: Another drug of the thiazolidinedione class, troglitazone, was associated with idiosyncratic hepatotoxicity, and very rare cases of liver failure, liver transplants, and death were reported during clinical use. In pre-approval controlled clinical trials in patients with type 2 diabetes, troglitazone was more frequently associated with clinically significant elevations in liver enzymes (ALT >3× upper limit of normal) compared to placebo. Very rare cases of reversible jaundice were also reported.

In pre-approval clinical studies in 4,598 patients treated with AVANDIA, encompassing approximately 3,600 patient years of exposure, there was no signal of drug-induced hepatotoxicity or elevation of ALT levels. In the pre-approval controlled trials, 0.2% of patients treated with AVANDIA had elevations in ALT >3× the upper limit of normal compared to 0.2% on placebo and 0.5% on active comparators. The ALT elevations in patients treated with AVANDIA were reversible and were not clearly causally related to therapy with AVANDIA.

In postmarketing experience with AVANDIA, reports of hepatitis and of hepatic enzyme elevations to 3 or more times the upper limit of normal have been received. Very rarely, these reports have involved hepatic failure with and without fatal outcome, although causality has not been established. Rosiglitazone is structurally related to troglitazone, a thiazolidinedione no longer marketed in the United States, which was associated with idiosyncratic hepatotoxicity and rare cases of liver failure, liver transplants, and death during clinical use. Pending the availability of the results of additional large, long-term controlled clinical trials and additional postmarketing safety data, it is recommended that patients treated with AVANDIA undergo periodic monitoring of liver enzymes.

Liver enzymes should be checked prior to the initiation of therapy with AVANDIA in all patients and periodically thereafter per the clinical judgement of the healthcare professional. Therapy with AVANDIA should not be initiated in patients with increased baseline liver enzyme levels (ALT >2.5× upper limit of normal). Patients with mildly elevated liver enzymes (ALT levels ≤2.5× upper limit of normal) at baseline or during therapy with AVANDIA should be evaluated to determine the cause of the liver enzyme elevation. Initiation of, or continuation of, therapy with AVANDIA in patients with mild liver enzyme elevations should proceed with caution and include close clinical follow-up, including more frequent liver enzyme monitoring, to determine if the liver enzyme elevations resolve or worsen. If at any time ALT levels increase to >3× the upper limit of normal in patients on therapy with AVANDIA, liver enzyme levels should be rechecked as soon as possible. If ALT levels remain >3× the upper limit of normal, therapy with AVANDIA should be discontinued.

Table 6. Glycemic Parameters in a 26-Week Combination Study of AVANDIA Plus Sulfonylurea and Metformin

	Sulfonylurea + metformin	AVANDIA 2 mg twice daily + sulfonylurea + metformin	AVANDIA 4 mg twice daily + sulfonylurea + metformin
N	273	276	277
FPG (mg/dL)			
Baseline (mean)	189	190	192
Change from baseline (mean)	14	-19	-40
Difference from sulfonylurea plus metformin (adjusted mean)	–	-30*	-52*
% of patients with ≥30 mg/dL decrease from baseline	16%	46%	62%
HbA1c (%)			
Baseline (mean)	8.7	8.6	8.7
Change from baseline (mean)	0.2	-0.4	-0.9
Difference from sulfonylurea plus metformin (adjusted mean)	–	-0.6*	-1.1*
% of patients with ≥0.7% decrease from baseline	16%	39%	63%

*<0.0001 compared to placebo.

Table 7. Weight Changes (kg) From Baseline During Clinical Trials With AVANDIA

		Control Group		AVANDIA 4 mg	AVANDIA 8 mg
Monotherapy	Duration		Median (25th, 75th percentile)	Median (25th, 75th percentile)	Median (25th, 75th percentile)
	26 weeks	placebo	-0.9 (-2.8, 0.9) n = 210	1.0 (-0.9, 3.6) n = 436	3.1 (1.1, 5.8) n = 439
	52 weeks	sulfonylurea	2.0 (0, 4.0) n = 173	2.0 (-0.6, 4.0) n = 150	2.6 (0, 5.3) n = 157
Combination therapy					
sulfonylurea	24-26 weeks	sulfonylurea	0 (-1.0, 1.3) n = 1,155	2.2 (0.5, 4.0) n = 613	3.5 (1.4, 5.9) n = 841
metformin	26 weeks	metformin	-1.4 (-3.2, 0.2) n = 175	0.8 (-1.0, 2.6) n = 100	2.1 (0, 4.3) n = 184
insulin	26 weeks	insulin	0.9 (-0.5, 2.7) n = 162	4.1 (1.4, 6.3) n = 164	5.4 (3.4, 7.3) n = 150
sulfonylurea + metformin	26 weeks	sulfonylurea + metformin	0.2 (-1.2, 1.6) n = 272	2.5 (0.8, 4.6) n = 275	4.5 (2.4, 7.3) n = 276

If any patient develops symptoms suggesting hepatic dysfunction, which may include unexplained nausea, vomiting, abdominal pain, fatigue, anorexia and/or dark urine, liver enzymes should be checked. The decision whether to continue the patient on therapy with AVANDIA should be guided by clinical judgment pending laboratory evaluations. If jaundice is observed, drug therapy should be discontinued.

There are no data available from clinical trials to evaluate the safety of AVANDIA in patients who experienced liver abnormalities, hepatic dysfunction, or jaundice while on troglitazone. AVANDIA should not be used in patients who experienced jaundice while taking troglitazone.

Laboratory Tests: Periodic fasting blood glucose and HbA1c measurements should be performed to monitor therapeutic response.

Liver enzyme monitoring is recommended prior to initiation of therapy with AVANDIA in all patients and periodically thereafter (see PRECAUTIONS, General, *Hepatic Effects* and ADVERSE REACTIONS, Laboratory Abnormalities, *Serum Transaminase Levels*).

Information for Patients: Patients should be informed of the following: Management of type 2 diabetes should include diet control. Caloric restriction, weight loss, and exercise are essential for the proper treatment of the diabetic patient because they help improve insulin sensitivity. This is important not only in the primary treatment of type 2 diabetes, but in maintaining the efficacy of drug therapy.

It is important to adhere to dietary instructions and to regularly have blood glucose and glycosylated hemoglobin tested. Patients should be advised that it can take 2 weeks to see a reduction in blood glucose and 2 to 3 months to see full effect. Patients should be informed that blood will be drawn to check their liver function prior to the start of therapy and periodically thereafter per the clinical judgement of the healthcare professional. Patients with unexplained symptoms of nausea, vomiting, abdominal pain, fatigue, anorexia, or dark urine should immediately report these symptoms to their physician. Patients who experience an unusually rapid increase in weight or edema or who develop shortness of breath or other symptoms of heart failure while on AVANDIA should immediately report these symptoms to their physician.

AVANDIA can be taken with or without meals.

When using AVANDIA in combination with other hypoglycemic agents, the risk of hypoglycemia, its symptoms and treatment, and conditions that predispose to its development should be explained to patients and their family members.

Therapy with AVANDIA, like other thiazolidinediones, may result in ovulation in some premenopausal anovulatory women. As a result, these patients may be at an increased risk for pregnancy while taking AVANDIA (see PRECAUTIONS, Pregnancy, *Pregnancy Category C*). Thus, adequate contraception in premenopausal women should be recommended. This possible effect has not been specifically investigated in clinical studies so the frequency of this occurrence is not known.

Drug Interactions: An inhibitor of CYP2C8 (such as gemfibrozil) may increase the AUC of rosiglitazone and an inducer of CYP2C8 (such as rifampin) may decrease the AUC of rosiglitazone. Therefore, if an inhibitor or an inducer of CYP2C8 is started or stopped during treatment with rosiglitazone, changes in diabetes treatment may be needed based upon clinical response. (See CLINICAL PHARMACOLOGY, Drug Interactions.)

Carcinogenesis, Mutagenesis, Impairment of Fertility:

Carcinogenesis: A 2-year carcinogenicity study was conducted in Charles River CD-1 mice at doses of 0.4, 1.5, and 6 mg/kg/day in the diet (highest dose equivalent to approximately 12 times human AUC at the maximum recommended human daily dose). Sprague-Dawley rats were dosed for 2 years by oral gavage at doses of 0.05, 0.3, and 2 mg/kg/day (highest dose equivalent to approximately 10 and 20 times human AUC at the maximum recommended human daily dose for male and female rats, respectively).

Rosiglitazone was not carcinogenic in the mouse. There was an increase in incidence of adipose hyperplasia in the mouse at doses ≥1.5 mg/kg/day (approximately 2 times human AUC at the maximum recommended human daily dose). In rats, there was a significant increase in the incidence of benign adipose tissue tumors (lipomas) at doses ≥0.3 mg/kg/day (approximately 2 times human AUC at the maximum recommended human daily dose). These proliferative changes in both species are considered due to the persistent pharmacological overstimulation of adipose tissue.

Mutagenesis: Rosiglitazone was not mutagenic or clastogenic in the in vitro bacterial assays for gene mutation, the in vitro chromosome aberration test in human lymphocytes, the in vivo mouse micronucleus test, and the in vivo/in vitro rat UDS assay. There was a small (about 2-fold) increase in mutation in the in vitro mouse lymphoma assay in the presence of metabolic activation.

Impairment of Fertility: Rosiglitazone had no effects on mating or fertility of male rats given up to 40 mg/kg/day (approximately 116 times human AUC at the maximum recommended human daily dose). Rosiglitazone altered estrous cyclicity (2 mg/kg/day) and reduced fertility (40 mg/kg/day) of female rats in association with lower plasma levels of progesterone and estradiol (approximately 20 and 200 times human AUC at the maximum recommended human daily dose, respectively). No such effects were noted at 0.2 mg/kg/day (approximately 3 times human AUC at the maximum recommended human daily dose). In monkeys, rosiglitazone (0.6 and 4.6 mg/kg/day; approximately 3 and 15 times human AUC at the maximum recommended human daily dose, respectively) diminished the follicular phase rise in serum estradiol with consequential reduction in the luteinizing hormone surge, lower luteal phase progesterone levels, and amenorrhea. The mechanism for these effects appears to be direct inhibition of ovarian steroidogenesis.

Animal Toxicology: Heart weights were increased in mice (3 mg/kg/day), rats (5 mg/kg/day), and dogs (2 mg/kg/day) with rosiglitazone treatments (approximately 5, 22, and 2 times human AUC at the maximum recommended human daily dose, respectively). Morphometric measurement indicated that there was hypertrophy in cardiac ventricular tissues, which may be due to increased heart work as a result of plasma volume expansion.

Pregnancy: ***Pregnancy Category C:*** There was no effect on implantation or the embryo with rosiglitazone treatment during early pregnancy in rats, but treatment during mid-late gestation was associated with fetal death and growth retardation in both rats and rabbits. Teratogenicity was not observed at doses up to 3 mg/kg in rats and 100 mg/kg in rabbits (approximately 20 and 75 times human AUC at the maximum recommended human daily dose, respectively). Rosiglitazone caused placental pathology in rats (3 mg/kg/day). Treatment of rats during gestation through lactation reduced litter size, neonatal viability, and postnatal growth, with growth retardation reversible after puberty. For effects on the placenta, embryo/fetus, and offspring, the no-effect dose was 0.2 mg/kg/day in rats and 15 mg/kg/day in rabbits. These no-effect levels are approximately 4 times human AUC at the maximum recommended human daily dose.

There are no adequate and well-controlled studies in pregnant women. AVANDIA should not be used during pregnancy unless the potential benefit justifies the potential risk to the fetus.

Because current information strongly suggests that abnormal blood glucose levels during pregnancy are associated with a higher incidence of congenital anomalies as well as increased neonatal morbidity and mortality, most experts recommend that insulin monotherapy be used during pregnancy to maintain blood glucose levels as close to normal as possible.

Labor and Delivery: The effect of rosiglitazone on labor and delivery in humans is not known.

Nursing Mothers: Drug-related material was detected in milk from lactating rats. It is not known whether AVANDIA is excreted in human milk. Because many drugs are excreted in human milk, AVANDIA should not be administered to a nursing woman.

Pediatric Use: The safety and effectiveness of AVANDIA in pediatric patients have not been established.

Geriatric Use: Results of the population pharmacokinetic analysis showed that age does not significantly affect the pharmacokinetics of rosiglitazone (see CLINICAL PHARMACOLOGY, Special Populations). Therefore, no dosage adjustments are required for the elderly. In controlled clinical trials, no overall differences in safety and effectiveness between older (≥65 years) and younger (<65 years) patients were observed.

ADVERSE REACTIONS

In clinical trials, approximately 8,400 patients with type 2 diabetes have been treated with AVANDIA; 6,000 patients were treated for 6 months or longer and 3,000 patients were treated for 12 months or longer.

Trials of AVANDIA as Monotherapy and in Combination With Other Hypoglycemic Agents: The incidence and types of adverse events reported in clinical trials of AVANDIA as monotherapy are shown in Table 8.

[See table 8 above]

Table 8. Adverse Events (≥5% in Any Treatment Group) Reported by Patients in Double-blind Clinical Trials With AVANDIA as Monotherapy

Preferred Term	AVANDIA Monotherapy N = 2,526	Placebo N = 601	Metformin N = 225	Sulfonylureas* N = 626
	%	%	%	%
Upper respiratory tract infection	9.9	8.7	8.9	7.3
Injury	7.6	4.3	7.6	6.1
Headache	5.9	5.0	8.9	5.4
Back pain	4.0	3.8	4.0	5.0
Hyperglycemia	3.9	5.7	4.4	8.1
Fatigue	3.6	5.0	4.0	1.9
Sinusitis	3.2	4.5	5.3	3.0
Diarrhea	2.3	3.3	15.6	3.0
Hypoglycemia	0.6	0.2	1.3	5.9

*Includes patients receiving glyburide (N = 514), gliclazide (N = 91) or glipizide (N = 21).

Overall, the types of adverse experiences reported when AVANDIA was used in combination with a sulfonylurea or metformin were similar to those during monotherapy with AVANDIA. Events of anemia and edema tended to be reported more frequently at higher doses, and were generally mild to moderate in severity and usually did not require discontinuation of treatment with AVANDIA.

In double-blind studies, anemia was reported in 1.9% of patients receiving AVANDIA as monotherapy compared to 0.7% on placebo, 0.6% on sulfonylureas, and 2.2% on metformin. Reports of anemia were greater in patients treated with a combination of AVANDIA and metformin (7.1%) and with a combination of AVANDIA and a sulfonylurea plus metformin (6.7%) compared to monotherapy with AVANDIA or in combination with a sulfonylurea (2.3%). Lower pre-treatment hemoglobin/hematocrit levels in patients enrolled in the metformin combination clinical trials may have contributed to the higher reporting rate of anemia in these studies (see ADVERSE REACTIONS, Laboratory Abnormalities, *Hematologic*).

In clinical trials, edema was reported in 4.8% of patients receiving AVANDIA as monotherapy compared to 1.3% on placebo, 1.0% on sulfonylureas, and 2.2% on metformin. The reporting rate of edema was higher for AVANDIA 8 mg in sulfonylurea combinations (12.4%) compared to other combinations, with the exception of insulin. Edema was reported in 14.7% of patients receiving AVANDIA in the insulin combination trials compared to 5.4% on insulin alone. Reports of new onset or exacerbation of congestive heart failure occurred at rates of 1% for insulin alone, and 2% (4 mg) and 3% (8 mg) for insulin in combination with AVANDIA.

In postmarketing experience in patients receiving thiazolidinedione therapy, serious adverse events with or without a fatal outcome, potentially related to volume expansion (e.g., congestive heart failure, pulmonary edema, and pleural effusions) have been reported. (See WARNINGS, Cardiac Failure and Other Cardiac Effects.)

In controlled combination therapy studies with sulfonylureas, mild to moderate hypoglycemic symptoms, which appear to be dose related, were reported. Few patients were withdrawn for hypoglycemia (<1%) and few episodes of hypoglycemia were considered to be severe (<1%). Hypoglycemia was the most frequently reported adverse event in the fixed-dose insulin combination trials, although few patients withdrew for hypoglycemia (4 of 408 for AVANDIA plus insulin and 1 of 203 for insulin alone). Rates of hypoglycemia, confirmed by capillary blood glucose concentration ≤50 mg/dL, were 6% for insulin alone and 12% (4 mg) and 14% (8 mg) for insulin in combination with AVANDIA. (See PRECAUTIONS, General, *Hypoglycemia* and DOSAGE AND ADMINISTRATION, Combination Therapy.)

In postmarketing experience with AVANDIA, angioedema and urticaria have been reported rarely.

Laboratory Abnormalities: ***Hematologic:*** Decreases in mean hemoglobin and hematocrit occurred in a dose-related fashion in patients treated with AVANDIA (mean decreases in individual studies up to 1.0 gram/dL hemoglobin and up to 3.3% hematocrit). The time course and magnitude of decreases were similar in patients treated with a combination of AVANDIA and other hypoglycemic agents or AVANDIA monotherapy. Pre-treatment levels of hemoglobin and hematocrit were lower in patients in metformin combination studies and may have contributed to the higher reporting rate of anemia. White blood cell counts also decreased slightly in patients treated with AVANDIA. Decreases in hematologic parameters may be related to increased plasma volume observed with treatment with AVANDIA.

Lipids: Changes in serum lipids have been observed following treatment with AVANDIA (see CLINICAL STUDIES).

Serum Transaminase Levels: In clinical studies in 4,598 patients treated with AVANDIA encompassing approximately 3,600 patient years of exposure, there was no evidence of drug-induced hepatotoxicity or elevated ALT levels. In controlled trials, 0.2% of patients treated with AVANDIA had reversible elevations in ALT >3× the upper limit of normal compared to 0.2% on placebo and 0.5% on active comparators. Hyperbilirubinemia was found in 0.3% of patients treated with AVANDIA compared with 0.9% treated with placebo and 1% in patients treated with active comparators. In the clinical program including long-term, open-label experience, the rate per 100 patient years exposure of ALT increase to >3× the upper limit of normal was 0.35 for patients treated with AVANDIA, 0.59 for placebo-treated patients, and 0.78 for patients treated with active comparator agents.

In pre-approval clinical trials, there were no cases of idiosyncratic drug reactions leading to hepatic failure. In postmarketing experience with AVANDIA, reports of hepatic enzyme elevations 3 or more times the upper limit of normal and hepatitis have been received (see PRECAUTIONS, General, *Hepatic Effects*).

OVERDOSAGE

Limited data are available with regard to overdosage in humans. In clinical studies in volunteers, AVANDIA has been administered at single oral doses of up to 20 mg and was well-tolerated. In the event of an overdose, appropriate supportive treatment should be initiated as dictated by the patient's clinical status.

DOSAGE AND ADMINISTRATION

The management of antidiabetic therapy should be individualized. AVANDIA may be administered either at a starting dose of 4 mg as a single daily dose or divided and administered in the morning and evening. For patients who respond inadequately following 8 to 12 weeks of treatment, as determined by reduction in FPG, the dose may be increased to 8 mg daily as monotherapy or in combination with metformin, sulfonylurea, or sulfonylurea plus metformin. Reductions in glycemic parameters by dose and regimen are described under CLINICAL STUDIES. AVANDIA may be taken with or without food.

Monotherapy: The usual starting dose of AVANDIA is 4 mg administered either as a single dose once daily or in divided doses twice daily. In clinical trials, the 4 mg twice daily regimen resulted in the greatest reduction in FPG and HbA1c.

Combination Therapy: When AVANDIA is added to existing therapy, the current dose(s) of the agent(s) can be continued upon initiation of AVANDIA therapy.

Sulfonylurea: When used in combination with sulfonylurea, the usual starting dose of AVANDIA is 4 mg administered as either a single dose once daily or in divided doses twice daily. If patients report hypoglycemia, the dose of the sulfonylurea should be decreased.

Metformin: The usual starting dose of AVANDIA in combination with metformin is 4 mg administered as either a single dose once daily or in divided doses twice daily. It is unlikely that the dose of metformin will require adjustment due to hypoglycemia during combination therapy with AVANDIA.

Insulin: For patients stabilized on insulin, the insulin dose should be continued upon initiation of therapy with AVANDIA. AVANDIA should be dosed at 4 mg daily. Doses of AVANDIA greater than 4 mg daily in combination with insulin are not currently indicated. It is recommended that the insulin dose be decreased by 10% to 25% if the patient reports hypoglycemia or if FPG concentrations decrease to less than 100 mg/dL. Further adjustments should be individualized based on glucose-lowering response.

Sulfonylurea Plus Metformin: The usual starting dose of AVANDIA in combination with a sulfonylurea plus metformin is 4 mg administered as either a single dose once daily or divided doses twice daily. If patients report hypoglycemia, the dose of the sulfonylurea should be decreased.

Maximum Recommended Dose: The dose of AVANDIA should not exceed 8 mg daily, as a single dose or divided twice daily. The 8 mg daily dose has been shown to be safe and effective in clinical studies as monotherapy and in combination with metformin, sulfonylurea, or sulfonylurea plus metformin. Doses of AVANDIA greater than 4 mg daily in combination with insulin are not currently indicated.

AVANDIA may be taken with or without food.

No dosage adjustments are required for the elderly.

No dosage adjustment is necessary when AVANDIA is used as monotherapy in patients with renal impairment. Since metformin is contraindicated in such patients, concomitant administration of metformin and AVANDIA is also contraindicated in patients with renal impairment.

Therapy with AVANDIA should not be initiated if the patient exhibits clinical evidence of active liver disease or increased serum transaminase levels (ALT >2.5× upper limit of normal at start of therapy) (see PRECAUTIONS, General, *Hepatic Effects* and CLINICAL PHARMACOLOGY, Special Populations, *Hepatic Impairment*). Liver enzyme monitoring is recommended in all patients prior to initiation of therapy with AVANDIA and periodically thereafter (see PRECAUTIONS, General, *Hepatic Effects*).

There are no data on the use of AVANDIA in patients younger than 18 years; therefore, use of AVANDIA in pediatric patients is not recommended.

HOW SUPPLIED

Tablets: Each pentagonal film-coated TILTAB tablet contains rosiglitazone as the maleate as follows: 2 mg–pink, debossed with SB on one side and 2 on the other; 4 mg–orange, debossed with SB on one side and 4 on the other; 8 mg–red-brown, debossed with SB on one side and 8 on the other.

2 mg bottles of 30: NDC 0029-3158-13
2 mg bottles of 60: NDC 0029-3158-18
2 mg bottles of 100: NDC 0029-3158-20
2 mg bottles of 500: NDC 0029-3158-25
2 mg SUP 100s: NDC 0029-3158-21
4 mg bottles of 30: NDC 0029-3159-13
4 mg bottles of 60: NDC 0029-3159-18

Continued on next page

Avandia—Cont.

4 mg bottles of 100: NDC 0029-3159-20
4 mg bottles of 500: NDC 0029-3159-25
4 mg SUP 100s: NDC 0029-3159-21
8 mg bottles of 30: NDC 0029-3160-13
8 mg bottles of 100: NDC 0029-3160-20
8 mg bottles of 500: NDC 0029-3160-25
8 mg SUP 100s: NDC 0029-3160-21

STORAGE

Store at 25°C (77°F); excursions 15°–30°C (59°–86°F). Dispense in a tight, light-resistant container.

REFERENCE

1. Park JY, Kim KA, Kang MH, et al. Effect of rifampin on the pharmacokinetics of rosiglitazone in healthy subjects. *Clin Pharmacol Ther* 2004;75:157–162.

GlaxoSmithKline, Research Triangle Park, NC 27709
AVANDIA and TILTAB are registered trademarks of GlaxoSmithKline.
©2005, GlaxoSmithKline. All rights reserved.
March 2005/AV:L12, AV:L13

AVODART® ℞

[av' ō dart]
(dutasteride)
Soft Gelatin Capsules

Prescribing information for this product, which appears on pages 1443–1446 of the 2005 PDR, has been revised as follows. Please write "See Supplement A" next to the product heading.

CLINICAL PHARMACOLOGY: Pharmacokinetics: *Metabolism and Elimination has been revised as follows.*

Dutasteride is extensively metabolized in humans. In vitro studies showed that dutasteride is metabolized by the CYP3A4 and CYP3A5 isoenzymes. Both of these isoenzymes produced the 4′-hydroxydutasteride, 6-hydroxydutasteride, and the 6,4′-dihydroxydutasteride metabolites. In addition, the 15-hydroxydutasteride metabolite was formed by CYP3A4. Dutasteride is not metabolized in vitro by human cytochrome P450 isoenzymes CYP1A2, CYP2A6, CYP2B6, CYP2C8, CYP2C9, CYP2C19, CYP2D6, and CYP2E1. In human serum, following dosing to steady state, unchanged dutasteride, 3 major metabolites (4′-hydroxydutasteride, 1,2-dihydrodutasteride, and 6-hydroxydutasteride), and 2 minor metabolites (6,4′-dihydroxydutasteride and 15-hydroxydutasteride), as assessed by mass spectrometric response, have been detected. The absolute stereochemistry of the hydroxyl additions in the 6 and 15 positions is not known. In vitro, the 4′-hydroxydutasteride and 1, 2-dihydrodutasteride metabolites are much less potent than dutasteride against both isoforms of human 5AR. The activity of 6β-hydroxydutasteride is comparable to that of dutasteride.

Dutasteride and its metabolites were excreted mainly in feces. As a percent of dose, there was approximately 5% unchanged dutasteride (~1% to ~15%) and 40% as dutasteride-related metabolites (~2% to ~90%). Only trace amounts of unchanged dutasteride were found in urine (<1%). Therefore, on average, the dose unaccounted for approximated 55% (range 5% to 97%).

The terminal elimination half-life of dutasteride is approximately 5 weeks at steady state. The average steady-state serum dutasteride concentration was 40 ng/mL following 0.5 mg/day for 1 year. Following daily dosing, dutasteride serum concentrations achieve 65% of steady-state concentration after 1 month and approximately 90% after 3 months. Due to the long half-life of dutasteride, serum concentrations remain detectable (greater than 0.1 ng/mL) for up to 4 to 6 months after discontinuation of treatment.

CLINICAL PHARMACOLOGY: Drug Interactions *has been revised as follows.*

In vitro drug metabolism studies reveal that dutasteride is metabolized by the human cytochrome P450 isoenzymes CYP3A4 and CYP3A5. In a human mass balance analysis (n = 8), dutasteride was extensively metabolized. Less than 20% of the dose was excreted unchanged in the feces. No clinical drug interaction studies have been performed to evaluate the impact of CYP3A enzyme inhibitors on dutasteride pharmacokinetics. However, based on the in vitro data, blood concentrations of dutasteride may increase in the presence of inhibitors of CYP3A4/5 such as ritonavir, ketoconazole, verapamil, diltiazem, cimetidine, troleandomycin, and ciprofloxacin. Dutasteride is not metabolized in vitro by human cytochrome P450 isoenzymes CYP1A2, CYP2A6, CYP2B6, CYP2C8, CYP2C9, CYP2C19, CYP2D6, and CYP2E1.

Clinical drug interaction studies have shown no pharmacokinetic or pharmacodynamic interactions between dutasteride and tamsulosin, terazosin, warfarin, digoxin, and cholestyramine (see PRECAUTIONS: Drug Interactions).

Dutasteride does not inhibit the in vitro metabolism of model substrates for the major human cytochrome P450 isoenzymes (CYP1A2, CYP2C9, CYP2C19, CYP2D6, and CYP3A4) at a concentration of 1,000 ng/mL, 25 times greater than steady-state serum concentrations in humans.

HOW SUPPLIED *has been revised as follows.*

AVODART Soft Gelatin Capsules 0.5 mg are oblong, opaque, dull yellow, gelatin capsules imprinted with "GX CE2" in red ink on one side packaged in bottles of 30 (NDC 0173-0712-15) and 90 (NDC 0173-0712-04) with child-resistant closures.

Manufactured by Cardinal Health
Beinheim, France for GlaxoSmithKline
Research Triangle Park, NC 27709
©2004, GlaxoSmithKline. All rights reserved.
September 2004/RL-2072, RL-2102

CEFTIN® Tablets ℞

[sĕf' tin]
(cefuroxime axetil tablets)

CEFTIN® for Oral Suspension ℞

(cefuroxime axetil powder for oral suspension)

Prescribing information for this product, which appears on pages 1450–1454 of the 2005 PDR, has been revised as follows. Please write "See Supplement A" next to the product heading.

The following paragraph has been revised in the DESCRIPTION *section.*

CEFTIN Tablets are film-coated and contain the equivalent of 250 or 500 mg of cefuroxime as cefuroxime axetil. CEFTIN Tablets contain the inactive ingredients colloidal silicon dioxide, croscarmellose sodium, hydrogenated vegetable oil, hypromellose, methylparaben, microcrystalline cellulose, propylene glycol, propylparaben, sodium benzoate, sodium lauryl sulfate, and titanium dioxide.

The HOW SUPPLIED *section has been revised as follows for CEFTIN Tablets.*

CEFTIN Tablets: CEFTIN Tablets, 250 mg of cefuroxime (as cefuroxime axetil), are white, capsule-shaped, film-coated tablets engraved with "GX ES7" on one side and blank on the other side as follows:

20 Tablets/Bottle	NDC 0173-0387-00
60 Tablets/Bottle	NDC 0173-0387-42

CEFTIN Tablets, 500 mg of cefuroxime (as cefuroxime axetil), are white, capsule-shaped, film-coated tablets engraved with "GX EG2" on one side and blank on the other side as follows:

20 Tablets/Bottle	NDC 0173-0394-00
60 Tablets/Bottle	NDC 0173-0394-42

Store the tablets between 15° and 30°C (59° and 86°F). Replace cap securely after each opening.

GlaxoSmithKline, Research Triangle Park, NC 27709
©2003, GlaxoSmithKline. All rights reserved.
December 2003/RL-2058

ENGERIX-B® ℞

[in' jə-rix]
[Hepatitis B Vaccine (Recombinant)]

Prescribing information for this product, which appears on pages 1470–1473 of the 2005 PDR, has been revised as follows. Please write "See Supplement A" next to the product heading.

The following PRECAUTIONS: Geriatric Use *section has been added.*

Clinical studies of ENGERIX-B did not include sufficient numbers of subjects 65 years of age and older to determine whether they respond differently from younger subjects. Other reports from the clinical literature indicate that hepatitis B vaccines are less immunogenic in adults 65 years of age and older than in younger individuals. Other reported clinical experience has not identified differences in overall safety between these subjects and younger adult subjects.

Manufactured by GlaxoSmithKline Biologicals
Rixensart, Belgium, US License No. 1617
Distributed by GlaxoSmithKline
Research Triangle Park, NC 27709
©2004, GlaxoSmithKline. All rights reserved.
August 2004/EB:L35

EPIVIR® Tablets ℞

[ĕp' ə-vir]
(lamivudine tablets)

EPIVIR® Oral Solution ℞

(lamivudine oral solution)

Prescribing information for this product, which appears on pages 1473–1477 of the 2005 PDR, has been revised as follows. Please write "See Supplement A" next to the product heading.

The following paragraphs have been revised in the CLINICAL PHARMACOLOGY: Special Populations: *Adults with Impaired Renal Function section.*

Based on a study in otherwise healthy subjects with impaired renal function, hemodialysis increased lamivudine clearance from a mean of 64 to 88 mL/min; however, the length of time of hemodialysis (4 hours) was insufficient to significantly alter mean lamivudine exposure after a single-dose administration. Continuous ambulatory peritoneal dialysis and automated peritoneal dialysis have negligible effects on lamivudine clearance. Therefore, it is recommended, following correction of dose for creatinine clearance, that no additional dose modification be made after routine hemodialysis or peritoneal dialysis.

It is not known whether lamivudine can be removed by continuous (24-hour) hemodialysis.

The OVERDOSAGE *section has been revised as follows.*

There is no known antidote for EPIVIR. One case of an adult ingesting 6 g of EPIVIR was reported; there were no clinical signs or symptoms noted and hematologic tests remained normal. Two cases of pediatric overdose were reported in ACTG300. One case was a single dose of 7 mg/kg of EPIVIR; the second case involved use of 5 mg/kg of EPIVIR twice daily for 30 days. There were no clinical signs or symptoms noted in either case. Because a negligible amount of lamivudine was removed via (4-hour) hemodialysis, continuous ambulatory peritoneal dialysis, and automated peritoneal dialysis, it is not known if continuous hemodialysis would provide clinical benefit in a lamivudine overdose event. If overdose occurs, the patient should be monitored, and standard supportive treatment applied as required.

The DOSAGE AND ADMINISTRATION: Dose Adjustment *section has been revised as follows.*

It is recommended that doses of EPIVIR be adjusted in accordance with renal function (see Table 9) (see CLINICAL PHARMACOLOGY).

Table 9. Adjustment of Dosage of EPIVIR in Adults and Adolescents in Accordance With Creatinine Clearance

Creatinine Clearance (mL/min)	Recommended Dosage of EPIVIR
≥50	150 mg twice daily or 300 mg once daily
30–49	150 mg once daily
15–29	150 mg first dose, then 100 mg once daily
5–14	150 mg first dose, then 50 mg once daily
<5	50 mg first dose, then 25 mg once daily

No additional dosing of EPIVIR is required after routine (4-hour) hemodialysis or peritoneal dialysis.

Although there are insufficient data to recommend a specific dose adjustment of EPIVIR in pediatric patients with renal impairment, a reduction in the dose and/or an increase in the dosing interval should be considered.

GlaxoSmithKline, Research Triangle Park, NC 27709
Manufactured under agreement from
Shire Pharmaceuticals Group plc, Basingstoke, UK
©2004, GlaxoSmithKline. All rights reserved.
December 2004/RL-2152

EPIVIR-HBV® ℞

[ĕp' ə-vir]
(lamivudine)
Tablets

EPIVIR-HBV® ℞

(lamivudine)
Oral Solution

Prescribing information for this product, which appears on pages 1477–1481 of the 2005 PDR, has been revised as follows. Please write "See Supplement A" next to the product heading.

The following paragraphs have been revised in the CLINICAL PHARMACOLOGY: Special Populations: *Adults with Impaired Renal Function section.*

Hemodialysis increases lamivudine clearance from a mean of 64 to 88 mL/min; however, the length of time of hemodialysis (4 hours) was insufficient to significantly alter mean lamivudine exposure after a single-dose administration. Continuous ambulatory peritoneal dialysis and automated peritoneal dialysis have negligible effects on lamivudine clearance. Therefore, it is recommended, following correction of dose for creatinine clearance, that no additional dose modification be made after routine hemodialysis or peritoneal dialysis.

It is not known whether lamivudine can be removed by continuous (24-hour) hemodialysis.

The OVERDOSAGE *section has been revised as follows.*

There is no known antidote for EPIVIR-HBV. One case of an adult ingesting 6 g of EPIVIR was reported; there were no clinical signs or symptoms noted and hematologic tests remained normal. Because a negligible amount of lamivudine was removed via (4-hour) hemodialysis, continuous ambulatory peritoneal dialysis, and automated peritoneal dialysis, it is not known if continuous hemodialysis would provide clinical benefit in a lamivudine overdose event. If overdose occurs, the patient should be monitored, and standard supportive treatment applied as required.

The DOSAGE AND ADMINISTRATION: Dose Adjustment *section has been revised as follows.*

It is recommended that doses of EPIVIR-HBV be adjusted in accordance with renal function (Table 8) (see CLINICAL PHARMACOLOGY: Special Populations).

Table 8. Adjustment of Adult Dosage of EPIVIR-HBV in Accordance With Creatinine Clearance

Creatinine Clearance (mL/min)	Recommended Dosage of EPIVIR-HBV
≥50	100 mg once daily
30–49	100 mg first dose, then 50 mg once daily
15–29	100 mg first dose, then 25 mg once daily
5–14	35 mg first dose, then 15 mg once daily
<5	35 mg first dose, then 10 mg once daily

No additional dosing of EPIVIR-HBV is required after routine (4-hour) hemodialysis or peritoneal dialysis.

Although there are insufficient data to recommend a specific dose adjustment of EPIVIR-HBV in pediatric patients with renal impairment, a dose reduction should be considered. GlaxoSmithKline, Research Triangle Park, NC 27709 Manufactured under agreement from Shire Pharmaceuticals Group plc, Basingstoke, UK ©2004, GlaxoSmithKline. All rights reserved. December 2004/RL-2153

IMITREX®   ℞
[ĭm'ĭ-trĕx]
(sumatriptan succinate)
Injection

For Subcutaneous Use Only.

Prescribing information for this product, which appears on pages 1513–1517 of the 2005 PDR, has been revised as follows. Please write "See Supplement A" next to the product heading.
The WARNINGS: Other Vasospasm-Related Events *section has been revised as follows.*
Sumatriptan may cause vasospastic reactions other than coronary artery vasospasm. Both peripheral vascular ischemia and colonic ischemia with abdominal pain and bloody diarrhea have been reported. Very rare reports of transient and permanent blindness and significant partial vision loss have been reported with the use of sumatriptan. Visual disorders may also be part of a migraine attack.
The PRECAUTIONS: Binding to Melanin-Containing Tissues *section has been revised as follows.*
Because sumatriptan binds to melanin, it could accumulate in melanin-rich tissues (such as the eye) over time. This raises the possibility that sumatriptan could cause toxicity in these tissues after extended use. However, no effects on the retina related to treatment with sumatriptan were noted in any of the toxicity studies. Although no systematic monitoring of ophthalmologic function was undertaken in clinical trials, and no specific recommendations for ophthalmologic monitoring are offered, prescribers should be aware of the possibility of long-term ophthalmologic effects (see CLINICAL PHARMACOLOGY).
The PRECAUTIONS: Pediatric Use *section has been revised as follows.*
Safety and effectiveness of IMITREX Injection in pediatric patients under 18 years of age have not been established; therefore, IMITREX Injection is not recommended for use in patients under 18 years of age.
Two controlled clinical trials evaluating sumatriptan nasal spray (5 to 20 mg) in pediatric patients aged 12 to 17 years enrolled a total of 1,248 adolescent migraineurs who treated a single attack. The studies did not establish the efficacy of sumatriptan nasal spray compared to placebo in the treatment of migraine in adolescents. Adverse events observed in these clinical trials were similar in nature to those reported in clinical trials in adults.
Five controlled clinical trials (2 single attack studies, 3 multiple attack studies) evaluating oral sumatriptan (25 to 100 mg) in pediatric patients aged 12 to 17 years enrolled a total of 701 adolescent migraineurs. These studies did not establish the efficacy of oral sumatriptan compared to placebo in the treatment of migraine in adolescents. Adverse events observed in these clinical trials were similar in nature to those reported in clinical trials in adults. The frequency of all adverse events in these patients appeared to be both dose- and age-dependent, with younger patients reporting events more commonly than older adolescents.
Postmarketing experience documents that serious adverse events have occurred in the pediatric population after use of subcutaneous, oral, and/or intranasal sumatriptan. These reports include events similar in nature to those reported rarely in adults, including stroke, visual loss, and death. A myocardial infarction has been reported in a 14-year-old male following the use of oral sumatriptan; clinical signs occurred within 1 day of drug administration. Since clinical data to determine the frequency of serious adverse events in pediatric patients who might receive injectable, oral, or intranasal sumatriptan are not presently available, the use of sumatriptan in patients aged younger than 18 years is not recommended.
GlaxoSmithKline, Research Triangle Park, NC 27709 ©2004, GlaxoSmithKline. All rights reserved. November 2004/RL-2120, RL-2145

IMITREX®   ℞
[ĭm' ĭ-trĕx]
(sumatriptan)
Nasal Spray

Prescribing information for this product, which appears on pages 1517–1521 of the 2005 PDR, has been revised as follows. Please write "See Supplement A" next to the product heading.
The WARNINGS: Other Vasospasm-Related Events *section has been revised as follows.*
Sumatriptan may cause vasospastic reactions other than coronary artery vasospasm. Both peripheral vascular ischemia and colonic ischemia with abdominal pain and bloody diarrhea have been reported. Very rare reports of transient

and permanent blindness and significant partial vision loss have been reported with the use of sumatriptan. Visual disorders may also be part of a migraine attack.
The PRECAUTIONS: Pediatric Use *section has been revised as follows.*
Safety and effectiveness of IMITREX Nasal Spray in pediatric patients under 18 years of age have not been established; therefore, IMITREX Nasal Spray is not recommended for use in patients under 18 years of age.
Two controlled clinical trials evaluating sumatriptan nasal spray (5 to 20 mg) in pediatric patients aged 12 to 17 years enrolled a total of 1,248 adolescent migraineurs who treated a single attack. The studies did not establish the efficacy of sumatriptan nasal spray compared to placebo in the treatment of migraine in adolescents. Adverse events observed in these clinical trials were similar in nature to those reported in clinical trials in adults.
Five controlled clinical trials (2 single attack studies, 3 multiple attack studies) evaluating oral sumatriptan (25 to 100 mg) in pediatric patients aged 12 to 17 years enrolled a total of 701 adolescent migraineurs. These studies did not establish the efficacy of oral sumatriptan compared to placebo in the treatment of migraine in adolescents. Adverse events observed in these clinical trials were similar in nature to those reported in clinical trials in adults. The frequency of all adverse events in these patients appeared to be both dose- and age-dependent, with younger patients reporting events more commonly than older adolescents.
Postmarketing experience documents that serious adverse events have occurred in the pediatric population after use of subcutaneous, oral, and/or intranasal sumatriptan. These reports include events similar in nature to those reported rarely in adults, including stroke, visual loss, and death. A myocardial infarction has been reported in a 14-year-old male following the use of oral sumatriptan; clinical signs occurred within 1 day of drug administration. Since clinical data to determine the frequency of serious adverse events in pediatric patients who might receive injectable, oral, or intranasal sumatriptan are not presently available, the use of sumatriptan in patients aged younger than 18 years is not recommended.
GlaxoSmithKline, Research Triangle Park, NC 27709 ©2004, GlaxoSmithKline. All rights reserved. October 2004/RL-2121, RL-2134

IMITREX®   ℞
[ĭm'ĭ-trĕx]
(sumatriptan succinate)
Tablets

Prescribing information for this product, which appears on pages 1521–1526 of the 2005 PDR, has been revised as follows. Please write "See Supplement A" next to the product heading.
The WARNINGS: Other Vasospasm-Related Events *section has been revised as follows.*
Sumatriptan may cause vasospastic reactions other than coronary artery vasospasm. Both peripheral vascular ischemia and colonic ischemia with abdominal pain and bloody diarrhea have been reported. Very rare reports of transient and permanent blindness and significant partial vision loss have been reported with the use of sumatriptan. Visual disorders may also be part of a migraine attack.
The PRECAUTIONS: Pediatric Use *section has been revised as follows.*
Safety and effectiveness of IMITREX Tablets in pediatric patients under 18 years of age have not been established; therefore, IMITREX Tablets are not recommended for use in patients under 18 years of age.
Two controlled clinical trials evaluating sumatriptan nasal spray (5 to 20 mg) in pediatric patients aged 12 to 17 years enrolled a total of 1,248 adolescent migraineurs who treated a single attack. The studies did not establish the efficacy of sumatriptan nasal spray compared to placebo in the treatment of migraine in adolescents. Adverse events observed in these clinical trials were similar in nature to those reported in clinical trials in adults.
Five controlled clinical trials (2 single attack studies, 3 multiple attack studies) evaluating oral sumatriptan (25 to 100 mg) in pediatric patients aged 12 to 17 years enrolled a total of 701 adolescent migraineurs. These studies did not establish the efficacy of oral sumatriptan compared to placebo in the treatment of migraine in adolescents. Adverse events observed in these clinical trials were similar in nature to those reported in clinical trials in adults. The frequency of all adverse events in these patients appeared to be both dose- and age-dependent, with younger patients reporting events more commonly than older adolescents.
Postmarketing experience documents that serious adverse events have occurred in the pediatric population after use of subcutaneous, oral, and/or intranasal sumatriptan. These reports include events similar in nature to those reported rarely in adults, including stroke, visual loss, and death. A myocardial infarction has been reported in a 14-year-old male following the use of oral sumatriptan; clinical signs occurred within 1 day of drug administration. Since clinical data to determine the frequency of serious adverse events in pediatric patients who might receive injectable, oral, or intranasal sumatriptan are not presently available, the use of sumatriptan in patients aged younger than 18 years is not recommended.
Two hospital unit dose packs have been added to the HOW SUPPLIED *section as follows.*

IMITREX Tablets, 50 mg are white, triangular-shaped, film-coated tablets debossed with "IMITREX 50" on one side and a chevron shape (^) on the other in blister packs of 9 tablets (NDC 0173-0736-01) and hospital unit dose packs of 18 tablets (NDC 0173-0736-02).
IMITREX Tablets, 100 mg, are pink, triangular-shaped, film-coated tablets debossed with "IMITREX 100" on one side and a chevron shape (^) on the other in blister packs of 9 tablets (NDC 0173-0737-01) and hospital unit dose packs of 18 tablets (NDC 0173-0737-02).
GlaxoSmithKline. Research Triangle Park, NC 27709 ©2004, GlaxoSmithKline. All rights reserved. December 2004/RL-2122, RL-2146, RL-2157

LAMICTAL®   ℞
[la-mĭk' tal]
(lamotrigine)
Tablets

LAMICTAL®   ℞
(lamotrigine)
Chewable Dispersible Tablets

Prescribing information for this product, which appears on pages 1531–1540 of the 2005 PDR, has been revised as follows. Please write "See Supplement A" next to the product heading.
The following Table 1 footnote has been revised in the CLINICAL PHARMACOLOGY: Pharmacokinetics and Drug Metabolism *section.*
† Carbamazepine, phenobarbital, phenytoin, and primidone have been shown to increase the apparent clearance of lamotrigine. Oral contraceptives and rifampin have also been shown to increase the apparent clearance of lamotrigine (see CLINICAL PHARMACOLOGY: Drug Interactions and PRECAUTIONS: Drug Interactions).
The following paragraph has been added to the CLINICAL PHARMACOLOGY: Pharmacokinetics and Drug Metabolism: *Drug Interactions section.*
Oral contraceptives and rifampin have also been shown to increase the apparent clearance of lamotrigine (see PRECAUTIONS: Drug Interactions).
The following Table 2 footnote has been revised in the CLINICAL PHARMACOLOGY: Pharmacokinetics and Drug Metabolism: *Age: Pediatric Patients section.*
* Carbamazepine, phenobarbital, phenytoin, and primidone have been shown to increase the apparent clearance of lamotrigine. Oral contraceptives and rifampin have also been shown to increase the apparent clearance of lamotrigine (see CLINICAL PHARMACOLOGY: Drug Interactions and PRECAUTIONS: Drug Interactions).
The following paragraph has been added to the PRECAUTIONS: Information for Patients *section.*
Women should be advised to notify their physician if they plan to start or stop use of oral contraceptives or other female hormonal preparations. They should also be advised to promptly notify their physician if they experience changes in menstrual pattern (e.g., break-through bleeding) while receiving LAMICTAL in combination with these medications.
The following paragraph has been revised in the PRECAUTIONS: Laboratory Tests *section.*
The value of monitoring plasma concentrations of LAMICTAL has not been established. Because of the possible pharmacokinetic interactions between LAMICTAL and other drugs including AEDs, (see Table 3), monitoring of the plasma levels of LAMICTAL and concomitant drugs may be indicated, particularly during dosage adjustments. In general, clinical judgment should be exercised regarding monitoring of plasma levels of LAMICTAL and other drugs and whether or not dosage adjustments are necessary.
The PRECAUTIONS: Drug Interactions: *Interactions With Oral Contraceptives section has been revised as follows.*
Effect of Oral Contraceptives on LAMICTAL: In a study in 16 female volunteers, an oral contraceptive preparation containing 30 mcg ethinylestradiol and 150 mcg levonorgestrel increased the apparent clearance of lamotrigine (300 mg/day) by approximately two fold with a mean decrease in AUC of 52% and in C_{max} of 39%. In this study, trough serum lamotrigine concentrations gradually increased and were approximately 2-fold higher on average at the end of the week of the inactive preparation compared to trough lamotrigine concentrations at the end of the active hormone cycle.
Gradual transient increases in lamotrigine levels will occur during the week of no active hormone preparation (pill-free week) for women not also taking a drug that increases the clearance of lamotrigine (carbamazepine, phenytoin, phenobarbital, primidone, or rifampin). The increase in lamotrigine levels will be greater if the dose of LAMICTAL is increased in the few days before or during the pill-free week.
Dosage adjustments may be necessary for women receiving oral contraceptive preparations (see DOSAGE AND ADMINISTRATION: Women and Oral Contraceptives).
Effect of LAMICTAL on Oral Contraceptives: Co-administration of LAMICTAL (300 mg/day) in 16 female volunteers did not affect the pharmacokinetics of the ethinylestradiol component of an oral contraceptive preparation containing 30 mcg ethinylestradiol and 150 mcg levonorgestrel. There was a mean decrease in the AUC and C_{max} of the levonorgestrel component of 19% and 12%, respectively. Measure-

Continued on next page

Lamictal—Cont.

ment of serum progesterone indicated that there was no hormonal evidence of ovulation in any of the 16 volunteers, although measurement of serum FSH, LH, and estradiol indicated that there was some loss of suppression of the hypothalamic-pituitary-ovarian axis.
The effects of doses of LAMICTAL other than 300 mg/day have not been studied.
The clinical significance of the observed hormonal changes on ovulatory activity is unknown. However, the possibility of decreased contraceptive efficacy in some patients cannot be excluded. Therefore, patients should be instructed to promptly report changes in their menstrual pattern (e.g., break-through bleeding).
Interactions With Other Hormonal Contraceptives or Hormone Replacement Therapy: The effect of other hormonal contraceptive preparations or hormone replacement therapy on the pharmacokinetics of lamotrigine has not been evaluated, although the effect may be similar to oral contraceptive preparations. Therefore, as for oral contraceptives, dosage adjustments may be necessary (see DOSAGE AND ADMINISTRATION: Women and Oral Contraceptives).
The net effects of drug interactions with LAMICTAL are summarized in Table 3.

Table 3. Summary of Drug Interactions With LAMICTAL

Drug	Drug Plasma Concentration With Adjunctive LAMICTAL*	Lamotrigine Plasma Concentration With Adjunctive Drugs†
Phenytoin (PHT)	↔	↓
Carbamazepine (CBZ)	↔	↓
CBZ epoxide‡	?	
Valproate	↓	↑
Valproate + PHT and/or CBZ	Not assessed	↔
Oxcarbazepine	↔	↔
10-monohydroxy oxcarbazepine metabolite§	↔	
Levetiracetam	↔	↔
Lithium	↔	Not assessed
Bupropion	Not assessed	↔
Olanzapine	↔	↔‖
Rifampin	Not assessed	↓
Ethinylestradiol/ levonorgesterol¶	↔#	↓

*From adjunctive clinical trials and volunteer studies.
† Net effects were estimated by comparing the mean clearance values obtained in adjunctive clinical trials and volunteers studies.
‡ Not administered, but an active metabolite of carbamazepine.
§ Not administered, but an active metabolite of oxcarbazepine.
↔ = No significant effect.
? = Conflicting data.
‖ Slight decrease, not expected to be clinically relevant.
¶ The effect of other hormonal contraceptive preparations or hormone replacement therapy on the pharmacokinetics of lamotrigine has not been evaluated, although the effect may be similar.
# Modest decrease in levonorgesterol (see PRECAUTIONS: Drug Interactions: Effect of LAMICTAL on Oral Contraceptives).

The following paragraphs have been added to the DOSAGE AND ADMINISTRATION: General Dosing Considerations for Epilepsy and Bipolar Disorder Patients *section.*
Women and Oral Contraceptives: Starting LAMICTAL in Women Taking Oral Contraceptives: Although oral contraceptives have been shown to increase the clearance of lamotrigine (see PRECAUTIONS: Drug Interactions), no adjustments to the recommended dose escalation guidelines for LAMICTAL should be necessary solely based on the use of oral contraceptives. Therefore, dose escalation should follow the recommended guidelines based on whether LAMICTAL is added to valproate, whether LAMICTAL is added to carbamazepine, phenytoin, phenobarbital, primidone, or rifampin, or whether LAMICTAL is added in the absence of valproate, carbamazepine, phenytoin, phenobarbital, primidone, or rifampin.
Adjustments to the Maintenance Dose of LAMICTAL: (1) Taking or Starting Oral Contraceptives: For women not taking carbamazepine, phenytoin, phenobarbital, primidone, or rifampin, the maintenance dose of LAMICTAL may need to be increased, by as much as 2 fold over the recommended target maintenance dose, according to clinical response (see PRECAUTIONS: Drug Interactions). For women taking LAMICTAL in addition to carbamazepine, phenytoin, phenobarbital, primidone, or rifampin, no adjustment should be necessary. ***(2) Stopping Oral Contraceptives:*** For women not taking carbamazepine, phenytoin, phenobarbital, primidone, or rifampin, the maintenance dose of LAMICTAL may need to be decreased by as much as 50% of the maintenance dose with concurrent oral contraceptives, according to clinical response (see PRECAUTIONS: Drug Interactions). For women taking LAMICTAL in addition to carbamazepine, phenytoin, phenobarbital, primidone or rifampin, no adjustment should be necessary.
Women and Other Hormonal Contraceptive Preparations or Hormone Replacement Therapy: Although the effect of other hormonal contraceptive preparations or hormone replacement therapy on the pharmacokinetics of lamotrigine has not been evaluated, the effect may be similar to oral contraceptives (see PRECAUTIONS: Drug Interactions). Therefore, similar adjustments to the dosage of LAMICTAL may be needed, based on clinical response.
The PATIENT INFORMATION *section has been revised as follows.*
The following wording is contained in a separate leaflet provided for patients.

Information for the Patient
LAMICTAL® (lamotrigine) Tablets
LAMICTAL® (lamotrigine) Chewable Dispersible Tablets
ALWAYS CHECK THAT YOU RECEIVE LAMICTAL

Patients prescribed LAMICTAL (lah-**MICK**-tall) have sometimes been given the wrong medicine in error because many medicines have names similar to LAMICTAL. Taking the wrong medication can cause serious health problems. When your healthcare provider gives you a prescription for LAMICTAL
- make sure you can read it clearly.
- talk to your pharmacist to check that you are given the correct medicine.
- check the tablets you receive against the pictures of the tablets below. The pictures show actual tablet shape and size and the wording describes the color and printing that is on each strength of LAMICTAL Tablets and Chewable Dispersible Tablets.

LAMICTAL (lamotrigine) Tablets

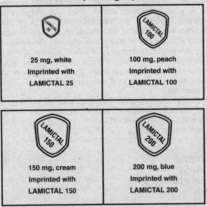

25 mg, white Imprinted with LAMICTAL 25

100 mg, peach Imprinted with LAMICTAL 100

150 mg, cream Imprinted with LAMICTAL 150

200 mg, blue Imprinted with LAMICTAL 200

LAMICTAL (lamotrigine) Chewable Dispersible Tablets

2 mg, white Imprinted with LTG 2

5 mg, white Imprinted with GX CL2

25 mg, white Imprinted with GX CL5

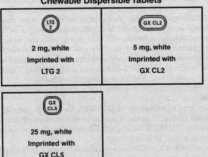

Please read this leaflet carefully before you take LAMICTAL and read the leaflet provided with any refill, in case any information has changed. This leaflet provides a summary of the information about your medicine. Please do not throw away this leaflet until you have finished your medicine. This leaflet does not contain all the information about LAMICTAL and is not meant to take the place of talking with your doctor. If you have any questions about LAMICTAL, ask your doctor or pharmacist.
Information About Your Medicine:
The name of your medicine is LAMICTAL (lamotrigine). The decision to use LAMICTAL is one that you and your doctor should make together. When taking lamotrigine, it is important to follow your doctor's instructions.
1. The Purpose of Your Medicine:
For Patients With Epilepsy: LAMICTAL is intended to be used either alone or in combination with other medicines to treat seizures in people aged 2 years or older.
For Patients With Bipolar Disorder: LAMICTAL is used as maintenance treatment of Bipolar I Disorder to delay the time to occurrence of mood episodes in people aged 18 years or older treated for acute mood episodes with standard therapy.
2. Who Should Not Take LAMICTAL:
You should not take LAMICTAL if you had an allergic reaction to it in the past.
3. Side Effects to Watch for:
- Most people who take LAMICTAL tolerate it well. Common side effects with LAMICTAL include dizziness, headache, blurred or double vision, lack of coordination, sleepiness, nausea, vomiting, insomnia, and rash. LAMICTAL may cause other side effects not listed in this leaflet. If you develop any side effects or symptoms you are concerned about or need more information, call your doctor.
- Although most patients who develop rash while receiving LAMICTAL have mild to moderate symptoms, some individuals may develop a serious skin reaction that requires hospitalization. Rarely, deaths have been reported. These serious skin reactions are most likely to happen within the first 8 weeks of treatment with LAMICTAL. Serious skin reactions occur more often in children than in adults.
- Rashes may be more likely to occur if you: (1) take LAMICTAL in combination with valproate [DEPAKENE® (valproic acid) or DEPAKOTE® (divalproex sodium)], (2) take a higher starting dose of LAMICTAL than your doctor prescribed, or (3) increase your dose of LAMICTAL faster than prescribed.
- It is not possible to predict whether a mild rash will develop into a more serious reaction. **Therefore, if you experience a skin rash, hives, fever, swollen lymph glands, painful sores in the mouth or around the eyes, or swelling of lips or tongue, tell a doctor immediately, since these symptoms may be the first signs of a serious reaction. A doctor should evaluate your condition and decide if you should continue taking LAMICTAL.**

4. The Use of LAMICTAL During Pregnancy and Breast-feeding:
The effects of LAMICTAL during pregnancy are not known at this time. If you are pregnant or are planning to become pregnant, talk to your doctor. Some LAMICTAL passes into breast milk and the effects of this on infants are unknown. Therefore, if you are breast-feeding, you should discuss this with your doctor to determine if you should continue to take LAMICTAL.
5. Use of Birth Control Pills or Other Female Hormonal Preparations:
- Do not start or stop using birth control pills or other female hormonal products until you have consulted your doctor.
- Tell your doctor as soon as possible if you experience changes in your menstrual pattern (e.g., break-through bleeding) while taking LAMICTAL and birth control pills or other female hormonal products.

6. How to Use LAMICTAL:
- It is important to take LAMICTAL exactly as instructed by your doctor. The dose of LAMICTAL must be increased slowly. It may take several weeks or months before your final dosage can be determined by your doctor, based on your response.
- Do not increase your dose of LAMICTAL or take more frequent doses than those indicated by your doctor. Contact your doctor, if you stop taking LAMICTAL for any reason. Do not restart without consulting your doctor.
- If you miss a dose of LAMICTAL, do not double your next dose.
- Always tell your doctor and pharmacist if you are taking any other prescription or over-the-counter medicines. Tell your doctor before you start any other medicines.
- Do NOT stop taking LAMICTAL or any of your other medicines unless instructed by your doctor.
- Use caution before driving a car or operating complex, hazardous machinery until you know if LAMICTAL affects your ability to perform these tasks.
- If you have epilepsy, tell your doctor if your seizures get worse or if you have any new types of seizures.

7. How to Take LAMICTAL:
LAMICTAL Tablets should be swallowed whole. Chewing the tablets may leave a bitter taste.
LAMICTAL Chewable Dispersible Tablets may be swallowed whole, chewed, or mixed in water or diluted fruit juice. If the tablets are chewed, consume a small amount of water or diluted fruit juice to aid in swallowing.
To disperse LAMICTAL Chewable Dispersible Tablets, add the tablets to a small amount of liquid (1 teaspoon, or enough to cover the medication) in a glass or spoon. Approximately 1 minute later, when the tablets are completely dispersed, mix the solution and take the entire amount immediately.
8. Storing Your Medicine:
Store LAMICTAL at room temperature away from heat and light. Always keep your medicines out of the reach of children.
This medicine was prescribed for your use only to treat seizures or to treat Bipolar Disorder. Do not give the drug to others.
If your doctor decides to stop your treatment, do not keep any leftover medicine unless your doctor tells you to. Throw away your medicine as instructed.
Manufactured for GlaxoSmithKline
Research Triangle Park, NC 27709
by DSM Pharmaceuticals, Inc.
Greenville, NC 27834 or
GlaxoSmithKline, Research Triangle Park, NC 27709
DEPAKENE and DEPAKOTE are registered trademarks of Abbott Laboratories.

August 2004/RL-2111, RL-2119

LEUKERAN® ℞
[*lū' kŭh-răn*]
(chlorambucil)
Tablets

Prescribing information for this product, which appears on pages 1556–1558 of the 2005 PDR, has been revised as follows. Please write "See Supplement A" next to the product heading.

The following has been added to the end of the PRECAUTIONS: General *section.*
Administration of live vaccines to immunocompromised patients should be avoided.
GlaxoSmithKline, Research Triangle Park, NC 27709
©2004, GlaxoSmithKline. All rights reserved.
November 2004/RL-2143

LEXIVA® ℞
[lex-ē'-va]
(fosamprenavir calcium)
Tablets

Prescribing information for this product, which appears on pages 1558–1564 of the 2005 PDR, has been revised as follows. Please write "See Supplement A" next to the product heading.

The following paragraph has been added to the PRECAUTIONS: Hepatic Impairment and Toxicity *section.*
Use of LEXIVA with ritonavir at higher-than-recommended dosages may result in transaminase elevations and should not be used (see OVERDOSAGE and DOSAGE AND ADMINISTRATION).

The following paragraph has been added to the OVERDOSAGE *section.*
In a healthy volunteer repeat-dose pharmacokinetic study evaluating high-dose combinations of LEXIVA plus ritonavir, an increased frequency of Grade 2/3 ALT elevations (>2.5 × ULN) was observed with LEXIVA 1,400 mg twice daily plus ritonavir 200 mg twice daily (4 of 25 subjects). Concurrent Grade 1/2 elevations in AST (>1.25 × ULN) were noted in 3 of these 4 subjects. These transaminase elevations resolved following discontinuation of dosing.

The following paragraph has been added to the DOSAGE AND ADMINISTRATION *section.*
High-Dose Combinations of LEXIVA plus Ritonavir: Higher-than-approved dose combinations of LEXIVA plus ritonavir are not recommended for use (see PRECAUTIONS and OVERDOSAGE).
GlaxoSmithKline, Research Triangle Park, NC 27709
Vertex Pharmaceuticals Incorporated, Cambridge, MA 02139
©2004, GlaxoSmithKline. All rights reserved.
December 2004/RL-2156

LOTRONEX® ℞
[lō' trə-nĕx]
(alosetron hydrochloride)
Tablets

Prescribing information for this product, which appears on pages 1564–1568 of the 2005 PDR, has been revised as follows. Please write "See Supplement A" next to the product heading.

WARNING: Infrequent but serious gastrointestinal adverse events have been reported with the use of LOTRONEX. These events, including ischemic colitis and serious complications of constipation, have resulted in hospitalization, and rarely, blood transfusion, surgery, and death.

- **The Prescribing Program for LOTRONEX™ was implemented to help reduce risks of serious gastrointestinal adverse events. Only physicians who have enrolled in GlaxoSmithKline's Prescribing Program for LOTRONEX, based on their understanding of the benefits and risks, should prescribe LOTRONEX (see PRECAUTIONS: Prescribing Program for LOTRONEX).**
- **LOTRONEX is indicated only for women with severe diarrhea-predominant IBS who have not responded adequately to conventional therapy (see INDICATIONS AND USAGE). Before receiving the initial prescription for LOTRONEX, the patient must read and sign the Patient-Physician Agreement for LOTRONEX (see PRECAUTIONS: Information for Patients).**
- **LOTRONEX should be discontinued immediately in patients who develop constipation or symptoms of ischemic colitis. Patients should immediately report constipation or symptoms of ischemic colitis to their physician. LOTRONEX should not be resumed in patients who develop ischemic colitis. Patients who have constipation should immediately contact their physician if the constipation does not resolve after LOTRONEX is discontinued. Patients with resolved constipation should resume LOTRONEX only on the advice of their treating physician.**

DESCRIPTION

The active ingredient in LOTRONEX Tablets is alosetron hydrochloride (HCl), a potent and selective antagonist of the serotonin 5-HT3 receptor type. Chemically, alosetron is designated as 2,3,4,5-tetrahydro-5-methyl-2-[(5-methyl-1H-imidazol-4-yl)methyl]-1H-pyrido[4,3-b]indol-1-one, monohydrochloride. Alosetron is achiral and has the empirical formula: $C_{17}H_{18}N_4O \bullet HCl$, representing a molecular weight of 330.8. Alosetron is a white to beige solid that has a solubility of 61 mg/mL in water, 42 mg/mL in 0.1M hydrochloric acid, 0.3 mg/mL in pH 6 phosphate buffer, and <0.1 mg/mL in pH 8 phosphate buffer.

LOTRONEX Tablets are supplied for oral administration as 0.5-mg (white) and 1-mg (blue) tablets. The 0.5-mg tablet contains 0.562 mg alosetron HCl equivalent to 0.5 mg alosetron and the 1-mg tablet contains 1.124 mg alosetron HCl equivalent to 1 mg of alosetron. Each tablet also contains the inactive ingredients: lactose (anhydrous), magnesium stearate, microcrystalline cellulose, and pregelatinized starch. The white film-coat for the 0.5-mg tablet contains hypromellose, titanium dioxide, and triacetin. The blue film-coat for the 1-mg tablet contains hypromellose, titanium dioxide, triacetin, and indigo carmine.

CLINICAL PHARMACOLOGY

Pharmacodynamics: ***Mechanism of Action:*** Alosetron is a potent and selective 5-HT3 receptor antagonist. 5-HT3 receptors are ligand-gated cation channels that are extensively distributed on enteric neurons in the human gastrointestinal tract, as well as other peripheral and central locations. Activation of these channels and the resulting neuronal depolarization affect the regulation of visceral pain, colonic transit and gastrointestinal secretions, processes that relate to the pathophysiology of irritable bowel syndrome (IBS). 5-HT3 receptor antagonists such as alosetron inhibit activation of non-selective cation channels which results in the modulation of the enteric nervous system.

The cause of IBS is unknown. IBS is characterized by visceral hypersensitivity and hyperactivity of the gastrointestinal tract, which lead to abnormal sensations of pain and motor activity. Following distention of the rectum, IBS patients exhibit pain and discomfort at lower volumes than healthy volunteers. Following such distention, alosetron reduced pain and exaggerated motor responses, possibly due to blockade of 5-HT3 receptors.

In healthy volunteers and IBS patients, alosetron (2 mg orally, twice daily for 8 days) increased colonic transit time without affecting orocecal transit time. In healthy volunteers, alosetron also increased basal jejunal water and sodium absorption after a single 4-mg dose. In IBS patients, multiple oral doses of alosetron (4 mg twice daily for 6.5 days) significantly increased colonic compliance.

Single oral doses of alosetron administered to healthy men produced a dose-dependent reduction in the flare response seen after intradermal injection of serotonin. Urinary 6-β-hydroxycortisol excretion decreased by 52% in elderly subjects after 27.5 days of alosetron 2 mg orally twice daily. This decrease was not statistically significant. In another study utilizing alosetron 1 mg orally twice daily for 4 days, there was a significant decrease in urinary 6-β-hydroxycortisol excretion. However, there was no change in the ratio of 6-β-hydroxycortisol to cortisol, indicating a possible decrease in cortisol production. The clinical significance of these findings is unknown.

Pharmacokinetics: The pharmacokinetics of alosetron have been studied after single oral doses ranging from 0.05 mg to 16 mg in healthy men. The pharmacokinetics of alosetron have also been evaluated in healthy women and men and in patients with IBS after repeated oral doses ranging from 1 mg twice daily to 8 mg twice daily.

Absorption: Alosetron is rapidly absorbed after oral administration with a mean absolute bioavailability of approximately 50% to 60% (approximate range 30% to >90%). After administration of radiolabeled alosetron, only 1% of the dose was recovered in the feces as unchanged drug. Following oral administration of a 1-mg alosetron dose to young men, a peak plasma concentration of approximately 5 ng/mL occurs at 1 hour. In young women, the mean peak plasma concentration is approximately 9 ng/mL, with a similar time to peak.

Food Effects: Alosetron absorption is decreased by approximately 25% by co-administration with food, with a mean delay in time to peak concentration of 15 minutes (see DOSAGE AND ADMINISTRATION).

Distribution: Alosetron demonstrates a volume of distribution of approximately 65 to 95 L. Plasma protein binding is 82% over a concentration range of 20 to 4,000 ng/mL.

Metabolism and Elimination: Plasma concentrations of alosetron increase proportionately with increasing single oral doses up to 8 mg and more than proportionately at a single oral dose of 16 mg. Twice-daily oral dosing of alosetron does not result in accumulation. The terminal elimination half-life of alosetron is approximately 1.5 hours (plasma clearance is approximately 600 mL/min). Population pharmacokinetic analysis in IBS patients confirmed that alosetron clearance is minimally influenced by doses up to 8 mg.

Renal elimination of unchanged alosetron accounts for only 6% of the dose. Renal clearance is approximately 94 mL/min.

Alosetron is extensively metabolized in humans. The biological activity of the metabolites is unknown. A mass balance study was performed utilizing an orally administered dose of unlabeled and ^{14}C-labeled alosetron. On a molar basis, alosetron metabolites reached additive peak plasma concentrations 9-fold greater than alosetron, and the additive metabolite AUCs were 13-fold greater than the alosetron AUC. Plasma radioactivity declined with a half-life 2-fold longer than that of alosetron, indicating the presence of circulating metabolites. Approximately 73% of the radiolabeled dose was recovered in urine with another 24% of the dose recovered in feces. Only 7% of the dose was recovered as unchanged drug. At least 13 metabolites have been detected in urine. The predominant product in urine was a 6-hydroxy metabolite (15% of the dose). This metabolite was secondarily metabolized to a glucuronide that was also present in urine (14% of the dose). Smaller amounts of the 6-hydroxy metabolite and the 6-O-glucuronide also appear to be present in feces. A bis-oxidized dicarbonyl accounted for 14% of the dose, and its monocarbonyl precursor accounted for another 4% in urine and 6% in feces. No other urinary metabolite accounted for more than 4% of the dose. Glucuronide or sulfate conjugates of unchanged alosetron were not detected in urine.

In studies of Japanese men, an N-desmethyl metabolite was found circulating in plasma in all subjects and accounted for up to 30% of the dose in one subject when alosetron was administered with food. The clinical significance of this finding is unknown.

Alosetron is metabolized by human microsomal cytochrome P450 (CYP), shown in vitro to involve enzymes 2C9 (30%), 3A4 (18%), and 1A2 (10%). Non-CYP-mediated Phase I metabolic conversion also contributes to an extent of about 11%. However, in vivo data suggest that CYP1A2 plays a more prominent role in alosetron metabolism, based on correlation of alosetron clearance with in vivo CYP1A2 activity measured by probe substrate, increased clearance induced by smoking, and inhibition of clearance by fluvoxamine (see CONTRAINDICATIONS and PRECAUTIONS: Drug Interactions).

Population Subgroups: ***Age:*** In some studies in healthy men or women, plasma concentrations were elevated by approximately 40% in individuals 65 years and older compared to young adults (see WARNINGS). However, this effect was not consistently observed in men.

Gender: Plasma concentrations are 30% to 50% lower and less variable in men compared to women given the same oral dose. Population pharmacokinetic analysis in IBS patients confirmed that alosetron concentrations were influenced by gender (27% lower in men).

Reduced Hepatic Function: No pharmacokinetic data are available in this patient group (see PRECAUTIONS: Hepatic Insufficiency and DOSAGE AND ADMINISTRATION: Patients with Hepatic Impairment).

Reduced Renal Function: Renal impairment (creatinine clearance 4 to 56 mL/min) has no effect on the renal elimination of alosetron due to the minor contribution of this pathway to elimination. The effect of renal impairment on metabolite kinetics and the effect of end-stage renal disease have not been assessed (see DOSAGE AND ADMINISTRATION: Patients with Renal Impairment).

Drug Interactions: See CONTRAINDICATIONS and PRECAUTIONS: Drug Interactions.

CLINICAL TRIALS

LOTRONEX 1 mg twice daily was studied in two 12-week U.S. multicenter, randomized, double-blind, placebo-controlled trials of identical design (Studies 1 and 2) in non-constipated women with IBS meeting the Rome Criteria[1] for at least 6 months. Women with severe pain or a history of severe constipation were excluded. A 2-week run-in period established baseline IBS symptoms.

Of the 633 women on LOTRONEX and 640 on placebo, about two thirds had diarrhea-predominant IBS. Compared with placebo, 10% to 19% more women with diarrhea-predominant IBS who received LOTRONEX had adequate relief of IBS abdominal pain and discomfort during each month of the study.

Clinical studies have not been performed to adequately confirm the benefits of LOTRONEX in men or patients under the age of 18.

Starting Dose: Data from a dose-ranging study of women (n = 85) who received 0.5 mg BID of alosetron, indicated that the incidence of constipation (14%) was lower than that experienced by women receiving 1 mg BID (29%). Therefore, to lower the risk of constipation, LOTRONEX should be started at a dosage of 0.5 mg twice a day. The efficacy of the 0.5-mg twice-daily dosage in treating severe diarrhea-predominant IBS has not been adequately evaluated in clinical trials.

Women with Severe Diarrhea-Predominant IBS: LOTRONEX is indicated only for women with severe diarrhea-predominant IBS (see INDICATIONS AND USAGE). The efficacy of LOTRONEX in this subset of the women studied in clinical trials is supported by prospective and retrospective analyses.

Prospective Analyses: In two 12-week, randomized, double-blind, placebo-controlled clinical trials of women with diarrhea-predominant IBS and bowel urgency on at least 50% of days at entry (Studies 3 and 4), a total of 778 women received LOTRONEX and 515 received placebo. Women receiving LOTRONEX had significant increases over placebo (13% to 16%) in the median percentage of days with urgency control.

The lower gastrointestinal functions of stool consistency, stool frequency, and sense of incomplete evacuation were also evaluated by patients' daily reports. Stool consistency was evaluated on a scale of 1 to 5 (1 = very hard, 2 = hard, 3 = formed, 4 = loose, and 5 = watery). At baseline, average stool consistency was approximately 4 (loose) for both treatment groups. During the 12 weeks of treatment, the average stool consistency decreased to approximately 3.0 (formed) for patients who received LOTRONEX and 3.5 for the patients who received placebo in the two studies.

At baseline, average stool frequency was approximately 3.2 per day for both treatment groups. During the 12 weeks of

Continued on next page

Lotronex—Cont.

treatment, the average daily stool frequency decreased to approximately 2.1 and 2.2 for patients receiving LOTRONEX and 2.7 and 2.8 for patients receiving placebo in the two studies.

There was no consistent effect upon the sense of incomplete evacuation during the 12 weeks of treatment for patients receiving LOTRONEX as compared to patients receiving placebo in either study.

Retrospective Analyses: In analyses of patients from Studies 1 and 2 who had diarrhea-predominant IBS and indicated their baseline run-in IBS symptoms were severe at the start of the trial, LOTRONEX provided greater adequate relief of IBS pain and discomfort than placebo. In further analyses of Studies 1 and 2, 57% of patients had urgency at baseline on 5 or more days per week. In this subset, 32% of patients on LOTRONEX had urgency no more than 1 day in the last week of the trial, compared to 19% of patients on placebo.

Patient-reported subjective outcomes related to IBS were assessed by questionnaires obtained at baseline and week 12. Patients in the more severe subset who received LOTRONEX reported less difficulty sleeping, less tiredness, fewer eating problems, and less interference with social activities and work/main activities due to IBS symptoms or problems compared to those who received placebo. Change in the impact of IBS symptoms and problems on emotional and mental distress, and on physical and sexual activity in women who received LOTRONEX were not statistically different from those reported by women who received placebo. In Studies 3 and 4, 66% of patients had urgency at baseline on 5 or more days per week. In this subset, 50% of patients on LOTRONEX had urgency no more than 1 day in the last week of the trial, compared to 29% of patients on placebo. Moreover, in the same subset, 12% on LOTRONEX had urgency no more than 2 days per week in any of the 12 weeks on treatment compared to 1% of placebo patients.

Figure 1. Percent of Patients With Urgency On >5 Days/Week At Baseline Who Improved to No More Than 1 Day in the Final Week

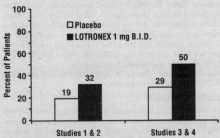

Long-Term Use: In a 48-week multinational, double-blind, placebo-controlled study, LOTRONEX 1 mg twice daily was evaluated in 714 women with non-constipated IBS. A retrospective analysis of the subset of women with severe diarrhea-predominant IBS (urgency on at least 10 days during the 2-week baseline period) was performed. Of the 417 patients with severe d-IBS enrolled, 62% completed the trial. LOTRONEX (n = 198) provided a greater average rate of adequate relief of IBS pain and discomfort (52% vs. 41%) and a greater average rate of satisfactory control of bowel urgency (60% vs. 48%) compared with placebo (n = 219). Significant improvement of these symptoms occurred for most of the 48-week treatment period with no evidence of tachyphylaxis.

INDICATIONS AND USAGE

LOTRONEX is indicated only for women with severe diarrhea-predominant irritable bowel syndrome (IBS) who have:
• chronic IBS symptoms (generally lasting 6 months or longer),
• had anatomic or biochemical abnormalities of the gastrointestinal tract excluded, and
• not responded adequately to conventional therapy.

Diarrhea-predominant IBS is severe if it includes diarrhea and one or more of the following:
• frequent and severe abdominal pain/discomfort
• frequent bowel urgency or fecal incontinence
• disability or restriction of daily activities due to IBS

Because of infrequent but serious gastrointestinal adverse events associated with LOTRONEX, the indication is restricted to those patients for whom the benefit-to-risk balance is most favorable.

Clinical studies have not been performed to adequately confirm the benefits of LOTRONEX in men.

CONTRAINDICATIONS

LOTRONEX **should not be initiated** in patients with constipation (see WARNINGS).

LOTRONEX is contraindicated in patients with a history of the following:
• chronic or severe constipation or sequelae from constipation
• intestinal obstruction, stricture, toxic megacolon, gastrointestinal perforation, and/or adhesions
• ischemic colitis, impaired intestinal circulation, thrombophlebitis, or hypercoagulable state
• Crohn's disease or ulcerative colitis
• diverticulitis
• hypersensitivity to any component of the product

LOTRONEX should not be used by patients who are unable to understand or comply with the Patient-Physician Agreement for LOTRONEX.

Concomitant administration of alosetron with fluvoxamine is contraindicated. Fluvoxamine, a known strong inhibitor of CYP1A2, has been shown to increase mean alosetron plasma concentrations (AUC) approximately 6 fold and prolong the half-life by approximately 3 fold (see PRECAUTIONS: Drug Interactions).

WARNINGS (SEE BOXED WARNING AND DOSAGE AND ADMINISTRATION.)

Some patients have experienced serious complications of constipation or ischemic colitis without warning.

Constipation: Serious complications of constipation including obstruction, ileus, impaction, toxic megacolon, and secondary bowel ischemia have been reported with use of LOTRONEX during clinical trials. In addition, rare cases of perforation and death have been reported from post-marketing clinical practice. In some cases, complications of constipation required intestinal surgery, including colectomy. **In IBS clinical trials, approximately 10% of patients on LOTRONEX withdrew prematurely because of constipation. The incidence of serious complications of constipation was approximately 0.1% (1 per 1,000 patients) in women receiving either LOTRONEX or placebo.** Patients who are elderly, debilitated, or taking additional medications that decrease gastrointestinal motility may be at greater risk for complications of constipation.

LOTRONEX should be discontinued immediately in patients who develop constipation (see BOXED WARNING).

Ischemic Colitis: Ischemic colitis has been reported in patients receiving LOTRONEX in clinical trials as well as during marketed use of the drug. **In IBS clinical trials, the cumulative incidence of ischemic colitis in women receiving LOTRONEX was 0.2% (2 per 1,000 patients, 95% confidence interval 1 to 3) through 3 months and was 0.3% (3 per 1,000 patients, 95% confidence interval 1 to 4) through 6 months. Ischemic colitis was not reported in women receiving placebo. The patient experience in controlled clinical trials is insufficient to estimate the incidence of ischemic colitis in patients taking LOTRONEX for longer than 6 months.**

LOTRONEX should be discontinued immediately in patients with signs of ischemic colitis such as rectal bleeding, bloody diarrhea, or new or worsening abdominal pain. Because ischemic colitis can be life-threatening, patients with signs or symptoms of ischemic colitis should be evaluated promptly and have appropriate diagnostic testing performed. Treatment with LOTRONEX should not be resumed in patients who develop ischemic colitis.

PRECAUTIONS

Prescribing Program for LOTRONEX: To prescribe LOTRONEX, the physician must be enrolled in the Prescribing Program for LOTRONEX. To enroll, physicians must understand the benefits and risks of treatment with LOTRONEX for severe diarrhea-predominant IBS, including the information in the Prescribing Information, Medication Guide, and Patient-Physician Agreement for LOTRONEX. Physicians need to be able to:
• Diagnose and manage IBS, ischemic colitis, constipation and complications of constipation, or refer patients to specialists as needed.
• Educate patients on the benefits and risks of treatment with LOTRONEX, provide them with the Medication Guide, instruct them to read it, and encourage them to ask questions when first considering LOTRONEX. Patients may be educated by the enrolled physician or a healthcare provider under a physician's direction.
• Prior to the initial prescription of LOTRONEX, obtain the patient's signature on the Patient-Physician Agreement form, sign it, place the original signed form in the patient's medical record, and give a copy to the patient.
• Affix program stickers to all prescriptions for LOTRONEX (i.e., the original and all subsequent prescriptions). Stickers will be provided as part of the GlaxoSmithKline Prescribing Program for LOTRONEX. No telephone, facsimile, or computerized prescriptions are permitted with this program. Refills are permitted to be written on prescriptions.
• Report all serious adverse events with LOTRONEX to GlaxoSmithKline at 1-888-825-5249 or to the Food and Drug Administration's MedWatch Program at 1-800-FDA-1088.

To enroll in the Prescribing Program for LOTRONEX call 1-888-825-5249 or visit www.lotronex.com to complete the Physician Enrollment Form.

Information for Patients: Patients should be fully counseled on and understand the risks and benefits of LOTRONEX before an initial prescription is written. The patient may be educated by the enrolled physician or a healthcare provider under a physician's direction.

PHYSICIANS MUST:
• Counsel patients for whom LOTRONEX is appropriate about the benefits and risks of LOTRONEX and discuss the impact of IBS symptoms on the patient's life.
• Give the patient a copy of the Medication Guide, which outlines the benefits and risks of LOTRONEX, and instruct the patient to read it carefully. Answer all questions the patient may have about LOTRONEX. The complete text of the Medication Guide is printed at the end of this document.
• Review the Patient-Physician Agreement for LOTRONEX with the patient, answer all questions, and give a copy of the signed agreement to the patient.

• Provide each patient with appropriate instructions for taking LOTRONEX.

Copies of the Patient-Physician Agreement for LOTRONEX and additional copies of the Medication Guide are available by contacting GlaxoSmithKline at 1-888-825-5249 or visiting www.lotronex.com.

PATIENTS WHO ARE PRESCRIBED LOTRONEX SHOULD BE INSTRUCTED TO:
• Read the Medication Guide before starting LOTRONEX and each time they refill their prescription.
• Not start taking LOTRONEX if they are constipated.
• Immediately discontinue LOTRONEX and contact their physician if they become constipated, or have symptoms of ischemic colitis such as new or worsening abdominal pain, bloody diarrhea, or blood in the stool. Contact their physician again if their constipation does not resolve after discontinuation of LOTRONEX. Resume LOTRONEX only if their constipation has resolved and after discussion with and the agreement of their treating physician.
• Stop taking LOTRONEX and contact their physician if LOTRONEX does not adequately control IBS symptoms after 4 weeks of taking 1 mg twice a day.

Drug Interactions: Because alosetron is metabolized by a variety of hepatic CYP drug-metabolizing enzymes, inducers or inhibitors of these enzymes may change the clearance of alosetron.

Fluvoxamine is a known strong inhibitor of CYP1A2 and also inhibits CYP3A4, CYP2C9, and CYP2C19. In a pharmacokinetic study, 40 healthy female subjects received fluvoxamine in escalating doses from 50 to 200 mg per day for 16 days, with coadministration of alosetron 1 mg on the last day. Fluvoxamine increased mean alosetron plasma concentrations (AUC) approximately 6 fold and prolonged the half-life by approximately 3 fold. Concomitant administration of alosetron and fluvoxamine is contraindicated (see CONTRAINDICATIONS).

Concomitant administration of alosetron and moderate CYP1A2 inhibitors, including quinolone antibiotics and cimetidine, has not been evaluated, but should be avoided unless clinically necessary because of similar potential drug interactions.

Ketoconazole is a known strong inhibitor of CYP3A4. In a pharmacokinetic study, 38 healthy female subjects received ketoconazole 200 mg twice daily for 7 days, with coadministration of alosetron 1 mg on the last day. Ketoconazole increased mean alosetron plasma concentrations (AUC) by 29%. Caution should be used when alosetron and ketoconazole are administered concomitantly. Coadministration of alosetron and strong CYP3A4 inhibitors, such as clarithromycin, telithromycin, protease inhibitors, voriconazole, and itraconazole has not been evaluated but should be undertaken with caution because of similar potential drug interactions. The effect of induction or inhibition of other pathways on exposure to alosetron and its metabolites is not known.

In vitro human liver microsome studies and an in vivo metabolic probe study demonstrated that alosetron did not inhibit CYP enzymes 2D6, 3A4, 2C9, or 2C19. In vitro, at total drug concentrations 27-fold higher than peak plasma concentrations observed with the 1-mg dosage, alosetron inhibited CYP enzymes 1A2 (60%) and 2E1 (50%). In an in vivo metabolic probe study, alosetron did not inhibit CYP2E1 but did produce 30% inhibition of both CYP1A2 and N-acetyltransferase. Although not studied with alosetron, inhibition of N-acetyltransferase may have clinically relevant consequences for drugs such as isoniazid, procainamide, and hydralazine. The effect on CYP1A2 was explored further in a clinical interaction study with theophylline and no effect on metabolism was observed. Another study showed that alosetron had no clinically significant effect on plasma concentrations of the oral contraceptive agents ethinyl estradiol and levonorgestrel (CYP3A4 substrates). A clinical interaction study was also conducted with alosetron and the CYP3A4 substrate cisapride. No significant effects on cisapride metabolism or QT interval were noted. The effects of alosetron on monoamine oxidases and on intestinal first pass secondary to high intraluminal concentrations have not been examined. Based on the above data from in vitro and in vivo studies, it is unlikely that alosetron will inhibit the hepatic metabolic clearance of drugs metabolized by the major CYP enzyme 3A4, as well as the CYP enzymes 2D6, 2C9, 2C19, 2E1, or 1A2.

Alosetron does not appear to induce the major cytochrome P450 (CYP) drug metabolizing enzyme 3A. Alosetron also does not appear to induce CYP enzymes 2E1 or 2C19. It is not known whether alosetron might induce other enzymes.

Hepatic Insufficiency: Due to the extensive hepatic metabolism of alosetron, increased exposure to alosetron and/or its metabolites is likely to occur in patients with hepatic insufficiency.

Carcinogenesis, Mutagenesis, Impairment of Fertility: In 2-year oral studies, alosetron was not carcinogenic in mice at doses up to 30 mg/kg/day or in rats at doses up to 40 mg/kg/day. These doses are, respectively, about 60 to 160 times the recommended human dose of alosetron of 2 mg/day (1 mg twice daily) based on body surface area. Alosetron was not genotoxic in the Ames tests, the mouse lymphoma cell (L5178Y/TK$^\pm$) forward gene mutation test, the human lymphocyte chromosome aberration test, the ex vivo rat hepatocyte unscheduled DNA synthesis (UDS) test, or the in vivo rat micronucleus test for mutagenicity. Alosetron at oral doses up to 40 mg/kg/day (about 160 times the recommended daily human dose based on body surface area) was found to have no effect on fertility and reproductive performance of male or female rats.

Pregnancy: *Teratogenic Effects:* Pregnancy Category B. Reproduction studies have been performed in rats at doses up to 40 mg/kg/day (about 160 times the recommended human dose based on body surface area) and rabbits at oral doses up to 30 mg/kg/day (about 240 times the recommended daily human dose based on body surface area). These studies have revealed no evidence of impaired fertility or harm to the fetus due to alosetron. There are, however, no adequate and well-controlled studies in pregnant women. Because animal reproduction studies are not always predictive of human response, LOTRONEX should be used during pregnancy only if clearly needed.

Nursing Mothers: Alosetron and/or metabolites of alosetron are excreted in the breast milk of lactating rats. It is not known whether alosetron is excreted in human milk. Because many drugs are excreted in human milk, caution should be exercised when LOTRONEX is administered to a nursing woman.

Pediatric Use: Safety and effectiveness in pediatric patients have not been established.

Geriatric Use: Postmarketing experience suggests that elderly patients may be at greater risk for complications of constipation (see WARNINGS).

ADVERSE REACTIONS

Table 1 summarizes adverse events from 22 repeat-dose studies in patients with IBS who were treated with 1 mg of LOTRONEX twice daily for 8 to 24 weeks. The adverse events in Table 1 were reported in 1% or more of patients who received LOTRONEX and occurred more frequently on LOTRONEX than on placebo. A statistically significant difference was observed for constipation in patients treated with LOTRONEX compared to placebo (p<0.0001).

Table 1. Adverse Events Reported in ≥1% of IBS Patients and More Frequently on LOTRONEX 1 mg B.I.D. than Placebo

Body System Adverse Event	LOTRONEX 1 mg B.I.D. (n = 8,328)	Placebo (n = 2,363)
Gastrointestinal		
Constipation	29%	6%
Abdominal discomfort and pain	7%	4%
Nausea	6%	5%
Gastrointestinal discomfort and pain	5%	3%
Abdominal distention	2%	1%
Regurgitation and reflux	2%	2%
Hemorrhoids	2%	1%

Gastrointestinal: Constipation is a frequent and dose-related side effect of treatment with LOTRONEX (see WARNINGS). In clinical studies constipation was reported in approximately 29% of IBS patients treated with LOTRONEX 1 mg twice daily (n = 9,316). This effect was statistically significant compared to placebo (p<0.0001). Eleven percent (11%) of patients treated with LOTRONEX 1 mg twice daily withdrew from the studies due to constipation. Although the number of IBS patients treated with LOTRONEX 0.5 mg twice daily is relatively small (n = 243), only 11% of those patients reported constipation and 4% withdrew from clinical studies due to constipation. Among the patients treated with LOTRONEX 1 mg twice daily who reported constipation, 75% reported a single episode and most reports of constipation (70%) occurred during the first month of treatment with the median time to first report of constipation onset of 8 days. Occurrences of constipation in clinical trials were generally mild to moderate in intensity, transient in nature, and resolved either spontaneously with continued treatment or with an interruption of treatment. However, serious complications of constipation have been reported in clinical studies and in postmarketing experience (see BOXED WARNING and WARNINGS). In Studies 1 and 2, 9% of patients treated with LOTRONEX reported constipation and 4 consecutive days with no bowel movement (see CLINICAL TRIALS). Following interruption of treatment, 78% of the affected patients resumed bowel movements within a 2-day period and were able to re-initiate treatment with LOTRONEX.

Hepatic: A similar incidence in elevation of ALT (>2 fold) was seen in patients receiving LOTRONEX or placebo (1.0% vs. 1.2%). A single case of hepatitis (elevated ALT, AST, alkaline phosphatase, and bilirubin) without jaundice was reported in a 12-week study. A causal association with LOTRONEX has not been established.

Long-Term Safety: Patient experience in controlled clinical trials is insufficient to estimate the incidence of ischemic colitis in patients taking LOTRONEX for longer than 6 months.

Other Events Observed During Clinical Evaluation of LOTRONEX: During its assessment in clinical trials, multiple and single doses of LOTRONEX were administered resulting in 11,874 subject-exposures in 86 completed clinical studies. The conditions, dosages, and duration of exposure to LOTRONEX varied between trials, and the studies included healthy male and female volunteers as well as male and female patients with IBS and other indications.

In the listing that follows, reported adverse events were classified using a standardized coding dictionary. Only those events that an investigator believed were possibly related to alosetron, occurred in at least 2 patients, and occurred at a greater frequency during treatment with LOTRONEX than

during placebo administration are presented. Serious adverse events occurring in at least 1 patient for an investigator believed there was reasonable possibility that the event was related to alosetron treatment and occurring at a greater frequency in LOTRONEX than placebo-treated patients are also presented.

In the following listing, events are categorized by body system. Within each body system, events are presented in descending order of frequency. The following definitions are used: *Infrequent* adverse events are those occurring on one or more occasion in 1/100 to 1/1,000 patients; *Rare* adverse events are those occurring on one or more occasion in fewer than 1/1,000 patients.

Although the events reported occurred during treatment with LOTRONEX, they were not necessarily caused by it.

Blood and Lymphatic: Rare: Quantitative red cell or hemoglobin defects, hemorrhage, and lymphatic signs and symptoms.

Cardiovascular: Infrequent: Tachyarrhythmias. *Rare:* Arrhythmias, increased blood pressure, and extrasystoles.

Drug Interaction, Overdose, and Trauma: Rare: Contusions and hematomas.

Ear, Nose, and Throat: Rare: Ear, nose, and throat infections; viral ear, nose, and throat infections; and laryngitis.

Endocrine and Metabolic: Rare: Disorders of calcium and phosphate metabolism, hyperglycemia, hypothalamus/pituitary hypofunction, hypoglycemia, and fluid disturbances.

Eye: Rare: Light sensitivity of eyes.

Gastrointestinal: Infrequent: Hyposalivation, dyspeptic symptoms, gastrointestinal spasms, ischemic colitis (see WARNINGS), and gastrointestinal lesions. *Rare:* Abnormal tenderness, colitis, gastrointestinal signs and symptoms, proctitis, diverticulitis, positive fecal occult blood, hyperacidity, decreased gastrointestinal motility and ileus, gastrointestinal obstructions, oral symptoms, gastrointestinal intussusception, gastritis, gastroduodenitis, gastroenteritis, and ulcerative colitis.

Hepatobiliary Tract and Pancreas: Rare: Abnormal bilirubin levels and cholecystitis.

Lower Respiratory: Infrequent: Breathing disorders. *Rare:* Viral respiratory infections.

Musculoskeletal: Rare: Muscle pain; muscle stiffness, tightness and rigidity; and bone and skeletal pain.

Neurological: Infrequent: Hypnagogic effects. *Rare:* Memory effects, tremors, dreams, cognitive function disorders, disturbances of sense of taste, disorders of equilibrium, confusion, sedation, and hypoesthesia.

Non-site Specific: Infrequent: Malaise and fatigue, cramps, pain, temperature regulation disturbances. *Rare:* General signs and symptoms, non-specific conditions, burning sensations, hot and cold sensations, cold sensations, and fungal infections.

Psychiatry: Infrequent: Anxiety. *Rare:* Depressive moods.

Reproduction: Rare: Sexual function disorders, female reproductive tract bleeding and hemorrhage, reproductive infections, and fungal reproductive infections.

Skin: Infrequent: Sweating and urticaria. *Rare:* Hair loss and alopecia; acne and folliculitis; disorders of sweat and sebum; allergic skin reaction; eczema; skin infections; dermatitis and dermatosis; and nail disorders.

Urology: Infrequent: Urinary frequency. *Rare:* Bladder inflammation; polyuria and diuresis; and urinary tract hemorrhage.

Postmarketing Experience: The following events have been identified during use of LOTRONEX in clinical practice. Because they were reported voluntarily from a population of unknown size, estimates of frequency cannot be made. These events have been chosen for inclusion due to a combination of their seriousness, frequency of reporting, or potential causal connection to LOTRONEX.

Gastrointestinal: Constipation, ileus, impaction, obstruction, perforation, ulceration, ischemic colitis, small bowel mesenteric ischemia (see WARNINGS).

Neurological: Headache.

Skin: Rash.

DRUG ABUSE AND DEPENDENCE

LOTRONEX has no known potential for abuse or dependence.

OVERDOSAGE

There is no specific antidote for overdose of LOTRONEX. Patients should be managed with appropriate supportive therapy. Individual oral doses as large as 16 mg have been administered in clinical studies without significant adverse events. This dose is 8 times higher than the recommended total daily dose. Inhibition of the metabolic elimination and reduced first pass of other drugs might occur with overdoses of alosetron (see PRECAUTIONS: Drug Interactions). Single oral doses of LOTRONEX at 15 mg/kg in female mice and 60 mg/kg in female rats (30 and 240 times, respectively, the recommended human dose based on body surface area) were lethal. Symptoms of acute toxicity were labored respiration, subdued behavior, ataxia, tremors, and convulsions.

DOSAGE AND ADMINISTRATION

For safety reasons, only physicians who enroll in the GlaxoSmithKline Program for LOTRONEX should prescribe LOTRONEX (see PRECAUTIONS: Prescribing Program for LOTRONEX).

Usual Dose in Adults: To lower the risk of constipation, LOTRONEX should be started at a dosage of 0.5 mg twice a day. Patients well controlled on 0.5 mg twice a day may be maintained on this regimen. If, after 4 weeks, the 0.5-mg twice-daily dosage is well tolerated but does not adequately control IBS symptoms, then the dosage can be increased to

up to 1 mg twice a day, the dose used in controlled clinical trials (see CLINICAL TRIALS). **LOTRONEX should be discontinued in patients who have not had adequate control of IBS symptoms after 4 weeks of treatment with 1 mg twice a day.**

LOTRONEX can be taken with or without food (see CLINICAL PHARMACOLOGY: Pharmacokinetics: Food Effects). LOTRONEX should be discontinued immediately in patients who develop constipation or signs of ischemic colitis. LOTRONEX should not be restarted in patients who develop ischemic colitis.

Clinical trial and postmarketing experience suggest that debilitated patients or patients taking additional medications that decrease gastrointestinal motility may be at greater risk of serious complications of constipation. Therefore, appropriate caution and follow-up should be exercised if LOTRONEX is prescribed for these patients (see also Geriatric Patients).

Pediatric Patients: Safety and effectiveness have not been established in pediatric patients.

Geriatric Patients: Postmarketing experience suggests that elderly patients may be at greater risk for complications of constipation; therefore, appropriate caution and follow-up should be exercised if LOTRONEX is prescribed for these patients (see WARNINGS).

Patients with Renal Impairment: There are insufficient data available on the biological activity of the metabolites of LOTRONEX. It is unknown if dosage adjustment is needed in patients with renal impairment (see CLINICAL PHARMACOLOGY: Reduced Renal Function).

Patients with Hepatic Impairment: No studies have been conducted in patients with hepatic impairment. LOTRONEX is extensively metabolized by the liver and increased exposure to LOTRONEX is likely to occur in patients with hepatic impairment. Increased drug exposure may increase the risk of serious adverse events. LOTRONEX should be used with caution in patients with hepatic impairment (see PRECAUTIONS: Hepatic Insufficiency and CLINICAL PHARMACOLOGY: Population Subgroups: Reduced Hepatic Function).

Information for Pharmacists: LOTRONEX may be dispensed only on presentation of a prescription for LOTRONEX with a sticker for the Prescribing Program for LOTRONEX attached. A Medication Guide for LOTRONEX must be given to the patient each time LOTRONEX is dispensed as required by law. No telephone, facsimile, or computerized prescriptions are permitted with this program. Refills are permitted to be written on prescriptions.

HOW SUPPLIED

LOTRONEX Tablets, 0.5 mg (0.562 mg alosetron HCl equivalent to 0.5 mg alosetron) are white, oval, film-coated tablets debossed with GX EX1 on one face.
Bottles of 30 (NDC 0173-0738-00) with child-resistant closures.
LOTRONEX Tablets, 1 mg (1.124 mg alosetron HCl equivalent to 1 mg alosetron), are blue, oval, film-coated tablets debossed with GX CT1 on one face.
Bottles of 30 (NDC 0173-0690-05) with child-resistant closures.

Store at 25°C (77°F); excursions permitted to 15-30°C (59-86°F) [see USP Controlled Room Temperature]. Protect from light and moisture.

REFERENCE

1. Thompson WG, Creed F, Drossman DA, et al. Functional bowel disease and functional abdominal pain. *Gastroenterol Int.* 1992;5:75-91.

MEDICATION GUIDE
LOTRONEX® (LOW-trah-nex) Tablets
(alosetron hydrochloride)

Before using LOTRONEX for the first time, you should:

- Understand that LOTRONEX has serious risks for some people.
- Read and follow the directions in this Medication Guide.
- Sign a Patient-Physician Agreement with your doctor.

Read this Medication Guide carefully before you sign the Patient-Physician Agreement. You must sign the Patient-Physician Agreement before you start LOTRONEX. Read the Medication Guide you get with each refill for LOTRONEX. There may be new information. This Medication Guide does not take the place of talking with your doctor.

1. What is the most important information I should know about LOTRONEX?
LOTRONEX is a medicine only for some women with severe chronic IBS whose:
  - main problem is diarrhea and
  - IBS symptoms have not been helped enough by other treatments.
A. Some patients have developed serious bowel side effects while taking LOTRONEX. Serious bowel (intestine) side effects can happen suddenly, including the following two:

  1. Serious complications of constipation: About 1 out of every 1,000 women who take LOTRONEX may get serious complications of constipation. These complications **may lead to a hospital stay, and in rare cases, blood transfusions, surgery, and death.** People who are older,

Continued on next page

Lotronex—Cont.

who are weak from illness, or who take other constipating medicines may be more likely to have serious constipation problems with LOTRONEX.

> To lower your chances of getting serious complications of constipation do the following:

> - **If you are constipated,** do not start taking LOTRONEX.
> - **If you get constipated while taking LOTRONEX,** stop taking it right away and call your doctor.
> - **If your constipation does not get better after stopping LOTRONEX,** call your doctor again.
> - **If you stopped taking LOTRONEX, do not start taking LOTRONEX again** unless your doctor tells you to do so.

2. **Ischemic colitis** (reduced blood flow to the bowel): About 3 out of every 1,000 women who take LOTRONEX over a 6-month period may get a serious problem where blood flow to parts of the large bowel is reduced. This is called ischemic colitis. The chance of getting ischemic colitis when you take LOTRONEX for more than 6 months is not known. Ischemic colitis may lead to a hospital stay, and in rare cases, blood transfusions, surgery, and death.

> To lower your chances of getting serious complications of ischemic colitis, stop taking LOTRONEX and call your doctor right away if you get:

> - new or worse pain in your stomach area (abdomen) or
> - blood in your bowel movements.

B. Is LOTRONEX right for you?

LOTRONEX may be right for you if all of these things are true about you:

- Your doctor has told you that your symptoms are due to IBS.
- Your IBS bowel problem is diarrhea.
- Your IBS has lasted for 6 months or longer.
- You tried other IBS treatments and they didn't give you the relief you need.
- Your IBS is severe.

You can tell if your IBS is severe if **at least 1** of the following is true for you:

- You have lots of painful stomach cramps or bloating.
- You often can't control the need to have a bowel movement, or you have "accidents" where your underwear gets dirty from diarrhea or bowel movements.
- You can't lead a normal home or work life because you need to be near a bathroom.

Enough testing has not been done to confirm LOTRONEX works in men or children under age 18.

C. There is a special prescribing program for LOTRONEX.

Only doctors who have signed up with the company that makes LOTRONEX should write prescriptions for LOTRONEX. As part of signing up, these doctors have said that they understand about IBS and the possible side effects of LOTRONEX. They have agreed to use a special sticker on all prescriptions for LOTRONEX, so the pharmacist will know that the doctors have signed up with the company.

You may be taught about LOTRONEX by your doctor or healthcare provider under a doctor's direction. Your doctor will ask you to sign a Patient-Physician Agreement after you read this Medication Guide for the first time. Signing the Agreement means that you understand the benefits and risks of LOTRONEX and that you have read and understand this Medication Guide.

2. What is LOTRONEX?

LOTRONEX is a medicine only for some women with severe chronic IBS whose:

- main problem is diarrhea and
- IBS symptoms have not been helped enough by other treatments.

LOTRONEX does not cure IBS, and it may not help every person who takes it. For those who are helped, LOTRONEX reduces lower stomach area (abdominal) pain and discomfort, the sudden need to have a bowel movement (bowel urgency), and diarrhea from IBS. If you stop taking LOTRONEX, your IBS symptoms may return within 1 or 2 weeks.

3. Who should not take LOTRONEX?

LOTRONEX is not right for everyone. **Do not take LOTRONEX if any of the following apply to you:**

- Your main IBS problem is constipation or you are constipated most of the time.
- You have had a serious problem from constipation.
- You have had serious bowel blockages.
- You have had blood flow problems to your bowels, such as ischemic colitis.
- You have had blood clots.
- You have had Crohn's disease, ulcerative colitis, or diverticulitis.
- You do not understand this Medication Guide or the Patient-Physician Agreement, or you are not willing to follow them.
- You are allergic to LOTRONEX or any of its ingredients. (See the list of ingredients at the end of this Medication Guide.)
- You are taking fluvoxamine (LUVOX®)

If you are constipated now, do not start taking LOTRONEX.

4. What should I talk about with my doctor before taking LOTRONEX?

Talk with your doctor:

- about the possible benefits and risks of LOTRONEX.

- about how much of a problem IBS is in your life and what treatments you have tried.
- about any other illnesses you have and medicines you take or plan to take. These include prescription and non-prescription medicines, supplements, and herbal remedies. Certain illnesses and medicines can increase your chance of getting serious side effects while taking LOTRONEX. Other medicines may interact with how the body handles LOTRONEX.
- if you are pregnant, planning to get pregnant, or breastfeeding.

5. How should I take LOTRONEX?

- **Take LOTRONEX exactly as your doctor prescribes it.** You can take LOTRONEX with or without food.
- **Begin with 0.5 mg two times a day for 4 weeks** to see how LOTRONEX affects you. You and your doctor may decide that you should keep taking this dose if you are doing well.
- **Check with your doctor 4 weeks after starting LOTRONEX:**
  - ➢ If you try 0.5 mg two times a day for 4 weeks, it may not control your symptoms. If you do not get constipation or other side effects from LOTRONEX, your doctor may increase your dose up to 1 mg two times a day.
  - ➢ If 1 mg two times a day does not work after 4 weeks, LOTRONEX is not likely to help you. You should stop taking it and call your doctor.
- **If you miss a dose of LOTRONEX,** just skip that dose. Do **not** take 2 doses the next time. Wait until the next time you are supposed to take it and then take your normal dose.
- **Follow the important instructions in the section "What is the most important information I should know about LOTRONEX?"** about when you must stop taking the drug and when you should call your doctor.
- **If you see other doctors** about your IBS or side effects from LOTRONEX, let the doctor who prescribed LOTRONEX know.

6. What are the possible side effects of LOTRONEX?

Constipation is the most common side effect among women with IBS who take LOTRONEX.

Some patients have developed serious bowel side effects while taking LOTRONEX. Read the section **"What is the most important information I should know about LOTRONEX?"** at the beginning of this Medication Guide for information about the serious side effects you may get with LOTRONEX.

This Medication Guide does not tell you about all the possible side effects of LOTRONEX. Your doctor or pharmacist can give you a more complete list.

7. General information about the safe and effective use of LOTRONEX

Medicines are sometimes prescribed for purposes other than those listed in a Medication Guide. If you have any questions or concerns about LOTRONEX, ask your doctor. Do not use LOTRONEX for a condition for which it was not prescribed. Do not share your medicine with other people. It may harm them.

Your doctor or pharmacist can give you more information about LOTRONEX that was written for healthcare professionals. You can also contact the company that makes LOTRONEX (toll free) at 1-888-825-5249 or at www.lotronex.com.

8. What are the ingredients of LOTRONEX?

Active Ingredient: alosetron hydrochloride

Inactive Ingredients: lactose (anhydrous), magnesium stearate, microcrystalline cellulose, and pregelatinized starch. The white film-coat for the 0.5-mg tablet contains hypromellose, titanium dioxide, and triacetin. The blue film-coat for the 1-mg tablet contains hypromellose, titanium dioxide, triacetin, and indigo carmine.

This Medication Guide has been approved by the US Food and Drug Administration.

February 2005   MG-030

PATIENT-PHYSICIAN AGREEMENT FOR LOTRONEX

LOTRONEX® (alosetron hydrochloride) is only for women with severe irritable bowel syndrome (IBS) whose main problem is diarrhea and who did not get the relief needed from other treatments. LOTRONEX has not been shown to help men with IBS or patients under age 18.

My doctor, or a healthcare provider under a doctor's direction, answered my questions about treatment with LOTRONEX. I have read and I understand the Medication Guide for LOTRONEX, and

- I understand that some patients using LOTRONEX have had serious bowel conditions (ischemic colitis and complications of constipation). I understand that these serious conditions can happen suddenly, and that they may lead to a hospital stay, and in rare cases, blood transfusions, surgery, and death. I also understand that certain patients may be more likely to develop a serious bowel condition while taking LOTRONEX. These include older patients, those who have other health problems and those who take other medicines that may cause constipation.
- My doctor and I agree that my IBS is severe and that other treatments have not given me the relief that I need. I also agree that I meet all of the requirements described in the section of the Medication Guide "What is the most important information I should know about LOTRONEX?" I understand that these requirements

help to make sure that LOTRONEX is used only by patients who are likely to have more benefit from treatment than risk.

- I don't have any problems listed in the section of the Medication Guide "Who should not take LOTRONEX?" that prevents me from taking LOTRONEX.
- I will follow instructions in the Medication Guide about:
  - ➢ **telling my doctor,** before taking LOTRONEX, about any illnesses I have, or other medicines I am taking or planning to take.
  - ➢ **taking LOTRONEX** exactly as my doctor prescribes it.
  - ➢ **stopping LOTRONEX** and calling my doctor right away if I get constipated, if I have new or worse pain in my abdomen, or if I see blood in my bowel movements.
  - ➢ **calling my doctor** again if the constipation I called about before has not gotten better.
  - ➢ **not starting LOTRONEX again** unless my doctor tells me to do so, if I stopped taking it because I got constipated.
  - ➢ **talking with my doctor 4 weeks after starting LOTRONEX** to recheck my IBS symptoms.
  - ➢ **stopping LOTRONEX and calling my doctor** if my IBS symptoms have not improved after 4 weeks of taking 1 mg 2 times a day.

I understand that LOTRONEX should be prescribed only by doctors who have signed up with the company that makes the drug. Doctors in the program must:

- fully discuss the drug's benefits and risks with each patient.
- sign this agreement with each patient before giving the initial prescription. It is not necessary to sign an agreement more than once.
- use a special sticker on all LOTRONEX prescriptions so that pharmacists know the doctor has signed up.

If I see other doctors about my IBS or possible side effects from LOTRONEX, I will let the doctor who prescribed LOTRONEX know.

My signature below indicates I have read, understood, and agree with all the statements made above. I would like to begin treatment with LOTRONEX.

Name of Patient (print)

Signature   Date

SECTION FOR THE PHYSICIAN

I am enrolled in the Prescribing Program for LOTRONEX, and I will continue to follow the requirements of the Program.

I, or a healthcare provider under a physician's direction, have given the patient named above:

- a copy of the Medication Guide for LOTRONEX, and instructed the patient to read it carefully before signing this Agreement, and to take it home.
- counseling about the benefits and risks of LOTRONEX.
- appropriate instructions for taking LOTRONEX.
- answers to all of the patient's questions about treatment with LOTRONEX.
- a prescription for LOTRONEX that has the program sticker affixed on it to alert pharmacists I am enrolled in the Prescribing Program for LOTRONEX.

The patient signed the Patient-Physician Agreement in my presence after I counseled the patient, asked if the patient had any questions about treatment with LOTRONEX, and answered all questions to the best of my ability.

Name of Patient (print)

Signature   Date

After the patient and the physician sign this Patient-Physician Agreement, give a copy to the patient and put the original signed form in the patient's medical record.

PRESCRIBING PROGRAM FOR LOTRONEX™:
PHYSICIAN ENROLLMENT FORM

The Prescribing Program for LOTRONEX was implemented to help reduce risks of serious gastrointestinal adverse events, some fatal, associated with this medicine. The program is intended to help physicians and their patients understand the benefits and risks of treatment with LOTRONEX in order to make fully informed decisions.

I wish to participate in the Prescribing Program for LOTRONEX (PPL) and acknowledge that I have read the complete Prescribing Information for LOTRONEX and understand and will follow the requirements of the PPL described below.

- For safety reasons, LOTRONEX is approved only for women with severe, diarrhea-predominant irritable bowel syndrome (D-IBS) who have:
  - ➢ Chronic IBS symptoms (generally lasting for 6 months or longer),
  - ➢ had anatomic or biochemical abnormalities of the gastrointestinal tract excluded, and
  - ➢ not responded adequately to conventional therapy.

Diarrhea-predominant IBS is severe if it includes diarrhea and one or more of the following:

  - ➢ Frequent and severe abdominal pain/discomfort
  - ➢ Frequent bowel urgency or fecal incontinence
  - ➢ Disability or restriction of daily activities due to IBS

- Physicians who enroll in the PPL should be able to diagnose and manage IBS, ischemic colitis, constipation, and complications of constipation, or refer patients to a specialist as needed.

- Patients considering treatment with LOTRONEX must be educated on the benefits and risks of the drug, given a copy of the Medication Guide, instructed to read it, and encouraged to ask questions. The patient may be educated by the enrolled physician or a healthcare provider under a physician's direction.
- After reviewing the Medication Guide prior to the initial prescription, the physician and the patient must both sign the Patient-Physician Agreement form. The original signed form must be placed in the patient's medical record, and a copy given to the patient.
- Program stickers must be affixed to all prescriptions for LOTRONEX (i.e., the original and all subsequent prescriptions). Stickers will be provided as part of the GlaxoSmithKline Prescribing Program for LOTRONEX. Refills are permitted to be written on prescriptions.
- All prescriptions for LOTRONEX must be written and not transmitted by telephone, facsimile, or computer.
- Prescribers must report all serious adverse events with LOTRONEX to GlaxoSmithKline at 1-888-825-5249 or to the Food and Drug Administration at 1-800-FDA-1088.

____
Name of Physician (print)

____________________ ____________________
Signature Date
DEA Number ____________________
Office Address: ____________________

Office Phone Number: ____________________
Office Fax Number: ____________________

Upon enrollment, you will receive a prescribing kit for LOTRONEX with the complete Prescribing Information, Prescribing Program for LOTRONEX stickers, multiple copies of the Medication Guide and Patient-Physician Agreement for LOTRONEX, and instructions for ordering additional supplies of Program materials.

You only need to enroll once, and you are under no obligation to prescribe LOTRONEX.

If you have any questions, please call the Prescribing Program for LOTRONEX at 1-888-825-5249 or visit www.lotronex.com.

TO ENROLL, VISIT WWW.LOTRONEX.COM OR PHONE 1-888-825-5249 OR COMPLETE THIS FORM IN ITS ENTIRETY AND MAIL OR FAX TO THE FOLLOWING ADDRESS:

Prescribing Program for Lotronex
Customer Response Center
Five Moore Drive
PO Box 13398
Research Triangle Park, NC 27709-3398
Fax Number: 1-866-698-7582

GlaxoSmithKline, Research Triangle Park, NC 27709
©2005, GlaxoSmithKline. All rights reserved.
February 2005/RL-2112, RL-2170, RL-2174

MALARONE® ℞
[*mal' ə-rōn*]
(atovaquone and proguanil hydrochloride)
Tablets

MALARONE® ℞
(atovaquone and proguanil hydrochloride)
Pediatric Tablets

Prescribing information for this product, which appears on pages 1568–1572 of the 2005 PDR, has been revised as follows. Please write "See Supplement A" next to the product heading.

The CLINICAL PHARMACOLOGY: Special Populations: *Renal Impairment section has been revised as follows.*

In patients with mild renal impairment (creatinine clearance 50 to 80 mL/min), oral clearance and/or AUC data for atovaquone, proguanil, and cycloguanil are within the range of values observed in patients with normal renal function (creatinine clearance >80 mL/min). In patients with moderate renal impairment (creatinine clearance 30 to 50 mL/min), mean oral clearance for proguanil was reduced by approximately 35% compared with patients with normal renal function (creatinine clearance >80 mL/min) and the oral clearance of atovaquone was comparable between patients with normal renal function and mild renal impairment. No data exist on the use of MALARONE for long-term prophylaxis (over 2 months) in individuals with moderate renal failure. In patients with severe renal impairment (creatinine clearance <30 mL/min), atovaquone C_{max} and AUC are reduced but the elimination half-lives for proguanil and cycloguanil are prolonged, with corresponding increases in AUC, resulting in the potential of drug accumulation and toxicity with repeated dosing (see CONTRAINDICATIONS).

The first paragraph of the CONTRAINDICATIONS *section has been revised as follows.*

MALARONE is contraindicated in individuals with known hypersensitivity to atovaquone or proguanil hydrochloride or any component of the formulation. Rare cases of anaphylaxis following treatment with atovaquone/proguanil have been reported.

The PRECAUTIONS: Carcinogenesis, Mutagenesis, Impairment of Fertility *section has been revised as follows.*

Atovaquone: Carcinogenicity studies in rats were negative; 24-month studies in mice showed treatment-related increases in incidence of hepatocellular adenoma and hepatocellular carcinoma at all doses tested which ranged from approximately 5 to 8 times the average steady-state plasma concentrations in humans during prophylaxis of malaria. Atovaquone was negative with or without metabolic activation in the Ames *Salmonella* mutagenicity assay, the Mouse Lymphoma mutagenesis assay, and the Cultured Human Lymphocyte cytogenetic assay. No evidence of genotoxicity was observed in the in vivo Mouse Micronucleus assay.

Proguanil: No evidence of a carcinogenic effect was observed in studies conducted in CD-1 mice (doses up to 1.51 times the average systemic human exposure based on AUC) and in Wistar Hannover rats (doses up to 1.12 times the average systemic human exposure).

Proguanil was negative with or without metabolic activation in the Ames *Salmonella* mutagenicity assay and the Mouse Lymphoma mutagenesis assay. No evidence of genotoxicity was observed in the in vivo Mouse Micronucleus assay.

Cycloguanil, the active metabolite of proguanil, was also negative in the Ames test, but was positive in the Mouse Lymphoma assay and the Mouse Micronucleus assay. These positive effects with cycloguanil, a dihydrofolate reductase inhibitor, were significantly reduced or abolished with folinic acid supplementation.

Genotoxicity studies have not been performed with atovaquone in combination with proguanil. Effects of MALARONE on male and female reproductive performance are unknown.

The ADVERSE REACTIONS: Post-Marketing Adverse Reactions: *Skin section has been revised as follows.*

Skin/Hypersensitivity: Cutaneous reactions ranging from rash, photosensitivity, angioedema, and urticaria to rare cases of anaphylaxis, erythema multiforme, and Stevens-Johnson syndrome.

The first paragraph of the OVERDOSAGE *section has been revised as follows.*

There is no information on overdoses of MALARONE substantially higher than the doses recommended for treatment.

The DOSAGE AND ADMINISTRATION: Patients With Renal Impairment *section has been revised as follows.*

MALARONE should not be used for malaria prophylaxis in patients with severe renal impairment (creatinine clearance <30 mL/min). MALARONE may be used with caution for the treatment of malaria in patients with severe renal impairment (creatinine clearance <30 mL/min), only if the benefits of the 3-day treatment regimen outweigh the potential risks associated with increased drug exposure (see CLINICAL PHARMACOLOGY: Special Populations: Renal Impairment). No dosage adjustments are needed in patients with mild (creatinine clearance 50 to 80 mL/min) and moderate (creatinine clearance 30 to 50 mL/min) renal impairment (see CLINICAL PHARMACOLOGY: Special Populations).

GlaxoSmithKline, Research Triangle Park, NC 27709
©2004, GlaxoSmithKline. All rights reserved.
November 2004/RL-2124, RL-2133

PARNATE® ℞
[*par' nāt*]
tranylcypromine sulfate
tablets 10 mg

Prescribing information for this product, which appears on pages 1583–1585 of the 2005 PDR, has been completely revised as follows. Please write "See Supplement A" next to the product heading.

Suicidality in Children and Adolescents
Antidepressants increased the risk of suicidal thinking and behavior (suicidality) in short-term studies in children and adolescents with Major Depressive Disorder (MDD) and other psychiatric disorders. Anyone considering the use of *Parnate* or any other antidepressant in a child or adolescent must balance this risk with the clinical need. Patients who are started on therapy should be observed closely for clinical worsening, suicidality, or unusual changes in behavior. Families and caregivers should be advised of the need for close observation and communication with the prescriber. *Parnate* is not approved for use in pediatric patients. (See WARNINGS and PRECAUTIONS—Pediatric Use.)
Pooled analyses of short-term (4 to 16 weeks) placebo-controlled trials of 9 antidepressant drugs (SSRIs and others) in children and adolescents with major depressive disorder (MDD), obsessive compulsive disorder (OCD), or other psychiatric disorders (a total of 24 trials involving over 4,400 patients) have revealed a greater risk of adverse events representing suicidal thinking or behavior (suicidality) during the first few months of treatment in those receiving antidepressants. The average risk of such events in patients receiving antidepressants was 4%, twice the placebo risk of 2%. No suicides occurred in these trials.

DESCRIPTION
Chemically, tranylcypromine sulfate is (±)-*trans*-2-phenylcyclopropylamine sulfate (2:1).

Each round, rose-red, film-coated tablet is imprinted with the product name PARNATE and SB and contains tranylcypromine sulfate equivalent to 10 mg of tranylcypromine. Inactive ingredients consist of cellulose, citric acid, croscarmellose sodium, D&C Red No. 7, FD&C Blue No. 2, FD&C Red No. 40, FD&C Yellow No. 6, gelatin, iron oxide, lactose, magnesium stearate, talc, titanium dioxide and trace amounts of other inactive ingredients.

ACTION
Tranylcypromine is a non-hydrazine monoamine oxidase inhibitor with a rapid onset of activity. It increases the concentration of epinephrine, norepinephrine and serotonin in storage sites throughout the nervous system and, in theory, this increased concentration of monoamines in the brain stem is the basis for its antidepressant activity. When tranylcypromine is withdrawn, monoamine oxidase activity is recovered in 3 to 5 days, although the drug is excreted in 24 hours.

INDICATIONS
For the treatment of Major Depressive Episode Without Melancholia.

Parnate (tranylcypromine sulfate) should be used in adult patients who can be closely supervised. It should rarely be the first antidepressant drug given. Rather, the drug is suited for patients who have failed to respond to the drugs more commonly administered for depression.

The effectiveness of *Parnate* has been established in adult outpatients, most of whom had a depressive illness which would correspond to a diagnosis of Major Depressive Episode Without Melancholia. As described in the American Psychiatric Association's Diagnostic and Statistical Manual, third edition (DSM III), Major Depressive Episode implies a prominent and relatively persistent (nearly every day for at least 2 weeks) depressed or dysphoric mood that usually interferes with daily functioning and includes at least 4 of the following 8 symptoms: change in appetite, change in sleep, psychomotor agitation or retardation, loss of interest in usual activities or decrease in sexual drive, increased fatigability, feelings of guilt or worthlessness, slowed thinking or impaired concentration and suicidal ideation or attempts.

The effectiveness of *Parnate* in patients who meet the criteria for Major Depressive Episode with Melancholia (endogenous features) has not been established.

SUMMARY OF CONTRAINDICATIONS
Parnate (tranylcypromine sulfate) should not be administered in combination with any of the following: MAO inhibitors or dibenzazepine derivatives; sympathomimetics (including amphetamines); some central nervous system depressants (including narcotics and alcohol); antihypertensive, diuretic, antihistaminic, sedative or anesthetic drugs; bupropion HCl; buspirone HCl; dextromethorphan; cheese or other foods with a high tyramine content; or excessive quantities of caffeine.

Parnate (tranylcypromine sulfate) should not be administered to any patient with a confirmed or suspected cerebrovascular defect or to any patient with cardiovascular disease, hypertension or history of headache.

(For complete discussion of contraindications and warnings, see below.)

CONTRAINDICATIONS
Parnate (tranylcypromine sulfate) is contraindicated:

1. In patients with cerebrovascular defects or cardiovascular disorders
Parnate should not be administered to any patient with a confirmed or suspected cerebrovascular defect or to any patient with cardiovascular disease or hypertension.

2. In the presence of pheochromocytoma
Parnate should not be used in the presence of pheochromocytoma since such tumors secrete pressor substances.

3. In combination with MAO inhibitors or with dibenzazepine-related entities
Parnate (tranylcypromine sulfate) should not be administered together or in rapid succession with other MAO inhibitors or with dibenzazepine-related entities. Hypertensive crises or severe convulsive seizures may occur in patients receiving such combinations.

In patients being transferred to *Parnate* from another MAO inhibitor or from a dibenzazepine-related entity, allow a medication-free interval of at least a week, then initiate *Parnate* using half the normal starting dosage for at least the first week of therapy. Similarly, at least a week should elapse between the discontinuance of *Parnate* and the administration of another MAO inhibitor or a dibenzazepine-related entity, or the readministration of *Parnate*.

The following list includes some other MAO inhibitors, dibenzazepine-related entities and tricyclic antidepressants, and the companies which market them.

Other MAO Inhibitors

Generic Name	**Source**
Furazolidone	
Isocarboxazid	Marplan® (Oxford Pharm Services)
Pargyline HCl	
Pargyline HCl and methyclothiazide	
Phenelzine sulfate	Nardil® (Parke-Davis)
Procarbazine HCl	Matulane® (Sigma Tau)

Dibenzazepine-Related and Other Tricyclics

Generic Name	**Source**
Amitriptyline HCl	Elavil® (Zeneca)
Perphenazine and amitriptyline HCl	Etrafon® (Schering) Triavil® (Lotus Biochemical)

Continued on next page

Parnate—Cont.

Clomipramine hydrochloride	Anafranil® (Geneva)
Desipramine HCl	Norpramin® (Aventis)
Imipramine HCl	Janimine™ (Geneva)
	Tofranil® (Novartis)
Nortriptyline HCl	(Geneva)
	Pamelor® (Mallinckrodt)
Protriptyline HCl	Vivactil® (Merck & Co., Inc.)
Doxepin HCl	Sinequan® (Pfizer)
Carbamazepine	Tegretol® (Novartis)
Cyclobenzaprine HCl	Flexeril® (Merck & Co., Inc.)
Amoxapine	(Geneva)
Maprotiline HCl	(Mylan)
Trimipramine maleate	Surmontil® (Wyeth-Ayerst Pharmaceuticals)

4. In combination with bupropion

The concurrent administration of a MAO inhibitor and bupropion hydrochloride (Wellbutrin®, Wellbutrin SR®, Zyban®, GlaxoSmithKline) is contraindicated. At least 14 days should elapse between discontinuation of a MAO inhibitor and initiation of treatment with bupropion hydrochloride.

5. In combination with dexfenfluramine hydrochloride

Because dexfenfluramine hydrochloride is a serotonin releaser and reuptake inhibitor, it should not be used concomitantly with Parnate (tranylcypromine sulfate).

6. In combination with selective serotonin reuptake inhibitors (SSRIs)

As a general rule, Parnate should not be administered in combination with any SSRI. There have been reports of serious, sometimes fatal, reactions (including hyperthermia, rigidity, myoclonus, autonomic instability with possible rapid fluctuations of vital signs, and mental status changes that include extreme agitation progressing to delirium and coma) in patients receiving fluoxetine (Prozac®, Eli Lilly and Company) in combination with a monoamine oxidase inhibitor (MAOI), and in patients who have recently discontinued fluoxetine and are then started on a MAOI. Some cases presented with features resembling neuroleptic malignant syndrome. Therefore, fluoxetine and other SSRIs should not be used in combination with a MAOI, or within 14 days of discontinuing therapy with a MAOI. Since fluoxetine and its major metabolite have very long elimination half-lives, at least 5 weeks should be allowed after stopping fluoxetine before starting a MAOI.

At least 2 weeks should be allowed after stopping sertraline (Zoloft®, Pfizer) or paroxetine (Paxil®, GlaxoSmithKline) before starting a MAOI.

7. In combination with buspirone

Parnate (tranylcypromine sulfate) should not be used in combination with buspirone HCl (BuSpar®, Bristol-Myers Squibb), since several cases of elevated blood pressure have been reported in patients taking MAO inhibitors who were then given buspirone HCl. At least 10 days should elapse between the discontinuation of Parnate and the institution of buspirone HCl.

8. In combination with sympathomimetics

Parnate (tranylcypromine sulfate) should not be administered in combination with sympathomimetics, including amphetamines, and over-the-counter drugs such as cold, hay fever or weight-reducing preparations that contain vasoconstrictors.

During Parnate therapy, it appears that certain patients are particularly vulnerable to the effects of sympathomimetics when the activity of certain enzymes is inhibited. Use of sympathomimetics and compounds such as guanethidine, methyldopa, reserpine, dopamine, levodopa and tryptophan with Parnate may precipitate hypertension, headache and related symptoms. The combination of MAOIs and tryptophan has been reported to cause behavioral and neurologic syndromes including disorientation, confusion, amnesia, delirium, agitation, hypomanic signs, ataxia, myoclonus, hyperreflexia, shivering, ocular oscillations and Babinski's signs.

9. In combination with meperidine

Do not use meperidine concomitantly with MAO inhibitors or within 2 or 3 weeks following MAOI therapy. Serious reactions have been precipitated with concomitant use, including coma, severe hypertension or hypotension, severe respiratory depression, convulsions, malignant hyperpyrexia, excitation, peripheral vascular collapse and death. It is thought that these reactions may be mediated by accumulation of 5-HT (serotonin) consequent to MAO inhibition.

10. In combination with dextromethorphan

The combination of MAO inhibitors and dextromethorphan has been reported to cause brief episodes of psychosis or bizarre behavior.

11. In combination with cheese or other foods with a high tyramine content

Hypertensive crises have sometimes occurred during Parnate therapy after ingestion of foods with a high tyramine content. In general, the patient should avoid protein foods in which aging or protein breakdown is used to increase flavor. In particular, patients should be instructed not to take foods such as cheese (particularly strong or aged varieties), sour cream, Chianti wine, sherry, beer (including nonalcoholic beer), liqueurs, pickled herring, anchovies, caviar, liver, canned figs, dried fruits (raisins, prunes, etc.), bananas, raspberries, avocados, overripe fruit, chocolate, soy

sauce, sauerkraut, the pods of broad beans (fava beans), yeast extracts, yogurt, meat extracts or meat prepared with tenderizers.

12. In patients undergoing elective surgery

Patients taking Parnate should not undergo elective surgery requiring general anesthesia. Also, they should not be given cocaine or local anesthesia containing sympathomimetic vasoconstrictors. The possible combined hypotensive effects of Parnate and spinal anesthesia should be kept in mind. Parnate should be discontinued at least 10 days prior to elective surgery.

ADDITIONAL CONTRAINDICATIONS

In general, the physician should bear in mind the possibility of a lowered margin of safety when Parnate (tranylcypromine sulfate) is administered in combination with potent drugs.

1. Parnate should not be used in combination with some central nervous system depressants such as narcotics and alcohol, or with hypotensive agents. A marked potentiating effect on these classes of drugs has been reported.

2. Anti-parkinsonism drugs should be used with caution in patients receiving Parnate since severe reactions have been reported.

3. Parnate should not be used in patients with a history of liver disease or in those with abnormal liver function tests.

4. Excessive use of caffeine in any form should be avoided in patients receiving Parnate.

WARNINGS TO PHYSICIANS

Clinical Worsening and Suicide Risk: Patients with major depressive disorder (MDD), both adult and pediatric, may experience worsening of their depression and/or the emergence of suicidal ideation and behavior (suicidality) or unusual changes in behavior, whether or not they are taking antidepressant medications, and this risk may persist until significant remission occurs. There has been a long-standing concern that antidepressants may have a role in inducing worsening of depression and the emergence of suicidality in certain patients. Antidepressants increased the risk of suicidal thinking and behavior (suicidality) in short-term studies in children and adolescents with MDD and other psychiatric disorders.

Pooled analyses of short-term placebo-controlled trials of 9 antidepressant drugs (SSRIs and others) in children and adolescents with MDD, OCD, or other psychiatric disorders (a total of 24 trials involving over 4,400 patients) have revealed a greater risk of adverse events representing suicidal behavior or thinking (suicidality) during the first few months of treatment in those receiving antidepressants. The average risk of such events in patients receiving antidepressants was 4%, twice the placebo risk of 2%. There was considerable variation in risk among drugs, but a tendency toward an increase for almost all drugs studied. The risk of suicidality was most consistently observed in the MDD trials, but there were signals of risk arising from some trials in other psychiatric indications (obsessive compulsive disorder and social anxiety disorder) as well. **No suicides occurred in any of these trials.** It is unknown whether the suicidality risk in pediatric patients extends to longer-term use, i.e., beyond several months. It is also unknown whether the suicidality risk extends to adults.

All pediatric patients being treated with antidepressants for any indication should be observed closely for clinical worsening, suicidality, and unusual changes in behavior, especially during the initial few months of a course of drug therapy, or at times of dose changes, either increases or decreases. Such observation would generally include at least weekly face-to-face contact with patients or their family members or caregivers during the first 4 weeks of treatment, then every other week visits for the next 4 weeks, then at 12 weeks, and as clinically indicated beyond 12 weeks. Additional contact by telephone may be appropriate between face-to-face visits.

Adults with MDD or co-morbid depression in the setting of other psychiatric illness being treated with antidepressants should be observed similarly for clinical worsening and suicidality, especially during the initial few months of a course of drug therapy, or at times of dose changes, either increases or decreases.

The following symptoms, anxiety, agitation, panic attacks, insomnia, irritability, hostility, aggressiveness, impulsivity, akathisia (psychomotor restlessness), hypomania, and mania, have been reported in adult and pediatric patients being treated with antidepressants for major depressive disorder as well as for other indications, both psychiatric and nonpsychiatric. Although a causal link between the emergence of such symptoms and either the worsening of depression and/or the emergence of suicidal impulses has not been established, there is concern that such symptoms may represent precursors to emerging suicidality.

Consideration should be given to changing the therapeutic regimen, including possibly discontinuing the medication, in patients whose depression is persistently worse, or who are experiencing emergent suicidality or symptoms that might be precursors to worsening depression or suicidality, especially if these symptoms are severe, abrupt in onset, or were not part of the patient's presenting symptoms.

Families and caregivers of pediatric patients being treated with antidepressants for major depressive disorder or other indications, both psychiatric and nonpsychiatric, should be alerted about the need to monitor patients for the emergence of agitation, irritability, unusual changes in behavior, and the other symptoms described above, as well as the emergence of suicidality, and to report such symptoms immediately to health care providers. Such

monitoring should include daily observation by families and caregivers. Prescriptions for Parnate should be written for the smallest quantity of tablets consistent with good patient management, in order to reduce the risk of overdose. Families and caregivers of adults being treated for depression should be similarly advised.

Screening Patients for Bipolar Disorder: A major depressive episode may be the initial presentation of bipolar disorder. It is generally believed (though not established in controlled trials) that treating such an episode with an antidepressant alone may increase the likelihood of precipitation of a mixed/manic episode in patients at risk for bipolar disorder. Whether any of the symptoms described above represent such a conversion is unknown. However, prior to initiating treatment with an antidepressant, patients with depressive symptoms should be adequately screened to determine if they are at risk for bipolar disorder; such screening should include a detailed psychiatric history, including a family history of suicide, bipolar disorder, and depression. It should be noted that Parnate is not approved for use in treating bipolar depression.

Parnate (tranylcypromine sulfate) is a potent agent with the capability of producing serious side effects. Parnate is not recommended in those depressive reactions where other antidepressant drugs may be effective. **It should be reserved for patients who can be closely supervised and who have not responded satisfactorily to the drugs more commonly administered for depression.**

Before prescribing, the physician should be completely familiar with the full material on dosage, side effects and contraindications on these pages, with the principles of MAO inhibitor therapy and the side effects of this class of drugs. Also, the physician should be familiar with the symptomatology of mental depressions and alternate methods of treatment to aid in the careful selection of patients for Parnate therapy.

Pregnancy Warning: Use of any drug in pregnancy, during lactation or in women of childbearing age requires that the potential benefits of the drug be weighed against its possible hazards to mother and child.

Animal reproductive studies show that Parnate passes through the placental barrier into the fetus of the rat, and into the milk of the lactating dog. The absence of a harmful action of Parnate on fertility or on postnatal development by either prenatal treatment or from the milk of treated animals has not been demonstrated. Tranylcypromine is excreted in human milk.

WARNING TO THE PATIENT

Patients should be instructed to report promptly the occurrence of headache or other unusual symptoms, i.e., palpitation and/or tachycardia, a sense of constriction in the throat or chest, sweating, dizziness, neck stiffness, nausea or vomiting.

Patients should be warned against eating the foods listed in Section 11 under Contraindications while on Parnate (tranylcypromine sulfate) therapy. Also, they should be told not to drink alcoholic beverages. The patient should also be warned about the possibility of hypotension and faintness, as well as drowsiness sufficient to impair performance of potentially hazardous tasks such as driving a car or operating machinery.

Patients should also be cautioned not to take concomitant medications, whether prescription or over-the-counter drugs such as cold, hay fever or weight-reducing preparations, without the advice of a physician. They should be advised not to consume excessive amounts of caffeine in any form. Likewise, they should inform other physicians, and their dentist, about their use of Parnate.

See PRECAUTIONS—Information for Patients for information regarding clinical worsening and suicide risk.

WARNINGS

HYPERTENSIVE CRISES: The most important reaction associated with Parnate (tranylcypromine sulfate) is the occurrence of hypertensive crises which have sometimes been fatal.

These crises are characterized by some or all of the following symptoms: occipital headache which may radiate frontally, palpitation, neck stiffness or soreness, nausea or vomiting, sweating (sometimes with fever and sometimes with cold, clammy skin) and photophobia. Either tachycardia or bradycardia may be present, and associated constricting chest pain and dilated pupils may occur. **Intracranial bleeding, sometimes fatal in outcome, has been reported in association with the paradoxical increase in blood pressure.** In all patients taking Parnate blood pressure should be followed closely to detect evidence of any pressor response. It is emphasized that full reliance should not be placed on blood pressure readings, but that the patient should also be observed frequently.

Therapy should be discontinued immediately upon the occurrence of palpitation or frequent headaches during Parnate therapy. These signs may be prodromal of a hypertensive crisis.

Important:
Recommended treatment in hypertensive crises

If a hypertensive crisis occurs, Parnate (tranylcypromine sulfate) should be discontinued and therapy to lower blood pressure should be instituted immediately. Headache tends to abate as blood pressure is lowered. On the basis of present evidence, phentolamine is recommended. (The dosage reported for phentolamine is 5 mg I.V.) Care should be taken to administer this drug slowly in order to avoid producing an excessive hypotensive effect. Fever should be managed by means of external cooling. Other symptomatic and supportive measures may be desirable in particular cases. Do not use parenteral reserpine.

PRECAUTIONS

Hypotension

Hypotension has been observed during Parnate (tranylcypromine sulfate) therapy. Symptoms of postural hypotension are seen most commonly but not exclusively in patients with pre-existent hypertension; blood pressure usually returns rapidly to pretreatment levels upon discontinuation of the drug. At doses above 30 mg daily, postural hypotension is a major side effect and may result in syncope. Dosage increases should be made more gradually in patients showing a tendency toward hypotension at the beginning of therapy. Postural hypotension may be relieved by having the patient lie down until blood pressure returns to normal.

Also, when *Parnate* is combined with those phenothiazine derivatives or other compounds known to cause hypotension, the possibility of additive hypotensive effects should be considered.

There have been reports of drug dependency in patients using doses of tranylcypromine significantly in excess of the therapeutic range. Some of these patients had a history of previous substance abuse. The following withdrawal symptoms have been reported: restlessness, anxiety, depression, confusion, hallucinations, headache, weakness and diarrhea.

Drugs which lower the seizure threshold, including MAO inhibitors, should not be used with Amipaque®. As with other MAO inhibitors, Parnate (tranylcypromine sulfate) should be discontinued at least 48 hours before myelography and should not be resumed for at least 24 hours postprocedure.

MAO inhibitors may have the capacity to suppress anginal pain that would otherwise serve as a warning of myocardial ischemia.

The usual precautions should be observed in patients with impaired renal function since there is a possibility of cumulative effects in such patients.

Older patients may suffer more morbidity than younger patients during and following an episode of hypertension or malignant hyperthermia. Older patients have less compensatory reserve to cope with any serious adverse reaction. Therefore, *Parnate* should be used with caution in the elderly population.

Although excretion of *Parnate* is rapid, inhibition of MAO may persist up to 10 days following discontinuation.

Because the influence of *Parnate* on the convulsive threshold is variable in animal experiments, suitable precautions should be taken if epileptic patients are treated.

Some MAO inhibitors have contributed to hypoglycemic episodes in diabetic patients receiving insulin or oral hypoglycemic agents. Therefore, *Parnate* should be used with caution in diabetics using these drugs.

Parnate may aggravate coexisting symptoms in depression, such as anxiety and agitation.

Use Parnate (tranylcypromine sulfate) with caution in hyperthyroid patients because of their increased sensitivity to pressor amines.

Parnate should be administered with caution to patients receiving Antabuse®†. In a single study, rats given high intraperitoneal doses of *d* or *l* isomers of tranylcypromine sulfate plus disulfiram experienced severe toxicity including convulsions and death. Additional studies in rats given high oral doses of racemic tranylcypromine sulfate (*Parnate*) and disulfiram produced no adverse interaction.

Information for Patients: Prescribers or other health professionals should inform patients, their families, and their caregivers about the benefits and risks associated with treatment with *Parnate* and should counsel them in its appropriate use. A patient Medication Guide About Using Antidepressants in Children and Teenagers is available for *Parnate*. The prescriber or health professional should instruct patients, their families, and their caregivers to read the Medication Guide and should assist them in understanding its contents. Patients should be given the opportunity to discuss the contents of the Medication Guide and to obtain answers to any questions they may have. The complete text of the Medication Guide is reprinted at the end of this document.

Patients should be advised of the following issues and asked to alert their prescriber if these occur while taking *Parnate*.

Clinical Worsening and Suicide Risk: Patients, their families, and their caregivers should be encouraged to be alert to the emergence of anxiety, agitation, panic attacks, insomnia, irritability, hostility, aggressiveness, impulsivity, akathisia (psychomotor restlessness), hypomania, mania, other unusual changes in behavior, worsening of depression, and suicidal ideation, especially early during antidepressant treatment and when the dose is adjusted up or down. Families and caregivers of patients should be advised to observe for the emergence of such symptoms on a day-to-day basis, since changes may be abrupt. Such symptoms should be reported to the patient's prescriber or health professional, especially if they are severe, abrupt in onset, or were not part of the patient's presenting symptoms. Symptoms such as these may be associated with an increased risk for suicidal thinking and behavior and indicate a need for very close monitoring and possibly changes in the medication.

Pediatric Use: Safety and effectiveness in the pediatric population have not been established (see BOX WARNING and WARNINGS—Clinical Worsening and Suicide Risk). Anyone considering the use of *Parnate* in a child or adolescent must balance the potential risks with the clinical need.

ADVERSE REACTIONS

Overstimulation which may include increased anxiety, agitation and manic symptoms is usually evidence of excessive therapeutic action. Dosage should be reduced, or a phenothiazine tranquilizer should be administered concomitantly.

Patients may experience restlessness or insomnia; may notice some weakness, drowsiness, episodes of dizziness or dry mouth; or may report nausea, diarrhea, abdominal pain or constipation. Most of these effects can be relieved by lowering the dosage or by giving suitable concomitant medication.

Tachycardia, significant anorexia, edema, palpitation, blurred vision, chills and impotence have each been reported.

Headaches without blood pressure elevation have occurred.

Rare instances of hepatitis, skin rash and alopecia have been reported.

Impaired water excretion compatible with the syndrome of inappropriate secretion of antidiuretic hormone (SIADH) has been reported.

Tinnitus, muscle spasm, tremors, myoclonic jerks, numbness, paresthesia, urinary retention and retarded ejaculation have been reported.

Hematologic disorders including anemia, leukopenia, agranulocytosis and thrombocytopenia have been reported.

Post-Introduction Reports

The following are spontaneously reported adverse events temporally associated with *Parnate* therapy. No clear relationship between *Parnate* and these events has been established. Localized scleroderma, flare-up of cystic acne, ataxia, confusion, disorientation, memory loss, urinary frequency, urinary incontinence, urticaria, fissuring in corner of mouth, akinesia.

DOSAGE AND ADMINISTRATION

Dosage should be adjusted to the requirements of the individual patient. Improvement should be seen within 48 hours to 3 weeks after starting therapy.

The usual effective dosage is 30 mg per day, usually given in divided doses. If there are no signs of improvement after a reasonable period (up to 2 weeks), then the dosage may be increased in 10 mg per day increments at intervals of 1 to 3 weeks; the dosage range may be extended to a maximum of 60 mg per day from the usual 30 mg per day.

OVERDOSAGE

SYMPTOMS: The characteristic symptoms that may be caused by overdosage are usually those described above.

However, an intensification of these symptoms and sometimes severe additional manifestations may be seen, depending on the degree of overdosage and on individual susceptibility. Some patients exhibit insomnia, restlessness and anxiety, progressing in severe cases to agitation, mental confusion and incoherence. Hypotension, dizziness, weakness and drowsiness may occur, progressing in severe cases to extreme dizziness and shock. A few patients have displayed hypertension with severe headache and other symptoms. Rare instances have been reported in which hypertension was accompanied by twitching or myoclonic fibrillation of skeletal muscles with hyperpyrexia, sometimes progressing to generalized rigidity and coma.

TREATMENT: Gastric lavage is helpful if performed early. Treatment should normally consist of general supportive measures, close observation of vital signs and steps to counteract specific symptoms as they occur, since MAO inhibition may persist. The management of hypertensive crises is described under WARNINGS in the HYPERTENSIVE CRISES section.

External cooling is recommended if hyperpyrexia occurs. Barbiturates have been reported to help relieve myoclonic reactions, but frequency of administration should be controlled carefully because Parnate (tranylcypromine sulfate) may prolong barbiturate activity. When hypotension requires treatment, the standard measures for managing circulatory shock should be initiated. If pressor agents are used, the rate of infusion should be regulated by careful observation of the patient because an exaggerated pressor response sometimes occurs in the presence of MAO inhibition. Remember that the toxic effect of *Parnate* may be delayed or prolonged following the last dose of the drug. Therefore, the patient should be closely observed for at least a week. It is not known if tranylcypromine is dialyzable.

HOW SUPPLIED

Parnate is supplied as round, rose-red, film-coated tablets imprinted with the product name PARNATE and SB and contains tranylcypromine sulfate equivalent to 10 mg of tranylcypromine, in bottles of 100 with a desiccant, manufactured by Abbott Laboratories, North Chicago, IL 60064.

10 mg 100's: NDC 0007-4471-20

Store between 15° and 30°C (59° and 86°F).

* metrizamide, Sanofi-Synthelabo Inc.

†disulfiram, Wyeth-Ayerst Pharmaceuticals.

Medication Guide

PARNATE® (PAR-nate) (tranylcypromine sulfate) Tablets About Using Antidepressants in Children and Teenagers

What is the most important information I should know if my child is being prescribed an antidepressant?

Parents or guardians need to think about 4 important things when their child is prescribed an antidepressant:

1. There is a risk of suicidal thoughts or actions
2. How to try to prevent suicidal thoughts or actions in your child
3. You should watch for certain signs if your child is taking an antidepressant
4. There are benefits and risks when using antidepressants

1. There is a Risk of Suicidal Thoughts or Actions

Children and teenagers sometimes think about suicide, and many report trying to kill themselves.

Antidepressants increase suicidal thoughts and actions in some children and teenagers. But suicidal thoughts and actions can also be caused by depression, a serious medical condition that is commonly treated with antidepressants. Thinking about killing yourself or trying to kill yourself is called *suicidality* or being *suicidal*.

A large study combined the results of 24 different studies of children and teenagers with depression or other illnesses. In these studies, patients took either a placebo (sugar pill) or an antidepressant for 1 to 4 months. ***No one committed suicide in these studies,*** but some patients became suicidal. On sugar pills, 2 out of every 100 became suicidal. On the antidepressants, 4 out of every 100 patients became suicidal.

For some children and teenagers, the risks of suicidal actions may be especially high. These include patients with

- Bipolar illness (sometimes called manic-depressive illness)
- A family history of bipolar illness
- A personal or family history of attempting suicide

If any of these are present, make sure you tell your healthcare provider before your child takes an antidepressant.

2. How to Try to Prevent Suicidal Thoughts and Actions

To try to prevent suicidal thoughts and actions in your child, pay close attention to changes in her or his moods or actions, especially if the changes occur suddenly. Other important people in your child's life can help by paying attention as well (e.g., your child, brothers and sisters, teachers, and other important people). The changes to look out for are listed in Section 3, on what to watch for.

Whenever an antidepressant is started or its dose is changed, pay close attention to your child. After starting an antidepressant, your child should generally see his or her healthcare provider:

- Once a week for the first 4 weeks
- Every 2 weeks for the next 4 weeks
- After taking the antidepressant for 12 weeks
- After 12 weeks, follow your healthcare provider's advice about how often to come back
- More often if problems or questions arise (see Section 3)

You should call your child's healthcare provider between visits if needed.

3. You Should Watch for Certain Signs If Your Child is Taking an Antidepressant

Contact your child's healthcare provider ***right away*** if your child exhibits any of the following signs for the first time, or if they seem worse, or worry you, your child, or your child's teacher:

- Thoughts about suicide or dying
- Attempts to commit suicide
- New or worse depression
- New or worse anxiety
- Feeling very agitated or restless
- Panic attacks
- Difficulty sleeping (insomnia)
- New or worse irritability
- Acting aggressive, being angry, or violent
- Acting on dangerous impulses
- An extreme increase in activity and talking
- Other unusual changes in behavior or mood

Never let your child stop taking an antidepressant without first talking to his or her healthcare provider. Stopping an antidepressant suddenly can cause other symptoms.

4. There are Benefits and Risks When Using Antidepressants

Antidepressants are used to treat depression and other illnesses. Depression and other illnesses can lead to suicide. In some children and teenagers, treatment with an antidepressant increases suicidal thinking or actions. It is important to discuss all the risks of treating depression and also the risks of not treating it. You and your child should discuss all treatment choices with your healthcare provider, not just the use of antidepressants.

Other side effects can occur with antidepressants (see section below).

Of all the antidepressants, only fluoxetine (Prozac®)* has been FDA approved to treat pediatric depression.

For obsessive compulsive disorder in children and teenagers, FDA has approved only fluoxetine (Prozac®)*, sertraline (Zoloft®)*, fluvoxamine, and clomipramine (Anafranil®)*.

Your healthcare provider may suggest other antidepressants based on the past experience of your child or other family members.

Is this all I need to know if my child is being prescribed an antidepressant?

No. This is a warning about the risk for suicidality. Other side effects can occur with antidepressants. Be sure to ask your healthcare provider to explain all the side effects of the particular drug he or she is prescribing. Also ask about drugs to avoid when taking an antidepressant. Ask your healthcare provider or pharmacist where to find more information.

Continued on next page

Parnate—Cont.

*The following are registered trademarks of their respective manufacturers: Prozac®/Eli Lilly and Company; Zoloft®/Pfizer Pharmaceuticals; Anafranil®/Mallinckrodt Inc. This Medication Guide has been approved by the U.S. Food and Drug Administration for all antidepressants.
January 2005/MG-PT:1
GlaxoSmithKline, Research Triangle Park, NC 27709
©2005, GlaxoSmithKline. All rights reserved.
January 2005/PT:L67

PAXIL®
[pax'il]
(paroxetine hydrochloride)
Tablets and Oral Suspension

℞

Prescribing information for this product, which appears on pages 1585–1592 of the 2005 PDR, has been completely revised as follows. Please write "See Supplement A" next to the product heading.

Suicidality in Children and Adolescents
Antidepressants increased the risk of suicidal thinking and behavior (suicidality) in short-term studies in children and adolescents with Major Depressive Disorder (MDD) and other psychiatric disorders. Anyone considering the use of PAXIL or any other antidepressant in a child or adolescent must balance this risk with the clinical need. Patients who are started on therapy should be observed closely for clinical worsening, suicidality, or unusual changes in behavior. Families and caregivers should be advised of the need for close observation and communication with the prescriber. PAXIL is not approved for use in pediatric patients. (See WARNINGS and PRECAUTIONS—Pediatric Use.)
Pooled analyses of short-term (4 to 16 weeks) placebo-controlled trials of 9 antidepressant drugs (SSRIs and others) in children and adolescents with major depressive disorder (MDD), obsessive compulsive disorder (OCD), or other psychiatric disorders (a total of 24 trials involving over 4,400 patients) have revealed a greater risk of adverse events representing suicidal thinking or behavior (suicidality) during the first few months of treatment in those receiving antidepressants. The average risk of such events in patients receiving antidepressants was 4%, twice the placebo risk of 2%. No suicides occurred in these trials.

DESCRIPTION

PAXIL (paroxetine hydrochloride) is an orally administered psychotropic drug. It is the hydrochloride salt of a phenylpiperidine compound identified chemically as (-)-*trans*-4R-(4'-fluorophenyl)-3S-[(3',4'-methylenedioxyphenoxy) methyl] piperidine hydrochloride hemihydrate and has the empirical formula of $C_{19}H_{20}FNO_3 \cdot HCl \cdot 1/2H_2O$. The molecular weight is 374.8 (329.4 as free base). The structural formula of paroxetine hydrochloride is:

Paroxetine hydrochloride is an odorless, off-white powder, having a melting point range of 120° to 138°C and a solubility of 5.4 mg/mL in water.
Tablets: Each film-coated tablet contains paroxetine hydrochloride equivalent to paroxetine as follows: 10 mg—yellow (scored); 20 mg—pink (scored); 30 mg—blue, 40 mg—green. Inactive ingredients consist of dibasic calcium phosphate dihydrate, hypromellose, magnesium stearate, polyethylene glycols, polysorbate 80, sodium starch glycolate, titanium dioxide, and 1 or more of the following: D&C Red No. 30, D&C Yellow No. 10, FD&C Blue No. 2, FD&C Yellow No. 6.

Suspension for Oral Administration: Each 5 mL of orange-colored, orange-flavored liquid contains paroxetine hydrochloride equivalent to paroxetine, 10 mg. Inactive ingredients consist of polacrilin potassium, microcrystalline cellulose, propylene glycol, glycerin, sorbitol, methyl paraben, propyl paraben, sodium citrate dihydrate, citric acid anhydrate, sodium saccharin, flavorings, FD&C Yellow No. 6, and simethicone emulsion, USP.

CLINICAL PHARMACOLOGY

Pharmacodynamics: The efficacy of paroxetine in the treatment of major depressive disorder, social anxiety disorder, obsessive compulsive disorder (OCD), panic disorder (PD), generalized anxiety disorder (GAD), and posttraumatic stress disorder (PTSD) is presumed to be linked to potentiation of serotonergic activity in the central nervous system resulting from inhibition of neuronal reuptake of serotonin (5-hydroxy-tryptamine, 5-HT). Studies at clinically relevant doses in humans have demonstrated that paroxetine blocks the uptake of serotonin into human platelets. In vitro studies in animals also suggest that paroxetine is a potent and highly selective inhibitor of neuronal serotonin reuptake and has only very weak effects on norepinephrine and dopamine neuronal reuptake. In vitro radioligand binding studies indicate that paroxetine has little affinity for muscarinic, alpha$_1$-, alpha$_2$-, beta-adrenergic-, dopamine (D$_2$)-, 5-HT$_1$-, 5-HT$_2$-, and histamine (H$_1$)-receptors; antagonism of muscarinic, histaminergic, and alpha$_1$-adrenergic receptors has been associated with various anticholinergic, sedative, and cardiovascular effects for other psychotropic drugs.
Because the relative potencies of paroxetine's major metabolites are at most 1/50 of the parent compound, they are essentially inactive.
Pharmacokinetics: Paroxetine is equally bioavailable from the oral suspension and tablet.
Paroxetine hydrochloride is completely absorbed after oral dosing of a solution of the hydrochloride salt. In a study in which normal male subjects (n = 15) received 30 mg tablets daily for 30 days, steady-state paroxetine concentrations were achieved by approximately 10 days for most subjects, although it may take substantially longer in an occasional patient. At steady state, mean values of C_{max}, T_{max}, C_{min}, and $T_{1/2}$ were 61.7 ng/mL (CV 45%), 5.2 hr. (CV 10%), 30.7 ng/mL (CV 67%), and 21.0 hr. (CV 32%), respectively. The steady-state C_{max} and C_{min} values were about 6 and 14 times what would be predicted from single-dose studies. Steady-state drug exposure based on AUC_{0-24} was about 8 times greater than would have been predicted from single-dose data in these subjects. The excess accumulation is a consequence of the fact that 1 of the enzymes that metabolizes paroxetine is readily saturable.
In steady-state dose proportionality studies involving elderly and nonelderly patients, at doses of 20 mg to 40 mg daily for the elderly and 20 mg to 50 mg daily for the nonelderly, some nonlinearity was observed in both populations, again reflecting a saturable metabolic pathway. In comparison to C_{min} values after 20 mg daily, values after 40 mg daily were only about 2 to 3 times greater than doubled.
The effects of food on the bioavailability of paroxetine were studied in subjects administered a single dose with and without food. AUC was only slightly increased (6%) when drug was administered with food but the C_{max} was 29% greater, while the time to reach peak plasma concentration decreased from 6.4 hours post-dosing to 4.9 hours.
Paroxetine is extensively metabolized after oral administration. The principal metabolites are polar and conjugated products of oxidation and methylation, which are readily cleared. Conjugates with glucuronic acid and sulfate predominate, and major metabolites have been isolated and identified. Data indicate that the metabolites have no more than 1/50 the potency of the parent compound at inhibiting serotonin uptake. The metabolism of paroxetine is accomplished in part by cytochrome $P_{450}IID_6$. Saturation of this enzyme at clinical doses appears to account for the nonlinearity of paroxetine kinetics with increasing dose and increasing duration of treatment. The role of this enzyme in paroxetine metabolism also suggests potential drug-drug interactions (see PRECAUTIONS).
Approximately 64% of a 30-mg oral solution dose of paroxetine was excreted in the urine with 2% as the parent compound and 62% as metabolites over a 10-day post-dosing period. About 36% was excreted in the feces (probably via the bile), mostly as metabolites and less than 1% as the parent compound over the 10-day post-dosing period.

Distribution: Paroxetine distributes throughout the body, including the CNS, with only 1% remaining in the plasma.
Protein Binding: Approximately 95% and 93% of paroxetine is bound to plasma protein at 100 ng/mL and 400 ng/mL, respectively. Under clinical conditions, paroxetine concentrations would normally be less than 400 ng/mL. Paroxetine does not alter the in vitro protein binding of phenytoin or warfarin.
Renal and Liver Disease: Increased plasma concentrations of paroxetine occur in subjects with renal and hepatic impairment. The mean plasma concentrations in patients with creatinine clearance below 30 mL/min. was approximately 4 times greater than seen in normal volunteers. Patients with creatinine clearance of 30 to 60 mL/min. and patients with hepatic functional impairment had about a 2-fold increase in plasma concentrations (AUC, C_{max}).
The initial dosage should therefore be reduced in patients with severe renal or hepatic impairment, and upward titration, if necessary, should be at increased intervals (see DOSAGE AND ADMINISTRATION).
Elderly Patients: In a multiple-dose study in the elderly at daily paroxetine doses of 20, 30, and 40 mg, C_{min} concentrations were about 70% to 80% greater than the respective C_{min} concentrations in nonelderly subjects. Therefore the initial dosage in the elderly should be reduced (see DOSAGE AND ADMINISTRATION).

CLINICAL TRIALS

Major Depressive Disorder: The efficacy of PAXIL as a treatment for major depressive disorder has been established in 6 placebo-controlled studies of patients with major depressive disorder (aged 18 to 73). In these studies, PAXIL was shown to be significantly more effective than placebo in treating major depressive disorder by at least 2 of the following measures: Hamilton Depression Rating Scale (HDRS), the Hamilton depressed mood item, and the Clinical Global Impression (CGI)-Severity of Illness. PAXIL was significantly better than placebo in improvement of the HDRS sub-factor scores, including the depressed mood item, sleep disturbance factor, and anxiety factor.
A study of outpatients with major depressive disorder who had responded to PAXIL (HDRS total score <8) during an initial 8-week open-treatment phase and were then randomized to continuation on PAXIL or placebo for 1 year demonstrated a significantly lower relapse rate for patients taking PAXIL (15%) compared to those on placebo (39%). Effectiveness was similar for male and female patients.
Obsessive Compulsive Disorder: The effectiveness of PAXIL in the treatment of obsessive compulsive disorder (OCD) was demonstrated in two 12-week multicenter placebo-controlled studies of adult outpatients (Studies 1 and 2). Patients in all studies had moderate to severe OCD (DSM-IIIR) with mean baseline ratings on the Yale Brown Obsessive Compulsive Scale (YBOCS) total score ranging from 23 to 26. Study 1, a dose-range finding study where patients were treated with fixed doses of 20, 40, or 60 mg of paroxetine/day demonstrated that daily doses of paroxetine 40 and 60 mg are effective in the treatment of OCD. Patients receiving doses of 40 and 60 mg paroxetine experienced a mean reduction of approximately 6 and 7 points, respectively, on the YBOCS total score which was significantly greater than the approximate 4-point reduction at 20 mg and a 3-point reduction in the placebo-treated patients. Study 2 was a flexible-dose study comparing paroxetine (20 to 60 mg daily) with clomipramine (25 to 250 mg daily). In this study, patients receiving paroxetine experienced a mean reduction of approximately 7 points on the YBOCS total score, which was significantly greater than the mean reduction of approximately 4 points in placebo-treated patients.
The following table provides the outcome classification by treatment group on Global Improvement items of the Clinical Global Impression (CGI) scale for Study 1.
[See table below]
Subgroup analyses did not indicate that there were any differences in treatment outcomes as a function of age or gender.
The long-term maintenance effects of PAXIL in OCD were demonstrated in a long-term extension to Study 1. Patients who were responders on paroxetine during the 3-month double-blind phase and a 6-month extension on open-label paroxetine (20 to 60 mg/day) were randomized to either paroxetine or placebo in a 6-month double-blind relapse prevention phase. Patients randomized to paroxetine were significantly less likely to relapse than comparably treated patients who were randomized to placebo.
Panic Disorder: The effectiveness of PAXIL in the treatment of panic disorder was demonstrated in three 10- to 12-week multicenter, placebo-controlled studies of adult outpatients (Studies 1-3). Patients in all studies had panic disorder (DSM-IIIR), with or without agoraphobia. In these studies, PAXIL was shown to be significantly more effective than placebo in treating panic disorder by at least 2 out of 3 measures of panic attack frequency and on the Clinical Global Impression Severity of Illness score.
Study 1 was a 10-week dose-range finding study; patients were treated with fixed paroxetine doses of 10, 20, or 40 mg/day or placebo. A significant difference from placebo was observed only for the 40 mg/day group. At endpoint, 76% of patients receiving paroxetine 40 mg/day were free of panic attacks, compared to 44% of placebo-treated patients.
Study 2 was a 12-week flexible-dose study comparing paroxetine (10 to 60 mg daily) and placebo. At endpoint, 51% of paroxetine patients were free of panic attacks compared to 32% of placebo-treated patients.

Outcome Classification (%) on CGI-Global Improvement Item for Completers in Study 1				
Outcome Classification	Placebo (n = 74)	PAXIL 20 mg (n = 75)	PAXIL 40 mg (n = 66)	PAXIL 60 mg (n = 66)
Worse	14%	7%	7%	3%
No Change	44%	35%	22%	19%
Minimally Improved	24%	33%	29%	34%
Much Improved	11%	18%	22%	24%
Very Much Improved	7%	7%	20%	20%

Study 3 was a 12-week flexible-dose study comparing paroxetine (10 to 60 mg daily) to placebo in patients concurrently receiving standardized cognitive behavioral therapy. At endpoint, 33% of the paroxetine-treated patients showed a reduction to 0 or 1 panic attacks compared to 14% of placebo patients.

In both Studies 2 and 3, the mean paroxetine dose for completers at endpoint was approximately 40 mg/day of paroxetine.

Long-term maintenance effects of PAXIL in panic disorder were demonstrated in an extension to Study 1. Patients who were responders during the 10-week double-blind phase and during a 3-month double-blind extension phase were randomized to either paroxetine (10, 20, or 40 mg/day) or placebo in a 3-month double-blind relapse prevention phase. Patients randomized to paroxetine were significantly less likely to relapse than comparably treated patients who were randomized to placebo.

Subgroup analyses did not indicate that there were any differences in treatment outcomes as a function of age or gender.

Social Anxiety Disorder: The effectiveness of PAXIL in the treatment of social anxiety disorder was demonstrated in three 12-week, multicenter, placebo-controlled studies (Studies 1, 2, and 3) of adult outpatients with social anxiety disorder (DSM-IV). In these studies, the effectiveness of PAXIL compared to placebo was evaluated on the basis of (1) the proportion of responders, as defined by a Clinical Global Impression (CGI) Improvement score of 1 (very much improved) or 2 (much improved), and (2) change from baseline in the Liebowitz Social Anxiety Scale (LSAS).

Studies 1 and 2 were flexible-dose studies comparing paroxetine (20 to 50 mg daily) and placebo. Paroxetine demonstrated statistically significant superiority over placebo on both the CGI Improvement responder criterion and the Liebowitz Social Anxiety Scale (LSAS). In Study 1, for patients who completed to week 12, 69% of paroxetine-treated patients compared to 29% of placebo-treated patients were CGI Improvement responders. In Study 2, CGI Improvement responders were 77% and 42% for the paroxetine- and placebo-treated patients, respectively.

Study 3 was a 12-week study comparing fixed paroxetine doses of 20, 40, or 60 mg/day with placebo. Paroxetine 20 mg was demonstrated to be significantly superior to placebo on both the LSAS Total Score and the CGI Improvement responder criterion; there were trends for superiority over placebo for the 40 mg and 60 mg/day dose groups. There was no indication in this study of any additional benefit for doses higher than 20 mg/day.

Subgroup analyses generally did not indicate differences in treatment outcomes as a function of age, race, or gender.

Generalized Anxiety Disorder: The effectiveness of PAXIL in the treatment of Generalized Anxiety Disorder (GAD) was demonstrated in two 8-week, multicenter, placebo-controlled studies (Studies 1 and 2) of adult outpatients with Generalized Anxiety Disorder (DSM-IV).

Study 1 was an 8-week study comparing fixed paroxetine doses of 20 mg or 40 mg/day with placebo. Doses of 20 mg or 40 mg of PAXIL were both demonstrated to be significantly superior to placebo on the Hamilton Rating Scale for Anxiety (HAM-A) total score. There was not sufficient evidence in this study to suggest a greater benefit for the 40 mg/day dose compared to the 20 mg/day dose.

Study 2 was a flexible-dose study comparing paroxetine (20 mg to 50 mg daily) and placebo. PAXIL demonstrated statistically significant superiority over placebo on the Hamilton Rating Scale for Anxiety (HAM-A) total score. A third study, also flexible-dose comparing paroxetine (20 mg to 50 mg daily), did not demonstrate statistically significant superiority of PAXIL over placebo on the Hamilton Rating Scale for Anxiety (HAM-A) total score, the primary outcome. Subgroup analyses did not indicate differences in treatment outcomes as a function of race or gender. There were insufficient elderly patients to conduct subgroup analyses on the basis of age.

In a longer-term trial, 566 patients meeting DSM-IV criteria for Generalized Anxiety Disorder, who had responded during a single-blind, 8-week acute treatment phase with 20 to 50 mg/day of PAXIL, were randomized to continuation of PAXIL at their same dose, or to placebo, for up to 24 weeks of observation for relapse. Response during the single-blind phase was defined by having a decrease of ≥2 points compared to baseline on the CGI-Severity of Illness scale, to a score of ≤3. Relapse during the double-blind phase was defined as an increase of ≥2 points compared to baseline on the CGI-Severity of Illness scale to a score of ≥4, or withdrawal due to lack of efficacy. Patients receiving continued PAXIL experienced a significantly lower relapse rate over the subsequent 24 weeks compared to those receiving placebo.

Posttraumatic Stress Disorder: The effectiveness of PAXIL in the treatment of Posttraumatic Stress Disorder (PTSD) was demonstrated in two 12-week, multicenter, placebo-controlled studies (Studies 1 and 2) of adult outpatients who met DSM-IV criteria for PTSD. The mean duration of PTSD symptoms for the 2 studies combined was 13 years (ranging from .1 year to 57 years). The percentage of patients with secondary major depressive disorder or non-PTSD anxiety disorders in the combined 2 studies was 41% (356 out of 858 patients) and 40% (345 out of 858 patients), respectively. Study outcome was assessed by (i) the Clinician-Administered PTSD Scale Part 2 (CAPS-2) score and (ii) the Clinical Global Impression-Global Improvement Scale (CGI-I). The CAPS-2 is a multi-item instrument that measures 3 aspects of PTSD with the following symptom clusters: Reexperienc-

ing/intrusion, avoidance/numbing and hyperarousal. The 2 primary outcomes for each trial were (i) change from baseline to endpoint on the CAPS-2 total score (17 items), and (ii) proportion of responders on the CGI-I, where responders were defined as patients having a score of 1 (very much improved) or 2 (much improved).

Study 1 was a 12-week study comparing fixed paroxetine doses of 20 mg or 40 mg/day to placebo. Doses of 20 mg and 40 mg of PAXIL were demonstrated to be significantly superior to placebo on change from baseline for the CAPS-2 total score and on proportion of responders on the CGI-I. There was not sufficient evidence in this study to suggest a greater benefit for the 40 mg/day dose compared to the 20 mg/day dose.

Study 2 was a 12-week flexible-dose study comparing paroxetine (20 to 50 mg daily) to placebo. PAXIL was demonstrated to be significantly superior to placebo on change from baseline for the CAPS-2 total score and on proportion of responders on the CGI-I.

A third study, also a flexible-dose study comparing paroxetine (20 to 50 mg daily) to placebo, demonstrated PAXIL to be significantly superior to placebo on change from baseline for CAPS-2 total score, but not on proportion of responders on the CGI-I.

The majority of patients in these trials were women (68% women: 377 out of 551 subjects in Study 1 and 66% women: 202 out of 303 subjects in Study 2). Subgroup analyses did not indicate differences in treatment outcomes as a function of gender. There were an insufficient number of patients who were 65 years and older or were non-Caucasian to conduct subgroup analyses on the basis of age or race, respectively.

INDICATIONS AND USAGE

Major Depressive Disorder: PAXIL is indicated for the treatment of major depressive disorder.

The efficacy of PAXIL in the treatment of a major depressive episode was established in 6-week controlled trials of outpatients whose diagnoses corresponded most closely to the DSM-III category of major depressive disorder (see CLINICAL PHARMACOLOGY—Clinical Trials). A major depressive episode implies a prominent and relatively persistent depressed or dysphoric mood that usually interferes with daily functioning (nearly every day for at least 2 weeks); it should include at least 4 of the following 8 symptoms: Change in appetite, change in sleep, psychomotor agitation or retardation, loss of interest in usual activities or decrease in sexual drive, increased fatigue, feelings of guilt or worthlessness, slowed thinking or impaired concentration, and a suicide attempt or suicidal ideation.

The effects of PAXIL in hospitalized depressed patients have not been adequately studied.

The efficacy of PAXIL in maintaining a response in major depressive disorder for up to 1 year was demonstrated in a placebo-controlled trial (see CLINICAL PHARMACOLOGY—Clinical Trials). Nevertheless, the physician who elects to use PAXIL for extended periods should periodically re-evaluate the long-term usefulness of the drug for the individual patient.

Obsessive Compulsive Disorder: PAXIL is indicated for the treatment of obsessions and compulsions in patients with obsessive compulsive disorder (OCD) as defined in the DSM-IV. The obsessions or compulsions cause marked distress, are time-consuming, or significantly interfere with social or occupational functioning.

The efficacy of PAXIL was established in two 12-week trials with obsessive compulsive outpatients whose diagnoses corresponded most closely to the DSM-IIIR category of obsessive compulsive disorder (see CLINICAL PHARMACOLOGY—Clinical Trials).

Obsessive compulsive disorder is characterized by recurrent and persistent ideas, thoughts, impulses, or images (obsessions) that are ego-dystonic and/or repetitive, purposeful, and intentional behaviors (compulsions) that are recognized by the person as excessive or unreasonable.

Long-term maintenance of efficacy was demonstrated in a 6-month relapse prevention trial. In this trial, patients assigned to paroxetine showed a lower relapse rate compared to patients on placebo (see CLINICAL PHARMACOLOGY—Clinical Trials). Nevertheless, the physician who elects to use PAXIL for extended periods should periodically re-evaluate the long-term usefulness of the drug for the individual patient (see DOSAGE AND ADMINISTRATION).

Panic Disorder: PAXIL is indicated for the treatment of panic disorder, with or without agoraphobia, as defined in DSM-IV. Panic disorder is characterized by the occurrence of unexpected panic attacks and associated concern about having additional attacks, worry about the implications or consequences of the attacks, and/or a significant change in behavior related to the attacks.

The efficacy of PAXIL was established in three 10- to 12-week trials in panic disorder patients whose diagnoses corresponded to the DSM-IIIR category of panic disorder (see CLINICAL PHARMACOLOGY—Clinical Trials).

Panic disorder (DSM-IV) is characterized by recurrent unexpected panic attacks, i.e., a discrete period of intense fear or discomfort in which 4 (or more) of the following symptoms develop abruptly and reach a peak within 10 minutes: (1) palpitations, pounding heart, or accelerated heart rate; (2) sweating; (3) trembling or shaking; (4) sensations of shortness of breath or smothering; (5) feeling of choking; (6) chest pain or discomfort; (7) nausea or abdominal distress; (8) feeling dizzy, unsteady, lightheaded, or faint; (9) derealization (feelings of unreality) or depersonalization (being de-

tached from oneself); (10) fear of losing control; (11) fear of dying; (12) paresthesias (numbness or tingling sensations); (13) chills or hot flushes.

Long-term maintenance of efficacy was demonstrated in a 3-month relapse prevention trial. In this trial, patients with panic disorder assigned to paroxetine demonstrated a lower relapse rate compared to patients on placebo (see CLINICAL PHARMACOLOGY—Clinical Trials). Nevertheless, the physician who prescribes PAXIL for extended periods should periodically re-evaluate the long-term usefulness of the drug for the individual patient.

Social Anxiety Disorder: PAXIL is indicated for the treatment of social anxiety disorder, also known as social phobia, as defined in DSM-IV (300.23). Social anxiety disorder is characterized by a marked and persistent fear of 1 or more social or performance situations in which the person is exposed to unfamiliar people or to possible scrutiny by others. Exposure to the feared situation almost invariably provokes anxiety, which may approach the intensity of a panic attack. The feared situations are avoided or endured with intense anxiety or distress. The avoidance, anxious anticipation, or distress in the feared situation(s) interferes significantly with the person's normal routine, occupational or academic functioning, or social activities or relationships, or there is marked distress about having the phobias. Lesser degrees of performance anxiety or shyness generally do not require psychopharmacological treatment.

The efficacy of PAXIL was established in three 12-week trials in adult patients with social anxiety disorder (DSM-IV). PAXIL has not been studied in children or adolescents with social phobia (see CLINICAL PHARMACOLOGY—Clinical Trials).

The effectiveness of PAXIL in long-term treatment of social anxiety disorder, i.e., for more than 12 weeks, has not been systematically evaluated in adequate and well-controlled trials. Therefore, the physician who elects to prescribe PAXIL for extended periods should periodically re-evaluate the long-term usefulness of the drug for the individual patient (see DOSAGE AND ADMINISTRATION).

Generalized Anxiety Disorder: PAXIL is indicated for the treatment of Generalized Anxiety Disorder (GAD), as defined in DSM-IV. Anxiety or tension associated with the stress of everyday life usually does not require treatment with an anxiolytic.

The efficacy of PAXIL in the treatment of GAD was established in two 8-week placebo-controlled trials in adults with GAD. PAXIL has not been studied in children or adolescents with Generalized Anxiety Disorder (see CLINICAL PHARMACOLOGY—Clinical Trials).

Generalized Anxiety Disorder (DSM-IV) is characterized by excessive anxiety and worry (apprehensive expectation) that is persistent for at least 6 months and which the person finds difficult to control. It must be associated with at least 3 of the following 6 symptoms: Restlessness or feeling keyed up or on edge, being easily fatigued, difficulty concentrating or mind going blank, irritability, muscle tension, sleep disturbance.

The efficacy of PAXIL in maintaining a response in patients with Generalized Anxiety Disorder, who responded during an 8-week acute treatment phase while taking PAXIL and were then observed for relapse during a period of up to 24 weeks, was demonstrated in a placebo-controlled trial (see CLINICAL PHARMACOLOGY—Clinical Trials). Nevertheless, the physician who elects to use PAXIL for extended periods should periodically re-evaluate the long-term usefulness of the drug for the individual patient (see DOSAGE AND ADMINISTRATION).

Posttraumatic Stress Disorder: PAXIL is indicated for the treatment of Posttraumatic Stress Disorder (PTSD).

The efficacy of PAXIL in the treatment of PTSD was established in two 12-week placebo-controlled trials in adults with PTSD (DSM-IV) (see CLINICAL PHARMACOLOGY—Clinical Trials).

PTSD, as defined by DSM-IV, requires exposure to a traumatic event that involved actual or threatened death or serious injury, or threat to the physical integrity of self or others, and a response that involves intense fear, helplessness, or horror. Symptoms that occur as a result of exposure to the traumatic event include reexperiencing of the event in the form of intrusive thoughts, flashbacks or dreams, and intense psychological distress and physiological reactivity on exposure to cues to the event; avoidance of situations reminiscent of the traumatic event, inability to recall details of the event, and/or numbing of general responsiveness manifested as diminished interest in significant activities, estrangement from others, restricted range of affect, or sense of foreshortened future; and symptoms of autonomic arousal including hypervigilance, exaggerated startle response, sleep disturbance, impaired concentration, and irritability or outbursts of anger. A PTSD diagnosis requires that the symptoms are present for at least a month and that they cause clinically significant distress or impairment in social, occupational, or other important areas of functioning. The efficacy of PAXIL in longer-term treatment of PTSD, i.e., for more than 12 weeks, has not been systematically evaluated in placebo-controlled trials. Therefore, the physician who elects to prescribe PAXIL for extended periods should periodically re-evaluate the long-term usefulness of the drug for the individual patient (see DOSAGE AND ADMINISTRATION).

CONTRAINDICATIONS

Concomitant use in patients taking either monoamine oxidase inhibitors (MAOIs) or thioridazine is contraindicated (see WARNINGS and PRECAUTIONS).

Continued on next page

Paxil—Cont.

PAXIL is contraindicated in patients with a hypersensitivity to paroxetine or any of the inactive ingredients in PAXIL.

WARNINGS

Clinical Worsening and Suicide Risk: Patients with major depressive disorder (MDD), both adult and pediatric, may experience worsening of their depression and/or the emergence of suicidal ideation and behavior (suicidality) or unusual changes in behavior, whether or not they are taking antidepressant medications, and this risk may persist until significant remission occurs. There has been a long-standing concern that antidepressants may have a role in inducing worsening of depression and the emergence of suicidality in certain patients. Antidepressants increased the risk of suicidal thinking and behavior (suicidality) in short-term studies in children and adolescents with Major Depressive Disorder (MDD) and other psychiatric disorders.

Pooled analyses of short-term placebo-controlled trials of 9 antidepressant drugs (SSRIs and others) in children and adolescents with MDD, OCD, or other psychiatric disorders (a total of 24 trials involving over 4,400 patients) have revealed a greater risk of adverse events representing suicidal behavior or thinking (suicidality) during the first few months of treatment in those receiving antidepressants. The average risk of such events in patients receiving antidepressants was 4%, twice the placebo risk of 2%. There was considerable variation in risk among drugs, but a tendency toward an increase for almost all drugs studied. The risk of suicidality was most consistently observed in the MDD trials, but there were signals of risk arising from some trials in other psychiatric indications (obsessive compulsive disorder and social anxiety disorder) as well. No suicides occurred in any of these trials. It is unknown whether the suicidality risk in pediatric patients extends to longer-term use, i.e., beyond several months. It is also unknown whether the suicidality risk extends to adults.

All pediatric patients being treated with antidepressants for any indication should be observed closely for clinical worsening, suicidality, and unusual changes in behavior, especially during the initial few months of a course of drug therapy, or at times of dose changes, either increases or decreases. Such observation would generally include at least weekly face-to-face contact with patients or their family members or caregivers during the first 4 weeks of treatment, then every other week visits for the next 4 weeks, then at 12 weeks, and as clinically indicated beyond 12 weeks. Additional contact by telephone may be appropriate between face-to-face visits.

Adults with MDD or co-morbid depression in the setting of other psychiatric illness being treated with antidepressants should be observed similarly for clinical worsening and suicidality, especially during the initial few months of a course of drug therapy, or at times of dose changes, either increases or decreases.

The following symptoms, anxiety, agitation, panic attacks, insomnia, irritability, hostility, aggressiveness, impulsivity, akathisia (psychomotor restlessness), hypomania, and mania, have been reported in adult and pediatric patients being treated with antidepressants for major depressive disorder as well as for other indications, both psychiatric and nonpsychiatric. Although a causal link between the emergence of such symptoms and either the worsening of depression and/or the emergence of suicidal impulses has not been established, there is concern that such symptoms may represent precursors to emerging suicidality.

Consideration should be given to changing the therapeutic regimen, including possibly discontinuing the medication, in patients whose depression is persistently worse, or who are experiencing emergent suicidality or symptoms that might be precursors to worsening depression or suicidality, especially if these symptoms are severe, abrupt in onset, or were not part of the patient's presenting symptoms.

If the decision has been made to discontinue treatment, medication should be tapered, as rapidly as feasible, but with recognition that abrupt discontinuation can be associated with certain symptoms (see PRECAUTIONS and DOSAGE AND ADMINISTRATION—Discontinuation of Treatment With PAXIL, for a description of the risks of discontinuation of PAXIL).

Families and caregivers of pediatric patients being treated with antidepressants for major depressive disorder or other indications, both psychiatric and nonpsychiatric, should be alerted about the need to monitor patients for the emergence of agitation, irritability, unusual changes in behavior, and the other symptoms described above, as well as the emergence of suicidality, and to report such symptoms immediately to health care providers. Such monitoring should include daily observation by families and caregivers. Prescriptions for PAXIL should be written for the smallest quantity of tablets consistent with good patient management, in order to reduce the risk of overdose. Families and caregivers of adults being treated for depression should be similarly advised.

Screening Patients for Bipolar Disorder: A major depressive episode may be initial presentation of bipolar disorder. It is generally believed (though not established in controlled trials) that treating such an episode with an antidepressant alone may increase the likelihood of precipitation of a mixed/manic episode in patients at risk for bipolar disorder. Whether any of the symptoms described above represent such a conversion is unknown. However, prior to initiating with an antidepressant, patients with depressive symptoms should be adequately screened to determine if they are at risk for bipolar disorder; such screening should include a detailed psychiatric history, including a family history of suicide, bipolar disorder, and depression. It should be noted that PAXIL is not approved for use in treating bipolar depression.

Potential for Interaction With Monoamine Oxidase Inhibitors: In patients receiving another serotonin reuptake inhibitor drug in combination with a monoamine oxidase inhibitor (MAOI), there have been reports of serious, sometimes fatal, reactions including hyperthermia, rigidity, myoclonus, autonomic instability with possible rapid fluctuations of vital signs, and mental status changes that include extreme agitation progressing to delirium and coma. These reactions have also been reported in patients who have recently discontinued that drug and have been started on an MAOI. Some cases presented with features resembling neuroleptic malignant syndrome. While there are no human data showing such an interaction with PAXIL, limited animal data on the effects of combined use of paroxetine and MAOIs suggest that these drugs may act synergistically to elevate blood pressure and evoke behavioral excitation. Therefore, it is recommended that PAXIL not be used in combination with an MAOI, or within 14 days of discontinuing treatment with an MAOI. At least 2 weeks should be allowed after stopping PAXIL before starting an MAOI.

Potential Interaction With Thioridazine: Thioridazine administration alone produces prolongation of the QTc interval, which is associated with serious ventricular arrhythmias, such as torsade de pointes–type arrhythmias, and sudden death. This effect appears to be dose related.

An in vivo study suggests that drugs which inhibit $P_{450}IID_6$, such as paroxetine, will elevate plasma levels of thioridazine. Therefore, it is recommended that paroxetine not be used in combination with thioridazine (see CONTRAINDICATIONS and PRECAUTIONS).

PRECAUTIONS

General: *Activation of Mania/Hypomania:* During premarketing testing, hypomania or mania occurred in approximately 1.0% of unipolar patients treated with PAXIL compared to 1.1% of active-control and 0.3% of placebo-treated unipolar patients. In a subset of patients classified as bipolar, the rate of manic episodes was 2.2% for PAXIL and 11.6% for the combined active-control groups. As with all drugs effective in the treatment of major depressive disorder, PAXIL should be used cautiously in patients with a history of mania.

Seizures: During premarketing testing, seizures occurred in 0.1% of patients treated with PAXIL, a rate similar to that associated with other drugs effective in the treatment of major depressive disorder. PAXIL should be used cautiously in patients with a history of seizures. It should be discontinued in any patient who develops seizures.

Discontinuation of Treatment With PAXIL: Recent clinical trials supporting the various approved indications for PAXIL employed a taper-phase regimen, rather than an abrupt discontinuation of treatment. The taper-phase regimen used in GAD and PTSD clinical trials involved an incremental decrease in the daily dose by 10 mg/day at weekly intervals. When a daily dose of 20 mg/day was reached, patients were continued on this dose for 1 week before treatment was stopped.

With this regimen in those studies, the following adverse events were reported at an incidence of 2% or greater for PAXIL and were at least twice that reported for placebo: Abnormal dreams, paresthesia, and dizziness. In the majority of patients, these events were mild to moderate and were self-limiting and did not require medical intervention.

During marketing of PAXIL and other SSRIs and SNRIs (serotonin and norepinephrine reuptake inhibitors), there have been spontaneous reports of adverse events occurring, upon the discontinuation of these drugs (particularly when abrupt), including the following: Dysphoric mood, irritability, agitation, dizziness, sensory disturbances (e.g., paresthesias such as electric shock sensations), anxiety, confusion, headache, lethargy, emotional lability, insomnia, and hypomania. While these events are generally self-limiting, there have been reports of serious discontinuation symptoms.

Patients should be monitored for these symptoms when discontinuing treatment with PAXIL. A gradual reduction in the dose rather than abrupt cessation is recommended whenever possible. If intolerable symptoms occur following a decrease in the dose or upon discontinuation of treatment, then resuming the previously prescribed dose may be considered. Subsequently, the physician may continue decreasing the dose but at a more gradual rate (see DOSAGE AND ADMINISTRATION).

See also PRECAUTIONS—Pediatric Use, for adverse events reported upon discontinuation of treatment with PAXIL in pediatric patients.

Akathisia: The use of paroxetine or other SSRIs has been associated with the development of akathisia, which is characterized by an inner sense of restlessness and psychomotor agitation such as an inability to sit or stand still usually associated with subjective distress. This is most likely to occur within the first few weeks of treatment.

Hyponatremia: Several cases of hyponatremia have been reported. The hyponatremia appeared to be reversible when PAXIL was discontinued. The majority of these occurrences have been in elderly individuals, some in patients taking diuretics or who were otherwise volume depleted.

Serotonin Syndrome: The development of a serotonin syndrome may occur in association with treatment with paroxetine, particularly with concomitant use of serotonergic drugs and with drugs which may have impaired metabolism of paroxetine. Symptoms have included agitation, confusion, diaphoresis, hallucinations, hyperreflexia, myoclonus, shivering, tachycardia, and tremor. The concomitant use of PAXIL with serotonin precursors (such as tryptophan) is not recommended (see WARNINGS—Potential for Interaction with Monoamine Oxidase Inhibitors and PRECAUTIONS—Drug Interactions).

Abnormal Bleeding: Published case reports have documented the occurrence of bleeding episodes in patients treated with psychotropic agents that interfere with serotonin reuptake. Subsequent epidemiological studies, both of the case-control and cohort design, have demonstrated an association between use of psychotropic drugs that interfere with serotonin reuptake and the occurrence of upper gastrointestinal bleeding. In 2 studies, concurrent use of a nonsteroidal anti-inflammatory drug (NSAID) or aspirin potentiated the risk of bleeding (see Drug Interactions). Although these studies focused on upper gastrointestinal bleeding, there is reason to believe that bleeding at other sites may be similarly potentiated. Patients should be cautioned regarding the risk of bleeding associated with the concomitant use of paroxetine with NSAIDs, aspirin, or other drugs that affect coagulation.

Use in Patients With Concomitant Illness: Clinical experience with PAXIL in patients with certain concomitant systemic illness is limited. Caution is advisable in using PAXIL in patients with diseases or conditions that could affect metabolism or hemodynamic responses.

As with other SSRIs, mydriasis has been infrequently reported in premarketing studies with PAXIL. A few cases of acute angle closure glaucoma associated with paroxetine therapy have been reported in the literature. As mydriasis can cause acute angle closure in patients with narrow angle glaucoma, caution should be used when PAXIL is prescribed for patients with narrow angle glaucoma.

PAXIL has not been evaluated or used to any appreciable extent in patients with a recent history of myocardial infarction or unstable heart disease. Patients with these diagnoses were excluded from clinical studies during the product's premarket testing. Evaluation of electrocardiograms of 682 patients who received PAXIL in double-blind, placebo-controlled trials, however, did not indicate that PAXIL is associated with the development of significant ECG abnormalities. Similarly, PAXIL does not cause any clinically important changes in heart rate or blood pressure.

Increased plasma concentrations of paroxetine occur in patients with severe renal impairment (creatinine clearance <30 mL/min.) or severe hepatic impairment. A lower starting dose should be used in such patients (see DOSAGE AND ADMINISTRATION).

Information for Patients: Prescribers or other health professionals should inform patients, their families, and their caregivers about the benefits and risks associated with treatment with PAXIL and should counsel them in its appropriate use. A patient Medication Guide About Using Antidepressants in Children and Teenagers is available for PAXIL. The prescriber or health professional should instruct patients, their families, and their caregivers to read the Medication Guide and should assist them in understanding its contents. Patients should be given the opportunity to discuss the contents of the Medication Guide and to obtain answers to any questions they may have. The complete text of the Medication Guide is reprinted at the end of this document.

Patients should be advised of the following issues and asked to alert their prescriber if these occur while taking PAXIL.

Clinical Worsening and Suicide Risk: Patients, their families, and their caregivers should be encouraged to be alert to the emergence of anxiety, agitation, panic attacks, insomnia, irritability, hostility, aggressiveness, impulsivity, akathisia (psychomotor restlessness), hypomania, mania, other unusual changes in behavior, worsening of depression, and suicidal ideation, especially early during antidepressant treatment and when the dose is adjusted up or down. Families and caregivers of patients should be advised to observe for the emergence of such symptoms on a day-to-day basis, since changes may be abrupt. Such symptoms should be reported to the patient's prescriber or health professional, especially they are severe, abrupt in onset, or were not part of the patient's presenting symptoms. Symptoms such as these may be associated with an increased risk for suicidal thinking and behavior and indicate a need for very close monitoring and possibly changes in the medication.

Drugs That Interfere With Hemostasis (NSAIDs, Aspirin, Warfarin, etc.): Patients should be cautioned about the concomitant use of paroxetine and NSAIDs, aspirin, or other drugs that affect coagulation since the combined use of psychotropic drugs that interfere with serotonin reuptake and these agents has been associated with an increased risk of bleeding.

Interference With Cognitive and Motor Performance: Any psychoactive drug may impair judgment, thinking, or motor skills. Although in controlled studies PAXIL has not been shown to impair psychomotor performance, patients should be cautioned about operating hazardous machinery, including automobiles, until they are reasonably certain that therapy with PAXIL does not affect their ability to engage in such activities.

Completing Course of Therapy: While patients may notice improvement with treatment with PAXIL in 1 to 4 weeks, they should be advised to continue therapy as directed.

Concomitant Medication: Patients should be advised to inform their physician if they are taking, or plan to take, any prescription or over-the-counter drugs, since there is a potential for interactions.

Alcohol: Although PAXIL has not been shown to increase the impairment of mental and motor skills caused by alcohol, patients should be advised to avoid alcohol while taking PAXIL.

Pregnancy: Patients should be advised to notify their physician if they become pregnant or intend to become pregnant during therapy.

Nursing: Patients should be advised to notify their physician if they are breast-feeding an infant (see PRECAUTIONS—Nursing Mothers).

Laboratory Tests: There are no specific laboratory tests recommended.

Drug Interactions: Tryptophan: As with other serotonin re-uptake inhibitors, an interaction between paroxetine and tryptophan may occur when they are coadministered. Adverse experiences, consisting primarily of headache, nausea, sweating, and dizziness, have been reported when tryptophan was administered to patients taking PAXIL. Consequently, concomitant use of PAXIL with tryptophan is not recommended (see Serotonin Syndrome).

Monoamine Oxidase Inhibitors: See CONTRAINDICATIONS and WARNINGS.

Serotonergic Drugs: Based on the mechanism of action of paroxetine and the potential for serotonin syndrome, caution is advised when PAXIL is coadministered with other drugs or agents that may affect the serotonergic neurotransmitter systems, such as tryptophan, triptans, serotonin reuptake inhibitors, linezolid (an antibiotic which is a reversible non-selective MAOI), lithium, tramadol, or St. John's Wort (see Serotonin Syndrome).

Thioridazine: See CONTRAINDICATIONS and WARNINGS.

Warfarin: Preliminary data suggest that there may be a pharmacodynamic interaction (that causes an increased bleeding diathesis in the face of unaltered prothrombin time) between paroxetine and warfarin. Since there is little clinical experience, the concomitant administration of PAXIL and warfarin should be undertaken with caution (see Drugs That Interfere With Hemostasis).

Triptans: There have been rare postmarketing reports describing patients with weakness, hyperreflexia, and incoordination following the use of a selective serotonin reuptake inhibitor (SSRI) and sumatriptan. If concomitant treatment with a triptan and an SSRI (e.g., fluoxetine, fluvoxamine, paroxetine, sertraline) is clinically warranted, appropriate observation of the patient is advised (see Serotonin Syndrome).

Drugs Affecting Hepatic Metabolism: The metabolism and pharmacokinetics of paroxetine may be affected by the induction or inhibition of drug-metabolizing enzymes.

Cimetidine: Cimetidine inhibits many cytochrome P_{450} (oxidative) enzymes. In a study where PAXIL (30 mg once daily) was dosed orally for 4 weeks, steady-state plasma concentrations of paroxetine were increased by approximately 50% during coadministration with oral cimetidine (300 mg three times daily) for the final week. Therefore, when these drugs are administered concurrently, dosage adjustment of PAXIL after the 20-mg starting dose should be guided by clinical effect. The effect of paroxetine on cimetidine's pharmacokinetics was not studied.

Phenobarbital: Phenobarbital induces many cytochrome P_{450} (oxidative) enzymes. When a single oral 30-mg dose of PAXIL was administered at phenobarbital steady state (100 mg once daily for 14 days), paroxetine AUC and $T_{1/2}$ were reduced (by an average of 25% and 38%, respectively) compared to paroxetine administered alone. The effect of paroxetine on phenobarbital pharmacokinetics was not studied. Since PAXIL exhibits nonlinear pharmacokinetics, the results of this study may not address the case where the 2 drugs are both being chronically dosed. No initial dosage adjustment of PAXIL is considered necessary when coadministered with phenobarbital; any subsequent adjustment should be guided by clinical effect.

Phenytoin: When a single oral 30-mg dose of PAXIL was administered at phenytoin steady state (300 mg once daily for 14 days), paroxetine AUC and $T_{1/2}$ were reduced (by an average of 50% and 35%, respectively) compared to PAXIL administered alone. In a separate study, when a single oral 300-mg dose of phenytoin was administered at paroxetine steady state (30 mg once daily for 14 days), phenytoin AUC was slightly reduced (12% on average) compared to phenytoin administered alone. Since both drugs exhibit nonlinear pharmacokinetics, the above studies may not address the case where the 2 drugs are both being chronically dosed. No initial dosage adjustments are considered necessary when these drugs are coadministered; any subsequent adjustments should be guided by clinical effect (see ADVERSE REACTIONS—Postmarketing Reports).

Drugs Metabolized by Cytochrome $P_{450}IID_6$: Many drugs, including most drugs effective in the treatment of major depressive disorder (paroxetine, other SSRIs and many tricyclics), are metabolized by the cytochrome P_{450} isozyme $P_{450}IID_6$. Like other agents that are metabolized by $P_{450}IID_6$, paroxetine may significantly inhibit the activity of this isozyme. In most patients (>90%), this $P_{450}IID_6$ isozyme is saturated early during dosing with PAXIL. In 1 study, daily dosing of PAXIL (20 mg once daily) under steady-state conditions increased single dose desipramine (100 mg) C_{max}, AUC, and $T_{1/2}$ by an average of approximately 2-, 5-, and

3-fold, respectively. Concomitant use of PAXIL with other drugs metabolized by cytochrome $P_{450}IID_6$ has not been formally studied but may require lower doses than usually prescribed for either PAXIL or the other drug.

Therefore, coadministration of PAXIL with other drugs that are metabolized by this isozyme, including certain drugs effective in the treatment of major depressive disorder (e.g., nortriptyline, amitriptyline, imipramine, desipramine, and fluoxetine), phenothiazines, risperidone, and Type 1C antiarrhythmics (e.g., propafenone, flecainide, and encainide), or that inhibit this enzyme (e.g., quinidine), should be approached with caution.

However, due to the risk of serious ventricular arrhythmias and sudden death potentially associated with elevated plasma levels of thioridazine, paroxetine and thioridazine should not be coadministered (see CONTRAINDICATIONS and WARNINGS).

At steady state, when the $P_{450}IID_6$ pathway is essentially saturated, paroxetine clearance is governed by alternative P_{450} isozymes that, unlike $P_{450}IID_6$, show no evidence of saturation (see PRECAUTIONS—Tricyclic Antidepressants).

Drugs Metabolized by Cytochrome $P_{450}IIIA_4$: An in vivo interaction study involving the coadministration under steady-state conditions of paroxetine and terfenadine, a substrate for cytochrome $P_{450}IIIA_4$, revealed no effect of paroxetine on terfenadine pharmacokinetics. In addition, in vitro studies have shown ketoconazole, a potent inhibitor of $P_{450}IIIA_4$ activity, to be at least 100 times more potent than paroxetine as an inhibitor of the metabolism of several substrates for this enzyme, including terfenadine, astemizole, cisapride, triazolam, and cyclosporine. Based on the assumption that the relationship between paroxetine's in vitro K_i and its lack of effect on terfenadine's in vivo clearance predicts its effect on other IIA$_4$ substrates, paroxetine's extent of inhibition of IIIA$_4$ activity is not likely to be of clinical significance.

Tricyclic Antidepressants (TCAs): Caution is indicated in the coadministration of tricyclic antidepressants (TCAs) with PAXIL, because paroxetine may inhibit TCA metabolism. Plasma TCA concentrations may need to be monitored, and the dose of TCA may need to be reduced, if a TCA is coadministered with PAXIL (see PRECAUTIONS—Drugs Metabolized by Cytochrome $P_{450}IID_6$).

Drugs Highly Bound to Plasma Protein: Because paroxetine is highly bound to plasma protein, administration of PAXIL to a patient taking another drug that is highly protein bound may cause increased free concentrations of the other drug, potentially resulting in adverse events. Conversely, adverse effects could result from displacement of paroxetine by other highly bound drugs.

Drugs That Interfere With Hemostasis (NSAIDs, Aspirin, Warfarin, etc.): Serotonin release by platelets plays an important role in hemostasis. Epidemiological studies of the case-control and cohort design that have demonstrated an association between use of psychotropic drugs that interfere with serotonin reuptake and the occurrence of upper gastrointestinal bleeding have also shown that concurrent use of an NSAID or aspirin potentiated the risk of bleeding. Thus, patients should be cautioned about the use of such drugs concurrently with paroxetine.

Alcohol: Although PAXIL does not increase the impairment of mental and motor skills caused by alcohol, patients should be advised to avoid alcohol while taking PAXIL.

Lithium: A multiple-dose study has shown that there is no pharmacokinetic interaction between PAXIL and lithium carbonate. However, due to the potential for serotonin syndrome, caution is advised when PAXIL is coadministered with lithium.

Digoxin: The steady-state pharmacokinetics of paroxetine was not altered when administered with digoxin at steady state. Mean digoxin AUC at steady state decreased by 15% in the presence of paroxetine. Since there is little clinical experience, the concurrent administration of paroxetine and digoxin should be undertaken with caution.

Diazepam: Under steady-state conditions, diazepam does not appear to affect paroxetine kinetics. The effects of paroxetine on diazepam were not evaluated.

Procyclidine: Daily oral dosing of PAXIL (30 mg once daily) increased steady-state AUC_{0-24}, C_{max}, and C_{min} values of procyclidine (5 mg oral once daily) by 35%, 37%, and 67%, respectively, compared to procyclidine alone at steady state. If anticholinergic effects are seen, the dose of procyclidine should be reduced.

Beta-Blockers: In a study where propranolol (80 mg twice daily) was dosed orally for 18 days, the established steady-state plasma concentrations of propranolol were unaltered during coadministration with PAXIL (30 mg once daily) for the final 10 days. The effects of propranolol on paroxetine have not been evaluated (see ADVERSE REACTIONS—Postmarketing Reports).

Theophylline: Reports of elevated theophylline levels associated with treatment with PAXIL have been reported. While this interaction has not been formally studied, it is recommended that theophylline levels be monitored when these drugs are concurrently administered.

Electroconvulsive Therapy (ECT): There are no clinical studies of the combined use of ECT and PAXIL.

Carcinogenesis, Mutagenesis, Impairment of Fertility:
Carcinogenesis: Two-year carcinogenicity studies were conducted in rodents given paroxetine in the diet at 1, 5, and 25 mg/kg/day (mice) and 1, 5, and 20 mg/kg/day (rats). These doses are up to 2.4 (mouse) and 3.9 (rat) times the maximum recommended human dose (MRHD) for major depressive disorder, social anxiety disorder, GAD, and PTSD

on a mg/m^2 basis. Because the MRHD for major depressive disorder is slightly less than that for OCD (50 mg versus 60 mg), the doses used in these carcinogenicity studies were only 2.0 (mouse) and 3.2 (rat) times the MRHD for OCD. There was a significantly greater number of male rats in the high-dose group with reticulum cell sarcomas (1/100, 0/50, 0/50, and 4/50 for control, low-, middle-, and high-dose groups, respectively) and a significantly increased linear trend across dose groups for the occurrence of lymphoreticular tumors in male rats. Female rats were not affected. Although there was a dose-related increase in the number of tumors in mice, there was no drug-related increase in the number of mice with tumors. The relevance of these findings to humans is unknown.

Mutagenesis: Paroxetine produced no genotoxic effects in a battery of 5 in vitro and 2 in vivo assays that included the following: Bacterial mutation assay, mouse lymphoma mutation assay, unscheduled DNA synthesis assay, and tests for cytogenetic aberrations in vivo in mouse bone marrow and in vitro in human lymphocytes and in a dominant lethal test in rats.

Impairment of Fertility: A reduced pregnancy rate was found in reproduction studies in rats at a dose of paroxetine of 15 mg/kg/day, which is 2.9 times the MRHD for major depressive disorder, social anxiety disorder, GAD, and PTSD or 2.4 times the MRHD for OCD on a mg/m^2 basis. Irreversible lesions occurred in the reproductive tract of male rats after dosing in toxicity studies for 2 to 52 weeks. These lesions consisted of vacuolation of epididymal tubular epithelium at 50 mg/kg/day and atrophic changes in the seminiferous tubules of the testes with arrested spermatogenesis at 25 mg/kg/day (9.8 and 4.9 times the MRHD for major depressive disorder, social anxiety disorder, and GAD; 8.2 and 4.1 times the MRHD for OCD and PD on a mg/m^2 basis).

Pregnancy: *Teratogenic Effects:* Pregnancy Category C. Reproduction studies were performed at doses up to 50 mg/kg/day in rats and 6 mg/kg/day in rabbits administered during organogenesis. These doses are equivalent to 9.7 (rat) and 2.2 (rabbit) times the maximum recommended human dose (MRHD) for major depressive disorder, social anxiety disorder, GAD, and PTSD (50 mg) and 8.1 (rat) and 1.9 (rabbit) times the MRHD for OCD, on an mg/m^2 basis. These studies have revealed no evidence of teratogenic effects. However, in rats, there was an increase in pup deaths during the first 4 days of lactation when dosing occurred during the last trimester of gestation and continued throughout lactation. This effect occurred at a dose of 1 mg/kg/day or 0.19 times (mg/m^2) the MRHD for major depressive disorder, social anxiety disorder, GAD, and PTSD; and at 0.16 times (mg/m^2) the MRHD for OCD. The no-effect dose for rat pup mortality was not determined. The cause of these deaths is not known. There are no adequate and well-controlled studies in pregnant women. Because animal reproduction studies are not always predictive of human response, this drug should be used during pregnancy only if the potential benefit justifies the potential risk to the fetus.

Nonteratogenic Effects: Neonates exposed to PAXIL and other SSRIs or SNRIs, late in the third trimester have developed complications requiring prolonged hospitalization, respiratory support, and tube feeding. Such complications can arise immediately upon delivery. Reported clinical findings have included respiratory distress, cyanosis, apnea, seizures, temperature instability, feeding difficulty, vomiting, hypoglycemia, hypotonia, hypertonia, hyperreflexia, tremor, jitteriness, irritability, and constant crying. These features are consistent with either a direct toxic effect of SSRIs and SNRIs or, possibly, a drug discontinuation syndrome. It should be noted, in some cases, the clinical picture is consistent with serotonin syndrome (see WARNINGS—Potential for Interaction With Monoamine Oxidase Inhibitors).

There have also been postmarketing reports of premature births in pregnant women exposed to paroxetine or other SSRIs.

When treating a pregnant woman with paroxetine during the third trimester, the physician should carefully consider the potential risks and benefits of treatment (see DOSAGE AND ADMINISTRATION).

Labor and Delivery: The effect of paroxetine on labor and delivery in humans is unknown.

Nursing Mothers: Like many other drugs, paroxetine is secreted in human milk, and caution should be exercised when PAXIL is administered to a nursing woman.

Pediatric Use: Safety and effectiveness in the pediatric population have not been established (see BOX WARNING and WARNINGS—Clinical Worsening and Suicide Risk). Three placebo-controlled trials in 752 pediatric patients with MDD have been conducted with PAXIL, and the data were not sufficient to support a claim for use in pediatric patients. Anyone considering the use of PAXIL in a child or adolescent must balance the potential risks with the clinical need.

In placebo-controlled clinical trials conducted with pediatric patients, the following adverse events were reported in at least 2% of pediatric patients treated with PAXIL and occurred at a rate at least twice that for pediatric patients receiving placebo: emotional lability (including self-harm, suicidal thoughts, attempted suicide, crying, and mood fluctuations), hostility, decreased appetite, tremor, sweating, hyperkinesia, and agitation.

Continued on next page

Paxil—Cont.

Events reported upon discontinuation of treatment with PAXIL in the pediatric clinical trials that included a taper phase regimen, which occurred in at least 2% of patients who received PAXIL and which occurred at a rate at least twice that of placebo, were: emotional lability (including suicidal ideation, suicide attempt, mood changes, and tearfulness), nervousness, dizziness, nausea, and abdominal pain (see Discontinuation of Treatment With PAXIL).

Geriatric Use: In worldwide premarketing clinical trials with PAXIL, 17% of patients treated with PAXIL (approximately 700) were 65 years of age or older. Pharmacokinetic studies revealed a decreased clearance in the elderly, and a lower starting dose is recommended; there were, however, no overall differences in the adverse event profile between elderly and younger patients, and effectiveness was similar in younger and older patients (see CLINICAL PHARMACOLOGY and DOSAGE AND ADMINISTRATION).

ADVERSE REACTIONS

Associated With Discontinuation of Treatment: Twenty percent (1,199/6,145) of patients treated with PAXIL in worldwide clinical trials in major depressive disorder and 16.1% (84/522), 11.8% (64/542), 9.4% (44/469), 10.7% (79/735), and 11.7% (79/676) of patients treated with PAXIL in worldwide trials in social anxiety disorder, OCD, panic disorder, GAD, and PTSD, respectively, discontinued treatment due to an adverse event. The most common events (≥1%) associated with discontinuation and considered to be drug related (i.e., those events associated with dropout at a rate approximately twice or greater for PAXIL compared to placebo) included the following:

[See first table at right]

Commonly Observed Adverse Events: *Major Depressive Disorder:* The most commonly observed adverse events associated with the use of paroxetine (incidence of 5% or greater and incidence for PAXIL at least twice that for placebo, derived from Table 1) were: Asthenia, sweating, nausea, decreased appetite, somnolence, dizziness, insomnia, tremor, nervousness, ejaculatory disturbance, and other male genital disorders.

Obsessive Compulsive Disorder: The most commonly observed adverse events associated with the use of paroxetine (incidence of 5% or greater and incidence for PAXIL at least twice that of placebo, derived from Table 2) were: Nausea, dry mouth, decreased appetite, constipation, dizziness, somnolence, tremor, sweating, impotence, and abnormal ejaculation.

Panic Disorder: The most commonly observed adverse events associated with the use of paroxetine (incidence of 5% or greater and incidence for PAXIL at least twice that for placebo, derived from Table 2) were: Asthenia, sweating, decreased appetite, libido decreased, tremor, abnormal ejaculation, female genital disorders, and impotence.

Social Anxiety Disorder: The most commonly observed adverse events associated with the use of paroxetine (incidence of 5% or greater and incidence for PAXIL at least twice that for placebo, derived from Table 2) were: Sweating, nausea, dry mouth, constipation, decreased appetite, somnolence, tremor, libido decreased, yawn, abnormal ejaculation, female genital disorders, and impotence.

Generalized Anxiety Disorder: The most commonly observed adverse events associated with the use of paroxetine (incidence of 5% or greater and incidence for PAXIL at least twice that for placebo, derived from Table 3) were: Asthenia, infection, constipation, decreased appetite, dry mouth, nausea, libido decreased, somnolence, tremor, sweating, and abnormal ejaculation.

Posttraumatic Stress Disorder: The most commonly observed adverse events associated with the use of paroxetine (incidence of 5% or greater and incidence for PAXIL at least twice that for placebo, derived from Table 3) were: Asthenia, sweating, nausea, dry mouth, diarrhea, decreased appetite, somnolence, libido decreased, abnormal ejaculation, female genital disorders, and impotence.

Incidence in Controlled Clinical Trials: The prescriber should be aware that the figures in the tables following cannot be used to predict the incidence of side effects in the course of usual medical practice where patient characteristics and other factors differ from those that prevailed in the clinical trials. Similarly, the cited frequencies cannot be compared with figures obtained from other clinical investigations involving different treatments, uses, and investigators. The cited figures, however, do provide the prescribing physician with some basis for estimating the relative contribution of drug and nondrug factors to the side effect incidence rate in the populations studied.

Major Depressive Disorder: Table 1 enumerates adverse events that occurred at an incidence of 1% or more among paroxetine-treated patients who participated in short-term (6-week) placebo-controlled trials in which patients were dosed in a range of 20 mg to 50 mg/day. Reported adverse events were classified using a standard COSTART-based Dictionary terminology.

[See table 1 at right]

Obsessive Compulsive Disorder, Panic Disorder, and Social Anxiety Disorder: Table 2 enumerates adverse events that occurred at a frequency of 2% or more among OCD patients on PAXIL who participated in placebo-controlled trials of 12-weeks duration in which patients were dosed in a range of 20 mg to 60 mg/day or among patients with panic disorder on PAXIL who participated in placebo-controlled trials of 10- to 12-weeks duration in which patients were dosed in a range of 10 mg to 60 mg/day or among patients with social anxiety disorder on PAXIL who participated in placebo-controlled trials of 12-weeks duration in which patients were dosed in a range of 20 mg to 50 mg/day.

	Major Depressive Disorder		OCD		Panic Disorder		Social Anxiety Disorder		Generalized Anxiety Disorder		PTSD	
	PAXIL	Placebo	PAXIL	Placebo	PAXIL	Placebo	PAXIL	Placebo	PAXIL	Placebo	PAXIL	Placebo
CNS												
Somnolence	2.3%	0.7%	—		1.9%	0.3%	3.4%	0.3%	2.0%	0.2%	2.8%	0.6%
Insomnia	—	—	1.7%	0%	1.3%	0.3%	3.1%	0%	—	—	—	—
Agitation	1.1%	0.5%	—								—	—
Tremor	1.1%	0.3%	—				1.7%	0%			1.0%	0.2%
Anxiety	—	—	—				1.1%	0%			—	—
Dizziness	—	—	1.5%	0%			1.9%	0%	1.0%	0.2%	—	—
Gastrointestinal												
Constipation	—	—	1.1%	0%							—	—
Nausea	3.2%	1.1%	1.9%	0%	3.2%	1.2%	4.0%	0.3%	2.0%	0.2%	2.2%	0.6%
Diarrhea	1.0%	0.3%	—								—	—
Dry mouth	1.0%	0.3%	—								—	—
Vomiting	1.0%	0.3%	—				1.0%	0%			—	—
Flatulence	—	—	—				1.0%	0.3%			—	—
Other												
Asthenia	1.6%	0.4%	1.9%	0.4%			2.5%	0.6%	1.8%	0.2%	1.6%	0.2%
Abnormal ejaculation[1]	1.6%	0%	2.1%	0%			4.9%	0.6%	2.5%	0.5%	—	—
Sweating	1.0%	0.3%	—				1.1%	0%	1.1%	0.2%	—	—
Impotence[1]	—	—	1.5%	0%							—	—
Libido Decreased	—	—	—				1.0%	0%			—	—

Where numbers are not provided the incidence of the adverse events in patients treated with PAXIL was not >1% or was not greater than or equal to 2 times the incidence of placebo.
1. Incidence corrected for gender.

Table 1. Treatment-Emergent Adverse Experience Incidence in Placebo-Controlled Clinical Trials for Major Depressive Disorder[1]

Body System	Preferred Term	PAXIL (n = 421)	Placebo (n = 421)
Body as a Whole	Headache	18%	17%
	Asthenia	15%	6%
Cardiovascular	Palpitation	3%	1%
	Vasodilation	3%	1%
Dermatologic	Sweating	11%	2%
	Rash	2%	1%
Gastrointestinal	Nausea	26%	9%
	Dry Mouth	18%	12%
	Constipation	14%	9%
	Diarrhea	12%	8%
	Decreased Appetite	6%	2%
	Flatulence	4%	2%
	Oropharynx Disorder[2]	2%	0%
	Dyspepsia	2%	1%
Musculoskeletal	Myopathy	2%	1%
	Myalgia	2%	1%
	Myasthenia	1%	0%
Nervous System	Somnolence	23%	9%
	Dizziness	13%	6%
	Insomnia	13%	6%
	Tremor	8%	2%
	Nervousness	5%	3%
	Anxiety	5%	3%
	Paresthesia	4%	2%
	Libido Decreased	3%	0%
	Drugged Feeling	2%	1%
	Confusion	1%	0%
Respiration	Yawn	4%	0%
Special Senses	Blurred Vision	4%	1%
	Taste Perversion	2%	0%
Urogenital System	Ejaculatory Disturbance[3,4]	13%	0%
	Other Male Genital Disorders[3,5]	10%	0%
	Urinary Frequency	3%	1%
	Urination Disorder[6]	3%	0%
	Female Genital Disorders[3,7]	2%	0%

1. Events reported by at least 1% of patients treated with PAXIL are included, except the following events which had an incidence on placebo ≥ PAXIL: Abdominal pain, agitation, back pain, chest pain, CNS stimulation, fever, increased appetite, myoclonus, pharyngitis, postural hypotension, respiratory disorder (includes mostly "cold symptoms" or "URI"), trauma, and vomiting.
2. Includes mostly "lump in throat" and "tightness in throat."
3. Percentage corrected for gender.
4. Mostly "ejaculatory delay."
5. Includes "anorgasmia," "erectile difficulties," "delayed ejaculation/orgasm," and "sexual dysfunction," and "impotence."
6. Includes mostly "difficulty with micturition" and "urinary hesitancy."
7. Includes mostly "anorgasmia" and "difficulty reaching climax/orgasm."

[See table 2 on next page]

Generalized Anxiety Disorder and Posttraumatic Stress Disorder: Table 3 enumerates adverse events that occurred at a frequency of 2% or more among GAD patients on PAXIL who participated in placebo-controlled trials of 8-weeks duration in which patients were dosed in a range of 10 mg/day to 50 mg/day or among PTSD patients on PAXIL who participated in placebo-controlled trials of 12-weeks duration in which patients were dosed in a range of 20 mg/day to 50 mg/day.

[See table 3 at top of page 204]

Dose Dependency of Adverse Events: A comparison of adverse event rates in a fixed-dose study comparing 10, 20, 30, and 40 mg/day of PAXIL with placebo in the treatment of major depressive disorder revealed a clear dose dependency for some of the more common adverse events associated with use of PAXIL, as shown in the following table:

[See table 4 on next page]

In a fixed-dose study comparing placebo and 20, 40, and 60 mg of PAXIL in the treatment of OCD, there was no clear relationship between adverse events and the dose of PAXIL to which patients were assigned. No new adverse events were observed in the group treated with 60 mg of PAXIL compared to any of the other treatment groups.

In a fixed-dose study comparing placebo and 10, 20, and 40 mg of PAXIL in the treatment of panic disorder, there was no clear relationship between adverse events and the dose of PAXIL to which patients were assigned, except for asthenia, dry mouth, anxiety, libido decreased, tremor, and abnormal ejaculation. In flexible-dose studies, no new adverse events were observed in patients receiving 60 mg of PAXIL compared to any of the other treatment groups.

In a fixed-dose study comparing placebo and 20, 40, and 60 mg of PAXIL in the treatment of social anxiety disorder, for most of the adverse events, there was no clear relationship between adverse events and the dose of PAXIL to which patients were assigned.

In a fixed-dose study comparing placebo and 20 and 40 mg of PAXIL in the treatment of generalized anxiety disorder, for most of the adverse events, there was no clear relationship between adverse events and the dose of PAXIL to which patients were assigned, except for the following adverse events: Asthenia, constipation, and abnormal ejaculation.

In a fixed-dose study comparing placebo and 20 and 40 mg of PAXIL in the treatment of posttraumatic stress disorder, for most of the adverse events, there was no clear relationship between adverse events and the dose of PAXIL to which patients were assigned, except for impotence and abnormal ejaculation.

Adaptation to Certain Adverse Events: Over a 4- to 6-week period, there was evidence of adaptation to some adverse events with continued therapy (e.g., nausea and dizziness), but less to other effects (e.g., dry mouth, somnolence, and asthenia).

Male and Female Sexual Dysfunction With SSRIs: Although changes in sexual desire, sexual performance, and sexual satisfaction often occur as manifestations of a psychiatric disorder, they may also be a consequence of pharmacologic treatment. In particular, some evidence suggests that selective serotonin reuptake inhibitors (SSRIs) can cause such untoward sexual experiences.

Reliable estimates of the incidence and severity of untoward experiences involving sexual desire, performance, and satisfaction are difficult to obtain, however, in part because patients and physicians may be reluctant to discuss them. Accordingly, estimates of the incidence of untoward sexual experience and performance cited in product labeling, are likely to underestimate their actual incidence.

In placebo-controlled clinical trials involving more than 3,200 patients, the ranges for the reported incidence of sexual side effects in males and females with major depressive disorder, OCD, panic disorder, social anxiety disorder, GAD, and PTSD are displayed in Table 5.

Table 2. Treatment-Emergent Adverse Experience Incidence in Placebo-Controlled Clinical Trials for Obsessive Compulsive Disorder, Panic Disorder, and Social Anxiety Disorder[1]

		Obsessive Compulsive Disorder		Panic Disorder		Social Anxiety Disorder	
Body System	**Preferred Term**	**PAXIL (n = 542)**	**Placebo (n = 265)**	**PAXIL (n = 469)**	**Placebo (n = 324)**	**PAXIL (n = 425)**	**Placebo (n = 339)**
Body as a Whole	Asthenia	22%	14%	14%	5%	22%	14%
	Abdominal Pain	—	—	4%	3%	—	—
	Chest Pain	3%	2%	—	—	—	—
	Back Pain	—	—	3%	2%	—	—
	Chills	2%	1%	2%	1%	—	—
	Trauma	—	—	—	—	3%	1%
Cardiovascular	Vasodilation	4%	1%	—	—	—	—
	Palpitation	2%	0%	—	—	—	—
Dermatologic	Sweating	9%	3%	14%	6%	9%	2%
	Rash	3%	2%	—	—	—	—
Gastrointestinal	Nausea	23%	10%	23%	17%	25%	7%
	Dry Mouth	18%	9%	18%	11%	9%	3%
	Constipation	16%	6%	8%	5%	5%	2%
	Diarrhea	10%	10%	12%	7%	9%	6%
	Decreased Appetite	9%	3%	7%	3%	8%	2%
	Dyspepsia	—	—	—	—	4%	2%
	Flatulence	—	—	—	—	4%	2%
	Increased Appetite	4%	3%	2%	1%	—	—
	Vomiting	—	—	—	—	2%	1%
Musculoskeletal	Myalgia	—	—	—	—	4%	3%
Nervous System	Insomnia	24%	13%	18%	10%	21%	16%
	Somnolence	24%	7%	19%	11%	22%	5%
	Dizziness	12%	6%	14%	10%	11%	7%
	Tremor	11%	1%	9%	1%	9%	1%
	Nervousness	9%	8%	—	—	8%	7%
	Libido Decreased	7%	4%	9%	1%	12%	1%
	Agitation	—	—	5%	4%	3%	1%
	Anxiety	—	—	5%	4%	5%	4%
	Abnormal Dreams	4%	1%	—	—	—	—
	Concentration Impaired	3%	2%	—	—	4%	1%
	Depersonalization	3%	0%	—	—	—	—
	Myoclonus	3%	0%	3%	2%	2%	1%
	Amnesia	2%	1%	—	—	—	—
Respiratory System	Rhinitis	—	—	3%	0%	—	—
	Pharyngitis	—	—	—	—	4%	2%
	Yawn	—	—	—	—	5%	1%
Special Senses	Abnormal Vision	4%	2%	—	—	4%	1%
	Taste Perversion	2%	0%	—	—	—	—
Urogenital System	Abnormal Ejaculation[2]	23%	1%	21%	1%	28%	1%
	Dysmenorrhea	—	—	—	—	5%	4%
	Female Genital Disorder[2]	3%	0%	9%	1%	9%	1%
	Impotence[2]	8%	1%	5%	0%	5%	1%
	Urinary Frequency	3%	1%	2%	0%	—	—
	Urination Impaired	3%	0%	—	—	—	—
	Urinary Tract Infection	2%	1%	2%	1%	—	—

1. Events reported by at least 2% of OCD, panic disorder, and social anxiety disorder in patients treated with PAXIL are included, except the following events which had an incidence on placebo ≥PAXIL: [OCD]: Abdominal pain, agitation, anxiety, back pain, cough increased, depression, headache, hyperkinesia, infection, paresthesia, pharyngitis, respiratory disorder, rhinitis, and sinusitis. [panic disorder]: Abnormal dreams, abnormal vision, chest pain, cough increased, depersonalization, depression, dysmenorrhea, dyspepsia, flu syndrome, headache, infection, myalgia, nervousness, palpitation, paresthesia, pharyngitis, rash, respiratory disorder, sinusitis, taste perversion, trauma, urination impaired, and vasodilation. [social anxiety disorder]: Abdominal pain, depression, headache, infection, respiratory disorder, and sinusitis.
2. Percentage corrected for gender.

[See table 5 at top of page 205]

There are no adequate and well-controlled studies examining sexual dysfunction with paroxetine treatment.

Paroxetine treatment has been associated with several cases of priapism. In those cases with a known outcome, patients recovered without sequelae.

While it is difficult to know the precise risk of sexual dysfunction associated with the use of SSRIs, physicians should routinely inquire about such possible side effects.

Weight and Vital Sign Changes: Significant weight loss may be an undesirable result of treatment with PAXIL for some patients but, on average, patients in controlled trials had minimal (about 1 pound) weight loss versus smaller changes on placebo and active control. No significant changes in vital signs (systolic and diastolic blood pressure, pulse and temperature) were observed in patients treated with PAXIL in controlled clinical trials.

ECG Changes: In an analysis of ECGs obtained in 682 patients treated with PAXIL and 415 patients treated with placebo in controlled clinical trials, no clinically significant changes were seen in the ECGs of either group.

Liver Function Tests: In placebo-controlled clinical trials, patients treated with PAXIL exhibited abnormal values on liver function tests at no greater rate than that seen in placebo-treated patients. In particular, the PAXIL-versus-placebo comparisons for alkaline phosphatase, SGOT, SGPT, and bilirubin revealed no differences in the percentage of patients with marked abnormalities.

Other Events Observed During the Premarketing Evaluation of PAXIL: During its premarketing assessment in major depressive disorder, multiple doses of PAXIL were administered to 6,145 patients in phase 2 and 3 studies. The conditions and duration of exposure to PAXIL varied greatly and included (in overlapping categories) open and double-blind studies, uncontrolled and controlled studies, inpatient and outpatient studies, and fixed-dose, and titration studies. During premarketing clinical trials in OCD, panic disorder, social anxiety disorder, generalized anxiety disorder, and posttraumatic stress disorder, 542, 469, 522, 735, and 676 patients, respectively, received multiple doses of PAXIL. Untoward events associated with this exposure were recorded by clinical investigators using terminology of their own choosing. Consequently, it is not possible to provide a meaningful estimate of the proportion of individuals experiencing adverse events without first grouping similar types of untoward events into a smaller number of standardized event categories.

In the tabulations that follow, reported adverse events were classified using a standard COSTART-based Dictionary terminology. The frequencies presented, therefore, represent the proportion of the 9,089 patients exposed to multiple doses of PAXIL who experienced an event of the type cited on at least 1 occasion while receiving PAXIL. All reported events are included except those already listed in Tables 1 to 3, those reported in terms so general as to be uninformative and those events where a drug cause was remote. It is important to emphasize that although the events reported occurred during treatment with paroxetine, they were not necessarily caused by it.

Events are further categorized by body system and listed in order of decreasing frequency according to the following definitions: Frequent adverse events are those occurring on 1 or more occasions in at least 1/100 patients (only those not already listed in the tabulated results from placebo-controlled trials appear in this listing); infrequent adverse events are those occurring in 1/100 to 1/1,000 patients; rare events are those occurring in fewer than 1/1,000 patients. Events of major clinical importance are also described in the PRECAUTIONS section.

Body as a Whole: *Infrequent:* Allergic reaction, chills, face edema, malaise, neck pain; *rare:* Adrenergic syndrome, cellulitis, moniliasis, neck rigidity, pelvic pain, peritonitis, sepsis, ulcer.

Cardiovascular System: *Frequent:* Hypertension, tachycardia; *infrequent:* Bradycardia, hematoma, hypotension, migraine, syncope; *rare:* Angina pectoris, arrhythmia nodal, atrial fibrillation, bundle branch block, cerebral ischemia, cerebrovascular accident, congestive heart failure, heart block, low cardiac output, myocardial infarct, myocardial ischemia, pallor, phlebitis, pulmonary embolus, supraventricular extrasystoles, thrombophlebitis, thrombosis, varicose vein, vascular headache, ventricular extrasystoles.

Digestive System: *Infrequent:* Bruxism, colitis, dysphagia, eructation, gastritis, gastroenteritis, gingivitis, glossitis, increased salivation, liver function tests abnormal, rectal hemorrhage, ulcerative stomatitis; *rare:* Aphthous stomatitis, bloody diarrhea, bulimia, cardiospasm, cholelithiasis, duodenitis, enteritis, esophagitis, fecal impactions, fecal incontinence, gum hemorrhage, hematemesis, hepatitis, ileitis, ileus, intestinal obstruction, jaundice, melena, mouth ulceration, peptic ulcer, salivary gland enlargement, sialadenitis, stomach ulcer, stomatitis, tongue discoloration, tongue edema, tooth caries.

Endocrine System: *Rare:* Diabetes mellitus, goiter, hyperthyroidism, hypothyroidism, thyroiditis.

Hemic and Lymphatic Systems: *Infrequent:* Anemia, leukopenia, lymphadenopathy, purpura; *rare:* Abnormal eryth-

Continued on next page

Paxil—Cont.

rocytes, basophilia, bleeding time increased, eosinophilia, hypochromic anemia, iron deficiency anemia, leukocytosis, lymphedema, abnormal lymphocytes, lymphocytosis, microcytic anemia, monocytosis, normocytic anemia, thrombocythemia, thrombocytopenia.

Metabolic and Nutritional: *Frequent:* Weight gain; *infrequent:* Edema, peripheral edema, SGOT increased, SGPT increased, thirst, weight loss; *rare:* Alkaline phosphatase increased, bilirubinemia, BUN increased, creatinine phosphokinase increased, dehydration, gamma globulins increased, gout, hypercalcemia, hypercholesteremia, hyperglycemia, hyperkalemia, hyperphosphatemia, hypocalcemia, hypoglycemia, hypokalemia, hyponatremia, ketosis, lactic dehydrogenase increased, non-protein nitrogen (NPN) increased.

Musculoskeletal System: *Frequent:* Arthralgia; *infrequent:* Arthritis, arthrosis; *rare:* Bursitis, myositis, osteoporosis, generalized spasm, tenosynovitis, tetany.

Nervous System: *Frequent:* Emotional lability, vertigo; *infrequent:* Abnormal thinking, alcohol abuse, ataxia, dystonia, dyskinesia, euphoria, hallucinations, hostility, hypertonia, hypesthesia, hypokinesia, incoordination, lack of emotion, libido increased, manic reaction, neurosis, paralysis, paranoid reaction; *rare:* Abnormal gait, akinesia, antisocial reaction, aphasia, choreoathetosis, circumoral paresthesias, convulsion, delirium, delusions, diplopia, drug dependence, dysarthria, extrapyramidal syndrome, fasciculations, grand mal convulsion, hyperalgesia, hysteria, manic-depressive reaction, meningitis, myelitis, neuralgia, neuropathy, nystagmus, peripheral neuritis, psychotic depression, psychosis, reflexes decreased, reflexes increased, stupor, torticollis, trismus, withdrawal syndrome.

Respiratory System: *Infrequent:* Asthma, bronchitis, dyspnea, epistaxis, hyperventilation, pneumonia, respiratory flu; *rare:* Emphysema, hemoptysis, hiccups, lung fibrosis, pulmonary edema, sputum increased, stridor, voice alteration.

Skin and Appendages: *Frequent:* Pruritus; *infrequent:* Acne, alopecia, contact dermatitis, dry skin, ecchymosis, eczema, herpes simplex, photosensitivity, urticaria; *rare:* Angioedema, erythema nodosum, erythema multiforme, exfoliative dermatitis, fungal dermatitis, furunculosis; herpes zoster, hirsutism, maculopapular rash, seborrhea, skin discoloration, skin hypertrophy, skin ulcer, sweating decreased, vesiculobullous rash.

Special Senses: *Frequent:* Tinnitus; *infrequent:* Abnormality of accommodation, conjunctivitis, ear pain, eye pain, keratoconjunctivitis, mydriasis, otitis media; *rare:* Amblyopia, anisocoria, blepharitis, cataract, conjunctival edema, corneal ulcer, deafness, exophthalmos, eye hemorrhage, glaucoma, hyperacusis, night blindness, otitis externa, parosmia, photophobia, ptosis, retinal hemorrhage, taste loss, visual field defect.

Urogenital System: *Infrequent:* Amenorrhea, breast pain, cystitis, dysuria, hematuria, menorrhagia, nocturia, polyuria, pyuria, urinary incontinence, urinary retention, urinary urgency, vaginitis; *rare:* Abortion, breast atrophy, breast enlargement, endometrial disorder, epididymitis, female lactation, fibrocystic breast, kidney calculus, kidney pain, leukorrhea, mastitis, metrorrhagia, nephritis, oliguria, salpingitis, urethritis, urinary casts, uterine spasm, urolith, vaginal hemorrhage, vaginal moniliasis.

Postmarketing Reports: Voluntary reports of adverse events in patients taking PAXIL that have been received since market introduction and not listed above that may have no causal relationship with the drug include acute pancreatitis, elevated liver function tests (the most severe cases were deaths due to liver necrosis, and grossly elevated transaminases associated with severe liver dysfunction), Guillain-Barré syndrome, toxic epidermal necrolysis, priapism, syndrome of inappropriate ADH secretion, symptoms suggestive of prolactinemia and galactorrhea, neuroleptic malignant syndrome-like events, serotonin syndrome; extrapyramidal symptoms which have included akathisia, bradykinesia, cogwheel rigidity, dystonia, hypertonia, oculogyric crisis which has been associated with concomitant use of pimozide; tremor and trismus; status epilepticus, acute renal failure, pulmonary hypertension, allergic alveolitis, anaphylaxis, eclampsia, laryngismus, optic neuritis, porphyria, ventricular fibrillation, ventricular tachycardia (including torsade de pointes), thrombocytopenia, hemolytic anemia, events related to impaired hematopoiesis (including aplastic anemia, pancytopenia, bone marrow aplasia, and agranulocytosis), and vasculitic syndromes (such as Henoch-Schönlein purpura). There has been a case report of an elevated phenytoin level after 4 weeks of PAXIL and phenytoin coadministration. There has been a case report of severe hypotension when PAXIL was added to chronic metoprolol treatment.

DRUG ABUSE AND DEPENDENCE

Controlled Substance Class: PAXIL is not a controlled substance.

Physical and Psychologic Dependence: PAXIL has not been systematically studied in animals or humans for its potential for abuse, tolerance or physical dependence. While the clinical trials did not reveal any tendency for any drug-seeking behavior, these observations were not systematic and it is not possible to predict on the basis of this limited experience the extent to which a CNS-active drug will be misused, diverted, and/or abused once marketed. Consequently, patients should be evaluated carefully for history of drug abuse, and such patients should be observed closely for signs of misuse or abuse of PAXIL (e.g., development of tolerance, incrementations of dose, drug-seeking behavior).

Table 3. Treatment-Emergent Adverse Experience Incidence in Placebo-Controlled Clinical Trials for Generalized Anxiety Disorder and Posttraumatic Stress Disorder[1]

Body System	Preferred Term	Generalized Anxiety Disorder		Posttraumatic Stress Disorder	
		PAXIL (n = 735)	Placebo (n = 529)	PAXIL (n = 676)	Placebo (n = 504)
Body as a Whole	Asthenia	14%	6%	12%	4%
	Headache	17%	14%	—	—
	Infection	6%	3%	5%	4%
	Abdominal Pain			4%	3%
	Trauma			6%	5%
Cardiovascular	Vasodilation	3%	1%	2%	1%
Dermatologic	Sweating	6%	2%	5%	1%
Gastrointestinal	Nausea	20%	5%	19%	8%
	Dry Mouth	11%	5%	10%	5%
	Constipation	10%	2%	5%	3%
	Diarrhea	9%	7%	11%	5%
	Decreased Appetite	5%	1%	6%	3%
	Vomiting	3%	2%	3%	2%
	Dyspepsia	—	—	5%	3%
Nervous System	Insomnia	11%	8%	12%	11%
	Somnolence	15%	5%	16%	5%
	Dizziness	6%	5%	6%	5%
	Tremor	5%	1%	4%	1%
	Nervousness	4%	3%	—	—
	Libido Decreased	9%	2%	5%	2%
	Abnormal Dreams			3%	2%
Respiratory System	Respiratory Disorder	7%	5%	—	—
	Sinusitis	4%	3%	—	—
	Yawn	4%	—	2%	<1%
Special Senses	Abnormal Vision	2%	1%	3%	1%
Urogenital System	Abnormal Ejaculation[2]	25%	2%	13%	2%
	Female Genital Disorder[2]	4%	1%	5%	1%
	Impotence[2]	4%	3%	9%	1%

1. Events reported by at least 2% of GAD and PTSD in patients treated with PAXIL are included, except the following events which had an incidence on placebo ≥PAXIL [GAD]: Abdominal pain, back pain, trauma, dyspepsia, myalgia, and pharyngitis. [PTSD]: Back pain, headache, anxiety, depression, nervousness, respiratory disorder, pharyngitis, and sinusitis.
2. Percentage corrected for gender.

Table 4. Treatment-Emergent Adverse Experience Incidence in a Dose-Comparison Trial in the Treatment of Major Depressive Disorder*

Body System/Preferred Term	Placebo n = 51	PAXIL			
		10 mg n = 102	20 mg n = 104	30 mg n = 101	40 mg n = 102
Body as a Whole					
Asthenia	0.0%	2.9%	10.6%	13.9%	12.7%
Dermatology					
Sweating	2.0%	1.0%	6.7%	8.9%	11.8%
Gastrointestinal					
Constipation	5.9%	4.9%	7.7%	9.9%	12.7%
Decreased Appetite	2.0%	2.0%	5.8%	4.0%	4.9%
Diarrhea	7.8%	9.8%	19.2%	7.9%	14.7%
Dry Mouth	2.0%	10.8%	18.3%	15.8%	20.6%
Nausea	13.7%	14.7%	26.9%	34.7%	36.3%
Nervous System					
Anxiety	0.0%	2.0%	5.8%	5.9%	5.9%
Dizziness	3.9%	6.9%	6.7%	8.9%	12.7%
Nervousness	0.0%	5.9%	5.8%	4.0%	2.9%
Paresthesia	0.0%	2.9%	1.0%	5.0%	5.9%
Somnolence	7.8%	12.7%	18.3%	20.8%	21.6%
Tremor	0.0%	0.0%	7.7%	7.9%	14.7%
Special Senses					
Blurred Vision	2.0%	2.9%	2.9%	2.0%	7.8%
Urogenital System					
Abnormal Ejaculation	0.0%	5.8%	6.5%	10.6%	13.0%
Impotence	0.0%	1.9%	4.3%	6.4%	1.9%
Male Genital Disorders	0.0%	3.8%	8.7%	6.4%	3.7%

*Rule for including adverse events in table: Incidence at least 5% for 1 of paroxetine groups and ≥ twice the placebo incidence for at least 1 paroxetine group.

OVERDOSAGE

Human Experience: Since the introduction of PAXIL in the United States, 342 spontaneous cases of deliberate or accidental overdosage during paroxetine treatment have been reported worldwide (circa 1999). These include overdoses with paroxetine alone and in combination with other substances. Of these, 48 cases were fatal and of the fatalities, 17 appeared to involve paroxetine alone. Eight fatal cases that documented the amount of paroxetine ingested were generally confounded by the ingestion of other drugs or alcohol or the presence of significant comorbid conditions. Of 145 non-fatal cases with known outcome, most recovered without sequelae. The largest known ingestion involved 2,000 mg of paroxetine (33 times the maximum recommended daily dose) in a patient who recovered.

Commonly reported adverse events associated with paroxetine overdosage include somnolence, coma, nausea, tremor, tachycardia, confusion, vomiting, and dizziness. Other notable signs and symptoms observed with overdoses involving paroxetine (alone or with other substances) include mydriasis, convulsions (including status epilepticus), ventricular dysrhythmias (including torsade de pointes), hypertension, aggressive reactions, syncope, hypotension, stupor, bradycardia, dystonia, rhabdomyolysis, symptoms of hepatic dysfunction (including hepatic failure, hepatic necrosis, jaundice, hepatitis, and hepatic steatosis), serotonin syndrome, manic reactions, myoclonus, acute renal failure, and urinary retention.

Overdosage Management: Treatment should consist of those general measures employed in the management of overdosage with any drugs effective in the treatment of major depressive disorder.

Ensure an adequate airway, oxygenation, and ventilation. Monitor cardiac rhythm and vital signs. General supportive and symptomatic measures are also recommended. Induction of emesis is not recommended. Gastric lavage with a large-bore orogastric tube with appropriate airway protection, if needed, may be indicated if performed soon after ingestion, or in symptomatic patients.
Activated charcoal should be administered. Due to the large volume of distribution of this drug, forced diuresis, dialysis, hemoperfusion, and exchange transfusion are unlikely to be of benefit. No specific antidotes for paroxetine are known.
A specific caution involves patients who are taking or have recently taken paroxetine who might ingest excessive quantities of a tricyclic antidepressant. In such a case, accumulation of the parent tricyclic and/or an active metabolite may increase the possibility of clinically significant sequelae and extend the time needed for close medical observation (see PRECAUTIONS—*Drugs Metabolized by Cytochrome* $P_{450}IID_6$).
In managing overdosage, consider the possibility of multiple drug involvement. The physician should consider contacting a poison control center for additional information on the treatment of any overdose. Telephone numbers for certified poison control centers are listed in the *Physicians' Desk Reference* (PDR).

DOSAGE AND ADMINISTRATION

Major Depressive Disorder: ***Usual Initial Dosage:*** PAXIL should be administered as a single daily dose with or without food, usually in the morning. The recommended initial dose is 20 mg/day. Patients were dosed in a range of 20 to 50 mg/day in the clinical trials demonstrating the effectiveness of PAXIL in the treatment of major depressive disorder. As with all drugs effective in the treatment of major depressive disorder, the full effect may be delayed. Some patients not responding to a 20-mg dose may benefit from dose increases, in 10-mg/day increments, up to a maximum of 50 mg/day. Dose changes should occur at intervals of at least 1 week.
Maintenance Therapy: There is no body of evidence available to answer the question of how long the patient treated with PAXIL should remain on it. It is generally agreed that acute episodes of major depressive disorder require several months or longer of sustained pharmacologic therapy. Whether the dose needed to induce remission is identical to the dose needed to maintain and/or sustain euthymia is unknown.
Systematic evaluation of the efficacy of PAXIL has shown that efficacy is maintained for periods of up to 1 year with doses that averaged about 30 mg.
Obsessive Compulsive Disorder: ***Usual Initial Dosage:*** PAXIL should be administered as a single daily dose with or without food, usually in the morning. The recommended dose of PAXIL in the treatment of OCD is 40 mg daily. Patients should be started on 20 mg/day and the dose can be increased in 10-mg/day increments. Dose changes should occur at intervals of at least 1 week. Patients were dosed in a range of 20 to 60 mg/day in the clinical trials demonstrating the effectiveness of PAXIL in the treatment of OCD. The maximum dosage should not exceed 60 mg/day.
Maintenance Therapy: Long-term maintenance of efficacy was demonstrated in a 6-month relapse prevention trial. In this trial, patients with OCD assigned to paroxetine demonstrated a lower relapse rate compared to patients on placebo (see CLINICAL PHARMACOLOGY—Clinical Trials). OCD is a chronic condition, and it is reasonable to consider continuation for a responding patient. Dosage adjustments should be made to maintain the patient on the lowest effective dosage, and patients should be periodically reassessed to determine the need for continued treatment.
Panic Disorder: ***Usual Initial Dosage:*** PAXIL should be administered as a single daily dose with or without food, usually in the morning. The target dose of PAXIL in the treatment of panic disorder is 40 mg/day. Patients should be started on 10 mg/day. Dose changes should occur in 10-mg/day increments and at intervals of at least 1 week. Patients were dosed in a range of 10 to 60 mg/day in the clinical trials demonstrating the effectiveness of PAXIL. The maximum dosage should not exceed 60 mg/day.
Maintenance Therapy: Long-term maintenance of efficacy was demonstrated in a 3-month relapse prevention trial. In this trial, patients with panic disorder assigned to paroxetine demonstrated a lower relapse rate compared to patients on placebo (see CLINICAL PHARMACOLOGY—Clinical Trials). Panic disorder is a chronic condition, and it is reasonable to consider continuation for a responding patient. Dosage adjustments should be made to maintain the patient on the lowest effective dosage, and patients should be periodically reassessed to determine the need for continued treatment.
Social Anxiety Disorder: ***Usual Initial Dosage:*** PAXIL should be administered as a single daily dose with or without food, usually in the morning. The recommended and initial dosage is 20 mg/day. In clinical trials the effectiveness of PAXIL was demonstrated in patients dosed in a range of 20 to 60 mg/day. While the safety of PAXIL has been evaluated in patients with social anxiety disorder at doses up to 60 mg/day, available information does not suggest any additional benefit for doses above 20 mg/day. (see CLINICAL PHARMACOLOGY—Clinical Trials).
Maintenance Therapy: There is no body of evidence available to answer the question of how long the patient treated with PAXIL should remain on it. Although the efficacy of PAXIL beyond 12 weeks of dosing has not been demonstrated in controlled clinical trials, social anxiety disorder is recognized as a chronic condition, and it is reasonable to consider continuation of treatment for a responding patient. Dosage adjustments should be made to maintain the patient on the lowest effective dosage, and patients should be periodically reassessed to determine the need for continued treatment.

Table 5. Incidence of Sexual Adverse Events in Controlled Clinical Trials

	PAXIL	Placebo
n (males)	**1446**	**1042**
Decreased Libido	6-15%	0-5%
Ejaculatory Disturbance	13-28%	0-2%
Impotence	2-9%	0-3%
n (females)	**1822**	**1340**
Decreased Libido	0-9%	0-2%
Orgasmic Disturbance	2-9%	0-1%

Generalized Anxiety Disorder: ***Usual Initial Dosage:*** PAXIL should be administered as a single daily dose with or without food, usually in the morning. In clinical trials the effectiveness of PAXIL was demonstrated in patients dosed in a range of 20 to 50 mg/day. The recommended starting dosage and the established effective dosage is 20 mg/day. There is not sufficient evidence to suggest a greater benefit to doses higher than 20 mg/day. Dose changes should occur in 10-mg/day increments and at intervals of at least 1 week.
Maintenance Therapy: Systematic evaluation of continuing PAXIL for periods of up to 24 weeks in patients with Generalized Anxiety Disorder who had responded while taking PAXIL during an 8-week acute treatment phase has demonstrated a benefit of such maintenance (see CLINICAL PHARMACOLOGY—Clinical Trials). Nevertheless, patients should be periodically reassessed to determine the need for maintenance treatment.
Posttraumatic Stress Disorder: ***Usual Initial Dosage:*** PAXIL should be administered as a single daily dose with or without food, usually in the morning. The recommended starting dosage and the established effective dosage is 20 mg/day. In 1 clinical trial, the effectiveness of PAXIL was demonstrated in patients dosed in a range of 20 to 50 mg/day. However, in a fixed dose study, there was not sufficient evidence to suggest a greater benefit for a dose of 40 mg/day compared to 20 mg/day. Dose changes, if indicated, should occur in 10 mg/day increments and at intervals of at least 1 week.
Maintenance Therapy: There is no body of evidence available to answer the question of how long the patient treated with PAXIL should remain on it. Although the efficacy of PAXIL beyond 12 weeks of dosing has not been demonstrated in controlled clinical trials, PTSD is recognized as a chronic condition, and it is reasonable to consider continuation of treatment for a responding patient. Dosage adjustments should be made to maintain the patient on the lowest effective dosage, and patients should be periodically reassessed to determine the need for continued treatment.
Special Populations: ***Treatment of Pregnant Women During the Third Trimester:*** Neonates exposed to PAXIL and other SSRIs or SNRIs, late in the third trimester have developed complications requiring prolonged hospitalization, respiratory support, and tube feeding (see PRECAUTIONS). When treating pregnant women with paroxetine during the third trimester, the physician should carefully consider the potential risks and benefits of treatment. The physician may consider tapering paroxetine in the third trimester.
Dosage for Elderly or Debilitated Patients, and Patients With Severe Renal or Hepatic Impairment: The recommended initial dose is 10 mg/day for elderly patients, debilitated patients, and/or patients with severe renal or hepatic impairment. Increases may be made if indicated. Dosage should not exceed 40 mg/day.
Switching Patients to or From a Monoamine Oxidase Inhibitor: At least 14 days should elapse between discontinuation of an MAOI and initiation of therapy with PAXIL. Similarly, at least 14 days should be allowed after stopping PAXIL before starting an MAOI.
Discontinuation of Treatment With PAXIL: Symptoms associated with discontinuation of PAXIL have been reported (see PRECAUTIONS). Patients should be monitored for these symptoms when discontinuing treatment, regardless of the indication for which PAXIL is being prescribed. A gradual reduction in the dose rather than abrupt cessation is recommended whenever possible. If intolerable symptoms occur following a decrease in the dose or upon discontinuation of treatment, then resuming the previously prescribed dose may be considered. Subsequently, the physician may continue decreasing the dose but at a more gradual rate.
NOTE: SHAKE SUSPENSION WELL BEFORE USING.

HOW SUPPLIED

Tablets: Film-coated, modified-oval as follows:
10-mg yellow, scored tablets engraved on the front with PAXIL and on the back with 10.
NDC 0029-3210-13 Bottles of 30
20-mg pink, scored tablets engraved on the front with PAXIL and on the back with 20.
NDC 0029-3211-13 Bottles of 30
NDC 0029-3211-20 Bottles of 100
NDC 0029-3211-21 SUP 100s (intended for institutional use only)
30-mg blue tablets engraved on the front with PAXIL and on the back with 30.
NDC 0029-3212-13 Bottles of 30
40-mg green tablets engraved on the front with PAXIL and on the back with 40.
NDC 0029-3213-13 Bottles of 30
Store tablets between 15° and 30°C (59° and 86°F).
Oral Suspension: Orange-colored, orange-flavored, 10 mg/5 mL, in 250 mL white bottles.
NDC 0029-3215-48
Store suspension at or below 25°C (77°F).
PAXIL is a registered trademark of GlaxoSmithKline.

Medication Guide

PAXIL® (PAX-il) (paroxetine hydrochloride) Tablets and Oral Solution

About Using Antidepressants in Children and Teenagers

What is the most important information I should know if my child is being prescribed an antidepressant?

Parents or guardians need to think about 4 important things when their child is prescribed an antidepressant:
1. There is a risk of suicidal thoughts or actions
2. How to try to prevent suicidal thoughts or actions in your child
3. You should watch for certain signs if your child is taking an antidepressant
4. There are benefits and risks when using antidepressants

1. There is a Risk of Suicidal Thoughts or Actions

Children and teenagers sometimes think about suicide, and many report trying to kill themselves.
Antidepressants increase suicidal thoughts and actions in some children and teenagers. But suicidal thoughts and actions can also be caused by depression, a serious medical condition that is commonly treated with antidepressants. Thinking about killing yourself or trying to kill yourself is called *suicidality or being suicidal*.
A large study combined the results of 24 different studies of children and teenagers with depression or other illnesses. In these studies, patients took either a placebo (sugar pill) or an antidepressant for 1 to 4 months. ***No one committed suicide in these studies,*** but some patients became suicidal. On sugar pills, 2 out of every 100 became suicidal. On the antidepressants, 4 out of every 100 patients became suicidal.
For some children and teenagers, the risks of suicidal actions may be especially high. These include patients with
- Bipolar illness (sometimes called manic-depressive illness)
- A family history of bipolar illness
- A personal or family history of attempting suicide

If any of these are present, make sure you tell your healthcare provider before your child takes an antidepressant.

2. How to Try to Prevent Suicidal Thoughts and Actions

To try to prevent suicidal thoughts and actions in your child, pay close attention to changes in her or his moods or actions, especially if the changes occur suddenly. Other important people in your child's life can help by paying attention as well (e.g., your child, brothers and sisters, teachers, and other important people). The changes to look out for are listed in Section 3, on what to watch for.
Whenever an antidepressant is started or its dose is changed, pay close attention to your child. After starting an antidepressant, your child should generally see his or her healthcare provider:
- Once a week for the first 4 weeks
- Every 2 weeks for the next 4 weeks
- After taking the antidepressant for 12 weeks
- After 12 weeks, follow your healthcare provider's advice about how often to come back
- More often if problems or questions arise (see Section 3)

You should call your child's healthcare provider between visits if needed.

3. You Should Watch for Certain Signs If Your Child is Taking an Antidepressant

Contact your child's healthcare provider ***right away*** if your child exhibits any of the following signs for the first time, or if they seem worse, or worry you, your child, or your child's teacher:
- Thoughts about suicide or dying
- Attempts to commit suicide
- New or worse depression
- New or worse anxiety

Continued on next page

Paxil—Cont.

- Feeling very agitated or restless
- Panic attacks
- Difficulty sleeping (insomnia)
- New or worse irritability
- Acting aggressive, being angry, or violent
- Acting on dangerous impulses
- An extreme increase in activity and talking
- Other unusual changes in behavior or mood

Never let your child stop taking an antidepressant without first talking to his or her healthcare provider. Stopping an antidepressant suddenly can cause other symptoms.

4. There are Benefits and Risks When Using Antidepressants

Antidepressants are used to treat depression and other illnesses. Depression and other illnesses can lead to suicide. In some children and teenagers, treatment with an antidepressant increases suicidal thinking or actions. It is important to discuss all the risks of treating depression and also the risks of not treating it. You and your child should discuss all treatment choices with your healthcare provider, not just the use of antidepressants.

Other side effects can occur with antidepressants (see section below).

Of all the antidepressants, only fluoxetine (Prozac®)* has been FDA approved to treat pediatric depression.

For obsessive compulsive disorder in children and teenagers, FDA has approved only fluoxetine (Prozac®)*, sertraline (Zoloft®)*, fluvoxamine, and clomipramine (Anafranil®)*.

Your healthcare provider may suggest other antidepressants based on the past experience of your child or other family members.

Is this all I need to know if my child is being prescribed an antidepressant?

No. This is a warning about the risk for suicidality. Other side effects can occur with antidepressants. Be sure to ask your healthcare provider to explain all the side effects of the particular drug he or she is prescribing. Also ask about drugs to avoid when taking an antidepressant. Ask your healthcare provider or pharmacist where to find more information.

*The following are registered trademarks of their respective manufacturers: Prozac®/Eli Lilly and Company; Zoloft®/Pfizer Pharmaceuticals; Anafranil®/Mallinckrodt Inc.

This Medication Guide has been approved by the U.S. Food and Drug Administration for all antidepressants.

MG-PX:1

GlaxoSmithKline, Research Triangle Park, NC 27709
©2005, GlaxoSmithKline. All rights reserved.
January 2005/PX:L34

PAXIL CR® ℞
[pax'il]
(paroxetine hydrochloride)
Controlled-Release Tablets

Prescribing information for this product, which appears on pages 1592–1599 of the 2005 PDR, has been completely revised as follows. Please write "See Supplement A" next to the product heading.

Suicidality in Children and Adolescents
Antidepressants increased the risk of suicidal thinking and behavior (suicidality) in short-term studies in children and adolescents with Major Depressive Disorder (MDD) and other psychiatric disorders. Anyone considering the use of PAXIL CR or any other antidepressant in a child or adolescent must balance this risk with the clinical need. Patients who are started on therapy should be observed closely for clinical worsening, suicidality, or unusual changes in behavior. Families and caregivers should be advised of the need for close observation and communication with the prescriber. PAXIL CR is not approved for use in pediatric patients. (See WARNINGS and PRECAUTIONS—Pediatric Use.)

Pooled analyses of short-term (4 to 16 weeks) placebo-controlled trials of 9 antidepressant drugs (SSRIs and others) in children and adolescents with major depressive disorder (MDD), obsessive compulsive disorder (OCD), or other psychiatric disorders (a total of 24 trials involving over 4,400 patients) have revealed a greater risk of adverse events representing suicidal thinking or behavior (suicidality) during the first few months of treatment in those receiving antidepressants. The average risk of such events in patients receiving antidepressants was 4%, twice the placebo risk of 2%. No suicides occurred in these trials.

DESCRIPTION

PAXIL CR (paroxetine hydrochloride) is an orally administered psychotropic drug with a chemical structure unrelated to other selective serotonin reuptake inhibitors or to tricyclic, tetracyclic, or other available antidepressant or antipanic agents. It is the hydrochloride salt of a phenylpiperidine compound identified chemically as (-)-*trans*-4R-(4'-fluorophenyl)-3S-[(3',4'-methylenedioxyphenoxy) methyl] piperidine hydrochloride hemihydrate and has the empirical formula of $C_{19}H_{20}FNO_3 \cdot HCl \cdot 1/2H_2O$. The molecular weight is 374.8 (329.4 as free base). The structural formula of paroxetine hydrochloride is:

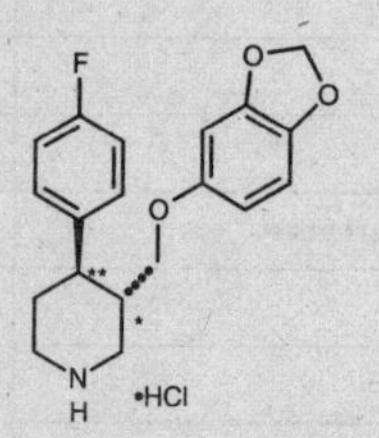

Paroxetine hydrochloride is an odorless, off-white powder, having a melting point range of 120° to 138°C and a solubility of 5.4 mg/mL in water.

Each enteric, film-coated, controlled-release tablet contains paroxetine hydrochloride equivalent to paroxetine as follows: 12.5 mg–yellow, 25 mg–pink, 37.5 mg–blue. One layer of the tablet consists of a degradable barrier layer and the other contains the active material in a hydrophilic matrix. Inactive ingredients consist of hypromellose, polyvinylpyrrolidone, lactose monohydrate, magnesium stearate, colloidal silicon dioxide, glyceryl behenate, methacrylic acid copolymer type C, sodium lauryl sulfate, polysorbate 80, talc, triethyl citrate, and 1 or more of the following colorants: Yellow ferric oxide, red ferric oxide, D&C Red No. 30, D&C Yellow No. 6, D&C Yellow No. 10, FD&C Blue No. 2.

CLINICAL PHARMACOLOGY

Pharmacodynamics: The efficacy of paroxetine in the treatment of major depressive disorder, panic disorder, social anxiety disorder, and premenstrual dysphoric disorder (PMDD) is presumed to be linked to potentiation of serotonergic activity in the central nervous system resulting from inhibition of neuronal reuptake of serotonin (5-hydroxytryptamine, 5-HT). Studies at clinically relevant doses in humans have demonstrated that paroxetine blocks the uptake of serotonin into human platelets. In vitro studies in animals also suggest that paroxetine is a potent and highly selective inhibitor of neuronal serotonin reuptake and has only very weak effects on norepinephrine and dopamine neuronal reuptake. In vitro radioligand binding studies indicate that paroxetine has little affinity for muscarinic, alpha$_1$-, alpha$_2$-, beta-adrenergic-, dopamine (D$_2$)-, 5-HT$_1$-, 5-HT$_2$-, and histamine (H$_1$)-receptors; antagonism of muscarinic, histaminergic, and alpha$_1$-adrenergic receptors has been associated with various anticholinergic, sedative, and cardiovascular effects for other psychotropic drugs.

Because the relative potencies of paroxetine's major metabolites are at most 1/50 of the parent compound, they are essentially inactive.

Pharmacokinetics: Tablets of PAXIL CR contain a degradable polymeric matrix (GEOMATRIX™) designed to control the dissolution rate of paroxetine over a period of approximately 4 to 5 hours. In addition to controlling the rate of drug release in vivo, an enteric coat delays the start of drug release until tablets of PAXIL CR have left the stomach.

Paroxetine hydrochloride is completely absorbed after oral dosing of a solution of the hydrochloride salt. In a study in which normal male and female subjects (n = 23) received single oral doses of PAXIL CR at 4 dosage strengths (12.5 mg, 25 mg, 37.5 mg, and 50 mg), paroxetine C_{max} and AUC_{0-inf} increased disproportionately with dose (as seen also with immediate-release formulations). Mean C_{max} and AUC_{0-inf} values at these doses were 2.0, 5.5, 9.0, and 12.5 ng/mL, and 121, 261, 338, and 540 ng•hr./mL, respectively. T_{max} was observed typically between 6 and 10 hours post-dose, reflecting a reduction in absorption rate compared with immediate-release formulations. The mean elimination half-life of paroxetine was 15 to 20 hours throughout this range of single doses of PAXIL CR. The bioavailability of 25 mg PAXIL CR is not affected by food.

During repeated administration of PAXIL CR (25 mg once daily), steady state was reached within 2 weeks (i.e., comparable to immediate-release formulations). In a repeat-dose study in which normal male and female subjects (n = 23) received PAXIL CR (25 mg daily), mean steady state C_{max}, C_{min}, and AUC_{0-24} values were 30 ng/mL, 20 ng/mL, and 550 ng•hr./mL, respectively.

Based on studies using immediate-release formulations, steady-state drug exposure based on AUC_{0-24} was several-fold greater than would have been predicted from single-dose data. The excess accumulation is a consequence of the fact that 1 of the enzymes that metabolizes paroxetine is readily saturable.

In steady-state dose proportionality studies involving elderly and nonelderly patients, at doses of the immediate-release formulation of 20 mg to 40 mg daily for the elderly and 20 mg to 50 mg daily for the nonelderly, some nonlinearity was observed in both populations, again reflecting a saturable metabolic pathway. In comparison to C_{min} values after 20 mg daily, values after 40 mg daily were only about 2 to 3 times greater than doubled.

Paroxetine is extensively metabolized after oral administration. The principal metabolites are polar and conjugated products of oxidation and methylation, which are readily cleared. Conjugates with glucuronic acid and sulfate predominate, and major metabolites have been isolated and identified. Data indicate that the metabolites have no more than 1/50 the potency of the parent compound at inhibiting serotonin uptake. The metabolism of paroxetine is accomplished in part by cytochrome P$_{450}$IID$_6$. Saturation of this enzyme at clinical doses appears to account for the nonlin-earity of paroxetine kinetics with increasing dose and increasing duration of treatment. The role of this enzyme in paroxetine metabolism also suggests potential drug-drug interactions (see PRECAUTIONS).

Approximately 64% of a 30-mg oral solution dose of paroxetine was excreted in the urine with 2% as the parent compound and 62% as metabolites over a 10-day post-dosing period. About 36% was excreted in the feces (probably via the bile), mostly as metabolites and less than 1% as the parent compound over the 10-day post-dosing period.

Distribution: Paroxetine distributes throughout the body, including the CNS, with only 1% remaining in the plasma.

Protein Binding: Approximately 95% and 93% of paroxetine is bound to plasma protein at 100 ng/mL and 400 ng/mL, respectively. Under clinical conditions, paroxetine concentrations would normally be less than 400 ng/mL. Paroxetine does not alter the in vitro protein binding of phenytoin or warfarin.

Renal and Liver Disease: Increased plasma concentrations of paroxetine occur in subjects with renal and hepatic impairment. The mean plasma concentrations in patients with creatinine clearance below 30 mL/min. was approximately 4 times greater than seen in normal volunteers. Patients with creatinine clearance of 30 to 60 mL/min. and patients with hepatic functional impairment had about a 2-fold increase in plasma concentrations (AUC, C_{max}).

The initial dosage should therefore be reduced in patients with severe renal or hepatic impairment, and upward titration, if necessary, should be at increased intervals (see DOSAGE AND ADMINISTRATION).

Elderly Patients: In a multiple-dose study in the elderly at daily doses of 20, 30, and 40 mg of the immediate-release formulation, C_{min} concentrations were about 70% to 80% greater than the respective C_{min} concentrations in non-elderly subjects. Therefore the initial dosage in the elderly should be reduced (see DOSAGE AND ADMINISTRATION).

Clinical Trials

Major Depressive Disorder: The efficacy of PAXIL CR controlled-release tablets as a treatment for major depressive disorder has been established in two 12-week, flexible-dose, placebo-controlled studies of patients with DSM-IV Major Depressive Disorder. One study included patients in the age range 18 to 65 years, and a second study included elderly patients, ranging in age from 60 to 88. In both studies, PAXIL CR was shown to be significantly more effective than placebo in treating major depressive disorder as measured by the following: Hamilton Depression Rating Scale (HDRS), the Hamilton depressed mood item, and the Clinical Global Impression (CGI)–Severity of Illness score.

A study of outpatients with major depressive disorder who had responded to immediate-release paroxetine tablets (HDRS total score <8) during an initial 8-week open-treatment phase and were then randomized to continuation on immediate-release paroxetine tablets or placebo for 1 year demonstrated a significantly lower relapse rate for patients taking immediate-release paroxetine tablets (15%) compared to those on placebo (39%). Effectiveness was similar for male and female patients.

Panic Disorder: The effectiveness of PAXIL CR in the treatment of panic disorder was evaluated in three 10-week, multicenter, flexible-dose studies (Studies 1, 2, and 3) comparing paroxetine controlled-release (12.5 to 75 mg daily) to placebo in adult outpatients who had panic disorder (DSM-IV), with or without agoraphobia. These trials were assessed on the basis of their outcomes on 3 variables: (1) the proportions of patients free of full panic attacks at endpoint; (2) change from baseline to endpoint in the mean number of full panic attacks; and (3) change from baseline to endpoint in the median Clinical Global Impression Severity score. For Studies 1 and 2, PAXIL CR was consistently superior to placebo on 2 of these 3 variables. Study 3 failed to consistently demonstrate a significant difference between PAXIL CR and placebo on any of these variables.

For all 3 studies, the mean dose of PAXIL CR for completers at endpoint was approximately 50 mg/day. Subgroup analyses did not indicate that there were any differences in treatment outcomes as a function of age or gender.

Long-term maintenance effects of the immediate-release formulation of paroxetine in panic disorder were demonstrated in an extension study. Patients who were responders during a 10-week double-blind phase with immediate-release paroxetine and during a 3-month double-blind extension phase were randomized to either immediate-release paroxetine or placebo in a 3-month double-blind relapse prevention phase. Patients randomized to paroxetine were significantly less likely to relapse than comparably treated patients who were randomized to placebo.

Social Anxiety Disorder: The efficacy of PAXIL CR as a treatment for social anxiety disorder has been established, in part, on the basis of extrapolation from the established effectiveness of the immediate-release formulation of paroxetine. In addition, the effectiveness of PAXIL CR in the treatment of social anxiety disorder was demonstrated in a 12-week, multicenter, double-blind, flexible-dose, placebo-controlled study of adult outpatients with a primary diagnosis of social anxiety disorder (DSM-IV). In the study, the effectiveness of PAXIL CR (12.5 to 37.5 mg daily) compared to placebo was evaluated on the basis of (1) change from baseline in the Liebowitz Social Anxiety Scale (LSAS) total score and (2) the proportion of responders who scored 1 or 2 (very much improved or much improved) on the Clinical Global Impression (CGI) Global Improvement score.

PAXIL CR demonstrated statistically significant superiority over placebo on both the LSAS total score and the CGI Improvement responder criterion. For patients who completed the trial, 64% of patients treated with PAXIL CR compared to 34.7% of patients treated with placebo were CGI Improvement responders.

Subgroup analyses did not indicate that there were any differences in treatment outcomes as a function of gender. Subgroup analyses of studies utilizing the immediate-release formulation of paroxetine generally did not indicate differences in treatment outcomes as a function of age, race, or gender.

Premenstrual Dysphoric Disorder: The effectiveness of PAXIL CR for the treatment of PMDD utilizing a continuous dosing regimen has been established in 2 placebo-controlled trials. Patients in these trials met DSM-IV criteria for PMDD. In a pool of 1,030 patients, treated with daily doses of PAXIL CR 12.5 or 25 mg/day, or placebo the mean duration of the PMDD symptoms was approximately 11 ± 7 years. Patients on systemic hormonal contraceptives were excluded from these trials. Therefore, the efficacy of PAXIL CR in combination with systemic (including oral) hormonal contraceptives for the continuous daily treatment of PMDD is unknown. In both positive studies, patients (N = 672) were treated with 12.5 mg/day or 25 mg/day of PAXIL CR or placebo continuously throughout the menstrual cycle for a period of 3 menstrual cycles. The VAS-Total score is a patient-rated instrument that mirrors the diagnostic criteria of PMDD as identified in the DSM-IV, and includes assessments for mood, physical symptoms, and other symptoms. 12.5 mg/day and 25 mg/day of PAXIL CR were significantly more effective than placebo as measured by change from baseline to the endpoint on the luteal phase VAS-Total score.

In a third study employing intermittent dosing, patients (N = 366) were treated for the 2 weeks prior to the onset of menses (luteal phase dosing, also known as intermittent dosing) with 12.5 mg/day or 25 mg/day of PAXIL CR or placebo for a period of 3 months. 12.5 mg/day and 25 mg/day of PAXIL CR, as luteal phase dosing, was significantly more effective than placebo as measured by change from baseline luteal phase VAS total score.

There is insufficient information to determine the effect of race or age on outcome in these studies.

INDICATIONS AND USAGE

Major Depressive Disorder: PAXIL CR is indicated for the treatment of major depressive disorder.

The efficacy of PAXIL CR in the treatment of a major depressive episode was established in two 12-week controlled trials of outpatients whose diagnoses corresponded to the DSM-IV category of major depressive disorder (see CLINICAL PHARMACOLOGY—Clinical Trials).

A major depressive episode (DSM-IV) implies a prominent and relatively persistent (nearly every day for at least 2 weeks) depressed mood or loss of interest or pleasure in nearly all activities, representing a change from previous functioning, and includes the presence of at least 5 of the following 9 symptoms during the same 2-week period: Depressed mood, markedly diminished interest or pleasure in usual activities, significant change in weight and/or appetite, insomnia or hypersomnia, psychomotor agitation or retardation, increased fatigue, feelings of guilt or worthlessness, slowed thinking or impaired concentration, a suicide attempt, or suicidal ideation.

The antidepressant action of paroxetine in hospitalized depressed patients has not been adequately studied.

PAXIL CR has not been systematically evaluated beyond 12 weeks in controlled clinical trials; however, the effectiveness of immediate-release paroxetine hydrochloride in maintaining a response in major depressive disorder for up to 1 year has been demonstrated in a placebo-controlled trial (see CLINICAL PHARMACOLOGY—Clinical Trials). The physician who elects to use PAXIL CR for extended periods should periodically re-evaluate the long-term usefulness of the drug for the individual patient.

Panic Disorder: PAXIL CR is indicated for the treatment of panic disorder, with or without agoraphobia, as defined in DSM-IV. Panic disorder is characterized by the occurrence of unexpected panic attacks and associated concern about having additional attacks, worry about the implications or consequences of the attacks, and/or a significant change in behavior related to the attacks.

The efficacy of PAXIL CR controlled-release tablets was established in two 10-week trials in panic disorder patients whose diagnoses corresponded to the DSM-IV category of panic disorder (see CLINICAL PHARMACOLOGY—Clinical Trials).

Panic disorder (DSM-IV) is characterized by recurrent unexpected panic attacks, i.e., a discrete period of intense fear or discomfort in which 4 (or more) of the following symptoms develop abruptly and reach a peak within 10 minutes: (1) palpitations, pounding heart, or accelerated heart rate; (2) sweating; (3) trembling or shaking; (4) sensations of shortness of breath or smothering; (5) feeling of choking; (6) chest pain or discomfort; (7) nausea or abdominal distress; (8) feeling dizzy, unsteady, lightheaded, or faint; (9) derealization (feelings of unreality) or depersonalization (being detached from oneself); (10) fear of losing control; (11) fear of dying; (12) paresthesias (numbness or tingling sensations); (13) chills or hot flushes.

Long-term maintenance of efficacy with the immediate-release formulation of paroxetine was demonstrated in a 3-month relapse prevention trial. In this trial, patients with panic disorder assigned to immediate-release paroxetine demonstrated a lower relapse rate compared to patients on placebo (see CLINICAL PHARMACOLOGY—Clinical Trials). Nevertheless, the physician who prescribes PAXIL CR for extended periods should periodically re-evaluate the long-term usefulness of the drug for the individual patient.

Social Anxiety Disorder: PAXIL CR is indicated for the treatment of social anxiety disorder, also known as social phobia, as defined in DSM-IV (300.23). Social anxiety disorder is characterized by a marked and persistent fear of 1 or more social or performance situations in which the person is exposed to unfamiliar people or to possible scrutiny by others. Exposure to the feared situation almost invariably provokes anxiety, which may approach the intensity of a panic attack. The feared situations are avoided or endured with intense anxiety or distress. The avoidance, anxious anticipation, or distress in the feared situation(s) interferes significantly with the person's normal routine, occupational or academic functioning, or social activities or relationships, or there is marked distress about having the phobias. Lesser degrees of performance anxiety or shyness generally do not require psychopharmacological treatment.

The efficacy of PAXIL CR as a treatment for social anxiety disorder has been established, in part, on the basis of extrapolation from the established effectiveness of the immediate-release formulation of paroxetine. In addition, the efficacy of PAXIL CR was established in a 12-week trial, in adult outpatients with social anxiety disorder (DSM-IV). PAXIL CR has not been studied in children or adolescents with social phobia (see CLINICAL PHARMACOLOGY—Clinical Trials).

The effectiveness of PAXIL CR in long-term treatment of social anxiety disorder, i.e., for more than 12 weeks, has not been systematically evaluated in adequate and well-controlled trials. Therefore, the physician who elects to prescribe PAXIL CR for extended periods should periodically re-evaluate the long-term usefulness of the drug for the individual patient (see DOSAGE AND ADMINISTRATION).

Premenstrual Dysphoric Disorder: PAXIL CR is indicated for the treatment of PMDD.

The efficacy of PAXIL CR in the treatment of PMDD has been established in 3 placebo-controlled trials (see CLINICAL PHARMACOLOGY—Clinical Trials).

The essential features of PMDD, according to DSM-IV, include markedly depressed mood, anxiety or tension, affective lability, and persistent anger or irritability. Other features include decreased interest in usual activities, difficulty concentrating, lack of energy, change in appetite or sleep, and feeling out of control. Physical symptoms associated with PMDD include breast tenderness, headache, joint and muscle pain, bloating, and weight gain. These symptoms occur regularly during the luteal phase and remit within a few days following the onset of menses; the disturbance markedly interferes with work or school or with usual social activities and relationships with others. In making the diagnosis, care should be taken to rule out other cyclical mood disorders that may be exacerbated by treatment with an antidepressant.

The effectiveness of PAXIL CR in long-term use, that is, for more than 3 menstrual cycles, has not been systematically evaluated in controlled trials. Therefore, the physician who elects to use PAXIL CR for extended periods should periodically re-evaluate the long-term usefulness of the drug for the individual patient.

CONTRAINDICATIONS

Concomitant use in patients taking either monoamine oxidase inhibitors (MAOIs) or thioridazine is contraindicated (see WARNINGS and PRECAUTIONS).

PAXIL CR is contraindicated in patients with a hypersensitivity to paroxetine or to any of the inactive ingredients in PAXIL CR.

WARNINGS

Clinical Worsening and Suicide Risk: Patients with major depressive disorder (MDD), both adult and pediatric, may experience worsening of their depression and/or the emergence of suicidal ideation and behavior (suicidality) or unusual changes in behavior, whether or not they are taking antidepressant medications, and this risk may persist until significant remission occurs. There has been a long-standing concern that antidepressants may have a role in inducing worsening of depression and the emergence of suicidality in certain patients. Antidepressants increased the risk of suicidal thinking and behavior (suicidality) in short-term studies in children and adolescents with Major Depressive Disorder (MDD) and other psychiatric disorders.

Pooled analyses of short-term placebo-controlled trials of 9 antidepressant drugs (SSRIs and others) in children and adolescents with MDD, OCD, or other psychiatric disorders (a total of 24 trials involving over 4,400 patients) have revealed a greater risk of adverse events representing suicidal behavior or thinking (suicidality) during the first few months of treatment in those receiving antidepressants. The average risk of such events in patients receiving antidepressants was 4%, twice the placebo risk of 2%. There was considerable variation in risk among drugs, but a tendency toward an increase for almost all drugs studied. The risk of suicidality was most consistently observed in the MDD trials, but there were signals of risk arising from some trials in other psychiatric indications (obsessive compulsive disorder and social anxiety disorder) as well. **No suicides occurred in any of these trials.** It is unknown whether the suicidality risk in pediatric patients extends to longer-term use, i.e., beyond several months. It is also unknown whether the suicidality risk extends to adults.

All pediatric patients being treated with antidepressants for any indication should be observed closely for clinical worsening, suicidality, and unusual changes in behavior, especially during the initial few months of a course of drug therapy, or at times of dose changes, either increases or decreases. Such observation would generally include at least weekly face-to-face contact with patients or their family members or caregivers during the first 4 weeks of treatment, then every other week visits for the next 4 weeks, then at 12 weeks, and as clinically indicated beyond 12 weeks. Additional contact by telephone may be appropriate between face-to-face visits.

Adults with MDD or co-morbid depression in the setting of other psychiatric illness being treated with antidepressants should be observed similarly for clinical worsening and suicidality, especially during the initial few months of a course of drug therapy, or at times of dose changes, either increases or decreases.

The following symptoms, anxiety, agitation, panic attacks, insomnia, irritability, hostility, aggressiveness, impulsivity, akathisia (psychomotor restlessness), hypomania, and mania, have been reported in adult and pediatric patients being treated with antidepressants for major depressive disorder as well as for other indications, both psychiatric and nonpsychiatric. Although a causal link between the emergence of such symptoms and either the worsening of depression and/or the emergence of suicidal impulses has not been established, there is concern that such symptoms may represent precursors to emerging suicidality.

Consideration should be given to changing the therapeutic regimen, including possibly discontinuing the medication, in patients whose depression is persistently worse, or who are experiencing emergent suicidality or symptoms that might be precursors to worsening depression or suicidality, especially if these symptoms are severe, abrupt in onset, or were not part of the patient's presenting symptoms.

If the decision has been made to discontinue treatment, medication should be tapered, as rapidly as is feasible, but with recognition that abrupt discontinuation can be associated with certain symptoms (see PRECAUTIONS and DOSAGE AND ADMINISTRATION—Discontinuation of Treatment With PAXIL CR, for a description of the risks of discontinuation of PAXIL CR).

Families and caregivers of pediatric patients being treated with antidepressants for major depressive disorder or other indications, both psychiatric and nonpsychiatric, should be alerted about the need to monitor patients for the emergence of agitation, irritability, unusual changes in behavior, and the other symptoms described above, as well as the emergence of suicidality, and to report such symptoms immediately to health care providers. Such monitoring should include daily observation by families and caregivers. Prescriptions for PAXIL CR should be written for the smallest quantity of tablets consistent with good patient management, in order to reduce the risk of overdose. Families and caregivers of adults being treated for depression should be similarly advised.

Screening Patients for Bipolar Disorder: A major depressive episode may be the initial presentation of bipolar disorder. It is generally believed (though not established in controlled trials) that treating such an episode with an antidepressant alone may increase the likelihood of precipitation of a mixed/manic episode in patients at risk for bipolar disorder. Whether any of the symptoms described above represent such a conversion is unknown. However, prior to initiating treatment with an antidepressant, patients with depressive symptoms should be adequately screened to determine if they are at risk for bipolar disorder; such screening should include a detailed psychiatric history, including a family history of suicide, bipolar disorder, and depression. It should be noted that PAXIL CR is not approved for use in treating bipolar depression.

Potential for Interaction With Monoamine Oxidase Inhibitors: In patients receiving another serotonin reuptake inhibitor drug in combination with an MAOI, there have been reports of serious, sometimes fatal, reactions including hyperthermia, rigidity, myoclonus, autonomic instability with possible rapid fluctuations of vital signs, and mental status changes that include extreme agitation progressing to delirium and coma. These reactions have also been reported in patients who have recently discontinued that drug and have been started on an MAOI. Some cases presented with features resembling neuroleptic malignant syndrome. While there are no human data showing such an interaction with paroxetine hydrochloride, limited animal data on the effects of combined use of paroxetine and MAOIs suggest that these drugs may act synergistically to elevate blood pressure and evoke behavioral excitation. Therefore, it is recommended that PAXIL CR not be used in combination with an MAOI, or within 14 days of discontinuing treatment with an MAOI. At least 2 weeks should be allowed after stopping PAXIL CR before starting an MAOI.

Potential Interaction With Thioridazine: Thioridazine administration alone produces prolongation of the QTc interval, which is associated with serious ventricular arrhythmias, such as torsade de pointes–type arrhythmias, and sudden death. This effect appears to be dose related.

An in vivo study suggests that drugs which inhibit $P_{450}IID_6$, such as paroxetine, will elevate plasma levels of thioridazine. Therefore, it is recommended that paroxetine not be used in combination with thioridazine (see CONTRAINDICATIONS and PRECAUTIONS).

PRECAUTIONS

General: ***Activation of Mania/Hypomania:*** During premarketing testing of immediate-release paroxetine hydrochlo-

Continued on next page

Paxil CR—Cont.

ride, hypomania or mania occurred in approximately 1.0% of paroxetine-treated unipolar patients compared to 1.1% of active-control and 0.3% of placebo-treated unipolar patients. In a subset of patients classified as bipolar, the rate of manic episodes was 2.2% for immediate-release paroxetine and 11.6% for the combined active-control groups. Among 1,627 patients with major depressive disorder, panic disorder, social anxiety disorder, or PMDD treated with PAXIL CR in controlled clinical studies, there were no reports of mania or hypomania. As with all drugs effective in the treatment of major depressive disorder, PAXIL CR should be used cautiously in patients with a history of mania.

Seizures: During premarketing testing of immediate-release paroxetine hydrochloride, seizures occurred in 0.1% of paroxetine-treated patients, a rate similar to that associated with other drugs effective in the treatment of major depressive disorder. Among 1,627 patients who received PAXIL CR in controlled clinical trials in major depressive disorder, panic disorder, social anxiety disorder, or PMDD, 1 patient (0.1%) experienced a seizure. PAXIL CR should be used cautiously in patients with a history of seizures. It should be discontinued in any patient who develops seizures.

Discontinuation of Treatment With PAXIL CR: Adverse events while discontinuing therapy with PAXIL CR were not systematically evaluated in most clinical trials; however, in recent placebo-controlled clinical trials utilizing daily doses of PAXIL CR up to 37.5 mg/day, spontaneously reported adverse events while discontinuing therapy with PAXIL CR were evaluated. Patients receiving 37.5 mg/day underwent an incremental decrease in the daily dose by 12.5 mg/day to a dose of 25 mg/day for 1 week before treatment was stopped. For patients receiving 25 mg/day or 12.5 mg/day, treatment was stopped without an incremental decrease in dose. With this regimen in those studies, the following adverse events were reported for PAXIL CR, at an incidence of 2% or greater for PAXIL CR and were at least twice that reported for placebo: Dizziness, nausea, nervousness, and additional symptoms described by the investigator as associated with tapering or discontinuing PAXIL CR (e.g., emotional lability, headache, agitation, electric shock sensations, fatigue, and sleep disturbances). These events were reported as serious in 0.3% of patients who discontinued therapy with PAXIL CR.

During marketing of PAXIL CR and other SSRIs and SNRIs (serotonin and norepinephrine reuptake inhibitors), there have been spontaneous reports of adverse events occurring upon discontinuation of these drugs, (particularly when abrupt), including the following: Dysphoric mood, irritability, agitation, dizziness, sensory disturbances (e.g., paresthesias such as electric shock sensations), anxiety, confusion, headache, lethargy, emotional lability, insomnia, and hypomania. While these events are generally self-limiting, there have been reports of serious discontinuation symptoms.

Patients should be monitored for these symptoms when discontinuing treatment with PAXIL CR. A gradual reduction in the dose rather than abrupt cessation is recommended whenever possible. If intolerable symptoms occur following a decrease in the dose or upon discontinuation of treatment, then resuming the previously prescribed dose may be considered. Subsequently, the physician may continue decreasing the dose but at a more gradual rate (see DOSAGE AND ADMINISTRATION).

See also PRECAUTIONS—Pediatric Use, for adverse events reported upon discontinuation of treatment with paroxetine in pediatric patients.

Akathisia: The use of paroxetine or other SSRIs has been associated with the development of akathisia, which is characterized by an inner sense of restlessness and psychomotor agitation such as an inability to sit or stand still usually associated with subjective distress. This is most likely to occur within the first few weeks of treatment.

Hyponatremia: Several cases of hyponatremia have been reported with immediate-release paroxetine hydrochloride. The hyponatremia appeared to be reversible when paroxetine was discontinued. The majority of these occurrences have been in elderly individuals, some in patients taking diuretics or who were otherwise volume depleted.

Serotonin Syndrome: The development of a serotonin syndrome may occur in association with treatment with paroxetine, particularly with concomitant use of serotonergic drugs and with drugs which may have impaired metabolism of immediate-release paroxetine hydrochloride. Symptoms have included agitation, confusion, diaphoresis, hallucinations, hyperreflexia, myoclonus, shivering, tachycardia, and tremor. The concomitant use of PAXIL CR with serotonin precursors (such as tryptophan) is not recommended (see WARNINGS—Potential for Interaction With Monoamine Oxidase Inhibitors and PRECAUTIONS—Drug Interactions).

Abnormal Bleeding: Published case reports have documented the occurrence of bleeding episodes in patients treated with psychotropic drugs that interfere with serotonin reuptake. Subsequent epidemiological studies, both of the case-control and cohort design, have demonstrated an association between use of psychotropic drugs that interfere with serotonin reuptake and the occurrence of upper gastrointestinal bleeding. In 2 studies, concurrent use of a nonsteroidal anti-inflammatory drug (NSAID) or aspirin potentiated the risk of bleeding (see Drug Interactions). Although

these studies focused on upper gastrointestinal bleeding, there is reason to believe that bleeding at other sites may be similarly potentiated. Patients should be cautioned regarding the risk of bleeding associated with the concomitant use of paroxetine with NSAIDs, aspirin, or other drugs that affect coagulation.

Use in Patients With Concomitant Illness: Clinical experience with immediate-release paroxetine hydrochloride in patients with certain concomitant systemic illness is limited. Caution is advisable in using PAXIL CR in patients with diseases or conditions that could affect metabolism or hemodynamic responses.

As with other SSRIs, mydriasis has been infrequently reported in premarketing studies with paroxetine hydrochloride. A few cases of acute angle closure glaucoma associated with therapy with immediate-release paroxetine have been reported in the literature. As mydriasis can cause acute angle closure in patients with narrow angle glaucoma, caution should be used when PAXIL CR is prescribed for patients with narrow angle glaucoma.

PAXIL CR or the immediate-release formulation has not been evaluated or used to any appreciable extent in patients with a recent history of myocardial infarction or unstable heart disease. Patients with these diagnoses were excluded from clinical studies during premarket testing. Evaluation of electrocardiograms of 682 patients who received immediate-release paroxetine hydrochloride in double-blind, placebo-controlled trials, however, did not indicate that paroxetine is associated with the development of significant ECG abnormalities. Similarly, paroxetine hydrochloride does not cause any clinically important changes in heart rate or blood pressure.

Increased plasma concentrations of paroxetine occur in patients with severe renal impairment (creatinine clearance <30 mL/min.) or severe hepatic impairment. A lower starting dose should be used in such patients (see DOSAGE AND ADMINISTRATION).

Information for Patients: Prescribers or other health professionals should inform patients, their families, and their caregivers about the benefits and risks associated with treatment with PAXIL CR and should counsel them in its appropriate use. A patient Medication Guide About Using Antidepressants in Children and Teenagers is available for PAXIL CR. The prescriber or health professional should instruct patients, their families, and their caregivers to read the Medication Guide and should assist them in understanding its contents. Patients should be given the opportunity to discuss the contents of the Medication Guide and to obtain answers to any questions they may have. The complete text of the Medication Guide is reprinted at the end of this document.

Patients should be advised of the following issues and asked to alert their prescriber if these occur while taking PAXIL CR.

Clinical Worsening and Suicide Risk: Patients, their families, and their caregivers should be encouraged to be alert to the emergence of anxiety, agitation, panic attacks, insomnia, irritability, hostility, aggressiveness, impulsivity, akathisia (psychomotor restlessness), hypomania, mania, other unusual changes in behavior, worsening of depression, and suicidal ideation, especially early during antidepressant treatment and when the dose is adjusted up or down. Families and caregivers of patients should be advised to observe for the emergence of such symptoms on a day-to-day basis, since changes may be abrupt. Such symptoms should be reported to the patient's prescriber or health professional, especially if they are severe, abrupt in onset, or were not part of the patient's presenting symptoms. Symptoms such as these may be associated with an increased risk for suicidal thinking and behavior and indicate a need for very close monitoring and possibly changes in the medication.

PAXIL CR should not be chewed or crushed, and should be swallowed whole.

Drugs That Interfere With Hemostasis (NSAIDs, Aspirin, Warfarin, etc.): Patients should be cautioned about the concomitant use of paroxetine and NSAIDs, aspirin, or other drugs that affect coagulation since the combined use of psychotropic drugs that interfere with serotonin reuptake and these agents has been associated with an increased risk of bleeding.

Interference With Cognitive and Motor Performance: Any psychoactive drug may impair judgment, thinking, or motor skills. Although in controlled studies immediate-release paroxetine hydrochloride has not been shown to impair psychomotor performance, patients should be cautioned about operating hazardous machinery, including automobiles, until they are reasonably certain that therapy with PAXIL CR does not affect their ability to engage in such activities.

Completing Course of Therapy: While patients may notice improvement with use of PAXIL CR in 1 to 4 weeks, they should be advised to continue therapy as directed.

Concomitant Medications: Patients should be advised to inform their physician if they are taking, or plan to take, any prescription or over-the-counter drugs, since there is a potential for interactions.

Alcohol: Although immediate-release paroxetine hydrochloride has not been shown to increase the impairment of mental and motor skills caused by alcohol, patients should be advised to avoid alcohol while taking PAXIL CR.

Pregnancy: Patients should be advised to notify their physician if they become pregnant or intend to become pregnant during therapy.

Nursing: Patients should be advised to notify their physician if they are breast-feeding an infant (see PRECAUTIONS—Nursing Mothers).

Laboratory Tests: There are no specific laboratory tests recommended.

Drug Interactions: Tryptophan: As with other serotonin reuptake inhibitors, an interaction between paroxetine and tryptophan may occur when they are coadministered. Adverse experiences, consisting primarily of headache, nausea, sweating, and dizziness, have been reported when tryptophan was administered to patients taking immediate-release paroxetine. Consequently, concomitant use of PAXIL CR with tryptophan is not recommended (see Serotonin Syndrome).

Monoamine Oxidase Inhibitors: See CONTRAINDICATIONS and WARNINGS.

Serotonergic Drugs: Based on the mechanism of action of paroxetine and the potential for serotonin syndrome, caution is advised when PAXIL CR is coadministered with other drugs or agents that may affect the serotonergic neurotransmitter systems, such as tryptophan, triptans, serotonin reuptake inhibitors, linezolid (an antibiotic which is a reversible non-selective MAOI), lithium, tramadol, or St. John's Wort (see Serotonin Syndrome).

Thioridazine: See CONTRAINDICATIONS and WARNINGS.

Warfarin: Preliminary data suggest that there may be a pharmacodynamic interaction (that causes an increased bleeding diathesis in the face of unaltered prothrombin time) between paroxetine and warfarin. Since there is little clinical experience, the concomitant administration of PAXIL CR and warfarin should be undertaken with caution (see Drugs That Interfere With Hemostasis).

Triptans: There have been rare postmarketing reports describing patients with weakness, hyperreflexia, and incoordination following the use of an SSRI and sumatriptan. If concomitant treatment with a triptan and an SSRI (e.g., fluoxetine, fluvoxamine, paroxetine, sertraline) is clinically warranted, appropriate observation of the patient is advised (see Serotonin Syndrome).

Drugs Affecting Hepatic Metabolism: The metabolism and pharmacokinetics of paroxetine may be affected by the induction or inhibition of drug-metabolizing enzymes.

Cimetidine: Cimetidine inhibits many cytochrome P_{450} (oxidative) enzymes. In a study where immediate-release paroxetine (30 mg once daily) was dosed orally for 4 weeks, steady-state plasma concentrations of paroxetine were increased by approximately 50% during coadministration with oral cimetidine (300 mg three times daily) for the final week. Therefore, when these drugs are administered concurrently, dosage adjustment of PAXIL CR after the starting dose should be guided by clinical effect. The effect of paroxetine on cimetidine's pharmacokinetics was not studied.

Phenobarbital: Phenobarbital induces many cytochrome P_{450} (oxidative) enzymes. When a single oral 30-mg dose of immediate-release paroxetine was administered at phenobarbital steady state (100 mg once daily for 14 days), paroxetine AUC and $T_{1/2}$ were reduced (by an average of 25% and 38%, respectively) compared to paroxetine administered alone. The effect of paroxetine on phenobarbital pharmacokinetics was not studied. Since paroxetine exhibits nonlinear pharmacokinetics, the results of this study may not address the case where the 2 drugs are both being chronically dosed. No initial dosage adjustment with PAXIL CR is considered necessary when coadministered with phenobarbital; any subsequent adjustment should be guided by clinical effect.

Phenytoin: When a single oral 30-mg dose of immediate-release paroxetine was administered at phenytoin steady state (300 mg once daily for 14 days), paroxetine AUC and $T_{1/2}$ were reduced (by an average of 50% and 35%, respectively) compared to immediate-release paroxetine administered alone. In a separate study, when a single oral 300-mg dose of phenytoin was administered at paroxetine steady state (30 mg once daily for 14 days), phenytoin AUC was slightly reduced (12% on average) compared to phenytoin administered alone. Since both drugs exhibit nonlinear pharmacokinetics, the above studies may not address the case where the 2 drugs are both being chronically dosed. No initial dosage adjustments are considered necessary when PAXIL CR is coadministered with phenytoin; any subsequent adjustments should be guided by clinical effect (see ADVERSE REACTIONS—Postmarketing Reports).

Drugs Metabolized by Cytochrome $P_{450}IID_6$: Many drugs, including most drugs effective in the treatment of major depressive disorder (paroxetine, other SSRIs, and many tricyclics), are metabolized by the cytochrome P_{450} isozyme $P_{450}IID_6$. Like other agents that are metabolized by $P_{450}IID_6$, paroxetine may significantly inhibit the activity of this isozyme. In most patients (>90%), this $P_{450}IID_6$ isozyme is saturated early during paroxetine dosing. In 1 study, daily dosing of immediate-release paroxetine (20 mg once daily) under steady-state conditions increased single-dose desipramine (100 mg) C_{max}, AUC, and $T_{1/2}$ by an average of approximately 2-, 5-, and 3-fold, respectively. Concomitant use of PAXIL CR with other drugs metabolized by cytochrome $P_{450}IID_6$ has not been formally studied but may require lower doses than usually prescribed for either PAXIL CR or the other drug.

Therefore, coadministration of PAXIL CR with other drugs that are metabolized by this isozyme, including certain drugs effective in the treatment of major depressive disorder (e.g., nortriptyline, amitriptyline, imipramine, desipramine, and fluoxetine), phenothiazines, risperidone, and Type 1C antiarrhythmics (e.g., propafenone, flecainide, and encainide), or that inhibit this enzyme (e.g., quinidine), should be approached with caution.

However, due to the risk of serious ventricular arrhythmias and sudden death potentially associated with elevated plasma levels of thioridazine, paroxetine and thioridazine should not be coadministered (see CONTRAINDICATIONS and WARNINGS).

At steady state, when the $P_{450}IID_6$ pathway is essentially saturated, paroxetine clearance is governed by alternative P_{450} isozymes that, unlike $P_{450}IID_6$, show no evidence of saturation (see PRECAUTIONS—Tricyclic Antidepressants).

Drugs Metabolized by Cytochrome $P_{450}IIIA_4$: An in vivo interaction study involving the coadministration under steady-state conditions of paroxetine and terfenadine, a substrate for $P_{450}IIIA_4$, revealed no effect of paroxetine on terfenadine pharmacokinetics. In addition, in vitro studies have shown ketoconazole, a potent inhibitor of $P_{450}IIIA_4$ activity, to be at least 100 times more potent than paroxetine as an inhibitor of the metabolism of several substrates for this enzyme, including terfenadine, astemizole, cisapride, triazolam, and cyclosporine. Based on the assumption that the relationship between paroxetine's in vitro K_i and its lack of effect on terfenadine's in vivo clearance predicts its effect on other $IIIA_4$ substrates, paroxetine's extent of inhibition of $IIIA_4$ activity is not likely to be of clinical significance.

Tricyclic Antidepressants (TCAs): Caution is indicated in the coadministration of TCAs with PAXIL CR, because paroxetine may inhibit TCA metabolism. Plasma TCA concentrations may need to be monitored, and the dose of TCA may need to be reduced, if a TCA is coadministered with PAXIL CR (see PRECAUTIONS—Drugs Metabolized by Cytochrome $P_{450}IID_6$).

Drugs Highly Bound to Plasma Protein: Because paroxetine is highly bound to plasma protein, administration of PAXIL CR to a patient taking another drug that is highly protein bound may cause increased free concentrations of the other drug, potentially resulting in adverse events. Conversely, adverse effects could result from displacement of paroxetine by other highly bound drugs.

Drugs That Interfere With Hemostasis (NSAIDs, Aspirin, Warfarin, etc.): Serotonin release by platelets plays an important role in hemostasis. Epidemiological studies of the case-control and cohort design that have demonstrated an association between use of psychotropic drugs that interfere with serotonin reuptake and the occurrence of upper gastrointestinal bleeding have also shown that concurrent use of an NSAID or aspirin potentiated the risk of bleeding. Thus, patients should be cautioned about the use of such drugs concurrently with paroxetine.

Alcohol: Although paroxetine does not increase the impairment of mental and motor skills caused by alcohol, patients should be advised to avoid alcohol while taking PAXIL CR.

Lithium: A multiple-dose study with immediate-release paroxetine hydrochloride has shown that there is no pharmacokinetic interaction between paroxetine and lithium carbonate. However, due to the potential for serotonin syndrome, caution is advised when immediate-release paroxetine hydrochloride is coadministered with lithium.

Digoxin: The steady-state pharmacokinetics of paroxetine was not altered when administered with digoxin at steady state. Mean digoxin AUC at steady state decreased by 15% in the presence of paroxetine. Since there is little clinical experience, the concurrent administration of PAXIL CR and digoxin should be undertaken with caution.

Diazepam: Under steady-state conditions, diazepam does not appear to affect paroxetine kinetics. The effects of paroxetine on diazepam were not evaluated.

Procyclidine: Daily oral dosing of immediate-release paroxetine (30 mg once daily) increased steady-state AUC_{0-24}, C_{max}, and C_{min} values of procyclidine (5 mg oral once daily) by 35%, 37%, and 67%, respectively, compared to procyclidine alone at steady state. If anticholinergic effects are seen, the dose of procyclidine should be reduced.

Beta-Blockers: In a study where propranolol (80 mg twice daily) was dosed orally for 18 days, the established steady-state plasma concentrations of propranolol were unaltered during coadministration with immediate-release paroxetine (30 mg once daily) for the final 10 days. The effects of propranolol on paroxetine have not been evaluated (see ADVERSE REACTIONS—Postmarketing Reports).

Theophylline: Reports of elevated theophylline levels associated with immediate-release paroxetine treatment have been reported. While this interaction has not been formally studied, it is recommended that theophylline levels be monitored when these drugs are concurrently administered.

Electroconvulsive Therapy (ECT): There are no clinical studies of the combined use of ECT and PAXIL CR.

Carcinogenesis, Mutagenesis, Impairment of Fertility:

Carcinogenesis: Two-year carcinogenicity studies were conducted in rodents given paroxetine in the diet at 1, 5, and 25 mg/kg/day (mice) and 1, 5, and 20 mg/kg/day (rats). These doses are up to approximately 2 (mouse) and 3 (rat) times the maximum recommended human dose (MRHD) on a mg/m^2 basis. There was a significantly greater number of male rats in the high-dose group with reticulum cell sarcomas (1/100, 0/50, 0/50, and 4/50 for control, low-, middle-, and high-dose groups, respectively) and a significantly increased linear trend across dose groups for the occurrence of lymphoreticular tumors in male rats. Female rats were not affected. Although there was a dose-related increase in the number of tumors in mice, there was no drug-related increase in the number of mice with tumors. The relevance of these findings to humans is unknown.

Mutagenesis: Paroxetine produced no genotoxic effects in a battery of 5 in vitro and 2 in vivo assays that included the following: Bacterial mutation assay, mouse lymphoma mutation assay, unscheduled DNA synthesis assay, and tests for cytogenetic aberrations in vivo in mouse bone marrow and in vitro in human lymphocytes and in a dominant lethal test in rats.

	PAXIL CR 25 mg (n = 348)	PAXIL CR 12.5 mg (n = 333)	Placebo (n = 349)
TOTAL	15%	9.9%	6.3%
Nausea*	6.0%	2.4%	0.9%
Asthenia	4.9%	3.0%	1.4%
Somnolence*	4.3%	1.8%	0.3%
Insomnia	2.3%	1.5%	0.0%
Concentration Impaired*	2.0%	0.6%	0.3%
Dry mouth*	2.0%	0.6%	0.3%
Dizziness*	1.7%	0.6%	0.6%
Decreased Appetite*	1.4%	0.6%	0.0%
Sweating*	1.4%	0.0%	0.3%
Tremor*	1.4%	0.3%	0.0%
Yawn*	1.1%	0.0%	0.0%
Diarrhea	0.9%	1.2%	0.0%

*Events considered to be dose dependent are defined as events having an incidence rate with 25 mg of PAXIL CR that was at least twice that with 12.5 mg of PAXIL CR (as well as the placebo group).

Impairment of Fertility: A reduced pregnancy rate was found in reproduction studies in rats at a dose of paroxetine of 15 mg/kg/day, which is approximately twice the MRHD on a mg/m^2 basis. Irreversible lesions occurred in the reproductive tract of male rats after dosing in toxicity studies for 2 to 52 weeks. These lesions consisted of vacuolation of epididymal tubular epithelium at 50 mg/kg/day and atrophic changes in the seminiferous tubules of the testes with arrested spermatogenesis at 25 mg/kg/day (approximately 8 and 4 times the MRHD on a mg/m^2 basis).

Pregnancy: Pregnancy Category C. Reproduction studies were performed at doses up to 50 mg/kg/day in rats and 6 mg/kg/day in rabbits administered during organogenesis. These doses are approximately 8 (rat) and 2 (rabbit) times the MRHD on an mg/m^2 basis. These studies have revealed no evidence of teratogenic effects. However, in rats, there was an increase in pup deaths during the first 4 days of lactation when dosing occurred during the last trimester of gestation and continued throughout lactation. This effect occurred at a dose of 1 mg/kg/day or approximately one-sixth of the MRHD on an mg/m^2 basis. The no-effect dose for rat pup mortality was not determined. The cause of these deaths is not known. There are no adequate and well-controlled studies in pregnant women. This drug should be used during pregnancy only if the potential benefit justifies the potential risk to the fetus.

Nonteratogenic Effects: Neonates exposed to PAXIL CR and other SSRIs or SNRIs, late in the third trimester have developed complications requiring prolonged hospitalization, respiratory support, and tube feeding. Such complications can arise immediately upon delivery. Reported clinical findings have included respiratory distress, cyanosis, apnea, seizures, temperature instability, feeding difficulty, vomiting, hypoglycemia, hypotonia, hypertonia, hyperreflexia, tremor, jitteriness, irritability, and constant crying. These features are consistent with either a direct toxic effect of SSRIs and SNRIs or, possibly, a drug discontinuation syndrome. It should be noted that, in some cases, the clinical picture is consistent with serotonin syndrome (see WARNINGS—Potential for Interaction With Monoamine Oxidase Inhibitors).

There have also been postmarketing reports of premature births in pregnant women exposed to paroxetine or other SSRIs.

When treating a pregnant woman with paroxetine during the third trimester, the physician should carefully consider the potential risks and benefits of treatment (see DOSAGE AND ADMINISTRATION).

Labor and Delivery: The effect of paroxetine on labor and delivery in humans is unknown.

Nursing Mothers: Like many other drugs, paroxetine is secreted in human milk, and caution should be exercised when PAXIL CR is administered to a nursing woman.

Pediatric Use: Safety and effectiveness in the pediatric population have not been established (see BOX WARNING and WARNINGS—Clinical Worsening and Suicide Risk). Three placebo-controlled trials in 752 pediatric patients with MDD have been conducted with PAXIL, and the data were not sufficient to support a claim for use in pediatric patients. Anyone considering the use of PAXIL CR in a child or adolescent must balance the potential risks with the clinical need.

In placebo-controlled clinical trials conducted with pediatric patients, the following adverse events were reported in at least 2% of pediatric patients treated with immediate-release paroxetine hydrochloride and occurred at a rate at least twice that for pediatric patients receiving placebo: emotional lability (including self-harm, suicidal thoughts, attempted suicide, crying, and mood fluctuations), hostility, decreased appetite, tremor, sweating, hyperkinesia, and agitation.

Events reported upon discontinuation of treatment with immediate-release paroxetine hydrochloride in the pediatric clinical trials that included a taper phase regimen, which occurred in at least 2% of patients who received immediate-release paroxetine hydrochloride and which occurred at a rate at least twice that of placebo, were: emotional lability (including suicidal ideation, suicide attempt, mood changes, and tearfulness), nervousness, dizziness, nausea, and abdominal pain (see Discontinuation of Treatment With PAXIL CR).

Geriatric Use: In worldwide premarketing clinical trials with immediate-release paroxetine hydrochloride, 17% of paroxetine-treated patients (approximately 700) were 65 years or older. Pharmacokinetic studies revealed a decreased clearance in the elderly, and a lower starting dose is recommended; there were, however, no overall differences in the adverse event profile between elderly and younger patients, and effectiveness was similar in younger and older patients (see CLINICAL PHARMACOLOGY and DOSAGE AND ADMINISTRATION).

In a controlled study focusing specifically on elderly patients with major depressive disorder, PAXIL CR was demonstrated to be safe and effective in the treatment of elderly patients (>60 years) with major depressive disorder. (See CLINICAL PHARMACOLOGY—Clinical Trials and ADVERSE REACTIONS—Table 2.)

ADVERSE REACTIONS

The information included under the "Adverse Findings Observed in Short-Term, Placebo-Controlled Trials With PAXIL CR" subsection of ADVERSE REACTIONS is based on data from 11 placebo-controlled clinical trials. Three of these studies were conducted in patients with major depressive disorder, 3 studies were done in patients with panic disorder, 1 study was conducted in patients with social anxiety disorder, and 4 studies were done in female patients with PMDD. Two of the studies in major depressive disorder, which enrolled patients in the age range 18 to 65 years, are pooled. Information from a third study of major depressive disorder, which focused on elderly patients (60 to 88 years), is presented separately as is the information from the panic disorder studies and the information from the PMDD studies. Information on additional adverse events associated with PAXIL CR and the immediate-release formulation of paroxetine hydrochloride is included in a separate subsection (see Other Events).

Adverse Findings Observed in Short-Term, Placebo-Controlled Trials With PAXIL CR:

Adverse Events Associated With Discontinuation of Treatment: ***Major Depressive Disorder:*** Ten percent (21/212) of patients treated with PAXIL CR discontinued treatment due to an adverse event in a pool of 2 studies of patients with major depressive disorder. The most common events (≥1%) associated with discontinuation and considered to be drug related (i.e., those events associated with dropout at a rate approximately twice or greater for PAXIL CR compared to placebo) included the following:

	PAXIL CR (n = 212)	Placebo (n = 211)
Nausea	3.7%	0.5%
Asthenia	1.9%	0.5%
Dizziness	1.4%	0.0%
Somnolence	1.4%	0.0%

In a placebo-controlled study of elderly patients with major depressive disorder, 13% (13/104) of patients treated with PAXIL CR discontinued due to an adverse event. Events meeting the above criteria included the following:

	PAXIL CR (n = 104)	Placebo (n = 109)
Nausea	2.9%	0.0%
Headache	1.9%	0.9%
Depression	1.9%	0.0%
LFT's abnormal	1.9%	0.0%

Panic Disorder: Eleven percent (50/444) of patients treated with PAXIL CR in panic disorder studies discontinued treatment due to an adverse event. Events meeting the above criteria included the following:

	PAXIL CR (n = 444)	Placebo (n = 445)
Nausea	2.9%	0.4%
Insomnia	1.8%	0.0%
Headache	1.4%	0.2%
Asthenia	1.1%	0.0%

Social Anxiety Disorder: Three percent (5/186) of patients treated with PAXIL CR in the social anxiety disorder study discontinued treatment due to an adverse event. Events meeting the above criteria included the following:

	PAXIL CR (n = 186)	Placebo (n = 184)
Nausea	2.2%	0.5%
Headache	1.6%	0.5%
Diarrhea	1.1%	0.5%

Continued on next page

Paxil CR—Cont.

Premenstrual Dysphoric Disorder: Spontaneously reported adverse events were monitored in studies of both continuous and intermittent dosing of PAXIL CR in the treatment of PMDD. Generally, there were few differences in the adverse event profiles of the 2 dosing regimens. Thirteen percent (88/681) of patients treated with PAXIL CR in PMDD studies of continuous dosing discontinued treatment due to an adverse event.

The most common events (≥1%) associated with discontinuation in either group treated with PAXIL CR with an incidence rate that is at least twice that of placebo in PMDD trials that employed a continuous dosing regimen are shown in the following table. This table also shows those events that were dose dependent (indicated with an asterisk) as defined as events having an incidence rate with 25 mg of PAXIL CR that was at least twice that with 12.5 mg of PAXIL CR (as well as the placebo group).

[See table at top of previous page]

Commonly Observed Adverse Events: *Major Depressive Disorder:* The most commonly observed adverse events associated with the use of PAXIL CR in a pool of 2 trials (incidence of 5.0% or greater and incidence for PAXIL CR at least twice that for placebo, derived from Table 1) were: Abnormal ejaculation, abnormal vision, constipation, decreased libido, diarrhea, dizziness, female genital disorders, nausea, somnolence, sweating, trauma, tremor, and yawning.

Using the same criteria, the adverse events associated with the use of PAXIL CR in a study of elderly patients with major depressive disorder were: Abnormal ejaculation, constipation, decreased appetite, dry mouth, impotence, infection, libido decreased, sweating, and tremor.

Panic Disorder: In the pool of panic disorder studies, the adverse events meeting these criteria were: Abnormal ejaculation, somnolence, impotence, libido decreased, tremor, sweating, and female genital disorders (generally anorgasmia or difficulty achieving orgasm).

Social Anxiety Disorder: In the social anxiety disorder study, the adverse events meeting these criteria were: Nausea, asthenia, abnormal ejaculation, sweating, somnolence, impotence, insomnia, and libido decreased.

Premenstrual Dysphoric Disorder: The most commonly observed adverse events associated with the use of PAXIL CR either during continuous dosing or luteal phase dosing (incidence of 5% or greater and incidence for PAXIL CR at least twice that for placebo, derived from Table 5) were: Nausea, asthenia, libido decreased, somnolence, insomnia, female genital disorders, sweating, dizziness, diarrhea, and constipation.

In the luteal phase dosing PMDD trial, which employed dosing of 12.5 mg/day or 25 mg/day of PAXIL CR limited to the 2 weeks prior to the onset of menses over 3 consecutive menstrual cycles, adverse events were evaluated during the first 14 days of each off-drug phase. When the 3 off-drug phases were combined, the following adverse events were reported at an incidence of 2% or greater for PAXIL CR and were at least twice the rate of that reported for placebo: Infection (5.3% versus 2.5%), depression (2.8% versus 0.8%), insomnia (2.4% versus 0.8%), sinusitis (2.4% versus 0%), and asthenia (2.0% versus 0.8%).

Incidence in Controlled Clinical Trials: Table 1 enumerates adverse events that occurred at an incidence of 1% or more among patients treated with PAXIL CR, aged 18 to 65, who participated in 2 short-term (12-week) placebo-controlled trials in major depressive disorder in which patients were dosed in a range of 25 mg to 62.5 mg/day. Table 2 enumerates adverse events reported at an incidence of 5% or greater among elderly patients (ages 60 to 88) treated with PAXIL CR who participated in a short-term (12-week) placebo-controlled trial in major depressive disorder in which patients were dosed in a range of 12.5 mg to 50 mg/day. Table 3 enumerates adverse events reported at an incidence of 1% or greater among patients (19 to 72 years) treated with PAXIL CR who participated in short-term (10-week) placebo-controlled trials in panic disorder in which patients were dosed in a range of 12.5 mg to 75 mg/day. Table 4 enumerates adverse events reported at an incidence of 1% or greater among adult patients treated with PAXIL CR who participated in a short-term (12-week), double-blind, placebo-controlled trial in social anxiety disorder in which patients were dosed in a range of 12.5 to 37.5 mg/day. Table 5 enumerates adverse events that occurred at an incidence of 1% or more among patients treated with PAXIL CR who participated in three, 12-week, placebo-controlled trials in PMDD in which patients were dosed at 12.5 mg/day or 25 mg/day and in one 12-week placebo-controlled trial in which patients were dosed for 2 weeks prior to the onset of menses (luteal phase dosing) at 12.5 mg/day or 25 mg/day. Reported adverse events were classified using a standard COSTART-based Dictionary terminology.

The prescriber should be aware that these figures cannot be used to predict the incidence of side effects in the course of usual medical practice where patient characteristics and other factors differ from those that prevailed in the clinical trials. Similarly, the cited frequencies cannot be compared with figures obtained from other clinical investigations involving different treatments, uses, and investigators. The cited figures, however, do provide the prescribing physician with some basis for estimating the relative contribution of drug and nondrug factors to the side effect incidence rate in the population studied.

[See table 1 above]

Table 1. Treatment-Emergent Adverse Events Occurring in ≥1% of Patients Treated With PAXIL CR in a Pool of 2 Studies in Major Depressive Disorder[1,2]

Body System/Adverse Event	% Reporting Event	
	PAXIL CR (n = 212)	Placebo (n = 211)
Body as a Whole		
Headache	27%	20%
Asthenia	14%	9%
Infection[3]	8%	5%
Abdominal Pain	7%	4%
Back Pain	5%	3%
Trauma[4]	5%	1%
Pain[5]	3%	1%
Allergic Reaction[6]	2%	1%
Cardiovascular System		
Tachycardia	1%	0%
Vasodilatation[7]	2%	0%
Digestive System		
Nausea	22%	10%
Diarrhea	18%	7%
Dry Mouth	15%	8%
Constipation	10%	4%
Flatulence	6%	4%
Decreased Appetite	4%	2%
Vomiting	2%	1%
Nervous System		
Somnolence	22%	8%
Insomnia	17%	9%
Dizziness	14%	4%
Libido Decreased	7%	3%
Tremor	7%	1%
Hypertonia	3%	1%
Paresthesia	3%	1%
Agitation	2%	1%
Confusion	1%	0%
Respiratory System		
Yawn	5%	0%
Rhinitis	4%	1%
Cough Increased	2%	1%
Bronchitis	1%	0%
Skin and Appendages		
Sweating	6%	2%
Photosensitivity	2%	0%
Special Senses		
Abnormal Vision[8]	5%	1%
Taste Perversion	2%	0%
Urogenital System		
Abnormal Ejaculation[9,10]	26%	1%
Female Genital Disorder[9,11]	10%	<1%
Impotence[9]	5%	3%
Urinary Tract Infection	3%	1%
Menstrual Disorder[9]	2%	<1%
Vaginitis[9]	2%	0%

1. Adverse events for which the PAXIL CR reporting incidence was less than or equal to the placebo incidence are not included. These events are: Abnormal dreams, anxiety, arthralgia, depersonalization, dysmenorrhea, dyspepsia, hyperkinesia, increased appetite, myalgia, nervousness, pharyngitis, purpura, rash, respiratory disorder, sinusitis, urinary frequency, and weight gain.
2. <1% means greater than zero and less than 1%.
3. Mostly flu.
4. A wide variety of injuries with no obvious pattern.
5. Pain in a variety of locations with no obvious pattern.
6. Most frequently seasonal allergic symptoms.
7. Usually flushing.
8. Mostly blurred vision.
9. Based on the number of males or females.
10. Mostly anorgasmia or delayed ejaculation.
11. Mostly anorgasmia or delayed orgasm.

[See table 2 at top of next page]
[See table 3 on pages 211 and 212]
[See table 4 on page 212]
[See table 5 at top of page 213]

Dose Dependency of Adverse Events: The following table shows results in PMDD trials of common adverse events, defined as events with an incidence of ≥1% with 25 mg of PAXIL CR that was at least twice that with 12.5 mg of PAXIL CR and with placebo.

Incidence of Common Adverse Events in Placebo, 12.5 mg and 25 mg of PAXIL CR in a Pool of 3 Fixed-Dose PMDD Trials

Common Adverse Event	PAXIL CR 25 mg (n = 348)	PAXIL CR 12.5 mg (n = 333)	Placebo (n = 349)
Sweating	8.9%	4.2%	0.9%
Tremor	6.0%	1.5%	0.3%
Concentration Impaired	4.3%	1.5%	0.6%
Yawn	3.2%	0.9%	0.3%
Paresthesia	1.4%	0.3%	0.3%
Hyperkinesia	1.1%	0.3%	0.0%
Vaginitis	1.1%	0.3%	0.3%

A comparison of adverse event rates in a fixed-dose study comparing immediate-release paroxetine with placebo in the treatment of major depressive disorder revealed a clear dose dependency for some of the more common adverse events associated with the use of immediate-release paroxetine.

Male and Female Sexual Dysfunction With SSRIs: Although changes in sexual desire, sexual performance, and sexual satisfaction often occur as manifestations of a psychiatric disorder, they may also be a consequence of pharmacologic treatment. In particular, some evidence suggests that SSRIs can cause such untoward sexual experiences.

Reliable estimates of the incidence and severity of untoward experiences involving sexual desire, performance, and satisfaction are difficult to obtain; however, in part because patients and physicians may be reluctant to discuss them. Accordingly, estimates of the incidence of untoward sexual experience and performance cited in product labeling, are likely to underestimate their actual incidence.

The percentage of patients reporting symptoms of sexual dysfunction in the pool of 2 placebo-controlled trials in nonelderly patients with major depressive disorder, in the pool of 3 placebo-controlled trials in patients with panic disorder, in the placebo-controlled trial in patients with social anxiety disorder, and in the intermittent dosing and the pool of 3 placebo-controlled continuous dosing trials in female patients with PMDD are as follows:
[See table at top of page 214]
There are no adequate, controlled studies examining sexual dysfunction with paroxetine treatment.

Paroxetine treatment has been associated with several cases of priapism. In those cases with a known outcome, patients recovered without sequelae.

While it is difficult to know the precise risk of sexual dysfunction associated with the use of SSRIs, physicians should routinely inquire about such possible side effects.

Weight and Vital Sign Changes: Significant weight loss may be an undesirable result of treatment with paroxetine for some patients but, on average, patients in controlled trials with PAXIL CR or the immediate-release formulation, had minimal weight loss (about 1 pound). No significant changes in vital signs (systolic and diastolic blood pressure, pulse, and temperature) were observed in patients treated with PAXIL CR, or immediate-release paroxetine hydrochloride, in controlled clinical trials.

ECG Changes: In an analysis of ECGs obtained in 682 patients treated with immediate-release paroxetine and 415 patients treated with placebo in controlled clinical trials, no clinically significant changes were seen in the ECGs of either group.

Liver Function Tests: In a pool of 2 placebo-controlled clinical trials, patients treated with PAXIL CR or placebo exhibited abnormal values on liver function tests at comparable rates. In particular, the controlled-release paroxetine-versus-placebo comparisons for alkaline phosphatase, SGOT, SGPT, and bilirubin revealed no differences in the percentage of patients with marked abnormalities.

In a study of elderly patients with major depressive disorder, 3 of 104 patients treated with PAXIL CR and none of 109 placebo patients experienced liver transaminase elevations of potential clinical concern.

Two of the patients treated with PAXIL CR dropped out of the study due to abnormal liver function tests; the third patient experienced normalization of transaminase levels with continued treatment. Also, in the pool of 3 studies of patients with panic disorder, 4 of 444 patients treated with PAXIL CR and none of 445 placebo patients experienced liver transaminase elevations of potential clinical concern. Elevations in all 4 patients decreased substantially after discontinuation of PAXIL CR. The clinical significance of these findings is unknown.

In placebo-controlled clinical trials with the immediate-release formulation of paroxetine, patients exhibited abnormal values on liver function tests at no greater rate than that seen in placebo-treated patients.

Other Events Observed During the Clinical Development of Paroxetine: The following adverse events were reported during the clinical development of PAXIL CR and/or the clinical development of the immediate-release formulation of paroxetine.

Adverse events for which frequencies are provided below occurred in clinical trials with the controlled-release formulation of paroxetine. During its premarketing assessment in major depressive disorder, panic disorder, social anxiety disorder, and PMDD multiple doses of PAXIL CR were administered to 1,627 patients in phase 3 double-blind, controlled, outpatient studies. Untoward events associated with this exposure were recorded by clinical investigators using terminology of their own choosing. Consequently, it is not possible to provide a meaningful estimate of the proportion of individuals experiencing adverse events without first grouping similar types of untoward events into a smaller number of standardized event categories.

In the tabulations that follow, reported adverse events were classified using a COSTART-based dictionary. The frequencies presented, therefore, represent the proportion of the 1,627 patients exposed to PAXIL CR who experienced an event of the type cited on at least 1 occasion while receiving PAXIL CR. All reported events are included except those already listed in Tables 1 through 5 and those events where a drug cause was remote. If the COSTART term for an event was so general as to be uninformative, it was deleted or, when possible, replaced with a more informative term. It is important to emphasize that although the events reported occurred during treatment with paroxetine, they were not necessarily caused by it.

Events are further categorized by body system and listed in order of decreasing frequency according to the following definitions: Frequent adverse events are those occurring on 1 or more occasions in at least 1/100 patients (only those not already listed in the tabulated results from placebo-controlled trials appear in this listing); infrequent adverse events are those occurring in 1/100 to 1/1,000 patients; rare events are those occurring in fewer than 1/1,000 patients.

Adverse events for which frequencies are not provided occurred during the premarketing assessment of immediate-release paroxetine in phase 2 and 3 studies of major depressive disorder, obsessive compulsive disorder, panic disorder, social anxiety disorder, generalized anxiety disorder, and posttraumatic stress disorder. The conditions and duration of exposure to immediate-release paroxetine varied greatly and included (in overlapping categories) open and double-blind studies, uncontrolled and controlled studies, inpatient and outpatient studies, and fixed-dose and titration studies. Only those events not previously listed for controlled-release paroxetine are included. The extent to which these events may be associated with PAXIL CR is unknown. Events are listed alphabetically within the respective body system. Events of major clinical importance are also described in the PRECAUTIONS section.

Body as a Whole: Infrequent were chills, face edema, fever, flu syndrome, malaise; rare were abscess, anaphylactoid reaction, anticholinergic syndrome, hypothermia; also observed were adrenergic syndrome, neck rigidity, sepsis.

Cardiovascular System: Infrequent were angina pectoris, bradycardia, hematoma, hypertension, hypotension, palpitation, postural hypotension, supraventricular tachycardia, syncope; rare were bundle branch block; also observed were arrhythmia nodal, atrial fibrillation, cerebrovascular accident, congestive heart failure, low cardiac output, myocardial infarct, myocardial ischemia, pallor, phlebitis, pulmonary embolus, supraventricular extrasystoles, thrombophlebitis, thrombosis, vascular headache, ventricular extrasystoles.

Digestive System: Infrequent were bruxism, dysphagia, eructation, gastritis, gastroenteritis, gastroesophageal reflux, gingivitis, hemorrhoids, liver function test abnormal, melena, pancreatitis, rectal hemorrhage, toothache, ulcerative stomatitis; rare were colitis, glossitis, gum hyperplasia, hepatosplenomegaly, increased salivation, intestinal obstruction, peptic ulcer, stomach ulcer, throat tightness; also observed were aphthous stomatitis, bloody diarrhea, bu-

Table 2. Treatment-Emergent Adverse Events Occurring in ≥5% of Patients Treated With PAXIL CR in a Study of Elderly Patients With Major Depressive Disorder[1,2]

Body System/Adverse Event	% Reporting Event	
	PAXIL CR (n = 104)	Placebo (n = 109)
Body as a Whole		
Headache	17%	13%
Asthenia	15%	14%
Trauma	8%	5%
Infection	6%	2%
Digestive System		
Dry Mouth	18%	7%
Diarrhea	15%	9%
Constipation	13%	5%
Dyspepsia	13%	10%
Decreased Appetite	12%	5%
Flatulence	8%	7%
Nervous System		
Somnolence	21%	12%
Insomnia	10%	8%
Dizziness	9%	5%
Libido Decreased	8%	<1%
Tremor	7%	0%
Skin and Appendages		
Sweating	10%	<1%
Urogenital System		
Abnormal Ejaculation[3,4]	17%	3%
Impotence[3]	9%	3%

1. Adverse events for which the PAXIL CR reporting incidence was less than or equal to the placebo incidence are not included. These events are nausea and respiratory disorder.
2. <1% means greater than zero and less than 1%.
3. Based on the number of males.
4. Mostly anorgasmia or delayed ejaculation.

Table 3. Treatment-Emergent Adverse Events Occurring in ≥1% of Patients Treated With PAXIL CR in a Pool of 3 Panic Disorder Studies[1,2]

Body System/Adverse Event	% Reporting Event	
	PAXIL CR (n = 444)	Placebo (n = 445)
Body as a Whole		
Asthenia	15%	10%
Abdominal Pain	6%	4%
Trauma[3]	5%	4%
Cardiovascular System		
Vasodilation[4]	3%	2%
Digestive System		
Nausea	23%	17%
Dry Mouth	13%	9%
Diarrhea	12%	9%
Constipation	9%	6%
Decreased Appetite	8%	6%
Metabolic/Nutritional Disorders		
Weight Loss	1%	0%
Musculoskeletal System		
Myalgia	5%	3%
Nervous System		
Insomnia	20%	11%
Somnolence	20%	9%
Libido Decreased	9%	4%
Nervousness	8%	7%
Tremor	8%	2%
Anxiety	5%	4%
Agitation	3%	2%
Hypertonia[5]	2%	<1%
Myoclonus	2%	<1%
Respiratory System		
Sinusitis	8%	5%
Yawn	3%	0%
Skin and Appendages		
Sweating	7%	2%
Special Senses		
Abnormal Vision[6]	3%	<1%

(Table continued on next page)

Continued on next page

Paxil CR—Cont.

limia, cardiospasm, cholelithiasis, duodenitis, enteritis, esophagitis, fecal impactions, fecal incontinence, gum hemorrhage, hematemesis, hepatitis, ileitis, ileus, jaundice, mouth ulceration, salivary gland enlargement, sialadenitis, stomatitis, tongue discoloration, tongue edema.

Endocrine System: Infrequent were ovarian cyst, testes pain; rare were diabetes mellitus, hyperthyroidism; also observed were goiter, hypothyroidism, thyroiditis.

Hemic and Lymphatic System: Infrequent were anemia, eosinophilia, hypochromic anemia, leukocytosis, leukopenia, lymphadenopathy, purpura; rare were thrombocytopenia; also observed were anisocytosis, basophilia, bleeding time increased, lymphedema, lymphocytosis, lymphopenia, microcytic anemia, monocytosis, normocytic anemia, thrombocythemia.

Metabolic and Nutritional Disorders: Infrequent were generalized edema, hyperglycemia, hypokalemia, peripheral edema, SGOT increased, SGPT increased, thirst; rare were bilirubinemia, dehydration, hyperkalemia, obesity; also observed were alkaline phosphatase increased, BUN increased, creatinine phosphokinase increased, gamma globulins increased, gout, hypercalcemia, hypercholesteremia, hyperphosphatemia, hypocalcemia, hypoglycemia, hyponatremia, ketosis, lactic dehydrogenase increased, non-protein nitrogen (NPN) increased.

Musculoskeletal System: Infrequent were arthritis, bursitis, tendonitis; rare were myasthenia, myopathy, myositis; also observed were generalized spasm, osteoporosis, tenosynovitis, tetany.

Nervous System: Frequent were depression; infrequent were amnesia, convulsion, depersonalization, dystonia, emotional lability, hallucinations, hyperkinesia, hypesthesia, hypokinesia, incoordination, libido increased, neuralgia, neuropathy, nystagmus, paralysis, vertigo; rare were ataxia, coma, diplopia, dyskinesia, hostility, paranoid reaction, torticollis, withdrawal syndrome; also observed were abnormal gait, akathisia, akinesia, aphasia, choreoathetosis, circumoral paresthesia, delirium, delusions, dysarthria, euphoria, extrapyramidal syndrome, fasciculations, grand mal convulsion, hyperalgesia, irritability, manic reaction, manic-depressive reaction, meningitis, myelitis, peripheral neuritis, psychosis, psychotic depression, reflexes decreased, reflexes increased, stupor, trismus.

Respiratory System: Frequent were pharyngitis; infrequent were asthma, dyspnea, epistaxis, laryngitis, pneumonia; rare were stridor; also observed were dysphonia, emphysema, hemoptysis, hiccups, hyperventilation, lung fibrosis, pulmonary edema, respiratory flu, sputum increased.

Skin and Appendages: Frequent were rash; infrequent were acne, alopecia, dry skin, eczema, pruritus, urticaria; rare were exfoliative dermatitis, furunculosis, pustular rash, seborrhea; also observed were angioedema, ecchymosis, erythema multiforme, erythema nodosum, hirsutism, maculopapular rash, skin discoloration, skin hypertrophy, skin ulcer, sweating decreased, vesiculobullous rash.

Special Senses: Infrequent were conjunctivitis, earache, keratoconjunctivitis, mydriasis, photophobia, retinal hemorrhage, tinnitus; rare were blepharitis, visual field defect; also observed were amblyopia, anisocoria, blurred vision, cataract, conjunctival edema, corneal ulcer, deafness, exophthalmos, glaucoma, hyperacusis, night blindness, parosmia, ptosis, taste loss.

Urogenital System: Frequent were dysmenorrhea*; infrequent were albuminuria, amenorrhea*, breast pain*, cystitis, dysuria, prostatitis*, urinary retention; rare were breast enlargement*, breast neoplasm*, female lactation, hematuria, kidney calculus, metrorrhagia*, nephritis, nocturia, pregnancy and puerperal disorders*, salpingitis, urinary incontinence, uterine fibroids enlarged*; also observed were breast atrophy, ejaculatory disturbance, endometrial disorder, epididymitis, fibrocystic breast, leukorrhea, mastitis, oliguria, polyuria, pyuria, urethritis, urinary casts, urinary urgency, urolith, uterine spasm, vaginal hemorrhage.

* Based on the number of men and women as appropriate.

Postmarketing Reports: Voluntary reports of adverse events in patients taking immediate-release paroxetine hydrochloride that have been received since market introduction and not listed above that may have no causal relationship with the drug include acute pancreatitis, elevated liver function tests (the most severe cases were deaths due to liver necrosis, and grossly elevated transaminases associated with severe liver dysfunction), Guillain-Barré syndrome, toxic epidermal necrolysis, priapism, syndrome of inappropriate ADH secretion, symptoms suggestive of prolactinemia and galactorrhea, neuroleptic malignant syndrome–like events, serotonin syndrome; extrapyramidal symptoms which have included akathisia, bradykinesia, cogwheel rigidity, dystonia, hypertonia, oculogyric crisis which has been associated with concomitant use of pimozide; tremor and trismus; status epilepticus, acute renal failure, pulmonary hypertension, allergic alveolitis, anaphylaxis, eclampsia, laryngismus, optic neuritis, porphyria, ventricular fibrillation, ventricular tachycardia (including torsade de pointes), thrombocytopenia, hemolytic anemia, events related to impaired hematopoiesis (including aplastic anemia, pancytopenia, bone marrow aplasia, and agranulocytosis), and vasculitic syndromes (such as Henoch-Schönlein purpura). There has been a case report of an elevated phenytoin level after 4 weeks of immediate-release paroxetine and phenytoin coadministration. There has been

Table 3 (cont.). Treatment-Emergent Adverse Events Occurring in ≥1% of Patients Treated With PAXIL CR in a Pool of 3 Panic Disorder Studies[1,2]

Body System/Adverse Event	% Reporting Event	
	PAXIL CR (n = 444)	Placebo (n = 445)
Urogenital System		
Abnormal Ejaculation[7,8]	27%	3%
Impotence[7]	10%	1%
Female Genital Disorders[9,10]	7%	1%
Urinary Frequency	2%	<1%
Urination Impaired	2%	<1%
Vaginitis[9]	1%	<1%

1. Adverse events for which the reporting rate for PAXIL CR was less than or equal to the placebo rate are not included. These events are: Abnormal dreams, allergic reaction, back pain, bronchitis, chest pain, concentration impaired, confusion, cough increased, depression, dizziness, dysmenorrhea, dyspepsia, fever, flatulence, headache, increased appetite, infection, menstrual disorder, migraine, pain, paresthesia, pharyngitis, respiratory disorder, rhinitis, tachycardia, taste perversion, thinking abnormal, urinary tract infection, and vomiting.
2. <1% means greater than zero and less than 1%.
3. Various physical injuries.
4. Mostly flushing.
5. Mostly muscle tightness or stiffness.
6. Mostly blurred vision.
7. Based on the number of male patients.
8. Mostly anorgasmia or delayed ejaculation.
9. Based on the number of female patients.
10. Mostly anorgasmia or difficulty achieving orgasm.

Table 4. Treatment-Emergent Adverse Effects Occurring in ≥1% of Patients Treated With PAXIL CR in a Social Anxiety Disorder Study[1,2]

Body System/Adverse Event	% Reporting Event	
	PAXIL CR (n = 186)	Placebo (n = 184)
Body as a Whole		
Headache	23%	17%
Asthenia	18%	7%
Abdominal Pain	5%	4%
Back Pain	4%	1%
Trauma[3]	3%	<1%
Allergic Reaction[4]	2%	<1%
Chest Pain	1%	<1%
Cardiovascular System		
Hypertension	2%	0%
Migraine	2%	1%
Tachycardia	2%	1%
Digestive System		
Nausea	22%	6%
Diarrhea	9%	8%
Constipation	5%	2%
Dry Mouth	3%	2%
Dyspepsia	2%	<1%
Decreased Appetite	1%	<1%
Tooth Disorder	1%	0%
Metabolic/Nutritional Disorders		
Weight Gain	3%	1%
Weight Loss	1%	0%
Nervous System		
Insomnia	9%	4%
Somnolence	9%	4%
Libido Decreased	8%	1%
Dizziness	7%	4%
Tremor	4%	2%
Anxiety	2%	1%
Concentration Impaired	2%	0%
Depression	2%	1%
Myoclonus	1%	<1%
Paresthesia	1%	<1%
Respiratory System		
Yawn	2%	0%
Skin and Appendages		
Sweating	14%	3%
Eczema	1%	0%
Special Senses		
Abnormal Vision[5]	2%	0%
Abnormality of Accommodation	2%	0%
Urogenital System		
Abnormal Ejaculation[6,7]	15%	1%
Impotence[6]	9%	0%
Female Genital Disorders[8,9]	3%	0%

1. Adverse events for which the reporting rate for PAXIL CR was less than or equal to the placebo rate are not included. These events are: Dysmenorrhea, flatulence, gastroenteritis, hypertonia, infection, pain, pharyngitis, rash, respiratory disorder, rhinitis, and vomiting.
2. <1% means greater than zero and less than 1%.
3. Various physical injuries.
4. Most frequently seasonal allergic symptoms.
5. Mostly blurred vision.
6. Based on the number of male patients.
7. Mostly anorgasmia or delayed ejaculation.
8. Based on the number of female patients.
9. Mostly anorgasmia or difficulty achieving orgasm.

a case report of severe hypotension when immediate-release paroxetine was added to chronic metoprolol treatment.

DRUG ABUSE AND DEPENDENCE

Controlled Substance Class: PAXIL CR is not a controlled substance.

Physical and Psychologic Dependence: PAXIL CR has not been systematically studied in animals or humans for its potential for abuse, tolerance or physical dependence. While the clinical trials did not reveal any tendency for any drug-seeking behavior, these observations were not systematic and it is not possible to predict on the basis of this limited experience the extent to which a CNS-active drug will be misused, diverted, and/or abused once marketed. Consequently, patients should be evaluated carefully for history of drug abuse, and such patients should be observed closely for signs of misuse or abuse of PAXIL CR (e.g., development of tolerance, incrementations of dose, drug-seeking behavior).

OVERDOSAGE

Human Experience: Since the introduction of immediate-release paroxetine hydrochloride in the United States, 342 spontaneous cases of deliberate or accidental overdosage during paroxetine treatment have been reported worldwide (circa 1999). These include overdoses with paroxetine alone and in combination with other substances. Of these, 48 cases were fatal and of the fatalities, 17 appeared to involve paroxetine alone. Eight fatal cases that documented the amount of paroxetine ingested were generally confounded by the ingestion of other drugs or alcohol or the presence of significant comorbid conditions. Of 145 non-fatal cases with known outcome, most recovered without sequelae. The largest known ingestion involved 2,000 mg of paroxetine (33 times the maximum recommended daily dose) in a patient who recovered.

Commonly reported adverse events associated with paroxetine overdosage include somnolence, coma, nausea, tremor, tachycardia, confusion, vomiting, and dizziness. Other notable signs and symptoms observed with overdoses involving paroxetine (alone or with other substances) include mydriasis, convulsions (including status epilepticus), ventricular dysrhythmias (including torsade de pointes), hypertension, aggressive reactions, syncope, hypotension, stupor, bradycardia, dystonia, rhabdomyolysis, symptoms of hepatic dysfunction (including hepatic failure, hepatic necrosis, jaundice, hepatitis, and hepatic steatosis), serotonin syndrome, manic reactions, myoclonus, acute renal failure, and urinary retention.

Overdosage Management: Treatment should consist of those general measures employed in the management of overdosage with any drugs effective in the treatment of major depressive disorder.

Ensure an adequate airway, oxygenation, and ventilation. Monitor cardiac rhythm and vital signs. General supportive and symptomatic measures are also recommended. Induction of emesis is not recommended. Gastric lavage with a large-bore orogastric tube with appropriate airway protection, if needed, may be indicated if performed soon after ingestion, or in symptomatic patients.

Activated charcoal should be administered. Due to the large volume of distribution of this drug, forced diuresis, dialysis, hemoperfusion, and exchange transfusion are unlikely to be of benefit. No specific antidotes for paroxetine are known.

A specific caution involves patients taking or recently having taken paroxetine who might ingest excessive quantities of a tricyclic antidepressant. In such a case, accumulation of the parent tricyclic and an active metabolite may increase the possibility of clinically significant sequelae and extend the time needed for close medical observation (see PRECAUTIONS—Drugs Metabolized by Cytochrome $P_{450}IID_6$). In managing overdosage, consider the possibility of multiple-drug involvement. The physician should consider contacting a poison control center for additional information on the treatment of any overdose. Telephone numbers for certified poison control centers are listed in the *Physicians' Desk Reference* (PDR).

DOSAGE AND ADMINISTRATION

Major Depressive Disorder: *Usual Initial Dosage:* PAXIL CR should be administered as a single daily dose, usually in the morning, with or without food. The recommended initial dose is 25 mg/day. Patients were dosed in a range of 25 mg to 62.5 mg/day in the clinical trials demonstrating the effectiveness of PAXIL CR in the treatment of major depressive disorder. As with all drugs effective in the treatment of major depressive disorder, the full effect may be delayed. Some patients not responding to a 25-mg dose may benefit from dose increases, in 12.5-mg/day increments, up to a maximum of 62.5 mg/day. Dose changes should occur at intervals of at least 1 week.

Patients should be cautioned that PAXIL CR should not be chewed or crushed, and should be swallowed whole.

Maintenance Therapy: There is no body of evidence available to answer the question of how long the patient treated with PAXIL CR should remain on it. It is generally agreed that acute episodes of major depressive disorder require several months or longer of sustained pharmacologic therapy. Whether the dose of an antidepressant needed to induce remission is identical to the dose needed to maintain and/or sustain euthymia is unknown.

Systematic evaluation of the efficacy of immediate-release paroxetine hydrochloride has shown that efficacy is maintained for periods of up to 1 year with doses that averaged about 30 mg, which corresponds to a 37.5-mg dose of PAXIL CR, based on relative bioavailability considerations (see CLINICAL PHARMACOLOGY—Pharmacokinetics).

Table 5. Treatment-Emergent Adverse Events Occurring in ≥1% of Patients Treated With PAXIL CR in a Pool of 3 Premenstrual Dysphoric Disorder Studies with Continuous Dosing or in 1 Premenstrual Dysphoric Disorder Study with Luteal Phase Dosing[1,2,3]

Body System/Adverse Event	% Reporting Event			
	Continuous Dosing		Luteal Phase Dosing	
	PAXIL CR (n = 681)	Placebo (n = 349)	PAXIL CR (n = 246)	Placebo (n = 120)
Body as a Whole				
Asthenia	17%	6%	15%	4%
Headache	15%	12%	—	—
Infection	6%	4%	—	—
Abdominal pain	—	—	3%	0%
Cardiovascular System				
Migraine	1%	<1%	—	—
Digestive System				
Nausea	17%	7%	18%	2%
Diarrhea	6%	2%	6%	0%
Constipation	5%	1%	2%	<1%
Dry Mouth	4%	2%	2%	<1%
Increased Appetite	3%	<1%	—	—
Decreased Appetite	2%	<1%	2%	0%
Dyspepsia	2%	1%	2%	2%
Gingivitis	—	—	1%	0%
Metabolic and Nutritional Disorders				
Generalized Edema	—	—	1%	<1%
Weight Gain	—	—	1%	<1%
Musculoskeletal System				
Arthralgia	2%	1%	—	—
Nervous System				
Libido Decreased	12%	5%	9%	6%
Somnolence	9%	2%	3%	<1%
Insomnia	8%	2%	7%	3%
Dizziness	7%	3%	6%	3%
Tremor	4%	<1%	5%	0%
Concentration Impaired	3%	<1%	1%	0%
Nervousness	2%	<1%	3%	2%
Anxiety	2%	1%	—	—
Lack of Emotion	2%	<1%	—	—
Depression	—	—	2%	<1%
Vertigo	—	—	2%	<1%
Abnormal Dreams	1%	<1%	—	—
Amnesia	—	—	1%	0%
Respiratory System				
Sinusitis	—	—	4%	2%
Yawn	2%	<1%	—	—
Bronchitis	—	—	2%	0%
Cough Increased	1%	<1%	—	—
Skin and Appendages				
Sweating	7%	<1%	6%	<1%
Special Senses				
Abnormal Vision	—	—	1%	0%
Urogenital System				
Female Genital Disorders[4]	8%	1%	2%	0%
Menorrhagia	1%	<1%	—	—
Vaginal Moniliasis	1%	<1%	—	—
Menstrual Disorder	—	—	1%	0%

1. Adverse events for which the reporting rate of PAXIL CR was less than or equal to the placebo rate are not included. These events for continuous dosing are: Abdominal pain, back pain, pain, trauma, weight gain, myalgia, pharyngitis, respiratory disorder, rhinitis, sinusitis, pruritis, dysmenorrhea, menstrual disorder, urinary tract infection, and vomiting. The events for luteal phase dosing are: Allergic reaction, back pain, headache, infection, pain, trauma, myalgia, anxiety, pharyngitis, respiratory disorder, cystitis, and dysmenorrhea.
2. <1% means greater than zero and less than 1%.
3. The luteal phase and continuous dosing PMDD trials were not designed for making direct comparisons between the 2 dosing regimens. Therefore, a comparison between the 2 dosing regimens of the PMDD trials of incidence rates shown in Table 5 should be avoided.
4. Mostly anorgasmia or difficulty achieving orgasm.

Panic Disorder: *Usual Initial Dosage:* PAXIL CR should be administered as a single daily dose, usually in the morning. Patients should be started on 12.5 mg/day. Dose changes should occur in 12.5-mg/day increments and at intervals of at least 1 week. Patients were dosed in a range of 12.5 to 75 mg/day in the clinical trials demonstrating the effectiveness of PAXIL CR. The maximum dosage should not exceed 75 mg/day.

Patients should be cautioned that PAXIL CR should not be chewed or crushed, and should be swallowed whole.

Maintenance Therapy: Long-term maintenance of efficacy with the immediate-release formulation of paroxetine was demonstrated in a 3-month relapse prevention trial. In this trial, patients with panic disorder assigned to immediate-release paroxetine demonstrated a lower relapse rate compared to patients on placebo. Panic disorder is a chronic condition, and it is reasonable to consider continuation for a responding patient. Dosage adjustments should be made to maintain the patient on the lowest effective dose, and patients should be periodically reassessed to determine the need for continued treatment.

Social Anxiety Disorder: *Usual Initial Dosage:* PAXIL CR should be administered as a single daily dose, usually in the morning, with or without food. The recommended initial dose is 12.5 mg/day. Patients were dosed in a range of

12.5 mg to 37.5 mg/day in the clinical trial demonstrating the effectiveness of PAXIL CR in the treatment of social anxiety disorder. If the dose is increased, this should occur at intervals of at least 1 week, in increments of 12.5 mg/day, up to a maximum of 37.5 mg/day.

Patients should be cautioned that PAXIL CR should not be chewed or crushed, and should be swallowed whole.

Maintenance Therapy: There is no body of evidence available to answer the question of how long the patient treated with PAXIL CR should remain on it. Although the efficacy of PAXIL CR beyond 12 weeks of dosing has not been demonstrated in controlled clinical trials, social anxiety disorder is recognized as a chronic condition, and it is reasonable to consider continuation of treatment for a responding patient. Dosage adjustments should be made to maintain the patient on the lowest effective dosage, and patients should be periodically reassessed to determine the need for continued treatment.

Premenstrual Dysphoric Disorder: *Usual Initial Dosage:* PAXIL CR should be administered as a single daily dose, usually in the morning, with or without food. PAXIL CR may be administered either daily throughout the menstrual cycle or limited to the luteal phase of the menstrual cycle,

Continued on next page

	Major Depressive Disorder		Panic Disorder		Social Anxiety Disorder		PMDD Continuous Dosing		PMDD Luteal Phase Dosing	
	PAXIL CR	Placebo	PAXIL CR	Placebo	PAXIL CR	Placebo	PAXIL CR	Placebo	PAXIL CR	Placebo
n (males)	**78**	**78**	**162**	**194**	**88**	**97**	**n/a**	**n/a**	**n/a**	**n/a**
Decreased Libido	10%	5%	9%	6%	13%	1%	n/a	n/a	n/a	n/a
Ejaculatory Disturbance	26%	1%	27%	3%	15%	1%	n/a	n/a	n/a	n/a
Impotence	5%	3%	10%	1%	9%	0%	n/a	n/a	n/a	n/a
n (females)	**134**	**133**	**282**	**251**	**98**	**87**	**681**	**349**	**246**	**120**
Decreased Libido	4%	2%	8%	2%	4%	1%	12%	5%	9%	6%
Orgasmic Disturbance	10%	<1%	7%	1%	3%	0%	8%	1%	2%	0%

Paxil CR—Cont.

depending on physician assessment. The recommended initial dose is 12.5 mg/day. In clinical trials, both 12.5 mg/day and 25 mg/day were shown to be effective. Dose changes should occur at intervals of at least 1 week.
Patients should be cautioned that PAXIL CR should not be chewed or crushed, and should be swallowed whole.
Maintenance/Continuation Therapy: The effectiveness of PAXIL CR for a period exceeding 3 menstrual cycles has not been systematically evaluated in controlled trials. However, women commonly report that symptoms worsen with age until relieved by the onset of menopause. Therefore, it is reasonable to consider continuation of a responding patient. Patients should be periodically reassessed to determine the need for continued treatment.
Special Populations: *Treatment of Pregnant Women During the Third Trimester:* Neonates exposed to PAXIL CR and other SSRIs or SNRIs, late in the third trimester have developed complications requiring prolonged hospitalization, respiratory support, and tube feeding (see PRECAUTIONS). When treating pregnant women with paroxetine during the third trimester, the physician should carefully consider the potential risks and benefits of treatment. The physician may consider tapering paroxetine in the third trimester.
Dosage for Elderly or Debilitated Patients, and Patients With Severe Renal or Hepatic Impairment: The recommended initial dose of PAXIL CR is 12.5 mg/day for elderly patients, debilitated patients, and/or patients with severe renal or hepatic impairment. Increases may be made if indicated. Dosage should not exceed 50 mg/day.
Switching Patients to or From a Monoamine Oxidase Inhibitor: At least 14 days should elapse between discontinuation of an MAOI and initiation of therapy with PAXIL CR. Similarly, at least 14 days should be allowed after stopping PAXIL CR before starting an MAOI.
Discontinuation of Treatment With PAXIL CR: Symptoms associated with discontinuation of immediate-release paroxetine hydrochloride or PAXIL CR have been reported (see PRECAUTIONS). Patients should be monitored for these symptoms when discontinuing treatment, regardless of the indication for which PAXIL CR is being prescribed. A gradual reduction in the dose rather than abrupt cessation is recommended whenever possible. If intolerable symptoms occur following a decrease in the dose or upon discontinuation of treatment, then resuming the previously prescribed dose may be considered. Subsequently, the physician may continue decreasing the dose but at a more gradual rate.

HOW SUPPLIED

PAXIL CR is supplied as an enteric film-coated, controlled-release, round tablet, as follows:
12.5-mg yellow tablets, engraved with PAXIL CR and 12.5
NDC 0029-3206-13 Bottles of 30
NDC 0029-3206-20 Bottles of 100
25-mg pink tablets, engraved with PAXIL CR and 25
NDC 0029-3207-13 Bottles of 30
NDC 0029-3207-20 Bottles of 100
NDC 0029-3207-21 SUP 100s (intended for institutional use only)
37.5-mg blue tablets, engraved with PAXIL CR and 37.5
NDC 0029-3208-13 Bottles of 30
Store at or below 25°C (77°F) [see USP].
PAXIL CR is a registered trademark of GlaxoSmithKline.
GEOMATRIX is a trademark of Jago Pharma, Muttenz, Switzerland.

Medication Guide
PAXIL CR® (PAX-il) (paroxetine hydrochloride)
Controlled-Release Tablets
About Using Antidepressants in Children and Teenagers
What is the most important information I should know if my child is being prescribed an antidepressant?
Parents or guardians need to think about 4 important things when their child is prescribed an antidepressant:
1. There is a risk of suicidal thoughts or actions
2. How to try to prevent suicidal thoughts or actions in your child

3. You should watch for certain signs if your child is taking an antidepressant
4. There are benefits and risks when using antidepressants

1. There is a Risk of Suicidal Thoughts or Actions
Children and teenagers sometimes think about suicide, and many report trying to kill themselves.
Antidepressants increase suicidal thoughts and actions in some children and teenagers. But suicidal thoughts and actions can also be caused by depression, a serious medical condition that is commonly treated with antidepressants. Thinking about killing yourself or trying to kill yourself is called *suicidality* or *being suicidal.*
A large study combined the results of 24 different studies of children and teenagers with depression or other illnesses. In these studies, patients took either a placebo (sugar pill) or an antidepressant for 1 to 4 months. **No one committed suicide in these studies,** but some patients became suicidal. On sugar pills, 2 out of every 100 became suicidal. On the antidepressants, 4 out of every 100 patients became suicidal.
For some children and teenagers, the risks of suicidal actions may be especially high. These include patients with
- Bipolar illness (sometimes called manic-depressive illness)
- A family history of bipolar illness
- A personal or family history of attempting suicide
If any of these are present, make sure you tell your healthcare provider before your child takes an antidepressant.
2. How to Try to Prevent Suicidal Thoughts and Actions
To try to prevent suicidal thoughts and actions in your child, pay close attention to changes in her or his moods or actions, especially if the changes occur suddenly. Other important people in your child's life can help by paying attention as well (e.g., your child, brothers and sisters, teachers, and other important people). The changes to look out for are listed in Section 3, on what to watch for.
Whenever an antidepressant is started or its dose is changed, pay close attention to your child. After starting an antidepressant, your child should generally see his or her healthcare provider:
- Once a week for the first 4 weeks
- Every 2 weeks for the next 4 weeks
- After taking the antidepressant for 12 weeks
- After 12 weeks, follow your healthcare provider's advice about how often to come back
- More often if problems or questions arise (see Section 3)
You should call your child's healthcare provider between visits if needed.
3. You Should Watch for Certain Signs If Your Child is Taking an Antidepressant
Contact your child's healthcare provider *right away* if your child exhibits any of the following signs for the first time, or if they seem worse, or worry you, your child, or your child's teacher:
- Thoughts about suicide or dying
- Attempts to commit suicide
- New or worse depression
- New or worse anxiety
- Feeling very agitated or restless
- Panic attacks
- Difficulty sleeping (insomnia)
- New or worse irritability
- Acting aggressive, being angry, or violent
- Acting on dangerous impulses
- An extreme increase in activity and talking
- Other unusual changes in behavior or mood
Never let your child stop taking an antidepressant without first talking to his or her healthcare provider. Stopping an antidepressant suddenly can cause other symptoms.
4. There are Benefits and Risks When Using Antidepressants
Antidepressants are used to treat depression and other illnesses. Depression and other illnesses can lead to suicide. In some children and teenagers, treatment with an antidepressant increases suicidal thinking or actions. It is important to discuss all the risks of treating depression and also the risks of not treating it. You and your child should discuss all treatment choices with your healthcare provider, not just the use of antidepressants.

Other side effects can occur with antidepressants (see section below).
Of all the antidepressants, only fluoxetine (Prozac®)* has been FDA approved to treat pediatric depression.
For obsessive compulsive disorder in children and teenagers, FDA has approved only fluoxetine (Prozac®)*, sertraline (Zoloft®)*, fluvoxamine, and clomipramine (Anafranil®)*.
Your healthcare provider may suggest other antidepressants based on the past experience of your child or other family members.
Is this all I need to know if my child is being prescribed an antidepressant?
No. This is a warning about the risk for suicidality. Other side effects can occur with antidepressants. Be sure to ask your healthcare provider to explain all the side effects of the particular drug he or she is prescribing. Also ask about drugs to avoid when taking an antidepressant. Ask your healthcare provider or pharmacist where to find more information.
*The following are registered trademarks of their respective manufacturers: Prozac®/Eli Lilly and Company; Zoloft®/Pfizer Pharmaceuticals; Anafranil®/Mallinckrodt Inc.
This Medication Guide has been approved by the U.S. Food and Drug Administration for all antidepressants.
January 2005/MG-PC:1
GlaxoSmithKline, Research Triangle Park, NC 27709
©2005, GlaxoSmithKline. All rights reserved.
January 2005/PC:L12, PC:L13

RELAFEN®   ℞
[rel'ə-fen]
(nabumetone)
Tablets

Prescribing information for this product, which appears on pages 1604–1606 of the 2005 PDR, has been revised as follows. Please write "See Supplement A" next to the product heading.
In the DESCRIPTION section, "hydroxypropyl methylcellulose" has been changed to "hypromellose."
The CLINICAL PHARMACOLOGY: Pharmacokinetics: *Renal Insufficiency section has been revised as follows.*
In studies of patients with renal insufficiency, the mean terminal half-life of 6MNA was increased in patients with severe renal dysfunction (creatinine clearance <30 mL/min/1.73 m²). In moderate renal insufficiency (creatinine clearance 30 to 49 mL/min), the terminal half-life of 6-MNA is increased and there is a 50% increase in the plasma levels of unbound 6-MNA. In patients undergoing hemodialysis, steady-state plasma concentrations of the active metabolite were similar to those observed in healthy subjects. Due to extensive protein binding, 6MNA is not dialyzable (see PRECAUTIONS: Renal Effects).
The following paragraph was revised in the WARNINGS: Risk of G.I. Ulceration, Bleeding, and Perforation with NSAID Therapy *section.*
Studies to date have not identified any subset of patients not at risk of developing peptic ulceration and bleeding. Except for a prior history of serious G.I. events and other risk factors known to be associated with peptic ulcer disease, such as alcoholism, smoking, other medications known to increase the risk of gastrointestinal ulcer (e.g., oral corticosteroids), etc., no risk factors (e.g., age, sex) have been associated with increased risk. Elderly or debilitated patients seem to tolerate ulceration or bleeding less well than other individuals and most spontaneous reports of fatal G.I. events are in this population.
The following paragraph was revised in the PRECAUTIONS: General: *Renal Effects section.*
Because nabumetone undergoes extensive hepatic metabolism, no adjustment of the dosage of RELAFEN is generally necessary in patients with renal insufficiency; however, as with all NSAIDs, patients with impaired renal function should be monitored more closely than patients with normal renal function (see CLINICAL PHARMACOLOGY: Renal Insufficiency). In patients with severe renal impairment (creatinine clearance ≤30 mL/min), laboratory tests should be performed at baseline and within weeks of starting therapy. Further tests should be carried out as necessary; if the impairment worsens, discontinuation of therapy may be warranted. In subjects with moderate renal impairment (creatinine clearance 30 to 49 mL/min) there is a 50% increase in unbound plasma 6-MNA and dose adjustment may be warranted. The oxidized and conjugated metabolites of 6MNA are eliminated primarily by the kidneys. The extent to which these largely inactive metabolites may accumulate in patients with renal failure has not been studied. As with other drugs whose metabolites are excreted by the kidneys, the possibility that adverse reactions (not listed in ADVERSE REACTIONS) may be attributable to these metabolites should be considered (see CLINICAL PHARMACOLOGY: Renal Insufficiency).
GlaxoSmithKline, Research Triangle Park, NC 27709
©2004, GlaxoSmithKline. All rights reserved.
August 2004/RL:L13

SEREVENT® DISKUS®   ℞
[ser' ə-vent disk' us]
(salmeterol xinafoate inhalation powder)
FOR ORAL INHALATION ONLY

Prescribing information for this product, which appears on pages 1620–1624 of the 2005 PDR, has been revised as follows. Please write "See Supplement A" next to the product heading.

The boxed warning at the beginning of the package insert has been revised as follows.

> **WARNING:** Data from a large placebo-controlled US study that compared the safety of salmeterol (SEREVENT® Inhalation Aerosol) or placebo added to usual asthma therapy showed a small but significant increase in asthma-related deaths in patients receiving salmeterol (13 deaths out of 13,176 patients treated for 28 weeks) versus those on placebo (3 of 13,179) (see WARNINGS and CLINICAL TRIALS: Asthma: *Salmeterol Multi-center Asthma Research Trial*).

The CLINICAL TRIALS: Asthma: *Salmeterol Multi-center Asthma Research Trial section has been revised as follows.* The Salmeterol Multi-center Asthma Research Trial (SMART) was a randomized, double-blind study that enrolled long-acting beta$_2$-agonist–naive patients with asthma (average age of 39 years, 71% Caucasian, 18% African American, 8% Hispanic) to assess the safety of salmeterol (SEREVENT Inhalation Aerosol, 42 mcg twice daily over 28 weeks) compared to placebo when added to usual asthma therapy. The primary endpoint was the combined number of respiratory-related deaths or respiratory-related life-threatening experiences (intubation and mechanical ventilation). Secondary endpoints included combined asthma-related deaths or life-threatening experiences and asthma-related deaths. A planned interim analysis was conducted when approximately half of the intended number of patients had been enrolled (N = 26,355).

Due to the low rate of primary events in the study, the findings of the planned interim analysis were not conclusive. However, analyses of secondary endpoints suggested that patients receiving salmeterol may be at increased risk for some of these events compared to patients receiving placebo. The analysis for the total population showed a relative risk of 1.40 (95% CI 0.91, 2.14) for the primary endpoint in the salmeterol group relative to the placebo group (50 out of 13,176 vs. 36 out of 13,179, respectively). In the total population, a higher number of asthma-related deaths (13 vs. 3, RR 4.37, 95% CI 1.25, 15.34) and combined asthma-related deaths or life-threatening experiences (37 vs. 22, RR 1.71, 95% CI 1.01, 2.89) occurred in patients treated with salmeterol than those treated with placebo. The analysis of the African American subgroup showed a relative risk of 4.10 (95% CI 1.54, 10.90) for the primary endpoint in patients treated with salmeterol relative to those treated with placebo (20 out of 2,366 vs. 5 out of 2,319, respectively). In African Americans, a higher number of asthma-related deaths (7 vs. 1, RR 7.26, 95% CI 0.89, 58.94) and combined asthma-related deaths or life-threatening experiences (19 vs. 4, RR 4.92, 95% CI 1.68, 14.45) occurred in patients treated with salmeterol than those treated with placebo. Analysis of the Caucasian population showed a relative risk of 1.05 (95% CI 0.62, 1.76) for the primary endpoint for those treated with salmeterol relative to those treated with placebo (29 out of 9,281 vs. 28 out of 9,361, respectively). In Caucasians, a higher number of asthma-related deaths (6 vs. 1, RR 5.82, 95% CI 0.70, 48.37) occurred in patients treated with salmeterol than in patients treated with placebo. In Caucasians, the relative risk was 1.08 (17 vs. 16, 95% CI 0.55, 2.14) for combined asthma-related deaths or life-threatening experiences in patients treated with salmeterol relative to placebo. The numbers of patients from other ethnic groups were too small to draw any conclusions in these populations. Even though SMART did not reach predetermined stopping criteria for the total population, the study was stopped due to the findings in African American patients and difficulties in enrollment.

The first paragraph of the WARNINGS section has been revised as follows.
DATA FROM A LARGE PLACEBO-CONTROLLED SAFETY STUDY THAT WAS STOPPED EARLY SUGGEST THAT SALMETEROL MAY BE ASSOCIATED WITH RARE SERIOUS ASTHMA EPISODES OR ASTHMA-RELATED DEATHS. Data from this study, called the Salmeterol Multi-center Asthma Research Trial (SMART), further suggest that the risk might be greater in African American patients. These results led to stopping the study prematurely (see CLINICAL TRIALS: Asthma: *Salmeterol Multi-center Asthma Research Trial*). The data from the SMART study are not adequate to determine whether concurrent use of inhaled corticosteroids provides protection from this risk. Given the similar basic mechanisms of action of beta$_2$-agonists, it is possible that the findings seen in the SMART study may be consistent with a class effect.
GlaxoSmithKline, Research Triangle Park, NC 27709
©2004, GlaxoSmithKline. All rights reserved.
September 2004/RL-2129

TABLOID® brand Thioguanine   ℞
[*tab' loid*]
40-mg Scored Tablets

Prescribing information for this product, which appears on pages 1624–1626 of the 2005 PDR, has been revised as follows. Please write "See Supplement A" next to the product heading.
The INDICATIONS AND USAGE section has been revised as follows.
a) Acute Nonlymphocytic Leukemias: TABLOID brand Thioguanine is indicated for remission induction and remission consolidation treatment of acute nonlymphocytic

leukemias. However, it is not recommended for use during maintenance therapy or similar long term continuous treatments due to the high risk of liver toxicity (see WARNINGS and ADVERSE REACTIONS).
The response to this agent depends upon the age of the patient (younger patients faring better than older) and whether thioguanine is used in previously treated or previously untreated patients. Reliance upon thioguanine alone is seldom justified for initial remission induction of acute nonlymphocytic leukemias because combination chemotherapy including thioguanine results in more frequent remission induction and longer duration of remission than thioguanine alone.
b) Other Neoplasms: TABLOID brand Thioguanine is not effective in chronic lymphocytic leukemia, Hodgkin's lymphoma, multiple myeloma, or solid tumors. Although thioguanine is one of several agents with activity in the treatment of the chronic phase of chronic myelogenous leukemia, more objective responses are observed with MYLERAN® (busulfan), and therefore busulfan is usually regarded as the preferred drug.
The following paragraphs have been added to the WARNINGS section.
THIOGUANINE IS NOT RECOMMENDED FOR MAINTENANCE THERAPY OR SIMILAR LONG TERM CONTINUOUS TREATMENTS DUE TO THE HIGH RISK OF LIVER TOXICITY ASSOCIATED WITH VASCULAR ENDOTHELIAL DAMAGE (see DOSAGE AND ADMINISTRATION and ADVERSE REACTIONS). This liver toxicity has been observed in a high proportion of children receiving thioguanine as part of maintenance therapy for acute lymphoblastic leukemia and in other conditions associated with continuous use of thioguanine. This liver toxicity is particularly prevalent in males. Liver toxicity usually presents as the clinical syndrome of hepatic veno-occlusive disease (hyperbilirubinemia, tender hepatomegaly, weight gain due to fluid retention, and ascites) or with signs of portal hypertension (splenomegaly, thrombocytopenia, and oesophageal varices). Histopathological features associated with this toxicity include hepatoportal sclerosis, nodular regenerative hyperplasia, peliosis hepatitis, and periportal fibrosis.
Thioguanine therapy should be discontinued in patients with evidence of liver toxicity as reversal of signs and symptoms of liver toxicity have been reported upon withdrawal. Patients must be carefully monitored (see PRECAUTIONS, Laboratory Tests). Early indications of liver toxicity are signs associated with portal hypertension such as thrombocytopenia out of proportion with neutropenia and splenomegaly. Elevations of liver enzymes have also been reported in association with liver toxicity but do not always occur.
The following paragraph has been added to the PRECAUTIONS: General section.
Administration of live vaccines to immunocompromised patients should be avoided.
The PRECAUTIONS: Drug Interactions section has been revised as follows.
There is usually complete cross-resistance between PURINETHOL (mercaptopurine) and TABLOID brand Thioguanine.
As there is in vitro evidence that aminosalicylate derivatives (e.g., olsalazine, mesalazine, or sulphasalazine) inhibit the TPMT enzyme, they should be administered with caution to patients receiving concurrent thioguanine therapy (see WARNINGS).
The ADVERSE REACTIONS: Hepatic Effects section has been revised as follows.
Liver toxicity associated with vascular endothelial damage has been reported when thioguanine is used in maintenance or similar long term continuous therapy which is not recommended (see WARNINGS and DOSAGE AND ADMINISTRATION). This usually presents as the clinical syndrome of hepatic veno-occlusive disease (hyperbilirubinemia, tender hepatomegaly, weight gain due to fluid retention, and ascites) or signs and symptoms of portal hypertension (splenomegaly, thrombocytopenia, and esophageal varices). Elevation of liver transaminases, alkaline phosphatase, and gamma glutamyl transferase and jaundice may also occur. Histopathological features associated with this toxicity include hepatoportal sclerosis, nodular regenerative hyperplasia, peliosis hepatitis, and periportal fibrosis.
Liver toxicity during short term cyclical therapy presents as veno-occlusive disease. Reversal of signs and symptoms of this liver toxicity has been reported upon withdrawal of short term or long term continuous therapy.
Centrilobular hepatic necrosis has been reported in a few cases; however, the reports are confounded by the use of high doses of thioguanine, other chemotherapeutic agents, and oral contraceptives and chronic alcohol abuse.
Manufactured by DSM Pharmaceuticals, Inc.
Greenville, NC 27834
for GlaxoSmithKline, Research Triangle Park, NC 27709
©2004, GlaxoSmithKline. All rights reserved.
December 2004/RL-2154

TIMENTIN®   ℞
[*tī-mĕn'tin*]
(sterile ticarcillin disodium and clavulanate potassium) for Intravenous Administration

Prescribing information for this product, which appears on pages 1632–1635 of the 2005 PDR, has been revised as follows. Please write "See Supplement A" next to the product heading.

The following paragraph was revised in the INDICATIONS AND USAGE section.
Appropriate culture and susceptibility tests should be performed before treatment in order to isolate and identify organisms causing infection and to determine their susceptibility to ticarcillin/clavulanic acid. Because of its broad spectrum of bactericidal activity against gram-positive and gram-negative bacteria, TIMENTIN is particularly useful for the treatment of mixed infections and for presumptive therapy prior to the identification of the causative organisms. TIMENTIN has been shown to be effective as single drug therapy in the treatment of some serious infections where normally combination antibiotic therapy might be employed. Therapy with TIMENTIN may be initiated before results of such tests are known when there is reason to believe the infection may involve any of the β-lactamase–producing organisms listed above.
GlaxoSmithKline, Research Triangle Park, NC 27709
©2004, GlaxoSmithKline. All rights reserved.
December 2004/TI:L14IV

TIMENTIN®   ℞
[*tī-mĕn'tin*]
(sterile ticarcillin disodium and clavulanate potassium) for Intravenous Administration
ADD-VANTAGE® ANTIBIOTIC VIAL

Prescribing information for this product, which appears on pages 1635–1639 of the 2005 PDR, has been revised as follows. Please write "See Supplement A" next to the product heading.
The following paragraph was revised in the INDICATIONS AND USAGE section.
Appropriate culture and susceptibility tests should be performed before treatment in order to isolate and identify organisms causing infection and to determine their susceptibility to ticarcillin/clavulanic acid. Because of its broad spectrum of bactericidal activity against gram-positive and gram-negative bacteria, TIMENTIN is particularly useful for the treatment of mixed infections and for presumptive therapy prior to the identification of the causative organisms. TIMENTIN has been shown to be effective as single drug therapy in the treatment of some serious infections where normally combination antibiotic therapy might be employed. Therapy with TIMENTIN may be initiated before results of such tests are known when there is reason to believe the infection may involve any of the β-lactamase–producing organisms listed above.
GlaxoSmithKline, Research Triangle Park, NC 27709
©2004, GlaxoSmithKline. All rights reserved.
December 2004/TI:L13AV

TIMENTIN®   ℞
[*tī-mĕn'tin*]
(sterile ticarcillin disodium and clavulanate potassium) for Intravenous Administration

> **PHARMACY BULK PACKAGE**
> **NOT FOR DIRECT INFUSION**

RECONSTITUTED STOCK SOLUTION MUST BE TRANSFERRED AND FURTHER DILUTED FOR IV INFUSION.
Prescribing information for this product, which appears on pages 1639–1642 of the 2005 PDR, has been revised as follows. Please write "See Supplement A" next to the product heading.
The following paragraph was revised in the INDICATIONS AND USAGE section.
Appropriate culture and susceptibility tests should be performed before treatment in order to isolate and identify organisms causing infection and to determine their susceptibility to ticarcillin/clavulanic acid. Because of its broad spectrum of bactericidal activity against gram-positive and gram-negative bacteria, TIMENTIN is particularly useful for the treatment of mixed infections and for presumptive therapy prior to the identification of the causative organisms. TIMENTIN has been shown to be effective as single drug therapy in the treatment of some serious infections where normally combination antibiotic therapy might be employed. Therapy with TIMENTIN may be initiated before results of such tests are known when there is reason to believe the infection may involve any of the β-lactamase–producing organisms listed above.
GlaxoSmithKline, Research Triangle Park, NC 27709
©2004, GlaxoSmithKline. All rights reserved.
December 2004/TI:L14PB

VALTREX®   ℞
[*val'trĕx*]
(valacyclovir hydrochloride) Caplets

Prescribing information for this product, which appears on pages 1650–1653 of the 2005 PDR, has been revised as follows. Please write "See Supplement A" next to the product heading.

Continued on next page

Valtrex—Cont.

The following has been added to the CLINICAL TRIALS: Genital Herpes Infections *section.*

Reduction of Transmission of Genital Herpes: A double-blind, placebo-controlled study to assess transmission of genital herpes was conducted in 1,484 monogamous, heterosexual, immunocompetent adult couples. The couples were discordant for HSV-2 infection. The source partner had a history of 9 or fewer genital herpes episodes per year. Both partners were counseled on safer sex practices and were advised to use condoms throughout the study period. Source partners were randomized to treatment with either VALTREX 500 mg once daily or placebo once daily for 8 months. The primary efficacy endpoint was symptomatic acquisition of HSV-2 in susceptible partners. Overall HSV-2 acquisition was defined as symptomatic HSV-2 acquisition and/or HSV-2 seroconversion in susceptible partners. The efficacy results are summarized in Table 3.

Table 3. Percentage of Susceptible Partners Who Acquired HSV-2 Defined by the Primary and Selected Secondary Endpoints

	VALTREX* (n = 743)	Placebo (n = 741)
Symptomatic HSV-2 acquisition	4 (0.5%)	16 (2.2%)
HSV-2 seroconversion	12 (1.6%)	24 (3.2%)
Overall HSV-2 acquisition	14 (1.9%)	27 (3.6%)

*Results show reductions in risk of 75% (symptomatic HSV-2 acquisition), 50% (HSV-2 seroconversion), and 48% (overall HSV-2 acquisition) with VALTREX versus placebo. Individual results may vary based on consistency of safer sex practices.

The following has been added to the INDICATIONS AND USAGE: Genital Herpes *section.*

When VALTREX is used as suppressive therapy in immunocompetent individuals with genital herpes, the risk of heterosexual transmission to susceptible partners is reduced. Safer sex practices should be used with suppressive therapy (see current Centers for Disease Control and Prevention (CDC) *Sexually Transmitted Diseases Treatment Guidelines*).

The PRECAUTIONS *section has been revised as follows.*

Dosage reduction is recommended when administering VALTREX to patients with renal impairment (see DOSAGE AND ADMINISTRATION). Acute renal failure and central nervous system symptoms have been reported in patients with underlying renal disease who have received inappropriately high doses of VALTREX for their level of renal function. Similar caution should be exercised when administering VALTREX to geriatric patients (see Geriatric Use) and patients receiving potentially nephrotoxic agents.

Given the dosage recommendations for treatment of cold sores, special attention should be paid when prescribing VALTREX for cold sores in patients who are elderly or who have impaired renal function (see DOSAGE AND ADMINISTRATION and Geriatric Use). Treatment should not exceed 1 day (2 doses of 2 grams in 24 hours). Therapy beyond 1 day does not provide additional clinical benefit.

Precipitation of acyclovir in renal tubules may occur when the solubility (2.5 mg/mL) is exceeded in the intratubular fluid. In the event of acute renal failure and anuria, the patient may benefit from hemodialysis until renal function is restored (see DOSAGE AND ADMINISTRATION).

The safety and efficacy of VALTREX have not been established in immunocompromised patients other than for the suppression of genital herpes in HIV-infected patients. The safety and efficacy of VALTREX for suppression of recurrent genital herpes in patients with advanced HIV disease (CD4 cell count <100 cells/mm[3]) have not been established. The efficacy of VALTREX for the treatment of genital herpes in HIV-infected patients has not been established. The safety and efficacy of VALTREX have not been established for the treatment of disseminated herpes zoster.

The efficacy of VALTREX for reducing transmission of genital herpes has not been established in individuals with multiple partners and non-heterosexual couples.

Information for Patients: *Herpes Zoster:* There are no data on treatment initiated more than 72 hours after onset of the zoster rash. Patients should be advised to initiate treatment as soon as possible after a diagnosis of herpes zoster.

Genital Herpes: Patients should be informed that VALTREX is not a cure for genital herpes. Because genital herpes is a sexually transmitted disease, patients should avoid contact with lesions or intercourse when lesions and/or symptoms are present to avoid infecting partners. Genital herpes is frequently transmitted in the absence of symptoms through asymptomatic viral shedding. Therefore, patients should be counseled to use safer sex practices in combination with suppressive therapy with VALTREX. Sex partners of infected persons should be advised that they might be infected even if they have no symptoms. Type-specific serologic testing of asymptomatic partners of persons with genital herpes can determine whether risk for HSV-2 acquisition exists.

VALTREX has not been shown to reduce transmission of sexually transmitted infections other than HSV-2.

If medical management of a genital herpes recurrence is indicated, patients should be advised to initiate therapy at the first sign or symptom of an episode.

There are no data on the effectiveness of treatment initiated more than 72 hours after the onset of signs and symptoms of a first episode of genital herpes or more than 24 hours after the onset of signs and symptoms of a recurrent episode.

There are no data on the safety or effectiveness of chronic suppressive therapy of more than 1 year's duration in otherwise healthy patients. There are no data on the safety or effectiveness of chronic suppressive therapy of more than 6 months' duration in HIV-infected patients.

Cold Sores (Herpes Labialis): Patients should be advised to initiate treatment at the earliest symptom of a cold sore (e.g., tingling, itching, or burning). There are no data on the effectiveness of treatment initiated after the development of clinical signs of a cold sore (e.g., papule, vesicle, or ulcer). Patients should be instructed that treatment for cold sores should not exceed 1 day (2 doses) and that their doses should be taken about 12 hours apart. Patients should be informed that VALTREX is not a cure for cold sores (herpes labialis).

Drug Interactions: See CLINICAL PHARMACOLOGY: Pharmacokinetics.

Carcinogenesis, Mutagenesis, Impairment of Fertility: The data presented below include references to the steady-state acyclovir AUC observed in humans treated with 1 gram VALTREX given orally 3 times a day to treat herpes zoster. Plasma drug concentrations in animal studies are expressed as multiples of human exposure to acyclovir (see CLINICAL PHARMACOLOGY: Pharmacokinetics).

Valacyclovir was noncarcinogenic in lifetime carcinogenicity bioassays at single daily doses (gavage) of valacyclovir giving plasma acyclovir concentrations equivalent to human levels in the mouse bioassay and 1.4 to 2.3 times human levels in the rat bioassay. There was no significant difference in the incidence of tumors between treated and control animals, nor did valacyclovir shorten the latency of tumors. Valacyclovir was tested in 5 genetic toxicity assays. An Ames assay was negative in the absence or presence of metabolic activation. Also negative were an in vitro cytogenetic study with human lymphocytes and a rat cytogenetic study. In the mouse lymphoma assay, valacyclovir was not mutagenic in the absence of metabolic activation. In the presence of metabolic activation (76% to 88% conversion to acyclovir), valacyclovir was mutagenic.

Valacyclovir was mutagenic in a mouse micronucleus assay. Valacyclovir did not impair fertility or reproduction in rats at 6 times human plasma levels.

Pregnancy: *Teratogenic Effects:* Pregnancy Category B. Valacyclovir was not teratogenic in rats or rabbits at 10 and 7 times human plasma levels, respectively, during the period of major organogenesis.

There are no adequate and well-controlled studies of VALTREX or ZOVIRAX in pregnant women. A prospective epidemiologic registry of acyclovir use during pregnancy was established in 1984 and completed in April 1999. There were 749 pregnancies followed in women exposed to systemic acyclovir during the first trimester of pregnancy resulting in 756 outcomes. The occurrence rate of birth defects approximates that found in the general population. However, the small size of the registry is insufficient to evaluate the risk for less common defects or to permit reliable or definitive conclusions regarding the safety of acyclovir in pregnant women and their developing fetuses. VALTREX should be used during pregnancy only if the potential benefit justifies the potential risk to the fetus.

Nursing Mothers: Following oral administration of a 500-mg dose of VALTREX to 5 nursing mothers, peak acyclovir concentrations (C_{max}) in breast milk ranged from 0.5 to 2.3 times (median 1.4) the corresponding maternal acyclovir serum concentrations. The acyclovir breast milk AUC ranged from 1.4 to 2.6 times (median 2.2) maternal serum AUC. A 500-mg maternal dosage of VALTREX twice daily would provide a nursing infant with an oral acyclovir dosage of approximately 0.6 mg/kg/day. This would result in less than 2% of the exposure obtained after administration of a standard neonatal dose of 30 mg/kg/day of intravenous acyclovir to the nursing infant. Unchanged valacyclovir was not detected in maternal serum, breast milk, or infant urine. VALTREX should be administered to a nursing mother with caution and only when indicated.

Pediatric Use: Safety and effectiveness of VALTREX in pre-pubertal pediatric patients have not been established.

Geriatric Use: Of the total number of subjects in clinical studies of VALTREX, 906 were 65 and over, and 352 were 75 and over. In a clinical study of herpes zoster, the duration of pain after healing (post-herpetic neuralgia) was longer in patients 65 and older compared with younger adults. Elderly patients are more likely to have reduced renal function and require dose reduction. Elderly patients are also more likely to have renal or CNS adverse events. With respect to CNS adverse events observed during clinical practice, agitation, hallucinations, confusion, delirium, and encephalopathy were reported more frequently in elderly patients (see CLINICAL PHARMACOLOGY, ADVERSE REACTIONS: Observed During Clinical Practice, and DOSAGE AND ADMINISTRATION).

The following has been added to the ADVERSE REACTIONS *section.*

Reduction of Transmission: In a clinical study for the reduction of transmission of genital herpes, the adverse events reported by patients receiving VALTREX 500 mg once daily (n = 743) or placebo once daily (n = 741) included headache (VALTREX 29%, placebo 26%), nasopharyngitis

(VALTREX 16%, placebo 15%), and upper respiratory tract infection (VALTREX 9%, placebo 10%). In this 8-month study, there were no clinically significant changes from baseline laboratory parameters in subjects receiving VALTREX compared with placebo.

The following has been added to the DOSAGE AND ADMINISTRATION: Genital Herpes *section.*

Reduction of Transmission: The recommended dosage of VALTREX for reduction of transmission of genital herpes in patients with a history of 9 or fewer recurrences per year is 500 mg once daily for the source partner. Patients should be counseled to use safer sex practices in combination with suppressive therapy with VALTREX. The efficacy of reducing transmission beyond 8 months in discordant couples has not been established.

GlaxoSmithKline, Research Triangle Park, NC 27709
©2004, GlaxoSmithKline. All rights reserved.
November 2004/RL-2037, RL-2148

WELLBUTRIN® ℞

[*wel'byü-trin*]
(bupropion hydrochloride)
Tablets

Prescribing information for this product, which appears on pages 1655–1659 of the 2005 PDR, has been revised as follows. Please write "See Supplement A" next to the product heading.

The following boxed warning has been added to the beginning of the package insert.

Suicidality in Children and Adolescents

Antidepressants increased the risk of suicidal thinking and behavior (suicidality) in short-term studies in children and adolescents with Major Depressive Disorder (MDD) and other psychiatric disorders. Anyone considering the use of WELLBUTRIN or any other antidepressant in a child or adolescent must balance this risk with the clinical need. Patients who are started on therapy should be observed closely for clinical worsening, suicidality, or unusual changes in behavior. Families and caregivers should be advised of the need for close observation and communication with the prescriber. WELLBUTRIN is not approved for use in pediatric patients. (See WARNINGS and PRECAUTIONS: Pediatric Use.)

Pooled analyses of short-term (4 to 16 weeks) placebo-controlled trials of 9 antidepressant drugs (SSRIs and others) in children and adolescents with major depressive disorder (MDD), obsessive compulsive disorder (OCD), or other psychiatric disorders (a total of 24 trials involving over 4,400 patients) have revealed a greater risk of adverse events representing suicidal thinking or behavior (suicidality) during the first few months of treatment in those receiving antidepressants. The average risk of such events in patients receiving antidepressants was 4%, twice the placebo risk of 2%. No suicides occurred in these trials.

The WARNINGS *section has been revised as follows.*

Clinical Worsening and Suicide Risk: Patients with major depressive disorder (MDD), both adult and pediatric, may experience worsening of their depression and/or the emergence of suicidal ideation and behavior (suicidality) or unusual changes in behavior, whether or not they are taking antidepressant medications, and this risk may persist until significant remission occurs. There has been a long-standing concern that antidepressants may have a role in inducing worsening of depression and the emergence of suicidality in certain patients. Antidepressants increased the risk of suicidal thinking and behavior (suicidality) in short-term studies in children and adolescents with Major Depressive Disorder (MDD) and other psychiatric disorders.

Pooled analyses of short-term placebo-controlled trials of 9 antidepressant drugs (SSRIs and others) in children and adolescents with MDD, OCD, or other psychiatric disorders (a total of 24 trials involving over 4,400 patients) have revealed a greater risk of adverse events representing suicidal behavior or thinking (suicidality) during the first few months of treatment in those receiving antidepressants. The average risk of such events in patients receiving antidepressants was 4%, twice the placebo risk of 2%. There was considerable variation in risk among drugs, but a tendency toward an increase for almost all drugs studied. The risk of suicidality was most consistently observed in the MDD trials, but there were signals of risk arising from some trials in other psychiatric indications (obsessive compulsive disorder and social anxiety disorder) as well. **No suicides occurred in any of these trials.** It is unknown whether the suicidality risk in pediatric patients extends to longer-term use, i.e., beyond several months. It is also unknown whether the suicidality risk extends to adults.

All pediatric patients being treated with antidepressants for any indication should be observed closely for clinical worsening, suicidality, and unusual changes in behavior, especially during the initial few months of a course of drug therapy, or at times of dose changes, either increases or decreases. Such observation would generally include at least weekly face-to-face contact with patients or their family members or caregivers during the first 4 weeks of treatment, then every other week visits for the next 4 weeks, then at 12 weeks, and as clinically indicated beyond 12 weeks. Additional contact by telephone may be appropriate between face-to-face visits.

Adults with MDD or co-morbid depression in the setting of other psychiatric illness being treated with antidepressants should be observed similarly for clinical worsening and suicidality, especially during the initial few months of a course of drug therapy, or at times of dose changes, either increases or decreases.

The following symptoms, anxiety, agitation, panic attacks, insomnia, irritability, hostility, aggressiveness, impulsivity, akathisia (psychomotor restlessness), hypomania, and mania, have been reported in adult and pediatric patients being treated with antidepressants for major depressive disorder as well as for other indications, both psychiatric and nonpsychiatric. Although a causal link between the emergence of such symptoms and either the worsening of depression and/or the emergence of suicidal impulses has not been established, there is concern that such symptoms may represent precursors to emerging suicidality.

Consideration should be given to changing the therapeutic regimen, including possibly discontinuing the medication, in patients whose depression is persistently worse, or who are experiencing emergent suicidality or symptoms that might be precursors to worsening depression or suicidality, especially if these symptoms are severe, abrupt in onset, or were not part of the patient's presenting symptoms.

Families and caregivers of pediatric patients being treated with antidepressants for major depressive disorder or other indications, both psychiatric and nonpsychiatric, should be alerted about the need to monitor patients for the emergence of agitation, irritability, unusual changes in behavior, and the other symptoms described above, as well as the emergence of suicidality, and to report such symptoms immediately to health care providers. Such monitoring should include daily observation by families and caregivers. Prescriptions for WELLBUTRIN should be written for the smallest quantity of tablets consistent with good patient management, in order to reduce the risk of overdose. Families and caregivers of adults being treated for depression should be similarly advised.

Screening Patients for Bipolar Disorder: A major depressive episode may be the initial presentation of bipolar disorder. It is generally believed (though not established in controlled trials) that treating such an episode with an antidepressant alone may increase the likelihood of precipitation of a mixed/manic episode in patients at risk for bipolar disorder. Whether any of the symptoms described above represent such a conversion is unknown. However, prior to initiating treatment with an antidepressant, patients with depressive symptoms should be adequately screened to determine if they are at risk for bipolar disorder; such screening should include a detailed psychiatric history, including a family history of suicide, bipolar disorder, and depression. It should be noted that WELLBUTRIN is not approved for use in treating bipolar depression.

Patients should be made aware that WELLBUTRIN contains the same active ingredient found in ZYBAN, used as an aid to smoking cessation treatment, and that WELLBUTRIN should not be used in combination with ZYBAN, or any other medications that contain bupropion.

Seizures: Bupropion is associated with seizures in approximately 0.4% (4/1,000) of patients treated at doses up to 450 mg/day. This incidence of seizures may exceed that of other marketed antidepressants by as much as 4-fold. This relative risk is only an approximate estimate because no direct comparative studies have been conducted. The estimated seizure incidence for WELLBUTRIN increases almost tenfold between 450 and 600 mg/day, which is twice the usually required daily dose (300 mg) and one and one-third the maximum recommended daily dose (450 mg). Given the wide variability among individuals and their capacity to metabolize and eliminate drugs this disproportionate increase in seizure incidence with dose incrementation calls for caution in dosing.

During the initial development, 25 among approximately 2,400 patients treated with WELLBUTRIN experienced seizures. At the time of seizure, 7 patients were receiving daily doses of 450 mg or below for an incidence of 0.33% (3/1,000) within the recommended dose range. Twelve patients experienced seizures at 600 mg/day (2.3% incidence); 6 additional patients had seizures at daily doses between 600 and 900 mg (2.8% incidence).

A separate, prospective study was conducted to determine the incidence of seizure during an 8-week treatment exposure in approximately 3,200 additional patients who received daily doses of up to 450 mg. Patients were permitted to continue treatment beyond 8 weeks if clinically indicated. Eight seizures occurred during the initial 8-week treatment period and 5 seizures were reported in patients continuing treatment beyond 8 weeks, resulting in a total seizure incidence of 0.4%.

The risk of seizure appears to be strongly associated with dose. Sudden and large increments in dose may contribute to increased risk. While many seizures occurred early in the course of treatment, some seizures did occur after several weeks at fixed dose. WELLBUTRIN should be discontinued and not restarted in patients who experience a seizure while on treatment.

The risk of seizure is also related to patient factors, clinical situations, and concomitant medications, which must be considered in selection of patients for therapy with WELLBUTRIN.

- **Patient factors:** Predisposing factors that may increase the risk of seizure with bupropion use include

history of head trauma or prior seizure, CNS tumor, the presence of severe hepatic cirrhosis, and concomitant medications that lower seizure threshold.

- **Clinical situations:** Circumstances associated with an increased seizure risk include, among others, excessive use of alcohol or sedatives (including benzodiazepines); addiction to opiates, cocaine, or stimulants; use of over-the-counter stimulants and anorectics; and diabetes treated with oral hypoglycemics or insulin.

- **Concomitant medications:** Many medications (e.g., antipsychotics, antidepressants, theophylline, systemic steroids) are known to lower seizure threshold.

Recommendations for Reducing the Risk of Seizure: Retrospective analysis of clinical experience gained during the development of WELLBUTRIN suggests that the risk of seizure may be minimized if

- **the total daily dose of WELLBUTRIN does *not* exceed 450 mg,**
- **the daily dose is administered 3 times daily, with each single dose *not* to exceed 150 mg to avoid high peak concentrations of bupropion and/or its metabolites, and**
- **the rate of incrementation of dose is very gradual.**

Extreme caution should be used when WELLBUTRIN is administered to patients with a history of seizure, cranial trauma, or other predisposition(s) toward seizure, or prescribed with other agents (e.g., antipsychotics, other antidepressants, theophylline, systemic steroids, etc.) that lower seizure threshold.

Hepatic Impairment: WELLBUTRIN should be used with extreme caution in patients with severe hepatic cirrhosis. In these patients a reduced dose and/or frequency is required, as peak bupropion, as well as AUC, levels are substantially increased and accumulation is likely to occur in such patients to a greater extent than usual. The dose should not exceed 75 mg once a day in these patients (see **CLINICAL PHARMACOLOGY, PRECAUTIONS, and DOSAGE AND ADMINISTRATION**).

Potential for Hepatotoxicity: In rats receiving large doses of bupropion chronically, there was an increase in incidence of hepatic hyperplastic nodules and hepatocellular hypertrophy. In dogs receiving large doses of bupropion chronically, various histologic changes were seen in the liver, and laboratory tests suggesting mild hepatocellular injury were noted.

The PRECAUTIONS: Information for Patients *section has been revised as follows.*

Information for Patients: Prescribers or other health professionals should inform patients, their families, and their caregivers about the benefits and risks associated with treatment with WELLBUTRIN and should counsel them in its appropriate use. A patient Medication Guide About Using Antidepressants in Children and Teenagers is available for WELLBUTRIN. The prescriber or health professional should instruct patients, their families, and their caregivers to read the Medication Guide and should assist them in understanding its contents. Patients should be given the opportunity to discuss the contents of the Medication Guide and to obtain answers to any questions they may have. The complete text of the Medication Guide is reprinted at the end of this document. Additional important information concerning WELLBUTRIN is provided in a tear-off leaflet entitled "Patient Information" at the end of this labeling.

Patients should be advised of the following issues and asked to alert their prescriber if these occur while taking WELLBUTRIN.

Clinical Worsening and Suicide Risk: Patients, their families, and their caregivers should be encouraged to be alert to the emergence of anxiety, agitation, panic attacks, insomnia, irritability, hostility, aggressiveness, impulsivity, akathisia (psychomotor restlessness), hypomania, mania, other unusual changes in behavior, worsening of depression, and suicidal ideation, especially early during antidepressant treatment and when the dose is adjusted up or down. Families and caregivers of patients should be advised to observe for the emergence of such symptoms on a day-to-day basis, since changes may be abrupt. Such symptoms should be reported to the patient's prescriber or health professional, especially if they are severe, abrupt in onset, or were not part of the patient's presenting symptoms. Symptoms such as these may be associated with an increased risk for suicidal thinking and behavior and indicate a need for very close monitoring and possibly changes in the medication.

Patients should be made aware that WELLBUTRIN contains the same active ingredient found in ZYBAN, used as an aid to smoking cessation, and that WELLBUTRIN should not be used in combination with ZYBAN or any other medications that contain bupropion hydrochloride.

Patients should be instructed to take WELLBUTRIN in equally divided doses 3 or 4 times a day to minimize the risk of seizure.

Patients should be told that WELLBUTRIN should be discontinued and not restarted if they experience a seizure while on treatment.

Patients should be told that any CNS-active drug like WELLBUTRIN may impair their ability to perform tasks requiring judgment or motor and cognitive skills. Consequently, until they are reasonably certain that WELLBUTRIN does not adversely affect their performance, they should refrain from driving an automobile or operating complex, hazardous machinery.

Patients should be told that the excessive use or abrupt discontinuation of alcohol or sedatives (including benzodiazepines) may alter the seizure threshold. Some patients have

reported lower alcohol tolerance during treatment with WELLBUTRIN. Patients should be advised that the consumption of alcohol should be minimized or avoided.

Patients should be advised to inform their physicians if they are taking or plan to take any prescription or over-the-counter drugs. Concern is warranted because WELLBUTRIN and other drugs may affect each other's metabolism.

Patients should be advised to notify their physicians if they become pregnant or intend to become pregnant during therapy.

The PRECAUTIONS: Pediatric Use *section has been revised as follows.*

Safety and effectiveness in the pediatric population have not been established. (see BOX WARNING and WARNINGS: Clinical Worsening and Suicide Risk). Anyone considering the use of WELLBUTRIN in a child or adolescent must balance the potential risks with the clinical need.

The following section has been added to the end of the package insert.

Medication Guide
WELLBUTRIN® (WELL byu-trin)
(bupropion hydrochloride) Tablets
About Using Antidepressants in Children and Teenagers
What is the most important information I should know if my child is being prescribed an antidepressant?
Parents or guardians need to think about 4 important things when their child is prescribed an antidepressant:
1. There is a risk of suicidal thoughts or actions
2. How to try to prevent suicidal thoughts or actions in your child
3. You should watch for certain signs if your child is taking an antidepressant
4. There are benefits and risks when using antidepressants

1. There is a Risk of Suicidal Thoughts or Actions
Children and teenagers sometimes think about suicide, and many report trying to kill themselves.

Antidepressants increase suicidal thoughts and actions in some children and teenagers. But suicidal thoughts and actions can also be caused by depression, a serious medical condition that is commonly treated with antidepressants. Thinking about killing yourself or trying to kill yourself is called *suicidality* or *being suicidal.*

A large study combined the results of 24 different studies of children and teenagers with depression or other illnesses. In these studies, patients took either a placebo (sugar pill) or an antidepressant for 1 to 4 months. *No one committed suicide in these studies,* but some patients became suicidal. On sugar pills, 2 out of every 100 became suicidal. On the antidepressants, 4 out of every 100 patients became suicidal.

For some children and teenagers, the risks of suicidal actions may be especially high. These include patients with
- Bipolar illness (sometimes called manic-depressive illness)
- A family history of bipolar illness
- A personal or family history of attempting suicide

If any of these are present, make sure you tell your healthcare provider before your child takes an antidepressant.

2. How to Try to Prevent Suicidal Thoughts and Actions
To try to prevent suicidal thoughts and actions in your child, pay close attention to changes in her or his moods or actions, especially if the changes occur suddenly. Other important people in your child's life can help by paying attention as well (e.g., your child, brothers and sisters, teachers, and other important people). The changes to look out for are listed in Section 3, on what to watch for.

Whenever an antidepressant is started or its dose is changed, pay close attention to your child.

After starting an antidepressant, your child should generally see his or her healthcare provider:
- Once a week for the first 4 weeks
- Every 2 weeks for the next 4 weeks
- After taking the antidepressant for 12 weeks
- After 12 weeks, follow your healthcare provider's advice about how often to come back
- More often if problems or questions arise (see Section 3)

You should call your child's healthcare provider between visits if needed.

3. You Should Watch For Certain Signs if Your Child is Taking an Antidepressant
Contact your child's healthcare provider *right away* if your child exhibits any of the following signs for the first time, or they seem worse, or worry you, your child, or your child's teacher:
- Thoughts about suicide or dying
- Attempts to commit suicide
- New or worse depression
- New or worse anxiety
- Feeling very agitated or restless
- Panic attacks
- Difficulty sleeping (insomnia)
- New or worse irritability
- Acting aggressive, being angry, or violent
- Acting on dangerous impulses
- An extreme increase in activity and talking
- Other unusual changes in behavior or mood

Never let your child stop taking an antidepressant without first talking to his or her healthcare provider. Stopping an antidepressant suddenly can cause other symptoms.

Continued on next page

Wellbutrin—Cont.

4. There are Benefits and Risks When Using Antidepressants

Antidepressants are used to treat depression and other illnesses. Depression and other illnesses can lead to suicide. In some children and teenagers, treatment with an antidepressant increases suicidal thinking or actions. It is important to discuss all the risks of treating depression and also the risks of not treating it. You and your child should discuss all treatment choices with your healthcare provider, not just the use of antidepressants.

Other side effects can occur with antidepressants (see section below).

Of all antidepressants, only fluoxetine (Prozac®)* has been FDA approved to treat pediatric depression.

For obsessive compulsive disorder in children and teenagers, FDA has approved only fluoxetine (Prozac®)*, sertraline (Zoloft®)*, fluvoxamine, and clomipramine (Anafranil®)*.

Your healthcare provider may suggest other antidepressants based on the past experience of your child or other family members.

Is this all I need to know if my child is being prescribed an antidepressant?

No. This is a warning about the risk of suicidality. Other side effects can occur with antidepressants. Be sure to ask your healthcare provider to explain all the side effects of the particular drug he or she is prescribing. Also ask about drugs to avoid when taking an antidepressant. Ask your healthcare provider or pharmacist where to find more information.

*The following are registered trademarks of their respective manufacturers: Prozac®/Eli Lilly and Company; Zoloft®/Pfizer Pharmaceuticals; Anafranil®/Mallinckrodt Inc.

This Medication Guide has been approved by the U.S. Food and Drug Administration for all antidepressants.

January 2005/MG-WT:1
Manufactured by DSM Pharmaceuticals, Inc.
Greenville, NC 27834 for
GlaxoSmithKline, Research Triangle Park, NC 27709
©2005, GlaxoSmithKline. All rights reserved.
January 2005/RL-2137, RL-2165

WELLBUTRIN SR® ℞
[wel'byü-trin]
(bupropion hydrochloride)
Sustained-Release Tablets

Prescribing information for this product, which appears on pages 1659–1663 of the 2005 PDR, has been revised as follows. Please write "See Supplement A" next to the product heading.

The following boxed warning has been added to the beginning of the package insert.

Suicidality in Children and Adolescents
Antidepressants increased the risk of suicidal thinking and behavior (suicidality) in short-term studies in children and adolescents with Major Depressive Disorder (MDD) and other psychiatric disorders. Anyone considering the use of WELLBUTRIN SR or any other antidepressant in a child or adolescent must balance this risk with the clinical need. Patients who are started on therapy should be observed closely for clinical worsening, suicidality, or unusual changes in behavior. Families and caregivers should be advised of the need for close observation and communication with the prescriber. WELLBUTRIN SR is not approved for use in pediatric patients. (See WARNINGS and PRECAUTIONS: Pediatric Use.)
Pooled analyses of short-term (4 to 16 weeks) placebo-controlled trials of 9 antidepressant drugs (SSRIs and others) in children and adolescents with major depressive disorder (MDD), obsessive compulsive disorder (OCD), or other psychiatric disorders (a total of 24 trials involving over 4,400 patients) have revealed a greater risk of adverse events representing suicidal thinking or behavior (suicidality) during the first few months of treatment in those receiving antidepressants. The average risk of such events in patients receiving antidepressants was 4%, twice the placebo risk of 2%. No suicides occurred in these trials.

The WARNINGS section has been revised as follows.
Clinical Worsening and Suicide Risk: Patients with major depressive disorder (MDD), both adult and pediatric, may experience worsening of their depression and/or the emergence of suicidal ideation and behavior (suicidality) or unusual changes in behavior, whether or not they are taking antidepressant medications, and this risk may persist until significant remission occurs. There has been a long-standing concern that antidepressants may have a role in inducing worsening of depression and the emergence of suicidality in certain patients. Antidepressants increased the risk of suicidal thinking and behavior (suicidality) in short-term studies in children and adolescents with Major Depressive Disorder (MDD) and other psychiatric disorders.

Pooled analyses of short-term placebo-controlled trials of 9 antidepressant drugs (SSRIs and others) in children and adolescents with MDD, OCD, or other psychiatric disorders (a total of 24 trials involving over 4,400 patients) have re-

vealed a greater risk of adverse events representing suicidal behavior or thinking (suicidality) during the first few months of treatment in those receiving antidepressants. The average risk of such events in patients receiving antidepressants was 4%, twice the placebo risk of 2%. There was considerable variation in risk among drugs, but a tendency toward an increase for almost all drugs studied. The risk of suicidality was most consistently observed in the MDD trials, but there were signals of risk arising from some trials in other psychiatric indications (obsessive compulsive disorder and social anxiety disorder) as well. **No suicides occurred in any of these trials.** It is unknown whether the suicidality risk in pediatric patients extends to longer-term use, i.e., beyond several months. It is also unknown whether the suicidality risk extends to adults.

All pediatric patients being treated with antidepressants for any indication should be observed closely for clinical worsening, suicidality, and unusual changes in behavior, especially during the initial few months of a course of drug therapy, or at times of dose changes, either increases or decreases. Such observation would generally include at least weekly face-to-face contact with patients or their family members or caregivers during the first 4 weeks of treatment, then every other week visits for the next 4 weeks, then at 12 weeks, and as clinically indicated beyond 12 weeks. Additional contact by telephone may be appropriate between face-to-face visits.

Adults with MDD or co-morbid depression in the setting of other psychiatric illness being treated with antidepressants should be observed similarly for clinical worsening and suicidality, especially during the initial few months of a course of drug therapy, or at times of dose changes, either increases or decreases.

The following symptoms, anxiety, agitation, panic attacks, insomnia, irritability, hostility, aggressiveness, impulsivity, akathisia (psychomotor restlessness), hypomania, and mania, have been reported in adult and pediatric patients being treated with antidepressants for major depressive disorder as well as for other indications, both psychiatric and nonpsychiatric. Although a causal link between the emergence of such symptoms and either the worsening of depression and/or the emergence of suicidal impulses has not been established, there is concern that such symptoms may represent precursors to emerging suicidality.

Consideration should be given to changing the therapeutic regimen, including possibly discontinuing the medication, in patients whose depression is persistently worse, or who are experiencing emergent suicidality or symptoms that might be precursors to worsening depression or suicidality, especially if these symptoms are severe, abrupt in onset, or were not part of the patient's presenting symptoms.

Families and caregivers of pediatric patients being treated with antidepressants for major depressive disorder or other indications, both psychiatric and nonpsychiatric, should be alerted about the need to monitor patients for the emergence of agitation, irritability, unusual changes in behavior, and the other symptoms described above, as well as the emergence of suicidality, and to report such symptoms immediately to health care providers. Such monitoring should include daily observation by families and caregivers. Prescriptions for WELLBUTRIN SR should be written for the smallest quantity of tablets consistent with good patient management, in order to reduce the risk of overdose. Families and caregivers of adults being treated for depression should be similarly advised.

Screening Patients for Bipolar Disorder: A major depressive episode may be the initial presentation of bipolar disorder. It is generally believed (though not established in controlled trials) that treating such an episode with an antidepressant alone may increase the likelihood of precipitation of a mixed/manic episode in patients at risk for bipolar disorder. Whether any of the symptoms described above represent such a conversion is unknown. However, prior to initiating treatment with an antidepressant, patients with depressive symptoms should be adequately screened to determine if they are at risk for bipolar disorder; such screening should include a detailed psychiatric history, including a family history of suicide, bipolar disorder, and depression. It should be noted that WELLBUTRIN SR is not approved for use in treating bipolar depression.

Patients should be made aware that WELLBUTRIN SR contains the same active ingredient found in ZYBAN, used as an aid to smoking cessation treatment, and that WELLBUTRIN SR should not be used in combination with ZYBAN, or any other medications that contain bupropion.
Seizures: Bupropion is associated with a dose-related risk of seizures. The risk of seizures is also related to patient factors, clinical situations, and concomitant medications, which must be considered in selection of patients for therapy with WELLBUTRIN SR.
WELLBUTRIN SR should be discontinued and not restarted in patients who experience a seizure while on treatment.

• **Dose:** At doses of WELLBUTRIN SR up to a dose of 300 mg/day, the incidence of seizure is approximately 0.1% (1/1,000) and increases to approximately 0.4% (4/1,000) at the maximum recommended dose of 400 mg/day.
Data for the immediate-release formulation of bupropion revealed a seizure incidence of approximately 0.4% (i.e., 13 of 3,200 patients followed prospectively) in patients treated at doses in a range of 300 to 450 mg/day. The 450-mg/day upper limit of this dose range is close to the currently recommended maximum dose of 400 mg/day for WELLBUTRIN SR Tablets. This seizure incidence (0.4%) may exceed that of other marketed antidepres-

sants and WELLBUTRIN SR Tablets up to 300 mg/day by as much as 4-fold. This relative risk is only an approximate estimate because no direct comparative studies have been conducted.

Additional data accumulated for the immediate-release formulation of bupropion suggested that the estimated seizure incidence increases almost tenfold between 450 and 600 mg/day, which is twice the usual adult dose and one and one-half the maximum recommended daily dose (400 mg) of WELLBUTRIN SR Tablets. This disproportionate increase in seizure incidence with dose incrementation calls for caution in dosing.

Data for WELLBUTRIN SR Tablets revealed a seizure incidence of approximately 0.1% (i.e., 3 of 3,100 patients followed prospectively) in patients treated at doses in a range of 100 to 300 mg/day. It is not possible to know if the lower seizure incidence observed in this study involving the sustained-release formulation of bupropion resulted from the different formulation or the lower dose used. However, as noted above, the immediate-release and sustained-release formulations are bioequivalent with regard to both rate and extent of absorption during steady state (the most pertinent condition to estimating seizure incidence), since most observed seizures occur under steady-state conditions.

• **Patient factors:** Predisposing factors that may increase the risk of seizure with bupropion use include history of head trauma or prior seizure, central nervous system (CNS) tumor, the presence of severe hepatic cirrhosis, and concomitant medications that lower seizure threshold.

• **Clinical situations:** Circumstances associated with an increased seizure risk include, among others, excessive use of alcohol or sedatives (including benzodiazepines); addiction to opiates, cocaine, or stimulants; use of over-the-counter stimulants and anorectics; and diabetes treated with oral hypoglycemics or insulin.

• **Concomitant medications:** Many medications (e.g., antipsychotics, antidepressants, theophylline, systemic steroids) are known to lower seizure threshold.

Recommendations for Reducing the Risk of Seizure: Retrospective analysis of clinical experience gained during the development of bupropion suggests that the risk of seizure may be minimized if

• the total daily dose of WELLBUTRIN SR Tablets does *not* exceed 400 mg,
• the daily dose is administered twice daily, and
• the rate of incrementation of dose is gradual.
• No single dose should exceed 200 mg to avoid high peak concentrations of bupropion and/or its metabolites.

WELLBUTRIN SR should be administered with extreme caution to patients with a history of seizure, cranial trauma, or other predisposition(s) toward seizure, or patients treated with other agents (e.g., antipsychotics, other antidepressants, theophylline, systemic steroids, etc.) that lower seizure threshold.

Hepatic Impairment: WELLBUTRIN SR should be used with extreme caution in patients with severe hepatic cirrhosis. In these patients a reduced frequency and/or dose is required, as peak bupropion, as well as AUC, levels are substantially increased and accumulation is likely to occur in such patients to a greater extent than usual. The dose should not exceed 100 mg every day or 150 mg every other day in these patients (see CLINICAL PHARMACOLOGY, PRECAUTIONS, and DOSAGE AND ADMINISTRATION).

Potential for Hepatotoxicity: In rats receiving large doses of bupropion chronically, there was an increase in incidence of hepatic hyperplastic nodules and hepatocellular hypertrophy. In dogs receiving large doses of bupropion chronically, various histologic changes were seen in the liver, and laboratory tests suggesting mild hepatocellular injury were noted.

The PRECAUTIONS: Information for Patients section has been revised as follows.
Information for Patients: Prescribers or other health professionals should inform patients, their families, and their caregivers about the benefits and risks associated with treatment with WELLBUTRIN SR and should counsel them in its appropriate use. A patient Medication Guide About Using Antidepressants in Children and Teenagers is available for WELLBUTRIN SR. The prescriber or health professional should instruct patients, their families, and their caregivers to read the Medication Guide and should assist them in understanding its contents. Patients should be given the opportunity to discuss the contents of the Medication Guide and to obtain answers to any questions they may have. The complete text of the Medication Guide is reprinted at the end of this document. Additional important information concerning WELLBUTRIN SR is provided in a tear-off leaflet entitled "Patient Information" at the end of this labeling.

Patients should be advised of the following issues and asked to alert their prescriber if these occur while taking WELLBUTRIN SR.

Clinical Worsening and Suicide Risk: Patients, their families, and their caregivers should be encouraged to be alert to the emergence of anxiety, agitation, panic attacks, insomnia, irritability, hostility, aggressiveness, impulsivity, akathisia (psychomotor restlessness), hypomania, mania, other unusual changes in behavior, worsening of depression, and suicidal ideation, especially early during antidepressant treatment and when the dose is adjusted up or down. Families and caregivers of patients should be advised to observe for the emergence of such symptoms on a day-to-day basis, since changes may be abrupt. Such symptoms should be reported to the patient's prescriber or health professional, especially if they are severe, abrupt in onset, or were not part of the patient's presenting symptoms. Symptoms such as these may be associated with an increased risk for suicidal thinking and behavior and indicate a need for very close monitoring and possibly changes in the medication.

Patients should be made aware that WELLBUTRIN SR contains the same active ingredient found in ZYBAN, used as an aid to smoking cessation treatment, and that WELLBUTRIN SR should not be used in combination with ZYBAN or any other medications that contain bupropion hydrochloride.

As dose is increased during initial titration to doses above 150 mg/day, patients should be instructed to take WELLBUTRIN SR Tablets in 2 divided doses, preferably with at least 8 hours between successive doses, to minimize the risk of seizures.

Patients should be told that WELLBUTRIN SR should be discontinued and not restarted if they experience a seizure while on treatment.

Patients should be told that any CNS-active drug like WELLBUTRIN SR Tablets may impair their ability to perform tasks requiring judgment or motor and cognitive skills. Consequently, until they are reasonably certain that WELLBUTRIN SR Tablets do not adversely affect their performance, they should refrain from driving an automobile or operating complex, hazardous machinery.

Patients should be told that the excessive use or abrupt discontinuation of alcohol or sedatives (including benzodiazepines) may alter the seizure threshold. Some patients have reported lower alcohol tolerance during treatment with WELLBUTRIN SR. Patients should be advised that the consumption of alcohol should be minimized or avoided.

Patients should be advised to inform their physicians if they are taking or plan to take any prescription or over-the-counter drugs. Concern is warranted because WELLBUTRIN SR Tablets and other drugs may affect each other's metabolism.

Patients should be advised to notify their physicians if they become pregnant or intend to become pregnant during therapy.

Patients should be advised to swallow WELLBUTRIN SR Tablets whole so that the release rate is not altered. Do not chew, divide, or crush tablets.

The PRECAUTIONS: Pediatric Use section has been revised as follows.

Safety and effectiveness in the pediatric population have not been established (see BOX WARNING and WARNINGS: Clinical Worsening and Suicide Risk). Anyone considering the use of WELLBUTRIN SR in a child or adolescent must balance the potential risks with the clinical need.

The following section has been added to the end of the package insert.

Medication Guide
WELLBUTRIN SR® (WELL byu-trin)
(bupropion hydrochloride) Sustained-Release Tablets
About Using Antidepressants in Children and Teenagers
What is the most important information I should know if my child is being prescribed an antidepressant?
Parents or guardians need to think about 4 important things when their child is prescribed an antidepressant:
1. There is a risk of suicidal thoughts or actions
2. How to try to prevent suicidal thoughts or actions in your child
3. You should watch for certain signs if your child is taking an antidepressant
4. There are benefits and risks when using antidepressants

1. There is a Risk of Suicidal Thoughts or Actions
Children and teenagers sometimes think about suicide, and many report trying to kill themselves.
Antidepressants increase suicidal thoughts and actions in some children and teenagers. But suicidal thoughts and actions can also be caused by depression, a serious medical condition that is commonly treated with antidepressants. Thinking about killing yourself or trying to kill yourself is called *suicidality* or *being suicidal*.
A large study combined the results of 24 different studies of children and teenagers with depression or other illnesses. In these studies, patients took either a placebo (sugar pill) or an antidepressant for 1 to 4 months. *No one committed suicide in these studies*, but some patients became suicidal. On sugar pills, 2 out of every 100 became suicidal. On the antidepressants, 4 out of every 100 patients became suicidal.
For some children and teenagers, the risks of suicidal actions may be especially high. These include patients with
• Bipolar illness (sometimes called manic-depressive illness)
• A family history of bipolar illness
• A personal or family history of attempting suicide
If any of these are present, make sure you tell your healthcare provider before your child takes an antidepressant.

2. How to Try to Prevent Suicidal Thoughts and Actions
To try to prevent suicidal thoughts and actions in your child, pay close attention to changes in her or his moods or actions, especially if the changes occur suddenly. Other important people in your child's life can help by paying attention as well (e.g., your child, brothers and sisters, teachers, and other important people). The changes to look out for are listed in Section 3, on what to watch for. Whenever an antidepressant is started or its dose is changed, pay close attention to your child.

After starting an antidepressant, your child should generally see his or her healthcare provider:
• Once a week for the first 4 weeks
• Every 2 weeks for the next 4 weeks
• After taking the antidepressant for 12 weeks
• After 12 weeks, follow your healthcare provider's advice about how often to come back
• More often if problems or questions arise (see Section 3)
You should call your child's healthcare provider between visits if needed.

3. You Should Watch For Certain Signs if Your Child is Taking an Antidepressant
Contact your child's healthcare provider *right away* if your child exhibits any of the following signs for the first time, or they seem worse, or worry you, your child, or your child's teacher:
• Thoughts about suicide or dying
• Attempts to commit suicide
• New or worse depression
• New or worse anxiety
• Feeling very agitated or restless
• Panic attacks
• Difficulty sleeping (insomnia)
• New or worse irritability
• Acting aggressive, being angry, or violent
• Acting on dangerous impulses
• An extreme increase in activity and talking
• Other unusual changes in behavior or mood
    Never let your child stop taking an antidepressant without first talking to his or her healthcare provider. Stopping an antidepressant suddenly can cause other symptoms.

4. There are Benefits and Risks When Using Antidepressants
Antidepressants are used to treat depression and other illnesses. Depression and other illnesses can lead to suicide. In some children and teenagers, treatment with an antidepressant increases suicidal thinking or actions. It is important to discuss all the risks of treating depression and also the risks of not treating it. You and your child should discuss all treatment choices with your healthcare provider, not just the use of antidepressants.
Other side effects can occur with antidepressants (see section below).
Of all antidepressants, only fluoxetine (Prozac®)* has been FDA approved to treat pediatric depression.
For obsessive compulsive disorder in children and teenagers, FDA has approved only fluoxetine (Prozac®)*, sertraline (Zoloft®)*, fluvoxamine, and clomipramine (Anafranil®)*. Your healthcare provider may suggest other antidepressants based on the past experience of your child or other family members.
Is this all I need to know if my child is being prescribed an antidepressant?
No. This is a warning about the risk of suicidality. Other side effects can occur with antidepressants. Be sure to ask your healthcare provider to explain all the side effects of the particular drug he or she is prescribing. Also ask about drugs to avoid when taking an antidepressant. Ask your healthcare provider or pharmacist where to find more information.
*The following are registered trademarks of their respective manufacturers: Prozac®/Eli Lilly and Company; Zoloft®/Pfizer Pharmaceuticals; Anafranil®/Mallinckrodt Inc.
This Medication Guide has been approved by the U.S. Food and Drug Administration for all antidepressants.
January 2005/MG-MS:1
Distributed by:
GlaxoSmithKline, Research Triangle Park, NC 27709
Manufactured by:
GlaxoSmithKline, Research Triangle Park, NC 27709
or DSM Pharmaceuticals, Inc., Greenville, NC 27834
©2005, GlaxoSmithKline. All rights reserved.
January 2005/RL-2136, RL-2164

WELLBUTRIN XL®   ℞
[wel'byü-trin]
(bupropion hydrochloride extended-release tablets)

Prescribing information for this product, which appears on pages 1663–1668 of the 2005 PDR, has been revised as follows. Please write "See Supplement A" next to the product heading.
The following boxed warning has been added to the beginning of the package insert.

Suicidality in Children and Adolescents
Antidepressants increased the risk of suicidal thinking and behavior (suicidality) in short-term studies in children and adolescents with Major Depressive Disorder (MDD) and other psychiatric disorders. Anyone considering the use of WELLBUTRIN XL or any other antidepressant in a child or adolescent must balance this risk with the clinical need. Patients who are started on therapy should be observed closely for clinical worsening, suicidality, or unusual changes in behavior. Families and caregivers should be advised of the need for close observation and communication with the prescriber. WELLBUTRIN XL is not approved for use in pediatric patients. (See WARNINGS and PRECAUTIONS: Pediatric Use.)
Pooled analyses of short-term (4 to 16 weeks) placebo-controlled trials of 9 antidepressant drugs (SSRIs and

---

others) in children and adolescents with major depressive disorder (MDD), obsessive compulsive disorder (OCD), or other psychiatric disorders (a total of 24 trials involving over 4,400 patients) have revealed a greater risk of adverse events representing suicidal thinking or behavior (suicidality) during the first few months of treatment in those receiving antidepressants. The average risk of such events in patients receiving antidepressants was 4%, twice the placebo risk of 2%. No suicides occurred in these trials.

The following paragraph has been revised in the CLINICAL PHARMACOLOGY: Pharmacokinetics section.
In a study comparing 14-day dosing with WELLBUTRIN XL Tablets 300 mg once daily to the immediate-release formulation of bupropion at 100 mg 3 times daily, equivalence was demonstrated for peak plasma concentration and area under the curve for bupropion and the 3 metabolites (hydroxybupropion, threohydrobupropion, and erythrohydrobupropion). Additionally, in a study comparing 14-day dosing with WELLBUTRIN XL Tablets 300 mg once daily to the sustained-release formulation of bupropion at 150 mg 2 times daily, equivalence was demonstrated for peak plasma concentration and area under the curve for bupropion and the 3 metabolites.
The WARNINGS section has been revised as follows.
Clinical Worsening and Suicide Risk: Patients with major depressive disorder (MDD), both adult and pediatric, may experience worsening of their depression and/or the emergence of suicidal ideation and behavior (suicidality) or unusual changes in behavior, whether or not they are taking antidepressant medications, and this risk may persist until significant remission occurs. There has been a long-standing concern that antidepressants may have a role in inducing worsening of depression and the emergence of suicidality in certain patients. Antidepressants increased the risk of suicidal thinking and behavior (suicidality) in short-term studies in children and adolescents with Major Depressive Disorder (MDD) and other psychiatric disorders.
Pooled analyses of short-term placebo-controlled trials of 9 antidepressant drugs (SSRIs and others) in children and adolescents with MDD, OCD, or other psychiatric disorders (a total of 24 trials involving over 4,400 patients) have revealed a greater risk of adverse events representing suicidal behavior or thinking (suicidality) during the first few months of treatment in those receiving antidepressants. The average risk of such events in patients receiving antidepressants was 4%, twice the placebo risk of 2%. There was considerable variation in risk among drugs, but a tendency toward an increase for almost all drugs studied. The risk of suicidality was most consistently observed in the MDD trials, but there were signals of risk arising from some trials in other psychiatric indications (obsessive compulsive disorder and social anxiety disorder) as well. **No suicides occurred in any of these trials.** It is unknown whether the suicidality risk in pediatric patients extends to longer-term use, i.e., beyond several months. It is also unknown whether the suicidality risk extends to adults.
All pediatric patients being treated with antidepressants for any indication should be observed closely for clinical worsening, suicidality, and unusual changes in behavior, especially during the initial few months of a course of drug therapy, or at times of dose changes, either increases or decreases. Such observation would generally include at least weekly face-to-face contact with patients or their family members or caregivers during the first 4 weeks of treatment, then every other week visits for the next 4 weeks, then at 12 weeks, and as clinically indicated beyond 12 weeks. Additional contact by telephone may be appropriate between face-to-face visits.
Adults with MDD or co-morbid depression in the setting of other psychiatric illness being treated with antidepressants should be observed similarly for clinical worsening and suicidality, especially during the initial few months of a course of drug therapy, or at times of dose changes, either increases or decreases.
The following symptoms, anxiety, agitation, panic attacks, insomnia, irritability, hostility, aggressiveness, impulsivity, akathisia (psychomotor restlessness), hypomania, and mania, have been reported in adult and pediatric patients being treated with antidepressants for major depressive disorder as well as for other indications, both psychiatric and nonpsychiatric. Although a causal link between the emergence of such symptoms and either the worsening of depression and/or the emergence of suicidal impulses has not been established, there is concern that such symptoms may represent precursors to emerging suicidality.
Consideration should be given to changing the therapeutic regimen, including possibly discontinuing the medication, in patients whose depression is persistently worse, or who are experiencing emergent suicidality or symptoms that might be precursors to worsening depression or suicidality, especially if these symptoms are severe, abrupt in onset, or were not part of the patient's presenting symptoms.
Families and caregivers of pediatric patients being treated with antidepressants for major depressive disorder or other indications, both psychiatric and nonpsychiatric, should be alerted about the need to monitor patients for the emergence of agitation, irritability, unusual changes in behavior, and the other symptoms described above, as well as the emergence of suicidality, and to report such symptoms immediately to health care providers. Such

Continued on next page

Wellbutrin XL—Cont.

monitoring should include daily observation by families and caregivers. Prescriptions for WELLBUTRIN XL should be written for the smallest quantity of tablets consistent with good patient management, in order to reduce the risk of overdose. Families and caregivers of adults being treated for depression should be similarly advised.

Screening Patients for Bipolar Disorder: A major depressive episode may be the initial presentation of bipolar disorder. It is generally believed (though not established in controlled trials) that treating such an episode with an antidepressant alone may increase the likelihood of precipitation of a mixed/manic episode in patients at risk for bipolar disorder. Whether any of the symptoms described above represent such a conversion is unknown. However, prior to initiating treatment with an antidepressant, patients with depressive symptoms should be adequately screened to determine if they are at risk for bipolar disorder; such screening should include a detailed psychiatric history, including a family history of suicide, bipolar disorder, and depression. It should be noted that WELLBUTRIN XL is not approved for use in treating bipolar depression.

Patients should be made aware that WELLBUTRIN XL contains the same active ingredient found in ZYBAN, used as an aid to smoking cessation treatment, and that WELLBUTRIN XL should not be used in combination with ZYBAN, or any other medications that contain bupropion, such as WELLBUTRIN SR (bupropion hydrochloride), the sustained-release formulation or WELLBUTRIN (bupropion hydrochloride), the immediate-release formulation.

Seizures: Bupropion is associated with a dose-related risk of seizures. The risk of seizures is also related to patient factors, clinical situations, and concomitant medications, which must be considered in selection of patients for therapy with WELLBUTRIN XL. WELLBUTRIN XL should be discontinued and not restarted in patients who experience a seizure while on treatment.

As WELLBUTRIN XL is bioequivalent to both the immediate-release formulation of bupropion and to the sustained-release formulation of bupropion, the seizure incidence with WELLBUTRIN XL, while not formally evaluated in clinical trials, may be similar to that presented below for the immediate-release and sustained-release formulations of bupropion.

- **Dose:** At doses up to 300 mg/day of the sustained-release formulation of bupropion (WELLBUTRIN SR), the incidence of seizure is approximately 0.1% (1/1,000).
  Data for the immediate-release formulation of bupropion revealed a seizure incidence of approximately 0.4% (i.e., 13 of 3,200 patients followed prospectively) in patients treated at doses in a range of 300 to 450 mg/day. This seizure incidence (0.4%) may exceed that of some other marketed antidepressants.
  Additional data accumulated for the immediate-release formulation of bupropion suggested that the estimated seizure incidence increases almost tenfold between 450 and 600 mg/day. The 600 mg dose is twice the usual adult dose and one and one-third the maximum recommended daily dose (450 mg) of WELLBUTRIN XL Tablets. This disproportionate increase in seizure incidence with dose incrementation calls for caution in dosing.
- **Patient factors:** Predisposing factors that may increase the risk of seizure with bupropion use include history of head trauma or prior seizure, central nervous system (CNS) tumor, the presence of severe hepatic cirrhosis, and concomitant medications that lower seizure threshold.
- **Clinical situations:** Circumstances associated with an increased seizure risk include, among others, excessive use of alcohol or sedatives (including benzodiazepines); addiction to opiates, cocaine, or stimulants; use of over-the-counter stimulants and anorectics; and diabetes treated with oral hypoglycemics or insulin.
- **Concomitant medications:** Many medications (e.g., antipsychotics, antidepressants, theophylline, systemic steroids) are known to lower seizure threshold.

Recommendations for Reducing the Risk of Seizure: Retrospective analysis of clinical experience gained during the development of bupropion suggests that the risk of seizure may be minimized if

- the total daily dose of WELLBUTRIN XL Tablets does *not* exceed 450 mg,
- the rate of incrementation of dose is gradual.

WELLBUTRIN XL should be administered with extreme caution to patients with a history of seizure, cranial trauma, or other predisposition(s) toward seizure, or patients treated with other agents (e.g., antipsychotics, other antidepressants, theophylline, systemic steroids, etc.) that lower seizure threshold.

Hepatic Impairment: WELLBUTRIN XL should be used with extreme caution in patients with severe hepatic cirrhosis. In these patients a reduced frequency and/or dose is required, as peak bupropion, as well as AUC, levels are substantially increased and accumulation is likely to occur in such patients to a greater extent than usual. The dose should not exceed 150 mg every other day in these patients (see CLINICAL PHARMACOLOGY, PRECAUTIONS, and DOSAGE AND ADMINISTRATION).

Potential for Hepatotoxicity: In rats receiving large doses of bupropion chronically, there was an increase in incidence of hepatic hyperplastic nodules and hepatocellular hypertrophy. In dogs receiving large doses of bupropion chroni-

cally, various histologic changes were seen in the liver, and laboratory tests suggesting mild hepatocellular injury were noted.

The PRECAUTIONS: Information for Patients *section has been revised as follows.*

Prescribers or other health professionals should inform patients, their families, and their caregivers about the benefits and risks associated with treatment with WELLBUTRIN XL and should counsel them in its appropriate use. A patient Medication Guide About Using Antidepressants in Children and Teenagers is available for WELLBUTRIN XL. The prescriber or health professional should instruct patients, their families, and their caregivers to read the Medication Guide and should assist them in understanding its contents. Patients should be given the opportunity to discuss the contents of the Medication Guide and to obtain answers to any questions they may have. The complete text of the Medication Guide is reprinted at the end of this document. Additional important information concerning WELLBUTRIN XL is provided in a tear-off leaflet entitled "Patient Information" at the end of this labeling.

Patients should be advised of the following issues and asked to alert their prescriber if these occur while taking WELLBUTRIN XL.

Clinical Worsening and Suicide Risk: Patients, their families, and their caregivers should be encouraged to be alert to the emergence of anxiety, agitation, panic attacks, insomnia, irritability, hostility, aggressiveness, impulsivity, akathisia (psychomotor restlessness), hypomania, mania, other unusual changes in behavior, worsening of depression, and suicidal ideation, especially early during antidepressant treatment and when the dose is adjusted up or down. Families and caregivers of patients should be advised to observe for the emergence of such symptoms on a day-to-day basis, since changes may be abrupt. Such symptoms should be reported to the patient's prescriber or health professional, especially if they are severe, abrupt in onset, or were not part of the patient's presenting symptoms. Symptoms such as these may be associated with an increased risk for suicidal thinking and behavior and indicate a need for very close monitoring and possibly changes in the medication.

Patients should be made aware that WELLBUTRIN XL contains the same active ingredient found in ZYBAN, used as an aid to smoking cessation treatment, and that WELLBUTRIN XL should not be used in combination with ZYBAN or any other medications that contain bupropion hydrochloride (such as WELLBUTRIN SR, the sustained-release formulation, and WELLBUTRIN, the immediate-release formulation).

Patients should be told that WELLBUTRIN XL should be discontinued and not restarted if they experience a seizure while on treatment.

Patients should be told that any CNS-active drug like WELLBUTRIN XL Tablets may impair their ability to perform tasks requiring judgment or motor and cognitive skills. Consequently, until they are reasonably certain that WELLBUTRIN XL Tablets do not adversely affect their performance, they should refrain from driving an automobile or operating complex, hazardous machinery.

Patients should be told that the excessive use or abrupt discontinuation of alcohol or sedatives (including benzodiazepines) may alter the seizure threshold. Some patients have reported lower alcohol tolerance during treatment with WELLBUTRIN XL. Patients should be advised that the consumption of alcohol should be minimized or avoided.

Patients should be advised to inform their physicians if they are taking or plan to take any prescription or over-the-counter drugs. Concern is warranted because WELLBUTRIN XL Tablets and other drugs may affect each other's metabolism.

Patients should be advised to notify their physicians if they become pregnant or intend to become pregnant during therapy.

Patients should be advised to swallow WELLBUTRIN XL Tablets whole so that the release rate is not altered. Do not chew, divide, or crush tablets.

Patients should be advised that they may notice in their stool something that looks like a tablet. This is normal. The medication in WELLBUTRIN XL is contained in a non-absorbable shell that has been specially designed to slowly release drug in the body. When this process is completed, the empty shell is eliminated from the body.

The PRECAUTIONS: Pediatric Use *section has been revised as follows.*

Safety and effectiveness in the pediatric population have not been established (see BOX WARNING and WARNINGS: Clinical Worsening and Suicide Risk). Anyone considering the use of WELLBUTRIN XL in a child or adolescent must balance the potential risks with the clinical need.

The first paragraph of the ADVERSE REACTIONS *section has been revised as follows.*

WELLBUTRIN XL has been demonstrated to have similar bioavailability both to the immediate-release formulation of bupropion and to the sustained-release formulation of bupropion (see CLINICAL PHARMACOLOGY). The information included under the Incidence in Controlled Trials subsection of ADVERSE REACTIONS is based primarily on data from controlled clinical trials with WELLBUTRIN SR Tablets, the sustained-release formulation of bupropion. WELLBUTRIN XL has not been studied in placebo-controlled trials, although it has been studied in non-placebo-controlled clinical bioavailability studies. Information on additional adverse events associated with the sustained-release formulation of bupropion in smoking cessation trials, as well as the immediate-release formulation of

bupropion, is included in a separate section (see Other Events Observed During the Clinical Development and Postmarketing Experience of Bupropion).

The following section has been added to the end of the package insert.

Medication Guide
WELLBUTRIN SR® (WELL byu-trin)
(bupropion hydrochloride) Sustained-Release Tablets
About Using Antidepressants in Children and Teenagers

What is the most important information I should know if my child is being prescribed an antidepressant?

Parents or guardians need to think about 4 important things when their child is prescribed an antidepressant:

1. There is a risk of suicidal thoughts or actions
2. How to try to prevent suicidal thoughts or actions in your child
3. You should watch for certain signs if your child is taking an antidepressant
4. There are benefits and risks when using antidepressants

1. There is a Risk of Suicidal Thoughts or Actions

Children and teenagers sometimes think about suicide, and many report trying to kill themselves.

Antidepressants increase suicidal thoughts and actions in some children and teenagers. But suicidal thoughts and actions can also be caused by depression, a serious medical condition that is commonly treated with antidepressants. Thinking about killing yourself or trying to kill yourself is called *suicidality* or *being suicidal.*

A large study combined the results of 24 different studies of children and teenagers with depression or other illnesses. In these studies, patients took either a placebo (sugar pill) or an antidepressant for 1 to 4 months. *No one committed suicide in these studies,* but some patients became suicidal. On sugar pills, 2 out of every 100 became suicidal. On the antidepressants, 4 out of every 100 patients became suicidal.

For some children and teenagers, the risks of suicidal actions may be especially high. These include patients with

- Bipolar illness (sometimes called manic-depressive illness)
- A family history of bipolar illness
- A personal or family history of attempting suicide

If any of these are present, make sure you tell your healthcare provider before your child takes an antidepressant.

2. How to Try to Prevent Suicidal Thoughts and Actions

To try to prevent suicidal thoughts and actions in your child, pay close attention to changes in her or his moods or actions, especially if the changes occur suddenly. Other important people in your child's life can help by paying attention as well (e.g., your child, brothers and sisters, teachers, and other important people). The changes to look out for are listed in Section 3, on what to watch for.

Whenever an antidepressant is started or its dose is changed, pay close attention to your child.

After starting an antidepressant, your child should generally see his or her healthcare provider:

- Once a week for the first 4 weeks
- Every 2 weeks for the next 4 weeks
- After taking the antidepressant for 12 weeks
- After 12 weeks, follow your healthcare provider's advice about how often to come back
- More often if problems or questions arise (see Section 3)

You should call your child's healthcare provider between visits if needed.

3. You Should Watch For Certain Signs if Your Child is Taking an Antidepressant

Contact your child's healthcare provider *right away* if your child exhibits any of the following signs for the first time, or they seem worse, or worry you, your child, or your child's teacher:

- Thoughts about suicide or dying
- Attempts to commit suicide
- New or worse depression
- New or worse anxiety
- Feeling very agitated or restless
- Panic attacks
- Difficulty sleeping (insomnia)
- New or worse irritability
- Acting aggressive, being angry, or violent
- Acting on dangerous impulses
- An extreme increase in activity and talking
- Other unusual changes in behavior or mood

Never let your child stop taking an antidepressant without first talking to his or her healthcare provider. Stopping an antidepressant suddenly can cause other symptoms.

4. There are Benefits and Risks When Using Antidepressants

Antidepressants are used to treat depression and other illnesses. Depression and other illnesses can lead to suicide. In some children and teenagers, treatment with an antidepressant increases suicidal thinking or actions. It is important to discuss all the risks of treating depression and also the risks of not treating it. You and your child should discuss all treatment choices with your healthcare provider, not just the use of antidepressants.

Other side effects can occur with antidepressants (see section below).

Of all antidepressants, only fluoxetine (Prozac®)* has been FDA approved to treat pediatric depression.

For obsessive compulsive disorder in children and teenagers, FDA has approved only fluoxetine (Prozac®)*, sertraline (Zoloft®)*, fluvoxamine, and clomipramine (Anafranil®)*.

Your healthcare provider may suggest other antidepressants based on the past experience of your child or other family members.

Is this all I need to know if my child is being prescribed an antidepressant?

No. This is a warning about the risk of suicidality. Other side effects can occur with antidepressants. Be sure to ask your healthcare provider to explain all the side effects of the particular drug he or she is prescribing. Also ask about drugs to avoid when taking an antidepressant. Ask your healthcare provider or pharmacist where to find more information.

* The following are registered trademarks of their respective manufacturers: Prozac®/Eli Lilly and Company; Zoloft®/Pfizer Pharmaceuticals; Anafranil®/Mallinckrodt Inc.

This Medication Guide has been approved by the U.S. Food and Drug Administration for all antidepressants.

January 2005/MG-WX:1

Manufactured by:
Biovail Corporation
Mississauga, ON L5N 8M5, Canada for
GlaxoSmithKline, Research Triangle Park, NC 27709
©2005, GlaxoSmithKline. All rights reserved.
January 2005/RL-2135, RL-2146, RL-2163

ZANTAC® 150 ℞
[zan'tak]
(ranitidine hydrochloride)
Tablets, USP

ZANTAC® 300 ℞
(ranitidine hydrochloride)
Tablets, USP

ZANTAC® 25 ℞
(ranitidine hydrochloride effervescent)
EFFERdose® Tablets

ZANTAC® 150 ℞
(ranitidine hydrochloride effervescent)
EFFERdose® Tablets

ZANTAC® ℞
(ranitidine hydrochloride)
Syrup, USP

Prescribing information for this product, which appears on pages 1670–1673 of the 2005 PDR, has been revised as follows. Please write "See Supplement A" next to the product heading.

The following paragraph has been revised in the PRECAUTIONS: Information for Patients *section.*

Phenylketonurics: ZANTAC 25 EFFERdose Tablets contain phenylalanine 2.81 mg per 25 mg of ranitidine. ZANTAC 150 EFFERdose Tablets contain phenylalanine 16.84 mg per 150 mg of ranitidine. ZANTAC EFFERdose Tablets should not be chewed, swallowed whole, or dissolved on the tongue.

The following paragraphs have been revised in the DOSAGE AND ADMINISTRATION *section.*

Preparation of ZANTAC 25 EFFERdose Tablets: Tablets should not be chewed, swallowed whole, or dissolved on the tongue. Dissolve 1 tablet in no less than 5 mL (1 teaspoonful) of water in an appropriate measuring cup. Wait until the tablet is completely dissolved before administering the solution to the infant/child. The solution may be administered by medicine dropper or oral syringe for infants.

Preparation of ZANTAC 150 EFFERdose Tablets: Tablets should not be chewed, swallowed whole, or dissolved on the tongue. Dissolve each dose in approximately 6 to 8 oz of water before drinking.

GlaxoSmithKline, Research Triangle Park, NC 27709
©2004, GlaxoSmithKline. All rights reserved.
October 2004/RL-2131

ZIAGEN® ℞
[zī'ə-jin]
(abacavir sulfate)
Tablets

ZIAGEN® ℞
(abacavir sulfate)
Oral Solution

Prescribing information for this product, which appears on pages 1673–1676 of the 2005 PDR, has been completely revised as follows. Please write "See Supplement A" next to the product heading.

WARNINGS

Hypersensitivity Reactions: Serious and sometimes fatal hypersensitivity reactions have been associated with ZIAGEN (abacavir sulfate). Hypersensitivity to abacavir is a multi-organ clinical syndrome usually characterized by a sign or symptom in 2 or more of the following groups: (1) fever, (2) rash, (3) gastrointestinal (including nausea, vomiting, diarrhea, or abdominal pain), (4) constitutional (including generalized malaise, fatigue, or achiness), and (5) respiratory (including dyspnea, cough, or pharyngitis). Discontinue ZIAGEN as soon as a hypersensitivity reaction is suspected. Permanently discontinue ZIAGEN if hypersensitivity cannot be ruled out, even when other diagnoses are possible.

Following a hypersensitivity reaction to abacavir, NEVER restart ZIAGEN or any other abacavir-containing product because more severe symptoms can occur within hours and may include life-threatening hypotension and death.

Reintroduction of ZIAGEN or any other abacavir-containing product, even in patients who have no identified history or unrecognized symptoms of hypersensitivity to abacavir therapy, can result in serious or fatal hypersensitivity reactions. Such reactions can occur within hours (see WARNINGS and PRECAUTIONS: Information for Patients).

Lactic Acidosis and Severe Hepatomegaly: Lactic acidosis and severe hepatomegaly with steatosis, including fatal cases, have been reported with the use of nucleoside analogues alone or in combination, including ZIAGEN and other antiretrovirals (see WARNINGS).

DESCRIPTION

ZIAGEN is the brand name for abacavir sulfate, a synthetic carbocyclic nucleoside analogue with inhibitory activity against HIV. The chemical name of abacavir sulfate is *(1S,cis)*-4-[2-amino-6-(cyclopropylamino)-9*H*-purin-9-yl]-2-cyclopentene-1-methanol sulfate (salt) (2:1). Abacavir sulfate is the enantiomer with *1S, 4R* absolute configuration on the cyclopentene ring. It has a molecular formula of $(C_{14}H_{18}N_6O)_2 \cdot H_2SO_4$ and a molecular weight of 670.76 daltons. It has the following structural formula:

Abacavir sulfate is a white to off-white solid with a solubility of approximately 77 mg/mL in distilled water at 25°C. It has an octanol/water (pH 7.1 to 7.3) partition coefficient (log *P*) of approximately 1.20 at 25°C.

ZIAGEN Tablets are for oral administration. Each tablet contains abacavir sulfate equivalent to 300 mg of abacavir as active ingredient and the following inactive ingredients: colloidal silicon dioxide, magnesium stearate, microcrystalline cellulose, and sodium starch glycolate. The tablets are coated with a film that is made of hypromellose, polysorbate 80, synthetic yellow iron oxide, titanium dioxide, and triacetin.

ZIAGEN Oral Solution is for oral administration. Each milliliter (1 mL) of ZIAGEN Oral Solution contains abacavir sulfate equivalent to 20 mg of abacavir (i.e., 20 mg/mL) as active ingredient and the following inactive ingredients: artificial strawberry and banana flavors, citric acid (anhydrous), methylparaben and propylparaben (added as preservatives), propylene glycol, saccharin sodium, sodium citrate (dihydrate), sorbitol solution, and water.

In vivo, abacavir sulfate dissociates to its free base, abacavir. All dosages for ZIAGEN are expressed in terms of abacavir.

MICROBIOLOGY

Mechanism of Action: Abacavir is a carbocyclic synthetic nucleoside analogue. Abacavir is converted intracellularly by cellular enzymes to the active metabolite, carbovir triphosphate, an analogue of deoxyguanosine-5′-triphosphate (dGTP). Carbovir triphosphate inhibits the activity of HIV-1 reverse transcriptase (RT) both by competing with the natural substrate dGTP and by its incorporation into viral DNA. The lack of a 3′-OH group in the incorporated nucleoside analogue prevents the formation of the 5′ to 3′ phosphodiester linkage essential for DNA chain elongation, and therefore, the viral DNA growth is terminated. Abacavir is a weak inhibitor of cellular DNA polymerases α, β, and γ.

Antiviral Activity: The in vitro anti–HIV-1 activity of abacavir was evaluated against a T-cell tropic laboratory strain HIV-1_{IIIB} in lymphoblastic cell lines, a monocyte/macrophage tropic laboratory strain HIV-1_{BaL} in primary monocytes/macrophages, and clinical isolates in peripheral blood mononuclear cells. The concentration of drug necessary to inhibit viral replication by 50 percent (IC_{50}) ranged from 3.7 to 5.8 µM (1 µM = 0.28 mcg/mL) and 0.07 to 1.0 µM against HIV-1_{IIIB} and HIV-1_{BaL}, respectively, and was 0.26 ± 0.18 µM against 8 clinical isolates. The IC_{50} values of abacavir against different HIV-1 clades (A-E) ranged from 0.0015 to 1.0 µM, and against HIV-2 isolates, from 0.024 to 0.49 µM Abacavir had synergistic activity in vitro in combination with amprenavir, nevirapine, and zidovudine, and additive activity in combination with didanosine, lamivudine, stavudine, tenofovir, and zalcitabine. Ribavirin had no effect on the in vitro anti–HIV-1 activity of abacavir.

Resistance: HIV-1 isolates with reduced susceptibility to abacavir have been selected in vitro and were also obtained from patients treated with abacavir. Genetic analysis of isolates from patients failing an abacavir-containing regimen demonstrated that amino acid substitutions K65R, L74V, Y115F, and M184V in HIV-1 RT contributed to abacavir resistance. In a study of therapy-naive adults receiving ZIAGEN 600 mg once daily (n = 384) or 300 mg twice daily (n = 386), in a background regimen of lamivudine 300 mg once daily and efavirenz 600 mg once daily (Study CNA30021), the incidence of virologic failure at 48 weeks was similar between the 2 groups (11% in both arms). Genotypic (n = 38) and phenotypic analyses (n = 35) of virologic failure isolates from this study showed that the RT mutations that emerged during abacavir once-daily and twice-daily therapy were K65R, L74V, Y115F, and M184V/I. The mutation M184V/I was the most commonly observed mutation in virologic failure isolates from patients receiving abacavir once daily (56%, 10/18) and twice daily (40%, 8/20).

Thirty-nine percent (7/18) of the isolates from patients who experienced virologic failure in the abacavir once-daily arm had a >2.5-fold decrease in abacavir susceptibility with a median-fold decrease of 1.3 (range 0.5 to 11) compared with 29% (5/17) of the failure isolates in the twice-daily arm with a median-fold decrease of 0.92 (range 0.7 to 13).

Cross-Resistance: Cross-resistance has been observed among nucleoside reverse transcriptase inhibitors (NRTIs). Recombinant laboratory strains of HIV-1_{HXB2} containing multiple abacavir resistance-associated mutations, namely, K65R, L74V, M184V, and Y115F, exhibited cross-resistance to didanosine, emtricitabine, lamivudine, tenofovir, and zalcitabine in vitro. The K65R mutation can confer resistance to abacavir, didanosine, emtricitabine, lamivudine, stavudine, tenofovir, and zalcitabine; the L74V mutation can confer resistance to abacavir, didanosine, and zalcitabine; and the M184V mutation can confer resistance to abacavir, didanosine, emtricitabine, lamivudine, and zalcitabine. An increasing number of thymidine analogue mutations (TAMs: M41L, D67N, K70R, L210W, T215Y/F, K219E/R/H/Q/N) is associated with a progressive reduction in abacavir susceptibility.

CLINICAL PHARMACOLOGY

Pharmacokinetics in Adults: The pharmacokinetic properties of abacavir have been studied in asymptomatic, HIV-infected adult patients after administration of a single intravenous (IV) dose of 150 mg and after single and multiple oral doses. The pharmacokinetic properties of abacavir were independent of dose over the range of 300 to 1,200 mg/day.

Absorption and Bioavailability: Abacavir was rapidly and extensively absorbed after oral administration. The geometric mean absolute bioavailability of the tablet was 83%. After oral administration of 300 mg twice daily in 20 patients, the steady-state peak serum abacavir concentration (C_{max}) was 3.0 ± 0.89 mcg/mL (mean ± SD) and $AUC_{(0-12\ hr)}$ was 6.02 ± 1.73 mcg•hr/mL. After oral administration of a single dose of 600 mg of abacavir in 20 patients, C_{max} was 4.26 ± 1.19 mcg/mL (mean ± SD) and AUC_{∞} was 11.95 ± 2.51 mcg•hr/mL. Bioavailability of abacavir tablets was assessed in the fasting and fed states. There was no significant difference in systemic exposure (AUC_{∞}) in the fed and fasting states; therefore, ZIAGEN Tablets may be administered with or without food. Systemic exposure to abacavir was comparable after administration of ZIAGEN Oral Solution and ZIAGEN Tablets. Therefore, these products may be used interchangeably.

Distribution: The apparent volume of distribution after IV administration of abacavir was 0.86 ± 0.15 L/kg, suggesting that abacavir distributes into extravascular space. In 3 subjects, the CSF $AUC_{(0-6\ hr)}$ to plasma abacavir $AUC_{(0-6\ hr)}$ ratio ranged from 27% to 33%.

Binding of abacavir to human plasma proteins is approximately 50%. Binding of abacavir to plasma proteins was independent of concentration. Total blood and plasma drug-related radioactivity concentrations are identical, demonstrating that abacavir readily distributes into erythrocytes.

Metabolism: In humans, abacavir is not significantly metabolized by cytochrome P450 enzymes. The primary routes of elimination of abacavir are metabolism by alcohol dehydrogenase (to form the 5′-carboxylic acid) and glucuronyl transferase (to form the 5′-glucuronide). The metabolites do not have antiviral activity. In vitro experiments reveal that abacavir does not inhibit human CYP3A4, CYP2D6, or CYP2C9 activity at clinically relevant concentrations.

Elimination: Elimination of abacavir was quantified in a mass balance study following administration of a 600-mg dose of ^{14}C-abacavir: 99% of the radioactivity was recovered, 1.2% was excreted in the urine as abacavir, 30% as the 5′-carboxylic acid metabolite, 36% as the 5′-glucuronide metabolite, and 15% as unidentified minor metabolites in the urine. Fecal elimination accounted for 16% of the dose.

In single-dose studies, the observed elimination half-life ($t_{1/2}$) was 1.54 ± 0.63 hours. After intravenous administration, total clearance was 0.80 ± 0.24 L/hr/kg (mean ± SD).

Special Populations: ***Adults With Impaired Renal Function:*** The pharmacokinetic properties of ZIAGEN have not been determined in patients with impaired renal function. Renal excretion of unchanged abacavir is a minor route of elimination in humans.

Adults With Impaired Hepatic Function: The pharmacokinetics of abacavir have been studied in patients with mild hepatic impairment (Child-Pugh score 5 to 6). Results showed that there was a mean increase of 89% in the abacavir AUC, and an increase of 58% in the half-life of abacavir after a single dose of 600 mg of abacavir. The AUCs of the metabolites were not modified by mild liver disease; however, the rates of formation and elimination of the metabolites were decreased. A dose of 200 mg (provided by 10 mL of ZIAGEN Oral Solution) administered twice daily is recommended for patients with mild liver disease. The safety, efficacy, and pharmacokinetics of abacavir have not been studied in patients with moderate or severe hepatic impairment, therefore ZIAGEN is contraindicated in these patients.

Pediatric Patients: The pharmacokinetics of abacavir have been studied after either single or repeat doses of ZIAGEN in 68 pediatric patients. Following multiple-dose administration of ZIAGEN 8 mg/kg twice daily, steady-state $AUC_{(0-12\ hr)}$ and C_{max} were 9.8 ± 4.56 mcg•hr/mL and 3.71 ± 1.36 mcg/mL (mean ± SD), respectively (see PRECAUTIONS: Pediatric Use).

Geriatric Patients: The pharmacokinetics of ZIAGEN have not been studied in patients over 65 years of age.

Continued on next page

Ziagen—Cont.

Gender: A population pharmacokinetic analysis in HIV-infected male (n = 304) and female (n = 67) patients showed no gender differences in abacavir AUC normalized for lean body weight.

Race: There are no significant differences between blacks and Caucasians in abacavir pharmacokinetics.

Drug Interactions: In human liver microsomes, abacavir did not inhibit cytochrome P450 isoforms (2C9, 2D6, 3A4). Based on these data, it is unlikely that clinically significant drug interactions will occur between abacavir and drugs metabolized through these pathways.

Due to the common metabolic pathways of abacavir and zidovudine via glucuronyl transferase, 15 HIV-infected patients were enrolled in a crossover study evaluating single doses of abacavir (600 mg), lamivudine (150 mg), and zidovudine (300 mg) alone or in combination. Analysis showed no clinically relevant changes in the pharmacokinetics of abacavir with the addition of lamivudine or zidovudine or the combination of lamivudine and zidovudine. Lamivudine exposure (AUC decreased 15%) and zidovudine exposure (AUC increased 10%) did not show clinically relevant changes with concurrent abacavir.

Due to their common metabolic pathways via alcohol dehydrogenase, the pharmacokinetic interaction between abacavir and ethanol was studied in 24 HIV-infected male patients. Each patient received the following treatments on separate occasions: a single 600-mg dose of abacavir, 0.7 g/kg ethanol (equivalent to 5 alcoholic drinks), and abacavir 600 mg plus 0.7 g/kg ethanol. Coadministration of ethanol and abacavir resulted in a 41% increase in abacavir AUC_∞ and a 26% increase in abacavir $t_{1/2}$. In males, abacavir had no effect on the pharmacokinetic properties of ethanol, so no clinically significant interaction is expected in men. This interaction has not been studied in females.

Methadone: In a study of 11 HIV-infected patients receiving methadone-maintenance therapy (40 mg and 90 mg daily), with 600 mg of ZIAGEN twice daily (twice the currently recommended dose), oral methadone clearance increased 22% (90% CI 6% to 42%). This alteration will not result in a methadone dose modification in the majority of patients; however, an increased methadone dose may be required in a small number of patients.

INDICATIONS AND USAGE

ZIAGEN Tablets and Oral Solution, in combination with other antiretroviral agents, are indicated for the treatment of HIV-1 infection.

Additional important information on the use of ZIAGEN for treatment of HIV-1 infection:

• ZIAGEN is one of multiple products containing abacavir. Before starting ZIAGEN, review medical history for prior exposure to any abacavir-containing product in order to avoid reintroduction in a patient with a history of hypersensitivity to abacavir.

• In one controlled study (CNA30021), more patients taking ZIAGEN 600 mg once daily had severe hypersensitivity reactions than patients taking ZIAGEN 300 mg twice daily. See WARNINGS, ADVERSE REACTIONS, and Description of Clinical Studies.

Description of Clinical Studies: ***Therapy-Naive Adults:*** CNA30024 was a multicenter, double-blind, controlled study in which 649 HIV-infected, therapy-naive adults were randomized and received either ZIAGEN (300 mg twice daily), lamivudine (150 mg twice daily), and efavirenz (600 mg once daily) or zidovudine (300 mg twice daily), lamivudine (150 mg twice daily), and efavirenz (600 mg once daily). The duration of double-blind treatment was at least 48 weeks. Study participants were: male (81%), Caucasian (51%), black (21%), and Hispanic (26%). The median age was 35 years, the median pretreatment CD4+ cell count was 264 cells/mm³, and median plasma HIV-1 RNA was 4.79 $\log_{10}$ copies/mL. The outcomes of randomized treatment are provided in Table 1.

[See table 1 above]

After 48 weeks of therapy, the median CD4+ cell count increases from baseline were 209 cells/mm³ in the group receiving ZIAGEN and 155 cells/mm³ in the zidovudine group. Through Week 48, 8 subjects (2%) in the group receiving ZIAGEN (5 CDC classification C events and 3 deaths) and 5 subjects (2%) on the zidovudine arm (3 CDC classification C events and 2 deaths) experienced clinical disease progression.

CNA3005 was a multicenter, double-blind, controlled study in which 562 HIV-infected, therapy-naive adults with a pre-entry plasma HIV-1 RNA >10,000 copies/mL were randomized to receive either ZIAGEN (300 mg twice daily) plus COMBIVIR (lamivudine 150 mg/zidovudine 300 mg twice daily), or indinavir (800 mg 3 times a day) plus COMBIVIR twice daily. Study participants were male (87%), Caucasian (73%), black (15%), and Hispanic (9%). At baseline the median age was 36 years, the median baseline CD4+ cell count was 360 cells/mm³, and median baseline plasma HIV-1 RNA was 4.8 $\log_{10}$ copies/mL. Proportions of patients with plasma HIV-1 RNA <400 copies/mL through 48 weeks of treatment are summarized in Table 2.

[See table 2 above]

Through Week 48, an overall mean increase in CD4+ cell count of about 150 cells/mm³ was observed in both treatment arms.

CNA30021 was an international, multicenter, double-blind, controlled study in which 770 HIV-infected, therapy-naive adults were randomized and received either abacavir

Table 1. Outcomes of Randomized Treatment Through Week 48 (CNA30024)

Outcome	ZIAGEN plus Lamivudine plus Efavirenz (n = 324)	Zidovudine plus Lamivudine plus Efavirenz (n = 325)
Responder*	69% (73%)	69% (71%)
Virologic failures†	6%	4%
Discontinued due to adverse reactions	14%	16%
Discontinued due to other reasons‡	10%	11%

*Patients achieved and maintained confirmed HIV-1 RNA ≤50 copies/mL (<400 copies/mL) through Week 48 (Roche® AMPLICOR Ultrasensitive HIV-1 MONITOR standard test 1.0 PCR).
† Includes viral rebound, insufficient viral response according to the investigator, and failure to achieve confirmed ≤50 copies/mL by Week 48.
‡ Includes consent withdrawn, lost to follow up, protocol violations, those with missing data, clinical progression, and other.

Table 2. Outcomes of Randomized Treatment Through Week 48 (CNA3005)

Outcome	ZIAGEN plus Lamivudine/Zidovudine (n = 282)	Indinavir plus Lamivudine/Zidovudine (n = 280)
HIV-1 RNA <400 copies/mL	46%	47%
HIV-1 RNA ≥400 copies/mL*	29%	28%
Discontinued due to adverse reactions	10%	13%
Discontinued due to other reasons†	8%	8%
Randomized but never initiated treatment	7%	5%

*Includes viral rebound and failure to achieve confirmed <400 copies/mL by Week 48 (Roche AMPLICOR HIV-1 MONITOR Test).
† Includes consent withdrawn, lost to follow up, protocol violations, those with missing data, clinical progression, and other.

Table 3. Outcomes of Randomized Treatment Through Week 48 (CNA30021)

Outcome	ZIAGEN 600 mg q.d. plus EPIVIR plus Efavirenz (n = 384)	ZIAGEN 300 mg b.i.d. plus EPIVIR plus Efavirenz (n = 386)
Responder*	64% (71%)	65% (72%)
Virologic failure†	11% (5%)	11% (5%)
Discontinued due to adverse reactions	13%	11%
Discontinued due to other reasons‡	11%	13%

*Patients achieved and maintained confirmed HIV-1 RNA <50 copies/mL (<400 copies/mL through Week 48 (Roche AMPLICOR Ultrasensitive HIV-1 MONITOR standard test version 1.0).
† Includes viral rebound, failure to achieve confirmed <50 copies/mL (<400 copies/mL) by Week 48, and insufficient viral load response.
‡ Includes consent withdrawn, lost to follow up, protocol violations, clinical progression, and other.

600 mg once daily or abacavir 300 mg twice daily, both in combination with lamivudine 300 mg once daily and efavirenz 600 mg once daily. The double-blind treatment duration was at least 48 weeks. Study participants had a mean age of 37 years, were: male (81%), Caucasian (54%), black (27%), and American Hispanic (15%). The median baseline CD4+ cell count was 262 cells/mm³ (range 21 to 918 cells/mm³) and the median baseline plasma HIV-1 RNA was 4.89 $\log_{10}$ copies/mL (range: 2.60 to 6.99 $\log_{10}$ copies/mL).

The outcomes of randomized treatment are provided in Table 3.

[See table 3 above]

After 48 weeks of therapy, the median CD4+ cell count increases from baseline were 188 cells/mm³ in the group receiving abacavir 600 mg once daily and 200 cells/mm³ in the group receiving abacavir 300 mg twice daily. Through Week 48, 6 subjects (2%) in the group receiving ZIAGEN 600 mg once daily (4 CDC classification C events and 2 deaths) and 10 subjects (3%) in the group receiving ZIAGEN 300 mg twice daily (7 CDC classification C events and 3 deaths) experienced clinical disease progression. None of the deaths were attributed to study medications.

CONTRAINDICATIONS

ZIAGEN Tablets and Oral Solution are contraindicated in patients with previously demonstrated hypersensitivity to abacavir or any other component of the products (see WARNINGS). Following a hypersensitivity reaction to abacavir, NEVER restart ZIAGEN or any other abacavir-containing product. Fatal rechallenge reactions have been associated with readministration of abacavir to patients with a prior history of a hypersensitivity reaction to abacavir (see WARNINGS and PRECAUTIONS).

ZIAGEN Tablets and Oral Solution are contraindicated in patients with moderate or severe hepatic impairment.

WARNINGS

Hypersensitivity Reaction: Serious and sometimes fatal hypersensitivity reactions have been associated with ZIAGEN and other abacavir-containing products. To minimize the risk of a life-threatening hypersensitivity reaction, permanently discontinue ZIAGEN if hypersensitivity cannot be ruled out, even when other diagnoses are possible. Important information on signs and symptoms of hypersensitivity, as well as clinical management, is presented below.

Signs and Symptoms of Hypersensitivity: Hypersensitivity to abacavir is a multi-organ clinical syndrome usually characterized by a sign or symptom in 2 or more of the following groups.

  Group 1: Fever
  Group 2: Rash

  Group 3: Gastrointestinal (including nausea, vomiting, diarrhea, or abdominal pain)
  Group 4: Constitutional (including generalized malaise, fatigue, or achiness)
  Group 5: Respiratory (including dyspnea, cough, or pharyngitis)

Hypersensitivity to abacavir following the presentation of a single sign or symptom has been reported infrequently.

Hypersensitivity to abacavir was reported in approximately 8% of 2,670 patients (n = 206) in 9 clinical trials (range: 2% to 9%) with enrollment from November 1999 to February 2002. Data on time to onset and symptoms of suspected hypersensitivity were collected on a detailed data collection module. The frequencies of symptoms are shown in Figure 1. Symptoms usually appeared within the first 6 weeks of treatment with abacavir, although the reaction may occur at any time during therapy. Median time to onset was 9 days; 89% appeared within the first 6 weeks; 95% of patients reported symptoms from 2 or more of the 5 groups listed above.

Figure 1. Hypersensitivity-Related Symptoms Reported with ≥10% Frequency in Clinical Trials (n = 206 Patients)

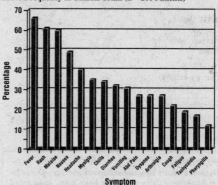

Other less common signs and symptoms of hypersensitivity include lethargy, myolysis, edema, abnormal chest x-ray findings (predominantly infiltrates, which can be localized), and paresthesia. Anaphylaxis, liver failure, renal failure, hypotension, adult respiratory distress syndrome, respiratory failure, and death have occurred in association with hypersensitivity reactions. In one study, 4 patients (11%) receiving ZIAGEN 600 mg once daily experienced hypotension with a hypersensitivity reaction compared with 0 patients receiving ZIAGEN 300 mg twice daily.

Physical findings associated with hypersensitivity to abacavir in some patients include lymphadenopathy, mucous membrane lesions (conjunctivitis and mouth ulcerations), and rash. The rash usually appears maculopapular or urticarial, but may be variable in appearance. There have been reports of erythema multiforme. Hypersensitivity reactions have occurred without rash.

Laboratory abnormalities associated with hypersensitivity to abacavir in some patients include elevated liver function tests, elevated creatine phosphokinase, elevated creatinine, and lymphopenia.

Clinical Management of Hypersensitivity: **Discontinue ZIAGEN as soon as a hypersensitivity reaction is suspected. To minimize the risk of a life-threatening hypersensitivity reaction, permanently discontinue ZIAGEN if hypersensitivity cannot be ruled out, even when other diagnoses are possible (e.g., acute onset respiratory diseases such as pneumonia, bronchitis, pharyngitis, or influenza; gastroenteritis; or reactions to other medications). Following a hypersensitivity reaction to abacavir, NEVER restart ZIAGEN or any other abacavir-containing product because more severe symptoms can occur within hours and may include life-threatening hypotension and death.**

When therapy with ZIAGEN has been discontinued for reasons other than symptoms of a hypersensitivity reaction, and if reinitiation of ZIAGEN or any other abacavir-containing product is under consideration, carefully evaluate the reason for discontinuation of ZIAGEN to ensure that the patient did not have symptoms of a hypersensitivity reaction. If hypersensitivity cannot be ruled out, DO NOT reintroduce ZIAGEN or any other abacavir-containing product. If symptoms consistent with hypersensitivity are not identified, reintroduction can be undertaken with continued monitoring for symptoms of a hypersensitivity reaction. Make patients aware that a hypersensitivity reaction can occur with reintroduction of ZIAGEN or any other abacavir-containing product and that reintroduction of ZIAGEN or any other abacavir-containing product needs to be undertaken only if medical care can be readily accessed by the patient or others.

Abacavir Hypersensitivity Reaction Registry: To facilitate reporting of hypersensitivity reactions and collection of information on each case, an Abacavir Hypersensitivity Registry has been established. **Physicians should register patients by calling 1-800-270-0425.**

Lactic Acidosis/Severe Hepatomegaly with Steatosis: Lactic acidosis and severe hepatomegaly with steatosis, including fatal cases, have been reported with the use of nucleoside analogues alone or in combination, including abacavir and other antiretrovirals. A majority of these cases have been in women. Obesity and prolonged nucleoside exposure may be risk factors. Particular caution should be exercised when administering ZIAGEN to any patient with known risk factors for liver disease; however, cases have also been reported in patients with no known risk factors. Treatment with ZIAGEN should be suspended in any patient who develops clinical or laboratory findings suggestive of lactic acidosis or pronounced hepatotoxicity (which may include hepatomegaly and steatosis even in the absence of marked transaminase elevations).

PRECAUTIONS

General: Abacavir should always be used in combination with other antiretroviral agents. Abacavir should not be added as a single agent when antiretroviral regimens are changed due to loss of virologic response.

Therapy-Experienced Patients: In clinical trials, patients with prolonged prior NRTI exposure or who had HIV-1 isolates that contained multiple mutations conferring resistance to NRTIs had limited response to abacavir. The potential for cross-resistance between abacavir and other NRTIs should be considered when choosing new therapeutic regimens in therapy-experienced patients (see MICROBIOLOGY: Cross-Resistance).

Fat Redistribution: Redistribution/accumulation of body fat including central obesity, dorsocervical fat enlargement (buffalo hump), peripheral wasting, facial wasting, breast enlargement, and "cushingoid appearance" have been observed in patients receiving antiretroviral therapy. The mechanism and long-term consequences of these events are currently unknown. A causal relationship has not been established.

Information for Patients: ***Hypersensitivity Reaction:*** Inform patients:

- **that a Medication Guide and Warning Card summarizing the symptoms of the abacavir hypersensitivity reaction and other product information will be dispensed by the pharmacist with each new prescription and refill of ZIAGEN, and encourage the patient to read the Medication Guide and Warning Card every time to obtain any new information that may be present about ZIAGEN. (The complete text of the Medication Guide is reprinted at the end of this document.)**
- **to carry the Warning Card with them.**
- how to identify a hypersensitivity reaction (see WARNINGS and MEDICATION GUIDE).
- that if they develop symptoms consistent with a hypersensitivity reaction to discontinue treatment with ZIAGEN and seek medical evaluation immediately.
- that a hypersensitivity reaction can worsen and lead to hospitalization or death if ZIAGEN is not immediately discontinued.
- that in one study, more severe hypersensitivity reactions were seen when ZIAGEN was dosed 600 mg once daily.

Table 4. Treatment-Emergent (All Causality) Adverse Reactions of at Least Moderate Intensity (Grades 2-4, ≥5% Frequency) in Therapy-Naive Adults (CNA30024*) Through 48 Weeks of Treatment

Adverse Reaction	ZIAGEN plus Lamivudine plus Efavirenz (n = 324)	Zidovudine plus Lamivudine plus Efavirenz (n = 325)
Dreams/sleep disorders	10%	10%
Drug hypersensitivity	9%	<1%†
Headaches/migraine	7%	11%
Nausea	7%	11%
Fatigue/malaise	7%	10%
Diarrhea	7%	6%
Rashes	6%	12%
Abdominal pain/gastritis/ gastrointestinal signs and symptoms	6%	8%
Depressive disorders	6%	6%
Dizziness	6%	6%
Musculoskeletal pain	6%	5%
Bronchitis	4%	5%
Vomiting	2%	9%

*This study used double-blind ascertainment of suspected hypersensitivity reactions. During the blinded portion of the study, suspected hypersensitivity to abacavir was reported by investigators in 9% of 324 patients in the abacavir group and 3% of 325 patients in the zidovudine group.

† Ten (3%) cases of suspected drug hypersensitivity were reclassified as not being due to abacavir following unblinding.

- **to not restart ZIAGEN or any other abacavir-containing product following a hypersensitivity reaction because more severe symptoms can occur within hours and may include life-threatening hypotension and death.**
- that a hypersensitivity reaction is usually reversible if it is detected promptly and ZIAGEN is stopped right away.
- that if they have interrupted ZIAGEN for reasons other than symptoms of hypersensitivity (for example, those who have an interruption in drug supply), a serious or fatal hypersensitivity reaction may occur with reintroduction of abacavir.
- to not restart ZIAGEN or any other abacavir-containing product without medical consultation and that restarting abacavir needs to be undertaken only if medical care can be readily accessed by the patient or others.

General: Inform patients that some HIV medicines, including ZIAGEN, can cause a rare, but serious condition called lactic acidosis with liver enlargement (hepatomegaly).

ZIAGEN is not a cure for HIV infection and patients may continue to experience illnesses associated with HIV infection, including opportunistic infections. Patients should remain under the care of a physician when using ZIAGEN. Advise patients that the use of ZIAGEN has not been shown to reduce the risk of transmission of HIV to others through sexual contact or blood contamination.

Inform patients that redistribution or accumulation of body fat may occur in patients receiving antiretroviral therapy and that the cause and long-term health effects of these conditions are not known at this time.

ZIAGEN Tablets and Oral Solution are for oral ingestion only.

Patients should be advised of the importance of taking ZIAGEN exactly as it is prescribed.

Drug Interactions: Pharmacokinetic properties of abacavir were not altered by the addition of either lamivudine or zidovudine or the combination of lamivudine and zidovudine. No clinically significant changes to lamivudine or zidovudine pharmacokinetics were observed following concomitant administration of abacavir.

Abacavir has no effect on the pharmacokinetic properties of ethanol. Ethanol decreases the elimination of abacavir causing an increase in overall exposure (see CLINICAL PHARMACOLOGY: Drug Interactions).

The addition of methadone has no clinically significant effect on the pharmacokinetic properties of abacavir. In a study of 11 HIV-infected patients receiving methadone-maintenance therapy (40 mg and 90 mg daily) with 600 mg of ZIAGEN twice daily (twice the currently recommended dose), oral methadone clearance increased 22% (90% CI 6% to 42%). This alteration will not result in a methadone dose modification in the majority of patients; however, an increased methadone dose may be required in a small number of patients.

Carcinogenesis, Mutagenesis, and Impairment of Fertility: Abacavir was administered orally at 3 dosage levels to separate groups of mice and rats in 2-year carcinogenicity studies. Results showed an increase in the incidence of malignant and non-malignant tumors. Malignant tumors occurred in the preputial gland of males and the clitoral gland of females of both species, and in the liver of female rats. In addition, non-malignant tumors also occurred in the liver and thyroid gland of female rats. These observations were made at systemic exposures in the range of 6 to 32 times the human exposure at the recommended dose. It is not known how predictive the results of rodent carcinogenicity studies may be for humans.

Abacavir induced chromosomal aberrations both in the presence and absence of metabolic activation in an in vitro cytogenetic study in human lymphocytes. Abacavir was mutagenic in the absence of metabolic activation, although it was not mutagenic in the presence of metabolic activation in an L5178Y mouse lymphoma assay. Abacavir was clastogenic in males and not clastogenic in females in an in vivo mouse bone marrow micronucleus assay.

Abacavir was not mutagenic in bacterial mutagenicity assays in the presence and absence of metabolic activation.

Abacavir had no adverse effects on the mating performance or fertility of male and female rats at a dose approximately 8 times the human exposure at the recommended dose based on body surface area comparisons.

Pregnancy: Pregnancy Category C. Studies in pregnant rats showed that abacavir is transferred to the fetus through the placenta. Fetal malformations (increased incidences of fetal anasarca and skeletal malformations) and developmental toxicity (depressed fetal body weight and reduced crown-rump length) were observed in rats at a dose which produced 35 times the human exposure, based on AUC. Embryonic and fetal toxicities (increased resorptions, decreased fetal body weights) and toxicities to the offspring (increased incidence of stillbirth and lower body weights) occurred at half of the above-mentioned dose in separate fertility studies conducted in rats. In the rabbit, no developmental toxicity and no increases in fetal malformations occurred at doses that produced 8.5 times the human exposure at the recommended dose based on AUC.

There are no adequate and well-controlled studies in pregnant women. ZIAGEN should be used during pregnancy only if the potential benefits outweigh the risk.

Antiretroviral Pregnancy Registry: To monitor maternal-fetal outcomes of pregnant women exposed to ZIAGEN, an Antiretroviral Pregnancy Registry has been established. Physicians are encouraged to register patients by calling 1-800-258-4263.

Nursing Mothers: The Centers for Disease Control and Prevention recommend that HIV-infected mothers not breastfeed their infants to avoid risking postnatal transmission of HIV infection.

Although it is not known if abacavir is excreted in human milk, abacavir is secreted into the milk of lactating rats. Because of both the potential for HIV transmission and the potential for serious adverse reactions in nursing infants, **mothers should be instructed not to breastfeed if they are receiving ZIAGEN.**

Pediatric Use: The safety and effectiveness of ZIAGEN have been established in pediatric patients 3 months to 13 years of age. Use of ZIAGEN in these age groups is supported by pharmacokinetic studies and evidence from adequate and well-controlled studies of ZIAGEN in adults and pediatric patients (see CLINICAL PHARMACOLOGY: Pharmacokinetics: Special Populations: Pediatric Patients, WARNINGS, ADVERSE REACTIONS, and DOSAGE AND ADMINISTRATION).

CNA3006 was a randomized, double-blind study comparing ZIAGEN 8 mg/kg twice daily plus lamivudine 4 mg/kg twice daily plus zidovudine 180 mg/m^2 twice daily versus lamivudine 4 mg/kg twice daily plus zidovudine 180 mg/m^2 twice daily. Two hundred and five therapy-experienced pediatric patients were enrolled: female (56%), Caucasian (17%), black (50%), Hispanic (30%), median age of 5.4 years, baseline CD4+ cell percent >15% (median = 27%), and median baseline plasma HIV-1 RNA of 4.6 log_{10} copies/mL. Eighty percent and 55% of patients had prior therapy with zidovudine and lamivudine, respectively, most often in combination. The median duration of prior nucleoside analogue therapy was 2 years. At 16 weeks the proportion of patients responding based on plasma HIV-1 RNA ≤400 copies/mL was significantly higher in patients receiving ZIAGEN plus lamivudine plus zidovudine compared with patients receiving lamivudine plus zidovudine, 13% versus 2%, respectively. Median plasma HIV-1 RNA changes from baseline were -0.53 log_{10} copies/mL in the group receiving ZIAGEN plus lamivudine plus zidovudine compared with -0.21 log_{10} copies/mL in the group receiving lamivudine plus zidovudine. Median CD4+ cell count increases from baseline were 69 $cells/mm^3$ in the group receiving ZIAGEN plus lamivudine plus zidovudine and 9 $cells/mm^3$ in the group receiving lamivudine plus zidovudine.

Geriatric Use: Clinical studies of ZIAGEN did not include sufficient numbers of patients aged 65 and over to determine whether they respond differently from younger patients. In general, dose selection for an elderly patient

Continued on next page

Ziagen—Cont.

should be cautious, reflecting the greater frequency of decreased hepatic, renal, or cardiac function, and of concomitant disease or other drug therapy.

ADVERSE REACTIONS

Hypersensitivity Reaction: Serious and sometimes fatal hypersensitivity reactions have been associated with ZIAGEN (abacavir sulfate). In one study, once-daily dosing of ZIAGEN was associated with more severe hypersensitivity reactions (see WARNINGS and PRECAUTIONS: Information for Patients).

Therapy-Naive Adults: Treatment-emergent clinical adverse reactions (rated by the investigator as moderate or severe) with a ≥5% frequency during therapy with ZIAGEN 300 mg twice daily, lamivudine 150 mg twice daily, and efavirenz 600 mg daily compared with zidovudine 300 mg twice daily, lamivudine 150 mg twice daily, and efavirenz 600 mg daily from CNA30024 are listed in Table 4.
[See table 4 at top of previous page]

Treatment-emergent clinical adverse reactions (rated by the investigator as moderate or severe) with a ≥5% frequency during therapy with ZIAGEN 300 mg twice daily, lamivudine 150 mg twice daily, and zidovudine 300 mg twice daily compared with indinavir 800 mg 3 times daily, lamivudine 150 mg twice daily, and zidovudine 300 mg twice daily from CNA3005 are listed in Table 5.
[See table 5 at right]

Five patients receiving ZIAGEN in Study CNA3005 experienced worsening of pre-existing depression compared to none in the indinavir arm. The background rates of pre-existing depression were similar in the 2 treatment arms.

ZIAGEN Once Daily versus ZIAGEN Twice Daily (Study CNA30021): Treatment-emergent clinical adverse reactions (rated by the investigator as at least moderate) with a ≥5% frequency during therapy with ZIAGEN 600 mg once daily or ZIAGEN 300 mg twice daily both in combination with lamivudine 300 mg once daily and efavirenz 600 mg once daily from Study CNA30021 were similar. (For hypersensitivity reactions, patients receiving ZIAGEN once daily showed a rate of 9% in comparison to a rate of 7% for patients receiving ZIAGEN twice daily.) However, patients receiving ZIAGEN 600 mg once daily, experienced a significantly higher incidence of severe drug hypersensitivity reactions and severe diarrhea compared to patients who received ZIAGEN 300 mg twice daily. Five percent (5%) of patients receiving ZIAGEN 600 mg once daily had severe drug hypersensitivity reactions compared to 2% of patients receiving ZIAGEN 300 mg twice daily. Two percent (2%) of patients receiving ZIAGEN 600 mg once daily had severe diarrhea while none of the patients receiving ZIAGEN 300 mg twice daily had this event.

Therapy-Experienced Pediatric Patients: Treatment-emergent clinical adverse reactions (rated by the investigator as moderate or severe) with a ≥5% frequency during therapy with ZIAGEN 8 mg/kg twice daily, lamivudine 4 mg/kg twice daily, and zidovudine 180 mg/m^2 twice daily compared with lamivudine 4 mg/kg twice daily and zidovudine 180 mg/m^2 twice daily from CNA3006 are listed in Table 6.
[See table 6 above]

Laboratory Abnormalities: Laboratory abnormalities (Grades 3-4) in therapy-naive adults during therapy with ZIAGEN 300 mg twice daily, lamivudine 150 mg twice daily, and efavirenz 600 mg daily compared with zidovudine 300 mg twice daily, lamivudine 150 mg twice daily, and efavirenz 600 mg daily from CNA30024 are listed in Table 7.
[See table 7 above]

In another study of therapy-naive adults (CNA3005), hyperglycemia and disorders of lipid metabolism occurred with similar frequency in patients treated with ZIAGEN and patients treated with indinavir.

In a study of therapy-experienced pediatric patients (CNA3006), laboratory abnormalities (anemia, neutropenia, liver function test abnormalities, and CPK elevations) were observed with similar frequencies as in a study of therapy-naive adults (CNA30024). Mild elevations of blood glucose were more frequent in pediatric patients receiving ZIAGEN (CNA3006) as compared to adult patients (CNA30024).

The frequencies of treatment-emergent laboratory abnormalities were comparable between treatment groups in Study CNA30021.

Other Adverse Events: In addition to adverse reactions in Tables 4, 5, 6, and 7, other adverse events observed in the expanded access program were pancreatitis and increased GGT.

Observed During Clinical Practice: In addition to adverse reactions reported from clinical trials, the following events have been identified during use of abacavir in clinical practice. Because they are reported voluntarily from a population of unknown size, estimates of frequency cannot be made. These events have been chosen for inclusion due to either their seriousness, frequency of reporting, potential causal connection to abacavir, or a combination of these factors.

Body as a Whole: Redistribution/accumulation of body fat (see PRECAUTIONS: Fat Redistribution).

Hepatic: Lactic acidosis and hepatic steatosis (see WARNINGS and PRECAUTIONS).

Skin: Suspected Stevens-Johnson syndrome (SJS) and toxic epidermal necrolysis (TEN) have been reported in patients receiving abacavir primarily in combination with medications known to be associated with SJS and TEN, respectively. Because of the overlap of clinical signs and symptoms

between hypersensitivity to abacavir and SJS and TEN, and the possibility of multiple drug sensitivities in some patients, abacavir should be discontinued and not restarted in such cases.

There have also been reports of erythema multiforme with abacavir use.

OVERDOSAGE

There is no known antidote for ZIAGEN. It is not known whether abacavir can be removed by peritoneal dialysis or hemodialysis.

DOSAGE AND ADMINISTRATION

A Medication Guide and Warning Card that provide information about recognition of hypersensitivity reactions should be dispensed with each new prescription and refill. To facilitate reporting of hypersensitivity reactions and collection of information on each case, an Abacavir Hypersensitivity Registry has been established. **Physicians should register patients by calling 1-800-270-0425.**

ZIAGEN may be taken with or without food.

Adults: The recommended oral dose of ZIAGEN for adults is 600 mg daily, administered as either 300 mg twice daily or 600 mg once daily, in combination with other antiretroviral agents.

Adolescents and Pediatric Patients: The recommended oral dose of ZIAGEN for adolescents and pediatric patients 3 months to up to 16 years of age is 8 mg/kg twice daily (up to a maximum of 300 mg twice daily) in combination with other antiretroviral agents.

Dose Adjustment in Hepatic Impairment: The recommended dose of ZIAGEN in patients with mild hepatic impairment (Child-Pugh score 5 to 6) is 200 mg twice daily. To enable dose reduction, ZIAGEN Oral Solution (10 mL twice daily) should be used for the treatment of these patients. The safety, efficacy, and pharmacokinetic properties of abacavir have not been established in patients with moderate to severe hepatic impairment, therefore ZIAGEN is contraindicated in these patients.

HOW SUPPLIED

ZIAGEN is available as tablets and oral solution.

ZIAGEN Tablets: Each tablet contains abacavir sulfate equivalent to 300 mg abacavir. The tablets are yellow, biconvex, capsule-shaped, film-coated, and imprinted with "GX 623" on one side with no marking on the reverse side. They are packaged as follows:
Bottles of 60 tablets (NDC 0173-0661-01).
Unit dose blister packs of 60 tablets (NDC 0173-0661-00).
Each pack contains 6 blister cards of 10 tablets each.
Store at controlled room temperature of 20° to 25°C (68° to 77°F) (see USP).

ZIAGEN Oral Solution: It is a clear to opalescent, yellowish, strawberry-banana-flavored liquid. Each mL of the solution contains abacavir sulfate equivalent to 20 mg of abacavir. It is packaged in plastic bottles as follows:
Bottles of 240 mL (NDC 0173-0664-00) with child-resistant closure. This product does not require reconstitution.
Store at controlled room temperature of 20° to 25°C (68° to 77°F) (see USP). DO NOT FREEZE. May be refrigerated.

ANIMAL TOXICOLOGY

Myocardial degeneration was found in mice and rats following administration of abacavir for 2 years. The systemic exposures were equivalent to 7 to 24 times the expected systemic exposure in humans. The clinical relevance of this finding has not been determined.

GlaxoSmithKline, Research Triangle Park, NC 27709
©2004, GlaxoSmithKline. All rights reserved.
August 2004/RL-2115

MEDICATION GUIDE

ZIAGEN® (ZY-uh-jen) Tablets
ZIAGEN® Oral Solution
Generic name: abacavir (uh-BACK-ah-veer) sulfate tablets and oral solution

Read the Medication Guide that comes with Ziagen before you start taking it and each time you get a refill because there may be new information. This information does not take the place of talking to your doctor about your medical condition or your treatment. Be sure to carry your Ziagen Warning Card with you at all times.

What is the most important information I should know about Ziagen?

- **Serious Allergic Reaction to Abacavir.** Ziagen contains abacavir (also contained in Epzicom™ and Trizivir®). Patients taking Ziagen may have a serious allergic reaction (hypersensitivity reaction) that can cause death.

  If you get a symptom from 2 or more of the following groups while taking Ziagen, stop taking Ziagen and call your doctor right away.

	Symptom(s)
Group 1	Fever
Group 2	Rash
Group 3	Nausea, vomiting, diarrhea, abdominal (stomach area) pain

Table 5. Treatment-Emergent (All Causality) Adverse Reactions of at Least Moderate Intensity (Grades 2-4, ≥5% Frequency) in Therapy-Naive Adults (CNA3005) Through 48 Weeks of Treatment

Adverse Reaction	ZIAGEN plus Lamivudine/Zidovudine (n = 262)	Indinavir plus Lamivudine/Zidovudine (n = 264)
Nausea	19%	17%
Headache	13%	9%
Malaise and fatigue	12%	12%
Nausea and vomiting	10%	10%
Diarrhea	7%	5%
Fever and/or chills	6%	3%
Depressive disorders	6%	4%
Musculoskeletal pain	5%	7%
Skin rashes	5%	4%
Ear/nose/throat infections	5%	4%
Viral respiratory infections	5%	5%
Anxiety	5%	3%
Renal sign/symptoms	<1%	5%
Pain (non-site-specific)	<1%	5%

Table 6. Treatment-Emergent (All Causality) Adverse Reactions of at Least Moderate Intensity (Grades 2-4, ≥5% Frequency) in Therapy-Experienced Pediatric Patients (CNA3006) Through 16 Weeks of Treatment

Adverse Reaction	ZIAGEN plus Lamivudine plus Zidovudine (n = 102)	Lamivudine plus Zidovudine (n = 103)
Fever and/or chills	9%	7%
Nausea and vomiting	9%	2%
Skin rashes	7%	1%
Ear/nose/throat infections	5%	1%
Pneumonia	4%	5%
Headache	1%	5%

Table 7. Laboratory Abnormalities (Grades 3-4) in Therapy-Naive Adults (CNA30024) Through 48 Weeks of Treatment

Grade 3/4 Laboratory Abnormalities	ZIAGEN plus Lamivudine plus Efavirenz (n = 324)	Zidovudine plus Lamivudine plus Efavirenz (n = 325)
Elevated CPK (>4 X ULN)	8%	8%
Elevated ALT (>5 X ULN)	6%	6%
Elevated AST (>5 X ULN)	6%	5%
Hypertriglyceridemia (>750 mg/dL)	6%	5%
Hyperamylasemia (>2 X ULN)	4%	5%
Neutropenia (ANC <750/mm^3)	2%	4%
Anemia (Hgb ≤6.9 gm/dL)	<1%	2%
Thrombocytopenia (Plt <50,000/mm^3)	1%	<1%
Leukopenia (WBC ≤1,500/mm^3)	<1%	2%

Group 4	Generally ill feeling, extreme tiredness, or achiness
Group 5	Shortness of breath, cough, sore throat

A list of these symptoms is on the Warning Card your pharmacist gives you. Carry this Warning Card with you.

If you stop Ziagen because of an allergic reaction, NEVER take Ziagen (abacavir sulfate) or any other abacavir-containing medicine (Epzicom and Trizivir) again. If you take Ziagen or any other abacavir-containing medicine again after you have had an allergic reaction, **WITHIN HOURS** you may get **life-threatening symptoms** that may include **very low blood pressure** or **death.**

If you stop Ziagen for any other reason, even for a few days and you are not allergic to Ziagen, talk with your doctor before taking it again. Taking Ziagen again can cause a serious allergic or life-threatening reaction, even if you never had an allergic reaction to it before. If your doctor tells you that you can take Ziagen again, start taking it when you are around medical help or people who can call a doctor if you need one.

• **Lactic Acidosis.** Some HIV medicines, including Ziagen, can cause a rare but serious condition called **lactic acidosis with liver enlargement (hepatomegaly).** Nausea and tiredness that don't get better may be symptoms of lactic acidosis. In some cases this condition can cause death. Women, overweight people, and people who have taken HIV medicines like Ziagen for a long time have a higher chance of getting lactic acidosis and liver enlargement. Lactic acidosis is a medical emergency and must be treated in the hospital.

Ziagen can have other serious side effects. Be sure to read the section below entitled "What are the possible side effects of Ziagen?"

What is Ziagen?
Ziagen is a prescription medicine used to treat HIV infection. Ziagen is taken by mouth as a tablet or a strawberry-banana-flavored liquid. Ziagen is a medicine called a nucleoside analogue reverse transcriptase inhibitor (NRTI). Ziagen is always used with other anti-HIV medicines. When used in combination with these other medicines, Ziagen helps lower the amount of HIV found in your blood. This helps to keep your immune system as healthy as possible so that it can help fight infection.

Different combinations of medicines are used to treat HIV infection. You and your doctor should discuss which combination of medicines is best for you.

• **Ziagen does not cure HIV infection or AIDS.** We do not know if Ziagen will help you live longer or have fewer of the medical problems that people get with HIV or AIDS. It is very important that you see your doctor regularly while you are taking Ziagen.

• **Ziagen does not lower the risk of passing HIV to other people through sexual contact, sharing needles, or being exposed to your blood.** For your health and the health of others, it is important to always practice safe sex by using a latex or polyurethane condom or other barrier method to lower the chance of sexual contact with semen, vaginal secretions, or blood. Never use or share dirty needles.

Ziagen has not been studied in children under 3 months of age or in adults over 65 years of age.

Who should not take Ziagen?
Do not take Ziagen if you:
• **have ever had a serious allergic reaction (a hypersensitivity reaction) to Ziagen or any other medicine that has abacavir as one of its ingredients (Epzicom and Trizivir).** See the end of this Medication Guide for a complete list of ingredients in Ziagen. If you have had such a reaction, return all of your unused Ziagen to your doctor or pharmacist.
• **have a liver that does not function properly.**

Before starting Ziagen, tell your doctor about all your medical conditions, including if you:
• **are pregnant or planning to become pregnant.** We do not know if Ziagen will harm your unborn child. You and your doctor will need to decide if Ziagen is right for you. If you use Ziagen while you are pregnant, talk to your doctor about how you can be on the Antiviral Pregnancy Registry for Ziagen.
• **are breastfeeding.** We do not know if Ziagen can be passed to your baby in your breast milk and whether it could harm your baby. Also, mothers with HIV should not breastfeed because HIV can be passed to the baby in the breast milk.

Tell your doctor about all the medicines you take, including prescription and nonprescription medicines, vitamins, and herbal supplements. Especially tell your doctor if you take:
• **methadone**
• **Epzicom (abacavir sulfate and lamivudine) and Trizivir (abacavir sulfate, lamivudine, and zidovudine).**

How should I take Ziagen?
• **Take Ziagen by mouth exactly as your doctor prescribes it.** Your doctor will tell you the right dose to take. The usual doses are 1 tablet twice a day or 2 tablets once a day. Do not skip doses.
• **You can take Ziagen with or without food.**
• **If you miss a dose of Ziagen, take the missed dose right away. Then, take the next dose at the usual time.**
• **Do not let your Ziagen run out.**
• **Starting Ziagen again can cause a serious allergic or life-threatening reaction, even if you never had an al-**

lergic reaction to it before. If you run out of Ziagen even for a few days, you must ask your doctor if you can start Ziagen again. If your doctor tells you that you can take Ziagen again, start taking it when you are around medical help or people who can call a doctor if you need one.
• If you stop your anti-HIV drugs, even for a short time, the amount of virus in your blood may increase and the virus may become harder to treat.
• **If you take too much Ziagen, call your doctor or poison control center right away.**

What should I avoid while taking Ziagen?
• Do not take Epzicom (**abacavir sulfate and lamivudine**) or Trizivir (**abacavir sulfate, lamivudine, and zidovudine**) while taking Ziagen. Some of these medicines are already in Ziagen.

Avoid doing things that can spread HIV infection, as Ziagen does not stop you from passing the HIV infection to others.
• **Do not share needles or other injection equipment.**
• **Do not share personal items that can have blood or body fluids on them, like toothbrushes and razor blades.**
• **Do not have any kind of sex without protection.** Always practice safe sex by using a latex or polyurethane condom or other barrier method to lower the chance of sexual contact with semen, vaginal secretions, or blood.
• **Do not breastfeed.** We do not know if Ziagen can be passed to your baby in your breast milk and whether it could harm your baby. Also, mothers with HIV should not breastfeed because HIV can be passed to the baby in the breast milk.

What are the possible side effects of Ziagen?
Ziagen can cause the following serious side effects:
• **Serious allergic reaction that can cause death.** (See "What is the most important information I should know about Ziagen?" at the beginning of this Medication Guide.)
• **Lactic acidosis with liver enlargement (hepatomegaly) that can cause death.** (See "What is the most important information I should know about Ziagen?" at the beginning of this Medication Guide.)
• **Changes in body fat.** These changes have happened in patients taking antiretroviral medicines like Ziagen. The changes may include an increased amount of fat in the upper back and neck ("buffalo hump"), breast, and around the back, chest, and stomach area. Loss of fat from the legs, arms, and face may also happen. The cause and long-term health effects of these conditions are not known.

The most common side effects of Ziagen include nausea, vomiting, tiredness, headache, diarrhea, trouble sleeping, fever and chills, and loss of appetite. Most of these side effects did not cause people to stop taking Ziagen.

This list of side effects is not complete. Ask your doctor or pharmacist for more information.

How should I store Ziagen?
• Store Ziagen at room temperature, between 68° to 77°F (20° to 25°C). Do not freeze Ziagen.
• Return your unused Ziagen to your doctor or pharmacist for proper disposal.
• **Keep Ziagen and all medicines out of the reach of children.**

General information for safe and effective use of Ziagen
Medicines are sometimes prescribed for conditions that are not mentioned in Medication Guides.

Do not use Ziagen for a condition for which it was not prescribed. Do not give Ziagen to other people, even if they have the same symptoms that you have. It may harm them. This Medication Guide summarizes the most important information about Ziagen. If you would like more information, talk with your doctor. You can ask your doctor or pharmacist for the information that is written for healthcare professionals or call 1-888-825-5249.

What are the ingredients in Ziagen?
Tablets: Each tablet contains abacavir sulfate equivalent to 300 mg of abacavir as active ingredient and the following inactive ingredients: colloidal silicon dioxide, magnesium stearate, microcrystalline cellulose, and sodium starch glycolate. The film-coating is made of hypromellose, polysorbate 80, synthetic yellow iron oxide, titanium dioxide, and triacetin.
Oral Solution: Each milliliter (1 mL) of Ziagen Oral Solution contains abacavir sulfate equivalent to 20 mg of abacavir (i.e., 20 mg/mL) as active ingredient and the following inactive ingredients: artificial strawberry and banana flavors, citric acid (anhydrous), methylparaben and propylparaben (added as preservatives), propylene glycol, saccharin sodium, sodium citrate (dihydrate), sorbitol solution, and water.

GlaxoSmithKline, Research Triangle Park, NC 27709
©2004, GlaxoSmithKline. All rights reserved.

August 2004/MG-028
This Medication Guide has been approved by the US Food and Drug Administration.

ZYBAN®   ℞
[zī' ban]
(bupropion hydrochloride)
Sustained-Release Tablets

Prescribing information for this product, which appears on pages 1691–1696 of the 2005 PDR, has been revised as follows. Please write "See Supplement A" next to the product heading.

The following boxed warning has been added to the beginning of the package insert.

Suicidality in Children and Adolescents
Although ZYBAN is not indicated for treatment of depression, it contains the same active ingredient as the antidepressant medications WELLBUTRIN®, WELLBUTRIN SR®, and WELLBUTRIN XL®. Antidepressants increased the risk of suicidal thinking and behavior (suicidality) in short-term studies in children and adolescents with Major Depressive Disorder (MDD) and other psychiatric disorders. Anyone considering the use of ZYBAN or any other antidepressant in a child or adolescent must balance this risk with the clinical need. Patients who are started on therapy should be observed closely for clinical worsening, suicidality, or unusual changes in behavior. Families and caregivers should be advised of the need for close observation and communication with the prescriber. ZYBAN is not approved for use in pediatric patients. (See WARNINGS and PRECAUTIONS: Pediatric Use.)
Pooled analyses of short-term (4 to 16 weeks) placebo-controlled trials of 9 antidepressant drugs (SSRIs and others) in children and adolescents with major depressive disorder (MDD), obsessive compulsive disorder (OCD), or other psychiatric disorders (a total of 24 trials involving over 4,400 patients) have revealed a greater risk of adverse events representing suicidal thinking or behavior (suicidality) during the first few months of treatment in those receiving antidepressants. The average risk of such events in patients receiving antidepressants was 4%, twice the placebo risk of 2%. No suicides occurred in these trials.

The WARNINGS section has been revised as follows.
Clinical Worsening and Suicide Risk: Patients with major depressive disorder (MDD), both adult and pediatric, may experience worsening of their depression and/or the emergence of suicidal ideation and behavior (suicidality) or unusual changes in behavior, whether or not they are taking antidepressant medications, and this risk may persist until significant remission occurs. There has been a long-standing concern that antidepressants may have a role in inducing worsening of depression and the emergence of suicidality in certain patients. Antidepressants increased the risk of suicidal thinking and behavior (suicidality) in short-term studies in children and adolescents with Major Depressive Disorder (MDD) and other psychiatric disorders.

Pooled analyses of short-term placebo-controlled trials of 9 antidepressant drugs (SSRIs and others) in children and adolescents with MDD, OCD, or other psychiatric disorders (a total of 24 trials involving over 4,400 patients) have revealed a greater risk of adverse events representing suicidal behavior or thinking (suicidality) during the first few months of treatment in those receiving antidepressants. The average risk of such events in patients receiving antidepressants was 4%, twice the placebo risk of 2%. There was considerable variation in risk among drugs, but a tendency toward an increase for almost all drugs studied. The risk of suicidality was most consistently observed in the MDD trials, but there were signals of risk arising from some trials in other psychiatric indications (obsessive compulsive disorder and social anxiety disorder) as well. **No suicides occurred in any of these trials.** It is unknown whether the suicidality risk in pediatric patients extends to longer-term use, i.e., beyond several months. It is also unknown whether the suicidality risk extends to adults.

All pediatric patients being treated with antidepressants for any indication should be observed closely for clinical worsening, suicidality, and unusual changes in behavior, especially during the initial few months of a course of drug therapy, or at times of dose changes, either increases or decreases. Such observation would generally include at least weekly face-to-face contact with patients or their family members or caregivers during the first 4 weeks of treatment, then every other week visits for the next 4 weeks, then at 12 weeks, and as clinically indicated beyond 12 weeks. Additional contact by telephone may be appropriate between face-to-face visits.

Adults with MDD or co-morbid depression in the setting of other psychiatric illness being treated with antidepressants should be observed similarly for clinical worsening and suicidality, especially during the initial few months of a course of drug therapy, or at times of dose changes, either increases or decreases.

The following symptoms, anxiety, agitation, panic attacks, insomnia, irritability, hostility, aggressiveness, impulsivity, akathisia (psychomotor restlessness), hypomania, and mania, have been reported in adult and pediatric patients being treated with antidepressants for major depressive disorder as well as for other indications, both psychiatric and nonpsychiatric. Although a causal link between the emergence of such symptoms and either the worsening of depression and/or the emergence of suicidal impulses has not been established, there is concern that such symptoms may represent precursors to emerging suicidality.

Consideration should be given to changing the therapeutic regimen, including possibly discontinuing the medication, in patients whose depression is persistently worse, or who are experiencing emergent suicidality or symptoms that might be precursors to worsening depression or suicidality, especially if these symptoms are severe, abrupt in onset, or were not part of the patient's presenting symptoms.

Continued on next page

Zyban—Cont.

Families and caregivers of pediatric patients being treated with antidepressants for major depressive disorder or other indications, both psychiatric and nonpsychiatric, should be alerted about the need to monitor patients for the emergence of agitation, irritability, unusual changes in behavior, and the other symptoms described above, as well as the emergence of suicidality, and to report such symptoms immediately to health care providers. Such monitoring should include daily observation by families and caregivers. Prescriptions for ZYBAN should be written for the smallest quantity of tablets consistent with good patient management, in order to reduce the risk of overdose. Families and caregivers of adults being treated for depression should be similarly advised.

Screening Patients for Bipolar Disorder: A major depressive episode may be the initial presentation of bipolar disorder. It is generally believed (though not established in controlled trials) that treating such an episode with an antidepressant alone may increase the likelihood of precipitation of a mixed/manic episode in patients at risk for bipolar disorder. Whether any of the symptoms described above represent such a conversion is unknown. However, prior to initiating treatment with an antidepressant, patients with depressive symptoms should be adequately screened to determine if they are at risk for bipolar disorder; such screening should include a detailed psychiatric history, including a family history of suicide, bipolar disorder, and depression. It should be noted that ZYBAN is not approved for use in treating bipolar depression.

Patients should be made aware that ZYBAN contains the same active ingredient found in WELLBUTRIN, WELLBUTRIN SR, and WELLBUTRIN XL used to treat depression, and that ZYBAN should not be used in combination with WELLBUTRIN, WELLBUTRIN SR, WELLBUTRIN XL, or any other medications that contain bupropion.

Because the use of bupropion is associated with a dose-dependent risk of seizures, *clinicians should not prescribe doses over 300 mg/day for smoking cessation.* The risk of seizures is also related to patient factors, clinical situation, and concurrent medications, which must be considered in selection of patients for therapy with ZYBAN. ZYBAN should be discontinued and not restarted in patients who experience a seizure while on treatment.

- **Dose:** *For smoking cessation, doses above 300 mg/day should not be used.* The seizure rate associated with doses of sustained-release bupropion up to 300 mg/day is approximately 0.1% (1/1,000). This incidence was prospectively determined during an 8-week treatment exposure in approximately 3,100 depressed patients. Data for the immediate-release formulation of bupropion revealed a seizure incidence of approximately 0.4% (4/1,000) in depressed patients treated at doses in a range of 300 to 450 mg/day. In addition, the estimated seizure incidence increases almost tenfold between 450 and 600 mg/day.
- **Patient factors:** Predisposing factors that may increase the risk of seizure with bupropion use include history of head trauma or prior seizure, central nervous system (CNS) tumor, the presence of severe hepatic cirrhosis, and concomitant medications that lower seizure threshold.
- **Clinical situations:** Circumstances associated with an increased seizure risk include, among others, excessive use of alcohol or sedatives (including benzodiazepines); addiction to opiates, cocaine, or stimulants; use of over-the-counter stimulants and anorectics; and diabetes treated with oral hypoglycemics or insulin.
- **Concomitant medications:** Many medications (e.g., antipsychotics, antidepressants, theophylline, systemic steroids) are known to lower seizure threshold.

Recommendations for Reducing the Risk of Seizure: Retrospective analysis of clinical experience gained during the development of bupropion suggests that the risk of seizure may be minimized if

- the total daily dose of ZYBAN does *not* exceed 300 mg (the maximum recommended dose for smoking cessation), and
- the recommended daily dose for most patients (300 mg/day) is administered in divided doses (150 mg twice daily).
- No single dose should exceed 150 mg to avoid high peak concentrations of bupropion and/or its metabolites.

ZYBAN should be administered with extreme caution to patients with a history of seizure, cranial trauma, or other predisposition(s) toward seizure, or patients treated with other agents (e.g., antipsychotics, antidepressants, theophylline, systemic steroids, etc.) that lower seizure threshold.

Hepatic Impairment: ZYBAN should be used with extreme caution in patients with severe hepatic cirrhosis. In these patients a reduced frequency of dosing is required, as peak bupropion levels are substantially increased and accumulation is likely to occur in such patients to a greater extent than usual. The dose should not exceed 150 mg every other day in these patients (see CLINICAL PHARMACOLOGY, PRECAUTIONS, and DOSAGE AND ADMINISTRATION).

Potential for Hepatotoxicity: In rats receiving large doses of bupropion chronically, there was an increase in incidence of hepatic hyperplastic nodules and hepatocellular hypertrophy. In dogs receiving large doses of bupropion chronically, various histologic changes were seen in the liver, and laboratory tests suggesting mild hepatocellular injury were noted.

The PRECAUTIONS: Information for Patients section has been revised as follows.

Information for Patients: Although ZYBAN is not indicated for treatment of depression, it contains the same active ingredient as the antidepressant medications WELLBUTRIN, WELLBUTRIN SR, and WELLBUTRIN XL. Prescribers or other health professionals should inform patients, their families, and their caregivers about the benefits and risks associated with treatment with ZYBAN and should counsel them in its appropriate use. A patient Medication Guide About Using Antidepressants in Children and Teenagers is available for ZYBAN. The prescriber or health professional should instruct patients, their families, and their caregivers to read the Medication Guide and should assist them in understanding its contents. Patients should be given the opportunity to discuss the contents of the Medication Guide and to obtain answers to any questions they may have. The complete text of the Medication Guide is reprinted at the end of this document. Additional important information concerning ZYBAN is provided in a tear-off leaflet entitled "Information for the Patient" at the end of this labeling.

Patients should be advised of the following issues and asked to alert their prescriber if these occur while taking ZYBAN.

Clinical Worsening and Suicide Risk: Patients, their families, and their caregivers should be encouraged to be alert to the emergence of anxiety, agitation, panic attacks, insomnia, irritability, hostility, aggressiveness, impulsivity, akathisia (psychomotor restlessness), hypomania, mania, other unusual changes in behavior, worsening of depression, and suicidal ideation, especially early during antidepressant treatment and when the dose is adjusted up or down. Families and caregivers of patients should be advised to observe for the emergence of such symptoms on a day-to-day basis, since changes may be abrupt. Such symptoms should be reported to the patient's prescriber or health professional, especially if they are severe, abrupt in onset, or were not part of the patient's presenting symptoms. Symptoms such as these may be associated with an increased risk for suicidal thinking and behavior and indicate a need for very close monitoring and possibly changes in the medication.

Patients should be made aware that ZYBAN contains the same active ingredient found in WELLBUTRIN, WELLBUTRIN SR, and WELLBUTRIN XL used to treat depression and that ZYBAN should not be used in conjunction with WELLBUTRIN, WELLBUTRIN SR, WELLBUTRIN XL, or any other medications that contain bupropion hydrochloride.

The PRECAUTIONS: Pediatric Use section has been revised as follows.

Safety and effectiveness in the pediatric population have not been established (see BOX WARNING and WARNINGS: Clinical Worsening and Suicide Risk). Anyone considering the use of ZYBAN in a child or adolescent must balance the potential risks with the clinical need.

The following section has been added to the end of the package insert.

Medication Guide
ZYBAN® (zi ban)
(bupropion hydrochloride) Sustained-Release Tablets
About Using Antidepressants in Children and Teenagers

What is the most important information I should know if my child is being prescribed an antidepressant?

Parents or guardians need to think about 4 important things when their child is prescribed an antidepressant:

1. There is a risk of suicidal thoughts or actions
2. How to try to prevent suicidal thoughts or actions in your child
3. You should watch for certain signs if your child is taking an antidepressant
4. There are benefits and risks when using antidepressants

1. There is a Risk of Suicidal Thoughts or Actions

Children and teenagers sometimes think about suicide, and many report trying to kill themselves.

Antidepressants increase suicidal thoughts and actions in some children and teenagers. But suicidal thoughts and actions can also be caused by depression, a serious medical condition that is commonly treated with antidepressants. Thinking about killing yourself or trying to kill yourself is called *suicidality* or *being suicidal.*

A large study combined the results of 24 different studies of children and teenagers with depression or other illnesses. In these studies, patients took either a placebo (sugar pill) or an antidepressant for 1 to 4 months. *No one committed suicide in these studies,* but some patients became suicidal. On sugar pills, 2 out of every 100 became suicidal. On the antidepressants, 4 out of every 100 patients became suicidal.

For some children and teenagers, the risks of suicidal actions may be especially high. These include patients with

- Bipolar illness (sometimes called manic-depressive illness)
- A family history of bipolar illness
- A personal or family history of attempting suicide

If any of these are present, make sure you tell your healthcare provider before your child takes an antidepressant.

2. How to Try to Prevent Suicidal Thoughts and Actions

To try to prevent suicidal thoughts and actions in your child, pay close attention to changes in her or his moods or actions, especially if the changes occur suddenly. Other important people in your child's life can help by paying attention as well (e.g., your child, brothers and sisters, teachers, and other important people). The changes to look out for are listed in Section 3, on what to watch for.

Whenever an antidepressant is started or its dose is changed, pay close attention to your child.

After starting an antidepressant, your child should generally see his or her healthcare provider:

- Once a week for the first 4 weeks
- Every 2 weeks for the next 4 weeks
- After taking the antidepressant for 12 weeks
- After 12 weeks, follow your healthcare provider's advice about how often to come back
- More often if problems or questions arise (see Section 3)

You should call your child's healthcare provider between visits if needed.

3. You Should Watch For Certain Signs if Your Child is Taking an Antidepressant

Contact your child's healthcare provider *right away* if your child exhibits any of the following signs for the first time, or they seem worse, or worry you, your child, or your child's teacher:

- Thoughts about suicide or dying
- Attempts to commit suicide
- New or worse depression
- New or worse anxiety
- Feeling very agitated or restless
- Panic attacks
- Difficulty sleeping (insomnia)
- New or worse irritability
- Acting aggressive, being angry, or violent
- Acting on dangerous impulses
- An extreme increase in activity and talking
- Other unusual changes in behavior or mood

Never let your child stop taking an antidepressant without first talking to his or her healthcare provider. Stopping an antidepressant suddenly can cause other symptoms.

4. There are Benefits and Risks When Using Antidepressants

Antidepressants are used to treat depression and other illnesses. Depression and other illnesses can lead to suicide. In some children and teenagers, treatment with an antidepressant increases suicidal thinking or actions. It is important to discuss all the risks of treating depression and also the risks of not treating it. You and your child should discuss all treatment choices with your healthcare provider, not just the use of antidepressants.

Other side effects can occur with antidepressants (see section below).

Of all antidepressants, only fluoxetine (Prozac®)* has been FDA approved to treat pediatric depression.

For obsessive compulsive disorder in children and teenagers, FDA has approved only fluoxetine (Prozac®)*, sertraline (Zoloft®)*, fluvoxamine, and clomipramine (Anafranil®)*.

Your healthcare provider may suggest other antidepressants based on the past experience of your child or other family members.

Is this all I need to know if my child is being prescribed an antidepressant?

No. This is a warning about the risk of suicidality. Other side effects can occur with antidepressants. Be sure to ask your healthcare provider to explain all the side effects of the particular drug he or she is prescribing. Also ask about drugs to avoid when taking an antidepressant. Ask your healthcare provider or pharmacist where to find more information.

*The following are registered trademarks of their respective manufacturers: Prozac®/Eli Lilly and Company; Zoloft®/Pfizer Pharmaceuticals; Anafranil®/Mallinckrodt Inc.

This Medication Guide has been approved by the U.S. Food and Drug Administration for all antidepressants.

January 2005/MG-ZY:1

Manufactured by DSM Pharmaceuticals, Inc.

Greenville, NC 27834 for

GlaxoSmithKline, Research Triangle Park, NC 27709

©2005, GlaxoSmithKline. All rights reserved.

January 2005/RL-2138, RL-2166

In the PDR annual,
the **Brand and Generic Name Index**
(PINK section)
alphabetizes drugs under both
brand and generic names.

Janssen Pharmaceutica Products, L.P.

1125 TRENTON-HARBOURTON ROAD
P.O. BOX 200
TITUSVILLE, NJ 08560-0200

For Medical Information Monday through Friday 9 am-5 pm EST Contact:
(800) JANSSEN
FAX: (609) 730-2461
After Hours and Weekends:
(800) JANSSEN

RISPERDAL® ℞
[rĭs-pər-dăl]
(risperidone)
Tablets/Oral Solution
RISPERDAL® M-TAB®
(risperidone)
Orally Disintegrating Tablets

Prescribing information for this product, which appears on pages 1742–1747 of the 2004 PDR, has been revised as follows. Please write "See Supplement A" next to the product heading.

The following **WARNING** *statement was added to the beginning of the full prescribing information:*

> **Increased Mortality in Elderly Patients with Dementia–Related Psychosis**
> **Elderly patients with dementia-related psychosis treated with atypical antipsychotic drugs are at an increased risk of death compared to placebo. Analyses of seventeen placebo controlled trials (modal duration of 10 weeks) in these patients revealed a risk of death in the drug-treated patients of between 1.6 to 1.7 times that seen in placebo-treated patients. Over the course of a typical 10 week controlled trial, the rate of death in drug-treated patients was about 4.5%, compared to a rate of about 2.6% in the placebo group. Although the causes of death were varied, most of the deaths appeared to be either cardiovascular (e.g., heart failure, sudden death) or infectious (e.g., pneumonia) in nature. RISPERDAL® (risperidone) is not approved for the treatment of patients with Dementia-Related Psychosis.**

In **WARNINGS** *section, the following paragraph was added as the first paragraph before* ***Neuroleptic Malignant Syndrome (NMS):***

Increased Mortality in Elderly Patients with Dementia-Related Psychosis Elderly patients with dementia-related psychosis treated with atypical antipsychotic drugs are at an increased risk of death compared to placebo. RISPERAL® (risperidone) is not approved for the treatment of dementia-related psychosis (see Boxed Warning).

In **WARNINGS** *section, the following subsection paragraph was revised:*

Cerebrovascular Adverse Events, Including Stroke, in Elderly Patients With Dementia-Related Psychosis

Cerebrovascular adverse events (e.g., stroke, transient ischemic attack), including fatalities, were reported in patients (mean age 85 years; range 73–97) in trials of risperidone in elderly patients with dementia-related psychosis. In placebo-controlled trials, there was a significantly higher incidence of cerebrovascular adverse events in patients treated with risperidone compared to patients treated with placebo. RISPERDAL® is not approved for the treatment of patients with dementia-related psychosis. (See also **Boxed WARNING, WARNINGS: Increased Mortality in Elderly Patients with Dementia-Related Psychosis.)**

In **PRECAUTIONS** *section the following sentence was added to the end of* **Dysphagia** *paragraph:*

(See also **Boxed WARNING, WARNINGS**: Increased Mortality in Elderly Patients with Dementia-Related Psychosis.)

In **PRECAUTIONS: Drug Interactions, Geriatric Use,** *the following 2 paragraphs were added as a subsection:*

Concomitant use with Furosemide in Elderly Patients with Dementia-Related Psychosis

In placebo-controlled trials in elderly patients with dementia-related psychosis, a higher incidence of mortality was observed in patients treated with furosemide plus risperidone (7.3%; mean age 89 years, range 75–97) when compared to patients treated with risperidone alone (3.1%; mean age 84 years, range 70–96) or furosemide alone (4.1%; mean age 80 years, range 67–90). The increase in mortality in patients treated with furosemide plus risperidone was observed in two of the four clinical trials.

No pathophysiological mechanism has been identified to explain this finding, and no consistent pattern for cause of death observed. Nevertheless, caution should be exercised and the risks and benefits of this combination should be considered prior to the decision to use. There was no increased incidence of mortality among patients taking other diuretics as concomitant medication with risperidone. Irrespective of treatment, dehydration was an overall risk factor for mortality and should therefore be carefully avoided in elderly patients with dementia-related psychosis. RISPERDAL® is not approved for the treatment of patients with dementia-related psychosis. (See also **Boxed WARNING, WARNINGS: Increased Mortality in Elderly Patients with Dementia- Related Psychosis.)**

7503229
US Patent 4,804,663
Revised April 2005

RISPERDAL® CONSTA® ℞
[rĭs-pər-dăl cŏn-stă]
(RISPERIDONE)
LONG-ACTING INJECTION

Prescribing information for this product, which appears on pages 1747–1753 of the 2004 PDR, has been revised as follows. Please write "See Supplement A" next to the product heading.

The following **WARNING** *statement was added to the beginning of the full prescribing information:*

> **Increased Mortality in Elderly Patients with Dementia –Related Psychosis**
> **Elderly patients with dementia-related psychosis treated with atypical antipsychotic drugs are at an increased risk of death compared to placebo. Analyses of seventeen placebo controlled trials (modal duration of 10 weeks) in these patients revealed a risk of death in the drug-treated patients of between 1.6 to 1.7 times that seen in placebo-treated patients. Over the course of a typical 10 week controlled trial, the rate of death in drug-treated patients was about 4.5%, compared to a rate of about 2.6% in the placebo group. Although the causes of death were varied, most of the deaths appeared to be either cardiovascular (e.g., heart failure, sudden death) or infectious (e.g., pneumonia) in nature. RISPERDAL® CONSTA® (risperidone) is not approved for the treatment of patients with Dementia-Related Psychosis.**

In **WARNINGS** *section, the following paragraph was added as the first paragraph before* **Neuroleptic Malignant Syndrome (NMS):**

Increased Mortality in Elderly Patients with Dementia-Related Psychosis

Elderly patients with dementia-related psychosis treated with atypical antipsychotic drugs are at an increased risk of death compared to placebo. RISPERDAL® CONSTA® (risperidone) is not approved for the treatment of dementia-related psychosis (see Boxed Warning).

In **WARNINGS** *section, the following subsection paragraph was revised:*

Cerebrovascular Adverse Events, Including Stroke, in Elderly Patients with Dementia-Related Psychosis

Cerebrovascular adverse events (e.g., stroke, transient ischemic attack), including fatalities, were reported in patients (mean age 85 years; range 73–97) in trials of oral risperidone in elderly patients with dementia-related psychosis. In placebo-controlled trials, there was a significantly higher incidence of cerebrovascular adverse events in patients treated with oral risperidone compared to patients treated with placebo. RISPERDAL® CONSTA® is not approved for the treatment of patients with dementia-related psychosis. (See also **Boxed WARNING, WARNINGS: Increased Mortality in Elderly Patients with Dementia-Related Psychosis.)**

In **PRECAUTIONS** *section the following sentence was added to the end of* **Dysphagia** *paragraph:*

(See also **Boxed WARNING, WARNINGS: Increased Mortality in Elderly Patients with Dementia-Related Psychosis.)**

In **PRECAUTIONS: Drug Interactions, Geriatric Use,** *the following 2 paragraphs were added as a subsection:*

Concomitant use with Furosemide in Elderly Patients with Dementia-Related Psychosis

In placebo-controlled trials in elderly patients with dementia-related psychosis, a higher incidence of mortality was observed in patients treated with furosemide plus oral risperidone (7.3%; mean age 89 years, range 75–97) when compared to patients treated with oral risperidone alone (3.1%; mean age 84 years, range 70–96) or furosemide alone (4.1%; mean age 80 years, range 67–90). The increase in mortality in patients treated with furosemide plus oral risperidone was observed in two of the four clinical trials.

No pathophysiological mechanism has been identified to explain this finding, and no consistent pattern for cause of death observed. Nevertheless, caution should be exercised and the risks and benefits of this combination should be considered prior to the decision to use. There was no increased incidence of mortality among patients taking other diuretics as concomitant medication with risperidone. Irrespective of treatment, dehydration was an overall risk factor for mortality and should therefore be carefully avoided in elderly patients with dementia-related psychosis. RISPERDAL® CONSTA® is not approved for the treatment of patients with dementia-related psychosis. (See also **Boxed WARNING, WARNINGS: Increased Mortality in Elderly Patients with Dementia-Related Psychosis.)**

7519504
US Patent 4,804,663
Revised April 2005

Eli Lilly and Company

LILLY CORPORATE CENTER
INDIANAPOLIS, IN 46285

Direct Inquiries to:
Lilly Corporate Center
Indianapolis, IN 46285
(317) 276-2000
www.lilly.com
For Medical Information Contact:
Lilly Research Laboratories
Lilly Corporate Center
Indianapolis, IN 46285
(800) 545-5979

SYMBYAX® ℞
[sim-bee-ax]
(olanzapine and fluoxetine HCl capsules)

Prescribing information for this product, which appears on pages 1888–1896 of the 2005 PDR, has been completely revised as follows. Please write "See Supplement A" next to the product heading.

WARNING

> **Suicidality in Children and Adolescents—Antidepressants increased the risk of suicidal thinking and behavior (suicidality) in short-term studies in children and adolescents with major depressive disorder (MDD) and other psychiatric disorders. Anyone considering the use of SYMBYAX or any other antidepressant in a child or adolescent must balance this risk with the clinical need. Patients who are started on therapy should be observed closely for clinical worsening, suicidality, or unusual changes in behavior. Families and caregivers should be advised of the need for close observation and communication with the prescriber. SYMBYAX is not approved for use in pediatric patients. (*See* WARNINGS *and* PRECAUTIONS, Pediatric Use.)**
> **Pooled analyses of short-term (4 to 16 weeks) placebo-controlled trials of 9 antidepressant drugs (SSRIs and others) in children and adolescents with major depressive disorder (MDD), obsessive compulsive disorder (OCD), or other psychiatric disorders (a total of 24 trials involving over 4400 patients) have revealed a greater risk of adverse events representing suicidal thinking or behavior (suicidality) during the first few months of treatment in those receiving antidepressants. The average risk of such events in patients receiving antidepressants was 4%, twice the placebo risk of 2%. No suicides occurred in these trials.**
> **Increased Mortality in Elderly Patients with Dementia-Related Psychosis—Elderly patients with dementia-related psychosis treated with atypical antipsychotic drugs are at an increased risk of death compared to placebo. Analyses of seventeen placebo-controlled trials (modal duration of 10 weeks) in these patients revealed a risk of death in the drug-treated patients of between 1.6 to 1.7 times that seen in placebo-treated patients. Over the course of a typical 10-week controlled trial, the rate of death in drug-treated patients was about 4.5%, compared to a rate of about 2.6% in the placebo group. Although the causes of death were varied, most of the deaths appeared to be either cardiovascular (e.g., heart failure, sudden death) or infections (e.g., pneumonia) in nature. SYMBYAX (olanzapine and fluoxetine HCl) is not approved for the treatment of patients with dementia-related psychosis (*see* WARNINGS).**

DESCRIPTION

SYMBYAX® (olanzapine and fluoxetine HCl capsules) combines 2 psychotropic agents, olanzapine (the active ingredient in Zyprexa®, and Zyprexa Zydis®) and fluoxetine hydrochloride (the active ingredient in Prozac®, Prozac Weekly™, and Sarafem®).

Olanzapine belongs to the thienobenzodiazepine class. The chemical designation is 2-methyl-4-(4-methyl-1-piperazinyl)-10*H*-thieno[2,3-*b*] [1,5]benzodiazepine. The molecular formula is $C_{17}H_{20}N_4S$, which corresponds to a molecular weight of 312.44.

Fluoxetine hydrochloride is a selective serotonin reuptake inhibitor (SSRI). The chemical designation is (±)-N-methyl-3-phenyl-3-[(α,α,α-trifluoro-*p*-tolyl)oxy]propylamine hydrochloride. The molecular formula is $C_{17}H_{18}F_3NO \cdot HCl$, which corresponds to a molecular weight of 345.79.

The chemical structures are:

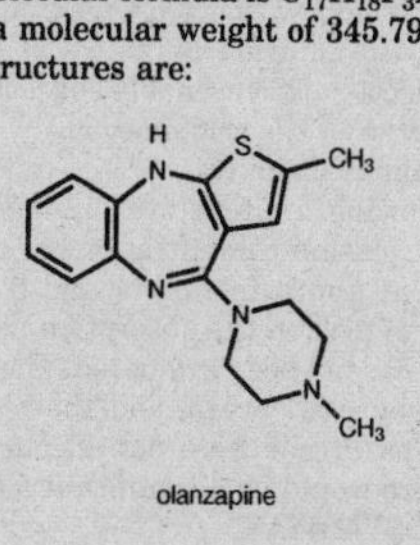

olanzapine

Continued on next page

Symbyax—Cont.

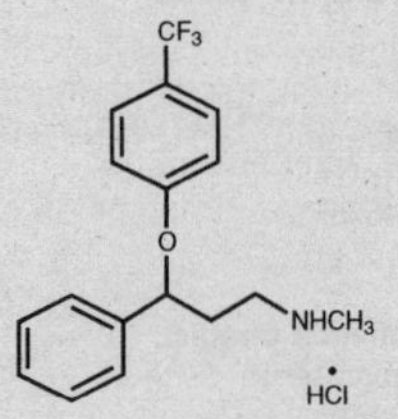

fluoxetine hydrochloride

Olanzapine is a yellow crystalline solid, which is practically insoluble in water.
Fluoxetine hydrochloride is a white to off-white crystalline solid with a solubility of 14 mg/mL in water.
SYMBYAX capsules are available for oral administration in the following strength combinations:

	6 mg/ 25 mg	6 mg/ 50 mg	12 mg/ 25 mg	12 mg/ 50 mg
olanzapine equivalent	6	6	12	12
fluoxetine base equivalent	25	50	25	50

Each capsule also contains pregelatinized starch, gelatin, dimethicone, titanium dioxide, sodium lauryl sulfate, edible black ink, red iron oxide, yellow iron oxide, and/or black iron oxide.

CLINICAL PHARMACOLOGY

Pharmacodynamics

Although the exact mechanism of SYMBYAX is unknown, it has been proposed that the activation of 3 monoaminergic neural systems (serotonin, norepinephrine, and dopamine) is responsible for its enhanced antidepressant effect. This is supported by animal studies in which the olanzapine/fluoxetine combination has been shown to produce synergistic increases in norepinephrine and dopamine release in the prefrontal cortex compared with either component alone, as well as increases in serotonin.
Olanzapine is a psychotropic agent with high affinity binding to the following receptors: serotonin $5HT_{2A/2C}$ (K_i=4 and 11 nM, respectively), dopamine D_{1-4} (K_i=11 to 31 nM), muscarinic M_{1-5} (K_i=1.9 to 25 nM), histamine H_1 (K_i=7 nM), and adrenergic α_1 receptors (K_i=19 nM). Olanzapine binds weakly to $GABA_A$, BZD, and β-adrenergic receptors (K_i>10 μM). Fluoxetine is an inhibitor of the serotonin transporter and is a weak inhibitor of the norepinephrine and dopamine transporters.
Antagonism at receptors other than dopamine and $5HT_2$ with similar receptor affinities may explain some of the other therapeutic and side effects of olanzapine. Olanzapine's antagonism of muscarinic M_{1-5} receptors may explain its anticholinergic effects. The antagonism of histamine H_1 receptors by olanzapine may explain the somnolence observed with this drug. The antagonism of α_1-adrenergic receptors by olanzapine may explain the orthostatic hypotension observed with this drug. Fluoxetine has relatively low affinity for muscarinic, α_1-adrenergic, and histamine H_1 receptors.

Pharmacokinetics

Fluoxetine (administered as a 60-mg single dose or 60 mg daily for 8 days) caused a small increase in the mean maximum concentration of olanzapine (16%) following a 5-mg dose, an increase in the mean area under the curve (17%) and a small decrease in mean apparent clearance of olanzapine (16%). In another study, a similar decrease in apparent clearance of olanzapine of 14% was observed following olanzapine doses of 6 or 12 mg with concomitant fluoxetine doses of 25 mg or more. The decrease in clearance reflects an increase in bioavailability. The terminal half-life is not affected, and therefore the time to reach steady state should not be altered. The overall steady-state plasma concentrations of olanzapine and fluoxetine when given as the combination in the therapeutic dose ranges were comparable with those typically attained with each of the monotherapies. The small change in olanzapine clearance, observed in both studies, likely reflects the inhibition of a minor metabolic pathway for olanzapine via CYP2D6 by fluoxetine, a potent CYP2D6 inhibitor, and was not deemed clinically significant. Therefore, the pharmacokinetics of the individual components is expected to reasonably characterize the overall pharmacokinetics of the combination.

Absorption and Bioavailability

SYMBYAX—Following a single oral 12-mg/50-mg dose of SYMBYAX, peak plasma concentrations of olanzapine and fluoxetine occur at approximately 4 and 6 hours, respectively. The effect of food on the absorption and bioavailability of SYMBYAX has not been evaluated. The bioavailability of olanzapine given as Zyprexa, and the bioavailability of fluoxetine given as Prozac were not affected by food. It is unlikely that there would be a significant food effect on the bioavailability of SYMBYAX.
Olanzapine—Olanzapine is well absorbed and reaches peak concentration approximately 6 hours following an oral dose. Food does not affect the rate or extent of olanzapine absorption when olanzapine is given as Zyprexa. It is eliminated extensively by first pass metabolism, with approximately 40% of the dose metabolized before reaching the systemic circulation.
Fluoxetine—Following a single oral 40-mg dose, peak plasma concentrations of fluoxetine from 15 to 55 ng/mL are observed after 6 to 8 hours. Food does not appear to affect the systemic bioavailability of fluoxetine given as Prozac, although it may delay its absorption by 1 to 2 hours, which is probably not clinically significant.

Distribution

SYMBYAX—The in vitro binding to human plasma proteins of the olanzapine/fluoxetine combination is similar to the binding of the individual components.
Olanzapine—Olanzapine is extensively distributed throughout the body, with a volume of distribution of approximately 1000 L. It is 93% bound to plasma proteins over the concentration range of 7 to 1100 ng/mL, binding primarily to albumin and α_1-acid glycoprotein.
Fluoxetine—Over the concentration range from 200 to 1000 ng/mL, approximately 94.5% of fluoxetine is bound in vitro to human serum proteins, including albumin and α_1-glycoprotein. The interaction between fluoxetine and other highly protein-bound drugs has not been fully evaluated (*see* PRECAUTIONS, Drugs tightly bound to plasma proteins).

Metabolism and Elimination

SYMBYAX—SYMBYAX therapy yielded steady-state concentrations of norfluoxetine similar to those seen with fluoxetine in the therapeutic dose range.
Olanzapine—Olanzapine displays linear pharmacokinetics over the clinical dosing range. Its half-life ranges from 21 to 54 hours (5th to 95th percentile; mean of 30 hr), and apparent plasma clearance ranges from 12 to 47 L/hr (5th to 95th percentile; mean of 25 L/hr). Administration of olanzapine once daily leads to steady-state concentrations in about 1 week that are approximately twice the concentrations after single doses. Plasma concentrations, half-life, and clearance of olanzapine may vary between individuals on the basis of smoking status, gender, and age (*see* Special Populations).
Following a single oral dose of ^{14}C-labeled olanzapine, 7% of the dose of olanzapine was recovered in the urine as unchanged drug, indicating that olanzapine is highly metabolized. Approximately 57% and 30% of the dose was recovered in the urine and feces, respectively. In the plasma, olanzapine accounted for only 12% of the AUC for total radioactivity, indicating significant exposure to metabolites. After multiple dosing, the major circulating metabolites were the 10-N-glucuronide, present at steady state at 44% of the concentration of olanzapine, and 4′-N-desmethyl olanzapine, present at steady state at 31% of the concentration of olanzapine. Both metabolites lack pharmacological activity at the concentrations observed.
Direct glucuronidation and CYP450-mediated oxidation are the primary metabolic pathways for olanzapine. In vitro studies suggest that CYP1A2, CYP2D6, and the flavin-containing monooxygenase system are involved in olanzapine oxidation. CYP2D6-mediated oxidation appears to be a minor metabolic pathway in vivo, because the clearance of olanzapine is not reduced in subjects who are deficient in this enzyme.
Fluoxetine—Fluoxetine is a racemic mixture (50/50) of *R*-fluoxetine and *S*-fluoxetine enantiomers. In animal models, both enantiomers are specific and potent serotonin uptake inhibitors with essentially equivalent pharmacologic activity. The *S*-fluoxetine enantiomer is eliminated more slowly and is the predominant enantiomer present in plasma at steady state.
Fluoxetine is extensively metabolized in the liver to its only identified active metabolite, norfluoxetine, via the CYP2D6 pathway. A number of unidentified metabolites exist.
In animal models, *S*-norfluoxetine is a potent and selective inhibitor of serotonin uptake and has activity essentially equivalent to *R*- or *S*-fluoxetine. *R*-norfluoxetine is significantly less potent than the parent drug in the inhibition of serotonin uptake. The primary route of elimination appears to be hepatic metabolism to inactive metabolites excreted by the kidney.

Clinical Issues Related to Metabolism and Elimination—The complexity of the metabolism of fluoxetine has several consequences that may potentially affect the clinical use of SYMBYAX.
Variability in metabolism — A subset (about 7%) of the population has reduced activity of the drug metabolizing enzyme CYP2D6. Such individuals are referred to as "poor metabolizers" of drugs such as debrisoquin, dextromethorphan, and the tricyclic antidepressants (TCAs). In a study involving labeled and unlabeled enantiomers administered as a racemate, these individuals metabolized *S*-fluoxetine at a slower rate and thus achieved higher concentrations of *S*-fluoxetine. Consequently, concentrations of *S*-norfluoxetine at steady state were lower. The metabolism of *R*-fluoxetine in these poor metabolizers appears normal. When compared with normal metabolizers, the total sum at steady state of the plasma concentrations of the 4 enantiomers was not significantly greater among poor metabolizers. Thus, the net pharmacodynamic activities were essentially the same. Alternative nonsaturable pathways (non-CYP2D6) also contribute to the metabolism of fluoxetine. This explains how fluoxetine achieves a steady-state concentration rather than increasing without limit.
Because the metabolism of fluoxetine, like that of a number of other compounds including TCAs and other selective serotonin antidepressants, involves the CYP2D6 system, concomitant therapy with drugs also metabolized by this enzyme system (such as the TCAs) may lead to drug interactions (*see* PRECAUTIONS, Drug Interactions).
Accumulation and slow elimination — The relatively slow elimination of fluoxetine (elimination half-life of 1 to 3 days after acute administration and 4 to 6 days after chronic administration) and its active metabolite, norfluoxetine (elimination half-life of 4 to 16 days after acute and chronic administration), leads to significant accumulation of these active species in chronic use and delayed attainment of steady state, even when a fixed dose is used. After 30 days of dosing at 40 mg/day, plasma concentrations of fluoxetine in the range of 91 to 302 ng/mL and norfluoxetine in the range of 72 to 258 ng/mL have been observed. Plasma concentrations of fluoxetine were higher than those predicted by single-dose studies, because the metabolism of fluoxetine is not proportional to dose. However, norfluoxetine appears to have linear pharmacokinetics. Its mean terminal half-life after a single dose was 8.6 days and after multiple dosing was 9.3 days. Steady-state levels after prolonged dosing are similar to levels seen at 4 to 5 weeks.
The long elimination half-lives of fluoxetine and norfluoxetine assure that, even when dosing is stopped, active drug substance will persist in the body for weeks (primarily depending on individual patient characteristics, previous dosing regimen, and length of previous therapy at discontinuation). This is of potential consequence when drug discontinuation is required or when drugs are prescribed that might interact with fluoxetine and norfluoxetine following the discontinuation of fluoxetine.

Special Populations

Geriatric—Based on the individual pharmacokinetic profiles of olanzapine and fluoxetine, the pharmacokinetics of SYMBYAX may be altered in geriatric patients. Caution should be used in dosing the elderly, especially if there are other factors that might additively influence drug metabolism and/or pharmacodynamic sensitivity.
In a study involving 24 healthy subjects, the mean elimination half-life of olanzapine was about 1.5 times greater in elderly subjects (>65 years of age) than in non-elderly subjects (≤65 years of age).
The disposition of single doses of fluoxetine in healthy elderly subjects (>65 years of age) did not differ significantly from that in younger normal subjects. However, given the long half-life and nonlinear disposition of the drug, a single-dose study is not adequate to rule out the possibility of altered pharmacokinetics in the elderly, particularly if they have systemic illness or are receiving multiple drugs for concomitant diseases. The effects of age upon the metabolism of fluoxetine have been investigated in 260 elderly but otherwise healthy depressed patients (≥60 years of age) who received 20 mg fluoxetine for 6 weeks. Combined fluoxetine plus norfluoxetine plasma concentrations were 209.3 ± 85.7 ng/mL at the end of 6 weeks. No unusual age-associated pattern of adverse events was observed in those elderly patients.
Renal Impairment—The pharmacokinetics of SYMBYAX has not been studied in patients with renal impairment. However, olanzapine and fluoxetine individual pharmacokinetics do not differ significantly in patients with renal impairment. SYMBYAX dosing adjustment based upon renal impairment is not routinely required.
Because olanzapine is highly metabolized before excretion and only 7% of the drug is excreted unchanged, renal dysfunction alone is unlikely to have a major impact on the pharmacokinetics of olanzapine. The pharmacokinetic characteristics of olanzapine were similar in patients with severe renal impairment and normal subjects, indicating that dosage adjustment based upon the degree of renal impairment is not required. In addition, olanzapine is not removed by dialysis. The effect of renal impairment on olanzapine metabolite elimination has not been studied.
In depressed patients on dialysis (N=12), fluoxetine administered as 20 mg once daily for 2 months produced steady-state fluoxetine and norfluoxetine plasma concentrations comparable with those seen in patients with normal renal function. While the possibility exists that renally excreted metabolites of fluoxetine may accumulate to higher levels in patients with severe renal dysfunction, use of a lower or less frequent dose is not routinely necessary in renally impaired patients.
Hepatic Impairment—Based on the individual pharmacokinetic profiles of olanzapine and fluoxetine, the pharmacokinetics of SYMBYAX may be altered in patients with hepatic impairment. The lowest starting dose should be considered for patients with hepatic impairment (*see* PRECAUTIONS, Use in Patients with Concomitant Illness *and* DOSAGE AND ADMINISTRATION, Special Populations).
Although the presence of hepatic impairment may be expected to reduce the clearance of olanzapine, a study of the effect of impaired liver function in subjects (N=6) with clinically significant cirrhosis (Childs-Pugh Classification A and B) revealed little effect on the pharmacokinetics of olanzapine.
As might be predicted from its primary site of metabolism, liver impairment can affect the elimination of fluoxetine. The elimination half-life of fluoxetine was prolonged in a study of cirrhotic patients, with a mean of 7.6 days compared with the range of 2 to 3 days seen in subjects without liver disease; norfluoxetine elimination was also delayed, with a mean duration of 12 days for cirrhotic patients compared with the range of 7 to 9 days in normal subjects.
Gender—Clearance of olanzapine is approximately 30% lower in women than in men. There were, however, no apparent differences between men and women in effectiveness or adverse effects. Dosage modifications based on gender should not be needed.

Smoking Status—Olanzapine clearance is about 40% higher in smokers than in nonsmokers, although dosage modifications are not routinely required.

Race—No SYMBYAX pharmacokinetic study was conducted to investigate the effects of race. Results from an olanzapine cross-study comparison between data obtained in Japan and data obtained in the US suggest that exposure to olanzapine may be about 2-fold greater in the Japanese when equivalent doses are administered. Olanzapine clinical study safety and efficacy data, however, did not suggest clinically significant differences among Caucasian patients, patients of African descent, and a 3rd pooled category including Asian and Hispanic patients. Dosage modifications for race, therefore, are not routinely required.

Combined Effects—The combined effects of age, smoking, and gender could lead to substantial pharmacokinetic differences in populations. The clearance of olanzapine in young smoking males, for example, may be 3 times higher than that in elderly nonsmoking females. SYMBYAX dosing modification may be necessary in patients who exhibit a combination of factors that may result in slower metabolism of the olanzapine component (see DOSAGE AND ADMINISTRATION, Special Populations).

CLINICAL STUDIES

The efficacy of SYMBYAX for the treatment of depressive episodes associated with bipolar disorder was established in 2 identically designed, 8-week, randomized, double-blind, controlled studies of patients who met Diagnostic and Statistical Manual 4th edition (DSM-IV) criteria for Bipolar I Disorder, Depressed utilizing flexible dosing of SYMBYAX (6/25, 6/50, or 12/50 mg/day), olanzapine (5 to 20 mg/day), and placebo. These studies included patients (≥18 years of age) with or without psychotic symptoms and with or without a rapid cycling course.

The primary rating instrument used to assess depressive symptoms in these studies was the Montgomery-Asberg Depression Rating Scale (MADRS), a 10-item clinician-rated scale with total scores ranging from 0 to 60. The primary outcome measure of these studies was the change from baseline to endpoint in the MADRS total score. In both studies, SYMBYAX was statistically significantly superior to both olanzapine monotherapy and placebo in reduction of the MADRS total score. The results of the studies are summarized below (Table 1).

Table 1: MADRS Total Score
Mean Change from Baseline to Endpoint

	Treatment Group	Baseline Mean	Change to Endpoint Mean[1]
Study 1	SYMBYAX (N=40)	30	−16[a]
	Olanzapine (N=182)	32	−12
	Placebo (N=181)	31	−10
Study 2	SYMBYAX (N=42)	32	−18[a]
	Olanzapine (N=169)	33	−14
	Placebo (N=174)	31	−9

[1] Negative number denotes improvement from baseline.
[a] Statistically significant compared to both olanzapine and placebo.

INDICATIONS AND USAGE

SYMBYAX is indicated for the treatment of depressive episodes associated with bipolar disorder. The efficacy of SYMBYAX was established in 2 identically designed, 8-week, randomized, double-blind clinical studies.

Unlike with unipolar depression, there are no established guidelines for the length of time patients with bipolar disorder experiencing a major depressive episode should be treated with agents containing antidepressant drugs.

The effectiveness of SYMBYAX for maintaining antidepressant response in this patient population beyond 8 weeks has not been established in controlled clinical studies. Physicians who elect to use SYMBYAX for extended periods should periodically reevaluate the benefits and long-term risks of the drug for the individual patient.

CONTRAINDICATIONS

Hypersensitivity—SYMBYAX is contraindicated in patients with a known hypersensitivity to the product or any component of the product.

Monoamine Oxidase Inhibitors (MAOI)—There have been reports of serious, sometimes fatal reactions (including hyperthermia, rigidity, myoclonus, autonomic instability with possible rapid fluctuations of vital signs, and mental status changes that include extreme agitation progressing to delirium and coma) in patients receiving fluoxetine in combination with an MAOI, and in patients who have recently discontinued fluoxetine and are then started on an MAOI. Some cases presented with features resembling neuroleptic malignant syndrome. Therefore, SYMBYAX should not be used in combination with an MAOI, or within a minimum of

14 days of discontinuing therapy with an MAOI. Since fluoxetine and its major metabolite have very long elimination half-lives, at least 5 weeks [perhaps longer, especially if fluoxetine has been prescribed chronically and/or at higher doses (see CLINICAL PHARMACOLOGY, Accumulation and slow elimination)] should be allowed after stopping SYMBYAX before starting an MAOI.

Thioridazine—Thioridazine should not be administered with SYMBYAX or administered within a minimum of 5 weeks after discontinuation of SYMBYAX (see WARNINGS, Thioridazine).

WARNINGS

Clinical Worsening and Suicide Risk—Patients with major depressive disorder (MDD), both adult and pediatric, may experience worsening of their depression and/or the emergence of suicidal ideation and behavior (suicidality) or unusual changes in behavior, whether or not they are taking antidepressant medications, and this risk may persist until significant remission occurs. There has been a long-standing concern that antidepressants may have a role in inducing worsening of depression and the emergence of suicidality in certain patients. Antidepressants increased the risk of suicidal thinking and behavior (suicidality) in short-term studies in children and adolescents with major depressive disorder (MDD) and other psychiatric disorders.

Pooled analyses of short-term placebo-controlled trials of 9 antidepressant drugs (SSRIs and others) in children and adolescents with MDD, OCD, or other psychiatric disorders (a total of 24 trials involving over 4400 patients) have revealed a greater risk of adverse events representing suicidal behavior or thinking (suicidality) during the first few months of treatment in those receiving antidepressants. The average risk of such events in patients receiving antidepressants was 4%, twice the placebo risk of 2%. There was considerable variation in risk among drugs, but a tendency toward an increase for almost all drugs studied. The risk of suicidality was most consistently observed in the MDD trials, but there were signals of risk arising from some trials in other psychiatric indications (obsessive compulsive disorder and social anxiety disorder) as well. **No suicides occurred in any of these trials.** It is unknown whether the suicidality risk in pediatric patients extends to longer-term use, i.e., beyond several months. It is also unknown whether the suicidality risk extends to adults.

All pediatric patients being treated with antidepressants for any indication should be observed closely for clinical worsening, suicidality, and unusual changes in behavior, especially during the initial few months of a course of drug therapy, or at times of dose changes, either increases or decreases. Such observation would generally include at least weekly face-to-face contact with patients or their family members or caregivers during the first 4 weeks of treatment, then every other week visits for the next 4 weeks, then at 12 weeks, and as clinically indicated beyond 12 weeks. Additional contact by telephone may be appropriate between face-to-face visits.

Adults with MDD or co-morbid depression in the setting of other psychiatric illness being treated with antidepressants should be observed similarly for clinical worsening and suicidality, especially during the initial few months of a course of drug therapy, or at times of dose changes, either increases or decreases.

The following symptoms, anxiety, agitation, panic attacks, insomnia, irritability, hostility, aggressiveness, impulsivity, akathisia (psychomotor restlessness), hypomania, and mania, have been reported in adult and pediatric patients being treated with antidepressants for major depressive disorder as well as for other indications, both psychiatric and nonpsychiatric. Although a causal link between the emergence of such symptoms and either the worsening of depression and/or the emergence of suicidal impulses has not been established, there is concern that such symptoms may represent precursors to emerging suicidality.

Consideration should be given to changing the therapeutic regimen, including possibly discontinuing the medication, in patients whose depression is persistently worse, or who are experiencing emergent suicidality or symptoms that might be precursors to worsening depression or suicidality, especially if these symptoms are severe, abrupt in onset, or were not part of the patient's presenting symptoms.

If the decision has been made to discontinue treatment, medication should be tapered, as rapidly as is feasible, but with recognition that abrupt discontinuation can be associated with certain symptoms (see PRECAUTIONS and DOSAGE AND ADMINISTRATION, Discontinuation of Treatment with SYMBYAX, for a description of the risks of discontinuation of SYMBYAX).

Families and caregivers of pediatric patients being treated with antidepressants for major depressive disorder or other indications, both psychiatric and nonpsychiatric, should be alerted about the need to monitor patients for the emergence of agitation, irritability, unusual changes in behavior, and the other symptoms described above, as well as the emergence of suicidality, and to report such symptoms immediately to health care providers. Such monitoring should include daily observation by families and caregivers. Prescriptions for SYMBYAX should be written for the smallest quantity of capsules consistent with good patient management, in order to reduce the risk of overdose. Families and caregivers of adults being treated for depression should be similarly advised.

It should be noted that SYMBYAX is not approved for use in treating any indications in the pediatric population.

Screening Patients for Bipolar Disorder—A major depressive episode may be the initial presentation of bipolar dis-

order. It is generally believed (though not established in controlled trials) that treating such an episode with an antidepressant alone may increase the likelihood of precipitation of a mixed/manic episode in patients at risk for bipolar disorder. Whether any of the symptoms described above represent such a conversion is unknown. However, prior to initiating treatment with an antidepressant, patients with depressive symptoms should be adequately screened to determine if they are at risk for bipolar disorder; such screening should include a detailed psychiatric history, including a family history of suicide, bipolar disorder, and depression. It should be noted that SYMBYAX is approved for use in treating bipolar depression.

Increased Mortality in Elderly Patients with Dementia-Related Psychosis—Elderly patients with dementia-related psychosis treated with atypical antipsychotic drugs are at an increased risk of death compared to placebo. SYMBYAX (olanzapine and fluoxetine HCl) is not approved for the treatment of patients with dementia-related psychosis (see BOX WARNING).

In olanzapine placebo-controlled clinical trials of elderly patients with dementia-related psychosis, the incidence of death in olanzapine-treated patients was significantly greater than placebo-treated patients (3.5% vs 1.5%, respectively). Risk factors that may predispose this patient population to increased mortality when treated with olanzapine include age ≥80 years, sedation, concomitant use of benzodiazepines or presence of pulmonary conditions (e.g., pneumonia, with or without aspiration).

Cerebrovascular Adverse Events (CVAE), Including Stroke, in Elderly Patients with Dementia-Related Psychosis—Cerebrovascular Cerebrovascular adverse events (e.g., stroke, transient ischemic attack), including fatalities, were reported in patients in trials of olanzapine in elderly patients with dementia-related psychosis. In placebo-controlled trials, there was a significantly higher incidence of cerebrovascular adverse events in patients treated with olanzapine compared to patients treated with placebo. Olanzapine is not approved for the treatment of patients with dementia-related psychosis.

Hyperglycemia and Diabetes Mellitus—Hyperglycemia, in some cases extreme and associated with ketoacidosis or hyperosmolar coma or death, has been reported in patients treated with atypical antipsychotics, including olanzapine alone, as well as olanzapine taken concomitantly with fluoxetine. Assessment of the relationship between atypical antipsychotic use and glucose abnormalities is complicated by the possibility of an increased background risk of diabetes mellitus in patients with schizophrenia and the increasing incidence of diabetes mellitus in the general population. Given these confounders, the relationship between atypical antipsychotic use and hyperglycemia-related adverse events is not completely understood. However, epidemiological studies suggest an increased risk of treatment-emergent hyperglycemia-related adverse events in patients treated with the atypical antipsychotics. Precise risk estimates for hyperglycemia-related adverse events in patients treated with atypical antipsychotics are not available.

Patients with an established diagnosis of diabetes mellitus who are started on atypical antipsychotics should be monitored regularly for worsening of glucose control. Patients with risk factors for diabetes mellitus (e.g., obesity, family history of diabetes) who are starting treatment with atypical antipsychotics should undergo fasting blood glucose testing at the beginning of treatment and periodically during treatment. Any patient treated with atypical antipsychotics should be monitored for symptoms of hyperglycemia including polydipsia, polyuria, polyphagia, and weakness. Patients who develop symptoms of hyperglycemia during treatment with atypical antipsychotics should undergo fasting blood glucose testing. In some cases, hyperglycemia has resolved when the atypical antipsychotic was discontinued; however, some patients required continuation of anti-diabetic treatment despite discontinuation of the suspect drug.

Orthostatic Hypotension—SYMBYAX may induce orthostatic hypotension associated with dizziness, tachycardia, bradycardia, and, in some patients, syncope, especially during the initial dose-titration period.

In the bipolar depression studies, statistically significantly more orthostatic changes occurred with the SYMBYAX group compared to placebo and olanzapine groups. Orthostatic systolic blood pressure decrease of at least 30 mm Hg occurred in 7.3% (6/82), 1.4% (5/346), and 1.4% (5/352) of the SYMBYAX, olanzapine and placebo groups, respectively. Among the group of controlled clinical studies with SYMBYAX, an orthostatic systolic blood pressure decrease of ≥30 mm Hg occurred in 4% (21/512) of SYMBYAX-treated patients, 5% (10/204) of fluoxetine-treated patients, 2% (16/644) of olanzapine-treated patients, and 2% (8/445) of placebo-treated patients. In this group of studies, the incidence of syncope in SYMBYAX-treated patients was 0.4% (2/571) compared to placebo 0.2% (1/477).

In a clinical pharmacology study of SYMBYAX, three healthy subjects were discontinued from the trial after experiencing severe, but self-limited, hypotension and bradycardia that occurred 2 to 9 hours following a single 12-mg/50-mg dose of SYMBYAX. Reactions consisting of this combination of hypotension and bradycardia (and also accompanied by sinus pause) have been observed in at least three other healthy subjects treated with various formulations of olanzapine (one oral, two intramuscular). In controlled clinical studies, the incidence of patients with a

Continued on next page

Symbyax—Cont.

≥20 bpm decrease in orthostatic pulse concomitantly with a ≥20 mm Hg decrease in orthostatic systolic blood pressure was 0.4% (2/549) in the SYMBYAX group, 0.2% (1/455) in the placebo group, 0.8% (5/659) in the olanzapine group, and 0% (0/241) in the fluoxetine group.

SYMBYAX should be used with particular caution in patients with known cardiovascular disease (history of myocardial infarction or ischemia, heart failure, or conduction abnormalities), cerebrovascular disease, or conditions that would predispose patients to hypotension (dehydration, hypovolemia, and treatment with antihypertensive medications).

Allergic Events and Rash—In SYMBYAX premarketing controlled clinical studies, the overall incidence of rash or allergic events in SYMBYAX-treated patients [4.6% (26/571)] was similar to that of placebo [5.2% (25/477)]. The majority of the cases of rash and/or urticaria were mild; however, three patients discontinued (one due to rash, which was moderate in severity, and two due to allergic events, one of which included face edema).

In fluoxetine US clinical studies, 7% of 10,782 fluoxetine-treated patients developed various types of rashes and/or urticaria. Among the cases of rash and/or urticaria reported in premarketing clinical studies, almost a third were withdrawn from treatment because of the rash and/or systemic signs or symptoms associated with the rash. Clinical findings reported in association with rash include fever, leukocytosis, arthralgias, edema, carpal tunnel syndrome, respiratory distress, lymphadenopathy, proteinuria, and mild transaminase elevation. Most patients improved promptly with discontinuation of fluoxetine and/or adjunctive treatment with antihistamines or steroids, and all patients experiencing these events were reported to recover completely. In fluoxetine premarketing clinical studies, 2 patients are known to have developed a serious cutaneous systemic illness. In neither patient was there an unequivocal diagnosis, but 1 was considered to have a leukocytoclastic vasculitis, and the other, a severe desquamating syndrome that was considered variously to be a vasculitis or erythema multiforme. Other patients have had systemic syndromes suggestive of serum sickness.

Since the introduction of fluoxetine, systemic events, possibly related to vasculitis, have developed in patients with rash. Although these events are rare, they may be serious, involving the lung, kidney, or liver. Death has been reported to occur in association with these systemic events.

Anaphylactoid events, including bronchospasm, angioedema, and urticaria alone and in combination, have been reported.

Pulmonary events, including inflammatory processes of varying histopathology and/or fibrosis, have been reported rarely. These events have occurred with dyspnea as the only preceding symptom.

Whether these systemic events and rash have a common underlying cause or are due to different etiologies or pathogenic processes is not known. Furthermore, a specific underlying immunologic basis for these events has not been identified. Upon the appearance of rash or of other possible allergic phenomena for which an alternative etiology cannot be identified, SYMBYAX should be discontinued.

Neuroleptic Malignant Syndrome (NMS)—A potentially fatal symptom complex sometimes referred to as NMS has been reported in association with administration of antipsychotic drugs, including olanzapine. Clinical manifestations of NMS are hyperpyrexia, muscle rigidity, altered mental status, and evidence of autonomic instability (irregular pulse or blood pressure, tachycardia, diaphoresis, and cardiac dysrhythmia). Additional signs may include elevated creatinine phosphokinase, myoglobinuria (rhabdomyolysis), and acute renal failure.

The diagnostic evaluation of patients with this syndrome is complicated. In arriving at a diagnosis, it is important to exclude cases where the clinical presentation includes both serious medical illness (e.g., pneumonia, systemic infection, etc.) and untreated or inadequately treated extrapyramidal signs and symptoms (EPS). Other important considerations in the differential diagnosis include central anticholinergic toxicity, heat stroke, drug fever, and primary central nervous system pathology.

The management of NMS should include: 1) immediate discontinuation of antipsychotic drugs and other drugs not essential to concurrent therapy, 2) intensive symptomatic treatment and medical monitoring, and 3) treatment of any concomitant serious medical problems for which specific treatments are available. There is no general agreement about specific pharmacological treatment regimens for NMS.

If after recovering from NMS, a patient requires treatment with an antipsychotic, the patient should be carefully monitored, since recurrences of NMS have been reported.

Tardive Dyskinesia—A syndrome of potentially irreversible, involuntary, dyskinetic movements may develop in patients treated with antipsychotic drugs. Although the prevalence of the syndrome appears to be highest among the elderly, especially elderly women, it is impossible to rely upon prevalence estimates to predict, at the inception of antipsychotic treatment, which patients are likely to develop the syndrome. Whether antipsychotic drug products differ in their potential to cause tardive dyskinesia is unknown.

The risk of developing tardive dyskinesia and the likelihood that it will become irreversible are believed to increase as the duration of treatment and the total cumulative dose of antipsychotic drugs administered to the patient increase. However, the syndrome can develop, although much less commonly, after relatively brief treatment periods at low doses or may even arise after discontinuation of treatment. There is no known treatment for established cases of tardive dyskinesia, although the syndrome may remit, partially or completely, if antipsychotic treatment is withdrawn. Antipsychotic treatment itself, however, may suppress (or partially suppress) the signs and symptoms of the syndrome and thereby may possibly mask the underlying process. The effect that symptomatic suppression has upon the long-term course of the syndrome is unknown.

The incidence of dyskinetic movement in SYMBYAX-treated patients was infrequent. The mean score on the Abnormal Involuntary Movement Scale (AIMS) across clinical studies involving SYMBYAX-treated patients decreased from baseline. Nonetheless, SYMBYAX should be prescribed in a manner that is most likely to minimize the risk of tardive dyskinesia. If signs and symptoms of tardive dyskinesia appear in a patient on SYMBYAX, drug discontinuation should be considered. However, some patients may require treatment with SYMBYAX despite the presence of the syndrome. The need for continued treatment should be reassessed periodically.

Thioridazine—In a study of 19 healthy male subjects, which included 6 slow and 13 rapid hydroxylators of debrisoquin, a single 25-mg oral dose of thioridazine produced a 2.4-fold higher C_{max} and a 4.5-fold higher AUC for thioridazine in the slow hydroxylators compared with the rapid hydroxylators. The rate of debrisoquin hydroxylation is felt to depend on the level of CYP2D6 isozyme activity. Thus, this study suggests that drugs that inhibit CYP2D6, such as certain SSRIs, including fluoxetine, will produce elevated plasma levels of thioridazine (see PRECAUTIONS).

Thioridazine administration produces a dose-related prolongation of the QT_c interval, which is associated with serious ventricular arrhythmias, such as torsades de pointes-type arrhythmias and sudden death. This risk is expected to increase with fluoxetine-induced inhibition of thioridazine metabolism (see CONTRAINDICATIONS, Thioridazine).

PRECAUTIONS

General

Concomitant Use of Olanzapine and Fluoxetine Products—SYMBYAX contains the same active ingredients that are in Zyprexa and Zyprexa Zydis (olanzapine) and in Prozac, Prozac Weekly, and Sarafem (fluoxetine HCl). Caution should be exercised when prescribing these medications concomitantly with SYMBYAX.

Abnormal Bleeding—Published case reports have documented the occurrence of bleeding episodes in patients treated with psychotropic drugs that interfere with serotonin reuptake. Subsequent epidemiological studies, both of the case-control and cohort design, have demonstrated an association between use of psychotropic drugs that interfere with serotonin reuptake and the occurrence of upper gastrointestinal bleeding. In two studies, concurrent use of a nonsteroidal anti-inflammatory drug (NSAID) or aspirin potentiated the risk of bleeding (see DRUG INTERACTIONS). Although these studies focused on upper gastrointestinal bleeding, there is reason to believe that bleeding at other sites may be similarly potentiated. Patients should be cautioned regarding the risk of bleeding associated with the concomitant use of SYMBYAX with NSAIDs, aspirin, or other drugs that affect coagulation.

Mania/Hypomania—In the two controlled bipolar depression studies there was no statistically significant difference in the incidence of manic events (manic reaction or manic depressive reaction) between SYMBYAX- and placebo-treated patients. In one of the studies, the incidence of manic events was (7% [3/43]) in SYMBYAX-treated patients compared to (3% [5/184]) in placebo-treated patients. In the other study, the incidence of manic events was (2% [1/43]) in SYMBYAX-treated patients compared to (8% [15/193]) in placebo-treated patients. This limited controlled trial experience of SYMBYAX in the treatment of bipolar depression makes it difficult to interpret these findings until additional data is obtained. Because of this and the cyclical nature of bipolar disorder, patients should be monitored closely for the development of symptoms of mania/hypomania during treatment with SYMBYAX.

Body Temperature Regulation—Disruption of the body's ability to reduce core body temperature has been attributed to antipsychotic drugs. Appropriate care is advised when prescribing SYMBYAX for patients who will be experiencing conditions which may contribute to an elevation in core body temperature (e.g., exercising strenuously, exposure to extreme heat, receiving concomitant medication with anticholinergic activity, or being subject to dehydration).

Cognitive and Motor Impairment—Somnolence was a commonly reported adverse event associated with SYMBYAX treatment, occurring at an incidence of 22% in SYMBYAX patients compared with 11% in placebo patients. Somnolence led to discontinuation in 2% (10/571) of patients in the premarketing controlled clinical studies.

As with any CNS-active drug, SYMBYAX has the potential to impair judgment, thinking, or motor skills. Patients should be cautioned about operating hazardous machinery, including automobiles, until they are reasonably certain that SYMBYAX therapy does not affect them adversely.

Discontinuation of Treatment with SYMBYAX

During marketing of fluoxetine, a component of SYMBYAX, and other SSRIs and SNRIs (serotonin and norepinephrine reuptake inhibitors), there have been spontaneous reports of adverse events occurring upon discontinuation of these drugs, particularly when abrupt, including the following: dysphoric mood, irritability, agitation, dizziness, sensory disturbances (e.g., paresthesias such as electric shock sensations), anxiety, confusion, headache, lethargy, emotional lability, insomnia, and hypomania. While these events are generally self-limiting, there have been reports of serious discontinuation symptoms. Patients should be monitored for these symptoms when discontinuing treatment with fluoxetine. A gradual reduction in the dose rather than abrupt cessation is recommended whenever possible. If intolerable symptoms occur following a decrease in the dose or upon discontinuation of treatment, then resuming the previously prescribed dose may be considered. Subsequently, the physician may continue decreasing the dose but at a more gradual rate. Plasma fluoxetine and norfluoxetine concentration decrease gradually at the conclusion of therapy, which may minimize the risk of discontinuation symptoms with this drug (see DOSAGE AND ADMINISTRATION).

Dysphagia—Dysphagia was observed infrequently in SYMBYAX-treated patients in premarketing clinical studies. Nonetheless, like other psychotropic drugs, SYMBYAX should be used cautiously in patients at risk for aspiration pneumonia.

Esophageal dysmotility and aspiration have been associated with antipsychotic drug use. Aspiration pneumonia is a common cause of morbidity and mortality in patients with advanced Alzheimer's disease.

Half-Life—Because of the long elimination half-lives of fluoxetine and its major active metabolite, changes in dose will not be fully reflected in plasma for several weeks, affecting both strategies for titration to final dose and withdrawal from treatment (see CLINICAL PHARMACOLOGY, Accumulation and slow elimination).

Hyperprolactinemia—As with other drugs that antagonize dopamine D_2 receptors, SYMBYAX elevates prolactin levels, and a modest elevation persists during administration; however, possibly associated clinical manifestations (e.g., galactorrhea and breast enlargement) were infrequently observed.

Tissue culture experiments indicate that approximately one-third of human breast cancers are prolactin dependent in vitro, a factor of potential importance if the prescription of these drugs is contemplated in a patient with previously detected breast cancer of this type. Although disturbances such as galactorrhea, amenorrhea, gynecomastia, and impotence have been reported with prolactin-elevating compounds, the clinical significance of elevated serum prolactin levels is unknown for most patients. As is common with compounds that increase prolactin release, an increase in mammary gland neoplasia was observed in the olanzapine carcinogenicity studies conducted in mice and rats (see Carcinogenesis). However, neither clinical studies nor epidemiologic studies have shown an association between chronic administration of this class of drugs and tumorigenesis in humans; the available evidence is considered too limited to be conclusive.

Hyponatremia—Hyponatremia has been observed in SYMBYAX premarketing clinical studies. In controlled trials, no SYMBYAX-treated patients had a treatment-emergent serum sodium below 130 mmol/L; however, a lowering of serum sodium below the reference range occurred at an incidence of 2% (10/500) of SYMBYAX patients compared with 0.5% (2/380) of placebo patients. In open label studies, 0.3% (5/1889) of these SYMBYAX-treated patients had a treatment-emergent serum sodium below 130 mmol/L.

Cases of hyponatremia (some with serum sodium lower than 110 mmol/L) have been reported with fluoxetine. The hyponatremia appeared to be reversible when fluoxetine was discontinued. Although these cases were complex with varying possible etiologies, some were possibly due to the syndrome of inappropriate antidiuretic hormone secretion (SIADH). The majority of these occurrences have been in older patients and in patients taking diuretics or who were otherwise volume depleted. In two 6-week controlled studies in patients ≥60 years of age, 10 of 323 fluoxetine patients and 6 of 327 placebo recipients had a lowering of serum sodium below the reference range; this difference was not statistically significant. The lowest observed concentration was 129 mmol/L. The observed decreases were not clinically significant.

Seizures—Seizures occurred in 0.2% (4/2066) of SYMBYAX-treated patients during open-label premarketing clinical studies. No seizures occurred in the premarketing controlled SYMBYAX studies. Seizures have also been reported with both olanzapine and fluoxetine monotherapy. Therefore, SYMBYAX should be used cautiously in patients with a history of seizures or with conditions that potentially lower the seizure threshold. Conditions that lower the seizure threshold may be more prevalent in a population of ≥65 years of age.

Transaminase Elevations—As with olanzapine, asymptomatic elevations of hepatic transaminases [ALT (SGPT), AST (SGOT), and GGT] and alkaline phosphatase have been observed with SYMBYAX. In the SYMBYAX-controlled database, ALT (SGPT) elevations (≥3 times the upper limit of the normal range) were observed in 6.3% (31/495) of patients exposed to SYMBYAX compared with 0.5% (2/384) of the placebo patients and 4.5% (25/560) of olanzapine-treated patients. The difference between SYMBYAX and placebo was statistically significant. None of these 31 SYMBYAX-treated patients experienced jaundice and three had transient elevations >200 IU/L.

In olanzapine placebo-controlled studies, clinically significant ALT (SGPT) elevations (≥3 times the upper limit of the normal range) were observed in 2% (6/243) of patients exposed to olanzapine compared with 0% (0/115) of the placebo patients. None of these patients experienced jaundice. In 2 of these patients, liver enzymes decreased toward normal despite continued treatment, and in 2 others, enzymes decreased upon discontinuation of olanzapine. In the remaining 2 patients, 1, seropositive for hepatitis C, had persistent enzyme elevations for 4 months after discontinuation, and the other had insufficient follow-up to determine if enzymes normalized.

Within the larger olanzapine premarketing database of about 2400 patients with baseline SGPT ≤90 IU/L, the incidence of SGPT elevation to >200 IU/L was 2% (50/2381). Again, none of these patients experienced jaundice or other symptoms attributable to liver impairment and most had transient changes that tended to normalize while olanzapine treatment was continued. Among all 2500 patients in olanzapine clinical studies, approximately 1% (23/2500) discontinued treatment due to transaminase increases.

Caution should be exercised in patients with signs and symptoms of hepatic impairment, in patients with pre-existing conditions associated with limited hepatic functional reserve, and in patients who are being treated with potentially hepatotoxic drugs. Periodic assessment of transaminases is recommended in patients with significant hepatic disease (see Laboratory Tests).

Weight Gain—In clinical studies, the mean weight increase for SYMBYAX-treated patients was statistically significantly greater than placebo-treated (3.6 kg vs -0.3 kg) and fluoxetine-treated (3.6 kg vs -0.7 kg) patients, but was not statistically significantly different from olanzapine-treated patients (3.6 kg vs 3.0 kg). Fourteen percent of SYMBYAX-treated patients met criterion for having gained >10% of their baseline weight. This was statistically significantly greater than placebo-treated (<1%) and fluoxetine-treated patients (<1%) but was not statistically significantly different than olanzapine-treated patients (11%).

Use in Patients with Concomitant Illness

Clinical experience with SYMBYAX in patients with concomitant systemic illnesses is limited (see CLINICAL PHARMACOLOGY, Renal Impairment and Hepatic Impairment). The following precautions for the individual components may be applicable to SYMBYAX.

Olanzapine exhibits in vitro muscarinic receptor affinity. In premarketing clinical studies, SYMBYAX was associated with constipation, dry mouth, and tachycardia, all adverse events possibly related to cholinergic antagonism. Such adverse events were not often the basis for study discontinuations; SYMBYAX should be used with caution in patients with clinically significant prostatic hypertrophy, narrow angle glaucoma, a history of paralytic ileus, or related conditions.

In five placebo-controlled studies of olanzapine in elderly patients with dementia-related psychosis (n=1184), the following treatment-emergent adverse events were reported in olanzapine-treated patients at an incidence of at least 2% and significantly greater than placebo-treated patients: falls, somnolence, peripheral edema, abnormal gait, urinary incontinence, lethargy, increased weight, asthenia, pyrexia, pneumonia, dry mouth and visual hallucinations. The rate of discontinuation due to adverse events was significantly greater with olanzapine than placebo (13% vs 7%).

As with other CNS-active drugs, SYMBYAX should be used with caution in elderly patients with dementia. Olanzapine is not approved for the treatment of patients with dementia-related psychosis. If the prescriber elects to treat elderly patients with dementia-related psychosis, vigilance should be exercised (see BOX WARNING and WARNINGS).

SYMBYAX has not been evaluated or used to any appreciable extent in patients with a recent history of myocardial infarction or unstable heart disease. Patients with these diagnoses were excluded from clinical studies during the premarket testing.

Caution is advised when using SYMBYAX in cardiac patients and in patients with diseases or conditions that could affect hemodynamic responses (see WARNINGS, Orthostatic Hypotension).

In subjects with cirrhosis of the liver, the clearances of fluoxetine and its active metabolite, norfluoxetine, were decreased, thus increasing the elimination half-lives of these substances. A lower dose of the fluoxetine-component of SYMBYAX should be used in patients with cirrhosis. Caution is advised when using SYMBYAX in patients with diseases or conditions that could affect its metabolism (see CLINICAL PHARMACOLOGY, Hepatic Impairment and DOSING AND ADMINISTRATION, Special Populations).

Olanzapine and fluoxetine individual pharmacokinetics do not differ significantly in patients with renal impairment. SYMBYAX dosing adjustment based upon renal impairment is not routinely required (see CLINICAL PHARMACOLOGY, Renal Impairment).

Information for Patients

Prescribers or other health professionals should inform patients, their families, and their caregivers about the benefits and risks associated with treatment with SYMBYAX and should counsel them in its appropriate use. A patient Medication Guide About Using Antidepressants in Children and Teenagers is available for SYMBYAX. The prescriber or health professional should instruct patients, their families, and their caregivers to read the Medication Guide and should assist them in understanding its contents. Patients should be given the opportunity to discuss the contents of the Medication Guide and to obtain answers to any questions they may have. The complete text of the Medication Guide is reprinted at the end of this document. Patients should be advised of the following issues and asked to alert their prescriber if these occur while taking SYMBYAX.

Clinical Worsening and Suicide Risk—Patients their families, and their caregivers should be encouraged to be alert to the emergence of anxiety, agitation, panic attacks, insomnia, irritability, hostility, aggressiveness, impulsivity, akathisia (psychomotor restlessness), hypomania, mania, other unusual changes in behavior, worsening of depression, and suicidal ideation, especially early during antidepressant treatment and when the dose is adjusted up or down. Families and caregivers of patients should be advised to observe for the emergence of such symptoms on a day-to-day basis, since changes may be abrupt. Such symptoms should be reported to the patient's prescriber or health professional, especially if they are severe, abrupt in onset, or were not part of the patient's presenting symptoms. Symptoms such as these may be associated with an increased risk for suicidal thinking and behavior and indicate a need for very close monitoring and possibly changes in the medication.

Abnormal Bleeding—Patients should be cautioned about the concomitant use of SYMBYAX and NSAIDs, aspirin, or other drugs that affect coagulation since the combined use of psychotropic drugs that interfere with serotonin reuptake and these agents has been associated with an increased risk of bleeding (see PRECAUTIONS, Abnormal Bleeding).

Alcohol—Patients should be advised to avoid alcohol while taking SYMBYAX.

Cognitive and Motor Impairment—As with any CNS-active drug, SYMBYAX has the potential to impair judgment, thinking, or motor skills. Patients should be cautioned about operating hazardous machinery, including automobiles, until they are reasonably certain that SYMBYAX therapy does not affect them adversely.

Concomitant Medication—Patients should be advised to inform their physician if they are taking Prozac®, Prozac Weekly™, Sarafem®, fluoxetine, Zyprexa®, or Zyprexa Zydis®. Patients should also be advised to inform their physicians if they are taking or plan to take any prescription or over-the-counter drugs, including herbal supplements, since there is a potential for interactions.

Heat Exposure and Dehydration—Patients should be advised regarding appropriate care in avoiding overheating and dehydration.

Nursing—Patients, if taking SYMBYAX, should be advised not to breast-feed.

Orthostatic Hypotension—Patients should be advised of the risk of orthostatic hypotension, especially during the period of initial dose titration and in association with the use of concomitant drugs that may potentiate the orthostatic effect of olanzapine, e.g., diazepam or alcohol (see WARNINGS and Drug Interactions).

Pregnancy—Patients should be advised to notify their physician if they become pregnant or intend to become pregnant during SYMBYAX therapy.

Rash—Patients should be advised to notify their physician if they develop a rash or hives while taking SYMBYAX.

Treatment Adherence—Patients should be advised to take SYMBYAX exactly as prescribed, and to continue taking SYMBYAX as prescribed even after their mood symptoms improve. Patients should be advised that they should not alter their dosing regimen, or stop taking SYMBYAX, without consulting their physician.

Patient information is printed at the end of this insert. Physicians should discuss this information with their patients and instruct them to read the Medication Guide before starting therapy with SYMBYAX and each time their prescription is refilled.

Laboratory Tests

Periodic assessment of transaminases is recommended in patients with significant hepatic disease (see Transaminase Elevations).

Drug Interactions

The risks of using SYMBYAX in combination with other drugs have not been extensively evaluated in systematic studies. The drug-drug interactions of the individual components are applicable to SYMBYAX. As with all drugs, the potential for interaction by a variety of mechanisms (e.g., pharmacodynamic, pharmacokinetic drug inhibition or enhancement, etc.) is a possibility. Caution is advised if the concomitant administration of SYMBYAX and other CNS-active drugs is required. In evaluating individual cases, consideration should be given to using lower initial doses of the concomitantly administered drugs, using conservative titration schedules, and monitoring of clinical status (see CLINICAL PHARMACOLOGY, Accumulation and slow elimination).

Antihypertensive agents—Because of the potential for olanzapine to induce hypotension, SYMBYAX may enhance the effects of certain antihypertensive agents (see WARNINGS, Orthostatic Hypotension).

Anti-Parkinsonian—The olanzapine component of SYMBYAX may antagonize the effects of levodopa and dopamine agonists.

Benzodiazepines—Multiple doses of olanzapine did not influence the pharmacokinetics of diazepam and its active metabolite N-desmethyldiazepam. However, the coadministration of diazepam with olanzapine potentiated the orthostatic hypotension observed with olanzapine.

When concurrently administered with fluoxetine, the half-life of diazepam may be prolonged in some patients (see CLINICAL PHARMACOLOGY, Accumulation and slow elimination). Coadministration of alprazolam and fluoxetine has resulted in increased alprazolam plasma concentrations and in further psychomotor performance decrement due to increased alprazolam levels.

Biperiden—Multiple doses of olanzapine did not influence the pharmacokinetics of biperiden.

Carbamazepine—Carbamazepine therapy (200 mg BID) causes an approximate 50% increase in the clearance of olanzapine. This increase is likely due to the fact that carbamazepine is a potent inducer of CYP1A2 activity. Higher daily doses of carbamazepine may cause an even greater increase in olanzapine clearance.

Patients on stable doses of carbamazepine have developed elevated plasma anticonvulsant concentrations and clinical anticonvulsant toxicity following initiation of concomitant fluoxetine treatment.

Clozapine—Elevation of blood levels of clozapine has been observed in patients receiving concomitant fluoxetine.

Electroconvulsive therapy (ECT)—There are no clinical studies establishing the benefit of the combined use of ECT and fluoxetine. There have been rare reports of prolonged seizures in patients on fluoxetine receiving ECT treatment (see Seizures).

Ethanol—Ethanol (45 mg/70 kg single dose) did not have an effect on olanzapine pharmacokinetics. The coadministration of ethanol with SYMBYAX may potentiate sedation and orthostatic hypotension.

Fluvoxamine—Fluvoxamine, a CYP1A2 inhibitor, decreases the clearance of olanzapine. This results in a mean increase in olanzapine C_{max} following fluvoxamine administration of 54% in female nonsmokers and 77% in male smokers. The mean increase in olanzapine AUC is 52% and 108%, respectively. Lower doses of the olanzapine component of SYMBYAX should be considered in patients receiving concomitant treatment with fluvoxamine.

Haloperidol—Elevation of blood levels of haloperidol has been observed in patients receiving concomitant fluoxetine.

Lithium—Multiple doses of olanzapine did not influence the pharmacokinetics of lithium.

There have been reports of both increased and decreased lithium levels when lithium was used concomitantly with fluoxetine. Cases of lithium toxicity and increased serotonergic effects have been reported. Lithium levels should be monitored in patients taking SYMBYAX concomitantly with lithium.

Monoamine oxidase inhibitors—See CONTRAINDICATIONS.

Phenytoin—Patients on stable doses of phenytoin have developed elevated plasma levels of phenytoin with clinical phenytoin toxicity following initiation of concomitant fluoxetine.

Pimozide—A single case report has suggested possible additive effects of pimozide and fluoxetine leading to bradycardia.

Sumatriptan—There have been rare postmarketing reports describing patients with weakness, hyperreflexia, and incoordination following the use of an SSRI and sumatriptan. If concomitant treatment with sumatriptan and an SSRI (e.g., fluoxetine, fluvoxamine, paroxetine, sertraline, or citalopram) is clinically warranted, appropriate observation of the patient is advised.

Theophylline—Multiple doses of olanzapine did not affect the pharmacokinetics of theophylline or its metabolites.

Thioridazine—See CONTRAINDICATIONS and WARNINGS, Thioridazine.

Tricyclic antidepressants (TCAs)—Single doses of olanzapine did not affect the pharmacokinetics of imipramine or its active metabolite desipramine.

In two fluoxetine studies, previously stable plasma levels of imipramine and desipramine have increased >2- to 10-fold when fluoxetine has been administered in combination. This influence may persist for three weeks or longer after fluoxetine is discontinued. Thus, the dose of TCA may need to be reduced and plasma TCA concentrations may need to be monitored temporarily when SYMBYAX is coadministered or has been recently discontinued (see Drugs metabolized by CYP2D6 and CLINICAL PHARMACOLOGY, Accumulation and slow elimination).

Tryptophan—Five patients receiving fluoxetine in combination with tryptophan experienced adverse reactions, including agitation, restlessness, and gastrointestinal distress.

Valproate—In vitro studies using human liver microsomes determined that olanzapine has little potential to inhibit the major metabolic pathway, glucuronidation, of valproate. Further, valproate has little effect on the metabolism of olanzapine in vitro. Thus, a clinically significant pharmacokinetic interaction between olanzapine and valproate is unlikely.

Warfarin—Warfarin (20-mg single dose) did not affect olanzapine pharmacokinetics. Single doses of olanzapine did not affect the pharmacokinetics of warfarin.

Altered anticoagulant effects, including increased bleeding, have been reported when fluoxetine is coadministered with warfarin (see PRECAUTIONS, Abnormal Bleeding). Patients receiving warfarin therapy should receive careful coagulation monitoring when SYMBYAX is initiated or stopped.

Drugs that interfere with hemostasis (NSAIDs, aspirin, warfarin, etc.)—Serotonin release by platelets plays an important role in hemostasis. Epidemiological studies of the case-control and cohort design that have demonstrated an association between use of psychotropic drugs that interfere with serotonin reuptake and the occurrence of upper gastrointestinal bleeding have also shown that concurrent use of an NSAID or aspirin potentiated the risk of bleeding (see PRECAUTIONS, Abnormal Bleeding). Thus, patients should be cautioned about the use of such drugs concurrently with SYMBYAX.

Continued on next page

Symbyax—Cont.

Drugs metabolized by CYP2D6—In vitro studies utilizing human liver microsomes suggest that olanzapine has little potential to inhibit CYP2D6. Thus, olanzapine is unlikely to cause clinically important drug interactions mediated by this enzyme.

Approximately 7% of the normal population has a genetic variation that leads to reduced levels of activity of CYP2D6. Such individuals have been referred to as poor metabolizers of drugs such as debrisoquin, dextromethorphan, and TCAs. Many drugs, such as most antidepressants, including fluoxetine and other selective uptake inhibitors of serotonin, are metabolized by this isoenzyme; thus, both the pharmacokinetic properties and relative proportion of metabolites are altered in poor metabolizers. However, for fluoxetine and its metabolite, the sum of the plasma concentrations of the 4 enantiomers is comparable between poor and extensive metabolizers (*see* CLINICAL PHARMACOLOGY, Variability in metabolism).

Fluoxetine, like other agents that are metabolized by CYP2D6, inhibits the activity of this isoenzyme, and thus may make normal metabolizers resemble poor metabolizers. Therapy with medications that are predominantly metabolized by the CYP2D6 system and that have a relatively narrow therapeutic index should be initiated at the low end of the dose range if a patient is receiving fluoxetine concurrently or has taken it in the previous five weeks. If fluoxetine is added to the treatment regimen of a patient already receiving a drug metabolized by CYP2D6, the need for a decreased dose of the original medication should be considered. Drugs with a narrow therapeutic index represent the greatest concern (including but not limited to, flecainide, vinblastine, and TCAs). Due to the risk of serious ventricular arrhythmias and sudden death potentially associated with elevated thioridazine plasma levels, thioridazine should not be administered with fluoxetine or within a minimum of five weeks after fluoxetine has been discontinued (*see* CONTRAINDICATIONS, Monoamine Oxidase Inhibitors (MAOI) *and* WARNINGS, Thioridazine).

Drugs metabolized by CYP3A—In vitro studies utilizing human liver microsomes suggest that olanzapine has little potential to inhibit CYP3A. Thus, olanzapine is unlikely to cause clinically important drug interactions mediated by these enzymes.

In an in vivo interaction study involving the coadministration of fluoxetine with single doses of terfenadine (a CYP3A substrate), no increase in plasma terfenadine concentrations occurred with concomitant fluoxetine. In addition, in vitro studies have shown ketoconazole, a potent inhibitor of CYP3A activity, to be at least 100 times more potent than fluoxetine or norfluoxetine as an inhibitor of the metabolism of several substrates for this enzyme, including astemizole, cisapride, and midazolam. These data indicate that fluoxetine's extent of inhibition of CYP3A activity is not likely to be of clinical significance.

Effect of olanzapine on drugs metabolized by other CYP enzymes—In vitro studies utilizing human liver microsomes suggest that olanzapine has little potential to inhibit CYP1A2, CYP2C9, and CYP2C19. Thus, olanzapine is unlikely to cause clinically important drug interactions mediated by these enzymes.

The effect of other drugs on olanzapine—Fluoxetine, an inhibitor of CYP2D6, decreases olanzapine clearance a small amount (*see* CLINICAL PHARMACOLOGY, Pharmacokinetics). Agents that induce CYP1A2 or glucuronyl transferase enzymes, such as omeprazole and rifampin, may cause an increase in olanzapine clearance. Fluvoxamine, an inhibitor of CYP1A2, decreases olanzapine clearance (*see* Drug Interactions, Fluvoxamine). The effect of CYP1A2 inhibitors, such as fluvoxamine and some fluoroquinolone antibiotics, on SYMBYAX has not been evaluated. Although olanzapine is metabolized by multiple enzyme systems, induction or inhibition of a single enzyme may appreciably alter olanzapine clearance. Therefore, a dosage increase (for induction) or a dosage decrease (for inhibition) may need to be considered with specific drugs.

Drugs tightly bound to plasma proteins—The in vitro binding of SYMBYAX to human plasma proteins is similar to the individual components. The interaction between SYMBYAX and other highly protein-bound drugs has not been fully evaluated. Because fluoxetine is tightly bound to plasma protein, the administration of fluoxetine to a patient taking another drug that is tightly bound to protein (e.g., Coumadin, digitoxin) may cause a shift in plasma concentrations potentially resulting in an adverse effect. Conversely, adverse effects may result from displacement of protein-bound fluoxetine by other tightly bound drugs (*see* CLINICAL PHARMACOLOGY, Distribution *and* PRECAUTIONS, Drug Interactions).

Carcinogenesis, Mutagenesis, Impairment of Fertility

No carcinogenicity, mutagenicity, or fertility studies were conducted with SYMBYAX. The following data are based on findings in studies performed with the individual components.

Carcinogenesis

Olanzapine—Oral carcinogenicity studies were conducted in mice and rats. Olanzapine was administered to mice in two 78-week studies at doses of 3, 10, and 30/20 mg/kg/day [equivalent to 0.8 to 5 times the maximum recommended human daily dose (MRHD) on a mg/m^2 basis] and 0.25, 2, and 8 mg/kg/day (equivalent to 0.06 to 2 times the MRHD on a mg/m^2 basis). Rats were dosed for 2 years at doses of 0.25, 1, 2.5, and 4 mg/kg/day (males) and 0.25, 1, 4, and 8 mg/kg/day (females) (equivalent to 0.1 to 2 and 0.1 to 4 times the MRHD on a mg/m^2 basis, respectively). The incidence of liver hemangiomas and hemangiosarcomas was significantly increased in one mouse study in females dosed at 8 mg/kg/day (2 times the MRHD on a mg/m^2 basis). These tumors were not increased in another mouse study in females dosed at 10 or 30/20 mg/kg/day (2 to 5 times the MRHD on a mg/m^2 basis); in this study, there was a high incidence of early mortalities in males of the 30/20 mg/kg/day group. The incidence of mammary gland adenomas and adenocarcinomas was significantly increased in female mice dosed at ≥2 mg/kg/day and in female rats dosed at ≥4 mg/kg/day (0.5 and 2 times the MRHD on a mg/m^2 basis, respectively). Antipsychotic drugs have been shown to chronically elevate prolactin levels in rodents. Serum prolactin levels were not measured during the olanzapine carcinogenicity studies; however, measurements during subchronic toxicity studies showed that olanzapine elevated serum prolactin levels up to 4-fold in rats at the same doses used in the carcinogenicity study. An increase in mammary gland neoplasms has been found in rodents after chronic administration of other antipsychotic drugs and is considered to be prolactin-mediated. The relevance for human risk of the finding of prolactin-mediated endocrine tumors in rodents is unknown (*see* PRECAUTIONS, Hyperprolactinemia).

Fluoxetine—The dietary administration of fluoxetine to rats and mice for two years at doses of up to 10 and 12 mg/kg/day, respectively (approximately 1.2 and 0.7 times, respectively, the MRHD on a mg/m^2 basis), produced no evidence of carcinogenicity.

Mutagenesis

Olanzapine—No evidence of mutagenic potential for olanzapine was found in the Ames reverse mutation test, in vivo micronucleus test in mice, the chromosomal aberration test in Chinese hamster ovary cells, unscheduled DNA synthesis test in rat hepatocytes, induction of forward mutation test in mouse lymphoma cells, or in vivo sister chromatid exchange test in bone marrow of Chinese hamsters.

Fluoxetine—Fluoxetine and norfluoxetine have been shown to have no genotoxic effects based on the following assays: bacterial mutation assay, DNA repair assay in cultured rat hepatocytes, mouse lymphoma assay, and in vivo sister chromatid exchange assay in Chinese hamster bone marrow cells.

Impairment of Fertility

SYMBYAX—Fertility studies were not conducted with SYMBYAX. However, in a repeat-dose rat toxicology study of three months duration, ovary weight was decreased in females treated with the low-dose [2 and 4 mg/kg/day (1 and 0.5 times the MRHD on a mg/m^2 basis), respectively] and high-dose [4 and 8 mg/kg/day (2 and 1 times the MRHD on a mg/m^2 basis), respectively] combinations of olanzapine and fluoxetine. Decreased ovary weight, and corpora luteal depletion and uterine atrophy were observed to a greater extent in the females receiving the high-dose combination than in females receiving either olanzapine or fluoxetine alone. In a 3-month repeat-dose dog toxicology study, reduced epididymal sperm and reduced testicular and prostate weights were observed with the high-dose combination of olanzapine and fluoxetine [5 and 5 mg/kg/day (9 and 2 times the MRHD on a mg/m^2 basis), respectively] and with olanzapine alone (5 mg/kg/day or 9 times the MRHD on a mg/m^2 basis).

Olanzapine—In a fertility and reproductive performance study in rats, male mating performance, but not fertility, was impaired at a dose of 22.4 mg/kg/day and female fertility was decreased at a dose of 3 mg/kg/day (11 and 1.5 times the MRHD on a mg/m^2 basis, respectively). Discontinuance of olanzapine treatment reversed the effects on male-mating performance. In female rats, the precoital period was increased and the mating index reduced at 5 mg/kg/day (2.5 times the MRHD on a mg/m^2 basis). Diestrous was prolonged and estrous was delayed at 1.1 mg/kg/day (0.6 times the MRHD on a mg/m^2 basis); therefore, olanzapine may produce a delay in ovulation.

Fluoxetine—Two fertility studies conducted in adult rats at doses of up to 7.5 and 12.5 mg/kg/day (approximately 0.9 and 1.5 times the MRHD on a mg/m^2 basis) indicated that fluoxetine had no adverse effects on fertility (*see* ANIMAL TOXICOLOGY).

Pregnancy — Pregnancy Category C

SYMBYAX

Embryo fetal development studies were conducted in rats and rabbits with olanzapine and fluoxetine in low-dose and high-dose combinations. In rats, the doses were: 2 and 4 mg/kg/day (low-dose) [1 and 0.5 times the MRHD on a mg/m^2 basis, respectively], and 4 and 8 mg/kg/day (high-dose) [2 and 1 times the MRHD on a mg/m^2 basis, respectively]. In rabbits, the doses were 4 and 4 mg/kg/day (low-dose) [4 and 1 times the MRHD on a mg/m^2 basis, respectively], and 8 and 8 mg/kg/day (high-dose) [9 and 2 times the MRHD on a mg/m^2 basis, respectively]. In these studies, olanzapine and fluoxetine were also administered alone at the high-doses (4 and 8 mg/kg/day, respectively, in the rat; 8 and 8 mg/kg/day, respectively, in the rabbit). In the rabbit, there was no evidence of teratogenicity; however, the high-dose combination produced decreases in fetal weight and retarded skeletal ossification in conjunction with maternal toxicity. Similarly, in the rat there was no evidence of teratogenicity; however, a decrease in fetal weight was observed with the high-dose combination.

In a pre- and postnatal study conducted in rats, olanzapine and fluoxetine were administered during pregnancy and throughout lactation in combination (low-dose: 2 and 4 mg/kg/day [1 and 0.5 times the MRHD on a mg/m^2 basis], respectively, high-dose: 4 and 8 mg/kg/day [2 and 1 times the MRHD on a mg/m^2 basis], respectively, and alone: 4 and 8 mg/kg/day [2 and 1 times the MRHD on a mg/m^2 basis], respectively). Administration of the high-dose combination resulted in a marked elevation in offspring mortality and growth retardation in comparison to the same doses of olanzapine and fluoxetine administered alone. These effects were not observed with the low-dose combination; however, there were a few cases of testicular degeneration and atrophy, depletion of epididymal sperm and infertility in the male progeny. The effects of the high-dose combination on postnatal endpoints could not be assessed due to high progeny mortality.

There are no adequate and well-controlled studies with SYMBYAX in pregnant women.

SYMBYAX should be used during pregnancy only if the potential benefit justifies the potential risk to the fetus.

Olanzapine

In reproduction studies in rats at doses up to 18 mg/kg/day and in rabbits at doses up to 30 mg/kg/day (9 and 30 times the MRHD on a mg/m^2 basis, respectively), no evidence of teratogenicity was observed. In a rat teratology study, early resorptions and increased numbers of nonviable fetuses were observed at a dose of 18 mg/kg/day (9 times the MRHD on a mg/m^2 basis). Gestation was prolonged at 10 mg/kg/day (5 times the MRHD on a mg/m^2 basis). In a rabbit teratology study, fetal toxicity (manifested as increased resorptions and decreased fetal weight) occurred at a maternally toxic dose of 30 mg/kg/day (30 times the MRHD on a mg/m^2 basis).

Placental transfer of olanzapine occurs in rat pups.

There are no adequate and well-controlled clinical studies with olanzapine in pregnant women. Seven pregnancies were observed during premarketing clinical studies with olanzapine, including two resulting in normal births, one resulting in neonatal death due to a cardiovascular defect, three therapeutic abortions, and one spontaneous abortion.

Fluoxetine

In embryo fetal development studies in rats and rabbits, there was no evidence of teratogenicity following administration of up to 12.5 and 15 mg/kg/day, respectively (1.5 and 3.6 times the MRHD on a mg/m^2 basis, respectively) throughout organogenesis. However, in rat reproduction studies, an increase in stillborn pups, a decrease in pup weight, and an increase in pup deaths during the first 7 days postpartum occurred following maternal exposure to 12 mg/kg/day (1.5 times the MRHD on a mg/m^2 basis) during gestation or 7.5 mg/kg/day (0.9 times the MRHD on a mg/m^2 basis) during gestation and lactation. There was no evidence of developmental neurotoxicity in the surviving offspring of rats treated with 12 mg/kg/day during gestation. The no-effect dose for rat pup mortality was 5 mg/kg/day (0.6 times the MRHD on a mg/m^2 basis).

Nonteratogenic Effects—Neonates exposed to fluoxetine and other SSRIs or serotonin and norepinephrine reuptake inhibitors (SNRIs), late in the third trimester have developed complications requiring prolonged hospitalization, respiratory support, and tube feeding. Such complications can arise immediately upon delivery. Reported clinical findings have included respiratory distress, cyanosis, apnea, seizures, temperature instability, feeding difficulty, vomiting, hypoglycemia, hypotonia, hypertonia, hyperreflexia, tremor, jitteriness, irritability, and constant crying. These features are consistent with either a direct toxic effect of SSRIs and SNRIs or, possibly, a drug discontinuation syndrome. It should be noted that, in some cases, the clinical picture is consistent with serotonin syndrome (*see* CONTRAINDICATIONS, Monoamine Oxidase Inhibitors). When treating a pregnant woman with fluoxetine during the third trimester, the physician should carefully consider the potential risks and benefits of treatment (*see* DOSAGE AND ADMINISTRATION).

Labor and Delivery

SYMBYAX

The effect of SYMBYAX on labor and delivery in humans is unknown. Parturition in rats was not affected by SYMBYAX. SYMBYAX should be used during labor and delivery only if the potential benefit justifies the potential risk.

Olanzapine

Parturition in rats was not affected by olanzapine. The effect of olanzapine on labor and delivery in humans is unknown.

Fluoxetine

The effect of fluoxetine on labor and delivery in humans is unknown. Fluoxetine crosses the placenta; therefore, there is a possibility that fluoxetine may have adverse effects on the newborn.

Nursing Mothers

SYMBYAX

There are no adequate and well-controlled studies with SYMBYAX in nursing mothers or infants. No studies have been conducted to examine the excretion of olanzapine or fluoxetine in breast milk following SYMBYAX treatment. It is recommended that women not breast-feed when receiving SYMBYAX.

Olanzapine

Olanzapine was excreted in milk of treated rats during lactation.

Fluoxetine

Fluoxetine is excreted in human breast milk. In one breast milk sample, the concentration of fluoxetine plus norfluoxetine was 70.4 ng/mL. The concentration in the mother's plasma was 295.0 ng/mL. No adverse effects on the infant were reported. In another case, an infant nursed by a mother on fluoxetine developed crying, sleep disturbance, vomiting, and watery stools. The infant's plasma drug levels were 340 ng/mL of fluoxetine and 208 ng/mL of norfluoxetine on the 2nd day of feeding.

Pediatric Use

Safety and effectiveness in the pediatric population have not been established (*see* BOX WARNING *and* WARNINGS, Clinical Worsening and Suicide Risk *and* ANIMAL TOXICOLOGY). Anyone considering the use of SYMBYAX in a child or adolescent must balance the potential risks with the clinical need.

Geriatric Use

SYMBYAX

Clinical studies of SYMBYAX did not include sufficient numbers of patients ≥65 years of age to determine whether they respond differently from younger patients. Other reported clinical experience has not identified differences in responses between the elderly and younger patients. In general, dose selection for an elderly patient should be cautious, usually starting at the low end of the dosing range, reflecting the greater frequency of decreased hepatic, renal, or cardiac function, and of concomitant disease or other drug therapy (*see* DOSAGE AND ADMINISTRATION).

Olanzapine

Of the 2500 patients in premarketing clinical studies with olanzapine, 11% (263 patients) were ≥65 years of age. In patients with schizophrenia, there was no indication of any different tolerability of olanzapine in the elderly compared with younger patients. Studies in patients with dementia-related psychosis have suggested that there may be a different tolerability profile in this population compared with younger patients with schizophrenia. In placebo-controlled studies of olanzapine in elderly patients with dementia-related psychosis, there was a significantly higher incidence of cerebrovascular adverse events (e.g., stroke, transient ischemic attack) in patients treated with olanzapine compared to patients treated with placebo. Olanzapine is not approved for the treatment of patients with dementia-related psychosis. If the prescriber elects to treat elderly patients with dementia-related psychosis, vigilance should be exercised (*see* BOX WARNING, WARNINGS, PRECAUTIONS, Use in Patients with Concomitant Illness *and* DOSAGE AND ADMINISTRATION, Special Populations).

As with other CNS-active drugs, olanzapine should be used with caution in elderly patients with dementia. Also, the presence of factors that might decrease pharmacokinetic clearance or increase the pharmacodynamic response to olanzapine should lead to consideration of a lower starting dose for any geriatric patient.

Fluoxetine

US fluoxetine clinical studies (10,782 patients) included 687 patients ≥65 years of age and 93 patients ≥75 years of age. No overall differences in safety or effectiveness were observed between these subjects and younger subjects, and other reported clinical experience has not identified differences in responses between the elderly and younger patients, but greater sensitivity of some older individuals cannot be ruled out. As with other SSRIs, fluoxetine has been associated with cases of clinically significant hyponatremia in elderly patients.

ADVERSE REACTIONS

The information below is derived from a premarketing clinical study database for SYMBYAX consisting of 2066 patients with various diagnoses with approximately 1061 patient-years of exposure. The conditions and duration of treatment with SYMBYAX varied greatly and included (in overlapping categories) open-label and double-blind phases of studies, inpatients and outpatients, fixed-dose and dose-titration studies, and short-term or long-term exposure.

Adverse events were recorded by clinical investigators using descriptive terminology of their own choosing. Consequently, it is not possible to provide a meaningful estimate of the proportion of individuals experiencing adverse events without first grouping similar types of events into a limited (i.e., reduced) number of standardized event categories.

In the tables and tabulations that follow, COSTART Dictionary terminology has been used to classify reported adverse events. The data in the tables represent the proportion of individuals who experienced, at least once, a treatment-emergent adverse event of the type listed. An event was considered treatment-emergent if it occurred for the first time or worsened while receiving therapy following baseline evaluation. It is possible that events reported during therapy were not necessarily related to drug exposure.

The prescriber should be aware that the figures in the tables and tabulations cannot be used to predict the incidence of side effects in the course of usual medical practice where patient characteristics and other factors differ from those that prevailed in the clinical studies. Similarly, the cited frequencies cannot be compared with figures obtained from other clinical investigations involving different treatments, uses, and investigators. The cited figures, however, do provide the prescribing clinician with some basis for estimating the relative contribution of drug and non-drug factors to the side effect incidence rate in the population studied.

Incidence in Controlled Clinical Studies

The following findings are based on the short-term, controlled premarketing studies in various diagnoses including bipolar depression.

Adverse events associated with discontinuation of treatment—Overall, 10% of the patients in the SYMBYAX group discontinued due to adverse events compared with 4.6% for placebo. Table 2 enumerates the adverse events leading to discontinuation associated with the use of SYMBYAX (incidence of at least 1% for SYMBYAX and greater than that for placebo). The bipolar depression column shows the incidence of adverse events with SYMBYAX in the bipolar depression studies and the "SYMBYAX-Controlled" column shows the incidence in the controlled SYMBYAX studies; the placebo column shows the incidence in the pooled controlled studies that included a placebo arm.

Table 2: Adverse Events Associated with Discontinuation*

Adverse Event	Percentage of Patients Reporting Event		
	SYMBYAX		Placebo
	Bipolar Depression (N=86)	SYMBYAX-Controlled (N=571)	(N=477)
Asthenia	0	1	0
Somnolence	0	2	0
Weight gain	0	2	0
Chest pain	1	0	0

*Table includes events associated with discontinuation of at least 1% and greater than placebo

Commonly observed adverse events in controlled clinical studies—The most commonly observed adverse events associated with the use of SYMBYAX (incidence of ≥5% and at least twice that for placebo in the SYMBYAX-controlled database) were: asthenia, edema, increased appetite, peripheral edema, pharyngitis, somnolence, thinking abnormal, tremor, and weight gain.

Adverse events occurring at an incidence of 2% or more in controlled clinical studies—Table 3 enumerates the treatment-emergent adverse events associated with the use of SYMBYAX (incidence of at least 2% for SYMBYAX and twice or more that for placebo).

Table 3: Treatment-Emergent Adverse Events: Incidence in Controlled Clinical Studies

Body System/ Adverse Event[1]	Percentage of Patients Reporting Event		
	SYMBYAX		Placebo
	Bipolar Depression (N=86)	SYMBYAX-Controlled (N=571)	(N=477)
Body as a Whole			
Asthena	13	15	3
Accidental injury	5	3	2
Fever	4	3	1
Cardiovascular System			
Hypertension	2	2	1
Tachycardia	2	2	0
Digestive System			
Diarrhea	19	8	7
Dry Mouth	16	11	6
Increased appetite	13	16	4
Tooth disorder	1	2	1
Metabolic and Nutritional Disorders			
Weight gain	17	21	3
Peripheral edema	4	8	1
Edema	0	5	0
Musculoskeletal System			
Joint disorder	1	2	1
Twitching	6	2	1
Arthralgia	5	3	1
Nervous System			
Somnolence	21	22	11
Tremor	9	8	3
Thinking abnormal	6	6	3
Libido decreased	4	2	1
Hyperkinesia	2	1	1
Personality disorder	2	1	1
Sleep disorder	2	1	1
Amnesia	1	3	0
Respiratory System			
Pharyngitis	4	6	3
Dyspnea	1	2	1
Special Senses			
Ambylopia	5	4	2
Ear pain	2	1	1
Otitis media	2	0	0
Speech disorder	0	2	0
Urogenital System			
Abnormal ejaculation[2]	7	2	1
Impotence[2]	4	2	1
Anorgasmia	3	1	0

[1] Included are events reported by at least 2% of patients taking SYMBYAX except the following events, which had an incidence on placebo ≥SYMBYAX: abdominal pain, abnormal dreams, agitation, akathisia, anorexia, anxiety, apathy, back pain, chest pain, constipation, cough increased, depression, dizziness, dysmenorrhea[2], dyspepsia, flatulence, flu syndrome, headache, hypertonia, insomnia, manic reaction, myalgia, nausea, nervousness, pain, palpitation, paresthesia, rash, rhinitis, sinusitis, sweating, vomiting.

[2] Adjusted for gender.

Additional Findings Observed in Clinical Studies

The following findings are based on clinical studies.

Effect on cardiac repolarization—The mean increase in QT_c interval for SYMBYAX-treated patients (4.9 msec) in clinical studies was significantly greater than that for placebo-treated (-0.9 msec) and olanzapine-treated (0.6 msec) patients, but was not significantly different from fluoxetine-treated (3.7 msec) patients. There were no differences between patients treated with SYMBYAX, placebo, olanzapine, or fluoxetine in the incidence of QT_c outliers (>500 msec).

Laboratory changes—In SYMBYAX clinical studies, SYMBYAX was associated with asymptomatic mean increases in alkaline phosphatase, cholesterol, GGT, and uric acid compared with placebo (*see* PRECAUTIONS, Transaminase Elevations).

SYMBYAX was associated with a slight decrease in hemoglobin that was statistically significantly greater than that seen with placebo, olanzapine, and fluoxetine.

An elevation in serum prolactin was observed with SYMBYAX. This elevation was not statistically different than that seen with olanzapine (*see* PRECAUTIONS, Hyperprolactinemia).

In olanzapine clinical studies among olanzapine-treated patients with random triglyceride levels of <150 mg/dL at baseline (N=485), 0.6% of patients experienced triglyceride levels of ≥500 mg/dL anytime during the studies. In these same studies, olanzapine-treated patients (N=962) had a mean increase of 27 mg/dL in triglycerides from a mean baseline value of 185 mg/dL.

In olanzapine placebo-controlled studies, olanzapine-treated patients with random cholesterol levels of <200 mg/dL at baseline (N=1439) experienced cholesterol levels of ≥240 mg/dL anytime during the studies significantly more often than placebo-treated patients (N=836) (8.1% vs 3.8%, respectively). In these same studies, olanzapine-treated patients (N=2528) had a mean increase of 1 mg/dL in cholesterol from a mean baseline value of 203 mg/dL, which was significantly different compared to placebo-treated patients (N=1420) with a mean decrease of 4 mg/dL from a mean baseline value of 203 mg/dL.

Sexual dysfunction—In the pool of controlled SYMBYAX studies, there were higher rates of the treatment–emergent adverse events decreased libido, anorgasmia, impotence and abnormal ejaculation in the SYMBYAX group than in the placebo group. One case of decreased libido led to discontinuation in the SYMBYAX group. In the controlled studies that contained a fluoxetine arm, the rates of decreased libido and abnormal ejaculation in the SYMBYAX group were less than the rates in the fluoxetine group. None of the differences were statistically significant.

Sexual dysfunction, including priapism, has been reported with all SSRIs. While it is difficult to know the precise risk of sexual dysfunction associated with the use of SSRIs, physicians should routinely inquire about such possible side effects.

Continued on next page

Symbyax—Cont.

Vital signs—Tachycardia, bradycardia, and orthostatic hypotension have occurred in SYMBYAX-treated patients (*see* WARNINGS, Orthostatic Hypotension). The mean pulse of SYMBYAX-treated patients was reduced by 1.6 beats/min.

Other Events Observed in Clinical Studies

Following is a list of all treatment-emergent adverse events reported at anytime by individuals taking SYMBYAX in clinical studies except (1) those listed in the body or footnotes of Tables 2 and 3 above or elsewhere in labeling, (2) those for which the COSTART terms were uninformative or misleading, (3) those events for which a causal relationship to SYMBYAX use was considered remote, and (4) events occurring in only 1 patient treated with SYMBYAX and which did not have a substantial probability of being acutely life-threatening.

Events are classified within body system categories using the following definitions: frequent adverse events are defined as those occurring on 1 or more occasions in at least 1/100 patients, infrequent adverse events are those occurring in 1/100 to 1/1000 patients, and rare events are those occurring in <1/1000 patients.

Body as a Whole—*Frequent:* chills, infection, neck pain, neck rigidity, photosensitivity reaction; *Infrequent:* cellulitis, cyst, hernia, intentional injury, intentional overdose, malaise, moniliasis, overdose, pelvic pain, suicide attempt; *Rare:* death, tolerance decreased.

Cardiovascular System—*Frequent:* migraine, vasodilatation; *Infrequent:* arrhythmia, bradycardia, cerebral ischemia, electrocardiogram abnormal, hypotension, QT-interval prolonged; *Rare:* angina pectoris, atrial arrhythmia, atrial fibrillation, bundle branch block, congestive heart failure, myocardial infarct, peripheral vascular disorder, T-wave inverted.

Digestive System—*Frequent:* increased salivation, thirst; *Infrequent:* cholelithiasis, colitis, eructation, esophagitis, gastritis, gastroenteritis, gingivitis, hepatomegaly, nausea and vomiting, peptic ulcer, periodontal abscess, stomatitis, tooth caries; *Rare:* aphthous stomatitis, fecal incontinence, gastrointestinal hemorrhage, gum hemorrhage, intestinal obstruction, liver fatty deposit, pancreatitis.

Endocrine System—*Infrequent:* hypothyroidism.

Hemic and Lymphatic System—*Frequent:* ecchymosis; *Infrequent:* anemia, leukocytosis, lymphadenopathy; *Rare:* coagulation disorder, leukopenia, purpura, thrombocythemia.

Metabolic and Nutritional—*Frequent:* generalized edema, weight loss; *Infrequent:* alcohol intolerance, dehydration, glycosuria, hyperlipemia, hypoglycemia, hypokalemia, obesity; *Rare:* acidosis, bilirubinemia, creatinine increased, gout, hyperkalemia, hypoglycemic reaction.

Musculoskeletal System—*Infrequent:* arthritis, bone disorder, generalized spasm, leg cramps, tendinous contracture, tenosynovitis; *Rare:* arthrosis, bursitis, myasthenia, myopathy, osteoporosis, rheumatoid arthritis.

Nervous System—*Infrequent:* abnormal gait, ataxia, buccoglossal syndrome, cogwheel rigidity, coma, confusion, depersonalization, dysarthria, emotional lability, euphoria, extrapyramidal syndrome, hostility, hypesthesia, hypokinesia, incoordination, movement disorder, myoclonus, neuralgia, neurosis, vertigo; *Rare:* acute brain syndrome, aphasia, dystonia, libido increased, subarachnoid hemorrhage, withdrawal syndrome.

Respiratory System—*Frequent:* bronchitis, lung disorder; *Infrequent:* apnea, asthma, epistaxis, hiccup, hyperventilation, laryngitis, pneumonia, voice alteration, yawn; *Rare:* emphysema, hemoptysis, laryngismus.

Skin and Appendages—*Infrequent:* acne, alopecia, contact dermatitis, dry skin, eczema, pruritis, psoriasis, skin discoloration, vesiculobullous rash; *Rare:* exfoliative dermatitis, maculopapular rash, seborrhea, skin ulcer.

Special Senses—*Frequent:* abnormal vision, taste perversion, tinnitus; *Infrequent:* abnormality of accommodation, conjunctivitis, deafness, diplopia, dry eyes, eye pain, miosis; *Rare:* eye hemorrhage.

Urogenital System—*Frequent:* breast pain, menorrhagia[1], urinary frequency, urinary incontinence, urinary tract infection; *Infrequent:* amenorrhea[1], breast enlargement, breast neoplasm, cystitis, dysuria, female lactation[1], fibrocystic breast[1], hematuria, hypomenorrhea[1], leukorrhea[1], menopause[1], metrorrhagia[1], oliguria, ovarian disorder[1], polyuria, urinary retention, urinary urgency, urination impaired, vaginal hemorrhage[1], vaginal moniliasis[1], vaginitis[1]; *Rare:* breast carcinoma, breast engorgement, endometrial disorder[1], gynecomastia[1], kidney calculus, uterine fibroids enlarged[1].

[1] Adjusted for gender.

Other Events Observed with Olanzapine or Fluoxetine Monotherapy

The following adverse events were not observed in SYMBYAX-treated patients during premarketing clinical studies but have been reported with olanzapine or fluoxetine monotherapy: aplastic anemia, cholestatic jaundice, diabetic coma, dyskinesia, eosinophilic pneumonia, hepatitis, idiosyncratic hepatitis, priapism, pulmonary embolism, rhabdomyolysis, serotonin syndrome, serum sickness-like reaction, sudden unexpected death, suicidal ideation, vasculitis, venous thromboembolic events (including pulmonary embolism and deep venous thrombosis), violent behaviors. Random cholesterol levels of ≥240 mg/dL and random triglyceride levels of ≥1000 mg/dL have been rarely reported.

DRUG ABUSE AND DEPENDENCE

Controlled Substance Class—SYMBYAX is not a controlled substance.

Physical and Psychological—SYMBYAX, as with fluoxetine and olanzapine, has not been systematically studied in humans for its potential for abuse, tolerance, or physical dependence. While the clinical studies did not reveal any tendency for any drug-seeking behavior, these observations were not systematic, and it is not possible to predict on the basis of this limited experience the extent to which a CNS-active drug will be misused, diverted, and/or abused once marketed. Consequently, physicians should carefully evaluate patients for history of drug abuse and follow such patients closely, observing them for signs of misuse or abuse of SYMBYAX (e.g., development of tolerance, incrementation of dose, drug-seeking behavior).

In studies in rats and rhesus monkeys designed to assess abuse and dependence potential, olanzapine alone was shown to have acute depressive CNS effects but little or no potential of abuse or physical dependence at oral doses up to 15 (rat) and 8 (monkey) times the MRHD (20 mg) on a mg/m^2 basis.

OVERDOSAGE

SYMBYAX

During premarketing clinical studies of the olanzapine/fluoxetine combination, overdose of both fluoxetine and olanzapine were reported in five study subjects. Four of the five subjects experienced loss of consciousness (3) or coma (1). No fatalities occurred.

Since the market introduction of olanzapine in October 1996, adverse event cases involving combination use of fluoxetine and olanzapine have been reported to Eli Lilly and Company. An overdose of combination therapy is defined as confirmed or suspected ingestion of a dose of olanzapine 20 mg or greater in combination with a dose of fluoxetine 80 mg or greater. As of 1 February 2002, 12 cases of combination therapy overdose were reported, most of which involved additional substances. Adverse events associated with these reports included somnolence; impaired consciousness (coma, lethargy); impaired neurologic function (ataxia, confusion, convulsions, dysarthria); arrhythmias; and fatality. Fatalities have been confounded by exposure to additional substances including alcohol, thioridazine, oxycodone, and propoxyphene.

Olanzapine

In postmarketing reports of overdose with olanzapine alone, symptoms have been reported in the majority of cases. In symptomatic patients, symptoms with ≥10% incidence included agitation/aggressiveness, dysarthria, tachycardia, various extrapyramidal symptoms, and reduced level of consciousness ranging from sedation to coma. Among less commonly reported symptoms were the following potentially medically serious events: aspiration, cardiopulmonary arrest, cardiac arrhythmias (such as supraventricular tachycardia as well as a patient that experienced sinus pause with spontaneous resumption of normal rhythm), delirium, possible neuroleptic malignant syndrome, respiratory depression/arrest, convulsion, hypertension, and hypotension. Eli Lilly and Company has received reports of fatality in association with overdose of olanzapine alone. In 1 case of death, the amount of acutely ingested olanzapine was reported to be possibly as low as 450 mg; however, in another case, a patient was reported to survive an acute olanzapine ingestion of 1500 mg.

Fluoxetine

Worldwide exposure to fluoxetine is estimated to be over 38 million patients (circa 1999). Of the 1578 cases of overdose involving fluoxetine, alone or with other drugs, reported from this population, there were 195 deaths.

Among 633 adult patients who overdosed on fluoxetine alone, 34 resulted in a fatal outcome, 378 completely recovered, and 15 patients experienced sequelae after overdose, including abnormal accommodation, abnormal gait, confusion, unresponsiveness, nervousness, pulmonary dysfunction, vertigo, tremor, elevated blood pressure, impotence, movement disorder, and hypomania. The remaining 206 patients had an unknown outcome. The most common signs and symptoms associated with non-fatal overdose were seizures, somnolence, nausea, tachycardia, and vomiting. The largest known ingestion of fluoxetine in adult patients was 8 grams in a patient who took fluoxetine alone and who subsequently recovered. However, in an adult patient who took fluoxetine alone, an ingestion as low as 520 mg has been associated with lethal outcome, but causality has not been established.

Among pediatric patients (ages 3 months to 17 years), there were 156 cases of overdose involving fluoxetine alone or in combination with other drugs. Six patients died, 127 patients completely recovered, 1 patient experienced renal failure, and 22 patients had an unknown outcome. One of the 6 fatalities was a 9-year-old boy who had a history of OCD, Tourette's Syndrome with tics, attention deficit disorder, and fetal alcohol syndrome. He had been receiving 100 mg of fluoxetine daily for 6 months in addition to clonidine, methylphenidate, and promethazine. Mixed-drug ingestion or other methods of suicide complicated all 6 overdoses in children that resulted in fatalities. The largest ingestion in pediatric patients was 3 grams, which was nonlethal.

Other important adverse events reported with fluoxetine overdose (single or multiple drugs) included coma, delirium, ECG abnormalities (such as QT-interval prolongation and ventricular tachycardia, including torsades de pointes-type arrhythmias), hypotension, mania, neuroleptic malignant syndrome-like events, pyrexia, stupor, and syncope.

Management of Overdose—In managing overdose, the possibility of multiple drug involvement should be considered. In case of acute overdose, establish and maintain an airway and ensure adequate ventilation, which may include intubation. Induction of emesis is not recommended as the possibility of obtundation, seizures, or dystonic reactions of the head and neck following overdose may create a risk for aspiration. Gastric lavage (after intubation, if patient is unconscious) and administration of activated charcoal together with a laxative should be considered. Cardiovascular monitoring should commence immediately and should include continuous electrocardiographic monitoring to detect possible arrhythmias.

A specific precaution involves patients who are taking or have recently taken SYMBYAX and may have ingested excessive quantities of a TCA (tricyclic antidepressant). In such cases, accumulation of the parent TCA and/or an active metabolite may increase the possibility of serious sequelae and extend the time needed for close medical observation.

Due to the large volume of distribution of olanzapine and fluoxetine, forced diuresis, dialysis, hemoperfusion, and exchange transfusion are unlikely to be of benefit. No specific antidote for either fluoxetine or olanzapine overdose is known. Hypotension and circulatory collapse should be treated with appropriate measures such as intravenous fluids and/or sympathomimetic agents. Do not use epinephrine, dopamine, or other sympathomimetics with β-agonist activity, since beta stimulation may worsen hypotension in the setting of olanzapine-induced alpha blockade.

The physician should consider contacting a poison control center for additional information on the treatment of any overdose. Telephone numbers for certified poison control centers are listed in the *Physicians' Desk Reference (PDR)*.

DOSAGE AND ADMINISTRATION

SYMBYAX should be administered once daily in the evening, generally beginning with the 6-mg/25-mg capsule. While food has no appreciable effect on the absorption of olanzapine and fluoxetine given individually, the effect of food on the absorption of SYMBYAX has not been studied. Dosage adjustments, if indicated, can be made according to efficacy and tolerability. Antidepressant efficacy was demonstrated with SYMBYAX in a dose range of olanzapine 6 to 12 mg and fluoxetine 25 to 50 mg (*see* CLINICAL STUDIES).

The safety of doses above 18 mg/75 mg has not been evaluated in clinical studies.

Special Populations

The starting dose of SYMBYAX 6 mg/25 mg should be used for patients with a predisposition to hypotensive reactions, patients with hepatic impairment, or patients who exhibit a combination of factors that may slow the metabolism of SYMBYAX (female gender, geriatric age, nonsmoking status). When indicated, dose escalation should be performed with caution in these patients. SYMBYAX has not been systematically studied in patients over 65 years of age or in patients <18 years of age (*see* WARNINGS, Orthostatic Hypotension, PRECAUTIONS, Pediatric Use, *and* Geriatric Use, *and* CLINICAL PHARMACOLOGY, Pharmacokinetics).

Treatment of Pregnant Women During the Third Trimester

Neonates exposed to fluoxetine, a component of SYMBYAX, and other SSRIs or SNRIs, late in the third trimester have developed complications requiring prolonged hospitalization, respiratory support, and tube feeding (*see* PRECAUTIONS). When treating pregnant women with fluoxetine during the third trimester, the physician should carefully consider the potential risks and benefits of treatment. The physician may consider tapering fluoxetine in the third trimester.

Discontinuation of Treatment with SYMBYAX

Symptoms associated with discontinuation of fluoxetine, a component of SYMBYAX, and other SSRIs and SNRIs, have been reported (*see* PRECAUTIONS). Patients should be monitored for these symptoms when discontinuing treatment. A gradual reduction in the dose rather than abrupt cessation is recommended whenever possible. If intolerable symptoms occur following a decrease in the dose or upon discontinuation of treatment, then resuming the previously prescribed dose may be considered. Subsequently, the physician may continue decreasing the dose but at a more gradual rate. Plasma fluoxetine and norfluoxetine concentration decrease gradually at the conclusion of therapy which may minimize the risk of discontinuation symptoms with this drug.

HOW SUPPLIED

SYMBYAX capsules are supplied in 6/25-, 6/50-, 12/25-, and 12/50-mg (mg equivalent olanzapine/mg equivalent fluoxetine[a]) strengths.

[See table at top of next page]

Store at 25°C (77°F); excursions permitted to 15–30°C (59–86°F) [see USP Controlled Room Temperature].

Keep tightly closed and protect from moisture.

ANIMAL TOXICOLOGY

Fluoxetine—In a juvenile toxicology study in CD rats, administration of 30 mg/kg of fluoxetine hydrochloride on postnatal days 21 through 90 resulted in increased serum activities of creatine kinase (CK) and aspartate aminotransferase (AST), which were accompanied microscopically by skeletal muscle degeneration, necrosis and regeneration. Other findings in rats administered 30 mg/kg included degeneration and necrosis of seminiferous tubules of the testis, epididymal epithelial vacuolation, and immaturity and inactivity of the female reproductive tract. Plasma levels

SYMBYAX	CAPSULE STRENGTH			
	6 mg/25 mg	6 mg/50 mg	12 mg/25 mg	12 mg/50 mg
Color	Mustard Yellow & Light Yellow	Mustard Yellow & Light Grey	Red & Light Yellow	Red & Light Grey
Capsule No.	PU3231	PU3233	PU3232	PU3234
Identification	Lilly 3231 6/25	Lilly 3233 6/50	Lilly 3232 12/25	Lilly 3234 12/50
NDC Codes				
Bottles 30	0002-3231-30	0002-3233-30	0002-3232-30	0002-3234-30
Bottles 100	0002-3231-02	0002-3233-02	0002-3232-02	0002-3234-02
Bottles 1000	0002-3231-04	0002-3233-04	0002-3232-04	0002-3234-04
Blisters ID[b] 100	0002-3231-33	0002-3233-33	0002-3232-33	0002-3234-33

[a] Fluoxetine base equivalent.
[b] IDENTI-DOSE®, Unit Dose Medication, Lilly.

achieved in these animals at 30 mg/kg were approximately 5- to 8-fold (fluoxetine) and 18- to 20-fold (norfluoxetine), and at 10 mg/kg approximately 2-fold (fluoxetine) and 8-fold (norfluoxetine) higher compared to plasma concentrations usually achieved in pediatric patients. Following an approximate 11-week recovery period, sperm 32 assessments in the 30-mg/kg males only, indicated an approximately 30% decrease in sperm concentrations without affecting sperm morphology or motility. Microscopic evaluation of testes and epididymides of these 30-mg/kg males indicated that testicular degeneration was irreversible. Delays in sexual maturation occurred in the 10-mg/kg males and in the 30-mg/kg males and females. The significance of these findings in humans is unknown. Femur lengths at 30 mg/kg increased to a lesser extent compared with control rats.

Medication Guide

About Using Antidepressants in Children and Teenagers

What is the most important information I should know if my child is being prescribed an antidepressant?

Parents or guardians need to think about 4 important things when their child is prescribed an antidepressant:

1. There is a risk of suicidal thoughts or actions
2. How to try to prevent suicidal thoughts or actions in your child
3. You should watch for certain signs if your child is taking an antidepressant
4. There are benefits and risks when using antidepressants

1. There is a Risk of Suicidal Thoughts or Actions

Children and teenagers sometimes think about suicide, and many report trying to kill themselves.

Antidepressants increase suicidal thoughts and actions in some children and teenagers. But suicidal thoughts and actions can also be caused by depression, a serious medical condition that is commonly treated with antidepressants. Thinking about killing yourself or trying to kill yourself is called *suicidality* or *being suicidal*.

A large study combined the results of 24 different studies of children and teenagers with depression or other illnesses. In these studies, patients took either a placebo (sugar pill) or an antidepressant for 1 to 4 months. ***No one committed suicide in these studies,*** but some patients became suicidal. On sugar pills, 2 out of every 100 became suicidal. On the antidepressants, 4 out of every 100 patients became suicidal.

For some children and teenagers, the risks of suicidal actions may be especially high. These include patients with

- Bipolar illness (sometimes called manic-depressive illness)
- A family history of bipolar illness
- A personal or family history of attempting suicide

If any of these are present, make sure you tell your health care provider before your child takes an antidepressant.

2. How to Try to Prevent Suicidal Thoughts and Actions

To try to prevent suicidal thoughts and actions in your child, pay close attention to changes in her or his moods or actions, especially if the changes occur suddenly. Other important people in your child's life can help by paying attention as well (e.g., your child, brothers and sisters, teachers, and other important people). The changes to look out for are listed in Section 3, on what to watch for.

Whenever an antidepressant is started or its dose is changed, pay close attention to your child.

After starting an antidepressant, your child should generally see his or her health care provider

- Once a week for the first 4 weeks
- Every 2 weeks for the next 4 weeks
- After taking the antidepressant for 12 weeks
- After 12 weeks, follow your health care provider's advice about how often to come back
- More often if problems or questions arise (see Section 3)

You should call your child's health care provider between visits if needed.

3. You Should Watch for Certain Signs If Your Child is Taking an Antidepressant

Contact your child's health care provider ***right away*** if your child exhibits any of the following signs for the first time, or if they seem worse, or worry you, your child, or your child's teacher:

- Thoughts about suicide or dying
- Attempts to commit suicide
- New or worse depression
- New or worse anxiety
- Feeling very agitated or restless
- Panic attacks
- Difficulty sleeping (insomnia)
- New or worse irritability
- Acting aggressive, being angry, or violent
- Acting on dangerous impulses
- An extreme increase in activity and talking
- Other unusual changes in behavior or mood

Never let your child stop taking an antidepressant without first talking to his or her health care provider. Stopping an antidepressant suddenly can cause other symptoms.

4. There are Benefits and Risks When Using Antidepressants

Antidepressants are used to treat depression and other illnesses. Depression and other illnesses can lead to suicide. In some children and teenagers, treatment with an antidepressant increases suicidal thinking or actions. It is important to discuss all the risks of treating depression and also the risks of not treating it. You and your child should discuss all treatment choices with your health care provider, not just the use of antidepressants.

Other side effects can occur with antidepressants (see section below).

Of all the antidepressants, only fluoxetine (Prozac®) has been FDA approved to treat pediatric depression.

For obsessive compulsive disorder in children and teenagers, FDA has approved only fluoxetine (Prozac®), sertraline (Zoloft®), fluvoxamine, and clomipramine (Anafranil®).

Your health care provider may suggest other antidepressants based on the past experience of your child or other family members.

Is this all I need to know if my child is being prescribed an antidepressant?

No. This is a warning about the risk for suicidality. Other side effects can occur with antidepressants. Be sure to ask your health care provider to explain all the side effects of the particular drug he or she is prescribing. Also ask about drugs to avoid when taking an antidepressant. Ask your health care provider or pharmacist where to find more information.

Prozac® is a registered trademark of Eli Lilly and Company.
Zoloft® is a registered trademark of Pfizer Pharmaceuticals.
Anafranil® is a registered trademark of Mallinckrodt Inc.

This Medication Guide has been approved by the US Food and Drug Administration for all antidepressants.

Rx only

Literature revised April 26, 2005
Eli Lilly and Company
Indianapolis, IN 46285
www.SYMBYAX.com
8.01 PV 4208 AMP PRINTED IN USA

ZYPREXA® ℞

[zī-prex-ah]

Olanzapine Tablets

ZYPREXA® ZYDIS®

Olanzapine Orally Disintegrating Tablets

ZYPREXA® IntraMuscular

Olanzapine for Injection

Prescribing information for this product, which appears on pages 1899–1906 of the 2005 PDR, has been completely revised as follows. Please write "See Supplement A" next to the product heading.

WARNING

Increased Mortality in Elderly Patients with Dementia-Related Psychosis — Elderly patients with dementia-related psychosis treated with atypical antipsychotic drugs are at an increased risk of death compared to placebo. Analyses of seventeen placebo-controlled trials (modal duration of 10 weeks) in these patients revealed a risk of death in the drug-treated patients of between 1.6 to 1.7 times that seen in placebo-treated patients. Over the course of a typical 10-week controlled trial, the rate of death in drug-treated patients was about 4.5%, compared to a rate of about 2.6% in the placebo group. Although the causes of death were varied, most of the deaths appeared to be either cardiovascular (e.g., heart failure, sudden death) or infectious (e.g., pneumonia) in nature. ZYPREXA (olanzapine) is not approved for the treatment of patients with dementia-related psychosis (*see* WARNINGS).

DESCRIPTION

ZYPREXA (olanzapine) is a psychotropic agent that belongs to the thienobenzodiazepine class. The chemical designation is 2-methyl-4-(4-methyl-1-piperazinyl)-10*H*-thieno[2,3-*b*][1,5]benzodiazepine. The molecular formula is $C_{17}H_{20}N_4S$, which corresponds to a molecular weight of 312.44. The chemical structure is:

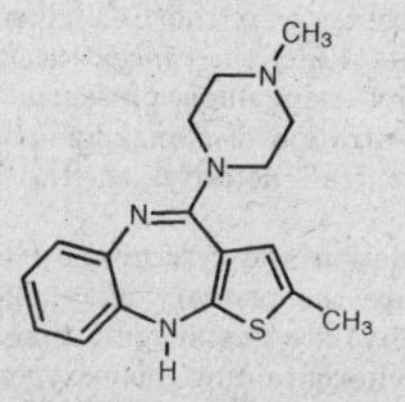

Olanzapine is a yellow crystalline solid, which is practically insoluble in water.

ZYPREXA tablets are intended for oral administration only.

Each tablet contains olanzapine equivalent to 2.5 mg (8 μmol), 5 mg (16 μmol), 7.5 mg (24 μmol), 10 mg (32 μmol), 15 mg (48 μmol), or 20 mg (64 μmol). Inactive ingredients are carnauba wax, crospovidone, hydroxypropyl cellulose, hypromellose, lactose, magnesium stearate, microcrystalline cellulose, and other inactive ingredients. The color coating contains Titanium Dioxide (all strengths), FD&C Blue No. 2 Aluminum Lake (15 mg), or Synthetic Red Iron Oxide (20 mg). The 2.5, 5.0, 7.5, and 10 mg tablets are imprinted with edible ink which contains FD&C Blue No. 2 Aluminum Lake.

ZYPREXA ZYDIS (olanzapine orally disintegrating tablets) is intended for oral administration only.

Each orally disintegrating tablet contains olanzapine equivalent to 5 mg (16 μmol), 10 mg (32 μmol), 15 mg (48 μmol) or 20 mg (64 μmol). It begins disintegrating in the mouth within seconds, allowing its contents to be subsequently swallowed with or without liquid. ZYPREXA ZYDIS (olanzapine orally disintegrating tablets) also contains the following inactive ingredients: gelatin, mannitol, aspartame, sodium methyl paraben and sodium propyl paraben.

ZYPREXA IntraMuscular (olanzapine for injection) is intended for intramuscular use only. Each vial provides for the administration of 10 mg (32 μmol) olanzapine with inactive ingredients 50 mg lactose monohydrate and 3.5 mg tartaric acid. Hydrochloric acid and/or sodium hydroxide may have been added during manufacturing to adjust pH.

CLINICAL PHARMACOLOGY

Pharmacodynamics

Olanzapine is a selective monoaminergic antagonist with high affinity binding to the following receptors: serotonin $5HT_{2A/2C}$ (K_i=4 and 11 nM, respectively), dopamine D_{1-4} (K_i=11-31 nM), muscarinic M_{1-5} (K_i=1.9-25 nM), histamine H_1 (K_i=7 nM), and adrenergic α_1 receptors (K_i=19 nM). Olanzapine binds weakly to $GABA_A$, BZD, and β adrenergic receptors (K_i>10 μM).

The mechanism of action of olanzapine, as with other drugs having efficacy in schizophrenia, is unknown. However, it has been proposed that this drug's efficacy in schizophrenia is mediated through a combination of dopamine and serotonin type 2 ($5HT_2$) antagonism. The mechanism of action of olanzapine in the treatment of acute manic episodes associated with Bipolar I Disorder is unknown.

Antagonism at receptors other than dopamine and $5HT_2$ with similar receptor affinities may explain some of the other therapeutic and side effects of olanzapine. Olanzapine's antagonism of muscarinic M_{1-5} receptors may explain its anticholinergic effects. Olanzapine's antagonism of histamine H_1 receptors may explain the somnolence observed with this drug. Olanzapine's antagonism of adrenergic α_1 receptors may explain the orthostatic hypotension observed with this drug.

Pharmacokinetics

Oral Administration

Olanzapine is well absorbed and reaches peak concentrations in approximately 6 hours following an oral dose. It is eliminated extensively by first pass metabolism, with approximately 40% of the dose metabolized before reaching the systemic circulation. Food does not affect the rate or extent of olanzapine absorption. Pharmacokinetic studies showed that ZYPREXA tablets and ZYPREXA ZYDIS (olanzapine orally disintegrating tablets) dosage forms of olanzapine are bioequivalent.

Olanzapine displays linear kinetics over the clinical dosing range. Its half-life ranges from 21 to 54 hours (5th to 95th percentile; mean of 30 hr), and apparent plasma clearance ranges from 12 to 47 L/hr (5th to 95th percentile; mean of 25 L/hr).

Administration of olanzapine once daily leads to steady-state concentrations in about one week that are approxi-

Continued on next page

Zyprexa—Cont.

mately twice the concentrations after single doses. Plasma concentrations, half-life, and clearance of olanzapine may vary between individuals on the basis of smoking status, gender, and age (see Special Populations).

Olanzapine is extensively distributed throughout the body, with a volume of distribution of approximately 1000 L. It is 93% bound to plasma proteins over the concentration range of 7 to 1100 ng/mL, binding primarily to albumin and α_1-acid glycoprotein.

Metabolism and Elimination — Following a single oral dose of ^{14}C labeled olanzapine, 7% of the dose of olanzapine was recovered in the urine as unchanged drug, indicating that olanzapine is highly metabolized. Approximately 57% and 30% of the dose was recovered in the urine and feces, respectively. In the plasma, olanzapine accounted for only 12% of the AUC for total radioactivity, indicating significant exposure to metabolites. After multiple dosing, the major circulating metabolites were the 10-N-glucuronide, present at steady state at 44% of the concentration of olanzapine, and 4'-N-desmethyl olanzapine, present at steady state at 31% of the concentration of olanzapine. Both metabolites lack pharmacological activity at the concentrations observed.

Direct glucuronidation and cytochrome P450 (CYP) mediated oxidation are the primary metabolic pathways for olanzapine. In vitro studies suggest that CYPs 1A2 and 2D6, and the flavin-containing monooxygenase system are involved in olanzapine oxidation. CYP2D6 mediated oxidation appears to be a minor metabolic pathway in vivo, because the clearance of olanzapine is not reduced in subjects who are deficient in this enzyme.

Intramuscular Administration

ZYPREXA IntraMuscular results in rapid absorption with peak plasma concentrations occurring within 15 to 45 minutes. Based upon a pharmacokinetic study in healthy volunteers, a 5 mg dose of intramuscular olanzapine for injection produces, on average, a maximum plasma concentration approximately 5 times higher than the maximum plasma concentration produced by a 5 mg dose of oral olanzapine. Area under the curve achieved after an intramuscular dose is similar to that achieved after oral administration of the same dose. The half-life observed after intramuscular administration is similar to that observed after oral dosing. The pharmacokinetics are linear over the clinical dosing range. Metabolic profiles after intramuscular administration are qualitatively similar to metabolic profiles after oral administration.

Special Populations

Renal Impairment — Because olanzapine is highly metabolized before excretion and only 7% of the drug is excreted unchanged, renal dysfunction alone is unlikely to have a major impact on the pharmacokinetics of olanzapine. The pharmacokinetic characteristics of olanzapine were similar in patients with severe renal impairment and normal subjects, indicating that dosage adjustment based upon the degree of renal impairment is not required. In addition, olanzapine is not removed by dialysis. The effect of renal impairment on metabolite elimination has not been studied.

Hepatic Impairment — Although the presence of hepatic impairment may be expected to reduce the clearance of olanzapine, a study of the effect of impaired liver function in subjects (n=6) with clinically significant (Childs Pugh Classification A and B) cirrhosis revealed little effect on the pharmacokinetics of olanzapine.

Age — In a study involving 24 healthy subjects, the mean elimination half-life of olanzapine was about 1.5 times greater in elderly (>65 years) than in non-elderly subjects (≤65 years). Caution should be used in dosing the elderly, especially if there are other factors that might additively influence drug metabolism and/or pharmacodynamic sensitivity (see DOSAGE AND ADMINISTRATION).

Gender — Clearance of olanzapine is approximately 30% lower in women than in men. There were, however, no apparent differences between men and women in effectiveness or adverse effects. Dosage modifications based on gender should not be needed.

Smoking Status — Olanzapine clearance is about 40% higher in smokers than in nonsmokers, although dosage modifications are not routinely recommended.

Race — In vivo studies have shown that exposures are similar among Japanese, Chinese and Caucasians, especially after normalization for body weight differences. Dosage modifications for race are, therefore, not recommended.

Combined Effects — The combined effects of age, smoking, and gender could lead to substantial pharmacokinetic differences in populations. The clearance in young smoking males, for example, may be 3 times higher than that in elderly nonsmoking females. Dosing modification may be necessary in patients who exhibit a combination of factors that may result in slower metabolism of olanzapine (see DOSAGE AND ADMINISTRATION).

For specific information about the pharmacology of lithium or valproate, refer to the CLINICAL PHARMACOLOGY section of the package inserts for these other products.

Clinical Efficacy Data

Schizophrenia

The efficacy of oral olanzapine in the treatment of schizophrenia was established in 2 short-term (6-week) controlled trials of inpatients who met DSM III-R criteria for schizophrenia. A single haloperidol arm was included as a comparative treatment in one of the two trials, but this trial did not compare these two drugs on the full range of clinically relevant doses for both.

Several instruments were used for assessing psychiatric signs and symptoms in these studies, among them the Brief Psychiatric Rating Scale (BPRS), a multi-item inventory of general psychopathology traditionally used to evaluate the effects of drug treatment in schizophrenia. The BPRS psychosis cluster (conceptual disorganization, hallucinatory behavior, suspiciousness, and unusual thought content) is considered a particularly useful subset for assessing actively psychotic schizophrenic patients. A second traditional assessment, the Clinical Global Impression (CGI), reflects the impression of a skilled observer, fully familiar with the manifestations of schizophrenia, about the overall clinical state of the patient. In addition, two more recently developed scales were employed; these included the 30-item Positive and Negative Symptoms Scale (PANSS), in which are embedded the 18 items of the BPRS, and the Scale for Assessing Negative Symptoms (SANS). The trial summaries below focus on the following outcomes: PANSS total and/or BPRS total; BPRS psychosis cluster; PANSS negative subscale or SANS; and CGI Severity. The results of the trials follow:

(1) In a 6-week, placebo-controlled trial (n=149) involving two fixed olanzapine doses of 1 and 10 mg/day (once daily schedule), olanzapine, at 10 mg/day (but not at 1 mg/day), was superior to placebo on the PANSS total score (also on the extracted BPRS total), on the BPRS psychosis cluster, on the PANSS Negative subscale, and on CGI Severity.

(2) In a 6-week, placebo-controlled trial (n=253) involving 3 fixed dose ranges of olanzapine (5.0 ± 2.5 mg/day, 10.0 ± 2.5 mg/day, and 15.0 ± 2.5 mg/day) on a once daily schedule, the two highest olanzapine dose groups (actual mean doses of 12 and 16 mg/day, respectively) were superior to placebo on BPRS total score, BPRS psychosis cluster, and CGI severity score; the highest olanzapine dose group was superior to placebo on the SANS. There was no clear advantage for the high dose group over the medium dose group.

Examination of population subsets (race and gender) did not reveal any differential responsiveness on the basis of these subgroupings.

In a longer-term trial, adult outpatients (n=326) who predominantly met DSM-IV criteria for schizophrenia and who remained stable on olanzapine during open label treatment for at least 8 weeks were randomized to continuation on their current olanzapine doses (ranging from 10 to 20 mg/day) or to placebo. The follow-up period to observe patients for relapse, defined in terms of increases in BPRS positive symptoms or hospitalization, was planned for 12 months, however, criteria were met for stopping the trial early due to an excess of placebo relapses compared to olanzapine relapses, and olanzapine was superior to placebo on time to relapse, the primary outcome for this study. Thus, olanzapine was more effective than placebo at maintaining efficacy in patients stabilized for approximately 8 weeks and followed for an observation period of up to 8 months.

Bipolar Disorder

Monotherapy — The efficacy of oral olanzapine in the treatment of acute manic or mixed episodes was established in 2 short-term (one 3-week and one 4-week) placebo-controlled trials in patients who met the DSM-IV criteria for Bipolar I Disorder with manic or mixed episodes. These trials included patients with or without psychotic features and with or without a rapid-cycling course.

The primary rating instrument used for assessing manic symptoms in these trials was the Young Mania Rating Scale (Y-MRS), an 11-item clinician-rated scale traditionally used to assess the degree of manic symptomatology (irritability, disruptive/aggressive behavior, sleep, elevated mood, speech, increased activity, sexual interest, language/thought disorder, thought content, appearance, and insight) in a range from 0 (no manic features) to 60 (maximum score). The primary outcome in these trials was change from baseline in the Y-MRS total score. The results of the trials follow:

(1) In one 3-week placebo-controlled trial (n=67) which involved a dose range of olanzapine (5-20 mg/day, once daily, starting at 10 mg/day), olanzapine was superior to placebo in the reduction of Y-MRS total score. In an identically designed trial conducted simultaneously with the first trial, olanzapine demonstrated a similar treatment difference, but possibly due to sample size and site variability, was not shown to be superior to placebo on this outcome.

(2) In a 4-week placebo-controlled trial (n=115) which involved a dose range of olanzapine (5-20 mg/day, once daily, starting at 15 mg/day), olanzapine was superior to placebo in the reduction of Y-MRS total score.

(3) In another trial, 361 patients meeting DSM-IV criteria for a manic or mixed episode of bipolar disorder who had responded during an initial open-label treatment phase for about two weeks, on average, to olanzapine 5 to 20 mg/day were randomized to either continuation of olanzapine at their same dose (n=225) or to placebo (n=136), for observation of relapse. Approximately 50% of the patients had discontinued from the olanzapine group by day 59 and 50% of the placebo group had discontinued by day 23 of double-blind treatment. Response during the open-label phase was defined by having a decrease of the Y-MRS total score to ≤12 and HAM-D 21 to ≤8. Relapse during the double-blind phase was defined as an increase of the Y-MRS or HAM-D 21 total score to ≥15, or being hospitalized for either mania or depression. In the randomized phase, patients receiving continued olanzapine experienced a significantly longer time to relapse.

Combination Therapy — The efficacy of oral olanzapine with concomitant lithium or valproate in the treatment of acute manic episodes was established in two controlled trials in patients who met the DSM-IV criteria for Bipolar I Disorder with manic or mixed episodes. These trials included patients with or without psychotic features and with or without a rapid-cycling course. The results of the trials follow:

(1) In one 6-week placebo-controlled combination trial, 175 outpatients on lithium or valproate therapy with inadequately controlled manic or mixed symptoms (Y-MRS ≥16) were randomized to receive either olanzapine or placebo, in combination with their original therapy. Olanzapine (in a dose range of 5-20 mg/day, once daily, starting at 10 mg/day) combined with lithium or valproate (in a therapeutic range of 0.6 mEq/L to 1.2 mEq/L or 50 µg/mL to 125 µg/mL, respectively) was superior to lithium or valproate alone in the reduction of Y-MRS total score.

(2) In a second 6-week placebo-controlled combination trial, 169 outpatients on lithium or valproate therapy with inadequately controlled manic or mixed symptoms (Y-MRS ≥16) were randomized to receive either olanzapine or placebo, in combination with their original therapy. Olanzapine (in a dose range of 5-20 mg/day, once daily, starting at 10 mg/day) combined with lithium or valproate (in a therapeutic range of 0.6 mEq/L to 1.2 mEq/L or 50 µg/mL to 125 µg/mL, respectively) was superior to lithium or valproate alone in the reduction of Y-MRS total score.

Agitation Associated with Schizophrenia and Bipolar I Mania

The efficacy of intramuscular olanzapine for injection for the treatment of agitation was established in 3 short-term (24 hours of IM treatment) placebo-controlled trials in agitated inpatients from two diagnostic groups: schizophrenia and Bipolar I Disorder (manic or mixed episodes). Each of the trials included a single active comparator treatment arm of either haloperidol injection (schizophrenia studies) or lorazepam injection (bipolar mania study). Patients enrolled in the trials needed to be: (1) judged by the clinical investigators as clinically agitated and clinically appropriate candidates for treatment with intramuscular medication, and (2) exhibiting a level of agitation that met or exceeded a threshold score of ≥14 on the five items comprising the Positive and Negative Syndrome Scale (PANSS) Excited Component (i.e., poor impulse control, tension, hostility, uncooperativeness and excitement items) with at least one individual item score ≥4 using a 1-7 scoring system (1=absent, 4=moderate, 7=extreme). In the studies, the mean baseline PANSS Excited Component score was 18.4, with scores ranging from 13 to 32 (out of a maximum score of 35), thus suggesting predominantly moderate levels of agitation with some patients experiencing mild or severe levels of agitation. The primary efficacy measure used for assessing agitation signs and symptoms in these trials was the change from baseline in the PANSS Excited Component at 2 hours post-injection. Patients could receive up to three injections during the 24 hour IM treatment periods; however, patients could not receive the second injection until after the initial 2 hour period when the primary efficacy measure was assessed. The results of the trials follow:

(1) In a placebo-controlled trial in agitated inpatients meeting DSM-IV criteria for schizophrenia (n=270), four fixed intramuscular olanzapine for injection doses of 2.5 mg, 5 mg, 7.5 mg and 10 mg were evaluated. All doses were statistically superior to placebo on the PANSS Excited Component at 2 hours post-injection. However, the effect was larger and more consistent for the three highest doses. There were no significant pairwise differences for the 7.5 and 10 mg doses over the 5 mg dose.

(2) In a second placebo-controlled trial in agitated inpatients meeting DSM-IV criteria for schizophrenia (n=311), one fixed intramuscular olanzapine for injection dose of 10 mg was evaluated. Olanzapine for injection was statistically superior to placebo on the PANSS Excited Component at 2 hours post-injection.

(3) In a placebo-controlled trial in agitated inpatients meeting DSM-IV criteria for Bipolar I Disorder (and currently displaying an acute manic or mixed episode with or without psychotic features) (n=201), one fixed intramuscular olanzapine for injection dose of 10 mg was evaluated. Olanzapine for injection was statistically superior to placebo on the PANSS Excited Component at 2 hours post-injection.

Examination of population subsets (age, race, and gender) did not reveal any differential responsiveness on the basis of these subgroupings.

INDICATIONS AND USAGE

Schizophrenia

Oral ZYPREXA is indicated for the treatment of schizophrenia.

The efficacy of ZYPREXA was established in short-term (6-week) controlled trials of schizophrenic inpatients (see CLINICAL PHARMACOLOGY).

The effectiveness of oral ZYPREXA at maintaining a treatment response in schizophrenic patients who had been stable on ZYPREXA for approximately 8 weeks and were then followed for a period of up to 8 months has been demonstrated in a placebo-controlled trial (see CLINICAL PHARMACOLOGY). Nevertheless, the physician who elects to use ZYPREXA for extended periods should periodically re-evaluate the long-term usefulness of the drug for the individual patient (see DOSAGE AND ADMINISTRATION).

Bipolar Disorder

Acute Monotherapy — Oral ZYPREXA is indicated for the treatment of acute mixed or manic episodes associated with Bipolar I Disorder.

The efficacy of ZYPREXA was established in two placebo-controlled trials (one 3-week and one 4-week) with patients meeting DSM-IV criteria for Bipolar I Disorder who currently displayed an acute manic or mixed episode with or without psychotic features (see CLINICAL PHARMACOLOGY).

Maintenance Monotherapy — The benefit of maintaining bipolar patients on monotherapy with oral ZYPREXA after achieving a responder status for an average duration of two weeks was demonstrated in a controlled trial (see Clinical Efficacy Data under CLINICAL PHARMACOLOGY). The physician who elects to use ZYPREXA for extended periods should periodically re-evaluate the long-term usefulness of the drug for the individual patient (see DOSAGE AND ADMINISTRATION).

Combination Therapy — The combination of oral ZYPREXA with lithium or valproate is indicated for the short-term treatment of acute manic episodes associated with Bipolar I Disorder.

The efficacy of ZYPREXA in combination with lithium or valproate was established in two placebo-controlled (6-week) trials with patients meeting DSM-IV criteria for Bipolar I Disorder who currently displayed an acute manic or mixed episode with or without psychotic features (see CLINICAL PHARMACOLOGY).

Agitation Associated with Schizophrenia and Bipolar I Mania

ZYPREXA IntraMuscular is indicated for the treatment of agitation associated with schizophrenia and bipolar I mania. "Psychomotor agitation" is defined in DSM-IV as "excessive motor activity associated with a feeling of inner tension." Patients experiencing agitation often manifest behaviors that interfere with their diagnosis and care, e.g., threatening behaviors, escalating or urgently distressing behavior, or self-exhausting behavior, leading clinicians to the use of intramuscular antipsychotic medications to achieve immediate control of the agitation.

The efficacy of ZYPREXA IntraMuscular for the treatment of agitation associated with schizophrenia and bipolar I mania was established in 3 short-term (24 hours) placebo-controlled trials in agitated inpatients with schizophrenia or Bipolar I Disorder (manic or mixed episodes) (see CLINICAL PHARMACOLOGY).

CONTRAINDICATIONS

ZYPREXA is contraindicated in patients with a known hypersensitivity to the product.

For specific information about the contraindications of lithium or valproate, refer to the CONTRAINDICATIONS section of the package inserts for these other products.

WARNINGS

Increased Mortality in Elderly Patients with Dementia-Related Psychosis — **Elderly patients with dementia-related psychosis treated with atypical antipsychotic drugs are at an increased risk of death compared to placebo. ZYPREXA is not approved for the treatment of patients with dementia-related psychosis (see BOX WARNING).**

In placebo-controlled clinical trials of elderly patients with dementia-related psychosis, the incidence of death in olanzapine-treated patients was significantly greater than placebo-treated patients (3.5% vs 1.5%, respectively). Risk factors that may predispose this patient population to increased mortality when treated with olanzapine include age ≥80 years, sedation, concomitant use of benzodiazepines or presence of pulmonary conditions (e.g., pneumonia, with or without aspiration).

Cerebrovascular Adverse Events, Including Stroke, in Elderly Patients with Dementia-Related Psychosis — Cerebrovascular adverse events (e.g., stroke, transient ischemic attack), including fatalities, were reported in patients in trials of olanzapine in elderly patients with dementia-related psychosis. In placebo-controlled trials, there was a significantly higher incidence of cerebrovascular adverse events in patients treated with olanzapine compared to patients treated with placebo. Olanzapine is not approved for the treatment of patients with dementia-related psychosis.

Hyperglycemia and Diabetes Mellitus — Hyperglycemia, in some cases extreme and associated with ketoacidosis or hyperosmolar coma or death, has been reported in patients treated with atypical antipsychotics including olanzapine. Assessment of the relationship between atypical antipsychotic use and glucose abnormalities is complicated by the possibility of an increased background risk of diabetes mellitus in patients with schizophrenia and the increasing incidence of diabetes mellitus in the general population. Given these confounders, the relationship between atypical antipsychotic use and hyperglycemia-related adverse events is not completely understood. However, epidemiological studies suggest an increased risk of treatment-emergent hyperglycemia-related adverse events in patients treated with the atypical antipsychotics. Precise risk estimates for hyperglycemia-related adverse events in patients treated with atypical antipsychotics are not available.

Patients with an established diagnosis of diabetes mellitus who are started on atypical antipsychotics should be monitored regularly for worsening of glucose control. Patients with risk factors for diabetes mellitus (e.g., obesity, family history of diabetes) who are starting treatment with atypical antipsychotics should undergo fasting blood glucose testing at the beginning of treatment and periodically during treatment. Any patient treated with atypical antipsychotics should be monitored for symptoms of hyperglycemia including polydipsia, polyuria, polyphagia, and weakness. Patients who develop symptoms of hyperglycemia during treatment with atypical antipsychotics should undergo fast-

ing blood glucose testing. In some cases, hyperglycemia has resolved when the atypical antipsychotic was discontinued; however, some patients required continuation of anti-diabetic treatment despite discontinuation of the suspect drug.

Neuroleptic Malignant Syndrome (NMS) — A potentially fatal symptom complex sometimes referred to as Neuroleptic Malignant Syndrome (NMS) has been reported in association with administration of antipsychotic drugs, including olanzapine. Clinical manifestations of NMS are hyperpyrexia, muscle rigidity, altered mental status and evidence of autonomic instability (irregular pulse or blood pressure, tachycardia, diaphoresis and cardiac dysrhythmia). Additional signs may include elevated creatinine phosphokinase, myoglobinuria (rhabdomyolysis), and acute renal failure.

The diagnostic evaluation of patients with this syndrome is complicated. In arriving at a diagnosis, it is important to exclude cases where the clinical presentation includes both serious medical illness (e.g., pneumonia, systemic infection, etc.) and untreated or inadequately treated extrapyramidal signs and symptoms (EPS). Other important considerations in the differential diagnosis include central anticholinergic toxicity, heat stroke, drug fever, and primary central nervous system pathology.

The management of NMS should include: 1) immediate discontinuation of antipsychotic drugs and other drugs not essential to concurrent therapy; 2) intensive symptomatic treatment and medical monitoring; and 3) treatment of any concomitant serious medical problems for which specific treatments are available. There is no general agreement about specific pharmacological treatment regimens for NMS.

If a patient requires antipsychotic drug treatment after recovery from NMS, the potential reintroduction of drug therapy should be carefully considered. The patient should be carefully monitored, since recurrences of NMS have been reported.

Tardive Dyskinesia — A syndrome of potentially irreversible, involuntary, dyskinetic movements may develop in patients treated with antipsychotic drugs. Although the prevalence of the syndrome appears to be highest among the elderly, especially elderly women, it is impossible to rely upon prevalence estimates to predict, at the inception of antipsychotic treatment, which patients are likely to develop the syndrome. Whether antipsychotic drug products differ in their potential to cause tardive dyskinesia is unknown.

The risk of developing tardive dyskinesia and the likelihood that it will become irreversible are believed to increase as the duration of treatment and the total cumulative dose of antipsychotic drugs administered to the patient increase. However, the syndrome can develop, although much less commonly, after relatively brief treatment periods at low doses.

There is no known treatment for established cases of tardive dyskinesia, although the syndrome may remit, partially or completely, if antipsychotic treatment is withdrawn. Antipsychotic treatment, itself, however, may suppress (or partially suppress) the signs and symptoms of the syndrome and thereby may possibly mask the underlying process. The effect that symptomatic suppression has upon the long-term course of the syndrome is unknown.

Given these considerations, olanzapine should be prescribed in a manner that is most likely to minimize the occurrence of tardive dyskinesia. Chronic antipsychotic treatment should generally be reserved for patients (1) who suffer from a chronic illness that is known to respond to antipsychotic drugs, and (2) for whom alternative, equally effective, but potentially less harmful treatments are not available or appropriate. In patients who do require chronic treatment, the smallest dose and the shortest duration of treatment producing a satisfactory clinical response should be sought. The need for continued treatment should be reassessed periodically.

If signs and symptoms of tardive dyskinesia appear in a patient on olanzapine, drug discontinuation should be considered. However, some patients may require treatment with olanzapine despite the presence of the syndrome.

For specific information about the warnings of lithium or valproate, refer to the WARNINGS section of the package inserts for these other products.

PRECAUTIONS
General

Hemodynamic Effects — Olanzapine may induce orthostatic hypotension associated with dizziness, tachycardia, and in some patients, syncope, especially during the initial dose-titration period, probably reflecting its α_1-adrenergic antagonistic properties. Hypotension, bradycardia with or without hypotension, tachycardia, and syncope were also reported during the clinical trials with intramuscular olanzapine for injection. In an open-label clinical pharmacology study in non-agitated patients with schizophrenia in which the safety and tolerability of intramuscular olanzapine were evaluated under a maximal dosing regimen (three 10 mg doses administered 4 hours apart), approximately one-third of these patients experienced a significant orthostatic decrease in systolic blood pressure (i.e., decrease ≥30 mmHg) (see DOSAGE AND ADMINISTRATION). Syncope was reported in 0.6% (15/2500) of olanzapine-treated patients in phase 2-3 oral olanzapine studies and in 0.3% (2/722) of olanzapine-treated patients with agitation in the intramuscular olanzapine for injection studies. Three normal volunteers in phase 1 studies with

intramuscular olanzapine experienced hypotension, bradycardia, and sinus pauses of up to 6 seconds that spontaneously resolved (in 2 cases the events occurred on intramuscular olanzapine, and in 1 case, on oral olanzapine). The risk for this sequence of hypotension, bradycardia, and sinus pause may be greater in nonpsychiatric patients compared to psychiatric patients who are possibly more adapted to certain effects of psychotropic drugs.

For oral olanzapine therapy, the risk of orthostatic hypotension and syncope may be minimized by initiating therapy with 5 mg QD (see DOSAGE AND ADMINISTRATION). A more gradual titration to the target dose should be considered if hypotension occurs.

For intramuscular olanzapine for injection therapy, patients should remain recumbent if drowsy or dizzy after injection until examination has indicated that they are not experiencing postural hypotension, bradycardia, and/or hypoventilation.

Olanzapine should be used with particular caution in patients with known cardiovascular disease (history of myocardial infarction or ischemia, heart failure, or conduction abnormalities), cerebrovascular disease, and conditions which would predispose patients to hypotension (dehydration, hypovolemia, and treatment with antihypertensive medications) where the occurrence of syncope, or hypotension and/or bradycardia might put the patient at increased medical risk.

Caution is necessary in patients who receive treatment with other drugs having effects that can induce hypotension, bradycardia, respiratory or central nervous system depression (see Drug Interactions). Concomitant administration of intramuscular olanzapine and parenteral benzodiazepine has not been studied and is therefore not recommended. If use of intramuscular olanzapine in combination with parenteral benzodiazepines is considered, careful evaluation of clinical status for excessive sedation and cardiorespiratory depression is recommended.

Seizures — During premarketing testing, seizures occurred in 0.9% (22/2500) of olanzapine-treated patients. There were confounding factors that may have contributed to the occurrence of seizures in many of these cases. Olanzapine should be used cautiously in patients with a history of seizures or with conditions that potentially lower the seizure threshold, e.g., Alzheimer's dementia. Conditions that lower the seizure threshold may be more prevalent in a population of 65 years or older.

Hyperprolactinemia — As with other drugs that antagonize dopamine D_2 receptors, olanzapine elevates prolactin levels, and a modest elevation persists during chronic administration. Tissue culture experiments indicate that approximately one-third of human breast cancers are prolactin dependent in vitro, a factor of potential importance if the prescription of these drugs is contemplated in a patient with previously detected breast cancer of this type. Although disturbances such as galactorrhea, amenorrhea, gynecomastia, and impotence have been reported with prolactin-elevating compounds, the clinical significance of elevated serum prolactin levels is unknown for most patients. As is common with compounds which increase prolactin release, an increase in mammary gland neoplasia was observed in the olanzapine carcinogenicity studies conducted in mice and rats (see Carcinogenesis). However, neither clinical studies nor epidemiologic studies have shown an association between chronic administration of this class of drugs and tumorigenesis in humans; the available evidence is considered too limited to be conclusive.

Transaminase Elevations — In placebo-controlled studies, clinically significant ALT (SGPT) elevations (≥3 times the upper limit of the normal range) were observed in 2% (6/243) of patients exposed to olanzapine compared to none (0/115) of the placebo patients. None of these patients experienced jaundice. In two of these patients, liver enzymes decreased toward normal despite continued treatment and in two others, enzymes decreased upon discontinuation of olanzapine. In the remaining two patients, one, seropositive for hepatitis C, had persistent enzyme elevation for four months after discontinuation, and the other had insufficient follow-up to determine if enzymes normalized.

Within the larger premarketing database of about 2400 patients with baseline SGPT ≤90 IU/L, the incidence of SGPT elevation to >200 IU/L was 2% (50/2381). Again, none of these patients experienced jaundice or other symptoms attributable to liver impairment and most had transient changes that tended to normalize while olanzapine treatment was continued.

Among 2500 patients in oral olanzapine clinical trials, about 1% (23/2500) discontinued treatment due to transaminase increases.

Caution should be exercised in patients with signs and symptoms of hepatic impairment, in patients with pre-existing conditions associated with limited hepatic functional reserve, and in patients who are being treated with potentially hepatotoxic drugs. Periodic assessment of transaminases is recommended in patients with significant hepatic disease (see Laboratory Tests).

Potential for Cognitive and Motor Impairment — Somnolence was a commonly reported adverse event associated with olanzapine treatment, occurring at an incidence of 26% in olanzapine patients compared to 15% in placebo patients. This adverse event was also dose related. Somnolence led to discontinuation in 0.4% (9/2500) of patients in the premarketing database.

Since olanzapine has the potential to impair judgment, thinking, or motor skills, patients should be cautioned

Continued on next page

Zyprexa—Cont.

about operating hazardous machinery, including automobiles, until they are reasonably certain that olanzapine therapy does not affect them adversely.

Body Temperature Regulation — Disruption of the body's ability to reduce core body temperature has been attributed to antipsychotic agents. Appropriate care is advised when prescribing olanzapine for patients who will be experiencing conditions which may contribute to an elevation in core body temperature, e.g., exercising strenuously, exposure to extreme heat, receiving concomitant medication with anticholinergic activity, or being subject to dehydration.

Dysphagia — Esophageal dysmotility and aspiration have been associated with antipsychotic drug use. Aspiration pneumonia is a common cause of morbidity and mortality in patients with advanced Alzheimer's disease. Olanzapine and other antipsychotic drugs should be used cautiously in patients at risk for aspiration pneumonia.

Suicide — The possibility of a suicide attempt is inherent in schizophrenia and in bipolar disorder, and close supervision of high-risk patients should accompany drug therapy. Prescriptions for olanzapine should be written for the smallest quantity of tablets consistent with good patient management, in order to reduce the risk of overdose.

Use in Patients with Concomitant Illness — Clinical experience with olanzapine in patients with certain concomitant systemic illnesses (see Renal Impairment and Hepatic Impairment under CLINICAL PHARMACOLOGY, Special Populations) is limited.

Olanzapine exhibits in vitro muscarinic receptor affinity. In premarketing clinical trials with olanzapine, olanzapine was associated with constipation, dry mouth, and tachycardia, all adverse events possibly related to cholinergic antagonism. Such adverse events were not often the basis for discontinuations from olanzapine, but olanzapine should be used with caution in patients with clinically significant prostatic hypertrophy, narrow angle glaucoma, or a history of paralytic ileus.

In five placebo-controlled studies of olanzapine in elderly patients with dementia-related psychosis (n=1184), the following treatment-emergent adverse events were reported in olanzapine-treated patients at an incidence of at least 2% and significantly greater than placebo-treated patients: falls, somnolence, peripheral edema, abnormal gait, urinary incontinence, lethargy, increased weight, asthenia, pyrexia, pneumonia, dry mouth and visual hallucinations. The rate of discontinuation due to adverse events was significantly greater with olanzapine than placebo (13% vs 7%). As with other CNS-active drugs, olanzapine should be used with caution in elderly patients with dementia. Olanzapine is not approved for the treatment of patients with dementia-related psychosis. If the prescriber elects to treat elderly patients with dementia-related psychosis, vigilance should be exercised (see BOX WARNING and WARNINGS).

Olanzapine has not been evaluated or used to any appreciable extent in patients with a recent history of myocardial infarction or unstable heart disease. Patients with these diagnoses were excluded from premarketing clinical studies. Because of the risk of orthostatic hypotension with olanzapine, caution should be observed in cardiac patients (see Hemodynamic Effects).

For specific information about the precautions of lithium or valproate, refer to the PRECAUTIONS section of the package inserts for these other products.

Information for Patients

Physicians are advised to discuss the following issues with patients for whom they prescribe olanzapine:

Orthostatic Hypotension — Patients should be advised of the risk of orthostatic hypotension, especially during the period of initial dose titration and in association with the use of concomitant drugs that may potentiate the orthostatic effect of olanzapine, e.g., diazepam or alcohol (see Drug Interactions).

Interference with Cognitive and Motor Performance — Because olanzapine has the potential to impair judgment, thinking, or motor skills, patients should be cautioned about operating hazardous machinery, including automobiles, until they are reasonably certain that olanzapine therapy does not affect them adversely.

Pregnancy — Patients should be advised to notify their physician if they become pregnant or intend to become pregnant during therapy with olanzapine.

Nursing — Patients should be advised not to breast-feed an infant if they are taking olanzapine.

Concomitant Medication — Patients should be advised to inform their physicians if they are taking, or plan to take, any prescription or over-the-counter drugs, since there is a potential for interactions.

Alcohol — Patients should be advised to avoid alcohol while taking olanzapine.

Heat Exposure and Dehydration — Patients should be advised regarding appropriate care in avoiding overheating and dehydration.

Phenylketonurics — ZYPREXA ZYDIS (olanzapine orally disintegrating tablets) contains phenylalanine (0.34, 0.45, 0.67, or 0.90 mg per 5, 10, 15, or 20 mg tablet, respectively).

Laboratory Tests

Periodic assessment of transaminases is recommended in patients with significant hepatic disease (see Transaminase Elevations).

Drug Interactions

The risks of using olanzapine in combination with other drugs have not been extensively evaluated in systematic studies. Given the primary CNS effects of olanzapine, caution should be used when olanzapine is taken in combination with other centrally acting drugs and alcohol.

Because of its potential for inducing hypotension, olanzapine may enhance the effects of certain antihypertensive agents.

Olanzapine may antagonize the effects of levodopa and dopamine agonists.

The Effect of Other Drugs on Olanzapine — Agents that induce CYP1A2 or glucuronyl transferase enzymes, such as omeprazole and rifampin, may cause an increase in olanzapine clearance. Inhibitors of CYP1A2 could potentially inhibit olanzapine clearance. Although olanzapine is metabolized by multiple enzyme systems, induction or inhibition of a single enzyme may appreciably alter olanzapine clearance. Therefore, a dosage increase (for induction) or a dosage decrease (for inhibition) may need to be considered with specific drugs.

Charcoal — The administration of activated charcoal (1 g) reduced the Cmax and AUC of oral olanzapine by about 60%. As peak olanzapine levels are not typically obtained until about 6 hours after dosing, charcoal may be a useful treatment for olanzapine overdose.

Cimetidine and Antacids — Single doses of cimetidine (800 mg) or aluminum- and magnesium-containing antacids did not affect the oral bioavailability of olanzapine.

Carbamazepine — Carbamazepine therapy (200 mg bid) causes an approximately 50% increase in the clearance of olanzapine. This increase is likely due to the fact that carbamazepine is a potent inducer of CYP1A2 activity. Higher daily doses of carbamazepine may cause an even greater increase in olanzapine clearance.

Ethanol — Ethanol (45 mg/70 kg single dose) did not have an effect on olanzapine pharmacokinetics.

Fluoxetine — Fluoxetine (60 mg single dose or 60 mg daily for 8 days) causes a small (mean 16%) increase in the maximum concentration of olanzapine and a small (mean 16%) decrease in olanzapine clearance. The magnitude of the impact of this factor is small in comparison to the overall variability between individuals, and therefore dose modification is not routinely recommended.

Fluvoxamine — Fluvoxamine, a CYP1A2 inhibitor, decreases the clearance of olanzapine. This results in a mean increase in olanzapine Cmax following fluvoxamine of 54% in female nonsmokers and 77% in male smokers. The mean increase in olanzapine AUC is 52% and 108%, respectively. Lower doses of olanzapine should be considered in patients receiving concomitant treatment with fluvoxamine.

Warfarin — Warfarin (20 mg single dose) did not affect olanzapine pharmacokinetics.

Effect of Olanzapine on Other Drugs — In vitro studies utilizing human liver microsomes suggest that olanzapine has little potential to inhibit CYP1A2, CYP2C9, CYP2C19, CYP2D6, and CYP3A. Thus, olanzapine is unlikely to cause clinically important drug interactions mediated by these enzymes.

Lithium — Multiple doses of olanzapine (10 mg for 8 days) did not influence the kinetics of lithium. Therefore, concomitant olanzapine administration does not require dosage adjustment of lithium.

Valproate — Studies in vitro using human liver microsomes determined that olanzapine has little potential to inhibit the major metabolic pathway, glucuronidation, of valproate. Further, valproate has little effect on the metabolism of olanzapine in vitro. In vivo administration of olanzapine (10 mg daily for 2 weeks) did not affect the steady state plasma concentrations of valproate. Therefore, concomitant olanzapine administration does not require dosage adjustment of valproate.

Single doses of olanzapine did not affect the pharmacokinetics of imipramine or its active metabolite desipramine, and warfarin. Multiple doses of olanzapine did not influence the kinetics of diazepam and its active metabolite N-desmethyldiazepam, ethanol, or biperiden. However, the co-administration of either diazepam or ethanol with olanzapine potentiated the orthostatic hypotension observed with olanzapine. Multiple doses of olanzapine did not affect the pharmacokinetics of theophylline or its metabolites.

Lorazepam — Administration of intramuscular lorazepam (2 mg) 1 hour after intramuscular olanzapine for injection (5 mg) did not significantly affect the pharmacokinetics of olanzapine, unconjugated lorazepam, or total lorazepam. However, this co-administration of intramuscular lorazepam and intramuscular olanzapine for injection added to the somnolence observed with either drug alone (see Hemodynamic Effects).

Carcinogenesis, Mutagenesis, Impairment of Fertility

Carcinogenesis — Oral carcinogenicity studies were conducted in mice and rats. Olanzapine was administered to mice in two 78-week studies at doses of 3, 10, 30/20 mg/kg/day (equivalent to 0.8-5 times the maximum recommended human daily oral dose on a mg/m² basis) and 0.25, 2, 8 mg/kg/day (equivalent to 0.06-2 times the maximum recommended human daily oral dose on a mg/m² basis). Rats were dosed for 2 years at doses of 0.25, 1, 2.5, 4 mg/kg/day (males) and 0.25, 1, 4, 8 mg/kg/day (females) (equivalent to 0.13-2 and 0.13-4 times the maximum recommended human daily oral dose on a mg/m² basis, respectively). The incidence of liver hemangiomas and hemangiosarcomas was significantly increased in one mouse study in female mice dosed at 8 mg/kg/day (2 times the maximum recommended human daily oral dose on a mg/m² basis). These tumors were not increased in another mouse study in females dosed at 10 or 30/20 mg/kg/day (2-5 times the maximum recommended human daily oral dose on a mg/m² basis); in this study, there was a high incidence of early mortalities in males of the 30/20 mg/kg/day group. The incidence of mammary gland adenomas and adenocarcinomas was significantly increased in female mice dosed at ≥2 mg/kg/day and in female rats dosed at ≥4 mg/kg/day (0.5 and 2 times the maximum recommended human daily oral dose on a mg/m² basis, respectively). Antipsychotic drugs have been shown to chronically elevate prolactin levels in rodents. Serum prolactin levels were not measured during the olanzapine carcinogenicity studies; however, measurements during subchronic toxicity studies showed that olanzapine elevated serum prolactin levels up to 4-fold in rats at the same doses used in the carcinogenicity study. An increase in mammary gland neoplasms has been found in rodents after chronic administration of other antipsychotic drugs and is considered to be prolactin mediated. The relevance for human risk of the finding of prolactin mediated endocrine tumors in rodents is unknown (see Hyperprolactinemia under PRECAUTIONS, General).

Mutagenesis — No evidence of mutagenic potential for olanzapine was found in the Ames reverse mutation test, in vivo micronucleus test in mice, the chromosomal aberration test in Chinese hamster ovary cells, unscheduled DNA synthesis test in rat hepatocytes, induction of forward mutation test in mouse lymphoma cells, or in vivo sister chromatid exchange test in bone marrow of Chinese hamsters.

Impairment of Fertility — In an oral fertility and reproductive performance study in rats, male mating performance, but not fertility, was impaired at a dose of 22.4 mg/kg/day and female fertility was decreased at a dose of 3 mg/kg/day (11 and 1.5 times the maximum recommended human daily oral dose on a mg/m² basis, respectively). Discontinuance of olanzapine treatment reversed the effects on male mating performance. In female rats, the precoital period was increased and the mating index reduced at 5 mg/kg/day (2.5 times the maximum recommended human daily oral dose on a mg/m² basis). Diestrous was prolonged and estrous delayed at 1.1 mg/kg/day (0.6 times the maximum recommended human daily oral dose on a mg/m² basis); therefore olanzapine may produce a delay in ovulation.

Pregnancy

Pregnancy Category C — In oral reproduction studies in rats at doses up to 18 mg/kg/day and in rabbits at doses up to 30 mg/kg/day (9 and 30 times the maximum recommended human daily oral dose on a mg/m² basis, respectively) no evidence of teratogenicity was observed. In an oral rat teratology study, early resorptions and increased numbers of nonviable fetuses were observed at a dose of 18 mg/kg/day (9 times the maximum recommended human daily oral dose on a mg/m² basis). Gestation was prolonged at 10 mg/kg/day (5 times the maximum recommended human daily oral dose on a mg/m² basis). In an oral rabbit teratology study, fetal toxicity (manifested as increased resorptions and decreased fetal weight) occurred at a maternally toxic dose of 30 mg/kg/day (30 times the maximum recommended human daily oral dose on a mg/m² basis).

Placental transfer of olanzapine occurs in rat pups.

There are no adequate and well-controlled trials with olanzapine in pregnant females. Seven pregnancies were observed during clinical trials with olanzapine, including 2 resulting in normal births, 1 resulting in neonatal death due to a cardiovascular defect, 3 therapeutic abortions, and 1 spontaneous abortion. Because animal reproduction studies are not always predictive of human response, this drug should be used during pregnancy only if the potential benefit justifies the potential risk to the fetus.

Labor and Delivery

Parturition in rats was not affected by olanzapine. The effect of olanzapine on labor and delivery in humans is unknown.

Nursing Mothers

Olanzapine was excreted in milk of treated rats during lactation. It is not known if olanzapine is excreted in human milk. It is recommended that women receiving olanzapine should not breast-feed.

Pediatric Use

Safety and effectiveness in pediatric patients have not been established.

Geriatric Use

Of the 2500 patients in premarketing clinical studies with oral olanzapine, 11% (263) were 65 years of age or over. In patients with schizophrenia, there was no indication of any different tolerability of olanzapine in the elderly compared to younger patients. Studies in elderly patients with dementia-related psychosis have suggested that there may be a different tolerability profile in this population compared to younger patients with schizophrenia. As with other CNS-active drugs, olanzapine should be used with caution in elderly patients with dementia. Olanzapine is not approved for the treatment of patients with dementia-related psychosis. If the prescriber elects to treat elderly patients with dementia-related psychosis, vigilance should be exercised. Also, the presence of factors that might decrease pharmacokinetic clearance or increase the pharmacodynamic response to olanzapine should lead to consideration of a lower starting dose for any geriatric patient (see BOX WARNING, WARNINGS, PRECAUTIONS and DOSAGE AND ADMINISTRATION).

ADVERSE REACTIONS

The information below is derived from a clinical trial database for olanzapine consisting of 8661 patients with approximately 4165 patient-years of exposure to oral olanzapine and 722 patients with exposure to intramuscular olanzapine for injection. This database includes: (1) 2500 patients who participated in multiple-dose oral olanzapine premarketing trials in schizophrenia and Alzheimer's disease representing approximately 1122 patient-years of exposure as of February 14, 1995; (2) 182 patients who participated in oral olanzapine premarketing bipolar mania trials representing approximately 66 patient-years of exposure; (3) 191 patients who participated in an oral olanzapine trial of patients having various psychiatric symptoms in association with Alzheimer's disease representing approximately 29 patient-years of exposure; (4) 5788 patients from 88 additional oral olanzapine clinical trials as of December 31, 2001; and (5) 722 patients who participated in intramuscular olanzapine for injection premarketing trials in agitated patients with schizophrenia, Bipolar I Disorder (manic or mixed episodes), or dementia. In addition, information from the premarketing 6-week clinical study database for olanzapine in combination with lithium or valproate, consisting of 224 patients who participated in bipolar mania trials with approximately 22 patient-years of exposure, is included below.

The conditions and duration of treatment with olanzapine varied greatly and included (in overlapping categories) open-label and double-blind phases of studies, inpatients and outpatients, fixed-dose and dose-titration studies, and short-term or longer-term exposure. Adverse reactions were assessed by collecting adverse events, results of physical examinations, vital signs, weights, laboratory analytes, ECGs, chest x-rays, and results of ophthalmologic examinations. Certain portions of the discussion below relating to objective or numeric safety parameters, namely, dose-dependent adverse events, vital sign changes, weight gain, laboratory changes, and ECG changes are derived from studies in patients with schizophrenia and have not been duplicated for bipolar mania or agitation. However, this information is also generally applicable to bipolar mania and agitation. Adverse events during exposure were obtained by spontaneous report and recorded by clinical investigators using terminology of their own choosing. Consequently, it is not possible to provide a meaningful estimate of the proportion of individuals experiencing adverse events without first grouping similar types of events into a smaller number of standardized event categories. In the tables and tabulations that follow, standard COSTART dictionary terminology has been used initially to classify reported adverse events.

The stated frequencies of adverse events represent the proportion of individuals who experienced, at least once, a treatment-emergent adverse event of the type listed. An event was considered treatment emergent if it occurred for the first time or worsened while receiving therapy following baseline evaluation. The reported events do not include those event terms that were so general as to be uninformative. Events listed elsewhere in labeling may not be repeated below. It is important to emphasize that, although the events occurred during treatment with olanzapine, they were not necessarily caused by it. The entire label should be read to gain a complete understanding of the safety profile of olanzapine.

The prescriber should be aware that the figures in the tables and tabulations cannot be used to predict the incidence of side effects in the course of usual medical practice where patient characteristics and other factors differ from those that prevailed in the clinical trials. Similarly, the cited frequencies cannot be compared with figures obtained from other clinical investigations involving different treatments, uses, and investigators. The cited figures, however, do provide the prescribing physician with some basis for estimating the relative contribution of drug and nondrug factors to the adverse event incidence in the population studied.

Incidence of Adverse Events in Short-Term, Placebo-Controlled and Combination Trials

The following findings are based on premarketing trials of (1) oral olanzapine for schizophrenia, bipolar mania, a subsequent trial of patients having various psychiatric symptoms in association with Alzheimer's disease, and premarketing combination trials, and (2) intramuscular olanzapine for injection in agitated patients with schizophrenia or bipolar mania.

Adverse Events Associated with Discontinuation of Treatment in Short-Term, Placebo-Controlled Trials

Schizophrenia — Overall, there was no difference in the incidence of discontinuation due to adverse events (5% for oral olanzapine vs 6% for placebo). However, discontinuations due to increases in SGPT were considered to be drug related (2% for oral olanzapine vs 0% for placebo) (see PRECAUTIONS).

Bipolar Mania Monotherapy — Overall, there was no difference in the incidence of discontinuation due to adverse events (2% for oral olanzapine vs 2% for placebo).

Agitation — Overall, there was no difference in the incidence of discontinuation due to adverse events (0.4% for intramuscular olanzapine for injection vs 0% for placebo).

Adverse Events Associated with Discontinuation of Treatment in Short-Term Combination Trials

Bipolar Mania Combination Therapy — In a study of patients who were already tolerating either lithium or valproate as monotherapy, discontinuation rates due to adverse events were 11% for the combination of oral olanzapine with lithium or valproate compared to 2% for patients who remained on lithium or valproate monotherapy. Discontinuations with the combination of oral olanzapine and lithium or valproate that occurred in more than 1 patient were somnolence (3%), weight gain (1%), and peripheral edema (1%).

Commonly Observed Adverse Events in Short-Term, Placebo-Controlled Trials

The most commonly observed adverse events associated with the use of oral olanzapine (incidence of 5% or greater) and not observed at an equivalent incidence among placebo-treated patients (olanzapine incidence at least twice that for placebo) were:

Common Treatment-Emergent Adverse Events Associated with the Use of Oral Olanzapine in 6-Week Trials — SCHIZOPHRENIA

Adverse Event	Percentage of Patients Reporting Event	
	Olanzapine (N=248)	Placebo (N=118)
Postural hypotension	5	2
Constipation	9	3
Weight gain	6	1
Dizziness	11	4
Personality disorder[1]	8	4
Akathisia	5	1

[1] Personality disorder is the COSTART term for designating non-aggressive objectionable behavior.

Common Treatment-Emergent Adverse Events Associated with the Use of Oral Olanzapine in 3-Week and 4-Week Trials — BIPOLAR MANIA

Adverse Event	Percentage of Patients Reporting Event	
	Olanzapine (N=125)	Placebo (N=129)
Asthenia	15	6
Dry mouth	22	7
Constipation	11	5
Dyspepsia	11	5
Increased appetite	6	3
Somnolence	35	13
Dizziness	18	6
Tremor	6	3

There was one adverse event (somnolence) observed at an incidence of 5% or greater among intramuscular olanzapine for injection-treated patients and not observed at an equivalent incidence among placebo-treated patients (olanzapine incidence at least twice that for placebo) during the placebo-controlled premarketing studies. The incidence of somnolence during the 24 hour IM treatment period in clinical trials in agitated patients with schizophrenia or bipolar mania was 6% for intramuscular olanzapine for injection and 3% for placebo.

Adverse Events Occurring at an Incidence of 2% or More Among Oral Olanzapine-Treated Patients in Short-Term, Placebo-Controlled Trials

Table 1 enumerates the incidence, rounded to the nearest percent, of treatment-emergent adverse events that occurred in 2% or more of patients treated with oral olanzapine (doses ≥2.5 mg/day) and with incidence greater than placebo who participated in the acute phase of placebo-controlled trials.

Table 1
Treatment-Emergent Adverse Events: Incidence in Short-Term, Placebo-Controlled Clinical Trials[1] with Oral Olanzapine

Body System/Adverse Event	Percentage of Patients Reporting Event	
	Olanzapine (N=532)	Placebo (N=294)
Body as a Whole		
Accidental injury	12	8
Asthenia	10	9
Fever	6	2
Back pain	5	2
Chest pain	3	1
Cardiovascular System		
Postural hypotension	3	1
Tachycardia	3	1
Hypertension	2	1
Digestive System		
Dry mouth	9	5
Constipation	9	4
Dyspepsia	7	5
Vomiting	4	3
Increased appetite	3	2
Hemic and Lymphatic System		
Ecchymosis	5	3
Metabolic and Nutritional Disorders		
Weight gain	5	3
Peripheral edema	3	1
Musculoskeletal System		
Extremity pain (other than joint)	5	3
Joint pain	5	3
Nervous System		
Somnolence	29	13
Insomnia	12	11
Dizziness	11	4
Abnormal gait	6	1
Tremor	4	3
Akathisia	3	2
Hypertonia	3	2
Articulation impairment	2	1
Respiratory System		
Rhinitis	7	6
Cough increased	6	3
Pharyngitis	4	3
Special Senses		
Amblyopia	3	2
Urogenital System		
Urinary incontinence	2	1
Urinary tract infection	2	1

[1] Events reported by at least 2% of patients treated with olanzapine, except the following events which had an incidence equal to or less than placebo: abdominal pain, agitation, anorexia, anxiety, apathy, confusion, depression, diarrhea, dysmenorrhea[2], hallucinations, headache, hostility, hyperkinesia, myalgia, nausea, nervousness, paranoid reaction, personality disorder[3], rash, thinking abnormal, weight loss.

[2] Denominator used was for females only (olanzapine, N=201; placebo, N=114).

[3] Personality disorder is the COSTART term for designating non-aggressive objectionable behavior.

Commonly Observed Adverse Events in Short-Term Combination Trials

In the bipolar mania combination placebo-controlled trials, the most commonly observed adverse events associated with the combination of olanzapine and lithium or valproate (incidence of ≥5% and at least twice placebo) were:

Common Treatment-Emergent Adverse Events Associated with the Use of Oral Olanzapine in 6-Week Combination Trials — BIPOLAR MANIA

Adverse Event	Percentage of Patients Reporting Event	
	Olanzapine with lithium or valproate (N=229)	Placebo with lithium or valproate (N=115)
Dry mouth	32	9
Weight gain	26	7
Increased appetite	24	8
Dizziness	14	7
Back pain	8	4
Constipation	8	4
Speech disorder	7	1
Increased salivation	6	2
Amnesia	5	2
Paresthesia	5	2

Adverse Events Occurring at an Incidence of 2% or More Among Oral Olanzapine-Treated Patients in Short-Term Combination Trials

Table 2 enumerates the incidence, rounded to the nearest percent, of treatment-emergent adverse events that occurred in 2% or more of patients treated with the combination of olanzapine (doses ≥5 mg/day) and lithium or valproate and with incidence greater than lithium or valproate alone who participated in the acute phase of placebo-controlled combination trials.

Continued on next page

TREATMENT-EMERGENT EXTRAPYRAMIDAL SYMPTOMS ASSESSED BY RATING SCALES INCIDENCE IN A FIXED DOSAGE RANGE, PLACEBO-CONTROLLED CLINICAL TRIAL OF ORAL OLANZAPINE IN SCHIZOPHRENIA — ACUTE PHASE*

	Percentage of Patients Reporting Event			
	Placebo	Olanzapine 5 ± 2.5 mg/day	Olanzapine 10 ± 2.5 mg/day	Olanzapine 15 ± 2.5 mg/day
Parkinsonism[1]	15	14	12	14
Akathisia[2]	23	16	19	27

* No statistically significant differences.
[1] Percentage of patients with a Simpson-Angus Scale total score >3.
[2] Percentage of patients with a Barnes Akathisia Scale global score ≥2.

TREATMENT-EMERGENT EXTRAPYRAMIDAL SYMPTOMS ASSESSED BY ADVERSE EVENTS INCIDENCE IN A FIXED DOSAGE RANGE, PLACEBO-CONTROLLED CLINICAL TRIAL OF ORAL OLANZAPINE IN SCHIZOPHRENIA — ACUTE PHASE

	Percentage of Patients Reporting Event			
	Placebo (N=68)	Olanzapine 5 ± 2.5 mg/day (N=65)	Olanzapine 10± 2.5 mg/day (N=64)	Olanzapine 15 ± 2.5 mg/day (N=69)
Dystonic events[1]	1	3	2	3
Parkinsonism events[2]	10	8	14	20
Akathisia events[3]	1	5	11*	10*
Dyskinetic events[4]	4	0	2	1
Residual events[5]	1	2	5	1
Any extrapyramidal event	16	15	25	32*

* Statistically significantly different from placebo.
[1] Patients with the following COSTART terms were counted in this category: dystonia, generalized spasm, neck rigidity, oculogyric crisis, opisthotonos, torticollis.
[2] Patients with the following COSTART terms were counted in this category: akinesia, cogwheel rigidity, extrapyramidal syndrome, hypertonia, hypokinesia, masked facies, tremor.
[3] Patients with the following COSTART terms were counted in this category: akathisia, hyperkinesia.
[4] Patients with the following COSTART terms were counted in this category: buccoglossal syndrome, choreoathetosis, dyskinesia, tardive dyskinesia.
[5] Patients with the following COSTART terms were counted in this category: movement disorder, myoclonus, twitching.

Zyprexa—Cont.

Table 2
Treatment-Emergent Adverse Events: Incidence in Short-Term, Placebo-Controlled Combination Clinical Trials[1] with Oral Olanzapine

	Percentage of Patients Reporting Event	
Body System/Adverse Event	Olanzapine with lithium or valproate (N=229)	Placebo with lithium or valproate (N=115)
Body as a Whole		
Asthenia	18	13
Back pain	8	4
Accidental injury	4	2
Chest pain	3	2
Cardiovascular System		
Hypertension	2	1
Digestive System		
Dry mouth	32	9
Increased appetite	24	8
Thirst	10	6
Constipation	8	4
Increased salivation	6	2
Metabolic and Nutritional Disorders		
Weight gain	26	7
Peripheral edema	6	4
Edema	2	1
Nervous System		
Somnolence	52	27
Tremor	23	13
Depression	18	17
Dizziness	14	7
Speech disorder	7	1
Amnesia	5	2
Paresthesia	5	2
Apathy	4	3
Confusion	4	1
Euphoria	3	2
Incoordination	2	0
Respiratory System		
Pharyngitis	4	1
Dyspnea	3	1
Skin and Appendages		
Sweating	3	1
Acne	2	0
Dry skin	2	0
Special Senses		
Amblyopia	9	5
Abnormal vision	2	0
Urogenital System		
Dysmenorrhea[2]	2	0
Vaginitis[2]	2	0

[1] Events reported by at least 2% of patients treated with olanzapine, except the following events which had an incidence equal to or less than placebo: abdominal pain, abnormal dreams, abnormal ejaculation, agitation, akathisia, anorexia, anxiety, arthralgia, cough increased, diarrhea, dyspepsia, emotional lability, fever, flatulence, flu syndrome, headache, hostility, insomnia, libido decreased, libido increased, menstrual disorder[2], myalgia, nausea, nervousness, pain, paranoid reaction, personality disorder, rash, rhinitis, sleep disorder, thinking abnormal, vomiting.
[2] Denominator used was for females only (olanzapine, N=128; placebo, N=51).

For specific information about the adverse reactions observed with lithium or valproate, refer to the ADVERSE REACTIONS section of the package inserts for these other products.

Adverse Events Occurring at an Incidence of 1% or More Among Intramuscular Olanzapine for Injection-Treated Patients in Short-Term, Placebo-Controlled Trials
Table 3 enumerates the incidence, rounded to the nearest percent, of treatment-emergent adverse events that occurred in 1% or more of patients treated with intramuscular olanzapine for injection (dose range of 2.5-10.0 mg/injection) and with incidence greater than placebo who participated in the short-term, placebo-controlled trials in agitated patients with schizophrenia or bipolar mania.

Table 3
Treatment-Emergent Adverse Events: Incidence in Short-Term (24 Hour), Placebo-Controlled Clinical Trials with Intramuscular Olanzapine for Injection in Agitated Patients with Schizophrenia or Bipolar Mania[1]

	Percentage of Patients Reporting Event	
Body System/Adverse Event	Olanzapine (N=415)	Placebo (N=150)
Body as a Whole		
Asthenia	2	1
Cardiovascular System		
Hypotension	2	0
Postural hypotension	1	0
Nervous System		
Somnolence	6	3
Dizziness	4	2
Tremor	1	0

[1] Events reported by at least 1% of patients treated with olanzapine for injection, except the following events which had an incidence equal to or less than placebo: agitation, anxiety, dry mouth, headache, hypertension, insomnia, nervousness.

Additional Findings Observed in Clinical Trials
The following findings are based on clinical trials.
Dose Dependency of Adverse Events in Short-Term, Placebo-Controlled Trials
Extrapyramidal Symptoms — The following table enumerates the percentage of patients with treatment-emergent extrapyramidal symptoms as assessed by categorical analyses of formal rating scales during acute therapy in a controlled clinical trial comparing oral olanzapine at 3 fixed doses with placebo in the treatment of schizophrenia.
[See first table at left]
The following table enumerates the percentage of patients with treatment-emergent extrapyramidal symptoms as assessed by spontaneously reported adverse events during acute therapy in the same controlled clinical trial comparing olanzapine at 3 fixed doses with placebo in the treatment of schizophrenia.
[See second table at left]
The following table enumerates the percentage of patients with treatment-emergent extrapyramidal symptoms as assessed by categorical analyses of formal rating scales during controlled clinical trials comparing fixed doses of intramuscular olanzapine for injection with placebo in agitation. Patients in each dose group could receive up to three injections during the trials (see CLINICAL PHARMACOLOGY). Patient assessments were conducted during the 24 hours following the initial dose of intramuscular olanzapine for injection. There were no statistically significant differences from placebo.
[See first table on next page]
The following table enumerates the percentage of patients with treatment-emergent extrapyramidal symptoms as assessed by spontaneously reported adverse events in the same controlled clinical trial comparing fixed doses of intramuscular olanzapine for injection with placebo in agitated patients with schizophrenia. There were no statistically significant differences from placebo.
[See second table on next page]
Other Adverse Events — The following table addresses dose relatedness for other adverse events using data from a schizophrenia trial involving fixed dosage ranges of oral olanzapine. It enumerates the percentage of patients with treatment-emergent adverse events for the three fixed-dose range groups and placebo. The data were analyzed using the Cochran-Armitage test, excluding the placebo group, and the table includes only those adverse events for which there was a statistically significant trend.
[See third table at bottom of next page]
Vital Sign Changes — Oral olanzapine was associated with orthostatic hypotension and tachycardia in clinical trials. Intramuscular olanzapine for injection was associated with bradycardia, hypotension, and tachycardia in clinical trials (see PRECAUTIONS).
Weight Gain — In placebo-controlled, 6-week studies, weight gain was reported in 5.6% of olanzapine patients compared to 0.8% of placebo patients. Olanzapine patients gained an average of 2.8 kg, compared to an average 0.4 kg weight loss in placebo patients; 29% of olanzapine patients gained greater than 7% of their baseline weight, compared to 3% of placebo patients. A categorization of patients at baseline on the basis of body mass index (BMI) revealed a significantly greater effect in patients with low BMI compared to normal or overweight patients; nevertheless, weight gain was greater in all 3 olanzapine groups compared to the placebo group. During long-term continuation therapy with olanzapine (238 median days of exposure), 56% of olanzapine patients met the criterion for having gained greater than 7% of their baseline weight. Average weight gain during long-term therapy was 5.4 kg.
Laboratory Changes — An assessment of the premarketing experience for olanzapine revealed an association with asymptomatic increases in SGPT, SGOT, and GGT (see PRECAUTIONS). Olanzapine administration was also associated with increases in serum prolactin (see PRECAUTIONS), with an asymptomatic elevation of the eosinophil count in 0.3% of patients, and with an increase in CPK.
Given the concern about neutropenia associated with other psychotropic compounds and the finding of leukopenia associated with the administration of olanzapine in several animal models (see ANIMAL TOXICOLOGY), careful attention was given to examination of hematologic parameters in premarketing studies with olanzapine. There was no indication of a risk of clinically significant neutropenia associated with olanzapine treatment in the premarketing database for this drug.
In clinical trials among olanzapine-treated patients with random triglyceride levels of <150 mg/dL at baseline (N=485), 0.6% of patients experienced triglyceride levels of ≥500 mg/dL anytime during the trials. In these same trials, olanzapine-treated patients (N=962) had a mean increase of 27 mg/dL in triglycerides from a mean baseline value of 185 mg/dL.
In placebo-controlled trials, olanzapine-treated patients with random cholesterol levels of <200 mg/dL baseline (N=1439) experienced cholesterol levels of ≥240 mg/dL any-

time during the trials significantly more often than placebo-treated patients (N=836) (8.1% vs 3.8%, respectively). In these same trials, olanzapine-treated patients (N=2528) had a mean increase of 1 mg/dL in cholesterol from a mean baseline value of 203 mg/dL, which was significantly different compared to placebo-treated patients (N=1420) with a mean decrease of 4 mg/dL from a mean baseline value of 203 mg/dL.

ECG Changes — Between-group comparisons for pooled placebo-controlled trials revealed no statistically significant olanzapine/placebo differences in the proportions of patients experiencing potentially important changes in ECG parameters, including QT, QTc, and PR intervals. Olanzapine use was associated with a mean increase in heart rate of 2.4 beats per minute compared to no change among placebo patients. This slight tendency to tachycardia may be related to olanzapine's potential for inducing orthostatic changes (*see* PRECAUTIONS).

Other Adverse Events Observed During the Clinical Trial Evaluation of Olanzapine

Following is a list of terms that reflect treatment-emergent adverse events reported by patients treated with oral olanzapine (at multiple doses ≥1 mg/day) in clinical trials (8661 patients, 4165 patient-years of exposure). This listing may not include those events already listed in previous tables or elsewhere in labeling, those events for which a drug cause was remote, those event terms which were so general as to be uninformative, and those events reported only once or twice which did not have a substantial probability of being acutely life-threatening.

Events are further categorized by body system and listed in order of decreasing frequency according to the following definitions: frequent adverse events are those occurring in at least 1/100 patients (only those not already listed in the tabulated results from placebo-controlled trials appear in this listing); infrequent adverse events are those occurring in 1/100 to 1/1000 patients; rare events are those occurring in fewer than 1/1000 patients.

Body as a Whole — *Frequent:* dental pain and flu syndrome; *Infrequent:* abdomen enlarged, chills, face edema, intentional injury, malaise, moniliasis, neck pain, neck rigidity, pelvic pain, photosensitivity reaction, and suicide attempt; *Rare:* chills and fever, hangover effect, and sudden death.
Cardiovascular System — *Frequent:* hypotension; *Infrequent:* atrial fibrillation, bradycardia, cerebrovascular accident, congestive heart failure, heart arrest, hemorrhage, migraine, pallor, palpitation, vasodilatation, and ventricular extrasystoles; *Rare:* arteritis, heart failure, and pulmonary embolus.
Digestive System — *Frequent:* flatulence, increased salivation, and thirst; *Infrequent:* dysphagia, esophagitis, fecal impaction, fecal incontinence, gastritis, gastroenteritis, gingivitis, hepatitis, melena, mouth ulceration, nausea and vomiting, oral moniliasis, periodontal abscess, rectal hemorrhage, stomatitis, tongue edema, and tooth caries; *Rare:* aphthous stomatitis, enteritis, eructation, esophageal ulcer, glossitis, ileus, intestinal obstruction, liver fatty deposit, and tongue discoloration.
Endocrine System — *Infrequent:* diabetes mellitus; *Rare:* diabetic acidosis and goiter.
Hemic and Lymphatic System — *Infrequent:* anemia, cyanosis, leukocytosis, leukopenia, lymphadenopathy, and thrombocytopenia; *Rare:* normocytic anemia and thrombocythemia.
Metabolic and Nutritional Disorders — *Infrequent:* acidosis, alkaline phosphatase increased, bilirubinemia, dehydration, hypercholesteremia, hyperglycemia, hyperlipemia, hyperuricemia, hypoglycemia, hypokalemia, hyponatremia, lower extremity edema, and upper extremity edema; *Rare:* gout, hyperkalemia, hypernatremia, hypoproteinemia, ketosis, and water intoxication.
Musculoskeletal System — *Frequent:* joint stiffness and twitching; *Infrequent:* arthritis, arthrosis, leg cramps, and myasthenia; *Rare:* bone pain, bursitis, myopathy, osteoporosis, and rheumatoid arthritis.
Nervous System — *Frequent:* abnormal dreams, amnesia, delusions, emotional lability, euphoria, manic reaction, paresthesia, and schizophrenic reaction; *Infrequent:* akinesia, alcohol misuse, antisocial reaction, ataxia, CNS stimulation, cogwheel rigidity, delirium, dementia, depersonalization, dysarthria, facial paralysis, hypesthesia, hypokinesia, hypotonia, incoordination, libido decreased, libido increased, obsessive compulsive symptoms, phobias, somatization, stimulant misuse, stupor, stuttering, tardive dyskinesia, vertigo, and withdrawal syndrome; *Rare:* circumoral paresthesia, coma, encephalopathy, neuralgia, neuropathy, nystagmus, paralysis, subarachnoid hemorrhage, and tobacco misuse.
Respiratory System — *Frequent:* dyspnea; *Infrequent:* apnea, asthma, epistaxis, hemoptysis, hyperventilation, hypoxia, laryngitis, and voice alteration; *Rare:* atelectasis, hiccup, hypoventilation, lung edema, and stridor.
Skin and Appendages — *Frequent:* sweating; *Infrequent:* alopecia, contact dermatitis, dry skin, eczema, maculopapular rash, pruritus, seborrhea, skin discoloration, skin ulcer, urticaria, and vesiculobullous rash; *Rare:* hirsutism and pustular rash.
Special Senses — *Frequent:* conjunctivitis; *Infrequent:* abnormality of accommodation, blepharitis, cataract, deafness, diplopia, dry eyes, ear pain, eye hemorrhage, eye inflammation, eye pain, ocular muscle abnormality, taste perversion, and tinnitus; *Rare:* corneal lesion, glaucoma, keratoconjunctivitis, macular hypopigmentation, miosis, mydriasis, and pigment deposits lens.
Urogenital System — *Frequent:* vaginitis*; *Infrequent:* abnormal ejaculation*, amenorrhea*, breast pain, cystitis, decreased menstruation*, dysuria, female lactation*, glycosuria, gynecomastia, hematuria, impotence*, increased menstruation*, menorrhagia*, metrorrhagia*, polyuria, premenstrual syndrome*, pyuria, urinary frequency, urinary retention, urinary urgency, urination impaired, uterine fibroids enlarged*, and vaginal hemorrhage*; *Rare:* albuminuria, breast enlargement, mastitis, and oliguria.

* Adjusted for gender.

Following is a list of terms that reflect treatment-emergent adverse events reported by patients treated with intramuscular olanzapine for injection (at one or more doses ≥2.5 mg/injection) in clinical trials (722 patients). This listing may not include those events already listed in previous tables or elsewhere in labeling, those events for which a drug cause was remote, those event terms which were so general as to be uninformative, and those events reported only once which did not have a substantial probability of being acutely life-threatening.

Events are further categorized by body system and listed in order of decreasing frequency according to the following definitions: frequent adverse events are those occurring in at least 1/100 patients (only those not already listed in the tabulated results from placebo-controlled trials appear in this listing); infrequent adverse events are those occurring in 1/100 to 1/1000 patients.

Body as a Whole — *Frequent:* injection site pain; *Infrequent:* abdominal pain and fever.
Cardiovascular System — *Infrequent:* AV block, heart block, and syncope.
Digestive System — *Infrequent:* diarrhea and nausea.
Hemic and Lymphatic System — *Infrequent:* anemia.
Metabolic and Nutritional Disorders — *Infrequent:* creatine phosphokinase increased, dehydration, and hyperkalemia.
Musculoskeletal System — *Infrequent:* twitching.
Nervous System — *Infrequent:* abnormal gait, akathisia, articulation impairment, confusion, and emotional lability.
Skin and Appendages — *Infrequent:* sweating.

Postintroduction Reports

Adverse events reported since market introduction that were temporally (but not necessarily causally) related to ZYPREXA therapy include the following: allergic reaction (e.g., anaphylactoid reaction, angioedema, pruritus or urticaria), diabetic coma, pancreatitis, priapism, rhabdomyolysis, and venous thromboembolic events (including pulmonary embolism and deep venous thrombosis). Random cholesterol levels of ≥240 mg/dL and random triglyceride levels of ≥1000 mg/dL have been rarely reported.

DRUG ABUSE AND DEPENDENCE

Controlled Substance Class

Olanzapine is not a controlled substance.

Physical and Psychological Dependence

In studies prospectively designed to assess abuse and dependence potential, olanzapine was shown to have acute depressive CNS effects but little or no potential of abuse or physical dependence in rats administered oral doses up to 15 times the maximum recommended human daily oral dose (20 mg) and rhesus monkeys administered oral doses up to 8 times the maximum recommended human daily oral dose on a mg/m^2 basis.

Olanzapine has not been systematically studied in humans for its potential for abuse, tolerance, or physical dependence. While the clinical trials did not reveal any tendency for any drug-seeking behavior, these observations were not systematic, and it is not possible to predict on the basis of this limited experience the extent to which a CNS-active drug will be misused, diverted, and/or abused once marketed. Consequently, patients should be evaluated carefully for a history of drug abuse, and such patients should be observed closely for signs of misuse or abuse of olanzapine (e.g., development of tolerance, increases in dose, drug-seeking behavior).

TREATMENT-EMERGENT EXTRAPYRAMIDAL SYMPTOMS ASSESSED BY RATING SCALES INCIDENCE IN A FIXED DOSE, PLACEBO-CONTROLLED CLINICAL TRIAL OF INTRAMUSCULAR OLANZAPINE FOR INJECTION IN AGITATED PATIENTS WITH SCHIZOPHRENIA*

	Percentage of Patients Reporting Event				
	Placebo	Olanzapine IM 2.5 mg	Olanzapine IM 5 mg	Olanzapine IM 7.5 mg	Olanzapine IM 10 mg
Parkinsonism[1]	0	0	0	0	3
Akathisia[2]	0	0	5	0	0

* No statistically significant differences.
[1] Percentage of patients with a Simpson-Angus total score >3.
[2] Percentage of patients with a Barnes Akathisia Scale global score ≥2.

TREATMENT-EMERGENT EXTRAPYRAMIDAL SYMPTOMS ASSESSED BY ADVERSE EVENTS INCIDENCE IN A FIXED DOSE, PLACEBO-CONTROLLED CLINICAL TRIAL OF INTRAMUSCULAR OLANZAPINE FOR INJECTION IN AGITATED PATIENTS WITH SCHIZOPHRENIA*

	Percentage of Patients Reporting Event				
	Placebo (N=45)	Olanzapine IM 2.5 mg (N=48)	Olanzapine IM 5 mg (N=45)	Olanzapine IM 7.5 mg (N=46)	Olanzapine IM 10 mg (N=46)
Dystonic events[1]	0	0	0	0	0
Parkinsonism events[2]	0	4	2	0	0
Akathisia events[3]	0	2	0	0	0
Dyskinetic events[4]	0	0	0	0	0
Residual events[5]	0	0	0	0	0
Any extrapyramidal event	0	4	2	0	0

* No statistically significant differences.
[1] Patients with the following COSTART terms were counted in this category: dystonia, generalized spasm, neck rigidity, oculogyric crisis, opisthotonos, torticollis.
[2] Patients with the following COSTART terms were counted in this category: akinesia, cogwheel rigidity, extrapyramidal syndrome, hypertonia, hypokinesia, masked facies, tremor.
[3] Patients with the following COSTART terms were counted in this category: akathisia, hyperkinesia.
[4] Patients with the following COSTART terms were counted in this category: buccoglossal syndrome, choreoathetosis, dyskinesia, tardive dyskinesia.
[5] Patients with the following COSTART terms were counted in this category: movement disorder, myoclonus, twitching.

Adverse Event	Percentage of Patients Reporting Event			
	Placebo (N=68)	Olanzapine 5 ± 2.5 mg/day (N=65)	Olanzapine 10 ± 2.5 mg/day (N=64)	Olanzapine 15 ± 2.5 mg/day (N=69)
Asthenia	15	8	9	20
Dry mouth	4	3	5	13
Nausea	9	0	2	9
Somnolence	16	20	30	39
Tremor	3	0	5	7

Continued on next page

Zyprexa—Cont.

	TABLET STRENGTH					
	2.5 mg	5 mg	7.5 mg	10 mg	15 mg	20 mg
Tablet No.	4112	4115	4116	4117	4415	4420
Identification	LILLY 4112	LILLY 4115	LILLY 4116	LILLY 4117	LILLY 4415	LILLY 4420
NDC Codes:						
Bottles 60	NDC 0002-4112-60	NDC 0002-4115-60	NDC 0002-4116-60	NDC 0002-4117-60	NDC 0002-4415-60	NDC 0002-4420-60
Blisters - ID* 100	NDC 0002-4112-33	NDC 0002-4115-33	NDC 0002-4116-33	NDC 0002-4117-33	NDC 0002-4415-33	NDC 0002-4420-33
Bottles 1000	NDC 0002-4112-04	NDC 0002-4115-04	NDC 0002-4116-04	NDC 0002-4117-04	NDC 0002-4415-04	NDC 0002-4420-04

* Identi-Dose® (unit dose medication, Lilly)

ZYPREXA ZYDIS Tablets*	TABLET STRENGTH			
	5 mg	10 mg	15 mg	20 mg
Tablet No.	4453	4454	4455	4456
Debossed	5	10	15	20
NDC Codes:				
Dose Pack 30 (Child-Resistant)	NDC 0002-4453-85	NDC 0002-4454-85	NDC 0002-4455-85	NDC 0002-4456-85

ZYPREXA is a registered trademark of Eli Lilly and Company.
ZYDIS is a registered trademark of Cardinal Health, Inc. or one of its subsidiaries.
*ZYPREXA ZYDIS (olanzapine orally disintegrating tablets) is manufactured for Eli Lilly and Company by Cardinal Health, United Kingdom, SN5 8RU.

OVERDOSAGE

Human Experience

In premarketing trials involving more than 3100 patients and/or normal subjects, accidental or intentional acute overdosage of olanzapine was identified in 67 patients. In the patient taking the largest identified amount, 300 mg, the only symptoms reported were drowsiness and slurred speech. In the limited number of patients who were evaluated in hospitals, including the patient taking 300 mg, there were no observations indicating an adverse change in laboratory analytes or ECG. Vital signs were usually within normal limits following overdoses.

In postmarketing reports of overdose with olanzapine alone, symptoms have been reported in the majority of cases. In symptomatic patients, symptoms with ≥10% incidence included agitation/aggressiveness, dysarthria, tachycardia, various extrapyramidal symptoms, and reduced level of consciousness ranging from sedation to coma. Among less commonly reported symptoms were the following potentially medically serious events: aspiration, cardiopulmonary arrest, cardiac arrhythmias (such as supraventricular tachycardia and one patient experiencing sinus pause with spontaneous resumption of normal rhythm), delirium, possible neuroleptic malignant syndrome, respiratory depression/arrest, convulsion, hypertension, and hypotension. Eli Lilly and Company has received reports of fatality in association with overdose of olanzapine alone. In one case of death, the amount of acutely ingested olanzapine was reported to be possibly as low as 450 mg; however, in another case, a patient was reported to survive an acute olanzapine ingestion of 1500 mg.

Overdosage Management

The possibility of multiple drug involvement should be considered. In case of acute overdosage, establish and maintain an airway and ensure adequate oxygenation and ventilation, which may include intubation. Gastric lavage (after intubation, if patient is unconscious) and administration of activated charcoal together with a laxative should be considered. The possibility of obtundation, seizures, or dystonic reaction of the head and neck following overdose may create a risk of aspiration with induced emesis. Cardiovascular monitoring should commence immediately and should include continuous electrocardiographic monitoring to detect possible arrhythmias.

There is no specific antidote to olanzapine. Therefore, appropriate supportive measures should be initiated. Hypotension and circulatory collapse should be treated with appropriate measures such as intravenous fluids and/or sympathomimetic agents. (Do not use epinephrine, dopamine, or other sympathomimetics with beta-agonist activity, since beta stimulation may worsen hypotension in the setting of olanzapine-induced alpha blockade.) Close medical supervision and monitoring should continue until the patient recovers.

DOSAGE AND ADMINISTRATION

Schizophrenia

Usual Dose — Oral olanzapine should be administered on a once-a-day schedule without regard to meals, generally beginning with 5 to 10 mg initially, with a target dose of 10 mg/day within several days. Further dosage adjustments, if indicated, should generally occur at intervals of not less than 1 week, since steady state for olanzapine would not be achieved for approximately 1 week in the typical patient. When dosage adjustments are necessary, dose increments/decrements of 5 mg QD are recommended.

Efficacy in schizophrenia was demonstrated in a dose range of 10 to 15 mg/day in clinical trials. However, doses above 10 mg/day were not demonstrated to be more efficacious than the 10 mg/day dose. An increase to a dose greater than the target dose of 10 mg/day (i.e., to a dose of 15 mg/day or greater) is recommended only after clinical assessment. The safety of doses above 20 mg/day has not been evaluated in clinical trials.

Dosing in Special Populations — The recommended starting dose is 5 mg in patients who are debilitated, who have a predisposition to hypotensive reactions, who otherwise exhibit a combination of factors that may result in slower metabolism of olanzapine (e.g., nonsmoking female patients ≥65 years of age), or who may be more pharmacodynamically sensitive to olanzapine (*see* CLINICAL PHARMACOLOGY; also *see* Use in Patients with Concomitant Illness and Drug Interactions *under* PRECAUTIONS). When indicated, dose escalation should be performed with caution in these patients.

Maintenance Treatment — While there is no body of evidence available to answer the question of how long the patient treated with olanzapine should remain on it, the effectiveness of oral olanzapine, 10 mg/day to 20 mg/day, in maintaining treatment response in schizophrenic patients who had been stable on ZYPREXA for approximately 8 weeks and were then followed for a period of up to 8 months has been demonstrated in a placebo-controlled trial (*see* CLINICAL PHARMACOLOGY). Patients should be periodically reassessed to determine the need for maintenance treatment with appropriate dose.

Bipolar Disorder

Usual Monotherapy Dose — Oral olanzapine should be administered on a once-a-day schedule without regard to meals, generally beginning with 10 or 15 mg. Dosage adjustments, if indicated, should generally occur at intervals of not less than 24 hours, reflecting the procedures in the placebo-controlled trials. When dosage adjustments are necessary, dose increments/decrements of 5 mg QD are recommended.

Short-term (3-4 weeks) antimanic efficacy was demonstrated in a dose range of 5 mg to 20 mg/day in clinical trials. The safety of doses above 20 mg/day has not been evaluated in clinical trials.

Maintenance Monotherapy — The benefit of maintaining bipolar patients on monotherapy with oral ZYPREXA at a dose of 5 to 20 mg/day, after achieving a responder status for an average duration of two weeks, was demonstrated in a controlled trial (*see* Clinical Efficacy Data *under* CLINICAL PHARMACOLOGY). The physician who elects to use ZYPREXA for extended periods should periodically re-evaluate the long-term usefulness of the drug for the individual patient.

Bipolar Mania Usual Dose in Combination with Lithium or Valproate — When administered in combination with lithium or valproate, oral olanzapine dosing should generally begin with 10 mg once-a-day without regard to meals.

Short-term (6 weeks) antimanic efficacy was demonstrated in a dose range of 5 mg to 20 mg/day in clinical trials. The safety of doses above 20 mg/day has not been evaluated in clinical trials.

Dosing in Special Populations — *See* Dosing in Special Populations *under* DOSAGE AND ADMINISTRATION, Schizophrenia.

Administration of ZYPREXA ZYDIS (olanzapine orally disintegrating tablets)

After opening sachet, peel back foil on blister. Do not push tablet through foil. Immediately upon opening the blister, using dry hands, remove tablet and place entire ZYPREXA ZYDIS in the mouth. Tablet disintegration occurs rapidly in saliva so it can be easily swallowed with or without liquid.

Agitation Associated with Schizophrenia and Bipolar I Mania

Usual Dose for Agitated Patients with Schizophrenia or Bipolar Mania — The efficacy of intramuscular olanzapine for injection in controlling agitation in these disorders was demonstrated in a dose range of 2.5 mg to 10 mg. The recommended dose in these patients is 10 mg. A lower dose of 5 or 7.5 mg may be considered when clinical factors warrant (*see* CLINICAL PHARMACOLOGY). If agitation warranting additional intramuscular doses persists following the initial dose, subsequent doses up to 10 mg may be given. However, the efficacy of repeated doses of intramuscular olanzapine for injection in agitated patients has not been systematically evaluated in controlled clinical trials. Also, the safety of total daily doses greater than 30 mg, or 10 mg injections given more frequently than 2 hours after the initial dose, and 4 hours after the second dose have not been evaluated in clinical trials. Maximal dosing of intramuscular olanzapine (e.g., three doses of 10 mg administered 2-4 hours apart) may be associated with a substantial occurrence of significant orthostatic hypotension (*see* PRECAUTIONS, Hemodynamic Effects). Thus, it is recommended that patients requiring subsequent intramuscular injections be assessed for orthostatic hypotension prior to the administration of any subsequent doses of intramuscular olanzapine for injection. The administration of an additional dose to a patient with a clinically significant postural change in systolic blood pressure is not recommended.

If ongoing olanzapine therapy is clinically indicated, oral olanzapine may be initiated in a range of 5-20 mg/day as soon as clinically appropriate (*see* Schizophrenia or Bipolar Disorder *under* DOSAGE AND ADMINISTRATION).

Intramuscular Dosing in Special Populations — A dose of 5 mg per injection should be considered for geriatric patients or when other clinical factors warrant. A lower dose of 2.5 mg per injection should be considered for patients who otherwise might be debilitated, be predisposed to hypotensive reactions, or be more pharmacodynamically sensitive to olanzapine (*see* CLINICAL PHARMACOLOGY; also *see* Use in Patients with Concomitant Illness and Drug Interactions *under* PRECAUTIONS).

Administration of ZYPREXA IntraMuscular

ZYPREXA IntraMuscular is intended for intramuscular use only. Do not administer intravenously or subcutaneously. Inject slowly, deep into the muscle mass.

Parenteral drug products should be inspected visually for particulate matter and discoloration prior to administration, whenever solution and container permit.

Directions for preparation of ZYPREXA IntraMuscular with Sterile Water for Injection

Dissolve the contents of the vial using 2.1 mL of Sterile Water for Injection to provide a solution containing approximately 5 mg/mL of olanzapine. The resulting solution should appear clear and yellow. ZYPREXA IntraMuscular reconstituted with Sterile Water for Injection should be used immediately (within 1 hour) after reconstitution. **Discard any unused portion.**

The following table provides injection volumes for delivering various doses of intramuscular olanzapine for injection reconstituted with Sterile Water for Injection.

Dose, mg Olanzapine	Volume of Injection, mL
10.0	Withdraw total contents of vial
7.5	1.5
5.0	1.0
2.5	0.5

Physical Incompatibility Information

ZYPREXA IntraMuscular should be reconstituted only with Sterile Water for Injection. ZYPREXA IntraMuscular should not be combined in a syringe with diazepam injection because precipitation occurs when these products are mixed. Lorazepam injection should not be used to reconstitute ZYPREXA IntraMuscular as this combination results in a delayed reconstitution time. ZYPREXA IntraMuscular should not be combined in a syringe with haloperidol injection because the resulting low pH has been shown to degrade olanzapine over time.

HOW SUPPLIED

The ZYPREXA 2.5 mg, 5 mg, 7.5 mg, and 10 mg tablets are white, round, and imprinted in blue ink with LILLY and tablet number. The 15 mg tablets are elliptical, blue, and debossed with LILLY and tablet number. The 20 mg tablets are elliptical, pink, and debossed with LILLY and tablet number. The tablets are available as follows:

[See first table above]

ZYPREXA ZYDIS (olanzapine orally disintegrating tablets) are yellow, round, and debossed with the tablet strength. The tablets are available as follows:

[See second table above]

ZYPREXA IntraMuscular is available in:

NDC 0002-7597-01 (No. VL7597) – 10 mg vial (1s)

Store ZYPREXA tablets, ZYPREXA ZYDIS, and ZYPREXA IntraMuscular vials (before reconstitution) at controlled room temperature, 20° to 25°C (68° to 77°F) [*see* USP]. Reconstituted ZYPREXA IntraMuscular may be stored at controlled room temperature, 20° to 25°C (68° to 77°F) [*see* USP] for up to 1 hour if necessary. **Discard any unused portion of reconstituted ZYPREXA IntraMuscular.** The USP defines controlled room temperature as a temperature maintained thermostatically that encompasses the usual and customary working environment of 20° to 25°C (68° to 77°F); that results in a mean kinetic temperature calculated to be not more than 25°C; and that allows for excursions between 15° and 30°C (59° and 86°F) that are experienced in pharmacies, hospitals, and warehouses.

Protect ZYPREXA tablets and ZYPREXA ZYDIS from light and moisture. Protect ZYPREXA IntraMuscular from light, do not freeze.

ANIMAL TOXICOLOGY

In animal studies with olanzapine, the principal hematologic findings were reversible peripheral cytopenias in individual dogs dosed at 10 mg/kg (17 times the maximum recommended human daily oral dose on a mg/m^2 basis), dose-related decreases in lymphocytes and neutrophils in mice, and lymphopenia in rats. A few dogs treated with 10 mg/kg developed reversible neutropenia and/or reversible hemolytic anemia between 1 and 10 months of treatment. Dose-related decreases in lymphocytes and neutrophils were seen in mice given doses of 10 mg/kg (equal to 2 times the maximum recommended human daily oral dose on a mg/m² basis) in studies of 3 months' duration. Nonspecific lymphopenia, consistent with decreased body weight gain, occurred in rats receiving 22.5 mg/kg (11 times the maximum recommended human daily oral dose on a mg/m² basis) for 3 months or 16 mg/kg (8 times the maximum recommended human daily oral dose on a mg/m² basis) for 6 or 12 months. No evidence of bone marrow cytotoxicity was found in any of the species examined. Bone marrows were normocellular or hypercellular, indicating that the reductions in circulating blood cells were probably due to peripheral (non-marrow) factors.

Literature revised April 14, 2005

Eli Lilly and Company
Indianapolis, IN 46285, USA
www.ZYPREXA.com

PV 3518 AMP PRINTED IN USA

Copyright © 1997, 2005, Eli Lilly and Company. All rights reserved.

Merck & Co., Inc.
PO BOX 4 WP39-206
WEST POINT, PA 19486-0004

For Medical Information Contact:
Generally:
Product and service information:
Call the Merck National Service Center, 8:00 AM to 7:00 PM (ET), Monday through Friday:
(800) NSC-MERCK
(800) 672-6372
FAX: (800) MERCK-68
FAX: (800) 637-2568
Adverse Drug Experiences:
Call the Merck National Service Center, 8:00 AM to 7:00 PM (ET), Monday through Friday:
(800) NSC-MERCK
(800) 672-6372
Pregnancy Registries
(800) 986-8999
In Emergencies:
24-hour emergency information for healthcare professionals:
(800) NSC-MERCK
(800) 672-6372
Sales and Ordering:
For product orders and direct account inquiries only, call the Order Management Center,
8:00 AM to 7:00 PM (ET), Monday through Friday:
(800) MERCK RX
(800) 637-2579

AMINOHIPPURATE SODIUM "PAH" ℞
Injection

Prescribing information for this product, which appears on page 1992 of the 2005 PDR, has been revised as follows. Please write "See Supplement A" next to the product heading.

In the **ADVERSE REACTIONS** section, in the 1st paragraph, delete the parentheses and add the word "anaphylaxis" after the word "including," so that the paragraph reads:

Hypersensitivity reactions including anaphylaxis, angioedema, and urticaria, vasomotor disturbances....

Revisions based on 9051024, issued October 2004.

INTRAVENOUS INFUSION (not for IV Bolus Injection)
CANCIDAS® ℞
[kan-si-das]
(caspofungin acetate) FOR INJECTION

Prescribing information for this product, which appears on pages 1999–2004 of the 2005 PDR, has been completely revised as follows. Please write "See Supplement A" next to the product heading.

DESCRIPTION

CANCIDAS* is a sterile, lyophilized product for intravenous (IV) infusion that contains a semisynthetic lipopeptide (echinocandin) compound synthesized from a fermentation product of *Glarea lozoyensis*. CANCIDAS is the first of a new class of antifungal drugs (echinocandins) that inhibit the synthesis of β (1,3)-D-glucan, an integral component of the fungal cell wall.

CANCIDAS (caspofungin acetate) is 1-[(4*R*,5*S*)-5-[(2-aminoethyl)amino]-N^2-(10,12-dimethyl-1-oxotetradecyl)-4-hydroxy-L-ornithine]-5-[(3*R*)-3-hydroxy-L-ornithine] pneumocandin B_0 diacetate (salt). In addition to the active ingredient caspofungin acetate, CANCIDAS contains the following inactive ingredients: sucrose, mannitol, acetic acid, and sodium hydroxide. Caspofungin acetate is a hygroscopic, white to off-white powder. It is freely soluble in water and methanol, and slightly soluble in ethanol. The pH of a saturated aqueous solution of caspofungin acetate is approximately 6.6. The empirical formula is $C_{52}H_{88}N_{10}O_{15}•2C_2H_4O_2$ and the formula weight is 1213.42. The structural formula is:

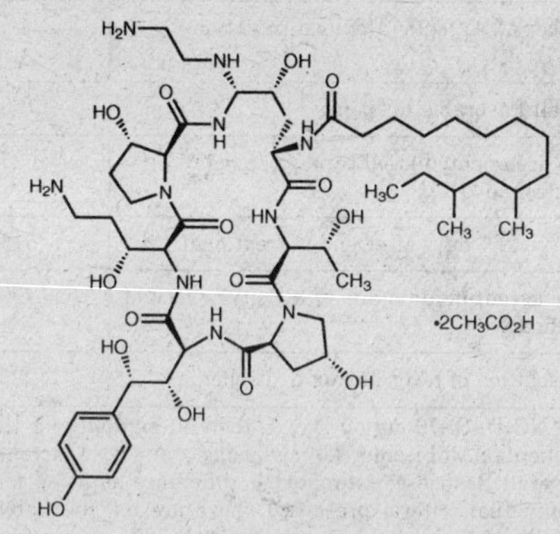

*Registered trademark of MERCK & CO., Inc.

COPYRIGHT © MERCK & CO., Inc., 2001
All rights reserved

CLINICAL PHARMACOLOGY

Pharmacokinetics

Distribution

Plasma concentrations of caspofungin decline in a polyphasic manner following single 1-hour IV infusions. A short α-phase occurs immediately postinfusion, followed by a β-phase (half-life of 9 to 11 hours) that characterizes much of the profile and exhibits clear log-linear behavior from 6 to 48 hours postdose during which the plasma concentration decreases 10-fold. An additional, longer half-life phase, γ-phase, (half-life of 40-50 hours), also occurs. Distribution, rather than excretion or biotransformation, is the dominant mechanism influencing plasma clearance. Caspofungin is extensively bound to albumin (~97%), and distribution into red blood cells is minimal. Mass balance results showed that approximately 92% of the administered radioactivity was distributed to tissues by 36 to 48 hours after a single 70-mg dose of [³H] caspofungin acetate. There is little excretion or biotransformation of caspofungin during the first 30 hours after administration.

Metabolism

Caspofungin is slowly metabolized by hydrolysis and N-acetylation. Caspofungin also undergoes spontaneous chemical degradation to an open-ring peptide compound, L-747969. At later time points (≥5 days postdose), there is a low level (≤7 picomoles/mg protein, or ≤1.3% of administered dose) of covalent binding of radiolabel in plasma following single-dose administration of [³H] caspofungin acetate, which may be due to two reactive intermediates formed during the chemical degradation of caspofungin to L-747969. Additional metabolism involves hydrolysis into constitutive amino acids and their degradates, including dihydroxyhomotyrosine and N-acetyl-dihydroxyhomotyrosine. These two tyrosine derivatives are found only in urine, suggesting rapid clearance of these derivatives by the kidneys.

Excretion

Two single-dose radiolabeled pharmacokinetic studies were conducted. In one study, plasma, urine, and feces were collected over 27 days, and in the second study plasma was collected over 6 months. Plasma concentrations of radioactivity and of caspofungin were similar during the first 24 to 48 hours postdose; thereafter drug levels fell more rapidly. In plasma, caspofungin concentrations fell below the limit of quantitation after 6 to 8 days postdose, while radiolabel fell below the limit of quantitation at 22.3 weeks postdose. After single intravenous administration of [³H] caspofungin acetate, excretion of caspofungin and its metabolites in humans was 35% of dose in feces and 41% of dose in urine. A small amount of caspofungin is excreted unchanged in urine (~1.4% of dose). Renal clearance of parent drug is low (~0.15 mL/min) and total clearance of caspofungin is 12 mL/min.

Special Populations

Gender

Plasma concentrations of caspofungin in healthy men and women were similar following a single 70-mg dose. After 13 daily 50-mg doses, caspofungin plasma concentrations in women were elevated slightly (approximately 22% in area under the curve [AUC]) relative to men. No dosage adjustment is necessary based on gender.

Geriatric

Plasma concentrations of caspofungin in healthy older men and women (≥65 years of age) were increased slightly (approximately 28% AUC) compared to young healthy men after a single 70-mg dose of caspofungin. In patients who were treated empirically or who had candidemia or other *Candida* infections (intra-abdominal abscesses, peritonitis, or pleural space infections), a similar modest effect of age was seen in older patients relative to younger patients. No dosage adjustment is necessary for the elderly (see PRECAUTIONS, *Geriatric Use*).

Race

Regression analyses of patient pharmacokinetic data indicated that no clinically significant differences in the pharmacokinetics of caspofungin were seen among Caucasians, Blacks, and Hispanics. No dosage adjustment is necessary on the basis of race.

Renal Insufficiency

In a clinical study of single 70-mg doses, caspofungin pharmacokinetics were similar in volunteers with mild renal insufficiency (creatinine clearance 50 to 80 mL/min) and control subjects. Moderate (creatinine clearance 31 to 49 mL/min), advanced (creatinine clearance 5 to 30 mL/min), and end-stage (creatinine clearance <10 mL/min and dialysis dependent) renal insufficiency moderately increased caspofungin plasma concentrations after single-dose administration (range: 30 to 49% for AUC). However, in patients with invasive aspergillosis, candidemia, or other *Candida* infections (intra-abdominal abscesses, peritonitis, or pleural space infections) who received multiple daily doses of CANCIDAS 50 mg, there was no significant effect of mild to end-stage renal impairment on caspofungin concentrations. No dosage adjustment is necessary for patients with renal insufficiency. Caspofungin is not dialyzable, thus supplementary dosing is not required following hemodialysis.

Hepatic Insufficiency

Plasma concentrations of caspofungin after a single 70-mg dose in patients with mild hepatic insufficiency (Child-Pugh score 5 to 6) were increased by approximately 55% in AUC compared to healthy control subjects. In a 14-day multiple-dose study (70 mg on Day 1 followed by 50 mg daily thereafter), plasma concentrations in patients with mild hepatic insufficiency were increased modestly (19 to 25% in AUC) on Days 7 and 14 relative to healthy control subjects. No dosage adjustment is recommended for patients with mild hepatic insufficiency. Patients with moderate hepatic insufficiency (Child-Pugh score 7 to 9) who received a single 70-mg dose of CANCIDAS had an average plasma caspofungin increase of 76% in AUC compared to control subjects. A dosage reduction is recommended for patients with moderate hepatic insufficiency (see DOSAGE AND ADMINISTRATION). There is no clinical experience in patients with severe hepatic insufficiency (Child-Pugh score >9).

Pediatric Patients

CANCIDAS has not been adequately studied in patients under 18 years of age.

MICROBIOLOGY

Mechanism of Action

Caspofungin acetate, the active ingredient of CANCIDAS, inhibits the synthesis of β (1,3)-D-glucan, an essential component of the cell wall of susceptible *Aspergillus* species and *Candida* species. β (1,3)-D-glucan is not present in mammalian cells. Caspofungin has shown activity against *Candida* species and in regions of active cell growth of the hyphae of *Aspergillus fumigatus*.

Activity in vitro

Caspofungin exhibits *in vitro* activity against *Aspergillus* species (*Aspergillus fumigatus, Aspergillus flavus*, and *Aspergillus terreus*) and *Candida* species (*Candida albicans, Candida glabrata, Candida guilliermondii, Candida krusei, Candida parapsilosis*, and *Candida tropicalis*). Susceptibility testing was performed according to the National Committee for Clinical Laboratory Standards (NCCLS) method M38-A (for *Aspergillus* species) and M27-A (for *Candida* species). Standardized susceptibility testing methods for echinocandins have not been established for yeasts and filamentous fungi, and results of susceptibility studies do not correlate with clinical outcome.

Activity in vivo

Caspofungin was active when parenterally administered to immunocompetent and immunosuppressed mice as long as 24 hours after disseminated infections with *C. albicans*, in which the endpoints were prolonged survival of infected mice and reduction of *C. albicans* from target organs. Caspofungin, administered parenterally to immunocompetent and immunosuppressed rodents, as long as 24 hours after disseminated or pulmonary infection with *Aspergillus fumigatus*, has shown prolonged survival, which has not been consistently associated with a reduction in mycological burden.

Drug Resistance

Mutants of *Candida* with reduced susceptibility to caspofungin have been identified in some patients during treatment. Similar observations were made in a study in mice infected with *C. albicans* and treated with orally administered doses of caspofungin. MIC values for caspofungin should not be used to predict clinical outcome, since a correlation between MIC values and clinical outcome has not been established. The incidence of drug resistance by various clinical isolates of *Candida* and *Aspergillus* species is unknown.

Drug Interactions

Studies *in vitro* and *in vivo* of caspofungin, in combination with amphotericin B, suggest no antagonism of antifungal activity against either *A. fumigatus* or *C. albicans*. The clinical significance of these results is unknown.

CLINICAL STUDIES

Empirical Therapy in febrile, neutropenic patients

A double-blind study enrolled 1111 febrile, neutropenic (<500 cells/mm³) patients who were randomized to treat-

Continued on next page

Information on the Merck & Co., Inc., products listed on these pages is from the full prescribing information in use April 1, 2004.

Cancidas—Cont.

ment with daily doses of CANCIDAS (50 mg/day following a 70-mg loading dose on Day 1) or AmBisome®[1] (amphotericin B liposome for injection, 3.0 mg/kg/day). Patients were stratified based on risk category (high-risk patients had undergone allogeneic stem cell transplantation or had relapsed acute leukemia) and on receipt of prior antifungal prophylaxis. Twenty-four percent of patients were high risk and 56% had received prior antifungal prophylaxis. Patients who remained febrile or clinically deteriorated following 5 days of therapy could receive 70 mg/day of CANCIDAS or 5.0 mg/kg/day of AmBisome. Treatment was continued to resolution of neutropenia (but not beyond 28 days unless a fungal infection was documented).

An overall favorable response required meeting each of the following criteria: no documented breakthrough fungal infections up to 7 days after completion of treatment, survival for 7 days after completion of study therapy, no discontinuation of the study drug because of drug-related toxicity or lack of efficacy, resolution of fever during the period of neutropenia, and successful treatment of any documented baseline fungal infection.

[1] Registered trademark of Gilead Sciences, Inc.

Based on the composite response rates, CANCIDAS was as effective as AmBisome in empirical therapy of persistent febrile neutropenia (see Table 1).
[See table 1 at right]
The rate of successful treatment of documented baseline infections, a component of the primary endpoint, was not statistically different between treatment groups.
The response rates did not differ between treatment groups based on either of the stratification variables: risk category or prior antifungal prophylaxis.
Candidemia and the following other Candida infections: intra-abdominal abscesses, peritonitis and pleural space infections
In a Phase III randomized, double-blind study, patients with a proven diagnosis of invasive candidiasis received daily doses of CANCIDAS (50 mg/day following a 70-mg loading dose on Day 1) or amphotericin B deoxycholate (0.6 to 0.7 mg/kg/day for non-neutropenic and 0.7 to 1.0 mg/kg/day for neutropenic patients). Patients were stratified by both neutropenic status and APACHE II score. Patients with *Candida* endocarditis, meningitis, or osteomyelitis were excluded from this study.
Patients who met the entry criteria and received one or more doses of IV study therapy were included in the primary (modified intention-to-treat [MITT]) analysis of response at the end of IV study therapy. A favorable response at this time point required both symptom/sign resolution/improvement and microbiological clearance of the *Candida* infection.
Two hundred thirty-nine patients were enrolled. Patient disposition is shown in Table 2.
[See table 2 at right]
Of the 239 patients enrolled, 224 met the criteria for inclusion in the MITT population (109 treated with CANCIDAS and 115 treated with amphotericin B). Of these 224 patients, 186 patients had candidemia (92 treated with CANCIDAS and 94 treated with amphotericin B). The majority of the patients with candidemia were non-neutropenic (87%) and had an APACHE II score less than or equal to 20 (77%) in both arms. Most candidemia infections were caused by *C. albicans* (39%), followed by *C. parapsilosis* (20%), *C. tropicalis* (17%), *C. glabrata* (8%), and *C. krusei* (3%).
At the end of IV study therapy, CANCIDAS was comparable to amphotericin B in the treatment of candidemia in the MITT population. For the other efficacy time points (Day 10 of IV study therapy, end of all antifungal therapy, 2-week post-therapy follow-up, and 6- to 8-week post-therapy follow-up), CANCIDAS was as effective as amphotericin B. Outcome, relapse and mortality data are shown in Table 3.
[See table 3 at right]
In this study, the efficacy of CANCIDAS in patients with intra-abdominal abscesses, peritonitis and pleural space *Candida* infections was evaluated in 19 non-neutropenic patients. Two of these patients had concurrent candidemia. *Candida* was part of a polymicrobial infection that required adjunctive surgical drainage in 11 of these 19 patients. A favorable response was seen in 9 of 9 patients with peritonitis, 3 of 4 with abscesses (liver, parasplenic, and urinary bladder abscesses), 2 of 2 with pleural space infections, 1 of 2 with mixed peritoneal and pleural infection, 1 of 1 with mixed abdominal abscess and peritonitis, and 0 of 1 with *Candida* pneumonia.
Overall, across all sites of infection included in the study, the efficacy of CANCIDAS was comparable to that of amphotericin B for the primary endpoint.
In this study, the efficacy data for CANCIDAS in neutropenic patients with candidemia were limited. In a separate compassionate use study, 4 patients with hepatosplenic candidiasis received prolonged therapy with CANCIDAS following other long-term antifungal therapy; three of these patients had a favorable response.
Esophageal Candidiasis (and information on oropharyngeal candidiasis)
The safety and efficacy of CANCIDAS in the treatment of esophageal candidiasis was evaluated in one large, controlled, noninferiority, clinical trial and two smaller dose-response studies.

TABLE 1
Favorable Response of Patients with Persistent Fever and Neutropenia

	CANCIDAS*	AmBisome*	% Difference (Confidence Interval)**
Number of Patients (Modified Intention-To-Treat)	556	539	
Overall Favorable Response	190 (33.9%)	181 (33.7%)	0.2 (-5.6, 6.0)
No documented breakthrough fungal infection	527 (94.8%)	515 (95.5%)	-0.8
Survival 7 days after end of treatment	515 (92.6%)	481 (89.2%)	3.4
No discontinuation due to toxicity or lack of efficacy	499 (89.7%)	461 (85.5%)	4.2
Resolution of fever during neutropenia	229 (41.2%)	223 (41.4%)	-0.2

* CANCIDAS: 70 mg on Day 1, then 50 mg daily for the remainder of treatment (daily dose increased to 70 mg for 73 patients); AmBisome: 3.0 mg/kg/day (daily dose increased to 5.0 mg/kg for 74 patients).
** Overall Response: estimated % difference adjusted for strata and expressed as CANCIDAS – AmBisome (95.2% CI); Individual criteria presented above are not mutually exclusive. The percent difference calculated as CANCIDAS – AmBisome.

TABLE 2
Disposition in Candidemia and Other *Candida* Infections
(Intra-abdominal abscesses, peritonitis, and pleural space infections)

	CANCIDAS*	Amphotericin B
Randomized patients	114	125
Patients completing study**	63 (55.3%)	69 (55.2%)
DISCONTINUATIONS OF STUDY**		
All Study Discontinuations	51 (44.7%)	56 (44.8%)
Study Discontinuations due to clinical adverse events	39 (34.2%)	43 (34.4%)
Study Discontinuations due to laboratory adverse events	0 (0%)	1 (0.8%)
DISCONTINUATIONS OF STUDY THERAPY		
All Study Therapy Discontinuations	48 (42.1%)	58 (46.4%)
Study Therapy Discontinuations due to clinical adverse events	30 (26.3%)	37 (29.6%)
Study Therapy Discontinuations due to laboratory adverse events	1 (0.9%)	7 (5.6%)
Study Therapy Discontinuations due to all drug-related*** adverse events	3 (2.6%)	29 (23.2%)

*Patients received CANCIDAS 70 mg on Day 1, then 50 mg daily for the remainder of their treatment.
**Study defined as study treatment period and 6-8 week follow-up period.
***Determined by the investigator to be possibly, probably, or definitely drug-related.

TABLE 3
Outcomes, Relapse, & Mortality in Candidemia and Other *Candida* Infections (Intra-abdominal abscesses, peritonitis, and pleural space infections)

	CANCIDAS*	Amphotericin B	% Difference** after adjusting for strata (Confidence Interval)***
Number of MITT[+] patients	109	115	
FAVORABLE OUTCOMES (MITT) AT THE END OF IV STUDY THERAPY			
All MITT patients	81/109 (74.3%)	78/115 (67.8%)	7.5 (-5.4, 20.3)
Candidemia	67/92 (72.8%)	63/94 (67.0%)	7.0 (-7.0, 21.1)
Neutropenic	6/14 (43%)	5/10 (50%)	
Non-neutropenic	61/78 (78%)	58/84 (69%)	
Endophthalmitis	0/1	2/3	
Multiple Sites	4/5	4/4	
Blood / Pleural	1/1	1/1	
Blood / Peritoneal	1/1	1/1	
Blood / Urine	–	1/1	
Peritoneal / Pleural	1/2	–	
Abdominal / Peritoneal	–	1/1	
Subphrenic / Peritoneal	1/1	–	
DISSEMINATED INFECTIONS, RELAPSES AND MORTALITY			
Disseminated Infections in neutropenic patients	4/14 (28.6%)	3/10 (30.0%)	
All relapses[++]	7/81 (8.6%)	8/78 (10.3%)	
Culture-confirmed relapse	5/81 (6%)	2/78 (3%)	
Overall study*** mortality in MITT	36/109 (33.0%)	35/115 (30.4%)	
Mortality during study therapy	18/109 (17%)	13/115 (11%)	
Mortality attributed to *Candida*	4/109 (4%)	7/115 (6%)	

*Patients received CANCIDAS 70 mg on Day 1, then 50 mg daily for the remainder of their treatment.
**Calculated as CANCIDAS – amphotericin B
***95% CI for candidemia, 95.6% for all patients
[+]Modified intention-to-treat
[++]Includes all patients who either developed a culture-confirmed recurrence of *Candida* infection or required antifungal therapy for the treatment of a proven or suspected *Candida* infection in the follow-up period.
***Study defined as study treatment period and 6-8 week follow-up period.

In all 3 studies, patients were required to have symptoms and microbiological documentation of esophageal candidiasis; most patients had advanced AIDS (with CD4 counts <50/mm³).

Of the 166 patients in the large study who had culture-confirmed esophageal candidiasis at baseline, 120 had *Candida albicans* and 2 had *Candida tropicalis* as the sole baseline pathogen whereas 44 had mixed baseline cultures containing *C. albicans* and one or more additional *Candida* species.

In the large, randomized, double-blind study comparing CANCIDAS 50 mg/day versus intravenous fluconazole 200 mg/day for the treatment of esophageal candidiasis, patients were treated for an average of 9 days (range 7-21 days). The primary endpoint was favorable overall response at 5 to 7 days following discontinuation of study therapy, which required both complete resolution of symptoms and significant endoscopic improvement. The definition of endoscopic response was based on severity of disease at baseline using a 4-grade scale and required at least a two-grade reduction from baseline endoscopic score or reduction to grade 0 for patients with a baseline score of 2 or less.

The proportion of patients with a favorable overall response for the primary endpoint was comparable for CANCIDAS and fluconazole as shown in Table 4.

[See table 4 at right]

The proportion of patients with a favorable symptom response was also comparable (90.1% and 89.4% for CANCIDAS and fluconazole, respectively). In addition, the proportion of patients with a favorable endoscopic response was comparable (85.2% and 86.2% for CANCIDAS and fluconazole, respectively).

As shown in Table 5, the esophageal candidiasis relapse rates at the Day 14 post-treatment visit were similar for the two groups. At the Day 28 post-treatment visit, the group treated with CANCIDAS had a numerically higher incidence of relapse, however, the difference was not statistically significant.

[See table 5 at right]

In this trial, which was designed to establish noninferiority of CANCIDAS to fluconazole for the treatment of esophageal candidiasis, 122 (70%) patients also had oropharyngeal candidiasis. A favorable response was defined as complete resolution of all symptoms of oropharyngeal disease and all visible oropharyngeal lesions. The proportion of patients with a favorable oropharyngeal response at the 5- to 7-day post-treatment visit was numerically lower for CANCIDAS, however, the difference was not statistically significant. The results are shown in Table 6.

[See table 6 at right]

As shown in Table 7, the oropharyngeal candidiasis relapse rates at the Day 14 and the Day 28 post-treatment visits were statistically significantly higher for CANCIDAS than for fluconazole.

[See table 7 at right]

The results from the two smaller dose-ranging studies corroborate the efficacy of CANCIDAS for esophageal candidiasis that was demonstrated in the larger study.

CANCIDAS was associated with favorable outcomes in 7 of 10 esophageal *C. albicans* infections refractory to at least 200 mg of fluconazole given for 7 days, although the *in vitro* susceptibility of the infecting isolates to fluconazole was not known.

Invasive Aspergillosis

Sixty-nine patients between the ages of 18 and 80 with invasive aspergillosis (IA) were enrolled in an open-label, noncomparative study to evaluate the safety, tolerability, and efficacy of CANCIDAS. Enrolled patients had previously been refractory to or intolerant of other antifungal therapy(ies). Refractory patients were classified as those who had disease progression or failed to improve despite therapy for at least 7 days with amphotericin B, lipid formulations of amphotericin B, itraconazole, or an investigational azole with reported activity against *Aspergillus*. Intolerance to previous therapy was defined as a doubling of creatinine (or creatinine ≥2.5 mg/dL while on therapy), other acute reactions, or infusion-related toxicity. To be included in the study, patients with pulmonary disease must have had definite (positive tissue histopathology or positive culture from tissue obtained by an invasive procedure) or probable (positive radiographic or computed tomography evidence with supporting culture from bronchoalveolar lavage or sputum, galactomannan enzyme-linked immunosorbent assay, and/or polymerase chain reaction) invasive aspergillosis. Patients with extrapulmonary disease had to have definite invasive aspergillosis. The definitions were modeled after the Mycoses Study Group Criteria.[2] Patients were administered a single 70-mg loading dose of CANCIDAS and subsequently dosed with 50 mg daily. The mean duration of therapy was 33.7 days, with a range of 1 to 162 days.

[2] Denning DW, Lee JY, Hostetler JS, et al. NIAID Mycoses Study Group multicenter trial of oral itraconazole therapy for invasive aspergillosis. *Am J Med* 1994; 97:135-144.

An independent expert panel evaluated patient data, including diagnosis of invasive aspergillosis, response and tolerability to previous antifungal therapy, treatment course on CANCIDAS, and clinical outcome.

A favorable response was defined as either complete resolution (complete response) or clinically meaningful improvement (partial response) of all signs and symptoms and attributable radiographic findings. Stable, nonprogressive disease was considered to be an unfavorable response.

Among the 69 patients enrolled in the study, 63 met entry diagnostic criteria and had outcome data; and of these, 52 patients received treatment for >7 days. Fifty-three (84%) were refractory to previous antifungal therapy and 10 (16%) were intolerant. Forty-five patients had pulmonary disease and 18 had extrapulmonary disease. Underlying conditions were hematologic malignancy (N=24), allogeneic bone marrow transplant or stem cell transplant (N=18), organ transplant (N=8), solid tumor (N=3), or other conditions (N=10).

TABLE 4
Favorable Response Rates for Patients with Esophageal Candidiasis

	CANCIDAS	Fluconazole	% Difference* (95% CI)
Day 5-7 post-treatment	66/81 (81.5%)	80/94 (85.1%)	-3.6 (-14.7, 7.5)

*calculated as CANCIDAS – fluconazole

TABLE 5
Relapse Rates at 14 and 28 Days Post-Therapy in Patients with Esophageal Candidiasis at Baseline

	CANCIDAS	Fluconazole	% Difference* (95% CI)
Day 14 post-treatment	7/66 (10.6%)	6/76 (7.9%)	2.7 (-6.9, 12.3)
Day 28 post-treatment	18/64 (28.1%)	12/72 (16.7%)	11.5 (-2.5, 25.4)

*calculated as CANCIDAS – fluconazole

TABLE 6
Oropharyngeal Candidiasis Response Rates at 5 to 7 Days Post-Therapy in Patients with Oropharyngeal and Esophageal Candidiasis at Baseline

	CANCIDAS	Fluconazole	% Difference* (95% CI)
Day 5-7 post-treatment	40/56 (71.4%)	55/66 (83.3%)	-11.9 (-26.8, 3.0)

*calculated as CANCIDAS – fluconazole

TABLE 7
Oropharyngeal Candidiasis Relapse Rates at 14 and 28 Days Post-Therapy in Patients with Oropharyngeal and Esophageal Candidiasis at Baseline

	CANCIDAS	Fluconazole	% Difference* (95% CI)
Day 14 post-treatment	17/40 (42.5%)	7/53 (13.2%)	29.3 (11.5, 47.1)
Day 28 post-treatment	23/39 (59.0%)	18/51 (35.3%)	23.7 (3.4, 43.9)

*calculated as CANCIDAS – fluconazole

All patients in the study received concomitant therapies for their other underlying conditions. Eighteen patients received tacrolimus and CANCIDAS concomitantly, of whom 8 also received mycophenolate mofetil.

Overall, the expert panel determined that 41% (26/63) of patients receiving at least one dose of CANCIDAS had a favorable response. For those patients who received >7 days of therapy with CANCIDAS, 50% (26/52) had a favorable response. The favorable response rates for patients who were either refractory to or intolerant of previous therapies were 36% (19/53) and 70% (7/10), respectively. The response rates among patients with pulmonary disease and extrapulmonary disease were 47% (21/45) and 28% (5/18), respectively. Among patients with extrapulmonary disease, 2 of 8 patients who also had definite, probable, or possible CNS involvement had a favorable response. Two of these 8 patients had progression of disease and manifested CNS involvement while on therapy.

There is substantial evidence that CANCIDAS is well tolerated and effective for the treatment of invasive aspergillosis in patients who are refractory to or intolerant of itraconazole, amphotericin B, and/or lipid formulations of amphotericin B. However, the efficacy of CANCIDAS has not been evaluated in concurrently controlled clinical studies, with other antifungal therapies.

INDICATIONS AND USAGE

CANCIDAS is indicated for:

- Empirical therapy for presumed fungal infections in febrile, neutropenic patients.
- Treatment of Candidemia and the following *Candida* infections: intra-abdominal abscesses, peritonitis and pleural space infections. CANCIDAS has not been studied in endocarditis, osteomyelitis, and meningitis due to *Candida*.
- Treatment of Esophageal Candidiasis (see CLINICAL STUDIES).
- Treatment of Invasive Aspergillosis in patients who are refractory to or intolerant of other therapies (i.e., amphotericin B, lipid formulations of amphotericin B, and/or itraconazole). CANCIDAS has not been studied as initial therapy for invasive aspergillosis.

CONTRAINDICATIONS

CANCIDAS is contraindicated in patients with hypersensitivity to any component of this product.

WARNINGS

Concomitant use of CANCIDAS with cyclosporine is not recommended unless the potential benefit outweighs the potential risk to the patient. In one clinical study, 3 of 4 healthy subjects who received CANCIDAS 70 mg on Days 1 through 10, and also received two 3 mg/kg doses of cyclosporine 12 hours apart on Day 10, developed transient elevations of alanine transaminase (ALT) on Day 11 that were 2 to 3 times the upper limit of normal (ULN). In a separate panel of subjects in the same study, 2 of 8 who received CANCIDAS 35 mg daily for 3 days and cyclosporine (two 3 mg/kg doses administered 12 hours apart) on Day 1 had small increases in ALT (slightly above the ULN) on Day 2. In both groups, elevations in aspartate transaminase (AST) paralleled ALT elevations, but were of lesser magnitude (see ADVERSE REACTIONS). Hence, concomitant use of CANCIDAS with cyclosporine is not recommended until multiple-dose use in patients is studied.

PRECAUTIONS

General

The efficacy of a 70-mg dose regimen in patients with invasive aspergillosis who are not clinically responding to the 50-mg daily dose is not known. Limited safety data suggest that an increase in dose to 70 mg daily is well tolerated. The safety and efficacy of doses above 70 mg have not been adequately studied in patients with Candida infections. However, CANCIDAS was generally well tolerated at a dose of 100 mg once daily for 21 days when administered to 15 healthy subjects.

The safety information on treatment durations longer than 4 weeks is limited; however, available data suggest that CANCIDAS continues to be well tolerated with longer courses of therapy (up to 162 days).

Hepatic Effects

Laboratory abnormalities in liver function tests have been seen in healthy volunteers and patients treated with CANCIDAS. In some patients with serious underlying conditions who were receiving multiple concomitant medications along with CANCIDAS, clinical hepatic abnormalities have also occurred. Isolated cases of significant hepatic dysfunction, hepatitis, or worsening hepatic failure have been reported in patients; a causal relationship to CANCIDAS has not been established. Patients who develop abnormal liver function tests during CANCIDAS therapy should be monitored for evidence of worsening hepatic function and evaluated for risk/benefit of continuing CANCIDAS therapy.

Drug Interactions

Studies *in vitro* show that caspofungin acetate is not an inhibitor of any enzyme in the cytochrome P450 (CYP) system. In clinical studies, caspofungin did not induce the CYP3A4 metabolism of other drugs. Caspofungin is not a substrate for P-glycoprotein and is a poor substrate for cytochrome P450 enzymes.

Clinical studies in healthy volunteers show that the pharmacokinetics of CANCIDAS are not altered by itraconazole, amphotericin B, mycophenolate, nelfinavir, or tacrolimus. CANCIDAS has no effect on the pharmacokinetics of itraconazole, amphotericin B, or the active metabolite of mycophenolate.

CANCIDAS reduced the blood AUC_{0-12} of tacrolimus (FK-506, Prograf®[3]) by approximately 20%, peak blood concentration (C_{max}) by 16%, and 12-hour blood concentration (C_{12hr}) by 26% in healthy subjects when tacrolimus (2 doses of 0.1 mg/kg 12 hours apart) was administered on the 10th day of CANCIDAS 70 mg daily, as compared to results from a control period in which tacrolimus was administered

Continued on next page

Information on the Merck & Co., Inc., products listed on these pages is from the full prescribing information in use April 1, 2004.

Cancidas—Cont.

alone. For patients receiving both therapies, standard monitoring of tacrolimus blood concentrations and appropriate tacrolimus dosage adjustments are recommended.

[3] Registered trademark of Fujisawa Healthcare, Inc.

In two clinical studies, cyclosporine (one 4 mg/kg dose or two 3 mg/kg doses) increased the AUC of caspofungin by approximately 35%. CANCIDAS did not increase the plasma levels of cyclosporine. There were transient increases in liver ALT and AST when CANCIDAS and cyclosporine were co-administered (see WARNINGS and ADVERSE REACTIONS).

A drug-drug interaction study with rifampin in healthy volunteers has shown a 30% decrease in caspofungin trough concentrations. Patients on rifampin should receive 70 mg of CANCIDAS daily. In addition, results from regression analyses of patient pharmacokinetic data suggest that co-administration of other inducers of drug clearance (efavirenz, nevirapine, phenytoin, dexamethasone, or carbamazepine) with CANCIDAS may result in clinically meaningful reductions in caspofungin concentrations. It is not known which drug clearance mechanism involved in caspofungin disposition may be inducible. When CANCIDAS is co-administered with inducers of drug clearance, such as efavirenz, nevirapine, phenytoin, dexamethasone, or carbamazepine, use of a daily dose of 70 mg of CANCIDAS should be considered.

Carcinogenesis, Mutagenesis, Impairment of Fertility

No long-term studies in animals have been performed to evaluate the carcinogenic potential of caspofungin.

Caspofungin did not show evidence of mutagenic or genotoxic potential when evaluated in the following *in vitro* assays: bacterial (Ames) and mammalian cell (V79 Chinese hamster lung fibroblasts) mutagenesis assays, the alkaline elution/rat hepatocyte DNA strand break test, and the chromosome aberration assay in Chinese hamster ovary cells. Caspofungin was not genotoxic when assessed in the mouse bone marrow chromosomal test at doses up to 12.5 mg/kg (equivalent to a human dose of 1 mg/kg based on body surface area comparisons), administered intravenously.

Fertility and reproductive performance were not affected by the intravenous administration of caspofungin to rats at doses up to 5 mg/kg. At 5 mg/kg exposures were similar to those seen in patients treated with the 70-mg dose.

Pregnancy

Pregnancy Category C. CANCIDAS was shown to be embryotoxic in rats and rabbits. Findings included incomplete ossification of the skull and torso and an increased incidence of cervical rib in rats. An increased incidence of incomplete ossifications of the talus/calcaneus was seen in rabbits. Caspofungin also produced increases in resorptions in rats and rabbits and periimplantation losses in rats. These findings were observed at doses which produced exposures similar to those seen in patients treated with a 70-mg dose. Caspofungin crossed the placental barrier in rats and rabbits and was detected in the plasma of fetuses of pregnant animals dosed with CANCIDAS. There are no adequate and well-controlled studies in pregnant women. CANCIDAS should be used during pregnancy only if the potential benefit justifies the potential risk to the fetus.

Nursing Mothers

Caspofungin was found in the milk of lactating, drug-treated rats. It is not known whether caspofungin is excreted in human milk. Because many drugs are excreted in human milk, caution should be exercised when caspofungin is administered to a nursing woman.

Patients with Hepatic Insufficiency

Patients with mild hepatic insufficiency (Child-Pugh score 5 to 6) do not need a dosage adjustment. For patients with moderate hepatic insufficiency (Child-Pugh score 7 to 9), CANCIDAS 35 mg daily is recommended. However, where recommended, a 70-mg loading dose should still be administered on Day 1 (see DOSAGE AND ADMINISTRATION). There is no clinical experience in patients with severe hepatic insufficiency (Child-Pugh score >9).

Pediatric Use

Safety and effectiveness in pediatric patients have not been established.

Geriatric Use

Clinical studies of CANCIDAS did not include sufficient numbers of patients aged 65 and over to determine whether they respond differently from younger patients. Although the number of elderly patients was not large enough for a statistical analysis, no overall differences in safety or efficacy were observed between these and younger patients. Plasma concentrations of caspofungin in healthy older men and women (≥65 years of age) were increased slightly (approximately 28% in AUC) compared to young healthy men. A similar effect of age on pharmacokinetics was seen in patients with candidemia or other *Candida* infections (intra-abdominal abscesses, peritonitis, or pleural space infections). No dose adjustment is recommended for the elderly; however, greater sensitivity of some older individuals cannot be ruled out.

ADVERSE REACTIONS

General

Possible histamine-mediated symptoms have been reported including reports of rash, facial swelling, pruritus, sensation of warmth, or bronchospasm. Anaphylaxis has been reported during administration of CANCIDAS.

Clinical Adverse Experiences

The overall safety of caspofungin was assessed in 1440 individuals who received single or multiple doses of caspofungin acetate: 564 febrile, neutropenic patients (empirical therapy study); 125 patients with candidemia and/or intra-abdominal abscesses, peritonitis, or pleural space infections (including 4 patients with chronic disseminated candidiasis); 285 patients with esophageal and/or oropharyngeal candidiasis; 72 patients with invasive aspergillosis; and 394 individuals in phase I studies. In the empirical therapy study patients had undergone hematopoietic stem-cell transplantation or chemotherapy. In the studies involving patients with documented *Candida* infections, the majority of the patients had serious underlying medical conditions (e.g., hematologic or other malignancy, recent major surgery, HIV) requiring multiple concomitant medications. Patients in the noncomparative *Aspergillus* study often had serious predisposing medical conditions (e.g., bone marrow or peripheral stem cell transplants, hematologic malignancy, solid tumors or organ transplants) requiring multiple concomitant medications.

Empirical Therapy

In the randomized, double-blinded empirical therapy study, patients received either CANCIDAS 50 mg/day (following a 70-mg loading dose) or AmBisome (3.0 mg/kg/day). In this study clinical or laboratory hepatic adverse events were reported in 39% and 45% of patients in the CANCIDAS and AmBisome groups, respectively, regardless of causality. Also reported was an isolated, serious adverse experience of hyperbilirubinemia considered possibly related to CANCIDAS. Drug-related clinical adverse experiences occurring in ≥2% of the patients in either treatment group are presented in Table 8.

TABLE 8
Drug-Related* Clinical Adverse Experiences Among Patients with Persistent Fever and Neutropenia
Incidence ≥2% for at least one treatment group by Body System

	CANCIDAS** N=564 (percent)	AmBisome*** N=547 (percent)
Body as a Whole		
Abdominal Pain	1.4	2.4
Chills	13.8	24.7
Fever	17.0	19.4
Flushing	1.8	4.2
Perspiration/Diaphoresis	2.8	2.2
Cardiovascular System		
Hypertension	1.1	2.0
Tachycardia	1.4	2.4
Digestive System		
Diarrhea	2.7	2.4
Nausea	3.5	11.3
Vomiting	3.5	8.6
Metabolism and Nutrition		
Hypokalemia	3.7	4.2
Musculoskeletal System		
Back Pain	0.7	2.7
Nervous System & Psychiatric		
Headache	4.3	5.7
Respiratory System		
Dyspnea	2.0	4.2
Tachypnea	0.4	2.0
Skin & Skin Appendage		
Rash	6.2	5.3

* Determined by the investigator to be possibly, probably, or definitely drug-related.
** 70 mg on Day 1, then 50 mg daily for the remainder of treatment; daily dose was increased to 70 mg for 73 patients.
*** 3.0 mg/kg/day; daily dose was increased to 5.0 mg/kg for 74 patients.

The proportion of patients who experienced an infusion-related adverse event was significantly lower in the group treated with CANCIDAS (35.1%) than in the group treated with AmBisome (51.6%).

Drug-related laboratory adverse experiences occurring in ≥2% of the patients in either treatment group are presented in Table 9.

[See table 9 below]

The percentage of patients with either a drug-related clinical or a drug-related laboratory adverse experience was significantly lower among patients receiving CANCIDAS (54.4%) than among patients receiving AmBisome (69.3%). Furthermore, the incidence of discontinuation due to a drug-related clinical or laboratory adverse experience was significantly lower among patients treated with CANCIDAS (5.0%) than among patients treated with AmBisome (8.0%). To evaluate the effect of CANCIDAS and AmBisome on renal function, nephrotoxicity was defined as doubling of serum creatinine relative to baseline or an increase of ≥1 mg/dL in serum creatinine if baseline serum creatinine was above the upper limit of the normal range. Among patients whose baseline creatinine clearance was >30 mL/min, the incidence of nephrotoxicity was significantly lower in the group treated with CANCIDAS (2.6%) than in the group treated with AmBisome (11.5%). Serious clinical renal events, regardless of causality, were similar between CANCIDAS (11/564, 2.0%) and AmBisome (12/547, 2.2%).

Candidemia and other Candida infections (see CLINICAL STUDIES)

In the randomized, double-blinded invasive candidiasis study, patients received either CANCIDAS 50 mg/day (following a 70-mg loading dose) or amphotericin B 0.6 to 1.0 mg/kg/day. Drug-related clinical adverse experiences occurring in ≥2% of the patients in either treatment group are presented in Table 10.

TABLE 10
Drug-Related* Clinical Adverse Experiences Among Patients with Candidemia or other *Candida* Infections**
Incidence ≥2% for at least one treatment group by Body System

	CANCIDAS 50 mg*** N=114 (percent)	Amphotericin B N=125 (percent)
Body as a Whole		
Chills	5.3	26.4
Fever	7.0	23.2
Cardiovascular System		
Hypertension	1.8	6.4
Hypotension	0.9	2.4
Tachycardia	1.8	10.4
Peripheral Vascular System		
Phlebitis/thrombophlebitis	3.5	4.8
Digestive System		
Diarrhea	2.6	0.8
Jaundice	0.9	3.2
Nausea	1.8	5.6
Vomiting	3.5	8.0
Metabolic/Nutritional/ Immune		
Hypokalemia	0.9	5.6
Nervous System & Psychiatric		
Tremor	1.8	2.4
Respiratory System		
Tachypnea	0.0	10.4
Skin & Skin Appendage		
Erythema	0.0	2.4
Rash	0.9	3.2
Sweating	0.9	3.2
Urogenital System		
Renal insufficiency	0.9	5.6
Renal insufficiency, acute	0.0	5.6

*Determined by the investigator to be possibly, probably, or definitely drug-related.
**Intra-abdominal abscesses, peritonitis and pleural space infections
***Patients received CANCIDAS 70 mg on Day 1, then 50 mg daily for the remainder of their treatment.

The incidence of drug-related clinical adverse experiences was significantly lower among patients treated with CANCIDAS (28.9%) than among patients treated with B (58.4%). Also, the proportion of patients who experienced an

TABLE 9
Drug-Related* Laboratory Adverse Experiences Among Patients with Persistent Fever and Neutropenia
Incidence ≥2% for at least one treatment group by Laboratory Test Category

	CANCIDAS** N=564 (percent)	AmBisome*** N=547 (percent)
Blood Chemistry		
Alanine aminotransferase increased	8.7	8.9
Alkaline phosphatase increased	7.0	12.0
Aspartate aminotransferase increased	7.0	7.6
Direct serum bilirubin increased	2.6	5.2
Total serum bilirubin increased	3.0	5.2
Hypokalemia	7.3	11.8
Hypomagnesemia	2.3	2.6
Serum creatinine increased	1.2	5.5

* Determined by the investigator to be possibly, probably, or definitely drug-related.
** 70 mg on Day 1, then 50 mg daily for the remainder of treatment; daily dose was increased to 70 mg for 73 patients.
*** 3.0 mg/kg/day; daily dose was increased to 5.0 mg/kg for 74 patients.

infusion-related adverse event was significantly lower in the group treated with CANCIDAS (20.2%) than in the group treated with amphotericin B (48.8%).

Drug-related laboratory adverse experiences occurring in ≥2% of the patients in either treatment group are presented in Table 11.

TABLE 11
Drug-Related* Laboratory Adverse Experiences Among Patients with Candidemia or other *Candida* Infections**
Incidence ≥2% for at least one treatment group by Laboratory Test Category

	CANCIDAS 50 mg*** N=114 (percent)	Amphotericin B N=125 (percent)
Blood Chemistry		
ALT increased	3.7	8.1
AST increased	1.9	9.0
Blood urea increased	1.9	15.8
Direct serum bilirubin increased	3.8	8.4
Serum alkaline phosphatase increased	8.3	15.6
Serum bicarbonate decreased	0.0	3.6
Serum creatinine increased	3.7	22.6
Serum phosphate increased	0.0	2.7
Serum potassium decreased	9.9	23.4
Serum potassium increased	0.9	2.4
Total serum bilirubin increased	2.8	8.9
Hematology		
Hematocrit decreased	0.9	7.3
Hemoglobin decreased	0.9	10.5
Urinalysis		
Urine protein increased	0.0	3.7

*Determined by the investigator to be possibly, probably, or definitely drug-related.

**Intra-abdominal abscesses, peritonitis and pleural space infections

***Patients received CANCIDAS 70 mg on Day 1, then 50 mg daily for the remainder of their treatment.

The incidence of drug-related laboratory adverse experiences was significantly lower among patients receiving CANCIDAS (24.3%) than among patients receiving amphotericin B (54.0%).

The percentage of patients with either a drug-related clinical adverse experience or a drug-related laboratory adverse experience was significantly lower among patients receiving CANCIDAS (42.1%) than among patients receiving amphotericin B (75.2%). Furthermore, a significant difference between the two treatment groups was observed with regard to incidence of discontinuation due to drug-related clinical or laboratory adverse experience; incidences were 3/114 (2.6%) in the group treated with CANCIDAS and 29/125 (23.2%) in the group treated with amphotericin B.

To evaluate the effect of CANCIDAS and amphotericin B on renal function, nephrotoxicity was defined as doubling of serum creatinine relative to baseline or an increase of ≥1 mg/dL in serum creatinine if baseline serum creatinine was above the upper limit of the normal range. In a subgroup of patients whose baseline creatinine clearance was >30 mL/min, the incidence of nephrotoxicity was significantly lower in the group treated with CANCIDAS than in the group treated with amphotericin B.

Esophageal Candidiasis and Oropharyngeal Candidiasis
Drug-related clinical adverse experiences occurring in ≥2% of patients with esophageal and/or oropharyngeal candidiasis are presented in Table 12.

[See table 12 above]

Laboratory abnormalities occurring in ≥2% of patients with esophageal and/or oropharyngeal candidiasis are presented in Table 13.

[See table 13 at top of next page]

Invasive Aspergillosis
In the open-label, noncomparative aspergillosis study, in which 69 patients received CANCIDAS (70-mg loading dose on Day 1 followed by 50 mg daily), the following drug-related clinical adverse experiences were observed with an incidence of ≥2%: fever (2.9%), infused-vein complications (2.9%), nausea (2.9%), vomiting (2.9%) and flushing (2.9%). Also reported infrequently in this patient population were pulmonary edema, ARDS, and radiographic infiltrates.

Drug-related laboratory abnormalities reported with an incidence ≥2% in patients treated with CANCIDAS in the noncomparative aspergillosis study were: serum alkaline phosphatase increased (2.9%), serum potassium decreased (2.9%), eosinophils increased (3.2%), urine protein increased (4.9%), and urine RBCs increased (2.2%).

Postmarketing Experience:
The following postmarketing adverse events have been reported:

TABLE 12
Drug-Related Clinical Adverse Experiences Among Patients with Esophageal and/or Oropharyngeal Candidiasis*
Incidence ≥2% for at least one treatment dose (per comparison) by Body System

	CANCIDAS 50 mg** N=83 (percent)	Fluconazole IV 200 mg** N=94 (percent)	CANCIDAS 50 mg*** N=80 (percent)	CANCIDAS 70 mg*** N=65 (percent)	Amphotericin B 0.5 mg/kg*** N=89 (percent)
Body as a Whole					
Asthenia/fatigue	0.0	0.0	0.0	0.0	6.7
Chills	0.0	0.0	2.5	1.5	75.3
Edema/swelling	0.0	0.0	0.0	0.0	5.6
Edema, facial	0.0	0.0	0.0	3.1	0.0
Fever	3.6	1.1	21.3	26.2	69.7
Flu-like illness	0.0	0.0	0.0	3.1	0.0
Malaise	0.0	0.0	0.0	0.0	5.6
Pain	0.0	0.0	1.3	4.6	5.6
Pain, abdominal	3.6	2.1	2.5	0.0	9.0
Warm sensation	0.0	0.0	0.0	1.5	4.5
Peripheral Vascular System					
Infused vein complication	12.0	8.5	2.5	1.5	0.0
Phlebitis/thrombophlebitis	15.7	8.5	11.3	13.8	22.5
Cardiovascular System					
Tachycardia	0.0	0.0	1.3	0.0	4.5
Vasculitis	0.0	0.0	0.0	0.0	3.4
Digestive System					
Anorexia	0.0	0.0	1.3	0.0	3.4
Diarrhea	3.6	2.1	1.3	3.1	11.2
Gastritis	0.0	2.1	0.0	0.0	0.0
Nausea	6.0	6.4	2.5	3.1	21.3
Vomiting	1.2	3.2	1.3	3.1	13.5
Hemic & Lymphatic System					
Anemia	0.0	0.0	3.8	0.0	9.0
Metabolic/Nutritional/ Immune					
Anaphylaxis	0.0	0.0	0.0	0.0	2.2
Musculoskeletal System					
Myalgia	1.2	0.0	0.0	3.1	2.2
Pain, back	0.0	0.0	0.0	0.0	2.2
Pain, musculoskeletal	0.0	0.0	1.3	0.0	4.5
Nervous System & Psychiatric					
Dizziness	0.0	2.1	0.0	1.5	1.1
Headache	6.0	1.1	11.3	7.7	19.1
Insomnia	1.2	0.0	0.0	0.0	2.2
Paresthesia	0.0	0.0	1.3	3.1	1.1
Tremor	0.0	0.0	0.0	0.0	7.9
Respiratory System					
Tachypnea	0.0	0.0	1.3	0.0	4.5
Skin & Skin Appendage					
Erythema	1.2	0.0	1.3	1.5	7.9
Induration	0.0	0.0	0.0	3.1	6.7
Pruritus	1.2	0.0	2.5	1.5	0.0
Rash	0.0	0.0	1.3	4.6	3.4
Sweating	0.0	0.0	1.3	0.0	3.4

*Relationship to drug was determined by the investigator to be possibly, probably or definitely drug-related.

**Derived from a Phase III comparator-controlled clinical study.

***Derived from Phase II comparator-controlled clinical studies.

Hepatobiliary: rare cases of clinically significant hepatic dysfunction

Cardiovascular: swelling and peripheral edema

Metabolic: hypercalcemia

Concomitant Therapy
In one clinical study, 3 of 4 subjects who received CANCIDAS 70 mg daily on Days 1 through 10, and also received two 3 mg/kg doses of cyclosporine 12 hours apart on Day 10, developed transient elevations of ALT on Day 11 that were 2 to 3 times the upper limit of normal (ULN). In a separate panel of subjects in the same study, 2 of 8 subjects who received CANCIDAS 35 mg daily for 3 days and cyclosporine (two 3 mg/kg doses administered 12 hours apart) on Day 1 had small increases in ALT (slightly above the ULN) on Day 2. In another clinical study, 2 of 8 healthy men developed transient ALT elevations of less than 2× ULN. In this study, cyclosporine (4 mg/kg) was administered on Days 1 and 12, and CANCIDAS was administered (70 mg) daily on Days 3 through 13. In one subject, the ALT elevation occurred on Days 7 and 9 and, in the other subject, the ALT elevation occurred on Day 19. These elevations returned to normal by Day 27. In all groups, elevations in AST paralleled ALT elevations but were of lesser magnitude. In these clinical studies, cyclosporine (one 4 mg/kg dose or two 3 mg/kg doses) increased the AUC of caspofungin by approximately 35% (see WARNINGS).

OVERDOSAGE

In clinical studies the highest dose was 210 mg, administered as a single dose to 6 healthy subjects. This dose was generally well tolerated. In addition, 100 mg once daily for 21 days has been administered to 15 healthy subjects and was generally well tolerated. Caspofungin is not dialyzable. The minimum lethal dose of caspofungin in rats was 50 mg/kg, a dose which is equivalent to 10 times the recommended daily dose based on relative body surface area comparison.

ANIMAL PHARMACOLOGY AND TOXICOLOGY

In one 5-week study in monkeys at doses which produced exposures approximately 4 to 6 times those seen in patients treated with a 70-mg dose, scattered small foci of subcapsular necrosis were observed microscopically in the livers of some animals (2/8 monkeys at 5 mg/kg and 4/8 monkeys at 8 mg/kg); however, this histopathological finding was not seen in another study of 27 weeks duration at similar doses.

DOSAGE AND ADMINISTRATION

Do not mix or co-infuse CANCIDAS with other medications, as there are no data available on the compatibility of CANCIDAS with other intravenous substances, additives, or medications. DO NOT USE DILUENTS CONTAINING DEXTROSE (α-D-GLUCOSE), as CANCIDAS is not stable in diluents containing dextrose. CANCIDAS should be administered by slow IV infusion over approximately 1 hour.

Empirical Therapy
A single 70-mg loading dose should be administered on Day 1, followed by 50 mg daily thereafter. Duration of treatment should be based on the patient's clinical response. Empirical therapy should be continued until resolution of neutropenia. Patients found to have a fungal infection should be treated for a minimum of 14 days; treatment should continue for at least 7 days after both neutropenia and clinical symptoms are resolved. If the 50-mg dose is well tolerated but does not provide an adequate clinical response, the daily dose can be increased to 70 mg. Although an increase in efficacy with 70 mg daily has not been demonstrated, limited safety data suggest that an increase in dose to 70 mg daily is well tolerated.

Candidemia and other Candida infections (see CLINICAL STUDIES)
A single 70-mg loading dose should be administered on Day 1, followed by 50 mg daily thereafter. Duration of treatment should be dictated by the patient's clinical and microbiological response. In general, antifungal therapy should continue for at least 14 days after the last positive culture.

Continued on next page

TABLE 13
Drug-Related Laboratory Abnormalities Reported Among Patients with Esophageal and/or Oropharyngeal Candidiasis*
Incidence ≥2% (for at least one treatment dose) by Laboratory Test Category

	CANCIDAS 50 mg** N=163 (percent)	CANCIDAS 70 mg*** N=65 (percent)	Fluconazole IV 200 mg** N=94 (percent)	Amphotericin B 0.5 mg/kg*** N=89 (percent)
Blood Chemistry				
ALT increased	10.6	10.8	11.8	22.7
AST increased	13.0	10.8	12.9	22.7
Blood urea increased	0.0	0.0	1.2	10.3
Direct serum bilirubin increased	0.6	0.0	3.3	2.5
Serum albumin decreased	8.6	4.6	5.4	14.9
Serum alkaline phosphatase increased	10.5	7.7	11.8	19.3
Serum bicarbonate decreased	0.9	0.0	0.0	6.6
Serum calcium decreased	1.9	0.0	3.2	1.1
Serum creatinine increased	0.0	1.5	2.2	28.1
Serum potassium decreased	3.7	10.8	4.3	31.5
Serum potassium increased	0.6	0.0	2.2	1.1
Serum sodium decreased	1.9	1.5	3.2	1.1
Serum uric acid increased	0.6	0.0	0.0	3.4
Total serum bilirubin increased	0.0	0.0	3.2	4.5
Total serum protein decreased	3.1	0.0	3.2	3.4
Hematology				
Eosinophils increased	3.1	3.1	1.1	1.1
Hematocrit decreased	11.1	1.5	5.4	32.6
Hemoglobin decreased	12.3	3.1	5.4	37.1
Lymphocytes increased	0.0	1.6	2.2	0.0
Neutrophils decreased	1.9	3.1	3.2	1.1
Platelet count decreased	3.1	1.5	2.2	3.4
Prothrombin time increased	1.3	1.5	0.0	2.3
WBC count decreased	6.2	4.6	8.6	7.9
Urinalysis				
Urine blood increased	0.0	0.0	0.0	4.0
Urine casts increased	0.0	0.0	0.0	8.0
Urine pH increased	0.8	0.0	0.0	3.6
Urine protein increased	1.2	0.0	3.3	4.5
Urine RBCs increased	1.1	3.8	5.1	12.0
Urine WBCs increased	0.0	7.7	0.0	24.0

*Relationship to drug was determined by the investigator to be possibly, probably or definitely drug-related.
**Derived from Phase II and Phase III comparator-controlled clinical studies.
***Derived from Phase II comparator-controlled clinical studies.

TABLE 14
CANCIDAS Concentrations

Dose	Reconstituted Solution Concentration	Infusion Volume	Infusion Solution Concentration
70-mg initial dose	7.2 mg/mL	260 mL	0.28 mg/mL
50-mg daily dose	5.2 mg/mL	260 mL	0.20 mg/mL
70-mg initial dose* (from two 50 mg vials)	5.2 mg/mL	264 mL	0.28 mg/mL
50-mg daily dose* (reduced volume)	5.2 mg/mL	110 mL	0.47 mg/mL
35-mg daily dose* (from one 50 mg vial) for Moderate Hepatic Insufficiency	5.2 mg/mL or 5.2 mg/mL	257 mL or 107 mL	0.14 mg/mL or 0.34 mg/mL

*See preceding text for these special situations.

Cancidas—Cont.

Patients who remain persistently neutropenic may warrant a longer course of therapy pending resolution of the neutropenia.

Esophageal Candidiasis
The dose should be 50 mg daily. Because of the risk of relapse of oropharyngeal candidiasis in patients with HIV infections, suppressive oral therapy could be considered (see CLINICAL STUDIES). A 70-mg loading dose has not been studied with this indication.

Invasive Aspergillosis
A single 70-mg loading dose should be administered on Day 1, followed by 50 mg daily thereafter. Duration of treatment should be based upon the severity of the patient's underlying disease, recovery from immunosuppression, and clinical response. The efficacy of a 70-mg dose regimen in patients who are not clinically responding to the 50-mg daily dose is not known. Limited safety data suggest that an increase in dose to 70 mg daily is well tolerated. The safety and efficacy of doses above 70 mg have not been adequately studied.

Hepatic Insufficiency
Patients with mild hepatic insufficiency (Child-Pugh score 5 to 6) do not need a dosage adjustment. For patients with moderate hepatic insufficiency (Child-Pugh score 7 to 9), CANCIDAS 35 mg daily is recommended. However, where recommended, a 70-mg loading dose should still be administered on Day 1. There is no clinical experience in patients with severe hepatic insufficiency (Child-Pugh score >9).

Concomitant Medication with Inducers of Drug Clearance
Patients on rifampin should receive 70 mg of CANCIDAS daily. Patients on nevirapine, efavirenz, carbamazepine, dexamethasone, or phenytoin may require an increase in dose to 70 mg of CANCIDAS daily (see PRECAUTIONS, *Drug Interactions*).

Preparation of CANCIDAS for use:
Do not mix or co-infuse CANCIDAS with other medications, as there are no data available on the compatibility of CANCIDAS with other intravenous substances, additives, or medications. DO NOT USE DILUENTS CONTAINING DEXTROSE (α-D-GLUCOSE), as CANCIDAS is not stable in diluents containing dextrose.

Preparation of the 70-mg infusion
1. Equilibrate the refrigerated vial of CANCIDAS to room temperature.
2. Aseptically add 10.5 mL of 0.9% Sodium Chloride Injection, Sterile Water for Injection, Bacteriostatic Water for Injection with methylparaben and propylparaben, or Bacteriostatic Water for Injection with 0.9% benzyl alcohol to the vial.[a] This reconstituted solution may be stored for up to one hour at ≤25°C (≤77°F).[b]
3. Aseptically transfer 10 mL[c] of reconstituted CANCIDAS to an IV bag (or bottle) containing 250 mL 0.9%, 0.45%, or 0.225% Sodium Chloride Injection, or Lactated Ringer's Injection. This infusion solution must be used within 24 hours if stored at ≤25°C (≤77°F) or within 48 hours if stored refrigerated at 2 to 8°C (36 to 46°F). (If a 70-mg vial is unavailable, see below: *Alternative Infusion Preparation Methods, Preparation of 70-mg dose from two 50-mg vials.*)

Preparation of the daily 50-mg infusion
1. Equilibrate the refrigerated vial of CANCIDAS to room temperature.
2. Aseptically add 10.5 mL of 0.9% Sodium Chloride Injection, Sterile Water for Injection, Bacteriostatic Water for Injection with methylparaben and propylparaben, or Bacteriostatic Water for Injection with 0.9% benzyl alcohol to the vial.[a] This reconstituted solution may be stored for up to one hour at ≤25°C (≤77°F).[b]
3. Aseptically transfer 10 mL[c] of reconstituted CANCIDAS to an IV bag (or bottle) containing 250 mL 0.9%, 0.45%, or 0.225% Sodium Chloride Injection, or Lactated Ringer's Injection. This infusion solution must be used within 24 hours if stored at ≤25°C (≤77°F) or within 48 hours if stored refrigerated at 2 to 8°C (36 to 46°F). (If a reduced infusion

volume is medically necessary, see below: *Alternative Infusion Preparation Methods, Preparation of 50-mg daily doses at reduced volume.*)

Alternative Infusion Preparation Methods
Preparation of 70-mg dose from two 50-mg vials
Reconstitute two 50-mg vials with 10.5 mL of diluent each (see *Preparation of the daily 50-mg infusion*). Aseptically transfer a total of 14 mL of the reconstituted CANCIDAS from the two vials to 250 mL of 0.9%, 0.45%, or 0.225% Sodium Chloride Injection, or Lactated Ringer's Injection.

Preparation of 50-mg daily doses at reduced volume
When medically necessary, the 50-mg daily doses can be prepared by adding 10 mL of reconstituted CANCIDAS to 100 mL of 0.9%, 0.45%, or 0.225% Sodium Chloride Injection, or Lactated Ringer's Injection (see *Preparation of the daily 50-mg infusion*).

Preparation of a 35-mg daily dose for patients with moderate Hepatic Insufficiency
Reconstitute one 50-mg vial (see above: *Preparation of the daily 50-mg infusion*). Aseptically transfer 7 mL of the reconstituted CANCIDAS from the vial to 250 mL or, if medically necessary, to 100 mL of 0.9%, 0.45%, or 0.225% Sodium Chloride Injection, or Lactated Ringer's Injection.

> *Preparation notes:*
> [a]The white to off-white cake will dissolve completely. Mix gently until a clear solution is obtained.
> [b]Visually inspect the reconstituted solution for particulate matter or discoloration during reconstitution and prior to infusion. Do not use if the solution is cloudy or has precipitated.
> [c]CANCIDAS is formulated to provide the full labeled vial dose (70 mg or 50 mg) when 10 mL is withdrawn from the vial.

[See table 14 at left]

HOW SUPPLIED

No. 3822 — CANCIDAS 50 mg is a white to off-white powder/cake for infusion in a vial with a red aluminum band and a plastic cap.
NDC 0006-3822-10 supplied as one single-use vial.
No. 3823 — CANCIDAS 70 mg is a white to off-white powder/cake for infusion in a vial with a yellow/orange aluminum band and a plastic cap.
NDC 0006-3823-10 supplied as one single-use vial.
Storage
Vials
The lyophilized vials should be stored refrigerated at 2° to 8°C (36° to 46°F).
Reconstituted Concentrate
Reconstituted CANCIDAS may be stored at ≤25°C (≤77°F) for one hour prior to the preparation of the patient infusion solution.
Diluted Product
The final patient infusion solution in the IV bag or bottle can be stored at ≤25°C (≤77°F) for 24 hours or at 2 to 8°C (36 to 46°F) for 48 hours.
Manufactured for:
MERCK & CO., INC., Whitehouse Station, NJ 08889, USA
Manufactured by:
MERCK & CO., INC., Whitehouse Station, NJ 08889, USA
or
Cardinal Health
Albuquerque, NM 87109
Issued September 2004
Printed in USA
Revisions based on 9344305, issued May 2004, and 9344306, issued September 2004.

COMVAX® ℞
[Haemophilus b conjugate (meningococcal protein conjugate) and hepatitis b (recombinant) vaccine]

Prescribing information for this product, which appears on pages 2007–2011 of the 2005 PDR, has been revised as follows. Please write "See Supplement A" next to the product heading.
In the **ADVERSE REACTIONS** section, under ADVERSE EVENT REPORTING, change NVICP number to "1-800-338-2382."
Revisions based on 9376602, issued August 2004.

COSMEGEN® for Injection ℞
(Dactinomycin for Injection)
(Actinomycin D)

Prescribing information for this product, which appears on pages 2011–2013 of the 2005 PDR, has been revised as follows. Please write "See Supplement A" next to the product heading.
In the **CONTRAINDICATIONS** section, before the first paragraph, as a new paragraph, add the following text:
Hypersensitivity to any component of this product.
In the **PRECAUTIONS** section, under *General*, in the second paragraph, after the second sentence, add the following text:
As such, live virus vaccines should not be administered during therapy with COSMEGEN.

In the **ADVERSE REACTIONS** section, in the fifth paragraph, in the first sentence, after "hepatic veno-occlusive disease" insert "which may be associated with intravascular clotting disorder and multi-organ failure".
Revisions based on 9000834, issued August 2004.

COZAAR® ℞
(losartan potassium tablets)

Prescribing information for this product, which appears on pages 2016–2021 of the 2005 PDR, has been revised as follows. Please write "See Supplement A" next to the product heading.
Under the **ADVERSE REACTIONS** section, under the subhead *Post-Marketing Experience,* after the 3rd paragraph, insert the following new paragraph: *Musculoskeletal:* Rare cases of rhabdomyolysis have been reported in patients receiving angiotensin II receptor blockers.
In the **HOW SUPPLIED** section:
delete the 5th line: "**NDC** 0006-0951-58 unit of use bottles of 100".
delete the period at the end of the 7th line and add the following new line: "**NDC** 0006-0951-87 bottles of 10,000."
delete the 13th line: "**NDC** 0006-0952-58 unit of use bottles of 100".
delete the period at the end of the 15th line and add the following new line: "**NDC** 0006-0952-87 bottles of 10,000."
delete the 21st line: "**NDC** 0006-0960-58 unit of use bottles of 100".
Delete the period at the end of the 23rd line and add the following new line: "**NDC** 0006-0960-86 bottles of 5,000."
Below the *Storage* section, after the 3rd line, add the following new line: "Manufactured for:"
Revisions based on 9573528, issued October 2004.

CUPRIMINE® Capsules ℞
(PENICILLAMINE)

Prescribing information for this product, which appears on pages 2028–2031 of the 2005 PDR, has been revised as follows. Please write "See Supplement A" next to the product heading.
In the **CLINICAL PHARMACOLOGY** section, in the seventh paragraph, at the end of the first sentence, delete "or milk." and replace with "milk, antacid, zinc or iron-containing preparation."
In the **CLINICAL PHARMACOLOGY** section, under *Pharmacokinetics*, in the second paragraph, at the end of the first sentence after "bound to proteins" add ", especially albumin and ceruloplasmin." At the end of the third sentence, replace "s-methyl-D-penicillamine." with "S-methyl-D-penicillamine." Change the last sentence in that paragraph to "Excretion is mainly renal, mainly as disulfides."
In the **WARNINGS** section, change the subhead *"Pregnancy"* to *"Pregnancy Category D"*.
At the beginning of the first paragraph, add the following sentence: Penicillamine can cause fetal harm when administered to a pregnant woman.
In the **WARNINGS** section, under *Pregnancy* in the second paragraph, at the end, add the following sentence: If this drug is used during pregnancy, or if the patient becomes pregnant while taking this drug, the patient should be apprised of the potential hazard to the fetus.
In the **PRECAUTIONS** section, change the subhead *"Carcinogenesis"* to *"Carcinogenesis, Mutagenesis, Impairment of Fertility"*. After the first paragraph, add the following paragraphs: Penicillamine is directly mutagenic to *S. typhimurium* strain TA92 in the Ames test; mutagenicity is enhanced by kidney postmitochondrial subcellular fraction 9. Penicillamine does not induce gene mutations in Chinese hamster V79 cells.
Penicillamine induces sister-chromatid exchanges and chromosome aberrations in cultivated mammalian cells. No studies on the effect of penicillamine on fertility are available.
Pregnancy
Pregnancy Category D
(see WARNINGS, *Pregnancy*)
At the end of the **PRECAUTIONS** section, add the following text:
Geriatric Use
Clinical studies of CUPRIMINE are limited in subjects aged 65 and over; they did not include sufficient numbers of elderly subjects aged 65 and over to adequately determine whether they respond differently from younger subjects. Review of reported clinical trials with penicillamine in the elderly suggest greater risk than in younger patients for overall skin rash and abnormality of taste. In general, dose selection for an elderly patient should be cautious, starting at the low end of the dosing range, reflecting the greater frequency of decreased hepatic, renal or cardiac function, and of concomitant disease or other drugs.
This drug is known to be substantially excreted by the kidney, and the risk of toxic reactions to this drug may be greater in patients with impaired renal function. Because elderly patients are more likely to have decreased renal function, care should be taken in dose selection, and careful monitoring of renal function is recommended.
Revisions based on 7873244, issued October 2004.

DECADRON® TABLETS ℞
(DEXAMETHASONE TABLETS, USP)

Prescribing information for this product, which appears on pages 2032–2033 of the 2005 PDR, has been completely revised as follows. Please write "See Supplement A" next to the product heading.

DESCRIPTION

DECADRON* (dexamethasone tablets, USP) tablets, for oral administration, are supplied in two potencies, 0.5 mg and 0.75 mg. Inactive ingredients are calcium phosphate, lactose, magnesium stearate, and starch. Tablets DECADRON 0.5 mg also contain D&C Yellow 10 and FD&C Yellow 6. Tablets DECADRON 0.75 mg also contain FD&C Blue 1.
The molecular weight for dexamethasone is 392.47. It is designated chemically as 9-fluoro-11β,17,21-trihydroxy-16α-methylpregna-1,4-diene-3,20-dione. The empirical formula is $C_{22}H_{29}FO_5$ and the structural formula is:

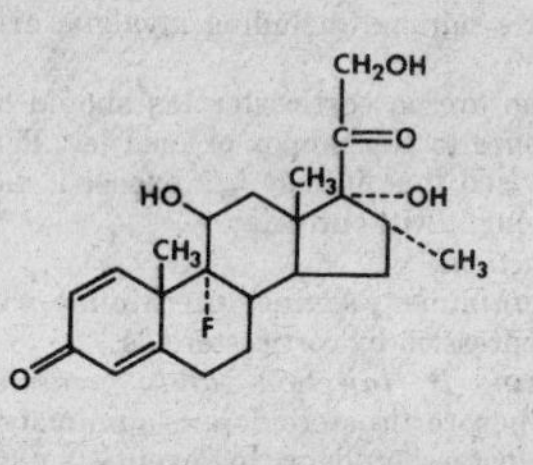

Dexamethasone, a synthetic adrenocortical steroid, is a white to practically white, odorless, crystalline powder. It is stable in air. It is practically insoluble in water.

*Registered trademark of MERCK & CO., Inc.

CLINICAL PHARMACOLOGY

Glucocorticoids, naturally occurring and synthetic, are adrenocortical steroids that are readily absorbed from the gastrointestinal tract. Glucocorticoids cause varied metabolic effects. In addition, they modify the body's immune responses to diverse stimuli. Naturally occurring glucocorticoids (hydrocortisone and cortisone), which also have sodium-retaining properties, are used as replacement therapy in adrenocortical deficiency states. Their synthetic analogs including dexamethasone are primarily used for their anti-inflammatory effects in disorders of many organ systems.
At equipotent anti-inflammatory doses, dexamethasone almost completely lacks the sodium-retaining property of hydrocortisone and closely related derivatives of hydrocortisone.

INDICATIONS AND USAGE

Allergic states: Control of severe or incapacitating allergic conditions intractable to adequate trials of conventional treatment in asthma, atopic dermatitis, contact dermatitis, drug hypersensitivity reactions, perennial or seasonal allergic rhinitis, and serum sickness.
Dermatologic diseases: Bullous dermatitis herpetiformis, exfoliative erythroderma, mycosis fungoides, pemphigus, and severe erythema multiforme (Stevens-Johnson syndrome).
Endocrine disorders: Primary or secondary adrenocortical insufficiency (hydrocortisone or cortisone is the drug of choice; may be used in conjunction with synthetic mineralocorticoid analogs where applicable; in infancy mineralocorticoid supplementation is of particular importance), congenital adrenal hyperplasia, hypercalcemia associated with cancer, and nonsuppurative thyroiditis.
Gastrointestinal diseases: To tide the patient over a critical period of the disease in regional enteritis and ulcerative colitis.
Hematologic disorders: Acquired (autoimmune) hemolytic anemia, congenital (erythroid) hypoplastic anemia (Diamond-Blackfan anemia), idiopathic thrombocytopenic purpura in adults, pure red cell aplasia, and selected cases of secondary thrombocytopenia.
Miscellaneous: Diagnostic testing of adrenocortical hyperfunction, trichinosis with neurologic or myocardial involvement, tuberculous meningitis with subarachnoid block or impending block when used with appropriate antituberculous chemotherapy.
Neoplastic diseases: For the palliative management of leukemias and lymphomas.
Nervous system: Acute exacerbations of multiple sclerosis, cerebral edema associated with primary or metastatic brain tumor, craniotomy, or head injury.
Ophthalmic diseases: Sympathetic ophthalmia, temporal arteritis, uveitis, and ocular inflammatory conditions unresponsive to topical corticosteroids.
Renal diseases: To induce a diuresis or remission of proteinuria in idiopathic nephrotic syndrome or that due to lupus erythematosus.
Respiratory diseases: Berylliosis, fulminating or disseminated pulmonary tuberculosis when used concurrently with appropriate antituberculous chemotherapy, idiopathic eosinophilic pneumonias, symptomatic sarcoidosis.
Rheumatic disorders: As adjunctive therapy for short-term administration (to tide the patient over an acute episode or exacerbation) in acute gouty arthritis, acute rheumatic carditis, ankylosing spondylitis, psoriatic arthritis, rheumatoid arthritis, including juvenile rheumatoid arthritis (selected cases may require low-dose maintenance therapy). For the treatment of dermatomyositis, polymyositis, and systemic lupus erythematosus.

CONTRAINDICATIONS

Systemic fungal infections (see WARNINGS, *Fungal infections*).
DECADRON tablets are contraindicated in patients who are hypersensitive to any components of this product.

WARNINGS

General
Rare instances of anaphylactoid reactions have occurred in patients receiving corticosteroid therapy (see ADVERSE REACTIONS).
Increased dosage of rapidly acting corticosteroids is indicated in patients on corticosteroid therapy subjected to any unusual stress before, during, and after the stressful situation.
Cardio-renal
Average and large doses of corticosteroids can cause elevation of blood pressure, sodium and water retention, and increased excretion of potassium. These effects are less likely to occur with the synthetic derivatives except when used in large doses. Dietary salt restriction and potassium supplementation may be necessary. All corticosteroids increase calcium excretion.
Literature reports suggest an apparent association between use of corticosteroids and left ventricular free wall rupture after a recent myocardial infarction; therefore, therapy with corticosteroids should be used with great caution in these patients.
Endocrine
Corticosteroids can produce reversible hypothalamic-pituitary adrenal (HPA) axis suppression with the potential for glucocorticosteroid insufficiency after withdrawal of treatment. Adrenocortical insufficiency may result from too rapid withdrawal of corticosteroids and may be minimized by gradual reduction of dosage. This type of relative insufficiency may persist for months after discontinuation of therapy; therefore, in any situation of stress occurring during that period, hormone therapy should be reinstituted. If the patient is receiving steroids already, dosage may have to be increased.
Metabolic clearance of corticosteroids is decreased in hypothyroid patients and increased in hyperthyroid patients. Changes in thyroid status of the patient may necessitate adjustment in dosage.
Infections
General
Patients who are on corticosteroids are more susceptible to infections than are healthy individuals. There may be decreased resistance and inability to localize infection when corticosteroids are used. Infection with any pathogen (viral, bacterial, fungal, protozoan or helminthic) in any location of the body may be associated with the use of corticosteroids alone or in combination with other immunosuppressive agents. These infections may be mild to severe. With increasing doses of corticosteroids, the rate of occurrence of infectious complications increases. Corticosteroids may also mask some signs of current infection.
Fungal Infections
Corticosteroids may exacerbate systemic fungal infections and therefore should not be used in the presence of such infections unless they are needed to control life-threatening drug reactions. There have been cases reported in which concomitant use of amphotericin B and hydrocortisone was followed by cardiac enlargement and congestive heart failure (see PRECAUTIONS, *Drug Interactions, Amphotericin B injection and potassium-depleting agents*).
Special Pathogens
Latent disease may be activated or there may be an exacerbation of intercurrent infections due to pathogens, including those caused by *Amoeba, Candida, Cryptococcus, Mycobacterium, Nocardia, Pneumocystis, Toxoplasma.*
It is recommended that latent amebiasis or active amebiasis be ruled out before initiating corticosteroid therapy in any patient who has spent time in the tropics or any patient with unexplained diarrhea.
Similarly, corticosteroids should be used with great care in patients with known or suspected Strongyloides (threadworm) infestation. In such patients, corticosteroid-induced immunosuppression may lead to Strongyloides hyperinfection and dissemination with widespread larval migration, often accompanied by severe enterocolitis and potentially fatal gram-negative septicemia.
Corticosteroids should not be used in cerebral malaria.
Tuberculosis
The use of corticosteroids in active tuberculosis should be restricted to those cases of fulminating or disseminated tuberculosis in which the corticosteroid is used for the management of the disease in conjunction with an appropriate antituberculous regimen.

Continued on next page

Information on the Merck & Co., Inc., products listed on these pages is from the full prescribing information in use April 1, 2004.

Decadron Tablets—Cont.

If corticosteroids are indicated in patients with latent tuberculosis or tuberculin reactivity, close observation is necessary as reactivation of the disease may occur. During prolonged corticosteroid therapy, these patients should receive chemoprophylaxis.

Vaccination
Administration of live or live, attenuated vaccines is contraindicated in patients receiving immunosuppressive doses of corticosteroids. Killed or inactivated vaccines may be administered. However, the response to such vaccines cannot be predicted. Immunization procedures may be undertaken in patients who are receiving corticosteroids as replacement therapy, e.g., for Addison's disease.

Viral Infections
Chickenpox and measles can have a more serious or even fatal course in pediatric and adult patients on corticosteroids. In pediatric and adult patients who have not had these diseases, particular care should be taken to avoid exposure. The contribution of the underlying disease and/or prior corticosteroid treatment to the risk is also not known. If exposed to chickenpox, prophylaxis with varicella zoster immune globulin (VZIG) may be indicated. If exposed to measles, prophylaxis with immune globulin (IG) may be indicated. (See the respective package inserts for VZIG and IG for complete prescribing information.) If chickenpox develops, treatment with antiviral agents should be considered.

Ophthalmic
Use of corticosteroids may produce posterior subcapsular cataracts, glaucoma with possible damage to the optic nerves, and may enhance the establishment of secondary ocular infections due to bacteria, fungi, or viruses. The use of oral corticosteroids is not recommended in the treatment of optic neuritis and may lead to an increase in the risk of new episodes. Corticosteroids should not be used in active ocular herpes simplex.

PRECAUTIONS

General
The lowest possible dose of corticosteroids should be used to control the condition under treatment. When reduction in dosage is possible, the reduction should be gradual.
Since complications of treatment with corticosteroids are dependent on the size of the dose and the duration of treatment, a risk/benefit decision must be made in each individual case as to dose and duration of treatment and as to whether daily or intermittent therapy should be used.
Kaposi's sarcoma has been reported to occur in patients receiving corticosteroid therapy, most often for chronic conditions. Discontinuation of corticosteroids may result in clinical improvement.

Cardio-renal
As sodium retention with resultant edema and potassium loss may occur in patients receiving corticosteroids, these agents should be used with caution in patients with congestive heart failure, hypertension, or renal insufficiency.

Endocrine
Drug-induced secondary adrenocortical insufficiency may be minimized by gradual reduction of dosage. This type of relative insufficiency may persist for months after discontinuation of therapy; therefore, in any situation of stress occurring during that period, hormone therapy should be reinstituted. Since mineralocorticoid secretion may be impaired, salt and/or a mineralocorticoid should be administered concurrently.

Gastrointestinal
Steroids should be used with caution in active or latent peptic ulcers, diverticulitis, fresh intestinal anastomoses, and nonspecific ulcerative colitis, since they may increase the risk of a perforation.
Signs of peritoneal irritation following gastrointestinal perforation in patients receiving corticosteroids may be minimal or absent.
There is an enhanced effect due to decreased metabolism of corticosteroids in patients with cirrhosis.

Musculoskeletal
Corticosteroids decrease bone formation and increase bone resorption both through their effect on calcium regulation (i.e., decreasing absorption and increasing excretion) and inhibition of osteoblast function. This, together with a decrease in the protein matrix of the bone secondary to an increase in protein catabolism, and reduced sex hormone production, may lead to inhibition of bone growth in pediatric patients and the development of osteoporosis at any age. Special consideration should be given to patients at increased risk of osteoporosis (e.g., postmenopausal women) before initiating corticosteroid therapy.

Neuro-psychiatric
Although controlled clinical trials have shown corticosteroids to be effective in speeding the resolution of acute exacerbations of multiple sclerosis, they do not show that they affect the ultimate outcome or natural history of the disease. The studies do show that relatively high doses of corticosteroids are necessary to demonstrate a significant effect. (See DOSAGE AND ADMINISTRATION.)
An acute myopathy has been observed with the use of high doses of corticosteroids, most often occurring in patients with disorders of neuromuscular transmission (e.g., myasthenia gravis), or in patients receiving concomitant therapy with neuromuscular blocking drugs (e.g., pancuronium). This acute myopathy is generalized, may involve ocular and respiratory muscles, and may result in quadriparesis. Ele-

vation of creatinine kinase may occur. Clinical improvement or recovery after stopping corticosteroids may require weeks to years.
Psychic derangements may appear when corticosteroids are used, ranging from euphoria, insomnia, mood swings, personality changes, and severe depression, to frank psychotic manifestations. Also, existing emotional instability or psychotic tendencies may be aggravated by corticosteroids.

Ophthalmic
Intraocular pressure may become elevated in some individuals. If steroid therapy is continued for more than 6 weeks, intraocular pressure should be monitored.

Information for Patients
Patients should be warned not to discontinue the use of corticosteroids abruptly or without medical supervision. As prolonged use may cause adrenal insufficiency and make patients dependent on corticosteroids, they should advise any medical attendants that they are taking corticosteroids and they should seek medical advice at once should they develop an acute illness including fever or other signs of infection. Following prolonged therapy, withdrawal of corticosteroids may result in symptoms of the corticosteroid withdrawal syndrome including myalgia, arthralgia, and malaise.
Persons who are on corticosteroids should be warned to avoid exposure to chickenpox or measles. Patients should also be advised that if they are exposed, medical advice should be sought without delay.

Drug Interactions
Aminoglutethimide: Aminoglutethimide may diminish adrenal suppression by corticosteroids.
Amphotericin B injection and potassium-depleting agents: When corticosteroids are administered concomitantly with potassium-depleting agents (e.g., amphotericin B, diuretics), patients should be observed closely for development of hypokalemia. In addition, there have been cases reported in which concomitant use of amphotericin B and hydrocortisone was followed by cardiac enlargement and congestive heart failure.
Antibiotics: Macrolide antibiotics have been reported to cause a significant decrease in corticosteroid clearance (see Drug Interactions, Hepatic Enzyme Inducers, Inhibitors and Substrates).
Anticholinesterases: Concomitant use of anticholinesterase agents and corticosteroids may produce severe weakness in patients with myasthenia gravis. If possible, anticholinesterase agents should be withdrawn at least 24 hours before initiating corticosteroid therapy.
Anticoagulants, oral: Co-administration of corticosteroids and warfarin usually results in inhibition of response to warfarin, although there have been some conflicting reports. Therefore, coagulation indices should be monitored frequently to maintain the desired anticoagulant effect.
Antidiabetics: Because corticosteroids may increase blood glucose concentrations, dosage adjustments of antidiabetic agents may be required.
Antitubercular drugs: Serum concentrations of isoniazid may be decreased.
Cholestyramine: Cholestyramine may increase the clearance of corticosteroids.
Cyclosporine: Increased activity of both cyclosporine and corticosteroids may occur when the two are used concurrently. Convulsions have been reported with this concurrent use.
Dexamethasone suppression test (DST): False-negative results in the dexamethasone suppression test (DST) in patients being treated with indomethacin have been reported. Thus, results of the DST should be interpreted with caution in these patients.
Digitalis glycosides: Patients on digitalis glycosides may be at increased risk of arrhythmias due to hypokalemia.
Ephedrine: Ephedrine may enhance the metabolic clearance of corticosteroids, resulting in decreased blood levels and lessened physiologic activity, thus requiring an increase in corticosteroid dosage.
Estrogens, including oral contraceptives: Estrogens may decrease the hepatic metabolism of certain corticosteroids, thereby increasing their effect.
Hepatic Enzyme Inducers, Inhibitors and Substrates: Drugs which induce cytochrome P450 3A4 (CYP 3A4) enzyme activity (e.g., barbiturates, phenytoin, carbamazepine, rifampin) may enhance the metabolism of corticosteroids and require that the dosage of the corticosteroid be increased. Drugs which inhibit CYP 3A4 (e.g., ketoconazole, macrolide antibiotics such as erythromycin) have the potential to result in increased plasma concentrations of corticosteroids. Dexamethasone is a moderate inducer of CYP 3A4. Co-administration with other drugs that are metabolized by CYP 3A4 (e.g., indinavir, erythromycin) may increase their clearance, resulting in decreased plasma concentration.
Ketoconazole: Ketoconazole has been reported to decrease the metabolism of certain corticosteroids by up to 60%, leading to increased risk of corticosteroid side effects. In addition, ketoconazole alone can inhibit adrenal corticosteroid synthesis and may cause adrenal insufficiency during corticosteroid withdrawal.
Nonsteroidal anti-inflammatory agents (NSAIDS): Concomitant use of aspirin (or other nonsteroidal antiinflammatory agents) and corticosteroids increases the risk of gastrointestinal side effects. Aspirin should be used cautiously in conjunction with corticosteroids in hypoprothrombinemia. The clearance of salicylates may be increased with concurrent use of corticosteroids.
Phenytoin: In post-marketing experience, there have been reports of both increases and decreases in phenytoin levels

with dexamethasone co-administration, leading to alterations in seizure control.
Skin tests: Corticosteroids may suppress reactions to skin tests.
Thalidomide: Co-administration with thalidomide should be employed cautiously, as toxic epidermal necrolysis has been reported with concomitant use.
Vaccines: Patients on corticosteroid therapy may exhibit a diminished response to toxoids and live or inactivated vaccines due to inhibition of antibody response. Corticosteroids may also potentiate the replication of some organisms contained in live attenuated vaccines. Routine administration of vaccines or toxoids should be deferred until corticosteroid therapy is discontinued if possible (see WARNINGS, Infections, Vaccination).

Carcinogenesis, Mutagenesis, Impairment of Fertility
No adequate studies have been conducted in animals to determine whether corticosteroids have a potential for carcinogenesis or mutagenesis.
Steroids may increase or decrease motility and number of spermatozoa in some patients.

Pregnancy
Teratogenic Effects: Pregnancy Category C.
Corticosteroids have been shown to be teratogenic in many species when given in doses equivalent to the human dose. Animal studies in which corticosteroids have been given to pregnant mice, rats, and rabbits have yielded an increased incidence of cleft palate in the offspring. There are no adequate and well-controlled studies in pregnant women. Corticosteroids should be used during pregnancy only if the potential benefit justifies the potential risk to the fetus. Infants born to mothers who have received substantial doses of corticosteroids during pregnancy should be carefully observed for signs of hypoadrenalism.

Nursing Mothers
Systemically administered corticosteroids appear in human milk and could suppress growth, interfere with endogenous corticosteroid production, or cause other untoward effects. Because of the potential for serious adverse reactions in nursing infants from corticosteroids, a decision should be made whether to discontinue nursing or to discontinue the drug, taking into account the importance of the drug to the mother.

Pediatric Use
The efficacy and safety of corticosteroids in the pediatric population are based on the well-established course of effect of corticosteroids, which is similar in pediatric and adult populations. Published studies provide evidence of efficacy and safety in pediatric patients for the treatment of nephrotic syndrome (patients >2 years of age), and aggressive lymphomas and leukemias (patients >1 month of age). Other indications for pediatric use of corticosteroids, e.g., severe asthma and wheezing, are based on adequate and well-controlled trials conducted in adults, on the premises that the course of the diseases and their pathophysiology are considered to be substantially similar in both populations.
The adverse effects of corticosteroids in pediatric patients are similar to those in adults (see ADVERSE REACTIONS). Like adults, pediatric patients should be carefully observed with frequent measurements of blood pressure, weight, height, intraocular pressure, and clinical evaluation for the presence of infection, psychosocial disturbances, thromboembolism, peptic ulcers, cataracts, and osteoporosis. Pediatric patients who are treated with corticosteroids by any route, including systemically administered corticosteroids, may experience a decrease in their growth velocity. This negative impact of corticosteroids on growth has been observed at low systemic doses and in the absence of laboratory evidence of hypothalamic-pituitary-adrenal (HPA) axis suppression (i.e., cosyntropin stimulation and basal cortisol plasma levels). Growth velocity may therefore be a more sensitive indicator of systemic corticosteroid exposure in pediatric patients than some commonly used tests of HPA axis function. The linear growth of pediatric patients treated with corticosteroids should be monitored, and the potential growth effects of prolonged treatment should be weighed against clinical benefits obtained and the availability of treatment alternatives. In order to minimize the potential growth effects of corticosteroids, pediatric patients should be titrated to the lowest effective dose.

Geriatric Use
Clinical studies did not include sufficient numbers of subjects aged 65 and over to determine whether they respond differently from younger subjects. Other reported clinical experience has not identified differences in responses between the elderly and younger patients. In general, dose selection for an elderly patient should be cautious, usually starting at the low end of the dosing range, reflecting the greater frequency of decreased hepatic, renal, or cardiac function, and of concomitant disease or other drug therapy. In particular, the increased risk of diabetes mellitus, fluid retention and hypertension in elderly patients treated with corticosteroids should be considered.

ADVERSE REACTIONS (listed alphabetically, under each subsection)

The following adverse reactions have been reported with DECADRON or other corticosteroids.
Allergic reactions: Anaphylactoid reaction, anaphylaxis, angioedema.
Cardiovascular: Bradycardia, cardiac arrest, cardiac arrhythmias, cardiac enlargement, circulatory collapse, congestive heart failure, fat embolism, hypertension, hyper-

trophic cardiomyopathy in premature infants, myocardial rupture following recent myocardial infarction (see WARNINGS, *Cardio-renal*), edema, pulmonary edema, syncope, tachycardia, thromboembolism, thrombophlebitis, vasculitis.

Dermatologic: Acne, allergic dermatitis, dry scaly skin, ecchymoses and petechiae, erythema, impaired wound healing, increased sweating, rash, striae, suppression of reactions to skin tests, thin fragile skin, thinning scalp hair, urticaria.

Endocrine: Decreased carbohydrate and glucose tolerance, development of cushingoid state, hyperglycemia, glycosuria, hirsutism, hypertrichosis, increased requirements for insulin or oral hypoglycemic agents in diabetes, manifestations of latent diabetes mellitus, menstrual irregularities, secondary adrenocortical and pituitary unresponsiveness (particularly in times of stress, as in trauma, surgery, or illness), suppression of growth in pediatric patients.

Fluid and electrolyte disturbances: Congestive heart failure in susceptible patients, fluid retention, hypokalemic alkalosis, potassium loss, sodium retention.

Gastrointestinal: Abdominal distention, elevation in serum liver enzyme levels (usually reversible upon discontinuation), hepatomegaly, increased appetite, nausea, pancreatitis, peptic ulcer with possible perforation and hemorrhage, perforation of the small and large intestine (particularly in patients with inflammatory bowel disease), ulcerative esophagitis.

Metabolic: Negative nitrogen balance due to protein catabolism.

Musculoskeletal: Aseptic necrosis of femoral and humeral heads, loss of muscle mass, muscle weakness, osteoporosis, pathologic fracture of long bones, steroid myopathy, tendon rupture, vertebral compression fractures.

Neurological/Psychiatric: Convulsions, depression, emotional instability, euphoria, headache, increased intracranial pressure with papilledema (pseudotumor cerebri) usually following discontinuation of treatment, insomnia, mood swings, neuritis, neuropathy, paresthesia, personality changes, psychic disorders, vertigo.

Ophthalmic: Exophthalmos, glaucoma, increased intraocular pressure, posterior subcapsular cataracts.

Other: Abnormal fat deposits, decreased resistance to infection, hiccups, increased or decreased motility and number of spermatozoa, malaise, moon face, weight gain.

OVERDOSAGE

Treatment of overdosage is by supportive and symptomatic therapy. In the case of acute overdosage, according to the patient's condition, supportive therapy may include gastric lavage or emesis.

DOSAGE AND ADMINISTRATION

For oral administration

The initial dosage varies from 0.75 to 9 mg a day depending on the disease being treated.

It Should Be Emphasized That Dosage Requirements Are Variable And Must Be Individualized On The Basis Of The Disease Under Treatment And The Response Of The Patient.

After a favorable response is noted, the proper maintenance dosage should be determined by decreasing the initial drug dosage in small decrements at appropriate time intervals until the lowest dosage that maintains an adequate clinical response is reached.

Situations which may make dosage adjustments necessary are changes in clinical status secondary to remissions or exacerbations in the disease process, the patient's individual drug responsiveness, and the effect of patient exposure to stressful situations not directly related to the disease entity under treatment. In this latter situation it may be necessary to increase the dosage of the corticosteroid for a period of time consistent with the patient's condition. If after long-term therapy the drug is to be stopped, it is recommended that it be withdrawn gradually rather than abruptly.

In the treatment of acute exacerbations of multiple sclerosis, daily doses of 30 mg of dexamethasone for a week followed by 4 to 12 mg every other day for one month have been shown to be effective (see PRECAUTIONS, *Neuro-psychiatric*).

In pediatric patients, the initial dose of dexamethasone may vary depending on the specific disease entity being treated. The range of initial doses is 0.02 to 0.3 mg/kg/day in three or four divided doses (0.6 to 9 mg/m^{2}bsa/day).

For the purpose of comparison, the following is the equivalent milligram dosage of the various corticosteroids:

Cortisone, 25	*Triamcinolone, 4*
Hydrocortisone, 20	*Paramethasone, 2*
Prednisolone, 5	*Betamethasone, 0.75*
Prednisone, 5	*Dexamethasone, 0.75*
Methylprednisolone, 4	

These dose relationships apply only to oral or intravenous administration of these compounds. When these substances or their derivatives are injected intramuscularly or into joint spaces, their relative properties may be greatly altered.

In acute, self-limited allergic disorders or acute exacerbations of chronic allergic disorders, the following dosage schedule combining parenteral and oral therapy is suggested:

Dexamethasone Sodium Phosphate injection, USP 4 mg per mL:
First Day
1 or 2 mL, intramuscularly
DECADRON tablets, 0.75 mg:
Second Day
4 tablets in two divided doses
Third Day
4 tablets in two divided doses
Fourth Day
2 tablets in two divided doses
Fifth Day
1 tablet
Sixth Day
1 tablet
Seventh Day
No treatment
Eighth Day
Follow-up visit

This schedule is designed to ensure adequate therapy during acute episodes, while minimizing the risk of overdosage in chronic cases.

In *cerebral edema*, Dexamethasone Sodium Phosphate injection, USP is generally administered initially in a dosage of 10 mg intravenously followed by 4 mg every six hours intramuscularly until the symptoms of cerebral edema subside. Response is usually noted within 12 to 24 hours and dosage may be reduced after two to four days and gradually discontinued over a period of five to seven days. For palliative management of patients with recurrent or inoperable brain tumors, maintenance therapy with either Dexamethasone Sodium Phosphate injection, USP or DECADRON tablets in a dosage of 2 mg two or three times daily may be effective.

Dexamethasone suppression tests

1. Tests for Cushing's syndrome

Give 1.0 mg of DECADRON orally at 11:00 p.m. Blood is drawn for plasma cortisol determination at 8:00 a.m. the following morning.

For greater accuracy, give 0.5 mg of DECADRON orally every 6 hours for 48 hours. Twenty-four hour urine collections are made for determination of 17-hydroxycorticosteroid excretion.

2. Test to distinguish Cushing's syndrome due to pituitary ACTH excess from Cushing's syndrome due to other causes.

Give 2.0 mg of DECADRON orally every 6 hours for 48 hours. Twenty-four hour urine collections are made for determination of 17-hydroxycorticosteroid excretion.

HOW SUPPLIED

Tablets DECADRON are compressed, pentagonal-shaped tablets, colored to distinguish potency. They are scored and coded on one side and embossed with DECADRON on the other. They are available as follows:

No. 7601 — 0.75 mg, bluish-green in color and coded MSD 63.
NDC 0006-0063-12 5-12 PAK* (package of 12)
NDC 0006-0063-68 bottles of 100.
No. 7598 — 0.5 mg, yellow in color and coded MSD 41.
NDC 0006-0041-68 bottles of 100.

Storage

Store at controlled room temperature 20 to 25°C (68 to 77°F).

Rx only

MERCK & CO., INC., Whitehouse Station, NJ 08889, USA
Issued May 2004
Printed in USA

DIURIL® Sodium Intravenous ℞
(Chlorothiazide Sodium)

Prescribing information for this product, which appears on pages 2037–2038 of the 2005 PDR, has been revised as follows. Please write "See Supplement A" next to the product heading.

In the **PRECAUTIONS** section, at the end, add the following subheading and text:

Geriatric Use

Clinical studies of Intravenous Sodium DIURIL did not include sufficient numbers of subjects aged 65 and over to determine whether they respond differently from younger subjects. Other reported clinical experience has not identified differences in responses between the elderly and younger patients. In general, dose selection for an elderly patient should be cautious, usually starting at the low end of the dosing range, reflecting the greater frequency of decreased hepatic, renal, or cardiac function, and of concomitant disease or other drug therapy.

This drug is known to be substantially excreted by the kidney, and the risk of toxic reactions to this drug may be greater in patients with impaired renal function. Because elderly patients are more likely to have decreased renal function, care should be taken in dose selection, and it may be useful to monitor renal function (see WARNINGS).

Revisions based on 9273239, issued September 2004.

DIURIL® Tablets ℞
(Chlorothiazide)
DIURIL® Oral Suspension ℞
(Chlorothiazide)

Prescribing information for this product, which appears on pages 2038–2039 of the 2005 PDR, has been revised as follows. Please write "See Supplement A" next to the product heading.

In the **PRECAUTIONS** section, at the end, add the following subheading and text:

Geriatric Use

Clinical studies of DIURIL did not include sufficient numbers of subjects aged 65 and over to determine whether they respond differently from younger subjects. Other reported clinical experience has not identified differences in responses between the elderly and younger patients. In general, dose selection for an elderly patient should be cautious, usually starting at the low end of the dosing range, reflecting the greater frequency of decreased hepatic, renal, or cardiac function, and of concomitant disease or other drug therapy.

This drug is known to be substantially excreted by the kidney, and the risk of toxic reactions to this drug may be greater in patients with impaired renal function. Because elderly patients are more likely to have decreased renal function, care should be taken in dose selection, and it may be useful to monitor renal function (see WARNINGS).

In the **HOW SUPPLIED** section, after the sixth paragraph, delete "(6505-01-156-1600, 250 mg/5 mL, 237 mL).".

Revisions based on 7897960, issued December 2003.

EMEND® ℞
[*ē′mĕnd*]
(aprepitant)
CAPSULES

Prescribing information for this product, which appears on pages 2045–2049 of the 2005 PDR, has been revised as follows. Please write "See Supplement A" next to the product heading.

In the **PRECAUTIONS** section, under the *General* subhead, after the second paragraph, add the following new paragraph:

In a separate pharmacokinetic study in patients receiving docetaxel, which is also metabolized by CYP3A4, EMEND did not influence the pharmacokinetics of docetaxel.

In the third paragraph, delete "docetaxel."

The language in the sixth paragraph has been changed as follows:

Upon coadministration with EMEND, the efficacy of hormonal contraceptives during and for 28 days following the last dose of EMEND may be reduced. Alternative or back-up methods of contraception should be used during treatment with EMEND and for 1 month following the last dose of EMEND (see PRECAUTIONS, *Drug Interactions*).

In the last paragraph, change the word "oral" to "hormonal."

Following the word "contraception" in the last sentence, add "during treatment with EMEND and for 1 month following the last dose of EMEND".

After the *Chemotherapeutic agents* subhead, add the following new subhead and text:

Docetaxel: In a pharmacokinetic study, EMEND did not influence the pharmacokinetics of docetaxel.

Under the *Oral contraceptives* subhead, delete all text after "8%." Then add the following new paragraph:

In another study, a daily dose of an oral contraceptive containing ethinyl estradiol and norethindrone was administered on Days 1 through 21, and EMEND was given as a 3-day regimen of 125 mg on Day 8 and 80 mg/day on Days 9 and 10 with ondansetron 32 mg IV on Day 8 and oral dexamethasone given as 12 mg on Day 8 and 8 mg/day on Days 9, 10, and 11. In the study, the AUC of ethinyl estradiol decreased by 19% on Day 10 and there was as much as a 64% decrease in ethinyl estradiol trough concentrations during Days 9 through 21. While there was no effect of EMEND on the AUC of norethindrone on Day 10, there was as much as a 60% decrease in norethindrone trough concentrations during Days 9 through 21. The coadministration of EMEND may reduce the efficacy of hormonal contraceptives during and for 28 days after administration of the last dose of EMEND. Alternative or back-up methods of contraception should be used during treatment with EMEND and for 1 month following the last dose of EMEND.

Revisions based on 9565002, issued December 2004.

In the **Patient Information**, in the **What should I tell my doctor before and during treatment with EMEND?** section, the language in the last paragraph has been changed as follows:

Women who use birth control medicines during treatment with EMEND and for up to 1 month after using EMEND should also use a back-up method of contraception to avoid pregnancy.

Revisions based on 9565101, issued December 2004.

FOSAMAX® ℞
[*foss-ah-max*]
(alendronate sodium)
Tablets and Oral Solution

Prescribing information for this product, which appears on pages 2049–2057 of the 2005 PDR, has been revised as follows. Please write "See Supplement A" next to the product heading.

Continued on next page

Information on the Merck & Co., Inc., products listed on these pages is from the full prescribing information in use April 1, 2004.

Fosamax—Cont.

In the **PRECAUTIONS** section, after *General* and before *Renal insufficiency,* add the following new subheading and two paragraphs:
Musculoskeletal Pain
In post marketing experience, severe and occasionally incapacitating bone, joint, and/or muscle pain has been reported in patients taking bisphosphonates that are approved for the prevention and treatment of osteoporosis (see ADVERSE REACTIONS). However, such reports have been infrequent. This category of drugs includes FOSAMAX (alendronate). Most of the patients were postmenopausal women. The time to onset of symptoms varied from one day to several months after starting the drug. Most patients had relief of symptoms after stopping. A subset had recurrence of symptoms when rechallenged with the same drug or another bisphosphonate.
In placebo-controlled clinical studies of FOSAMAX, the percentages of patients with these symptoms were similar in the FOSAMAX and placebo groups.
In the **ADVERSE REACTIONS** section, under *Post-Marketing Experience,* add the following new paragraph after the *Gastrointestinal* subentry:
Musculoskeletal: bone, joint, and/or muscle pain, occasionally severe, and rarely incapacitating (see PRECAUTIONS, *Musculoskeletal Pain*).
In the **ADVERSE REACTIONS** section, under *Post-Marketing Experience, Special Senses,* replace "rarely scleritis" with "scleritis or episcleritis."
Revisions based on 7957026, issued August 2004; and 7957027, issued December 2004.
Replace the *Patient Information about FOSAMAX for Osteoporosis* with the following:

Patient Information
FOSAMAX® (alendronate sodium) Tablets

Read this information before you start taking FOSAMAX* (FOSS-ah-max). Also, read the leaflet each time you refill your prescription, just in case anything has changed. This leaflet does not take the place of discussions with your doctor. You and your doctor should discuss FOSAMAX when you start taking your medicine and at regular checkups.
_____
* Registered trademark of MERCK & CO., Inc.
 COPYRIGHT © MERCK & CO., Inc., 1995, 1997, 2000
 All rights reserved.
What is the most important information I should know about FOSAMAX?
- **You must take FOSAMAX exactly as directed to help make sure it works and to help lower the chance of harmful side effects.**
- **After getting up for the day and before taking your first food, drink, or other medicine, swallow your FOSAMAX tablet with a full glass (6-8 oz) of <u>plain water</u> only.**
  - **Not** mineral water
  - **Not** coffee or tea
  - **Not** juice
- **Do not chew or suck on a tablet of FOSAMAX.**
- **After swallowing your FOSAMAX tablet, do not lie down – stay fully upright (sitting, standing, or walking) for at least 30 minutes. Do not lie down until after your first food of the day.** This will help the FOSAMAX tablet reach your stomach quickly and help reduce the chance that FOSAMAX might irritate your esophagus, the tube that connects your mouth with your stomach.
- **After swallowing your FOSAMAX tablet, wait at least 30 minutes before taking your first food, drink, or other medicine of the day,** including antacids, calcium, and other supplements and vitamins. FOSAMAX is effective only if it is taken when your stomach is empty.
- **Do not take FOSAMAX at bedtime or before getting up for the day.**
- **If you have chest pain, new or worsening heartburn, or have trouble or pain when you swallow, stop taking FOSAMAX and call your doctor.**
What is FOSAMAX?
FOSAMAX is for:
- The treatment or prevention of osteoporosis (thinning of bone) in women after menopause. It reduces the chance of having a hip or spinal fracture (break).
- Treatment to increase bone mass in men with osteoporosis.
- The treatment of osteoporosis in either men or women receiving corticosteroid medicines (for example, prednisone).
Improvement in bone density may be seen as early as 3 months after you start taking FOSAMAX. For FOSAMAX to continue to work, you need to keep taking it.
FOSAMAX is not a hormone.
There is more information about osteoporosis at the end of this leaflet.
Who should not take FOSAMAX?
Do not take FOSAMAX if you:
- Have certain problems with your esophagus, the tube that connects your mouth with your stomach
- Cannot stand or sit upright for at least 30 minutes
- Have low levels of calcium in your blood
- Have severe kidney disease
- Are allergic to FOSAMAX or any of its ingredients. A list of ingredients is at the end of this leaflet.
If you are pregnant or nursing, talk to your doctor about whether taking FOSAMAX is right for you based on possible risk to you and your child.
Talk to your doctor about any:

- Problems with swallowing
- Stomach or digestive problems
- Other medical problems you have or have had in the past
- Medicines you take, including prescription and non-prescription medicines, vitamins, and herbal supplements
How should I take FOSAMAX?
See "What is the most important information I should know about FOSAMAX?" for important information about how to take the medicine and to help make sure it works for you. In addition, follow these instructions:
- After getting up for the day and before taking your first food, drink, or other medicine, swallow your FOSAMAX tablet with a full glass (6-8 oz) of plain water only.
- Take 1 FOSAMAX tablet once a day, every day.
- It is important that you keep taking FOSAMAX for as long as your doctor says to take it. For FOSAMAX to continue to work, you need to keep taking it.
- If you miss a dose, do not take it later in the day. Continue your usual schedule of 1 tablet once a day the next morning.
- If you think you took more than the prescribed dose of FOSAMAX, drink a full glass of milk and contact your local poison control center or emergency room right away. Do not try to vomit. Do not lie down.
What should I avoid while taking FOSAMAX?
- **Do not eat, drink, or take other medicines or supplements before taking FOSAMAX.**
- **Wait for at least 30 minutes after taking FOSAMAX to eat, drink, or take other medicines or supplements.**
- **Do not lie down for at least 30 minutes after taking FOSAMAX. Do not lie down until after your first food of the day.**
What are the possible side effects of FOSAMAX?
Some patients may get severe digestive reactions from FOSAMAX. (See "What is the most important information I should know about FOSAMAX?") These reactions include irritation, inflammation, or ulcers of the esophagus, which may sometimes bleed. This may occur especially if patients do not drink a full glass of water with FOSAMAX or if they lie down in less than 30 minutes or before their first food of the day. Esophagus reactions may get worse if patients continue to take FOSAMAX after developing symptoms of an irritated esophagus.
Stop taking FOSAMAX and call your doctor right away if you get any of these signs of possible serious problems:
- Chest pain
- Heartburn
- Trouble or pain when swallowing
Side effects in patients taking FOSAMAX usually have been mild. They generally have not caused patients to stop taking FOSAMAX.
The most common side effect is abdominal (stomach area) pain. Less common side effects are nausea, vomiting, a full or bloated feeling in the stomach, constipation, diarrhea, black or bloody stools (bowel movements), gas, headache, a changed sense of taste, and bone, muscle, and/or joint pain. Severe bone, joint, and/or muscle pain has been reported in patients taking, by mouth, bisphosphonates drugs that are used to treat osteoporosis (thin bones). However, such reports have been rare. This group of drugs includes FOSAMAX. Most of the patients were postmenopausal women (women who had stopped having periods). Patients developed pain within one day to several months after starting the drug. Most patients experienced relief after stopping the drug. Patients who develop severe bone, joint, and/or muscle pain after starting FOSAMAX should contact their physician.
Transient flu-like symptoms (rarely with fever), typically at the start of treatment, have occurred.
In rare cases, patients taking FOSAMAX may get itching or eye pain, or a rash that may be made worse by sunlight. Rarely, severe skin reactions may occur. Patients may get allergic reactions, such as hives or, in rare cases, swelling that can be of their face, lips, tongue, or throat, which may cause trouble in breathing or swallowing. Mouth ulcers (sores) may occur if FOSAMAX is chewed or dissolved in the mouth.
Anytime you have a medical problem you think may be from FOSAMAX, talk to your doctor.
What should I know about osteoporosis?
Normally your bones are being rebuilt all the time. First, old bone is removed (resorbed). Then a similar amount of new bone is formed. This balanced process keeps your skeleton healthy and strong.
Osteoporosis is a thinning and weakening of the bones. It is common in women after menopause, and may also occur in men. In osteoporosis, bone is removed faster than it is formed, so overall bone mass is lost and bones become weaker. Therefore, keeping bone mass is important to keep your bones healthy. In both men and women, osteoporosis may also be caused by certain medicines called corticosteroids.
At first, osteoporosis usually has no symptoms, but it can cause fractures (broken bones). Fractures usually cause pain. Fractures of the bones of the spine may not be painful, but over time they can make you shorter. Eventually, your spine can curve and your body can become bent over. Fractures may happen during normal, everyday activity, such as lifting, or from minor injury that would normally not cause bones to break. Fractures most often occur at the hip, spine, or wrist. This can lead to pain, severe disability, or loss of ability to move around (mobility).
Who is at risk for osteoporosis?
Many things put people at risk of osteoporosis. The following people have a higher chance of getting osteoporosis:

Women who:
- Are going through or who are past menopause
Men who:
- Are elderly
People who:
- Are white (Caucasian) or oriental (Asian)
- Are thin
- Have family member with osteoporosis
- Do not get enough calcium or vitamin D
- Do not exercise
- Smoke
- Drink alcohol often
- Take bone thinning medicines (like prednisone or other corticosteroids) for a long time
What can I do to help prevent or treat osteoporosis?
In addition to FOSAMAX, your doctor may suggest one or more of the following lifestyle changes:
- **Stop smoking.** Smoking may increase your chance of getting osteoporosis.
- **Reduce the use of alcohol.** Too much alcohol may increase the risk of osteoporosis and injuries that can cause fractures.
- **Exercise regularly.** Like muscles, bones need exercise to stay strong and healthy. Exercise must be safe to prevent injuries, including fractures. Talk with your doctor before you begin any exercise program.
- **Eat a balanced diet.** Having enough calcium in your diet is important. Your doctor can advise you whether you need to change your diet or take any dietary supplements, such as calcium or vitamin D.
What are the ingredients in FOSAMAX?
FOSAMAX contains alendronate sodium as the active ingredient and the following inactive ingredients: cellulose, lactose, croscarmellose sodium and magnesium stearate. The 10 mg tablet also contains carnauba wax.
How do I store FOSAMAX?
Store FOSAMAX at room temperature, 59-86°F (15-30°C). Discard all expired medicines. Keep all medicines out of the reach of children.
General information about using FOSAMAX safely and effectively
Medicines are sometimes prescribed for conditions that are not mentioned in patient information leaflets. This medicine was prescribed for your particular condition. FOSAMAX acts specifically on your bones. Do not use it for another condition or give it to others.
This leaflet is a summary of information about FOSAMAX. If you have any questions or concerns about FOSAMAX or osteoporosis, talk to your doctor, pharmacist, or other health care provider. You can ask your doctor or pharmacist for information about FOSAMAX written for health care providers. For more information, call 1-877-408-4699 (toll-free) or visit the following website: www.fosamax.com.
Revisions based on 7969414, issued April 2004; and 7969415, issued December 2004.
Replace the *Patient Information about Once Weekly FOSAMAX for Osteoporosis* with the following:
Patient Information
Once Weekly FOSAMAX® (alendronate sodium)
Tablets and Oral Solution
Read this information before you start taking FOSAMAX* (FOSS-ah-max). Also, read the leaflet each time you refill your prescription, just in case anything has changed. This leaflet does not take the place of discussions with your doctor. You and your doctor should discuss FOSAMAX when you start taking your medicine and at regular checkups.
_____
* Registered trademark of MERCK & CO., Inc.
 COPYRIGHT © MERCK & CO., Inc., 2000
 All rights reserved.
What is the most important information I should know about once weekly FOSAMAX?
- **You must take once weekly FOSAMAX exactly as directed to help make sure it works and to help lower the chance of harmful side effects.**
- **Choose the day of the week that best fits your schedule. Every week, take 1 dose of FOSAMAX (one tablet or one entire bottle of solution) on your chosen day.**
- **After getting up for the day and before taking your first food, drink, or other medicine, take your FOSAMAX with plain water only as follows:**
  - **TABLETS: Swallow one tablet with a full glass (6-8 oz) of plain water.**
  - **ORAL SOLUTION: Drink one entire bottle of solution followed by at least 2 ounces (a quarter of a cup) of plain water.**
  Do **not** take FOSAMAX with:
  Mineral water
  Coffee or tea
  Juice
- **Do not chew or suck on a tablet of FOSAMAX.**
- **After taking your FOSAMAX, do not lie down – stay fully upright (sitting, standing, or walking) for at least 30 minutes. Do not lie down until after your first food of the day.** This will help FOSAMAX reach your stomach quickly and help reduce the chance that FOSAMAX might irritate your esophagus, the tube that connects your mouth with your stomach.
- **After taking your FOSAMAX, wait at least 30 minutes before taking your first food, drink, or other medicine of the day,** including antacids, calcium, and other supplements and vitamins. FOSAMAX is effective only if it is taken when your stomach is empty.
- **Do not take FOSAMAX at bedtime or before getting up for the day.**

- **If you have chest pain, new or worsening heartburn, or have trouble or pain when you swallow, stop taking FOSAMAX and call your doctor.**

What is FOSAMAX?

FOSAMAX is for:

- The treatment or prevention of osteoporosis (thinning of bone) in women after menopause. It reduces the chance of having a hip or spinal fracture (break).
- Treatment to increase bone mass in men with osteoporosis.

FOSAMAX tablets are for treatment and prevention, and FOSAMAX oral solution is for treatment of osteoporosis.

Improvement in bone density may be seen as early as 3 months after you start taking FOSAMAX. For FOSAMAX to continue to work, you need to keep taking it.

FOSAMAX is not a hormone.

There is more information about osteoporosis at the end of this leaflet.

Who should not take FOSAMAX?

Do not take FOSAMAX (tablets or oral solution) if you:

- Have certain problems with your esophagus, the tube that connects your mouth with your stomach
- Cannot stand or sit upright for at least 30 minutes
- Have low levels of calcium in your blood
- Have severe kidney disease
- Are allergic to FOSAMAX or any of its ingredients. A list of ingredients is at the end of this leaflet.

Do not take FOSAMAX oral solution if you have difficulty swallowing liquids.

If you are pregnant or nursing, talk to your doctor about whether taking FOSAMAX is right for you based on possible risk to you and your child.

Talk to your doctor about any:

- Problems with swallowing
- Stomach or digestive problems
- Other medical problems you have or have had in the past
- Medicines you take, including prescription and non-prescription medicines, vitamins, and herbal supplements

How should I take once weekly FOSAMAX?

See "What is the most important information I should know about once weekly FOSAMAX?" for important information about how to take the medicine and to help make sure it works for you. In addition, follow these instructions:

- Take 1 dose of FOSAMAX **once a week**.
- Choose the day of the week that best fits your schedule. Every week take 1 dose of FOSAMAX on your chosen day.
- After getting up for the day and before taking your first food, drink, or other medicine, take your FOSAMAX with plain water only as follows:
  - TABLETS: Swallow one tablet with a full glass (6-8 oz) of plain water.
  - ORAL SOLUTION: Drink one entire bottle of solution followed by at least 2 ounces (a quarter of a cup) of plain water.
- It is important that you keep taking FOSAMAX for as long as your doctor says to take it. For FOSAMAX to continue to work, you need to keep taking it.
- If you miss a dose, take only 1 dose of FOSAMAX on the morning after you remember. Do not take 2 doses on the same day. Continue your usual schedule of 1 dose once a week on your chosen day.
- If you think you took more than the prescribed dose of FOSAMAX, drink a full glass of milk and contact your local poison control center or emergency room right away. Do not try to vomit. Do not lie down.

What should I avoid while taking FOSAMAX?

- **Do not eat, drink, or take other medicines or supplements before taking FOSAMAX.**
- **Wait for at least 30 minutes after taking FOSAMAX to eat, drink, or take other medicines or supplements.**
- **Do not lie down for at least 30 minutes after taking FOSAMAX. Do not lie down until after your first food of the day.**

What are the possible side effects of FOSAMAX?

Some patients may get severe digestive reactions from FOSAMAX. (See "What is the most important information I should know about once weekly FOSAMAX?") These reactions include irritation, inflammation, or ulcers of the esophagus, which may sometimes bleed. This may occur especially if patients do not drink the recommended amount of water with FOSAMAX or if they lie down in less than 30 minutes or before their first food of the day. Esophagus reactions may get worse if patients continue to take FOSAMAX after developing symptoms of an irritated esophagus.

Stop taking FOSAMAX and call your doctor right away if you get any of these signs of possible serious problems:

- Chest pain
- Heartburn
- Trouble or pain when swallowing

Side effects in patients taking FOSAMAX usually have been mild. They generally have not caused patients to stop taking FOSAMAX.

The most common side effect is abdominal (stomach area) pain. Less common side effects are nausea, vomiting, a full or bloated feeling in the stomach, constipation, diarrhea, black or bloody stools (bowel movements), gas, headache, a changed sense of taste, and bone, muscle, and/or joint pain. Severe bone, joint, and/or muscle pain has been reported in patients taking, by mouth, bisphosphonates drugs that are used to treat osteoporosis (thin bones). However, such reports have been rare. This group of drugs includes FOSAMAX. Most of the patients were postmenopausal women (women who had stopped having periods). Patients developed pain within one day to several months after starting the drug. Most patients experienced relief after stopping the drug. Patients who develop severe bone, joint, and/or muscle pain after starting FOSAMAX should contact their physician.

Transient flu-like symptoms (rarely with fever), typically at the start of treatment, have occurred.

In rare cases, patients taking FOSAMAX may get itching or eye pain, or a rash that may be made worse by sunlight. Rarely, severe skin reactions may occur. Patients may get allergic reactions, such as hives or, in rare cases, swelling that can be of their face, lips, tongue, or throat, which may cause trouble in breathing or swallowing. Mouth ulcers (sores) may occur if the FOSAMAX tablet is chewed or dissolved in the mouth.

Anytime you have a medical problem you think may be from FOSAMAX, talk to your doctor.

What should I know about osteoporosis?

Normally your bones are being rebuilt all the time. First, old bone is removed (resorbed). Then a similar amount of new bone is formed. This balanced process keeps your skeleton healthy and strong.

Osteoporosis is a thinning and weakening of the bones. It is common in women after menopause, and may also occur in men. In osteoporosis, bone is removed faster than it is formed, so overall bone mass is lost and bones become weaker. Therefore, keeping bone mass is important to keep your bones healthy. In both men and women, osteoporosis may also be caused by certain medicines called corticosteroids.

At first, osteoporosis usually has no symptoms, but it can cause fractures (broken bones). Fractures usually cause pain. Fractures of the bones of the spine may not be painful, but over time they can make you shorter. Eventually, your spine can curve and your body can become bent over. Fractures may happen during normal, everyday activity, such as lifting, or from minor injury that would normally not cause bones to break. Fractures most often occur at the hip, spine, or wrist. This can lead to pain, severe disability, or loss of ability to move around (mobility).

Who is at risk for osteoporosis?

Many things put people at risk of osteoporosis. The following people have a higher chance of getting osteoporosis:

Women who:

- Are going through or who are past menopause

Men who:

- Are elderly

People who:

- Are white (Caucasian) or oriental (Asian)
- Are thin
- Have family member with osteoporosis
- Do not get enough calcium or vitamin D
- Do not exercise
- Smoke
- Drink alcohol often
- Take bone thinning medicines (like prednisone or other corticosteroids) for a long time

What can I do to help prevent or treat osteoporosis?

In addition to FOSAMAX, your doctor may suggest one or more of the following lifestyle changes:

- **Stop smoking.** Smoking may increase your chance of getting osteoporosis.
- **Reduce the use of alcohol.** Too much alcohol may increase the risk of osteoporosis and injuries that can cause fractures.
- **Exercise regularly.** Like muscles, bones need exercise to stay strong and healthy. Exercise must be safe to prevent injuries, including fractures. Talk with your doctor before you begin any exercise program.
- **Eat a balanced diet.** Having enough calcium in your diet is important. Your doctor can advise you whether you need to change your diet or take any dietary supplements, such as calcium or vitamin D.

What are the ingredients in FOSAMAX?

Tablets

FOSAMAX tablets contain alendronate sodium as the active ingredient and the following inactive ingredients: cellulose, lactose, croscarmellose sodium and magnesium stearate.

Oral Solution

Fosamax oral solution contains alendronate sodium as the active ingredient and the following inactive ingredients: sodium citrate, citric acid, sodium saccharin, artificial raspberry flavor, purified water, sodium propylparaben and sodium butylparaben.

How do I store FOSAMAX?

Tablets

Store at room temperature, 59-86°F (15-30°C).

Oral Solution

Store at 77°F (25°C). Occasional storage between 59-86°F (15-30°C) is allowed. Do not freeze.

Discard all expired medicines. Keep all medicines out of the reach of children.

General information about using FOSAMAX safely and effectively

Medicines are sometimes prescribed for conditions that are not mentioned in patient information leaflets. This medicine was prescribed for your particular condition. FOSAMAX acts specifically on your bones. Do not use it for another condition or give it to others.

This leaflet is a summary of information about FOSAMAX. If you have any questions or concerns about FOSAMAX or osteoporosis, talk to your doctor, pharmacist, or other health care provider. You can ask your doctor or pharmacist for information about FOSAMAX written for health care providers. For more information, call 1-877-408-4699 (toll-free) or visit the following website: www.fosamax.com.

Revisions based on 9364106, issued April 2004; and 9364107, issued December 2004.

HYZAAR® 50-12.5 ℞

(losartan potassium-hydrochlorothiazide tablets)

HYZAAR® 100-25

(losartan potassium-hydrochlorothiazide tablets)

Prescribing information for this product, which appears on pages 2061–2065 of the 2005 PDR, has been revised as follows. Please write "See Supplement A" next to the product heading.

Under the **ADVERSE REACTIONS** section, under the subhead *Post-Marketing Experience*, after the 3rd paragraph, insert the following new paragraph: *Musculoskeletal:* Rare cases of rhabdomyolysis have been reported in patients receiving angiotensin II receptor blockers.

In the **HOW SUPPLIED** section:

delete the 8th line: "**NDC** 0006-0717-58 unit of use bottles of 100".

delete the period at the end of the 10th line and add the following new line: "**NDC** 0006-0717-86 bottles of 5,000."

delete the 18th line: "**NDC** 0006-0747-58 unit of use bottles of 100".

delete the period at the end of the 20th line and add the following new line: "**NDC** 0006-0747-81 bottles of 4,000."

Below the *Storage* section, on the 4th line, delete the words "Dist. By:" and add "Manufactured for:"

Revisions based on 9573625, issued October 2004.

INDOCIN® ℞

Capsules, Oral Suspension and Suppositories

[*in-do-sin*]

(Indomethacin)

Prescribing information for this product, which appears on pages 2065–2068 of the 2005 PDR, has been revised as follows. Please write "See Supplement A" next to the product heading.

In the **PRECAUTIONS** section, under *Drug Interactions*, at the end of the fourth paragraph, add the following text: In post-marketing experience, bleeding has been reported in patients on concomitant treatment with anticoagulants and INDOCIN. Caution should be exercised when INDOCIN and anticoagulants are administered concomitantly.

Revisions based on 7873329, issued July 2004.

STERILE

INDOCIN® I.V. ℞

(INDOMETHACIN FOR INJECTION)

Prescribing information for this product, which appears on pages 2068–2069 of the 2005 PDR, has been revised as follows. Please write "See Supplement A" next to the product heading.

In the **ADVERSE REACTIONS** section, under *Gastrointestinal*, after "transient ileus," add the following text: gastric perforation,

In the **DOSAGE AND ADMINISTRATION** section, under *Directions for Use*, second paragraph, first sentence, change "*sterile*" to "*Sterile*".

Revisions based on 9408720, issued July 2004.

INVANZ® ℞

(ertapenem for injection)

Prescribing information for this product, which appears on pages 2069–2074 of the 2005 PDR, has been revised as follows. Please write "See Supplement A" next to the product heading.

In the **CLINICAL PHARMACOLOGY** section, under *Microbiology*, **Aerobic gram-positive microorganisms**:, before *Streptococcus pneumoniae* (penicillin-intermediate strains only), add the following:

Staphylococcus epidermidis (methicillin susceptible strains only)

In the **CLINICAL PHARMACOLOGY** section, under *Microbiology*, **Aerobic gram-negative microorganisms**:, after *Proteus vulgaris*, add the following:

Providencia rettgeri

Providencia stuartii

In the **CLINICAL PHARMACOLOGY** section, under *Microbiology*, **Anaerobic microorganisms**:, before *Clostridium perfringens*, add the following:

Bacteroides vulgatus

Revisions based on 9500004, issued September 2004.

Continued on next page

Information on the Merck & Co., Inc., products listed on these pages is from the full prescribing information in use April 1, 2004.

MEFOXIN® ℞
(Cefoxitin for Injection)

Prescribing information for this product, which appears on pages 2081–2084 of the 2005 PDR, has been revised as follows. Please write "See Supplement A" next to the product heading.

In the **CLINICAL PHARMACOLOGY** section, beneath the *Clinical Pharmacology* subhead, add the following paragraph after the second paragraph:

In a published study of geriatric patients ranging in age from 64 to 88 years with normal renal function for their age (creatinine clearance ranging from 31.5 to 174.0 mL/min), the half-life for cefoxitin ranged from 51 to 90 minutes, resulting in higher plasma concentrations than in younger adults. These changes were attributed to decreased renal function associated with the aging process.

In the **PRECAUTIONS** section, after the *Pediatric Use* section, add the following section:

Geriatric Use

Of the 1,775 subjects who received cefoxitin in clinical studies, 424 (24%) were 65 and over, while 124 (7%) were 75 and over. No overall differences in safety or effectiveness were observed between these subjects and younger subjects, and other reported clinical experience has not identified differences in responses between the elderly and younger patients, but greater sensitivity of some older individuals cannot be ruled out (see CLINICAL PHARMACOLOGY).

This drug is known to be substantially excreted by the kidney, and the risk of toxic reactions to this drug may be greater in patients with impaired renal function. Because elderly patients are more likely to have decreased renal function, care should be taken in dose selection, and it may be useful to monitor renal function (see DOSAGE AND ADMINISTRATION and PRECAUTIONS).

Revisions based on 7882342, issued June 2004.

MEFOXIN® PREMIXED INTRAVENOUS SOLUTION ℞
(Cefoxitin Injection)

Prescribing information for this product, which appears on pages 2084–2087 of the 2005 PDR, has been revised as follows. Please write "See Supplement A" next to the product heading.

In the **CLINICAL PHARMACOLOGY** section, beneath the *Clinical Pharmacology* subhead, add the following paragraph after the second paragraph:

In a published study of geriatric patients ranging in age from 64 to 88 years with normal renal function for their age (creatinine clearance ranging from 31.5 to 174.0 mL/min), the half-life for cefoxitin ranged from 51 to 90 minutes, resulting in higher plasma concentrations than in younger adults. These changes were attributed to decreased renal function associated with the aging process.

In the **PRECAUTIONS** section, after the *Pediatric Use* section, add the following section:

Geriatric Use

Of the 1,775 subjects who received cefoxitin in clinical studies, 424 (24%) were 65 and over, while 124 (7%) were 75 and over. No overall differences in safety or effectiveness were observed between these subjects and younger subjects, and other reported clinical experience has not identified differences in responses between the elderly and younger patients, but greater sensitivity of some older individuals cannot be ruled out (see CLINICAL PHARMACOLOGY).

This drug is known to be substantially excreted by the kidney, and the risk of toxic reactions to this drug may be greater in patients with impaired renal function. Because elderly patients are more likely to have decreased renal function, care should be taken in dose selection, and it may be useful to monitor renal function (see DOSAGE AND ADMINISTRATION and PRECAUTIONS).

Revisions based on 7948526, issued June 2004.

MEPHYTON® Tablets ℞
(phytonadione)
Vitamin K_1

Prescribing information for this product, which appears on pages 2087–2088 of the 2005 PDR, has been revised as follows. Please write "See Supplement A" next to the product heading.

In the **CONTRAINDICATIONS** section, add an "S" to the end of the heading "**CONTRAINDICATION**".

In the **ADVERSE REACTIONS** section, at the beginning, add the following paragraph: "Severe hypersensitivity reactions, including anaphylactoid reactions and deaths have been reported following parenteral administration. The majority of these reported events occurred following intravenous administration."

In the **HOW SUPPLIED** section, under ***Storage:***, at the end of the first sentence, in the bracketed statement, change "**See**" to "**see**".

At the end, replace the copyright line with "COPYRIGHT © 1986, 1991, MERCK & CO., Inc."

Revisions based on 7918719, issued April 2004.

MEVACOR® Tablets ℞
(Lovastatin)

Prescribing information for this product, which appears on pages 2090–2094 of the 2005 PDR, has been revised as follows. Please write "See Supplement A" next to the product heading.

In the **WARNINGS** section, under ***Myopathy/Rhabdomyolysis:***

In the first subparagraph under the first bulleted paragraph, titled **"Potent inhibitors of CYP3A4,"** add **"telithromycin,"** in bold type between **"clarithromycin"** and **"HIV protease inhibitors"**.

Following the second subparagraph in the first bulleted paragraph, add the following new third subparagraph (use bold and italic type where indicated):

Danazol, particularly with higher doses of lovastatin (see below; PRECAUTIONS, *Drug Interactions, Other drug interactions*).

In paragraph no. **1** under **CONSEQUENTLY:**

In the first sentence, add **"telithromycin"** between **"clarithromycin"** and **"HIV protease inhibitors"**. In the second sentence, delete "or" between "erythromycin," and "clarithromycin" and add ", or telithromycin" after "clarithromycin".

Following paragraph no. **2** under **CONSEQUENTLY**, add the following new paragraph:

3. The dose of lovastatin should not exceed 20 mg daily in patients receiving concomitant medication with danazol. The benefits of the use of lovastatin in patients receiving danazol should be carefully weighed against the risk of this combination.

Renumber the numbered paragraphs following the above new paragraph from **3**, **4**, and **5** to **4**, **5**, and **6**.

In the **PRECAUTIONS** section, under *Drug Interactions, CYP3A4 Interactions:*

In the second paragraph, add **"Telithromycin"** between **"Clarithromycin"** and **"HIV protease inhibitors"** in the list.

In the **PRECAUTIONS** section, under *Other drug interactions:*

Add the following new first paragraph:

Danazol: The risk of myopathy/rhabdomyolysis is increased by concomitant administration of danazol particularly with higher doses of lovastatin (see WARNINGS, *Myopathy/Rhabdomyolysis*).

In the **DOSAGE AND ADMINISTRATION** section:

Change the subhead *Dosage in Patients taking Cyclosporine* to the following: *Dosage in Patients taking Cyclosporine or Danazol*

In the first paragraph of the same subsection, add "or danazol" after "In patients taking cyclosporine".

Revisions based on 7825352, issued November 2004.

NOROXIN® Tablets ℞
(norfloxacin)

Prescribing information for this product, which appears on pages 2103–2106 of the 2005 PDR, has been revised as follows. Please write "See Supplement A" next to the product heading.

In the **WARNINGS** section, delete the second paragraph.

In the **ADVERSE REACTIONS** section, set the subhead "***Post Marketing***" in boldface type. Also, under *Cardiovascular*, delete the parentheses in the sentence.

Revisions based on 7898535, issued July 2004.

PNEUMOVAX® 23 ℞
(Pneumococcal Vaccine Polyvalent)

Prescribing information for this product, which appears on pages 2114–2116 of the 2005 PDR, has been revised as follows. Please write "See Supplement A" next to the product heading.

In the **INDICATIONS AND USAGE** section, under *Revaccination*, please delete the first paragraph beginning at "Early studies" and ending with "side effects."

Same section, in second paragraph, please delete first word "Routine" so that the sentence begins with "Revaccination." Same sentence, please insert "routinely" between "not" and "recommended" so that the sentence reads "Revaccination of immunocompetent persons previously vaccinated with 23-valent polysaccharide vaccine is not routinely recommended."

In the **ADVERSE REACTIONS** section, second paragraph, please delete "Very rarely, cellulitis-like reactions were reported. These cellulitis-like reactions, reported in post-marketing experience, show short onset time from vaccine administration and were transient in nature."

Please replace with the following: "In post-marketing experience, injection site cellulitis-like reactions were reported rarely; between 1989 and 2002, when approximately 43 million doses were distributed, the annual reporting rate was < 2/100,000 doses. These cellulitis-like reactions occurred with initial and repeat vaccination at a median onset time of 2 days after vaccine administration and were transient in nature." In the same section, following paragraph above, please insert new paragraph: "Compared with primary vaccination, an increased rate of self limited local reactions has been observed with revaccination at 3–5 years following primary vaccination."

Revisions based on 7999823, issued December 2004.

PRINIVIL® TABLETS ℞
(LISINOPRIL)

Prescribing information for this product, which appears on pages 2123–2127 of the 2005 PDR, has been revised as follows. Please write "See Supplement A" next to the product heading.

In the **DESCRIPTION** section, in the third paragraph, first sentence, delete "2.5 mg,".

In the **PRECAUTIONS** section, after *Pediatric Use* section, insert the following text:

Geriatric Use

Clinical studies of PRINIVIL in patients with hypertension and congestive heart failure did not include sufficient numbers of subjects aged 65 and over to determine whether they respond differently from younger subjects. Other clinical experience in this population has not identified differences in responses between the elderly and younger patients. In general, dose selection for an elderly patient should be cautious, usually starting at the low end of the dosing range, reflecting the greater frequency of decreased hepatic, renal, or cardiac function, and of concomitant disease or other drug therapy.

In a clinical study of PRINIVIL in patients with myocardial infarctions 4413 (47 percent) were 65 and over, while 1656 (18 percent) were 75 and over. No overall differences in safety or efficacy were observed between elderly and younger patients.

Other reported clinical experience has not identified differences in responses between elderly and younger patients, but greater sensitivity of some older individuals cannot be ruled out.

Pharmacokinetic studies indicate that maximum blood levels and area under plasma concentration time curve (AUC) are doubled in elderly patients.

This drug is known to be substantially excreted by the kidney, and the risk of toxic reactions to this drug may be greater in patients with impaired renal function. Because elderly patients are more likely to have decreased renal function, care should be taken in dose selection. Evaluation of patients with hypertension, congestive heart failure, or myocardial infarction should always include assessment of renal function. (See DOSAGE AND ADMINISTRATION.)

In the **HOW SUPPLIED** section, delete first paragraph: "No. 3658 – Tablets PRINIVIL, 2.5 mg, are white, round, flat-faced, beveled edge, compressed tablets, coded MSD on one side and 15 on the other. They are supplied as follows: **NDC** 0006 0015 58 unit of use bottles of 100." On line 10 beneath heading, delete "**NDC** 0006 0019 87 bottles of 10,000." On line 16, delete "**NDC** 0006 0106 87 bottles of 10,000." On line 21, delete "**NDC** 0006 0207 87 bottles of 10,000."

Revisions based on 7825250, issued May 2004.

PROPECIA® ℞
[*prō-pē-sha*]
(finasteride)
Tablets, 1 mg

Prescribing information for this product, which appears on pages 2130–2133 of the 2005 PDR, has been revised as follows. Please write "See Supplement A" next to the product heading.

In the **DESCRIPTION** section, in the fourth paragraph, replace "docusate sodium" with "hydroxypropyl methylcellulose, hydroxypropyl cellulose LF, titanium dioxide,", delete "hydroxypropyl methylcellulose 2910, hydroxypropyl cellulose, titanium dioxide," and after "talc,", insert "docusate sodium,".

In the **CLINICAL PHARMACOLOGY** section, in the third paragraph, add the following at the end:

Mean circulating levels of testosterone and estradiol were increased by approximately 15% as compared to baseline, but these remained within the physiologic range.

In the **CLINICAL PHARMACOLOGY** section, delete the sixth paragraph and under the *Pharmacokinetics* section, replace all copy before the *Clinical Studies* section with the following:

Absorption

In a study in 15 healthy young male subjects, the mean bioavailability of finasteride 1-mg tablets was 65% (range 26–170%), based on the ratio of area under the curve (AUC) relative to an intravenous (IV) reference dose. At steady state following dosing with 1 mg/day (n=12), maximum finasteride plasma concentration averaged 9.2 ng/mL (range, 4.9–13.7 ng/mL) and was reached 1 to 2 hours postdose; $AUC_{(0-24\ hr)}$ was 53 ng•hr/mL (range, 20–154 ng•hr/mL). Bioavailability of finasteride was not affected by food.

Distribution

Mean steady-state volume of distribution was 76 liters (range, 44–96 liters; n=15).

Approximately 90% of circulating finasteride is bound to plasma proteins. There is a slow accumulation phase for finasteride after multiple dosing.

Finasteride has been found to cross the blood-brain barrier. Semen levels have been measured in 35 men taking finasteride 1 mg/day for 6 weeks. In 60% (21 of 35) of the samples, finasteride levels were undetectable (<0.2 ng/mL). The mean finasteride level was 0.26 ng/mL and the highest level measured was 1.52 ng/mL. Using the highest semen level measured and assuming 100% absorption from a 5-mL ejaculate per day, human exposure through vaginal absorption would be up to 7.6 ng per day, which is 750 times lower than the exposure from the no-effect dose for developmental abnormalities in Rhesus monkeys and 650-fold less than the dose of finasteride (5 µg) that had no effect on circulating DHT levels in men (see PRECAUTIONS, *Pregnancy*).

Metabolism

Finasteride is extensively metabolized in the liver, primarily via the cytochrome P450 3A4 enzyme subfamily. Two metabolites, the t-butyl side chain monohydroxylated and monocarboxylic acid metabolites, have been identified that possess no more than 20% of the 5α-reductase inhibitory activity of finasteride.

Excretion

Following intravenous infusion in healthy young subjects (n=15), mean plasma clearance of finasteride was 165 mL/min (range, 70–279 mL/min). Mean terminal half-life in plasma was 4.5 hours (range, 3.3–13.4 hours; n=12). Following an oral dose of ^{14}C-finasteride in man (n=6), a mean of 39% (range, 32–46%) of the dose was excreted in the urine in the form of metabolites; 57% (range, 51–64%) was excreted in the feces. Mean terminal half-life is approximately 5–6 hours in men 18–60 years of age and 8 hours in men more than 70 years of age.

Special Populations

Pediatric: Finasteride pharmacokinetics have not been investigated in patients <18 years of age.

Gender: PROPECIA is not indicated for use in women.

Geriatric: No dosage adjustment is necessary in the elderly. Although the elimination rate of finasteride is decreased in the elderly, these findings are of no clinical significance. See also *Pharmacokinetics, Excretion,* and PRECAUTIONS, *Geriatric Use* sections.

Race: The effect of race on finasteride pharmacokinetics has not been studied.

Renal Insufficiency: No dosage adjustment is necessary in patients with renal insufficiency. In patients with chronic renal impairment, with creatinine clearances ranging from 9.0 to 55 mL/min, AUC, maximum plasma concentration, half-life, and protein binding after a single dose of ^{14}C-finasteride were similar to those obtained in healthy volunteers. Urinary excretion of metabolites was decreased in patients with renal impairment. This decrease was associated with an increase in fecal excretion of metabolites. Plasma concentrations of metabolites were significantly higher in patients with renal impairment (based on a 60% increase in total radioactivity AUC). However, finasteride has been well tolerated in men with normal renal function receiving up to 80 mg/day for 12 weeks where exposure of these patients to metabolites would presumably be much greater.

Hepatic Insufficiency: The effect of hepatic insufficiency on finasteride pharmacokinetics has not been studied. Caution should be used in the administration of PROPECIA in patients with liver function abnormalities, as finasteride is metabolized extensively in the liver.

Drug Interactions (also see PRECAUTIONS, *Drug Interactions*)

No drug interactions of clinical importance have been identified. Finasteride does not appear to affect the cytochrome P450-linked drug-metabolizing enzyme system. Compounds that have been tested in man include antipyrine, digoxin, propranolol, theophylline, and warfarin and no clinically meaningful interactions were found.

Mean (SD) Pharmacokinetic Parameters
in Healthy Men (ages 18-26)

	Mean (± SD) n=15
Bioavailability	65% (26-170%)*
Clearance (mL/min)	165 (55)
Volume of Distribution (L)	76 (14)

*Range

Mean (SD) Noncompartmental Pharmacokinetic
Parameters After Multiple Doses of 1 mg/day in
Healthy Men (ages 19-42)

	Mean (± SD) (n=12)
AUC (ng•hr/mL)	53 (33.8)
Peak Concentration (ng/mL)	9.2 (2.6)
Time to Peak (hours)	1.3 (0.5)
Half-Life (hours)*	4.5 (1.6)

*First-dose values; all other parameters are last-dose values

In the **CONTRAINDICATIONS** section, in the second paragraph, in the second sentence, after "Because of the ability of", add "Type II".

In the **WARNINGS** section, in the first paragraph, after "(see also", add "WARNINGS, EXPOSURE OF WOMEN - RISK TO MALE FETUS;".

In the **PRECAUTIONS** section, under *Information for Patients*, add the following paragraph at the end:

Physicians should instruct their patients to read the patient package insert before starting therapy with PROPECIA and

to read it again each time the prescription is renewed so that they are aware of current information for patients regarding PROPECIA.

In the **PRECAUTIONS** section, under *Drug/Laboratory Test Interactions*, replace the existing paragraph with the following paragraphs:

Finasteride had no effect on circulating levels of cortisol, thyroid-stimulating hormone, or thyroxine, nor did it affect the plasma lipid profile (e.g., total cholesterol, low-density lipoproteins, high-density lipoproteins and triglycerides) or bone mineral density. In studies with finasteride, no clinically meaningful changes in luteinizing hormone (LH), follicle-stimulating hormone (FSH) or prolactin were detected. In healthy volunteers, treatment with finasteride did not alter the response of LH and FSH to gonadotropin- releasing hormone indicating that the hypothalamic-pituitary-testicular axis was not affected.

In clinical studies with PROPECIA (finasteride, 1 mg) in men 18–41 years of age, the mean value of serum prostate-specific antigen (PSA) decreased from 0.7 ng/mL at baseline to 0.5 ng/mL at Month 12. Further, in clinical studies with PROSCAR (finasteride, 5 mg) when used in older men who have benign prostatic hyperplasia (BPH), PSA levels are decreased by approximately 50%. These findings should be taken into account for proper interpretation of serum PSA when evaluating men treated with finasteride.

In the **PRECAUTIONS** section, under *Drug Interactions*, in the first paragraph, in the second sentence, after "warfarin and no", add "clinically meaningful".

In the **PRECAUTIONS** section, under *Drug Interactions*, in the second paragraph, after "acetaminophen,", add "acetylsalicylic acid,".

In the **PRECAUTIONS** section, under *Carcinogenesis, Mutagenesis, Impairment of Fertility*, in the third paragraph, replace the second, third, and fourth sentences with the following sentence:

In an *in vitro* chromosome aberration assay, using Chinese hamster ovary cells, there was a slight increase in chromosome aberrations.

In the **PRECAUTIONS** section, under *Pregnancy, Teratogenic Effects: Pregnancy Category X*, in the third paragraph, replace the first sentence with the following:

Administration of finasteride to pregnant rats on gestational days 6–20 at doses ranging from 100 µg/kg/day to 100 mg/kg/day (1–684 times the human exposure, estimated) resulted in dose-dependent development of hypospadias in 3.6 to 100% of male offspring.

In the **PRECAUTIONS** section, under *Pregnancy, Teratogenic Effects: Pregnancy Category X*, in the third paragraph, in the second sentence, replace "(≥ 1.5 times the recommended human dose of 1 mg/day" with "(0.2 times the human exposure, estimated" and replace "one-fifth the recommended human dose of 1 mg/day" with "0.02 times the human exposure, estimated". In the fourth paragraph, in the second sentence, replace "150 times the recommended human dose of 1 mg/day" with "(20 times the human exposure, estimated)". In the fifth paragraph, in the first sentence, replace "5000" with "1908" and after "1 mg/day", insert ", based on body surface area comparison". In the sixth paragraph, in the second sentence, replace "as high as" with "up to", replace "750" with "250", and after "1 mg/day", insert ", based on body surface area comparison". Replace the third sentence with the following:

In confirmation of the relevance of the rhesus model for human fetal development, oral administration of a 2 mg/kg/day dose of finasteride to pregnant monkeys resulted in external genital abnormalities in male fetuses.

In the **ADVERSE REACTIONS** section, under *Clinical Studies for PROPECIA (finasteride 1 mg) in the Treatment of Male Pattern Hair Loss*, replace the first two paragraphs with the following:

In three controlled clinical trials for PROPECIA of 12-month duration, 1.4% of patients taking PROPECIA (n=945) were discontinued due to adverse experiences that were considered to be possibly, probably or definitely drug-related (1.6% for placebo; n=934). Clinical adverse experiences that were reported as possibly, probably or definitely drug-related in ≥1% of patients treated with PROPECIA or placebo are presented in Table 1.

TABLE 2
Drug-Related Adverse Experiences for PROSCAR (finasteride 5 mg)
BENIGN PROSTATIC HYPERPLASIA

	Year 1 (%)		Years 2, 3 and 4* (%)	
	Finasteride, 5 mg	Placebo	Finasteride, 5 mg	Placebo
Impotence	8.1	3.7	5.1	5.1
Decreased Libido	6.4	3.4	2.6	2.6
Decreased Volume of Ejaculate	3.7	0.8	1.5	0.5
Ejaculation Disorder	0.8	0.1	0.2	0.1
Breast Enlargement	0.5	0.1	1.8	1.1
Breast Tenderness	0.4	0.1	0.7	0.3
Rash	0.5	0.2	0.5	0.1

*Combined Years 2–4
N = 1524 and 1516, finasteride vs placebo, respectively

TABLE 1
Drug-Related Adverse Experiences for PROPECIA
(finasteride 1 mg) in Year 1 (%)
MALE PATTERN HAIR LOSS

	PROPECIA N=945	Placebo N=934
Decreased Libido	1.8	1.3
Erectile Dysfunction	1.3	0.7
Ejaculation Disorder *(Decreased Volume of Ejaculate)*	1.2 *(0.8)*	0.7 *(0.4)*
Discontinuation due to drug-related sexual adverse experiences	1.2	0.9

In the **ADVERSE REACTIONS** section, under *Postmarketing Experience for PROPECIA (finasteride 1 mg)*, after the first sentence, add "See *Controlled Clinical Trials and Long-Term Open Extension Studies for PROSCAR* (finasteride 5 mg) in the Treatment of Benign Prostatic Hyperplasia*."

In the **ADVERSE REACTIONS** section, under *Controlled Clinical Trials and Long-Term Open Extension Studies for PROSCAR* (finasteride 5 mg) in the Treatment of Benign Prostatic Hyperplasia*, replace the first paragraph with the following:

In the PROSCAR Long-Term Efficacy and Safety Study (PLESS), a 4-year controlled clinical study, 3040 patients between the ages of 45 and 78 with symptomatic BPH and an enlarged prostate were evaluated for safety over a period of 4 years (1524 on PROSCAR 5 mg/day and 1516 on placebo). 3.7% (57 patients) treated with PROSCAR 5 mg and 2.1% (32 patients) treated with placebo discontinued therapy as a result of adverse reactions related to sexual function, which are the most frequently reported adverse reactions.

Table 2 presents the only clinical adverse reactions considered possibly, probably or definitely drug related by the investigator, for which the incidence on PROSCAR was ≥1% and greater than placebo over the 4 years of the study. In years 2–4 of the study, there was no significant difference between treatment groups in the incidences of impotence, decreased libido and ejaculation disorder.

[See table 2 above]

The adverse experience profiles in the 1-year, placebo-controlled, Phase III BPH studies and the 5-year open extensions with PROSCAR 5 mg and PLESS were similar. There is no evidence of increased adverse experiences with increased duration of treatment with PROSCAR 5 mg. New reports of drug-related sexual adverse experiences decreased with duration of therapy.

Also in the **ADVERSE REACTIONS** section, under *Controlled Clinical Trials and Long-Term Open Extension Studies for PROSCAR* (finasteride 5 mg) in the Treatment of Benign Prostatic Hyperplasia*, at the end of the third paragraph, add the following:

This information from the literature (Thompson IM, Goodman PJ, Tangen CM, et al. The influence of finasteride on the development of prostate cancer. *N Engl J Med* 2003;349:213–22) is provided for consideration by physicians when PROSCAR is used as indicated. PROSCAR is not approved to reduce the risk of developing prostate cancer.

Continued on next page

Propecia—Cont.

In the **DOSAGE AND ADMINISTRATION** section, in the first sentence, after "1 mg", add "orally".
In the **HOW SUPPLIED** section, at the end of the second and third paragraphs, add "(with desiccant)", and after the third paragraph, add the following:
NDC 0006-0071-54 PROPAK - carton of 1 unit of use bottle of 90 (with desiccant).
Revisions based on 9328505, issued October 2004.

RECOMBIVAX HB® ℞
Hepatitis B Vaccine (Recombinant)

Prescribing information for this product, which appears on pages 2138–2141 of the 2005 PDR, has been revised as follows. Please write "See Supplement A" next to the product heading.
In the **DESCRIPTION** section, in the third paragraph, sentence beginning "Each lot of..." please delete the words "safety, in mice and guinea pigs, and for."
In the **PRECAUTIONS** section, under *General*, under "Information for Vaccine Recipients and Parents/Guardians," the third paragraph, the sentence beginning "Patients, parents and guardians" please change NVICP phone number to "1-800-338-2382."
Revisions based on 7994328, issued August 2004.

VAQTA® ℞
(Hepatitis A Vaccine, Inactivated)

Prescribing information for this product, which appears on pages 2160–2163 of the 2005 PDR, has been revised as follows. Please write "See Supplement A" next to the product heading.
In the **ADVERSE REACTIONS** section, under the *Marketed Experience* paragraph, under *NERVOUS SYSTEM* please add ", encephalitis" after ataxia.
Revisions based on 9413406, issued July 2004.

ZOCOR® Tablets ℞
[*zō'kŏr*]
(simvastatin)

Prescribing information for this product, which appears on pages 2178–2183 of the 2005 PDR, has been revised as follows. Please write "See Supplement A" next to the product heading.
In the **WARNINGS** section, under ***Myopathy/Rhabdomyolysis,*** after "**Potent inhibitors of CYP3A4: Cyclosporine, itraconazole, ketoconazole, erythromycin, clarithromycin,**" insert "**telithromycin,**".
In the **WARNINGS** section, under ***Myopathy/Rhabdomyolysis***, under **Other drugs:**, above the paragraph beginning "**Amiodarone or verapamil with higher doses of simvastatin,**" insert a new paragraph: "**Danazol particularly with higher doses of simvastatin** (see below; PRECAUTIONS, *Drug Interactions, Other drug interactions*)."
In the **WARNINGS** section, under ***Myopathy/Rhabdomyolysis***, under **Consequently:**, after "**1. Use of simvastatin concomitantly with itraconazole, ketoconazole, erythromycin, clarithromycin,**" insert "**telithromycin,**". Then, in the next sentence, change "or clarithromycin is" to "clarithromycin, or telithromycin is".
In the **WARNINGS** section, under ***Myopathy/Rhabdomyolysis***, under **Consequently:**, after "**3. The dose of simvastatin should not exceed 10 mg daily in patients receiving concomitant medication with cyclosporine**" insert "**or danazol**". Then, change the next sentence to read as follows: "The benefits of the use of simvastatin in patients receiving cyclosporine or danazol should be carefully weighed against the risks of these combinations."
In the **PRECAUTIONS** section, under *Other Interactions, CYP3A4 Interactions*, in the vertical list of boldfaced drug names, insert "**Telithromycin**" between "**Clarithromycin**" and "**HIV protease inhibitors**".
In the **PRECAUTIONS** section, under *Other drug interactions*, above the paragraph beginning "*Amiodarone or Verapamil:* The risk of myopathy/rhabdomyolysis is increased", insert a new paragraph: "*Danazol:* The risk of myopathy/rhabdomyolysis is increased by concomitant administration of danazol particularly with higher doses of simvastatin (see WARNINGS, *Myopathy/Rhabdomyolysis*)." Then, in the next sentence after "administration of amiodarone or verapamil", insert "with higher doses of simvastatin".
In the **DOSAGE AND ADMINISTRATION** section, at the end of the second paragraph, after "(i.e., cyclosporine," insert "danazol,".
In the **DOSAGE AND ADMINISTRATION** section, at the end of the subhead title "*Patients taking Cyclosporine*" insert "or *Danazol*". Then, in the first sentence under that, between "In patients taking cyclosporine" and "concomitantly with ZOCOR", insert "or danazol".
Revisions based on 9556648, issued November 2004.

Merck/Schering-Plough Pharmaceuticals

PO BOX 1000
UG4B–75A
351 N. SUMNEYTOWN PIKE
NORTH WALES, PA 19454

For Product and Service Information, Medical Information, and Adverse Drug Experience Reporting:
Call: Merck/Schering-Plough National Service Center Monday through Friday, 8:00 AM to 7:00 PM (ET) 866-637-2501
Fax: 800-637-2568
For 24-hour emergency information, healthcare professionals should call:
Merck/Schering-Plough National Service Center at 866-637-2501
For Product Ordering,
Call: Order Management Center Monday through Friday, 8:00 AM to 7:00 PM (ET) 800-637-2579

VYTORIN™ 10/10 ℞
(EZETIMIBE 10 MG/SIMVASTATIN 10 MG TABLETS)

VYTORIN™ 10/20
(EZETIMIBE 10 MG/SIMVASTATIN 20 MG TABLETS)

VYTORIN™ 10/40
(EZETIMIBE 10 MG/SIMVASTATIN 40 MG TABLETS)

VYTORIN™ 10/80
(EZETIMIBE 10 MG/SIMVASTATIN 80 MG TABLETS)

Prescribing information for this product, which appears on pages 2183–2189 of the 2005 PDR, has been revised as follows. Please write "See Supplement A" next to the product heading.
In the **WARNINGS** section, under ***Myopathy/Rhabdomyolysis:***
In the first subparagraph under the first bulleted paragraph, titled "**Potent inhibitors of CYP3A4:**" add "**telithromycin,**" between "**clarithromycin,**" and "**HIV protease inhibitors**".
In the second subsection under the first bulleted paragraph, titled "**Other drugs:**" following the second subparagraph, add the following new paragraph:
Danazol particularly with higher doses of VYTORIN (see below; CLINICAL PHARMACOLOGY, *Pharmacokinetics*; PRECAUTIONS, *Drug Interactions, Other drug interactions*).
In paragraph no. **1.** under "**Consequently:**" replace the first and second sentences with the following:
Use of VYTORIN concomitantly with itraconazole, ketoconazole, erythromycin, clarithromycin, telithromycin, HIV protease inhibitors, nefazodone, or large quantities of grapefruit juice (>1 quart daily) should be avoided. If treatment with itraconazole, ketoconazole, erythromycin, clarithromycin or telithromycin is unavoidable, therapy with VYTORIN should be suspended during the course of treatment.
Under "**Consequently:**" replace paragraph no. **4.** with the following:
4. The dose of VYTORIN should not exceed 10/10 mg daily in patients receiving concomitant medication with cyclosporine or danazol. The benefits of the use of VYTORIN in patients receiving cyclosporine or danazol should be carefully weighed against the risks of these combinations. **(See PRECAUTIONS, *Drug Interactions, Other Drug Interactions, Cyclosporine.*)**
In the **PRECAUTIONS** section, under ***Drug Interactions* (See also CLINICAL PHARMACOLOGY, *Drug Interactions*)**, *VYTORIN*, **CYP3A4 Interactions**, add "**Telithromycin**" between "**Clarithromycin**" and "**HIV protease inhibitors**" in the list.
Under ***Other drug interactions***, add the following new first paragraph:
Danazol: The risk of myopathy/rhabdomyolysis is increased by concomitant administration of danazol particularly with higher doses of VYTORIN (see CLINICAL PHARMACOLOGY, *Pharmacokinetics;* WARNINGS, *Myopathy/Rhabdomyolysis*).
Under ***Other drug interactions***, replace the paragraph titled *Amiodarone or Verapamil* with the following paragraph:
Amiodarone or Verapamil: The risk of myopathy/rhabdomyolysis is increased by concomitant administration of amiodarone or verapamil with higher doses of VYTORIN (see WARNINGS, *Myopathy/Rhabdomyolysis*).
In the **ADVERSE REACTIONS** section, under *Post-marketing Experience*, replace the second paragraph with the following paragraph:
Hypersensitivity reactions, including angioedema and rash; increased CPK; elevations in liver transaminases; hepatitis; thrombocytopenia; pancreatitis; nausea; cholelithiasis; cholecystitis; and, very rarely in patients taking an HMG-CoA reductase inhibitor with ezetimibe, rhabdomyolysis (see WARNINGS, *Myopathy/Rhabdomyolysis*).
In the **DOSAGE AND ADMINISTRATION** section, change the subhead ***Patients taking Cyclosporine*** to ***Patients taking Cyclosporine or Danazol***. In the second sentence, add "or danazol" after "In patients taking cyclosporine".
In the **HOW SUPPLIED** section, under the paragraph beginning "No. 3873," insert the following sentence between the sentence beginning "**NDC** 66582-311-82" and the sentence beginning "**NDC** 66582-311-28":
NDC 66582-311-87 bottles of 10,000 (If repackaged in blisters, then opaque or light-resistant blisters should be used.)
Under the paragraph beginning "No. 3874," insert the following sentence between the sentence beginning "**NDC** 66582-312-82" and the sentence beginning "**NDC** 66582-312-28":
NDC 66582-312-87 bottles of 10,000 (If repackaged in blisters, then opaque or light-resistant blisters should be used.)
Add the following new subsection at the end of the **HOW SUPPLIED** section:
Storage of 10,000 count bottles
Store bottle of 10,000 VYTORIN 10/10 and 10/20 capsule-shaped tablets at 20-25° C (68-77° F). [See USP Controlled Room Temperature.] Store in original container until time of use. When product container is subdivided, repackage into a tightly-closed, light-resistant container. Entire contents must be repackaged immediately upon opening.
Under "By:
MSD Technology Singapore Pte. Ltd.
Singapore 637766"
add the following new copy at the end:
Or
Merck Sharp & Dohme (Italia) S.p.A.
Via Emilia, 21
27100 – Pavia
Italy
Revisions based on 9619601, issued August 2004, and 9619602, issued November 2004.
In the Patient Information about VYTORIN, under **What should I tell my doctor before and while taking VYTORIN?** add "• danazol" in the bulleted list between "• cyclosporine" and "• antifungal agents (such as itraconazole or ketoconazole)". In the same bulleted list, replace "• the antibiotics erythromycin and clarithromycin" with "• the antibiotics erythromycin, clarithromycin, and telithromycin".
Under **What are the possible side effects of VYTORIN?** replace the bulleted subparagraph with the following:
- allergic reactions including swelling of the face, lips, tongue, and/or throat that may cause difficulty in breathing or swallowing (which may require treatment right away), and rash; alterations in some laboratory blood tests; liver problems; inflammation of the pancreas; nausea; gallstones; inflammation of the gallbladder.

Under "By:
MSD Technology Singapore Pte. Ltd.
Singapore 637766"
add the following new copy at the end:
Or
Merck Sharp & Dohme (Italia) S.p.A.
Via Emilia, 21
27100 – Pavia
Italy
Revisions based on 9621001, issued August 2004, and 9621002, issued November 2004.

ZETIA® ℞
(EZETIMIBE)
TABLETS

Prescribing information for this product, which appears on pages 2189–2194 of the 2005 PDR, has been revised as follows. Please write "See Supplement A" next to the product heading.
In the **PRECAUTIONS** section, under *Skeletal Muscle*, at the end of the first paragraph, add: (See also ADVERSE REACTIONS for post-marketing experience.)
In the **ADVERSE REACTIONS** section, under *Post-marketing Experience*, replace the second paragraph with the following:
Hypersensitivity reactions, including angioedema and rash; myalgia; increased CPK; elevations in liver transaminases; hepatitis; thrombocytopenia; pancreatitis; nausea; cholelithiasis; cholecystitis; and, very rarely, myopathy/rhabdomyolysis (see PRECAUTIONS, *Skeletal Muscle*).
Revisions based on 25751876T, Rev 05, issued November 2004, and 25751884T, Rev 06, issued January 2005.
In the Patient Information about ZETIA, replace the second paragraph under **What are the possible side effects of ZETIA?** with the following paragraphs: Additionally, the following side effects have been reported in general use: allergic reactions (which may require treatment right away) including swelling of the face, lips, tongue, and/or throat that may cause difficulty in breathing or swallowing, and rash; muscle aches; alterations in some laboratory blood tests; liver problems; inflammation of the pancreas; nausea; gallstones; inflammation of the gallbladder.
Contact your doctor promptly if you experience unexplained muscle pain, tenderness, or weakness while taking ZETIA. This is because on rare occasions, muscle problems can be serious, including muscle breakdown resulting in kidney damage.
Revisions based on 25751779T, Rev 05, issued November 2004, and 25751787T, Rev 06, issued January 2005.

Ortho-McNeil Pharmaceutical
RARITAN, NJ 08869-0602

www.ortho-mcneil.com
For Medical Information Contact:
(800) 682-6532
In Emergencies:
(908) 218-7325
For Patient Education Materials Contact:
877-323-2200
For Customer Service (Sales and Ordering):
800-631-5273

DITROPAN XL®   ℞
[dĭ-trō-păn]
(oxybutynin chloride)
Extended Release Tablets

Prescribing information for this product, which appears on pages 2491–2493 of the 2005 PDR, has been completely revised as follows. Please write "See Supplement A" next to the product heading.
Prescribing Information

DESCRIPTION

DITROPAN XL® (oxybutynin chloride) is an antispasmodic, anticholinergic agent. Each DITROPAN XL Extended Release Tablet contains 5 mg, 10 mg, or 15 mg of oxybutynin chloride USP, formulated as a once-a-day controlled-release tablet for oral administration. Oxybutynin chloride is administered as a racemate of R- and S-enantiomers.
Chemically, oxybutynin chloride is d,l (racemic) 4-diethylamino-2-butynyl phenylcyclohexylglycolate hydrochloride. The empirical formula of oxybutynin chloride is $C_{22}H_{31}NO_3$ • HCl.

Its structural formula is:

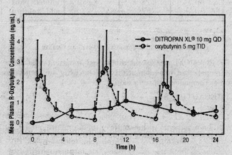

Oxybutynin chloride is a white crystalline solid with a molecular weight of 393.9. It is readily soluble in water and acids, but relatively insoluble in alkalis.
DITROPAN XL also contains the following inert ingredients: cellulose acetate, hypromellose, lactose, magnesium stearate, polyethylene glycol, polyethylene oxide, synthetic iron oxides, titanium dioxide, polysorbate 80, sodium chloride, and butylated hydroxytoluene.

System Components and Performance

DITROPAN XL uses osmotic pressure to deliver oxybutynin chloride at a controlled rate over approximately 24 hours. The system, which resembles a conventional tablet in appearance, comprises an osmotically active bilayer core surrounded by a semipermeable membrane. The bilayer core is composed of a drug layer containing the drug and excipients, and a push layer containing osmotically active components. There is a precision-laser drilled orifice in the semipermeable membrane on the drug-layer side of the tablet. In an aqueous environment, such as the gastrointestinal tract, water permeates through the membrane into the tablet core, causing the drug to go into suspension and the push layer to expand. This expansion pushes the suspended drug out through the orifice. The semipermeable membrane controls the rate at which water permeates into the tablet core, which in turn controls the rate of drug delivery. The controlled rate of drug delivery into the gastrointestinal lumen is thus independent of pH or gastrointestinal motility. The function of DITROPAN XL depends on the existence of an osmotic gradient between the contents of the bilayer core and the fluid in the gastrointestinal tract. Since the osmotic gradient remains constant, drug delivery remains essentially constant. The biologically inert components of the tablet remain intact during gastrointestinal transit and are eliminated in the feces as an insoluble shell.

CLINICAL PHARMACOLOGY

Oxybutynin chloride exerts a direct antispasmodic effect on smooth muscle and inhibits the muscarinic action of acetylcholine on smooth muscle. Oxybutynin chloride exhibits only one-fifth of the anticholinergic activity of atropine on the rabbit detrusor muscle, but four to ten times the antispasmodic activity. No blocking effects occur at skeletal neuromuscular junctions or autonomic ganglia (antinicotinic effects).
Oxybutynin chloride relaxes bladder smooth muscle. In patients with conditions characterized by involuntary bladder contractions, cystometric studies have demonstrated that oxybutynin increases bladder (vesical) capacity, diminishes the frequency of uninhibited contractions of the detrusor muscle, and delays the initial desire to void. Oxybutynin thus decreases urgency and the frequency of both incontinent episodes and voluntary urination.
Antimuscarinic activity resides predominantly in the R-isomer. A metabolite, desethyloxybutynin, has pharmacolog-

ical activity similar to that of oxybutynin in *in vitro* studies.

Pharmacokinetics
Absorption

Following the first dose of DITROPAN XL® (oxybutynin chloride), oxybutynin plasma concentrations rise for 4 to 6 hours; thereafter steady concentrations are maintained for up to 24 hours, minimizing fluctuations between peak and trough concentrations associated with oxybutynin.
The relative bioavailabilities of R- and S-oxybutynin from DITROPAN XL are 156% and 187%, respectively, compared with oxybutynin. The mean pharmacokinetic parameters for R- and S-oxybutynin are summarized in Table 1. The plasma concentration-time profiles for R- and S-oxybutynin are similar in shape; Figure 1 shows the profile for R-oxybutynin.

Table 1
Mean (SD) R- and S-Oxybutynin Pharmacokinetic Parameters Following a Single Dose of DITROPAN XL 10 mg (n=43)

Parameters (units)	R-Oxybutynin		S-Oxybutynin	
C_{max} (ng/mL)	1.0	(0.6)	1.8	(1.0)
T_{max} (h)	12.7	(5.4)	11.8	(5.3)
$t_{1/2}$ (h)	13.2	(6.2)	12.4	(6.1)
$AUC_{(0-48)}$ (ng•h/mL)	18.4	(10.3)	34.2	(16.9)
AUC_{inf} (ng•h/mL)	21.3	(12.2)	39.5	(21.2)

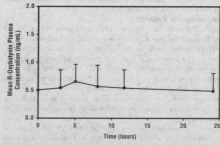

Figure 1. *Mean R-oxybutynin plasma concentrations following a single dose of DITROPAN XL 10 mg and oxybutynin 5 mg administered every 8 hours (n=23 for each treatment).*

Steady-state oxybutynin plasma concentrations are achieved by Day 3 of repeated DITROPAN XL dosing, with no observed drug accumulation or change in oxybutynin and desethyloxybutynin pharmacokinetic parameters.
DITROPAN XL steady-state pharmacokinetics was studied in 19 children aged 5-15 years with detrusor overactivity associated with a neurological condition (e.g., spina bifida). The children were on DITROPAN XL total daily dose ranging from 5 to 20 mg (0.10 to 0.77 mg/kg). Sparse sampling technique was used to obtain serum samples. When all available data are normalized to an equivalent of 5 mg per day DITROPAN XL, the mean pharmacokinetic parameters derived for R- and S-oxybutynin and R- and S-desethyloxybutynin are summarized in Table 2. The plasma-time concentration profiles for R- and S-oxybutynin are similar in shape; Figure 2 shows the profile for R-oxybutynin when all available data are normalized to an equivalent of 5 mg per day.
[See table 2 above]

Food Effects
The rate and extent of absorption and metabolism of oxybutynin are similar under fed and fasted conditions.

Distribution
Plasma concentrations of oxybutynin decline biexponentially following intravenous or oral administration. The volume of distribution is 193 L after intravenous administration of 5 mg oxybutynin chloride.
Metabolism
Oxybutynin is metabolized primarily by the cytochrome P450 enzyme systems, particularly CYP3A4 found mostly in the liver and gut wall. Its metabolic products include phenylcyclohexylglycolic acid, which is pharmacologically inactive, and desethyloxybutynin, which is pharmacologically active. Following DITROPAN XL administration, plasma concentrations of R- and S-desethyloxybutynin are 73% and 92%, respectively, of concentrations observed with oxybutynin.
Excretion
Oxybutynin is extensively metabolized by the liver, with less than 0.1% of the administered dose excreted unchanged in the urine. Also, less than 0.1% of the administered dose is excreted as the metabolite desethyloxybutynin.
Dose Proportionality
Pharmacokinetic parameters of oxybutynin and desethyloxybutynin (C_{max} and AUC) following administration of 5–20 mg of DITROPAN XL are dose proportional.
Special Populations
Geriatric: The pharmacokinetics of DITROPAN XL were similar in all patients studied (up to 78 years of age).
Pediatric: The pharmacokinetics of DITROPAN XL were evaluated in 19 children aged 5-15 years with detrusor overactivity associated with a neurological condition (e.g., spina bifida). The pharmacokinetics of DITROPAN XL in these pediatric patients were consistent with those reported for adults (see Tables 1 and 2, and Figures 1 and 2 above).
Gender: There are no significant differences in the pharmacokinetics of oxybutynin in healthy male and female volunteers following administration of DITROPAN XL.
Race: Available data suggest that there are no significant differences in the pharmacokinetics of oxybutynin based on race in healthy volunteers following administration of DITROPAN XL.
Renal Insufficiency: There is no experience with the use of DITROPAN XL in patients with renal insufficiency.
Hepatic Insufficiency: There is no experience with the use of DITROPAN XL in patients with hepatic insufficiency.
Drug-Drug Interactions: See **PRECAUTIONS:** Drug Interactions.

CLINICAL STUDIES

DITROPAN XL® (oxybutynin chloride) was evaluated for the treatment of patients with overactive bladder with symptoms of urge urinary incontinence, urgency, and frequency in three controlled studies and one open label study. The majority of patients were Caucasian (89.0%) and female (91.9%) with a mean age of 59 years (range, 18 to 98 years). Entry criteria required that patients have urge or mixed incontinence (with a predominance of urge) as evidenced by ≥ 6 urge incontinence episodes per week and ≥ 10 micturitions per day. Study 1 was a fixed dose escalation design, whereas the other studies used a dose adjustment design in which each patient's final dose was adjusted to a balance between improvement of incontinence symptoms and tolerability of side effects. Controlled studies included patients known to be responsive to oxybutynin or other anticholinergic medications, and these patients were maintained on a final dose for up to 2 weeks.
The efficacy results for the three controlled trials are presented in the following tables and figures.

Number of Urge Urinary Incontinence Episodes Per Week

Study 1	n	DITROPAN XL®	n	Placebo
Mean Baseline	34	15.9	16	-20.9
Mean (SD) Change from Baseline†	34	-15.8 (8.9)	16	-7.6 (8.6)
95% Confidence Interval for Difference (DITROPAN XL® - Placebo)		(-13.6, -2.8)*		

*The difference between DITROPAN XL® and placebo was statistically significant.
†Covariate adjusted mean with missing observations set to baseline values

Table 2
Mean ± SD R- and S-Oxybutynin and R- and S-Desethyloxybutynin Pharmacokinetic Parameters in Children Aged 5–15 Following Administration of 5 to 20 mg DITROPAN XL Once Daily (n=19) All Available Data Normalized to an Equivalent of DITROPAN XL 5 mg Once Daily

	R-Oxybutynin	S-Oxybutynin	R-Desethyloxybutynin	S-Desethyloxybutynin
C_{max} (ng/mL)	0.7 ± 0.4	1.3 ± 0.8	7.8 ± 3.7	4.2 ± 2.3
T_{max} (hr)	5.0	5.0	5.0	5.0
AUC (ng.hr/mL)	12.8 ± 7.0	23.7 ± 14.4	125.1 ± 66.7	73.6 ± 47.7

Figure 2. *Mean steady-state (± SD) R-oxybutynin plasma concentrations following administration of 5 to 20 mg DITROPAN XL once daily in children 5-15. Plot represents all available data normalized to an equivalent of DITROPAN XL 5 mg once daily.*

Continued on next page

Ditropan XL—Cont.

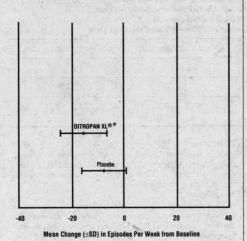

Mean Change (±SD) in Episodes Per Week from Baseline

Table 3
Incidence (%) of Adverse Events Reported by ≥ 5% of Patients Using DITROPAN XL (5–30 mg/day) and % of Corresponding Adverse Events in Two Fixed Dose (10mg/day) Studies

Body System	Adverse Event	DITROPAN XL 5–30 mg/day (n=429)	DITROPAN XL 10 mg/day (n=576)
General	headache	10	6
	asthenia	7	3
	pain	7	4
Digestive	dry mouth	61	29
	constipation	13	7
	diarrhea	9	7
	nausea	9	2
	dyspepsia	7	5
Nervous	somnolence	12	2
	dizziness	6	4
Respiratory	rhinitis	6	2
Special senses	blurred vision	8	1
	dry eyes	6	3
Urogenital	urinary tract infection	5	5

Study 2	n	DITROPAN XL®	n	oxybutynin
Mean Baseline	53	27.6	52	23.0
Mean (SD) Change from Baseline†	53	-17.6 (11.9)	52	-19.4 (11.9)
95% Confidence Interval for Difference (DITROPAN XL® - oxybutynin)		(-2.8, 6.5)		

† Covariate adjusted mean with missing observations set to baseline values

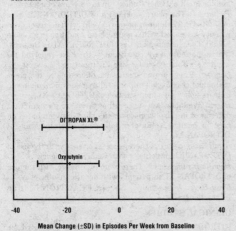

Mean Change (±SD) in Episodes Per Week from Baseline

Number of Urge Urinary Incontinence Episodes Per Week (continued)

Study 3	n	DITROPAN XL®	n	oxybutynin
Mean Baseline	111	18.9	115	19.5
Mean (SD) Change from Baseline†	111	-14.5 (8.7)	115	-13.8 (8.6)
95% Confidence Interval for Difference (DITROPAN XL® - oxybutynin)		(-3.0, 1.6)**		

** The difference between DITROPAN XL® and oxybutynin fulfilled the criteria for comparable efficacy.

† Covariate adjusted mean with missing observations set to baseline values

[See figure at top of next column]

INDICATIONS AND USAGE

DITROPAN XL® (oxybutynin chloride) is a once-daily controlled-release tablet indicated for the treatment of overactive bladder with symptoms of urge urinary incontinence, urgency, and frequency.

DITROPAN XL is also indicated in the treatment of pediatric patients aged 6 years and older with symptoms of detrusor overactivity associated with a neurological condition (e.g., spina bifida).

CONTRAINDICATIONS

DITROPAN XL® (oxybutynin chloride) is contraindicated in patients with urinary retention, gastric retention and other severe decreased gastrointestinal motility conditions, uncontrolled narrow-angle glaucoma and in patients who are at risk for these conditions.

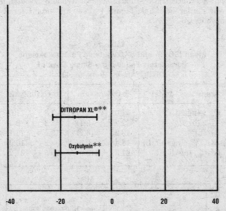

Mean Change (±SD) in Episodes Per Week from Baseline

DITROPAN XL is also contraindicated in patients who have demonstrated hypersensitivity to the drug substance or other components of the product.

PRECAUTIONS
General
DITROPAN XL® (oxybutynin chloride) should be used with caution in patients with hepatic or renal impairment and in patients with myasthenia gravis due to the risk of symptom aggravation.

Urinary Retention
DITROPAN XL should be administered with caution to patients with clinically significant bladder outflow obstruction because of the risk of urinary retention (see **CONTRAINDICATIONS**).

Gastrointestinal Disorders
DITROPAN XL should be administered with caution to patients with gastrointestinal obstructive disorders because of the risk of gastric retention (see **CONTRAINDICATIONS**).

DITROPAN XL, like other anticholinergic drugs, may decrease gastrointestinal motility and should be used with caution in patients with conditions such as ulcerative colitis and intestinal atony.

DITROPAN XL should be used with caution in patients who have gastro-esophageal reflux and/or who are concurrently taking drugs (such as bisphosphonates) that can cause or exacerbate esophagitis.

As with any other nondeformable material, caution should be used when administering DITROPAN XL to patients with preexisting severe gastrointestinal narrowing (pathologic or iatrogenic). There have been rare reports of obstructive symptoms in patients with known strictures in association with the ingestion of other drugs in nondeformable controlled-release formulations.

Information for Patients
Patients should be informed that heat prostration (fever and heat stroke due to decreased sweating) can occur when anticholinergics such as oxybutynin chloride are administered in the presence of high environmental temperature.

Because anticholinergic agents such as oxybutynin may produce drowsiness (somnolence) or blurred vision, patients should be advised to exercise caution.

Patients should be informed that alcohol may enhance the drowsiness caused by anticholinergic agents such as oxybutynin.

Patients should be informed that DITROPAN XL should be swallowed whole with the aid of liquids. Patients should not chew, divide, or crush tablets. The medication is contained within a nonabsorbable shell designed to release the drug at a controlled rate. The tablet shell is eliminated from the body; patients should not be concerned if they occasionally notice in their stool something that looks like a tablet.

DITROPAN XL should be taken at approximately the same time each day.

Drug Interactions
The concomitant use of oxybutynin with other anticholinergic drugs or with other agents which produce dry mouth, constipation, somnolence (drowsiness), and/or other anticholinergic-like effects may increase the frequency and/or severity of such effects.

Anticholinergic agents may potentially alter the absorption of some concomitantly administered drugs due to anticholinergic effects on gastrointestinal motility. This may be of concern for drugs with a narrow therapeutic index.

Mean oxybutynin chloride plasma concentrations were approximately 2 fold higher when DITROPAN XL was administered with ketoconazole, a potent CYP3A4 inhibitor. Other inhibitors of the cytochrome P450 3A4 enzyme system, such as antimycotic agents (e.g., itraconazole and miconazole) or macrolide antibiotics (e.g., erythromycin and clarithromycin), may alter oxybutynin mean pharmacokinetic parameters (i.e., C_{max} and AUC). The clinical relevance of such potential interactions is not known. Caution should be used when such drugs are co-administered.

Concurrent ingestion of antacid (20 mL of antacid containing aluminum hydroxide, magnesium hydroxide, and simethicone) did not significantly affect the exposure of oxybutynin or desethyloxybutynin.

Carcinogenesis, Mutagenesis, Impairment of Fertility
A 24-month study in rats at dosages of oxybutynin chloride of 20, 80, and 160 mg/kg/day showed no evidence of carcinogenicity. These doses are approximately 6, 25, and 50 times the maximum human exposure, based on surface area.

Oxybutynin chloride showed no increase of mutagenic activity when tested in *Schizosaccharomyces pompholiciformis*, *Saccharomyces cerevisiae*, and *Salmonella typhimurium* test systems.

Reproduction studies with oxybutynin chloride in the mouse, rat, hamster, and rabbit showed no definite evidence of impaired fertility.

Pregnancy: Teratogenic Effects
Pregnancy Category B
Reproduction studies with oxybutynin chloride in the mouse, rat, hamster, and rabbit showed no definite evidence of impaired fertility or harm to the animal fetus. The safety of DITROPAN XL administration to women who are or who may become pregnant has not been established. Therefore, DITROPAN XL should not be given to pregnant women unless, in the judgment of the physician, the probable clinical benefits outweigh the possible hazards.

Nursing Mothers
It is not known whether oxybutynin is excreted in human milk. Because many drugs are excreted in human milk, caution should be exercised when DITROPAN XL is administered to a nursing woman.

Pediatric Use
The safety and efficacy of DITROPAN XL were studied in 60 children in a 24-week, open-label trial. Patients were aged 6-15 years, all had symptoms of detrusor overactivity in association with a neurological condition (e.g., spina bifida), all used clean intermittent catheterization, and all were current users of oxybutynin chloride. Study results demonstrated that administration of DITROPAN XL 5 to 20 mg/day was associated with an increase from baseline in mean urine volume per catheterization from 108 mL to 136 mL, an increase from baseline in mean urine volume after morning awakening from 148 mL to 189 mL, and an increase from baseline in the mean percentage of catheterizations without a leaking episode from 34% to 51%.

Urodynamic results were consistent with clinical results. Administration of DITROPAN XL resulted in an increase from baseline in mean maximum cystometric capacity from 185 mL to 254 mL, a decrease from baseline in mean detrusor pressure at maximum cystometric capacity from 44 cm H_2O to 33 cm H_2O, and a reduction in the percentage of patients demonstrating uninhibited detrusor contractions (of at least 15 cm H_2O) from 60% to 28%.

DITROPAN XL is not recommended in pediatric patients who can not swallow the tablet whole without chewing, dividing, or crushing, or in children under the age of 6 (See **DOSAGE AND ADMINISTRATION**).

Geriatric Use
The rate and severity of anticholinergic effects reported by patients less than 65 years old and those 65 years and older were similar (see **CLINICAL PHARMACOLOGY**, **Pharmacokinetics**, ***Special Populations:*** *Gender*).

ADVERSE REACTIONS

Adverse Events with DITROPAN XL
The safety and efficacy of DITROPAN XL® (oxybutynin chloride) was evaluated in a total of 580 participants who received DITROPAN XL in 4 clinical trials (429 patients, 151 healthy volunteers). These participants were treated with 5-30 mg/day for up to 4.5 months. Three of these studies allowed dose adjustments based on efficacy and adverse events and one was a fixed dose escalation design. Safety information is provided for 429 patients from these three controlled clinical studies and one open label study in the first column of Table 3 below. Adverse events from two additional fixed dose, active controlled, 12 week treatment duration, postmarketing studies, in which 576 patients were treated with DITROPAN XL 10 mg/day, are also listed in Table 3 (second column). The adverse events are reported regardless of causality.
[See table 3 at top of previous page]
The most common adverse events reported by patients receiving 5-30 mg/day DITROPAN XL were the expected side effects of anticholinergic agents. The incidence of dry mouth was dose-related.
The discontinuation rate for all adverse events was 6.8% in the 429 patients from the 4 studies of efficacy and safety who received 5-30 mg/day. The most frequent adverse event causing early discontinuation of study medication was nausea (1.9%), while discontinuation due to dry mouth was 1.2%.
In addition, the following adverse events were reported by 2 to < 5% of the 429 patients who received 5-30 mg/day of DITROPAN XL in the 4 efficacy and safety studies. *General:* abdominal pain, dry nasal and sinus mucous membranes, accidental injury, back pain, flu syndrome; *Cardiovascular:* hypertension, palpitation, vasodilatation; *Digestive:* flatulence, gastroesophageal reflux; *Musculoskeletal:* arthritis; *Nervous:* insomnia, nervousness, confusion; *Respiratory:* upper respiratory tract infection, cough, sinusitis, bronchitis, pharyngitis; *Skin:* dry skin, rash; *Urogenital:* impaired urination (hesitancy), increased post void residual volume, urinary retention, cystitis.
Additional rare adverse events reported from worldwide postmarketing experience with DITROPAN XL include: peripheral edema, cardiac arrhythmia, tachycardia, hallucinations, convulsions, and impotence.
Additional adverse events reported with some other oxybutynin chloride formulations include: cycloplegia, mydriasis, and suppression of lactation.

OVERDOSAGE

The continuous release of oxybutynin from DITROPAN XL® (oxybutynin chloride) should be considered in the treatment of overdosage. Patients should be monitored for at least 24 hours. Treatment should be symptomatic and supportive. Activated charcoal as well as a cathartic may be administered.
Overdosage with oxybutynin chloride has been associated with anticholinergic effects including central nervous system excitation, flushing, fever, dehydration, cardiac arrhythmia, vomiting, and urinary retention.
Ingestion of 100 mg oxybutynin chloride in association with alcohol has been reported in a 13-year-old boy who experienced memory loss, and a 34-year-old woman who developed stupor, followed by disorientation and agitation on awakening, dilated pupils, dry skin, cardiac arrhythmia, and retention of urine. Both patients fully recovered with symptomatic treatment.

DOSAGE AND ADMINISTRATION

DITROPAN XL® (oxybutynin chloride) must be swallowed whole with the aid of liquids, and must not be chewed, divided, or crushed.
DITROPAN XL may be administered with or without food.
Adults: The recommended starting dose of DITROPAN XL is 5 or 10 mg once daily at approximately the same time each day. Dosage may be adjusted in 5-mg increments to achieve a balance of efficacy and tolerability (up to a maximum of 30 mg/day). In general, dosage adjustment may proceed at approximately weekly intervals.
Pediatric patients aged 6 years of age and older: The recommended starting dose of DITROPAN XL is 5 mg once daily. Dosage may be adjusted in 5-mg increments to achieve a balance of efficacy and tolerability (up to a maximum of 20 mg/day).

HOW SUPPLIED

DITROPAN XL® (oxybutynin chloride) Extended Release Tablets are available in three dosage strengths, 5 mg (pale yellow), 10 mg (pink), and 15 mg (gray) and are imprinted with "5 XL", "10 XL", or "15 XL". DITROPAN XL Extended Release Tablets are supplied in bottles of 100 tablets.

5 mg	100 count bottle	NDC 17314-8500-1
10 mg	100 count bottle	NDC 17314-8501-1
15 mg	100 count bottle	NDC 17314-8502-1

Storage
Store at 25°C (77°F); excursions permitted to 15-30°C (59-86°F) [see USP Controlled Room Temperature]. Protect from moisture and humidity.
Rx Only
For more information call 1-888-395-1232 or visit www.DITROPANXL.com

Manufactured by ALZA Corporation, Mountain View, CA 94043
An ALZA OROS®
Technology Product
DITROPAN XL® and OROS® are registered trademarks of ALZA Corporation.
Distributed and Marketed by Ortho-McNeil Pharmaceutical, Inc., Raritan, NJ 08869.
ORTHO-McNEIL
631-10-800-2 Revised June 2004

ELMIRON® -100 mg ℞

[ĕl-mī-rŏn]
(pentosan polysulfate sodium) Capsules

Prescribing information for this product, which appears on pages 2493–2495 of the 2005 PDR, has been completely revised as follows. Please write "See Supplement A" next to the product heading.
Prescribing Information

DESCRIPTION

Pentosan polysulfate sodium is a semi-synthetically produced heparin-like macromolecular carbohydrate derivative, which chemically and structurally resembles glycosaminoglycans. It is a white odorless powder, slightly hygroscopic and soluble in water to 50% at pH 6. It has a molecular weight of 4000 to 6000 Dalton with the following structural formula:

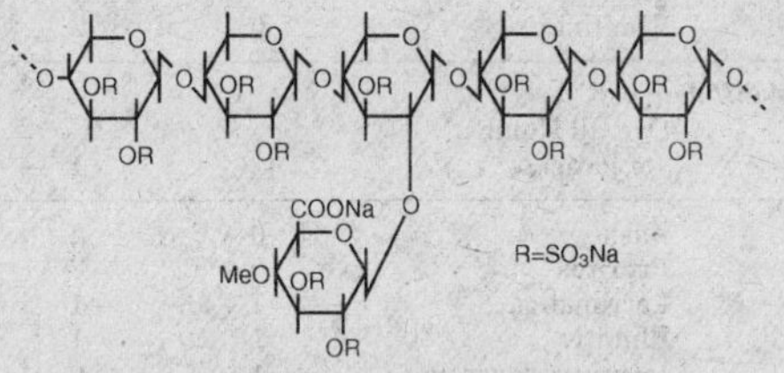

ELMIRON® is supplied in white opaque hard gelatin capsules containing 100 mg pentosan polysulfate sodium, microcrystalline cellulose, and magnesium stearate. It also contains pharmaceutical glaze, synthetic black iron oxide, FD&C Blue No. 2 aluminum lake, FD&C Red No. 40 aluminum lake, FD&C Blue No. 1 aluminum lake, D&C Yellow No. 10 aluminum lake, m-butyl alcohol, propylene glycol, alcohol (SD-3A), lecithin, ethylene glycol, monoethyl ether, and ammonium hydroxide. It is formulated for oral use.

CLINICAL PHARMACOLOGY

General: Pentosan polysulfate sodium is a low molecular weight heparin-like compound. It has anticoagulant and fibrinolytic effects. The mechanism of action of pentosan polysulfate sodium in interstitial cystitis is not known.
Pharmacokinetics:
Absorption: In preliminary clinical studies with different doses of radiolabeled pentosan polysulfate sodium, absorption was approximately 3% of the administered dose (n=3).
Distribution: Preclinical studies with parenterally administered radiolabeled pentosan polysulfate sodium showed distribution to the uroepithelium of the genitourinary tract with lesser amounts found in the liver, spleen, lung, skin, periosteum, and bone marrow. Erythrocyte penetration is low in animals.
Metabolism: Preliminary literature studies of metabolism in 5 healthy volunteers with radiolabeled drug suggest that 68% of the dose, at about 1 hour after IV administration, undergoes partial desulfation in the liver and spleen. In another study of 3 healthy volunteers, partial depolymerization occurs in the kidney. Both the desulfation and depolymerization can be saturated with continued dosing.
Excretion: In preliminary clinical studies in 8 healthy male volunteers, the elimination half-life of pentosan polysulfate sodium had a mean value at 24 hours after IV injection of 40 mg.
The elimination half-life in urine following orally administered radiolabeled pentosan polysulfate sodium was determined to be 4.8 hours for the unchanged drug.
In preliminary human studies in 3 healthy male volunteers, after single doses of radiolabeled drug, urinary excretion averaged 3.5% of the administered dose. After multiple doses of pentosan polysulfate sodium, urine excretion of radioactivity averaged 11% of the administered dose.
Further analyses of the urinary fraction obtained after repeated dosing showed that about 3% of the dose may be unchanged pentosan polysulfate sodium.
Special Populations: Dose adjustments in geriatric patients and in patients with hepatic or renal impairment were not studied.
Pharmacodynamics:
The mechanism by which pentosan polysulfate sodium achieves its effects in patients is unknown. In preliminary clinical models, pentosan polysulfate sodium adhered to the bladder wall mucosal membrane. The drug may act as a buffer to control cell permeability preventing irritating solutes in the urine from reaching the cells.
Food effects: The effect of food on absorption of pentosan polysulfate sodium is not known. In clinical trials, ELMIRON was administered with water 1 hour before or 2 hours after meals.
Drug-Drug Interactions: Not studied.

CLINICAL TRIALS

ELMIRON was evaluated in two clinical trials for the relief of pain in patients with chronic interstitial cystitis (IC). All patients met the NIH definition of IC based upon the results of cystoscopy, cytology, and biopsy. One blinded, randomized, placebo controlled study evaluated 151 patients (145 women, 5 men, 1 unknown) with a mean age of 44 years (range 18 to 81). Approximately equal numbers of patients received either placebo or ELMIRON 100 mg three times a day for 3 months. Clinical improvement in bladder pain was based upon the patient's own assessment. In this study, 28/74 (38%) of patients who received ELMIRON and 13/74 (18%) of patients who received placebo, showed greater than 50% improvement in bladder pain (p=0.005).
A second clinical trial, the physician's usage study, was a prospectively designed retrospective analysis of 2499 patients who received ELMIRON 300 mg a day without blinding. Of the 2499 patients, 2220 were women, 254 were men, and 25 were of unknown sex. The patients had a mean age of 47 years and 23% were over 60 years of age. By 3 months, 1307 (52%) of the patients had dropped out or were ineligible for analysis, overall, 1192 (48%) received ELMIRON for 3 months; 892 (36%) received ELMIRON for 6 months; and 598 (24%) received ELMIRON for one year.
Patients had unblinded evaluations every 3 months for the patient's rating of overall change in pain in comparison to baseline and for the difference calculated in "pain/discomfort" scores. At baseline, pain/discomfort scores for the original 2499 patients were severe or unbearable in 60%, moderate in 33% and mild or none in 7% of patients. The extent of the patients' pain improvement is shown in Table 1.
At 3 months, 722/2499 (29%) of the patients originally in the study had pain scores that improved by one or two categories. By 6 months, in the 892 patients who continued taking ELMIRON, an additional 116/2499 (5%) of patients had improved pain scores. After 6 months, the percent of patients who reported the first onset of pain relief was less than 1.5% of patients who originally entered in the study (see Table 2).

Table 1:
Pain Scores in Reference to Baseline in Open Label Physician's Usage Study (N=2499)[1]

Efficacy Parameter	3 months[2]	6 months[2]
Patient Rating of Overall Change in Pain (Recollection of difference between current pain and baseline pain)[3]	N=1161 Median=3 Mean=3.44 CI: (3.37, 3.51)	N=724 Median=4 Mean=3.91 CI: (3.83, 3.99)
Change in Pain/Discomfort Score (Calculated difference in scores at the time point and baseline)[4]	N=1440 Median=1 Mean=0.51 CI: (0.45, 0.57)	N=904 Median=1 Mean=0.66 CI: (0.61, 0.71)

[1] Trial not designed to detect onset of pain relief.
[2] CI=95% confidence interval.
[3] 6-point-scale: 1 = worse, 2 = no better, 3 = slightly improved, 4 = moderately improved, 5 = greatly improved, 6=symptom gone.
[4] 3-point scale: 1=none or mild, 2=moderate, 3=severe or unbearable.

Table 2:
Number (%) of Patients with New Relief of Pain/Discomfort[1] in the Open-Label Physician's Usage Study (N=2499)

	at 3 months[2] (n=1192)	at 6 months[3] (n=892)
Considering only the patients who continued treatment	722/1192 (61%)	116/892 (13%)
Considering all the patients originally enrolled in the study	722/2499 (29%)	116/2499 (5%)

[1] First-time improvement in pain/discomfort score by 1 or 2 categories.
[2] Number (%) of patients with improvement of pain/discomfort score at 3 months when compared to baseline.
[3] Number (%) of patients without pain/discomfort improvement at 3 months who had improvement at 6 months.

INDICATIONS AND USAGE

ELMIRON (pentosan polysulfate sodium) is indicated for the relief of bladder pain or discomfort associated with interstitial cystitis.

Continued on next page

Elmiron—Cont.

CONTRAINDICATIONS

ELMIRON (pentosan polysulfate sodium) is contraindicated in patients with known hypersensitivity to the drug, structurally related compounds, or excipients.

WARNINGS

None.

PRECAUTIONS

General:
ELMIRON (pentosan polysulfate sodium) is a weak anticoagulant (1/15 the activity of heparin). At a daily dose of 300 mg (n = 128), rectal hemorrhage was reported as an adverse event in 6.3% of patients. Bleeding complications of ecchymosis, epistaxis, and gum hemorrhage have been reported (see **ADVERSE REACTIONS**). Patients undergoing invasive procedures or having signs/symptoms of underlying coagulopathy or other increased risk of bleeding (due to other therapies such as coumarin anticoagulants, heparin, t-PA, streptokinase, or high dose aspirin) should be evaluated for hemorrhage. Patients with diseases such as aneurysms, thrombocytopenia, hemophilia, gastrointestinal ulcerations, polyps, or diverticula should be carefully evaluated before starting ELMIRON.

A similar product that was given subcutaneously, sublingually, or intramuscularly (and not initially metabolized by the liver) is associated with delayed immunoallergic thrombocytopenia with symptoms of thrombosis and hemorrhage. Caution should be exercised when using ELMIRON in patients who have a history of heparin induced thrombocytopenia.

Hepatic Insufficiency: Pentosan polysulfate sodium is desulfated by both the liver and the spleen. The extent to which hepatic insufficiency or splenic disorders may increase the bioavailability of the parent or active metabolites of pentosan polysulfate sodium is not known. Caution should be exercised when using ELMIRON in these patients.

Mildly (<2.5 x normal) elevated transaminase, alkaline phosphatase, γ-glutamyl transpeptidase, and lactic dehydrogenase occurred in 1.2% of patients. The increases usually appeared 3 to 12 months after the start of ELMIRON therapy, and were not associated with jaundice or other clinical signs or symptoms. These abnormalities are usually transient, may remain essentially unchanged, or may rarely progress with continued use. Increases in PTT and PT (<1% for both) or thrombocytopenia (0.2%) were noted.

Alopecia is associated with pentosan polysulfate and with heparin products. In clinical trials of ELMIRON, alopecia could begin within the first 4 weeks of treatment. Ninety-seven percent (97%) of the cases of alopecia reported were alopecia areata, limited to a single area on the scalp.

Information for Patients: Patients should take the drug as prescribed, in the dosage prescribed, and no more frequently than prescribed. Patients should be reminded that ELMIRON has a weak anticoagulant effect. This effect may increase bleeding times.

Laboratory Test Findings: Pentosan polysulfate sodium did not affect prothrombin time (PT) or partial thromboplastin time (PTT) up to 1200 mg per day in 24 healthy male subjects treated for 8 days. Pentosan polysulfate sodium also inhibits the generation of factor Xa in plasma and inhibits thrombin-induced platelet aggregation in human platelet rich plasma *ex vivo*. (See **PRECAUTIONS**—Hepatic Insufficiency Section for additional information.)

Carcinogenicity, Mutagenesis, Impairment of Fertility: Long term studies in animals have not been performed to evaluate the carcinogenic potential of ELMIRON. Pentosan polysulfate sodium was not clastogenic or mutagenic when tested in the mouse micronucleus test or the Ames test (*S. typhimurium*). The effect of pentosan polysulfate sodium on spermatogenesis has not been investigated.

Pregnancy Category B: Reproduction studies have been performed in mice and rats with intravenous daily doses of 15 mg/kg, and in rabbits with 7.5 mg/kg. These doses are 0.42 and 0.14 times the daily oral human doses of ELMIRON when normalized to body surface area. These studies did not reveal evidence of impaired fertility or harm to the fetus from ELMIRON. Direct *in vitro* bathing of cultured mouse embryos with pentosan polysulfate sodium (PPS) at a concentration of 1mg/mL may cause reversible limb bud abnormalities. Adequate and well controlled studies have not been performed in pregnant women. Because animal studies are not always predictive of human response, this drug should be used in pregnancy only if clearly needed.

Nursing Mothers: It is not known whether this drug is excreted in human milk. Because many drugs are excreted in human milk, caution should be exercised when ELMIRON is administered to a nursing woman.

Pediatric Use: Safety and effectiveness in pediatric patients below the age of 16 years have not been established.

ADVERSE REACTIONS

ELMIRON was evaluated in clinical trials in a total of 2627 patients (2343 women, 262 men, 22 unknown) with a mean age of 47[range 18 to 88 with 581 (22%) over 60 years of age]. Of the 2627 patients, 128 patients were in a 3 month trial and the remaining 2499 patients were in a long term, unblinded trial.

Deaths occurred in 6/2627 (0.2%) patients who received the drug over a period of 3 to 75 months. The deaths appear to be related to other concurrent illnesses or procedures, except in one patient for whom the cause was not known.

Serious adverse events occurred in 33/2627 (1.3%) patients. Two patients had severe abdominal pain or diarrhea and dehydration that required hospitalization. Because there was not a control group of patients with interstitial cystitis who were concurrently evaluated, it is difficult to determine which events are associated with ELMIRON and which events are associated with concurrent illness, medicine, or other factors.

Adverse Experience In Placebo-Controlled Clinical Trials of ELMIRON 100 mg Three Times a Day for 3 Months

Body System/	Adverse Experience	Elmiron n=128	Placebo n=130
CNS	Overall Number of Patients*	3	5
	Insomnia	1	0
	Headache	1	3
	Severe Emotional Lability/Depression	2	1
	Nystagmus/Dizziness	1	1
	Hyperkinesia	1	1
GI	Overall Number of Patients*	7	7
	Nausea	3	3
	Diarrhea	3	6
	Dyspepsia	1	0
	Jaundice	0	1
	Vomiting	0	2
Skin/Allergic	Overall Number of Patients*	2	4
	Rash	0	2
	Pruritus	0	2
	Lacrimation	1	1
	Rhinitis	1	1
	Increased Sweating	1	0
Other	Overall Number of Patients*	1	3
	Amenorrhea	0	1
	Arthralgia	0	1
	Vaginitis	1	1
Total Events		17	27
Total Number of Patients Reporting Adverse Events		13	19

* Within a body system, the individual events do not sum to equal overall number of patients because a patient may have more than one event.

The adverse events described below were reported in an unblinded clinical trial of 2499 interstitial cystitis patients treated with ELMIRON. Of the original 2499 patients, 1192 (48%) received ELMIRON for 3 months; 892 (36%) received ELMIRON for 6 months; and 598 (24%) received ELMIRON for one year, 355 (14%) received ELMIRON for 2 years, and 145 (6%) for 4 years.

Frequency (1 to 4%): Alopecia (4%), diarrhea (4%), nausea (4%), headache (3%), rash (3%), dyspepsia (2%), abdominal pain (2%), liver function abnormalities (1%), dizziness (1%).

Frequency (≤1%):

Digestive: Vomiting, mouth ulcer, colitis, esophagitis, gastritis, flatulence, constipation, anorexia, gum hemorrhage.

Hematologic: Anemia, ecchymosis, increased prothrombin time, increased partial thromboplastin time, leukopenia, thrombocytopenia.

Hypersensitive Reactions: Allergic reaction, photosensitivity.

Respiratory System: Pharyngitis, rhinitis, epistaxis, dyspnea.

Skin and Appendages: Pruritus, urticaria.

Special Senses: Conjunctivitis, tinnitus, optic neuritis, amblyopia, retinal hemorrhage.

Post-Marketing Experience:

Rectal Hemorrhage: ELMIRON was evaluated in a randomized, double-blind, parallel group, Phase 4 study conducted in 380 patients with interstitial cystitis dosed for 32 weeks. At a daily dose of 300 mg (n = 128), rectal hemorrhage was reported as an adverse event in 6.3% of patients. The severity of the events was described as "mild" in most patients. Patients in that study who were administered ELMIRON 900 mg daily, a dose higher than the approved dose, experienced a higher incidence of rectal hemorrhage, 15%.

Liver Function Abnormality: A randomized, double-blind, parallel group, phase 2 study was conducted in 100 men (51 ELMIRON and 49 placebo) dosed for 16 weeks. At a daily dose of 900 mg, a dose higher than the approved dose, elevated liver function tests were reported as an adverse event in 11.8% (n = 6) of ELMIRON treated patients and 2% (n = 1) of placebo treated patients.

OVERDOSAGE

Overdose has not been reported. Based upon the pharmacodynamics of the drug, toxicity is likely to be reflected as anticoagulation, bleeding, thrombocytopenia, liver function abnormalities, and gastric distress. (See **CLINICAL PHARMACOLOGY** and **PRECAUTIONS** sections.) At a daily dose of 900 mg for 32 weeks (n = 127) in a clinical trial, rectal hemorrhage was reported as an adverse event in 15% of patients. At a daily dose of ELMIRON 900 mg for 16 weeks in a clinical trial that enrolled 51 patients in the ELMIRON group and 49 in the placebo group, elevated liver function tests were reported as an adverse event in 11.8% of patients in the ELMIRON group and 2% of patients in the placebo group. In the event of acute overdosage, the patient should be given gastric lavage if possible, carefully observed and given symptomatic and supportive treatment.

DOSAGE AND ADMINISTRATION

The recommended dose of ELMIRON is 300 mg/day taken as one 100 mg capsule orally three times daily. The capsules should be taken with water at least 1 hour before meals or 2 hours after meals.

Patients receiving ELMIRON should be reassessed after 3 months. If improvement has not occurred and if limiting adverse events are not present, ELMIRON may be continued for another 3 months.

The clinical value and risks of continued treatment in patients whose pain has not improved by 6 months is not known.

HOW SUPPLIED

ELMIRON® is supplied in white opaque hard gelatin capsules imprinted "BNP7600" containing 100 mg pentosan polysulfate sodium. Supplied in bottles of 100 capsules.
NDC NUMBER 17314-9300-1

STORAGE

Store at controlled room temperature 15°-30°C (59°-86°F).

Rx only

ELMIRON® is a Registered Trademark of IVAX Research, Inc. under license to ORTHO-McNEIL PHARMACEUTICAL, INC.

ORTHO-McNEIL
ORTHO-McNEIL PHARMACEUTICAL, INC.
Raritan, New Jersey, 08869

Manufactured by IVAX Pharmaceuticals, Inc. Miami, FL 33137	Distributed by: ORTHO-McNEIL PHARMACEUTICAL, INC Raritan, New Jersey, 08869-4043

Revised August 2004 633-20-506-2
U.S. Patent #5,180,715

LEVAQUIN® ℞

[*lĕvă-kwĭn*]
(levofloxacin) Tablets
LEVAQUIN®
(levofloxacin) Oral Solution
LEVAQUIN®
(levofloxacin) Injection
LEVAQUIN®
(levofloxacin in 5% dextrose) Injection

Prescribing information for this product, which appears on pages 2501–2507 of the 2005 PDR, has been completely revised as follows. Please write "See Supplement A" next to the product heading.

Prescribing Information

To reduce the development of drug-resistant bacteria and maintain the effectiveness of LEVAQUIN® (levofloxacin) and other antibacterial drugs, LEVAQUIN should be used only to treat or prevent infections that are proven or strongly suspected to be caused by bacteria.

DESCRIPTION

LEVAQUIN® (levofloxacin) is a synthetic broad spectrum antibacterial agent for oral and intravenous administration. Chemically, levofloxacin, a chiral fluorinated carboxyquinolone, is the pure (-)-(S)-enantiomer of the racemic drug substance ofloxacin. The chemical name is (-)-(S)-9-fluoro-2,3-dihydro-3-methyl-10-(4-methyl-1-piperazinyl)-7-oxo-7H-pyridol[1,2,3-de]-1,4-benzoxazine-6-carboxylic acid hemihydrate.

The chemical structure is:

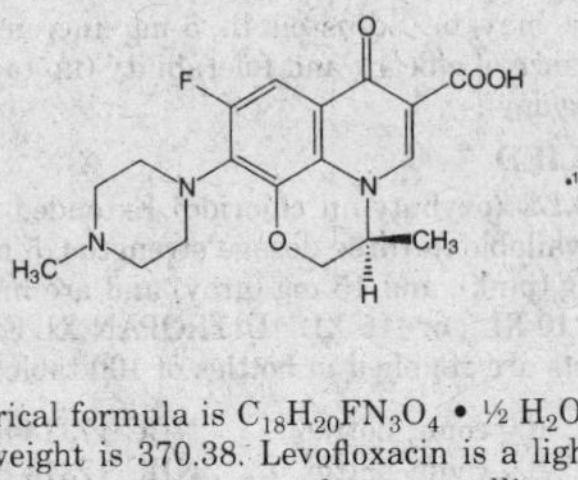

Its empirical formula is $C_{18}H_{20}FN_3O_4 \cdot ½ H_2O$ and its molecular weight is 370.38. Levofloxacin is a light yellowish-white to yellow-white crystal or crystalline powder. The molecule exists as a zwitterion at the pH conditions in the small intestine.

The data demonstrate that from pH 0.6 to 5.8, the solubility of levofloxacin is essentially constant (approximately 100 mg/mL). Levofloxacin is considered *soluble to freely soluble* in this pH range, as defined by USP nomenclature. Above pH 5.8, the solubility increases rapidly to its maximum at pH 6.7 (272 mg/mL) and is considered *freely soluble* in this range. Above pH 6.7, the solubility decreases and reaches a minimum value (about 50 mg/mL) at a pH of approximately 6.9.

Levofloxacin has the potential to form stable coordination compounds with many metal ions. This in vitro chelation potential has the following formation order: $Al^{+3}>Cu^{+2}>Zn^{+2}>Mg^{+2}>Ca^{+2}$.

LEVAQUIN Tablets are available as film-coated tablets and contain the following inactive ingredients:

250 mg (as expressed in the anhydrous form): hypromellose, crospovidone, microcrystalline cellulose, magnesium stearate, polyethylene glycol, titanium dioxide, polysorbate 80 and synthetic red iron oxide.

500 mg (as expressed in the anhydrous form): hypromellose, crospovidone, microcrystalline cellulose, magnesium stearate, polyethylene glycol, titanium dioxide, polysorbate 80 and synthetic red and yellow iron oxides.

750 mg (as expressed in the anhydrous form): hypromellose, crospovidone, microcrystalline cellulose, magnesium stearate, polyethylene glycol, titanium dioxide, polysorbate 80.

LEVAQUIN Oral Solution, 25 mg/mL is a multi-use self-preserving aqueous solution of levofloxacin with pH ranging from 5.0-6.0. The appearance of LEVAQUIN Oral Solution may range from clear yellow to clear greenish-yellow. This does not adversely affect product potency.

LEVAQUIN Oral Solution contains the following inactive ingredients: sucrose, glycerin, sucralose, hydrochloric acid, purified water, propylene glycol, artificial and natural flavors, benzyl alcohol, ascorbic acid, and caramel color. It may also contain a solution of sodium hydroxide for pH adjustment.

LEVAQUIN Injection in Single-Use Vials is a sterile, preservative-free aqueous solution of levofloxacin with pH ranging from 3.8 to 5.8. LEVAQUIN Injection in Premix Flexible Containers is a sterile, preservative-free aqueous solution of levofloxacin with pH ranging from 3.8 to 5.8. The appearance of LEVAQUIN Injection may range from a clear yellow to a greenish-yellow solution. This does not adversely affect product potency.

LEVAQUIN Injection in Single-Use Vials contains levofloxacin in Water for Injection. LEVAQUIN Injection in Premix Flexible Containers is a dilute, non-pyrogenic, nearly isotonic premixed solution that contains levofloxacin in 5% Dextrose (D_5W). Solutions of hydrochloric acid and sodium hydroxide may have been added to adjust the pH.

The flexible container is fabricated from a specially formulated non-plasticized, thermoplastic copolyester (CR3). The amount of water that can permeate from the container into the overwrap is insufficient to affect the solution significantly. Solutions in contact with the flexible container can leach out certain of the container's chemical components in very small amounts within the expiration period. The suitability of the container material has been confirmed by tests in animals according to USP biological tests for plastic containers.

CLINICAL PHARMACOLOGY

The mean ±SD pharmacokinetic parameters of levofloxacin determined under single and steady-state conditions following oral (p.o.) tablet, oral solution, or intravenous (i.v.) doses of levofloxacin are summarized in Table 1.

Absorption

Levofloxacin is rapidly and essentially completely absorbed after oral administration. Peak plasma concentrations are usually attained one to two hours after oral dosing. The absolute bioavailability of a 500 mg tablet and a 750 mg tablet of levofloxacin are both approximately 99%, demonstrating complete oral absorption of levofloxacin. Following a single intravenous dose of levofloxacin to healthy volunteers, the mean ±SD peak plasma concentration attained was 6.2 ±1.0 µg/mL after a 500 mg dose infused over 60 minutes and 11.5 ±4.0 µg/mL after a 750 mg dose infused over 90 minutes. Levofloxacin oral solution and tablet formulations are bioequivalent.

Levofloxacin pharmacokinetics are linear and predictable after single and multiple oral or i.v. dosing regimens. Steady-state conditions are reached within 48 hours following a 500 mg or 750 mg once-daily dosage regimen. The mean ±SD peak and trough plasma concentrations attained following multiple once-daily oral dosage regimens were approximately 5.7 ±1.4 and 0.5 ±0.2 µg/mL after the 500 mg doses, and 8.6 ±1.9 and 1.1 ±0.4 µg/mL after the 750 mg doses, respectively. The mean ±SD peak and trough plasma concentrations attained following multiple once-daily i.v. regimens were approximately 6.4 ±0.8 and 0.6 ±0.2 µg/mL after the 500 mg doses, and 12.1 ±4.1 and 1.3 ±0.71 µg/mL after the 750 mg doses, respectively.

Oral administration of a 500-mg LEVAQUIN with food prolongs the time to peak concentration by approximately 1 hour and decreases the peak concentration by approximately 14% following tablet and approximately 25% following oral solution administration. Therefore, levofloxacin tablets can be administered without regard to food. It is recommended that levofloxacin oral solution be taken 1 hour before, or 2 hours after eating.

The plasma concentration profile of levofloxacin after i.v. administration is similar and comparable in extent of exposure (AUC) to that observed for levofloxacin tablets when equal doses (mg/mg) are administered. Therefore, the oral and i.v. routes of administration can be considered interchangeable. (See following chart.)

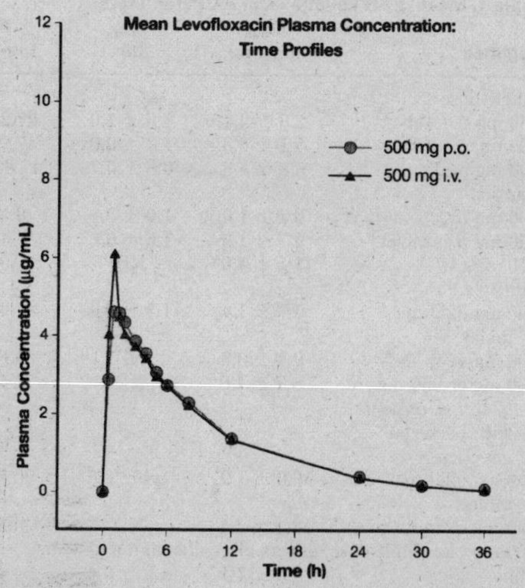
Mean Levofloxacin Plasma Concentration:
Time Profiles
500 mg p.o.
500 mg i.v.
Plasma Concentration (µg/mL)
Time (h)

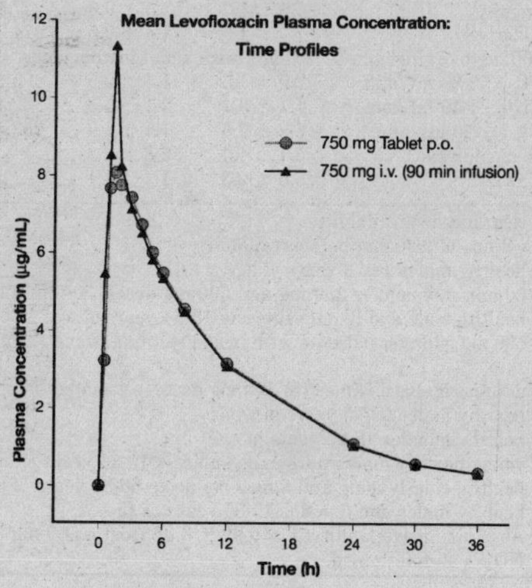
Mean Levofloxacin Plasma Concentration:
Time Profiles
750 mg Tablet p.o.
750 mg i.v. (90 min infusion)
Plasma Concentration (µg/mL)
Time (h)

Distribution

The mean volume of distribution of levofloxacin generally ranges from 74 to 112 L after single and multiple 500 mg or 750 mg doses, indicating widespread distribution into body tissues. Levofloxacin reaches its peak levels in skin tissues and in blister fluid of healthy subjects at approximately 3 hours after dosing. The skin tissue biopsy to plasma AUC ratio is approximately 2 and the blister fluid to plasma AUC ratio is approximately 1 following multiple once-daily oral administration of 750 mg and 500 mg levofloxacin, respectively, to healthy subjects. Levofloxacin also penetrates well into lung tissues. Lung tissue concentrations were generally 2- to 5- fold higher than plasma concentrations and ranged from approximately 2.4 to 11.3 µg/g over a 24-hour period after a single 500 mg oral dose.

In vitro, over a clinically relevant range (1 to 10 µg/mL) of serum/plasma levofloxacin concentrations, levofloxacin is approximately 24 to 38% bound to serum proteins across all species studied, as determined by the equilibrium dialysis method. Levofloxacin is mainly bound to serum albumin in humans. Levofloxacin binding to serum proteins is independent of the drug concentration.

Metabolism

Levofloxacin is stereochemically stable in plasma and urine and does not invert metabolically to its enantiomer, D-ofloxacin. Levofloxacin undergoes limited metabolism in humans and is primarily excreted as unchanged drug in the urine. Following oral administration, approximately 87% of an administered dose was recovered as unchanged drug in urine within 48 hours, whereas less than 4% of the dose was recovered in feces in 72 hours. Less than 5% of an administered dose was recovered in the urine as the desmethyl and N-oxide metabolites, the only metabolites identified in humans. These metabolites have little relevant pharmacological activity.

Excretion

Levofloxacin is excreted largely as unchanged drug in the urine. The mean terminal plasma elimination half-life of levofloxacin ranges from approximately 6 to 8 hours following single or multiple doses of levofloxacin given orally or intravenously. The mean apparent total body clearance and renal clearance range from approximately 144 to 226 mL/min and 96 to 142 mL/min, respectively. Renal clearance in excess of the glomerular filtration rate suggests that tubular secretion of levofloxacin occurs in addition to its glomerular filtration. Concomitant administration of either cimetidine or probenecid results in approximately 24% and 35% reduction in the levofloxacin renal clearance, respectively, indicating that secretion of levofloxacin occurs in the renal proximal tubule. No levofloxacin crystals were found in any of the urine samples freshly collected from subjects receiving levofloxacin.

Special Populations

Geriatric: There are no significant differences in levofloxacin pharmacokinetics between young and elderly subjects when the subjects' differences in creatinine clearance are taken into consideration. Following a 500 mg oral dose of levofloxacin to healthy elderly subjects (66–80 years of age), the mean terminal plasma elimination half-life of levofloxacin was about 7.6 hours, as compared to approximately 6 hours in younger adults. The difference was attributable to the variation in renal function status of the subjects and was not believed to be clinically significant. Drug absorption appears to be unaffected by age. Levofloxacin dose adjustment based on age alone is not necessary.

Pediatric: The pharmacokinetics of levofloxacin in pediatric subjects have not been studied.

Gender: There are no significant differences in levofloxacin pharmacokinetics between male and female subjects when subjects' differences in creatinine clearance are taken into consideration. Following a 500 mg oral dose of levofloxacin to healthy male subjects, the mean terminal plasma elimination half-life of levofloxacin was about 7.5 hours, as compared to approximately 6.1 hours in female subjects. This difference was attributable to the variation in renal function status of the male and female subjects and was not believed to be clinically significant. Drug absorption appears to be unaffected by the gender of the subjects. Dose adjustment based on gender alone is not necessary.

Race: The effect of race on levofloxacin pharmacokinetics was examined through a covariate analysis performed on data from 72 subjects: 48 white and 24 non-white. The apparent total body clearance and apparent volume of distribution were not affected by the race of the subjects.

Renal insufficiency: Clearance of levofloxacin is substantially reduced and plasma elimination half-life is substantially prolonged in patients with impaired renal function (creatinine clearance <50 mL/min), requiring dosage adjustment in such patients to avoid accumulation. Neither hemodialysis nor continuous ambulatory peritoneal dialysis (CAPD) is effective in removal of levofloxacin from the body, indicating that supplemental doses of levofloxacin are not required following hemodialysis or CAPD. (See **PRECAUTIONS: General** and **DOSAGE AND ADMINISTRATION**.)

Hepatic insufficiency: Pharmacokinetic studies in hepatically impaired patients have not been conducted. Due to the limited extent of levofloxacin metabolism, the pharmacokinetics of levofloxacin are not expected to be affected by hepatic impairment.

Bacterial infection: The pharmacokinetics of levofloxacin in patients with serious community-acquired bacterial infections are comparable to those observed in healthy subjects.

Drug-drug interactions: The potential for pharmacokinetic drug interactions between levofloxacin and theophylline, warfarin, cyclosporine, digoxin, probenecid, cimetidine, sucralfate, and antacids has been evaluated. (See **PRECAUTIONS: Drug Interactions**.)

[See table 1 at top of next page]

MICROBIOLOGY

Levofloxacin is the L-isomer of the racemate, ofloxacin, a quinolone antimicrobial agent. The antibacterial activity of ofloxacin resides primarily in the L-isomer. The mechanism of action of levofloxacin and other fluoroquinolone antimicrobials involves inhibition of bacterial topoisomerase IV and DNA gyrase (both of which are type II topoisomerases), enzymes required for DNA replication, transcription, repair and recombination.

Levofloxacin has in vitro activity against a wide range of gram-negative and gram-positive microorganisms. Levofloxacin is often bactericidal at concentrations equal to or slightly greater than inhibitory concentrations.

Fluoroquinolones, including levofloxacin, differ in chemical structure and mode of action from aminoglycosides, macrolides and β-lactam antibiotics, including penicillins. Fluoroquinolones may, therefore, be active against bacteria resistant to these antimicrobials.

Resistance to levofloxacin due to spontaneous mutation in vitro is a rare occurrence (range: 10^{-9} to 10^{-10}). Although cross-resistance has been observed between levofloxacin and some other fluoroquinolones, some microorganisms resistant to other fluoroquinolones may be susceptible to levofloxacin.

Levofloxacin has been shown to be active against most strains of the following microorganisms both in vitro and in clinical infections as described in the **INDICATIONS AND USAGE** section:

Aerobic gram-positive microorganisms

Enterococcus faecalis (many strains are only moderately susceptible)
Staphylococcus aureus (methicillin-susceptible strains)
Staphylococcus epidermidis (methicillin-susceptible strains)
Staphylococcus saprophyticus
Streptococcus pneumoniae (including multi-drug resistant strains [MDRSP]*)
Streptococcus pyogenes

*MDRSP (Multi-drug resistant *Streptococcus pneumoniae*) isolates are strains resistant to two or more of the following antibiotics: penicillin (MIC ≥2 µg/mL, 2nd generation cephalosporins, e.g., cefuroxime, macrolides, tetracyclines and trimethoprim/sulfamethoxazole.

Aerobic gram-negative microorganisms

Enterobacter cloacae
Escherichia coli

Continued on next page

Levaquin—Cont.

Haemophilus influenzae
Haemophilus parainfluenzae
Klebsiella pneumoniae
Legionella pneumophila
Moraxella catarrhalis
Proteus mirabilis
Pseudomonas aeruginosa
Serratia marcescens

As with other drugs in this class, some strains of *Pseudomonas aeruginosa* may develop resistance fairly rapidly during treatment with levofloxacin.

Other microorganisms
Chlamydia pneumoniae
Mycoplasma pneumoniae

Levofloxacin has been shown to be active against *Bacillus anthracis* both *in vitro* and by use of plasma levels as a surrogate marker in a rhesus monkey model for anthrax (postexposure). (See **INDICATIONS AND USAGE** and **ADDITIONAL INFORMATION - INHALATIONAL ANTHRAX**).

The following in vitro data are available, **but their clinical significance is unknown**.

Levofloxacin exhibits in vitro minimum inhibitory concentrations (MIC values) of 2 µg/mL or less against most (≥90%) strains of the following microorganisms; however, the safety and effectiveness of levofloxacin in treating clinical infections due to these microorganisms have not been established in adequate and well-controlled trials.

Aerobic gram-positive microorganisms
Staphylococcus haemolyticus
Streptococcus (Group G)
Streptococcus milleri
Streptococcus (Group C/F)
Streptococcus agalactiae
Viridans group streptococci
Aerobic gram-negative microorganisms
Acinetobacter baumannii
Enterobacter aerogenes
Proteus vulgaris
Acinetobacter lwoffii
Enterobacter sakazakii
Providencia rettgeri
Bordetella pertussis
Klebsiella oxytoca
Providencia stuartii
Citrobacter (diversus) koseri
Morganella morganii
Pseudomonas fluorescens
Citrobacter freundii
Pantoea (Enterobacter) agglomerans
Anaerobic gram-positive microorganisms
Clostridium perfringens
Susceptibility Tests
Susceptibility testing for levofloxacin should be performed, as it is the optimal predictor of activity.
Dilution techniques: Quantitative methods are used to determine antimicrobial minimal inhibitory concentrations (MIC values). These MIC values provide estimates of the susceptibility of bacteria to antimicrobial compounds. The MIC values should be determined using a standardized procedure. Standardized procedures are based on a dilution method[1] (broth or agar) or equivalent with standardized inoculum concentrations and standardized concentrations of levofloxacin powder. The MIC values should be interpreted according to the following criteria:
For testing *Enterobacteriaceae*, Enterococci, *Staphylococcus* species, and *Pseudomonas aeruginosa:*

MIC (µg/mL)	Interpretation
≤2	Susceptible (S)
4	Intermediate (I)
≥8	Resistant (R)

For testing *Haemophilus influenzae* and *Haemophilus parainfluenzae:*[a]

MIC (µg/mL)	Interpretation
≤2	Susceptible (S)

[a] These interpretive standards are applicable only to broth microdilution susceptibility testing with *Haemophilus influenzae* and *Haemophilus parainfluenzae* using Haemophilus Test Medium.[1]

The current absence of data on resistant strains precludes defining any categories other than "Susceptible." Strains yielding MIC results suggestive of a "nonsusceptible" category should be submitted to a reference laboratory for further testing.

For testing *Streptococcus* spp. including *S. pneumoniae:*[b]

MIC (µg/mL)	Interpretation
≤2	Susceptible (S)
4	Intermediate (I)
≥8	Resistant (R)

[b] These interpretive standards are applicable only to broth microdilution susceptibility tests using cation-adjusted Mueller-Hinton broth with 2-5% lysed horse blood.

A report of "Susceptible" indicates that the pathogen is likely to be inhibited if the antimicrobial compound in the

Table 1. Mean ± SD Levofloxacin PK Parameters

Regimen	C_{max} (µg/mL)	T_{max} (h)	AUC (µg·h/mL)	CL/F[1] (mL/min)	Vd/F[2] (L)	$t_{1/2}$ (h)	CL_R (mL/min)
Single dose							
250 mg p.o. tablet[3]	2.8 ± 0.4	1.6 ± 1.0	27.2 ± 3.9	156 ± 20	ND	7.3 ± 0.9	142 ± 21
500 mg p.o. tablet[3]*	5.1 ± 0.8	1.3 ± 0.6	47.9 ± 6.8	178 ± 28	ND	6.3 ± 0.6	103 ± 30
500 mg oral solution[12]	5.8 ± 1.8	0.8 ± 0.7	47.8 ± 10.8	1835 ± 40	112 ± 37.2	7.0 ± 1.47	ND
500 mg i.v.[3]	6.2 ± 1.0	1.0 ± 0.1	48.3 ± 5.4	175 ± 20	90 ± 11	6.4 ± 0.7	112 ± 25
750 mg p.o. tablet[5]*	9.3 ± 1.6	1.6 ± 0.8	101 ± 20	129 ± 24	83 ± 17	7.5 ± 0.9	ND
750 mg i.v.[5]	11.5 ± 4.0[4]	ND	110 ± 40	126 ± 39	75 ± 13	7.5 ± 1.6	ND
Multiple dose							
500 mg q24h p.o. tablet[3]	5.7 ± 1.4	1.1 ± 0.4	47.5 ± 6.7	175 ± 25	102 ± 22	7.6 ± 1.6	116 ± 31
500 mg q24h i.v.[3]	6.4 ± 0.8	ND	54.6 ± 11.1	158 ± 29	91 ± 12	7.0 ± 0.8	99 ± 28
500 mg or 250 mg q24h i.v., patients with bacterial infection[6]	8.7 ± 4.0[7]	ND	72.5 ± 51.2[7]	154 ± 72	111 ± 58	ND	ND
750 mg q24h p.o. tablet[5]	8.6 ± 1.9	1.4 ± 0.5	90.7 ± 17.6	143 ± 29	100 ± 16	8.8 ± 1.5	116 ± 28
750 mg q24h i.v.[5]	12.1 ± 4.1[4]	ND	108 ± 34	126 ± 37	80 ± 27	7.9 ± 1.9	ND
500 mg p.o. single dose, effects of gender and age:							
Male[8]	5.5 ± 1.1	1.2 ± 0.4	54.4 ± 18.9	166 ± 44	89 ± 13	7.5 ± 2.1	126 ± 38
Female[9]	7.0 ± 1.6	1.7 ± 0.5	67.7 ± 24.2	136 ± 44	62 ± 16	6.1 ± 0.8	106 ± 40
Young[10]	5.5 ± 1.0	1.5 ± 0.6	47.5 ± 9.8	182 ± 35	83 ± 18	6.0 ± 0.9	140 ± 33
Elderly[11]	7.0 ± 1.6	1.4 ± 0.5	74.7 ± 23.3	121 ± 33	67 ± 19	7.6 ± 2.0	91 ± 29
500 mg p.o. single dose, patients with renal insufficiency:							
CL_{CR} 50-80 mL/min	7.5 ± 1.8	1.5 ± 0.5	95.6 ± 11.8	88 ± 10	ND	9.1 ± 0.9	57 ± 8
CL_{CR} 20-49 mL/min	7.1 ± 3.1	2.1 ± 1.3	182.1 ± 62.6	51 ± 19	ND	27 ± 10	26 ± 13
CL_{CR} <20 mL/min	8.2 ± 2.6	1.1 ± 1.0	263.5 ± 72.5	33 ± 8	ND	35 ± 5	13 ± 3
Hemodialysis	5.7 ± 1.0	2.8 ± 2.2	ND	ND	ND	76 ± 42	ND
CAPD	6.9 ± 2.3	1.4 ± 1.1	ND	ND	ND	51 ± 24	ND

[1] clearance/bioavailability
[2] volume of distribution/bioavailability
[3] healthy males 18-53 years of age
[4] 60 min infusion for 250 mg and 500 mg doses, 90 min infusion for 750 mg dose
[5] healthy male and female subjects 18-54 years of age
[6] 500 mg q48h for patients with moderate renal impairment (CL_{CR} 20-50 mL/min) and infections of the respiratory tract or skin
[7] dose-normalized values (to 500 mg dose), estimated by population pharmacokinetic modeling
[8] healthy males 22-75 years of age
[9] healthy females 18-80 years of age
[10] young healthy male and female subjects 18-36 years of age
[11] healthy elderly male and female subjects 66-80 years of age
[12] healthy males and females 19-55 years of age
* Absolute bioavailability; F = 0.99 ± 0.08 from a 500-mg tablet and F=0.99 ± 0.06 from a 750-mg tablet; ND = not determined.

blood reaches the concentrations usually achievable. A report of "Intermediate" indicates that the result should be considered equivocal, and, if the microorganism is not fully susceptible to alternative, clinically feasible drugs, the test should be repeated. This category implies possible clinical applicability in body sites where the drug is physiologically concentrated or in situations where a high dosage of drug can be used. This category also provides a buffer zone which prevents small uncontrolled technical factors from causing major discrepancies in interpretation. A report of "Resistant" indicates that the pathogen is not likely to be inhibited if the antimicrobial compound in the blood reaches the concentrations usually achievable; other therapy should be selected.

Standardized susceptibility test procedures require the use of laboratory control microorganisms to control the technical aspects of the laboratory procedures. Standard levofloxacin powder should give the following MIC values:

Microorganism		MIC (µg/mL)
Enterococcus faecalis	ATCC 29212	0.25-2
Escherichia coli	ATCC 25922	0.008-0.06
Escherichia coli	ATCC 35218	0.015-0.06
Haemophilus influenzae	ATCC 49247[c]	0.008-0.03
Pseudomonas aeruginosa	ATCC 27853	0.5-4
Staphylococcus aureus	ATCC 29213	0.06-0.5
Streptococcus pneumoniae	ATCC 49619[d]	0.5-2

[c] This quality control range is applicable to only *H. influenzae* ATCC 49247 tested by a broth microdilution procedure using Haemophilus Test Medium (HTM).[1]
[d] This quality control range is applicable to only *S. pneumoniae* ATCC 49619 tested by a broth microdilution procedure using cation-adjusted Mueller-Hinton broth with 2-5% lysed horse blood.

Diffusion techniques: Quantitative methods that require measurement of zone diameters also provide reproducible estimates of the susceptibility of bacteria to antimicrobial compounds. One such standardized procedure[2] requires the use of standardized inoculum concentrations. This procedure uses paper disks impregnated with 5-µg levofloxacin to test the susceptibility of microorganisms to levofloxacin.

Reports from the laboratory providing results of the standard single-disk susceptibility test with a 5-µg levofloxacin disk should be interpreted according to the following criteria:
For testing *Enterobacteriaceae*, Enterococci, *Staphylococcus* species, and *Pseudomonas aeruginosa:*

Zone diameter (mm)	Interpretation
≥17	Susceptible (S)
14–16	Intermediate (I)
≤13	Resistant (R)

For *Haemophilus influenzae* and *Haemophilus parainfluenzae:*[e]

Zone diameter (mm)	Interpretation
≥17	Susceptible (S)

[e] These interpretive standards are applicable only to disk diffusion susceptibility testing with *Haemophilus influenzae* and *Haemophilus parainfluenzae* using Haemophilus Test Medium.[2]

The current absence of data on resistant strains precludes defining any categories other than "Susceptible." Strains yielding zone diameter results suggestive of a "nonsusceptible" category should be submitted to a reference laboratory for further testing.

For *Streptococcus* spp. including *S. pneumoniae:*[f]

Zone diameter (mm)	Interpretation
≥17	Susceptible (S)
14–16	Intermediate (I)
≤13	Resistant (R)

[f] These zone diameter standards for *Streptococcus* spp. including *S. pneumoniae* apply only to tests performed using Mueller-Hinton agar supplemented with 5% sheep blood and incubated in 5% CO_2.

Interpretation should be as stated above for results using dilution techniques. Interpretation involves correlation of the diameter obtained in the disk test with the MIC for levofloxacin.

As with standardized dilution techniques, diffusion methods require the use of laboratory control microorganisms to control the technical aspects of the laboratory procedures. For the diffusion technique, the 5-µg levofloxacin disk should provide the following zone diameters in these laboratory test quality control strains:

Microorganism		Zone Diameter (mm)
Escherichia coli	ATCC 25922	29-37
Haemophilus influenzae	ATCC 49247[g]	32-40
Pseudomonas aeruginosa	ATCC 27853	19-26
Staphylococcus aureus	ATCC 25923	25-30
Streptococcus pneumoniae	ATCC 49619[h]	20-25

[g] This quality control range is applicable to only *H. influenzae* ATCC 49247 tested by a disk diffusion procedure using Haemophilus Test Medium (HTM).[2]
[h] This quality control range is applicable to only *S. pneumoniae* ATCC 49619 tested by a disk diffusion procedure using Mueller-Hinton agar supplemented with 5% sheep blood and incubated in 5% CO_2.

INDICATIONS AND USAGE

To reduce the development of drug-resistant bacteria and maintain the effectiveness of LEVAQUIN® (levofloxacin) and other antibacterial drugs, LEVAQUIN should be used only to treat or prevent infections that are proven or strongly suspected to be caused by susceptible bacteria. When culture and susceptibility information are available, they should be considered in selecting or modifying antibacterial therapy. In the absence of such data, local epidemiology and susceptibility patterns may contribute to the empiric selection of therapy.

LEVAQUIN Tablets/Injection and Oral Solution are indicated for the treatment of adults (≥18 years of age) with mild, moderate, and severe infections caused by susceptible strains of the designated microorganisms in the conditions listed below. LEVAQUIN Injection is indicated when intravenous administration offers a route of administration advantageous to the patient (e.g., patient cannot tolerate an oral dosage form). Please see **DOSAGE AND ADMINISTRATION** for specific recommendations.

Acute maxillary sinusitis due to *Streptococcus pneumoniae, Haemophilus influenzae*, or *Moraxella catarrhalis*.

Acute bacterial exacerbation of chronic bronchitis due to *Staphylococcus aureus, Streptococcus pneumoniae, Haemophilus influenzae, Haemophilus parainfluenzae*, or *Moraxella catarrhalis*.

Nosocomial pneumonia due to methicillin-susceptible *Staphylococcus aureus, Pseudomonas aeruginosa, Serratia marcescens, Escherichia coli, Klebsiella pneumoniae, Haemophilus influenzae, or Streptococcus pneumoniae*. Adjunctive therapy should be used as clinically indicated. Where *Pseudomonas aeruginosa* is a documented or presumptive pathogen, combination therapy with an anti-pseudomonal β-lactam is recommended. (See **CLINICAL STUDIES**.)

Community-acquired pneumonia due to *Staphylococcus aureus, Streptococcus pneumoniae* (including multi-drug-resistant strains [MDRSP])*, Haemophilus influenzae, *Haemophilus parainfluenzae, Klebsiella pneumoniae, Moraxella catarrhalis, Chlamydia pneumoniae, Legionella pneumophila*, or *Mycoplasma pneumoniae*. (See **CLINICAL STUDIES**.)

*MDRSP (Multi-drug resistant *Streptococcus pneumoniae*) isolates are strains resistant to two or more of the following antibiotics: penicillin (MIC ≥2 μg/mL), 2nd generation cephalosporins, e.g., cefuroxime, macrolides, tetracyclines and trimethoprim/sulfamethoxazole.

Complicated skin and skin structure infections due to methicillin-susceptible *Staphylococcus aureus, Enterococcus faecalis, Streptococcus pyogenes*, or *Proteus mirabilis*.

Uncomplicated skin and skin structure infections (mild to moderate) including abscesses, cellulitis, furuncles, impetigo, pyoderma, wound infections, due to *Staphylococcus aureus* or *Streptococcus pyogenes*.

Chronic bacterial prostatitis due to *Escherichia coli, Enterococcus faecalis*, or *Staphylococcus epidermidis*.

Complicated urinary tract infections (mild to moderate) due to *Enterococcus faecalis, Enterobacter cloacae, Escherichia coli, Klebsiella pneumoniae, Proteus mirabilis*, or *Pseudomonas aeruginosa*.

Acute pyelonephritis (mild to moderate) caused by *Escherichia coli*.

Uncomplicated urinary tract infections (mild to moderate) due to *Escherichia coli, Klebsiella pneumoniae*, or *Staphylococcus saprophyticus*.

Inhalational anthrax (post-exposure): To prevent the development of inhalational anthrax following exposure to *Bacillus anthracis* (See **DOSAGE AND ADMINISTRATION** and **ADDITIONAL INFORMATION - INHALATIONAL ANTHRAX**).

Levofloxacin has not been tested in human for the post-exposure prevention of inhalation anthrax. However, plasma concentrations achieved in humans are reasonably likely to predict efficacy (See **ADDITIONAL INFORMATION - INHALATIONAL ANTHRAX**).

Appropriate culture and susceptibility tests should be performed before treatment in order to isolate and identify organisms causing the infection and to determine their susceptibility to levofloxacin. Therapy with levofloxacin may be initiated before results of these tests are known; once results become available, appropriate therapy should be selected.

As with other drugs in this class, some strains of *Pseudomonas aeruginosa* may develop resistance fairly rapidly during treatment with levofloxacin. Culture and susceptibility testing performed periodically during therapy will provide information about the continued susceptibility of the pathogens to the antimicrobial agent and also the possible emergence of bacterial resistance.

CONTRAINDICATIONS

Levofloxacin is contraindicated in persons with a history of hypersensitivity to levofloxacin, quinolone antimicrobial agents, or any other components of this product.

WARNINGS

THE SAFETY AND EFFICACY OF LEVOFLOXACIN IN PEDIATRIC PATIENTS, ADOLESCENTS (UNDER THE AGE OF 18 YEARS), PREGNANT WOMEN, AND NURSING WOMEN HAVE NOT BEEN ESTABLISHED. (See **PRECAUTIONS: Pediatric Use, Pregnancy,** and **Nursing Mothers** subsections.)

In immature rats and dogs, the oral and intravenous administration of levofloxacin resulted in increased osteochondrosis. Histopathological examination of the weight-bearing joints of immature dogs dosed with levofloxacin revealed persistent lesions of the cartilage. Other fluoroquinolones also produce similar erosions in the weight bearing joints and other signs of arthropathy in immature animals of various species. The relevance of these findings to the clinical use of levofloxacin is unknown. (See **ANIMAL PHARMACOLOGY**.)

Convulsions and toxic psychoses have been reported in patients receiving quinolones, including levofloxacin. Quinolones may also cause increased intracranial pressure and central nervous system stimulation which may lead to tremors, restlessness, anxiety, lightheadedness, confusion, hallucinations, paranoia, depression, nightmares, insomnia, and, rarely, suicidal thoughts or acts. These reactions may occur following the first dose. If these reactions occur in patients receiving levofloxacin, the drug should be discontinued and appropriate measures instituted. As with other quinolones, levofloxacin should be used with caution in patients with a known or suspected CNS disorder that may predispose to seizures or lower the seizure threshold (e.g., severe cerebral arteriosclerosis, epilepsy) or in the presence of other risk factors that may predispose to seizures or lower the seizure threshold (e.g., certain drug therapy, renal dysfunction.) (See **PRECAUTIONS: General, Information for Patients, Drug Interactions** and **ADVERSE REACTIONS**.)

Serious and occasionally fatal hypersensitivity and/or anaphylactic reactions have been reported in patients receiving therapy with quinolones, including levofloxacin. These reactions often occur following the first dose. Some reactions have been accompanied by cardiovascular collapse, hypotension/shock, seizure, loss of consciousness, tingling, angioedema (including tongue, laryngeal, throat, or facial edema/swelling), airway obstruction (including bronchospasm, shortness of breath, and acute respiratory distress), dyspnea, urticaria, itching, and other serious skin reactions. Levofloxacin should be discontinued immediately at the first appearance of a skin rash or any other sign of hypersensitivity. Serious acute hypersensitivity reactions may require treatment with epinephrine and other resuscitative measures, including oxygen, intravenous fluids, antihistamines, corticosteroids, pressor amines, and airway management, as clinically indicated. (See **PRECAUTIONS** and **ADVERSE REACTIONS**.)

Serious and sometimes fatal events, some due to hypersensitivity, and some due to uncertain etiology, have been reported rarely in patients receiving therapy with quinolones, including levofloxacin. These events may be severe and generally occur following the administration of multiple doses. Clinical manifestations may include one or more of the following: fever, rash or severe dermatologic reactions (e.g., toxic epidermal necrolysis, Stevens-Johnson Syndrome); vasculitis; arthralgia; myalgia; serum sickness; allergic pneumonitis; interstitial nephritis; acute renal insufficiency or failure; hepatitis; jaundice; acute hepatic necrosis or failure; anemia, including hemolytic and aplastic; thrombocytopenia, including thrombotic thrombocytopenic purpura; leukopenia; agranulocytosis; pancytopenia; and/or other hematologic abnormalities. The drug should be discontinued immediately at the first appearance of a skin rash or any other sign of hypersensitivity and supportive measures instituted. (See **PRECAUTIONS: Information for Patients** and **ADVERSE REACTIONS**.)

Peripheral Neuropathy: Rare cases of sensory or sensorimotor axonal polyneuropathy affecting small and/or large axons resulting in paresthesias, hypoesthesias, dysesthesias and weakness have been reported in patients receiving quinolones, including levofloxacin. Levofloxacin should be discontinued if the patient experiences symptoms of neuropathy including pain, burning, tingling, numbness, and/or weakness or other alterations of sensation including light touch, pain, temperature, position sense, and vibratory sensation in order to prevent the development of an irreversible condition.

Pseudomembranous colitis has been reported with nearly all antibacterial agents, including levofloxacin, and may range in severity from mild to life-threatening. Therefore, it is important to consider this diagnosis in patients who present with diarrhea subsequent to the administration of any antibacterial agent.

Treatment with antibacterial agents alters the normal flora of the colon and may permit overgrowth of clostridia. Studies indicate that a toxin produced by *Clostridium difficile* is one primary cause of "antibiotic-associated colitis."

After the diagnosis of pseudomembranous colitis has been established, therapeutic measures should be initiated. Mild cases of pseudomembranous colitis usually respond to drug discontinuation alone. In moderate to severe cases, consideration should be given to management with fluids and electrolytes, protein supplementation, and treatment with an antibacterial drug clinically effective against *C. difficile* colitis. (See **ADVERSE REACTIONS**.)

Tendon Effects: Ruptures of the hand, Achilles tendon, or other tendons that required surgical repair or resulted in prolonged disability have been reported in patients receiving quinolones, including levofloxacin. Post-marketing surveillance reports indicate that this risk may be increased in patients receiving concomitant corticosteroids, especially the elderly. Levofloxacin should be discontinued if the patient experiences pain, inflammation, or rupture of a tendon. Patients should rest and refrain from exercise until the diagnosis of tendonitis or tendon rupture has been confidently excluded. Tendon rupture can occur during or after therapy with quinolones, including levofloxacin.

PRECAUTIONS

General

Prescribing LEVAQUIN in the absence of a proven or strongly suspected bacterial infection or a prophylactic indication is unlikely to provide benefit to the patient and increases the risk of the development of drug-resistant bacteria.

Because a rapid or bolus intravenous injection may result in hypotension, LEVOFLOXACIN INJECTION SHOULD ONLY BE ADMINISTERED BY SLOW INTRAVENOUS INFUSION OVER A PERIOD OF 60 OR 90 MINUTES DEPENDING ON THE DOSAGE. (See **DOSAGE AND ADMINISTRATION**.)

Although levofloxacin is more soluble than other quinolones, adequate hydration of patients receiving levofloxacin should be maintained to prevent the formation of a highly concentrated urine.

Administer levofloxacin with caution in the presence of renal insufficiency. Careful clinical observation and appropriate laboratory studies should be performed prior to and during therapy since elimination of levofloxacin may be reduced. In patients with impaired renal function (creatinine clearance <50 mL/min), adjustment of the dosage regimen is necessary to avoid the accumulation of levofloxacin due to decreased clearance. (See **CLINICAL PHARMACOLOGY** and **DOSAGE AND ADMINISTRATION**.)

Moderate to severe phototoxicity reactions have been observed in patients exposed to direct sunlight while receiving drugs in this class. Excessive exposure to sunlight should be avoided. However, in clinical trials with levofloxacin, phototoxicity has been observed in less than 0.1% of patients. Therapy should be discontinued if phototoxicity (e.g., a skin eruption) occurs.

As with other quinolones, levofloxacin should be used with caution in any patient with a known or suspected CNS disorder that may predispose to seizures or lower the seizure threshold (e.g., severe cerebral arteriosclerosis, epilepsy) or in the presence of other risk factors that may predispose to seizures or lower the seizure threshold (e.g., certain drug therapy, renal dysfunction). (See **WARNINGS** and **Drug Interactions**.)

As with other quinolones, disturbances of blood glucose, including symptomatic hyper- and hypoglycemia, have been reported, usually in diabetic patients receiving concomitant treatment with an oral hypoglycemic agent (e.g., glyburide/glibenclamide) or with insulin. In these patients, careful monitoring of blood glucose is recommended. If a hypoglycemic reaction occurs in a patient being treated with levofloxacin, levofloxacin should be discontinued immediately and appropriate therapy should be initiated immediately. (See **Drug Interactions** and **ADVERSE REACTIONS**.)

Torsades de pointes: Some quinolones, including levofloxacin, have been associated with prolongation of the QT interval on the electrocardiogram and infrequent cases of arrhythmia. Rare cases of torsades de pointes have been spontaneously reported during post-marketing surveillance in patients receiving quinolones, including levofloxacin. Levofloxacin should be avoided in patients with known prolongation of the QT interval, patients with uncorrected hypokalemia, and patients receiving class IA (quinidine, procainamide), or class III (amiodarone, sotalol) antiarrhythmic agents.

As with any potent antimicrobial drug, periodic assessment of organ system functions, including renal, hepatic, and hematopoietic, is advisable during therapy. (See **WARNINGS** and **ADVERSE REACTIONS**.)

Information for Patients

Patients should be advised:

- Patients should be counseled that antibacterial drugs including LEVAQUIN® (levofloxacin) should only be used to treat bacterial infections. They do not treat viral infections (e.g., the common cold). When LEVAQUIN is prescribed to treat a bacterial infection, patients should be told that although it is common to feel better early in the course of therapy, the medication should be taken exactly as directed. Skipping doses or not completing the full course of therapy may (1) decrease the effectiveness of the immediate treatment and (2) increase the likelihood that bacteria will develop resistance and will not be treatable by LEVAQUIN or other antibacterial drugs in the future.
- that peripheral neuropathies have been associated with levofloxacin use. symptoms peripheral neuropathy including pain, burning, tingling, numbness, and/or weakness develop, they should discontinue treatment and contact their physicians;
- to drink fluids liberally;
- that antacids containing magnesium, or aluminum, as well as sucralfate, metal cations such as iron, and multivitamin preparations with zinc or Videx® (didanosine) should be taken at least two hours before or two hours after oral levofloxacin administration. (See **Drug Interactions**);
- that levofloxacin oral tablets can be taken without regard to meals;
- that levofloxacin oral solution should be taken 1 hour before or 2 hours after eating;
- that levofloxacin may cause neurologic adverse effects (e.g., dizziness, lightheadedness) and that patients should know how they react to levofloxacin before they operate an automobile or machinery or engage in other activities requiring mental alertness and coordination. (See **WARNINGS** and **ADVERSE REACTIONS**);

Continued on next page

Levaquin—Cont.

- to discontinue treatment and inform their physician if they experience pain, inflammation, or rupture of a tendon, and to rest and refrain from exercise until the diagnosis of tendinitis or tendon rupture has been confidently excluded;
- that levofloxacin may be associated with hypersensitivity reactions, even following the first dose, and to discontinue the drug at the first sign of a skin rash, hives or other skin reactions, a rapid heartbeat, difficulty in swallowing or breathing, any swelling suggesting angioedema (e.g., swelling of the lips, tongue, face, tightness of the throat, hoarseness), or other symptoms of an allergic reaction. (See **WARNINGS** and **ADVERSE REACTIONS**);
- to avoid excessive sunlight or artificial ultraviolet light while receiving levofloxacin and to discontinue therapy if phototoxicity (i.e., skin eruption) occurs;
- that if they are diabetic and are being treated with insulin or an oral hypoglycemic agent and a hypoglycemic reaction occurs, they should discontinue levofloxacin and consult a physician. (See **PRECAUTIONS: General** and **Drug Interactions.**);
- that concurrent administration of warfarin and levofloxacin has been associated with increases of the International Normalized Ratio (INR) or prothrombin time and clinical episodes of bleeding. Patients should notify their physician if they are taking warfarin.
- that convulsions have been reported in patients taking quinolones, including levofloxacin, and to notify their physician before taking this drug if there is a history of this condition.

Drug Interactions

Antacids, Sucralfate, Metal Cations, Multivitamins

LEVAQUIN Tablets: While the chelation by divalent cations is less marked than with other quinolones, concurrent administration of LEVAQUIN Tablets with antacids containing magnesium, or aluminum, as well as sucralfate, metal cations such as iron, and multivitamin preparations with zinc may interfere with the gastrointestinal absorption of levofloxacin, resulting in systemic levels considerably lower than desired. Tablets with antacids containing magnesium, aluminum, as well as sucralfate, metal cations such as iron, and multivitamins preparations with zinc or Videx® (didanosine) may substantially interfere with the gastrointestinal absorption of levofloxacin, resulting in systemic levels considerably lower than desired. These agents should be taken at least two hours before or two hours after levofloxacin administration.

LEVAQUIN Injection: There are no data concerning an interaction of **intravenous** quinolones with **oral** antacids, sucralfate, multivitamins, Videx® (didanosine), or metal cations. However, no quinolone should be co-administered with any solution containing multivalent cations, e.g., magnesium, through the same intravenous line. (See **DOSAGE AND ADMINISTRATION**.)

Theophylline: No significant effect of levofloxacin on the plasma concentrations, AUC, and other disposition parameters for theophylline was detected in a clinical study involving 14 healthy volunteers. Similarly, no apparent effect of theophylline on levofloxacin absorption and disposition was observed. However, concomitant administration of other quinolones with theophylline has resulted in prolonged elimination half-life, elevated serum theophylline levels, and a subsequent increase in the risk of theophylline-related adverse reactions in the patient population. Therefore, theophylline levels should be closely monitored and appropriate dosage adjustments made when levofloxacin is co-administered. Adverse reactions, including seizures, may occur with or without an elevation in serum theophylline levels. (See **WARNINGS** and **PRECAUTIONS: General.**)

Warfarin: No significant effect of levofloxacin on the peak plasma concentrations, AUC, and other disposition parameters for R- and S-warfarin was detected in a clinical study involving healthy volunteers. Similarly, no apparent effect of warfarin on levofloxacin absorption and disposition was observed. There have been reports during the post-marketing experience in patients that levofloxacin enhances the effects of warfarin. Elevations of the prothrombin time in the setting of concurrent warfarin and levofloxacin use have been associated with episodes of bleeding. Prothrombin time, International Normalized Ratio (INR), or other suitable anticoagulation tests should be closely monitored if levofloxacin is administered concomitantly with warfarin. Patients should also be monitored for evidence of bleeding.

Cyclosporine: No significant effect of levofloxacin on the peak plasma concentrations, AUC, and other disposition parameters for cyclosporine was detected in a clinical study involving healthy volunteers. However, elevated serum levels of cyclosporine have been reported in the patient population when co-administered with some other quinolones. Levofloxacin C_{max} and k_e were slightly lower while T_{max} and $t_{1/2}$ were slightly longer in the presence of cyclosporine than those observed in other studies without concomitant medication. The differences, however, are not considered to be clinically significant. Therefore, no dosage adjustment is required for levofloxacin or cyclosporine when administered concomitantly.

Digoxin: No significant effect of levofloxacin on the peak plasma concentrations, AUC, and other disposition parameters for digoxin was detected in a clinical study involving healthy volunteers. Levofloxacin absorption and disposition kinetics were similar in the presence or absence of digoxin. Therefore, no dosage adjustment for levofloxacin or digoxin is required when administered concomitantly.

Body as a Whole – General Disorders:	Ascites, allergic reaction, asthenia, drug level increase, edema, enlarged abdomen, fever, headache, hot flashes, influenza-like symptoms, leg pain, malaise, rigors, substernal chest pain, syncope, multiple organ failure, changed temperature sensation, withdrawal syndrome
Cardiovascular Disorders, General:	Cardiac failure, hypertension, hypertension aggravated hypotension, postural hypotension
Central and Peripheral Nervous System Disorders:	Convulsions (seizures), dysphonia, hyperesthesia, hyperkinesia, hypertonia, hypoesthesia, involuntary muscle contractions, migraine, paresthesia, paralysis, speech disorder, stupor, tremor, vertigo, encephalopathy, abnormal gait, leg cramps, intracranial hypertension, ataxia
Gastro-Intestinal System Disorders:	Dry mouth, dysphagia, esophagitis, gastritis, gastroenteritis, gastroesophageal reflux, G.I. hemorrhage, glossitis, hemorrhoids, intestinal obstruction, pancreatitis, tongue edema, melena, stomatitis
Hearing and Vestibular Disorders:	Earache, tinnitus
Heart Rate and Rhythm Disorders:	Arrhythmia, arrhythmia ventricular, atrial fibrillation, bradycardia, cardiac arrest, ventricular fibrillation, heart block, palpitation, supraventricular tachycardia, ventricular tachycardia, tachycardia
Liver and Biliary System Disorders:	Abnormal hepatic function, cholecystitis, cholelithiasis, elevated bilirubin, hepatic enzymes increased, hepatic failure, jaundice
Metabolic and Nutritional Disorders:	Hypomagnesemia, thirst, dehydration, electrolyte abnormality, fluid overload, gout, hyperglycemia, hyperkalemia, hypernatremia, hypoglycemia, hypokalemia, hyponatremia, hypophosphatemia, nonprotein nitrogen increase, weight decrease
Musculo-Skeletal System Disorders:	Arthralgia, arthritis, arthrosis, myalgia, osteomyelitis, skeletal pain, synovitis, tendonitis, tendon disorder
Myo, Endo, Pericardial and Valve Disorders:	Angina pectoris, endocarditis, myocardial infarction
Neoplasms:	Carcinoma, thrombocythemia
Other Special Senses Disorders:	Parosmia, taste perversion
Platelet, Bleeding and Clotting Disorders:	Hematoma, epistaxis, prothrombin decreased, pulmonary embolism, purpura, thrombocytopenia
Psychiatric Disorders:	Abnormal dreaming, agitation, anorexia, confusion, depression, hallucination, impotence, nervousness, paroniria, sleep disorder, somnolence
Red Blood Cell Disorders:	Anemia
Reproductive Disorders:	Dysmenorrhea, leukorrhea
Resistance Mechanism Disorders:	Abscess, bacterial infection, fungal infection, herpes simplex, moniliasis, otitis media, sepsis, viral infection
Respiratory System Disorders:	Airways obstruction, aspiration, asthma, bronchitis, bronchospasm, chronic obstructive airway disease, coughing, hemoptysis, epistaxis, hypoxia, laryngitis, pharyngitis, pleural effusion, pleurisy, pneumonitis, pneumonia, pneumothorax, pulmonary collapse, pulmonary edema, respiratory depression, respiratory insufficiency, upper respiratory tract infection
Skin and Appendages Disorders:	Alopecia, bullous eruption, dry skin, eczema, genital pruritus, increased sweating, rash, skin exfoliation, skin ulceration, urticaria
Urinary System Disorders:	Abnormal renal function, acute renal failure, dysuria, hematuria, oliguria, urinary incontinence, urinary retention, urinary tract infection
Vascular (Extracardiac) Disorders:	Flushing, gangrene, phlebitis, purpura, thrombophlebitis (deep)
Vision Disorders:	Abnormal vision, eye pain, conjunctivitis
White Cell and RES Disorders:	Agranulocytosis, granulocytopenia, leukocytosis, lymphadenopathy

Probenecid and Cimetidine: No significant effect of probenecid or cimetidine on the rate and extent of levofloxacin absorption was observed in a clinical study involving healthy volunteers. The AUC and $t_{1/2}$ of levofloxacin were 27-38% and 30% higher, respectively, while CL/F and CL_R were 21-35% lower during concomitant treatment with probenecid or cimetidine compared to levofloxacin alone. Although these differences were statistically significant, the changes were not high enough to warrant dosage adjustment for levofloxacin when probenecid or cimetidine is co-administered.

Non-steroidal anti-inflammatory drugs: The concomitant administration of a non-steroidal anti-inflammatory drug with a quinolone, including levofloxacin, may increase the risk of CNS stimulation and convulsive seizures. (See **WARNINGS** and **PRECAUTIONS: General.**)

Antidiabetic agents: Disturbances of blood glucose, including hyperglycemia and hypoglycemia, have been reported in patients treated concomitantly with quinolones and an antidiabetic agent. Therefore, careful monitoring of blood glucose is recommended when these agents are co-administered.

Carcinogenesis, Mutagenesis, Impairment of Fertility

In a lifetime bioassay in rats, levofloxacin exhibited no carcinogenic potential following daily dietary administration for 2 years; the highest dose (100 mg/kg/day) was 1.4 times the highest recommended human dose (750 mg) based upon relative body surface area. Levofloxacin did not shorten the time to tumor development of UV-induced skin tumors in hairless albino (Skh-1) mice at any levofloxacin dose level and was therefore not photo-carcinogenic under conditions of this study. Dermal levofloxacin concentrations in the hairless mice ranged from 25 to 42 μg/g at the highest levofloxacin dose level (300 mg/kg/day) used in the photo-carcinogenicity study. By comparison, dermal levofloxacin concentrations in human subjects receiving 750 mg of levofloxacin averaged approximately 11.8 μg/g at C_{max}.

Levofloxacin was not mutagenic in the following assays: Ames bacterial mutation assay (*S. typhimurium* and *E. coli*), CHO/HGPRT forward mutation assay, mouse micronucleus test, mouse dominant lethal test, rat unscheduled DNA synthesis assay, and the mouse sister chromatid exchange assay. It was positive in the in vitro chromosomal aberration (CHL cell line) and sister chromatid exchange (CHL/IU cell line) assays.

Levofloxacin caused no impairment of fertility or reproductive performance in rats at oral doses as high as 360 mg/kg/day, corresponding to 4.2 times the highest recommended human dose based upon relative body surface area and intravenous doses as high as 100 mg/kg/day, corresponding to 1.2 times the highest recommended human dose based upon relative body surface area.

Pregnancy: Teratogenic Effects. Pregnancy Category C.

Levofloxacin was not teratogenic in rats at oral doses as high as 810 mg/kg/day which corresponds to 9.4 times the highest recommended human dose based upon relative body surface area, or at intravenous doses as high as 160 mg/kg/day corresponding to 1.9 times the highest recommended human dose based upon relative body surface area. The oral dose of 810 mg/kg/day to rats caused decreased fetal body weight and increased fetal mortality. No teratogenicity was observed when rabbits were dosed orally as high as 50 mg/kg/day which corresponds to 1.1 times the highest recommended human dose based upon relative body surface area, or when dosed intravenously as high as 25 mg/kg/day, corresponding to 0.5 times the highest recommended human dose based upon relative body surface area.

There are, however, no adequate and well-controlled studies in pregnant women. Levofloxacin should be used during pregnancy only if the potential benefit justifies the potential risk to the fetus. (See **WARNINGS**.)

Nursing Mothers

Levofloxacin has not been measured in human milk. Based upon data from ofloxacin, it can be presumed that levofloxacin will be excreted in human milk. Because of the potential for serious adverse reactions from levofloxacin in nursing infants, a decision should be made whether to discontinue nursing or to discontinue the drug, taking into account the importance of the drug to the mother.

Pediatric Use

Safety and effectiveness in pediatric patients and adolescents below the age of 18 years have not been established. Quinolones, including levofloxacin, cause arthropathy and osteochondrosis in juvenile animals of several species. (See **WARNINGS**.)

Geriatric Use

In phase 3 clinical trials, 1,190 levofloxacin-treated patients (25%) were ≥65 years of age. Of these, 675 patients (14%) were between the ages of 65 and 74 and 515 patients (11%) were 75 years or older. No overall differences in safety or effectiveness were observed between these subjects and younger subjects, and other reported clinical experience has not identified differences in responses between the elderly and younger patients, but greater sensitivity of some older individuals cannot be ruled out.

Elderly patients may be more susceptible drug-associated effects on the QT interval. Therefore, precaution should be taken when using levofloxacin with concomitant drugs that can result in prolongation of the QT interval (e.g. class IA or class III antiarrhythmics) or in patients with risk factors for

Torsades de pointes (e.g. known QT prolongation, uncorrected hypokalemia). See **PRECAUTIONS: GENERAL: Torsades de Pointes.**

The pharmacokinetic properties of levofloxacin younger adults and elderly adults do not differ significantly when creatinine clearance is taken into consideration. However since the drug is known to be substantially excreted by the kidney, the risk of toxic reactions to this drug may be greater in patients with impaired renal function. Because elderly patients are more likely to have decreased renal function, care should be taken in dose selection, and it may be useful to monitor renal function.

ADVERSE REACTIONS

The incidence of drug-related adverse reactions in patients during Phase 3 clinical trials conducted in North America was 6.2%. Among patients receiving levofloxacin therapy, 4.3% discontinued levofloxacin therapy due to adverse experiences. The overall incidence, type and distribution of adverse events was similar in patients receiving levofloxacin doses of 750 mg once daily compared to patients receiving doses from 250 mg once daily to 500 mg twice daily.

In clinical trials, the following events were considered likely to be drug-related in patients receiving levofloxacin: nausea 1.2%, diarrhea 1.0%, vaginitis 0.6%, insomnia 0.4%, abdominal pain 0.4%, flatulence 0.3%, pruritus 0.3%, dizziness 0.3%, rash 0.3%, dyspepsia 0.2%, genital moniliasis 0.2%, moniliasis 0.2%, taste perversion 0.2%, vomiting 0.2%, injection site pain 0.2%, injection site reaction 0.2%, injection site inflammation 0.1%, constipation 0.1%, fungal infection 0.1%, genital pruritis 0.1%, headache 0.1%, nervousness 0.1%, rash erythematous 0.1%, urticaria 0.1%, anorexia 0.1%, somnolence 0.1%, agitation 0.1%, rash maculopapular 0.1%, tremor 0.1%, condition aggravated 0.1%, allergic reaction 0.1%.

In clinical trials, the following events occurred in >3% of patients, regardless of drug relationship:
nausea 7.1%, headache 6.2%, diarrhea 5.5%, insomnia 5.1%, constipation 3.5%.

In clinical trials, the following events occurred in 1 to 3% of patients, regardless of drug relationship:
abdominal pain 2.7%, dizziness 2.5%, vomiting 2.5%, dyspepsia 2.3%, vaginitis 1.7%, rash 1.6%, chest pain 1.4%, pruritus 1.3%, sinusitis 1.3%, dyspnea 1.4%, fatigue 1.4%, flatulence 1.2%, pain 1.6%, back pain 1.2%, rhinitis 1.2%, anxiety 1.2%, pharyngitis 1.2%.

In clinical trials, the following events, of potential medical importance, occurred at a rate of 0.1% to 0.9%, regardless of drug relationship:

[See table at top of previous page]

In clinical trials using multiple-dose therapy, ophthalmologic abnormalities, including cataracts and multiple punctate lenticular opacities, have been noted in patients undergoing treatment with other quinolones. The relationship of the drugs to these events is not presently established.

Crystalluria and cylindruria have been reported with other quinolones.

The following markedly abnormal laboratory values appeared in >2% of patients receiving levofloxacin. It is not known whether these abnormalities were caused by the drug or the underlying condition being treated.

Blood Chemistry: decreased glucose (2.2%)

Hematology: decreased lymphocytes (2.2%)

Post-Marketing Adverse Reactions

Additional adverse events reported from worldwide post-marketing experience with levofloxacin include: allergic pneumonitis, anaphylactic shock, anaphylactoid reaction, dysphonia, abnormal EEG, encephalopathy, eosinophilia, erythema multiforme, hemolytic anemia, multi-system organ failure, increased International Normalized Ratio (INR)/prothrombin time, peripheral neuropathy, rhabdomyolysis, Stevens-Johnson Syndrome, tendon rupture, torsades de pointes, vasodilation.

OVERDOSAGE

Levofloxacin exhibits a low potential for acute toxicity. Mice, rats, dogs and monkeys exhibited the following clinical signs after receiving a single high dose of levofloxacin: ataxia, ptosis, decreased locomotor activity, dyspnea, prostration, tremors, and convulsions. Doses in excess of 1500 mg/kg orally and 250 mg/kg i.v. produced significant mortality in rodents. In the event of an acute overdosage, the stomach should be emptied. The patient should be observed and appropriate hydration maintained. Levofloxacin is not efficiently removed by hemodialysis or peritoneal dialysis.

DOSAGE AND ADMINISTRATION

LEVAQUIN Injection should only be administered by intravenous infusion. It is not for intramuscular, intrathecal, intraperitoneal, or subcutaneous administration.

CAUTION: RAPID OR BOLUS INTRAVENOUS INFUSION MUST BE AVOIDED. Levofloxacin Injection should be infused intravenously slowly over a period of not less than 60 or 90 minutes, depending on the dosage. (See **PRECAUTIONS.**)

Single-use vials require dilution prior to administration. (See **PREPARATION FOR ADMINISTRATION.**)

The usual dose of LEVAQUIN Tablets or Oral Solution (25 mg/mL) is 250 mg or 500 mg or 750 mg administered orally every 24 hours, as indicated by infection and described in the following dosing chart. The usual dose of LEVAQUIN Injection is 250 mg or 500 mg administered by slow infusion over 60 minutes every 24 hours or 750 mg administered by slow infusion over 90 minutes every 24 hours, as indicated by infection and described in the following dosing chart. Levofloxacin tablets can be administered without regard to food. It is recommended that levofloxacin oral solution be taken 1 hour before or 2 hours after eating. These recommendations apply to patients with normal renal function (i.e., creatinine clearance > 80 mL/min). For patients with altered renal function see the **Patients with Impaired Renal Function** subsection. Oral doses should be administered at least two hours before or two hours after antacids containing magnesium, aluminum, as well as sucralfate, metal cations such as iron, and multivitamin preparations with zinc or Videx® (didanosine), chewable/buffered tablets or the pediatric powder for oral solution.

Patients with Normal Renal Function

Infection[1]	Unit Dose	Freq.	Duration[2]	Daily Dose
Comm. Acquired Pneumonia	500 mg	q24h	7–14 days	500 mg
Comm. Acquired Pneumonia	750 mg[3]	q24h	5 days	750 mg
Nosocomial Pneumonia	750 mg	q24h	7–14 days	750 mg
Complicated SSSI	750 mg	q24h	7–14 days	750 mg
Acute Bacterial Exacerbation of Chronic Bronchitis	500 mg	q24h	7 days	500 mg
Acute Maxillary Sinusitis	500 mg	q24h	10–14 days	500 mg
Uncomplicated SSSI	500 mg	q24h	7–10 days	500 mg
Chronic Bacterial Prostatitis	500 mg	q24h	28 days	500 mg
Complicated UTI	250 mg	q24h	10 days	250 mg
Acute pyelonephritis	250 mg	q24h	10 days	250 mg
Uncomplicated UTI	250 mg	q24h	3 days	250 mg
Inhalational anthrax (post-exposure)				
Adult[4,5]	500 mg	q24h	60 days[5]	500 mg

1 **DUE TO THE DESIGNATED PATHOGENS** (See **INDICATIONS AND USAGE.**)
2 Sequential therapy (intravenous to oral) may be instituted at the discretion of the physician.
3 Efficacy of this alternative regimen has only been documented for infections caused by penicillin-susceptible *Streptococcus pneumoniae, (excluding MDRSP), Haemophilius influenzae, Haemophilus parainfluenzae, Mycoplasma pneumoniae* and *Chlamydia pneumoniae*.
4 Drug administration should begin as soon as possible after suspected or confirmed exposure to aerosolized *B. anthracis*. This indication is based on a surrogate endpoint. Levofloxacin plasma concentrations achieved in humans are reasonably likely to predict clinical benefit (See **CLINICAL PHARMACOLOGY** and **ADDITIONAL INFORMATION – INHALATIONAL ANTHRAX**).
5 The safety of levofloxacin in adults for durations of therapy beyond 28 days has not been studied. Prolonged levofloxacin therapy in adults should only be used when the benefit outweighs the risk (See **ADDITIONAL INFORMATION – INHALATIONAL ANTHRAX**).

Patients with Impaired Renal Function

Renal Status	Initial Dose	Subsequent Dose
Acute Bacterial Exacerbation of Chronic Bronchitis/Comm. Acquired Pneumonia/Acute Maxillary Sinusitis/ Uncomplicated SSSI/Chronic Bacterial Prostatitis		
CL_{CR} from 50 to 80 mL/min	No dosage adjustment required	
CL_{CR} from 20 to 49 mL/min	500 mg	250 mg q24h
CL_{CR} from 10 to 19 mL/min	500 mg	250 mg q48h
Hemodialysis	500 mg	250 mg q48h
CAPD	500 mg	250 mg q48h
Complicated SSSI/Nosocomial Pneumonia/Comm. Acquired Pneumonia		
CL_{CR} from 50 to 80 mL/min	No dosage adjustment required	
CL_{CR} from 20 to 49 mL/min	750 mg	750 mg q48h
CL_{CR} from 10 to 19 mL/min	750 mg	500 mg q48h
Hemodialysis	750 mg	500 mg q48h
CAPD	750 mg	500 mg q48h
Complicated UTI/Acute Pyelonephritis		
CL_{CR} ≥20 mL/min	No dosage adjustment required	
CL_{CR} from 10 to 19 mL/min	250 mg	250 mg q48h
Uncomplicated UTI	No dosage adjustment required	

CL_{CR}=creatinine clearances
CAPD=chronic ambulatory peritoneal dialysis

[See first table above]
[See second table above]

When only the serum creatinine is known, the following formula may be used to estimate creatinine clearance.

Men: Creatinine Clearance (mL/min) =
$$\frac{\text{Weight (kg)} \times (140 - \text{age})}{72 \times \text{serum creatinine (mg/dL)}}$$
Women: 0.85 × the value calculated for men.

The serum creatinine should represent a steady state of renal function.

Preparation of Levofloxacin Injection for Administration

LEVAQUIN Injection in Single-Use Vials: LEVAQUIN Injection is supplied in single-use vials containing a concentrated levofloxacin solution with the equivalent of 500 mg (20 mL vial) and 750 mg (30 mL vial) of levofloxacin in Water for Injection, USP. The 20 mL and 30 mL vials each contain 25 mg of levofloxacin/mL. **THESE LEVAQUIN INJECTION SINGLE-USE VIALS MUST BE FURTHER DILUTED WITH AN APPROPRIATE SOLUTION PRIOR TO INTRAVENOUS ADMINISTRATION.** (See **COMPATIBLE INTRAVENOUS SOLUTIONS.**) The concentration of the resulting diluted solution should be 5 mg/mL prior to administration.

This intravenous drug product should be inspected visually for particulate matter prior to administration. Samples containing visible particles should be discarded.

Since no preservative or bacteriostatic agent is present in this product, aseptic technique must be used in preparation of the final intravenous solution. **Since the vials are for single-use only, any unused portion remaining in the vial should be discarded. When used to prepare two 250 mg doses from the 20 mL vial containing 500 mg of levofloxacin, the full content of the vial should be withdrawn at once using a single-entry procedure, and a second dose should be prepared and stored for subsequent use.** (See **Stability LEVAQUIN Injection Following Dilution.**)

Since only limited data are available on the compatibility of levofloxacin intravenous injection with other intravenous substances, **additives or other medications should not be added to LEVAQUIN Injection in single-use vials or infused simultaneously through the same intravenous line.** If the same intravenous line is used for sequential infusion of several different drugs, the line should be flushed before and after infusion of LEVAQUIN Injection with an infusion solution compatible with LEVAQUIN Injection and with any other drug(s) administered via this common line.

Prepare the desired dosage of levofloxacin according to the following chart:

[See first table at top of next page]

For example, to prepare a 500 mg dose using the 20 mL vial (25 mg/mL), withdraw 20 mL and dilute with a compatible intravenous solution to a total volume of 100 mL.

Compatible Intravenous Solutions: Any of the following intravenous solutions may be used to prepare a 5 mg/mL levofloxacin solution with the approximate pH values:

Intravenous Fluids	Final pH of LEVAQUIN Solution
0.9% Sodium Chloride Injection, USP	4.71
5% Dextrose Injection, USP	4.58
5% Dextrose/0.9% NaCl Injection	4.62
5% Dextrose in Lactated Ringers	4.92
Plasma-Lyte® 56/5% Dextrose Injection	5.03
5% Dextrose, 0.45% Sodium Chloride, and 0.15% Potassium Chloride Injection	4.61
Sodium Lactate Injection (M/6)	5.54

LEVAQUIN Injection Premix in Single-Use Flexible Containers (5 mg/mL): LEVAQUIN Injection is also supplied in flexible containers containing a premixed, ready-to-use levofloxacin solution in D_5W for single-use. The fill volume is either 50 or 100 mL for the 100 mL flexible container or 150 mL for the 150 mL container. **NO FURTHER DILUTION OF THESE PREPARATIONS IS NECESSARY. Consequently each 100 mL and 150 mL premix flexible container already contains a dilute solution with the equivalent of 250 mg or 500 mg (100 mL container), and 750 mg of levofloxacin**

Continued on next page

Levaquin—Cont.

(150 mL container) in 5% Dextrose (D₅W). The concentration of each presentation is 5 mg/mL of levofloxacin solution.

This parenteral drug product should be inspected visually for particulate matter prior to administration. Samples containing visible particles should be discarded.

Since the premix flexible containers are for single-use only, any unused portion should be discarded.

Since only limited data are available on the compatibility of levofloxacin intravenous injection with other intravenous substances, **additives or other medications should not be added to LEVAQUIN Injection in flexible containers or infused simultaneously through the same intravenous line.** If the same intravenous line is used for sequential infusion of several different drugs, the line should be flushed before and after infusion of LEVAQUIN Injection with an infusion solution compatible with LEVAQUIN Injection and with any other drug(s) administered via this common line.

Instructions for the Use of LEVAQUIN Injection Premix in Flexible Containers

To open:
1. Tear outer wrap at the notch and remove solution container.
2. Check the container for minute leaks by squeezing the inner bag firmly. If leaks are found, or if the seal is not intact, discard the solution, as the sterility may be compromised.
3. Do not use if the solution is cloudy or a precipitate is present.
4. Use sterile equipment.
5. **WARNING: Do not use flexible containers in series connections.** Such use could result in air embolism due to residual air being drawn from the primary container before administration of the fluid from the secondary container is complete.

Preparation for administration:
1. Close flow control clamp of administration set.
2. Remove cover from port at bottom of container.
3. Insert piercing pin of administration set into port with a twisting motion until the pin is firmly seated. **NOTE: See full directions on administration set carton.**
4. Suspend container from hanger.
5. Squeeze and release drip chamber to establish proper fluid level in chamber during infusion of LEVAQUIN Injection in Premix Flexible Containers.
6. Open flow control clamp to expel air from set. Close clamp.
7. Regulate rate of administration with flow control clamp.

Stability of LEVAQUIN Injection as Supplied
When stored under recommended conditions, LEVAQUIN Injection, as supplied in 20 mL and 30 mL vials, or 100 mL and 150 mL flexible containers, is stable through the expiration date printed on the label.

Stability of LEVAQUIN Injection Following Dilution
LEVAQUIN Injection, when diluted in a compatible intravenous fluid to a concentration of 5 mg/mL, is stable for 72 hours when stored at or below 25°C (77°F) and for 14 days when stored under refrigeration at 5°C (41°F) in plastic intravenous containers. Solutions that are diluted in a compatible intravenous solution and frozen in glass bottles or plastic intravenous containers are stable for 6 months when stored at -20°C (-4°F). **THAW FROZEN SOLUTIONS AT ROOM TEMPERATURE 25°C (77°F) OR IN A REFRIGERATOR 8°C (46°F). DO NOT FORCE THAW BY MICROWAVE IRRADIATION OR WATER BATH IMMERSION. DO NOT REFREEZE AFTER INITIAL THAWING.**

HOW SUPPLIED
LEVAQUIN Tablets
LEVAQUIN (levofloxacin) Tablets are supplied as 250, 500, and 750 mg capsule-shaped, coated tablets. LEVAQUIN Tablets are packaged in bottles and in unit-dose blister strips in the following configurations:

250 mg tablets are terra cotta pink and are imprinted: "LEVAQUIN" on one side and "250" on the other side.

    bottles of 50 (NDC 0045-1520-50)

    unit-dose/100 tablets (NDC 0045-1520-10)

500 mg tablets are peach and are imprinted: "LEVAQUIN" on one side and "500" on the other side.

    bottles of 50 (NDC 0045-1525-50)

    unit-dose/100 tablets (NDC 0045-1525-10)

750 mg tablets are white and are imprinted: "LEVAQUIN" on one side and "750" on the other side.

    bottles of 20 (NDC 0045-1530-20)

    unit-dose/100 tablets (NDC 0045-1530-10)

    LEVA-Pak 5 tablets (NDC 0045-1530-05)

LEVAQUIN Tablets should be stored at 15° to 30°C (59° to 86°F) in well-closed containers.

LEVAQUIN Tablets are manufactured for OMP DIVISION, ORTHO-McNEIL PHARMACEUTICAL, INC. by Janssen Ortho LLC, Gurabo, Puerto Rico 00778.

LEVAQUIN Oral Solution
LEVAQUIN Oral Solution is supplied in a 16 oz. multi-use bottle (NDC 0045-1515-01). Each bottle contains 480 mL of the 25-mg/mL-levofloxacin oral solution.

LEVAQUIN Oral Solution should be stored at 25°C (77°F); excursions permitted to 15°-30°C (59° to 86°F) [refer to USP controlled room temperature].

LEVAQUIN Oral Solution is manufactured for OMP DIVISION, ORTHO-McNEIL PHARMACEUTICAL, INC. by Ortho Pharmaceutical in Manati, Puerto Rico, 00674.

Desired Dosage Strength	From Appropriate Vial, Withdraw Volume	Volume of Diluent	Infusion Time
250 mg	10 mL (20 mL Vial)	40 mL	60 min
500 mg	20 mL (20 mL Vial)	80 mL	60 min
750 mg	30 mL (30 mL Vial)	120 mL	90 min

Pathogen	N	Levofloxacin No. (%) of Patients Microbiologic/Clinical Outcomes	N	Imipenem/Cilastatin No. (%) of Patients Microbiologic/Clinical Outcomes
MSSA[a]	21	14 (66.7)/ 13 (61.9)	19	13 (68.4)/ 15 (78.9)
P. aeruginosa[b]	17	10 (58.8)/ 11 (64.7)	17	5 (29.4)/ 7 (41.2)
S. marcescens	11	9 (81.8)/ 7 (63.6)	7	2 (28.6)/ 3 (42.9)
E. coli	12	10 (83.3)/ 7 (58.3)	11	7 (63.6)/ 8 (72.7)
K. pneumoniae[c]	11	9 (81.8)/ 5 (45.5)	7	6 (85.7)/ 3 (42.9)
H. influenzae	16	13 (81.3)/ 10 (62.5)	15	14 (93.3)/ 11 (73.3)
S. pneumoniae	4	3 (75.0)/ 3 (75.0)	7	5 (71.4)/ 4 (57.1)

[a]Methicillin-susceptible S. aureus
[b]See above text for use of combination therapy.
[c]The observed differences in rates for the clinical and microbiological outcomes may reflect other factors that were not accounted for in the study.

LEVAQUIN Injection
Single-Use Vials: LEVAQUIN (levofloxacin) Injection is supplied in single-use vials. Each vial contains a concentrated solution with the equivalent of 500 mg of levofloxacin in 20 mL vials and 750 mg of levofloxacin in 30 mL vials.
25 mg/mL, 20 mL vials (NDC 0045-0069-51)
25 mg/mL, 30 mL vials (NDC 0045-0065-55)
LEVAQUIN Injection in Single-Use Vials should be stored at controlled room temperature and protected from light.
LEVAQUIN Injection in Single-Use Vials is manufactured for OMP DIVISION, ORTHO-McNEIL PHARMACEUTICAL, INC. by OMJ Pharmaceuticals, Inc., San German, Puerto Rico 00683.
Premix in Flexible Containers: LEVAQUIN (levofloxacin in 5% dextrose) Injection is supplied as a single-use, premixed solution in flexible containers. Each bag contains a dilute solution with the equivalent of 250, 500, or 750 mg of levofloxacin, respectively, in 5% Dextrose (D₅W).
5 mg/mL (250 mg), 100 mL flexible container, (NDC 0045-0067-01)
5 mg/mL (500 mg), 100 mL flexible container, 100 mL fill (NDC 0045-0068-01)
5 mg/mL (750 mg), 150 mL flexible container, 150 mL fill (NDC 0045-0066-01)
LEVAQUIN Injection Premix in Flexible Containers should be stored at or below 25°C (77°F); however, brief exposure up to 40°C (104°F) does not adversely affect the product. Avoid excessive heat and protect from freezing and light.
LEVAQUIN Injection Premix in Flexible Containers is manufactured for OMP DIVISION, ORTHO-McNEIL PHARMACEUTICAL, INC. by ABBOTT Laboratories, North Chicago, IL 60064.

CLINICAL STUDIES
Nosocomial Pneumonia
Adult patients with clinically and radiologically documented nosocomial pneumonia were enrolled in a multi-center, randomized, open-label study comparing intravenous levofloxacin (750 mg once daily) followed by oral levofloxacin (750 mg once daily) for a total of 7-15 days to intravenous imipenem/cilastatin (500-1000 mg q6-8 hours daily) followed by oral ciprofloxacin (750 mg q12 hours daily) for a total of 7-15 days. Levofloxacin-treated patients received an average of 7 days of intravenous therapy (range: 1-16 days); comparator-treated patients received an average of 8 days of intravenous therapy (range: 1–19 days).
Overall, in the clinically and microbiologically evaluable population, adjunctive therapy was empirically initiated at study entry in 56 of 93 (60.2%) patients in the levofloxacin arm and 53 of 94 (56.4%) patients in the comparator arm. The average duration of adjunctive therapy was 7 days in the levofloxacin arm and 7 days in the comparator. In clinically and microbiologically evaluable patients with documented *Pseudomonas aeruginosa* infection, 15 of 17 (88.2%) received ceftazidime (N=11) or piperacillin/tazobactam (N=4) in the levofloxacin arm and 16 of 17 (94.1%) received an aminoglycoside in the comparator arm. Overall, in clinically and microbiologically evaluable patients, vancomycin was added to the treatment regimen of 37 of 93 (39.8%) patients in the levofloxacin arm and 28 of 94 (29.8%) patients in the comparator arm for suspected methicillin-resistant *S. aureus* infection.
Clinical success rates in clinically and microbiologically evaluable patients at the posttherapy visit (primary study endpoint assessed on day 3-15 after completing therapy) were 58.1% for levofloxacin and 60.6% for comparator. The 95% CI for the difference of response rates (levofloxacin minus comparator) was [-17.2, 12.0]. The microbiological eradication rates at the posttherapy visit were 66.7% for levofloxacin and 60.6% for comparator. The 95% CI for the difference of eradication rates (levofloxacin minus comparator) was [-8.3, 20.3]. Clinical success and microbiological eradication rates by pathogen were as follows:
[See second table above]
Community-Acquired Bacterial Pneumonia
7 to 14 Day Treatment Regimen
Adult inpatients and outpatients with a diagnosis of community-acquired bacterial pneumonia were evaluated in two pivotal clinical studies. In the first study, 590 patients were enrolled in a prospective, multi-center, unblinded randomized trial comparing levofloxacin 500 mg once daily orally or intravenously for 7 to 14 days to ceftriaxone 1 to 2 grams intravenously once or in equally divided doses twice daily followed by cefuroxime axetil 500 mg orally twice daily for a total of 7 to 14 days. Patients assigned to treatment with the control regimen were allowed to receive erythromycin (or doxycycline if intolerant of erythromycin) if an infection due to atypical pathogens was suspected or proven. Clinical and microbiologic evaluations were performed during treatment, 5 to 7 days posttherapy, and 3 to 4 weeks posttherapy. Clinical success (cure plus improvement) with levofloxacin at 5 to 7 days posttherapy, the primary efficacy variable in this study, was superior (95%) to the control group (83%). The 95% CI for the difference of response rates (levofloxacin minus comparator) was [-6, 19]. In the second study, 264 patients were enrolled in a prospective, multi-center, non-comparative trial of 500 mg levofloxacin administered orally or intravenously once daily for 7 to 14 days. Clinical success for clinically evaluable patients was 93%. For both studies, the clinical success rate in patients with atypical pneumonia due to *Chlamydia pneumoniae, Mycoplasma pneumoniae,* and *Legionella pneumophila* were 96%, 96%, and 70%, respectively. Microbiologic eradication rates across both studies were as follows:

Pathogen	No. Pathogens	Microbiologic Eradication Rate (%)
H. influenzae	55	98
S. pneumoniae	83	95
S. aureus	17	88
M. catarrhalis	18	94
H. parainfluenzae	19	95
K. pneumoniae	10	100.0

Community-Acquired Bacterial Pneumonia
5-Day Treatment Regimen
To evaluate the safety and efficacy of higher dose and shorter course of levofloxacin, 528 outpatient and hospitalized adults with clinically and radiologically determined mild to severe community-acquired pneumonia were evaluated in a double-blind, randomized, prospective, multi-center study comparing levofloxacin 750 mg, i.v. or p.o., q.d. for five days or levofloxacin 500 mg i.v. or p.o., q.d. for 10 days.
Clinical success rates (cure plus improvement) in the clinically evaluable population were 90.9% in the levofloxacin 750 mg group and 91.1% in the levofloxacin 500 mg group. The 95% CI for the difference of response rates (levofloxacin 750 minus levofloxacin 500) was [-5.9, 5.4]. In the clinically evaluable population (31-38 days after enrollment) pneumonia was observed in 7 out of 151 patients in the levofloxacin 750 mg group and 2 out of 147 patients in the levofloxacin 500 mg group. Given the small numbers observed, the significance of this finding can not be determined statistically. The microbiological efficacy of the 5-day regimen was documented for infections listed in the table below.

	Eradication rate
Penicillin susceptible S. pneumoniae	19/20
Haemophilus influenzae	12/12
Haemophilus parainfluenzae	10/10
Mycoplasma pneumoniae	26/27
Chlamydia pneumoniae	13/15

Community-Acquired Pneumonia Due to Multi-Drug Resistant Streptococcus pneumoniae (MDRSP)*
LEVAQUIN was effective for the treatment of community-acquired pneumonia caused by multi-drug resistant *Streptococcus pneumoniae* (MDRSP)*. Of 40 microbiologically evaluable patients with MDRSP isolates, 38 patients (95.0%) achieved clinical and bacteriologic success at posttherapy. The clinical and bacterial success rates are shown in the table below.
*MDRSP (Multi-drug resistant *Streptococcus pneumoniae*) isolates are strains resistant to two or more of the following

antibiotics: penicillin (MIC ≥2 μg/mL), 2nd generation cephalosporins, e.g., cefuroxime, macrolides, tetracyclines and trimethoprim/ sulfamethoxazole.
[See table above]
Not all isolates were resistant to all antimicrobial classes tested. Success and eradication rates are summarized in the table below.

Resistant *Streptococcus pneumoniae* clinical success and bacteriologic eradication rates

S. pn with MDRSP	Clinical Success	Bacteriologic Eradication
Resistant to 2	17/18 (94.4%)	17/18 (94.4%)
Resistant to 3	14/15 (93.3%)	14/15 (93.3%)
Resistant to 4	7/7 (100%)	7/7 (100%)
Resistant to 5	0	0
Bacteremias with MDRSP	8/9 (89%)	8/9 (89%)

Complicated Skin and Skin Structure Infections
Three hundred ninety-nine patients were enrolled in an open-label, randomized, comparative study for complicated skin and skin structure infections. The patients were randomized to receive either levofloxacin 750 mg QD (IV followed by oral), or an approved comparator for a median of 10 ± 4.7 days. As is expected in complicated skin and skin structure infections, surgical procedures were performed in the levofloxacin and comparator groups. Surgery (incision and drainage or debridement) was performed on 45% of the levofloxacin treated patients and 44% of the comparator treated patients, either shortly before or during antibiotic treatment and formed an integral part of therapy for this indication.
Among those who could be evaluated clinically 2-5 days after completion of study drug, overall success rates (improved or cured) were 116/138 (84.1%) for patients treated with levofloxacin and 106/132 (80.3%) for patients treated with the comparator.
Success rates varied with the type of diagnosis ranging from 68% in patients with infected ulcers to 90% in patients with infected wounds and abscesses. These rates were equivalent to those seen with comparator drugs.

Chronic Bacterial Prostatitis
Adult patients with a clinical diagnosis of prostatitis and microbiological culture results from urine sample collected after prostatic massage (VB_3) or expressed prostatic secretion (EPS) specimens obtained via the Meares-Stamey procedure were enrolled in a multicenter, randomized, double-blind study comparing oral levofloxacin 500 mg, once daily for a total of 28 days to oral ciprofloxacin 500 mg, twice daily for a total of 28 days. The primary efficacy endpoint was microbiologic efficacy in microbiologically evaluable patients. A total of 136 and 125 microbiologically evaluable patients were enrolled in the levofloxacin and ciprofloxacin groups, respectively. The microbiologic eradication rate by patient infection at 5-18 days after completion of therapy was 75.0% in the levofloxacin group and 76.8% in the ciprofloxacin group (95% CI [-12.58, 8.98] for levofloxacin minus ciprofloxacin). The overall eradication rates for pathogens of interest are presented below:

	Levofloxacin (N=136)		Ciprofloxacin (N=125)	
Pathogen	N	Eradication	N	Eradication
E. coli	15	14 (93.3%)	11	9 (81.8%)
E. faecalis	54	39 (72.2%)	44	33 (75.0%)
**S. epidermidis*	11	9 (81.8%)	14	11 (78.6%)

*Eradication rates shown are for patients who had a sole pathogen only; mixed cultures were excluded.

Eradication rates for *S. epidermidis* when found with other co-pathogens are consistent with rates seen in pure isolates.
Clinical success (cure + improvement with no need for further antibiotic therapy) rates in microbiologically evaluable population 5-18 days after completion of therapy were 75.0% for levofloxacin-treated patients and 72.8% for ciprofloxacin-treated patients (95% CI [-8.87, 13.27] for levofloxacin minus ciprofloxacin). Clinical long-term success (24-45 days after completion of therapy) rates were 66.7% for the levofloxacin-treated patients and 76.9% for the ciprofloxacin-treated patients (95% CI [-23.40, 2.89] for levofloxacin minus ciprofloxacin).

ADDITIONAL INFORMATION - INHALATION ANTHRAX
The mean plasma concentrations of levofloxacin associated with a statistically significant improvement in survival over placebo in the rhesus monkey model of inhalational anthrax are reached or exceeded in adult patients receiving oral and intravenous regimens (See DOSAGE AND ADMINISTRATION).
Levofloxacin pharmacokinetics were evaluated in various populations. Levofloxacin plasma concentrations achieved in humans serve as a surrogate endpoint reasonably likely to predict clinical benefit and provide the basis for this indication. The mean (±s.d.) steady-state peak plasma concentration in human adults receiving 500 mg orally or intravenously once daily is 5.1 ± 0.8 and 6.2 ± 1.0 μg/mL, respectively; and the corresponding total exposure is 47.9 ± 6.8 and 48.3 ± 5.4 μg•h/mL, respectively.
In adults, the safety of levofloxacin for treatment durations of up to 28 days is well characterized. However, information pertaining to extended use at 500 mg daily up to 60 days is limited.
A placebo-controlled animal study in rhesus monkeys exposed to an inhaled mean dose of 49 LD_{50} (~2.7 X 10^6) spores (range 17-118 LD_{50}) of *B. anthracis* (Ames strain) was conducted. The minimal inhibitory concentration (MIC) of levofloxacin for the anthrax strain used in this study was 0.125 μg/mL. In the animals studied, mean plasma concentrations of levofloxacin achieved at expected T_{max} (1 hour post-dose) following oral dosing to steady state ranged from 2.79 to 4.87 μg/mL. Mean steady state trough concentrations at 24 hours post-dose ranged from 0.107 to 0.164 μg/mL. Mortality due to anthrax for animals that received a 30 day regimen of oral levofloxacin beginning 24 hrs post exposure was significantly lower (1/10), compared to the placebo group (9/10) [P = 0.0011, 2-sided Fisher's Exact Test]. The one levofloxacin treated animal that died of anthrax did so following the 30-day drug administration period.

Clinical and Bacteriological Success Rates for Levofloxacin-Treated MDRSP* CAP Patients (Population: Valid for Efficacy)

Screening Susceptiblity	Clinical Success		Bacteriological Success**	
	n/N[a]	%	n/N[b]	%
Penicillin-resistant	16/17	94.1	16/17	94.1
2nd generation cephalosporin resistant	31/32	96.9	31/32	96.9
Macrolide-resistant	28/29	96.6	28/29	96.6
Trimethoprim/Sulfamethoxazole resistant	17/19	89.5	17/19	89.5
Tetracycline-resistant	12/12	100	12/12	100

[a] n = the number of microbiologically evaluable patients who were clinical successes; N = number of microbiologically evaluable patients in the designated resistance group.
[b] n = the number of MDRSP isolates eradicated or presumed eradicated in microbiologically evaluable patients; N = number of MDRSP isolates in a designated resistance group.
* MDRSP (Multi-drug resistant *Streptococcus pneumoniae*) isolates are strains resistant to two or more of the following antibiotics: penicillin (MIC ≥2 μg/mL), 2nd generation cephalosporins, e.g., cefuroxime, macrolides, tetracyclines and trimethoprim/ sulfamethoxazole.
** One patient had a respiratory isolate that was resistant to tetracycline, cefuroxime, macrolides and TMP/SMX and intermediate to penicillin and a blood isolate that was intermediate to penicillin and cefuroxime and resistant to the other classes. The patient is included in the database based on respiratory isolate.

ANIMAL PHARMACOLOGY
Levofloxacin and other quinolones have been shown to cause arthropathy in immature animals of most species tested. (See **WARNINGS**.) In immature dogs (4-5 months old), oral doses of 10 mg/kg/day for 7 days and intravenous doses of 4 mg/kg/day for 14 days of levofloxacin resulted in arthropathic lesions. Administration at oral doses of 300 mg/kg/day for 7 days and intravenous doses of 60 mg/kg/day for 4 weeks produced arthropathy in juvenile rats. Three-month old beagle dogs dosed orally with levofloxacin for 8 or 9 consecutive days, with an 18-week recovery period, exhibited musculoskeletal clinical signs by the final dose at dose levels ≥ 2.5 mg/kg (approximately >0.2-fold the potential therapeutic dose (1500 mg q24h) based upon plasma AUC comparisons). Synovitis and articular cartilage lesions were observed at the 10 and 40 mg/kg dose levels (equivalent to and 3-fold greater than the potential therapeutic dose, respectively). All musculoskeletal clinical signs were resolved by week 5 of recovery; synovitis was resolved by the end of the 18-week recovery period; whereas, articular cartilage erosions and chondropathy persisted.
When tested in a mouse ear swelling bioassay, levofloxacin exhibited phototoxicity similar in magnitude to ofloxacin, but less phototoxicity than other quinolones.
While crystalluria has been observed in some intravenous rat studies, urinary crystals are not formed in the bladder, being present only after micturition and are not associated with nephrotoxicity.
In mice, the CNS stimulatory effect of quinolones is enhanced by concomitant administration of non-steroidal anti-inflammatory drugs.
In dogs, levofloxacin administered at 6 mg/kg or higher by rapid intravenous injection produced hypotensive effects. These effects were considered to be related to histamine release.
In vitro and in vivo studies in animals indicate that levofloxacin is neither an enzyme inducer or inhibitor in the human therapeutic plasma concentration range; therefore, no drug metabolizing enzyme-related interactions with other drugs or agents are anticipated.

REFERENCES

1. National Committee for Clinical Laboratory Standards. Methods for Dilution Antimicrobial Susceptibility Tests for Bacteria That Grow Aerobically. Sixth Edition. Approved Standard NCCLS Document M7-A6,Vol. 23, No. 2, NCCLS, Wayne, PA, January, 2003.
2. National Committee for Clinical Laboratory Standards. Performance Standards for Antimicrobial Disk Susceptibility Tests. Eighth Edition. Approved Standard NCCLS Document M2-A8, Vol. 23, No. 1, NCCLS, Wayne, PA, January, 2003.

Patient Information About:
LEVAQUIN®
(levofloxacin) Tablets
250 mg Tablets, 500 mg Tablets, and 750 mg Tablets and LEVAQUIN® (levofloxacin) Oral Solution, 25 mg/mL

This leaflet contains important information about LEVAQUIN® (levofloxacin), and should be read completely before you begin treatment. This leaflet does not take the place of discussions with your doctor or health care professional about your medical condition or your treatment. This leaflet does not list all benefits and risks of LEVAQUIN®. The medicine described here can be prescribed only by a licensed health care professional. If you have any questions about LEVAQUIN® talk to your health care professional. Only your health care professional can determine if LEVAQUIN® is right for you.

What is LEVAQUIN®?
LEVAQUIN® is a quinolone antibiotic used to treat lung, sinus, skin, and urinary tract infections caused by certain germs called bacteria. LEVAQUIN® kills many of the types of bacteria that can infect the lungs, sinuses, skin, and urinary tract and has been shown in a large number of clinical trials to be safe and effective for the treatment of bacterial infections.
Sometimes viruses rather than bacteria may infect the lungs and sinuses (for example the common cold). LEVAQUIN®, like other antibiotics, does not kill viruses.
You should contact your health care professional if you think that your condition is not improving while taking LEVAQUIN®. LEVAQUIN® Tablets are terra cotta pink for the 250 mg tablet, peach colored for the 500 mg tablet, or white for the 750 mg tablet. The appearance of LEVAQUIN® Oral Solution may range from clear yellow to clear greenish-yellow.

How and when should I take LEVAQUIN®?
LEVAQUIN® should be taken once a day for 3, 5, 7, 10, 14 or 28 days depending on your prescription. LEVAQUIN® Tablets should be swallowed and may be taken with or without food. LEVAQUIN® Oral Solution should be taken 1 hour before or 2 hours after eating. Try to take the tablet and oral solution at the same time each day and drink fluids liberally.
You may begin to feel better quickly; however, in order to make sure that all bacteria are killed, you should complete the full course of medication. Do not take more than the prescribed dose of LEVAQUIN® even if you missed a dose by mistake. You should not take a double dose.

Who should not take LEVAQUIN®?
You should not take LEVAQUIN® if you have ever had a severe allergic reaction to any of the group of antibiotics known as "quinolones" such as ciprofloxacin. Serious and occasionally fatal allergic reactions have been reported in patients receiving therapy with quinolones, including LEVAQUIN®.
If you are pregnant or are planning to become pregnant while taking LEVAQUIN®, talk to your health care professional before taking this medication. LEVAQUIN® is not recommended for use during pregnancy or nursing, as the effects on the unborn child or nursing infant are unknown.
LEVAQUIN® is not recommended for children.

What are possible side effects of LEVAQUIN®?
LEVAQUIN® is generally well tolerated. The most common side effects caused by LEVAQUIN®, which are usually mild, include nausea, diarrhea, itching, abdominal pain, dizziness, flatulence, rash and vaginitis in women.
You should be careful about driving or operating machinery until you are sure LEVAQUIN® is not causing dizziness.
Allergic reactions have been reported in patients receiving quinolones including LEVAQUIN®, even after just one dose. If you develop hives, skin rash or other symptoms of an allergic reaction, you should stop taking this medication and call your health care professional.
Ruptures of shoulder, hand, or Achilles tendons have been reported in patients receiving quinolones, including LEVAQUIN®. If you develop pain, swelling, or rupture of a tendon you should stop taking LEVAQUIN® and contact your health care professional.
Some quinolone antibiotics have been associated with the development of phototoxicity ("sunburns" and "blistering sunburns") following exposure to sunlight or other sources of ultraviolet light such as artificial ultraviolet light used in tanning salons. LEVAQUIN® has been infrequently associated with phototoxicity. You should avoid excessive exposure to sunlight or artificial ultraviolet light while you are taking LEVAQUIN®.
If you have diabetes and you develop a hypoglycemic reaction while on LEVAQUIN®, you should stop taking LEVAQUIN® and call your health care professional.
Convulsions have been reported in patients receiving quinolone antibiotics including LEVAQUIN®. If you have experienced convulsions in the past, be sure to let your physician know that you have a history of convulsions.
Quinolones, including LEVAQUIN®, may also cause central nervous system stimulation which may lead to tremors, restlessness, anxiety, lightheadedness, confusion, hallucinations, paranoia, depression, nightmares, insomnia, and rarely, suicidal thoughts or acts.

Continued on next page

Levaquin—Cont.

If you notice any side effects not mentioned in this leaflet or you have concerns about the side effects you are experiencing, please inform your health care professional.
For more complete information regarding levofloxacin, please refer to the full prescribing information, which may be obtained from your health care professional, pharmacist, or the Physicians Desk Reference (PDR).

What about other medicines I am taking?
Taking warfarin (Coumadin®) and LEVAQUIN® together can further predispose you to the development of bleeding problems. If you take warfarin, be sure to tell your health care professional.
Many antacids and multivitamins may interfere with the absorption of LEVAQUIN® and may prevent it from working properly. You should take LEVAQUIN® either 2 hours before or 2 hours after taking these products.
It is important to let your health care professional know all of the medicines you are using.

Other information
Take your dose of LEVAQUIN® once a day.
Complete the course of medication even if you are feeling better.
Keep this medication out of the reach of children.
This information does not take the place of discussions with your doctor or health care professional about your medical condition or your treatment.

ORTHO-McNEIL
OMP DIVISION
ORTHO-McNEIL PHARMACEUTICAL, INC.
Raritan, New Jersey, USA 08869
U.S. Patent No. 5,053,407.
© OMP 2000 Revised November 2004 7518211

TOPAMAX® ℞
[*tō-pă-măks*]
(topiramate)
Tablets

TOPAMAX® ℞
(topiramate capsules)
Sprinkle Capsules

Prescribing Information

Prescribing information for this product, which appears on pages 2541–2548 of the 2005 PDR, has been completely revised as follows. Please write "See Supplement A" next to the product heading.

DESCRIPTION

Topiramate is a sulfamate-substituted monosaccharide. TOPAMAX® (topiramate) Tablets are available as 25 mg, 50 mg, 100 mg, and 200 mg round tablets for oral administration. TOPAMAX® (topiramate capsules) Sprinkle Capsules are available as 15 mg and 25 mg sprinkle capsules for oral administration as whole capsules or opened and sprinkled onto soft food.
Topiramate is a white crystalline powder with a bitter taste. Topiramate is most soluble in alkaline solutions containing sodium hydroxide or sodium phosphate and having a pH of 9 to 10. It is freely soluble in acetone, chloroform, dimethylsulfoxide, and ethanol. The solubility in water is 9.8 mg/mL. Its saturated solution has a pH of 6.3. Topiramate has the molecular formula $C_{12}H_{21}NO_8S$ and a molecular weight of 339.37. Topiramate is designated chemically as 2,3:4,5-Di-*O*-isopropylidene-β-D-fructopyranose sulfamate and has the following structural formula:

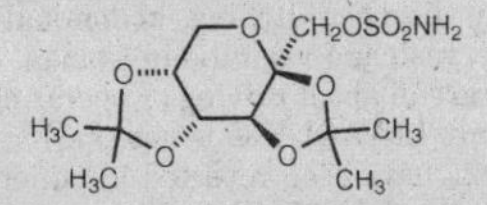

TOPAMAX® (topiramate) Tablets contain the following inactive ingredients: lactose monohydrate, pregelatinized starch, microcrystalline cellulose, sodium starch glycolate, magnesium stearate, purified water, carnauba wax, hypromellose, titanium dioxide, polyethylene glycol, synthetic iron oxide (50, 100, and 200 mg tablets) and polysorbate 80.
TOPAMAX® (topiramate capsules) Sprinkle Capsules contain topiramate coated beads in a hard gelatin capsule. The inactive ingredients are: sugar spheres (sucrose and starch), povidone, cellulose acetate, gelatin, silicone dioxide, sodium lauryl sulfate, titanium dioxide, and black pharmaceutical ink.

CLINICAL PHARMACOLOGY

Mechanism of Action:
The precise mechanisms by which topiramate exerts its anticonvulsant and migraine prophylaxis effects are unknown; however, preclinical studies have revealed four properties that may contribute to topiramate's efficacy for epilepsy and migraine prophylaxis. Electrophysiological and biochemical evidence suggests that topiramate, at pharmacologically relevant concentrations, blocks voltage-dependent sodium channels, augments the activity of the neurotransmitter gamma-aminobutyrate at some subtypes of the GABA-A receptor, antagonizes the AMPA/kainate subtype of the glutamate receptor, and inhibits the carbonic anhydrase enzyme, particularly isozymes II and IV.

Pharmacodynamics:
Topiramate has anticonvulsant activity in rat and mouse maximal electroshock seizure (MES) tests. Topiramate is only weakly effective in blocking clonic seizures induced by the $GABA_A$ receptor antagonist, pentylenetetrazole. Topiramate is also effective in rodent models of epilepsy, which include tonic and absence-like seizures in the spontaneous epileptic rat (SER) and tonic and clonic seizures induced in rats by kindling of the amygdala or by global ischemia.

Pharmacokinetics:
The sprinkle formulation is bioequivalent to the immediate release tablet formulation and, therefore, may be substituted as a therapeutic equivalent.
Absorption of topiramate is rapid, with peak plasma concentrations occurring at approximately 2 hours following a 400 mg oral dose. The relative bioavailability of topiramate from the tablet formulation is about 80% compared to a solution. The bioavailability of topiramate is not affected by food.
The pharmacokinetics of topiramate are linear with dose proportional increases in plasma concentration over the dose range studied (200 to 800 mg/day). The mean plasma elimination half-life is 21 hours after single or multiple doses. Steady state is thus reached in about 4 days in patients with normal renal function. Topiramate is 15-41% bound to human plasma proteins over the blood concentration range of 0.5-250 µg/mL. The fraction bound decreased as blood concentration increased.
Carbamazepine and phenytoin do not alter the binding of topiramate. Sodium valproate, at 500 µg/ml (a concentration 5-10 times higher than considered therapeutic for valproate) decreased the protein binding of topiramate from 23% to 13%. Topiramate does not influence the binding of sodium valproate.

Metabolism and Excretion:
Topiramate is not extensively metabolized and is primarily eliminated unchanged in the urine (approximately 70% of an administered dose). Six metabolites have been identified in humans, none of which constitutes more than 5% of an administered dose. The metabolites are formed via hydroxylation, hydrolysis, and glucuronidation. There is evidence of renal tubular reabsorption of topiramate. In rats, given probenecid to inhibit tubular reabsorption, along with topiramate, a significant increase in renal clearance of topiramate was observed. This interaction has not been evaluated in humans. Overall, oral plasma clearance (CL/F) is approximately 20 to 30 mL/min in humans following oral administration.

Pharmacokinetic Interactions (see also Drug Interactions):
Antiepileptic Drugs
Potential interactions between topiramate and standard AEDs were assessed in controlled clinical pharmacokinetic studies in patients with epilepsy. The effect of these interactions on mean plasma AUCs are summarized under **PRECAUTIONS (Table 3)**.

Special Populations:
Renal Impairment:
The clearance of topiramate was reduced by 42% in moderately renally impaired (creatinine clearance 30-69 mL/min/1.73m^2) and by 54% in severely renally impaired subjects (creatinine clearance <30 mL/min/1.73m^2) compared to normal renal function subjects (creatinine clearance >70 mL/min/1.73m^2). Since topiramate is presumed to undergo significant tubular reabsorption, it is uncertain whether this experience can be generalized to all situations of renal impairment. It is conceivable that some forms of renal disease could differentially affect glomerular filtration rate and tubular reabsorption resulting in a clearance of topiramate not predicted by creatinine clearance. In general, however, use of one-half the usual starting and maintenance dose is recommended in patients with moderate or severe renal impairment (see **PRECAUTIONS: General** and **DOSAGE AND ADMINISTRATION**).

Hemodialysis:
Topiramate is cleared by hemodialysis. Using a high efficiency, counterflow, single pass-dialysate hemodialysis procedure, topiramate dialysis clearance was 120 mL/min with blood flow through the dialyzer at 400 mL/min. This high clearance (compared to 20-30 mL/min total oral clearance in healthy adults) will remove a clinically significant amount of topiramate from the patient over the hemodialysis treatment period. Therefore, a supplemental dose may be required (see **DOSAGE AND ADMINISTRATION**).

Hepatic Impairment:
In hepatically impaired subjects, the clearance of topiramate may be decreased; the mechanism underlying the decrease is not well understood.

Age, Gender, and Race:
The pharmacokinetics of topiramate in elderly subjects (65-85 years of age, N=16) were evaluated in a controlled clinical study. The elderly subject population had reduced renal function [creatinine clearance (-20%)] compared to young adults. Following a single oral 100 mg dose, maximum plasma concentration for elderly and young adults was achieved at approximately 1-2 hours. Reflecting the primary renal elimination of topiramate, topiramate plasma and renal clearance were reduced 21% and 19%, respectively, in elderly subjects, compared to young adults. Similarly, topiramate half-life was longer (13%) in the elderly. Reduced topiramate clearance resulted in slightly higher maximum plasma concentration (23%) and AUC (25%) in elderly subjects than observed in young adults. Topiramate clearance is decreased in the elderly only to the extent that renal function is reduced. As recommended for all patients, dosage adjustment may be indicated in the elderly patient when impaired renal function (creatinine clearance rate ≤70 mL/min/1.73 m^2) is evident. It may be useful to monitor renal function in the elderly patient (see **Special Populations: Renal Impairment**, **PRECAUTIONS: General** and **DOSAGE AND ADMINISTRATION**).
Clearance of topiramate in adults was not affected by gender or race.

Pediatric Pharmacokinetics:
Pharmacokinetics of topiramate were evaluated in patients ages 4 to 17 years receiving one or two other antiepileptic drugs. Pharmacokinetic profiles were obtained after one week at doses of 1, 3, and 9 mg/kg/day. Clearance was independent of dose.
Pediatric patients have a 50% higher clearance and consequently shorter elimination half-life than adults. Consequently, the plasma concentration for the same mg/kg dose may be lower in pediatric patients compared to adults. As in adults, hepatic enzyme-inducing antiepileptic drugs decrease the steady state plasma concentrations of topiramate.

CLINICAL STUDIES

The studies described in the following sections were conducted using TOPAMAX® (topiramate) Tablets.

Epilepsy
The results of controlled clinical trials established the efficacy of TOPAMAX® (topiramate) Tablets and TOPAMAX® (topiramate capsules) Sprinkle Capsules as adjunctive therapy in adults and pediatric patients ages 2-16 years with partial onset seizures or primary generalized tonic-clonic seizures, and in patients 2 years of age and older with seizures associated with Lennox-Gastaut syndrome.

Controlled Trials in Patients With Partial Onset Seizures
Adults With Partial Onset Seizures
The effectiveness of topiramate as an adjunctive treatment for adults with partial onset seizures was established in six multicenter, randomized, double-blind, placebo-controlled trials, two comparing several dosages of topiramate and placebo and four comparing a single dosage with placebo, in patients with a history of partial onset seizures, with or without secondarily generalized seizures.
Patients in these studies were permitted a maximum of two antiepileptic drugs (AEDs) in addition to TOPAMAX® Tablets or placebo. In each study, patients were stabilized on optimum dosages of their concomitant AEDs during the baseline phase lasting between 4 and 12 weeks. Patients who experienced a prespecified minimum number of partial onset seizures, with or without secondary generalization, during the baseline phase (12 seizures for 12-week baseline, 8 for 8-week baseline, or 3 for 4-week baseline) were randomly assigned to placebo or a specified dose of TOPAMAX® Tablets in addition to their other AEDs.
Following randomization, patients began the double-blind phase of treatment. In five of the six studies, patients received active drug beginning at 100 mg per day; the dose was then increased by 100 mg or 200 mg/day increments weekly or every other week until the assigned dose was reached, unless intolerance prevented increases. In the sixth study (119), the 25 or 50 mg/day initial doses of topiramate were followed by respective weekly increments of 25 or 50 mg/day until the target dose of 200 mg/day was reached. After titration, patients entered a 4, 8, or 12-week stabilization period. The numbers of patients randomized to each dose, and the actual mean and median doses in the stabilization period are shown in Table 1.

Pediatric Patients Ages 2-16 Years With Partial Onset Seizures
The effectiveness of topiramate as an adjunctive treatment for pediatric patients ages 2-16 years with partial onset seizures was established in a multicenter, randomized, double-blind, placebo-controlled trial, comparing topiramate and placebo in patients with a history of partial onset seizures, with or without secondarily generalized seizures.
Patients in this study were permitted a maximum of two antiepileptic drugs (AEDs) in addition to TOPAMAX® Tablets or placebo. In this study, patients were stabilized on optimum dosages of their concomitant AEDs during an 8-week baseline phase. Patients who experienced at least six partial onset seizures, with or without secondarily generalized seizures, during the baseline phase were randomly assigned to placebo or TOPAMAX® Tablets in addition to their other AEDs.
Following randomization, patients began the double-blind phase of treatment. Patients received active drug beginning at 25 or 50 mg per day; the dose was then increased by 25 mg to 150 mg/day increments every other week until the assigned dosage of 125, 175, 225, or 400 mg/day based on patients' weight to approximate a dosage of 6 mg/kg per day was reached, unless intolerance prevented increases. After titration, patients entered an 8-week stabilization period.

Controlled Trials in Patients With Primary Generalized Tonic-Clonic Seizures
The effectiveness of topiramate as an adjunctive treatment for primary generalized tonic-clonic seizures in patients 2 years old and older was established in a multicenter, randomized, double-blind, placebo-controlled trial, comparing a single dosage of topiramate and placebo.
Patients in this study were permitted a maximum of two antiepileptic drugs (AEDs) in addition to TOPAMAX® or placebo. Patients were stabilized on optimum dosages of their concomitant AEDs during an 8-week baseline phase. Patients who experienced at least three primary generalized tonic-clonic seizures during the baseline phase were randomly assigned to placebo or TOPAMAX® in addition to their other AEDs.
Following randomization, patients began the double-blind phase of treatment. Patients received active drug beginning

at 50 mg per day for four weeks; the dose was then increased by 50 mg to 150 mg/day increments every other week until the assigned dose of 175, 225, or 400 mg/day based on patients' body weight to approximate a dosage of 6 mg/kg per day was reached, unless intolerance prevented increases. After titration, patients entered a 12-week stabilization period.

Controlled Trial in Patients With Lennox-Gastaut Syndrome

The effectiveness of topiramate as an adjunctive treatment for seizures associated with Lennox-Gastaut syndrome was established in a multicenter, randomized, double-blind, placebo-controlled trial comparing a single dosage of topiramate with placebo in patients 2 years of age and older. Patients in this study were permitted a maximum of two antiepileptic drugs (AEDs) in addition to TOPAMAX® or placebo. Patients who were experiencing at least 60 seizures per month before study entry were stabilized on optimum dosages of their concomitant AEDs during a four week baseline phase. Following baseline, patients were randomly assigned to placebo or TOPAMAX® in addition to their other AEDs. Active drug was titrated beginning at 1 mg/kg per day for a week; the dose was then increased to 3 mg/kg per day for one week then to 6 mg/kg per day. After titration, patients entered an 8-week stabilization period. The primary measures of effectiveness were the percent reduction in drop attacks and a parental global rating of seizure severity.

[See table 1 at right]

In all add-on trials, the reduction in seizure rate from baseline during the entire double-blind phase was measured. The median percent reductions in seizure rates and the responder rates (fraction of patients with at least a 50% reduction) by treatment group for each study are shown below in Table 2. As described above, a global improvement in seizure severity was also assessed in the Lennox-Gastaut trial. [See table 2 at right]

Subset analyses of the antiepileptic efficacy of TOPAMAX® Tablets in these studies showed no differences as a function of gender, race, age, baseline seizure rate, or concomitant AED.

Migraine

The results of 2 multicenter, randomized, double-blind, placebo-controlled, parallel-group clinical trials established the effectiveness of TOPAMAX® in the prophylactic treatment of migraine headache. The design of both trials (one study was conducted in the U.S. and one study was conducted in the U.S. and Canada) were identical, enrolling patients with a history of migraine, with or without aura, for at least 6 months, according to the International Headache Society diagnostic criteria. Patients with a history of cluster headaches or basilar, ophthalmoplegic, hemiplegic, or transformed migraine headaches were excluded from the trials. Patients were required to have completed up to a 2 week washout of any prior migraine preventive medications before starting the baseline phase.

Patients who experienced 3 to 12 migraine headaches over the 4-weeks in the baseline phase were equally randomized to either TOPAMAX® 50 mg/day, 100 mg/day, 200 mg/day, or placebo and treated for a total of 26 weeks (8-week titration period and 18-week maintenance period). Treatment was initiated at 25 mg/day for one week, and then the daily dosage was increased by 25-mg increments each week until reaching the assigned target dose or maximum tolerated dose (administered twice daily).

Effectiveness of treatment was assessed by the reduction in migraine headache frequency, as measured by the change in 4-week migraine rate from the baseline phase to double-blind treatment period in each TOPAMAX® treatment group compared to placebo in the intent to treat (ITT) population.

In the first study a total of 469 patients (416 females, 53 males), ranging in age from 13 to 70 years, were randomized and provided efficacy data. Two hundred sixty five patients completed the entire 26-week double-blind phase. The median average daily dosages were 47.8 mg/day, 88.3 mg/day, and 132.1 mg/day in the target dose groups of TOPAMAX® 50, 100, and 200 mg/day, respectively.

The mean migraine headache frequency rate at baseline was approximately 5.5 migraine headaches/28 days and was similar across treatment groups. The change in the mean 4-week migraine frequency from baseline to the double-blind phase was -1.3, -2.1, and -2.2 in the TOPAMAX® 50, 100, and 200 mg/day groups, respectively, versus -0.8 in the placebo group (see Figure 1). The differences between the TOPAMAX® 100 and 200 mg/day groups versus placebo were statistically significant (p<0.001 for both comparisons).

In the second study a total of 468 patients (406 females, 62 males), ranging in age from 12 to 65 years, were randomized and provided efficacy data. Two hundred fifty five patients completed the entire 26-week double-blind phase. The median average daily dosages were 46.5 mg/day, 85.6 mg/day, and 150.2 mg/day in the target dose groups of TOPAMAX® 50, 100, and 200 mg/day, respectively.

The mean migraine headache frequency rate at baseline was approximately 5.5 migraine headaches/28 days and was similar across treatment groups. The change in the mean 4-week migraine headache period frequency from baseline to the double-blind phase was -1.4, -2.1, and -2.4 in the TOPAMAX® 50, 100, and 200 mg/day groups, respectively, versus -1.1 in the placebo group (see Figure 1). The differences between the TOPAMAX® 100 and 200 mg/day groups versus placebo were statistically significant (p=0.008 and <0.001, respectively).

Table 1: Topiramate Dose Summary During the Stabilization Periods of Each of Six Double-Blind, Placebo-Controlled, Add-On Trials in Adults with Partial Onset Seizures[b]

Protocol	Stabilization Dose	Placebo[a]	Target Topiramate Dosage (mg/day) 200	400	600	800	1,000
YD	N	42	42	40	41	—	—
	Mean Dose	5.9	200	390	556	—	—
	Median Dose	6.0	200	400	600	—	—
YE	N	44	—	—	40	45	40
	Mean Dose	9.7	—	—	544	739	796
	Median Dose	10.0	—	—	600	800	1,000
Y1	N	23	19	—	—	—	—
	Mean Dose	3.8	395	—	—	—	—
	Median Dose	4.0	400	—	—	—	—
Y2	N	30	—	—	28	—	—
	Mean Dose	5.7	—	—	522	—	—
	Median Dose	6.0	—	—	600	—	—
Y3	N	28	—	—	—	25	—
	Mean Dose	7.9	—	—	—	568	—
	Median Dose	8.0	—	—	—	600	—
119	N	90	157	—	—	—	—
	Mean Dose	8	200	—	—	—	—
	Median Dose	8	200	—	—	—	—

[a] Placebo dosages are given as the number of tablets. Placebo target dosages were as follows: Protocol Y1, 4 tablets/day; Protocols YD and Y2, 6 tablets/day; Protocol Y3 and 119, 8 tablets/day; Protocol YE, 10 tablets/day.
[b] Dose-response studies were not conducted for other indications or pediatric partial onset seizures.

Table 2: Efficacy Results in Double-Blind, Placebo-Controlled, Add-On Epilepsy Trials

Protocol	Efficacy Results	Placebo	Target Topiramate Dosage (mg/day) 200	400	600	800	1,000	≈6 mg/kg/day*
Partial Onset Seizures								
Studies in Adults								
YD	N	45	45	45	46	—	—	—
	Median % Reduction	11.6	27.2[a]	47.5[b]	44.7[c]	—	—	—
	% Responders	18	24	44[d]	46[d]	—	—	—
YE	N	47	—	—	48	48	47	—
	Median % Reduction	1.7	—	—	40.8[c]	41.0[c]	36.0[c]	—
	% Responders	9	—	—	40[c]	41[c]	36[d]	—
Y1	N	24	—	23	—	—	—	—
	Median % Reduction	1.1	—	40.7[e]	—	—	—	—
	% Responders	8	—	35[d]	—	—	—	—
Y2	N	30	—	—	30	—	—	—
	Median % Reduction	-12.2	—	—	46.4[f]	—	—	—
	% Responders	10	—	—	47[c]	—	—	—
Y3	N	28	—	—	—	28	—	—
	Median % Reduction	-20.6	—	—	—	24.3[c]	—	—
	% Responders	0	—	—	—	43[c]	—	—
119	N	91	168	—	—	—	—	—
	Median % Reduction	20.0	44.2[c]	—	—	—	—	—
	% Responders	24	45[c]	—	—	—	—	—
Studies in Pediatric Patients								
YP	N	45	—	—	—	—	—	41
	Median % Reduction	10.5	—	—	—	—	—	33.1[d]
	% Responders	20	—	—	—	—	—	39
Primary Generalized Tonic-Clonic[h]								
YTC	N	40	—	—	—	—	—	39
	Median % Reduction	9.0	—	—	—	—	—	56.7[d]
	% Responders	20	—	—	—	—	—	56[c]
Lennox-Gastaut Syndrome[i]								
YL	N	49	—	—	—	—	—	46
	Median % Reduction	-5.1	—	—	—	—	—	14.8[d]
	% Responders	14	—	—	—	—	—	28[g]
	Improvement in Seizure Severity[j]	28	—	—	—	—	—	52[d]

Comparisons with placebo: [a]p=0.080; [b]p≤0.010; [c]p≤0.001; [d]p≤0.050; [e]p=0.065; [f]p≤0.005; [g]p=0.071; [h]Median % reduction and % responders are reported for PGTC Seizures; [i]Median % reduction and % responders for drop attacks, i.e., tonic or atonic seizures; [j]Percent of subjects who were minimally, much, or very much improved from baseline
* For Protocols YP and YTC, protocol-specified target dosages (<9.3 mg/kg/day) were assigned based on subject's weight to approximate a dosage of 6 mg/kg per day; these dosages corresponded to mg/day dosages of 125, 175, 225, and 400 mg/day.

In both studies, there were no apparent differences in treatment effect within age, or gender, subgroups. Because most patients were Caucasian, there were insufficient numbers of patients from other races to make a meaningful comparison of race.

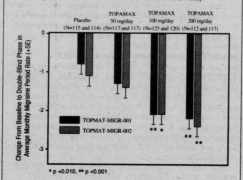

Figure 1: Reduction in 4-Week Migraine Headache Frequency (Studies TOPMAT-MIGR-001 and TOPMAT-MIGR-002)

INDICATIONS AND USAGE

Epilepsy

TOPAMAX® (topiramate) Tablets and TOPAMAX® (topiramate capsules) Sprinkle Capsules are indicated as adjunctive therapy for adults and pediatric patients ages 2-16 years with partial onset seizures, or primary generalized tonic-clonic seizures, and in patients 2 years of age and older with seizures associated with Lennox-Gastaut syndrome.

Migraine

TOPAMAX® (topiramate) Tablets and TOPAMAX® (topiramate capsules) Sprinkle Capsules are indicated for adults for the prophylaxis of migraine headache. The usefulness of TOPAMAX® in the acute treatment of migraine headache has not been studied.

CONTRAINDICATIONS

TOPAMAX® is contraindicated in patients with a history of hypersensitivity to any component of this product.

WARNINGS

Metabolic Acidosis

Hyperchloremic, non-anion gap, metabolic acidosis (i.e., decreased serum bicarbonate below the normal reference range in the absence of chronic respiratory alkalosis) is as-

Continued on next page

Topamax—Cont.

sociated with topiramate treatment. This metabolic acidosis is caused by renal bicarbonate loss due to the inhibitory effect of topiramate on carbonic anhydrase. Such electrolyte imbalance has been observed with the use of topiramate in placebo-controlled clinical trials and in the post-marketing period. Generally, topiramate-induced metabolic acidosis occurs early in treatment although cases can occur at any time during treatment. Bicarbonate decrements are usually mild-moderate (average decrease of 4 mEq/L at daily doses of 400 mg in adults and at approximately 6 mg/kg/day in pediatric patients); rarely, patients can experience severe decrements to values below 10 mEq/L. Conditions or therapies that predispose to acidosis (such as renal disease, severe respiratory disorders, status epilepticus, diarrhea, surgery, ketogenic diet, or drugs) may be additive to the bicarbonate lowering effects of topiramate.

In adults, the incidence of persistent treatment-emergent decreases in serum bicarbonate (levels of <20 mEq/L at two consecutive visits or at the final visit) in controlled clinical trials for adjunctive treatment of epilepsy was 32% for 400 mg/day, and 1% for placebo. Metabolic acidosis has been observed at doses as low as 50 mg/day. The incidence of a markedly abnormally low serum bicarbonate (i.e., absolute value <17 mEq/L and >5 mEq/L decrease from pretreatment) in these trials was 3% for 400 mg/day, and 0% for placebo. Serum bicarbonate levels have not been systematically evaluated at daily doses greater than 400 mg/day.

In pediatric patients (<16 years of age), the incidence of persistent treatment-emergent decreases in serum bicarbonate in placebo-controlled trials for adjunctive treatment of Lennox-Gastaut syndrome or refractory partial onset seizures was 67% for TOPAMAX® (at approximately 6 mg/kg/day), and 10% for placebo. The incidence of a markedly abnormally low serum bicarbonate (i.e., absolute value <17 mEq/L and >5 mEq/L decrease from pretreatment) in these trials was 11% for TOPAMAX® and 0% for placebo. Cases of moderately severe metabolic acidosis have been reported in patients as young as 5 months old, especially at daily doses above 5 mg/kg/day.

The incidence of persistent treatment-emergent decreases in serum bicarbonate in placebo-controlled trials for adults for prophylaxis of migraine was 44% for 200 mg/day, 39% for 100 mg/day, 23% for 50 mg/day, and 7% for placebo. The incidence of a markedly abnormally low serum bicarbonate (i.e., absolute value <17 mEq/L and >5 mEq/L decrease from pretreatment) in these trials was 11% for 200 mg/day, 9% for 100 mg/day, 2% for 50 mg/day, and <1% for placebo.

Some manifestations of acute or chronic metabolic acidosis may include hyperventilation, nonspecific symptoms such as fatigue and anorexia, or more severe sequelae including cardiac arrhythmias or stupor. Chronic, untreated metabolic acidosis may increase the risk for nephrolithiasis or nephrocalcinosis, and may also result in osteomalacia (referred to as rickets in pediatric patients) and/or osteoporosis with an increased risk for fractures. Chronic metabolic acidosis in pediatric patients may also reduce growth rates. A reduction in growth rate may eventually decrease the maximal height achieved. The effect of topiramate on growth and bone-related sequelae has not been systematically investigated.

Measurement of baseline and periodic serum bicarbonate during topiramate treatment is recommended. If metabolic acidosis develops and persists, consideration should be given to reducing the dose or discontinuing topiramate (using dose tapering). If the decision is made to continue patients on topiramate in the face of persistent acidosis, alkali treatment should be considered.

Acute Myopia and Secondary Angle Closure Glaucoma

A syndrome consisting of acute myopia associated with secondary angle closure glaucoma has been reported in patients receiving TOPAMAX®. Symptoms include acute onset of decreased visual acuity and/or ocular pain. Opthalmologic findings can include myopia, anterior chamber shallowing, ocular hyperemia (redness) and increased intraocular pressure. Mydriasis may or may not be present. This syndrome may be associated with supraciliary effusion resulting in anterior displacement of the lens and iris, with secondary angle closure glaucoma. Symptoms typically occur within 1 month of initiating TOPAMAX® therapy. In contrast to primary narrow angle glaucoma, which is rare under 40 years of age, secondary angle closure glaucoma associated with topiramate has been reported in pediatric patients as well as adults. The primary treatment to reverse symptoms is discontinuation of TOPAMAX® as rapidly as possible, according to the judgement of the treating physician. Other measures, in conjunction with discontinuation of TOPAMAX®, may be helpful.

Elevated intraocular pressure of any etiology, if left untreated, can lead to serious sequelae including permanent vision loss.

Oligohidrosis and Hyperthermia

Oligohidrosis (decreased sweating), infrequently resulting in hospitalization, has been reported in association with TOPAMAX® use. Decreased sweating and an elevation in body temperature above normal characterized these cases. Some of the cases were reported after exposure to elevated environmental temperatures.

The majority of the reports have been in children. Patients, especially pediatric patients, treated with TOPAMAX® should be monitored closely for evidence of decreased sweating and increased body temperature, especially in hot weather. Caution should be used when TOPAMAX® is pre-

scribed with other drugs that predispose patients to heat-related disorders; these drugs include, but are not limited to, other carbonic anhydrase inhibitors and drugs with anticholinergic activity.

Withdrawal of AEDs

Antiepileptic drugs, including TOPAMAX®, should be withdrawn gradually to minimize the potential of increased seizure frequency.

Cognitive/Neuropsychiatric Adverse Events

Adults

Adverse events most often associated with the use of TOPAMAX® were related to the central nervous system and were observed in both the epilepsy and migraine populations. In adults, the most frequent of these can be classified into three general categories: 1) Cognitive-related dysfunction (e.g., confusion, psychomotor slowing, difficulty with concentration/attention, difficulty with memory, speech or language problems, particularly word-finding difficulties); 2) Psychiatric/behavioral disturbances (e.g., depression or mood problems); and 3) Somnolence or fatigue.

Cognitive-Related Dysfunction

The majority of cognitive-related adverse events were mild to moderate in severity, and they frequently occurred in isolation. Rapid titration rate and higher initial dose were associated with higher incidences of these events. Many of these events contributed to withdrawal from treatment (see ADVERSE REACTIONS, Table 4 and Table 8).

In the original add on epilepsy controlled trials (using rapid titration such as 100-200 mg/day weekly increments), the proportion of patients who experienced one or more cognitive-related adverse events was 42% for 200 mg/day, 41% for 400 mg/day, 52% for 600 mg/day, 56% for 800 and 1000 mg/day, and 14% for placebo. These dose-related adverse reactions began with a similar frequency in the titration or in the maintenance phase, although in some patients the events began during titration and persisted into the maintenance phase. Some patients who experienced one or more cognitive-related adverse events in the titration phase had a dose-related recurrence of these events in the maintenance phase.

In the 6 month migraine prophylaxis controlled trials using a slower titration regimen (25 mg/day weekly increments), the proportion of patients who experienced one or more cognitive-related adverse events was 19% for TOPAMAX® 50 mg/day, 22% for 100 mg/day, 28% for 200 mg/day, and 10% for placebo. These dose-related adverse reactions typically began in the titration phase and often persisted into the maintenance phase, but infrequently began in the maintenance phase. Some patients experienced a recurrence of one or more of these cognitive adverse events and this recurrence was typically in the titration phase. A relatively small proportion of topiramate-treated patients experienced more than one concurrent cognitive adverse event. The most common cognitive adverse events occurring together included difficulty with memory along with difficulty with concentration/attention, difficulty with memory along with language problems, and difficulty with concentration/attention along with language problems. Rarely, topiramate-treated patients experienced three concurrent cognitive events.

Psychiatric/Behavioral Disturbances

Psychiatric/behavioral disturbances (depression or mood problems) were dose-related for both the add-on epilepsy and migraine populations.

In the double blind phases of clinical trials with topiramate in approved and investigational indications, suicide attempts occurred at a rate of 3/1000 patient years (13 events/3999 patient years) on topiramate versus 0 (0 events/1430 patient years) on placebo. One completed suicide was reported in a bipolar disorder trial in a patient on topiramate.

Somnolence/Fatigue

Somnolence and fatigue were the adverse events most frequently reported during clinical trials of TOPAMAX® for adjunctive epilepsy. For the epilepsy population, the incidence of somnolence did not differ substantially between 200 mg/day and 1000 mg/day, but the incidence of fatigue was dose-related and increased at dosages above 400 mg/day. For the migraine population, fatigue and somnolence were dose-related and more common in the titration phase. Additional nonspecific CNS events commonly observed with topiramate in the add-on epilepsy population include dizziness or ataxia.

Pediatric Patients

In double-blind clinical studies, the incidences of cognitive/neuro psychiatric adverse events in pediatric patients were generally lower than previously observed in adults. These events included psychomotor slowing, difficulty with concentration/attention, speech disorders/related speech problems and language problems. The most frequently reported neuropsychiatric events in this population were somnolence and fatigue. No patients discontinued treatment due to adverse events in double-blind trials.

Sudden Unexplained Death in Epilepsy (SUDEP)

During the course of premarketing development of TOPAMAX® (topiramate) Tablets, 10 sudden and unexplained deaths were recorded among a cohort of treated patients (2,796 subject years of exposure). This represents an incidence of 0.0035 deaths per patient year. Although this rate exceeds that expected in a healthy population matched for age and sex, it is within the range of estimates for the incidence of sudden unexplained deaths in patients with epilepsy not receiving TOPAMAX® (ranging from 0.0005 for the general population of patients with epilepsy, to 0.003 for a clinical trial population similar to that in the TOPAMAX® program, to 0.005 for patients with refractory epilepsy).

PRECAUTIONS

Hyperammonemia and Encephalopathy Associated with Concomitant Valproic Acid Use

Concomitant administration of topiramate and valproic acid has been associated with hyperammonemia with or without encephalopathy in patients who have tolerated either drug alone. Clinical symptoms of hyperammonemic encephalopathy often include acute alterations in level of consciousness and/or cognitive function with lethargy or vomiting. In most cases, symptoms and signs abated with discontinuation of either drug. This adverse event is not due to a pharmacokinetic interaction.

It is not known if topiramate monotherapy is associated with hyperammonemia.

Patients with inborn errors of metabolism or reduced hepatic mitochondrial activity may be at an increased risk for hyperammonemia with or without encephalopathy. Although not studied, an interaction of topiramate and valproic acid may exacerbate existing defects or unmask deficiencies in susceptible persons.

In patients who develop unexplained lethargy, vomiting, or changes in mental status, hyperammonemic encephalopathy should be considered and an ammonia level should be measured.

Kidney Stones

A total of 32/2,086 (1.5%) of adults exposed to topiramate during its development reported the occurrence of kidney stones, an incidence about 2-4 times greater than expected in a similar, untreated population. As in the general population, the incidence of stone formation among topiramate treated patients was higher in men. Kidney stones have also been reported in pediatric patients.

An explanation for the association of TOPAMAX® and kidney stones may lie in the fact that topiramate is a carbonic anhydrase inhibitor. Carbonic anhydrase inhibitors, e.g., acetazolamide or dichlorphenamide, promote stone formation by reducing urinary citrate excretion and by increasing urinary pH. The concomitant use of TOPAMAX® with other carbonic anhydrase inhibitors or potentially in patients on a ketogenic diet may create a physiological environment that increases the risk of kidney stone formation, and should therefore be avoided.

Increased fluid intake increases the urinary output, lowering the concentration of substances involved in stone formation. Hydration is recommended to reduce new stone formation.

Paresthesia

Paresthesia (usually tingling of the extremities), an effect associated with the use of other carbonic anhydrase inhibitors, appears to be a common effect of TOPAMAX®. Paresthesia was more frequently reported in the migraine prophylaxis trials versus the adjunctive therapy trials in epilepsy. In the majority of instances, paresthesia did not lead to treatment discontinuation.

Adjustment of Dose in Renal Failure

The major route of elimination of unchanged topiramate and its metabolites is via the kidney. Dosage adjustment may be required in patients with reduced renal function (see DOSAGE AND ADMINISTRATION).

Decreased Hepatic Function

In hepatically impaired patients, topiramate should be administered with caution as the clearance of topiramate may be decreased.

Information for Patients

Patients taking TOPAMAX® should be told to seek immediate medical attention if they experience blurred vision or periorbital pain.

Patients, especially pediatric patients, treated with TOPAMAX® should be monitored closely for evidence of decreased sweating and increased body temperature, especially in hot weather.

Patients, particularly those with predisposing factors, should be instructed to maintain an adequate fluid intake in order to minimize the risk of renal stone formation [see PRECAUTIONS: General, for support regarding hydration as a preventative measure].

Patients should be warned about the potential for somnolence, dizziness, confusion, and difficulty concentrating and advised not to drive or operate machinery until they have gained sufficient experience on topiramate to gauge whether it adversely affects their mental and/or motor performance.

Additional food intake may be considered if the patient is losing weight while on this medication.

Please refer to the end of the product labeling for important information on how to take TOPAMAX® (topiramate capsules) Sprinkle Capsules.

Laboratory Tests:

Measurement of baseline and periodic serum bicarbonate during topiramate treatment is recommended (see WARNINGS).

Drug Interactions:

In vitro studies indicate that topiramate does not inhibit enzyme activity for CYP1A2, CYP2A6, CYP2B6, CYP2C9, CYP2C19, CYP2D6, CYP2E1 and CYP3A4/5 isozymes.

Antiepileptic Drugs

Potential interactions between topiramate and standard AEDs were assessed in controlled clinical pharmacokinetic studies in patients with epilepsy. The effects of these interactions on mean plasma AUCs are summarized in Table 3. In Table 3, the second column (AED concentration) describes what happens to the concentration of the AED listed in the first column when topiramate is added.

The third column (topiramate concentration) describes how the coadministration of a drug listed in the first column modifies the the concentration of topiramate in experimental settings when TOPAMAX® was given alone.
[See table 3 at right]

In addition to the pharmacokinetic interaction described in the above table, concomitant administration of valproic acid and topiramate has been associated with hyperammonemia with and without encephalopathy (see **PRECAUTIONS**, Hyperammonemia and Encephalopathy Associated with Concomitant Valproic Acid Use).

Other Drug Interactions

Digoxin: In a single-dose study, serum digoxin AUC was decreased by 12% with concomitant TOPAMAX® administration. The clinical relevance of this observation has not been established.

CNS Depressants: Concomitant administration of TOPAMAX® and alcohol or other CNS depressant drugs has not been evaluated in clinical studies. Because of the potential of topiramate to cause CNS depression, as well as other cognitive and/or neuropsychiatric adverse events, topiramate should be used with extreme caution if used in combination with alcohol and other CNS depressants.

Oral Contraceptives: In a pharmacokinetic interaction study in healthy volunteers with a concomitantly administered combination oral contraceptive product containing 1 mg norethindrone (NET) plus 35 mcg ethinyl estradiol (EE), TOPAMAX® given in the absence of other medications at doses of 50 to 200 mg/day was not associated with statistically significant changes in mean exposure (AUC) to either component of the oral contraceptive. In another study, exposure to EE was statistically significantly decreased at doses of 200, 400, and 800 mg/day (18%, 21%, and 30%, respectively) when given as adjunctive therapy in patients taking valproic acid. In both studies, TOPAMAX® (50 mg/day to 800 mg/day) did not significantly affect exposure to NET. Although there was a dose dependent decrease in EE exposure for doses between 200-800 mg/day, there was no significant dose dependent change in EE exposure for doses of 50-200 mg/day. The clinical significance of the changes observed is not known. The possibility of decreased contraceptive efficacy and increased breakthrough bleeding should be considered in patients taking combination oral contraceptive products with TOPAMAX®. Patients taking estrogen containing contraceptives should be asked to report any change in their bleeding patterns. Contraceptive efficacy can be decreased even in the absence of breakthrough bleeding.

Metformin: A drug-drug interaction study conducted in healthy volunteers evaluated the steady-state pharmacokinetics of metformin and topiramate in plasma when metformin was given alone and when metformin and topiramate were given simultaneously. The results of this study indicated that metformin mean C_{max} and mean AUC_{0-12h} increased by 18% and 25%, respectively, while mean CL/F decreased 20% when metformin was co-administered with topiramate. Topiramate did not affect metformin t_{max}. The clinical significance of the effect of topiramate on metformin pharmacokinetics is unclear. Oral plasma clearance of topiramate appears to be reduced when administered with metformin. The extent of change in the clearance is unknown. The clinical significance of the effect of metformin on topiramate pharmacokinetics is unclear. When TOPAMAX® is added or withdrawn in patients on metformin therapy, careful attention should be given to the routine monitoring for adequate control of their diabetic disease state.

Lithium: Multiple dosing of topiramate 100 mg every 12 hrs decreased the AUC and C_{max} of Lithium (300 mg every 8 hrs) by 20% (N=12, 6 M; 6 F).

Haloperidol: The pharmacokinetics of a single dose of haloperidol (5 mg) were not affected following multiple dosing of topiramate (100 mg every 12 hr) in 13 healthy adults (6 M, 7 F).

Amitriptyline: There was a 12% increase in AUC and C_{max} for amitriptyline (25 mg per day) in 18 normal subjects (9 male; 9 female) receiving 200 mg/day of topiramate. Some subjects may experience a large increase in amitriptyline concentration in the presence of topiramate and any adjustments in amitriptyline dose should be made according to the patient's clinical response and not on the basis of plasma levels.

Sumatriptan: Multiple dosing of topiramate (100 mg every 12 hr) in 24 healthy volunteers (14 M, 10 F) did not affect the pharmacokinetics of single dose sumatriptan either orally (100 mg) or subcutaneously (6 mg).

Risperidone: There was a 25% decrease in exposure to risperidone (2 mg single dose) in 12 healthy volunteers (6 M, 6 F) receiving 200 mg/day of topiramate. Therefore, patients receiving risperidone in combination with topiramate should be closely monitored for clinical response.

Propranolol: Multiple dosing of topiramate (200 mg/day) in 34 healthy volunteers (17 M, 17 F) did not affect the pharmacokinetics of propranolol following daily 160 mg doses. Propranolol doses of 160 mg/day in 39 volunteers (27M, 12F) had no affect on the exposure to topiramate at a dose of 200 mg/day of topiramate.

Dihydroergotamine: Multiple dosing of topiramate (200 mg/day) in 24 healthy volunteers (12 M, 12 F) did not affect the pharmacokinetics of a 1 mg subcutaneous dose of dihydroergotamine. Similarly, a 1 mg subcutaneous dose of dihydroergotamine did not affect the pharmacokinetics of a 200 mg/day dose of topiramate in the same study.

Others: Concomitant use of TOPAMAX®, a carbonic anhydrase inhibitor, with other carbonic anhydrase inhibitors,

e.g., acetazolamide or dichlorphenamide, may create a physiological environment that increases the risk of renal stone formation, and should therefore be avoided.

Drug/Laboratory Test Interactions: There are no known interactions of topiramate with commonly used laboratory tests.

Table 3: Summary of AED Interactions with TOPAMAX®

AED Co-administered	AED Concentration	Topiramate Concentration
Phenytoin	NC or 25% increase[a]	48% decrease
Carbamazepine (CBZ)	NC	40% decrease
CBZ epoxide[b]	NC	NE
Valproic acid	11% decrease	14% decrease
Phenobarbital	NC	NE
Primidone	NC	NE
Lamotrigine	NC at TPM doses up to 400 mg/day	15% increase

[a] = Plasma concentration increased 25% in some patients, generally those on a b.i.d. dosing regimen of phenytoin.
[b] = is not administered but is an active metabolite of carbamazepine.
NC = Less than 10% change in plasma concentration.
AED = Antiepileptic drug.
NE = Not Evaluated.
TPM = Topiramate

Table 4: Incidence of Treatment-Emergent Adverse Events in Placebo-Controlled, Add-On Epilepsy Trials in Adults[a,b] Where Rate Was > 1% in Any Topiramate Group and Greater Than the Rate in Placebo-Treated Patients

Body System/ Adverse Event[c]	Placebo (N=291)	TOPAMAX® Dosage (mg/day) 200-400 (N=183)	600-1,000 (N=414)
Body as a Whole – General Disorders			
Fatigue	13	15	30
Asthenia	1	6	3
Back Pain	4	5	3
Chest Pain	3	4	2
Influenza-Like Symptoms	2	3	4
Leg Pain	2	2	4
Hot Flushes	1	2	1
Allergy	1	2	3
Edema	1	2	1
Body Odor	0	1	0
Rigors	0	1	<1
Central & Peripheral Nervous System Disorders			
Dizziness	15	25	32
Ataxia	7	16	14
Speech Disorders/Related Speech Problems	2	13	11
Paresthesia	4	11	19
Nystagmus	7	10	11
Tremor	6	9	9
Language Problems	1	6	10
Coordination Abnormal	2	4	4
Hypoaesthesia	1	2	1
Gait Abnormal	1	3	2
Muscle Contractions Involuntary	1	2	2
Stupor	0	2	1
Vertigo	1	1	2
Gastro-Intestinal System Disorders			
Nausea	8	10	12
Dyspepsia	6	7	6
Abdominal Pain	4	6	7
Constipation	2	4	3
Gastroenteritis	1	2	1
Dry Mouth	1	2	4
Gingivitis	<1	1	1
GI Disorder	<1	1	0
Hearing and Vestibular Disorders			
Hearing Decreased	1	2	1
Metabolic and Nutritional Disorders			
Weight Decrease	3	9	13
Muscle-Skeletal System Disorders			
Myalgia	1	2	2
Skeletal Pain	0	1	0
Platelet, Bleeding & Clotting Disorders			
Epistaxis	1	2	1
Psychiatric Disorders			
Somnolence	12	29	28
Nervousness	6	16	19
Psychomotor Slowing	2	13	21
Difficulty with Memory	3	12	14
Anorexia	4	10	12
Confusion	5	11	14
Depression	5	5	13
Difficulty with Concentration/Attention	2	6	14
Mood Problems	2	4	9
Agitation	2	3	3
Aggressive Reaction	2	3	3
Emotional Lability	1	3	3
Cognitive Problems	1	3	3
Libido Decreased	1	2	<1
Apathy	1	1	3
Depersonalization	1	1	2
Reproductive Disorders, Female			
Breast Pain	2	4	0
Amenorrhea	1	2	2
Menorrhagia	0	2	1
Menstrual Disorder	1	2	1

(Table continued on next page)

Carcinogenesis, Mutagenesis, Impairment of Fertility:
An increase in urinary bladder tumors was observed in mice given topiramate (20, 75, and 300 mg/kg) in the diet for 21 months. The elevated bladder tumor incidence, which was

Continued on next page

Topamax—Cont.

statistically significant in males and females receiving 300 mg/kg, was primarily due to the increased occurrence of a smooth muscle tumor considered histomorphologically unique to mice. Plasma exposures in mice receiving 300 mg/kg were approximately 0.5 to 1 times steady-state exposures measured in patients receiving topiramate monotherapy at the recommended human dose (RHD) of 400 mg, and 1.5 to 2 times steady-state topiramate exposures in patients receiving 400 mg of topiramate plus phenytoin. The relevance of this finding to human carcinogenic risk is uncertain. No evidence of carcinogenicity was seen in rats following oral administration of topiramate for 2 years at doses up to 120 mg/kg (approximately 3 times the RHD on a mg/m² basis).

Topiramate did not demonstrate genotoxic potential when tested in a battery of *in vitro* and *in vivo* assays. Topiramate was not mutagenic in the Ames test or the *in vitro* mouse lymphoma assay; it did not increase unscheduled DNA synthesis in rat hepatocytes *in vitro*; and it did not increase chromosomal aberrations in human lymphocytes *in vitro* or in rat bone marrow *in vivo*.

No adverse effects on male or female fertility were observed in rats at doses up to 100 mg/kg (2.5 times the RHD on a mg/m² basis).

Pregnancy: Pregnancy Category C.

Topiramate has demonstrated selective developmental toxicity, including teratogenicity, in experimental animal studies. When oral doses of 20, 100, or 500 mg/kg were administered to pregnant mice during the period of organogenesis, the incidence of fetal malformations (primarily craniofacial defects) was increased at all doses. The low dose is approximately 0.2 times the recommended human dose (RHD=400 mg/day) on a mg/m² basis. Fetal body weights and skeletal ossification were reduced at 500 mg/kg in conjunction with decreased maternal body weight gain.

In rat studies (oral doses of 20, 100, and 500 mg/kg or 0.2, 2.5, 30, and 400 mg/kg), the frequency of limb malformations (ectrodactyly, micromelia, and amelia) was increased among the offspring of dams treated with 400 mg/kg (10 times the RHD on a mg/m² basis) or greater during the organogenesis period of pregnancy. Embryotoxicity (reduced fetal body weights, increased incidence of structural variations) was observed at doses as low as 20 mg/kg (0.5 times the RHD on a mg/m² basis). Clinical signs of maternal toxicity were seen at 400 mg/kg and above, and maternal body weight gain was reduced during treatment with 100 mg/kg or greater.

In rabbit studies (20, 60, and 180 mg/kg or 10, 35, and 120 mg/kg orally during organogenesis), embryo/fetal mortality was increased at 35 mg/kg (2 times the RHD on a mg/m² basis) or greater, and teratogenic effects (primarily rib and vertebral malformations) were observed at 120 mg/kg (6 times the RHD on a mg/m² basis). Evidence of maternal toxicity (decreased body weight gain, clinical signs, and/or mortality) was seen at 35 mg/kg and above.

When female rats were treated during the latter part of gestation and throughout lactation (0.2, 4, 20, and 100 mg/kg or 2, 20, and 200 mg/kg), offspring exhibited decreased viability and delayed physical development at 200 mg/kg (5 times the RHD on a mg/m² basis) and reductions in pre- and/or postweaning body weight gain at 2 mg/kg (0.05 times the RHD on a mg/m² basis) and above. Maternal toxicity (decreased body weight gain, clinical signs) was evident at 100 mg/kg or greater.

In a rat embryo/fetal development study with a postnatal component (0.2, 2.5, 30, or 400 mg/kg during organogenesis; noted above), pups exhibited delayed physical development at 400 mg/kg (10 times the RHD on a mg/m² basis) and persistent reductions in body weight gain at 30 mg/kg (1 times the RHD on a mg/m² basis) and higher.

There are no studies using TOPAMAX® in pregnant women. TOPAMAX® should be used during pregnancy only if the potential benefit outweighs the potential risk to the fetus.

In post-marketing experience, cases of hypospadias have been reported in male infants exposed in utero to topiramate, with or without other anticonvulsants; however, a causal relationship with topiramate has not been established.

Labor and Delivery:

In studies of rats where dams were allowed to deliver pups naturally, no drug-related effects on gestation length or parturition were were observed at dosage levels up to 200 mg/kg/day.

The effect of TOPAMAX® on labor and delivery in humans is unknown.

Nursing Mothers:

Topiramate is excreted in the milk of lactating rats. The excretion of topiramate in human milk has not been evaluated in controlled studies. Limited observations in patients suggest an extensive secretion of topiramate into breast milk. Since many drugs are excreted in human milk, and because the potential for serious adverse reactions in nursing infants to TOPAMAX® is unknown, the potential benefit to the mother should be weighed against the potential risk to the infant when considering recommendations regarding nursing.

Pediatric Use:

Safety and effectiveness in patients below the age of 2 years have not been established for the adjunctive therapy treatment of partial onset seizures, primary generalized tonic-clonic seizures, or seizures associated with Lennox-Gastaut syndrome. Topiramate is associated with metabolic acidosis. Chronic untreated metabolic acidosis in pediatric patients may cause osteomalacia/rickets and may reduce growth rates. A reduction in growth rate may eventually decrease the maximal height achieved. The effect of topiramate on growth and bone-related sequelae has not been systematically investigated (see **WARNINGS**).

Safety and effectiveness in pediatric patients have not been established for the prophylaxis treatment of migraine headache.

Geriatric Use:

In clinical trials, 3% of patients were over 60. No age related difference in effectiveness or adverse effects were evident.

Table 4 (cont.): Incidence of Treatment-Emergent Adverse Events in Placebo-Controlled, Add-On Epilepsy Trials in Adults[a,b] Where Rate Was > 1% in Any Topiramate Group and Greater Than the Rate in Placebo-Treated Patients

Body System/ Adverse Event[c]	Placebo (N=291)	TOPAMAX® Dosage (mg/day)	
		200-400 (N=183)	600-1,000 (N=414)
Reproductive Disorders, Male			
Prostatic Disorder	<1	2	0
Resistance Mechanism Disorders			
Infection	1	2	1
Infection Viral	1	2	<1
Moniliasis	<1	1	0
Respiratory System Disorders			
Pharyngitis	2	6	3
Rhinitis	6	7	6
Sinusitis	4	5	6
Dyspnea	1	1	2
Skin and Appendages Disorders			
Skin Disorder	<1	2	1
Sweating Increased	<1	1	<1
Rash Erythematous	<1	1	<1
Special Sense Other, Disorders			
Taste Perversion	0	2	4
Urinary System Disorders			
Hematuria	1	2	<1
Urinary Tract Infection	1	2	3
Micturition Frequency	1	1	2
Urinary Incontinence	<1	2	1
Urine Abnormal	0	1	<1
Vision Disorders			
Vision Abnormal	2	13	10
Diplopia	5	10	10
White Cell and RES Disorders			
Leukopenia	1	2	1

[a] Patients in these add-on trials were receiving 1 to 2 concomitant antiepileptic drugs in addition to TOPAMAX® or placebo.
[b] Values represent the percentage of patients reporting a given adverse event. Patients may have reported more than one adverse event during the study and can be included in more than one adverse event category.
[c] Adverse events reported by at least 1% of patients in the TOPAMAX® 200-400 mg/day group and more common than in the placebo group are listed in this table.

Table 5: Incidence of Treatment-Emergent Adverse Events in Study 119[a,b] Where Rate Was ≥ 2% in the Topiramate Group and Greater Than the Rate in Placebo-Treated Patients

Body System/ Adverse Event[c]	Placebo (N=92)	TOPAMAX® Dosage (mg/day) 200 (N=171)
Body as a Whole – General Disorders		
Fatigue	4	9
Chest Pain	1	2
Cardiovascular Disorders, General		
Hypertension	0	2
Central & Peripheral Nervous System Disorders		
Paresthesia	2	9
Dizziness	4	7
Tremor	2	3
Hypoasthesia	0	2
Leg Cramps	0	2
Language Problems	0	2
Gastro-Intestinal System Disorders		
Abdominal Pain	3	5
Constipation	0	4
Diarrhea	1	2
Dyspepsia	0	2
Dry Mouth	0	2
Hearing and Vestibular Disorders		
Tinnitus	0	2
Metabolic and Nutritional Disorders		
Weight Decrease	4	8
Psychiatric Disorders		
Somnolence	9	15
Anorexia	7	9
Nervousness	2	9
Difficulty with Concentration/Attention	0	5
Insomnia	3	4
Difficulty with Memory	1	2
Aggressive Reaction	0	2
Respiratory System Disorders		
Rhinitis	0	4
Urinary System Disorders		
Cystitis	0	2
Vision Disorders		
Diplopia	0	2
Vision Abnormal	0	2

[a] Patients in these add-on trials were receiving 1 to 2 concomitant antiepileptic drugs in addition to TOPAMAX® or placebo.
[b] Values represent the percentage of patients reporting a given adverse event. Patients may have reported more than one adverse event during the study and can be included in more than one adverse event category.
[c] Adverse events reported by at least 2% of patients in the TOPAMAX® 200 mg/kg group and more common than in the placebo group are listed in this table.

Table 6: Incidence (%) of Dose-Related Adverse Events
From Placebo-Controlled, Add-On Trials in Adults with Partial Onset Seizures[a]

Adverse Event	Placebo (N=216)	TOPAMAX® Dosage (mg/day) 200 (N=45)	400 (N=68)	600-1,000 (N=414)
Fatigue	13	11	12	30
Nervousness	7	13	18	19
Difficulty with Concentration/Attention	1	7	9	14
Confusion	4	9	10	14
Depression	6	9	7	13
Anorexia	4	4	6	12
Language problems	<1	2	9	10
Anxiety	6	2	3	10
Mood problems	2	0	6	9
Weight decrease	3	4	9	13

[a] Dose-response studies were not conducted for other adult indications or for pediatric indications.

Table 7: Incidence (%) of Treatment-Emergent Adverse Events in Placebo-Controlled, Add-On Epilepsy Trials in Pediatric Patients Ages 2-16 Years[a,b] (Events That Occurred in at Least 1% of Topiramate-Treated Patients and Occurred More Frequently in Topiramate-Treated Than Placebo-Treated Patients)

Body System/ Adverse Event	Placebo (N=101)	Topiramate (N=98)
Body as a Whole – General Disorders		
Fatigue	5	16
Injury	13	14
Allergic Reaction	1	2
Back Pain	0	1
Pallor	0	1
Cardiovascular Disorders, General		
Hypertension	0	1
Central & Peripheral Nervous System Disorders		
Gait Abnormal	5	8
Ataxia	2	6
Hyperkinesia	4	5
Dizziness	2	4
Speech Disorders/Related Speech Problems	2	4
Hyporeflexia	0	2
Convulsions Grand Mal	0	1
Fecal Incontinence	0	1
Paresthesia	0	1
Gastro-Intestinal System Disorders		
Nausea	5	6
Saliva Increased	4	6
Constipation	4	5
Gastroenteritis	2	3
Dysphagia	0	1
Flatulence	0	1
Gastroesophageal Reflux	0	1
Glossitis	0	1
Gum Hyperplasia	0	1
Heart Rate and Rhythm Disorders		
Bradycardia	0	1
Metabolic and Nutritional Disorders		
Weight Decrease	1	9
Thirst	1	2
Hypoglycemia	0	1
Weight Increase	0	1
Platelet, Bleeding, & Clotting Disorders		
Purpura	4	8
Epistaxis	1	4
Hematoma	0	1
Prothrombin Increased	0	1
Thrombocytopenia	0	1
Psychiatric Disorders		
Somnolence	16	26
Anorexia	15	24
Nervousness	7	14
Personality Disorder (Behavior Problems)	9	11
Difficulty with Concentration/Attention	2	10
Aggressive Reaction	4	9
Insomnia	7	8
Difficulty with Memory NOS	0	5
Confusion	3	4
Psychomotor Slowing	2	3
Appetite Increased	0	1
Neurosis	0	1
Reproductive Disorders, Female		
Leukorrhoea	0	2
Resistance Mechanism Disorders		
Infection Viral	3	7
Respiratory System Disorders		
Pneumonia	1	5
Respiratory Disorder	0	1
Skin and Appendages Disorders		
Skin Disorder	2	3
Alopecia	1	2
Dermatitis	0	2
Hypertrichosis	1	2
Rash Erythematous	0	2
Eczema	0	1
Seborrhoea	0	1
Skin Discoloration	0	1

(Table continued on next page)

However, clinical studies of topiramate did not include sufficient numbers of subjects aged 65 and over to determine whether they respond differently than younger subjects. Dosage adjustment may be necessary for elderly with impaired renal function (creatinine clearance rate ≤70 mL/min/1.73 m^2) due to reduced clearance of topiramate (see **CLINICAL PHARMACOLOGY** and **DOSAGE AND ADMINISTRATION**).

Race and Gender Effects:
Evaluation of effectiveness and safety in clinical trials has shown no race or gender related effects.

ADVERSE REACTIONS
The data described in the following section were obtained using TOPAMAX® (topiramate) Tablets.

Epilepsy
The most commonly observed adverse events associated with the use of topiramate at dosages of 200 to 400 mg/day in controlled trials in adults with partial onset seizures, primary generalized tonic-clonic seizures, or Lennox-Gastaut syndrome, that were seen at greater frequency into piramate-treated patients and did not appear to be dose-related were: somnolence, dizziness, ataxia, speech disorders and related speech problems, psychomotor slowing, abnormal vision, difficulty with memory, paresthesia and diplopia [see Table 4]. The most common dose-related adverse events at dosages of 200 to 1,000 mg/day were: fatigue, nervousness, difficulty with concentration or attention, confusion, depression, anorexia, language problems, anxiety, mood problems, and weight decrease [see Table 6].

Adverse events associated with the use of topiramate at dosages of 5 to 9 mg/kg/day in controlled trials in pediatric patients with partial onset seizures, primary generalized tonic-clonic seizures, or Lennox-Gastaut syndrome, that were seen at greater frequency in topiramate-treated patients were: fatigue, somnolence, anorexia, nervousness, difficulty with concentration/attention, difficulty with memory, aggressive reaction, and weight decrease [see Table 7].

In controlled clinical trials in adults, 11% of patients receiving topiramate 200 to 400 mg/day as adjunctive therapy discontinued due to adverse events. This rate appeared to increase at dosages above 400 mg/day. Adverse events associated with discontinuing therapy included somnolence, dizziness, anxiety, difficulty with concentration or attention, fatigue, and paresthesia and increased at dosages above 400 mg/day. None of the pediatric patients who received topiramate adjunctive therapy at 5 to 9 mg/kg/day in controlled clinical trials discontinued due to adverse events.

Approximately 28% of the 1,757 adults with epilepsy who received topiramate at dosages of 200 to 1,600 mg/day in clinical studies discontinued treatment because of adverse events; an individual patient could have reported more than one adverse event. These adverse events were: psychomotor slowing (4.0%), difficulty with memory (3.2%), fatigue (3.2%), confusion (3.1%), somnolence (3.2%), difficulty with concentration/attention (2.9%), anorexia (2.7%), depression (2.6%), dizziness (2.5%), weight decrease (2.5%), nervousness (2.3%), ataxia (2.1%), and paresthesia (2.0%). Approximately 11% of the 310 pediatric patients who received topiramate at dosages up to 30 mg/kg/day discontinued due to adverse events. Adverse events associated with discontinuing therapy included aggravated convulsions (2.3%), difficulty with concentration/attention (1.6%), language problems (1.3%), personality disorder (1.3%), and somnolence (1.3%).

Incidence in Epilepsy Controlled Clinical Trials – Add-On Therapy – Partial Onset Seizures, Primary Generalized Tonic-Clonic Seizures, and Lennox-Gastaut Syndrome
Table 4 lists treatment-emergent adverse events that occurred in at least 1% of adults treated with 200 to 400 mg/day topiramate in controlled trials that were numerically more common at this dose than in the patients treated with placebo. In general, most patients who experienced adverse events during the first eight weeks of these trials no longer experienced them by their last visit. Table 7 lists treatment-emergent adverse events that occurred in at least 1% of pediatric patients treated with 5 to 9 mg/kg topiramate in controlled trials that were numerically more common than in patients treated with placebo.

The prescriber should be aware that these data were obtained when TOPAMAX® was added to concurrent antiepileptic drug therapy and cannot be used to predict the frequency of adverse events in the course of usual medical practice where patient characteristics and other factors may differ from those prevailing during clinical studies. Similarly, the cited frequencies cannot be directly compared with data obtained from other clinical investigations involving different treatments, uses, or investigators. Inspection of these frequencies, however, does provide the prescribing physician with a basis to estimate the relative contribution of drug and non-drug factors to the adverse event incidences in the population studied.

[See table 4 on pages 271 and 272]

Incidence in Study 119 – Add-On Therapy– Adults with Partial Onset Seizures
Study 119 was a randomized, double-blind, placebo-controlled, parallel group study with 3 treatment arms: 1) placebo; 2) topiramate 200 mg/day with a 25 mg/day starting dose, increased by 25 mg/day each week for 8 weeks until the 200 mg/day maintenance dose was reached; and 3) topiramate 200 mg/day with a 50 mg/day starting dose, increased by 50 mg/day each week for 4 weeks until the 200 mg/day maintenance dose was reached. All patients were maintained on concomitant carbamazepine with or without another concomitant antiepileptic drug.

The incidence of adverse events (Table 5) did not differ significantly between the 2 topiramate regimens. Because the frequencies of adverse events reported in this study were markedly lower than those reported in the previous epilepsy studies, they cannot be directly compared with data obtained in other studies.

Topamax—Cont.

[See table 5 on page 272]
[See table 6 at top of previous page]
[See table 7 on previous page and above]

Other Adverse Events Observed During Double-Blind Epilepsy Trials

Other events that occurred in more than 1% of adults treated with 200 to 400 mg of topiramate in placebo-controlled epilepsy trials but with equal or greater frequency in the placebo group were: headache, injury, anxiety, rash, pain, convulsions aggravated, coughing, fever, diarrhea, vomiting, muscle weakness, insomnia, personality disorder, dysmenorrhea, upper respiratory tract infection, and eye pain.

Other Adverse Events Observed During All Epilepsy Clinical Trials

Topiramate, initiated as adjunctive therapy, has been administered to 1,927 adults and 313 pediatric patients with epilepsy during all clinical studies. During these studies, all adverse events were recorded by the clinical investigators using terminology of their own choosing. To provide a meaningful estimate of the proportion of individuals having adverse events, similar types of events were grouped into a smaller number of standardized categories using modified WHOART dictionary terminology. The frequencies presented represent the proportion of patients who experienced an event of the type cited on at least one occasion while receiving topiramate. Reported events are included except those already listed in the previous tables or text, those too general to be informative, and those not reasonably associated with the use of the drug.

Events are classified within body system categories and enumerated in order of decreasing frequency using the following definitions: *frequent* occurring in at least 1/100 patients; *infrequent* occurring in 1/100 to 1/1000 patients; *rare* occurring in fewer than 1/1000 patients.

Autonomic Nervous System Disorders: *Infrequent:* vasodilation.

Body as a Whole: *Infrequent:* syncope, abdomen enlarged. *Rare:* alcohol intolerance.

Cardiovascular Disorders, General: *Infrequent:* hypotension, postural hypotension, angina pectoris.

Central & Peripheral Nervous System Disorders: *Frequent:* hypertonia. *Infrequent:* neuropathy, apraxia, hyperaesthesia, dyskinesia, dysphonia, scotoma, ptosis, dystonia, visual field defect, encephalopathy, EEG abnormal. *Rare:* upper motor neuron lesion, cerebellar syndrome, tongue paralysis.

Gastrointestinal System Disorders: *Frequent:* vomiting. *Infrequent:* hemorrhoids, stomatitis, melena, gastritis, tongue edema, esophagitis.

Heart Rate and Rhythm Disorders: *Infrequent:* AV block.

Liver and Biliary System Disorders: *Infrequent:* SGPT increased, SGOT increased, gamma-GT increased.

Metabolic and Nutritional Disorders: *Frequent:* dehydration. *Infrequent:* hypokalemia, alkaline phosphatase increased, hypocalcemia, hyperlipemia, acidosis, hyperglycemia, xerophthalmia. *Rare:* hyperchloremia, diabetes mellitus, hypernatremia, hyponatremia, hypocholesterolemia, hypophosphatemia, creatinine increased.

Musculoskeletal System Disorders: *Frequent:* arthralgia.

Neoplasms: *Infrequent:* thrombocythemia. *Rare:* polycythemia.

Platelet, Bleeding, and Clotting Disorders: *Infrequent:* gingival bleeding. *Rare:* pulmonary embolism.

Psychiatric Disorders: *Frequent:* impotence, hallucination, euphoria, psychosis, suicide attempt. *Infrequent:* paranoid reaction, delusion, paranoia, delirium, abnormal dreaming, neurosis. *Rare:* libido increased, manic reaction.

Red Blood Cell Disorders: *Frequent:* anemia. *Rare:* marrow depression, pancytopenia.

Reproductive Disorders, Male: *Infrequent:* ejaculation disorder, breast discharge.

Skin and Appendages Disorders: *Frequent:* acne. *Infrequent:* urticaria, photosensitivity reaction, abnormal hair texture. *Rare:* chloasma.

Special Senses Other, Disorders: *Infrequent:* taste loss, parosmia.

Urinary System Disorders: *Frequent:* dysuria, renal calculus. *Infrequent:* urinary retention, face edema, renal pain, albuminuria, polyuria, oliguria.

Vascular (Extracardiac) Disorders: *Infrequent:* flushing, deep vein thrombosis, phlebitis. *Rare:* vasospasm.

Vision Disorders: *Frequent:* conjunctivitis. *Infrequent:* abnormal accommodation, photophobia, strabismus. *Rare:* mydriasis, iritis.

White Cell and Reticuloendothelial System Disorders: *Infrequent:* lymphadenopathy, eosinophilia, lymphopenia, granulocytopenia. *Rare:* lymphocytosis.

Migraine

In the four multicenter, randomized, double-blind, placebo-controlled, parallel group migraine prophylaxis clinical trials, most of the adverse events with topiramate were mild or moderate in severity. Most adverse events occurred more frequently during the titration period than during the maintenance period.

Table 8 includes those adverse events reported for patients in the placebo-controlled trials where the incidence rate in any topiramate treatment group was at least 2 % and was greater than that for placebo patients.

[See table 8 at right and on next page]

Of the 1,135 patients exposed to topiramate in the placebo-controlled studies, 25% discontinued due to adverse events, compared to 10% of the 445 placebo patients. The adverse events associated with discontinuing therapy in the topiramate-treated patients included paresthesia (7%), fatigue (4%), nausea (4%), difficulty with concentration/attention (3%), insomnia (3%), anorexia (2%), and dizziness (2%). Patients treated with topiramate experienced mean percent reductions in body weight that were dose-dependent. This change was not seen in the placebo group. Mean changes of 0%, -2%, -3%, and -4% were seen for the placebo group, topiramate 50, 100, and 200 mg groups, respectively.

Table 9 shows adverse events that were dose-dependent. Several central nervous system adverse events, including some that represented cognitive dysfunction, were dose-related. The most common dose-related adverse events were

Table 7 *(cont.)*: Incidence (%) of Treatment-Emergent Adverse Events in Placebo-Controlled, Add-On Epilepsy Trials in Pediatric Patients Ages 2-16 Years[a,b] (Events That Occurred in at Least 1% of Topiramate-Treated Patients and Occurred More Frequently in Topiramate-Treated Than Placebo-Treated Patients)

Body System/ Adverse Event	Placebo (N=101)	Topiramate (N=98)
Urinary System Disorders		
Urinary Incontinence	2	4
Nocturia	0	1
Vision Disorders		
Eye Abnormality	1	2
Vision Abnormal	1	2
Diplopia	0	1
Lacrimation Abnormal	0	1
Myopia	0	1
White Cell and RES Disorders		
Leukopenia	0	2

[a] Patients in these add-on trials were receiving 1 to 2 concomitant antiepileptic drugs in addition to TOPAMAX® or placebo.
[b] Values represent the percentage of patients reporting a given adverse event. Patients may have reported more than one adverse event during the study and can be included in more than one adverse event category.

Table 8: Incidence of Treatment-Emergent Adverse Events in Placebo-Controlled, Migraine Trials Where Rate Was ≥2% in Any Topiramate Group and Greater than the Rate in Placebo-Treated Patients[a]

Body System/ Adverse Event	Placebo (N=445)	TOPAMAX® Dosage (mg/day) 50 (N=235)	100 (N=386)	200 (N=514)
Body as a Whole – General Disorders				
Fatigue	11	14	15	19
Injury	7	9	6	6
Asthenia	1	<1	2	2
Fever	1	1	1	2
Influenza-Like Symptoms	<1	<1	<1	2
Allergy	<1	2	<1	<1
Central & Peripheral Nervous System Disorders				
Paresthesia	6	35	51	49
Dizziness	10	8	9	12
Hypoaesthesia	2	6	7	8
Language Problems	2	7	6	7
Involuntary Muscle Contractions	1	2	2	4
Ataxia	<1	1	2	1
Speech Disorders/Related Speech Problems	<1	1	<1	2
Gastro-Intestinal System Disorders				
Nausea	8	9	13	14
Diarrhea	4	9	11	11
Abdominal Pain	5	6	6	7
Dyspepsia	3	4	5	3
Dry Mouth	2	2	3	5
Vomiting	2	1	2	3
Gastroenteritis	1	3	3	2
Hearing and Vestibular Disorders				
Tinnitus	1	<1	1	2
Metabolic and Nutritional Disorders				
Weight Decrease	1	6	9	11
Thirst	<1	2	2	1
Musculoskeletal System Disorders				
Arthralgia	2	7	3	1
Neoplasms				
Neoplasm NOS	<1	2	<1	<1
Psychiatric Disorders				
Anorexia	6	9	15	14
Somnolence	5	8	7	10
Difficulty with Memory NOS	2	7	7	11
Difficulty with Concentration/Attention	2	3	6	10
Insomnia	5	6	7	6
Anxiety	3	4	5	6
Mood Problems	2	3	6	5
Depression	4	3	4	6
Nervousness	2	4	4	4
Confusion	2	2	3	4
Psychomotor Slowing	1	3	2	4
Libido Decreased	1	1	1	2
Aggravated Depression	1	1	2	2
Agitation	1	2	2	1
Cognitive Problems NOS	1	<1	2	2
Reproductive Disorders, Female				
Menstrual Disorder	2	3	2	2
Reproductive Disorders, Male				
Ejaculation Premature	0	3	0	0
Resistance Mechanism Disorders				
Viral Infection	3	4	4	3
Otitis Media	<1	2	1	1
Respiratory System Disorders				
Upper Respiratory Tract Infection	12	13	14	12
Sinusitis	6	10	6	8
Pharyngitis	4	5	6	2
Coughing	2	2	4	3
Bronchitis	2	3	3	3
Dyspnea	2	1	3	2
Rhinitis	1	1	2	2

(Table continued on next page)

paresthesia, fatigue, nausea, anorexia, dizziness, difficulty with memory, diarrhea, weight decrease, difficulty with concentration/attention, and somnolence.

[See table 9 at right]

Other Adverse Events Observed During Migraine Clinical Trials

Topiramate, for the treatment of prophylaxis of migraine headache, has been administered to 1,367 patients in all clinical studies (includes double-blind and open-label extension). During these studies, all adverse events were recorded by the clinical investigators using terminology of their own choosing. To provide a meaningful estimate of the proportion of individuals having adverse events, similar types of events were grouped into a smaller number of standardized categories using modified WHOART dictionary terminology.

The following additional adverse events that were not described earlier were reported by greater than 1% of the 1,367 topiramate-treated patients in the controlled clinical trials:

Body as a Whole: Pain, chest pain, allergic reaction.
Central & Peripheral Nervous System Disorders: Headache, vertigo, tremor, sensory disturbance, migraine aggravated.
Gastrointestinal System Disorders: Constipation, gastroesophageal reflux, tooth disorder.
Musculoskeletal System Disorders: Myalgia.
Platelet, Bleeding, and Clotting Disorders: Epistaxis.
Reproductive Disorders, Female: Intermenstrual bleeding.
Resistance Mechanism Disorders: Infection, genital moniliasis.
Respiratory System Disorders: Pneumonia, asthma.
Skin and Appendages Disorders: Rash, alopecia.
Vision Disorders: Abnormal accommodation, eye pain.

Postmarketing and Other Experience

In addition to the adverse experiences reported during clinical testing of TOPAMAX®, the following adverse experiences have been reported worldwide in patients receiving topiramate post-approval. These adverse experiences have not been listed above and data are insufficient to support an estimate of their incidence or to establish causation. The listing is alphabetized: bullous skin reactions (including erythema multiforme, Stevens-Johnson syndrome, toxic epidermal necrolysis), hepatic failure (including fatalities), hepatitis, pancreatitis, pemphigus, and renal tubular acidosis.

DRUG ABUSE AND DEPENDENCE

The abuse and dependence potential of TOPAMAX® has not been evaluated in human studies.

OVERDOSAGE

Overdoses of TOPAMAX® have been reported. Signs and symptoms included convulsions, drowsiness, speech disturbance, blurred vision, diplopia, mentation impaired, lethargy, abnormal coordination, stupor, hypotension, abdominal pain, agitation, dizziness and depression. The clinical consequences were not severe in most cases, but deaths have been reported after poly-drug overdoses involving TOPAMAX®.

Topiramate overdose has resulted in severe metabolic acidosis (see **WARNINGS**).

A patient who ingested a dose between 96 and 110 g topiramate was admitted to hospital with coma lasting 20-24 hours followed by full recovery after 3 to 4 days.

In acute TOPAMAX® overdose, if the ingestion is recent, the stomach should be emptied immediately by lavage or by induction of emesis. Activated charcoal has been shown to adsorb topiramate *in vitro*. Treatment should be appropriately supportive. Hemodialysis is an effective means of removing topiramate from the body.

DOSAGE AND ADMINISTRATION

Epilepsy

TOPAMAX® has been shown to be effective in adults and pediatric patients ages 2-16 years with partial onset seizures or primary generalized tonic-clonic seizures, and in patients 2 years of age and older with seizures associated with Lennox-Gastaut syndrome. In the controlled add-on trials, no correlation has been demonstrated between trough plasma concentrations of topiramate and clinical efficacy. No evidence of tolerance has been demonstrated in humans. Doses above 400 mg/day (600, 800, or 1,000 mg/day) have not been shown to improve responses in dose-response studies in adults with partial onset seizures.

It is not necessary to monitor topiramate plasma concentrations to optimize TOPAMAX® therapy. On occasion, the addition of TOPAMAX® to phenytoin may require an adjustment of the dose of phenytoin to achieve optimal clinical outcome. Addition or withdrawal of phenytoin and/or carbamazepine during adjunctive therapy with TOPAMAX® may require adjustment of the dose of TOPAMAX®. Because of the bitter taste, tablets should not be broken.

TOPAMAX® can be taken without regard to meals.

Adults (17 Years of Age and Over) - Partial Seizures, Primary Generalized Tonic-Clonic Seizures, or Lennox-Gastaut Syndrome

The recommended total daily dose of TOPAMAX® as adjunctive therapy in adults with partial seizures is 200-400 mg/day in two divided doses, and 400 mg/day in two divided doses as adjunctive treatment in adults with primary generalized tonic-clonic seizures. It is recommended that therapy be initiated at 25-50 mg/day followed by titration to an effective dose in increments of 25-50 mg/week. Ti-

Table 8 (cont.): Incidence of Treatment-Emergent Adverse Events in Placebo-Controlled, Migraine Trials Where Rate Was ≥2% in Any Topiramate Group and Greater than the Rate in Placebo-Treated Patients[a]

Body System/ Adverse Event	Placebo (N=445)	TOPAMAX® Dosage (mg/day)		
		50 (N=235)	100 (N=386)	200 (N=514)
Skin and Appendages Disorders				
Pruritis	2	4	2	2
Special Sense Other, Disorders				
Taste Perversion	1	15	8	12
Taste Loss	<1	1	1	2
Urinary System Disorders				
Urinary Tract Infection	2	4	2	4
Renal Calculus	0	0	1	2
Vision Disorders				
Vision Abnormal	<1	1	2	3
Blurred Vision[b]	2	4	2	4
Conjunctivitis	1	1	2	1

[a] Values represent the percentage of patients reporting a given adverse event. Patients may have reported more than one adverse event during the study and can be included in more than one adverse event category.
[b] Blurred vision was the most common term considered as vision abnormal. Blurred vision was an included term that accounted for >50% of events coded as vision abnormal, a preferred term.

Table 9: Incidence (%) of Dose-Related Adverse Events From Placebo-Controlled, Migraine Trials[a]

Adverse Event	Placebo (N=445)	TOPAMAX® Dosage (mg/day)		
		50 (N=235)	100 (N=386)	200 (N=514)
Paresthesia	6	35	51	49
Fatigue	11	14	15	19
Nausea	8	9	13	14
Anorexia	6	9	15	14
Dizziness	10	8	9	12
Weight decrease	1	6	9	11
Difficulty with Memory NOS	2	7	7	11
Diarrhea	4	9	11	11
Difficulty with Concentration/Attention	2	3	6	10
Somnolence	5	8	7	10
Hypoaesthesia	2	6	7	8
Anxiety	3	4	5	6
Depression	4	3	4	6
Mood Problems	2	3	6	5
Dry Mouth	2	2	3	5
Confusion	2	2	3	4
Involuntary Muscle Contractions	1	2	2	4
Abnormal Vision	<1	1	2	3
Renal Calculus	0	0	1	2

[a] The incidence rate of the adverse event in the 200 mg/day group was ≥2% than the rate in both the placebo group and the 50 mg/day group.

trating in increments of 25 mg/week may delay the time to reach an effective dose. Daily doses above 1,600 mg have not been studied.

In the study of primary generalized tonic-clonic seizures the initial titration rate was slower than in previous studies; the assigned dose was reached at the end of 8 weeks (see **CLINICAL STUDIES, Controlled Trials in Patients With Primary Generalized Tonic-Clonic Seizures).**

Pediatric Patients (Ages 2-16 Years) - Partial Seizures, Primary Generalized Tonic-Clonic Seizures, or Lennox-Gastaut Syndrome

The recommended total daily dose of TOPAMAX® (topiramate) as adjunctive therapy for patients with partial seizures, primary generalized tonic-clonic seizures, or seizures associated with Lennox-Gastaut syndrome is approximately 5 to 9 mg/kg/day in two divided doses. Titration should begin at 25 mg (or less, based on a range of 1 to 3 mg/kg/day) nightly for the first week. The dosage should then be increased at 1- or 2-week intervals by increments of 1 to 3 mg/kg/day (administered in two divided doses), to achieve optimal clinical response. Dose titration should be guided by clinical outcome.

In the study of primary generalized tonic-clonic seizures the initial titration rate was slower than in previous studies; the assigned dose of 6 mg/kg/day was reached at the end of 8 weeks (see **CLINICAL STUDIES, Controlled Trials in Patients With Primary Generalized Tonic-Clonic Seizures).**

Migraine

The recommended total daily dose of TOPAMAX® as treatment for prophylaxis of migraine headache is 100 mg/day administered in two divided doses. The recommended titration rate for topiramate for migraine prophylaxis to 100 mg/day is:

	Morning Dose	Evening Dose
Week 1	None	25 mg
Week 2	25 mg	25 mg
Week 3	25 mg	50 mg
Week 4	50 mg	50 mg

Dose and titration rate should be guided by clinical outcome. If required, longer intervals between dose adjustments can be used.

Administration of TOPAMAX® Sprinkle Capsules

TOPAMAX® (topiramate capsules) Sprinkle Capsules may be swallowed whole or may be administered by carefully opening the capsule and sprinkling the entire contents on a small amount (teaspoon) of soft food. This drug/food mixture should be swallowed immediately and not chewed. It should not be stored for future use.

Patients with Renal Impairment:

In renally impaired subjects (creatinine clearance less than 70 mL/min/1.73m²), one half of the usual adult dose is recommended. Such patients will require a longer time to reach steady-state at each dose.

Geriatric Patients (Ages 65 Years and Over):

Dosage adjustment may be indicated in the elderly patient when impaired renal function (creatinine clearance rate ≤70 mL/min/1.73 m²) is evident (see **DOSAGE AND ADMINISTRATION: Patients with Renal Impairment** and **CLINICAL PHARMACOLOGY: Special Populations: Age, Gender, and Race).**

Patients Undergoing Hemodialysis:

Topiramate is cleared by hemodialysis at a rate that is 4 to 6 times greater than a normal individual. Accordingly, a prolonged period of dialysis may cause topiramate concentration to fall below that required to maintain an antiseizure effect. To avoid rapid drops in topiramate plasma concentration during hemodialysis, a supplemental dose of topiramate may be required. The actual adjustment should take into account 1) the duration of dialysis period, 2) the clearance rate of the dialysis system being used, and 3) the effective renal clearance of topiramate in the patient being dialyzed.

Patients with Hepatic Disease:

In hepatically impaired patients topiramate plasma concentrations may be increased. The mechanism is not well understood.

HOW SUPPLIED

TOPAMAX® (topiramate) Tablets is available as debossed, coated, round tablets in the following strengths and colors:
25 mg white (coded "TOP" on one side; "25" on the other)
50 mg light-yellow (coded "TOPAMAX" on one side; "50" on the other)
100 mg yellow (coded "TOPAMAX" on one side; "100" on the other)
200 mg salmon (coded "TOPAMAX" on one side; "200" on the other)

Continued on next page

Topamax—Cont.

They are supplied as follows:

25 mg tablets – bottles of 60 count with desiccant (NDC 0045-0639-65)

50 mg tablets – bottles of 60 count with desiccant (NDC 0045-0640-65)

100 mg tablets – bottles of 60 count with desiccant (NDC 0045-0641-65)

200 mg tablets – bottles of 60 count with desiccant (NDC 0045-0642-65)

TOPAMAX® (topiramate capsules) Sprinkle Capsules contain small, white to off white spheres. The gelatin capsules are white and clear.

They are marked as follows:

15 mg capsule with "TOP" and "15 mg" on the side
25 mg capsule with "TOP" and "25 mg" on the side
The capsules are supplied as follows:
15 mg capsules – bottles of 60 (NDC 0045-0647-65)
25 mg capsules – bottles of 60 (NDC 0045-0645-65)

TOPAMAX® (topiramate) Tablets should be stored in tightly-closed containers at controlled room temperature, (59 to 86°F, 15 to 30°C). Protect from moisture.

TOPAMAX® (topiramate capsules) Sprinkle Capsules should be stored in tightly-closed containers at or below 25°C (77°F). Protect from moisture.

TOPAMAX® (topiramate) and TOPAMAX® (topiramate capsules) are trademarks of Ortho-McNeil Pharmaceutical.

HOW TO TAKE
TOPAMAX® (topiramate capsules) SPRINKLE CAPSULES
A Guide for Patients and Their Caregivers

Your doctor has given you a prescription for TOPAMAX® (topiramate capsules) Sprinkle Capsules. Here are your instructions for taking this medication. Please read these instructions prior to use.

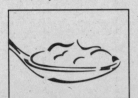

To Take With Food
You may sprinkle the contents of TOPAMAX® Sprinkle Capsules on a small amount (teaspoon) of soft food, such as applesauce, custard, ice cream, oatmeal, pudding, or yogurt.

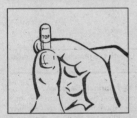

Hold the capsule upright so that you can read the word "TOP."

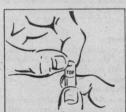

Carefully twist off the clear portion of the capsule. You may find it best to do this over the small portion of the food onto which you will be pouring the sprinkles.

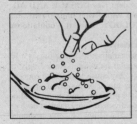

Sprinkle all of the capsule's contents onto a spoonful of soft food, taking care to see that the entire prescribed dosage is sprinkled onto the food.

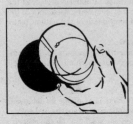

Be sure the patient swallows the entire spoonful of the sprinkle/food mixture immediately. Chewing should be avoided. It may be helpful to have the patient drink fluids immediately in order to make sure all of the mixture is swallowed. IMPORTANT: Never store any sprinkle/food mixture for use at a later time.

To Take Without Food
TOPAMAX® Sprinkle Capsules may also be swallowed as whole capsules.

For more information about TOPAMAX® Sprinkle Capsules, ask your doctor or pharmacist.

ORTHO-McNEIL
OMP DIVISION
ORTHO-McNEIL PHARMACEUTICAL, INC.
Raritan, NJ 08869
© OMP 1999   Revision Date October 2004   7517112

ULTRACET® ℞
[ŭl′tră-sĕt]
(tramadol hydrochloride/acetaminophen tablets)

Prescribing Information

Prescribing information for this product, which appears on pages 2549–2551 of the 2005 PDR, has been completely revised as follows. Please write "See Supplement A" next to the product heading.

DESCRIPTION

ULTRACET® (tramadol hydrochloride/acetaminophen) Tablets combines two analgesics, tramadol 37.5 mg and acetaminophen 325 mg.

The chemical name for tramadol hydrochloride is (±)*cis*-2-[(dimethylamino)methyl]-1-(3-methoxyphenyl) cyclohexanol hydrochloride. Its structural formula is:

The molecular weight of tramadol hydrochloride is 299.84. Tramadol hydrochloride is a white, bitter, crystalline and odorless powder.

The chemical name for acetaminophen is *N*-acetyl-*p*-aminophenol. Its structural formula is:

The molecular weight of acetaminophen is 151.17. Acetaminophen is an analgesic and antipyretic agent which occurs as a white, odorless, crystalline powder, possessing a slightly bitter taste.

ULTRACET tablets contain 37.5 mg tramadol hydrochloride and 325 mg acetaminophen and are light yellow in color. Inactive ingredients in the tablet are powdered cellulose, pregelatinized corn starch, sodium starch glycolate, starch, purified water, magnesium stearate, OPADRY® Light Yellow, and carnauba wax.

CLINICAL PHARMACOLOGY

The following information is based on studies of tramadol alone or acetaminophen alone, except where otherwise noted:

Pharmacodynamics
Tramadol is a centrally acting synthetic opioid analgesic. Although its mode of action is not completely understood, from animal tests, at least two complementary mechanisms appear applicable: binding of parent and M1 metabolite to μ-opioid receptors and weak inhibition of reuptake of norepinephrine and serotonin.

Opioid activity is due to both low affinity binding of the parent compound and higher affinity binding of the O-demethylated metabolite M1 to μ-opioid receptors. In animal models, M1 is up to 6 times more potent than tramadol in producing analgesia and 200 times more potent in μ-opioid binding. Tramadol-induced analgesia is only partially antagonized by the opiate antagonist naloxone in several animal tests. The relative contribution of both tramadol and M1 to human analgesia is dependent upon the plasma concentrations of each compound (see CLINICAL PHARMACOLOGY, Pharmacokinetics).

Tramadol has been shown to inhibit reuptake of norepinephrine and serotonin in vitro, as have some other opioid analgesics. These mechanisms may contribute independently to the overall analgesic profile of tramadol.

Apart from analgesia, tramadol administration may produce a constellation of symptoms (including dizziness, somnolence, nausea, constipation, sweating and pruritus) similar to that of other opioids.

Acetaminophen
Acetaminophen is a non-opiate, non-salicylate analgesic.

Pharmacokinetics
Tramadol is administered as a racemate and both the [-] and [+] forms of both tramadol and M1 are detected in the circulation. The pharmacokinetics of plasma tramadol and acetaminophen following oral administration of one ULTRACET tablet are shown in Table 1. Tramadol has a slower absorption and longer half-life when compared to acetaminophen.

[See table 1 at bottom of next page]

A single dose pharmacokinetic study of ULTRACET in volunteers showed no drug interactions between tramadol and acetaminophen. Upon multiple oral dosing to steady state, however, the bioavailability of tramadol and metabolite M1

was lower for the combination tablets compared to tramadol administered alone. The decrease in AUC was 14% for (+)-tramadol, 10.4% for (−)-tramadol, 11.9% for (+)-M1 and 24.2% for (−)-M1. The cause of this reduced bioavailability is not clear. Following single or multiple dose administration of ULTRACET, no significant change in acetaminophen pharmacokinetics was observed when compared to acetaminophen given alone.

Absorption:
The absolute bioavailability of tramadol from ULTRACET tablets has not been determined. Tramadol hydrochloride has a mean absolute bioavailability of approximately 75% following administration of a single 100 mg oral dose of ULTRAM® tablets. The mean peak plasma concentration of racemic tramadol and M1 after administration of two ULTRACET tablets occurs at approximately two and three hours, respectively, post-dose.

Peak plasma concentrations of acetaminophen occur within one hour and are not affected by co-administration with tramadol. Oral absorption of acetaminophen following administration of ULTRACET occurs primarily in the small intestine.

Food Effects:
When ULTRACET was administered with food, the time to peak plasma concentration was delayed for approximately 35 minutes for tramadol and almost one hour for acetaminophen. However, peak plasma concentration or the extent of absorption of either tramadol or acetaminophen were not affected. The clinical significance of this difference is unknown.

Distribution:
The volume of distribution of tramadol was 2.6 and 2.9 L/kg in male and female subjects, respectively, following a 100 mg intravenous dose. The binding of tramadol to human plasma proteins is approximately 20% and binding also appears to be independent of concentration up to 10 µg/mL. Saturation of plasma protein binding occurs only at concentrations outside the clinically relevant range.

Acetaminophen appears to be widely distributed throughout most body tissues except fat. Its apparent volume of distribution is about 0.9 L/kg. A relative small portion (~20%) of acetaminophen is bound to plasma protein.

Metabolism:
Following oral administration, tramadol is extensively metabolized by a number of pathways, including CYP2D6 and CYP3A4, as well as by conjugation of parent and metabolites. Approximately 30% of the dose is excreted in the urine as unchanged drug, whereas 60% of the dose is excreted as metabolites. The major metabolic pathways appear to be *N*- and *O*-demethylation and glucuronidation or sulfation in the liver. Metabolite M1 (*O*-desmethyltramadol) is pharmacologically active in animal models. Formation of M1 is dependent on CYP2D6 and as such is subject to inhibition, which may affect the therapeutic response (see PRECAUTIONS, Drug Interactions).

Approximately 7% of the population has reduced activity of the CYP2D6 isoenzyme of cytochrome P450. These individuals are "poor metabolizers" of debrisoquine, dextromethorphan, tricyclic antidepressants, among other drugs. Based on a population PK analysis of Phase 1 studies in healthy subjects, concentrations of tramadol were approximately 20% higher in "poor metabolizers" versus "extensive metabolizers," while M1 concentrations were 40% lower. In vitro drug interaction studies in human liver microsomes indicates that inhibitors of CYP2D6 such as fluoxetine and its metabolite norfluoxetine, amitriptyline and quinidine inhibit the metabolism of tramadol to various degrees. The full pharmacological impact of these alterations in terms of either efficacy or safety is unknown. Concomitant use of SEROTONIN re-uptake INHIBITORS and MAO INHIBITORS may enhance the risk of adverse events, including seizure (see WARNINGS) and serotonin syndrome.

Acetaminophen is primarily metabolized in the liver by first-order kinetics and involves three principal separate pathways:
a) conjugation with glucuronide;
b) conjugation with sulfate; and
c) oxidation via the cytochrome, P450-dependent, mixed-function oxidase enzyme pathway to form a reactive intermediate metabolite, which conjugates with glutathione and is then further metabolized to form cysteine and mercapturic acid conjugates. The principal cytochrome P450 isoenzyme involved appears to be CYP2E1, with CYP1A2 and CYP3A4 as additional pathways.

In adults, the majority of acetaminophen is conjugated with glucuronic acid and, to a lesser extent, with sulfate. These glucuronide-, sulfate-, and glutathione-derived metabolites lack biologic activity. In premature infants, newborns, and young infants, the sulfate conjugate predominates.

Elimination:
Tramadol is eliminated primarily through metabolism by the liver and the metabolites are eliminated primarily by the kidneys. The plasma elimination half-lives of racemic tramadol and M1 are approximately 5-6 and 7 hours, respectively, after administration of ULTRACET. The apparent plasma elimination half-life of racemic tramadol increased to 7-9 hours upon multiple dosing of ULTRACET. The half-life of acetaminophen is about 2 to 3 hours in adults. It is somewhat shorter in children and somewhat longer in neonates and in cirrhotic patients. Acetaminophen is eliminated from the body primarily by formation of glucuronide and sulfate conjugates in a dose-dependent manner. Less than 9% of acetaminophen is excreted unchanged in the urine.

Special Populations

Renal:
The pharmacokinetics of ULTRACET® in patients with renal impairment have not been studied. Based on studies using tramadol alone, excretion of tramadol and metabolite M1 is reduced in patients with creatinine clearance of less than 30 mL/min, adjustment of dosing regimen in this patient population is recommended. (See DOSAGE AND ADMINISTRATION.) The total amount of tramadol and M1 removed during a 4-hour dialysis period is less than 7% of the administered dose based on studies using tramadol alone.

Hepatic:
The pharmacokinetics and tolerability of ULTRACET in patients with impaired hepatic function has not been studied. Since tramadol and acetaminophen are both extensively metabolized by the liver, the use of ULTRACET in patients with hepatic impairment is not recommended (see PRECAUTIONS and DOSAGE AND ADMINISTRATION).

Geriatric:
A population pharmacokinetic analysis of data obtained from a clinical trial in patients with chronic pain treated with ULTRACET which included 55 patients between 65 and 75 years of age and 19 patients over 75 years of age, showed no significant changes in pharmacokinetics of tramadol and acetaminophen in elderly patients with normal renal and hepatic function (see PRECAUTIONS, Geriatric Use).

Gender:
Tramadol clearance was 20% higher in female subjects compared to males on four phase I studies of ULTRACET in 50 male and 34 female healthy subjects. The clinical significance of this difference is unknown.

Pediatric:
Pharmacokinetics of ULTRACET tablets have not been studied in pediatric patients below 16 years of age.

Clinical Studies
Single Dose Studies for Treatment of Acute Pain
In pivotal single-dose studies in acute pain, two tablets of ULTRACET® administered to patients with pain following oral surgical procedures provided greater relief than placebo or either of the individual components given at the same dose. The onset of pain relief after ULTRACET was faster than tramadol alone. Onset of analgesia occurred in less than one hour. The duration of pain relief after ULTRACET was longer than acetaminophen alone. Analgesia was generally comparable to that of the comparator, ibuprofen.

INDICATIONS AND USAGE
ULTRACET® is indicated for the short-term (five days or less) management of acute pain.

CONTRAINDICATIONS
ULTRACET® should not be administered to patients who have previously demonstrated hypersensitivity to tramadol, acetaminophen, any other component of this product or opioids. ULTRACET is contraindicated in any situation where opioids are contraindicated, including acute intoxication with any of the following: alcohol, hypnotics, narcotics, centrally acting analgesics, opioids or psychotropic drugs. ULTRACET may worsen central nervous system and respiratory depression in these patients.

WARNINGS
Seizure Risk
Seizures have been reported in patients receiving tramadol within the recommended dosage range. Spontaneous post-marketing reports indicate that seizure risk is increased with doses of tramadol above the recommended range. Concomitant use of tramadol increases the seizure risk in patients taking:
- Selective serotonin reuptake inhibitors (SSRI antidepressants or anorectics),
- Tricyclic antidepressants (TCAs), and other tricyclic compounds (e.g., cyclobenzaprine, promethazine, etc.), or
- Other opioids.
Administration of tramadol may enhance the seizure risk in patients taking:
- MAO inhibitors (see also WARNINGS—Use with MAO Inhibitors),
- Neuroleptics, or
- Other drugs that reduce the seizure threshold.
Risk of convulsions may also increase in patients with epilepsy, those with a history of seizures, or in patients with a recognized risk for seizure (such as head trauma, metabolic disorders, alcohol and drug withdrawal, CNS infections). In tramadol overdose, naloxone administration may increase the risk of seizure.

Anaphylactoid Reactions
Serious and rarely fatal anaphylactoid reactions have been reported in patients receiving therapy with tramadol. When these events do occur it is often following the first dose. Other reported allergic reactions include pruritus, hives, bronchospasm, angioedema, toxic epidermal necrolysis and Stevens-Johnson syndrome. Patients with a history of anaphylactoid reactions to codeine and other opioids may be at increased risk and therefore should not receive ULTRACET (see CONTRAINDICATIONS).

Respiratory Depression
Administer ULTRACET® cautiously in patients at risk for respiratory depression. In these patients, alternative non-opioid analgesics should be considered. When large doses of tramadol are administered with anesthetic medications or alcohol, respiratory depression may result. Respiratory depression should be treated as an overdose. If naloxone is to be administered, use cautiously because it may precipitate seizures (see WARNINGS, Seizure Risk and OVERDOSAGE).

Interaction With Central Nervous System (CNS) Depressants
ULTRACET® should be used with caution and in reduced dosages when administered to patients receiving CNS depressants such as alcohol, opioids, anesthetic agents, narcotics, phenothiazines, tranquilizers or sedative hypnotics. Tramadol increases the risk of CNS and respiratory depression in these patients.

Increased Intracranial Pressure or Head Trauma
ULTRACET® should be used with caution in patients with increased intracranial pressure or head injury. The respiratory depressant effects of opioids include carbon dioxide retention and secondary elevation of cerebrospinal fluid pressure and may be markedly exaggerated in these patients. Additionally, pupillary changes (miosis) from tramadol may obscure the existence, extent, or course of intracranial pathology. Clinicians should also maintain a high index of suspicion for adverse drug reaction when evaluating altered mental status in these patients if they are receiving ULTRACET (see Respiratory Depression).

Use in Ambulatory Patients
Tramadol may impair the mental and or physical abilities required for the performance of potentially hazardous tasks such as driving a car or operating machinery. The patient using this drug should be cautioned accordingly.

Use With MAO Inhibitors and Serotonin Re-uptake Inhibitors
Use ULTRACET® with great caution in patients taking monoamine oxidase inhibitors. Animal studies have shown increased deaths with combined administration of MAO inhibitors and tramadol. Concomitant use of tramadol with MAO inhibitors or SSRI's increases the risk of adverse events, including seizure and serotonin syndrome.

Use With Alcohol
ULTRACET® should not be used concomitantly with alcohol consumption. The use of ULTRACET in patients with liver disease is not recommended.

Use With Other Acetaminophen-containing Products
Due to the potential for acetaminophen hepatotoxicity at doses higher than the recommended dose, ULTRACET® should not be used concomitantly with other acetaminophen-containing products.

Withdrawal
Withdrawal symptoms may occur if ULTRACET® is discontinued abruptly. (See DRUG ABUSE AND DEPENDENCE.) These symptoms may include: anxiety, sweating, insomnia, rigors, pain, nausea, tremors, diarrhea, upper respiratory symptoms, piloerection, and rarely hallucinations. Other symptoms that have been seen less frequently with ULTRACET discontinuation include: panic attacks, severe anxiety, and paresthesias. Clinical experience suggests that withdrawal symptoms may be avoided by tapering ULTRACET at the time of discontinuation.

Physical Dependence and Abuse
Tramadol may induce psychic and physical dependence of the morphine-type (μ-opioid). (See DRUG ABUSE AND DEPENDENCE.) Tramadol should not be used in opioid-dependent patients. Tramadol has been shown to reinitiate physical dependence in some patients that have been previously dependent on other opioids. Dependence and abuse, including drug-seeking behavior and taking illicit actions to obtain the drug are not limited to those patients with prior history of opioid dependence.

Risk of Overdosage
Serious potential consequences of overdosage with tramadol are central nervous system depression, respiratory depression and death. In treating an overdose, primary attention should be given to maintaining adequate ventilation along with general supportive treatment. (See OVERDOSAGE.) Serious potential consequences of overdosage with acetaminophen are hepatic (centrilobular) necrosis, leading to hepatic failure and death. Emergency help should be sought immediately and treatment initiated immediately if overdose is suspected, even if symptoms are not apparent.

PRECAUTIONS
General
The recommended dose of ULTRACET® should not be exceeded.
Do not co-administer ULTRACET with other tramadol or acetaminophen-containing products. (See WARNINGS, Use With Other Acetaminophen-containing Products and Risk of Overdosage.)

Pediatric Use
The safety and effectiveness of ULTRACET® has not been studied in the pediatric population.

Geriatric Use
In general, dose selection for an elderly patient should be cautious, reflecting the greater frequency of decreased hepatic, renal, or cardiac function; of concomitant disease and multiple drug therapy.

Acute Abdominal Conditions
The administration of ULTRACET® may complicate the clinical assessment of patients with acute abdominal conditions.

Use in Renal Disease
ULTRACET® has not been studied in patients with impaired renal function. Experience with tramadol suggest that impaired renal function results in a decreased rate and extent of excretion of tramadol and its active metabolite, M1. In patients with creatinine clearances of less than 30 mL/min, it is recommended that the dosing interval of ULTRACET be increased not to exceed 2 tablets every 12 hours.

Use in Hepatic Disease
ULTRACET® has not been studied in patients with impaired hepatic function. The use of ULTRACET in patients with hepatic impairment is not recommended (see WARNINGS, Use With Alcohol).

Information for Patients
- ULTRACET® may impair mental or physical abilities required for the performance of potentially hazardous tasks such as driving a car or operating machinery.
- ULTRACET should not be taken with alcohol containing beverages.
- The patient should be instructed not to take ULTRACET in combination with other tramadol or acetaminophen-containing products, including over-the-counter preparations.
- ULTRACET should be used with caution when taking medications such as tranquilizers, hypnotics or other opiate containing analgesics.
- The patient should be instructed to inform the physician if they are pregnant, think they might become pregnant, or are trying to become pregnant (see PRECAUTIONS, Labor and Delivery).
- The patient should understand the single-dose and 24-hour dose limit and the time interval between doses, since exceeding these recommendations can result in respiratory depression, seizures, hepatic toxicity and death.

Drug Interactions
In vitro studies indicate that tramadol is unlikely to inhibit the CYP3A4-mediated metabolism of other drugs when tramadol is administered concomitantly at therapeutic doses. Tramadol does not appear to induce its own metabolism in humans, since observed maximal plasma concentrations after multiple oral doses are higher than expected based on single-dose data. Tramadol is a mild inducer of selected drug metabolism pathways measured in animals.

Use With Carbamazepine
Patients taking **carbamazepine** may have a significantly reduced analgesic effect of tramadol. Because carbamazepine increases tramadol metabolism and because of the seizure risk associated with tramadol, concomitant administration of ULTRACET® and carbamazepine is not recommended.

Use With Quinidine
Tramadol is metabolized to M1 by CYP2D6. **Quinidine** is a selective inhibitor of that isoenzyme; so that concomitant administration of quinidine and tramadol results in increased concentrations of tramadol and reduced concentrations of M1. The clinical consequences of these findings are unknown. In vitro drug interaction studies in human liver microsomes indicate that tramadol has no effect on quinidine metabolism.

Use With Inhibitors of CYP2D6
In vitro drug interaction studies in human liver microsomes indicate that concomitant administration with inhibitors of CYP2D6 such as fluoxetine, paroxetine, and amitriptyline could result in some inhibition of the metabolism of tramadol.

Use With Cimetidine
Concomitant administration of ULTRACET and **cimetidine** has not been studied. Concomitant administration of tramadol and cimetidine does not result in clinically significant changes in tramadol pharmacokinetics. Therefore, no alteration of the ULTRACET dosage regimen is recommended.

Use With MAO Inhibitors
Interactions with **MAO Inhibitors,** due to interference with detoxification mechanisms, have been reported for some centrally acting drugs (see WARNINGS, Use With MAO Inhibitors).

Use With Digoxin
Post-marketing surveillance of tramadol has revealed rare reports of **digoxin** toxicity.

Table 1: Summary of Mean (±SD) Pharmacokinetic Parameters of the (+)- and (−) Enantiomers of Tramadol and M1 and Acetaminophen Following A Single Oral Dose Of One Tramadol/Acetaminophen Combination Tablet (37.5 mg/ 325 mg) in Volunteers

Parameter[a]	(+)-Tramadol		(−)-Tramadol		(+)-M1		(−)-M1		acetaminophen	
C_{max} (ng/mL)	64.3	(9.3)	55.5	(8.1)	10.9	(5.7)	12.8	(4.2)	4.2	(0.8)
t_{max} (h)	1.8	(0.6)	1.8	(0.7)	2.1	(0.7)	2.2	(0.7)	0.9	(0.7)
CL/F (mL/min)	588	(226)	736	(244)	—	—	—	—	365	(84)
$t_{1/2}$ (h)	5.1	(1.4)	4.7	(1.2)	7.8	(3.0)	6.2	(1.6)	2.5	(0.6)

[a]For acetaminophen, C_{max} was measured as μg/mL.

Continued on next page

Ultracet—Cont.

Use With Warfarin Like Compounds
Post-marketing surveillance of both tramadol and acetaminophen individual products have revealed rare alterations of warfarin effect, including elevation of prothrombin times.

While such changes have been generally of limited clinical significance for the individual products, periodic evaluation of prothrombin time should be performed when ULTRACET and warfarin-like compounds are administered concurrently.

Carcinogenesis, Mutagenesis, Impairment of Fertility

There are no animal or laboratory studies on the combination product (tramadol and acetaminophen) to evaluate carcinogenesis, mutagenesis, or impairment of fertility.

A slight but statistically significant increase in two common murine tumors, pulmonary and hepatic, was observed in a mouse carcinogenicity study, particularly in aged mice. Mice were dosed orally up to 30 mg/kg (90 mg/m^2 or 0.5 times the maximum daily human tramadol dosage of 185 mg/m^2) for approximately two years, although the study was not done with the Maximum Tolerated Dose. This finding is not believed to suggest risk in humans. No such finding occurred in rat carcinogenicity study (dosing orally up to 30 mg/kg, 180 mg/m^2, or 1 time the maximum daily human tramadol dosage).

Tramadol was not mutagenic in the following assays: Ames *Salmonella* microsomal activation test, CHO/HPRT mammalian cell assay, mouse lymphoma assay (in the absence of metabolic activation), dominant lethal mutation tests in mice, chromosome aberration test in Chinese hamsters, and bone marrow micronucleus tests in mice and Chinese hamsters. Weakly mutagenic results occurred in the presence of metabolic activation in the mouse lymphoma assay and micronucleus test in rats. Overall, the weight of evidence from these tests indicates that tramadol does not pose a genotoxic risk to humans.

No effects on fertility were observed for tramadol at oral dose levels up to 50 mg/kg (350 mg/m^2) in male rats and 75 mg/kg (450 mg/m^2) in female rats. These dosages are 1.6 and 2.4 times the maximum daily human tramadol dosage of 185 mg/m^2.

Pregnancy

Teratogenic Effects: *Pregnancy Category C*
No drug-related teratogenic effects were observed in the progeny of rats treated orally with tramadol and acetaminophen. The tramadol/acetaminophen combination product was shown to be embryotoxic and fetotoxic in rats at a maternally toxic dose, 50/434 mg/kg tramadol/acetaminophen (300/2604 mg/m^2 or 1.6 times the maximum daily human tramadol/acetaminophen dosage of 185/1591 mg/m^2), but was not teratogenic at this dose level. Embryo and fetal toxicity consisted of decreased fetal weights and increased supernumerary ribs.

Non-teratogenic effects:
Tramadol alone was evaluated in peri- and post-natal studies in rats. Progeny of dams receiving oral (gavage) dose levels of 50 mg/kg (300 mg/m^2 or 1.6 times the maximum daily human tramadol dosage) or greater had decreased weights, and pup survival was decreased early in lactation at 80 mg/kg (480 mg/m^2 or 2.6 times the maximum daily human tramadol dosage).

There are no adequate and well-controlled studies in pregnant women. ULTRACET® should be used during pregnancy only if the potential benefit justifies the potential risk to the fetus. Neonatal seizures, neonatal withdrawal syndrome, fetal death and still birth have been reported with tramadol hydrochloride during post-marketing.

Labor and Delivery

ULTRACET® should not be used in pregnant women prior to or during labor unless the potential benefits outweigh the risks. Safe use in pregnancy has not been established. Chronic use during pregnancy may lead to physical dependence and post-partum withdrawal symptoms in the newborn. (See DRUG ABUSE AND DEPENDENCE.) Tramadol has been shown to cross the placenta. The mean ratio of serum tramadol in the umbilical veins compared to maternal veins was 0.83 for 40 women given tramadol during labor.

The effect of ULTRACET, if any, on the later growth, development, and functional maturation of the child is unknown.

Nursing Mothers

ULTRACET® is not recommended for obstetrical preoperative medication or for post-delivery analgesia in nursing mothers because its safety in infants and newborns has not been studied.

Following a single IV 100 mg dose of tramadol, the cumulative excretion in breast milk within 16 hours post-dose was 100 µg of tramadol (0.1% of the maternal dose) and 27 µg of M1.

ADVERSE REACTIONS

Table 2 reports the incidence rate of treatment-emergent adverse events over five days of ULTRACET® use in clinical trials (subjects took an average of at least 6 tablets per day).

Table 2: Incidence of Treatment-Emergent Adverse Events (≥2.0%)

Body System Preferred Term	ULTRACET (N = 142) %
Gastrointestinal System	
Constipation	6
Diarrhea	3
Nausea	3
Dry Mouth	2
Psychiatric Disorders	
Somnolence	6
Anorexia	3
Insomnia	2
Central & Peripheral Nervous System	
Dizziness	3
Skin and Appendages	
Sweating Increased	4
Pruritus	2
Reproductive Disorders, Male*	
Prostatic Disorder	2

*Number of males = 62

Incidence at least 1%, causal relationship at least possible or greater: the following lists adverse reactions that occurred with an incidence of at least 1% in single-dose or repeated-dose clinical trials of ULTRACET.
Body as a Whole—Asthenia, fatigue, hot flushes
Central and Peripheral Nervous System—Dizziness, headache, tremor
Gastrointestinal System—Abdominal pain, constipation, diarrhea, dyspepsia, flatulence, dry mouth, nausea, vomiting
Psychiatric Disorders—Anorexia, anxiety, confusion, euphoria, insomnia, nervousness, somnolence
Skin and Appendages—Pruritus, rash, increased sweating.
Selected Adverse events occurring at less than 1%: the following lists clinically relevant adverse reactions that occurred with an incidence of less than 1% in ULTRACET clinical trials.
Body as a Whole—Chest pain, rigors, syncope, withdrawal syndrome
Cardiovascular Disorders—Hypertension, aggravated hypertension, hypotension
Central and Peripheral Nervous System—Ataxia, convulsions, hypertonia, migraine, aggravated migraine, involuntary muscle contractions, stupor, vertigo
Gastrointestinal System—Dysphagia, melena, tongue edema
Hearing and Vestibular Disorders—Tinnitus
Heart Rate and Rhythm Disorders—Arrhythmia, palpitation, tachycardia
Liver and Biliary System—Hepatic function abnormal
Metabolic and Nutritional Disorders—Weight decrease
Psychiatric Disorders—Amnesia, depersonalization, depression, drug abuse, emotional lability, hallucination, impotence, paroniria, abnormal thinking
Red Blood Cell Disorders—Anemia
Respiratory System—Dyspnea
Urinary System—Albuminuria, micturition disorder, oliguria, urinary retention
Vision Disorders—Abnormal vision
Other clinically significant adverse experiences previously reported with tramadol hydrochloride.
Other events which have been reported with the use of tramadol products and for which a causal association has not been determined include: vasodilation, orthostatic hypotension, myocardial ischemia, pulmonary edema, allergic reactions (including anaphylaxis and urticaria, Stevens-Johnson syndrome/TENS), cognitive dysfunction, difficulty concentrating, depression, suicidal tendency, hepatitis liver failure and gastrointestinal bleeding. Reported laboratory abnormalities included elevated creatinine and liver function tests. Serotonin syndrome (whose symptoms may include mental status change, hyperreflexia, fever, shivering, tremor, agitation, diaphoresis, seizures and coma) has been reported with tramadol when used concomitantly with other serotonergic agents such as SSRIs and MAOIs.
Other clinically significant adverse experiences previously reported with acetaminophen.
Allergic reactions (primarily skin rash) or reports of hypersensitivity secondary to acetaminophen are rare and generally controlled by discontinuation of the drug and, when necessary, symptomatic treatment.

DRUG ABUSE AND DEPENDENCE

Tramadol may induce psychic and physical dependence of the morphine-type (μ-opioid). (See WARNINGS.) Dependence and abuse, including drug-seeking behavior and taking illicit actions to obtain the drug are not limited to those patients with a prior history of opioid dependence. The risk in patients with substance abuse has been observed to be higher. Tramadol is associated with craving and tolerance development. Withdrawal symptoms may occur if tramadol is discontinued abruptly. These symptoms may include: anxiety, sweating, insomnia, rigors, pain, nausea, tremors, diarrhea, upper respiratory symptoms, piloerection and rarely hallucinations. Other symptoms that have been seen less frequently with ULTRACET® discontinuation include: panic attacks, severe anxiety, and paresthesias. Clinical experience suggests that withdrawal symptoms may be relieved by reinstitution of opioid therapy followed by a gradual, tapered dose reduction of the medication combined with symptomatic support.

OVERDOSAGE

ULTRACET® is a combination product. The clinical presentation of overdose may include the signs and symptoms of tramadol toxicity, acetaminophen toxicity or both. The initial symptoms of tramadol overdosage may include respiratory depression and or seizures. The initial symptoms seen within the first 24 hours following an acetaminophen overdose are: anorexia, nausea, vomiting, malaise, pallor and diaphoresis.

Tramadol

Serious potential consequences of overdosage are respiratory depression, lethargy, coma, seizure, cardiac arrest and death. (See WARNINGS.) Fatalities have been reported in post marketing in association with both intentional and unintentional overdose with tramadol.

Acetaminophen

Serious potential consequences of overdosage with acetaminophen are hepatic centrilobular necrosis, leading to hepatic failure and death. Renal tubular necrosis, hypoglycemia and coagulation defects also may occur. Early symptoms following a potentially hepatotoxic overdose may include: nausea, vomiting, diaphoresis and general malaise. Clinical and laboratory evidence of hepatic toxicity may not be apparent until 48 to 72 hours post ingestion.

Treatment of Overdose

A single or multiple overdose with ULTRACET® may be a potentially lethal polydrug overdose, and consultation with a regional poison control center is recommended.

In treating an overdose of ULTRACET, primary attention should be given to maintaining adequate ventilation along with general supportive treatment. While naloxone will reverse some, but not all, symptoms caused by overdosage with tramadol, the risk of seizures is also increased with naloxone administration. In animals, convulsions following the administration of toxic doses of tramadol could be suppressed with barbiturates or benzodiazepines but were increased with naloxone. Naloxone administration did not change the lethality of an overdose in mice. Based on experience with tramadol, hemodialysis is not expected to be helpful in an overdose because it removes less than 7% of the administered dose in a 4-hour dialysis period.

Standard recommendations should be followed for the treatment of acetaminophen overdose.

DOSAGE AND ADMINISTRATION

For the short-term (five days or less) management of acute pain, the recommended dose of ULTRACET® is 2 tablets every 4 to 6 hours as needed for pain relief up to a maximum of 8 tablets per day.

Individualization of Dose

In patients with creatinine clearances of less than 30 mL/min, it is recommended that the dosing interval of ULTRACET® be increased not to exceed 2 tablets every 12 hours. Dose selection for an elderly patient should be cautious, in view of the potential for greater sensitivity to adverse events.

HOW SUPPLIED

ULTRACET® (tramadol hydrochloride/acetaminophen) Tablets are light yellow, coated, capsule-shaped tablets imprinted "O-M" on one side and "650" on the other are available as follows:
100's: NDC 0045 0650 60 (Bottles of 100 tablets)
500's: NDC 0045 0650 70 (Bottles of 500 tablets)
HUD 100's: NDC 0045 0650 10 (Packages of 100 unit doses in blister packs, 10 cards of 10 tablets each)
Dispense in a tight container. Store at 25°C (77°F); excursions permitted to 15 - 30°C (59 - 86°F).
ORTHO-McNEIL
OMP DIVISION
ORTHO-McNEIL PHARMACEUTICAL, INC.
Raritan, New Jersey 08869
U.S. Patent 5,336,691
© OMP 2004   Issued April 2004   7517201

To keep your **PDR** up to date throughout the year, note these revisions on the corresponding pages of the annual volume. Simply write **"See Supplement A"** next to the product heading.

Pfizer Inc.
235 EAST 42ND STREET
NEW YORK, NY 10017–5755

For updates to the product information listed below, please check the Pfizer Web site, http://www.pfizer.com, or call (800) 438-1985. For complete product listing, please see the Manufacturers' Index.

For Medical Information, Contact:
(800) 438-1985
24 hours a day, seven days a week.

Distribution:
1855 Shelby Oaks Drive North
Memphis, TN 38134
(901) 387-5200

Customer Service:
(800) 533-4535

Pfizer companies include:
Agouron Pharmaceuticals
Parke-Davis – (see Parke-Davis)
Pharmacia – (see Pharmacia & UpJohn)
G.D. Searle – (see G.D. Searle & Co.)

CADUET® ℞
[*kā-dew-ĕt*]
(amlodipine besylate/atorvastatin calcium)
Tablets

Prescribing information for this product, which appears on pages 2599–2605 of the 2005 PDR, has been completely revised as follows. Please write "See Supplement A" next to the product heading.

DESCRIPTION
CADUET® (amlodipine besylate and atorvastatin calcium) tablets combine the long-acting calcium channel blocker amlodipine besylate with the synthetic lipid-lowering agent atorvastatin calcium.
The amlodipine besylate component of CADUET is chemically described as 3-Ethyl-5-methyl (±)-2-[(2-aminoethoxy)methyl]-4-(o-chlorophenyl)-1,4-dihydro-6-methyl-3,5-pyridinedicarboxylate, monobenzenesulphonate. Its empirical formula is $C_{20}H_{25}ClN_2O_5 \bullet C_6H_6O_3S$.
The atorvastatin calcium component of CADUET is chemically described as [R-(R*, R*)]-2-(4-fluorophenyl)-β, δ-dihydroxy-5-(1-methylethyl)-3-phenyl-4-[(phenylamino)carbonyl]-1H-pyrrole-1-heptanoic acid, calcium salt (2:1) trihydrate. Its empirical formula is $(C_{33}H_{34}\ FN_2O_5)_2\ Ca \bullet 3H_2O$.
The structural formulae for amlodipine besylate and atorvastatin calcium are shown below.

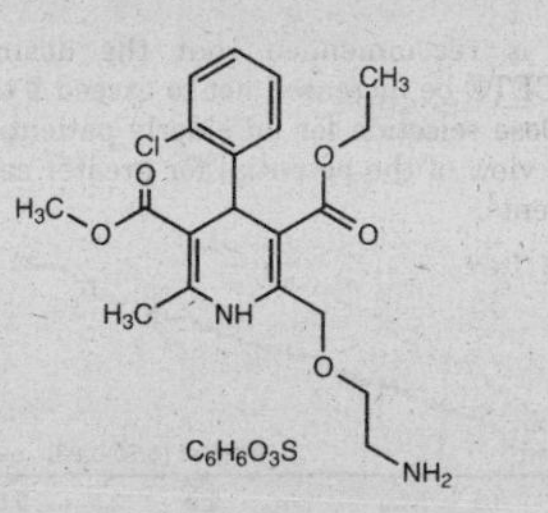

Amlodipine besylate

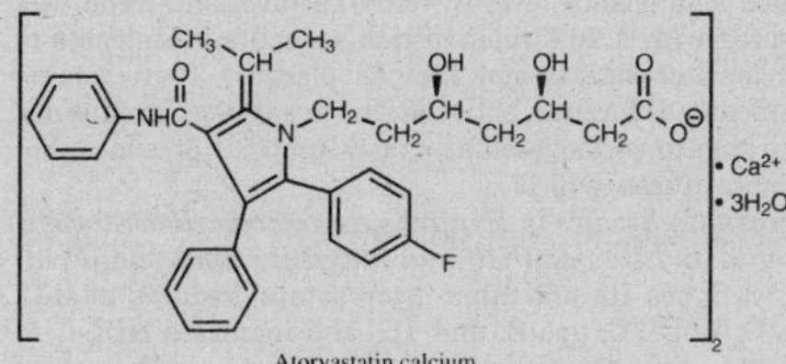

Atorvastatin calcium

CADUET contains amlodipine besylate, a white to off-white crystalline powder, and atorvastatin calcium, also a white to off-white crystalline powder. Amlodipine besylate has a molecular weight of 567.1 and atorvastatin calcium has a molecular weight of 1209.42. Amlodipine besylate is slightly soluble in water and sparingly soluble in ethanol. Atorvastatin calcium is insoluble in aqueous solutions of pH 4 and below. Atorvastatin calcium is very slightly soluble in distilled water, pH 7.4 phosphate buffer, and acetonitrile; slightly soluble in ethanol, and freely soluble in methanol.
CADUET tablets are formulated for oral administration in the following strength combinations:
[See table 1 above]
Each tablet also contains calcium carbonate, croscarmellose sodium, microcrystalline cellulose, pregelatinized starch, polysorbate 80, hydroxypropyl cellulose, purified water, colloidal silicon dioxide (anhydrous), magnesium stearate, Opadry® II White 85F28751 (polyvinyl alcohol, titanium dioxide, PEG 3000 and talc) or Opadry® II Blue 85F10919 (polyvinyl alcohol, titanium dioxide, PEG 3000, talc and FD&C blue #2). Combinations of atorvastatin with 2.5 mg and 5 mg amlodipine are film coated white, and combinations of atorvastatin with 10 mg amlodipine are film coated blue.

Table 1. CADUET Tablet Strengths

	2.5 mg/ 10 mg	2.5 mg/ 20 mg	2.5 mg/ 40 mg	5 mg/ 10 mg	5 mg/ 20 mg	5 mg/ 40 mg	5 mg/ 80 mg	10 mg/ 10 mg	10 mg/ 20 mg	10 mg/ 40 mg	10 mg/ 80 mg
amlodipine equivalent (mg)	2.5	2.5	2.5	5	5	5	5	10	10	10	10
atorvastatin equivalent (mg)	10	20	40	10	20	40	80	10	20	40	80

CLINICAL PHARMACOLOGY
Mechanism of Action
CADUET
CADUET is a combination of two drugs, a dihydropyridine calcium antagonist (calcium ion antagonist or slow-channel blocker) amlodipine (antihypertensive/antianginal agent) and an HMG-CoA reductase inhibitor atorvastatin (cholesterol lowering agent). The amlodipine component of CADUET inhibits the transmembrane influx of calcium ions into vascular smooth muscle and cardiac muscle. The atorvastatin component of CADUET is a selective, competitive inhibitor of HMG-CoA reductase, the rate-limiting enzyme that converts 3-hydroxy-3-methylglutaryl-coenzyme A to mevalonate, a precursor of sterols, including cholesterol.
The Amlodipine Component of CADUET
Experimental data suggest that amlodipine binds to both dihydropyridine and nondihydropyridine binding sites. The contractile processes of cardiac muscle and vascular smooth muscle are dependent upon the movement of extracellular calcium ions into these cells through specific ion channels. Amlodipine inhibits calcium ion influx across cell membranes selectively, with a greater effect on vascular smooth muscle cells than on cardiac muscle cells. Negative inotropic effects can be detected *in vitro* but such effects have not been seen in intact animals at therapeutic doses. Serum calcium concentration is not affected by amlodipine. Within the physiologic pH range, amlodipine is an ionized compound (pKa=8.6), and its kinetic interaction with the calcium channel receptor is characterized by a gradual rate of association and dissociation with the receptor binding site, resulting in a gradual onset of effect.
Amlodipine is a peripheral arterial vasodilator that acts directly on vascular smooth muscle to cause a reduction in peripheral vascular resistance and reduction in blood pressure.
The precise mechanisms by which amlodipine relieves angina have not been fully delineated, but are thought to include the following:
Exertional Angina: In patients with exertional angina, amlodipine reduces the total peripheral resistance (afterload) against which the heart works and reduces the rate pressure product, and thus myocardial oxygen demand, at any given level of exercise.
Vasospastic Angina: Amlodipine has been demonstrated to block constriction and restore blood flow in coronary arteries and arterioles in response to calcium, potassium epinephrine, serotonin, and thromboxane A_2 analog in experimental animal models and in human coronary vessels *in vitro*. This inhibition of coronary spasm is responsible for the effectiveness of amlodipine in vasospastic (Prinzmetal's or variant) angina.
The Atorvastatin Component of CADUET
Cholesterol and triglycerides circulate in the bloodstream as part of lipoprotein complexes. With ultracentrifugation, these complexes separate into HDL (high-density lipoprotein), IDL (intermediate-density lipoprotein), LDL (low-density lipoprotein), and VLDL (very-low-density lipoprotein) fractions. Triglycerides (TG) and cholesterol in the liver are incorporated into VLDL and released into the plasma for delivery to peripheral tissues. LDL is formed from VLDL and is catabolized primarily through the high-affinity LDL receptor.
Clinical and pathologic studies show that elevated plasma levels of total cholesterol (total-C), LDL-cholesterol (LDL-C), and apolipoprotein B (apo B) promote human atherosclerosis and are risk factors for developing cardiovascular disease, while increased levels of HDL-C are associated with a decreased cardiovascular risk.
Epidemiologic investigations have established that cardiovascular morbidity and mortality vary directly with the level of total-C and LDL-C, and inversely with the level of HDL-C.
In animal models, atorvastatin lowers plasma cholesterol and lipoprotein levels by inhibiting HMG-CoA reductase and cholesterol synthesis in the liver and by increasing the number of hepatic LDL receptors on the cell-surface to enhance uptake and catabolism of LDL; atorvastatin also reduces LDL production and the number of LDL particles.
Atorvastatin reduces total-C, LDL-C, and apo B in patients with homozygous and heterozygous familial hypercholesterolemia (FH), nonfamilial forms of hypercholesterolemia, and mixed dyslipidemia. Atorvastatin also reduces VLDL-C and TG and produces variable increases in HDL-C and apolipoprotein A-1. Atorvastatin reduces total-C, LDL-C, VLDL-C, apo B, TG, and non-HDL-C, and increases HDL-C in patients with isolated hypertriglyceridemia. Atorvastatin reduces intermediate density lipoprotein cholesterol (IDL-C) in patients with dysbetalipoproteinemia.
Like LDL, cholesterol-enriched triglyceride-rich lipoproteins, including VLDL, intermediate density lipoprotein (IDL), and remnants, can also promote atherosclerosis. Elevated plasma triglycerides are frequently found in a triad with low HDL-C levels and small LDL particles, as well as in association with non-lipid metabolic risk factors for coronary heart disease. As such, total plasma TG has not consistently been shown to be an independent risk factor for CHD. Furthermore, the independent effect of raising HDL or lowering TG on the risk of coronary and cardiovascular morbidity and mortality has not been determined.

Pharmacokinetics and Metabolism
Absorption
Studies with amlodipine: After oral administration of therapeutic doses of amlodipine alone, absorption produces peak plasma concentrations between 6 and 12 hours. Absolute bioavailability has been estimated to be between 64% and 90%. The bioavailability of amlodipine when administered alone is not altered by the presence of food.
Studies with atorvastatin: After oral administration alone, atorvastatin is rapidly absorbed; maximum plasma concentrations occur within 1 to 2 hours. Extent of absorption increases in proportion to atorvastatin dose. The absolute bioavailability of atorvastatin (parent drug) is approximately 14% and the systemic availability of HMG-CoA reductase inhibitory activity is approximately 30%. The low systemic availability is attributed to presystemic clearance in gastrointestinal mucosa and/or hepatic first-pass metabolism. Although food decreases the rate and extent of drug absorption by approximately 25% and 9%, respectively, as assessed by Cmax and AUC, LDL-C reduction is similar whether atorvastatin is given with or without food. Plasma atorvastatin concentrations are lower (approximately 30% for Cmax and AUC) following evening drug administration compared with morning. However, LDL-C reduction is the same regardless of the time of day of drug administration (see **DOSAGE AND ADMINISTRATION**).
Studies with CADUET: Following oral administration of CADUET peak plasma concentrations of amlodipine and atorvastatin are seen at 6 to 12 hours and 1 to 2 hours post dosing, respectively. The rate and extent of absorption (bioavailability) of amlodipine and atorvastatin from CADUET are not significantly different from the bioavailability of amlodipine and atorvastatin administered separately (see above).
The bioavailability of amlodipine from CADUET was not affected by food. Although food decreases the rate and extent of absorption of atorvastatin from CADUET by approximately 32% and 11%, respectively, as it does with atorvastatin when given alone. LDL-C reduction is similar whether atorvastatin is given with or without food.
Distribution
Studies with amlodipine: Ex vivo studies have shown that approximately 93% of the circulating amlodipine drug is bound to plasma proteins in hypertensive patients. Steady-state plasma levels of amlodipine are reached after 7 to 8 days of consecutive daily dosing.
Studies with atorvastatin: Mean volume of distribution of atorvastatin is approximately 381 liters. Atorvastatin is ≥98% bound to plasma proteins. A blood/plasma ratio of approximately 0.25 indicates poor drug penetration into red blood cells. Based on observations in rats, atorvastatin calcium is likely to be secreted in human milk (see **CONTRAINDICATIONS, Pregnancy and Lactation,** and **PRECAUTIONS, Nursing Mothers**).
Metabolism
Studies with amlodipine: Amlodipine is extensively (about 90%) converted to inactive metabolites via hepatic metabolism.
Studies with atorvastatin: Atorvastatin is extensively metabolized to ortho- and parahydroxylated derivatives and various beta-oxidation products. *In vitro* inhibition of HMG-CoA reductase by ortho- and parahydroxylated metabolites is equivalent to that of atorvastatin. Approximately 70% of circulating inhibitory activity for HMG-CoA reductase is attributed to active metabolites. *In vitro* studies suggest the importance of atorvastatin metabolism by cytochrome P450 3A4, consistent with increased plasma concentrations of atorvastatin in humans following coadministration with erythromycin, a known inhibitor of this isozyme (see **PRECAUTIONS, Drug Interactions**). In animals, the orthohydroxy metabolite undergoes further glucuronidation.
Excretion
Studies with amlodipine: Elimination from the plasma is biphasic with a terminal elimination half-life of about 30-50 hours. Ten percent of the parent amlodipine compound and 60% of the metabolites of amlodipine are excreted in the urine.

Continued on next page

Caduet—Cont.

Studies with atorvastatin: Atorvastatin and its metabolites are eliminated primarily in bile following hepatic and/or extra-hepatic metabolism; however, the drug does not appear to undergo enterohepatic recirculation. Mean plasma elimination half-life of atorvastatin in humans is approximately 14 hours, but the half-life of inhibitory activity for HMG-CoA reductase is 20 to 30 hours due to the contribution of active metabolites. Less than 2% of a dose of atorvastatin is recovered in urine following oral administration.

Special Populations

Geriatric
Studies with amlodipine: Elderly patients have decreased clearance of amlodipine with a resulting increase in AUC of approximately 40-60%, and a lower initial dose of amlodipine may be required.

Studies with atorvastatin: Plasma concentrations of atorvastatin are higher (approximately 40% for Cmax and 30% for AUC) in healthy elderly subjects (age ≥65 years) than in young adults. Clinical data suggest a greater degree of LDL-lowering at any dose of atorvastatin in the elderly population compared to younger adults (see **PRECAUTIONS** section, **Geriatric Use**).

Pediatric
Studies with amlodipine: Sixty-two hypertensive patients aged 6 to 17 years received doses of amlodipine between 1.25 mg and 20 mg. Weight-adjusted clearance and volume of distribution were similar to values in adults.
Studies with atorvastatin: Pharmacokinetic data in the pediatric population are not available.

Gender
Studies with atorvastatin: Plasma concentrations of atorvastatin in women differ from those in men (approximately 20% higher for Cmax and 10% lower for AUC); however, there is no clinically significant difference in LDL-C reduction with atorvastatin between men and women.

Renal Insufficiency
Studies with amlodipine: The pharmacokinetics of amlodipine are not significantly influenced by renal impairment. Patients with renal failure may therefore receive the usual initial amlodipine dose.
Studies with atorvastatin: Renal disease has no influence on the plasma concentrations or LDL-C reduction of atorvastatin; thus, dose adjustment of atorvastatin in patients with renal dysfunction is not necessary (see **DOSAGE AND ADMINISTRATION**).

Hemodialysis
While studies have not been conducted in patients with end-stage renal disease, hemodialysis is not expected to significantly enhance clearance of atorvastatin and/or amlodipine since both drugs are extensively bound to plasma proteins.

Hepatic Insufficiency
Studies with amlodipine: Elderly patients and patients with hepatic insufficiency have decreased clearance of amlodipine with a resulting increase in AUC of approximately 40-60%, and a lower initial dose may be required.
Studies with atorvastatin: In patients with chronic alcoholic liver disease, plasma concentrations of atorvastatin are markedly increased. Cmax and AUC are each 4-fold greater in patients with Childs-Pugh A disease. Cmax and AUC of atorvastatin are approximately 16-fold and 11-fold increased, respectively, in patients with Childs-Pugh B disease (see **CONTRAINDICATIONS**).

Heart Failure
Studies with amlodipine: In patients with moderate to severe heart failure, the increase in AUC for amlodipine was similar to that seen in the elderly and in patients with hepatic insufficiency.

Pharmacodynamics

Hemodynamic Effects of Amlodipine: Following administration of therapeutic doses to patients with hypertension, amlodipine produces vasodilation resulting in a reduction of supine and standing blood pressures. These decreases in blood pressure are not accompanied by a significant change in heart rate or plasma catecholamine levels with chronic dosing. Although the acute intravenous administration of amlodipine decreases arterial blood pressure and increases heart rate in hemodynamic studies of patients with chronic stable angina, chronic administration of oral amlodipine in clinical trials did not lead to clinically significant changes in heart rate or blood pressures in normotensive patients with angina.

With chronic once daily oral administration of amlodipine, antihypertensive effectiveness is maintained for at least 24 hours. Plasma concentrations correlate with effect in both young and elderly patients. The magnitude of reduction in blood pressure with amlodipine is also correlated with the height of pretreatment elevation; thus, individuals with moderate hypertension (diastolic pressure 105-114 mmHg) had about a 50% greater response than patients with mild hypertension (diastolic pressure 90-104 mmHg). Normotensive subjects experienced no clinically significant change in blood pressures (+1/-2 mmHg).

In hypertensive patients with normal renal function, therapeutic doses of amlodipine resulted in a decrease in renal vascular resistance and an increase in glomerular filtration rate and effective renal plasma flow without change in filtration fraction or proteinuria.

As with other calcium channel blockers, hemodynamic measurements of cardiac function at rest and during exercise (or pacing) in patients with normal ventricular function treated with amlodipine have generally demonstrated a small increase in cardiac index without significant influence on dP/dt or on left ventricular end diastolic pressure or volume. In hemodynamic studies, amlodipine has not been associated with a negative inotropic effect when administered in the therapeutic dose range to intact animals and man, even when co-administered with beta-blockers to man. Similar findings, however, have been observed in normals or well-compensated patients with heart failure with agents possessing significant negative inotropic effects.

Electrophysiologic Effects of Amlodipine: Amlodipine does not change sinoatrial nodal function or atrioventricular conduction in intact animals or man. In patients with chronic stable angina, intravenous administration of 10 mg did not significantly alter A-H and H-V conduction and sinus node recovery time after pacing. Similar results were obtained in patients receiving amlodipine and concomitant beta blockers. In clinical studies in which amlodipine was administered in combination with beta-blockers to patients with either hypertension or angina, no adverse effects on electrocardiographic parameters were observed. In clinical trials with angina patients alone, amlodipine therapy did not alter electrocardiographic intervals or produce higher degrees of AV blocks.

LDL-C Reduction with Atorvastatin: Atorvastatin as well as some of its metabolites are pharmacologically active in humans. The liver is the primary site of action and the principal site of cholesterol synthesis and LDL clearance. Drug dosage rather than systemic drug concentration correlates better with LDL-C reduction. Individualization of drug dosage should be based on therapeutic response (see **DOSAGE AND ADMINISTRATION**).

Clinical Studies

Clinical Studies with Amlodipine
Amlodipine Effects in Hypertension
Adult Patients: The antihypertensive efficacy of amlodipine has been demonstrated in a total of 15 double-blind, placebo-controlled, randomized studies involving 800 patients on amlodipine and 538 on placebo. Once daily administration produced statistically significant placebo-corrected reductions in supine and standing blood pressures at 24 hours postdose, averaging about 12/6 mmHg in the standing position and 13/7 mmHg in the supine position in patients with mild to moderate hypertension. Maintenance of the blood pressure effect over the 24-hour dosing interval was observed, with little difference in peak and trough effect. Tolerance was not demonstrated in patients studied for up to 1 year. The 3 parallel, fixed doses, dose response studies showed that the reduction in supine and standing blood pressures was dose-related within the recommended dosing range. Effects on diastolic pressure were similar in young and older patients. The effect on systolic pressure was greater in older patients, perhaps because of greater baseline systolic pressure. Effects were similar in black patients and in white patients.
Pediatric Patients: Two-hundred sixty-eight hypertensive patients aged 6 to 17 years were randomized first to amlodipine 2.5 or 5 mg once daily for 4 weeks and then randomized again to the same dose or to placebo for another 4 weeks. Patients receiving 5 mg amlodipine at the end of 8 weeks had lower blood pressure than those secondarily randomized to placebo. The magnitude of the treatment effect is difficult to interpret, but it is probably less than 5 mmHg systolic on the 5 mg dose. Adverse events were similar to those seen in adults.
Amlodipine Effects in Chronic Stable Angina: The effectiveness of 5-10 mg/day of amlodipine in exercise-induced angina has been evaluated in 8 placebo-controlled, double-blind clinical trials of up to 6 weeks duration involving 1038 patients (684 amlodipine, 354 placebo) with chronic stable angina. In 5 of the 8 studies, significant increases in exercise time (bicycle or treadmill) were seen with the 10 mg dose. Increases in symptom-limited exercise time averaged 12.8% (63 sec) for amlodipine 10 mg, and averaged 7.9% (38 sec) for amlodipine 5 mg. Amlodipine 10 mg also increased time to 1 mm ST segment deviation in several studies and decreased angina attack rate. The sustained efficacy of amlodipine in angina patients has been demonstrated over long-term dosing. In patients with angina, there were no clinically significant reductions in blood pressures (4/1 mmHg) or changes in heart rate (+0.3 bpm).
Amlodipine Effects in Vasospastic Angina: In a double-blind, placebo-controlled clinical trial of 4 weeks duration in 50 patients, amlodipine therapy decreased attacks by approximately 4/week compared with a placebo decrease of approximately 1/week (p<0.01). Two of 23 amlodipine and 7 of 27 placebo patients discontinued from the study due to lack of clinical improvement.
Amlodipine Effects in Patients with Congestive Heart Failure: Amlodipine has been compared to placebo in four 8-12 week studies of patients with NYHA class II/III heart failure, involving a total of 697 patients. In these studies, there was no evidence of worsened heart failure based on measures of exercise tolerance, NYHA classification, symptoms, or LVEF. In a long-term (follow-up at least 6 months, mean 13.8 months) placebo-controlled mortality/morbidity study of amlodipine 5-10 mg in 1153 patients with NYHA classes III (n=931) or IV (n=222) heart failure on stable doses of diuretics, digoxin, and ACE inhibitors, amlodipine had no effect on the primary endpoint of the study which was the combined endpoint of all-cause mortality and cardiac morbidity (as defined by life-threatening arrhythmia, acute myocardial infarction, or hospitalization for worsened heart failure), or on NYHA classification, or symptoms of heart failure. Total combined all-cause mortality and cardiac morbidity events were 222/571 (39%) for patients on amlodipine and 246/583 (42%) for patients on placebo; the cardiac morbid events represented about 25% of the endpoints in the study.

Another study (PRAISE-2) randomized patients with NYHA class III (80%) or IV (20%) heart failure without clinical symptoms or objective evidence of underlying ischemic disease, on stable doses of ACE inhibitor (99%), digitalis (99%) and diuretics (99%), to placebo (n=827) or amlodipine (n=827) and followed them for a mean of 33 months. There was no statistically significant difference between amlodipine and placebo in the primary endpoint of all cause mortality (95% confidence limits from 8% reduction to 29% increase on amlodipine). With amlodipine there were more reports of pulmonary edema.

Clinical Studies with Atorvastatin
Prevention of Cardiovascular Disease: In the Anglo-Scandinavian Cardiac Outcomes Trial (ASCOT), the effect of atorvastatin on fatal and non-fatal coronary heart disease was assessed in 10,305 hypertensive patients 40-80 years of age (mean of 63 years), without a previous myocardial infarction and with TC levels ≤251 mg/dl (6.5 mmol/l). Additionally all patients had at least 3 of the following cardiovascular risk factors: male gender (81.1%), age >55 years (84.5%), smoking (33.2%), diabetes (24.3%), history of CHD in a first-degree relative (26%), TC:HDL >6 (14.3%), peripheral vascular disease (5.1%), left ventricular hypertrophy (14.4%), prior cerebrovascular event (9.8%), specific ECG abnormality (14.3%), proteinuria/albuminuria (62.4%)]. In this double-blind, placebo-controlled study patients were treated with anti-hypertensive therapy (Goal BP <140/90 mm Hg for non-diabetic patients, <130/80 mm Hg for diabetic patients) and allocated to either atorvastatin 10 mg daily (n=5168) or placebo (n=5137), using a covariate adaptive method which took into account the distribution of nine baseline characteristics of patients already enrolled and minimized the imbalance of those characteristics across the groups. Patients were followed for a median duration of 3.3 years.

The effect of 10 mg/day of atorvastatin on lipid levels was similar to that seen in previous clinical trials.

Atorvastatin significantly reduced the rate of coronary events [either fatal coronary heart disease (46 events in the placebo group vs 40 events in the atorvastatin group) or nonfatal MI (108 events in the placebo group vs 60 events in the atorvastatin group)] with a relative risk reduction of 36% [(based on incidences of 1.9% for atorvastatin vs 3.0% for placebo), p=0.0005 (see Figure 1)]. The risk reduction was consistent regardless of age, smoking status, obesity or presence of renal dysfunction. The effect of atorvastatin was seen regardless of baseline LDL levels. Due to the small number of events, results for women were inconclusive.

Figure 1: Effect of Atorvastatin 10 mg/day on Cumulative Incidence of Nonfatal Myocardial Infarction or Coronary Heart Disease Death (in ASCOT-LLA)

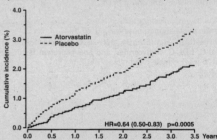

Atorvastatin also significantly decreased the relative risk for revascularization procedures by 42% Although the reduction of fatal and non-fatal strokes did not reach a pre-defined significance level (p=0.01), a favorable trend was observed with a 26% relative risk reduction (incidences of 1.7% for atorvastatin and 2.3% for placebo). There was no significant difference between the treatment groups for death due to cardiovascular causes (p=0.51) or noncardiovascular causes (p=0.17).

Atorvastatin Studies in Hypercholesterolemia (Heterozygous Familial and Nonfamilial) and Mixed Dyslipidemia (Fredrickson Types IIa and IIb): Atorvastatin reduces total-C, LDL-C, VLDL-C, apo B, and TG, and increases HDL-C in patients with hypercholesterolemia and mixed dyslipidemia. Therapeutic response is seen within 2 weeks, and maximum response is usually achieved within 4 weeks and maintained during chronic therapy.

Atorvastatin is effective in a wide variety of patient populations with hypercholesterolemia, with and without hypertriglyceridemia, in men and women, and in the elderly.

In two multicenter, placebo-controlled, dose-response studies in patients with hypercholesterolemia, atorvastatin given as a single dose over 6 weeks significantly reduced total-C, LDL-C, apo B, and TG (pooled results are provided in Table 2).

[See table 2 at top of next page]

In patients with *Fredrickson* Types IIa and IIb hyperlipoproteinemia pooled from 24 controlled trials, the median (25th and 75th percentile) percent changes from baseline in HDL-C for atorvastatin 10, 20, 40, and 80 mg were 6.4 (-1.4, 14), 8.7 (0, 17), 7.8 (0, 16), and 5.1 (-2.7, 15), respectively. Additionally, analysis of the pooled data demonstrated consistent and significant decreases in total-C, LDL-C, TG, total-C/HDL-C, and LDL-C/HDL-C.

In three multicenter, double-blind studies in patients with hypercholesterolemia, atorvastatin was compared to other

HMG-CoA reductase inhibitors. After randomization, patients were treated for 16 weeks with either atorvastatin 10 mg per day or a fixed dose of the comparative agent (Table 3).

[See table 3 at right]

The impact on clinical outcomes of the differences in lipid-altering effects between treatments shown in Table 3 is not known. Table 3 does not contain data comparing the effects of atorvastatin 10 mg and higher doses of lovastatin, pravastatin, and simvastatin. The drugs compared in the studies summarized in the table are not necessarily interchangeable.

Atorvastatin Effects in Hypertriglyceridemia (Fredrickson Type IV): The response to atorvastatin in 64 patients with isolated hypertriglyceridemia treated across several clinical trials is shown in the table below. For the atorvastatin-treated patients, median (min, max) baseline TG level was 565 (267-1502).

[See table 4 at right]

Atorvastatin Effects in Dysbetalipoproteinemia (Fredrickson Type III): The results of an open-label crossover study of atorvastatin in 16 patients (genotypes: 14 apo E2/E2 and 2 apo E3/E2) with dysbetalipoproteinemia (*Fredrickson* Type III) are shown in the table below.

[See table 5 below]

Atorvastatin Effects in Homozygous Familial Hypercholesterolemia: In a study without a concurrent control group, 29 patients ages 6 to 37 years with homozygous FH received maximum daily doses of 20 to 80 mg of atorvastatin. The mean LDL-C reduction in this study was 18%. Twenty-five patients with a reduction in LDL-C had a mean response of 20% (range of 7% to 53%, median of 24%); the remaining 4 patients had 7% to 24% increases in LDL-C. Five of the 29 patients had absent LDL-receptor function. Of these, 2 patients also had a portacaval shunt and had no significant reduction in LDL-C. The remaining 3 receptor-negative patients had a mean LDL-C reduction of 22%.

Atorvastatin Effects in Heterozygous Familial Hypercholesterolemic Pediatric Patients: In a double-blind, placebo-controlled study followed by an open-label phase, 187 boys and postmenarchal girls 10-17 years of age (mean age 14.1 years) with heterozygous FH or severe hypercholesterolemia were randomized to atorvastatin (n=140) or placebo (n=47) for 26 weeks and then all received atorvastatin for 26 weeks. Inclusion in the study required 1) a baseline LDL-C level ≥ 190 mg/dL or 2) a baseline LDL-C ≥ 160 mg/dL and positive family history of FH or documented premature cardiovascular disease in a first- or second-degree relative. The mean baseline LDL-C value was 218.6 mg/dL (range: 138.5-385.0 mg/dL) in the atorvastatin group compared to 230.0 mg/dL (range: 160.0-324.5 mg/dL) in placebo group. The dosage of atorvastatin (once daily) was 10 mg for the first 4 weeks and up-titrated to 20 mg if the LDL-C level was > 130 mg/dL. The number of atorvastatin-treated patients who required up-titration to 20 mg after Week 4 during the double-blind phase was 80 (57.1%).

Atorvastatin significantly decreased plasma levels of total-C, LDL-C, triglycerides, and apolipoprotein B during the 26 week double-blind phase (see Table 6).

[See table 6 at right]

The mean achieved LDL-C value was 130.7 mg/dL (range: 70.0-242.0 mg/dL) in the atorvastatin group compared to 228.5 mg/dL (range: 152.0-385.0 mg/dL) in the placebo group during the 26 week double-blind phase.

The safety and efficacy of atorvastatin doses above 20 mg have not been studied in controlled trials in children. The long-term efficacy of atorvastatin therapy in childhood to reduce morbidity and mortality in adulthood has not been established.

Clinical Study of Combined Amlodipine and Atorvastatin in Patients with Hypertension and Dyslipidemia

In a double-blind, placebo-controlled study, a total of 1660 patients with co-morbid hypertension and dyslipidemia received once daily treatment with eight dose combinations of amlodipine and atorvastatin (5/10, 10/10, 5/20, 10/20, 5/40, 10/40, 5/80, or 10/80 mg), amlodipine alone (5 mg or 10 mg), atorvastatin alone (10 mg, 20 mg, 40 mg, or 80 mg) or placebo. In addition to concomitant hypertension and dyslipidemia, 15% of the patients had diabetes mellitus, 22% were smokers and 14% had a positive family history of cardiovascular disease. At eight weeks, all eight combination-treatment groups of amlodipine and atorvastatin demonstrated statistically significant dose-related reductions in systolic blood pressure (SBP), diastolic blood pressure (DBP) and LDL-C compared to placebo, with no overall modification of effect of either component on SBP, DBP and LDL-C (Table 7).

[See table 7 at top of next page]

INDICATIONS AND USAGE

CADUET (amlodipine and atorvastatin) is indicated in patients for whom treatment with both amlodipine and atorvastatin is appropriate.

Amlodipine

1. *Hypertension:* Amlodipine is indicated for the treatment of hypertension. It may be used alone or in combination with other antihypertensive agents;

2. *Chronic Stable Angina:* Amlodipine is indicated for the treatment of chronic stable angina. Amlodipine may be used alone or in combination with other antianginal or antihypertensive agents;

3. *Vasospastic Angina (Prinzmetal's or Variant Angina):* Amlodipine is indicated for the treatment of confirmed or suspected vasospastic angina. Amlodipine may be used as monotherapy or in combination with other antianginal drugs.

AND

Atorvastatin

1. *Prevention of Cardiovascular Disease:* In adult patients without clinically evident coronary heart disease, but with multiple risk factors for coronary heart disease such as age ≥ 55 years, smoking, hypertension, low HDL-C, or a family history of early coronary heart disease, atorvastatin is indicated to:
— Reduce the risk of myocardial infarction
— Reduce the risk for revascularization procedures and angina

2. *Heterozygous Familial and Nonfamilial Hypercholesterolemia:* Atorvastatin is indicated as an adjunct to diet to reduce elevated total-C, LDL-C, apo B, and TG levels and to increase HDL-C in patients with primary hypercholesterolemia (heterozygous familial and nonfamilial) and mixed dyslipidemia (*Fredrickson* Types IIa and IIb);

3. *Elevated Serum TG Levels:* Atorvastatin is indicated as an adjunct to diet for the treatment of patients with elevated serum TG levels (*Fredrickson* Type IV);

4. *Primary Dysbetalipoproteinemia:* Atorvastatin is indicated for the treatment of patients with primary dysbetalipoproteinemia (*Fredrickson* Type III) who do not respond adequately to diet;

5. *Homozygous Familial Hypercholesterolemia:* Atorvastatin is indicated to reduce total-C and LDL-C in patients with homozygous familial hypercholesterolemia as an adjunct to other lipid-lowering treatments (e.g., LDL apheresis) or if such treatments are unavailable;

6. *Pediatric Patients:* Atorvastatin is indicated as an adjunct to diet to reduce total-C, LDL-C, and apo B levels in boys and postmenarchal girls, 10 to 17 years of age, with heterozygous familial hypercholesterolemia if after an adequate trial of diet therapy the following findings are present:
a. LDL-C remains ≥ 190 mg/dL or
b. LDL-C remains ≥ 160 mg/dL and:
• there is a positive family history of premature cardiovascular disease or
• two or more other CVD risk factors are present in the pediatric patients.

Continued on next page

Table 2. Dose-Response in Patients With Primary Hypercholesterolemia (Adjusted Mean Percent Change From Baseline)[a]

DOSE	N	TC	LDL-C	ApoB	TG	HDL-C	Non-HDL-C/HDL-C
Placebo	21	4	4	3	10	-3	7
10 mg	22	-29	-39	-32	-19	6	-34
20 mg	20	-33	-43	-35	-26	9	-41
40 mg	21	-37	-50	-42	-29	6	-45
80 mg	23	-45	-60	-50	-37	5	-53

[a]Results are pooled from 2 dose-response studies.

Table 3. Mean Percent Change From Baseline at Endpoint (Double-Blind, Randomized, Active-Controlled Trials)

Treatment (Daily Dose)	N	Total-C	LDL-C	Apo B	TG	HDL-C	Non-HDL-C/HDL-C
Study 1							
Atorvastatin 10 mg	707	-27[a]	-36[a]	-28[a]	-17[a]	+7	-37[a]
Lovastatin 20 mg	191	-19	-27	-20	-6	+7	-28
95% CI for Diff[1]		-9.2, -6.5	-10.7, -7.1	-10.0, -6.5	-15.2, -7.1	-1.7, 2.0	-11.1, -7.1
Study 2							
Atorvastatin 10 mg	222	-25[b]	-35[b]	-27[b]	-17[b]	+6	-36[b]
Pravastatin 20 mg	77	-17	-23	-17	-9	+8	-28
95% CI for Diff[1]		-10.8, -6.1	-14.5, -8.2	-13.4, -7.4	-14.1, -0.7	-4.9, 1.6	-11.5, -4.1
Study 3							
Atorvastatin 10 mg	132	-29[c]	-37[c]	-34[c]	-23[c]	+7	-39[c]
Simvastatin 10 mg	45	-24	-30	-30	-15	+7	-33
95% CI for Diff[1]		-8.7, -2.7	-10.1, -2.6	-8.0, -1.1	-15.1, -0.7	-4.3, 3.9	-9.6, -1.9

[1] A negative value for the 95% CI for the difference between treatments favors atorvastatin for all except HDL-C, for which a positive value favors atorvastatin. If the range does not include 0, this indicates a statistically significant difference.
[a] Significantly different from lovastatin, ANCOVA, p ≤0.05
[b] Significantly different from pravastatin, ANCOVA, p ≤0.05
[c] Significantly different from simvastatin, ANCOVA, p ≤0.05

Table 4. Combined Patients With Isolated Elevated TG: Median (min, max) Percent Changes From Baseline

	Placebo (N=12)	Atorvastatin 10 mg (N=37)	Atorvastatin 20 mg (N=13)	Atorvastatin 80 mg (N=14)
Triglycerides	-12.4 (-36.6, 82.7)	-41.0 (-76.2, 49.4)	-38.7 (-62.7, 29.5)	-51.8 (-82.8, 41.3)
Total-C	-2.3 (-15.4, 24.4)	-28.2 (-44.9, -6.8)	-34.9 (-49.6, -15.2)	-44.4 (-63.5, -3.8)
LDL-C	3.6 (-31.3, 31.6)	-26.5 (-57.7, 9.8)	-30.4 (-53.9, 0.3)	-40.5 (-60.6, -13.8)
HDL-C	3.8 (-18.6, 13.4)	13.8 (-9.7, 61.5)	11.0 (-3.2, 25.2)	7.5 (-10.8, 37.2)
VLDL-C	-1.0 (-31.9, 53.2)	-48.8 (-85.8, 57.3)	-44.6 (-62.2, -10.8)	-62.0 (-88.2, 37.6)
non-HDL-C	-2.8 (-17.6, 30.0)	-33.0 (-52.1, -13.3)	-42.7 (-53.7, -17.4)	-51.5 (-72.9, -4.3)

Table 5. Open-Label Crossover Study of 16 Patients With Dysbetalipoproteinemia (*Fredrickson* Type III)

	Median (min, max) at Baseline (mg/dL)	Median % Change (min, max) Atorvastatin 10 mg	Atorvastatin 80 mg
Total-C	442 (225, 1320)	-37 (-85, 17)	-58 (-90, -31)
Triglycerides	678 (273, 5990)	-39 (-92, -8)	-53 (-95, -30)
IDL-C + VLDL-C	215 (111, 613)	-32 (-76, 9)	-63 (-90, -8)
non-HDL-C	411 (218, 1272)	-43 (-87, -19)	-64 (-92, -36)

Table 6. Lipid-altering Effects of Atorvastatin in Adolescent Boys and Girls with Heterozygous Familial Hypercholesterolemia or Severe Hypercholesterolemia (Mean Percent Change from Baseline at Endpoint in Intention-to-Treat Population)

DOSAGE	N	Total-C	LDL-C	HDL-C	TG	Apolipoprotein B
Placebo	47	-1.5	-0.4	-1.9	1.0	0.7
Atorvastatin	140	-31.4	-39.6	2.8	-12.0	-34.0

Caduet—Cont.

Therapy with lipid-altering agents should be a component of multiple-risk-factor intervention in individuals at increased risk for atherosclerotic vascular disease due to hypercholesterolemia. Lipid-altering agents should be used, in addition to a diet restricted in saturated fat and cholesterol, only when the response to diet and other nonpharmacological measures has been inadequate (see *National Cholesterol Education Program (NCEP) Guidelines,* summarized in Table 8).

[See table 8 at right]

After the LDL-C goal has been achieved, if the TG is still ≥ 200 mg/dL, non-HDL-C (total-C minus HDL-C) becomes a secondary target of therapy. Non-HDL-C goals are set 30 mg/dL higher than LDL-C goals for each risk category. Prior to initiating therapy with atorvastatin, secondary causes for hypercholesterolemia (e.g., poorly controlled diabetes mellitus, hypothyroidism, nephrotic syndrome, dysproteinemias, obstructive liver disease, other drug therapy, and alcoholism) should be excluded, and a lipid profile performed to measure total-C, LDL-C, HDL-C, and TG. For patients with TG <400 mg/dL (<4.5 mmol/L), LDL-C can be estimated using the following equation: LDL-C = total-C - (0.20 x [TG] + HDL-C). For TG levels >400 mg/dL (>4.5 mmol/L), this equation is less accurate and LDL-C concentrations should be determined by ultracentrifugation.

The antidyslipidemic component of CADUET has not been studied in conditions where the major lipoprotein abnormality is elevation of chylomicrons (*Fredrickson* Types I and V). The NCEP classification of cholesterol levels in pediatric patients with a familial history of hypercholesterolemia or premature cardiovascular disease is summarized below:

Table 9. NCEP Classification of Cholesterol Levels in Pediatric Patients

Category	Total-C (mg/dL)	LDL-C (mg/dL)
Acceptable	<170	<110
Borderline	170-199	110-129
High	≥200	≥130

CONTRAINDICATIONS

CADUET contains atorvastatin and is therefore contraindicated in patients with active liver disease or unexplained persistent elevations of serum transaminases.

CADUET is contraindicated in patients with known hypersensitivity to any component of this medication.

Pregnancy and Lactation

Atherosclerosis is a chronic process and discontinuation of lipid-lowering drugs during pregnancy should have little impact on the outcome of long-term therapy of primary hypercholesterolemia. Cholesterol and other products of cholesterol biosynthesis are essential components for fetal development (including synthesis of steroids and cell membranes). Since HMG-CoA reductase inhibitors decrease cholesterol synthesis and possibly the synthesis of other biologically active substances derived from cholesterol, they may cause fetal harm when administered to pregnant women. Therefore, HMG-CoA reductase inhibitors are contraindicated during pregnancy and in nursing mothers. CADUET, WHICH INCLUDES ATORVASTATIN, SHOULD BE ADMINISTERED TO WOMEN OF CHILDBEARING AGE ONLY WHEN SUCH PATIENTS ARE HIGHLY UNLIKELY TO CONCEIVE AND HAVE BEEN INFORMED OF THE POTENTIAL HAZARDS. If the patient becomes pregnant while taking this drug, therapy should be discontinued and the patient apprised of the potential hazard to the fetus.

WARNINGS

Increased Angina and/or Myocardial Infarction

Rarely, patients, particularly those with severe obstructive coronary artery disease, have developed documented increased frequency, duration and/or severity of angina or acute myocardial infarction on starting calcium channel blocker therapy or at the time of dosage increase. The mechanism of this effect has not been elucidated.

Liver Dysfunction

HMG-CoA reductase inhibitors, like some other lipid-lowering therapies, have been associated with biochemical abnormalities of liver function. **Persistent elevations (>3 times the upper limit of normal [ULN] occurring on 2 or more occasions) in serum transaminases occurred in 0.7% of patients who received atorvastatin in clinical trials. The incidence of these abnormalities was 0.2%, 0.2%, 0.6%, and 2.3% for 10, 20, 40, and 80 mg, respectively.**

In clinical trials in patients taking atorvastatin the following has been observed. One patient in clinical trials developed jaundice. Increases in liver function tests (LFT) in other patients were not associated with jaundice or other clinical signs or symptoms. Upon dose reduction, drug interruption, or discontinuation, transaminase levels returned to or near pretreatment levels without sequelae. Eighteen of 30 patients with persistent LFT elevations continued treatment with a reduced dose of atorvastatin.

It is recommended that liver function tests be performed prior to and at 12 weeks following both the initiation of therapy and any elevation of dose, and periodically (e.g., semiannually) thereafter. Liver enzyme changes generally occur in the first 3 months of treatment with atorvastatin. Patients who develop increased transaminase levels should

Table 7. Efficacy in Terms of Reduction in Blood Pressure and LDL-C

Efficacy of the Combined Treatments in Reducing Systolic BP

Parameter / Analysis		ATO 0 mg	ATO 10 mg	ATO 20 mg	ATO 40 mg	ATO 80 mg
AML 0 mg	Mean Change (mmHg)	-3.0	-4.5	-6.2	-6.2	-6.4
	Difference versus placebo (mmHg)	-	-1.5	-3.2	-3.2	-3.4
AML 5 mg	Mean change (mmHg)	-12.8	-13.7	-15.3	-12.7	-12.2
	Difference versus placebo (mmHg)	-9.8	-10.7	-12.3	-9.7	-9.2
AML 10 mg	Mean change (mmHg)	-16.2	-15.9	-16.1	-16.3	-17.6
	Difference versus placebo (mmHg)	-13.2	-12.9	-13.1	-13.3	-14.6

Efficacy of the Combined Treatments in Reducing Diastolic BP

Parameter / Analysis		ATO 0 mg	ATO 10 mg	ATO 20 mg	ATO 40 mg	ATO 80 mg
AML 0 mg	Mean change (mmHg)	-3.3	-4.1	-3.9	-5.1	-1
	Difference versus placebo (mmHg)	-	-0.8	-0.6	-1.8	-0.8
AML 5 mg	Mean change (mmHg)	-7.6	-8.2	-9.4	-7.3	-8.4
	Difference versus placebo (mmHg)	-4.3	-4.9	-6.1	-4.0	-5.1
AML 10 mg	Mean change (mmHg)	-10.4	-9.1	-10.6	-9.8	-11.1
	Difference versus placebo (mmHg)	-7.1	-5.8	-7.3	-6.5	-7.8

Efficacy of the Combined Treatments in Reducing LDL-C (% change)

Parameter / Analysis		ATO 0 mg	ATO 10 mg	ATO 20 mg	ATO 40 mg	ATO 80 mg
AML 0 mg	Mean % change	-1.1	-33.4	-39.5	-43.1	-47.2
AML 5 mg	Mean % change	-0.1	-38.7	-42.3	-44.9	-48.4
AML 10 mg	Mean % change	-2.5	-36.6	-38.6	-43.2	-49.1

Table 8. NCEP Treatment Guidelines: LDL-C Goals and Cutpoints for Therapeutic Lifestyle Changes and Drug Therapy in Different Risk Categories

Risk Category	LDL-C Goal (mg/dL)	LDL-C Level at Which to Initiate Therapeutic Lifestyle Changes (mg/dL)	LDL-C Level at Which to Consider Drug Therapy (mg/dL)
CHD[a] or CHD risk equivalents (10-year risk >20%)	<100	≥100	≥130 (100-129: drug optional)[b]
2+ Risk Factors (10-year risk ≤20%)	<130	≥130	10-year risk 10%-20%: ≥130 10-year risk <10%: ≥ 160
0–1 Risk Factor[c]	<160	≥160	≥190 (160-189: LDL-lowering drug optional)

[a] CHD, coronary heart disease

[b] Some authorities recommend use of LDL-lowering drugs in this category if an LDL-C level of < 100 mg/dL cannot be achieved by therapeutic lifestyle changes. Others prefer use of drugs that primarily modify triglycerides and HDL-C, e.g., nicotinic acid or fibrate. Clinical judgement also may call for deferring drug therapy in this subcategory.

[c] Almost all people with 0-1 risk factor have 10-year risk <10%; thus, 10-year risk assessment in people with 0-1 risk factor is not necessary.

be monitored until the abnormalities resolve. Should an increase in ALT or AST of >3 times ULN persist, reduction of dose or withdrawal of CADUET is recommended.

CADUET should be used with caution in patients who consume substantial quantities of alcohol and/or have a history of liver disease. Active liver disease or unexplained persistent transaminase elevations are contraindications to the use of CADUET (see **CONTRAINDICATIONS**).

Skeletal Muscle

Rare cases of rhabdomyolysis with acute renal failure secondary to myoglobinuria have been reported with the atorvastatin component of CADUET and with other drugs in the HMG-CoA reductase inhibitor class.

Uncomplicated myalgia has been reported in atorvastatin-treated patients (see **ADVERSE REACTIONS**). Myopathy, defined as muscle aches or muscle weakness in conjunction with increases in creatine phosphokinase (CPK) values >10 times ULN, should be considered in any patient with diffuse myalgias, muscle tenderness or weakness, and/or marked elevation of CPK. Patients should be advised to report promptly unexplained muscle pain, tenderness or weakness, particularly if accompanied by malaise or fever.

CADUET therapy should be discontinued if markedly elevated CPK levels occur or myopathy is diagnosed or suspected.

The risk of myopathy during treatment with drugs in the HMG-CoA reductase inhibitor class is increased with concurrent administration of cyclosporine, fibric acid derivatives, erythromycin, niacin, or azole antifungals. Physicians considering combined therapy with CADUET and fibric acid derivatives, erythromycin, immunosuppressive drugs, azole antifungals, or lipid-lowering doses of niacin should carefully weigh the potential benefits and risks and should carefully monitor patients for any signs or symptoms of muscle pain, tenderness, or weakness, particularly during the initial months of therapy and during any periods of upward dosage titration of either drug. Periodic creatine phosphokinase (CPK) determinations may be considered in such situations, but there is no assurance that such monitoring will prevent the occurrence of severe myopathy.

In patients taking CADUET, therapy should be temporarily withheld or discontinued in any patient with an acute, serious condition suggestive of a myopathy or having a risk factor predisposing to the development of renal failure

secondary to rhabdomyolysis (e.g., severe acute infection, hypotension, major surgery, trauma, severe metabolic, endocrine and electrolyte disorders, and uncontrolled seizures).

PRECAUTIONS

General
Since the vasodilation induced by the amlodipine component of CADUET is gradual in onset, acute hypotension has rarely been reported after oral administration of amlodipine. Nonetheless, caution should be exercised when administering CADUET as with any other peripheral vasodilator particularly in patients with severe aortic stenosis.

Before instituting therapy with CADUET, an attempt should be made to control hypercholesterolemia with appropriate diet, exercise, and weight reduction in obese patients, and to treat other underlying medical problems (see **INDICATIONS AND USAGE**).

Use in Patients with Congestive Heart Failure
In general, calcium channel blockers should be used with caution in patients with heart failure. The amlodipine component of CADUET (5-10 mg per day) has been studied in a placebo-controlled trial of 1153 patients with NYHA Class III or IV heart failure (see **CLINICAL PHARMACOLOGY**) on stable doses of ACE inhibitor, digoxin, and diuretics. Follow-up was at least 6 months, with a mean of about 14 months. There was no overall adverse effect on survival or cardiac morbidity (as defined by life-threatening arrhythmia, acute myocardial infarction, or hospitalization for worsened heart failure). Amlodipine has been compared to placebo in four 8-12 week studies of patients with NYHA class II/III heart failure, involving a total of 697 patients. In these studies, there was no evidence of worsened heart failure based on measures of exercise tolerance, NYHA classification, symptoms, or LVEF.

Beta-Blocker Withdrawal
The amlodipine component of CADUET is not a beta-blocker and therefore gives no protection against the dangers of abrupt beta-blocker withdrawal; any such withdrawal should be by gradual reduction of the dose of beta-blocker.

Endocrine Function
HMG-CoA reductase inhibitors, such as the atorvastatin component of CADUET interfere with cholesterol synthesis and theoretically might blunt adrenal and/or gonadal steroid production. Clinical studies have shown that atorvastatin does not reduce basal plasma cortisol concentration or impair adrenal reserve. The effects of HMG-CoA reductase inhibitors on male fertility have not been studied in adequate numbers of patients. The effects, if any, on the pituitary-gonadal axis in premenopausal women are unknown. Caution should be exercised if an HMG-CoA reductase inhibitor is administered concomitantly with drugs that may decrease the levels or activity of endogenous steroid hormones, such as ketoconazole, spironolactone, and cimetidine.

CNS Toxicity
Studies with atorvastatin: Brain hemorrhage was seen in a female dog treated with atorvastatin calcium for 3 months at a dose equivalent to 120 mg atorvastatin/kg/day. Brain hemorrhage and optic nerve vacuolation were seen in another female dog that was sacrificed in moribund condition after 11 weeks of escalating doses of atorvastatin calcium equivalent to up to 280 mg atorvastatin/kg/day. The 120 mg/kg dose of atorvastatin resulted in a systemic exposure approximately 16 times the human plasma area-under-the-curve (AUC, 0-24 hours) based on the maximum human dose of 80 mg/day. A single tonic convulsion was seen in each of 2 male dogs (one treated with atorvastatin calcium at a dose equivalent to 10 mg atorvastatin/kg/day and one at a dose equivalent to 120 mg atorvastatin/kg/day) in a 2-year study. No CNS lesions have been observed in mice after chronic treatment for up to 2 years at doses of atorvastatin calcium equivalent to up to 400 mg atorvastatin/kg/day or in rats at doses equivalent to up to 100 mg atorvastatin/kg/day. These doses were 6 to 11 times (mouse) and 8 to 16 times (rat) the human AUC (0-24) based on the maximum recommended human dose of 80 mg atorvastatin/day.

CNS vascular lesions, characterized by perivascular hemorrhages, edema, and mononuclear cell infiltration of perivascular spaces, have been observed in dogs treated with other members of the HMG-CoA reductase class. A chemically similar drug in this class produced optic nerve degeneration (Wallerian degeneration of retinogeniculate fibers) in clinically normal dogs in a dose-dependent fashion at a dose that produced plasma drug levels about 30 times higher than the mean drug level in humans taking the highest recommended dose.

Information for Patients
Due to the risk of myopathy with drugs of the HMG-CoA reductase class, to which the atorvastatin component of CADUET belongs, patients should be advised to report promptly unexplained muscle pain, tenderness, or weakness, particularly if accompanied by malaise or fever.

Drug Interactions
Data from a drug-drug interaction study involving 10 mg of amlodipine and 80 mg of atorvastatin in healthy subjects indicate that the pharmacokinetics of amlodipine are not altered when the drugs are coadministered. The effect of amlodipine on the pharmacokinetics of atorvastatin showed no effect on the Cmax: 91% (90% confidence interval: 80 to 103%), but the AUC of atorvastatin increased by 18% (90% confidence interval: 109 to 127%) in the presence of amlodipine.

No drug interaction studies have been conducted with CADUET and other drugs, although studies have been conducted in the individual amlodipine and atorvastatin components, as described below:

Studies with Amlodipine:
In vitro data in human plasma indicate that amlodipine has no effect on the protein binding of drugs tested (digoxin, phenytoin, warfarin, and indomethacin).

Cimetidine: Co-administration of amlodipine with cimetidine did not alter the pharmacokinetics of amlodipine.

Maalox® (antacid): Co-administration of the antacid Maalox with a single dose of amlodipine had no significant effect on the pharmacokinetics of amlodipine.

Sildenafil: A single 100 mg dose of sildenafil (Viagra®) in subjects with essential hypertension had no effect on the pharmacokinetic parameters of amlodipine. When amlodipine and sildenafil were used in combination, each agent independently exerted its own blood pressure lowering effect.

Digoxin: Co-administration of amlodipine with digoxin did not change serum digoxin levels or digoxin renal clearance in normal volunteers.

Ethanol (alcohol): Single and multiple 10 mg doses of amlodipine had no significant effect on the pharmacokinetics of ethanol.

Warfarin: Co-administration of amlodipine with warfarin did not change the warfarin prothrombin response time.

In clinical trials, amlodipine has been safely administered with thiazide diuretics, beta-blockers, angiotensin-converting enzyme inhibitors, long-acting nitrates, sublingual nitroglycerin, digoxin, warfarin, non-steroidal anti-inflammatory drugs, antibiotics, and oral hypoglycemic drugs.

Studies with Atorvastatin:
The risk of myopathy during treatment with drugs of the HMG-CoA reductase class is increased with concurrent administration of cyclosporine, fibric acid derivatives, niacin (nicotinic acid), erythromycin, or azole antifungals (see **WARNINGS, Skeletal Muscle**).

Antacid: When atorvastatin and Maalox TC suspension were coadministered, plasma concentrations of atorvastatin decreased approximately 35%. However, LDL-C reduction was not altered.

Antipyrine: Because atorvastatin does not affect the pharmacokinetics of antipyrine, interactions with other drugs metabolized via the same cytochrome isozymes are not expected.

Colestipol: Plasma concentrations of atorvastatin decreased approximately 25% when colestipol and atorvastatin were coadministered. However, LDL-C reduction was greater when atorvastatin and colestipol were coadministered than when either drug was given alone.

Cimetidine: Atorvastatin plasma concentrations and LDL-C reduction were not altered by coadministration of cimetidine.

Digoxin: When multiple doses of atorvastatin and digoxin were coadministered, steady-state plasma digoxin concentrations increased by approximately 20%. Patients taking digoxin should be monitored appropriately.

Erythromycin: In healthy individuals, plasma concentrations of atorvastatin increased approximately 40% with co-administration of atorvastatin and erythromycin, a known inhibitor of cytochrome P450 3A4 (see **WARNINGS, Skeletal Muscle**).

Oral Contraceptives: Coadministration of atorvastatin and an oral contraceptive increased AUC values for norethindrone and ethinyl estradiol by approximately 30% and 20%. These increases should be considered when selecting an oral contraceptive for a woman taking CADUET.

Warfarin: Atorvastatin had no clinically significant effect on prothrombin time when administered to patients receiving chronic warfarin treatment.

Drug/Laboratory Test Interactions
None known.

Carcinogenesis, Mutagenesis, Impairment of Fertility
Studies with amlodipine: Rats and mice treated with amlodipine maleate in the diet for up to two years, at concentrations calculated to provide daily dosage levels of 0.5, 1.25, and 2.5 mg amlodipine/kg/day, showed no evidence of a carcinogenic effect of the drug. For the mouse, the highest dose was, on a mg/m² basis, similar to the maximum recommended human dose of 10 mg amlodipine/day*. For the rat, the highest dose level was, on a mg/m² basis, about twice the maximum recommended human dose*.

Mutagenicity studies conducted with amlodipine maleate revealed no drug related effects at either the gene or chromosome levels.

There was no effect on the fertility of rats treated orally with amlodipine maleate (males for 64 days and females for 14 days prior to mating) at doses up to 10 mg amlodipine/kg/day (8 times* the maximum recommended human dose of 10 mg/day on a mg/m² basis).

Studies with atorvastatin: In a 2-year carcinogenicity study with atorvastatin calcium in rats at dose levels equivalent to 10, 30, and 100 mg atorvastatin/kg/day, 2 rare tumors were found in muscle in high-dose females: in one, there was a rhabdomyosarcoma and, in another, there was a fibrosarcoma. This dose represents a plasma AUC (0-24) value of approximately 16 times the mean human plasma drug exposure after an 80 mg oral dose.

A 2-year carcinogenicity study in mice given atorvastatin calcium at dose levels equivalent to 100, 200, and 400 mg atorvastatin/kg/day resulted in a significant increase in liver adenomas in high-dose males and liver carcinomas in

high-dose females. These findings occurred at plasma AUC (0-24) values of approximately 6 times the mean human plasma drug exposure after an 80 mg oral dose.

In vitro, atorvastatin was not mutagenic or clastogenic in the following tests with and without metabolic activation: the Ames test with *Salmonella typhimurium* and *Escherichia coli*, the HGPRT forward mutation assay in Chinese hamster lung cells, and the chromosomal aberration assay in Chinese hamster lung cells. Atorvastatin was negative in the *in vivo* mouse micronucleus test.

There were no effects on fertility when rats were given atorvastatin calcium at doses equivalent to up to 175 mg atorvastatin/kg/day (15 times the human exposure). There was aplasia and aspermia in the epididymides of 2 of 10 rats treated with atorvastatin calcium at a dose equivalent to 100 mg atorvastatin/kg/day for 3 months (16 times the human AUC at the 80 mg dose); testis weights were significantly lower at 30 and 100 mg/kg/day and epididymal weight was lower at 100 mg/kg/day. Male rats given the equivalent of 100 mg atorvastatin/kg/day for 11 weeks prior to mating had decreased sperm motility, spermatid head concentration, and increased abnormal sperm. Atorvastatin caused no adverse effects on semen parameters, or reproductive organ histopathology in dogs given doses of atorvastatin calcium equivalent to 10, 40, or 120 mg atorvastatin/kg/day for two years.

Pregnancy
Pregnancy Category X (see CONTRAINDICATIONS)
Safety in pregnant women has not been established with CADUET. CADUET should be administered to women of child-bearing potential only when such patients are highly unlikely to conceive and have been informed of the potential hazards. If the woman becomes pregnant while taking CADUET, it should be discontinued and the patient advised again as to the potential hazards to the fetus.

Studies with amlodipine: No evidence of teratogenicity or other embryo/fetal toxicity was found when pregnant rats and rabbits were treated orally with amlodipine maleate at doses up to 10 mg amlodipine/kg/day (respectively 8 times* and 23 times* the maximum recommended human dose of 10 mg/day on a mg/m² basis) during their respective periods of major organogenesis. However, litter size was significantly decreased (by about 50%) and the number of intra-uterine deaths was significantly increased (about 5-fold) in rats receiving amlodipine maleate at 10 mg amlodipine/kg/day for 14 days before mating and throughout mating and gestation. Amlodipine maleate has been shown to prolong both the gestation period and the duration of labor in rats at this dose. There are no adequate and well-controlled studies in pregnant women.

*Based on patient weight of 50 kg.

Studies with atorvastatin: Atorvastatin crosses the rat placenta and reaches a level in fetal liver equivalent to that of maternal plasma. Atorvastatin was not teratogenic in rats at doses of atorvastatin calcium equivalent to up to 300 mg atorvastatin/kg/day or in rabbits at doses of atorvastatin calcium equivalent to up to 100 mg atorvastatin/kg/day. These doses resulted in multiples of about 30 times (rat) or 20 times (rabbit) the human exposure based on surface area (mg/m²).

In a study in rats given atorvastatin calcium at doses equivalent to 20, 100, or 225 mg atorvastatin/kg/day, from gestation day 7 through to lactation day 21 (weaning), there was decreased pup survival at birth, neonate, weaning, and maturity for pups of mothers dosed with 225 mg/kg/day. Body weight was decreased on days 4 and 21 for pups of mothers dosed at 100 mg/kg/day; pup body weight was decreased at birth and at days 4, 21, and 91 at 225 mg/kg/day. Pup development was delayed (rotorod performance at 100 mg/kg/day and acoustic startle at 225 mg/kg/day; pinnae detachment and eye opening at 225 mg/kg/day). These doses of atorvastatin correspond to 6 times (100 mg/kg) and 22 times (225 mg/kg) the human AUC at 80 mg/day.

Rare reports of congenital anomalies have been received following intrauterine exposure to HMG-CoA reductase inhibitors. There has been one report of severe congenital bony deformity, tracheo-esophageal fistula, and anal atresia (VATER association) in a baby born to a woman who took lovastatin with dextroamphetamine sulfate during the first trimester of pregnancy.

Labor and Delivery
No studies have been conducted in pregnant women on the effect of CADUET, amlodipine or atorvastatin on the mother or the fetus during labor or delivery, or on the duration of labor or delivery. Amlodipine has been shown to prolong the duration of labor in rats.

Nursing Mothers
It is not known whether the amlodipine component of CADUET is excreted in human milk. Nursing rat pups taking atorvastatin had plasma and liver drug levels of 50% and 40%, respectively, of that in their mother's milk. Because of the potential for adverse reactions in nursing infants, women taking CADUET should not breast-feed (see **CONTRAINDICATIONS**).

Pediatric Use
There have been no studies conducted to determine the safety or effectiveness of CADUET in pediatric populations.
Studies with amlodipine: The effect of amlodipine on blood pressure in patients less than 6 years of age is not known.
Studies with atorvastatin: Safety and effectiveness in patients 10-17 years of age with heterozygous familial hyper-

Continued on next page

Caduet—Cont.

cholesterolemia have been evaluated in controlled clinical trials of 6 months duration in adolescent boys and postmenarchal girls. Patients treated with atorvastatin had an adverse experience profile generally similar to that of patients treated with placebo, the most common adverse experiences observed in both groups, regardless of causality assessment, were infections. **Doses greater than 20 mg have not been studied in this patient population.** In this limited controlled study, there was no detectable effect on growth or sexual maturation in boys or on menstrual cycle length in girls. See **CLINICAL PHARMACOLOGY, Clinical Studies** section; **ADVERSE REACTIONS,** *Pediatric Patients*; and **DOSAGE AND ADMINISTRATION,** *Pediatric Patients (10-17 years of age) with Heterozygous Familial Hypercholesterolemia.* Adolescent females should be counseled on appropriate contraceptive methods while on atorvastatin therapy (see **CONTRAINDICATIONS** and **PRECAUTIONS, Pregnancy**). **Atorvastatin has not been studied in controlled clinical trials involving pre-pubertal patients or patients younger than 10 years of age.**

Clinical efficacy with doses of atorvastatin up to 80 mg/day for 1 year have been evaluated in an uncontrolled study of patients with homozygous FH including 8 pediatric patients. See **CLINICAL PHARMACOLOGY, Clinical Studies,** *Atorvastatin Effects in Homozygous Familial Hypercholesterolemia.*

Geriatric Use

There have been no studies conducted to determine the safety or effectiveness of CADUET in geriatric populations.

In studies with amlodipine: Clinical studies of amlodipine did not include sufficient numbers of subjects aged 65 and over to determine whether they respond differently from younger subjects. Other reported clinical experience has not identified differences in responses between the elderly and younger patients. In general, dose selection of the amlodipine component of CADUET for an elderly patient should be cautious, usually starting at the low end of the dosing range, reflecting the greater frequency of decreased hepatic, renal, or cardiac function, and of concomitant disease or other drug therapy. Elderly patients have decreased clearance of amlodipine with a resulting increase of AUC of approximately 40-60%, and a lower initial dose may be required (see **DOSAGE AND ADMINISTRATION**).

In studies with atorvastatin: The safety and efficacy of atorvastatin (10-80 mg) in the geriatric population (≥65 years of age) was evaluated in the ACCESS study. In this 54-week open-label trial 1,958 patients initiated therapy with atorvastatin calcium 10 mg. Of these, 835 were elderly (≥65 years) and 1,123 were non-elderly. The mean change in LDL-C from baseline after 6 weeks of treatment with atorvastatin calcium 10 mg was -38.2% in the elderly patients versus -34.6% in the non-elderly group.

The rates of discontinuation in patients on atorvastatin due to adverse events were similar between the two age groups. There were no differences in clinically relevant laboratory abnormalities between the age groups.

ADVERSE REACTIONS

CADUET

CADUET (amlodipine besylate/atorvastatin calcium) has been evaluated for safety in 1092 patients in double-blind placebo controlled studies treated for co-morbid hypertension and dyslipidemia. In general, treatment with CADUET was well tolerated. For the most part, adverse experiences have been mild or moderate in severity. In clinical trials with CADUET, no adverse experiences peculiar to this combination have been observed. Adverse experiences are similar in terms of nature, severity, and frequency to those reported previously with amlodipine and atorvastatin.

The following information is based on the clinical experience with amlodipine and atorvastatin.

The Amlodipine Component of CADUET

Amlodipine has been evaluated for safety in more than 11,000 patients in U.S. and foreign clinical trials. In general, treatment with amlodipine was well tolerated at doses up to 10 mg daily. Most adverse reactions reported during therapy with amlodipine were of mild or moderate severity. In controlled clinical trials directly comparing amlodipine (N=1730) in doses up to 10 mg to placebo (N=1250), discontinuation of amlodipine due to adverse reactions was required in only about 1.5% of patients and was not significantly different from placebo (about 1%). The most common side effects are headache and edema. The incidence (%) of side effects which occurred in a dose related manner are as follows:

Adverse Event	amlodipine 2.5 mg N=275	5.0 mg N=296	10.0 mg N=268	Placebo N=520
Edema	1.8	3.0	10.8	0.6
Dizziness	1.1	3.4	3.4	1.5
Flushing	0.7	1.4	2.6	0.0
Palpitation	0.7	1.4	4.5	0.6

Other adverse experiences which were not clearly dose related but which were reported with an incidence greater than 1.0% in placebo-controlled clinical trials include the following:

Placebo-Controlled Studies

Adverse Event	amlodipine (%) (N=1730)	Placebo (%) (N=1250)
Headache	7.3	7.8
Fatigue	4.5	2.8
Nausea	2.9	1.9
Abdominal Pain	1.6	0.3
Somnolence	1.4	0.6

For several adverse experiences that appear to be drug and dose related, there was a greater incidence in women than men associated with amlodipine treatment as shown in the following table:

Adverse Event	amlodipine M=% (N=1218)	F=% (N=512)	Placebo M=% (N=914)	F=% (N=336)
Edema	5.6	14.6	1.4	5.1
Flushing	1.5	4.5	0.3	0.9
Palpitations	1.4	3.3	0.9	0.9
Somnolence	1.3	1.6	0.8	0.3

The following events occurred in ≤1% but >0.1% of patients treated with amlodipine in controlled clinical trials or under conditions of open trials or marketing experience where a causal relationship is uncertain; they are listed to alert the physician to a possible relationship:

Cardiovascular: arrhythmia (including ventricular tachycardia and atrial fibrillation), bradycardia, chest pain, hypotension, peripheral ischemia, syncope, tachycardia, postural dizziness, postural hypotension, vasculitis.

Central and Peripheral Nervous System: hypoesthesia, neuropathy peripheral, paresthesia, tremor, vertigo.

Gastrointestinal: anorexia, constipation, dyspepsia,** dysphagia, diarrhea, flatulence, pancreatitis, vomiting, gingival hyperplasia.

General: allergic reaction, asthenia,** back pain, hot flushes, malaise, pain, rigors, weight gain, weight decrease.

Musculoskeletal System: arthralgia, arthrosis, muscle cramps,** myalgia.

Psychiatric: sexual dysfunction (male** and female), insomnia, nervousness, depression, abnormal dreams, anxiety, depersonalization.

Respiratory System: dyspnea,** epistaxis.

Skin and Appendages: angioedema, erythema multiforme, pruritus,** rash,** rash erythematous, rash maculopapular.

**These events occurred in less than 1% in placebo-controlled trials, but the incidence of these side effects was between 1% and 2% in all multiple dose studies.

Special Senses: abnormal vision, conjunctivitis, diplopia, eye pain, tinnitus.

Urinary System: micturition frequency, micturition disorder, nocturia.

Autonomic Nervous System: dry mouth, sweating increased.

Metabolic and Nutritional: hyperglycemia, thirst.

Hemopoietic: leukopenia, purpura, thrombocytopenia.

The following events occurred in ≤0.1% of patients treated with amlodipine in controlled clinical trials or under conditions of open trials or marketing experience: cardiac failure, pulse irregularity, extrasystoles, skin discoloration, urticaria, skin dryness, alopecia, dermatitis, muscle weakness, twitching, ataxia, hypertonia, migraine, cold and clammy skin, apathy, agitation, amnesia, gastritis, increased appetite, loose stools, coughing, rhinitis, dysuria, polyuria, parosmia, taste perversion, abnormal visual accommodation, and xerophthalmia.

Other reactions occurred sporadically and cannot be distinguished from medications or concurrent disease states such as myocardial infarction and angina.

Amlodipine therapy has not been associated with clinically significant changes in routine laboratory tests. No clinically relevant changes were noted in serum potassium, serum glucose, total triglycerides, total cholesterol, HDL cholesterol, uric acid, blood urea nitrogen, or creatinine.

The following postmarketing event has been reported infrequently with amlodipine treatment where a causal relationship is uncertain: gynecomastia. In postmarketing experience, jaundice and hepatic enzyme elevations (mostly consistent with cholestasis or hepatitis) in some cases severe enough to require hospitalization have been reported in association with use of amlodipine.

Amlodipine has been used safely in patients with chronic obstructive pulmonary disease, well-compensated congestive heart failure, peripheral vascular disease, diabetes mellitus, and abnormal lipid profiles.

The Atorvastatin Component of CADUET

Atorvastatin is generally well-tolerated. Adverse reactions have usually been mild and transient. In controlled clinical studies of 2502 patients, <2% of patients were discontinued due to adverse experiences attributable to atorvastatin calcium. The most frequent adverse events thought to be related to atorvastatin calcium were constipation, flatulence, dyspepsia, and abdominal pain.

Clinical Adverse Experiences

Adverse experiences reported in ≥2% of patients in placebo-controlled clinical studies of atorvastatin, regardless of causality assessment, are shown in Table 10.

[See table 10 at left]

Anglo-Scandinavian Cardiac Outcomes Trial (ASCOT)

In ASCOT (see **CLINICAL PHARMACOLOGY, Clinical Studies, *Clinical Studies with Atorvastatin***) involving 10,305 participants treated with atorvastatin 10 mg daily (n=5,168) or placebo (n=5,137), the safety and tolerability profile of the group treated with atorvastatin was comparable to that of the group treated with placebo during a median of 3.3 years of follow-up.

The following adverse events were reported, regardless of causality assessment, in patients treated with atorvastatin in clinical trials. The events in italics occurred in ≥2% of patients and the events in plain type occurred in <2% of patients.

Body as a Whole: *Chest pain*, face edema, fever, neck rigidity, malaise, photosensitivity reaction, generalized edema.

Digestive System: *Nausea*, gastroenteritis, liver function tests abnormal, colitis, vomiting, gastritis, dry mouth, rectal hemorrhage, esophagitis, eructation, glossitis, mouth ulceration, anorexia, increased appetite, stomatitis, biliary pain, cheilitis, duodenal ulcer, dysphagia, enteritis, melena, gum hemorrhage, stomach ulcer, tenesmus, ulcerative stomatitis, hepatitis, pancreatitis, cholestatic jaundice.

Respiratory System: *Bronchitis, rhinitis*, pneumonia, dyspnea, asthma, epistaxis.

Nervous System: *Insomnia, dizziness*, paresthesia, somnolence, amnesia, abnormal dreams, libido decreased, emotional lability, incoordination, peripheral neuropathy, torticollis, facial paralysis, hyperkinesia, depression, hypesthesia, hypertonia.

Musculoskeletal System: *Arthritis*, leg cramps, bursitis, tenosynovitis, myasthenia, tendinous contracture, myositis.

Skin and Appendages: Pruritus, contact dermatitis, alopecia, dry skin, sweating, acne, urticaria, eczema, seborrhea, skin ulcer.

Urogenital System: *Urinary tract infection*, urinary frequency, cystitis, hematuria, impotence, dysuria, kidney calculus, nocturia, epididymitis, fibrocystic breast, vaginal hemorrhage, albuminuria, breast enlargement, metrorrhagia, nephritis, urinary incontinence, urinary retention, urinary urgency, abnormal ejaculation, uterine hemorrhage.

Special Senses: Amblyopia, tinnitus, dry eyes, refraction disorder, eye hemorrhage, deafness, glaucoma, parosmia, taste loss, taste perversion.

Cardiovascular System: Palpitation, vasodilatation, syncope, migraine, postural hypotension, phlebitis, arrhythmia, angina pectoris, hypertension.

Metabolic and Nutritional Disorders: *Peripheral edema*, hyperglycemia, creatine phosphokinase increased, gout, weight gain, hypoglycemia.

Hemic and Lymphatic System: Ecchymosis, anemia, lymphadenopathy, thrombocytopenia, petechia.

Postintroduction Reports with Atorvastatin

Adverse events associated with atorvastatin therapy reported since market introduction, that are not listed above, regardless of causality assessment, include the following: anaphylaxis, angioneurotic edema, bullous rashes (including erythema multiforme, Stevens-Johnson syndrome, and toxic epidermal necrolysis), and rhabdomyolysis.

Table 10. Adverse Events in Placebo-Controlled Studies (% of Patients)

Body System/ Adverse Event	Placebo N=270	atorvastatin 10 mg N=863	20 mg N=36	40 mg N=79	80 mg N=94
BODY AS A WHOLE					
Infection	10.0	10.3	2.8	10.1	7.4
Headache	7.0	5.4	16.7	2.5	6.4
Accidental Injury	3.7	4.2	0.0	1.3	3.2
Flu Syndrome	1.9	2.2	0.0	2.5	3.2
Abdominal Pain	0.7	2.8	0.0	3.8	2.1
Back Pain	3.0	2.8	0.0	3.8	1.1
Allergic Reaction	2.6	0.9	2.8	1.3	0.0
Asthenia	1.9	2.2	0.0	3.8	0.0
DIGESTIVE SYSTEM					
Constipation	1.8	2.1	0.0	2.5	1.1
Diarrhea	1.5	2.7	0.0	3.8	5.3
Dyspepsia	4.1	2.3	2.8	1.3	2.1
Flatulence	3.3	2.1	2.8	1.3	1.1
RESPIRATORY SYSTEM					
Sinusitis	2.6	2.8	0.0	2.5	6.4
Pharyngitis	1.5	2.5	0.0	1.3	2.1
SKIN AND APPENDAGES					
Rash	0.7	3.9	2.8	3.8	1.1
MUSCULOSKELETAL SYSTEM					
Arthralgia	1.5	2.0	0.0	5.1	0.0
Myalgia	1.1	3.2	5.6	1.3	0.0

Pediatric Patients (ages 10-17 years)
In a 26-week controlled study in boys and postmenarchal girls (n=140), the safety and tolerability profile of atorvastatin 10 to 20 mg daily was generally similar to that of placebo (see **CLINICAL PHARMACOLOGY, Clinical Studies** section and **PRECAUTIONS, Pediatric Use**).

OVERDOSAGE

There is no information on overdosage with CADUET in humans.

Information on Amlodipine

Single oral doses of amlodipine maleate equivalent to 40 mg amlodipine/kg and 100 mg amlodipine/kg in mice and rats, respectively, caused deaths. Single oral amlodipine maleate doses equivalent to 4 or more mg amlodipine/kg in dogs (11 or more times the maximum recommended clinical dose on a mg/m^2 basis) caused a marked peripheral vasodilation and hypotension.

Overdosage might be expected to cause excessive peripheral vasodilation with marked hypotension and possibly a reflex tachycardia. In humans, experience with intentional overdosage of amlodipine is limited. Reports of intentional overdosage include a patient who ingested 250 mg and was asymptomatic and was not hospitalized; another (120 mg) was hospitalized, underwent gastric lavage and remained normotensive; the third (105 mg) was hospitalized and had hypotension (90/50 mmHg) which normalized following plasma expansion. A patient who took 70 mg amlodipine and an unknown quantity of benzodiazepine in a suicide attempt developed shock which was refractory to treatment and died the following day with abnormally high benzodiazepine plasma concentration. A case of accidental drug overdose has been documented in a 19-month-old male who ingested 30 mg amlodipine (about 2 mg/kg). During the emergency room presentation, vital signs were stable with no evidence of hypotension, but a heart rate of 180 bpm. Ipecac was administered 3.5 hours after ingestion and on subsequent observation (overnight) no sequelae were noted.

If massive overdose should occur, active cardiac and respiratory monitoring should be instituted. Frequent blood pressure measurements are essential. Should hypotension occur, cardiovascular support including elevation of the extremities and the judicious administration of fluids should be initiated. If hypotension remains unresponsive to these conservative measures, administration of vasopressors (such as phenylephrine) should be considered with attention to circulating volume and urine output. Intravenous calcium gluconate may help to reverse the effects of calcium entry blockade. As amlodipine is highly protein bound, hemodialysis is not likely to be of benefit.

Information on Atorvastatin

There is no specific treatment for atorvastatin overdosage. In the event of an overdose, the patient should be treated symptomatically, and supportive measures instituted as required. Due to extensive drug binding to plasma proteins, hemodialysis is not expected to significantly enhance atorvastatin clearance.

DOSAGE AND ADMINISTRATION

Dosage of CADUET must be individualized on the basis of both effectiveness and tolerance for each individual component in the treatment of hypertension/angina and hyperlipidemia.

Amlodipine (Hypertension or angina)

Adults: The usual initial antihypertensive oral dose of amlodipine is 5 mg once daily with a maximum dose of 10 mg once daily. Small, fragile, or elderly individuals, or patients with hepatic insufficiency may be started on 2.5 mg once daily and this dose may be used when adding amlodipine to other antihypertensive therapy.

Dosage should be adjusted according to each patient's need. In general, titration should proceed over 7 to 14 days so that the physician can fully assess the patient's response to each dose level. Titration may proceed more rapidly, however, if clinically warranted, provided the patient is assessed frequently.

The recommended dose of amlodipine for chronic stable or vasospastic angina is 5-10 mg, with the lower dose suggested in the elderly and in patients with hepatic insufficiency. Most patients will require 10 mg for adequate effect. See **ADVERSE REACTIONS** section for information related to dosage and side effects.

Children: The effective antihypertensive oral dose of amlodipine in pediatric patients ages 6-17 years is 2.5 mg to 5 mg once daily. Doses in excess of 5 mg daily have not been studied in pediatric patients. See **CLINICAL PHARMACOLOGY**.

Atorvastatin (Hyperlipidemia)

The patient should be placed on a standard cholesterol-lowering diet before receiving atorvastatin and should continue on this diet during treatment with atorvastatin.

Hypercholesterolemia (Heterozygous Familial and Nonfamilial) and Mixed Dyslipidemia (Fredrickson Types IIa and IIb)

The recommended starting dose of atorvastatin is 10 or 20 mg once daily. Patients who require a large reduction in LDL-C (more than 45%) may be started at 40 mg once daily. The dosage range of atorvastatin is 10 to 80 mg once daily. Atorvastatin can be administered as a single dose at any time of the day, with or without food. The starting dose and maintenance doses of atorvastatin should be individualized according to patient characteristics such as goal of therapy and response (see *NCEP Guidelines*, summarized in Table 8). After initiation and/or upon titration of atorvastatin, lipid levels should be analyzed within 2 to 4 weeks and dosage adjusted accordingly.

Since the goal of treatment is to lower LDL-C, the NCEP recommends that LDL-C levels be used to initiate and assess treatment response. Only if LDL-C levels are not available, should total-C be used to monitor therapy.

Heterozygous Familial Hypercholesterolemia in Pediatric Patients (10-17 years of age)

The recommended starting dose of atorvastatin is 10 mg/day; the maximum recommended dose is 20 mg/day (doses greater than 20 mg have not been studied in this patient population). Doses should be individualized according to the recommended goal of therapy (see NCEP Pediatric Panel Guidelines[1], **CLINICAL PHARMACOLOGY**, and **INDICATIONS AND USAGE**). Adjustments should be made at intervals of 4 weeks or more.

Homozygous Familial Hypercholesterolemia

The dosage of atorvastatin in patients with homozygous FH is 10 to 80 mg daily. Atorvastatin should be used as an adjunct to other lipid-lowering treatments (e.g., LDL apheresis) in these patients or if such treatments are unavailable. Note: a 2.5/80 mg CADUET tablet is not available. Management of patients needing a 2.5/80 mg combination requires individual assessments of dyslipidemia and therapy with the individual components as a 2.5/80 mg CADUET tablet is not available.

[1] National Cholesterol Education Program (NCEP): Highlights of the Report of the Expert Panel on Blood Cholesterol Levels in Children Adolescents. *Pediatrics*. 89(3):495-501. 1992.

Concomitant Therapy

Atorvastatin may be used in combination with a bile acid binding resin for additive effect. The combination of HMG-CoA reductase inhibitors and fibrates should generally be avoided (see **WARNINGS, Skeletal Muscle**, and **PRECAUTIONS, Drug Interactions** for other drug-drug interactions).

Dosage in Patients With Renal Insufficiency

Renal disease does not affect the plasma concentrations nor LDL-C reduction of atorvastatin; thus, dosage adjustment in patients with renal dysfunction is not necessary (see **CLINICAL PHARMACOLOGY, Pharmacokinetics**).

CADUET

CADUET may be substituted for its individually titrated components. Patients may be given the equivalent dose of CADUET or a dose of CADUET with increased amounts of amlodipine, atorvastatin or both for additional antianginal effects, blood pressure lowering, or lipid lowering effect.

CADUET may be used to provide additional therapy for patients already on one of its components. As initial therapy for one indication and continuation of treatment of the other, the recommended starting dose of CADUET should be selected based on the continuation of the component being used and the recommended starting dose for the added monotherapy.

CADUET may be used to initiate treatment in patients with hyperlipidemia and either hypertension or angina. The recommended starting dose of CADUET should be based on the appropriate combination of recommendations for the monotherapies. The maximum dose of the amlodipine component of CADUET is 10 mg once daily. The maximum dose of the atorvastatin component of CADUET is 80 mg once daily.

See above for detailed information related to the dosing and administration of amlodipine and atorvastatin.

HOW SUPPLIED

CADUET® tablets contain amlodipine besylate and atorvastatin calcium equivalent to amlodipine and atorvastatin in the dose strengths described below.

CADUET tablets are differentiated by tablet color/size and are engraved with "Pfizer" on one side and a unique number on the other side. CADUET tablets are supplied for oral administration in the following strengths and package configurations:

Table 11. CADUET Packaging Configurations

CADUET				
Package Configuration	Tablet Strength (amlodipine besylate/ atorvastatin calcium) mg	NDC #	Engraving	Tablet Color
Bottle of 30	2.5/10	0069-2960-30	CDT 251	White
Bottle of 30	2.5/20	0069-2970-30	CDT 252	White
Bottle of 30	2.5/40	0069-2980-30	CDT 254	White
Bottle of 30	5/10	0069-2150-30	CDT 051	White
Bottle of 30	5/20	0069-2170-30	CDT 052	White
Bottle of 30	5/40	0069-2190-30	CDT 054	White
Bottle of 30	5/80	0069-2260-30	CDT 058	White
Bottle of 30	10/10	0069-2160-30	CDT 101	Blue
Bottle of 30	10/20	0069-2180-30	CDT 102	Blue
Bottle of 30	10/40	0069-2250-30	CDT 104	Blue
Bottle of 30	10/80	0069-2270-30	CDT 108	Blue

[See table 11 above]

Store at 25°C (77°F); excursions permitted to 15-30°C (59-86°F) [see USP Controlled Room Temperature].

Rx only

Manufactured by:
Pfizer Ireland Pharmaceuticals
Dublin, Ireland
Distributed by
Pfizer Labs
Division of Pfizer Inc, NY, NY 10017
LAB-0276-3.0 **Revised October 2004**

GEODON® ℞

[*gē-ō-dŏn*]
(ziprasidone HCl)
Capsules
GEODON®
(ziprasidone mesylate)
for Injection
FOR IM USE ONLY

Prescribing information for this product, which appears on pages 2609–2615 of the 2005 PDR, has been completely revised as follows. Please write "See Supplement A" next to the product heading.

Increased Mortality in Elderly Patients with Dementia-Related Psychosis
Elderly patients with dementia-related psychosis treated with atypical antipsychotic drugs are at an increased risk of death compared to placebo. Analyses of seventeen placebo controlled trials (modal duration of 10 weeks) in these patients revealed a risk of death in the drug-treated patients of between 1.6 to 1.7 times that seen in placebo-treated patients. Over the course of a typical 10 week controlled trial, the rate of death in drug-treated patients was about 4.5%, compared to a rate of about 2.6% in the placebo group. Although the causes of death were varied, most of the deaths appeared to be either cardiovascular (e.g., heart failure, sudden death) or infectious (e.g., pneumonia) in nature. Geodon (ziprasidone) is not approved for the treatment of patients with Dementia-Related Psychosis.

DESCRIPTION

GEODON® is available as GEODON Capsules (ziprasidone hydrochloride) for oral administration and as GEODON for Injection (ziprasidone mesylate) for intramuscular injection. Ziprasidone is a psychotropic agent that is chemically unrelated to phenothiazine or butyrophenone antipsychotic agents. It has a molecular weight of 412.94 (free base), with the following chemical name: 5-[2-[4-(1,2-benzisothiazol-3-yl)-1-piperazinyl]ethyl]-6-chloro-1,3-dihydro-2*H*-indol-2-one. The empirical formula of $C_{21}H_{21}ClN_4OS$ (free base of ziprasidone) represents the following structural formula:

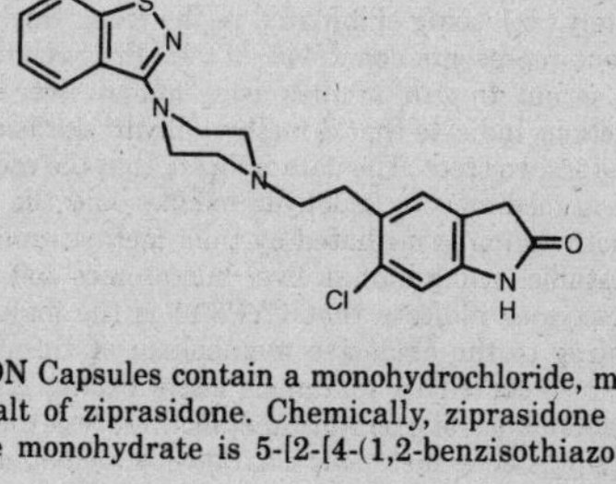

GEODON Capsules contain a monohydrochloride, monohydrate salt of ziprasidone. Chemically, ziprasidone hydrochloride monohydrate is 5-[2-[4-(1,2-benzisothiazol-3-yl)-

Continued on next page

Geodon—Cont.

1-piperazinyl]ethyl]-6-chloro-1,3-dihydro-2*H*-indol-2-one, monohydrochloride, monohydrate. The empirical formula is $C_{21}H_{21}ClN_4OS \cdot HCl \cdot H_2O$ and its molecular weight is 467.42. Ziprasidone hydrochloride monohydrate is a white to slightly pink powder.

GEODON Capsules are supplied for oral administration in 20 mg (blue/white), 40 mg (blue/blue), 60 mg (white/white), and 80 mg (blue/white) capsules. GEODON Capsules contain ziprasidone hydrochloride monohydrate, lactose, pregelatinized starch, and magnesium stearate.

GEODON for Injection contains a lyophilized form of ziprasidone mesylate trihydrate. Chemically, ziprasidone mesylate trihydrate is 5-[2-[4-(1,2-benzisothiazol-3-yl)-1-piperazinyl]ethyl]-6-chloro-1,3-dihydro-2*H*-indol-2-one, methanesulfonate, trihydrate. The empirical formula is $C_{21}H_{21}ClN_4OS \cdot CH_3SO_3H \cdot 3H_2O$ and its molecular weight is 563.09.

GEODON for Injection is available in a single dose vial as ziprasidone mesylate (20 mg ziprasidone/mL when reconstituted according to label instructions - see **Preparation for Administration**) for intramuscular administration. Each mL of ziprasidone mesylate for injection (when reconstituted) contains 20 mg of ziprasidone and 4.7 mg of methanesulfonic acid solubilized by 294 mg of sulfobutylether β-cyclodextrin sodium (SBECD).

CLINICAL PHARMACOLOGY

Pharmacodynamics

Ziprasidone exhibited high *in vitro* binding affinity for the dopamine D_2 and D_3, the serotonin $5HT_{2A}$, $5HT_{2C}$, $5HT_{1A}$, $5HT_{1D}$, and α_1-adrenergic receptors (K_i s of 4.8, 7.2, 0.4, 1.3, 3.4, 2, and 10 nM, respectively), and moderate affinity for the histamine H_1 receptor (K_i=47 nM). Ziprasidone functioned as an antagonist at the D_2, $5HT_{2A}$, and $5HT_{1D}$ receptors, and as an agonist at the $5HT_{1A}$ receptor. Ziprasidone inhibited synaptic reuptake of serotonin and norepinephrine. No appreciable affinity was exhibited for other receptor/binding sites tested, including the cholinergic muscarinic receptor (IC_{50} >1 μM).

The mechanism of action of ziprasidone, as with other drugs having efficacy in schizophrenia, is unknown. However, it has been proposed that this drug's efficacy in schizophrenia is mediated through a combination of dopamine type 2 (D_2) and serotonin type 2 ($5HT_2$) antagonism. As with other drugs having efficacy in bipolar disorder, the mechanism of action of ziprasidone in bipolar disorder is unknown.

Antagonism at receptors other than dopamine and $5HT_2$ with similar receptor affinities may explain some of the other therapeutic and side effects of ziprasidone. Ziprasidone's antagonism of histamine H_1 receptors may explain the somnolence observed with this drug. Ziprasidone's antagonism of α_1-adrenergic receptors may explain the orthostatic hypotension observed with this drug.

Oral Pharmacokinetics

Ziprasidone's activity is primarily due to the parent drug. The multiple-dose pharmacokinetics of ziprasidone are dose-proportional within the proposed clinical dose range, and ziprasidone accumulation is predictable with multiple dosing. Elimination of ziprasidone is mainly via hepatic metabolism with a mean terminal half-life of about 7 hours within the proposed clinical dose range. Steady-state concentrations are achieved within one to three days of dosing. The mean apparent systemic clearance is 7.5 mL/min/kg. Ziprasidone is unlikely to interfere with the metabolism of drugs metabolized by cytochrome P450 enzymes.

Absorption: Ziprasidone is well absorbed after oral administration, reaching peak plasma concentrations in 6 to 8 hours. The absolute bioavailability of a 20 mg dose under fed conditions is approximately 60%. The absorption of ziprasidone is increased up to two-fold in the presence of food.

Distribution: Ziprasidone has a mean apparent volume of distribution of 1.5 L/kg. It is greater than 99% bound to plasma proteins, binding primarily to albumin and α_1-acid glycoprotein. The *in vitro* plasma protein binding of ziprasidone was not altered by warfarin or propranolol, two highly protein-bound drugs, nor did ziprasidone alter the binding of these drugs in human plasma. Thus, the potential for drug interactions with ziprasidone due to displacement is minimal.

Metabolism and Elimination: Ziprasidone is extensively metabolized after oral administration with only a small amount excreted in the urine (<1%) or feces (<4%) as unchanged drug. Ziprasidone is primarily cleared via three metabolic routes to yield four major circulating metabolites, benzisothiazole (BITP) sulphoxide, BITP-sulphone, ziprasidone sulphoxide, and S-methyl-dihydroziprasidone. Approximately 20% of the dose is excreted in the urine, with approximately 66% being eliminated in the feces. Unchanged ziprasidone represents about 44% of total drug-related material in serum. *In vitro* studies using human liver subcellular fractions indicate that S-methyl-dihydroziprasidone is generated in two steps. The data indicate that the reduction reaction is mediated by aldehyde oxidase and the subsequent methylation is mediated by thiol methyltransferase. *In vitro* studies using human liver microsomes and recombinant enzymes indicate that CYP3A4 is the major CYP contributing to the oxidative metabolism of ziprasidone. CYP1A2 may contribute to a much lesser extent. Based on *in vivo* abundance of excretory metabolites, less than one-third of ziprasidone metabolic clearance is mediated by cytochrome P450 catalyzed oxidation and approximately two-thirds via reduction by aldehyde oxidase. There are no

known clinically relevant inhibitors or inducers of aldehyde oxidase.

Intramuscular Pharmacokinetics

Systemic Bioavailability: The bioavailability of ziprasidone administered intramuscularly is 100%. After intramuscular administration of single doses, peak serum concentrations typically occur at approximately 60 minutes post-dose or earlier and the mean half-life ($T_{1/2}$) ranges from two to five hours. Exposure increases in a dose-related manner and following three days of intramuscular dosing, little accumulation is observed.

Metabolism and Elimination: Although the metabolism and elimination of IM ziprasidone have not been systematically evaluated, the intramuscular route of administration would not be expected to alter the metabolic pathways.

Special Populations

Age and Gender Effects—In a multiple-dose (8 days of treatment) study involving 32 subjects, there was no difference in the pharmacokinetics of ziprasidone between men and women or between elderly (>65 years) and young (18 to 45 years) subjects. Additionally, population pharmacokinetic evaluation of patients in controlled trials has revealed no evidence of clinically significant age or gender-related differences in the pharmacokinetics of ziprasidone. Dosage modifications for age or gender are, therefore, not recommended.

Ziprasidone intramuscular has not been systematically evaluated in elderly patients (65 years and over).

Race—No specific pharmacokinetic study was conducted to investigate the effects of race. Population pharmacokinetic evaluation has revealed no evidence of clinically significant race-related differences in the pharmacokinetics of ziprasidone. Dosage modifications for race are, therefore, not recommended.

Smoking—Based on *in vitro* studies utilizing human liver enzymes, ziprasidone is not a substrate for CYP1A2; smoking should therefore not have an effect on the pharmacokinetics of ziprasidone. Consistent with these *in vitro* results, population pharmacokinetic evaluation has not revealed any significant pharmacokinetic differences between smokers and nonsmokers.

Renal Impairment—Because ziprasidone is highly metabolized, with less than 1% of the drug excreted unchanged, renal impairment alone is unlikely to have a major impact on the pharmacokinetics of ziprasidone. The pharmacokinetics of ziprasidone following 8 days of 20 mg BID dosing were similar among subjects with varying degrees of renal impairment (n=27), and subjects with normal renal function, indicating that dosage adjustment based upon the degree of renal impairment is not required. Ziprasidone is not removed by hemodialysis.

Hepatic Impairment—As ziprasidone is cleared substantially by the liver, the presence of hepatic impairment would be expected to increase the AUC of ziprasidone; a multiple-dose study at 20 mg BID for 5 days in subjects (n=13) with clinically significant (Childs-Pugh Class A and B) cirrhosis revealed an increase in AUC_{0-12} of 13% and 34% in Childs-Pugh Class A and B, respectively, compared to a matched control group (n=14). A half-life of 7.1 hours was observed in subjects with cirrhosis compared to 4.8 hours in the control group.

Intramuscular ziprasidone has not been systematically evaluated in elderly patients or in patients with hepatic or renal impairment. As the cyclodextrin excipient is cleared by renal filtration, ziprasidone intramuscular should be administered with caution to patients with impaired renal function.

Drug-Drug Interactions

An *in vitro* enzyme inhibition study utilizing human liver microsomes showed that ziprasidone had little inhibitory effect on CYP1A2, CYP2C9, CYP2C19, CYP2D6 and CYP3A4, and thus would not likely interfere with the metabolism of drugs primarily metabolized by these enzymes. *In vivo* studies have revealed no effect of ziprasidone on the pharmacokinetics of dextromethorphan, estrogen, progesterone, or lithium (see **Drug Interactions** under **PRECAUTIONS**).

In vivo studies have revealed an approximately 35% decrease in ziprasidone AUC by concomitantly administered carbamazepine, an approximately 35-40% increase in ziprasidone AUC by concomitantly administered ketoconazole, but no effect on ziprasidone's pharmacokinetics by cimetidine or antacid (see **Drug Interactions** under **PRECAUTIONS**).

Clinical Trials

Schizophrenia

The efficacy of oral ziprasidone in the treatment of schizophrenia was evaluated in 5 placebo-controlled studies, 4 short-term (4- and 6-week) trials and one long-term (52-week) trial. All trials were in inpatients, most of whom met DSM III-R criteria for schizophrenia. Each study included 2 to 3 fixed doses of ziprasidone as well as placebo. Four of the 5 trials were able to distinguish ziprasidone from placebo; one short-term study did not. Although a single fixed-dose haloperidol arm was included as a comparative treatment in one of the three short-term trials, this single study was inadequate to provide a reliable and valid comparison of ziprasidone and haloperidol.

Several instruments were used for assessing psychiatric signs and symptoms in these studies. The Brief Psychiatric Rating Scale (BPRS) and the Positive and Negative Syndrome Scale (PANSS) are both multi-item inventories of general psychopathology usually used to evaluate the effects of drug treatment in schizophrenia. The BPRS psychosis cluster (conceptual disorganization, hallucinatory behavior, suspiciousness, and unusual thought content) is

considered a particularly useful subset for assessing actively psychotic schizophrenic patients. A second widely used assessment, the Clinical Global Impression (CGI), reflects the impression of a skilled observer, fully familiar with the manifestations of schizophrenia, about the overall clinical state of the patient. In addition, the Scale for Assessing Negative Symptoms (SANS) was employed for assessing negative symptoms in one trial.

The results of the oral ziprasidone trials in schizophrenia follow:

(1) In a 4-week, placebo-controlled trial (n=139) comparing 2 fixed doses of ziprasidone (20 and 60 mg BID) with placebo, only the 60 mg BID dose was superior to placebo on the BPRS total score and the CGI severity score. This higher dose group was not superior to placebo on the BPRS psychosis cluster or on the SANS.

(2) In a 6-week, placebo-controlled trial (n=302) comparing 2 fixed doses of ziprasidone (40 and 80 mg BID) with placebo, both dose groups were superior to placebo on the BPRS total score, the BPRS psychosis cluster, the CGI severity score and the PANSS total and negative subscale scores. Although 80 mg BID had a numerically greater effect than 40 mg BID, the difference was not statistically significant.

(3) In a 6-week, placebo-controlled trial (n=419) comparing 3 fixed doses of ziprasidone (20, 60, and 100 mg BID) with placebo, all three dose groups were superior to placebo on the PANSS total score, the BPRS total score, the BPRS psychosis cluster, and the CGI severity score. Only the 100 mg BID dose group was superior to placebo on the PANSS negative subscale score. There was no clear evidence for a dose-response relationship within the 20 mg BID to 100 mg BID dose range.

(4) In a 4-week, placebo-controlled trial (n=200) comparing 3 fixed doses of ziprasidone (5, 20, and 40 mg BID), none of the dose groups was statistically superior to placebo on any outcome of interest.

(5) A study was conducted in chronic, symptomatically stable schizophrenic inpatients (n=294) randomized to 3 fixed doses of ziprasidone (20, 40, or 80 mg BID) or placebo and followed for 52 weeks. Patients were observed for "impending psychotic relapse," defined as CGI-improvement score of ≥6 (much worse or very much worse) and/or scores ≥6 (moderately severe) on the hostility or uncooperativeness items of the PANSS on two consecutive days. Ziprasidone was significantly superior to placebo in both time to relapse and rate of relapse, with no significant difference between the different dose groups.

There were insufficient data to examine population subsets based on age and race. Examination of population subsets based on gender did not reveal any differential responsiveness.

Bipolar Mania

The efficacy of ziprasidone in acute mania was established in 2 placebo-controlled, double-blind, 3-week studies in patients meeting DSM-IV criteria for Bipolar I Disorder with an acute manic or mixed episode with or without psychotic features.

Primary rating instruments used for assessing manic symptoms in these trials were: (1) the Mania Rating Scale (MRS), which is derived from the Schedule for Affective Disorders and Schizophrenia-Change Version (SADS-CB) with items grouped as the Manic Syndrome subscale (elevated mood, less need for sleep, excessive energy, excessive activity, grandiosity), the Behavior and Ideation subscale (irritability, motor hyperactivity, accelerated speech, racing thoughts, poor judgment) and impaired insight; and (2) the Clinical Global Impression - Severity of Illness Scale (CGI-S), which was used to assess the clinical significance of treatment response.

The results of the oral ziprasidone trials in bipolar mania follow:

(1) In a 3-week placebo-controlled trial (n=210), the dose of ziprasidone was 40 mg BID on Day 1 and 80 mg BID on Day 2. Titration within the range of 40-80 mg BID (in 20 mg BID increments) was permitted for the duration of the study. Ziprasidone was significantly more effective than placebo in reduction of the MRS total score and the CGI-S score. The mean daily dose of ziprasidone in this study was 132 mg.

(2) In a second 3-week placebo-controlled trial (n=205), the dose of ziprasidone was 40 mg on Day 1. Titration within the range of 40-80 mg BID (in 20 mg BID increments) was permitted for the duration of study (beginning on Day 2). Ziprasidone was significantly more effective than placebo in reduction of the MRS total score and the CGI-S score. The mean daily dose of ziprasidone in this study was 112 mg.

Acute Agitation in Schizophrenic Patients

The efficacy of intramuscular ziprasidone in the management of agitated schizophrenic patients was established in two short-term, double-blind trials of schizophrenic subjects who were considered by the investigators to be "acutely agitated" and in need of IM antipsychotic medication. In addition, patients were required to have a score of 3 or more on at least 3 of the following items of the PANSS: anxiety, tension, hostility and excitement. Efficacy was evaluated by analysis of the area under the curve (AUC) of the Behavioural Activity Rating Scale (BARS) and Clinical Global Impression (CGI) severity rating. The BARS is a seven point scale with scores ranging from 1 (difficult or unable to rouse) to 7 (violent, requires restraint). Patients' scores on the BARS at baseline were mostly 5 (signs of overt activity [physical or verbal], calms down with instructions) and as determined by investigators, exhibited a degree of agitation that warranted intramuscular therapy. There were few patients with a rating higher than 5 on the BARS, as the most severely agitated patients were generally unable to provide informed consent for participation in pre-marketing clinical trials.

Both studies compared higher doses of ziprasidone intramuscular with a 2 mg control dose. In one study, the higher dose was 20 mg, which could be given up to 4 times in the 24 hours of the study, at interdose intervals of no less than 4 hours. In the other study, the higher dose was 10 mg, which could be given up to 4 times in the 24 hours of the study, at interdose intervals of no less than 2 hours.

The results of the intramuscular ziprasidone trials follow:
(1) In a one-day, double-blind, randomized trial (n=79) involving doses of ziprasidone intramuscular of 20 mg or 2 mg, up to QID, ziprasidone intramuscular 20 mg was statistically superior to ziprasidone intramuscular 2 mg, as assessed by AUC of the BARS at 0 to 4 hours, and by CGI severity at 4 hours and study endpoint.
(2) In another one-day, double-blind, randomized trial (n=117) involving doses of ziprasidone intramuscular of 10 mg or 2 mg, up to QID, ziprasidone intramuscular 10 mg was statistically superior to ziprasidone intramuscular 2 mg, as assessed by AUC of the BARS at 0 to 2 hours, but not by CGI severity.

INDICATIONS AND USAGE
Schizophrenia
Ziprasidone is indicated for the treatment of schizophrenia. When deciding among the alternative treatments available for this condition, the prescriber should consider the finding of ziprasidone's greater capacity to prolong the QT/QTc interval compared to several other antipsychotic drugs (see **WARNINGS**). Prolongation of the QTc interval is associated in some other drugs with the ability to cause torsade de pointes-type arrhythmia, a potentially fatal polymorphic ventricular tachycardia, and sudden death. In many cases this would lead to the conclusion that other drugs should be tried first. Whether ziprasidone will cause torsade de pointes or increase the rate of sudden death is not yet known (see **WARNINGS**).

The efficacy of oral ziprasidone was established in short-term (4- and 6-week) controlled trials of schizophrenic inpatients (see **CLINICAL PHARMACOLOGY**).

In a placebo-controlled trial involving the follow-up for up to 52 weeks of stable schizophrenic inpatients, GEODON was demonstrated to delay the time to and rate of relapse. The physician who elects to use GEODON for extended periods should periodically re-evaluate the long-term usefulness of the drug for the individual patient.

Bipolar Mania
Ziprasidone is indicated for the treatment of acute manic or mixed episodes associated with bipolar disorder, with or without psychotic features. A manic episode is a distinct period of abnormally and persistently elevated, expansive, or irritable mood. A mixed episode is characterized by the criteria for a manic episode in conjunction with those for a major depressive episode (depressed mood, loss of interest or pleasure in nearly all activities).

The efficacy of ziprasidone in acute mania was established in 2 placebo-controlled, double-blind, 3-week studies in patients meeting DSM-IV criteria for Bipolar I Disorder who currently displayed an acute manic or mixed episode with or without psychotic features (see **CLINICAL PHARMACOLOGY**).

The effectiveness of ziprasidone for longer-term use and for prophylactic use in mania has not been systematically evaluated in controlled clinical trials. Therefore, physicians who elect to use ziprasidone for extended periods should periodically re-evaluate the long-term risks and benefits of the drug for the individual patient (see **DOSAGE AND ADMINISTRATION**).

Acute Agitation in Schizophrenic Patients
Ziprasidone intramuscular is indicated for the treatment of acute agitation in schizophrenic patients for whom treatment with ziprasidone is appropriate and who need intramuscular antipsychotic medication for rapid control of the agitation. "Psychomotor agitation" is defined in DSM-IV as "excessive motor activity associated with a feeling of inner tension." Schizophrenic patients experiencing agitation often manifest behaviors that interfere with their diagnosis and care, e.g., threatening behaviors, escalating or urgently distressing behavior, or self-exhausting behavior, leading clinicians to the use of intramuscular antipsychotic medications to achieve immediate control of the agitation. The efficacy of intramuscular ziprasidone for acute agitation in schizophrenia was established in single-day controlled trials of schizophrenic inpatients (see **CLINICAL PHARMACOLOGY**). Since there is no experience regarding the safety of administering ziprasidone intramuscular to schizophrenic patients already taking oral ziprasidone, the practice of co-administration is not recommended.

CONTRAINDICATIONS
QT Prolongation
Because of ziprasidone's dose-related prolongation of the QT interval and the known association of fatal arrhythmias with QT prolongation by some other drugs, ziprasidone is contraindicated in patients with a known history of QT prolongation (including congenital long QT syndrome), with recent acute myocardial infarction, or with uncompensated heart failure (see **WARNINGS**).

Pharmacokinetic/pharmacodynamic studies between ziprasidone and other drugs that prolong the QT interval have not been performed. An additive effect of ziprasidone and other drugs that prolong the QT interval cannot be excluded. Therefore, ziprasidone should not be given with dofetilide, sotalol, quinidine, other Class Ia and III anti-

arrhythmics, mesoridazine, thioridazine, chlorpromazine, droperidol, pimozide, sparfloxacin, gatifloxacin, moxifloxacin, halofantrine, mefloquine, pentamidine, arsenic trioxide, levomethadyl acetate, dolasetron mesylate, probucol or tacrolimus. Ziprasidone is also contraindicated with drugs that have demonstrated QT prolongation as one of their pharmacodynamic effects and have this effect described in the full prescribing information as a contraindication or a boxed or bolded warning (see **WARNINGS**).

Hypersensitivity
Ziprasidone is contraindicated in individuals with a known hypersensitivity to the product.

WARNINGS
Increased Mortality in Elderly Patients with Dementia-Related Psychosis
Elderly patients with dementia-related psychosis treated with atypical antipsychotic drugs are at an increased risk of death compared to placebo. Geodon (ziprasidone) is not approved for the treatment of patients with dementia-related psychosis (see Boxed Warning).

QT Prolongation and Risk of Sudden Death
Ziprasidone use should be avoided in combination with other drugs that are known to prolong the QTc interval (see CONTRAINDICATIONS, and see Drug Interactions under PRECAUTIONS). Additionally, clinicians should be alert to the identification of other drugs that have been consistently observed to prolong the QTc interval. Such drugs should not be prescribed with ziprasidone. Ziprasidone should also be avoided in patients with congenital long QT syndrome and in patients with a history of cardiac arrhythmias (see CONTRAINDICATIONS).

A study directly comparing the QT/QTc prolonging effect of oral ziprasidone with several other drugs effective in the treatment of schizophrenia was conducted in patient volunteers. In the first phase of the trial, ECGs were obtained at the time of maximum plasma concentration when the drug was administered alone. In the second phase of the trial, ECGs were obtained at the time of maximum plasma concentration while the drug was co-administered with an inhibitor of the CYP4503A4 metabolism of the drug.

In the first phase of the study, the mean change in QTc from baseline was calculated for each drug, using a sample-based correction that removes the effect of heart rate on the QT interval. The mean increase in QTc from baseline for ziprasidone ranged from approximately 9 to 14 msec greater than for four of the comparator drugs (risperidone, olanzapine, quetiapine, and haloperidol), but was approximately 14 msec less than the prolongation observed for thioridazine.

In the second phase of the study, the effect of ziprasidone on QTc length was not augmented by the presence of a metabolic inhibitor (ketoconazole 200 mg BID).

In placebo-controlled trials, oral ziprasidone increased the QTc interval compared to placebo by approximately 10 msec at the highest recommended daily dose of 160 mg. In clinical trials with oral ziprasidone, the electrocardiograms of 2/2988 (0.06%) patients who received GEODON and 1/440 (0.23%) patients who received placebo revealed QTc intervals exceeding the potentially clinically relevant threshold of 500 msec. In the ziprasidone-treated patients, neither case suggested a role of ziprasidone. One patient had a history of prolonged QTc and a screening measurement of 489 msec; QTc was 503 msec during ziprasidone treatment. The other patient had a QTc of 391 msec at the end of treatment with ziprasidone and upon switching to thioridazine experienced QTc measurements of 518 and 593 msec.

Some drugs that prolong the QT/QTc interval have been associated with the occurrence of torsade de pointes and with sudden unexplained death. The relationship of QT prolongation to torsade de pointes is clearest for larger increases (20 msec and greater) but it is possible that smaller QT/QTc prolongations may also increase risk, or increase it in susceptible individuals, such as those with hypokalemia, hypomagnesemia, or genetic predisposition. Although torsade de pointes has not been observed in association with the use of ziprasidone at recommended doses in premarketing studies, experience is too limited to rule out an increased risk (see ADVERSE REACTIONS; Other Events Observed During Post-marketing Use).

A study evaluating the QT/QTc prolonging effect of intramuscular ziprasidone, with intramuscular haloperidol as a control, was conducted in patient volunteers. In the trial, ECGs were obtained at the time of maximum plasma concentration following two injections of ziprasidone (20 mg then 30 mg) or haloperidol (7.5 mg then 10 mg) given four hours apart. Note that a 30 mg dose of intramuscular ziprasidone is 50% higher than the recommended therapeutic dose. The mean change in QTc from baseline was calculated for each drug, using a sample-based correction that removes the effect of heart rate on the QT interval. The mean increase in QTc from baseline for ziprasidone was 4.6 msec following the first injection and 12.8 msec following the second injection. The mean increase in QTc from baseline for haloperidol was 6.0 msec following the first injection and 14.7 msec following the second injection. In this study, no patients had a QTc interval exceeding 500 msec.

As with other antipsychotic drugs and placebo, sudden unexplained deaths have been reported in patients taking ziprasidone at recommended doses. The premarketing experience for ziprasidone did not reveal an excess risk of mortality for ziprasidone compared to other antipsychotic drugs or placebo, but the extent of exposure was limited,

especially for the drugs used as active controls and placebo. Nevertheless, ziprasidone's larger prolongation of QTc length compared to several other antipsychotic drugs raises the possibility that the risk of sudden death may be greater for ziprasidone than for other available drugs for treating schizophrenia. This possibility needs to be considered in deciding among alternative drug products (see INDICATIONS AND USAGE).

Certain circumstances may increase the risk of the occurrence of torsade de pointes and/or sudden death in association with the use of drugs that prolong the QTc interval, including (1) bradycardia; (2) hypokalemia or hypomagnesemia; (3) concomitant use of other drugs that prolong the QTc interval; and (4) presence of congenital prolongation of the QT interval.

It is recommended that patients being considered for ziprasidone treatment who are at risk for significant electrolyte disturbances, hypokalemia in particular, have baseline serum potassium and magnesium measurements. Hypokalemia (and/or hypomagnesemia) may increase the risk of QT prolongation and arrhythmia. Hypokalemia may result from diuretic therapy, diarrhea, and other causes. Patients with low serum potassium and/or magnesium should be repleted with those electrolytes before proceeding with treatment. It is essential to periodically monitor serum electrolytes in patients for whom diuretic therapy is introduced during ziprasidone treatment. Persistently prolonged QTc intervals may also increase the risk of further prolongation and arrhythmia, but it is not clear that routine screening ECG measures are effective in detecting such patients. Rather, ziprasidone should be avoided in patients with histories of significant cardiovascular illness, e.g., QT prolongation, recent acute myocardial infarction, uncompensated heart failure, or cardiac arrhythmia. Ziprasidone should be discontinued in patients who are found to have persistent QTc measurements >500 msec.

For patients taking ziprasidone who experience symptoms that could indicate the occurrence of torsade de pointes, e.g., dizziness, palpitations, or syncope, the prescriber should initiate further evaluation, e.g., Holter monitoring may be useful.

Neuroleptic Malignant Syndrome (NMS)
A potentially fatal symptom complex sometimes referred to as Neuroleptic Malignant Syndrome (NMS) has been reported in association with administration of antipsychotic drugs. Clinical manifestations of NMS are hyperpyrexia, muscle rigidity, altered mental status and evidence of autonomic instability (irregular pulse or blood pressure, tachycardia, diaphoresis, and cardiac dysrhythmia). Additional signs may include elevated creatinine phosphokinase, myoglobinuria (rhabdomyolysis), and acute renal failure.

The diagnostic evaluation of patients with this syndrome is complicated. In arriving at a diagnosis, it is important to exclude cases where the clinical presentation includes both serious medical illness (e.g., pneumonia, systemic infection, etc.) and untreated or inadequately treated extrapyramidal signs and symptoms (EPS). Other important considerations in the differential diagnosis include central anticholinergic toxicity, heat stroke, drug fever, and primary central nervous system (CNS) pathology.

The management of NMS should include: (1) immediate discontinuation of antipsychotic drugs and other drugs not essential to concurrent therapy; (2) intensive symptomatic treatment and medical monitoring; and (3) treatment of any concomitant serious medical problems for which specific treatments are available. There is no general agreement about specific pharmacological treatment regimens for NMS.

If a patient requires antipsychotic drug treatment after recovery from NMS, the potential reintroduction of drug therapy should be carefully considered. The patient should be carefully monitored, since recurrences of NMS have been reported.

Tardive Dyskinesia
A syndrome of potentially irreversible, involuntary, dyskinetic movements may develop in patients undergoing treatment with antipsychotic drugs. Although the prevalence of the syndrome appears to be highest among the elderly, especially elderly women, it is impossible to rely upon prevalence estimates to predict, at the inception of antipsychotic treatment, which patients are likely to develop the syndrome. Whether antipsychotic drug products differ in their potential to cause tardive dyskinesia is unknown.

The risk of developing tardive dyskinesia and the likelihood that it will become irreversible are believed to increase as the duration of treatment and the total cumulative dose of antipsychotic drugs administered to the patient increase. However, the syndrome can develop, although much less commonly, after relatively brief treatment periods at low doses.

There is no known treatment for established cases of tardive dyskinesia, although the syndrome may remit, partially or completely, if antipsychotic treatment is withdrawn. Antipsychotic treatment itself, however, may suppress (or partially suppress) the signs and symptoms of the syndrome and thereby may possibly mask the underlying process. The effect that symptomatic suppression has upon the long-term course of the syndrome is unknown.

Given these considerations, ziprasidone should be prescribed in a manner that is most likely to minimize the occurrence of tardive dyskinesia. Chronic antipsychotic treatment should generally be reserved for patients who suffer

Continued on next page

Geodon—Cont.

from a chronic illness that (1) is known to respond to antipsychotic drugs, and (2) for whom alternative, equally effective, but potentially less harmful treatments are not available or appropriate. In patients who do require chronic treatment, the smallest dose and the shortest duration of treatment producing a satisfactory clinical response should be sought. The need for continued treatment should be reassessed periodically.

If signs and symptoms of tardive dyskinesia appear in a patient on ziprasidone, drug discontinuation should be considered. However, some patients may require treatment with ziprasidone despite the presence of the syndrome.

Hyperglycemia and Diabetes Mellitus

Hyperglycemia, in some cases extreme and associated with ketoacidosis or hyperosmolar coma or death, has been reported in patients treated with atypical antipsychotics. There have been few reports of hyperglycemia or diabetes in patients treated with GEODON. Although fewer patients have been treated with GEODON, it is not known if this more limited experience is the sole reason for the paucity of such reports. Assessment of the relationship between atypical antipsychotic use and glucose abnormalities is complicated by the possibility of an increased background risk of diabetes mellitus in patients with schizophrenia and the increasing incidence of diabetes mellitus in the general population. Given these confounders, the relationship between atypical antipsychotic use and hyperglycemia-related adverse events is not completely understood. However, epidemiological studies, which did not include GEODON, suggest an increased risk of treatment-emergent hyperglycemia-related adverse events in patients treated with the atypical antipsychotics included in these studies. Because GEODON was not marketed at the time these studies were performed, it is not known if GEODON is associated with this increased risk. Precise risk estimates for hyperglycemia-related adverse events in patients treated with atypical antipsychotics are not available.

Patients with an established diagnosis of diabetes mellitus who are started on atypical antipsychotics should be monitored regularly for worsening of glucose control. Patients with risk factors for diabetes mellitus (e.g., obesity, family history of diabetes) who are starting treatment with atypical antipsychotics should undergo fasting blood glucose testing at the beginning of treatment and periodically during treatment. Any patient treated with atypical antipsychotics should be monitored for symptoms of hyperglycemia including polydipsia, polyuria, polyphagia, and weakness. Patients who develop symptoms of hyperglycemia during treatment with atypical antipsychotics should undergo fasting blood glucose testing. In some cases, hyperglycemia has resolved when the atypical antipsychotic was discontinued; however, some patients required continuation of antidiabetic treatment despite discontinuation of the suspect drug.

PRECAUTIONS

General

Rash—In premarketing trials with ziprasidone, about 5% of patients developed rash and/or urticaria, with discontinuation of treatment in about one-sixth of these cases. The occurrence of rash was related to dose of ziprasidone, although the finding might also be explained by the longer exposure time in the higher dose patients. Several patients with rash had signs and symptoms of associated systemic illness, e.g., elevated WBCs. Most patients improved promptly with adjunctive treatment with antihistamines or steroids and/or upon discontinuation of ziprasidone, and all patients experiencing these events were reported to recover completely. Upon appearance of rash for which an alternative etiology cannot be identified, ziprasidone should be discontinued.

Orthostatic Hypotension—Ziprasidone may induce orthostatic hypotension associated with dizziness, tachycardia, and, in some patients, syncope, especially during the initial dose-titration period, probably reflecting its α_1-adrenergic antagonist properties. Syncope was reported in 0.6% of the patients treated with ziprasidone.

Ziprasidone should be used with particular caution in patients with known cardiovascular disease (history of myocardial infarction or ischemic heart disease, heart failure or conduction abnormalities), cerebrovascular disease or conditions which would predispose patients to hypotension (dehydration, hypovolemia, and treatment with antihypertensive medications).

Seizures—During clinical trials, seizures occurred in 0.4% of patients treated with ziprasidone. There were confounding factors that may have contributed to the occurrence of seizures in many of these cases. As with other antipsychotic drugs, ziprasidone should be used cautiously in patients with a history of seizures or with conditions that potentially lower the seizure threshold, e.g., Alzheimer's dementia. Conditions that lower the seizure threshold may be more prevalent in a population of 65 years or older.

Hyperprolactinemia—As with other drugs that antagonize dopamine D_2 receptors, ziprasidone elevates prolactin levels in humans. Increased prolactin levels were also observed in animal studies with this compound, and were associated with an increase in mammary gland neoplasia in mice; a similar effect was not observed in rats (see **Carcinogenesis**). Tissue culture experiments indicate that approximately one-third of human breast cancers are prolactin-dependent in vitro, a factor of potential importance if the prescription of these drugs is contemplated in a patient with previously detected breast cancer. Although disturbances such as ga-

lactorrhea, amenorrhea, gynecomastia, and impotence have been reported with prolactin-elevating compounds, the clinical significance of elevated serum prolactin levels is unknown for most patients. Neither clinical studies nor epidemiologic studies conducted to date have shown an association between chronic administration of this class of drugs and tumorigenesis in humans; the available evidence is considered too limited to be conclusive at this time.

Potential for Cognitive and Motor Impairment—Somnolence was a commonly reported adverse event in patients treated with ziprasidone. In the 4- and 6-week placebo-controlled trials, somnolence was reported in 14% of patients on ziprasidone compared to 7% of placebo patients. Somnolence led to discontinuation in 0.3% of patients in short-term clinical trials. Since ziprasidone has the potential to impair judgment, thinking, or motor skills, patients should be cautioned about performing activities requiring mental alertness, such as operating a motor vehicle (including automobiles) or operating hazardous machinery until they are reasonably certain that ziprasidone therapy does not affect them adversely.

Priapism—One case of priapism was reported in the premarketing database. While the relationship of the event to ziprasidone use has not been established, other drugs with alpha-adrenergic blocking effects have been reported to induce priapism, and it is possible that ziprasidone may share this capacity. Severe priapism may require surgical intervention.

Body Temperature Regulation—Although not reported with ziprasidone in premarketing trials, disruption of the body's ability to reduce core body temperature has been attributed to antipsychotic agents. Appropriate care is advised when prescribing ziprasidone for patients who will be experiencing conditions which may contribute to an elevation in core body temperature, e.g., exercising strenuously, exposure to extreme heat, receiving concomitant medication with anticholinergic activity, or being subject to dehydration.

Dysphagia—Esophageal dysmotility and aspiration have been associated with antipsychotic drug use. Aspiration pneumonia is a common cause of morbidity and mortality in elderly patients, in particular those with advanced Alzheimer's dementia. Ziprasidone and other antipsychotic drugs should be used cautiously in patients at risk for aspiration pneumonia.

Suicide—The possibility of a suicide attempt is inherent in psychotic illness or bipolar disorder, and close supervision of high-risk patients should accompany drug therapy. Prescriptions for ziprasidone should be written for the smallest quantity of capsules consistent with good patient management in order to reduce the risk of overdose.

Use in Patients with Concomitant Illness—Clinical experience with ziprasidone in patients with certain concomitant systemic illnesses (see **Renal Impairment** and **Hepatic Impairment** under **CLINICAL PHARMACOLOGY, Special Populations**) is limited.

Ziprasidone has not been evaluated or used to any appreciable extent in patients with a recent history of myocardial infarction or unstable heart disease. Patients with these diagnoses were excluded from premarketing clinical studies. Because of the risk of QTc prolongation and orthostatic hypotension with ziprasidone, caution should be observed in cardiac patients (see **QTc Prolongation** under **WARNINGS** and **Orthostatic Hypotension** under **PRECAUTIONS**).

Information for Patients

Please refer to the patient package insert. To assure safe and effective use of GEODON, the information and instructions provided in the patient information should be discussed with patients.

Laboratory Tests

Patients being considered for ziprasidone treatment that are at risk of significant electrolyte disturbances should have baseline serum potassium and magnesium measurements. Low serum potassium and magnesium should be repleted before proceeding with treatment. Patients who are started on diuretics during ziprasidone therapy need periodic monitoring of serum potassium and magnesium. Ziprasidone should be discontinued in patients who are found to have persistent QTc measurements >500 msec (see **WARNINGS**).

Drug Interactions

Drug-drug interactions can be pharmacodynamic (combined pharmacologic effects) or pharmacokinetic (alteration of plasma levels). The risks of using ziprasidone in combination with other drugs have been evaluated as described below. All interactions studies have been conducted with oral ziprasidone. Based upon the pharmacodynamic and pharmacokinetic profile of ziprasidone, possible interactions could be anticipated:

Pharmacodynamic Interactions

(1) Ziprasidone should not be used with any drug that prolongs the QT interval (see **CONTRAINDICATIONS**).

(2) Given the primary CNS effects of ziprasidone, caution should be used when it is taken in combination with other centrally acting drugs.

(3) Because of its potential for inducing hypotension, ziprasidone may enhance the effects of certain antihypertensive agents.

(4) Ziprasidone may antagonize the effects of levodopa and dopamine agonists.

Pharmacokinetic Interactions

The Effect of Other Drugs on Ziprasidone

Carbamazepine—Carbamazepine is an inducer of CYP3A4; administration of 200 mg BID for 21 days resulted in a de-

crease of approximately 35% in the AUC of ziprasidone. This effect may be greater when higher doses of carbamazepine are administered.

Ketoconazole—Ketoconazole, a potent inhibitor of CYP3A4, at a dose of 400 mg QD for 5 days, increased the AUC and Cmax of ziprasidone by about 35-40%. Other inhibitors of CYP3A4 would be expected to have similar effects.

Cimetidine—Cimetidine at a dose of 800 mg QD for 2 days did not affect ziprasidone pharmacokinetics.

Antacid—The coadministration of 30 mL of Maalox® with ziprasidone did not affect the pharmacokinetics of ziprasidone.

In addition, population pharmacokinetic analysis of schizophrenic patients enrolled in controlled clinical trials has not revealed evidence of any clinically significant pharmacokinetic interactions with benztropine, propranolol, or lorazepam.

Effect of Ziprasidone on Other Drugs

In vitro studies revealed little potential for ziprasidone to interfere with the metabolism of drugs cleared primarily by CYP1A2, CYP2C9, CYP2C19, CYP2D6, and CYP3A4, and little potential for drug interactions with ziprasidone due to displacement (see **CLINICAL PHARMACOLOGY, Pharmacokinetics**).

Lithium—Ziprasidone at a dose of 40 mg BID administered concomitantly with lithium at a dose of 450 mg BID for 7 days did not affect the steady-state level or renal clearance of lithium.

Oral Contraceptives—Ziprasidone at a dose of 20 mg BID did not affect the pharmacokinetics of concomitantly administered oral contraceptives, ethinyl estradiol (0.03 mg) and levonorgestrel (0.15 mg).

Dextromethorphan—Consistent with in vitro results, a study in normal healthy volunteers showed that ziprasidone did not alter the metabolism of dextromethorphan, a CYP2D6 model substrate, to its major metabolite, dextrorphan. There was no statistically significant change in the urinary dextromethorphan/dextrorphan ratio.

Carcinogenesis, Mutagenesis, Impairment of Fertility

Carcinogenesis—Lifetime carcinogenicity studies were conducted with ziprasidone in Long Evans rats and CD-1 mice. Ziprasidone was administered for 24 months in the diet at doses of 2, 6, or 12 mg/kg/day to rats, and 50, 100, or 200 mg/kg/day to mice (0.1 to 0.6 and 1 to 5 times the maximum recommended human dose [MRHD] of 200 mg/day on a mg/m² basis, respectively). In the rat study, there was no evidence of an increased incidence of tumors compared to controls. In male mice, there was no increase in incidence of tumors relative to controls. In female mice, there were dose-related increases in the incidences of pituitary gland adenoma and carcinoma, and mammary gland adenocarcinoma at all doses tested (50 to 200 mg/kg/day or 1 to 5 times the MRHD on a mg/m² basis). Proliferative changes in the pituitary and mammary glands of rodents have been observed following chronic administration of other antipsychotic agents and are considered to be prolactin-mediated. Increases in serum prolactin were observed in a 1-month dietary study in female, but not male, mice at 100 and 200 mg/kg/day (or 2.5 and 5 times the MRHD on a mg/m² basis). Ziprasidone had no effect on serum prolactin in rats in a 5-week dietary study at the doses that were used in the carcinogenicity study. The relevance for human risk of the findings of prolactin-mediated endocrine tumors in rodents is unknown (see **Hyperprolactinemia** under **PRECAUTIONS, General**).

Mutagenesis—Ziprasidone was tested in the Ames bacterial mutation assay, the in vitro mammalian cell gene mutation mouse lymphoma assay, the in vitro chromosomal aberration assay in human lymphocytes, and the in vivo chromosomal aberration assay in mouse bone marrow. There was a reproducible mutagenic response in the Ames assay in one strain of S. typhimurium in the absence of metabolic activation. Positive results were obtained in both the in vitro mammalian cell gene mutation assay and the in vitro chromosomal aberration assay in human lymphocytes.

Impairment of Fertility—Ziprasidone was shown to increase time to copulation in Sprague-Dawley rats in two fertility and early embryonic development studies at doses of 10 to 160 mg/kg/day (0.5 to 8 times the MRHD of 200 mg/day on a mg/m² basis). Fertility rate was reduced at 160 mg/kg/day (8 times the MRHD on a mg/m² basis). There was no effect on fertility at 40 mg/kg/day (2 times the MRHD on a mg/m² basis). The effect on fertility appeared to be in the female since fertility was not impaired when males given 160 mg/kg/day (8 times the MRHD on a mg/m² basis) were mated with untreated females. In a 6-month study in male rats given 200 mg/kg/day (10 times the MRHD on a mg/m² basis) there were no treatment-related findings observed in the testes.

Pregnancy - Pregnancy Category C—In animal studies ziprasidone demonstrated developmental toxicity, including possible teratogenic effects at doses similar to human therapeutic doses. When ziprasidone was administered to pregnant rabbits during the period of organogenesis, an increased incidence of fetal structural abnormalities (ventricular septal defects and other cardiovascular malformations and kidney alterations) was observed at a dose of 30 mg/kg/day (3 times the MRHD of 200 mg/day on a mg/m² basis). There was no evidence to suggest that these developmental effects were secondary to maternal toxicity. The developmental no-effect dose was 10 mg/kg/day (equivalent to the MRHD on a mg/m² basis). In rats, embryofetal toxicity (decreased fetal weights, delayed skeletal ossification) was observed following administration of 10 to 160 mg/kg/day (0.5 to 8 times the MRHD on a mg/m² basis) during organogenesis or throughout gestation, but there was no evidence of teratogenicity. Doses of 40 and 160 mg/kg/day (2 and 8 times the MRHD on a mg/m² basis) were associated with maternal toxicity. The developmental no-effect dose was 5 mg/kg/day (0.2 times the MRHD on a mg/m² basis). There was an increase in the number of pups born dead and a decrease in postnatal survival through the first 4 days of lactation among the offspring of female rats treated during gestation and lactation with doses of 10 mg/kg/day (0.5 times the MRHD on a mg/m² basis) or greater. Offspring developmental delays and neurobehavioral functional impairment were observed at doses of 5 mg/kg/day (0.2 times the MRHD on a mg/m² basis) or greater. A no-effect level was not established for these effects.

There are no adequate and well-controlled studies in pregnant women. Ziprasidone should be used during pregnancy only if the potential benefit justifies the potential risk to the fetus.

Labor and Delivery—The effect of ziprasidone on labor and delivery in humans is unknown.

Nursing Mothers—It is not known whether, and if so in what amount, ziprasidone or its metabolites are excreted in human milk. It is recommended that women receiving ziprasidone should not breast feed.

Pediatric Use—The safety and effectiveness of ziprasidone in pediatric patients have not been established.

Geriatric Use—Of the approximately 4500 patients treated with ziprasidone in clinical studies, 2.4% (109) were 65 years of age or over. In general, there was no indication of any different tolerability of ziprasidone or for reduced clearance of ziprasidone in the elderly compared to younger adults. Nevertheless, the presence of multiple factors that might increase the pharmacodynamic response to ziprasidone, or cause poorer tolerance or orthostasis, should lead to consideration of a lower starting dose, slower titration, and careful monitoring during the initial dosing period for some elderly patients.

ADVERSE REACTIONS

Premarketing experience

The premarketing development program for oral ziprasidone included approximately 5700 patients and/or normal subjects exposed to one or more doses of ziprasidone. Of these 5700, over 4800 were patients who participated in multiple-dose effectiveness trials, and their experience corresponded to approximately 1831 patient-years. These patients include: (1) 4331 patients who participated in multiple-dose trials, predominantly in schizophrenia, representing approximately 1698 patient-years of exposure as of February 5, 2000; and (2) 472 patients who participated in bipolar mania trials representing approximately 133 patient-years of exposure. The conditions and duration of treatment with ziprasidone included open-label and double-blind studies, inpatient and outpatient studies, and short-term and longer-term exposure.

The premarketing development program for intramuscular ziprasidone included 570 patients and/or normal subjects who received one or more injections of ziprasidone. Over 325 of these subjects participated in trials involving the administration of multiple doses.

Adverse events during exposure were obtained by collecting voluntarily reported adverse experiences, as well as results of physical examinations, vital signs, weights, laboratory analyses, ECGs, and results of ophthalmologic examinations. Adverse experiences were recorded by clinical investigators using terminology of their own choosing. Consequently, it is not possible to provide a meaningful estimate of the proportion of individuals experiencing adverse events without first grouping similar types of events into a smaller number of standardized event categories. In the tables and tabulations that follow, standard COSTART dictionary terminology has been used to classify reported adverse events. The stated frequencies of adverse events represent the proportion of individuals who experienced, at least once, a treatment-emergent adverse event of the type listed. An event was considered treatment emergent if it occurred for the first time or worsened while receiving therapy following baseline evaluation.

The prescriber should be aware that these figures cannot be used to predict the incidence of side effects in the course of usual medical practice where patient characteristics and other factors differ from those which prevailed in the clinical trials. Similarly, the cited frequencies cannot be compared with figures obtained from other clinical investigations involving different treatments, uses, and investigators. The cited figures, however, do provide the prescribing physician with some basis for estimating the relative contribution of drug and non-drug factors to the side effect incidence rate in the population studied.

Adverse Findings Observed in Short-Term, Placebo-Controlled Trials with Oral Ziprasidone

The following findings are based on the short-term placebo-controlled premarketing trials for schizophrenia (a pool of two 6-week, and two 4-week fixed-dose trials) and bipolar mania (a pool of two 3-week flexible-dose trials) in which ziprasidone was administered in doses ranging from 10 to 200 mg/day.

Adverse Events Associated with Discontinuation of Treatment in Short-Term, Placebo-Controlled Trials of Oral Ziprasidone

Schizophrenia—Approximately 4.1% (29/702) of ziprasidone-treated patients in short-term, placebo-controlled studies discontinued treatment due to an adverse event, compared with about 2.2% (6/273) on placebo. The most common event associated with dropout was rash, including

7 dropouts for rash among ziprasidone patients (1%) compared to no placebo patients (see **PRECAUTIONS**).

Bipolar Mania—Approximately 6.5% (18/279) of ziprasidone-treated patients in short-term, placebo-controlled studies discontinued treatment due to an adverse event, compared with about 3.7% (5/136) on placebo. The most common events associated with dropout in the ziprasidone-treated patients were akathisia, anxiety, depression, dizziness, dystonia, rash and vomiting, with 2 dropouts for each of these events among ziprasidone patients (1%) compared to one placebo patient each for dystonia and rash (1%) and no placebo patients for the remaining adverse events.

Commonly Observed Adverse Events in Short-Term, Placebo-Controlled Trials—The most commonly observed adverse events associated with the use of ziprasidone (incidence of 5% or greater) and not observed at an equivalent incidence among placebo-treated patients (ziprasidone incidence at least twice that for placebo) are shown in Tables 1 and 2.

Table 1: Common Treatment-Emergent Adverse Events Associated with the Use of Ziprasidone in 4- and 6-Week Trials—SCHIZOPHRENIA

Adverse Event	Percentage of Patients Reporting Event	
	Ziprasidone (N=702)	Placebo (N=273)
Somnolence	14	7
Respiratory Tract Infection	8	3

Table 2: Common Treatment-Emergent Adverse Events Associated with the Use of Ziprasidone in 3-Week Trials—BIPOLAR MANIA

Adverse Event	Percentage of Patients Reporting Event	
	Ziprasidone (N=279)	Placebo (N=136)
Somnolence	31	12
Extrapyramidal Symptoms*	31	12
Dizziness**	16	7
Akathisia	10	5
Abnormal Vision	6	3
Asthenia	6	2
Vomiting	5	2

* Extrapyramidal Symptoms includes the following adverse event terms: extrapyramidal syndrome, hypertonia, dystonia, dyskinesia, hypokinesia, tremor, paralysis and twitching. None of these adverse events occurred individually at an incidence greater than 10% in bipolar mania trials.
** Dizziness includes the adverse event terms dizziness and lightheadedness.

Adverse Events Occurring at an Incidence of 2% or More Among Ziprasidone-Treated Patients in Short-Term, Oral, Placebo-Controlled Trials

Table 3 enumerates the incidence, rounded to the nearest percent, of treatment-emergent adverse events that occurred during acute therapy (up to 6 weeks) in predominantly patients with schizophrenia, including only those events that occurred in 2% or more of patients treated with ziprasidone and for which the incidence in patients treated with ziprasidone was greater than the incidence in placebo-treated patients.

Table 3. Treatment-Emergent Adverse Event Incidence In Short-Term Oral Placebo-Controlled Trials—SCHIZOPHRENIA

Body System/Adverse Event	Percentage of Patients Reporting Event	
	Ziprasidone (N=702)	Placebo (N=273)
Body as a Whole		
Asthenia	5	3
Accidental Injury	4	2
Chest Pain	3	2
Cardiovascular		
Tachycardia	2	1
Digestive		
Nausea	10	7
Constipation	9	8
Dyspepsia	8	7
Diarrhea	5	4
Dry Mouth	4	2
Anorexia	2	1
Nervous		
Extrapyramidal Symptoms*	14	8
Somnolence	14	7
Akathisia	8	7
Dizziness**	8	6
Respiratory		
Respiratory Tract Infection	8	3
Rhinitis	4	2
Cough Increased	3	1
Skin and Appendages		
Rash	4	3
Fungal Dermatitis	2	1
Special Senses		
Abnormal Vision	3	2

* Extrapyramidal Symptoms includes the following adverse event terms: extrapyramidal syndrome, hypertonia, dystonia, dyskinesia, hypokinesia, tremor, paralysis and twitching. None of these adverse events occurred individually at an incidence greater than 5% in schizophrenia trials.
** Dizziness includes the adverse event terms dizziness and lightheadedness.

Table 4 enumerates the incidence, rounded to the nearest percent, of treatment-emergent adverse events that occurred during acute therapy (up to 3 weeks) in patients with bipolar mania, including only those events that occurred in 2% or more of patients treated with ziprasidone and for which the incidence in patients treated with ziprasidone was greater than the incidence in placebo-treated patients.

Table 4. Treatment-Emergent Adverse Event Incidence In Short-Term Oral Placebo-Controlled Trials—BIPOLAR MANIA

Body System/Adverse Event	Percentage of Patients Reporting Event	
	Ziprasidone (N=279)	Placebo (N=136)
Body as a Whole		
Headache	18	17
Asthenia	6	2
Accidental Injury	4	1
Cardiovascular		
Hypertension	3	2
Digestive		
Nausea	10	7
Diarrhea	5	4
Dry Mouth	5	4
Vomiting	5	2
Increased Salivation	4	0
Tongue Edema	3	1
Dysphagia	2	0
Musculoskeletal		
Myalgia	2	0
Nervous		
Somnolence	31	12
Extrapyramidal Symptoms*	31	12
Dizziness**	16	7
Akathisia	10	5

Continued on next page

Geodon—Cont.

Anxiety	5	4
Hypesthesia	2	1
Speech Disorder	2	0
Respiratory		
Pharyngitis	3	1
Dyspnea	2	1
Skin and Appendages		
Fungal Dermatitis	2	1
Special Senses		
Abnormal Vision	6	3

* Extrapyramidal Symptoms includes the following adverse event terms: extrapyramidal syndrome, hypertonia, dystonia, dyskinesia, hypokinesia, tremor, paralysis and twitching. None of these adverse events occurred individually at an incidence greater than 10% in bipolar mania trials.

**Dizziness includes the adverse event terms dizziness and lightheadedness.

Explorations for interactions on the basis of gender did not reveal any clinically meaningful differences in the adverse event occurrence on the basis of this demographic factor.

Dose Dependency of Adverse Events in Short-Term, Fixed-Dose, Placebo-Controlled Trials

An analysis for dose response in the schizophrenia 4-study pool revealed an apparent relation of adverse event to dose for the following events: asthenia, postural hypotension, anorexia, dry mouth, increased salivation, arthralgia, anxiety, dizziness, dystonia, hypertonia, somnolence, tremor, rhinitis, rash, and abnormal vision.

Extrapyramidal Symptoms (EPS)—The incidence of reported EPS (which included the adverse event terms extrapyramidal syndrome, hypertonia, dystonia, dyskinesia, hypokinesia, tremor, paralysis and twitching) for ziprasidone-treated patients in the short-term, placebo-controlled schizophrenia trials was 14% vs. 8% for placebo. Objectively collected data from those trials on the Simpson-Angus Rating Scale (for EPS) and the Barnes Akathisia Scale (for akathisia) did not generally show a difference between ziprasidone and placebo.

Vital Sign Changes—Ziprasidone is associated with orthostatic hypotension (see **PRECAUTIONS**).

Weight Gain—The proportions of patients meeting a weight gain criterion of ≥7% of body weight were compared in a pool of four 4- and 6-week placebo-controlled schizophrenia clinical trials, revealing a statistically significantly greater incidence of weight gain for ziprasidone (10%) compared to placebo (4%). A median weight gain of 0.5 kg was observed in ziprasidone patients compared to no median weight change in placebo patients. In this set of clinical trials, weight gain was reported as an adverse event in 0.4% and 0.4% of ziprasidone and placebo patients, respectively. During long-term therapy with ziprasidone, a categorization of patients at baseline on the basis of body mass index (BMI) revealed the greatest mean weight gain and highest incidence of clinically significant weight gain (>7% of body weight) in patients with low BMI (<23) compared to normal (23-27) or overweight patients (>27). There was a mean weight gain of 1.4 kg for those patients with a "low" baseline BMI, no mean change for patients with a "normal" BMI, and a 1.3 kg mean weight loss for patients who entered the program with a "high" BMI.

ECG Changes—Ziprasidone is associated with an increase in the QTc interval (see **WARNINGS**). In the schizophrenia trials, ziprasidone was associated with a mean increase in heart rate of 1.4 beats per minute compared to a 0.2 beats per minute decrease among placebo patients.

Other Adverse Events Observed During the Premarketing Evaluation of Oral Ziprasidone

Following is a list of COSTART terms that reflect treatment-emergent adverse events as defined in the introduction to the **ADVERSE REACTIONS** section reported by patients treated with ziprasidone in schizophrenia trials at multiple doses >4 mg/day within the database of 3834 patients. All reported events are included except those already listed in Table 3 or elsewhere in labeling, those event terms that were so general as to be uninformative, events reported only once and that did not have a substantial probability of being acutely life-threatening, events that are part of the illness being treated or are otherwise common as background events, and events considered unlikely to be drug-related. It is important to emphasize that, although the events reported occurred during treatment with ziprasidone, they were not necessarily caused by it.

Events are further categorized by body system and listed in order of decreasing frequency according to the following definitions: frequent adverse events are those occurring in at least 1/100 patients (only those not already listed in the tabulated results from placebo-controlled trials appear in this listing); infrequent adverse events are those occurring in 1/100 to 1/1000 patients; rare events are those occurring in fewer than 1/1000 patients.

TABLE 5. Treatment-Emergent Adverse Event Incidence In Short-Term Fixed-Dose Intramuscular Trials

Body System/Adverse Event	Percentage of Patients Reporting Event		
	Ziprasidone 2 mg (N=92)	Ziprasidone 10 mg (N=63)	Ziprasidone 20 mg (N=41)
Body as a Whole			
Headache	3	13	5
Injection Site Pain	9	8	7
Asthenia	2	0	0
Abdominal Pain	0	2	0
Flu Syndrome	1	0	0
Back Pain	1	0	0
Cardiovascular			
Postural Hypotension	0	0	5
Hypertension	2	0	0
Bradycardia	0	0	2
Vasodilation	1	0	0
Digestive			
Nausea	4	8	12
Rectal Hemorrhage	0	0	2
Diarrhea	3	3	0
Vomiting	0	3	0
Dyspepsia	1	3	2
Anorexia	0	2	0
Constipation	0	0	2
Tooth Disorder	1	0	0
Dry Mouth	1	0	0
Nervous			
Dizziness	3	3	10
Anxiety	2	0	0
Insomnia	3	0	0
Somnolence	8	8	20
Akathisia	0	2	0
Agitation	2	2	0
Extrapyramidal Syndrome	2	0	0
Hypertonia	1	0	0
Cogwheel Rigidity	1	0	0
Paresthesia	0	2	0
Personality Disorder	0	2	0
Psychosis	1	0	0
Speech Disorder	0	2	0
Respiratory			
Rhinitis	1	0	0
Skin and Appendages			
Furunculosis	0	2	0
Sweating	0	0	2
Urogenital			
Dysmenorrhea	0	2	0
Priapism	1	0	0

Body as a Whole: *Frequent:* abdominal pain, flu syndrome, fever, accidental fall, face edema, chills, photosensitivity reaction, flank pain, hypothermia, motor vehicle accident.

Cardiovascular System: *Frequent:* tachycardia, hypertension, postural hypotension; *Infrequent:* bradycardia, angina pectoris, atrial fibrillation; *Rare:* first degree AV block, bundle branch block, phlebitis, pulmonary embolus, cardiomegaly, cerebral infarct, cerebrovascular accident, deep thrombophlebitis, myocarditis, thrombophlebitis.

Digestive System: *Frequent:* anorexia, vomiting; *Infrequent:* rectal hemorrhage, dysphagia, tongue edema; *Rare:* gum hemorrhage, jaundice, fecal impaction, gamma glutamyl transpeptidase increased, hematemesis, cholestatic jaundice, hepatitis, hepatomegaly, leukoplakia of mouth, fatty liver deposit, melena.

Endocrine: *Rare:* hypothyroidism, hyperthyroidism, thyroiditis.

Hemic and Lymphatic System: *Infrequent:* anemia, ecchymosis, leukocytosis, leukopenia, eosinophilia, lymphadenopathy; *Rare:* thrombocytopenia, hypochromic anemia, lymphocytosis, monocytosis, basophilia, lymphedema, polycythemia, thrombocythemia.

Metabolic and Nutritional Disorders: *Infrequent:* thirst, transaminase increased, peripheral edema, hyperglycemia, creatine phosphokinase increased, alkaline phosphatase increased, hypercholesteremia, dehydration, lactic dehydrogenase increased, albuminuria, hypokalemia; *Rare:* BUN increased, creatinine increased, hyperlipemia, hypocholesteremia, hyperkalemia, hypochloremia, hypoglycemia, hyponatremia, hypoproteinemia, glucose tolerance decreased, gout, hyperchloremia, hyperuricemia, hypocalcemia, hypoglycemic reaction, hypomagnesemia, ketosis, respiratory alkalosis.

Musculoskeletal System: *Frequent:* myalgia; *Infrequent:* tenosynovitis; *Rare:* myopathy.

Nervous System: *Frequent:* agitation, extrapyramidal syndrome, tremor, dystonia, hypertonia, dyskinesia, hostility, twitching, paresthesia, confusion, vertigo, hypokinesia, hyperkinesia, abnormal gait, oculogyric crisis, hypesthesia, ataxia, amnesia, cogwheel rigidity, delirium, hypotonia, akinesia, dysarthria, withdrawal syndrome, buccoglossal syndrome, choreoathetosis, diplopia, incoordination, neuropathy; *Infrequent:* paralysis; *Rare:* myoclonus, nystagmus, torticollis, circumoral paresthesia, opisthotonos, reflexes increased, trismus.

Respiratory System: *Frequent:* dyspnea; *Infrequent:* pneumonia, epistaxis; *Rare:* hemoptysis, laryngismus.

Skin and Appendages: *Infrequent:* maculopapular rash, urticaria, alopecia, eczema, exfoliative dermatitis, contact dermatitis, vesiculobullous rash.

Special Senses: *Frequent:* fungal dermatitis; *Infrequent:* conjunctivitis, dry eyes, tinnitus, blepharitis, cataract, photophobia; *Rare:* eye hemorrhage, visual field defect, keratitis, keratoconjunctivitis.

Urogenital System: *Infrequent:* impotence, abnormal ejaculation, amenorrhea, hematuria, menorrhagia, female lactation, polyuria, urinary retention, metrorrhagia, male sexual dysfunction, anorgasmia, glycosuria; *Rare:* gynecomastia, vaginal hemorrhage, nocturia, oliguria, female sexual dysfunction, uterine hemorrhage.

Adverse Findings Observed in Trials of Intramuscular Ziprasidone

Adverse Events Occurring at an Incidence of 1% or More Among Ziprasidone-Treated Patients in Short-Term Trials of Intramuscular Ziprasidone

Table 5 enumerates the incidence, rounded to the nearest percent, of treatment-emergent adverse events that occurred during acute therapy with intramuscular ziprasidone in 1% or more of patients.

In these studies, the most commonly observed adverse events associated with the use of intramuscular ziprasidone (incidence of 5% or greater) and observed at a rate on intramuscular ziprasidone (in the higher dose groups) at least twice that of the lowest intramuscular ziprasidone group were headache (13%), nausea (12%), and somnolence (20%). [See table 5 at top of previous page]

Other Events Observed During Post-marketing Use

Adverse event reports not listed above that have been received since market introduction include rare occurrences of the following (no causal relationship with ziprasidone has been established): *Cardiac Disorders:* Tachycardia, Torsade de Pointes (in the presence of multiple confounding factors - see **WARNINGS**); *Reproductive System and Breast Disorders:* galactorrhea; *Nervous System Disorders:* Neuroleptic malignant syndrome; *Psychiatric Disorders:* Insomnia; *Skin and subcutaneous Tissue Disorders:* Allergic reaction, rash; *Vascular Disorders:* Postural hypotension.

DRUG ABUSE AND DEPENDENCE

Controlled Substance Class—Ziprasidone is not a controlled substance.

Physical and Psychological Dependence—Ziprasidone has not been systematically studied, in animals or humans, for its potential for abuse, tolerance, or physical dependence. While the clinical trials did not reveal any tendency for drug-seeking behavior, these observations were not systematic and it is not possible to predict on the basis of this limited experience the extent to which ziprasidone will be misused, diverted, and/or abused once marketed. Consequently, patients should be evaluated carefully for a history of drug abuse, and such patients should be observed closely for signs of ziprasidone misuse or abuse (e.g., development of tolerance, increases in dose, drug-seeking behavior).

OVERDOSAGE

Human Experience—In premarketing trials involving more than 5400 patients and/or normal subjects, accidental or intentional overdosage of oral ziprasidone was documented in 10 patients. All of these patients survived without sequelae. In the patient taking the largest confirmed amount, 3240 mg, the only symptoms reported were minimal sedation, slurring of speech, and transitory hypertension (200/95).

In post-marketing use, adverse events reported in association with ziprasidone overdose generally included extrapyramidal symptoms, somnolence, tremor, and anxiety. The largest confirmed post-marketing single ingestion was 12,800 mg; extrapyramidal symptoms and a QTc interval of 446 msec were reported with no cardiac sequelae.

Management of Overdosage—In case of acute overdosage, establish and maintain an airway and ensure adequate oxygenation and ventilation. Intravenous access should be established and gastric lavage (after intubation, if patient is unconscious) and administration of activated charcoal together with a laxative should be considered. The possibility of obtundation, seizure, or dystonic reaction of the head and neck following overdose may create a risk of aspiration with induced emesis.

Cardiovascular monitoring should commence immediately and should include continuous electrocardiographic moni-

toring to detect possible arrhythmias. If antiarrhythmic therapy is administered, disopyramide, procainamide, and quinidine carry a theoretical hazard of additive QT-prolonging effects that might be additive to those of ziprasidone. Hypotension and circulatory collapse should be treated with appropriate measures such as intravenous fluids. If sympathomimetic agents are used for vascular support, epinephrine and dopamine should not be used, since beta stimulation combined with α_1 antagonism associated with ziprasidone may worsen hypotension. Similarly, it is reasonable to expect that the alpha-adrenergic-blocking properties of bretylium might be additive to those of ziprasidone, resulting in problematic hypotension.

In cases of severe extrapyramidal symptoms, anticholinergic medication should be administered. There is no specific antidote to ziprasidone, and it is not dialyzable. The possibility of multiple drug involvement should be considered. Close medical supervision and monitoring should continue until the patient recovers.

DOSAGE AND ADMINISTRATION

Schizophrenia

When deciding among the alternative treatments available for schizophrenia, the prescriber should consider the finding of ziprasidone's greater capacity to prolong the QT/QTc interval compared to several other antipsychotic drugs (see **WARNINGS**).

Initial Treatment

GEODON® Capsules should be administered at an initial daily dose of 20 mg BID with food. In some patients, daily dosage may subsequently be adjusted on the basis of individual clinical status up to 80 mg BID. Dosage adjustments, if indicated, should generally occur at intervals of not less than 2 days, as steady-state is achieved within 1 to 3 days. In order to ensure use of the lowest effective dose, ordinarily patients should be observed for improvement for several weeks before upward dosage adjustment.

Efficacy in schizophrenia was demonstrated in a dose range of 20 to 100 mg BID in short-term, placebo-controlled clinical trials. There were trends toward dose response within the range of 20 to 80 mg BID, but results were not consistent. An increase to a dose greater than 80 mg BID is not generally recommended. The safety of doses above 100 mg BID has not been systematically evaluated in clinical trials.

Maintenance Treatment

While there is no body of evidence available to answer the question of how long a patient treated with ziprasidone should remain on it, systematic evaluation of ziprasidone has shown that its efficacy in schizophrenia is maintained for periods of up to 52 weeks at a dose of 20 to 80 mg BID (see **CLINICAL PHARMACOLOGY**). No additional benefit was demonstrated for doses above 20 mg BID. Patients should be periodically reassessed to determine the need for maintenance treatment.

Bipolar Mania

Initial Treatment

Oral ziprasidone should be administered at an initial daily dose of 40 mg BID with food. The dose should then be increased to 60 mg or 80 mg BID on the second day of treatment and subsequently adjusted on the basis of toleration and efficacy within the range 40-80 mg BID. In the flexible-dose clinical trials, the mean daily dose administered was approximately 120 mg (see **CLINICAL PHARMACOLOGY**).

Maintenance Treatment

There is no body of evidence available from controlled trials to guide a clinician in the longer-term management of a patient who improves during treatment of mania with ziprasidone. While it is generally agreed that pharmacological treatment beyond an acute response in mania is desirable, both for maintenance of the initial response and for prevention of new manic episodes, there are no systematically obtained data to support the use of ziprasidone in such longer-term treatment (i.e., beyond 3 weeks).

Intramuscular Administration for Acute Agitation in Schizophrenia

The recommended dose is 10 to 20 mg administered as required up to a maximum dose of 40 mg per day. Doses of 10 mg may be administered every two hours; doses of 20 mg may be administered every four hours up to a maximum of 40 mg/day. Intramuscular administration of ziprasidone for more than three consecutive days has not been studied.

If long-term therapy is indicated, oral ziprasidone hydrochloride capsules should replace the intramuscular administration as soon as possible.

Since there is no experience regarding the safety of administering ziprasidone intramuscular to schizophrenic patients already taking oral ziprasidone, the practice of co-administration is not recommended.

Dosing in Special Populations

Oral: Dosage adjustments are generally not required on the basis of age, gender, race, or renal or hepatic impairment.

Intramuscular: Ziprasidone intramuscular has not been systematically evaluated in elderly patients or in patients with hepatic or renal impairment. As the cyclodextrin excipient is cleared by renal filtration, ziprasidone intramuscular should be administered with caution to patients with impaired renal function. Dosing adjustments are not required on the basis of gender or race.

Preparation for Administration

GEODON® for Injection (ziprasidone mesylate) should only be administered by intramuscular injection. Single-dose vials require reconstitution prior to administration; any unused portion should be discarded.

Add 1.2 mL of Sterile Water for Injection to the vial and shake vigorously until all the drug is dissolved. Each mL of reconstituted solution contains 20 mg ziprasidone. To administer a 10 mg dose, draw up 0.5 mL of the reconstituted solution. To administer a 20 mg dose, draw up 1.0 mL of the reconstituted solution. Since no preservative or bacteriostatic agent is present in this product, aseptic technique must be used in preparation of the final solution. This medicinal product must not be mixed with other medicinal products or solvents other than Sterile Water for Injection. Parenteral drug products should be inspected visually for particulate matter and discoloration prior to administration, whenever solution and container permit.

HOW SUPPLIED

GEODON® Capsules are differentiated by capsule color/size and are imprinted in black ink with "Pfizer" and a unique number. GEODON Capsules are supplied for oral administration in 20 mg (blue/white), 40 mg (blue/blue), 60 mg (white/white), and 80 mg (blue/white) capsules. They are supplied in the following strengths and package configurations:

Package Configuration	GEODON® Capsules Capsule Strength (mg)	NDC Code	Imprint
Bottles of 60	20	NDC-0049-3960-60	396
Bottles of 60	40	NDC-0049-3970-60	397
Bottles of 60	60	NDC-0049-3980-60	398
Bottles of 60	80	NDC-0049-3990-60	399
Unit dose/80	20	NDC-0049-3960-41	396
Unit dose/80	40	NDC-0049-3970-41	397
Unit dose/80	60	NDC-0049-3980-41	398
Unit dose/80	80	NDC-0049-3990-41	399

Storage and Handling—GEODON® Capsules should be stored at controlled room temperature, 15°-30°C (59°-86°F). GEODON® for Injection is available in a single dose vial as ziprasidone mesylate (20 mg ziprasidone/mL when reconstituted according to label instructions—see **Preparation for Administration**) for intramuscular administration. Each mL of ziprasidone mesylate for injection (when reconstituted) affords a colorless to pale pink solution that contains 20 mg of ziprasidone and 4.7 mg of methanesulfonic acid solubilized by 294 mg of sulfobutylether β-cyclodextrin sodium (SBECD).

GEODON® for Injection		
Package	Concentration	NDC Code
Single Use Vials	20 mg/mL	NDC-0049-3920-83

Storage and Handling—GEODON® for Injection should be stored at controlled room temperature, 15°-30°C (59°-86°F) in dry form. Protect from light. Following reconstitution, GEODON for Injection can be stored, when protected from light, for up to 24 hours at 15°-30°C (59°-86°F) or up to 7 days refrigerated, 2°-8°C (36°-46°F).

Rx only   ©2005 PFIZER INC
Distributed by
Pfizer Roerig
Division of Pfizer Inc, NY, NY 10017
LAB-0273-5.0   Revised April 2005

NORVASC®   ℞

[*nor'vask*]
(amlodipine besylate)
Tablets

Prescribing information for this product, which appears on pages 2621–2625 of the 2005 PDR, has been completely revised as follows. Please write "See Supplement A" next to the product heading.

DESCRIPTION

NORVASC® is the besylate salt of amlodipine, a long-acting calcium channel blocker.

Amlodipine besylate is chemically described as 3-Ethyl-5-methyl (±)-2-[(2-aminoethoxy)methyl]-4-(2-chlorophenyl)-1,4-dihydro-6-methyl-3,5-pyridinedicarboxylate, monobenzenesulphonate. Its empirical formula is $C_{20}H_{25}ClN_2O_5 \cdot C_6H_6O_3S$, and its structural formula is:

[See structural formula at top of next column]

Amlodipine besylate is a white crystalline powder with a molecular weight of 567.1. It is slightly soluble in water and sparingly soluble in ethanol. NORVASC (amlodipine besylate) tablets are formulated as white tablets equivalent to 2.5, 5 and 10 mg of amlodipine for oral administration. In addition to the active ingredient, amlodipine besylate, each

Continued on next page

Norvasc—Cont.

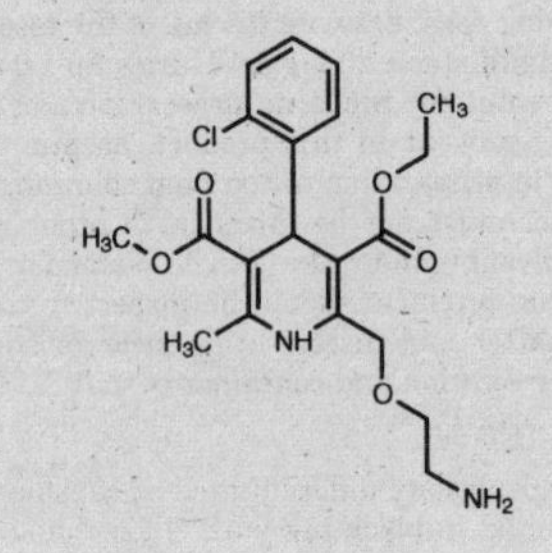

$C_6H_6O_3S$

tablet contains the following inactive ingredients: microcrystalline cellulose, dibasic calcium phosphate anhydrous, sodium starch glycolate, and magnesium stearate.

CLINICAL PHARMACOLOGY

Mechanism of Action

Amlodipine is a dihydropyridine calcium antagonist (calcium ion antagonist or slow-channel blocker) that inhibits the transmembrane influx of calcium ions into vascular smooth muscle and cardiac muscle. Experimental data suggest that amlodipine binds to both dihydropyridine and nondihydropyridine binding sites. The contractile processes of cardiac muscle and vascular smooth muscle are dependent upon the movement of extracellular calcium ions into these cells through specific ion channels. Amlodipine inhibits calcium ion influx across cell membranes selectively, with a greater effect on vascular smooth muscle cells than on cardiac muscle cells. Negative inotropic effects can be detected *in vitro* but such effects have not been seen in intact animals at therapeutic doses. Serum calcium concentration is not affected by amlodipine. Within the physiologic pH range, amlodipine is an ionized compound (pKa=8.6), and its kinetic interaction with the calcium channel receptor is characterized by a gradual rate of association and dissociation with the receptor binding site, resulting in a gradual onset of effect.

Amlodidpine is a peripheral arterial vasodilator that acts directly on vascular smooth muscle to cause a reduction in peripheral vascular resistance and reduction in blood pressure.

The precise mechanisms by which amlodipine relieves angina have not been fully delineated, but are thought to include the following:

Exertional Angina: In patients with exertional angina, NORVASC reduces the total peripheral resistance (afterload) against which the heart works and reduces the rate pressure product, and thus myocardial oxygen demand, at any given level of exercise.

Vasospastic Angina: NORVASC has been demonstrated to block constriction and restore blood flow in coronary arteries and arterioles in response to calcium, potassium epinephrine, serotonin, and thromboxane A_2 analog in experimental animal models and in human coronary vessels *in vitro*. This inhibition of coronary spasm is responsible for the effectiveness of NORVASC in vasospastic (Prinzmetal's or variant) angina.

Pharmacokinetics and Metabolism: After oral administration of therapeutic doses of NORVASC, absorption produces peak plasma concentrations between 6 and 12 hours. Absolute bioavailability has been estimated to be between 64 and 90%. The bioavailability of NORVASC is not altered by the presence of food.

Amlodipine is extensively (about 90%) converted to inactive metabolites via hepatic metabolism with 10% of the parent compound and 60% of the metabolites excreted in the urine. *Ex vivo* studies have shown that approximately 93% of the circulating drug is bound to plasma proteins in hypertensive patients. Elimination from the plasma is biphasic with a terminal elimination half-life of about 30-50 hours. Steady-state plasma levels of amlodipine are reached after 7 to 8 days of consecutive daily dosing.

The pharmacokinetics of amlodipine are not significantly influenced by renal impairment. Patients with renal failure may therefore receive the usual initial dose.

Elderly patients and patients with hepatic insufficiency have decreased clearance of amlodipine with a resulting increase in AUC of approximately 40-60%, and a lower initial dose may be required. A similar increase in AUC was observed in patients with moderate to severe heart failure.

Pediatric Patients: Sixty-two hypertensive patients aged 6 to 17 years received doses of NORVASC between 1.25 mg and 20 mg. Weight-adjusted clearance and volume of distribution were similar to values in adults.

Pharmacodynamics

Hemodynamics Following administration of therapeutic doses to patients with hypertension, NORVASC produces vasodilation resulting in a reduction of supine and standing blood pressures. These decreases in blood pressure are not accompanied by a significant change in heart rate or plasma catecholamine levels with chronic dosing. Although the acute intravenous administration of amlodipine decreases arterial blood pressure and increases heart rate in hemodynamic studies of patients with chronic stable angina, chronic oral administration of amlodipine in clinical trials did not lead to clinically significant changes in heart rate or blood pressures in normotensive patients with angina.

With chronic once daily oral administration, antihypertensive effectiveness is maintained for at least 24 hours. Plasma concentrations correlate with effect in both young and elderly patients. The magnitude of reduction in blood pressure with NORVASC is also correlated with the height of pretreatment elevation; thus, individuals with moderate hypertension (diastolic pressure 105-114 mmHg) had about a 50% greater response than patients with mild hypertension (diastolic pressure 90-104 mmHg). Normotensive subjects experienced no clinically significant change in blood pressures (+1/–2 mmHg).

In hypertensive patients with normal renal function, therapeutic doses of NORVASC resulted in a decrease in renal vascular resistance and an increase in glomerular filtration rate and effective renal plasma flow without change in filtration fraction or proteinuria.

As with other calcium channel blockers, hemodynamic measurements of cardiac function at rest and during exercise (or pacing) in patients with normal ventricular function treated with NORVASC have generally demonstrated a small increase in cardiac index without significant influence on dP/dt or on left ventricular end diastolic pressure or volume. In hemodynamic studies, NORVASC has not been associated with a negative inotropic effect when administered in the therapeutic dose range to intact animals and man, even when co-administered with beta-blockers to man. Similar findings, however, have been observed in normals or well-compensated patients with heart failure with agents possessing significant negative inotropic effects.

Electrophysiologic Effects: NORVASC does not change sinoatrial nodal function or atrioventricular conduction in intact animals or man. In patients with chronic stable angina, intravenous administration of 10 mg did not significantly alter A-H and H-V conduction and sinus node recovery time after pacing. Similar results were obtained in patients receiving NORVASC and concomitant beta blockers. In clinical studies in which NORVASC was administered in combination with beta-blockers to patients with either hypertension or angina, no adverse effects on electrocardiographic parameters were observed. In clinical trials with angina patients alone, NORVASC therapy did not alter electrocardiographic intervals or produce higher degrees of AV blocks.

Clinical Studies

Effects in Hypertension

Adult Patients: The antihypertensive efficacy of NORVASC has been demonstrated in a total of 15 double-blind, placebo-controlled, randomized studies involving 800 patients on NORVASC and 538 on placebo. Once daily administration produced statistically significant placebo-corrected reductions in supine and standing blood pressures at 24 hours postdose, averaging about 12/6 mmHg in the standing position and 13/7 mmHg in the supine position in patients with mild to moderate hypertension. Maintenance of the blood pressure effect over the 24-hour dosing interval was observed, with little difference in peak and trough effect. Tolerance was not demonstrated in patients studied for up to 1 year. The 3 parallel, fixed dose, dose response studies showed that the reduction in supine and standing blood pressures was dose-related within the recommended dosing range. Effects on diastolic pressure were similar in young and older patients. The effect on systolic pressure was greater in older patients, perhaps because of greater baseline systolic pressure. Effects were similar in black patients and in white patients.

Pediatric Patients: Two hundred sixty-eight hypertensive patients aged 6 to 17 years were randomized first to NORVASC 2.5 or 5 mg once daily for 4 weeks and then randomized again to the same dose or to placebo for another 4 weeks. Patients receiving 5 mg at the end of 8 weeks had lower blood pressure than those secondarily randomized to placebo. The magnitude of the treatment effect is difficult to interpret, but it is probably less than 5 mmHg systolic on the 5 mg dose. Adverse events were similar to those seen in adults.

Effects in Chronic Stable Angina:

The effectiveness of 5-10 mg/day of NORVASC in exercise-induced angina has been evaluated in 8 placebo-controlled, double-blind clinical trials of up to 6 weeks duration involving 1038 patients (684 NORVASC, 354 placebo) with chronic stable angina. In 5 of the 8 studies significant increases in exercise time (bicycle or treadmill) were seen with the 10 mg dose. Increases in symptom-limited exercise time averaged 12.8% (63 sec) for NORVASC 10 mg, and averaged 7.9% (38 sec) for NORVASC 5 mg. NORVASC 10 mg also increased time to 1 mm ST segment deviation in several studies and decreased angina attack rate. The sustained efficacy of NORVASC in angina patients has been demonstrated over long-term dosing. In patients with angina there were no clinically significant reductions in blood pressures (4/1 mmHg) or changes in heart rate (+0.3 bpm).

Effects in Vasospastic Angina:

In a double-blind, placebo-controlled clinical trial of 4 weeks duration in 50 patients, NORVASC therapy decreased attacks by approximately 4/week compared with a placebo decrease of approximately 1/week ($p<0.01$). Two of 23 NORVASC and 7 of 27 placebo patients discontinued from the study due to lack of clinical improvement.

Studies in Patients with Congestive Heart Failure:

NORVASC has been compared to placebo in four 8-12 week studies of patients with NYHA class II/III heart failure, involving a total of 697 patients. In these studies, there was no evidence of worsened heart failure based on measures of exercise tolerance, NYHA classification, symptoms, or left ventricular ejection fraction. In a long-term (follow-up at least 6 months, mean 13.8 months) placebo-controlled mortality/morbidity study of NORVASC 5-10 mg in 1153 patients with NYHA classes III (n=931) or IV (n=222) heart failure on stable doses of diuretics, digoxin, and ACE inhibitors, NORVASC had no effect on the primary endpoint of the study which was the combined endpoint of all-cause mortality and cardiac morbidity (as defined by life-threatening arrhythmia, acute myocardial infarction, or hospitalization for worsened heart failure), or on NYHA classification, or symptoms of heart failure. Total combined all-cause mortality and cardiac morbidity events were 222/571 (39%) for patients on NORVASC and 246/583 (42%) for patients on placebo; the cardiac morbid events represented about 25% of the endpoints in the study.

Another study (PRAISE-2) randomized patients with NYHA class III (80%) or IV (20%) heart failure without clinical symptoms or objective evidence of underlying ischemic disease, on stable doses of ACE inhibitor (99%), digitalis (99%) and diuretics (99%), to placebo (n=827) or NORVASC (n=827) and followed them for a mean of 33 months. There was no statistically significant difference between NORVASC and placebo in the primary endpoint of all cause mortality (95% confidence limits from 8% reduction to 29% increase on NORVASC). With NORVASC there were more reports of pulmonary edema.

INDICATIONS AND USAGE

1. Hypertension

NORVASC is indicated for the treatment of hypertension. It may be used alone or in combination with other antihypertensive agents.

2. Chronic Stable Angina

NORVASC is indicated for the treatment of chronic stable angina. NORVASC may be used alone or in combination with other antianginal agents.

3. Vasospastic Angina (Prinzmetal's or Variant Angina)

NORVASC is indicated for the treatment of confirmed or suspected vasospastic angina. NORVASC may be used as monotherapy or in combination with other antianginal drugs.

CONTRAINDICATIONS

NORVASC is contraindicated in patients with known sensitivity to amlodipine.

WARNINGS

Increased Angina and/or Myocardial Infarction: Rarely, patients, particularly those with severe obstructive coronary artery disease, have developed documented increased frequency, duration and/or severity of angina or acute myocardial infarction on starting calcium channel blocker therapy or at the time of dosage increase. The mechanism of this effect has not been elucidated.

PRECAUTIONS

General: Since the vasodilation induced by NORVASC is gradual in onset, acute hypotension has rarely been reported after oral administration. Nonetheless, caution, as with any other peripheral vasodilator, should be exercised when administering NORVASC, particularly in patients with severe aortic stenosis.

Use in Patients with Congestive Heart Failure: In general, calcium channel blockers should be used with caution in patients with heart failure. NORVASC (5-10 mg per day) has been studied in a placebo-controlled trial of 1153 patients with NYHA Class III or IV heart failure (see CLINICAL PHARMACOLOGY) on stable doses of ACE inhibitor, digoxin, and diuretics. Follow-up was at least 6 months, with a mean of about 14 months. There was no overall adverse effect on survival or cardiac morbidity (as defined by life-threatening arrhythmia, acute myocardial infarction, or hospitalization for worsened heart failure). NORVASC has been compared to placebo in four 8-12 week studies of patients with NYHA class II/III heart failure, involving a total of 697 patients. In these studies, there was no evidence of worsened heart failure based on measures of exercise tolerance, NYHA classification, symptoms, or LVEF.

Beta-Blocker Withdrawal: NORVASC is not a beta-blocker and therefore gives no protection against the dangers of abrupt beta-blocker withdrawal; any such withdrawal should be by gradual reduction of the dose of beta-blocker.

Patients with Hepatic Failure: Since NORVASC is extensively metabolized by the liver and the plasma elimination half-life (t 1/2) is 56 hours in patients with impaired hepatic function, caution should be exercised when administering NORVASC to patients with severe hepatic impairment.

Drug Interactions: *In vitro* data indicate that NORVASC has no effect on the human plasma protein binding of digoxin, phenytoin, warfarin, and indomethacin.

Effect of other agents on NORVASC.

CIMETIDINE: Co-administration of NORVASC with cimetidine did not alter the pharmacokinetics of NORVASC.

GRAPEFRUIT JUICE: Co-administration of 240 mL of grapefruit juice with a single oral dose of amlodipine 10 mg in 20 healthy volunteers had no significant effect on the pharmacokinetics of amlodipine.

MAALOX (antacid): Co-administration of the antacid Maalox with a single dose of NORVASC had no significant effect on the pharmacokinetics of NORVASC.

SILDENAFIL: A single 100 mg dose of sildenafil (Viagra®) in subjects with essential hypertension had no effect on the pharmacokinetic parameters of NORVASC. When NORVASC and sildenafil were used in combination, each agent independently exerted its own blood pressure lowering effect.

Effect of NORVASC on other agents.

ATORVASTATIN: Co-administration of multiple 10 mg doses of NORVASC with 80 mg of atorvastatin resulted in no significant change in the steady state pharmacokinetic parameters of atorvastatin.

DIGOXIN: Co-administration of NORVASC with digoxin did not change serum digoxin levels or digoxin renal clearance in normal volunteers.

ETHANOL (alcohol): Single and multiple 10 mg doses of NORVASC had no significant effect on the pharmacokinetics of ethanol.

WARFARIN: Co-administration of NORVASC with warfarin did not change the warfarin prothrombin response time.

In clinical trials, NORVASC has been safely administered with thiazide diuretics, beta-blockers, angiotensin-converting enzyme inhibitors, long-acting nitrates, sublingual nitroglycerin, digoxin, warfarin, non-steroidal anti-inflammatory drugs, antibiotics, and oral hypoglycemic drugs.

Drug/Laboratory Test Interactions: None known.

Carcinogenesis, Mutagenesis, Impairment of Fertility: Rats and mice treated with amlodipine maleate in the diet for up to two years, at concentrations calculated to provide daily dosage levels of 0.5, 1.25, and 2.5 amlodipine mg/kg/day showed no evidence of a carcinogenic effect of the drug. For the mouse, the highest dose was, on a mg/m^2 basis, similar to the maximum recommended human dose of 10 mg amlodipine/day*. For the rat, the highest dose was, on a mg/m^2 basis, about twice the maximum recommended human dose*.

Mutagenicity studies conducted with amlodipine maleate revealed no drug related effects at either the gene or chromosome levels.

There was no effect on the fertility of rats treated orally with amlodipine (males for 64 days and females for 14 days prior to mating) at doses up to 10 mg amlodipine/kg/day (8 times* the maximum recommended human dose of 10 mg/day on a mg/m^2 basis).

Pregnancy Category C: No evidence of teratogenicity or other embryo/fetal toxicity was found when pregnant rats and rabbits were treated orally with amlodipine maleate as doses up to 10 mg amlodipine/kg/day (respectively 8 times* and 23 times* the maximum recommended human dose of 10 mg on a mg/m^2 basis) during their respective periods of major organogenesis. However, litter size was significantly decreased (by about 50%) and the number of intrauterine deaths was significantly increased (about 5-fold) in rats receiving amlodipine maleate at a dose equivalent to 10 mg amlodipine/kg/day for 14 days before mating and throughout mating and gestation. Amlodipine maleate has been shown to prolong both the gestation period and the duration of labor in rats at this dose. There are no adequate and well-controlled studies in pregnant women. Amlodipine should be used during pregnancy only if the potential benefit justifies the potential risk to the fetus.

*Based on patient weight of 50 kg.

Nursing Mothers: It is not known whether amlodipine is excreted in human milk. In the absence of this information, it is recommended that nursing be discontinued while NORVASC is administered.

Pediatric Use: The effect of NORVASC on blood pressure in patients less than 6 years of age is not known.

Geriatric Use: Clinical studies of NORVASC did not include sufficient numbers of subjects aged 65 and over to determine whether they respond differently from younger subjects. Other reported clinical experience has not identified differences in responses between the elderly and younger patients. In general, dose selection for an elderly patient should be cautious, usually starting at the low end of the dosing range, reflecting the greater frequency of decreased hepatic, renal, or cardiac function, and of concomitant disease or other drug therapy. Elderly patients have decreased clearance of amlodipine with a resulting increase of AUC of approximately 40-60%, and a lower initial dose may be required (see **DOSAGE AND ADMINISTRATION**).

ADVERSE REACTIONS

NORVASC has been evaluated for safety in more than 11,000 patients in U.S. and foreign clinical trials. In general, treatment with NORVASC was well-tolerated at doses up to 10 mg daily. Most adverse reactions reported during therapy with NORVASC were of mild or moderate severity. In controlled clinical trials directly comparing NORVASC (N=1730) in doses up to 10 mg to placebo (N=1250), discontinuation of NORVASC due to adverse reactions was required in only about 1.5% of patients and was not significantly different from placebo (about 1%). The most common side effects are headache and edema. The incidence (%) of side effects which occurred in a dose related manner are as follows:

Adverse Event	2.5 mg N=275	5.0 mg N=296	10.0 mg N=268	Placebo N=520
Edema	1.8	3.0	10.8	0.6
Dizziness	1.1	3.4	3.4	1.5
Flushing	0.7	1.4	2.6	0.0
Palpitation	0.7	1.4	4.5	0.6

Other adverse experiences which were not clearly dose related but which were reported with an incidence greater than 1.0% in placebo-controlled clinical trials include the following:

Placebo-Controlled Studies

	NORVASC (%) (N=1730)	PLACEBO (%) (N=1250)
Headache	7.3	7.8
Fatigue	4.5	2.8
Nausea	2.9	1.9
Abdominal Pain	1.6	0.3
Somnolence	1.4	0.6

For several adverse experiences that appear to be drug and dose related, there was a greater incidence in women than men associated with amlodipine treatment as shown in the following table:

Adverse	NORVASC		PLACEBO	
Event	Male=% (N=1218)	Female=% (N=512)	Male=% (N=914)	Female=% (N=336)
Edema	5.6	14.6	1.4	5.1
Flushing	1.5	4.5	0.3	0.9
Palpitations	1.4	3.3	0.9	0.9
Somnolence	1.3	1.6	0.8	0.3

The following events occurred in <1% but >0.1% of patients in controlled clinical trials or under conditions of open trials or marketing experience where a causal relationship is uncertain; they are listed to alert the physician to a possible relationship:

Cardiovascular: arrhythmia (including ventricular tachycardia and atrial fibrillation), bradycardia, chest pain, hypotension, peripheral ischemia, syncope, tachycardia, postural dizziness, postural hypotension, vasculitis.

Central and Peripheral Nervous System: hypoesthesia, neuropathy peripheral, paresthesia, tremor, vertigo.

Gastrointestinal: anorexia, constipation, dyspepsia,** dysphagia, diarrhea, flatulence, pancreatitis, vomiting, gingival hyperplasia.

General: allergic reaction, asthenia,** back pain, hot flushes, malaise, pain, rigors, weight gain, weight decrease.

Musculoskeletal System: arthralgia, arthrosis, muscle cramps,** myalgia.

Psychiatric: sexual dysfunction (male** and female), insomnia, nervousness, depression, abnormal dreams, anxiety, depersonalization.

Respiratory System: dyspnea,** epistaxis.

Skin and Appendages: angioedema, erythema multiforme, pruritus,** rash,** rash erythematous, rash maculopapular.

**These events occurred in less than 1% in placebo-controlled trials, but the incidence of these side effects was between 1% and 2% in all multiple dose studies.

Special Senses: abnormal vision, conjunctivitis, diplopia, eye pain, tinnitus.

Urinary System: micturition frequency, micturition disorder, nocturia.

Autonomic Nervous System: dry mouth, sweating increased.

Metabolic and Nutritional: hyperglycemia, thirst.

Hemopoietic: leukopenia, purpura, thrombocytopenia.

The following events occurred in <0.1% of patients: cardiac failure, pulse irregularity, extrasystoles, skin discoloration, urticaria, skin dryness, alopecia, dermatitis, muscle weakness, twitching, ataxia, hypertonia, migraine, cold and clammy skin, apathy, agitation, amnesia, gastritis, increased appetite, loose stools, coughing, rhinitis, dysuria, polyuria, parosmia, taste perversion, abnormal visual accommodation, and xerophthalmia.

Other reactions occurred sporadically and cannot be distinguished from medications or concurrent disease states such as myocardial infarction and angina.

NORVASC therapy has not been associated with clinically significant changes in routine laboratory tests. No clinically relevant changes were noted in serum potassium, serum glucose, total triglycerides, total cholesterol, HDL cholesterol, uric acid, blood urea nitrogen, or creatinine.

The following postmarketing event has been reported infrequently where a causal relationship is uncertain: gynecomastia. In postmarketing experience, jaundice and hepatic enzyme elevations (mostly consistent with cholestasis or hepatitis) in some cases severe enough to require hospitalization have been reported in association with use of amlodipine.

NORVASC has been used safely in patients with chronic obstructive pulmonary disease, well-compensated congestive heart failure, peripheral vascular disease, diabetes mellitus, and abnormal lipid profiles.

OVERDOSAGE

Single oral doses of amlodipine equivalent to 40 mg amlodipine/kg and 100 mg amlodipine/kg in mice and rats, respectively, caused deaths. Single oral amlodipine maleate doses equivalent to 4 or more mg amlodipine/kg or higher in dogs (11 or more time times the maximum recommended human dose on a mg/m^2 basis) caused a marked peripheral vasodilation and hypotension.

Overdosage might be expected to cause excessive peripheral vasodilation with marked hypotension and possibly a reflex tachycardia. In humans, experience with intentional overdosage of NORVASC is limited. Reports of intentional overdosage include a patient who ingested 250 mg and was asymptomatic and was not hospitalized; another (120 mg) was hospitalized, underwent gastric lavage and remained normotensive; the third (105 mg) was hospitalized and had hypotension (90/50 mmHg) which normalized following plasma expansion. A case of accidental drug overdose has been documented in a 19-month-old male who ingested 30 mg amlodipine (about 2 mg/kg). During the emergency room presentation, vital signs were stable with no evidence of hypotension, but a heart rate of 180 bpm. Ipecac was administered 3.5 hours after ingestion and on subsequent observation (overnight) no sequelae were noted.

If massive overdose should occur, active cardiac and respiratory monitoring should be instituted. Frequent blood pressure measurements are essential. Should hypotension occur, cardiovascular support including elevation of the extremities and the judicious administration of fluids should be initiated. If hypotension remains unresponsive to these conservative measures, administration of vasopressors (such as phenylephrine) should be considered with attention to circulating volume and urine output. Intravenous calcium gluconate may help to reverse the effects of calcium entry blockade. As NORVASC is highly protein bound, hemodialysis is not likely to be of benefit.

DOSAGE AND ADMINISTRATION

Adults: The usual initial antihypertensive oral dose of NORVASC is 5 mg once daily with a maximum dose of 10 mg once daily. Small, fragile, or elderly individuals, or patients with hepatic insufficiency may be started on 2.5 mg once daily and this dose may be used when adding NORVASC to other antihypertensive therapy.

Dosage should be adjusted according to each patient's need. In general, titration should proceed over 7 to 14 days so that the physician can fully assess the patient's response to each dose level. Titration may proceed more rapidly, however, if clinically warranted, provided the patient is assessed frequently.

The recommended dose for chronic stable or vasospastic angina is 5-10 mg, with the lower dose suggested in the elderly and in patients with hepatic insufficiency. Most patients will require 10 mg for adequate effect. See ADVERSE REACTIONS section for information related to dosage and side effects.

Children: The effective antihypertensive oral dose in pediatric patients ages 6-17 years is 2.5 mg to 5 mg once daily. Doses in excess of 5 mg daily have not been studied in pediatric patients. See **CLINICAL PHARMACOLOGY**.

Co-administration with Other Antihypertensive and/or Antianginal Drugs: NORVASC has been safely administered with thiazides, ACE inhibitors, beta-blockers, long-acting nitrates, and/or sublingual nitroglycerin.

HOW SUPPLIED

NORVASC® –2.5 mg Tablets (amlodipine besylate equivalent to 2.5 mg of amlodipine per tablet) are supplied as white, diamond, flat-faced, beveled edged engraved with "NORVASC" on one side and "2.5" on the other side and supplied as follows:

NDC 0069-1520-68	Bottle of 90

NORVASC® –5 mg Tablets (amlodipine besylate equivalent to 5 mg of amlodipine per tablet) are white, elongated octagon, flat-faced, beveled edged engraved with both "NORVASC" and "5" on one side and plain on the other side and supplied as follows:

NDC 0069-1530-68	Bottle of 90
NDC 0069-1530-41	Unit Dose package of 100
NDC 0069-1530-72	Bottle of 300

NORVASC® –10 mg Tablets (amlodipine besylate equivalent to 10 mg of amlodipine per tablet) are white, round, flat-faced, beveled edged engraved with both "NORVASC" and "10" on one side and plain on the other side and supplied as follows:

NDC 0069-1540-68	Bottle of 90
NDC 0069-1540-41	Unit Dose package of 100

Store bottles at controlled room temperature, 59° to 86°F (15° to 30°C) and dispense in tight, light-resistant containers (USP).

Rx only

Pfizer Labs

Division of Pfizer Inc, NY, NY 10017

LAB-0014-4 Revised January 2005

RELPAX®

℞

[rĕl-păks]

(eletriptan hydrobromide)

Tablets

Prescribing information for this product, which appears on pages 2625–2629 of the 2005 PDR, has been completely revised as follows. Please write "See Supplement A" next to the product heading.

DESCRIPTION

RELPAX® (eletriptan) Tablets contain eletriptan hydrobromide, which is a selective 5-hydroxytryptamine 1B/1D (5-HT1B/1D) receptor agonist. Eletriptan is chemically designated as (R)-3-[(1-Methyl-2-pyrrolidinyl)methyl]-5-[2-(phenylsulfonyl)ethyl]-1H-indole, monohydrobromide, and it has the following chemical structure:

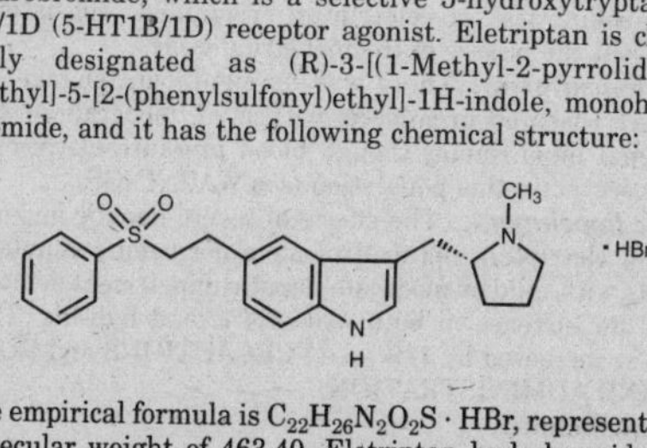

The empirical formula is $C_{22}H_{26}N_2O_2S \cdot HBr$, representing a molecular weight of 463.40. Eletriptan hydrobromide is a white to light pale colored powder that is readily soluble in water.

Continued on next page

Relpax—Cont.

Each RELPAX Tablet for oral administration contains 24.2 or 48.5 mg of eletriptan hydrobromide equivalent to 20 mg or 40 mg of eletriptan, respectively. Each tablet also contains the inactive ingredients microcrystalline cellulose NF, lactose NF, croscarmellose sodium NF, magnesium stearate NF, titanium dioxide USP, hypromellose, triacetin USP and FD&C Yellow No. 6 aluminum lake.

CLINICAL PHARMACOLOGY

Mechanism of Action: Eletriptan binds with high affinity to 5-HT_{1B}, 5-HT_{1D} and 5-HT_{1F} receptors, has modest affinity for 5-HT_{1A}, 5-HT_{1E}, 5-HT_{2B} and 5-HT_7 receptors, and little or no affinity for 5-HT_{2A}, 5-HT_{2C}, 5-HT_3, 5-HT_4, 5-HT_{5A} and 5-HT_6 receptors. Eletriptan has no significant affinity or pharmacological activity at adrenergic $alpha_1$, $alpha_2$, or beta; dopaminergic D_1 or D_2; muscarinic; or opioid receptors.

Two theories have been proposed to explain the efficacy of 5-HT receptor agonists in migraine. One theory suggests that activation of 5-HT_1 receptors located on intracranial blood vessels, including those on the arteriovenous anastomoses, leads to vasoconstriction, which is correlated with the relief of migraine headache. The other hypothesis suggests that activation of 5-HT_1 receptors on sensory nerve endings in the trigeminal system results in the inhibition of pro-inflammatory neuropeptide release.

In the anesthetized dog, eletriptan has been shown to reduce carotid arterial blood flow, with only a small increase in arterial blood pressure at high doses. While the effect on blood flow was selective for the carotid arterial bed, decreases in coronary artery diameter were observed. Eletriptan has also been shown to inhibit trigeminal nerve activity in the rat.

Pharmacokinetics:

Absorption: Eletriptan is well absorbed after oral administration with peak plasma levels occurring approximately 1.5 hours after dosing to healthy subjects. In patients with moderate to severe migraine the median T_{max} is 2.0 hours. The mean absolute bioavailability of eletriptan is approximately 50%. The oral pharmacokinetics are slightly more than dose proportional over the clinical dose range. The AUC and C_{max} of eletriptan are increased by approximately 20 to 30% following oral administration with a high fat meal.

Distribution: The volume of distribution of eletriptan following IV administration is 138L. Plasma protein binding is moderate and approximately 85%.

Metabolism: The N-demethylated metabolite of eletriptan is the only known active metabolite. This metabolite causes vasoconstriction similar to eletriptan in animal models. Though the half-life of the metabolite is estimated to be about 13 hours, the plasma concentration of the N-demethylated metabolite is 10-20% of parent drug and is unlikely to contribute significantly to the overall effect of the parent compound.

In vitro studies indicate that eletriptan is primarily metabolized by cytochrome P-450 enzyme CYP3A4 (see WARNINGS, DOSAGE AND ADMINISTRATION and CLINICAL PHARMACOLOGY: Drug Interactions).

Elimination: The terminal elimination half-life of eletriptan is approximately 4 hours. Mean renal clearance (CL_R) following oral administration is approximately 3.9 L/h. Non-renal clearance accounts for about 90% of the total clearance.

Special Populations:

Age: The pharmacokinetics of eletriptan are generally unaffected by age.

Eletriptan has been given to only 50 patients over the age of 65. Blood pressure was increased to a greater extent in elderly subjects than in young subjects. The pharmacokinetic disposition of eletriptan in the elderly is similar to that seen in younger adults (see PRECAUTIONS).

There is a statistically significant increased half-life (from about 4.4 hours to 5.7 hours) between elderly (65 to 93 years of age) and younger adult subjects (18 to 45 years of age) (see PRECAUTIONS).

Gender: The pharmacokinetics of eletriptan are unaffected by gender.

Race: A comparison of pharmacokinetic studies run in western countries with those run in Japan have indicated an approximate 35% reduction in the exposure of eletriptan in Japanese male volunteers compared to western males. Population pharmacokinetic analysis of two clinical studies indicates no evidence of pharmacokinetic differences between Caucasians and non Caucasian patients.

Menstrual Cycle: In a study of 16 healthy females, the pharmacokinetics of eletriptan remained consistent throughout the phases of the menstrual cycle.

Renal Impairment: There was no significant change in clearance observed in subjects with mild, moderate or severe renal impairment, though blood pressure elevations were observed in this population (see WARNINGS).

Hepatic Impairment: The effects of severe hepatic impairment on eletriptan metabolism have not been evaluated. Subjects with mild or moderate hepatic impairment demonstrated an increase in both AUC (34%) and half-life. The C_{max} was increased by 18% (see PRECAUTIONS and DOSAGE AND ADMINISTRATION).

Drug Interactions:

CYP3A4 inhibitors: *In vitro* studies have shown that eletriptan is metabolized by the CYP3A4 enzyme. A clinical study demonstrated about a 3-fold increase in C_{max} and about a 6-fold increase in the AUC of eletriptan when combined with ketoconazole. The half-life increased from 5 hours to 8 hours and the T_{max} increased from 2.8 hours to 5.4 hours. Another clinical study demonstrated about a 2-fold increase in C_{max} and about a 4-fold increase in AUC when erythromycin was co-administered with eletriptan. It has also been shown that co-administration of verapamil and eletriptan yields about a 2-fold increase in C_{max} and about a 3-fold increase in AUC of eletriptan, and that co-administration of fluconazole and eletriptan yields about a 1.4-fold increase in C_{max} and about a 2-fold increase in AUC of eletriptan.

Eletriptan should not be used within at least 72 hours of treatment with the following potent CYP3A4 inhibitors: ketoconazole, itraconazole, nefazodone, troleandomycin, clarithromycin, ritonavir and nelfinavir. Eletriptan should not be used within 72 hours with drugs that have demonstrated potent CYP3A4 inhibition and have this potent effect described in the CONTRAINDICATIONS, WARNINGS or PRECAUTIONS sections of their labeling (see WARNINGS and DOSAGE AND ADMINISTRATION).

Propranolol: The C_{max} and AUC of eletriptan were increased by 10 and 33% respectively in the presence of propranolol. No interactive increases in blood pressure were observed. No dosage adjustment appears to be needed for patients taking propranolol (see PRECAUTIONS).

The effect of eletriptan on other drugs: The effect of eletriptan on enzymes other than cytochrome P-450 has not been investigated. *In vitro* human liver microsome studies suggest that eletriptan has little potential to inhibit CYP1A2, 2C9, 2E1 and 3A4 at concentrations up to 100μM. While eletriptan has an effect on CYP2D6 at high concentration, this effect should not interfere with metabolism of other drugs wnen eletriptan is used at recommended doses. There is no *in vitro* or *in vivo* evidence that clinical doses of eletriptan will induce drug metabolizing enzymes. Therefore, eletriptan is unlikely to cause clinically important drug interactions mediated by these enzymes.

CLINICAL STUDIES

The efficacy of RELPAX in the acute treatment of migraines was evaluated in eight randomized, double-blind placebo-controlled studies. All eight studies used 40 mg. Seven studies evaluated an 80 mg dose and two studies included a 20 mg dose.

In all eight studies, randomized patients treated their headaches as outpatients. Seven studies enrolled adults and one study enrolled adolescents (age 11 to 17). Patients treated in the seven adult studies were predominantly female (85%) and Caucasian (94%) with a mean age of 40 years (range 18 to 78). In all studies, patients were instructed to treat a moderate to severe headache. Headache response, defined as a reduction in headache severity from moderate or severe pain to mild or no pain, was assessed up to 2 hours after dosing. Associated symptoms such as nausea, vomiting, photophobia and phonophobia were also assessed.

Maintenance of response was assessed for up to 24 hours post dose. In the adult studies, a second dose of RELPAX Tablets or other medication was allowed 2 to 24 hours after the initial treatment for both persistent and recurrent headaches. The incidence and time to use of these additional treatments were also recorded.

In the seven adult studies, the percentage of patients achieving headache response 2 hours after treatment was significantly greater among patients receiving RELPAX Tablets at all doses compared to those who received placebo. The two hour response rates from these controlled clinical studies are summarized in Table 1.

Table 1: Percentage of Patients with Headache Response (Mild or No Headache) 2 Hours Following Treatment

	Placebo	RELPAX 20 mg	RELPAX 40 mg	RELPAX 80 mg
Study 1	23.8% (n=126)	54.3%* (n=129)	65.0%* (n=117)	77.1%* (n=118)
Study 2	19.0% (n=232)	NA	61.6%* (n=430)	64.6%* (n=446)
Study 3	21.7% (n=276)	47.3%* (n=273)	61.9%* (n=281)	58.6%* (n=290)
Study 4	39.5% (n=86)	NA	62.3%* (n=175)	70.0%* (n=170)
Study 5	20.6% (n=102)	NA	53.9%* (n=206)	67.9%* (n=209)
Study 6	31.3% (n=80)	NA	63.9%* (n=169)	66.9%* (n=160)
Study 7	29.5% (n=122)	NA	57.5%* (n=492)	NA

* p value < 0.05 vs placebo
NA - Not Applicable

Comparisons of the performance of different drugs based upon results obtained in different clinical trials are never reliable. Because studies are generally conducted at different times, with different samples of patients, by different investigators, employing different criteria and/or different interpretations of the same criteria, under different conditions (dose, dosing regimen, etc.), quantitative estimates of treatment response and the timing of response may be expected to vary considerably from study to study.

The estimated probability of achieving an initial headache response within 2 hours following treatment is depicted in Figure 1.

Figure 1: Estimated Probability of Initial Headache Response Within 2 Hours*

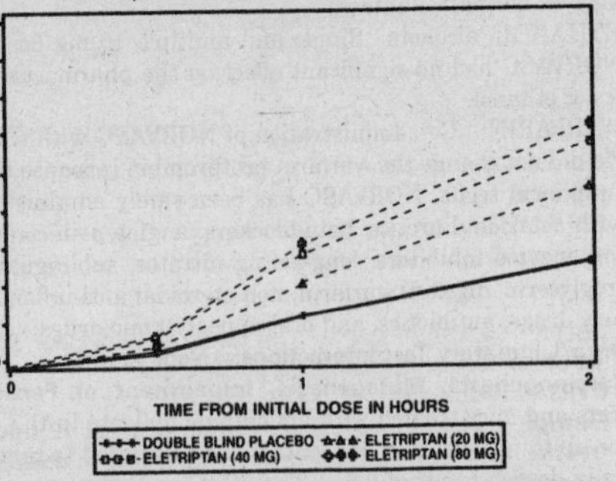

*Figure 1 shows the Kaplan-Meier plot of probability over time of obtaining headache response (no or mild pain) following treatment with eletriptan. The plot is based on 7 placebo-controlled, outpatient trials in adults providing evidence of efficacy (Studies 1 through 7). Patients not achieving headache response or taking additional treatment prior to 2 hours were censored at 2 hours.

For patients with migraine-associated photophobia, phonophobia, and nausea at baseline, there was a decreased incidence of these symptoms following administration of RELPAX as compared to placebo.

Two to 24 hours following the initial dose of study treatment, patients were allowed to use additional treatment for pain relief in the form of a second dose of study treatment or other medication. The estimated probability of taking a second dose or other medications for migraine over the 24 hours following the initial dose of study treatment is summarized in Figure 2.

Figure 2: Estimated Probability of Taking a Second Dose/ Other Medication Over the 24 Hours Following the First Dose*

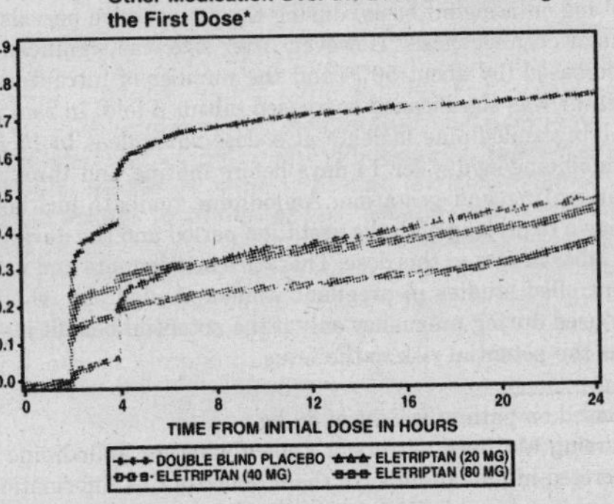

*This Kaplan-Meier plot is based on data obtained in 7 placebo-controlled trials in adults (Studies 1 through 7). Patients were instructed to take a second dose of study medication as follows: a) in the event of no response at 2 hours (studies 2 and 4-7) or at 4 hours (study 3); b) in the event of headache recurrence within 24 hours (studies 2-7). Patients not using additional treatments were censored at 24 hours. The plot includes both patients who had headache response at 2 hours and those who had no response to the initial dose. It should be noted that the protocols did not allow remedication within 2 hours post dose.

The efficacy of RELPAX was unaffected by the duration of attack; gender or age of the patient; relationship to menses; or concomitant use of estrogen replacement therapy/oral contraceptives or frequently used migraine prophylactic drugs.

In a single study in adolescents (n=274), there were no statistically significant differences between treatment groups. The headache response rate at 2 hours was 57% for both RELPAX 40 mg Tablets and placebo.

INDICATIONS AND USAGE

RELPAX is indicated for the acute treatment of migraine with or without aura in adults.

RELPAX is not intended for the prophylactic therapy of migraine or for use in the management of hemiplegic or basilar migraine (see CONTRAINDICATIONS). Safety and effectiveness of RELPAX Tablets have not been established for cluster headache, which is present in an older, predominantly male population.

CONTRAINDICATIONS

RELPAX Tablets should not be given to patients with ischemic heart disease (e.g., angina pectoris, history of myocardial infarction, or documented silent ischemia) or to patients who have symptoms, or findings consistent with ischemic heart disease, coronary artery vasospasm, including Prinzmetal's variant angina, or other significant underlying cardiovascular disease (see WARNINGS).

RELPAX Tablets should not be given to patients with cerebrovascular syndromes including (but not limited to) strokes of any type as well as transient ischemic attacks (see WARNINGS).

RELPAX Tablets should not be given to patients with peripheral vascular disease including (but not limited to) ischemic bowel disease (see WARNINGS).

Because RELPAX Tablets may increase blood pressure, it should not be given to patients with uncontrolled hypertension (see WARNINGS).

RELPAX Tablets should not be administered to patients with hemiplegic or basilar migraine.

RELPAX Tablets should not be used within 24 hours of treatment with another 5-HT₁ agonist, an ergotamine-containing or ergot-type medication such as dihydroergotamine (DHE) or methysergide.

RELPAX Tablets should not be used in patients with known hypersensitivity to eletriptan or any of its inactive ingredients.

RELPAX Tablets should not be given to patients with severe hepatic impairment.

WARNINGS

RELPAX Tablets should only be used where a clear diagnosis of migraine has been established.

CYP3A4 Inhibitors:

Eletriptan should not be used within at least 72 hours of treatment with the following potent CYP3A4 inhibitors: ketoconazole, itraconazole, nefazodone, troleandomycin, clarithromycin, ritonavir, and nelfinavir. Eletriptan should not be used within 72 hours with drugs that have demonstrated potent CYP3A4 inhibition and have this potent effect described in the CONTRAINDICATIONS, WARNINGS or PRECAUTIONS sections of their labeling (see CLINICAL PHARMACOLOGY: Drug Interactions and DOSAGE AND ADMINISTRATION).

In a coronary angiographic study of rapidly infused intravenous eletriptan to concentrations exceeding those achieved with 80 mg oral eletriptan in the presence of potent CYP3A4 inhibitors, a small dose-related decrease in coronary artery diameter similar to that seen with a 6 mg subcutaneous dose of sumatriptan was observed.

Risk of Myocardial Ischemia and/or Infarction and Other Cardiac Events: Because of the potential of 5-HT₁ agonists to cause coronary vasospasm, eletriptan should not be given to patients with documented ischemic or vasospastic coronary artery disease (CAD) (see CONTRAINDICATIONS). It is strongly recommended that eletriptan not be given to patients in whom unrecognized CAD is predicted by the presence of risk factors (e.g., hypertension, hypercholesterolemia, smoker, obesity, diabetes, strong family history of CAD, female with surgical or physiological menopause, or male over 40 years of age) unless a cardiovascular evaluation provides satisfactory clinical evidence that the patient is reasonably free of coronary artery and ischemic myocardial disease or other significant underlying cardiovascular disease. The sensitivity of cardiac diagnostic procedures to detect cardiovascular disease or predisposition to coronary artery vasospasm is modest, at best. If, during the cardiovascular evaluation, the patient's medical history, electrocardiographic, or other investigations reveal findings indicative of, or consistent with coronary artery vasospasm or myocardial ischemia, eletriptan should not be administered (see CONTRAINDICATIONS).

For patients with risk factors predictive of CAD, who are determined to have a satisfactory cardiovascular evaluation, it is strongly recommended that administration of the first dose of eletriptan take place in the setting of a physician's office or similar medically staffed and equipped facility unless the patient has previously received eletriptan. Because cardiac ischemia can occur in the absence of clinical symptoms, consideration should be given to obtaining on the first occasion of use an electrocardiogram (ECG) during the interval immediately following administration of RELPAX Tablets, in these patients with risk factors.

It is recommended that patients who are intermittent long-term users of 5-HT₁ agonists including RELPAX Tablets, and who have or acquire risk factors predictive of CAD, as described above, undergo periodic cardiovascular evaluation as they continue to use RELPAX Tablets.

The systematic approach described above is intended to reduce the likelihood that patients with unrecognized cardiovascular disease will be inadvertently exposed to eletriptan.

Cardiac Events and Fatalities Associated With 5-HT₁ Agonists: Serious adverse cardiac events, including acute myocardial infarction, life-threatening disturbances of cardiac rhythm, and death have been reported within a few hours following the administration of other 5-HT₁ agonists. Considering the extent of use of 5-HT₁ agonists in patients with migraine, the incidence of these events is extremely low.

Premarketing experience with eletriptan among the 7,143 unique individuals who received eletriptan during premarketing clinical trials: In a clinical pharmacology study, in subjects undergoing diagnostic coronary angiography, a subject with a history of angina, hypertension and hypercholesterolemia, receiving intravenous eletriptan (Cmax of 127 ng/mL equivalent to 60 mg oral eletriptan), reported chest tightness and experienced angiographically documented coronary vasospasm with no ECG changes of ischemia. There was also one report of atrial fibrillation in a patient with a past history of atrial fibrillation.

Postmarketing experience with eletriptan: There was one report of myocardial infarction and death in a patient with cardiovascular risk factors (hypertension, hyperlipidemia, strong family history of CAD) in association with inappropriate concomitant use of eletriptan and sumatriptan. The uncontrolled nature of postmarketing surveillance, however, makes it impossible to determine definitively if the case was actually caused by eletriptan or to reliably assess causation in individual cases.

Cerebrovascular Events and Fatalities Associated With 5-HT₁ Agonists: Cerebral hemorrhage, subarachnoid hemorrhage, stroke, and other cerebrovascular events have been reported in patients treated with 5-HT₁ agonists, and some have resulted in fatalities. In a number of cases, it appears possible that the cerebrovascular events were primary, the agonist having been administered in the incorrect belief that the symptoms experienced were a consequence of migraine, when they were not. It should be noted that patients with migraine may be at increased risk of certain cerebrovascular events (e.g., stroke, hemorrhage, and transient ischemic attack).

Other Vasospasm-Related Events: 5-HT₁ agonists may cause vasospastic reactions other than coronary artery vasospasm. Both peripheral vascular ischemia and colonic ischemia with abdominal pain and bloody diarrhea have been reported with 5-HT₁ agonists.

Increase in Blood Pressure: Significant elevation in blood pressure, including hypertensive crisis, has been reported on rare occasion in patients receiving 5-HT₁ agonists with and without a history of hypertension. In clinical pharmacology studies, oral eletriptan (at doses of 60 mg or more) was shown to cause small, transient dose-related increases in blood pressure, predominantly diastolic, consistent with its mechanism of action and with other 5-HT₁B/1D agonists. The effect was more pronounced in renally impaired and elderly subjects. A single patient with hepatic cirrhosis received eletriptan 80 mg and experienced a blood pressure of 220/96 mm Hg five hours after dosing. The treatment related event persisted for seven hours.

Eletriptan is contraindicated in patients with uncontrolled hypertension (see CONTRAINDICATIONS).

An 18% increase in mean pulmonary artery pressure was seen following dosing with another 5-HT₁ agonist in a study evaluating subjects undergoing cardiac catheterization.

PRECAUTIONS

General: As with other 5-HT₁ agonists, sensations of tightness, pain, pressure and heaviness have been reported after treatment with eletriptan in the precordium, throat, and jaw. Events that are localized to the chest, throat, neck and jaw have not been associated with arrhythmias or ischemic ECG changes in clinical trials; in a clinical pharmacology study of subjects undergoing diagnostic coronary angiography, one subject with a history of angina, hypertension and hypercholesterolemia, receiving intravenous eletriptan, reported chest tightness and experienced angiographically documented coronary vasospasm with no ECG changes of ischemia. Because 5-HT₁ agonists may cause coronary artery vasospasm, patients who experience signs or symptoms suggestive of angina following dosing should be evaluated for the presence of CAD or a predisposition to Prinzmetal's variant angina before receiving additional doses of medication, and should be monitored electrocardiographically if dosing is resumed and similar symptoms recur. Similarly, patients who experience other symptoms or signs suggestive of decreased arterial flow, such as ischemic bowel syndrome or Raynaud's syndrome following the use of any 5-HT₁ agonist are candidates for further evaluation (see CONTRAINDICATIONS and WARNINGS).

Hepatically Impaired Patients: The effects of severe hepatic impairment on eletriptan metabolism was not evaluated. Subjects with mild or moderate hepatic impairment demonstrated an increase in both AUC (34%) and half-life. The Cmax was increased by 18%. Eletriptan should not be used in patients with severe hepatic impairment. No dose adjustment is necessary in mild to moderate impairment (see DOSAGE AND ADMINISTRATION).

Binding to Melanin-Containing Tissues: In rats treated with a single intravenous (3 mg/kg) dose of radiolabeled eletriptan, elimination of radioactivity from the retina was prolonged, suggesting that eletriptan and/or its metabolites may bind to the melanin of the eye. Because there could be accumulation in melanin-rich tissues over time, this raises the possibility that eletriptan could cause toxicity in these tissues after extended use. Although no systematic monitoring of ophthalmologic function was undertaken in clinical trials, and no specific recommendations for ophthalmologic monitoring are offered, prescribers should be aware of the possibility of long-term ophthalmologic effects.

Corneal Opacities: Transient corneal opacities were seen in dogs receiving oral eletriptan at 5 mg/kg and above. They were observed during the first week of treatment, but were not present thereafter despite continued treatment. Exposure at the no-effect dose level of 2.5 mg/kg was approximately equal to that achieved in humans at the maximum recommended daily dose.

Information for Patients: See PATIENT INFORMATION at the end of this labeling for the text of the separate leaflet provided for patients.

Laboratory Tests: No specific laboratory tests are recommended.

Drug Interactions:

Ergot-containing drugs: Ergot-containing drugs have been reported to cause prolonged vasospastic reactions. Because these effects may be additive, use of ergotamine-containing or ergot-type medications (like dihydroergotamine [DHE] or methysergide) and eletriptan within 24 hours of each other is not recommended (see CONTRAINDICATIONS).

CYP3A4 Inhibitors: Eletriptan is metabolized primarily by CYP3A4 (see WARNINGS regarding use with potent CYP3A4 inhibitors).

Monoamine Oxidase Inhibitors: Eletriptan is not a substrate for monoamine oxidase (MAO) enzymes, therefore there is no expectation of an interaction between eletriptan and MAO inhibitors.

Propranolol: The Cmax and AUC of eletriptan were increased by 10 and 33% respectively in the presence of propranolol. No interactive increases in blood pressure were observed. No dosage adjustment appears to be needed for patients taking propranolol (see CLINICAL PHARMACOLOGY).

Selective serotonin reuptake inhibitors (SSRIs): SSRIs (e.g., fluoxetine, fluvoxamine, paroxetine, sertraline) have been reported, rarely, to cause weakness, hyperreflexia, and incoordination when coadministered with 5-HT₁ agonists. If concomitant treatment with eletriptan and an SSRI is clinically warranted, appropriate observation of the patient is advised.

Other 5-HT₁ agonists: Concomitant use of other 5-HT₁ agonists within 24 hours of RELPAX treatment is not recommended (see CONTRAINDICATIONS).

Drug/Laboratory Test Interactions: RELPAX Tablets are not known to interfere with commonly employed clinical laboratory tests.

Carcinogenesis: Lifetime carcinogenicity studies, 104 weeks in duration, were carried out in mice and rats by administering eletriptan in the diet. In rats, the incidence of testicular interstitial cell adenomas was increased at the high dose of 75 mg/kg/day. The estimated exposure (AUC) to parent drug at that dose was approximately 6 times that achieved in humans receiving the maximum recommended daily dose (MRDD) of 80 mg, and at the no-effect dose of 15 mg/kg/day it was approximately 2 times the human exposure at the MRDD. In mice, the incidence of hepatocellular adenomas was increased at the high dose of 400 mg/kg/day. The exposure to parent drug (AUC) at that dose was approximately 18 times that achieved in humans receiving the MRDD, and the AUC at the no-effect dose of 90 mg/kg/day was approximately 7 times the human exposure at the MRDD.

Mutagenesis: Eletriptan was not mutagenic in bacterial or mammalian cell assays *in vitro*, testing negative in the Ames reverse mutation test and the hypoxanthine-guanine phosphoribosyl transferase (HGPRT) mutation test in Chinese hamster ovary cells. It was not clastogenic in two *in vivo* mouse micronucleus assays. Results were equivocal in *in vitro* human lymphocyte clastogenicity tests, in which the incidence of polyploidy was increased in the absence of metabolic activation (-S9 conditions), but not in the presence of metabolic activation.

Impairment of Fertility: In a rat fertility and early embryonic development study, doses tested were 50, 100 and 200 mg/kg/day, resulting in systemic exposures to parent drug in rats, based on AUC, that were 4, 8 and 16 times MRDD, respectively, in males and 7, 14 and 28 times MRDD, respectively, in females. There was a prolongation of the estrous cycle at the 200 mg/kg/day dose due to an increase in duration of estrus, based on vaginal smears. There were also dose-related, statistically significant decreases in mean numbers of corpora lutea per dam at all 3 doses, resulting in decreases in mean numbers of implants and viable fetuses per dam. This suggests a partial inhibition of ovulation by eletriptan. There was no effect on fertility of males and no other effect on fertility of females.

Pregnancy: *Pregnancy Category C:* In reproductive toxicity studies in rats and rabbits, oral administration of eletriptan was associated with developmental toxicity (decreased fetal and pup weights and an increased incidence of fetal structural abnormalities). Effects on fetal and pup weights were observed at doses that were, on a mg/m² basis, 6 to 12 times greater than the clinical maximum recommended daily dose (MRDD) of 80 mg. The increase in structural alterations occurred in the rat and rabbit at doses that, on a mg/m² basis, were 12 times greater than (rat) and approximately equal to (rabbit) the MRDD.

When pregnant rats were administered eletriptan during the period of organogenesis at doses of 10, 30 or 100 mg/kg/day, fetal weights were decreased and the incidences of vertebral and sternebral variations were increased at 100 mg/kg/day (approximately 12 times the MRDD on a mg/m² basis). The 100 mg/kg dose was also maternally toxic, as evidenced by decreased maternal body weight gain during gestation. The no-effect dose for developmental toxicity in rats exposed during organogenesis was 30 mg/kg, which is approximately 4 times the MRDD on a mg/m² basis.

When doses of 5, 10 or 50 mg/kg/day were given to New Zealand White rabbits throughout organogenesis, fetal weights were decreased at 50 mg/kg, which is approximately 12 times the MRDD on a mg/m² basis. The incidences of fused sternebrae and vena cava deviations were increased in all treated groups. Maternal toxicity was not produced at any dose. A no-effect dose for developmental toxicity in rabbits exposed during organogenesis was not established, and the 5 mg/kg dose is approximately equal to the MRDD on a mg/m² basis.

There are no adequate and well-controlled studies in pregnant women; therefore, eletriptan should be used during pregnancy only if the potential benefit justifies the potential risk to the fetus.

Nursing Mothers: Eletriptan is excreted in human breast milk. In one study of 8 women given a single dose of 80 mg, the mean total amount of eletriptan in breast milk over 24 hours in this group was approximately 0.02% of the admin-

Continued on next page

Relpax—Cont.

istered dose. The ratio of eletriptan mean concentration in breast milk to plasma was 1:4, but there was great variability. The resulting eletriptan concentration-time profile was similar to that seen in the plasma over 24 hours, with very low concentrations of drug (mean 1.7 ng/mL) still present in the milk 18-24 hours post dose. The N-desmethyl active metabolite was not measured in the breast milk. Caution should be exercised when RELPAX is administered to nursing women.

Pediatric Use: Safety and effectiveness of RELPAX Tablets in pediatric patients have not been established; therefore, RELPAX is not recommended for use in patients under 18 years of age.

The efficacy of RELPAX Tablets (40 mg) in patients 11-17 was not established in a randomized, placebo-controlled trial of 274 adolescent migraineurs (see CLINICAL STUDIES). Adverse events observed were similar in nature to those reported in clinical trials in adults. Postmarketing experience with other triptans includes a limited number of reports that describe pediatric patients who have experienced clinically serious adverse events that are similar in nature to those reported rarely in adults. Long-term safety of eletriptan was studied in 76 adolescent patients who received treatment for up to one year. A similar profile of adverse events to that of adults was observed. The long-term safety of eletriptan in pediatric patients has not been established.

Geriatric Use: Eletriptan has been given to only 50 patients over the age of 65. Blood pressure was increased to a greater extent in elderly subjects than in young subjects. The pharmacokinetic disposition of eletriptan in the elderly is similar to that seen in younger adults (see CLINICAL PHARMACOLOGY). In clinical trials, there were no apparent differences in efficacy or the incidence of adverse events between patients under 65 years of age and those 65 and above (n=50).

There is a statistically significantly increased half-life (from about 4.4 hours to 5.7 hours) between elderly (65 to 93 years of age) and younger adult subjects (18 to 45 years of age) (see CLINICAL PHARMACOLOGY).

ADVERSE REACTIONS

Serious cardiac events, including some that have been fatal, have occurred following the use of 5-HT$_1$ agonists. These events are extremely rare and most have been reported in patients with risk factors predictive of CAD. Events reported have included coronary artery vasospasm, transient myocardial ischemia, myocardial infarction, ventricular tachycardia, and ventricular fibrillation (see CONTRAINDICATIONS, WARNINGS and PRECAUTIONS).

Incidence in Controlled Clinical Trials:

Among 4,597 patients who treated the first migraine headache with RELPAX in short-term placebo-controlled trials, the most common adverse events reported with treatment with RELPAX were asthenia, nausea, dizziness, and somnolence. These events appear to be dose related.

In long-term open-label studies where patients were allowed to treat multiple migraine attacks for up to 1 year, 128 (8.3%) out of 1,544 patients discontinued treatment due to adverse events.

Table 2 lists adverse events that occurred in the subset of 5,125 migraineurs who received eletriptan doses of 20 mg, 40 mg and 80 mg or placebo in worldwide placebo-controlled clinical trials. The events cited reflect experience gained under closely monitored conditions of clinical trials in a highly selected patient population. In actual clinical practice or in other clinical trials, those frequency estimates may not apply, as the conditions of use, reporting behavior, and the kinds of patients treated may differ.

Only adverse events that were more frequent in a RELPAX treatment group compared to the placebo group with an incidence greater than or equal to 2% are included in Table 2.

Table 2: Adverse Experience Incidence in Placebo-Controlled Migraine Clinical Trials: Events Reported by ≥ 2% Patients Treated with RELPAX and More Than Placebo

Adverse Event Type	Placebo (n=988)	RELPAX 20 mg (n=431)	RELPAX 40 mg (n=1774)	RELPAX 80 mg (n=1932)
ATYPICAL SENSATIONS				
Paresthesia	2%	3%	3%	4%
Flushing/feeling of warmth	2%	2%	2%	2%
PAIN AND PRESSURE SENSATIONS				
Chest – tightness/pain/pressure	1%	1%	2%	4%
Abdominal – pain/discomfort/stomach pain/cramps/pressure	1%	1%	2%	2%
DIGESTIVE				
Dry mouth	2%	2%	3%	4%
Dyspepsia	1%	1%	2%	2%
Dysphagia – throat tightness/difficulty swallowing	0.2%	1%	2%	2%
Nausea	5%	4%	5%	8%
NEUROLOGICAL				
Dizziness	3%	3%	6%	7%
Somnolence	4%	3%	6%	7%
Headache	3%	4%	3%	4%
OTHER				
Asthenia	3%	4%	5%	10%

RELPAX is generally well-tolerated. Across all doses, most adverse reactions were mild and transient. The frequency of adverse events in clinical trials did not increase when up to 2 doses of RELPAX were taken within 24 hours. The incidence of adverse events in controlled clinical trials was not affected by gender, age, or race of the patients. Adverse event frequencies were also unchanged by concomitant use of drugs commonly taken for migraine prophylaxis (e.g., SSRIs, beta blockers, calcium channel blockers, tricyclic antidepressants), estrogen replacement therapy and oral contraceptives.

Other Events Observed in Association With the Administration of RELPAX Tablets:

In the paragraphs that follow, the frequencies of less commonly reported adverse clinical events are presented. Because the reports include events observed in open studies, the role of RELPAX Tablets in their causation cannot be reliably determined. Furthermore, variability associated with adverse event reporting, the terminology used to describe adverse events, etc., limit the value of the quantitative frequency estimates provided. Event frequencies are calculated as the number of patients reporting an event divided by the total number of patients (N=4,719) exposed to RELPAX. All reported events are included except those already listed in Table 2, those too general to be informative, and those not reasonably associated with the use of the drug. Events are further classified within body system categories and enumerated in order of decreasing frequency using the following definitions: frequent adverse events are those occurring in at least 1/100 patients, infrequent adverse events are those occurring in 1/100 to 1/1000 patients and rare adverse events are those occurring in fewer than 1/1000 patients.

General: Frequent were back pain, chills and pain. Infrequent were face edema and malaise. Rare were abdomen enlarged, abscess, accidental injury, allergic reaction, fever, flu syndrome, halitosis, hernia, hypothermia, lab test abnormal, moniliasis, rheumatoid arthritis and shock.

Cardiovascular: Frequent was palpitation. Infrequent were hypertension, migraine, peripheral vascular disorder and tachycardia. Rare were angina pectoris, arrhythmia, atrial fibrillation, AV block, bradycardia, hypotension, syncope, thrombophlebitis, cerebrovascular disorder, vasospasm and ventricular arrhythmia.

Digestive: Infrequent were anorexia, constipation, diarrhea, eructation, esophagitis, flatulence, gastritis, gastrointestinal disorder, glossitis, increased salivation and liver function tests abnormal. Rare were gingivitis, hematemesis, increased appetite, rectal disorder, stomatitis, tongue disorder, tongue edema and tooth disorder.

Endocrine: Rare were goiter, thyroid adenoma and thyroiditis.

Hemic and Lymphatic: Rare were anemia, cyanosis, leukopenia, lymphadenopathy, monocytosis and purpura.

Metabolic: Infrequent were creatine phosphokinase increased, edema, peripheral edema and thirst. Rare were alkaline phosphatase increased, bilirubinemia, hyperglycemia, weight gain and weight loss.

Musculoskeletal: Infrequent were arthralgia, arthritis, arthrosis, bone pain, myalgia and myasthenia. Rare were bone neoplasm, joint disorder, myopathy and tenosynovitis.

Neurological: Frequent were hypertonia, hypesthesia and vertigo. Infrequent were abnormal dreams, agitation, anxiety, apathy, ataxia, confusion, depersonalization, depression, emotional lability, euphoria, hyperesthesia, hyperkinesia, incoordination, insomnia, nervousness, speech disorder, stupor, thinking abnormal and tremor. Rare were abnormal gait, amnesia, aphasia, catatonic reaction, dementia, diplopia, dystonia, hallucinations, hemiplegia, hyperalgesia, hypokinesia, hysteria, manic reaction, neuropathy, neurosis, oculogyric crisis, paralysis, psychotic depression, sleep disorder and twitching.

Respiratory: Frequent was pharyngitis. Infrequent were asthma, dyspnea, respiratory disorder, respiratory tract infection, rhinitis, voice alteration and yawn. Rare were bronchitis, choking sensation, cough increased, epistaxis, hiccup, hyperventilation, laryngitis, sinusitis and sputum increased.

Skin and Appendages: Frequent was sweating. Infrequent were pruritus, rash and skin disorder. Rare were alopecia, dry skin, eczema, exfoliative dermatitis, maculopapular rash, psoriasis, skin discoloration, skin hypertrophy and urticaria.

Special Senses: Infrequent was abnormal vision, conjunctivitis, ear pain, eye pain, lacrimation disorder, photophobia, taste perversion and tinnitus. Rare were abnormality of accommodation, dry eyes, ear disorder, eye hemorrhage, otitis media, parosmia and ptosis.

Urogenital: Infrequent were impotence, polyuria, urinary frequency and urinary tract disorder. Rare were breast pain, kidney pain, leukorrhea, menorrhagia, menstrual disorder and vaginitis.

DRUG ABUSE AND DEPENDENCE

Although the abuse potential of RELPAX has not been assessed, no abuse of, tolerance to, withdrawal from, or drug-seeking behavior was observed in patients who received RELPAX in clinical trials or their extensions. The 5-HT$_{1B/1D}$ agonists, as a class, have not been associated with drug abuse.

OVERDOSAGE

No significant overdoses in premarketing clinical trials have been reported. Volunteers (N=21) have received single doses of 120 mg without significant adverse effects. Daily doses of 160 mg were commonly employed in Phase III trials. Based on the pharmacology of the 5-HT$_{1B/1D}$ agonists, hypertension or other more serious cardiovascular symptoms could occur on overdose.

The elimination half-life of eletriptan is about 4 hours (see CLINICAL PHARMACOLOGY) and therefore monitoring of patients after overdose with eletriptan should continue for at least 20 hours, or longer should symptoms or signs persist.

There is no specific antidote to eletriptan. In cases of severe intoxication, intensive care procedures are recommended, including establishing and maintaining a patent airway, ensuring adequate oxygenation and ventilation, and monitoring and support of the cardiovascular system.

It is unknown what effect hemodialysis or peritoneal dialysis has on the serum concentration of eletriptan.

DOSAGE AND ADMINISTRATION

In controlled clinical trials, single doses of 20 mg and 40 mg were effective for the acute treatment of migraine in adults. A greater proportion of patients had a response following a 40 mg dose than following a 20 mg dose (see CLINICAL STUDIES). Individuals may vary in response to doses of RELPAX Tablets. The choice of dose should therefore be made on an individual basis. An 80 mg dose, although also effective, was associated with an increased incidence of adverse events. Therefore, the maximum recommended single dose is 40 mg.

If after the initial dose, headache improves but then returns, a repeat dose may be beneficial. If a second dose is required, it should be taken at least 2 hours after the initial dose. If the initial dose is ineffective, controlled clinical trials have not shown a benefit of a second dose to treat the same attack. The maximum daily dose should not exceed 80 mg.

The safety of treating an average of more than 3 headaches in a 30-day period has not been established.

CYP3A4 Inhibitors: Eletriptan is metabolized by the CYP3A4 enzyme. Eletriptan should not be used within at least 72 hours of treatment with the following potent CYP3A4 inhibitors: ketoconazole, itraconazole, nefazodone, troleandomycin, clarithromycin, ritonavir and nelfinavir. Eletriptan should not be used within 72 hours with drugs that have demonstrated potent CYP3A4 inhibition and have this potent effect described in the CONTRAINDICATIONS, WARNINGS or PRECAUTIONS sections of their labeling (see WARNINGS and CLINICAL PHARMACOLOGY: Drug Interactions).

Hepatic Impairment: The drug should not be given to patients with severe hepatic impairment since the effect of severe hepatic impairment on eletriptan metabolism was not evaluated. No dose adjustment is necessary in mild to mod-

Relpax Tablets

Package Configuration	Tablet Strength (mg)	NDC Code	Debossing
Heat Seal Card of 6 Tablets. Two Heat Seal Cards in a Display	20 mg	0049-2330-34	REP20 and Pfizer
Heat Seal Card of 6 Tablets. Two Heat Seal Cards in a Display	40 mg	0049-2340-34	REP40 and Pfizer
Blister of 6 Tablets	20 mg	0049-2330-45	REP20 and Pfizer
Blister of 6 Tablets	40 mg	0049-2340-45	REP40 and Pfizer

erate impairment (see CLINICAL PHARMACOLOGY, CONTRAINDICATIONS and PRECAUTIONS).

HOW SUPPLIED

RELPAX® Tablets of 20 mg and 40 mg eletriptan (base) as the hydrobromide. RELPAX Tablets are orange, round, convex shaped, film-coated tablets with appropriate debossing. They are supplied in the following strengths and package configurations:

[See table at top of previous page]

Store at 25°C (77°F); excursions permitted to 15-30°C (59-86°F) [see USP Controlled Room Temperature].

PATIENT SUMMARY OF INFORMATION

RELPAX®

(eletriptan hydrobromide)

Please read this information before you start taking RELPAX and each time you renew your prescription. Remember, this summary does not take the place of discussions with your doctor. You and your doctor should discuss RELPAX when you start taking your medication and at regular checkups.

What is RELPAX?

RELPAX is a prescription medicine used to treat migraine headaches in adults. RELPAX is not for other types of headaches.

What is a Migraine Headache?

Migraine is an intense, throbbing headache. You may have pain on one or both sides of your head. You may have nausea and vomiting, and be sensitive to light and noise. The pain and symptoms of a migraine headache can be worse than a common headache. Some women get migraines around the time of their menstrual period. Some people have visual symptoms before the headache, such as flashing lights or wavy lines, called an aura.

How Does RELPAX Work?

Treatment with RELPAX reduces swelling of blood vessels surrounding the brain. This swelling is associated with the headache pain of a migraine attack. RELPAX blocks the release of substances from nerve endings that cause more pain and other symptoms like nausea, and sensitivity to light and sound.

It is thought that these actions contribute to relief of your symptoms by RELPAX.

Who should not take RELPAX?

Do not take RELPAX if you:

- have uncontrolled high blood pressure.
- have heart disease or a history of heart disease.
- have hemiplegic or basilar migraine (if you are not sure about this, ask your doctor).
- have or had a stroke or problems with your blood circulation.
- have serious liver problems.
- have taken any of the following medicines in the last 24 hours: other "triptans" like almotriptan (Axert®), frovatriptan (Frova™), naratriptan (Amerge®), rizatriptan (Maxalt®), sumatriptan (Imitrex®), zolmitriptan (Zomig®); ergotamines like Bellergal-S®, Cafergot®, Ergomar®, Wigraine®; dihydroergotamine like D.H.E. 45® or Migranal®; or methysergide (Sansert®). These medicines have side effects similar to RELPAX.*
- have taken the following medicines within at least 72 hours: ketoconazole (Nizoral®), itraconazole (Sporanox®), nefazodone (Serzone®), troleandomycin (TAO®), clarithromycin (Biaxin®), ritonavir (Norvir®), and nelfinavir (Viracept®). These medicines may cause an increase in the amount of RELPAX in the blood.*
- are allergic to RELPAX or any of its ingredients. The active ingredient is eletriptan. The inactive ingredients are listed at the end of this leaflet.

Tell your doctor about all the medicines you take or plan to take, including prescription and non-prescription medicines, supplements, and herbal remedies. Your doctor will decide if you can take RELPAX with your other medicines.

Tell your doctor if you know that you have any of the following: risk factors for heart disease like high cholesterol, diabetes, smoking, obesity, menopause, or a family history of heart disease or stroke.

How should I take RELPAX?

RELPAX comes in 20 mg and 40 mg tablets. When you have a migraine headache, take your medicine as directed by your doctor.

- Take one RELPAX tablet as soon as you feel a migraine coming on.
- If your headache improves and then comes back after 2 hours, you can take a second tablet.
- If the first tablet did not help your headache at all, do not take a second tablet without talking with your doctor.
- Do not take more than two RELPAX tablets in any 24-hour period.

What are the possible side effects of RELPAX?

RELPAX is generally well tolerated. As with any medicine, people taking RELPAX may have side effects. The side effects are usually mild and do not last long.

The most common side effects of RELPAX are:

- dizziness
- nausea
- weakness
- tiredness
- pain or pressure sensation (e.g., in the chest or throat)

In very rare cases, patients taking triptans may experience serious side effects, including heart attacks. **Call your doctor right away** if you have:

- severe chest pains
- shortness of breath

This is not a complete list of side effects. Talk to your doctor if you develop any symptoms that concern you.

What to do in case of an overdose?

Call your doctor or poison control center or go to the ER.

General advice about RELPAX

Medicines are sometimes prescribed for conditions that are not mentioned in patient information leaflets. Do not use RELPAX for a condition for which it was not prescribed. Do not give RELPAX to other people, even if they have the same symptoms you have.

This leaflet summarizes the most important information about RELPAX. If you would like more information about RELPAX, talk with your doctor. You can ask your doctor or pharmacist for information on RELPAX that is written for health professionals. You can also call 1-866-4RELPAX (1-866-473-5729) or visit our web site at **www.RELPAX.com.**

What are the ingredients in RELPAX?

Active ingredient: eletriptan hydrobromide

Inactive ingredients: microcrystalline cellulose, lactose, croscarmellose sodium, magnesium stearate, titanium oxide, hypromellose, triacetin, and FD&C Yellow No. 6 aluminum lake.

Store RELPAX Tablets at room temperature 15-30°C (59-86°F).

*The brands listed are the trademarks of their respective owners and are not trademarks of Pfizer Inc.

Rx only

Distributed by

Roerig

Division of Pfizer Inc, NY, NY 10017

LAB-0076-45.0 Revised January 2005

VFEND® I.V. ℞

[vee'fənd]

(voriconazole) for Injection

VFEND® Tablets ℞

(voriconazole)

VFEND® (voriconazole) for Oral Suspension ℞

Prescribing information for this product, which appears on pages 2647–2656 of the 2005 PDR, has been completely revised as follows. Please write "See Supplement A" next to the product heading.

DESCRIPTION

VFEND® (voriconazole), a triazole antifungal agent, is available as a lyophilized powder for solution for intravenous infusion, film-coated tablets for oral administration, and as a powder for oral suspension. The structural formula is:

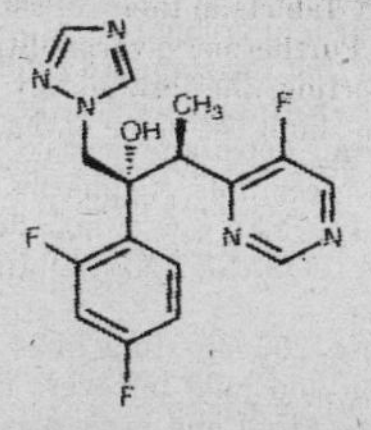

Voriconazole is designated chemically as (2R, 3S)-2-(2, 4-difluorophenyl)-3-(5-fluoro-4-pyrimidinyl)-1-(1*H*-1,2,4-triazol-1-yl)-2-butanol with an empirical formula of $C_{16}H_{14}F_3N_5O$ and a molecular weight of 349.3.

Voriconazole drug substance is a white to light-colored powder.

VFEND I.V. is a white lyophilized powder containing nominally 200 mg voriconazole and 3200 mg sulfobutyl ether beta-cyclodextrin sodium in a 30 mL Type I clear glass vial. VFEND I.V. is intended for administration by intravenous infusion. It is a single-dose, unpreserved product. Vials containing 200 mg lyophilized voriconazole are intended for reconstitution with Water for Injection to produce a solution containing 10 mg/mL VFEND and 160 mg/mL of sulfobutyl ether beta-cyclodextrin sodium. The resultant solution is further diluted prior to administration as an intravenous infusion (see DOSAGE AND ADMINISTRATION).

VFEND Tablets contain 50 mg or 200 mg of voriconazole. The inactive ingredients include lactose monohydrate, pregelatinized starch, croscarmellose sodium, povidone, magnesium stearate and a coating containing hypromellose, titanium dioxide, lactose monohydrate and triacetin.

VFEND for Oral Suspension is a white to off-white powder providing a white to off-white orange-flavored suspension when reconstituted. Bottles containing 45 g powder for oral suspension are intended for reconstitution with water to produce a suspension containing 40 mg/mL voriconazole. The inactive ingredients include colloidal silicon dioxide, titanium dioxide, xanthan gum, sodium citrate dihydrate, sodium benzoate, anhydrous citric acid, natural orange flavor, and sucrose.

CLINICAL PHARMACOLOGY

Pharmacokinetics

General Pharmacokinetic Characteristics

The pharmacokinetics of voriconazole have been characterized in healthy subjects, special populations and patients. The pharmacokinetics of voriconazole are non-linear due to saturation of its metabolism. The interindividual variability of voriconazole pharmacokinetics is high. Greater than proportional increase in exposure is observed with increasing dose. It is estimated that, on average, increasing the oral dose in healthy subjects from 200 mg Q12h to 300 mg Q12h leads to a 2.5-fold increase in exposure (AUC_τ), while increasing the intravenous dose from 3 mg/kg Q12h to 4 mg/kg Q12h produces a 2.3-fold increase in exposure (Table 1).

[See table 1 below]

During oral administration of 200 mg or 300 mg twice daily for 14 days in patients at risk of aspergillosis (mainly patients with malignant neoplasms of lymphatic or hematopoietic tissue), the observed pharmacokinetic characteristics were similar to those observed in healthy subjects (Table 2).

Table 2
Pharmacokinetic Parameters of Voriconazole in Patients at Risk for Aspergillosis

	200 mg Oral Q12h (n=9)	300 mg Oral Q12h (n=9)
AUC_τ* (µg•h/mL) (CV%)	20.31 (69%)	36.51 (45%)
C_{max}* (µg/mL) (CV%)	3.00 (51%)	4.66 (35%)

*Geometric mean values on Day 14 of multiple dosing in 2 cohorts of patients

Sparse plasma sampling for pharmacokinetics was conducted in the therapeutic studies in patients aged 12-18 years. In 11 adolescent patients who received a mean voriconazole maintenance dose of 4 mg/kg IV, the median of the calculated mean plasma concentrations was 1.60 µg/mL (inter-quartile range 0.28 to 2.73 µg/mL). In 17 adolescent patients for whom mean plasma concentrations were calculated following a mean oral maintenance dose of 200 mg Q12h, the median of the calculated mean plasma concentrations was 1.16 µg/mL (inter-quartile range 0.85 to 2.14 µg/mL).

When the recommended intravenous or oral loading dose regimens are administered to healthy subjects, peak plasma concentrations close to steady state are achieved within the first 24 hours of dosing. Without the loading dose, accumulation occurs during twice-daily multiple dosing with steady-state peak plasma voriconazole concentrations being achieved by day 6 in the majority of subjects (Table 3).

[See table 3 at top of next page]

Steady state trough plasma concentrations with voriconazole are achieved after approximately 5 days of oral or intravenous dosing without a loading dose regimen. However, when an intravenous loading dose regimen is used, steady state trough plasma concentrations are achieved within 1 day.

Absorption

The pharmacokinetic properties of voriconazole are similar following administration by the intravenous and oral routes. Based on a population pharmacokinetic analysis of pooled data in healthy subjects (N=207), the oral bioavailability of voriconazole is estimated to be 96% (CV 13%). Bioequivalence was established between the 200 mg tablet and the 40 mg/mL oral suspension when administered as a 400 mg Q12h loading dose followed by a 200 mg Q12h maintenance dose.

Maximum plasma concentrations (C_{max}) are achieved 1-2 hours after dosing. When multiple doses of voriconazole are administered with high-fat meals, the mean C_{max} and AUC_τ are reduced by 34% and 24%, respectively when administered as a tablet and by 58% and 37% respectively when administered as the oral suspension (see DOSAGE AND ADMINISTRATION).

In healthy subjects, the absorption of voriconazole is not affected by coadministration of oral ranitidine, cimetidine, or omeprazole, drugs that are known to increase gastric pH.

Distribution

The volume of distribution at steady state for voriconazole is estimated to be 4.6 L/kg, suggesting extensive distribution into tissues. Plasma protein binding is estimated to be 58% and was shown to be independent of plasma concentrations achieved following single and multiple oral doses of 200 mg or 300 mg (approximate range: 0.9-15 µg/mL). Varying degrees of hepatic and renal insufficiency do not affect the protein binding of voriconazole.

Continued on next page

Table 1
Population Pharmacokinetic Parameters of Voriconazole in Volunteers

	200 mg Oral Q12h	300 mg Oral Q12h	3 mg/kg IV Q12h	4 mg/kg IV Q12h
AUC_τ* (µg•h/mL) (CV%)	19.86 (94%)	50.32 (74%)	21.81 (100%)	50.40 (83%)

*Mean AUC_τ are predicted values from population pharmacokinetic analysis of data from 236 volunteers

VFEND—Cont.

Metabolism
In vitro studies showed that voriconazole is metabolized by the human hepatic cytochrome P450 enzymes, CYP2C19, CYP2C9 and CYP3A4 (see CLINICAL PHARMACOLOGY - Drug Interactions).
In vivo studies indicated that CYP2C19 is significantly involved in the metabolism of voriconazole. This enzyme exhibits genetic polymorphism. For example, 15-20% of Asian populations may be expected to be poor metabolizers. For Caucasians and Blacks, the prevalence of poor metabolizers is 3-5%. Studies conducted in Caucasian and Japanese healthy subjects have shown that poor metabolizers have, on average, 4-fold higher voriconazole exposure (AUC_τ) than their homozygous extensive metabolizer counterparts. Subjects who are heterozygous extensive metabolizers have, on average, 2-fold higher voriconazole exposure than their homozygous extensive metabolizer counterparts.
The major metabolite of voriconazole is the N-oxide, which accounts for 72% of the circulating radiolabelled metabolites in plasma. Since this metabolite has minimal antifungal activity, it does not contribute to the overall efficacy of voriconazole.

Excretion
Voriconazole is eliminated via hepatic metabolism with less than 2% of the dose excreted unchanged in the urine. After administration of a single radiolabelled dose of either oral or IV voriconazole, preceded by multiple oral or IV dosing, approximately 80% to 83% of the radioactivity is recovered in the urine. The majority (>94%) of the total radioactivity is excreted in the first 96 hours after both oral and intravenous dosing.
As a result of non-linear pharmacokinetics, the terminal half-life of voriconazole is dose dependent and therefore not useful in predicting the accumulation or elimination of voriconazole.

Pharmacokinetic-Pharmacodynamic Relationships
Clinical Efficacy and Safety
In 10 clinical trials, the median values for the average and maximum voriconazole plasma concentrations in individual patients across these studies (N=1121) was 2.51 μg/mL (inter-quartile range 1.21 to 4.44 μg/mL) and 3.79 μg/mL (inter-quartile range 2.06 to 6.31 μg/mL), respectively. A pharmacokinetic-pharmacodynamic analysis of patient data from 6 of these 10 clinical trials (N=280) could not detect a positive association between mean, maximum or minimum plasma voriconazole concentration and efficacy. However, PK/PD analyses of the data from all 10 clinical trials identified positive associations between plasma voriconazole concentrations and rate of both liver function test abnormalities and visual disturbances (see ADVERSE REACTIONS).
Electrocardiogram
A placebo-controlled, randomized, crossover study to evaluate the effect on the QT interval of healthy male and female volunteers was conducted with three single oral doses of voriconazole and ketoconazole. Serial ECGs and plasma samples were obtained at specified intervals over a 24-hour post dose observation period. The placebo-adjusted mean maximum increases in QTc from baseline after 800, 1200 and 1600 mg of voriconazole and after ketoconazole 800 mg were all <10 msec. Females exhibited a greater increase in QTc than males, although all mean changes were <10 msec. Age was not found to affect the magnitude of increase in QTc. No subject in any group had an increase in QTc of ≥60 msec from baseline. No subject experienced an interval exceeding the potentially clinically relevant threshold of 500 msec. However, the QT effect of voriconazole combined with drugs known to prolong the QT interval is unknown (see CONTRAINDICATIONS, PRECAUTIONS-Drug Interactions).

Pharmacokinetics in Special Populations
Gender
In a multiple oral dose study, the mean C_{max} and AUC_τ for healthy young females were 83% and 113% higher, respectively, than in healthy young males (18-45 years), after tablet dosing. In the same study, no significant differences in the mean C_{max} and AUC_τ were observed between healthy elderly males and healthy elderly females (≥65 years). In a similar study, after dosing with the oral suspension, the mean AUC for healthy young females was 45% higher than in healthy young males whereas the mean C_{max} was comparable between genders. The steady state trough voriconazole concentrations (C_{min}) seen in females were 100% and 91% higher than in males receiving the tablet and the oral suspension, respectively.
In the clinical program, no dosage adjustment was made on the basis of gender. The safety profile and plasma concentrations observed in male and female subjects were similar. Therefore, no dosage adjustment based on gender is necessary.
Geriatric
In an oral multiple dose study the mean C_{max} and AUC_τ in healthy elderly males (≥ 65 years) were 61% and 86% higher, respectively, than in young males (18-45 years). No significant differences in the mean C_{max} and AUC_τ were observed between healthy elderly females (≥ 65 years) and healthy young females (18-45 years).
In the clinical program, no dosage adjustment was made on the basis of age. An analysis of pharmacokinetic data obtained from 552 patients from 10 voriconazole clinical trials showed that the median voriconazole plasma concentrations in the elderly patients (>65 years) were approximately 80% to 90% higher than those in the younger patients (≤65 years) after either IV or oral administration. However, the safety profile of voriconazole in young and elderly subjects was similar and, therefore, no dosage adjustment is necessary for the elderly.

Table 3
Pharmacokinetic Parameters of Voriconazole from Loading Dose and Maintenance Dose Regimens (Individual Studies in Volunteers)

	400 mg Q12h on Day 1, 200 mg Q12h on Days 2 to 10 (n=17)		6 mg/kg IV** Q12h on Day 1, 3 mg/kg IV Q12h on Days 2 to 10 (n=9)	
	Day 1, 1st dose	Day 10	Day 1, 1st dose	Day 10
AUC_τ* (μg•h/mL) (CV%)	9.31 (38%)	11.13 (103%)	13.22 (22%)	13.25 (58%)
C_{max} (μg/mL) (CV%)	2.30 (19%)	2.08 (62%)	4.70 (22%)	3.06 (31%)

*AUC_τ values are calculated over dosing interval of 12 hours
Pharmacokinetic parameters for loading and maintenance doses summarized for same cohort of volunteers
**IV infusion over 60 minutes

Pediatric
A population pharmacokinetic analysis was conducted on pooled data from 35 immunocompromised pediatric patients aged 2 to <12 years old who were included in two pharmacokinetic studies of intravenous voriconazole (single dose and multiple dose). Twenty-four of these patients received multiple intravenous maintenance doses of 3 mg/kg and 4 mg/kg. A comparison of the pediatric and adult population pharmacokinetic data revealed that the predicted average steady state plasma concentrations were similar at the maintenance dose of 4 mg/kg every 12 hours in children and 3 mg/kg every 12 hours in adults (medians of 1.19 μg/mL and 1.16 μg/mL in children and adults, respectively) (see PRECAUTIONS, Pediatric Use).
Hepatic Insufficiency
After a single oral dose (200 mg) of voriconazole in 8 patients with mild (Child-Pugh Class A) and 4 patients with moderate (Child-Pugh Class B) hepatic insufficiency, the mean systemic exposure (AUC) was 3.2-fold higher than in age and weight matched controls with normal hepatic function. There was no difference in mean peak plasma concentrations (C_{max}) between the groups. When only the patients with mild (Child-Pugh Class A) hepatic insufficiency were compared to controls, there was still a 2.3-fold increase in the mean AUC in the group with hepatic insufficiency compared to controls.
In an oral multiple dose study, AUC_τ was similar in 6 subjects with moderate hepatic impairment (Child-Pugh Class B) given a lower maintenance dose of 100 mg twice daily compared to 6 subjects with normal hepatic function given the standard 200 mg twice daily maintenance dose. The mean peak plasma concentrations (C_{max}) were 20% lower in the hepatically impaired group.
It is recommended that the standard loading dose regimens be used but that the maintenance dose be halved in patients with mild to moderate hepatic cirrhosis (Child-Pugh Class A and B) receiving voriconazole. No pharmacokinetic data are available for patients with severe hepatic cirrhosis (Child-Pugh Class C) (see DOSAGE AND ADMINISTRATION).
Renal Insufficiency
In a single oral dose (200 mg) study in 24 subjects with normal renal function and mild to severe renal impairment, systemic exposure (AUC) and peak plasma concentration (C_{max}) of voriconazole were not significantly affected by renal impairment. Therefore, no adjustment is necessary for oral dosing in patients with mild to severe renal impairment.
In a multiple dose study of IV voriconazole (6 mg/kg IV loading dose × 2, then 3 mg/kg IV × 5.5 days) in 7 patients with moderate renal dysfunction (creatinine clearance 30-50 mL/min), the systemic exposure (AUC) and peak plasma concentrations (C_{max}) were not significantly different from those in 6 volunteers with normal renal function.
However, in patients with moderate renal dysfunction (creatinine clearance 30-50 mL/min), accumulation of the intravenous vehicle, SBECD, occurs. The mean systemic exposure (AUC) and peak plasma concentrations (C_{max}) of SBECD were increased 4-fold and almost 50%, respectively, in the moderately impaired group compared to the normal control group.
Intravenous voriconazole should be avoided in patients with moderate or severe renal impairment (creatinine clearance <50 mL/min), unless an assessment of the benefit/risk to the patient justifies the use of intravenous voriconazole (see DOSAGE AND ADMINISTRATION - Dosage Adjustment).
A pharmacokinetic study in subjects with renal failure undergoing hemodialysis showed that voriconazole is dialyzed with clearance of 121 mL/min. The intravenous vehicle, SBECD, is hemodialyzed with clearance of 55 mL/min. A 4-hour hemodialysis session does not remove a sufficient amount of voriconazole to warrant dose adjustment.

Drug Interactions
Effects of Other Drugs on Voriconazole
Voriconazole is metabolized by the human hepatic cytochrome P450 enzymes CYP2C19, CYP2C9, and CYP3A4. Results of *in vitro* metabolism studies indicate that the affinity of voriconazole is highest for CYP2C19, followed by CYP2C9, and is appreciably lower for CYP3A4. Inhibitors or inducers of these three enzymes may increase or decrease voriconazole systemic exposure (plasma concentrations), respectively.

The systemic exposure to voriconazole is significantly reduced or is expected to be reduced by the concomitant administration of the following agents and their use is contraindicated:
***Rifampin* (potent CYP450 inducer):** Rifampin (600 mg once daily) decreased the steady state C_{max} and AUC_τ of voriconazole (200 mg Q12h × 7 days) by an average of 93% and 96%, respectively, in healthy subjects. Doubling the dose of voriconazole to 400 mg Q12h does not restore adequate exposure to voriconazole during coadministration with rifampin.
Coadministration of voriconazole and rifampin is contraindicated (see CONTRAINDICATIONS, PRECAUTIONS - Drug Interactions).
***Ritonavir* (potent CYP450 inducer; CYP3A4 inhibitor and substrate):** Ritonavir (400 mg Q12h for 9 days) decreased the steady state C_{max} and AUC_τ of oral voriconazole (400 mg Q12h for 1 day, then 200 mg Q12h for 8 days) by an average of 66% and 82%, respectively, in healthy subjects. The effect of ritonavir (100 mg Q12h as used to inhibit CYP3A and increase concentrations of other antiretroviral drugs) on voriconazole concentrations has not been studied. Repeat oral administration of voriconazole (400 mg Q12h for 1 day, then 200 mg Q12h for 8 days) did not have a significant effect on steady state C_{max} and AUC_τ of ritonavir following repeat dose administration (400 mg Q12h for 9 days) in healthy subjects. **Coadministration of voriconazole and ritonavir (400 mg Q12h) is contraindicated** (see CONTRAINDICATIONS, PRECAUTIONS - Drug Interactions).
***Carbamazepine and long-acting barbiturates* (potent CYP450 inducers):** Although not studied *in vitro* or *in vivo*, carbamazepine and long-acting barbiturates (e.g., phenobarbital, mephobarbital) are likely to significantly decrease plasma voriconazole concentrations. **Coadministration of voriconazole with carbamazepine or long-acting barbiturates is contraindicated** (see CONTRAINDICATIONS, PRECAUTIONS - Drug Interactions).
Minor or no significant pharmacokinetic interactions that do not require dosage adjustment:
***Cimetidine* (non-specific CYP450 inhibitor and increases gastric pH):** Cimetidine (400 mg Q12h × 8 days) increased voriconazole steady state C_{max} and AUC_τ by an average of 18% (90% CI: 6%, 32%) and 23% (90% CI: 13%, 33%), respectively, following oral doses of 200 mg Q12h × 7 days to healthy subjects.
***Ranitidine* (increases gastric pH):** Ranitidine (150 mg Q12h) had no significant effect on voriconazole C_{max} and AUC_τ following oral doses of 200 mg Q12h × 7 days to healthy subjects.
Macrolide antibiotics: Co-administration of **erythromycin** (CYP3A4 inhibitor;1g Q12h for 7 days) or **azithromycin** (500 mg qd for 3 days) with voriconazole 200 mg Q12h for 14 days had no significant effect on voriconazole steady state C_{max} and AUC_τ in healthy subjects. The effects of voriconazole on the pharmacokinetics of either erythromycin or azithromycin are not known.

Effects of Voriconazole on Other Drugs
In vitro studies with human hepatic microsomes show that voriconazole inhibits the metabolic activity of the cytochrome P450 enzymes CYP2C19, CYP2C9, and CYP3A4. In these studies, the inhibition potency of voriconazole for CYP3A4 metabolic activity was significantly less than that of two other azoles, ketoconazole and itraconazole. *In vitro* studies also show that the major metabolite of voriconazole, voriconazole N-oxide, inhibits the metabolic activity of CYP2C9 and CYP3A4 to a greater extent than that of CYP2C19. Therefore, there is potential for voriconazole and its major metabolite to increase the systemic exposure (plasma concentrations) of other drugs metabolized by these CYP450 enzymes.
The systemic exposure of the following drugs is significantly increased or is expected to be significantly increased by coadministration of voriconazole and their use is contraindicated:
***Sirolimus* (CYP3A4 substrate):** Repeat dose administration of oral voriconazole (400 mg Q12h for 1 day, then 200 mg Q12h for 8 days) increased the C_{max} and AUC of sirolimus (2 mg single dose) an average of 7-fold (90% CI: 5.7, 7.5) and 11-fold (90% CI: 9.9, 12.6), respectively, in healthy subjects. **Coadministration of voriconazole and sirolimus is contraindicated** (see CONTRAINDICATIONS, PRECAUTIONS - Drug Interactions).
***Terfenadine, astemizole, cisapride, pimozide and quinidine* (CYP3A4 substrates):** Although not studied *in vitro* or *in vivo*, concomitant administration of voriconazole with terfenadine, astemizole, cisapride, pimozide or quinidine may

result in inhibition of the metabolism of these drugs. Increased plasma concentrations of these drugs can lead to QT prolongation and rare occurrences of *torsade de pointes*. **Coadministration of voriconazole and terfenadine, astemizole, cisapride, pimozide and quinidine is contraindicated** (see CONTRAINDICATIONS, PRECAUTIONS - Drug Interactions).

Ergot alkaloids: Although not studied *in vitro* or *in vivo*, voriconazole may increase the plasma concentration of ergot alkaloids (ergotamine and dihydroergotamine) and lead to ergotism. **Coadministration of voriconazole with ergot alkaloids is contraindicated** (see CONTRAINDICATIONS, PRECAUTIONS - Drug Interactions).

Coadministration of voriconazole with the following agents results in increased exposure or is expected to result in increased exposure to these drugs. Therefore, careful monitoring and/or dosage adjustment of these drugs is needed:

Cyclosporine (CYP3A4 substrate): In stable renal transplant recipients receiving chronic cyclosporine therapy, concomitant administration of oral voriconazole (200 mg Q12h for 8 days) increased cyclosporine C_{max} and AUC, an average of 1.1 times (90% CI: 0.9, 1.41) and 1.7 times (90% CI: 1.5, 2.0), respectively, as compared to when cyclosporine was administered without voriconazole. When initiating therapy with voriconazole in patients already receiving cyclosporine, it is recommended that the cyclosporine dose be reduced to one-half of the original dose and followed with frequent monitoring of the cyclosporine blood levels. Increased cyclosporine levels have been associated with nephrotoxicity. When voriconazole is discontinued, cyclosporine levels should be frequently monitored and the dose increased as necessary (see PRECAUTIONS - Drug Interactions).

Methadone (CYP3A4, CYP2C19, CYP2C9 substrate): Repeat dose administration of oral voriconazole (400mg Q12h for 1 day, then 200mg Q12h for 4 days) increased the C_{max} and AUC, of pharmacologically active R-methadone by 31% (90% CI: 22%, 40%) and 47% (90% CI: 38%, 57%), respectively, in subjects receiving a methadone maintenance dose (30-100 mg QD). The C_{max} and AUC of (S)-methadone increased by 65% (90% CI: 53%, 79%) and 103% (90% CI: 85%, 124%), respectively. Increased plasma concentrations of methadone have been associated with toxicity including QT prolongation. Frequent monitoring for adverse events and toxicity related to methadone is recommended during coadministration. Dose reduction of methadone may be needed (see PRECAUTIONS - Drug Interactions).

Tacrolimus (CYP3A4 substrate): Repeat oral dose administration of voriconazole (400 mg Q12h × 1 day, then 200 mg Q12h × 6 days) increased tacrolimus (0.1 mg/kg single dose) C_{max} and AUC, in healthy subjects by an average of 2-fold (90% CI: 1.9, 2.5) and 3-fold (90% CI: 2.7, 3.8), respectively. When initiating therapy with voriconazole in patients already receiving tacrolimus, it is recommended that the tacrolimus dose be reduced to one-third of the original dose and followed with frequent monitoring of the tacrolimus blood levels. Increased tacrolimus levels have been associated with nephrotoxicity. When voriconazole is discontinued, tacrolimus levels should be carefully monitored and the dose increased as necessary (see PRECAUTIONS - Drug Interactions).

Warfarin (CYP2C9 substrate): Coadministration of voriconazole (300 mg Q12h × 12 days) with warfarin (30 mg single dose) significantly increased maximum prothrombin time by approximately 2 times that of placebo in healthy subjects. Close monitoring of prothrombin time or other suitable anticoagulation tests is recommended if warfarin and voriconazole are coadministered and the warfarin dose adjusted accordingly (see PRECAUTIONS - Drug Interactions).

Oral Coumarin Anticoagulants (CYP2C9, CYP3A4 substrates): Although not studied *in vitro* or *in vivo*, voriconazole may increase the plasma concentrations of coumarin anticoagulants and therefore may cause an increase in prothrombin time. If patients receiving coumarin preparations are treated simultaneously with voriconazole, the prothrombin time or other suitable anti-coagulation tests should be monitored at close intervals and the dosage of anticoagulants adjusted accordingly (see PRECAUTIONS - Drug Interactions).

Statins (CYP3A4 substrates): Although not studied clinically, voriconazole has been shown to inhibit lovastatin metabolism *in vitro* (human liver microsomes). Therefore, voriconazole is likely to increase the plasma concentrations of statins that are metabolized by CYP3A4. It is recommended that dose adjustment of the statin be considered during coadministration. Increased statin concentrations in plasma have been associated with rhabdomyolysis (see PRECAUTIONS - Drug Interactions).

Benzodiazepines (CYP3A4 substrates): Although not studied clinically, voriconazole has been shown to inhibit midazolam metabolism *in vitro* (human liver microsomes). Therefore, voriconazole is likely to increase the plasma concentrations of benzodiazepines that are metabolized by CYP3A4 (e.g., midazolam, triazolam, and alprazolam) and lead to a prolonged sedative effect. It is recommended that dose adjustment of the benzodiazepine be considered during coadministration (see PRECAUTIONS - Drug Interactions).

Calcium Channel Blockers (CYP3A4 substrates): Although not studied clinically, voriconazole has been shown to inhibit felodipine metabolism *in vitro* (human liver microsomes). Therefore, voriconazole may increase the plasma concentrations of calcium channel blockers that are metabolized by CYP3A4. Frequent monitoring for adverse events and toxicity related to calcium channel blockers is recom-

mended during coadministration. Dose adjustment of the calcium channel blocker may be needed (see PRECAUTIONS - Drug Interactions).

Sulfonylureas (CYP2C9 substrates): Although not studied *in vitro* or *in vivo*, voriconazole may increase plasma concentrations of sulfonylureas (e.g., tolbutamide, glipizide, and glyburide) and therefore cause hypoglycemia. Frequent monitoring of blood glucose and appropriate adjustment (i.e., reduction) of the sulfonylurea dosage is recommended during coadministration (see PRECAUTIONS - Drug Interactions).

Vinca Alkaloids (CYP3A4 substrates): Although not studied *in vitro* or *in vivo*, voriconazole may increase the plasma concentrations of the vinca alkaloids (e.g., vincristine and vinblastine) and lead to neurotoxicity. Therefore, it is recommended that dose adjustment of the vinca alkaloid be considered.

No significant pharmacokinetic interactions were observed when voriconazole was coadministered with the following agents. Therefore, no dosage adjustment for these agents is recommended:

Prednisolone (CYP3A4 substrate): Voriconazole (200 mg Q12h × 30 days) increased C_{max} and AUC of prednisolone (60 mg single dose) by an average of 11% and 34%, respectively, in healthy subjects.

Digoxin (P-glycoprotein mediated transport): Voriconazole (200 mg Q12h × 12 days) had no significant effect on steady state C_{max} and AUC, of digoxin (0.25 mg once daily for 10 days) in healthy subjects.

Mycophenolic acid (UDP-glucuronyl transferase substrate): Voriconazole (200 mg Q12h × 5 days) had no significant effect on the C_{max} and AUC, of mycophenolic acid and its major metabolite, mycophenolic acid glucuronide after administration of a 1 g single oral dose of mycophenolate mofetil.

Two-Way Interactions

Concomitant use of the following agents with voriconazole is contraindicated:

Efavirenz, a non-nucleoside reverse transcriptase inhibitor (CYP450 inducer; CYP3A4 inhibitor and substrate): Steady state efavirenz (400 mg PO QD) decreased the steady state C_{max} and AUC, of voriconazole (400 mg PO Q12h for 1 day, then 200 mg PO Q12h for 8 days) by an average of 61% and 77%, respectively, in healthy subjects. Voriconazole at steady state (400 mg PO Q12h for 1 day, then 200 mg Q12h for 8 days) increased the steady state C_{max} and AUC, of efavirenz (400 mg PO QD for 9 days) by an average of 38% and 44%, respectively, in healthy subjects. **Coadministration of voriconazole and efavirenz is contraindicated** (see CONTRAINDICATIONS, PRECAUTIONS - Drug Interactions).

Rifabutin (potent CYP450 inducer): Rifabutin (300 mg once daily) decreased the C_{max} and AUC, of voriconazole at 200 mg twice daily by an average of 67% (90% CI: 58%, 73%) and 79% (90% CI: 71%, 84%), respectively, in healthy subjects. During coadministration with rifabutin (300 mg once daily), the steady state C_{max} and AUC, of voriconazole following an increased dose of 400 mg twice daily were on average approximately 2 times higher, compared with voriconazole alone at 200 mg twice daily. Coadministration of voriconazole at 400 mg twice daily with rifabutin 300 mg twice daily increased the C_{max} and AUC, of rifabutin by an average of 3-times (90% CI: 2.2, 4.0) and 4 times (90% CI: 3.5, 5.4), respectively, compared to rifabutin given alone. **Coadministration of voriconazole and rifabutin is contraindicated.**

Significant drug interactions that may require dosage adjustment, frequent monitoring of drug levels and/or frequent monitoring of drug-related adverse events/toxicity:

Phenytoin (CYP2C9 substrate and potent CYP450 inducer): Repeat dose administration of phenytoin .(300 mg once daily) decreased the steady state C_{max} and AUC, of orally administered voriconazole (200 mg Q12h × 14 days) by an average of 50% and 70%, respectively, in healthy subjects. Administration of a higher voriconazole dose (400 mg Q12h × 7 days) with phenytoin (300 mg once daily) resulted in comparable steady state voriconazole C_{max} and AUC, estimates as compared to when voriconazole was given at 200 mg Q12h without phenytoin.

Phenytoin may be coadministered with voriconazole if the maintenance dose of voriconazole is increased from 4 mg/kg to 5 mg/kg intravenously every 12 hours or from 200 mg to 400 mg orally, every 12 hours (100 mg to 200 mg orally, every 12 hours in patients less than 40 kg) (see DOSAGE AND ADMINISTRATION).

Repeat dose administration of voriconazole (400 mg Q12h × 10 days) increased the steady state C_{max} and AUC, of phenytoin (300 mg once daily) by an average of 70% and 80%, respectively, in healthy subjects. The increase in phenytoin C_{max} and AUC when coadministered with voriconazole may be expected to be as high as 2 times the C_{max} and AUC estimates when phenytoin is given without voriconazole. Therefore, frequent monitoring of plasma phenytoin concentrations and phenytoin-related adverse effects is recommended when phenytoin is coadministered with voriconazole (see PRECAUTIONS - Drug Interactions).

Omeprazole (CYP2C19 inhibitor; CYP2C19 and CYP3A4 substrate): Coadministration of omeprazole (40 mg once daily × 10 days) with oral voriconazole (400 mg Q12h × 1 day, then 200 mg Q12h × 9 days) increased the steady state C_{max} and AUC, of voriconazole by an average of 15% (90% CI: 5%, 25%) and 40% (90% CI: 29%, 55%), respectively, in healthy subjects. No dosage adjustment of voriconazole is recommended.

Coadministration of voriconazole (400 mg Q12h × 1 day, then 200 mg × 6 days) with omeprazole (40 mg once daily ×

7 days) to healthy subjects significantly increased the steady state C_{max} and AUC, of omeprazole an average of 2 times (90% CI: 1.8, 2.6) and 4 times (90% CI: 3.3, 4.4), respectively, as compared to when omeprazole is given without voriconazole. When initiating voriconazole in patients already receiving omeprazole doses of 40 mg or greater, it is recommended that the omeprazole dose be reduced by one-half (see PRECAUTIONS - Drug Interactions).

The metabolism of other proton pump inhibitors that are CYP2C19 substrates may also be inhibited by voriconazole and may result in increased plasma concentrations of these drugs.

No significant pharmacokinetic interaction was seen and no dosage adjustment of these drugs is recommended:

Indinavir (CYP3A4 inhibitor and substrate): Repeat dose administration of indinavir (800 mg TID for 10 days) had no significant effect on voriconazole C_{max} and AUC following repeat dose administration (200 mg Q12h for 17 days) in healthy subjects.

Repeat dose administration of voriconazole (200 mg Q12h for 7 days) did not have a significant effect on steady state C_{max} and AUC, of indinavir following repeat dose administration (800 mg TID for 7 days) in healthy subjects.

Other Two-Way Interactions Expected to be Significant Based on *In Vitro* and *In Vivo* Findings:

Other HIV Protease Inhibitors (CYP3A4 substrates and inhibitors): *In vitro* studies (human liver microsomes) suggest that voriconazole may inhibit the metabolism of HIV protease inhibitors (e.g., saquinavir, amprenavir and nelfinavir). *In vitro* studies (human liver microsomes) also show that the metabolism of voriconazole may be inhibited by HIV protease inhibitors (e.g., saquinavir and amprenavir). Patients should be frequently monitored for drug toxicity during the coadministration of voriconazole and HIV protease inhibitors (see PRECAUTIONS - Drug Interactions).

Other Non-Nucleoside Reverse Transcriptase Inhibitors (NNRTIs) (CYP3A4 substrates, inhibitors or CYP450 inducers): *In vitro* studies (human liver microsomes) show that the metabolism of voriconazole may be inhibited by a NNRTI (e.g., delavirdine). The findings of a clinical voriconazole-efavirenz drug interaction study in healthy volunteers suggest that the metabolism of voriconazole may be induced by a NNRTI. This *in vivo* study also showed that voriconazole may inhibit the metabolism of a NNRTI. Efavirenz and voriconazole coadministration is contraindicated (see CLINICAL PHARMACOLOGY – Drug Interactions, CONTRAINDICATIONS, PRECAUTIONS – Drug Interactions). Patients should be frequently monitored for drug toxicity during the coadministration of voriconazole and other NNRTIs (e.g., nevirapine and delavirdine) (see PRECAUTIONS - Drug Interactions).

MICROBIOLOGY

Mechanism of Action

Voriconazole is a triazole antifungal agent. The primary mode of action of voriconazole is the inhibition of fungal cytochrome P-450-mediated 14 alpha-lanosterol demethylation, an essential step in fungal ergosterol biosynthesis. The accumulation of 14 alpha-methyl sterols correlates with the subsequent loss of ergosterol in the fungal cell wall and may be responsible for the antifungal activity of voriconazole. Voriconazole has been shown to be more selective for fungal cytochrome P-450 enzymes than for various mammalian cytochrome P-450 enzyme systems.

Activity *In Vitro* and *In Vivo*

Voriconazole has demonstrated *in vitro* activity against *Aspergillus* species (*A. fumigatus, A. flavus, A. niger* and *A. terreus*), *Candida* species (*C. albicans, C. glabrata, C. krusei, C. parapsilosis* and *C. tropicalis*), *Scedosporium apiospermum* and *Fusarium* spp., including *Fusarium solani* (see INDICATIONS AND USAGE, CLINICAL STUDIES). *In vitro* susceptibility testing was performed according to the National Committee for Clinical Laboratory Standards (NCCLS) methods (M38-P for moulds and M27-A for yeasts). Voriconazole breakpoints have not been established for any fungi. The relationship between clinical outcome and *in vitro* susceptibility results remains to be elucidated. Voriconazole was active in normal and/or immunocompromised guinea pigs with systemic and/or pulmonary infections due to *A. fumigatus* (including an isolate with reduced susceptibility to itraconazole) or *Candida* species [*C.albicans* (including an isolate with reduced susceptibility to fluconazole), *C. krusei and C. glabrata*] in which the endpoints were prolonged survival of infected animals and/or reduction of mycological burden from target organs. In one experiment, voriconazole exhibited activity against *Scedosporium apiospermum* infections in immune competent guinea pigs.

Drug Resistance

Voriconazole drug resistance development has not been adequately studied *in vitro* against *Candida, Aspergillus, Scedosporium* and *Fusarium* species. The frequency of drug resistance development for the various fungi for which this drug is indicated is not known.

Fungal isolates exhibiting reduced susceptibility to fluconazole or itraconazole may also show reduced susceptibility to voriconazole, suggesting cross-resistance can occur among these azoles. The relevance of cross-resistance and clinical outcome has not been fully characterized. Clinical cases where azole cross-resistance is demonstrated may require alternative antifungal therapy.

INDICATIONS AND USAGE

VFEND is indicated for use in the treatment of the following fungal infections:

Continued on next page

VFEND—Cont.

Invasive aspergillosis. In clinical trials, the majority of isolates recovered were *Aspergillus fumigatus*. There was a small number of cases of culture-proven disease due to species of *Aspergillus* other than *A. fumigatus* (see CLINICAL STUDIES, MICROBIOLOGY).
Candidemia in nonneutropenic patients and the following *Candida* infections: disseminated infections in skin and infections in abdomen, kidney, bladder wall, and wounds (see CLINICAL STUDIES, MICROBIOLOGY).
Esophageal candidiasis (see CLINICAL STUDIES, MICROBIOLOGY).
Serious fungal infections caused by *Scedosporium apiospermum* (asexual form of *Pseudallescheria boydii*) and *Fusarium* spp. including *Fusarium solani*, in patients intolerant of, or refractory to, other therapy (see CLINICAL STUDIES, MICROBIOLOGY).
Specimens for fungal culture and other relevant laboratory studies (including histopathology) should be obtained prior to therapy to isolate and identify causative organism(s). Therapy may be instituted before the results of the cultures and other laboratory studies are known. However, once these results become available, antifungal therapy should be adjusted accordingly.

CLINICAL STUDIES

Voriconazole, administered orally or parenterally, has been evaluated as primary or salvage therapy in 520 patients aged 12 years and older with infections caused by *Aspergillus* spp., *Fusarium* spp., and *Scedosporium* spp.

Invasive Aspergillosis

Voriconazole was studied in patients for primary therapy of invasive aspergillosis (randomized, controlled study 307/602), for primary and salvage therapy of aspergillosis (noncomparative study 304) and for treatment of patients with invasive aspergillosis who were refractory to, or intolerant of, other antifungal therapy (non-comparative study 309/604).

Study 307/602

The efficacy of voriconazole compared to amphotericin B in the primary treatment of acute invasive aspergillosis was demonstrated in 277 patients treated for 12 weeks in Study 307/602. The majority of study patients had underlying hematologic malignancies, including bone marrow transplantation. The study also included patients with solid organ transplantation, solid tumors, and AIDS. The patients were mainly treated for definite or probable invasive aspergillosis of the lungs. Other aspergillosis infections included disseminated disease, CNS infections and sinus infections. Diagnosis of definite or probable invasive aspergillosis was made according to criteria modified from those established by the National Institute of Allergy and Infectious Diseases Mycoses Study Group/European Organisation for Research and Treatment of Cancer (NIAID MSG/EORTC).
Voriconazole was administered intravenously with a loading dose of 6 mg/kg every 12 hours for the first 24 hours followed by a maintenance dose of 4 mg/kg every 12 hours for a minimum of seven days. Therapy could then be switched to the oral formulation at a dose of 200 mg Q12h. Median duration of IV voriconazole therapy was 10 days (range 2-90 days). After IV voriconazole therapy, the median duration of PO voriconazole therapy was 76 days (range 2-232 days).
Patients in the comparator group received conventional amphotericin B as a slow infusion at a daily dose of 1.0-1.5 mg/kg/day. Median duration of IV amphotericin therapy was 12 days (range 1-85 days). Treatment was then continued with other licensed antifungal therapy (OLAT), including itraconazole and lipid amphotericin B formulations. Although initial therapy with conventional amphotericin B was to be continued for at least two weeks, actual duration of therapy was at the discretion of the investigator. Patients who discontinued initial randomized therapy due to toxicity or lack of efficacy were eligible to continue in the study with OLAT treatment.
A satisfactory global response at 12 weeks (complete or partial resolution of all attributable symptoms, signs, radiographic/bronchoscopic abnormalities present at baseline) was seen in 53% of voriconazole treated patients compared to 32% of amphotericin B treated patients (Table 4). A benefit of voriconazole compared to amphotericin B on patient survival at Day 84 was seen with a 71% survival rate on voriconazole compared to 58% on amphotericin B (Table 4). Table 4 also summarizes the response (success) based on mycological confirmation and species.
[See table 4 above]

Study 304

The results of this comparative trial (Study 307/602) confirmed the results of an earlier trial in the primary and salvage treatment of patients with acute invasive aspergillosis (Study 304). In this earlier study, an overall success rate of 52% (26/50) was seen in patients treated with voriconazole for primary therapy. Success was seen in 17/29 (59%) with *Aspergillus fumigatus* infections and 3/6 (50%) patients with infections due to non-*fumigatus* species [*A. flavus* (1/1); *A. nidulans* (0/2); *A. niger* (2/2); *A. terreus* (0/1)]. Success in patients who received voriconazole as salvage therapy is presented in Table 5.

Study 309/604

Additional data regarding response rates in patients who were refractory to, or intolerant of, other antifungal agents are also provided in Table 5. Overall mycological eradication for culture-documented infections due to *fumigatus* and

Table 4
Overall Efficacy and Success by Species in the Primary Treatment of Acute Invasive Aspergillosis Study 307/602

	Voriconazole	Ampho B[c]	Stratified Difference (95% CI)[d]
	n/N (%)	n/N (%)	
Efficacy as Primary Therapy			
Satisfactory Global Response[a]	76/144 (53)	42/133 (32)	21.8% (10.5%, 33.0%) p<0.0001
Survival at Day 84[b]	102/144 (71)	77/133 (58)	13.1% (2.1%, 24.2%)
Success by Species			
	Success n/N (%)		
Overall success	76/144 (53)	42/133 (32)	
Mycologically confirmed[e]	37/84 (44)	16/67 (24)	
Aspergillus spp.[f]			
A. fumigatus	28/63 (44)	12/47 (26)	
A. flavus	3/6	4/9	
A. terreus	2/3	0/3	
A. niger	1/4	0/9	
A. nidulans	1/1	0/0	

[a] Assessed by independent Data Review Committee (DRC)
[b] Proportion of subjects alive
[c] Amphotericin B followed by other licensed antifungal therapy
[d] Difference and corresponding 95% confidence interval are stratified by protocol
[e] Not all mycologically confirmed specimens were speciated
[f] Some patients had more than one species isolated at baseline

non-*fumigatus* species of *Aspergillus* was 36/82 (44%) and 12/30 (40%), respectively, in voriconazole treated patients. Patients had various underlying diseases and species other than *A. fumigatus* contributed to mixed infections in some cases.
For patients who were infected with a single pathogen and were refractory to, or intolerant of, other antifungal agents, the satisfactory response rates for voriconazole in studies 304 and 309/604 are presented in Table 5.

Table 5 Combined Response Data in Salvage Patients with Single Aspergillus Species (Studies 304 and 309/604)

	Success n/N
A. fumigatus	43/97 (44%)
A. flavus	5/12
A. nidulans	1/3
A. niger	4/5
A. terreus	3/8
A. versicolor	0/1

Nineteen patients had more than one species of *Aspergillus* isolated. Success was seen in 4/17 (24%) of these patients.

Candidemia in nonneutropenic patients and other deep tissue *Candida* infections

Voriconazole was compared to the regimen of amphotericin B followed by fluconazole in Study 608, an open label, comparative study in nonneutropenic patients with candidemia associated with clinical signs of infection. Patients were randomized in 2:1 ratio to receive either voriconazole (n=283) or the regimen of amphotericin B followed by fluconazole (n=139). Patients were treated with randomized study drug for a median of 15 days. Most of the candidemia in patients evaluated for efficacy was caused by *C. albicans* (46%), followed by *C. tropicalis* (19%), *C. parapsilosis* (17%), *C. glabrata* (15%), and *C. krusei* (1%).
An independent Data Review Committee (DRC), blinded to study treatment, reviewed the clinical and mycological data from this study, and generated one assessment of response for each patient. A successful response required all of the following: resolution or improvement in all clinical signs and symptoms of infection, blood cultures negative for *Candida*, infected deep tissue sites negative for *Candida* or resolution of all local signs of infection, and no systemic antifungal therapy other than study drug. The primary analysis, which counted DRC-assessed successes at the fixed time point (12 weeks after End of Therapy [EOT]), demonstrated that voriconazole was comparable to the regimen of amphotericin B followed by fluconazole (response rates of 41% and 41%, respectively) in the treatment of candidemia. Patients who did not have a 12-week assessment for any reason were considered a treatment failure.
The overall clinical and mycological success rates by *Candida* species in Study 150-608 are presented in Table 6.

Table 6
Overall Success Rates Sustained From EOT To The Fixed 12-Week Follow-Up Time Point By Baseline Pathogen[a,b]

Baseline Pathogen	Clinical and Mycological Success (%)	
	Voriconazole	Amphotericin B --> Fluconazole
C. albicans	46/107 (43%)	30/63 (48%)
C. tropicalis	17/53 (32%)	1/16 (6%)
C. parapsilosis	24/45 (53%)	10/19 (53%)
C. glabrata	12/36 (33%)	7/21 (33%)
C. krusei	1/4	0/1

[a] A few patients had more than one pathogen at baseline.
[b] Patients who did not have a 12-week assessment for any reason were considered a treatment failure.

In a secondary analysis, which counted DRC-assessed successes at any time point (EOT, or 2, 6, or 12 weeks after EOT), the response rates were 65% for voriconazole and 71% for the regimen of amphotericin B followed by fluconazole.
In Studies 608 and 309/604 (non-comparative study in patients with invasive fungal infections who were refractory to, or intolerant of, other antifungal agents), voriconazole was evaluated in 35 patients with deep tissue *Candida* infections. A favorable response was seen in 4 of 7 patients with intraabdominal infections, 5 of 6 patients with kidney and bladder wall infections, 3 of 3 patients with deep tissue abscess or wound infection, 1 of 2 patients with pneumonia/pleural space infections, 2 of 4 patients with skin lesions, 1 of 1 patients with mixed intraabdominal and pulmonary infection, 1 of 2 patients with suppurative phlebitis, 1 of 3 patients with hepatosplenic infection, 1 of 5 patients with osteomyelitis, 0 of 1 with liver infection, and 0 of 1 with cervical lymph node infection.

Esophageal Candidiasis

The efficacy of oral voriconazole 200 mg bid compared to oral fluconazole 200 mg od in the primary treatment of esophageal candidiasis was demonstrated in Study 150-305, a double-blind, double-dummy study in immunocompromised patients with endoscopically-proven esophageal candidiasis. Patients were treated for a median of 15 days (range 1 to 49 days). Outcome was assessed by repeat endoscopy at end of treatment (EOT). A successful response was defined as a normal endoscopy at EOT or at least a 1 grade improvement over baseline endoscopic score. For patients in the Intent to Treat (ITT) population with only a baseline endoscopy, a successful response was defined as symptomatic cure or improvement at EOT compared to baseline. Voriconazole and fluconazole (200 mg od) showed comparable efficacy rates against esophageal candidiasis, as presented in Table 7.
[See table 7 at top of next page]
Microbiologic success rates by *Candida* species are presented in Table 8.

[See table 8 at right]

Other Serious Fungal Pathogens

In pooled analyses of patients, voriconazole was shown to be effective against the following additional fungal pathogens: *Scedosporium apiospermum* - Successful response to voriconazole therapy was seen in 15 of 24 patients (63%). Three of these patients relapsed within 4 weeks, including 1 patient with pulmonary, skin and eye infections, 1 patient with cerebral disease, and 1 patient with skin infection. Ten patients had evidence of cerebral disease and 6 of these had a successful outcome (1 relapse). In addition, a successful response was seen in 1 of 3 patients with mixed organism infections.

Fusarium spp. - Nine of 21 (43%) patients were successfully treated with voriconazole. Of these 9 patients, 3 had eye infections, 1 had an eye and blood infection, 1 had a skin infection, 1 had a blood infection alone, 2 had sinus infections, and 1 had disseminated infection (pulmonary, skin, hepatosplenic). Three of these patients (1 with disseminated disease, 1 with an eye infection and 1 with a blood infection) had *Fusarium solani* and were complete successes. Two of these patients relapsed, 1 with a sinus infection and profound neutropenia and 1 post surgical patient with blood and eye infections.

CONTRAINDICATIONS

VFEND is contraindicated in patients with known hypersensitivity to voriconazole or its excipients. There is no information regarding cross-sensitivity between VFEND (voriconazole) and other azole antifungal agents. Caution should be used when prescribing VFEND to patients with hypersensitivity to other azoles.

Coadministration of the CYP3A4 substrates, terfenadine, astemizole, cisapride, pimozide or quinidine with VFEND are contraindicated since increased plasma concentrations of these drugs can lead to QT prolongation and rare occurrences of *torsade de pointes* (see CLINICAL PHARMACOLOGY - Drug Interactions, PRECAUTIONS - Drug Interactions).

Coadministration of VFEND with sirolimus is contraindicated because VFEND significantly increases sirolimus concentrations in healthy subjects (see CLINICAL PHARMACOLOGY - Drug Interactions, PRECAUTIONS - Drug Interactions).

Coadministration of VFEND with rifampin, carbamazepine and long-acting barbiturates is contraindicated since these drugs are likely to decrease plasma voriconazole concentrations significantly (see CLINICAL PHARMACOLOGY - Drug Interactions, PRECAUTIONS - Drug Interactions).

Coadministration of VFEND with ritonavir (400 mg Q12h) is contraindicated because ritonavir (400 mg Q12h) significantly decreases plasma voriconazole concentrations in healthy subjects. The effect of ritonavir (100 mg Q12h as used to inhibit CYP3A and increase concentrations of other antiretroviral drugs) on voriconazole concentrations has not been studied (see CLINICAL PHARMACOLOGY - Drug Interactions, PRECAUTIONS - Drug Interactions).

Coadministration of VFEND with efavirenz is contraindicated because efavirenz significantly decreases voriconazole plasma concentrations while VFEND also significantly increases efavirenz plasma concentrations (see CLINICAL PHARMACOLOGY - Drug Interactions, PRECAUTIONS - Drug Interactions).

Coadministration of VFEND with rifabutin is contraindicated since VFEND significantly increases rifabutin plasma concentrations and rifabutin also significantly decreases voriconazole plasma concentrations (see CLINICAL PHARMACOLOGY - Drug Interactions, PRECAUTIONS - Drug Interactions).

Coadministration of VFEND with ergot alkaloids (ergotamine and dihydroergotamine) is contraindicated because VFEND may increase the plasma concentration of ergot alkaloids, which may lead to ergotism.

WARNINGS

VISUAL DISTURBANCES: The effect of VFEND on visual function is not known if treatment continues beyond 28 days. If treatment continues beyond 28 days, visual function including visual acuity, visual field and color perception should be monitored **(see PRECAUTIONS – Information for Patients and ADVERSE EVENTS – Visual Disturbances).**

HEPATIC TOXICITY: In clinical trials, there have been uncommon cases of serious hepatic reactions during treatment with VFEND (including clinical hepatitis, cholestasis and fulminant hepatic failure, including fatalities). Instances of hepatic reactions were noted to occur primarily in patients with serious underlying medical conditions (predominantly hematological malignancy). Hepatic reactions, including hepatitis and jaundice, have occurred among patients with no other identifiable risk factors. Liver dysfunction has usually been reversible on discontinuation of therapy **(see PRECAUTIONS – Laboratory Tests and ADVERSE EVENTS – Clinical Laboratory Values).**

Monitoring of hepatic function: Liver function tests should be evaluated at the start of and during the course of VFEND therapy. Patients who develop abnormal liver function tests during VFEND therapy should be monitored for the development of more severe hepatic injury. Patient management should include laboratory evaluation of hepatic function (particularly liver function tests and bilirubin). Discontinuation of VFEND must be considered if clinical signs and symptoms consistent with liver disease develop that may be attributable to VFEND (see PRECAUTIONS - Laboratory Tests, DOSAGE AND ADMINISTRATION -

Table 7
Success Rates in Patients Treated for Esophageal Candidiasis

Population	Voriconazole	Fluconazole	Difference % (95% CI)[a]
PP[b]	113/115 (98.2%)	134/141 (95.0%)	3.2 (-1.1, 7.5)
ITT[c]	175/200 (87.5%)	171/191 (89.5%)	-2.0 (-8.3, 4.3)

[a] Confidence Interval for the difference (Voriconazole – Fluconazole) in success rates.
[b] PP (Per Protocol) patients had confirmation of *Candida* esophagitis by endoscopy, received at least 12 days of treatment, and had a repeat endoscopy at EOT (end of treatment).
[c] ITT (Intent to Treat) patients without endoscopy or clinical assessment at EOT were treated as failures.

Table 8
Clinical and mycological outcome by baseline pathogen in patients with esophageal candidiasis (Study 150-305).

Pathogen[a]	Voriconazole		Fluconazole	
	Favorable endoscopic response[b]	Mycological eradication[b]	Favorable endoscopic response[b]	Mycological eradication[b]
	Success/Total (%)	Eradication/Total (%)	Success/Total (%)	Eradication/Total (%)
C. albicans	134/140 (96%)	90/107 (84%)	147/156 (94%)	91/115 (79%)
C. glabrata	8/8 (100%)	4/7 (57%)	4/4 (100%)	1/4 (25%)
C. krusei	1/1	1/1	2/2 (100%)	0/0

[a]Some patients had more than one species isolated at baseline
[b]Patients with endoscopic and/or mycological assessment at end of therapy

Table 9 Effect of Other Drugs on Voriconazole Pharmacokinetics

Drug/Drug Class (Mechanism of Interaction by the Drug)	Voriconazole Plasma Exposure (C_{max} and AUC$_\tau$ after 200 mg Q12h)	Recommendations for Voriconazole Dosage Adjustment/Comments
Rifampin*, Efavirenz** and Rifabutin* (CYP450 Induction)	Significantly Reduced	Contraindicated
Ritonavir (400mg Q12h HIV Protease Inhibitor)** (CYP450 Induction)	Significantly Reduced	Contraindicated The effect of ritonavir (100 mg Q12h as used to inhibit CYP3A and increase concentrations of other antiretroviral drugs) on voriconazole concentrations has not been studied.
Carbamazepine (CYP450 Induction)	Not Studied *In Vivo* or *In Vitro*, but Likely to Result in Significant Reduction	Contraindicated
Long Acting Barbiturates (CYP450 Induction)	Not Studied *In Vivo* or *In Vitro*, but Likely to Result in Significant Reduction	Contraindicated
Phenytoin* (CYP450 Induction)	Significantly Reduced	Increase voriconazole maintenance dose from 4 mg/kg to 5 mg/kg IV every 12 hrs or from 200 mg to 400 mg orally every 12 hrs (100 mg to 200 mg orally every 12 hrs in patients weighing less than 40 kg)
Other HIV Protease Inhibitors (CYP3A4 Inhibition)	*In Vivo* Studies Showed No Significant Effects of Indinavir on Voriconazole Exposure *In Vitro* Studies Demonstrated Potential for Inhibition of Voriconazole Metabolism (Increased Plasma Exposure)	No dosage adjustment in the voriconazole dosage needed when coadministered with indinavir Frequent monitoring for adverse events and toxicity related to voriconazole when coadministered with other HIV protease inhibitors
Other NNRTIs*** (CYP3A4 Inhibition or CYP450 Induction)	*In Vitro* Studies Demonstrated Potential for Inhibition of Voriconazole Metabolism by Delavirdine and Other NNRTIs (Increased Plasma Exposure) A Voriconazole-Efavirenz Drug Interaction Study Demonstrated the Potential for the Metabolism of Voriconazole to be Induced by Efavirenz and Other NNRTIs (Decreased Plasma Exposure)	Frequent monitoring for adverse events and toxicity related to voriconazole Careful assessment of voriconazole effectiveness

*Results based on *in vivo* clinical studies generally following repeat oral dosing with 200 mg Q12h voriconazole to healthy subjects
**Results based on *in vivo* clinical study following repeat oral dosing with 400 mg Q12h for 1 day, then 200 mg Q12h for 8 days voriconazole to healthy subjects
*** Non-Nucleoside Reverse Transcriptase Inhibitors

Dosage Adjustment, ADVERSE EVENTS - Clinical Laboratory Tests).

Pregnancy Category D: Voriconazole can cause fetal harm when administered to a pregnant woman.

Voriconazole was teratogenic in rats (cleft palates, hydronephrosis/hydroureter) from 10 mg/kg (0.3 times the recommended maintenance dose (RMD) on a mg/m² basis) and embryotoxic in rabbits at 100 mg/kg (6 times the RMD). Other effects in rats included reduced ossification of sacral and caudal vertebrae, skull, pubic and hyoid bone, supernumerary ribs, anomalies of the sternebrae and dilatation of the ureter/renal pelvis. Plasma estradiol in pregnant rats was reduced at all dose levels. Voriconazole treatment in rats produced increased gestational length and dystocia, which were associated with increased perinatal pup mortality at the 10 mg/kg dose. The effects seen in rabbits were an increased embryomortality, reduced fetal weight and increased incidences of skeletal variations, cervical ribs and extrasternebral ossification sites.

If this drug is used during pregnancy, or if the patient becomes pregnant while taking this drug, the patient should be apprised of the potential hazard to the fetus.

Galactose intolerance: VFEND tablets contain lactose and should not be given to patients with rare hereditary problems of galactose intolerance, Lapp lactase deficiency or glucose-galactose malabsorption.

PRECAUTIONS

General

(See WARNINGS, DOSAGE AND ADMINISTRATION)

Continued on next page

VFEND—Cont.

Arrhythmias and QT Prolongation

Some azoles, including voriconazole, have been associated with prolongation of the QT interval on the electrocardiogram. During clinical development and post-marketing surveillance, there have been rare cases of arrhythmias, (including ventricular arrhythmias such as *torsade de pointes*), cardiac arrests and sudden deaths in patients taking voriconazole. These cases usually involved seriously ill patients with multiple confounding risk factors, such as history of cardiotoxic chemotherapy, cardiomyopathy, hypokalemia and concomitant medications that may have been contributory.

Voriconazole should be administered with caution to patients with these potentially proarrhythmic conditions.

Rigorous attempts to correct potassium, magnesium and calcium should be made before starting voriconazole (see CLINICAL PHARMACOLOGY - Pharmacokinetic-Pharmacodynamic Relationships - Electrocardiogram).

Infusion Related Reactions

During infusion of the intravenous formulation of voriconazole in healthy subjects, anaphylactoid-type reactions, including flushing, fever, sweating, tachycardia, chest tightness, dyspnea, faintness, nausea, pruritus and rash, have occurred uncommonly. Symptoms appeared immediately upon initiating the infusion. Consideration should be given to stopping the infusion should these reactions occur.

Information for Patients

Patients should be advised:

- that VFEND Tablets or Oral Suspension should be taken at least one hour before, or one hour following, a meal.
- **that they should not drive at night while taking VFEND. VFEND may cause changes to vision, including blurring and/or photophobia.**
- **that they should avoid potentially hazardous tasks, such as driving or operating machinery if they perceive any change in vision.**
- that strong, direct sunlight should be avoided during VFEND therapy.
- that VFEND for Oral Suspension contains sucrose and is not recommended for patients with rare hereditary problems of fructose intolerance, sucrase-isomaltase deficiency or glucose-galactose malabsorption.

Laboratory Tests

Electrolyte disturbances such as hypokalemia, hypomagnesemia and hypocalcemia should be corrected prior to initiation of VFEND therapy.

Patient management should include laboratory evaluation of renal (particularly serum creatinine) and hepatic function (particularly liver function tests and bilirubin).

Drug Interactions

Tables 9 and 10 provide a summary of significant drug interactions with voriconazole that either have been studied *in vivo* (clinically) or that may be expected to occur based on results of *in vitro* metabolism studies with human liver microsomes. For more details, see CLINICAL PHARMACOLOGY - Drug Interactions.

[See table 9 on previous page]

[See table 10 at right and on next page]

Patients with Hepatic Insufficiency

It is recommended that the standard loading dose regimens be used but that the maintenance dose be halved in patients with mild to moderate hepatic cirrhosis (Child-Pugh Class A and B) receiving VFEND (see CLINICAL PHARMACOLOGY - Hepatic Insufficiency, DOSAGE and ADMINISTRATION - Hepatic Insufficiency).

VFEND has not been studied in patients with severe cirrhosis (Child-Pugh Class C). VFEND has been associated with elevations in liver function tests and clinical signs of liver damage, such as jaundice, and should only be used in patients with severe hepatic insufficiency if the benefit outweighs the potential risk. Patients with hepatic insufficiency must be carefully monitored for drug toxicity.

Patients with Renal Insufficiency

In patients with moderate to severe renal dysfunction (creatinine clearance <50 mL/min), accumulation of the intravenous vehicle, SBECD, occurs. Oral voriconazole should be administered to these patients, unless an assessment of the benefit/risk to the patient justifies the use of intravenous voriconazole. Serum creatinine levels should be closely monitored in these patients, and if increases occur, consideration should be given to changing to oral voriconazole therapy (see CLINICAL PHARMACOLOGY - Renal Insufficiency, DOSAGE AND ADMINISTRATION - Renal Insufficiency).

Renal Adverse Events

Acute renal failure has been observed in severely ill patients undergoing treatment with VFEND. Patients being treated with voriconazole are likely to be treated concomitantly with nephrotoxic medications and have concurrent conditions that may result in decreased renal function.

Monitoring of Renal Function

Patients should be monitored for the development of abnormal renal function. This should include laboratory evaluation, particularly serum creatinine.

Dermatological Reactions

Patients have rarely developed serious cutaneous reactions, such as Stevens-Johnson syndrome, during treatment with VFEND. If patients develop a rash, they should be monitored closely and consideration given to discontinuation of VFEND. VFEND has been infrequently associated with

photosensitivity skin reaction, especially during long-term therapy. It is recommended that patients avoid strong, direct sunlight during VFEND therapy.

Carcinogenesis, Mutagenesis, Impairment of Fertility

Two-year carcinogenicity studies were conducted in rats and mice. Rats were given oral doses of 6, 18 or 50 mg/kg voriconazole, or 0.2, 0.6, or 1.6 times the recommended maintenance dose (RMD) on a mg/m^2 basis. Hepatocellular adenomas were detected in females at 50 mg/kg and hepatocellular carcinomas were found in males at 6 and 50 mg/kg. Mice were given oral doses of 10, 30 or 100 mg/kg voriconazole, or 0.1, 0.4, or 1.4 times the RMD on a mg/m^2

Table 10 Effect of Voriconazole on Pharmacokinetics of Other Drugs

Drug/Drug Class (Mechanism of Interaction by Voriconazole)	Drug Plasma Exposure (C_{max} and AUC_τ)	Recommendations for Drug Dosage Adjustment/Comments
Sirolimus* (CYP3A4 Inhibition)	Significantly Increased	**Contraindicated**
Rifabutin* and Efavirenz** (CYP3A4 Inhibition)	Significantly Increased	**Contraindicated**
Ritonavir (400 mg Q12h HIV Protease Inhibitor)** (CYP3A4 Inhibition)	No significant Effect of Voriconazole on Ritonavir C_{max} or AUC_τ	**Contraindicated** because of significant reduction of voriconazole C_{max} and AUC_τ
Terfenadine, Astemizole, Cisapride, Pimozide, Quinidine (CYP3A4 Inhibition)	Not Studied *In Vivo* or *In Vitro*, but Drug Plasma Exposure Likely to be Increased	**Contraindicated** because of potential for QT prolongation and rare occurrence of *torsade de pointes*
Ergot Alkaloids (CYP450 Inhibition)	Not Studied *In Vivo* or *In Vitro*, but Drug Plasma Exposure Likely to be Increased	**Contraindicated**
Cyclosporine* (CYP3A4 Inhibition)	AUC_τ Significantly Increased; No Significant Effect on C_{max}	When initiating therapy with VFEND in patients already receiving cyclosporine, reduce the cyclosporine dose to one-half of the starting dose and follow with frequent monitoring of cyclosporine blood levels. Increased cyclosporine levels have been associated with nephrotoxicity. When VFEND is discontinued, cyclosporine concentrations must be frequently monitored and the dose increased as necessary.
Methadone*** (CYP3A4 Inhibition)	Increased	Increased plasma concentrations of methadone have been associated with toxicity including QT prolongation. Frequent monitoring for adverse events and toxicity related to methadone is recommended during coadministration. Dose reduction of methadone may be needed
Tacrolimus* (CYP3A4 Inhibition)	Significantly Increased	When initiating therapy with VFEND in patients already receiving tacrolimus, reduce the tacrolimus dose to one-third of the starting dose and follow with frequent monitoring of tacrolimus blood levels. Increased tacrolimus levels have been associated with nephrotoxicity. When VFEND is discontinued, tacrolimus concentrations must be frequently monitored and the dose increased as necessary.
Phenytoin* (CYP2C9 Inhibition)	Significantly Increased	Frequent monitoring of phenytoin plasma concentrations and frequent monitoring of adverse effects related to phenytoin.
Warfarin* (CYP2C9 Inhibition)	Prothrombin Time Significantly Increased	Monitor PT or other suitable anticoagulation tests. Adjustment of warfarin dosage may be needed.
Omeprazole* (CYP2C19/3A4 Inhibition)	Significantly Increased	When initiating therapy with VFEND in patients already receiving omeprazole doses of 40 mg or greater, reduce the omeprazole dose by one-half. The metabolism of other proton pump inhibitors that are CYP2C19 substrates may also be inhibited by voriconazole and may result in increased plasma concentrations of other proton pump inhibitors.
Other HIV Protease Inhibitors (CYP3A4 Inhibition)	*In Vivo* Studies Showed No Significant Effects on Indinavir Exposure *In Vitro* Studies Demonstrated Potential for Voriconazole to Inhibit Metabolism (Increased Plasma Exposure)	No dosage adjustment for indinavir when coadministered with VFEND Frequent monitoring for adverse events and toxicity related to other HIV protease inhibitors
Other NNRTIs**** (CYP3A4 Inhibition)	A Voriconazole-Efavirenz Drug Interaction Study Demonstrated the Potential for Voriconazole to Inhibit Metabolism of Other NNRTIs (Increased Plasma Exposure)	Frequent monitoring for adverse events and toxicity related to NNRTI
Benzodiazepines (CYP3A4 Inhibition)	*In Vitro* Studies Demonstrated Potential for Voriconazole to Inhibit Metabolism (Increased Plasma Exposure)	Frequent monitoring for adverse events and toxicity (i.e., prolonged sedation) related to benzodiazepines metabolized by CYP3A4 (e.g., midazolam, triazolam, alprazolam). Adjustment of benzodiazepine dosage may be needed.

(Table continued on next page)

basis. In mice, hepatocellular adenomas were detected in males and females and hepatocellular carcinomas were detected in males at 1.4 times the RMD of voriconazole. Voriconazole demonstrated clastogenic activity (mostly chromosome breaks) in human lymphocyte cultures *in vitro*. Voriconazole was not genotoxic in the Ames assay, CHO assay, the mouse micronucleus assay or the DNA repair test (Unscheduled DNA Synthesis assay).

Voriconazole produced a reduction in the pregnancy rates of rats dosed at 50 mg/kg, or 1.6 times the RMD. This was statistically significant only in the preliminary study and not in a larger fertility study.

Teratogenic Effects

Pregnancy category D (see WARNINGS).

Women of Childbearing Potential

Women of childbearing potential should use effective contraception during treatment.

Nursing Mothers

The excretion of voriconazole in breast milk has not been investigated. VFEND should not be used by nursing mothers unless the benefit clearly outweighs the risk.

Pediatric Use

Safety and effectiveness in pediatric patients below the age of 12 years have not been established.

A total of 22 patients aged 12-18 years with invasive aspergillosis were included in the therapeutic studies. Twelve out of 22 (55%) patients had successful response after treatment with a maintenance dose of voriconazole 4 mg/kg Q12h.

Sparse plasma sampling for pharmacokinetics in adolescents was conducted in the therapeutic studies (see CLINICAL PHARMACOLOGY - Pharmacokinetics, General Pharmacokinetic Characteristics).

Geriatric Use

In multiple dose therapeutic trials of voriconazole, 9.2% of patients were $\geq$ 65 years of age and 1.8% of patients were $\geq$ 75 years of age. In a study in healthy volunteers, the systemic exposure (AUC) and peak plasma concentrations (C_{max}) were increased in elderly males compared to young males. Pharmacokinetic data obtained from 552 patients from 10 voriconazole therapeutic trials showed that voriconazole plasma concentrations in the elderly patients were approximately 80% to 90% higher than those in younger patients after either IV or oral administration. However, the overall safety profile of the elderly patients was similar to that of the young so no dosage adjustment is recommended (see CLINICAL PHARMACOLOGY - Pharmacokinetics in Special Populations).

ADVERSE REACTIONS

Overview

The most frequently reported adverse events (all causalities) in the therapeutic trials were visual disturbances, fever, rash, vomiting, nausea, diarrhea, headache, sepsis, peripheral edema, abdominal pain, and respiratory disorder. The treatment-related adverse events which most often led to discontinuation of voriconazole therapy were elevated liver function tests, rash, and visual disturbances (see hepatic toxicity under WARNINGS and discussion of Clinical Laboratory Values and dermatological and visual adverse events below).

Discussion of Adverse Reactions

The data described in Table 11 reflect exposure to voriconazole in 1655 patients in the therapeutic studies. This represents a heterogeneous population, including immunocompromised patients, e.g., patients with hematological malignancy or HIV and non-neutropenic patients. This subgroup does not include healthy volunteers and patients treated in the compassionate use and non-therapeutic studies. This patient population was 62% male, had a mean age of 46 years (range 11-90, including 51 patients aged 12-18 years), and was 78% white and 10% black. In the initial regulatory filing, 561 patients had a duration of voriconazole therapy of greater than 12 weeks, with 136 patients receiving voriconazole for over six months. Table 11 includes all adverse events which were reported at an incidence of $\geq$2% during voriconazole therapy in the all therapeutic studies population, studies 307/602 and 608 combined, or study 305, as well as events of concern which occurred at an incidence of <2%.

In study 307/602, 381 patients (196 on voriconazole, 185 on amphotericin B) were treated to compare voriconazole to amphotericin B followed by other licensed antifungal therapy in the primary treatment of patients with acute invasive aspergillosis. In study 608, 403 patients with candidemia were treated to compare voriconazole (272 patients) to the regimen of amphotericin B followed by fluconazole (131 patients). Study 305 evaluated the effects of oral voriconazole (200 patients) and oral fluconazole (191 patients) in the treatment of esophageal candidiasis. Laboratory test abnormalities for these studies are discussed under Clinical Laboratory Values below.

[See table 11 above and on next page]

VISUAL DISTURBANCES: Voriconazole treatment-related visual disturbances are common. In therapeutic trials, approximately 21% of patients experienced abnormal vision, color vision changes and/or photophobia. The visual disturbances were generally mild and rarely resulted in discontinuation. Visual disturbances may be associated with higher plasma concentrations and/or doses.

The mechanism of action of the visual disturbance is unknown, although the site of action is most likely to be within the retina. In a study in healthy volunteers investigating the effect of 28-day treatment with voriconazole on retinal function, voriconazole caused a decrease in the electroreti-

Table 10 *(cont.)* Effect of Voriconazole on Pharmacokinetics of Other Drugs

Drug/Drug Class (Mechanism of Interaction by Voriconazole)	Drug Plasma Exposure (C_{max} and AUC_{τ})	Recommendations for Drug Dosage Adjustment/Comments
HMG-CoA Reductase Inhibitors (Statins) (CYP3A4 Inhibition)	*In Vitro* Studies Demonstrated Potential for Voriconazole to Inhibit Metabolism (Increased Plasma Exposure)	Frequent monitoring for adverse events and toxicity related to statins. Increased statin concentrations in plasma have been associated with rhabdomyolysis. Adjustment of the statin dosage may be needed.
Dihydropyridine Calcium Channel Blockers (CYP3A4 Inhibition)	*In Vitro* Studies Demonstrated Potential for Voriconazole to Inhibit Metabolism (Increased Plasma Exposure)	Frequent monitoring for adverse events and toxicity related to calcium channel blockers. Adjustment of calcium channel blocker dosage may be needed.
Sulfonylurea Oral Hypoglycemics (CYP2C9 Inhibition)	Not Studied *In Vivo* or *In Vitro*, but Drug Plasma Exposure Likely to be Increased	Frequent monitoring of blood glucose and for signs and symptoms of hypoglycemia. Adjustment of oral hypoglycemic drug dosage may be needed.
Vinca Alkaloids (CYP3A4 Inhibition)	Not Studied *In Vivo* or *In Vitro*, but Drug Plasma Exposure Likely to be Increased	Frequent monitoring for adverse events and toxicity (i.e., neurotoxicity) related to vinca alkaloids. Adjustment of vinca alkaloid dosage may be needed.

* Results based on *in vivo* clinical studies generally following repeat oral dosing with 200 mg BID voriconazole to healthy subjects
** Results based on *in vivo* clinical study following repeat oral doing with 400 mg Q12h for 1 day, then 200 mg Q12h for 8 days voriconazole to healthy subjects
*** Results based on *in vivo* clinical study following repeat oral doing with 400 mg Q12h for 1 day, then 200 mg Q12h for 4 days voriconazole to subjects receiving a methadone maintenance dose (30-100 mg QD)
**** Non-Nucleoside Reverse Transcriptase Inhibitors

Table 11

Treatment Emergent Adverse Events

Rate $\geq$ 2% on Voriconazole or Adverse Events of Concern in All Therapeutic Studies Population, Studies 307/602-608 Combined, or Study 305. Possibly Related to Therapy or Causality Unknown†

	All Therapeutic Studies	Studies 307/602 and 608 (IV/oral therapy)			Study 305 (oral therapy)	
	Voriconazole N=1655	Voriconazole N=468	Ampho B* N=185	Ampho B → Fluconazole N=131	Voriconazole N=200	Fluconazole N=191
	N (%)	N (%)	N (%)	N (%)	N (%)	N (%)
Special Senses**						
Abnormal vision	310 (18.7)	63 (13.5)	1 (0.5)	0	31 (15.5)	8 (4.2)
Photophobia	37 (2.2)	8 (1.7)	0	0	5 (2.5)	2 (1.0)
Chromatopsia	20 (1.2)	2 (0.4)	0	0	2 (1.0)	0
Body as a Whole						
Fever	94 (5.7)	8 (1.7)	25 (13.5)	5 (3.8)	0	0
Chills	61 (3.7)	1 (0.2)	36 (19.5)	8 (6.1)	1 (0.5)	0
Headache	49 (3.0)	9 (1.9)	8 (4.3)	1 (0.8)	0	1 (0.5)
Cardiovascular System						
Tachycardia	39 (2.4)	6 (1.3)	5 (2.7)	0	0	0
Digestive System						
Nausea	89 (5.4)	18 (3.8)	29 (15.7)	2 (1.5)	2 (1.0)	3 (1.6)
Vomiting	72 (4.4)	15 (3.2)	18 (9.7)	1 (0.8)	2 (1.0)	1 (0.5)
Liver function tests abnormal	45 (2.7)	15 (3.2)	4 (2.2)	1 (0.8)	6 (3.0)	2 (1.0)
Cholestatic jaundice	17 (1.0)	8 (1.7)	0	1 (0.8)	3 (1.5)	0

(Table continued on next page)

nogram (ERG) waveform amplitude, a decrease in the visual field, and an alteration in color perception. The ERG measures electrical currents in the retina. The effects were noted early in administration of voriconazole and continued through the course of study drug dosing. Fourteen days after end of dosing, ERG, visual fields and color perception returned to normal (see WARNINGS, PRECAUTIONS – Information For Patients).

Dermatological Reactions: Dermatological reactions were common in the patients treated with voriconazole. The mechanism underlying these dermatologic adverse events remains unknown. In clinical trials, rashes considered related to therapy were reported by 7% (110/1655) of voriconazole-treated patients. The majority of rashes were of mild to moderate severity. Cases of photosensitivity reactions appear to be more likely to occur with long-term treatment. Patients have rarely developed serious cutaneous reactions, including Stevens-Johnson syndrome, toxic epidermal necrolysis and erythema multiforme during treatment with VFEND. If patients develop a rash, they should be monitored closely and consideration given to dis-

continuation of VFEND. It is recommended that patients avoid strong, direct sunlight during VFEND therapy.

Less Common Adverse Events

The following adverse events occurred in < 2% of all voriconazole-treated patients in all therapeutic studies (N=1655). This listing includes events where a causal relationship to voriconazole cannot be ruled out or those which may help the physician in managing the risks to the patients. The list does not include events included in Table 11 above and does not include every event reported in the voriconazole clinical program.

Body as a Whole: abdominal pain, abdomen enlarged, allergic reaction, anaphylactoid reaction (see PRECAUTIONS), ascites, asthenia, back pain, chest pain, cellulitis, edema, face edema, flank pain, flu syndrome, graft versus host reaction, granuloma, infection, bacterial infection, fungal infection, injection site pain, injection site infection/inflammation, mucous membrane disorder, multi-organ failure, pain, pelvic pain, peritonitis, sepsis, substernal chest pain

Continued on next page

VFEND—Cont.

Cardiovascular: atrial arrhythmia, atrial fibrillation, AV block complete, bigeminy, bradycardia, bundle branch block, cardiomegaly, cardiomyopathy, cerebral hemorrhage, cerebral ischemia, cerebrovascular accident, congestive heart failure, deep thrombophlebitis, endocarditis, extrasystoles, heart arrest, hypertension, hypotension, myocardial infarction, nodal arrhythmia, palpitation, phlebitis, postural hypotension, pulmonary embolus, QT interval prolonged, supraventricular extrasystoles, supraventricular tachycardia, syncope, thrombophlebitis, vasodilatation, ventricular arrhythmia, ventricular fibrillation, ventricular tachycardia (including *torsade de pointes*)

Digestive: anorexia, cheilitis, cholecystitis, cholelithiasis, constipation, diarrhea, duodenal ulcer perforation, duodenitis, dyspepsia, dysphagia, dry mouth, esophageal ulcer, esophagitis, flatulence, gastroenteritis, gastrointestinal hemorrhage, GGT/LDH elevated, gingivitis, glossitis, gum hemorrhage, gum hyperplasia, hematemesis, hepatic coma, hepatic failure, hepatitis, intestinal perforation, intestinal ulcer, jaundice, enlarged liver, melena, mouth ulceration, pancreatitis, parotid gland enlargement, periodontitis, proctitis, pseudomembranous colitis, rectal disorder, rectal hemorrhage, stomach ulcer, stomatitis, tongue edema

Endocrine: adrenal cortex insufficiency, diabetes insipidus, hyperthyroidism, hypothyroidism

Hemic and Lymphatic: agranulocytosis, anemia (macrocytic, megaloblastic, microcytic, normocytic), aplastic anemia, hemolytic anemia, bleeding time increased, cyanosis, DIC, ecchymosis, eosinophilia, hypervolemia, leukopenia, lymphadenopathy, lymphangitis, marrow depression, pancytopenia, petechia, purpura, enlarged spleen, thrombocytopenia, thrombotic thrombocytopenic purpura

Metabolic and Nutritional: albuminuria, BUN increased, creatine phosphokinase increased, edema, glucose tolerance decreased, hypercalcemia, hypercholesteremia, hyperglycemia, hyperkalemia, hypermagnesemia, hypernatremia, hyperuricemia, hypocalcemia, hypoglycemia, hypomagnesemia, hyponatremia, hypophosphatemia, peripheral edema, uremia

Musculoskeletal: arthralgia, arthritis, bone necrosis, bone pain, leg cramps, myalgia, myasthenia, myopathy, osteomalacia, osteoporosis

Nervous System: abnormal dreams, acute brain syndrome, agitation, akathisia, amnesia, anxiety, ataxia, brain edema, coma, confusion, convulsion, delirium, dementia, depersonalization, depression, diplopia, dizziness, encephalitis, encephalopathy, euphoria, Extrapyramidal Syndrome, grand mal convulsion, Guillain-Barré syndrome, hypertonia, hypesthesia, insomnia, intracranial hypertension, libido decreased, neuralgia, neuropathy, nystagmus, oculogyric crisis, paresthesia, psychosis, somnolence, suicidal ideation, tremor, vertigo

Respiratory System: cough increased, dyspnea, epistaxis, hemoptysis, hypoxia, lung edema, pharyngitis, pleural effusion, pneumonia, respiratory disorder, respiratory distress syndrome, respiratory tract infection, rhinitis, sinusitis, voice alteration

Skin and Appendages: alopecia, angioedema, contact dermatitis, discoid lupus erythematosis, eczema, erythema multiforme, exfoliative dermatitis, fixed drug eruption, furunculosis, herpes simplex, maculopapular rash, melanosis, photosensitivity skin reaction, pruritus, psoriasis, skin discoloration, skin disorder, skin dry, Stevens-Johnson syndrome, sweating, toxic epidermal necrolysis, urticaria

Special Senses: abnormality of accommodation, blepharitis, color blindness, conjunctivitis, corneal opacity, deafness, ear pain, eye pain, eye hemorrhage, dry eyes, hypoacusis, keratitis, keratoconjunctivitis, mydriasis, night blindness, optic atrophy, optic neuritis, otitis externa, papilledema, retinal hemorrhage, retinitis, scleritis, taste loss, taste perversion, tinnitus, uveitis, visual field defect

Urogenital: anuria, blighted ovum, creatinine clearance decreased, dysmenorrhea, dysuria, epididymitis, glycosuria, hemorrhagic cystitis, hematuria, hydronephrosis, impotence, kidney pain, kidney tubular necrosis, metrorrhagia, nephritis, nephrosis, oliguria, scrotal edema, urinary incontinence, urinary retention, urinary tract infection, uterine hemorrhage, vaginal hemorrhage

Clinical Laboratory Values

The overall incidence of clinically significant transaminase abnormalities in all therapeutic studies was 12.4% (206/1655) of patients treated with voriconazole. Increased incidence of liver function test abnormalities may be associated with higher plasma concentrations and/or doses. The majority of abnormal liver function tests either resolved during treatment without dose adjustment or following dose adjustment, including discontinuation of therapy.

Voriconazole has been infrequently associated with cases of serious hepatic toxicity including cases of jaundice and rare cases of hepatitis and hepatic failure leading to death. Most of these patients had other serious underlying conditions.

Liver function tests should be evaluated at the start of and during the course of VFEND therapy. Patients who develop abnormal liver function tests during VFEND therapy should be monitored for the development of more severe hepatic injury. Patient management should include laboratory evaluation of hepatic function (particularly liver function tests and bilirubin). Discontinuation of VFEND must be considered if clinical signs and symptoms consistent with liver disease develop that may be attributable to VFEND (see WARNINGS and PRECAUTIONS - Laboratory Tests).

Table 11 *(cont.)*
Treatment Emergent Adverse Events
Rate ≥ 2% on Voriconazole or Adverse Events of Concern in All Therapeutic Studies Population, Studies 307/602-608 Combined, or Study 305. Possibly Related to Therapy or Causality Unknown†

	All Therapeutic Studies	Studies 307/602 and 608 (IV/oral therapy)			Study 305 (oral therapy)	
	Voriconazole N=1655	Voriconazole N=468	Ampho B* N=185	Ampho B → Fluconazole N=131	Voriconazole N=200	Fluconazole N=191
	N (%)	N (%)	N (%)	N (%)	N (%)	N (%)
Metabolic and Nutritional Systems						
Alkaline phosphatase increased	59 (3.6)	19 (4.1)	4 (2.2)	3 (2.3)	10 (5.0)	3 (1.6)
Hepatic enzymes increased	30 (1.8)	11 (2.4)	5 (2.7)	1 (0.8)	3 (1.5)	0
SGOT increased	31 (1.9)	9 (1.9)	0	1 (0.8)	8 (4.0)	2 (1.0)
SGPT increased	29 (1.8)	9 (1.9)	1 (0.5)	2 (1.5)	6 (3.0)	2 (1.0)
Hypokalemia	26 (1.6)	3 (0.6)	36 (19.5)	16 (12.2)	0	0
Bilirubinemia	15 (0.9)	5 (1.1)	3 (1.6)	2 (1.5)	1 (0.5)	0
Creatinine increased	4 (0.2)	0	59 (31.9)	10 (7.6)	1 (0.5)	0
Nervous System						
Hallucinations	39 (2.4)	13 (2.8)	1 (0.5)	0	0	0
Skin and Appendages						
Rash	88 (5.3)	20 (4.3)	7 (3.8)	1 (0.8)	3 (1.5)	1 (0.5)
Urogenital						
Kidney function abnormal	10 (0.6)	6 (1.3)	40 (21.6)	9 (6.9)	1 (0.5)	1 (0.5)
Acute kidney failure	7 (0.4)	2 (0.4)	11 (5.9)	7 (5.3)	0	0

†Study 307/602: invasive aspergillosis; Study 608: candidemia; Study 305: esophageal candidiasis
*Amphotericin B followed by other licensed antifungal therapy
**See WARNINGS – Visual Disturbances, PRECAUTIONS – Information for Patients

Table 12
Protocol 305
Clinically Significant Laboratory Test Abnormalities

	Criteria*	Voriconazole	Fluconazole
		n/N (%)	n/N (%)
T. Bilirubin	>1.5× ULN	8/185 (4.3)	7/186 (3.8)
AST	>3.0× ULN	38/187 (20.3)	15/186 (8.1)
ALT	>3.0× ULN	20/187 (10.7)	12/186 (6.5)
Alk phos	>3.0× ULN	19/187 (10.2)	14/186 (7.5)

*   Without regard to baseline value
n   number of patients with a clinically significant abnormality while on study therapy
N   total number of patients with at least one observation of the given lab test while on study therapy
ULN upper limit of normal

Table 13
Protocol 307/602
Clinically Significant Laboratory Test Abnormalities

	Criteria*	Voriconazole	Amphotericin B**
		n/N (%)	n/N (%)
T. Bilirubin	>1.5× ULN	35/180 (19.4)	46/173 (26.6)
AST	>3.0× ULN	21/180 (11.7)	18/174 (10.3)
ALT	>3.0× ULN	34/180 (18.9)	40/173 (23.1)
Alk phos	>3.0× ULN	29/181 (16.0)	38/173 (22.0)
Creatinine	>1.3× ULN	39/182 (21.4)	102/177 (57.6)
Potassium	<0.9× LLN	30/181 (16.6)	70/178 (39.3)

*   Without regard to baseline value
**   Amphotericin B followed by other licensed antifungal therapy
n   number of patients with a clinically significant abnormality while on study therapy
N   total number of patients with at least one observation of the given lab test while on study therapy
ULN upper limit of normal
LLN lower limit of normal

Acute renal failure has been observed in severely ill patients undergoing treatment with VFEND. Patients being treated with voriconazole are likely to be treated concomitantly with nephrotoxic medications and have concurrent conditions that may result in decreased renal function. It is recommended that patients are monitored for the development of abnormal renal function. This should include laboratory evaluation, particularly serum creatinine.

Tables 12 and 13 and 14 show the number of patients with hypokalemia and clinically significant changes in renal and liver function tests in three randomized, comparative multicenter studies. In study 305, patients with esophageal candidiasis were randomized to either oral voriconazole or oral fluconazole. In study 307/602, patients with definite or probable invasive aspergillosis were randomized to either voriconazole or amphotericin B therapy. In study 608, patients with candidemia were randomized to either voriconazole or the regimen of amphotericin B followed by fluconazole.

[See table 12 on previous page]
[See table 13 on previous page]
[See table 14 at right]

OVERDOSE

In clinical trials, there were three cases of accidental overdose. All occurred in pediatric patients who received up to five times the recommended intravenous dose of voriconazole. A single adverse event of photophobia of 10 minutes duration was reported.

There is no known antidote to voriconazole.

Voriconazole is hemodialyzed with clearance of 121 mL/min. The intravenous vehicle, SBECD, is hemodialyzed with clearance of 55 mL/min. In an overdose, hemodialysis may assist in the removal of voriconazole and SBECD from the body.

The minimum lethal oral dose in mice and rats was 300 mg/kg (equivalent to 4 and 7 times the recommended maintenance dose (RMD), based on body surface area). At this dose, clinical signs observed in both mice and rats included salivation, mydriasis, titubation (loss of balance while moving), depressed behavior, prostration, partially closed eyes, and dyspnea. Other signs in mice were convulsions, corneal opacification and swollen abdomen.

DOSAGE AND ADMINISTRATION
Administration
VFEND Tablets or Oral Suspension should be taken at least one hour before, or one hour following, a meal.
VFEND I.V. for Injection requires reconstitution to 10 mg/mL and subsequent dilution to 5 mg/mL or less prior to administration as an infusion, at a maximum rate of 3 mg/kg per hour over 1-2 hours (see Intravenous Administration).

NOT FOR IV BOLUS INJECTION
Electrolyte disturbances such as hypokalemia, hypomagnesemia and hypocalcemia should be corrected prior to initiation of VFEND therapy (see PRECAUTIONS).
Use in Adults
Invasive aspergillosis and serious fungal infections due to *Fusarium* spp. and *Scedosporium apiospermum*:
For the treatment of adults with invasive aspergillosis and infections due to *Fusarium* spp. and *Scedosporium apiospermum*, therapy must be initiated with the specified loading dose regimen of intravenous VFEND to achieve plasma concentrations on Day 1 that are close to steady state. On the basis of high oral bioavailability, switching between intravenous and oral administration is appropriate when clinically indicated (see CLINICAL PHARMACOLOGY). Once the patient can tolerate medication given by mouth, the oral tablet form or oral suspension form of VFEND may be utilized. (See Table 15.)
Candidemia in nonneutropenic patients and other deep tissue *Candida* infections:
See Table 15. Patients should be treated for at least 14 days following resolution of symptoms or following last positive culture, whichever is longer.
Esophageal Candidiasis
See Table 15. Patients should be treated for a minimum of 14 days and for at least 7 days following resolution of symptoms.
[See table 15 above]
Dosage Adjustment
If patient response is inadequate, the oral maintenance dose may be increased from 200 mg every 12 hours to 300 mg every 12 hours. For adult patients weighing less than 40 kg, the oral maintenance dose may be increased from 100 mg every 12 hours to 150 mg every 12 hours. If patients are unable to tolerate 300 mg orally every 12 hours, reduce the oral maintenance dose by 50 mg steps to a minimum of 200 mg every 12 hours (or to 100 mg every 12 hours for adult patients weighing less than 40 kg).
If patients are unable to tolerate 4 mg/kg IV, reduce the intravenous maintenance dose to 3 mg/kg every 12 hours.
Phenytoin may be coadministered with VFEND if the intravenous maintenance dose of VFEND is increased to 5 mg/kg every 12 hours, or the oral maintenance dose is increased from 200 mg to 400 mg every 12 hours (100 mg to 200 mg every 12 hours in adult patients weighing less than 40 kg) (see CLINICAL PHARMACOLOGY, PRECAUTIONS - Drug Interactions).
Duration of therapy should be based on the severity of the patient's underlying disease, recovery from immunosuppression, and clinical response.
Use in Geriatric Patients
No dose adjustment is necessary for geriatric patients.
Use in Patients with Hepatic Insufficiency
In the clinical program, patients were included who had baseline liver function tests (ALT, AST) up to 5 times the upper limit of normal. No dose adjustment is necessary in patients with this degree of abnormal liver function, but continued monitoring of liver function tests for further elevations is recommended (see WARNINGS).
It is recommended that the standard loading dose regimens be used but that the maintenance dose be halved in patients with mild to moderate hepatic cirrhosis (Child-Pugh Class A and B).
VFEND has not been studied in patients with severe hepatic cirrhosis (Child-Pugh Class C) or in patients with chronic hepatitis B or chronic hepatitis C disease. VFEND has been associated with elevations in liver function tests and clinical signs of liver damage, such as jaundice, and should only be used in patients with severe hepatic insuffi-

Table 14
Protocol 608
Clinically Significant Laboratory Test Abnormalities

	Criteria*	Voriconazole	Amphotericin B followed by Fluconazole
		n/N (%)	n/N (%)
T. Bilirubin	>1.5× ULN	50/261 (19.2)	31/115 (27.0)
AST	>3.0× ULN	40/261 (15.3)	16/116 (13.8)
ALT	>3.0× ULN	22/261 (8.4)	15/116 (12.9)
Alk phos	>3.0× ULN	59/261 (22.6)	26/115 (22.6)
Creatinine	>1.3× ULN	39/260 (15.0)	32/118 (27.1)
Potassium	<0.9× LLN	43/258 (16.7)	35/118 (29.7)

* Without regard to baseline value
n number of patients with a clinically significant abnormality while on study therapy
N total number of patients with at least one observation of the given lab test while on study therapy
ULN upper limit of normal
LLN lower limit of normal

Table 15
Recommended Dosing Regimen

Infection	Loading Dose	Maintenance Dose	
	IV	IV	Oral[a]
Invasive Aspergillosis	6 mg/kg q12h for the first 24 hours	4 mg/kg q12h	200 mg q12h
Candidemia in nonneutropenic patients and other deep tissue *Candida* infections	6 mg/kg q12h for the first 24 hours	3-4 mg/kg q12h[b]	200 mg q12h
Esophageal Candidiasis	c	c	200 mg q12h
Scedosporiosis and Fusariosis	6 mg/kg q12h for the first 24 hours	4 mg/kg q12h	200 mg q12h

[a] Patients who weigh 40 kg or more should receive an oral maintenance dose of 200 mg VFEND every 12 hours. Adult patients who weigh less than 40 kg should receive an oral maintenance dose of 100 mg every 12 hours.
[b] In clinical trials, patients with candidemia received 3 mg/kg q12h as primary therapy, while patients with other deep tissue *Candida* infections received 4 mg/kg as salvage therapy. Appropriate dose should be based on the severity and nature of the infection.
[c] Not evaluated in patients with esophageal candidiasis.

Table 16 Required Volumes of 10 mg/mL VFEND Concentrate

Body Weight (kg)	Volume of VFEND Concentrate (10 mg/mL) required for:		
	3 mg/kg dose (number of vials)	4 mg/kg dose (number of vials)	6 mg/kg dose (number of vials)
30	9.0 mL (1)	12 mL (1)	18 mL (1)
35	10.5 mL (1)	14 mL (1)	21 mL (2)
40	12.0 mL (1)	16 mL (1)	24 mL (2)
45	13.5 mL (1)	18 mL (1)	27 mL (2)
50	15.0 mL (1)	20 mL (1)	30 mL (2)
55	16.5 mL (1)	22 mL (2)	33 mL (2)
60	18.0 mL (1)	24 mL (2)	36 mL (2)
65	19.5 mL (1)	26 mL (2)	39 mL (2)
70	21.0 mL (2)	28 mL (2)	42 mL (3)
75	22.5 mL (2)	30 mL (2)	45 mL (3)
80	24.0 mL (2)	32 mL (2)	48 mL (3)
85	25.5 mL (2)	34 mL (2)	51 mL (3)
90	27.0 mL (2)	36 mL (2)	54 mL (3)
95	28.5 mL (2)	38 mL (2)	57 mL (3)
100	30.0 mL (2)	40 mL (2)	60 mL (3)

ciency if the benefit outweighs the potential risk. Patients with hepatic insufficiency must be carefully monitored for drug toxicity.
Use in Patients with Renal Insufficiency
The pharmacokinetics of orally administered VFEND are not significantly affected by renal insufficiency. Therefore, no adjustment is necessary for oral dosing in patients with mild to severe renal impairment (see CLINICAL PHARMACOLOGY - Special Populations).
In patients with moderate or severe renal insufficiency (creatinine clearance <50 mL/min), accumulation of the intravenous vehicle, SBECD, occurs. Oral voriconazole should be administered to these patients, unless an assessment of the benefit/risk to the patient justifies the use of intravenous voriconazole. Serum creatinine levels should be closely mon-

itored in these patients, and, if increases occur, consideration should be given to changing to oral voriconazole therapy (see DOSAGE and ADMINISTRATION).
Voriconazole is hemodialyzed with clearance of 121 mL/min. The intravenous vehicle, SBECD, is hemodialyzed with clearance of 55 mL/min. A 4-hour hemodialysis session does not remove a sufficient amount of voriconazole to warrant dose adjustment.
Intravenous Administration
VFEND I.V. For Injection:
Reconstitution
The powder is reconstituted with 19 mL of Water For Injection to obtain an extractable volume of 20 mL of clear con-

Continued on next page

VFEND—Cont.

centrate containing 10 mg/mL of voriconazole. It is recommended that a standard 20 mL (non-automated) syringe be used to ensure that the exact amount (19.0 mL) of Water for Injection is dispensed. Discard the vial if a vacuum does not pull the diluent into the vial. Shake the vial until all the powder is dissolved.

Dilution

VFEND must be infused over 1-2 hours, at a concentration of 5 mg/mL or less. Therefore, the required volume of the 10 mg/mL VFEND concentrate should be further diluted as follows (appropriate diluents listed below):

1. Calculate the volume of 10 mg/mL VFEND concentrate required based on the patient's weight (see Table 16).
2. In order to allow the required volume of VFEND concentrate to be added, withdraw and discard at least an equal volume of diluent from the infusion bag or bottle to be used. The volume of diluent remaining in the bag or bottle should be such that when the 10 mg/mL VFEND concentrate is added, the final concentration is not less than 0.5 mg/mL nor greater than 5 mg/mL.
3. Using a suitable size syringe and aseptic technique, withdraw the required volume of VFEND concentrate from the appropriate number of vials and add to the infusion bag or bottle. **Discard Partially Used Vials.**

The final VFEND solution must be infused over 1-2 hours at a maximum rate of 3 mg/kg per hour.

[See table 16 on previous page]

VFEND I.V. for Injection is a single dose unpreserved sterile lyophile. Therefore, from a microbiological point of view, once reconstituted, the product should be used immediately. If not used immediately, in-use storage times and conditions prior to use are the responsibility of the user and should not be longer than 24 hours at 2° to 8°C (36° to 46°F). This medicinal product is for single use only and any unused solution should be discarded. Only clear solutions without particles should be used.

The reconstituted solution can be diluted with:
9 mg/mL (0.9%) Sodium Chloride USP
Lactated Ringers USP
5% Dextrose and Lactated Ringers USP
5% Dextrose and 0.45% Sodium Chloride USP
5% Dextrose USP
5% Dextrose and 20 mEq Potassium Chloride USP
0.45% Sodium Chloride USP
5% Dextrose and 0.9% Sodium Chloride USP

The compatibility of VFEND I.V. with diluents other than those described above is unknown (see Incompatibilities below).

Parenteral drug products should be inspected visually for particulate matter and discoloration prior to administration, whenever solution and container permit.

Incompatibilities:

VFEND I.V. must not be infused into the same line or cannula concomitantly with other drug infusions, including parenteral nutrition, e.g., Aminofusin 10% Plus. Aminofusin 10% Plus is physically incompatible, with an increase in subvisible particulate matter after 24 hours of storage at 4°C.

Infusions of blood products must not occur simultaneously with VFEND I.V.

Infusions of total parenteral nutrition can occur simultaneously with VFEND I.V.

VFEND I.V. must not be diluted with 4.2% Sodium Bicarbonate Infusion. The mildly alkaline nature of this diluent caused slight degradation of VFEND after 24 hours storage at room temperature. Although refrigerated storage is recommended following reconstitution, use of this diluent is not recommended as a precautionary measure. Compatibility with other concentrations is unknown.

VFEND for Oral Suspension

Reconstitution

Tap the bottle to release the powder. Add 46 mL of water to the bottle. Shake the closed bottle vigorously for about 1 minute. Remove child-resistant cap and push bottle adaptor into the neck of the bottle. Replace the cap. Write the date of expiration of the reconstituted suspension on the bottle label (the shelf-life of the reconstituted suspension is 14 days at controlled room temperature 15-30°C [59-86°F]).

Instructions for use

Shake the closed bottle of reconstituted suspension for approximately 10 seconds before each use. The reconstituted oral suspension should only be administered using the oral dispenser supplied with each pack.

Incompatibilities

VFEND for Oral Suspension and the 40 mg/mL reconstituted oral suspension should not be mixed with any other medication or additional flavoring agent. It is not intended that the suspension be further diluted with water or other vehicles.

HOW SUPPLIED

Powder for Solution for Injection

VFEND I.V. for Injection is supplied in a single use vial as a sterile lyophilized powder equivalent to 200 mg VFEND and 3200 mg sulfobutyl ether beta-cyclodextrin sodium (SBECD).

Individually packaged vials of 200 mg VFEND I.V.
(NDC 0049-3190-28)

Tablets

VFEND 50 mg tablets; white, film-coated, round, debossed with "Pfizer" on one side and "VOR50" on the reverse.
Bottles of 30 (NDC 0049-3170-30)

VFEND 200 mg tablets; white, film-coated, capsule shaped, debossed with "Pfizer" on one side and "VOR200" on the reverse.
Bottles of 30 (NDC 0049-3180-30)

Powder for Oral Suspension

VFEND for Oral Suspension is supplied in 100 mL high density polyethylene (HDPE) bottles. Each bottle contains 45 g of powder for oral suspension. Following reconstitution, the volume of the suspension is 75 mL, providing a usable volume of 70 mL (40 mg voriconazole/mL). A 5 mL oral dispenser and a press-in bottle adaptor are also provided.
(NDC 0049-3160-44)

STORAGE

VFEND I.V. for Injection unreconstituted vials should be stored at 15° - 30°C (59° - 86°F) [see USP Controlled Room Temperature]. VFEND is a single dose unpreserved sterile lyophile. From a microbiological point of view, following reconstitution of the lyophile with Water for Injection, the reconstituted solution should be used immediately. If not used immediately, in-use storage times and conditions prior to use are the responsibility of the user and should not be longer than 24 hours at 2° to 8°C (36° to 46°F). Chemical and physical in-use stability has been demonstrated for 24 hours at 2° to 8°C (36° to 46°F). This medicinal product is for single use only and any unused solution should be discarded. Only clear solutions without particles should be used (see DOSAGE AND ADMINISTRATION - Intravenous Administration).

VFEND Tablets should be stored at 15° - 30°C (59° - 86°F) [see USP Controlled Room Temperature].

VFEND Powder for Oral Suspension should be stored at 2° - 8°C (36° - 46° F) (in a refrigerator) before reconstitution. The shelf-life of the powder for oral suspension is 18 months. The reconstituted suspension should be stored at 15° - 30°C (59° - 86°F) [see USP Controlled Room Temperature]. Do not refrigerate or freeze. Keep the container tightly closed. The shelf-life of the reconstituted suspension is 14 days. Any remaining suspension should be discarded 14 days after reconstitution.

REFERENCES

1. National Committee for Clinical Laboratory Standards. Reference method for broth dilution antifungal susceptibility testing of conidium-forming filamentous fungi. Approved Standard M38-P. National Committee for Clinical Laboratory Standards, Villanova, Pa.
2. National Committee for Clinical Laboratory Standards. Reference method for broth dilution antifungal susceptibility testing of yeasts. Approved Standard M27-A. National Committee for Clinical Laboratory Standards, Villanova, Pa.

Rx only

Distributed by
Pfizer Roerig
Division of Pfizer Inc, NY, NY 10017
LAB-0271-12 Revised March 2005

VIRACEPT® ℞

[*vī-ră-cept*]
(nelfinavir mesylate)
TABLETS and ORAL POWDER

Prescribing information for this product, which appears on pages 2659–2665 of the 2005 PDR, has been completely revised as follows. Please write "See Supplement A" next to the product heading.

DESCRIPTION

VIRACEPT® (nelfinavir mesylate) is an inhibitor of the human immunodeficiency virus (HIV) protease. VIRACEPT Tablets are available for oral administration as a light blue, capsule-shaped tablet with a clear film coating in 250 mg strength (as nelfinavir free base) and as a white oval tablet with a clear film coating in 625 mg strength (as nelfinavir free base). Each tablet contains the following common inactive ingredients: calcium silicate, crospovidone, magnesium stearate, hypromellose, and triacetin. In addition, the 250 mg tablet contains FD&C blue #2 powder and the 625 mg tablet contains colloidal silicon dioxide. VIRACEPT Oral Powder is available for oral administration in a 50 mg/g strength (as nelfinavir free base) in bottles. The oral powder also contains the following inactive ingredients: microcrystalline cellulose, maltodextrin, dibasic potassium phosphate, crospovidone, hypromellose, aspartame, sucrose palmitate, and natural and artificial flavor. The chemical name for nelfinavir mesylate is [3*S*-[2(2*S**, 3*S**), 3α,4aβ,8aβ]]-*N*-(1,1-dimethylethyl)decahydro-2-[2-hydroxy-3-[(3-hydroxy-2-methylbenzoyl)amino]-4-(phenylthio)butyl]-3-isoquinoline carboxamide mono-methanesulfonate (salt) and the molecular weight is 663.90 (567.79 as the free base). Nelfinavir mesylate has the following structural formula:

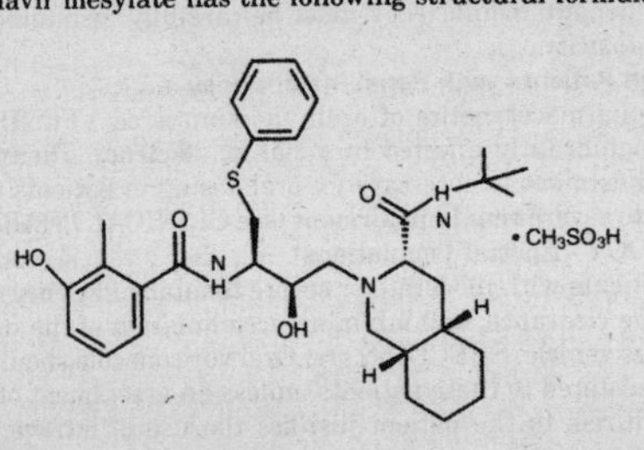

Nelfinavir mesylate is a white to off-white amorphous powder, slightly soluble in water at pH ≤4 and freely soluble in methanol, ethanol, 2-propanol and propylene glycol.

MICROBIOLOGY

Mechanism of Action: Nelfinavir is an inhibitor of the HIV-1 protease. Inhibition of the viral protease prevents cleavage of the *gag* and *gag-pol* polyprotein resulting in the production of immature, non-infectious virus.

Antiviral Activity In Vitro: The antiviral activity of nelfinavir *in vitro* has been demonstrated in both acute and/or chronic HIV infections in lymphoblastoid cell lines, peripheral blood lymphocytes and monocytes/macrophages. Nelfinavir was found to be active against several laboratory strains and clinical isolates of HIV-1 and the HIV-2 strain ROD. The EC_{95} (95% effective concentration) of nelfinavir ranged from 7 to 196 nM. Drug combination studies with protease inhibitors showed nelfinavir had antagonistic interactions with indinavir, additive interactions with ritonavir or saquinavir and synergistic interactions with amprenavir and lopinavir. Minimal to no cellular cytotoxicity was observed with any of these protease inhibitors alone or in combination with nelfinavir. In combination with reverse transcriptase inhibitors, nelfinavir demonstrated additive (didanosine or stavudine) to synergistic (abacavir, delavirdine, efavirenz, lamivudine, nevirapine, tenofovir, zalcitabine or zidovudine) antiviral activity *in vitro* without enhanced cytotoxicity.

Drug Resistance: HIV-1 isolates with reduced susceptibility to nelfinavir have been selected *in vitro.* HIV isolates from selected patients treated with nelfinavir alone or in combination with reverse transcriptase inhibitors were monitored for phenotypic (n=19) and genotypic (n=195, 157 of which were evaluable) changes in clinical trials over a period of 2 to 82 weeks. One or more viral protease mutations at amino acid positions 30, 35, 36, 46, 71, 77 and 88 were detected in the HIV-1 of >10% of patients with evaluable isolates. The overall incidence of the D30N mutation in the viral protease of evaluable isolates (n=157) from patients receiving nelfinavir monotherapy or nelfinavir in combination with zidovudine and lamivudine or stavudine was 54.8%. The overall incidence of other mutations associated with primary protease inhibitor resistance was 9.6% for the L90M substitution whereas substitutions at 48, 82, or 84 were not observed. Of the 19 clinical isolates for which both phenotypic and genotypic analyses were performed, 9 showed reduced susceptibility (5- to 93-fold) to nelfinavir *in vitro.* All 9 patient isolates possessed one or more mutations in the viral protease gene. Amino acid position 30 appeared to be the most frequent mutation site.

Cross-resistance: Non-clinical Studies- Patient-derived recombinant HIV isolates containing the D30N mutation (n=4) and demonstrating high-level (>10-fold) NFV-resistance remained susceptible (<2.5-fold resistance) to amprenavir, indinavir, lopinavir, and saquinavir, *in vitro.* Patient-derived recombinant HIV isolates containing the L90M mutation (n=8) demonstrated moderate to high-level resistance to NFV and had varying levels of susceptibility to amprenavir, indinavir, lopinavir, and saquinavir, *in vitro.* Most patient-derived recombinant isolates with phenotypic and genotypic evidence of reduced susceptibility (>2.5-fold) to amprenavir, indinavir, lopinavir, and/or saquinavir demonstrated high-level cross-resistance to nelfinavir, *in vitro.* Mutations associated with resistance to other PIs (e.g. G48V, V82A/F/T, I84V, L90M) appeared to confer high-level cross-resistance to NFV. Following ritonavir therapy 6 of 7 clinical isolates with decreased ritonavir susceptibility (8- to 113-fold) *in vitro* compared to baseline also exhibited decreased susceptibility to nelfinavir *in vitro* (5- to 40-fold). Cross-resistance between nelfinavir and reverse transcriptase inhibitors is unlikely because different enzyme targets are involved. Clinical isolates (n=5) with decreased susceptibility to lamivudine, nevirapine or zidovudine remain fully susceptible to nelfinavir *in vitro.*

Clinical Studies- There have been no controlled or comparative studies evaluating the virologic response to subsequent protease inhibitor-containing regimens in patients who have demonstrated loss of virologic response to a nelfinavir-containing regimen. However, virologic response was evaluated in a single-arm prospective study of 26 patients with extensive prior antiretroviral experience with reverse transcriptase inhibitors (mean 2.9) who had received VIRACEPT for a mean duration of 59.7 weeks and were switched to a ritonavir (400 mg BID)/saquinavir hard-gel (400 mg BID) containing regimen after a prolonged period of VIRACEPT failure (median 48 weeks). Sequence analysis of HIV-1 isolates prior to switch demonstrated a D30N or an L90M substitution in 18 and 6 patients, respectively. Subjects remained on therapy for a mean of 48 weeks (range 40 to 56 weeks) where 17 of 26 (65%) subjects and 13 of 26 (50%) subjects were treatment responders with HIV RNA below the assay limit of detection (<500 HIV RNA copies/mL, Chiron bDNA) at 24 and 48 weeks, respectively.

CLINICAL PHARMACOLOGY

Pharmacokinetics

The pharmacokinetic properties of nelfinavir were evaluated in healthy volunteers and HIV-infected patients; no substantial differences were observed between the two groups.

Absorption: Pharmacokinetic parameters of nelfinavir (area under the plasma concentration-time curve during a 24-hour period at steady-state [AUC_{24}], peak plasma concentrations [C_{max}], morning and evening trough concentrations [C_{trough}]) from a pharmacokinetic study in HIV-positive patients after multiple dosing with 1250 mg (five 250 mg tablets) twice daily (BID) for 28 days (10 patients) and 750 mg (three 250 mg tablets) three times daily (TID) for 28 days (11 patients) are summarized in Table 1.

Table 1
Summary of a Pharmacokinetic Study in HIV-positive Patients with Multiple Dosing of 1250 mg BID for 28 days and 750 mg TID for 28 days

Regimen	AUC_{24} mg.h/L	C_{max} mg/L	C_{trough} Morning mg/L	C_{trough} Afternoon or Evening mg/L
1250 mg BID	52.8 ± 15.7	4.0 ± 0.8	2.2 ± 1.3	0.7 ± 0.4
750 mg TID	43.6 ± 17.8	3.0 ± 1.6	1.4 ± 0.6	1.0 ± 0.5

data are mean ± SD

The difference between morning and afternoon or evening trough concentrations for the TID and BID regimens was also observed in healthy volunteers who were dosed at precisely 8- or 12-hour intervals.

In healthy volunteers receiving a single 1250 mg dose, the 625 mg tablet was not bioequivalent to the 250 mg tablet formulation. Under fasted conditions (n=27), the AUC and C_{max} were 34% and 24% higher, respectively, for the 625 mg tablets. In a relative bioavailability assessment under fed conditions (n=28), the AUC was 24% higher for the 625 mg tablet; the C_{max} was comparable for both formulations. (See ADVERSE REACTIONS.)

In healthy volunteers receiving a single 750 mg dose under fed conditions, nelfinavir concentrations were similar following administration of the 250 mg tablet and oral powder. *Effect of Food on Oral Absorption:* Food increases nelfinavir exposure and decreases nelfinavir pharmacokinetic variability relative to the fasted state. In one study, healthy volunteers received a single dose of 1250 mg of VIRACEPT 250 mg tablets (5 tablets) under fasted or fed conditions (three different meals). In a second study, healthy volunteers received single doses of 1250 mg VIRACEPT (5 × 250 mg tablets) under fasted or fed conditions (two different fat content meals). The results from the two studies are summarized in Table 2 and Table 3, respectively.

Table 2
Increase in AUC, C_{max} and T_{max} for Nelfinavir in Fed State Relative to Fasted State Following 1250 mg VIRACEPT (5 × 250 mg tablets)

Number of Kcal	% Fat	Number of subjects	AUC fold increase	C_{max} fold increase	Increase in T_{max} (hr)
125	20	n=21	2.2	2.0	1.00
500	20	n=22	3.1	2.3	2.00
1000	50	n=23	5.2	3.3	2.00

Table 3
Increase in Nelfinavir AUC, C_{max} and T_{max} in Fed Low Fat (20%) versus High fat (50%) State Relative to Fasted State Following 1250 mg VIRACEPT (5 × 250 mg tablets)

Number of Kcal	% Fat	Number of subjects	AUC fold increase	C_{max} fold increase	Increase in T_{max} (hr)
500	20	n=22	3.1	2.5	1.8
500	50	n=22	5.1	3.8	2.1

Nelfinavir exposure can be increased by increasing the calorie or fat content in meals taken with VIRACEPT.

A food effect study has not been conducted with the 625 mg tablet. However, based on a cross-study comparison (n=26 fed vs. n=26 fasted) following single dose administration of nelfinavir 1250 mg, the magnitude of the food effect for the 625 mg nelfinavir tablet appears comparable to that of the 250 mg tablets. VIRACEPT should be taken with a meal.
Distribution: The apparent volume of distribution following oral administration of nelfinavir was 2-7 L/kg. Nelfinavir in serum is extensively protein-bound (>98%).
Metabolism: Unchanged nelfinavir comprised 82-86% of the total plasma radioactivity after a single oral 750 mg dose of ¹⁴C-nelfinavir. *In vitro,* multiple cytochrome P-450 enzymes including CYP3A and CYP2C19 are responsible for metabolism of nelfinavir. One major and several minor oxidative metabolites were found in plasma. The major oxidative metabolite has *in vitro* antiviral activity comparable to the parent drug.
Elimination: The terminal half-life in plasma was typically 3.5 to 5 hours. The majority (87%) of an oral 750 mg dose containing ¹⁴C-nelfinavir was recovered in the feces; fecal radioactivity consisted of numerous oxidative metabolites (78%) and unchanged nelfinavir (22%). Only 1-2% of

Table 5: Drug Interactions:
Changes in Pharmacokinetic Parameters for Coadministered Drug in the Presence of VIRACEPT

Coadministered Drug	Nelfinavir Dose	N	% Change of Coadministered Drug Pharmacokinetic Parameters[1] (90% CI)		
			AUC	C_{max}	C_{min}
HIV-Protease Inhibitors					
Indinavir 800 mg Single Dose	750 mg q8h × 7 days	6	↑51% (↑29-↑77%)	↓10% (↓28-↑13%)	NA
Ritonavir 500 mg Single Dose	750 mg q8h × 5 doses	10	↔	↔	NA
Saquinavir 1200 mg Single Dose[2]	750 mg tid × 4 days	14	↑392% (↑291-↑521%)	↑179% (↑117-↑259%)	NA
Amprenavir 800 mg tid × 14 days	750 mg tid × 14 days	6	↔	↓14% (↓38-↑20%)	↑189% (↑52-↑448%)
Nucleoside Reverse Transcriptase Inhibitors					
Lamivudine 150 mg Single Dose	750 mg q8h × 7-10 days	11	↑10% (↑2-↑18%)	↑31% (↑9-↑56%)	NA
Stavudine 30-40 mg bid × 56 days	750 mg tid × 56 days	8	See footnote[3]		
Zidovudine 200 mg Single Dose	750 mg q8h × 7-10 days	11	↓35% (↓29-↓40%)	↓31% (↓13-↓46%)	NA
Non-Nucleoside Reverse Transcriptase Inhibitors					
Efavirenz 600 mg qd × 7 days	750 mg q8h × 7 days	10	↓12% (↓31-↑12%)	↓12% (↓29-↑8%)	↓22% (↓54-↑32%)
Nevirapine 200 mg qd × 14 days[3] Followed by 200 mg bid × 14 days	750 mg tid × 36 days	23	See footnote[3]		
Delavirdine 400 mg q8h × 14 days	750 mg q8h × 7 days	7	↓31% (↓57-↑10%)	↓27% (↓49-↑4%)	↓33% (↓70-↑49%)
Anti-infective Agents					
Rifabutin 150 mg qd × 8 days[4]	750 mg q8h × 7-8 days[5]	12	↑83% (↑72-↑96%)	↑19% (↑11-↑28%)	↑177% (↑144-↑215%)
Rifabutin 300 mg qd × 8 days	750 mg q8h × 7-8 days	10	↑207% (↑161-↑263%)	↑146% (↑118-↑178%)	↑305% (↑245-↑375%)
Azithromycin 1200 mg Single Dose	750 mg tid × 11 days	12	↑112% (↑80-↑150%)	↑136% (↑77-↑215%)	NA
HMG-CoA Reductase Inhibitors					
Atorvastatin 10 mg qd × 28 days	1250 mg bid × 14 days	15	↑74% (↑41-↑116%)	↑122% (↑68-↑193%)	↑39% (↓21-↑145%)
Simvastatin 20 mg qd × 28 days	1250 mg bid × 14 days	16	↑505% (↑393-↑643%)	↑517% (↑367-↑715%)	ND
Other Agents					
Ethinyl estradiol 35 µg qd × 15 days	750 mg q8h × 7 days	12	↓47% (↓42-↓52%)	↓28% (↓16-↓37%)	↓62% (↓57-↓67%)
Norethindrone 0.4 mg qd × 15 days	750 mg q8h × 7 days	12	↓18% (↓13-↓23%)	↔	↓46% (↓38-↓53%)

(Table continued on next page)

the dose was recovered in urine, of which unchanged nelfinavir was the major component.
Special Populations
Hepatic Insufficiency: The multi-dose pharmacokinetics of nelfinavir have not been studied in HIV-positive patients with hepatic insufficiency.
Renal Insufficiency: The pharmacokinetics of nelfinavir have not been studied in patients with renal insufficiency; however, less than 2% of nelfinavir is excreted in the urine, so the impact of renal impairment on nelfinavir elimination should be minimal.
Gender and Race: No significant pharmacokinetic differences have been detected between males and females. Pharmacokinetic differences due to race have not been evaluated.
Pediatrics: The pharmacokinetics of nelfinavir have been investigated in 5 studies in pediatric patients from birth to 13 years of age either receiving VIRACEPT three times or twice daily. The dosing regimens and associated AUC_{24} values are summarized in Table 4.

Table 4
Summary of Steady-state AUC_{24} of Nelfinavir in Pediatric Studies

Protocol no.	Dosing regimen[1]	N[2]	Age	AUC_{24} (mg.hr/L) arithmetic mean ± SD
AG1343-524	20 (19-28) mg/kg TID	14	2-13 years	56.1 ± 29.8
PACTG-725	55 (48-60) mg/kg BID	6	3-11 years	101.8 ± 56.1
PENTA 7	40 (34-43) mg/kg TID	4	2-9 months	33.8 ± 8.9
PENTA 7	75 (55-83) mg/kg BID	12	2-9 months	37.2 ± 19.2
PACTG-353	40 (14-56) mg/kg BID	10	6 weeks	44.1 ± 27.4
			1 week	45.8 ± 32.1

[1] Protocol specified dose (actual dose range)
[2] N: number of subjects with evaluable pharmacokinetic results
C_{trough} values are not presented in the table because they are not available for all studies

Pharmacokinetic data are also available for 86 patients (age 2 to 12 years) who received VIRACEPT 25-35 mg/kg TID in Study AG1343-556. The pharmacokinetic data from Study AG1343-556 were more variable than data from other studies conducted in the pediatric population; the 95% confidence interval for AUC_{24} was 9 to 121 mg.hr/L.
Overall, use of VIRACEPT in the pediatric population is associated with highly variable drug exposure. The high vari-

Viracept—Cont.

ability may be due to inconsistent food intake in pediatric patients. (See PRECAUTIONS: Pediatric Use, DOSAGE AND ADMINISTRATION.)

Geriatric Patients: The pharmacokinetics of nelfinavir have not been studied in patients over 65 years of age.

Drug Interactions (also see CONTRAINDICATIONS, WARNINGS, PRECAUTIONS: Drug Interactions)

CYP3A and CYP2C19 appear to be the predominant enzymes that metabolize nelfinavir in humans. The potential ability of nelfinavir to inhibit the major human cytochrome P450 enzymes (CYP3A, CYP2C19, CYP2D6, CYP2C9, CYP1A2 and CYP2E1) has been investigated *in vitro*. Only CYP3A was inhibited at concentrations in the therapeutic range. Specific drug interaction studies were performed with nelfinavir and a number of drugs. Table 5 summarizes the effects of nelfinavir on the geometric mean AUC, C_{max} and C_{min} of coadministered drugs. Table 6 shows the effects of coadministered drugs on the geometric mean AUC, C_{max} and C_{min} of nelfinavir.

[See table 5 on previous page and at right]

[See table 6 at right]

For information regarding clinical recommendations see CONTRAINDICATIONS, WARNINGS, PRECAUTIONS: Drug Interactions.

INDICATIONS AND USAGE

VIRACEPT in combination with other antiretroviral agents is indicated for the treatment of HIV infection.

Description of Studies

In the clinical studies described below, efficacy was evaluated by the percent of patients with plasma HIV RNA < 400 copies/mL (Studies 511 and 542) or < 500 copies/mL (Study ACTG 364), using the Roche RT-PCR (Amplicor) HIV-1 Monitor or < 50 copies/mL, using the Roche HIV-1 Ultrasensitive assay (Study Avanti 3). In the analysis presented in each figure, patients who terminated the study early for any reason, switched therapy due to inadequate efficacy or who had a missing HIV-RNA measurement that was either preceded or followed by a measurement above the limit of assay quantification were considered to have HIV-RNA above 400 copies/mL, above 500 copies/mL, or above 50 copies/mL at subsequent time points, depending on the assay that was used.

a. Studies in Antiretroviral Treatment Naïve Patients

Study 511: VIRACEPT + zidovudine + lamivudine versus zidovudine + lamivudine

Study 511 was a double-blind, randomized, placebo controlled trial comparing treatment with zidovudine (ZDV; 200 mg TID) and lamivudine (3TC; 150 mg BID) plus 2 doses of VIRACEPT (750 mg and 500 mg TID) to zidovudine (200 mg TID) and lamivudine (150 mg BID) alone in 297 antiretroviral naive HIV-1 infected patients (median age 35 years [range 21 to 63], 89% male and 78% Caucasian). Mean baseline CD4 cell count was 288 cells/mm³ and mean baseline plasma HIV RNA was 5.21 $\log_{10}$ copies/mL (160,394 copies/mL). The percent of patients with plasma HIV RNA < 400 copies/mL and mean changes in CD4 cell count are summarized in Figures 1 and 2, respectively.

Figure 1
Study 511: Percentage of Patients With HIV RNA Below 400 Copies/mL

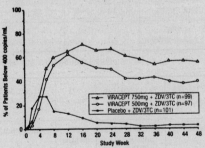

Figure 2
Study 511: Mean Change From Baseline in CD4 Cell Counts

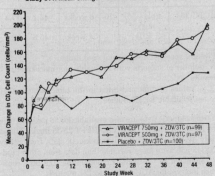

Study 542: VIRACEPT BID + stavudine + lamivudine compared to VIRACEPT TID + stavudine + lamivudine
Study 542 is an ongoing, randomized, open-label trial comparing the HIV RNA suppression achieved by VIRACEPT

Table 5 *(cont.)*: **Drug Interactions:**
Changes in Pharmacokinetic Parameters for Coadministered Drug in the Presence of VIRACEPT

Coadministered Drug	Nelfinavir Dose	N	% Change of Coadministered Drug Pharmacokinetic Parameters[1] (90% CI)		
			AUC	C_{max}	C_{min}
Methadone 80 mg +/- 21 mg qd[6] >1 month	1250 mg bid × 8 days	13	↓47% (↓42 - ↓51%)	↓46% (↓42 - ↓49%)	↓53% (↓49 - ↓57%)
Phenytoin 300 mg qd × 14 days[7]	1250 mg bid × 7 days	12	↓29% (↓17 - ↓39%)	↓21% (↓12- ↓29%)	↓39% (↓27- ↓49%)

NA: Not relevent for single-dose treatment; ND: Cannot be determined
[1] ↑ Indicates increase ↓ Indicates decrease ↔ Indicates no change (geometric mean exposure increased or decreased <10%)
[2] Using the soft-gelatin capsule formulation of saquinavir 1200 mg
[3] Based on non-definitive cross-study comparison, drug plasma concentrations appeared to be unaffected by coadministration
[4] Rifabutin 150 mg qd changes are relative to Rifabutin 300 mg qd × 8 days without coadministration with nelfinavir
[5] Comparable changes in rifabutin concentrations were observed with VIRACEPT 1250 mg q12h × 7 days
[6] Changes are reported for total plasma methadone; changes for the individual R-enantiomer and S-enantiomer were similar
[7] Phenytoin exposure measures are reported for total phenytoin exposure. The effect of nelfinavir on unbound phenytoin was similar

Table 6: Drug Interactions:
Changes in Pharmacokinetic Parameters for Nelfinavir in the Presence of the Coadministered Drug

Coadministered Drug	Nelfinavir Dose	N	% Change of Nelfinavir Pharmacokinetic Parameters[1] (90% CI)		
			AUC	C_{max}	C_{min}
HIV-Protease Inhibitors					
Indinavir 800 mg q8h × 7 days	750 mg Single Dose	6	↑83% (↑42- ↑137%)	↑31% (↑16- ↑48%)	NA
Ritonavir 500 mg q12h × 3 doses	750 mg Single Dose	10	↑152% (↑96- ↑224%)	↑44% (↑28- ↑63%)	NA
Saquinavir 1200 mg tid × 4 days[2]	750 mg Single Dose	14	↑18% (↑7- ↑30%)	↔	NA
Amprenavir 800 mg tid × 14 days	750 mg tid × 14 days	6	See footnote[3]		
Nucleoside Reverse Transcriptase Inhibitors					
Didanosine 200 mg Single Dose	750 mg Single Dose	9	↔		NA
Zidovudine 200 mg + Lamivudine 150 mg Single Dose	750 mg q8h × 7-10 days	11	↔	↔	↔
Non-Nucleoside Reverse Transcriptase Inhibitors					
Efavirenz 600 mg qd × 7 days	750 mg q8h × 7 days	7	↑20% (↑8- ↑34%)	↑21% (↑10- ↑33%)	↔
Nevirapine 200 mg qd × 14 days Followed by 200 mg bid × 14 days	750 mg tid × 36 days	23	↔	↔	↓32% (↓50- ↑5%)
Delavirdine 400 mg q8h × 7 days	750 mg q8h × 14 days	12	↑107% (↑83- ↑135%)	↑88% (↑66- ↑113%)	↑136% (↑103- ↑175%)
Anti-infective Agents					
Ketoconazole 400 mg qd × 7 days	500 mg q8h × 5-6 days	12	↑35% (↑24- ↑46%)	↑25% (↑11- ↑40%)	↑14% (↓23- ↑69%)
Rifabutin 150 mg qd × 8 days	750 mg q8h × 7-8 days	11	↓23% (↓14- ↓31%)	↓18% (↓8- ↓27%)	↓25% (↓8- ↓39%)
	1250 mg q12h × 7-8 days	11	↔	↔	↓15% (↓43- ↑27%)
Rifabutin 300 mg qd × 8 days	750 mg q8h × 7-8 days	10	↓32% (↓15- ↓46%)	↓24% (↓10- ↓36%)	↓53% (↓15- ↓73%)
Rifampin 600 mg qd × 7 days	750 mg q8h × 5-6 days	12	↓83% (↓79- ↓86%)	↓76% (↓69- ↓82%)	↓92% (↓86- ↓95%)
Azithromycin 1200 mg Single Dose	750 mg tid × 9 days	12	↓15% (↓7- ↓22%)	↓10% (↓19- ↑1%)	↓29% (↓19- ↓38%)
HMG-CoA Reductase Inhibitors					
Atorvastatin 10 mg qd × 28 days	1250 mg bid × 14 days	15	See footnote[3]		
Simvastatin 20 mg qd × 28 days	1250 mg bid × 14 days	16	See footnote[3]		
Other Agents					
Methadone 80 mg +/- 21 mg qd > 1 month	1250 mg bid × 8 days	13	See footnote[3]		
Phenytoin 300 mg qd × 7 days	1250 mg bid × 14 days	15	↔	↔	↓18% (↓45- ↑23%)

NA: Not relevent for single-dose treatment
[1] ↑ Indicates increase ↓ Indicates decrease ↔ Indicates no change (geometric mean exposure increased or decreased < 10%)
[2] Using the soft-gelatin capsule formulation of saquinavir 1200 mg
[3] Based on non-definitive cross-study comparison, nelfinavir plasma concentrations appeared to be unaffected by coadministration

1250 mg BID versus VIRACEPT 750 mg TID in patients also receiving stavudine (d4T; 30-40 mg BID) and lamivudine (3TC; 150 mg BID). Patients had a median age of 36 years (range 18 to 83), were 84% male, and were 91% Caucasian. Patients had received less than 6 months of therapy with nucleoside transcriptase inhibitors and were naïve to protease inhibitors. Mean baseline CD4 cell count was 296 cells/mm^3 and mean baseline plasma HIV RNA was 5.0 $\log_{10}$ copies/mL (100,706 copies/mL).

Results showed that there was no significant difference in mean CD4 cell count among treatment groups; the mean increases from baseline for the BID and TID arms were 150 cells/mm^3 at 24 weeks and approximately 200 cells/mm^3 at 48 weeks.

The percent of patients with HIV RNA < 400 copies/mL is summarized in Figure 3. The outcomes of patients through 48 weeks of treatment are summarized in Table 7.

Figure 3
Study 542: Percentage of Patients With HIV RNA Below 400 Copies/mL

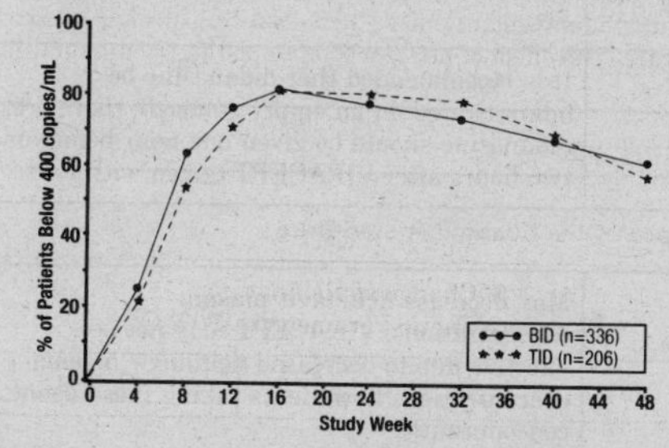

Table 7
Outcomes of Randomized Treatment Through 48 Weeks

Outcome	VIRACEPT 1250 mg BID Regimen	VIRACEPT 750 mg TID Regimen
Number of patients evaluable*	323	192
HIV RNA < 400 copies/mL	198 (61%)	111 (58%)
HIV RNA ≥ 400 copies/mL	46 (14%)	22 (11%)
Discontinued due to VIRACEPT toxicity**	9 (3%)	2 (1%)
Discontinued due to other antiretroviral agents' toxicity**	3 (1%)	3 (2%)
Others***	67 (21%)	54 (28%)

*Twelve patients in the BID arm and fourteen patients in the TID arm have not yet reached 48 weeks of therapy.
**These rates only reflect dose-limiting toxicities that were counted as the initial reason for treatment failure in the anlysis (see ADVERSE REACTIONS for a description of the safety profile of these regimens).
***Consent withdrawn, lost to follow-up, intercurrent illness, noncompliance or missing data; all assumed as failures.

Study Avanti 3: VIRACEPT TID + zidovudine + lamivudine compared to zidovudine + lamivudine

Study Avanti 3 was a placebo-controlled, randomized, double-blind study designed to evaluate the safety and efficacy of VIRACEPT (750 mg TID) in combination with zidovudine (ZDV; 300 mg BID) and lamivudine (3TC; 150 mg BID) (n=53) versus placebo in combination with ZDV and 3TC (n=52) administered to antiretroviral-naive patients with HIV infection and a CD4 cell count between 150 and 500 cells/µL. Patients had a mean age of 35 (range 22-59), were 89% male, and 88% Caucasian. Mean baseline CD4 cell count was 304 cells/mm^3 and mean baseline plasma HIV RNA was 4.8 $\log_{10}$ copies/mL (57,887 copies/mL). The percent of patients with plasma HIV RNA < 50 copies/mL at 52 weeks was 54% for the VIRACEPT + ZDV + 3TC treatment group and 13% for the ZDV + 3TC treatment group.

b. Studies in Antiretroviral Treatment Experienced Patients

Study ACTG 364: VIRACEPT TID + 2NRTIs compared to efavirenz + 2NRTIs compared to VIRACEPT + efavirenz + 2NRTIs

Study ACTG 364 was a randomized, double-blind study that evaluated the combination of VIRACEPT 750 mg TID and/or efavirenz 600 mg QD with 2 NRTIs (either didanosine [ddI] + d4T, ddI + 3TC, or d4T + 3TC) in patients with prolonged prior nucleoside exposure who had completed 2 previous ACTG studies. Patients had a mean age of 41 years (range 18 to 75), were 88% male, and were 74% Caucasian. Mean baseline CD4 cell count was 389 cells/mm^3 and mean baseline plasma HIV RNA was 3.9 $\log_{10}$ copies/mL (7,954 copies/mL).

The percent of patients with plasma HIV RNA < 500 copies/mL at 48 weeks was 42%, 62%, and 72% for the VIRACEPT (n=66), EFV (n=65), and VIRACEPT + EFV (n=64) treatment groups, respectively. The 4-drug combination of VIRACEPT + EFV + 2 NRTIs was more effective in suppressing plasma HIV RNA in these patients than either 3-drug regimen.

CONTRAINDICATIONS

VIRACEPT is contraindicated in patients with clinically significant hypersensitivity to any of its components.

Coadministration of VIRACEPT is contraindicated with drugs that are highly dependent on CYP3A for clearance and for which elevated plasma concentrations are associated with serious and/or life-threatening events. These drugs are listed in Table 8.

Table 8
Drugs That Are Contraindicated With VIRACEPT

Drug Class	Drugs Within Class That Are Contraindicated With VIRACEPT
Antiarrhythmics	Amiodarone, Quinidine
Ergot Derivatives	Dihydroergotamine, Ergonovine, Ergotamine, Methylergonovine
Neuroleptic	Pimozide
Sedative/Hypnotics	Midazolam, Triazolam

WARNINGS

ALERT: Find out about medicines that should not be taken with VIRACEPT. This statement is included on the product's bottle label.

Drug Interactions (also see PRECAUTIONS)

Nelfinavir is an inhibitor of the CYP3A enzyme. Coadministration of VIRACEPT and drugs primarily metabolized by CYP3A may result in increased plasma concentrations of the other drug that could increase or prolong its therapeutic and adverse effects. Caution should be exercised when inhibitors of CYP3A, including VIRACEPT, are coadministered with drugs that are metabolized by CYP3A and that prolong the QT interval. (See ADVERSE REACTIONS: Post-Marketing Experience.) Nelfinavir is metabolized by CYP3A and CYP2C19. Coadministration of VIRACEPT and drugs that induce CYP3A or CYP2C19 may decrease nelfinavir plasma concentrations and reduce its therapeutic effect. Coadministration of VIRACEPT and drugs that inhibit CYP3A or CYP2C19 may increase nelfinavir plasma concentrations. (Also see **PRECAUTIONS: Table 9: Drugs That Should Not Be Coadministered With VIRACEPT, Table 10: Established and Other Potentially Significant Drug Interactions.**)

Concomitant use of VIRACEPT with lovastatin or simvastatin is not recommended. Caution should be exercised if HIV protease inhibitors, including VIRACEPT, are used concurrently with other HMG-CoA reductase inhibitors that are also metabolized by the CYP3A pathway (e.g., atorvastatin). (Also see **Tables 5 and 6: Drug Interactions**). The risk of myopathy including rhabdomyolysis may be increased when protease inhibitors, including VIRACEPT, are used in combination with these drugs.

Particular caution should be used when prescribing sildenafil in patients receiving protease inhibitors, including VIRACEPT. Coadministration of a protease inhibitor with sildenafil is expected to substantially increase sildenafil concentrations and may result in an increase in sildenafil-associated adverse events, including hypotension, visual changes, and priapism. (See PRECAUTIONS, Drug Interactions and Information for Patients, and the complete prescribing information for sildenafil.)

Concomitant use of St. John's wort (hypericum perforatum) or St. John's wort containing products and VIRACEPT is not recommended. Coadministration of St. John's wort with protease inhibitors, including VIRACEPT, is expected to substantially decrease protease inhibitor concentrations and may result in sub-optimal levels of VIRACEPT and lead to loss of virologic response and possible resistance to VIRACEPT or to the class of protease inhibitors.

Patients with Phenylketonuria

Patients with Phenylketonuria: VIRACEPT Oral Powder contains 11.2 mg phenylalanine per gram of powder.

Diabetes mellitus/Hyperglycemia

New onset diabetes mellitus, exacerbation of pre-existing diabetes mellitus and hyperglycemia have been reported during post-marketing surveillance in HIV-infected patients receiving protease inhibitor therapy. Some patients required either initiation or dose adjustments of insulin or oral hypoglycemic agents for treatment of these events. In some cases diabetic ketoacidosis has occurred. In those patients who discontinued protease inhibitor therapy, hyperglycemia persisted in some cases. Because these events have been reported voluntarily during clinical practice, estimates of frequency cannot be made and a causal relationship between protease inhibitor therapy and these events has not been established.

PRECAUTIONS

General

Nelfinavir is principally metabolized by the liver. Therefore, caution should be exercised when administering this drug to patients with hepatic impairment.

Resistance/Cross Resistance

HIV cross-resistance between protease inhibitors has been observed. (See MICROBIOLOGY.)

Hemophilia

There have been reports of increased bleeding, including spontaneous skin hematomas and hemarthrosis, in patients with hemophilia type A and B treated with protease inhibitors. In some patients, additional factor VIII was given. In more than half of the reported cases, treatment with protease inhibitors was continued or reintroduced. A causal relationship has not been established.

Fat Redistribution

Redistribution/accumulation of body fat including central obesity, dorsocervical fat enlargement (buffalo hump), peripheral wasting, facial wasting, breast enlargement, and "cushingoid appearance" have been observed in patients receiving antiretroviral therapy. The mechanism and long-term consequences of these events are currently unknown. A causal relationship has not been established.

Information For Patients

"A statement to patients and healthcare providers is included on the product's bottle label: **ALERT: Find out about medicines that should NOT be taken with VIRACEPT.** A Patient Package Insert (PPI) for VIRACEPT is available for patient information."

For optimal absorption, patients should be advised to take VIRACEPT with food (see CLINICAL PHARMACOLOGY: Pharmacokinetics and DOSAGE AND ADMINISTRATION).

Patients should be informed that VIRACEPT is not a cure for HIV infection and that they may continue to acquire illnesses associated with advanced HIV infection, including opportunistic infections.

Patients should be told that there is currently no data demonstrating that VIRACEPT therapy can reduce the risk of transmitting HIV to others through sexual contact or blood contamination.

Patients should be told that sustained decreases in plasma HIV RNA have been associated with a reduced risk of progression to AIDS and death. Patients should be advised to take VIRACEPT and other concomitant antiretroviral therapy every day as prescribed. Patients should not alter the dose or discontinue therapy without consulting with their doctor. If a dose of VIRACEPT is missed, patients should take the dose as soon as possible and then return to their normal schedule. However, if a dose is skipped, the patient should not double the next dose.

Patients should be informed that VIRACEPT Tablets are film-coated and that this film-coating is intended to make the tablets easier to swallow.

The most frequent adverse event associated with VIRACEPT is diarrhea, which can usually be controlled with non-prescription drugs, such as loperamide, which slow gastrointestinal motility.

Patients should be informed that redistribution or accumulation of body fat may occur in patients receiving antiretroviral therapy and that the cause and long term health effects of these conditions are not known at this time.

VIRACEPT may interact with some drugs, therefore, patients should be advised to report to their doctor the use of any other prescription, non-prescription medication or herbal products, particularly St. John's wort.

Patients receiving oral contraceptives should be instructed that alternate or additional contraceptive measures should be used during therapy with VIRACEPT.

Patients receiving sildenafil and nelfinavir should be advised that they may be at an increased risk of sildenafil-associated adverse events including hypotension, visual changes, and prolonged penile erection, and should promptly report any symptoms to their doctor.

Drug Interactions (Also see CONTRAINDICATIONS, WARNINGS, CLINICAL PHARMACOLOGY: Drug Interactions)

Nelfinavir is an inhibitor of CYP3A. Coadministration of VIRACEPT and drugs primarily metabolized by CYP3A (e.g., dihydropyridine calcium channel blockers, HMG-CoA reductase inhibitors, immunosuppressants and sildenafil) may result in increased plasma concentrations of the other drug that could increase or prolong both its therapeutic and adverse effects. (See Tables 9 and 10). Nelfinavir is metabolized by CYP3A and CYP2C19. Coadministration of VIRACEPT and drugs that induce CYP3A or CYP2C19, such as rifampin, may decrease nelfinavir plasma concentrations and reduce its therapeutic effect. Coadministration of VIRACEPT and drugs that inhibit CYP3A or CYP2C19 may increase nelfinavir plasma concentrations.

Drug interaction studies reveal no clinically significant drug interactions between nelfinavir and didanosine, lamivudine, stavudine, zidovudine, efavirenz, nevirapine, or ketoconazole and no dose adjustments are needed. In the case of didanosine, it is recommended that didanosine be administered on an empty stomach; therefore, nelfinavir should be administered with food one hour after or more than 2 hours before didanosine.

Based on known metabolic profiles, clinically significant drug interactions are not expected between VIRACEPT and dapsone, trimethoprim/sulfamethoxazole, or itraconazole.

Table 9
Drugs That Should Not Be Coadministered With VIRACEPT

Drug Class: Drug Name	Clinical Comment
Antiarrhythmics: amiodarone, quinidine	CONTRAINDICATED due to potential for serious and/or life threatening reactions such as cardiac arrhythmias.

Continued on next page

Viracept—Cont.

Antimycobacterial: rifampin	May lead to loss of virologic response and possible resistance to VIRACEPT or other coadministered antiretroviral agents.
Ergot Derivatives: dihydroergotamine, ergonovine, ergotamine, methylergonovine	CONTRAINDICATED due to potential for serious and/or life threatening reactions such as acute ergot toxicity characterized by peripheral vasospasm and ischemia of the extremities and other tissues.
Herbal Products: St. John's wort (hypericum perforatum)	May lead to loss of virologic response and possible resistance to VIRACEPT or other coadministered antiretroviral agents.
HMG-CoA Reductase Inhibitors: lovastatin, simvastatin	Potential for serious reactions such as risk of myopathy including rhabdomyolysis.
Neuroleptic: pimozide	CONTRAINDICATED due to potential for serious and/or life threatening reactions such as cardiac arrhythmias.
Sedative/Hypnotics: midazolam, triazolam	CONTRAINDICTED due to potential for serious and/or life threatening reactions such as prolonged or increased sedation or respiratory depression.

[See table 10 at right]

Carcinogenesis, Mutagenesis, Impairment of Fertility
Carcinogenicity studies in mice and rats were conducted with nelfinavir at oral doses up to 1000 mg/kg/day. No evidence of a tumorigenic effect was noted in mice at systemic exposures (C_{max}) up to 9-fold those measured in humans at the recommended therapeutic dose (750 mg TID or 1250 mg BID). In rats, thyroid follicular cell adenomas and carcinomas were increased in males at 300 mg/kg/day and higher and in females at 1000 mg/kg/day. Systemic exposures (C_{max}) at 300 and 1000 mg/kg/day were 1- to 3-fold, respectively, those measured in humans at the recommended therapeutic dose. Repeated administration of nelfinavir to rats produced effects consistent with hepatic microsomal enzyme induction and increased thyroid hormone disposition; these effects predispose rats, but not humans, to thyroid follicular cell neoplasms. Nelfinavir showed no evidence of mutagenic or clastogenic activity in a battery of in vitro and in vivo genetic toxicology assays. These studies included bacterial mutation assays in *S. typhimurium* and *E. coli*, a mouse lymphoma tyrosine kinase assay, a chromosomal aberration assay in human lymphocytes, and an in vivo mouse bone marrow micronucleus assay.
Nelfinavir produced no effects on either male or female mating and fertility or embryo survival in rats at systemic exposures comparable to the human therapeutic exposure.

Pregnancy—Pregnancy Category B
There were no effects on fetal development or maternal toxicity when nelfinavir was administered to pregnant rats at systemic exposures (AUC) comparable to human exposure. Administration of nelfinavir to pregnant rabbits resulted in no fetal development effects up to a dose at which a slight decrease in maternal body weight was observed; however, even at the highest dose evaluated, systemic exposure in rabbits was significantly lower than human exposure. Additional studies in rats indicated that exposure to nelfinavir in females from mid-pregnancy through lactation had no effect on the survival, growth, and development of the offspring to weaning. Subsequent reproductive performance of these offspring was also not affected by maternal exposure to nelfinavir. However, there are no adequate and well-controlled studies in pregnant women taking VIRACEPT. Because animal reproduction studies are not always predictive of human response, VIRACEPT should be used during pregnancy only if clearly needed.

Antiretroviral Pregnancy Registry: (APR): To monitor maternal-fetal outcomes of pregnant women exposed to VIRACEPT and other antiretroviral agents, an Antiretroviral Pregnancy Registry has been established. Physicians are encouraged to register patients by calling (800) 258-4263.

Nursing Mothers
The Centers for Disease Control and Prevention recommends that HIV-infected mothers not breast-feed their infants to avoid risking postnatal transmission of HIV. Studies in lactating rats have demonstrated that nelfinavir is excreted in milk. Because of both the potential for HIV transmission and the potential for serious adverse reactions in nursing infants, **mothers should be instructed not to breast-feed if they are receiving VIRACEPT.**

Pediatric Use
The safety and effectiveness of VIRACEPT have been established in patients from 2 to 13 years of age. The use of

Table 10
Established and Other Potentially Significant Drug Interactions:
Alteration in Dose or Regimen May Be Recommended Based on Drug Interaction Studies
(see CLINICAL PHARMACOLOGY, for Magnitude of Interaction, Tables 5 and 6)

Concomitant Drug Class: Drug Name	Effect on Concentration	Clinical Comment
HIV-Antiviral Agents		
Protease Inhibitors: indinavir ritonavir saquinavir	↑ nelfinavir ↑ indinavir ↑ nelfinavir ↑ saquinavir	Appropriate doses for these combinations, with respect to safety and efficacy, have not been established.
Non-nucleoside Reverse Transcriptase Inhibitors: delavirdine nevirapine	↑ nelfinavir ↓ delavirdine ↓ nelfinavir (C_{min})	Appropriate doses for these combinations, with respect to safety and efficacy, have not been established.
Nucleoside Reverse Transcriptase Inhibitor: didanosine		It is recommended that didanosine be administered on an empty stomach; therefore, didanosine should be given one hour before or two hours after VIRACEPT (given with food).
Other Agents		
Anti-Convulsants: carbamazepine phenobarbital	↓ nelfinavir	May decrease nelfinavir plasma concentrations. VIRACEPT may not be effective due to decreased nelfinavir plasma concentrations in patients taking these agents concomitantly.
Anti-Convulsant: phenytoin	↓ phenytoin	Phenytoin plasma/serum concentrations should be monitored; phenytoin dose may require adjustment to compensate for altered phenytoin concentration.
Anti-Mycobacterial: rifabutin	↑ rifabutin ↓ nelfinavir (750 mg TID) ↔nelfinavir (1250 mg BID)	It is recommended that the dose of rifabutin be reduced to one-half the usual dose when administered with VIRACEPT; 1250 mg BID is the preferred dose of VIRACEPT when coadministered with rifabutin.
Erectile Dysfunction Agent: sildenafil	↑ sildenafil	Sildenafil should not exceed a maximum single dose of 25 mg in a 48 hour period.
HMG-CoA Reductase Inhibitor: atorvastatin	↑ atorvastatin	Use lowest possible dose of atorvastatin with careful monitoring, or consider other HMG-CoA reductase inhibitors such as pravastatin or fluvastatin in combination with VIRACEPT.
Immuno-suppressants: cyclosporine tacrolimus sirolimus	↑ immuno-suppressants	Plasma concentrations may be increased by VIRACEPT.
Narcotic Analgesic: methadone	↓ methadone	Dosage of methadone may need to be increased when coadministered with VIRACEPT.
Oral Contraceptive: ethinyl estradiol	↓ ethinyl estradiol	Alternative or additional contraceptive measures should be used when oral contraceptives and VIRACEPT are coadministered.
Macrolide Antibiotic: azithromycin	↑ azithromycin	Dose adjustment of azithromycin is not recommended, but close monitoring for known side effects such as liver enzyme abnormalities and hearing impairment is warranted.

VIRACEPT in these age groups is supported by evidence from adequate and well-controlled studies of VIRACEPT in adults and pharmacokinetic studies and studies supporting activity in pediatric patients. In patients less than 2 years of age, VIRACEPT was found to be safe at the doses studied, but a reliably effective dose could not be established (see CLINICAL PHARMACOLOGY: Special Populations, ADVERSE REACTIONS: Pediatric Population, and DOSAGE AND ADMINISTRATION: Pediatric Patients).
The following issues should be considered when initiating VIRACEPT in pediatric patients:
• In pediatric patients ≥ 2 years of age receiving VIRACEPT as part of triple combination antiretroviral therapy in randomized studies, the proportion of patients achieving a HIV RNA level <400 copies/mL through 48 weeks ranged from 26% to 42%.
• Response rates in children <2 years of age appeared to be poorer than those in patients ≥ 2 years of age in some studies.
• Highly variable drug exposure remains a significant problem in the use of VIRACEPT in pediatric patients. Unpredictable drug exposure may be exacerbated in pediatric patients because of increased clearance compared to adults and difficulties with compliance and adequate food intake with dosing. Pharmacokinetic results from the pediatric studies are reported in Table 4 (see CLINICAL PHARMACOLOGY, Special Populations).
Study 556 was a randomized, double-blind, placebo-controlled trial with VIRACEPT or placebo coadministered with ZDV and ddI in 141 HIV-positive children who had re-

ceived minimal antiretroviral therapy. The mean age of the children was 3.9 years. Ninety four (67%) children were between 2-12 years, and 47 (33%) were < 2 years of age. The mean baseline HIV RNA value was 5.0 log for all patients and the mean baseline CD4 cell count was 886 cells/mm³ for all patients. The efficacy of VIRACEPT measured by HIV RNA <400 at 48 weeks in children ≥ 2 years of age was 26% compared to 2% of placebo patients (p=0.0008). In the children < 2 years of age, only 1 of 27 and 2 of 20 maintained an undetectable HIV RNA level at 48 weeks for placebo and VIRACEPT patients, respectively.
PACTG 377 was an open-label study that randomized 181 HIV treatment-experienced pediatric patients to receive: d4T+NVP+RTV, d4T+3TC+NFV, or d4T+3TC+NVP+NFV with NFV given on a TID schedule. The median age was 5.9 years and 46% were male. At baseline the median HIV RNA was 4.4 log and median CD4 cell count was 690 cells/mm³. Substudy PACTG 725 evaluated d4T+3TC+NFV with NFV given on a BID schedule. The proportion of patients with detectable viral load at baseline achieving HIV RNA <400 copies/mL at 48 weeks was: 41% for d4T+NVP+RTV, 42% for d4T+3TC+NFV, 30% for d4T+NVP+NFV, and 52% for d4T+3TC+NVP+NFV. No significant clinical differences were identified between patients receiving VIRACEPT in BID or TID schedules.
VIRACEPT has been evaluated in 2 studies of young infants. The PENTA 7 study was an open-label study to evaluate the toxicity, tolerability, pharmacokinetics, and activity of NFV+d4T+ddI in 20 HIV-infected infants less than 12 weeks of age. PACTG 353 evaluated the pharmacokinetics and safety of VIRACEPT in infants born to HIV-infected women receiving NFV as part of combination therapy during pregnancy.

Table 11
Percentage of Patients with Treatment-Emergent[1] Adverse Events of Moderate or Severe Intensity Reported in ≥ 2% of Patients

Adverse Events	Study 511 24 weeks			Study 542 48 weeks	
	Placebo + ZDV/3TC (n=101)	500 mg TID VIRACEPT + ZDV/3TC (n=97)	750 mg TID VIRACEPT + ZDV/3TC (n=100)	1250 mg BID VIRACEPT + d4T/3TC (n=344)	750 mg TID VIRACEPT + d4T/3TC (n=210)
Digestive System					
Diarrhea	3%	14%	20%	20%	15%
Nausea	4%	3%	7%	3%	3%
Flatulence	0	5%	2%	1%	1%
Skin/Appendages					
Rash	1%	1%	3%	2%	1%

[1] Includes those adverse events at least possibly related to study drug or of unknown relationship and excludes concurrent HIV conditions

Table 12
Percentage of Patients by Treatment Group With Marked Laboratory Abnormalities[1] in > 2% of Patients

	Study 511			Study 542	
	Placebo + ZDV/3TC (n=101)	500 mg TID VIRACEPT + ZDV/3TC (n=97)	750 mg TID VIRACEPT + ZDV/3TC (n=100)	1250 mg BID VIRACEPT + d4T/3TC (n=344)	750 mg TID VIRACEPT + d4T/3TC (n=210)
Hematology					
Hemoglobin	6%	3%	2%	0	0
Neutrophils	4%	3%	5%	2%	1%
Lymphocytes	1%	6%	1%	1%	0
Chemistry					
ALT (SGPT)	6%	1%	1%	2%	1%
AST (SGOT)	4%	1%	0	2%	1%
Creatine Kinase	7%	2%	2%	NA	NA

[1] Marked laboratory abnormalities are defined as a shift from Grade 0 at baseline to at least Grade 3 or from Grade 1 to Grade 4

Table 14
Dosing Table for Children ≥2 years of age (powder)

Body weight		Twice daily (BID) 45-55 mg/kg		Three times daily (TID) 25-35 mg/kg	
Kg.	Lbs.	Scoops of powder (50 mg/1 g)	Teaspoons[1] of Powder	Scoops of powder (50 mg/1 g)	Teaspoons[1] of Powder
9.0 to < 10.5	20 to < 23	10	2½	6	1½
10.5 to < 12	23 to < 26.5	11	2¾	7	1¾
12 to < 14	26.5 to < 31	13	3¼	8	2
14 to < 16	31 to < 35	15	3¾	9	2¼
16 to < 18	35 to < 39.5	Not recommended[2]	Not recommended[2]	10	2½
18 to < 23	39.5 to < 50.5	Not recommended[2]	Not recommended[2]	12	3
≥23	≥50.5	Not recommended[2]	Not recommended[2]	15	3¾

[1] If a teaspoon is used to measure VIRACEPT oral powder, 1 level teaspoon contains 200 mg of VIRACEPT (4 level scoops equals 1 level teaspoon)
[2] Use VIRACEPT 250 mg tablet

Geriatric Use
Clinical studies of VIRACEPT did not include sufficient numbers of subjects aged 65 and over to determine whether they respond differently from younger subjects.

ADVERSE REACTIONS
The safety of VIRACEPT was studied in over 5000 patients who received drug either alone or in combination with nucleoside analogues. The majority of adverse events were of mild intensity. The most frequently reported adverse event among patients receiving VIRACEPT was diarrhea, which was generally of mild to moderate intensity. The frequency of nelfinavir-associated diarrhea may be increased in patients receiving the 625 mg tablet because of the increased bioavailability of this formulation.

Drug-related clinical adverse experiences of moderate or severe intensity in ≥ 2% of patients treated with VIRACEPT coadministered with d4T and 3TC (Study 542) for up to 48 weeks or with ZDV plus 3TC (Study 511) for up to 24 weeks are presented in Table 11.
[See table 11 above]
Adverse events occurring in less than 2% of patients receiving VIRACEPT in all phase II/III clinical trials and considered at least possibly related or of unknown relationship to treatment and of at least moderate severity are listed below.
Body as a Whole: abdominal pain, accidental injury, allergic reaction, asthenia, back pain, fever, headache, malaise, pain, and redistribution/accumulation of body fat (see PRECAUTIONS, Fat Redistribution).
Digestive System: anorexia, dyspepsia, epigastric pain, gastrointestinal bleeding, hepatitis, mouth ulceration, pancreatitis and vomiting.
Hemic/Lymphatic System: anemia, leukopenia and thrombocytopenia.
Metabolic/Nutritional System: increases in alkaline phosphatase, amylase, creatine phosphokinase, lactic dehydrogenase, SGOT, SGPT and gamma glutamyl transpeptidase; hyperlipemia, hyperuricemia, hyperglycemia, hypoglycemia, dehydration, and liver function tests abnormal.
Musculoskeletal System: arthralgia, arthritis, cramps, myalgia, myasthenia and myopathy.
Nervous System: anxiety, depression, dizziness, emotional lability, hyperkinesia, insomnia, migraine, paresthesia, seizures, sleep disorder, somnolence and suicide ideation.
Respiratory System: dyspnea, pharyngitis, rhinitis, and sinusitis.

Skin/Appendages: dermatitis, folliculitis, fungal dermatitis, maculopapular rash, pruritus, sweating, and urticaria.
Special Senses: acute iritis and eye disorder.
Urogenital System: kidney calculus, sexual dysfunction and urine abnormality.

Post-Marketing Experience
The following additional adverse experiences have been reported from postmarketing surveillance as at least possibly related or of unknown relationship to VIRACEPT:
Body as a Whole: hypersensitivity reactions (including bronchospasm, moderate to severe rash, fever and edema).
Cardiovascular System: QTc prolongation, torsades de pointes.
Digestive System: jaundice
Metabolic/Nutritional System: bilirubinemia, metabolic acidosis.

Laboratory Abnormalities
The percentage of patients with marked laboratory abnormalities in Studies 542 and 511 are presented in Table 12. Marked laboratory abnormalities are defined as a Grade 3 or 4 abnormality in a patient with a normal baseline value or a Grade 4 abnormality in a patient with a Grade 1 abnormality at baseline.
[See table 12 at left]

Pediatric Population
VIRACEPT has been studied in approximately 400 pediatric patients in clinical trials from birth to 13 years of age. The adverse event profile seen during pediatric clinical trials was similar to that for adults.
The most commonly reported drug-related, treatment-emergent adverse events reported in the pediatric studies included: diarrhea, leukopenia/neutropenia, rash, anorexia and abdominal pain. Diarrhea, regardless of assigned relationship to study drug, was reported in 39% to 47% of pediatric patients receiving VIRACEPT in 2 of the larger treatment trials. Leukopenia/neutropenia was the laboratory abnormality most commonly reported as a significant event across the pediatric studies.

OVERDOSAGE
Human experience of acute overdose with VIRACEPT is limited. There is no specific antidote for overdose with VIRACEPT. If indicated, elimination of unabsorbed drug should be achieved by emesis or gastric lavage. Administration of activated charcoal may also be used to aid removal of unabsorbed drug. Since nelfinavir is highly protein bound, dialysis is unlikely to significantly remove drug from blood.

DOSAGE AND ADMINISTRATION
Adults: The recommended dose is 1250 mg (five 250 mg tablets or two 625 mg tablets) twice daily or 750 mg (three 250 mg tablets) three times daily. VIRACEPT should be taken with a meal. Patients unable to swallow the 250 or 625 mg tablets may dissolve the tablets in a small amount of water. Once dissolved, patients should mix the cloudy liquid well, and consume it immediately. The glass should be rinsed with water and the rinse swallowed to ensure the entire dose is consumed.
Pediatric Patients (2-13 years): In children 2 years of age and older, the recommended oral dose of VIRACEPT Oral Powder or 250 mg tablets is 45 to 55 mg/kg twice daily or 25 to 35 mg/kg three times daily. All doses should be taken **with a meal.** Doses higher than the adult maximum dose of 2500 mg per day have not been studied in children. For children unable to take tablets, VIRACEPT Oral Powder may be administered. The oral powder may be mixed with a small amount of water, milk, formula, soy formula, soy milk or dietary supplements; once mixed, the entire contents must be consumed in order to obtain the full dose. If the mixture is not consumed immediately, it must be stored under refrigeration, but storage must not exceed 6 hours. Acidic food or juice (e.g., orange juice, apple juice or apple sauce) are not recommended to be used in combination with VIRACEPT, because the combination may result in a bitter taste. VIRACEPT Oral Powder should not be reconstituted with water in its original container.
The healthcare provider should assess appropriate formulation and dosage for each patient. Crushed 250 mg tablets can be used in lieu of powder. Tables 13 and 14 provide dosing guidelines for VIRACEPT tablets and powder based on age and body weight.

Table 13
Dosing Table for Children ≥ 2 years of age (tablets)

Body weight		Twice daily (BID) 45 - 55 mg/kg ≥2 years	Three times daily (TID) 25 - 35 mg/kg ≥2 years
Kg.	Lbs.	# of tablets (250 mg)	# of tablets (250 mg)
10-12	22-26.4	2	1
13-18	28.6-39.6	3	2
19-20	41.8-44	4	2
≥21	≥46.2	4-5[1]	3[2]

[1] For BID dosing, the maximum dose per day is 5 tablets BID
[2] For TID dosing, the maximum dose per day is 3 tablets TID

[See table 14 above]

Continued on next page

Viracept—Cont.

HOW SUPPLIED

VIRACEPT (nelfinavir mesylate) 250 mg: Light blue, capsule-shaped tablets with a clear film coating engraved with "VIRACEPT" on one side and "250 mg" on the other.
Bottles of 300, 250 mg tablets .... NDC 63010-010-30
VIRACEPT (nelfinavir mesylate) 625 mg: White oval tablet with a clear film coating engraved with "V" on one side and "625" on the other.
Bottles of 120, 625 mg tablets .... NDC 63010-027-70
VIRACEPT (nelfinavir mesylate) Oral Powder is available as a 50 mg/g off-white powder containing 50 mg (as nelfinavir free base) in each level scoopful (1 gram).
Multiple use bottles of 144 grams of powder with scoop .... NDC 63010-011-90
Viracept tablets and oral powder should be stored at 15° to 30°C (59° TO 86°F).
Keep container tightly closed. Dispense in original container.
Rx only
VIRACEPT and Agouron are registered trademarks of Agouron Pharmaceuticals, Inc.

LAB-0174-11 Revised September 2004

ZOLOFT® ℞
[*zō-lŏft*]
(sertraline hydrochloride)
Tablets and Oral Concentrate

Prescribing information for this product, which appears on pages 2681–2688 of the 2005 PDR, has been completely revised as follows. Please write "See Supplement A" next to the product heading.

Suicidality in Children and Adolescents
Antidepressants increased the risk of suicidal thinking and behavior (suicidality) in short-term studies in children and adolescents with Major Depressive Disorder (MDD) and other psychiatric disorders. Anyone considering the use of Zoloft or any other antidepressant in a child or adolescent must balance this risk with the clinical need. Patients who are started on therapy should be observed closely for clinical worsening, suicidality, or unusual changes in behavior. Families and caregivers should be advised of the need for close observation and communication with the prescriber. Zoloft is not approved for use in pediatric patients except for patients with obsessive compulsive disorder (OCD). (See Warnings and Precautions: Pediatric Use)
Pooled analyses of short-term (4 to 16 weeks) placebo-controlled trials of 9 antidepressant drugs (SSRIs and others) in children and adolescents with major depressive disorder (MDD), obsessive compulsive disorder (OCD), or other psychiatric disorders (a total of 24 trials involving over 4400 patients) have revealed a greater risk of adverse events representing suicidal thinking or behavior (suicidality) during the first few months of treatment in those receiving antidepressants. The average risk of such events in patients receiving antidepressants was 4%, twice the placebo risk of 2%. No suicides occurred in these trials.

DESCRIPTION

ZOLOFT® (sertraline hydrochloride) is a selective serotonin reuptake inhibitor (SSRI) for oral administration. It has a molecular weight of 342.7. Sertraline hydrochloride has the following chemical name: (1S-cis)-4-(3,4-dichlorophenyl)-1,2,3,4-tetrahydro-N-methyl-1-naphthalenamine hydrochloride. The empirical formula $C_{17}H_{17}NCl_2$•HCl is represented by the following structural formula:

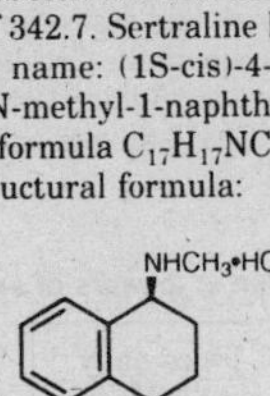

Sertraline hydrochloride is a white crystalline powder that is slightly soluble in water and isopropyl alcohol, and sparingly soluble in ethanol.
ZOLOFT is supplied for oral administration as scored tablets containing sertraline hydrochloride equivalent to 25, 50 and 100 mg of sertraline and the following inactive ingredients: dibasic calcium phosphate dihydrate, D & C Yellow #10 aluminum lake (in 25 mg tablet), FD & C Blue #1 aluminum lake (in 25 mg tablet), FD & C Red #40 aluminum lake (in 25 mg tablet), FD & C Blue #2 aluminum lake (in 50 mg tablet), hydroxypropyl cellulose, hypromellose, magnesium stearate, microcrystalline cellulose, polyethylene glycol, polysorbate 80, sodium starch glycolate, synthetic yellow iron oxide (in 100 mg tablet), and titanium dioxide.
ZOLOFT oral concentrate is available in a multidose 60 mL bottle. Each mL of solution contains sertraline hydrochloride equivalent to 20 mg of sertraline. The solution contains the following inactive ingredients: glycerin, alcohol (12%), menthol, butylated hydroxytoluene (BHT). The oral concentrate must be diluted prior to administration (see PRECAUTIONS, Information for Patients and DOSAGE AND ADMINISTRATION).

CLINICAL PHARMACOLOGY

Pharmacodynamics
The mechanism of action of sertraline is presumed to be linked to its inhibition of CNS neuronal uptake of serotonin (5HT). Studies at clinically relevant doses in man have demonstrated that sertraline blocks the uptake of serotonin into human platelets. *In vitro* studies in animals also suggest that sertraline is a potent and selective inhibitor of neuronal serotonin reuptake and has only very weak effects on norepinephrine and dopamine neuronal reuptake. *In vitro* studies have shown that sertraline has no significant affinity for adrenergic ($alpha_1$, $alpha_2$, beta), cholinergic, GABA, dopaminergic, histaminergic, serotonergic ($5HT_{1A}$, $5HT_{1B}$, $5HT_2$), or benzodiazepine receptors; antagonism of such receptors has been hypothesized to be associated with various anticholinergic, sedative, and cardiovascular effects for other psychotropic drugs. The chronic administration of sertraline was found in animals to downregulate brain norepinephrine receptors, as has been observed with other drugs effective in the treatment of major depressive disorder. Sertraline does not inhibit monoamine oxidase.

Pharmacokinetics
Systemic Bioavailability–In man, following oral once-daily dosing over the range of 50 to 200 mg for 14 days, mean peak plasma concentrations (Cmax) of sertraline occurred between 4.5 to 8.4 hours post-dosing. The average terminal elimination half-life of plasma sertraline is about 26 hours. Based on this pharmacokinetic parameter, steady-state sertraline plasma levels should be achieved after approximately one week of once-daily dosing. Linear dose-proportional pharmacokinetics were demonstrated in a single dose study in which the Cmax and area under the plasma concentration time curve (AUC) of sertraline were proportional to dose over a range of 50 to 200 mg. Consistent with the terminal elimination half-life, there is an approximately two-fold accumulation, compared to a single dose, of sertraline with repeated dosing over a 50 to 200 mg dose range. The single dose bioavailability of sertraline tablets is approximately equal to an equivalent dose of solution.
In a relative bioavailability study comparing the pharmacokinetics of 100 mg sertraline as the oral solution to a 100 mg sertraline tablet in 16 healthy adults, the solution to tablet ratio of geometric mean AUC and Cmax values were 114.8% and 120.6%, respectively. 90% confidence intervals (CI) were within the range of 80-125% with the exception of the upper 90% CI limit for Cmax which was 126.5%.
The effects of food on the bioavailability of the sertraline tablet and oral concentrate were studied in subjects administered a single dose with and without food. For the tablet, AUC was slightly increased when drug was administered with food but the Cmax was 25% greater, while the time to reach peak plasma concentration (Tmax) decreased from 8 hours post-dosing to 5.5 hours. For the oral concentrate, Tmax was slightly prolonged from 5.9 hours to 7.0 hours with food.
Metabolism–Sertraline undergoes extensive first pass metabolism. The principal initial pathway of metabolism for sertraline is N-demethylation. N-desmethylsertraline has a plasma terminal elimination half-life of 62 to 104 hours. Both *in vitro* biochemical and *in vivo* pharmacological testing have shown N-desmethylsertraline to be substantially less active than sertraline. Both sertraline and N-desmethylsertraline undergo oxidative deamination and subsequent reduction, hydroxylation, and glucuronide conjugation. In a study of radiolabeled sertraline involving two healthy male subjects, sertraline accounted for less than 5% of the plasma radioactivity. About 40-45% of the administered radioactivity was recovered in urine in 9 days. Unchanged sertraline was not detectable in the urine. For the same period, about 40-45% of the administered radioactivity was accounted for in feces, including 12-14% unchanged sertraline.
Desmethylsertraline exhibits time-related, dose dependent increases in AUC (0-24 hour), Cmax and Cmin, with about a 5-9 fold increase in these pharmacokinetic parameters between day 1 and day 14.
Protein Binding–*In vitro* protein binding studies performed with radiolabeled ^3H-sertraline showed that sertraline is highly bound to serum proteins (98%) in the range of 20 to 500 ng/mL. However, at up to 300 and 200 ng/mL concentrations, respectively, sertraline and N-desmethylsertraline did not alter the plasma protein binding of two other highly protein bound drugs, viz., warfarin and propranolol (see PRECAUTIONS).
Pediatric Pharmacokinetics–Sertraline pharmacokinetics were evaluated in a group of 61 pediatric patients (29 aged 6-12 years, 32 aged 13-17 years) with a DSM-III-R diagnosis of major depressive disorder or obsessive-compulsive disorder. Patients included both males (N=28) and females (N=33). During 42 days of chronic sertraline dosing, sertraline was titrated up to 200 mg/day and maintained at that dose for a minimum of 11 days. On the final day of sertraline 200 mg/day, the 6-12 year old group exhibited a mean sertraline AUC (0-24 hr) of 3107 ng-hr/mL, mean Cmax of 165 ng/mL, and mean half-life of 26.2 hr. The 13-17 year old group exhibited a mean sertraline AUC (0-24 hr) of 2296 ng-hr/mL, mean Cmax of 123 ng/mL, and mean half-life of 27.8 hr. Higher plasma levels in the 6-12 year old group were largely attributable to patients with lower body weights. No gender associated differences were observed. By comparison, a group of 22 separately studied adults between 18 and 45 years of age (11 male, 11 female) received 30 days of 200 mg/day sertraline and exhibited a mean sertraline AUC (0-24 hr) of 2570 ng-hr/mL, mean Cmax of 142 ng/mL, and mean half-life of 27.2 hr. Relative to the adults, both the 6-12 year olds and the 13-17 year olds showed about 22% lower AUC (0-24 hr) and Cmax values when plasma concentration was adjusted for weight. These data suggest that pediatric patients metabolize sertraline with slightly greater efficiency than adults. Nevertheless, lower doses may be advisable for pediatric patients given their lower body weights, especially in very young patients, in order to avoid excessive plasma levels (see DOSAGE AND ADMINISTRATION).
Age–Sertraline plasma clearance in a group of 16 (8 male, 8 female) elderly patients treated for 14 days at a dose of 100 mg/day was approximately 40% lower than in a similarly studied group of younger (25 to 32 y.o.) individuals. Steady-state, therefore, should be achieved after 2 to 3 weeks in older patients. The same study showed a decreased clearance of desmethylsertraline in older males, but not in older females.
Liver Disease–As might be predicted from its primary site of metabolism, liver impairment can affect the elimination of sertraline. In patients with chronic mild liver impairment (N=10, 8 patients with Child-Pugh scores of 5-6 and 2 patients with Child-Pugh scores of 7-8) who received 50 mg sertraline per day maintained for 21 days, sertraline clearance was reduced, resulting in approximately 3-fold greater exposure compared to age-matched volunteers with no hepatic impairment (N=10). The exposure to desmethylsertraline was approximately 2-fold greater compared to age-matched volunteers with no hepatic impairment. There were no significant differences in plasma protein binding observed between the two groups. The effects of sertraline in patients with moderate and severe hepatic impairment have not been studied. The results suggest that the use of sertraline in patients with liver disease must be approached with caution. If sertraline is administered to patients with liver impairment, a lower or less frequent dose should be used (see PRECAUTIONS and DOSAGE AND ADMINISTRATION).
Renal Disease–Sertraline is extensively metabolized and excretion of unchanged drug in urine is a minor route of elimination. In volunteers with mild to moderate (CLcr=30-60 mL/min), moderate to severe (CLcr=10-29 mL/min) or severe (receiving hemodialysis) renal impairment (N=10 each group), the pharmacokinetics and protein binding of 200 mg sertraline per day maintained for 21 days were not altered compared to age-matched volunteers (N=12) with no renal impairment. Thus sertraline multiple dose pharmacokinetics appear to be unaffected by renal impairment (see PRECAUTIONS).

Clinical Trials
Major Depressive Disorder–The efficacy of ZOLOFT as a treatment for major depressive disorder was established in two placebo-controlled studies in adult outpatients meeting DSM-III criteria for major depressive disorder. Study 1 was an 8-week study with flexible dosing of ZOLOFT in a range of 50 to 200 mg/day; the mean dose for completers was 145 mg/day. Study 2 was a 6-week fixed-dose study, including ZOLOFT doses of 50, 100, and 200 mg/day. Overall, these studies demonstrated ZOLOFT to be superior to placebo on the Hamilton Depression Rating Scale and the Clinical Global Impression Severity and Improvement scales. Study 2 was not readily interpretable regarding a dose response relationship for effectiveness.
Study 3 involved depressed outpatients who had responded by the end of an initial 8-week open treatment phase on ZOLOFT 50-200 mg/day. These patients (N=295) were randomized to continuation for 44 weeks on double-blind ZOLOFT 50-200 mg/day or placebo. A statistically significantly lower relapse rate was observed for patients taking ZOLOFT compared to those on placebo. The mean dose for completers was 70 mg/day.
Analyses for gender effects on outcome did not suggest any differential responsiveness on the basis of sex.
Obsessive-Compulsive Disorder (OCD)–The effectiveness of ZOLOFT in the treatment of OCD was demonstrated in three multicenter placebo-controlled studies of adult outpatients (Studies 1-3). Patients in all studies had moderate to severe OCD (DSM-III or DSM-III-R) with mean baseline ratings on the Yale-Brown Obsessive-Compulsive Scale (YBOCS) total score ranging from 23 to 25.
Study 1 was an 8-week study with flexible dosing of ZOLOFT in a range of 50 to 200 mg/day; the mean dose for completers was 186 mg/day. Patients receiving ZOLOFT experienced a mean reduction of approximately 4 points on the YBOCS total score which was significantly greater than the mean reduction of 2 points in placebo-treated patients.
Study 2 was a 12-week fixed-dose study, including ZOLOFT doses of 50, 100, and 200 mg/day. Patients receiving ZOLOFT doses of 50 and 200 mg/day experienced mean reductions of approximately 6 points on the YBOCS total score which were significantly greater than the approximately 3 point reduction in placebo-treated patients.
Study 3 was a 12-week study with flexible dosing of ZOLOFT in a range of 50 to 200 mg/day; the mean dose for completers was 185 mg/day. Patients receiving ZOLOFT experienced a mean reduction of approximately 7 points on the YBOCS total score which was significantly greater than the mean reduction of approximately 4 points in placebo-treated patients.

Analyses for age and gender effects on outcome did not suggest any differential responsiveness on the basis of age or sex.

The effectiveness of ZOLOFT for the treatment of OCD was also demonstrated in a 12-week, multicenter, placebo-controlled, parallel group study in a pediatric outpatient population (children and adolescents, ages 6-17). Patients receiving ZOLOFT in this study were initiated at doses of either 25 mg/day (children, ages 6-12) or 50 mg/day (adolescents, ages 13-17), and then titrated over the next four weeks to a maximum dose of 200 mg/day, as tolerated. The mean dose for completers was 178 mg/day. Dosing was once a day in the morning or evening. Patients in this study had moderate to severe OCD (DSM-III-R) with mean baseline ratings on the Children's Yale-Brown Obsessive-Compulsive Scale (CYBOCS) total score of 22. Patients receiving sertraline experienced a mean reduction of approximately 7 units on the CYBOCS total score which was significantly greater than the 3 unit reduction for placebo patients. Analyses for age and gender effects on outcome did not suggest any differential responsiveness on the basis of age or sex.

In a longer-term study, patients meeting DSM-III-R criteria for OCD who had responded during a 52-week single-blind trial on ZOLOFT 50-200 mg/day (n=224) were randomized to continuation of ZOLOFT or to substitution of placebo for up to 28 weeks of observation for discontinuation due to relapse or insufficient clinical response. Response during the single-blind phase was defined as a decrease in the YBOCS score of ≥ 25% compared to baseline and a CGI-I of 1 (very much improved), 2 (much improved) or 3 (minimally improved). Relapse during the double-blind phase was defined as the following conditions being met (on three consecutive visits for 1 and 2, and for visit 3 for condition 3): (1) YBOCS score increased by ≥ 5 points, to a minimum of 20, relative to baseline; (2) CGI-I increased by ≥ one point; and (3) worsening of the patient's condition in the investigator's judgment, to justify alternative treatment. Insufficient clinical response indicated a worsening of the patient's condition that resulted in study discontinuation, as assessed by the investigator. Patients receiving continued ZOLOFT treatment experienced a significantly lower rate of discontinuation due to relapse or insufficient clinical response over the subsequent 28 weeks compared to those receiving placebo. This pattern was demonstrated in male and female subjects.

Panic Disorder–The effectiveness of ZOLOFT in the treatment of panic disorder was demonstrated in three double-blind, placebo-controlled studies (Studies 1-3) of adult outpatients who had a primary diagnosis of panic disorder (DSM-III-R), with or without agoraphobia.

Studies 1 and 2 were 10-week flexible dose studies. ZOLOFT was initiated at 25 mg/day for the first week, and then patients were dosed in a range of 50-200 mg/day on the basis of clinical response and toleration. The mean ZOLOFT doses for completers to 10 weeks were 131 mg/day and 144 mg/day, respectively, for Studies 1 and 2. In these studies, ZOLOFT was shown to be significantly more effective than placebo on change from baseline in panic attack frequency and on the Clinical Global Impression Severity of Illness and Global Improvement scores. The difference between ZOLOFT and placebo in reduction from baseline in the number of full panic attacks was approximately 2 panic attacks per week in both studies.

Study 3 was a 12-week fixed-dose study, including ZOLOFT doses of 50, 100, and 200 mg/day. Patients receiving ZOLOFT experienced a significantly greater reduction in panic attack frequency than patients receiving placebo. Study 3 was not readily interpretable regarding a dose response relationship for effectiveness.

Subgroup analyses did not indicate that there were any differences in treatment outcomes as a function of age, race, or gender.

In a longer-term study, patients meeting DSM-III-R criteria for Panic Disorder who had responded during a 52-week open trial on ZOLOFT 50-200 mg/day (n=183) were randomized to continuation of ZOLOFT or to substitution of placebo for up to 28 weeks of observation for discontinuation due to relapse or insufficient clinical response. Response during the open phase was defined as a CGI-I score of 1 (very much improved) or 2 (much improved). Relapse during the double-blind phase was defined as the following conditions being met on three consecutive visits: (1) CGI-I ≥ 3; (2) meets DSM-III-R criteria for Panic Disorder; (3) number of panic attacks greater than at baseline. Insufficient clinical response indicated a worsening of the patient's condition that resulted in study discontinuation, as assessed by the investigator. Patients receiving continued ZOLOFT treatment experienced a significantly lower rate of discontinuation due to relapse or insufficient clinical response over the subsequent 28 weeks compared to those receiving placebo. This pattern was demonstrated in male and female subjects.

Posttraumatic Stress Disorder (PTSD)–The effectiveness of ZOLOFT in the treatment of PTSD was established in two multicenter placebo-controlled studies (Studies 1-2) of adult outpatients who met DSM-III-R criteria for PTSD. The mean duration of PTSD for these patients was 12 years (Studies 1 and 2 combined) and 44% of patients (169 of the 385 patients treated) had secondary depressive disorder.

Studies 1 and 2 were 12-week flexible dose studies. ZOLOFT was initiated at 25 mg/day for the first week, and patients were then dosed in the range of 50-200 mg/day on the basis of clinical response and toleration. The mean ZOLOFT dose for completers was 146 mg/day and 151 mg/day, respectively for Studies 1 and 2. Study outcome was assessed by the Clinician-Administered PTSD Scale Part 2 (CAPS) which is a multi-item instrument that measures the three PTSD diagnostic symptom clusters of reexperiencing/intrusion, avoidance/numbing, and hyperarousal as well as the patient-rated Impact of Event Scale (IES) which measures intrusion and avoidance symptoms. ZOLOFT was shown to be significantly more effective than placebo on change from baseline to endpoint on the CAPS, IES and on the Clinical Global Impressions (CGI) Severity of Illness and Global Improvement scores. In two additional placebo-controlled PTSD trials, the difference in response to treatment between patients receiving ZOLOFT and patients receiving placebo was not statistically significant. One of these additional studies was conducted in patients similar to those recruited for Studies 1 and 2, while the second additional study was conducted in predominantly male veterans.

As PTSD is a more common disorder in women than men, the majority (76%) of patients in these trials were women (152 and 139 women on sertraline and placebo versus 39 and 55 men on sertraline and placebo; Studies 1 and 2 combined). Post hoc exploratory analyses revealed a significant difference between ZOLOFT and placebo on the CAPS, IES and CGI in women, regardless of baseline diagnosis of comorbid major depressive disorder, but essentially no effect in the relatively smaller number of men in these studies. The clinical significance of this apparent gender interaction is unknown at this time. There was insufficient information to determine the effect of race or age on outcome.

In a longer-term study, patients meeting DSM-III-R criteria for PTSD who had responded during a 24-week open trial on ZOLOFT 50-200 mg/day (n=96) were randomized to continuation of ZOLOFT or to substitution of placebo for up to 28 weeks of observation for relapse. Response during the open phase was defined as a CGI-I of 1 (very much improved) or 2 (much improved), and a decrease in the CAPS-2 score of > 30% compared to baseline. Relapse during the double-blind phase was defined as the following conditions being met on two consecutive visits: (1) CGI-I ≥ 3; (2) CAPS-2 score increased by ≥ 30% and by ≥ 15 points relative to baseline; and (3) worsening of the patient's condition in the investigator's judgment. Patients receiving continued ZOLOFT treatment experienced significantly lower relapse rates over the subsequent 28 weeks compared to those receiving placebo. This pattern was demonstrated in male and female subjects.

Premenstrual Dysphoric Disorder (PMDD) – The effectiveness of ZOLOFT for the treatment of PMDD was established in two double-blind, parallel group, placebo-controlled flexible dose trials (Studies 1 and 2) conducted over 3 menstrual cycles. Patients in Study 1 met DSM-III-R criteria for Late Luteal Phase Dysphoric Disorder (LLPDD), the clinical entity now referred to as Premenstrual Dysphoric Disorder (PMDD) in DSM-IV. Patients in Study 2 met DSM-IV criteria for PMDD. Study 1 utilized daily dosing throughout the study, while Study 2 utilized luteal phase dosing for the 2 weeks prior to the onset of menses. The mean duration of PMDD symptoms for these patients was approximately 10.5 years in both studies. Patients on oral contraceptives were excluded from these trials; therefore, the efficacy of sertraline in combination with oral contraceptives for the treatment of PMDD is unknown.

Efficacy was assessed with the Daily Record of Severity of Problems (DRSP), a patient-rated instrument that mirrors the diagnostic criteria for PMDD as identified in the DSM-IV, and includes assessments for mood, physical symptoms, and other symptoms. Other efficacy assessments included the Hamilton Depression Rating Scale (HAMD-17), and the Clinical Global Impression Severity of Illness (CGI-S) and Improvement (CGI-I) scores.

In Study 1, involving n=251 randomized patients, ZOLOFT treatment was initiated at 50 mg/day and administered daily throughout the menstrual cycle. In subsequent cycles, patients were dosed in the range of 50-150 mg/day on the basis of clinical response and toleration. The mean dose for completers was 102 mg/day. ZOLOFT administered daily throughout the menstrual cycle was significantly more effective than placebo on change from baseline to endpoint on the DRSP total score, the HAMD-17 total score, and the CGI-S score, as well as the CGI-I score at endpoint.

In Study 2, involving n=281 randomized patients, ZOLOFT treatment was initiated at 50 mg/day in the late luteal phase (last 2 weeks) of each menstrual cycle and then discontinued at the onset of menses. In subsequent cycles, patients were dosed in the range of 50-100 mg/day in the luteal phase of each cycle, on the basis of clinical response and toleration. Patients who were titrated to 100 mg/day received 50 mg/day for the first 3 days of the cycle, then 100 mg/day for the remainder of the cycle. The mean ZOLOFT dose for completers was 74 mg/day. ZOLOFT administered in the late luteal phase of the menstrual cycle was significantly more effective than placebo on change from baseline to endpoint on the DRSP total score and the CGI-S score, as well as the CGI-I score at endpoint.

There was insufficient information to determine the effect of race or age on outcome in these studies.

Social Anxiety Disorder – The effectiveness of ZOLOFT in the treatment of social anxiety disorder (also known as social phobia) was established in two multicenter placebo-controlled studies (Study 1 and 2) of adult outpatients who met DSM-IV criteria for social anxiety disorder.

Study 1 was a 12-week, multicenter, flexible dose study comparing ZOLOFT (50-200 mg/day) to placebo, in which ZOLOFT was initiated at 25 mg/day for the first week. Study outcome was assessed by (a) the Liebowitz Social Anxiety Scale (LSAS), a 24-item clinician administered instrument that measures fear, anxiety and avoidance of social and performance situations, and by (b) the proportion of responders as defined by the Clinical Global Impression of Improvement (CGI-I) criterion of CGI-I ≤ 2 (very much or much improved). ZOLOFT was statistically significantly more effective than placebo as measured by the LSAS and the percentage of responders.

Study 2 was a 20-week, multicenter, flexible dose study that compared ZOLOFT (50-200 mg/day) to placebo. Study outcome was assessed by the (a) Duke Brief Social Phobia Scale (BSPS), a multi-item clinician-rated instrument that measures fear, avoidance and physiologic response to social or performance situations, (b) the Marks Fear Questionnaire Social Phobia Subscale (FQ-SPS), a 5-item patient-rated instrument that measures change in the severity of phobic avoidance and distress, and (c) the CGI-I responder criterion of ≤ 2. ZOLOFT was shown to be statistically significantly more effective than placebo as measured by the BSPS total score and fear, avoidance and physiologic factor scores, as well as the FQ-SPS total score, and to have significantly more responders than placebo as defined by the CGI-I.

Subgroup analyses did not suggest differences in treatment outcome on the basis of gender. There was insufficient information to determine the effect of race or age on outcome.

In a longer-term study, patients meeting DSM-IV criteria for social anxiety disorder who had responded while assigned to ZOLOFT (CGI-I of 1 or 2) during a 20-week placebo-controlled trial on ZOLOFT 50-200 mg/day were randomized to continuation of ZOLOFT or to substitution of placebo for up to 24 weeks of observation for relapse. Relapse was defined as ≥ 2 point increase in the Clinical Global Impression – Severity of Illness (CGI-S) score compared to baseline or study discontinuation due to lack of efficacy. Patients receiving ZOLOFT continuation treatment experienced a statistically significantly lower relapse rate over this 24-week study than patients randomized to placebo substitution.

INDICATIONS AND USAGE

Major Depressive Disorder–ZOLOFT® (sertraline hydrochloride) is indicated for the treatment of major depressive disorder in adults.

The efficacy of ZOLOFT in the treatment of a major depressive episode was established in six to eight week controlled trials of adult outpatients whose diagnoses corresponded most closely to the DSM-III category of major depressive disorder (see Clinical Trials under CLINICAL PHARMACOLOGY).

A major depressive episode implies a prominent and relatively persistent depressed or dysphoric mood that usually interferes with daily functioning (nearly every day for at least 2 weeks); it should include at least 4 of the following 8 symptoms: change in appetite, change in sleep, psychomotor agitation or retardation, loss of interest in usual activities or decrease in sexual drive, increased fatigue, feelings of guilt or worthlessness, slowed thinking or impaired concentration, and a suicide attempt or suicidal ideation.

The antidepressant action of ZOLOFT in hospitalized depressed patients has not been adequately studied.

The efficacy of ZOLOFT in maintaining an antidepressant response for up to 44 weeks following 8 weeks of open-label acute treatment (52 weeks total) was demonstrated in a placebo-controlled trial. The usefulness of the drug in patients receiving ZOLOFT for extended periods should be reevaluated periodically (see Clinical Trials under CLINICAL PHARMACOLOGY).

Obsessive-Compulsive Disorder–ZOLOFT is indicated for the treatment of obsessions and compulsions in patients with obsessive-compulsive disorder (OCD), as defined in the DSM-III-R; i.e., the obsessions or compulsions cause marked distress, are time-consuming, or significantly interfere with social or occupational functioning.

The efficacy of ZOLOFT was established in 12-week trials with obsessive-compulsive outpatients having diagnoses of obsessive-compulsive disorder as defined according to DSM-III or DSM-III-R criteria (see Clinical Trials under CLINICAL PHARMACOLOGY).

Obsessive-compulsive disorder is characterized by recurrent and persistent ideas, thoughts, impulses, or images (obsessions) that are ego-dystonic and/or repetitive, purposeful, and intentional behaviors (compulsions) that are recognized by the person as excessive or unreasonable.

The efficacy of ZOLOFT in maintaining a response, in patients with OCD who responded during a 52-week treatment phase while taking ZOLOFT and were then observed for relapse during a period of up to 28 weeks, was demonstrated in a placebo-controlled trial (see Clinical Trials under CLINICAL PHARMACOLOGY). Nevertheless, the physician who elects to use ZOLOFT for extended periods should periodically re-evaluate the long-term usefulness of the drug for the individual patient (see DOSAGE AND ADMINISTRATION).

Panic Disorder–ZOLOFT is indicated for the treatment of panic disorder in adults, with or without agoraphobia, as defined in DSM-IV. Panic disorder is characterized by the occurrence of unexpected panic attacks and associated concern about having additional attacks, worry about the im-

Continued on next page

Zoloft—Cont.

plications or consequences of the attacks, and/or a significant change in behavior related to the attacks.

The efficacy of ZOLOFT was established in three 10-12 week trials in adult panic disorder patients whose diagnoses corresponded to the DSM-III-R category of panic disorder (see Clinical Trials under CLINICAL PHARMACOLOGY).

Panic disorder (DSM-IV) is characterized by recurrent unexpected panic attacks, i.e., a discrete period of intense fear or discomfort in which four (or more) of the following symptoms develop abruptly and reach a peak within 10 minutes: (1) palpitations, pounding heart, or accelerated heart rate; (2) sweating; (3) trembling or shaking; (4) sensations of shortness of breath or smothering; (5) feeling of choking; (6) chest pain or discomfort; (7) nausea or abdominal distress; (8) feeling dizzy, unsteady, lightheaded, or faint; (9) derealization (feelings of unreality) or depersonalization (being detached from oneself); (10) fear of losing control; (11) fear of dying; (12) paresthesias (numbness or tingling sensations); (13) chills or hot flushes.

The efficacy of ZOLOFT in maintaining a response, in adult patients with panic disorder who responded during a 52-week treatment phase while taking ZOLOFT and were then observed for relapse during a period of up to 28 weeks, was demonstrated in a placebo-controlled trial (see Clinical Trials under CLINICAL PHARMACOLOGY). Nevertheless, the physician who elects to use ZOLOFT for extended periods should periodically re-evaluate the long-term usefulness of the drug for the individual patient (see DOSAGE AND ADMINISTRATION).

Posttraumatic Stress Disorder (PTSD)—ZOLOFT (sertraline hydrochloride) is indicated for the treatment of posttraumatic stress disorder in adults.

The efficacy of ZOLOFT in the treatment of PTSD was established in two 12-week placebo-controlled trials of adult outpatients whose diagnosis met criteria for the DSM-III-R category of PTSD (see Clinical Trials under CLINICAL PHARMACOLOGY).

PTSD, as defined by DSM-III-R/IV, requires exposure to a traumatic event that involved actual or threatened death or serious injury, or threat to the physical integrity of self or others, and a response which involves intense fear, helplessness, or horror. Symptoms that occur as a result of exposure to the traumatic event include reexperiencing of the event in the form of intrusive thoughts, flashbacks or dreams, and intense psychological distress and physiological reactivity on exposure to cues to the event; avoidance of situations reminiscent of the traumatic event, inability to recall details of the event, and/or numbing of general responsiveness manifested as diminished interest in significant activities, estrangement from others, restricted range of affect, or sense of foreshortened future; and symptoms of autonomic arousal including hypervigilance, exaggerated startle response, sleep disturbance, impaired concentration, and irritability or outbursts of anger. A PTSD diagnosis requires that the symptoms are present for at least a month and that they cause clinically significant distress or impairment in social, occupational, or other important areas of functioning.

The efficacy of ZOLOFT in maintaining a response in adult patients with PTSD for up to 28 weeks following 24 weeks of open-label treatment was demonstrated in a placebo-controlled trial. Nevertheless, the physician who elects to use ZOLOFT for extended periods should periodically re-evaluate the long-term usefulness of the drug for the individual patient (see DOSAGE AND ADMINISTRATION).

Premenstrual Dysphoric Disorder (PMDD) – ZOLOFT is indicated for the treatment of premenstrual dysphoric disorder (PMDD) in adults.

The efficacy of ZOLOFT in the treatment of PMDD was established in 2 placebo-controlled trials of female adult outpatients treated for 3 menstrual cycles who met criteria for the DSM-III-R/IV category of PMDD (see Clinical Trials under CLINICAL PHARMACOLOGY).

The essential features of PMDD include markedly depressed mood, anxiety or tension, affective lability, and persistent anger or irritability. Other features include decreased interest in activities, difficulty concentrating, lack of energy, change in appetite or sleep, and feeling out of control. Physical symptoms associated with PMDD include breast tenderness, headache, joint and muscle pain, bloating and weight gain. These symptoms occur regularly during the luteal phase and remit within a few days following onset of menses; the disturbance markedly interferes with work or school or with usual social activities and relationships with others. In making the diagnosis, care should be taken to rule out other cyclical mood disorders that may be exacerbated by treatment with an antidepressant.

The effectiveness of ZOLOFT in long-term use, that is, for more than 3 menstrual cycles, has not been systematically evaluated in controlled trials. Therefore, the physician who elects to use ZOLOFT for extended periods should periodically re-evaluate the long-term usefulness of the drug for the individual patient (see DOSAGE AND ADMINISTRATION).

Social Anxiety Disorder – ZOLOFT (sertraline hydrochloride) is indicated for the treatment of social anxiety disorder, also known as social phobia in adults.

The efficacy of ZOLOFT in the treatment of social anxiety disorder was established in two placebo-controlled trials of adult outpatients with a diagnosis of social anxiety disorder as defined by DSM-IV criteria (see Clinical Trials under CLINICAL PHARMACOLOGY).

Social anxiety disorder, as defined by DSM-IV, is characterized by marked and persistent fear of social or performance situations involving exposure to unfamiliar people or possible scrutiny by others and by fears of acting in a humiliating or embarrassing way. Exposure to the feared social situation almost always provokes anxiety and feared social or performance situations are avoided or else are endured with intense anxiety or distress. In addition, patients recognize that the fear is excessive or unreasonable and the avoidance and anticipatory anxiety of the feared situation is associated with functional impairment or marked distress.

The efficacy of ZOLOFT in maintaining a response in adult patients with social anxiety disorder for up to 24 weeks following 20 weeks of ZOLOFT treatment was demonstrated in a placebo-controlled trial. Physicians who prescribe ZOLOFT for extended periods should periodically re-evaluate the long-term usefulness of the drug for the individual patient (see Clinical Trials under CLINICAL PHARMACOLOGY).

CONTRAINDICATIONS

All Dosage Forms of ZOLOFT:

Concomitant use in patients taking monoamine oxidase inhibitors (MAOIs) is contraindicated (see WARNINGS). Concomitant use in patients taking pimozide is contraindicated (see PRECAUTIONS).

ZOLOFT is contraindicated in patients with a hypersensitivity to sertraline or any of the inactive ingredients in ZOLOFT.

Oral Concentrate:

ZOLOFT oral concentrate is contraindicated with ANTABUSE (disulfiram) due to the alcohol content of the concentrate.

WARNINGS

Cases of serious sometimes fatal reactions have been reported in patients receiving ZOLOFT® (sertraline hydrochloride), a selective serotonin reuptake inhibitor (SSRI), in combination with a monoamine oxidase inhibitor (MAOI). Symptoms of a drug interaction between an SSRI and an MAOI include: hyperthermia, rigidity, myoclonus, autonomic instability with possible rapid fluctuations of vital signs, mental status changes that include confusion, irritability, and extreme agitation progressing to delirium and coma. These reactions have also been reported in patients who have recently discontinued an SSRI and have been started on an MAOI. Some cases presented with features resembling neuroleptic malignant syndrome. Therefore, ZOLOFT should not be used in combination with an MAOI, or within 14 days of discontinuing treatment with an MAOI. Similarly, at least 14 days should be allowed after stopping ZOLOFT before starting an MAOI.

Clinical Worsening and Suicide Risk

Patients with major depressive disorder (MDD), both adult and pediatric, may experience worsening of their depression and/or the emergence of suicidal ideation and behavior (suicidality) or unusual changes in behavior, whether or not they are taking antidepressant medications, and this risk may persist until significant remission occurs. There has been a long-standing concern that antidepressants may have a role in inducing worsening of depression and the emergence of suicidality in certain patients. Antidepressants increased the risk of suicidal thinking and behavior (suicidality) in short-term studies in children and adolescents with Major Depressive Disorder (MDD) and other psychiatric disorders.

Pooled analyses of short-term placebo-controlled trials of 9 antidepressant drugs (SSRIs and others) in children and adolescents with MDD, OCD, or other psychiatric disorders (a total of 24 trials involving over 4400 patients) have revealed a greater risk of adverse events representing suicidal behavior or thinking (suicidality) during the first few months of treatment in those receiving antidepressants. The average risk of such events in patients receiving antidepressants was 4%, twice the placebo risk of 2%. There was considerable variation in risk among drugs, but a tendency toward an increase for almost all drugs studied. The risk of suicidality was most consistently observed in the MDD trials, but there were signals of risk arising from some trials in other psychiatric indications (obsessive-compulsive disorder and social anxiety disorder) as well. **No suicides occurred in any of these trials.** It is unknown whether the suicidality risk in pediatric patients extends to longer-term use, i.e., beyond several months. It is also unknown whether the suicidality risk extends to adults.

All pediatric patients being treated with antidepressants for any indication should be observed closely for clinical worsening, suicidality, and unusual changes in behavior, especially during the initial few months of a course of drug therapy, or at times of dose changes, either increases or decreases. Such observation would generally include at least weekly face-to-face contact with patients or their family members or caregivers during the first 4 weeks of treatment, then every other week visits for the next 4 weeks, then at 12 weeks, and as clinically indicated beyond 12 weeks. Additional contact by telephone may be appropriate between face-to-face visits.

Adults with MDD or co-morbid depression in the setting of other psychiatric illness being treated with antidepressants should be observed similarly for clinical worsening and suicidality, especially during the initial few months of a course of drug therapy, or at times of dose changes, either increases or decreases.

The following symptoms, anxiety, agitation, panic attacks, insomnia, irritability, hostility aggressiveness, impulsivity,

akathisia (psychomotor restlessness), hypomania, and mania, have been reported in adult and pediatric patients being treated with antidepressants for major depressive disorder as well as for other indications, both psychiatric and nonpsychiatric. Although a causal link between the emergence of such symptoms and either the worsening of depression and/or the emergence of suicidal impulses has not been established, there is concern that such symptoms may represent precursors to emerging suicidality.

Consideration should be given to changing the therapeutic regimen, including possibly discontinuing the medication, in patients whose depression is persistently worse, or who are experiencing emergent suicidality or symptoms that might be precursors to worsening depression or suicidality, especially if these symptoms are severe, abrupt in onset, or were not part of the patient's presenting symptoms.

If the decision has been made to discontinue treatment, medication should be tapered, as rapidly as is feasible, but with recognition that abrupt discontinuation can be associated with certain symptoms (see PRECAUTIONS and DOSAGE AND ADMINISTRATION—Discontinuation of Treatment with ZOLOFT, for a description of the risks of discontinuation of ZOLOFT).

Families and caregivers of pediatric patients being treated with antidepressants for major depressive disorder or other indications, both psychiatric and nonpsychiatric, should be alerted about the need to monitor patients for the emergence of agitation, irritability, unusual changes in behavior, and the other symptoms described above, as well as the emergence of suicidality, and to report such symptoms immediately to health care providers. Such monitoring should include daily observation by families and caregivers. Prescriptions for ZOLOFT should be written for the smallest quantity of tablets consistent with good patient management, in order to reduce the risk of overdose. Families and caregivers of adults being treated for depression should be similarly advised.

Screening Patients for Bipolar Disorder: A major depressive episode may be the initial presentation of bipolar disorder. It is generally believed (though not established in controlled trials) that treating such an episode with an antidepressant alone may increase the likelihood of precipitation of a mixed/manic episode in patients at risk for bipolar disorder. Whether any of the symptoms described above represent such a conversion is unknown. However, prior to initiating treatment with an antidepressant, patients with depressive symptoms should be adequately screened to determine if they are at risk for bipolar disorder; such screening should include a detailed psychiatric history, including a family history of suicide, bipolar disorder, and depression. It should be noted that ZOLOFT is not approved for use in treating bipolar depression.

PRECAUTIONS

General

Activation of Mania/Hypomania—During premarketing testing, hypomania or mania occurred in approximately 0.4% of ZOLOFT® (sertraline hydrochloride) treated patients.

Weight Loss—Significant weight loss may be an undesirable result of treatment with sertraline for some patients, but on average, patients in controlled trials had minimal, 1 to 2 pound weight loss, versus smaller changes on placebo. Only rarely have sertraline patients been discontinued for weight loss.

Seizure—ZOLOFT has not been evaluated in patients with a seizure disorder. These patients were excluded from clinical studies during the product's premarket testing. No seizures were observed among approximately 3000 patients treated with ZOLOFT in the development program for major depressive disorder. However, 4 patients out of approximately 1800 (220<18 years of age) exposed during the development program for obsessive-compulsive disorder experienced seizures, representing a crude incidence of 0.2%. Three of these patients were adolescents, two with a seizure disorder and one with a family history of seizure disorder, none of whom were receiving anticonvulsant medication. Accordingly, ZOLOFT should be introduced with care in patients with a seizure disorder.

Discontinuation of Treatment with Zoloft

During marketing of Zoloft and other SSRIs and SNRIs (Serotonin and Norepinephrine Reuptake Inhibitors), there have been spontaneous reports of adverse events occurring upon discontinuation of these drugs, particularly when abrupt, including the following: dysphoric mood, irritability, agitation, dizziness, sensory disturbances (e.g. paresthesias such as electric shock sensations), anxiety, confusion, headache, lethargy, emotional lability, insomnia, and hypomania. While these events are generally self-limiting, there have been reports of serious discontinuation symptoms.

Patients should be monitored for these symptoms when discontinuing treatment with Zoloft. A gradual reduction in the dose rather than abrupt cessation is recommended whenever possible. If intolerable symptoms occur following a decrease in the dose or upon discontinuation of treatment, then resuming the previously prescribed dose may be considered. Subsequently, the physician may continue decreasing the dose but at a more gradual rate (see DOSAGE AND ADMINISTRATION).

Abnormal Bleeding

Published case reports have documented the occurrence of bleeding episodes in patients treated with psychotropic drugs that interfere with serotonin reuptake. Subsequent epidemiological studies, both of the case-control and cohort design, have demonstrated an association between use of psychotropic drugs that interfere with serotonin reuptake and the occurrence of upper gastrointestinal bleeding. In two studies, concurrent use of a non-selective nonsteroidal anti-inflammatory drug (i.e., NSAIDs that inhibit both cyclooxygenase isoenzymes, COX 1 and 2) or aspirin potentiated the risk of bleeding (see DRUG INTERACTIONS). Although these studies focused on upper gastrointestinal bleeding, there is reason to believe that bleeding at other sites may be similarly potentiated. Patients should be cautioned regarding the risk of bleeding associated with the concomitant use of ZOLOFT with non-selective NSAIDs (i.e., NSAIDs that inhibit both cyclooxygenase isoenzymes, COX 1 and 2), aspirin, or other drugs that affect coagulation.

Weak Uricosuric Effect–ZOLOFT® (sertraline hydrochloride) is associated with a mean decrease in serum uric acid of approximately 7%. The clinical significance of this weak uricosuric effect is unknown.

Use in Patients with Concomitant Illness–Clinical experience with ZOLOFT in patients with certain concomitant systemic illness is limited. Caution is advisable in using ZOLOFT in patients with diseases or conditions that could affect metabolism or hemodynamic responses.

Patients with a recent history of myocardial infarction or unstable heart disease were excluded from clinical studies during the product's premarket testing. However, the electrocardiograms of 774 patients who received ZOLOFT in double-blind trials were evaluated and the data indicate that ZOLOFT is not associated with the development of significant ECG abnormalities.

ZOLOFT administered in a flexible dose range of 50 to 200 mg/day (mean dose of 89 mg/day) was evaluated in a post-marketing, placebo-controlled trial of 372 randomized subjects with a DSM-IV diagnosis of major depressive disorder and recent history of myocardial infarction or unstable angina requiring hospitalization. Exclusions from this trial included, among others, patients with uncontrolled hypertension, need for cardiac surgery, history of CABG within 3 months of index event, severe or symptomatic bradycardia, non-atherosclerotic cause of angina, clinically significant renal impairment (creatinine > 2.5 mg/dl), and clinically significant hepatic dysfunction. ZOLOFT treatment initiated during the acute phase of recovery (within 30 days post-MI or post-hospitalization for unstable angina) was indistinguishable from placebo in this study on the following week 16 treatment endpoints: left ventricular ejection fraction, total cardiovascular events (angina, chest pain, edema, palpitations, syncope, postural dizziness, CHF, MI, tachycardia, bradycardia, and changes in BP), and major cardiovascular events involving death or requiring hospitalization (for MI, CHF, stroke, or angina).

ZOLOFT is extensively metabolized by the liver. In patients with chronic mild liver impairment, sertraline clearance was reduced, resulting in increased AUC, Cmax and elimination half-life. The effects of sertraline in patients with moderate and severe hepatic impairment have not been studied. The use of sertraline in patients with liver disease must be approached with caution. If sertraline is administered to patients with liver impairment, a lower or less frequent dose should be used (see CLINICAL PHARMACOLOGY and DOSAGE AND ADMINISTRATION).

Since ZOLOFT is extensively metabolized, excretion of unchanged drug in urine is a minor route of elimination. A clinical study comparing sertraline pharmacokinetics in healthy volunteers to that in patients with renal impairment ranging from mild to severe (requiring dialysis) indicated that the pharmacokinetics and protein binding are unaffected by renal disease. Based on the pharmacokinetic results, there is no need for dosage adjustment in patients with renal impairment (see CLINICAL PHARMACOLOGY).

Interference with Cognitive and Motor Performance–In controlled studies, ZOLOFT did not cause sedation and did not interfere with psychomotor performance. (See **Information for Patients**.)

Hyponatremia–Several cases of hyponatremia have been reported and appeared to be reversible when ZOLOFT was discontinued. Some cases were possibly due to the syndrome of inappropriate antidiuretic hormone secretion. The majority of these occurrences have been in elderly individuals, some in patients taking diuretics or who were otherwise volume depleted.

Platelet Function–There have been rare reports of altered platelet function and/or abnormal results from laboratory studies in patients taking ZOLOFT. While there have been reports of abnormal bleeding or purpura in several patients taking ZOLOFT, it is unclear whether ZOLOFT had a causative role.

Information for Patients

Prescribers or other health professionals should inform patients, their families, and their caregivers about the benefits and risks associated with treatment with Zoloft and should counsel them in its appropriate use. A patient Medication Guide About Using Antidepressants in Children and Teenagers is available for ZOLOFT. The prescriber or health professional should instruct patients, their families, and their caregivers to read the Medication Guide and should assist them in understanding its contents. Patients should be given the opportunity to discuss the contents of the Medication Guide and to obtain answers to any questions they may have. The complete text of the Medication Guide is reprinted at the end of this document.

Patients should be advised of the following issues and asked to alert their prescriber if these occur while taking ZOLOFT.

Clinical Worsening and Suicide Risk: Patients, their families, and their caregivers should be encouraged to be alert to the emergence of anxiety, agitation, panic attacks, insomnia, irritability, hostility, aggressiveness, impulsivity, akathisia (psychomotor restlessness), hypomania, mania, other unusual changes in behavior, worsening of depression, and suicidal ideation, especially early during antidepressant treatment and when the dose is adjusted up or down. Families and caregivers of patients should be advised to observe for the emergence of such symptoms on a day-to-day basis, since changes may be abrupt. Such symptoms should be reported to the patient's prescriber or health professional, especially if they are severe, abrupt in onset, or were not part of the patient's presenting symptoms. Symptoms such as these may be associated with an increased risk for suicidal thinking and behavior and indicate a need for very close monitoring and possibly changes in the medication.

Patients should be told that although ZOLOFT has not been shown to impair the ability of normal subjects to perform tasks requiring complex motor and mental skills in laboratory experiments, drugs that act upon the central nervous system may affect some individuals adversely. Therefore, patients should be told that until they learn how they respond to ZOLOFT they should be careful doing activities when they need to be alert, such as driving a car or operating machinery.

Patients should be cautioned about the concomitant use of ZOLOFT and non-selective NSAIDs (i.e., NSAIDs that inhibit both cyclooxygenase isoenzymes, COX 1 and 2), aspirin, or other drugs that affect coagulation since the combined use of psychotropic drugs that interfere with serotonin reuptake and these agents has been associated with an increased risk of bleeding.

Patients should be told that although ZOLOFT has not been shown in experiments with normal subjects to increase the mental and motor skill impairments caused by alcohol, the concomitant use of ZOLOFT and alcohol is not advised.

Patients should be told that while no adverse interaction of ZOLOFT with over-the-counter (OTC) drug products is known to occur, the potential for interaction exists. Thus, the use of any OTC product should be initiated cautiously according to the directions of use given for the OTC product.

Patients should be advised to notify their physician if they become pregnant or intend to become pregnant during therapy.

Patients should be advised to notify their physician if they are breast feeding an infant.

ZOLOFT oral concentrate is contraindicated with ANTABUSE (disulfiram) due to the alcohol content of the concentrate.

ZOLOFT Oral Concentrate contains 20 mg/mL of sertraline (as the hydrochloride) as the active ingredient and 12% alcohol. ZOLOFT Oral Concentrate must be diluted before use. Just before taking, use the dropper provided to remove the required amount of ZOLOFT Oral Concentrate and mix with 4 oz (1/2 cup) of water, ginger ale, lemon/lime soda, lemonade or orange juice ONLY. Do not mix ZOLOFT Oral Concentrate with anything other than the liquids listed. The dose should be taken immediately after mixing. Do not mix in advance. At times, a slight haze may appear after mixing; this is normal. Note that caution should be exercised for persons with latex sensitivity, as the dropper dispenser contains dry natural rubber.

Laboratory Tests
None.

Drug Interactions
Potential Effects of Coadministration of Drugs Highly Bound to Plasma Proteins–Because sertraline is tightly bound to plasma protein, the administration of ZOLOFT® (sertraline hydrochloride) to a patient taking another drug which is tightly bound to protein (e.g., warfarin, digitoxin) may cause a shift in plasma concentrations potentially resulting in an adverse effect. Conversely, adverse effects may result from displacement of protein bound ZOLOFT by other tightly bound drugs.

In a study comparing prothrombin time AUC (0-120 hr) following dosing with warfarin (0.75 mg/kg) before and after 21 days of dosing with either ZOLOFT (50-200 mg/day) or placebo, there was a mean increase in prothrombin time of 8% relative to baseline for ZOLOFT compared to a 1% decrease for placebo (p<0.02). The normalization of prothrombin time for the ZOLOFT group was delayed compared to the placebo group. The clinical significance of this change is unknown. Accordingly, prothrombin time should be carefully monitored when ZOLOFT therapy is initiated or stopped.

Cimetidine–In a study assessing disposition of ZOLOFT (100 mg) on the second of 8 days of cimetidine administration (800 mg daily), there were significant increases in ZOLOFT mean AUC (50%), Cmax (24%) and half-life (26%) compared to the placebo group. The clinical significance of these changes is unknown.

CNS Active Drugs–In a study comparing the disposition of intravenously administered diazepam before and after 21 days of dosing with either ZOLOFT (50 to 200 mg/day escalating dose) or placebo, there was a 32% decrease relative to

baseline in diazepam clearance for the ZOLOFT group compared to a 19% decrease relative to baseline for the placebo group (p<0.03). There was a 23% increase in Tmax for desmethyldiazepam in the ZOLOFT group compared to a 20% decrease in the placebo group (p<0.03). The clinical significance of these changes is unknown.

In a placebo-controlled trial in normal volunteers, the administration of two doses of ZOLOFT did not significantly alter steady-state lithium levels or the renal clearance of lithium.

Nonetheless, at this time, it is recommended that plasma lithium levels be monitored following initiation of ZOLOFT therapy with appropriate adjustments to the lithium dose. In a controlled study of a single dose (2 mg) of pimozide, 200 mg sertraline (q.d.) co-administration to steady state was associated with a mean increase in pimozide AUC and Cmax of about 40%, but was not associated with any changes in EKG. Since the highest recommended pimozide dose (10 mg) has not been evaluated in combination with sertraline, the effect on QT interval and PK parameters at doses higher than 2 mg at this time are not known. While the mechanism of this interaction is unknown, due to the narrow therapeutic index of pimozide and due to the interaction noted at a low dose of pimozide, concomitant administration of ZOLOFT and pimozide should be contraindicated (see CONTRAINDICATIONS).

The risk of using ZOLOFT in combination with other CNS active drugs has not been systematically evaluated. Consequently, caution is advised if the concomitant administration of ZOLOFT and such drugs is required.

There is limited controlled experience regarding the optimal timing of switching from other drugs effective in the treatment of major depressive disorder, obsessive-compulsive disorder, panic disorder, posttraumatic stress disorder, premenstrual dysphoric disorder and social anxiety disorder to ZOLOFT. Care and prudent medical judgment should be exercised when switching, particularly from long-acting agents. The duration of an appropriate washout period which should intervene before switching from one selective serotonin reuptake inhibitor (SSRI) to another has not been established.

Monoamine Oxidase Inhibitors–See CONTRAINDICATIONS and WARNINGS.

Drugs Metabolized by P450 3A4–In three separate *in vivo* interaction studies, sertraline was co-administered with cytochrome P450 3A4 substrates, terfenadine, carbamazepine, or cisapride under steady-state conditions. The results of these studies indicated that sertraline did not increase plasma concentrations of terfenadine, carbamazepine, or cisapride. These data indicate that sertraline's extent of inhibition of P450 3A4 activity is not likely to be of clinical significance. Results of the interaction study with cisapride indicate that sertraline 200 mg (q.d.) induces the metabolism of cisapride (cisapride AUC and Cmax were reduced by about 35%).

Drugs Metabolized by P450 2D6–Many drugs effective in the treatment of major depressive disorder, e.g., the SSRIs, including sertraline, and most tricyclic antidepressant drugs effective in the treatment of major depressive disorder inhibit the biochemical activity of the drug metabolizing isozyme cytochrome P450 2D6 (debrisoquin hydroxylase), and, thus, may increase the plasma concentrations of co-administered drugs that are metabolized by P450 2D6. The drugs for which this potential interaction is of greatest concern are those metabolized primarily by 2D6 and which have a narrow therapeutic index, e.g., the tricyclic antidepressant drugs effective in the treatment of major depressive disorder and the Type 1C antiarrhythmics propafenone and flecainide. The extent to which this interaction is an important clinical problem depends on the extent of the inhibition of P450 2D6 by the antidepressant and the therapeutic index of the co-administered drug. There is variability among the drugs effective in the treatment of major depressive disorder in the extent of clinically important 2D6 inhibition, and in fact sertraline at lower doses has a less prominent inhibitory effect on 2D6 than some others in the class. Nevertheless, even sertraline has the potential for clinically important 2D6 inhibition. Consequently, concomitant use of a drug metabolized by P450 2D6 with ZOLOFT may require lower doses than usually prescribed for the other drug. Furthermore, whenever ZOLOFT is withdrawn from co-therapy, an increased dose of the co-administered drug may be required (see Tricyclic Antidepressant Drugs Effective in the Treatment of Major Depressive Disorder under PRECAUTIONS).

Sumatriptan–There have been rare postmarketing reports describing patients with weakness, hyperreflexia, and incoordination following the use of a selective serotonin reuptake inhibitor (SSRI) and sumatriptan. If concomitant treatment with sumatriptan and an SSRI (e.g., citalopram, fluoxetine, fluvoxamine, paroxetine, sertraline) is clinically warranted, appropriate observation of the patient is advised.

Tricyclic Antidepressant Drugs Effective in the Treatment of Major Depressive Disorder (TCAs)–The extent to which SSRI-TCA interactions may pose clinical problems will depend on the degree of inhibition and the pharmacokinetics of the SSRI involved. Nevertheless, caution is indicated in the co-administration of TCAs with ZOLOFT, because

Continued on next page

Zoloft—Cont.

sertraline may inhibit TCA metabolism. Plasma TCA concentrations may need to be reduced, and the dose of TCA may need to be monitored, and the dose of TCA may need to be reduced, if a TCA is co-administered with ZOLOFT (see Drugs Metabolized by P450 2D6 under PRECAUTIONS).

Hypoglycemic Drugs–In a placebo-controlled trial in normal volunteers, administration of ZOLOFT for 22 days (including 200 mg/day for the final 13 days) caused a statistically significant 16% decrease from baseline in the clearance of tolbutamide following an intravenous 1000 mg dose. ZOLOFT administration did not noticeably change either the plasma protein binding or the apparent volume of distribution of tolbutamide, suggesting that the decreased clearance was due to a change in the metabolism of the drug. The clinical significance of this decrease in tolbutamide clearance is unknown.

Atenolol–ZOLOFT (100 mg) when administered to 10 healthy male subjects had no effect on the beta-adrenergic blocking ability of atenolol.

Digoxin–In a placebo-controlled trial in normal volunteers, administration of ZOLOFT for 17 days (including 200 mg/day for the last 10 days) did not change serum digoxin levels or digoxin renal clearance.

Microsomal Enzyme Induction–Preclinical studies have shown ZOLOFT to induce hepatic microsomal enzymes. In clinical studies, ZOLOFT was shown to induce hepatic enzymes minimally as determined by a small (5%) but statistically significant decrease in antipyrine half-life following administration of 200 mg/day for 21 days. This small change in antipyrine half-life reflects a clinically insignificant change in hepatic metabolism.

Drugs That Interfere With Hemostasis (Non-selective NSAIDs, Aspirin, Warfarin, etc.)
Serotonin release by platelets plays an important role in hemostasis. Epidemiological studies of the case-control and cohort design that have demonstrated an association between the use of psychotropic drugs that interfere with serotonin reuptake and the occurrence of upper gastrointestinal bleeding have also shown that concurrent use of a non-selective NSAID (i.e., NSAIDs that inhibit both cyclooxygenase isoenzymes, COX 1 and 2) or aspirin potentiated the risk of bleeding. Thus, patients should be cautioned about the use of such drugs concurrently with ZOLOFT.

Electroconvulsive Therapy–There are no clinical studies establishing the risks or benefits of the combined use of electroconvulsive therapy (ECT) and ZOLOFT.

Alcohol–Although ZOLOFT did not potentiate the cognitive and psychomotor effects of alcohol in experiments with normal subjects, the concomitant use of ZOLOFT and alcohol is not recommended.

Carcinogenesis–Lifetime carcinogenicity studies were carried out in CD-1 mice and Long-Evans rats at doses up to 40 mg/kg/day. These doses correspond to 1 times (mice) and 2 times (rats) the maximum recommended human dose (MRHD) on a mg/m² basis. There was a dose-related increase of liver adenomas in male mice receiving sertraline at 10-40 mg/kg (0.25-1.0 times the MRHD on a mg/m² basis). No increase was seen in female mice or in rats of either sex receiving the same treatments, nor was there an increase in hepatocellular carcinomas. Liver adenomas have a variable rate of spontaneous occurrence in the CD-1 mouse and are of unknown significance to humans. There was an increase in follicular adenomas of the thyroid in female rats receiving sertraline at 40 mg/kg (2 times the MRHD on a mg/m² basis); this was not accompanied by thyroid hyperplasia. While there was an increase in uterine adenocarcinomas in rats receiving sertraline at 10-40 mg/kg (0.5-2.0

times the MRHD on a mg/m² basis) compared to placebo controls, this effect was not clearly drug related.

Mutagenesis–Sertraline had no genotoxic effects, with or without metabolic activation, based on the following assays: bacterial mutation assay; mouse lymphoma mutation assay; and tests for cytogenetic aberrations *in vivo* in mouse bone marrow and *in vitro* in human lymphocytes.

Impairment of Fertility–A decrease in fertility was seen in one of two rat studies at a dose of 80 mg/kg (4 times the maximum recommended human dose on a mg/m² basis).

Pregnancy–Pregnancy Category C–Reproduction studies have been performed in rats and rabbits at doses up to 80 mg/kg/day and 40 mg/kg/day, respectively. These doses correspond to approximately 4 times the maximum recommended human dose (MRHD) on a mg/m² basis. There was no evidence of teratogenicity at any dose level. When pregnant rats and rabbits were given sertraline during the period of organogenesis, delayed ossification was observed in fetuses at doses of 10 mg/kg (0.5 times the MRHD on a mg/m² basis) in rats and 40 mg/kg (4 times the MRHD on a mg/m² basis) in rabbits. When female rats received sertraline during the last third of gestation and throughout lactation, there was an increase in the number of stillborn pups and in the number of pups dying during the first 4 days after birth. Pup body weights were also decreased during the first four days after birth. These effects occurred at a dose of 20 mg/kg (1 times the MRHD on a mg/m² basis). The no effect dose for rat pup mortality was 10 mg/kg (0.5 times the MRHD on a mg/m² basis). The decrease in pup survival was shown to be due to *in utero* exposure to sertraline. The clinical significance of these effects is unknown. There are no adequate and well-controlled studies in pregnant women. ZOLOFT® (sertraline hydrochloride) should be used during pregnancy only if the potential benefit justifies the potential risk to the fetus.

Pregnancy-Nonteratogenic Effects–Neonates exposed to Zoloft and other SSRIs or SNRIs, late in the third trimester

---

TABLE 1
MOST COMMON TREATMENT-EMERGENT ADVERSE EVENTS: INCIDENCE IN PLACEBO-CONTROLLED CLINICAL TRIALS

Body System/ Adverse Event	Major Depressive Disorder/Other*		OCD		Panic Disorder		PTSD		PMDD Daily Dosing		PMDD Luteal Phase Dosing[2]		Social Anxiety Disorder	
	ZOLOFT (N=861)	Placebo (N=853)	ZOLOFT (N=533)	Placebo (N=373)	ZOLOFT (N=430)	Placebo (N=275)	ZOLOFT (N=374)	Placebo (N=376)	ZOLOFT (N=121)	Placebo (N=122)	ZOLOFT (N=136)	Placebo (N=127)	ZOLOFT (N=344)	Placebo (N=268)
Autonomic Nervous System Disorders														
Ejaculation Failure[1]	7	<1	17	2	19	1	11	1	N/A	N/A	N/A	N/A	14	–
Mouth Dry	16	9	14	9	15	10	11	6	6	3	10	3	12	4
Sweating Increased	8	3	6	1	5	1	4	1	6	<1	3	0	11	2
Centr. & Periph. Nerv. System Disorders														
Somnolence	13	6	15	8	15	9	13	9	7	<1	2	0	9	6
Tremor	11	3	8	1	5	1	5	1	2	0	<1	<1	9	3
Dizziness	12	7	17	9	10	10	8	5	6	3	7	5	14	6
General														
Fatigue	11	8	14	6	11	5	10	5	16	7	10	<1	12	6
Pain	1	2	3	1	3	3	4	6	6	<1	3	2	1	3
Malaise	<1	1	1	1	7	14	10	10	9	5	7	5	3	3
Gastrointestinal Disorders														
Abdominal Pain	2	2	5	5	6	7	6	5	7	<1	3	3	5	5
Anorexia	3	2	11	2	7	2	8	2	3	2	5	0	6	3
Constipation	8	6	6	4	7	3	3	3	2	3	1	2	5	3
Diarrhea/Loose Stools	18	9	24	10	20	9	24	15	13	3	13	7	21	8
Dyspepsia	6	3	10	4	10	8	6	6	7	2	7	3	13	5
Nausea	26	12	30	11	29	18	21	11	23	9	13	3	22	8
Psychiatric Disorders														
Agitation	6	4	6	3	6	2	5	5	2	<1	1	0	4	2
Insomnia	16	9	28	12	25	18	20	11	17	11	12	10	25	10
Libido Decreased	1	<1	11	2	7	1	7	2	11	2	4	2	9	3

[1] Primarily ejaculatory delay. Denominator used was for male patients only (N=271 ZOLOFT major depressive disorder/other*; N=271 placebo major depressive disorder/other*; N=296 ZOLOFT OCD; N=219 placebo OCD; N=216 ZOLOFT panic disorder; N=134 placebo panic disorder; N=130 ZOLOFT PTSD; N=149 placebo PTSD; No male patients in PMDD studies; N=205 ZOLOFT social anxiety disorder; N=153 placebo social anxiety disorder).

* Major depressive disorder and other premarketing controlled trials.

[2] The luteal phase and daily dosing PMDD trials were not designed for making direct comparisons between the two dosing regimens. Therefore, a comparison between the two dosing regimens of the PMDD trials of incidence rates shown in Table 1 should be avoided.

have developed complications requiring prolonged hospitalization, respiratory support, and tube feeding. These findings are based on postmarketing reports. Such complications can arise immediately upon delivery. Reported clinical findings have included respiratory distress, cyanosis, apnea, seizures, temperature instability, feeding difficulty, vomiting, hypoglycemia, hypotonia, hypertonia, hyperreflexia, tremor, jitteriness, irritability, and constant crying. These features are consistent with either a direct toxic effect of SSRIs and SNRIs or, possibly, a drug discontinuation syndrome. It should be noted that, in some cases, the clinical picture is consistent with serotonin syndrome (see WARNINGS).

When treating a pregnant woman with ZOLOFT during the third trimester, the physician should carefully consider the potential risks and benefits of treatment (see DOSAGE AND ADMINISTRATION).

Labor and Delivery–The effect of ZOLOFT on labor and delivery in humans is unknown.

Nursing Mothers–It is not known whether, and if so in what amount, sertraline or its metabolites are excreted in human milk. Because many drugs are excreted in human milk, caution should be exercised when ZOLOFT is administered to a nursing woman.

Pediatric Use–The efficacy of ZOLOFT for the treatment of obsessive-compulsive disorder was demonstrated in a 12-week, multicenter, placebo-controlled study with 187 outpatients ages 6-17 (see Clinical Trials under CLINICAL PHARMACOLOGY). Safety and effectiveness in the pediatric population other than pediatric patients with OCD have not been established (see BOX WARNING and WARNINGS-Clinical Worsening and Suicide Risk). Two placebo controlled trials (n=373) in pediatric patients with MDD have been conducted with Zoloft, and the data were not sufficient to support a claim for use in pediatric patients. Anyone considering the use of Zoloft in a child or adolescent must balance the potential risks with the clinical need.

The safety of ZOLOFT use in children and adolescents with OCD, ages 6-18, was evaluated in a 12-week, multicenter, placebo-controlled study with 187 outpatients, ages 6-17, and in a flexible dose, 52 week open extension study of 137 patients, ages 6-18, who had completed the initial 12-week, double-blind, placebo-controlled study. ZOLOFT was administered at doses of either 25 mg/day (children, ages 6-12) or 50 mg/day (adolescents, ages 13-18) and then titrated in weekly 25 mg/day or 50 mg/day increments, respectively, to a maximum dose of 200 mg/day based upon clinical response. The mean dose for completers was 157 mg/day. In the acute 12 week pediatric study and in the 52 week study, ZOLOFT had an adverse event profile generally similar to that observed in adults.

Sertraline pharmacokinetics were evaluated in 61 pediatric patients between 6 and 17 years of age with major depressive disorder or OCD and revealed similar drug exposures to those of adults when plasma concentration was adjusted for weight (see Pharmacokinetics under CLINICAL PHARMACOLOGY).

Approximately 600 patients with major depressive disorder or OCD between 6 and 17 years of age have received ZOLOFT in clinical trials, both controlled and uncontrolled. The adverse event profile observed in these patients was generally similar to that observed in adult studies with ZOLOFT (see ADVERSE REACTIONS). As with other SSRIs, decreased appetite and weight loss have been observed in association with the use of ZOLOFT. In a pooled analysis of two 10-week, double-blind, placebo-controlled, flexible dose (50-200 mg) outpatient trials for major depressive disorder (n=373), there was a difference in weight change between sertraline and placebo of roughly 1 kilogram, for both children (ages 6-11) and adolescents (ages 12-17), in both cases representing a slight weight loss for sertraline compared to a slight gain for placebo. At baseline the mean weight for children was 39.0 kg for sertraline and 38.5 kg for placebo. At baseline the mean weight for adolescents was 61.4 kg for sertraline and 62.5 kg for placebo. There was a bigger difference between sertraline and placebo in the proportion of outliers for clinically important weight loss in children than in adolescents. For children, about 7% had a weight loss > 7% of body weight compared to none of the placebo patients; for adolescents, about 2% had a weight loss > 7% of body weight compared to about 1% of the placebo patients. A subset of these patients who completed the randomized controlled trials (sertraline n=99, placebo n=122) were continued into a 24-week, flexible-dose, open-label, extension study. A mean weight loss of approximately 0.5 kg was seen during the first eight weeks of treatment for subjects with first exposure to sertraline during the open-label extension study, similar to mean weight loss observed among sertraline treated subjects during the first eight weeks of the randomized controlled trials. The subjects continuing in the open label study began gaining weight compared to baseline by week 12 of sertraline treatment. Those subjects who completed 34 weeks of sertraline treatment (10 weeks in a placebo controlled trial + 24 weeks open label, n=68) had weight gain that was similar to that expected using data from age-adjusted peers. Regular monitoring of weight and growth is recommended if treatment of a pediatric patient with an SSRI is to be continued long term. Safety and effectiveness in pediatric patients below the age of 6 have not been established.

The risks, if any, that may be associated with ZOLOFT's use beyond 1 year in children and adolescents with OCD or major depressive disorder have not been systematically assessed. The prescriber should be mindful that the evidence relied upon to conclude that sertraline is safe for use in children and adolescents derives from clinical studies that were 10 to 52 weeks in duration and from the extrapolation of experience gained with adult patients. In particular, there are no studies that directly evaluate the effects of long-term sertraline use on the growth, development, and maturation of children and adolescents. Although there is no affirmative finding to suggest that sertraline possesses a capacity to adversely affect growth, development or maturation, the absence of such findings is not compelling evidence of the absence of the potential of sertraline to have adverse effects in chronic use (see WARNINGS – Clinical Worsening and Suicide Risk).

Geriatric Use–U.S. geriatric clinical studies of ZOLOFT in major depressive disorder included 663 ZOLOFT-treated subjects ≥ 65 years of age, of those, 180 were ≥ 75 years of age. No overall differences in the pattern of adverse reactions were observed in the geriatric clinical trial subjects relative to those reported in younger subjects (see ADVERSE REACTIONS), and other reported experience has not identified differences in safety patterns between the elderly and younger subjects. As with all medications, greater sensitivity of some older individuals cannot be ruled out. There were 947 subjects in placebo-controlled geriatric clinical studies of ZOLOFT in major depressive disorder. No overall differences in the pattern of efficacy were observed in the geriatric clinical trial subjects relative to those reported in younger subjects.

Other Adverse Events in Geriatric Patients. In 354 geriatric subjects treated with ZOLOFT in placebo-controlled trials, the overall profile of adverse events was generally similar to that shown in Tables 1 and 2. Urinary tract infection was the only adverse event not appearing in Tables 1 and 2 and reported at an incidence of at least 2% and at a rate greater than placebo in placebo-controlled trials.

As with other SSRIs, ZOLOFT has been associated with cases of clinically significant hyponatremia in elderly patients (see Hyponatremia under PRECAUTIONS).

ADVERSE REACTIONS

During its premarketing assessment, multiple doses of ZOLOFT were administered to over 4000 adult subjects as of February 18, 2000. The conditions and duration of exposure to ZOLOFT varied greatly, and included (in overlapping categories) clinical pharmacology studies, open and double-blind studies, uncontrolled and controlled studies, inpatient and outpatient studies, fixed-dose and titration studies, and studies for multiple indications, including major depressive disorder, OCD, panic disorder, PTSD, PMDD and social anxiety disorder.

Untoward events associated with this exposure were recorded by clinical investigators using terminology of their own choosing. Consequently, it is not possible to provide a meaningful estimate of the proportion of individuals experiencing adverse events without first grouping similar types of untoward events into a smaller number of standardized event categories.

In the tabulations that follow, a World Health Organization dictionary of terminology has been used to classify reported adverse events. The frequencies presented, therefore, represent the proportion of the over 4000 adult individuals exposed to multiple doses of ZOLOFT who experienced a treatment-emergent adverse event of the type cited on at least one occasion while receiving ZOLOFT. An event was considered treatment-emergent if it occurred for the first time or worsened while receiving therapy following baseline evaluation. It is important to emphasize that events reported during therapy were not necessarily caused by it.

The prescriber should be aware that the figures in the tables and tabulations cannot be used to predict the incidence of side effects in the course of usual medical practice where patient characteristics and other factors differ from those that prevailed in the clinical trials. Similarly, the cited frequencies cannot be compared with figures obtained from other clinical investigations involving different treatments, uses, and investigators. The cited figures, however, do provide the prescribing physician with some basis for estimating the relative contribution of drug and nondrug factors to the side effect incidence rate in the population studied.

Incidence in Placebo-Controlled Trials–Table 1 enumerates the most common treatment-emergent adverse events associated with the use of ZOLOFT (incidence of at least 5% for ZOLOFT and at least twice that for placebo within at least one of the indications) for the treatment of adult patients with major depressive disorder/other*, OCD, panic disorder, PTSD, PMDD and social anxiety disorder in placebo-controlled clinical trials. Most patients in major depressive disorder/other*, OCD, panic disorder, PTSD and social anxiety disorder studies received doses of 50 to 200 mg/day. Patients in the PMDD study with daily dosing throughout the menstrual cycle received doses of 50 to 150 mg/day, and in the PMDD study with dosing during the luteal phase of the menstrual cycle received doses of 50 to 100 mg/day. Table 2 enumerates treatment-emergent adverse events that occurred in 2% or more of adult patients treated with ZOLOFT and with incidence greater than placebo who participated in controlled clinical trials comparing ZOLOFT with placebo in the treatment of major depressive disorder/other*, OCD, panic disorder, PTSD, PMDD and social anxiety disorder. Table 2 provides combined data for the pool of studies that are provided separately by indication in Table 1.

[See table 1 on previous page]

TABLE 2
TREATMENT-EMERGENT ADVERSE EVENTS: INCIDENCE IN PLACEBO-CONTROLLED CLINICAL TRIALS
Percentage of Patients Reporting Event
Major Depressive Disorder/Other*, OCD, Panic Disorder, PTSD, PMDD and Social Anxiety Disorder combined

Body System/Adverse Event**	ZOLOFT (N=2799)	Placebo (N=2394)
Autonomic Nervous System Disorders		
Ejaculation Failure[1]	14	1
Mouth Dry	14	8
Sweating Increased	7	2
Centr. & Periph. Nerv. System Disorders		
Somnolence	13	7
Dizziness	12	7
Headache	25	23
Paresthesia	2	1
Tremor	8	2
Disorders of Skin and Appendages		
Rash	3	2
Gastrointestinal Disorders		
Anorexia	6	2
Constipation	6	4
Diarrhea/Loose Stools	20	10
Dyspepsia	8	4
Nausea	25	11
Vomiting	4	2
General		
Fatigue	12	7
Psychiatric Disorders		
Agitation	5	3
Anxiety	4	3
Insomnia	21	11
Libido Decreased	6	2
Nervousness	5	4
Special Senses		
Vision Abnormal	3	2

[1]Primarily ejaculatory delay. Denominator used was for male patients only (N=1118 ZOLOFT; N=926 placebo).

*Major depressive disorder and other premarketing controlled trials.

**Included are events reported by at least 2% of patients taking ZOLOFT except the following events, which had an incidence on placebo greater than or equal to ZOLOFT: abdominal pain, back pain, flatulence, malaise, pain, pharyngitis, respiratory disorder, upper respiratory tract infection.

Associated with Discontinuation in Placebo-Controlled Clinical Trials

Table 3 lists the adverse events associated with discontinuation of ZOLOFT® (sertraline hydrochloride) treatment (incidence at least twice that for placebo and at least 1% for ZOLOFT in clinical trials) in major depressive disorder/other*, OCD, panic disorder, PTSD, PMDD and social anxiety disorder.

[See table 3 at top of next page]

Male and Female Sexual Dysfunction with SSRIs

Although changes in sexual desire, sexual performance and sexual satisfaction often occur as manifestations of a psychiatric disorder, they may also be a consequence of pharmacologic treatment. In particular, some evidence suggests that selective serotonin reuptake inhibitors (SSRIs) can cause such untoward sexual experiences. Reliable estimates of the incidence and severity of untoward experiences involving sexual desire, performance and satisfaction are difficult to obtain, however, in part because patients and physicians may be reluctant to discuss them. Accordingly, estimates of the incidence of untoward sexual experience and performance cited in product labeling, are likely to underestimate their actual incidence.

Continued on next page

Zoloft—Cont.

Table 4 below displays the incidence of sexual side effects reported by at least 2% of patients taking ZOLOFT in placebo-controlled trials.

TABLE 4

Adverse Event	ZOLOFT	Placebo
Ejaculation failure* (primarily delayed ejaculation)	14%	1%
Decreased libido**	6%	1%

* Denominator used was for male patients only (N=1118 ZOLOFT; N=926 placebo)

** Denominator used was for male and female patients (N=2799 ZOLOFT; N=2394 placebo)

There are no adequate and well-controlled studies examining sexual dysfunction with sertraline treatment.

Priapism has been reported with all SSRIs.

While it is difficult to know the precise risk of sexual dysfunction associated with the use of SSRIs, physicians should routinely inquire about such possible side effects.

Other Adverse Events in Pediatric Patients–In over 600 pediatric patients treated with ZOLOFT, the overall profile of adverse events was generally similar to that seen in adult studies. However, the following adverse events, from controlled trials, not appearing in Tables 1 and 2, were reported at an incidence of at least 2% and occurred at a rate of at least twice the placebo rate (N=281 patients treated with ZOLOFT): fever, hyperkinesia, urinary incontinence, aggressive reaction, sinusitis, epistaxis and purpura.

Other Events Observed During the Premarketing Evaluation of ZOLOFT® (sertraline hydrochloride)–Following is a list of treatment-emergent adverse events reported during premarketing assessment of ZOLOFT in clinical trials (over 4000 adult subjects) except those already listed in the previous tables or elsewhere in labeling.

In the tabulations that follow, a World Health Organization dictionary of terminology has been used to classify reported adverse events. The frequencies presented, therefore, represent the proportion of the over 4000 adult individuals exposed to multiple doses of ZOLOFT who experienced an event of the type cited on at least one occasion while receiving ZOLOFT. All events are included except those already listed in the previous tables or elsewhere in labeling and those reported in terms so general as to be uninformative and those for which a causal relationship to ZOLOFT treatment seemed remote. It is important to emphasize that although the events reported occurred during treatment with ZOLOFT, they were not necessarily caused by it. Events are further categorized by body system and listed in order of decreasing frequency according to the following definitions: frequent adverse events are those occurring on one or more occasions in at least 1/100 patients; infrequent adverse events are those occurring in 1/100 to 1/1000 patients; rare events are those occurring in fewer than 1/1000 patients. Events of major clinical importance are also described in the PRECAUTIONS section.

Autonomic Nervous System Disorders–*Frequent:* impotence; *Infrequent:* flushing, increased saliva, cold clammy skin, mydriasis; *Rare:* pallor, glaucoma, priapism, vasodilation.

Body as a Whole-General Disorders–*Rare:* allergic reaction, allergy.

Cardiovascular–*Frequent:* palpitations, chest pain; *Infrequent:* hypertension, tachycardia, postural dizziness, postural hypotension, periorbital edema, peripheral edema, hypotension, peripheral ischemia, syncope, edema, dependent edema; *Rare:* precordial chest pain, substernal chest pain, aggravated hypertension, myocardial infarction, cerebrovascular disorder.

Central and Peripheral Nervous System Disorders–*Frequent:* hypertonia, hypoesthesia; *Infrequent:* twitching, confusion, hyperkinesia, vertigo, ataxia, migraine, abnormal coordination, hyperesthesia, leg cramps, abnormal gait, nystagmus, hypokinesia; *Rare:* dysphonia, coma, dyskinesia, hypotonia, ptosis, choreoathetosis, hyporeflexia.

Disorders of Skin and Appendages–*Infrequent:* pruritus, acne, urticaria, alopecia, dry skin, erythematous rash, photosensitivity reaction, maculopapular rash; *Rare:* follicular rash, eczema, dermatitis, contact dermatitis, bullous eruption, hypertrichosis, skin discoloration, pustular rash.

Endocrine Disorders–*Rare:* exophthalmos, gynecomastia.

Gastrointestinal Disorders–*Frequent:* appetite increased; *Infrequent:* dysphagia, tooth caries aggravated, eructation, esophagitis, gastroenteritis; *Rare:* melena, glossitis, gum hyperplasia, hiccup, stomatitis, tenesmus, colitis, diverticulitis, fecal incontinence, gastritis, rectum hemorrhage, hemorrhagic peptic ulcer, proctitis, ulcerative stomatitis, tongue edema, tongue ulceration.

General–*Frequent:* back pain, asthenia, malaise, weight increase; *Infrequent:* fever, rigors, generalized edema; *Rare:* face edema, aphthous stomatitis.

Hearing and Vestibular Disorders–*Rare:* hyperacusis, labyrinthine disorder.

Hematopoietic and Lymphatic–*Rare:* anemia, anterior chamber eye hemorrhage.

Liver and Biliary System Disorders–*Rare:* abnormal hepatic function.

Metabolic and Nutritional Disorders–*Infrequent:* thirst; *Rare:* hypoglycemia, hypoglycemia reaction.

TABLE 3
MOST COMMON ADVERSE EVENTS ASSOCIATED WITH DISCONTINUATION IN PLACEBO-CONTROLLED CLINICAL TRIALS

Adverse Event	Major Depressive Disorder/ Other*, OCD, Panic Disorder, PTSD, PMDD and Social Anxiety Disorder combined (N=2799)	Major Depressive Disorder/ Other* (N=861)	OCD (N=533)	Panic Disorder (N=430)	PTSD (N=374)	PMDD Daily Dosing (N=121)	PMDD Luteal Phase Dosing (N=136)	Social Anxiety Disorder (N=344)
Abdominal Pain	–	–	–	–	–	–	–	1%
Agitation	–	1%	–	2%	–	–	–	–
Anxiety	–	–	–	–	–	–	–	2%
Diarrhea/Loose Stools	2%	2%	2%	1%	–	2%	–	–
Dizziness	–	–	1%	–	–	–	–	–
Dry Mouth	–	1%	–	–	–	–	–	–
Dyspepsia	–	–	–	1%	–	–	–	–
Ejaculation Failure[(1)]	1%	1%	1%	2%	–	N/A	N/A	2%
Fatigue	–	–	–	–	–	–	–	2%
Headache	1%	2%	–	–	1%	–	–	2%
Hot Flushes	–	–	–	–	–	–	1%	–
Insomnia	2%	1%	3%	2%	–	–	1%	3%
Nausea	3%	4%	3%	3%	2%	2%	1%	2%
Nervousness	–	–	–	–	–	2%	–	–
Palpitation	–	–	–	–	–	–	1%	–
Somnolence	1%	1%	2%	2%	–	–	–	–
Tremor	–	2%	–	–	–	–	–	–

[(1)]Primarily ejaculatory delay. Denominator used was for male patients only (N=271 major depressive disorder/other*; N=296 OCD; N=216 panic disorder; N=130 PTSD; No male patients in PMDD studies; N=205 social anxiety disorder).

*Major depressive disorder and other premarketing controlled trials.

Musculoskeletal System Disorders–*Frequent:* myalgia; *Infrequent:* arthralgia, dystonia, arthrosis, muscle cramps, muscle weakness.

Psychiatric Disorders–*Frequent:* yawning, other male sexual dysfunction, other female sexual dysfunction; *Infrequent:* depression, amnesia, paroniria, teeth-grinding, emotional lability, apathy, abnormal dreams, euphoria, paranoid reaction, hallucination, aggressive reaction, aggravated depression, delusions; *Rare:* withdrawal syndrome, suicide ideation, libido increased, somnambulism, illusion.

Reproductive–*Infrequent:* menstrual disorder, dysmenorrhea, intermenstrual bleeding, vaginal hemorrhage, amenorrhea, leukorrhea; *Rare:* female breast pain, menorrhagia, balanoposthitis, breast enlargement, atrophic vaginitis, acute female mastitis.

Respiratory System Disorders–*Frequent:* rhinitis; *Infrequent:* coughing, dyspnea, upper respiratory tract infection, epistaxis, bronchospasm, sinusitis; *Rare:* hyperventilation, bradypnea, stridor, apnea, bronchitis, hemoptysis, hypoventilation, laryngismus, laryngitis.

Special Senses–*Frequent:* tinnitus; *Infrequent:* conjunctivitis, earache, eye pain, abnormal accommodation; *Rare:* xerophthalmia, photophobia, diplopia, abnormal lacrimation, scotoma, visual field defect.

Urinary System Disorders–*Infrequent:* micturition frequency, polyuria, urinary retention, dysuria, nocturia, urinary incontinence; *Rare:* cystitis, oliguria, pyelonephritis, hematuria, renal pain, strangury.

Laboratory Tests–In man, asymptomatic elevations in serum transaminases (SGOT [or AST] and SGPT [or ALT]) have been reported infrequently (approximately 0.8%) in association with ZOLOFT® (sertraline hydrochloride) administration. These hepatic enzyme elevations usually occurred within the first 1 to 9 weeks of drug treatment and promptly diminished upon drug discontinuation.

ZOLOFT therapy was associated with small mean increases in total cholesterol (approximately 3%) and triglycerides (approximately 5%), and a small mean decrease in serum uric acid (approximately 7%) of no apparent clinical importance.

The safety profile observed with ZOLOFT treatment in patients with major depressive disorder, OCD, panic disorder, PTSD, PMDD and social anxiety disorder is similar.

Other Events Observed During the Postmarketing Evaluation of ZOLOFT–Reports of adverse events temporally associated with ZOLOFT that have been received since market introduction, that are not listed above and that may have no causal relationship with the drug, include the following: acute renal failure, anaphylactoid reaction, angioedema, blindness, optic neuritis, cataract, increased coagulation times, bradycardia, AV block, atrial arrhythmias, QT-interval prolongation, ventricular tachycardia (including torsade de pointes-type arrhythmias), hypothyroidism, agranulocytosis, aplastic anemia and pancytopenia, leukopenia, thrombocytopenia, lupus-like syndrome, serum sickness, hyperglycemia, galactorrhea, hyperprolactinemia, neuroleptic malignant syndrome-like events, extrapyramidal symptoms, oculogyric crisis, serotonin syndrome, psychosis, pulmonary hypertension, severe skin reactions, which potentially can be fatal, such as Stevens-Johnson syndrome, vasculitis, photosensitivity and other severe cutaneous disorders, rare reports of pancreatitis, and liver events—clinical features (which in the majority of cases appeared to be reversible with discontinuation of ZOLOFT) occurring in one or more patients include: elevated enzymes, increased bilirubin, hepatomegaly, hepatitis, jaundice, abdominal pain, vomiting, liver failure and death.

DRUG ABUSE AND DEPENDENCE

Controlled Substance Class–ZOLOFT® (sertraline hydrochloride) is not a controlled substance.

Physical and Psychological Dependence–In a placebo-controlled, double-blind, randomized study of the comparative abuse liability of ZOLOFT, alprazolam, and d-amphetamine in humans, ZOLOFT did not produce the positive subjective effects indicative of abuse potential, such as euphoria or drug liking, that were observed with the other two drugs. Premarketing clinical experience with ZOLOFT did not reveal any tendency for a withdrawal syndrome or any drug-seeking behavior. In animal studies ZOLOFT does not demonstrate stimulant or barbiturate-like (depressant) abuse potential. As with any CNS active drug, however, physicians should carefully evaluate patients for history of drug abuse and follow such patients closely, observing them for signs of ZOLOFT misuse or abuse (e.g., development of tolerance, incrementation of dose, drug-seeking behavior).

OVERDOSAGE

Human Experience–Of 1,027 cases of overdose involving sertraline hydrochloride worldwide, alone or with other drugs, there were 72 deaths (circa 1999).

Among 634 overdoses in which sertraline hydrochloride was the only drug ingested, 8 resulted in fatal outcome, 75 completely recovered, and 27 patients experienced sequelae after overdosage to include alopecia, decreased libido, diarrhea, ejaculation disorder, fatigue, insomnia, somnolence and serotonin syndrome. The remaining 524 cases had an unknown outcome. The most common signs and symptoms associated with non-fatal sertraline hydrochloride overdosage were somnolence, vomiting, tachycardia, nausea, dizziness, agitation and tremor.

The largest known ingestion was 13.5 grams in a patient who took sertraline hydrochloride alone and subsequently recovered. However, another patient who took 2.5 grams of sertraline hydrochloride alone experienced a fatal outcome. Other important adverse events reported with sertraline hydrochloride overdose (single or multiple drugs) include bradycardia, bundle branch block, coma, convulsions, delirium, hallucinations, hypertension, hypotension, manic reaction, pancreatitis, QT-interval prolongation, serotonin syndrome, stupor and syncope.

Overdose Management–Treatment should consist of those general measures employed in the management of overdosage with any antidepressant.

Ensure an adequate airway, oxygenation and ventilation. Monitor cardiac rhythm and vital signs. General supportive and symptomatic measures are also recommended. Induction of emesis is not recommended. Gastric lavage with a large-bore orogastric tube with appropriate airway protection, if needed, may be indicated if performed soon after ingestion, or in symptomatic patients.

Activated charcoal should be administered. Due to large volume of distribution of this drug, forced diuresis, dialysis, hemoperfusion and exchange transfusion are unlikely to be of benefit. No specific antidotes for sertraline are known.

In managing overdosage, consider the possibility of multiple drug involvement. The physician should consider contacting a poison control center on the treatment of any overdose. Telephone numbers for certified poison control centers are listed in the *Physicians' Desk Reference*® (PDR®).

DOSAGE AND ADMINISTRATION
Initial Treatment
Dosage for Adults
Major Depressive Disorder and Obsessive-Compulsive Disorder–ZOLOFT treatment should be administered at a dose of 50 mg once daily.

Panic Disorder, Posttraumatic Stress Disorder and Social Anxiety Disorder–ZOLOFT treatment should be initiated with a dose of 25 mg once daily. After one week, the dose should be increased to 50 mg once daily.

While a relationship between dose and effect has not been established for major depressive disorder, OCD, panic disorder, PTSD or social anxiety disorder, patients were dosed in a range of 50-200 mg/day in the clinical trials demonstrating the effectiveness of ZOLOFT for the treatment of these indications. Consequently, a dose of 50 mg, administered once daily, is recommended as the initial therapeutic dose. Patients not responding to a 50 mg dose may benefit from dose increases up to a maximum of 200 mg/day. Given the 24 hour elimination half-life of ZOLOFT, dose changes should not occur at intervals of less than 1 week.

Premenstrual Dysphoric Disorder–ZOLOFT treatment should be initiated with a dose of 50 mg/day, either daily throughout the menstrual cycle or limited to the luteal phase of the menstrual cycle, depending on physician assessment.

While a relationship between dose and effect has not been established for PMDD, patients were dosed in the range of 50-150 mg/day with dose increases at the onset of each new menstrual cycle (see Clinical Trials under CLINICAL PHARMACOLOGY). Patients not responding to a 50 mg/day dose may benefit from dose increases (at 50 mg increments/menstrual cycle) up to 150 mg/day when dosing daily throughout the menstrual cycle, or 100 mg/day when dosing during the luteal phase of the menstrual cycle. If a 100 mg/day dose has been established with luteal phase dosing, a 50 mg/day titration step for three days should be utilized at the beginning of each luteal phase dosing period.

ZOLOFT should be administered once daily, either in the morning or evening.

Dosage for Pediatric Population (Children and Adolescents)
Obsessive-Compulsive Disorder–ZOLOFT treatment should be initiated with a dose of 25 mg once daily in children (ages 6-12) and at a dose of 50 mg once daily in adolescents (ages 13-17).

While a relationship between dose and effect has not been established for OCD, patients were dosed in a range of 25-200 mg/day in the clinical trials demonstrating the effectiveness of ZOLOFT for pediatric patients (6-17 years) with OCD. Patients not responding to an initial dose of 25 or 50 mg/day may benefit from dose increases up to a maximum of 200 mg/day. For children with OCD, their generally lower body weights compared to adults should be taken into consideration in advancing the dose, in order to avoid excess dosing. Given the 24 hour elimination half-life of ZOLOFT, dose changes should not occur at intervals of less than 1 week.

ZOLOFT should be administered once daily, either in the morning or evening.

Maintenance/Continuation/Extended Treatment
Major Depressive Disorder–It is generally agreed that acute episodes of major depressive disorder require several months or longer of sustained pharmacologic therapy beyond response to the acute episode. Systematic evaluation of ZOLOFT has demonstrated that its antidepressant efficacy is maintained for periods of up to 44 weeks following 8 weeks of initial treatment at a dose of 50-200 mg/day (mean dose of 70 mg/day) (see Clinical Trials under CLINICAL PHARMACOLOGY). It is not known whether the dose of ZOLOFT needed for maintenance treatment is identical to the dose needed to achieve an initial response. Patients should be periodically reassessed to determine the need for maintenance treatment.

Posttraumatic Stress Disorder–It is generally agreed that PTSD requires several months or longer of sustained pharmacological therapy beyond response to initial treatment. Systematic evaluation of ZOLOFT has demonstrated that

its efficacy in PTSD is maintained for periods of up to 28 weeks following 24 weeks of treatment at a dose of 50-200 mg/day (see Clinical Trials under CLINICAL PHARMACOLOGY). It is not known whether the dose of ZOLOFT needed for maintenance treatment is identical to the dose needed to achieve an initial response. Patients should be periodically reassessed to determine the need for maintenance treatment.

Social Anxiety Disorder–Social anxiety disorder is a chronic condition that may require several months or longer of sustained pharmacological therapy beyond response to initial treatment. Systematic evaluation of ZOLOFT has demonstrated that its efficacy in social anxiety disorder is maintained for periods of up to 24 weeks following 20 weeks of treatment at a dose of 50-200 mg/day (see Clinical Trials under CLINICAL PHARMACOLOGY). Dosage adjustments should be made to maintain patients on the lowest effective dose and patients should be periodically reassessed to determine the need for long-term treatment.

Obsessive-Compulsive Disorder and Panic Disorder–It is generally agreed that OCD and Panic Disorder require several months or longer of sustained pharmacological therapy beyond response to initial treatment. Systematic evaluation of continuing ZOLOFT for periods of up to 28 weeks in patients with OCD and Panic Disorder who have responded while taking ZOLOFT during initial treatment phases of 24 to 52 weeks of treatment at a dose range of 50-200 mg/day has demonstrated a benefit of such maintenance treatment (see Clinical Trials under CLINICAL PHARMACOLOGY). It is not known whether the dose of ZOLOFT needed for maintenance treatment is identical to the dose needed to achieve an initial response. Nevertheless, patients should be periodically reassessed to determine the need for maintenance treatment.

Premenstrual Dysphoric Disorder–The effectiveness of ZOLOFT in long-term use, that is, for more than 3 menstrual cycles, has not been systematically evaluated in controlled trials. However, as women commonly report that symptoms worsen with age until relieved by the onset of menopause, it is reasonable to consider continuation of a responding patient. Dosage adjustments, which may include changes between dosage regimens (e.g., daily throughout the menstrual cycle versus during the luteal phase of the menstrual cycle), may be needed to maintain the patient on the lowest effective dosage and patients should be periodically reassessed to determine the need for continued treatment.

Switching Patients to or from a Monoamine Oxidase Inhibitor–At least 14 days should elapse between discontinuation of an MAOI and initiation of therapy with ZOLOFT. In addition, at least 14 days should be allowed after stopping ZOLOFT before starting an MAOI (see CONTRAINDICATIONS and WARNINGS).

Special Populations
Dosage for Hepatically Impaired Patients–The use of sertraline in patients with liver disease should be approached with caution. The effects of sertraline in patients with moderate and severe hepatic impairment have not been studied. If sertraline is administered to patients with liver impairment, a lower or less frequent dose should be used (see CLINICAL PHARMACOLOGY and PRECAUTIONS).

Treatment of Pregnant Women During the Third Trimester–Neonates exposed to ZOLOFT and other SSRIs or SNRIs, late in the third trimester have developed complications requiring prolonged hospitalization, respiratory support, and tube feeding (see PRECAUTIONS). When treating pregnant women with ZOLOFT during the third trimester, the physician should carefully consider the potential risks and benefits of treatment. The physician may consider tapering ZOLOFT in the third trimester.

Discontinuation of Treatment with Zoloft
Symptoms associated with discontinuation of ZOLOFT and other SSRIs and SNRIs, have been reported (see PRECAUTIONS). Patients should be monitored for these symptoms when discontinuing treatment. A gradual reduction in the dose rather than abrupt cessation is recommended whenever possible. If intolerable symptoms occur following a decrease in the dose or upon discontinuation of treatment, then resuming the previously prescribed dose may be considered. Subsequently, the physician may continue decreasing the dose but at a more gradual rate.

ZOLOFT Oral Concentrate
ZOLOFT Oral Concentrate contains 20 mg/mL of sertraline (as the hydrochloride) as the active ingredient and 12% alcohol. ZOLOFT Oral Concentrate must be diluted before use. Just before taking, use the dropper provided to remove the required amount of ZOLOFT Oral Concentrate and mix with 4 oz (1/2 cup) of water, ginger ale, lemon/lime soda, lemonade or orange juice ONLY. Do not mix ZOLOFT Oral Concentrate with anything other than the liquids listed. The dose should be taken immediately after mixing. Do not mix in advance. At times, a slight haze may appear after mixing; this is normal. Note that caution should be exercised for patients with latex sensitivity, as the dropper dispenser contains dry natural rubber.

ZOLOFT Oral Concentrate is contraindicated with ANTABUSE (disulfiram) due to the alcohol content of the concentrate.

HOW SUPPLIED

ZOLOFT® (sertraline hydrochloride) capsular-shaped scored tablets, containing sertraline hydrochloride equivalent to 25, 50 and 100 mg of sertraline, are packaged in bottles.

ZOLOFT® 25 mg Tablets: light green film coated tablets engraved on one side with ZOLOFT and on the other side scored and engraved with 25 mg.

| NDC 0049-4960-30 | Bottles of 30 |
| NDC 0049-4960-50 | Bottles of 50 |

ZOLOFT® 50 mg Tablets: light blue film coated tablets engraved on one side with ZOLOFT and on the other side scored and engraved with 50 mg.

NDC 0049-4900-30	Bottles of 30
NDC 0049-4900-66	Bottles of 100
NDC 0049-4900-73	Bottles of 500
NDC 0049-4900-94	Bottles of 5000
NDC 0049-4900-41	Unit Dose Packages of 100

ZOLOFT® 100 mg Tablets: light yellow film coated tablets engraved on one side with ZOLOFT and on the other side scored and engraved with 100 mg.

NDC 0049-4910-30	Bottles of 30
NDC 0049-4910-66	Bottles of 100
NDC 0049-4910-73	Bottles of 500
NDC 0049-4910-94	Bottles of 5000
NDC 0049-4910-41	Unit Dose Packages of 100

Store at 25°C (77°F); excursions permitted to 15° - 30°C (59° - 86°F) [see USP Controlled Room Temperature].

ZOLOFT® Oral Concentrate: ZOLOFT Oral Concentrate is a clear, colorless solution with a menthol scent containing sertraline hydrochloride equivalent to 20 mg of sertraline per mL and 12% alcohol. It is supplied as a 60 mL bottle with an accompanying calibrated dropper.

| NDC 0049-4940-23 | Bottles of 60 mL |

Store at 25°C (77°F); excursions permitted to 15° - 30°C (59° - 86°F) [see USP Controlled Room Temperature].

Rx only　　　　　　　　　　　　　　©2005 Pfizer Inc
Distributed by
Pfizer Roerig
Division of Pfizer Inc., NY, NY 10017
LAB-0218-9.0　　　　　　　　　　　　　Revised April 2005

Medication Guide
About Using Antidepressants in Children and Teenagers
What is the most important information I should know if my child is being prescribed an antidepressant?
Parents or guardians need to think about 4 important things when their child is prescribed an antidepressant:
1. There is a risk of suicidal thoughts or actions
2. How to try to prevent suicidal thoughts or actions in your child
3. You should watch for certain signs if your child is taking an antidepressant
4. There are benefits and risks when using antidepressants

1. There is a Risk of Suicidal Thoughts or Actions
Children and teenagers sometimes think about suicide, and many report trying to kill themselves.
Antidepressants increase suicidal thoughts and actions in some children and teenagers. But suicidal thoughts and actions can also be caused by depression, a serious medical condition that is commonly treated with antidepressants. Thinking about killing yourself or trying to kill yourself is called *suicidality* or *being suicidal*.
A large study combined the results of 24 different studies of children and teenagers with depression or other illnesses. In these studies, patients took either a placebo (sugar pill) or an antidepressant for 1 to 4 months. *No one committed suicide in these studies,* but some patients became suicidal. On sugar pills, 2 out of every 100 became suicidal. On the antidepressants, 4 out of every 100 patients became suicidal.
For some children and teenagers, the risks of suicidal actions may be especially high. These include patients with
- Bipolar illness (sometimes called manic-depressive illness)
- A family history of bipolar illness
- A personal or family history of attempting suicide
If any of these are present, make sure you tell your healthcare provider before your child takes an antidepressant.
2. How to Try to Prevent Suicidal Thoughts and Actions
To try to prevent suicidal thoughts and actions in your child, pay close attention to changes in her or his moods or actions, especially if the changes occur suddenly. Other important people in your child's life can help by paying attention as well (e.g., your child, brothers and sisters, teachers, and other important people). The changes to look out for are listed in Section 3, on what to watch for.
Whenever an antidepressant is started or its dose is changed, pay close attention to your child.
After starting an antidepressant, your child should generally see his or her healthcare provider:
- Once a week for the first 4 weeks
- Every 2 weeks for the next 4 weeks
- After taking the antidepressant for 12 weeks
- After 12 weeks, follow your healthcare provider's advice about how often to come back
- More often if problems or questions arise (see Section 3)
You should call your child's healthcare provider between visits if needed.
3. You Should Watch for Certain Signs If Your Child is Taking an Antidepressant
Contact your child's healthcare provider *right away* if your child exhibits any of the following signs for the first time, or if they seem worse, or worry you, your child, or your child's teacher:
- Thoughts about suicide or dying

Continued on next page

Zoloft—Cont.

- Attempts to commit suicide
- New or worse depression
- New or worse anxiety
- Feeling very agitated or restless
- Panic attacks
- Difficulty sleeping (insomnia)
- New or worse irritability
- Acting aggressive, being angry, or violent
- Acting on dangerous impulses
- An extreme increase in activity and talking
- Other unusual changes in behavior or mood

Never let your child stop taking an antidepressant without first talking to his or her healthcare provider. Stopping an antidepressant suddenly can cause other symptoms.

4. There are Benefits and Risks When Using Antidepressants

Antidepressants are used to treat depression and other illnesses. Depression and other illnesses can lead to suicide. In some children and teenagers, treatment with an antidepressant increases suicidal thinking or actions. It is important to discuss all the risks of treating depression and also the risks of not treating it. You and your child should discuss all treatment choices with your healthcare provider, not just the use of antidepressants.

Other side effects can occur with antdepressants (see section below).

Of all the antidepressants, only fluoxetine (Prozac®) has been FDA approved to treat pediatric depression.

For obsessive compulsive disorder in children and teenagers, FDA has approved only fluoxetine (Prozac®), sertraline (Zoloft®), fluvoxamine, and clomipramine (Anafranil®).

Your healthcare provider may suggest other antidepressants based on the past experience of your child or other family members.

Is this all I need to know if my child is being prescribed an antidepressant?

No. This is a warning about the risk for suicidality. Other side effects can occur with antidepressants. Be sure to ask your healthcare provider to explain all the side effects of the particular drug he or she is prescribing. Also ask about drugs to avoid when taking an antidepressant. Ask your healthcare provider or pharmacist where to find more information.

*Prozac® is a registered trademark of Eli Lilly and Company

*Zoloft® is a registered trademark of Pfizer Pharmaceuticals

*Anafranil® is a registered trademark of Mallinckrodt Inc.

This Medication Guide has been approved by the U.S. Food and Drug Administration for all antidepressants.

Pharmacia & Upjohn

A division of Pfizer
235 EAST 42ND STREET
NEW YORK, NY 10017-5755

For updates to the product information listed below, please check the Pfizer Web site, http://www.pfizer.com, or call (800) 438-1985. For complete product listing, please see the Manufacturers' Index.

For Medical Information, Contact:
(800) 438-1985
24 hours a day, seven days a week

Distribution:
1855 Shelby Oaks Drive North
Memphis, TN 38134
(901) 387-5200

Customer Service:
(800) 533-4535

CAMPTOSAR® ℞

[*kămp-tō-sär*]
irinotecan hydrochloride injection
For Intravenous Use Only

Prescribing information for this product, which appears on pages 2699–2707 of the 2005 PDR, has been completely revised as follows. Please write "See Supplement A" next to the product heading.

WARNINGS

CAMPTOSAR Injection should be administered only under the supervision of a physician who is experienced in the use of cancer chemotherapeutic agents. Appropriate management of complications is possible only when adequate diagnostic and treatment facilities are readily available. CAMPTOSAR can induce both early and late forms of diarrhea that appear to be mediated by different mechanisms. Both forms of diarrhea may be severe. Early diarrhea (occurring during or shortly after infusion of CAMPTOSAR) may be accompanied by cholinergic symptoms of rhinitis, increased salivation, miosis, lacrimation, diaphoresis, flushing, and intestinal hyperperistalsis that can cause abdominal cramping. Early diarrhea and other cholinergic symptoms may be prevented or ameliorated by atropine (see PRECAUTIONS, General). Late diarrhea (generally occurring more than 24 hours after administration of CAMPTOSAR) can be life threatening since it may be prolonged and may lead to dehydration, electrolyte imbalance, or sepsis. Late diarrhea should be treated promptly with loperamide. Patients with diarrhea should be carefully monitored and given fluid and electrolyte replacement if they become dehydrated or antibiotic therapy if they develop ileus, fever, or severe neutropenia (see WARNINGS). Administration of CAMPTOSAR should be interrupted and subsequent doses reduced if severe diarrhea occurs (see DOSAGE AND ADMINISTRATION).

Severe myelosuppression may occur (see WARNINGS).

Table 1.Summary of Mean (±Standard Deviation) Irinotecan and SN-38 Pharmacokinetic Parameters in Patients with Solid Tumors

Dose (mg/m^2)	Irinotecan					SN-38		
	C_{max} (ng/mL)	AUC_{0-24} (ng·h/mL)	$t_{1/2}$ (h)	V_z (L/m^2)	CL ($L/h/m^2$)	C_{max} (ng/mL)	AUC_{0-24} (ng·h/mL)	$t_{1/2}$ (h)
125 (N=64)	1,660 ±797	10,200 ±3,270	5.8[a] ±0.7	110 ±48.5	13.3 ±6.01	26.3 ±11.9	229 ±108	10.4[a] ±3.1
340 (N=6)	3,392 ±874	20,604 ±6,027	11.7[b] ±1.0	234 ±69.6	13.9 ±4.0	56.0 ±28.2	474 ±245	21.0[b] ±4.3

C_{max} - Maximum plasma concentration
AUC_{0-24} - Area under the plasma concentration-time curve from time 0 to 24 hours after the end of the 90-minute infusion
$t_{1/2}$ - Terminal elimination half-life
V_z - Volume of distribution of terminal elimination phase
CL - Total systemic clearance
[a] Plasma specimens collected for 24 hours following the end of the 90-minute infusion.
[b] Plasma specimens collected for 48 hours following the end of the 90-minute infusion. Because of the longer collection period, these values provide a more accurate reflection of the terminal elimination half-lives of irinotecan and SN-38.

DESCRIPTION

CAMPTOSAR Injection (irinotecan hydrochloride injection) is an antineoplastic agent of the topoisomerase I inhibitor class. Irinotecan hydrochloride was clinically investigated as CPT-11.

CAMPTOSAR is supplied as a sterile, pale yellow, clear, aqueous solution. It is available in two single-dose sizes: 2 mL-fill vials contain 40 mg irinotecan hydrochloride and 5 mL-fill vials contain 100 mg irinotecan hydrochloride. Each milliliter of solution contains 20 mg of irinotecan hydrochloride (on the basis of the trihydrate salt), 45 mg of sorbitol NF powder, and 0.9 mg of lactic acid, USP. The pH of the solution has been adjusted to 3.5 (range, 3.0 to 3.8) with sodium hydroxide or hydrochloric acid. CAMPTOSAR is intended for dilution with 5% Dextrose Injection, USP (D5W), or 0.9% Sodium Chloride Injection, USP, prior to intravenous infusion. The preferred diluent is 5% Dextrose Injection, USP.

Irinotecan hydrochloride is a semisynthetic derivative of camptothecin, an alkaloid extract from plants such as *Camptotheca acuminata*. The chemical name is (***S***)-4,11-diethyl-3,4,12,14-tetrahydro-4-hydroxy-3,14-dioxo1***H***-pyrano[3′,4′:6,7]-indolizino[1,2-b]quinolin-9-yl-[1,4′-bipiperidine]-1′-carboxylate, monohydrochloride, trihydrate. Its structural formula is as follows:

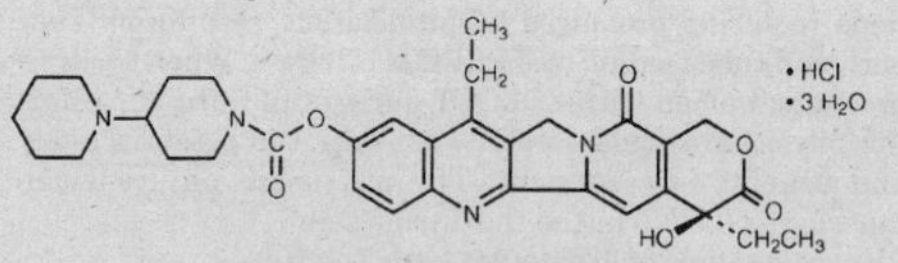

Irinotecan Hydrochloride

Irinotecan hydrochloride is a pale yellow to yellow crystalline powder, with the empirical formula $C_{33}H_{38}N_4O_6 \bullet HCl \bullet 3H_2O$ and a molecular weight of 677.19. It is slightly soluble in water and organic solvents.

CLINICAL PHARMACOLOGY

Irinotecan is a derivative of camptothecin. Camptothecins interact specifically with the enzyme topoisomerase I which relieves torsional strain in DNA by inducing reversible single-strand breaks. Irinotecan and its active metabolite SN-38 bind to the topoisomerase I-DNA complex and prevent religation of these single-strand breaks. Current research suggests that the cytotoxicity of irinotecan is due to double-strand DNA damage produced during DNA synthesis when replication enzymes interact with the ternary complex formed by topoisomerase I, DNA, and either irinotecan or SN-38. Mammalian cells cannot efficiently repair these double-strand breaks.

Irinotecan serves as a water-soluble precursor of the lipophilic metabolite SN-38. SN-38 is formed from irinotecan by carboxylesterase-mediated cleavage of the carbamate bond between the camptothecin moiety and the dipiperidino side chain. SN-38 is approximately 1000 times as potent as irinotecan as an inhibitor of topoisomerase I purified from human and rodent tumor cell lines. In vitro cytotoxicity assays show that the potency of SN-38 relative to irinotecan varies from 2- to 2000-fold. However, the plasma area under the concentration versus time curve (AUC) values for SN-38 are 2% to 8% of irinotecan and SN-38 is 95% bound to plasma proteins compared to approximately 50% bound to plasma proteins for irinotecan (see Pharmacokinetics). The precise contribution of SN-38 to the activity of CAMPTOSAR is thus unknown. Both irinotecan and SN-38 exist in an active lactone form and an inactive hydroxy acid anion form. A pH-dependent equilibrium exists between the two forms such that an acid pH promotes the formation of the lactone, while a more basic pH favors the hydroxy acid anion form.

Administration of irinotecan has resulted in antitumor activity in mice bearing cancers of rodent origin and in human carcinoma xenografts of various histological types.

Pharmacokinetics

After intravenous infusion of irinotecan in humans, irinotecan plasma concentrations decline in a multiexponential manner, with a mean terminal elimination half-life of about 6 to 12 hours. The mean terminal elimination half-life of the active metabolite SN-38 is about 10 to 20 hours. The half-lives of the lactone (active) forms of irinotecan and SN-38 are similar to those of total irinotecan and SN-38, as the lactone and hydroxy acid forms are in equilibrium.

Over the recommended dose range of 50 to 350 mg/m^2, the AUC of irinotecan increases linearly with dose; the AUC of SN-38 increases less than proportionally with dose. Maximum concentrations of the active metabolite SN-38 are generally seen within 1 hour following the end of a 90-minute infusion of irinotecan. Pharmacokinetic parameters for irinotecan and SN-38 following a 90-minute infusion of irinotecan at dose levels of 125 and 340 mg/m^2 determined in two clinical studies in patients with solid tumors are summarized in Table 1:

[See table 1 above]

Irinotecan exhibits moderate plasma protein binding (30% to 68% bound). SN-38 is highly bound to human plasma proteins (approximately 95% bound). The plasma protein to which irinotecan and SN-38 predominantly binds is albumin.

Metabolism and Excretion: The metabolic conversion of irinotecan to the active metabolite SN-38 is mediated by carboxylesterase enzymes and primarily occurs in the liver. SN-38 is subsequently conjugated predominantly by the enzyme UDP-glucuronosyl transferase 1A1 (UGT1A1) to form a glucuronide metabolite. UGT1A1 activity is reduced in individuals with genetic polymorphisms that lead to reduced enzyme activity such as the UGT1A1*28 polymorphism. Approximately 10% of the North American population is homozygous for the UGT1A1*28 allele. In a prospective study, in which irinotecan was administered as a single-agent on a once-every-3-week schedule, patients who were homozygous for UGT1A1*28 had a higher exposure to SN-38 than patients with the wild-type UGT1A1 allele (See WARNINGS and DOSAGE AND ADMINISTRATION). SN-38 glucuronide had 1/50 to 1/100 the activity of SN-38 in cytotoxicity assays using two cell lines in vitro. The disposition of irinotecan has not been fully elucidated in humans. The urinary excretion of irinotecan is 11% to 20%; SN-38, <1%; and SN-38 glucuronide, 3%. The cumulative biliary and urinary excretion of irinotecan and its metabolites (SN-38 and SN-38 glucuronide) over a period of 48 hours following administration of irinotecan in two patients ranged from approximately 25% (100 mg/m^2) to 50% (300 mg/m^2).

Pharmacokinetics in Special Populations

Geriatric: In studies using the weekly schedule, the terminal half-life of irinotecan was 6.0 hours in patients who were 65 years or older and 5.5 hours in patients younger than 65 years. Dose-normalized AUC_{0-24} for SN-38 in patients who were at least 65 years of age was 11% higher than in patients younger than 65 years. No change in the starting dose is recommended for geriatric patients receiving the weekly dosage schedule of irinotecan. The pharmacokinetics of irinotecan given once every 3 weeks has not been studied in the geriatric population; a lower starting dose is recommended in patients 70 years or older based on clinical toxicity experience with this schedule (see DOSAGE AND ADMINISTRATION).

Pediatric: See **Pediatric Use** under **PRECAUTIONS**.

Gender: The pharmacokinetics of irinotecan do not appear to be influenced by gender.

Race: The influence of race on the pharmacokinetics of irinotecan has not been evaluated.

Hepatic Insufficiency: The influence of hepatic insufficiency on the pharmacokinetic characteristics of irinotecan and its metabolites has not been formally studied. Among patients with known hepatic tumor involvement (a majority of patients), irinotecan and SN-38 AUC values were somewhat higher than values for patients without liver metastases (see PRECAUTIONS).

Renal Insufficiency: The influence of renal insufficiency on the pharmacokinetics of irinotecan has not been evaluated.

Drug-Drug Interactions

5-fluorouracil (5-FU) and leucovorin (LV): In a phase 1 clinical study involving irinotecan, 5-fluorouracil (5-FU), and leucovorin (LV) in 26 patients with solid tumors, the disposition of irinotecan was not substantially altered when the drugs were co-administered. Although the C_{max} and AUC_{0-24} of SN-38, the active metabolite, were reduced (by 14% and 8%, respectively) when irinotecan was followed by 5-FU and LV administration compared with when irinotecan was given alone, this sequence of administration was used in the combination trials and is recommended (see DOSAGE AND ADMINISTRATION). Formal in vivo or in vitro drug interaction studies to evaluate the influence of irinotecan on the disposition of 5-FU and LV have not been conducted.

Anticonvulsants: Exposure to irinotecan and its active metabolite SN-38 is substantially reduced in adult and pediatric patients concomitantly receiving the CYP3A4 enzyme-inducing anticonvulsants phenytoin, phenobarbital or carbamazepine. The appropriate starting dose for patients taking these anticonvulsants has not been formally defined. The following drugs are also CYP3A4 inducers: rifampin, rifabutin. For patients requiring anticonvulsant treatment, consideration should be given to substituting non-enzyme inducing anticonvulsants at least 2 weeks prior to initiation of irinotecan therapy. Dexamethasone does not appear to alter the pharmacokinetics of irinotecan.

St. John's Wort: St. John's Wort is an inducer of CYP3A4 enzymes. Exposure to the active metabolite SN-38 is reduced in patients receiving concomitant St. John's Wort. St. John's Wort should be discontinued at least 2 weeks prior to the first cycle of irinotecan, and St. John's Wort is contraindicated during irinotecan therapy.

Ketoconazole: Ketoconazole is a strong inhibitor of CYP3A4 enzymes. Patients receiving concomitant ketoconazole have increased exposure to irinotecan and its active metabolite SN-38. Patients should discontinue ketoconazole at least 1 week prior to starting irinotecan therapy and ketoconazole is contraindicated during irinotecan therapy.

CLINICAL STUDIES

Irinotecan has been studied in clinical trials in combination with 5-fluorouracil (5-FU) and leucovorin (LV) and as a single agent (see DOSAGE AND ADMINISTRATION). When given as a component of combination-agent treatment, irinotecan was either given with a weekly schedule of bolus 5-FU/LV or with an every-2-week schedule of infusional 5-FU/LV. Weekly and a once-every-3-week dosage schedules were used for the single-agent irinotecan studies. Clinical studies of combination and single-agent use are described below.

First-Line Therapy in Combination with 5-FU/LV for the Treatment of Metastatic Colorectal Cancer

Two phase 3, randomized, controlled, multinational clinical trials support the use of CAMPTOSAR Injection as first-line treatment of patients with metastatic carcinoma of the colon or rectum. In each study, combinations of irinotecan with 5-FU and LV were compared with 5-FU and LV alone. Study 1 compared combination irinotecan/bolus 5-FU/LV therapy given weekly with a standard bolus regimen of 5-FU/LV alone given daily for 5 days every 4 weeks; an irinotecan-alone treatment arm given on a weekly schedule was also included. Study 2 evaluated two different methods of administering infusional 5-FU/LV, with or without irinotecan. In both studies, concomitant medications such as antiemetics, atropine, and loperamide were given to patients for prophylaxis and/or management of symptoms from treatment. In Study 2, a 7-day course of fluoroquinolone antibiotic prophylaxis was given in patients whose diarrhea persisted for greater than 24 hours despite loperamide or if they developed a fever in addition to diarrhea. Treatment with oral fluoroquinolone was also initiated in patients who developed an absolute neutrophil count (ANC) <500/mm³, even in the absence of fever or diarrhea. Patients in both studies also received treatment with intravenous antibiotics if they had persistent diarrhea or fever or if ileus developed. In both studies, the combination of irinotecan/5-FU/LV therapy resulted in significant improvements in objective tumor response rates, time to tumor progression, and survival when compared with 5-FU/LV alone. These differences in survival were observed in spite of second-line therapy in a majority of patients on both arms, including crossover to irinotecan-containing regimens in the control arm. Patient characteristics and major efficacy results are shown in Table 2.

[See table 2 above]

Improvement was noted with irinotecan-based combination therapy relative to 5-FU/LV when response rates and time to tumor progression were examined across the following demographic and disease-related subgroups (age, gender, ethnic origin, performance status, extent of organ involvement with cancer, time from diagnosis of cancer, prior adjuvant therapy, and baseline laboratory abnormalities). Figures 1 and 2 illustrate the Kaplan-Meier survival curves for the comparison of irinotecan/5-FU/LV versus 5-FU/LV in Studies 1 and 2, respectively.

Table 2. Combination Dosage Schedule: Study Results

	Study 1			Study 2	
	Irinotecan + Bolus 5-FU/LV weekly × 4 q 6 weeks	Bolus 5-FU/LV daily × 5 q 4 weeks	Irinotecan weekly × 4 q 6 weeks	Irinotecan + Infusional 5-FU/LV	Infusional 5-FU/LV
Number of Patients	231	226	226	198	187
Demographics and Treatment Administration					
Female/Male (%)	34/65	45/54	35/64	33/67	47/53
Median Age in years (range)	62 (25-85)	61 (19-85)	61 (30-87)	62 (27-75)	59 (24-75)
Performance Status (%)					
0	39	41	46	51	51
1	46	45	46	42	41
2	15	13	8	7	8
Primary Tumor (%)					
Colon	81	85	84	55	65
Rectum	17	14	15	45	35
Median Time from Diagnosis to Randomization (months, range)	1.9 (0-161)	1.7 (0-203)	1.8 (0.1-185)	4.5 (0-88)	2.7 (0-104)
Prior Adjuvant 5-FU Therapy (%)					
No	89	92	90	74	76
Yes	11	8	10	26	24
Median Duration of Study Treatment[a] (months)	5.5	4.1	3.9	5.6	4.5
Median Relative Dose Intensity (%)[a]					
Irinotecan	72	—	75	87	—
5-FU	71	86	—	86	93
Efficacy Results					
Confirmed Objective Tumor Response Rate[b] (%)	39	21 ($p<0.0001$)[c]	18	35	22 ($p<0.005$)[c]
Median Time to Tumor Progression[d] (months)	7.0	4.3 ($p=0.004$)[d]	4.2	6.7	4.4 ($p<0.001$)[d]
Median Survival (months)	14.8	12.6 ($p<0.05$)[d]	12.0	17.4	14.1 ($p<0.05$)[d]

[a] Study 1: N=225 (irinotecan/5-FU/LV), N=219 (5-FU/LV), N=223 (irinotecan)
  Study 2: N=199 (irinotecan/5-FU/LV), N=186 (5-FU/LV)
[b] Confirmed ≥ 4 to 6 weeks after first evidence of objective response
[c] Chi-square test
[d] Log-rank test

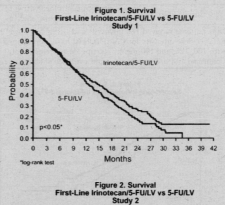

Figure 1. Survival
First-Line Irinotecan/5-FU/LV vs 5-FU/LV
Study 1

*log-rank test

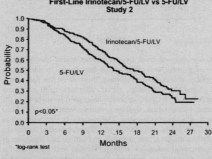

Figure 2. Survival
First-Line Irinotecan/5-FU/LV vs 5-FU/LV
Study 2

*log-rank test

Second-Line Treatment for Recurrent or Progressive Metastatic Colorectal Cancer After 5-FU-Based Treatment

Weekly Dosage Schedule

Data from three open-label, single-agent, clinical studies, involving a total of 304 patients in 59 centers, support the use of CAMPTOSAR in the treatment of patients with metastatic cancer of the colon or rectum that has recurred or progressed following treatment with 5-FU-based therapy. These studies were designed to evaluate tumor response rate and do not provide information on actual clinical benefit, such as effects on survival and disease-related symptoms. In each study, CAMPTOSAR was administered in repeated 6-week cycles consisting of a 90-minute intravenous infusion once weekly for 4 weeks, followed by a 2-week rest period. Starting doses of CAMPTOSAR in these trials were 100, 125, or 150 mg/m², but the 150-mg/m² dose was poorly tolerated (due to unacceptably high rates of grade 4 late diarrhea and febrile neutropenia). Study 1 enrolled 48 patients and was conducted by a single investigator at several regional hospitals. Study 2 was a multicenter study conducted by the North Central Cancer Treatment Group. All 90 patients enrolled in Study 2 received a starting dose of 125 mg/m². Study 3 was a multicenter study that enrolled 166 patients from 30 institutions. The initial dose in Study 3 was 125 mg/m² but was reduced to 100 mg/m² because the toxicity seen at the 125-mg/m² dose was perceived to be greater than that seen in previous studies. All patients in these studies had metastatic colorectal cancer, and the majority had disease that recurred or progressed following a 5-FU-based regimen administered for metastatic disease. The results of the individual studies are shown in Table 3. [See table 3 at top of next page]

In the intent-to-treat analysis of the pooled data across all three studies, 193 of the 304 patients began therapy at the recommended starting dose of 125 mg/m² Among these 193 patients, 2 complete and 27 partial responses were observed, for an overall response rate of 15.0% (95% Confidence Interval [CI], 10.0% to 20.1%) at this starting dose. A considerably lower response rate was seen with a starting dose of 100 mg/m². The majority of responses were observed within the first two cycles of therapy, but responses did occur in later cycles of treatment (one response was observed after the eighth cycle). The median response duration for patients beginning therapy at 125 mg/m² was 5.8 months (range, 2.6 to 15.1 months). Of the 304 patients treated in the three studies, response rates to CAMPTOSAR were similar in males and females and among patients older and younger than 65 years. Rates were also similar in patients with cancer of the colon or cancer of the rectum and in patients with single and multiple metastatic sites. The response rate was 18.5% in patients with a performance status of 0 and 8.2% in patients with a performance status of 1 or 2. Patients with a performance status of 3 or 4 have not been studied. Over half of the patients responding to CAMPTOSAR had not responded to prior 5-FU. Patients who had received previous irradiation to the pelvis responded to CAMPTOSAR at approximately the same rate as those who had not previously received irradiation.

Once-Every-3-Week Dosage Schedule

Single-Arm Studies: Data from an open-label, single-agent, single-arm, multicenter, clinical study involving a to-

Continued on next page

Camptosar—Cont.

tal of 132 patients support a once every-3-week dosage schedule of irinotecan in the treatment of patients with metastatic cancer of the colon or rectum that recurred or progressed following treatment with 5-FU. Patients received a starting dose of 350 mg/m^2 given by 30-minute intravenous infusion once every 3 weeks. Among the 132 previously treated patients in this trial, the intent-to-treat response rate was 12.1% (95% CI, 7.0% to 18.1%).

Randomized Trials: Two multicenter, randomized, clinical studies further support the use of irinotecan given by the once-every-3-week dosage schedule in patients with metastatic colorectal cancer whose disease has recurred or progressed following prior 5-FU therapy. In the first study, second-line irinotecan therapy plus best supportive care was compared with best supportive care alone. In the second study, second-line irinotecan therapy was compared with infusional 5-FU-based therapy. In both studies, irinotecan was administered intravenously at a starting dose of 350 mg/m^2 over 90 minutes once every 3 weeks. The starting dose was 300 mg/m^2 for patients who were 70 years and older or who had a performance status of 2. The highest total dose permitted was 700 mg. Dose reductions and/or administration delays were permitted in the event of severe hematologic and/or nonhematologic toxicities while on treatment. Best supportive care was provided to patients in both arms of Study 1 and included antibiotics, analgesics, corticosteroids, transfusions, psychotherapy, or any other symptomatic therapy as clinically indicated. In both studies, concomitant medications such as antiemetics, atropine, and loperamide were given to patients for prophylaxis and/or management of symptoms from treatment. If late diarrhea persisted for greater than 24 hours despite loperamide, a 7-day course of fluoroquinolone antibiotic prophylaxis was given. Patients in the control arm of the second study received one of the following 5-FU regimens: (1) LV, 200 mg/m^2 IV over 2 hours; followed by 5-FU, 400 mg/m^2 IV bolus; followed by 5-FU, 600 mg/m^2 continuous IV infusion over 22 hours on days 1 and 2 every 2 weeks; (2) 5-FU, 250 to 300 mg/m^2/day protracted continuous IV infusion until toxicity; (3) 5-FU, 2.6 to 3 g/m^2 IV over 24 hours every week for 6 weeks with or without LV, 20 to 500 mg/m^2/day every week IV for 6 weeks with 2-week rest between cycles. Patients were to be followed every 3 to 6 weeks for 1 year.

A total of 535 patients were randomized in the two studies at 94 centers. The primary endpoint in both studies was survival. The studies demonstrated a significant overall survival advantage for irinotecan compared with best supportive care (p=0.0001) and infusional 5-FU-based therapy (p=0.035) as shown in Figures 3 and 4. In Study 1, median survival for patients treated with irinotecan was 9.2 months compared with 6.5 months for patients receiving best supportive care. In Study 2, median survival for patients treated with irinotecan was 10.8 months compared with 8.5 months for patients receiving infusional 5-FU-based therapy. Multiple regression analyses determined that patients' baseline characteristics also had a significant effect on survival. When adjusted for performance status and other baseline prognostic factors, survival among patients treated with irinotecan remained significantly longer than in the control populations (p=0.001 for Study 1 and p=0.017 for Study 2). Measurements of pain, performance status, and weight loss were collected prospectively in the two studies; however, the plan for the analysis of these data was defined retrospectively. When comparing irinotecan with best supportive care in Study 1, this analysis showed a statistically significant advantage for irinotecan, with longer time to development of pain (6.9 months versus 2.0 months), time to performance status deterioration (5.7 months versus 3.3 months), and time to > 5% weight loss (6.4 months versus 4.2 months). Additionally, 33.3% (33/99) of patients with a baseline performance status of 1 or 2 showed an improvement in performance status when treated with irinotecan versus 11.3% (7/62) of patients receiving best supportive care (p=0.002). Because of the inclusion of patients with non-measurable disease, intent-to-treat response rates could not be assessed.

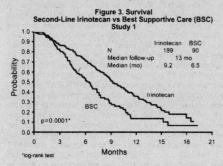

Figure 3. Survival
Second-Line Irinotecan vs Best Supportive Care (BSC)
Study 1

	Irinotecan	BSC
N	189	90
Median follow-up		13 mo
Median (mo)	9.2	6.5

*log-rank test

[See figure 4 in next column]

In the two randomized studies, the EORTC QLQ-C30 instrument was utilized. At the start of each cycle of therapy, patients completed a questionnaire consisting of 30 questions, such as "Did pain interfere with daily activities?" (1 = Not at All, to 4 = Very Much) and "Do you have any trouble taking a long walk?" (Yes or No). The answers from the 30 questions were converted into 15 subscales, that were scored from 0 to 100, and the global health status subscale

Table 3. Weekly Dosage Schedule: Study Results

	Study			
	1	2	3	
Number of Patients	48	90	64	102
Starting Dose (mg/m^2/wk × 4)	125[a]	125	125	100
Demographics and Treatment Administration				
Female/Male (%)	46/54	36/64	50/50	51/49
Median Age in years (range)	63 (29-78)	63 (32-81)	61 (42-84)	64 (25-84)
Ethnic Origin (%)				
White	79	96	81	91
African American	12	4	11	5
Hispanic	8	0	8	2
Oriental/Asian	0	0	0	2
Performance Status (%)				
0	60	38	59	44
1	38	48	33	51
2	2	14	8	5
Primary Tumor (%)				
Colon	100	71	89	87
Rectum	0	29	11	8
Unknown	0	0	0	5
Prior 5-FU Therapy (%)				
For Metastatic Disease	81	66	73	68
≤ 6 months after Adjuvant	15	7	27	28
> 6 months after Adjuvant	2	16	0	2
Classification Unknown	2	12	0	3
Prior Pelvic/Abdominal Irradiation (%)				
Yes	3	29	0	0
Other	0	9	2	4
None	97	62	98	96
Duration of Treatment with CAMPTOSAR (median, months)	5	4	4	3
Relative Dose Intensity[b] (median %)	74	67	73	81
Efficacy				
Confirmed Objective Response Rate (%)[c] (95% CI)	21 (9.3 - 32.3)	13 (6.3 - 20.4)	14 (5.5 - 22.6)	9 (3.3 - 14.3)
Time to Response (median, months)	2.6	1.5	2.8	2.8
Response Duration (median, months)	6.4	5.9	5.6	6.4
Survival (median, months)	10.4	8.1	10.7	9.3
1-Year Survival (%)	46	31	45	43

[a] Nine patients received 150 mg/m^2 as a starting dose; two (22.2%) responded to CAMPTOSAR.
[b] Relative dose intensity for CAMPTOSAR based on planned dose intensity of 100, 83.3, and 66.7 mg/m^2/wk corresponding with 150, 125, and 100 mg/m^2 starting doses, respectively.
[c] Confirmed ≥ 4 to 6 weeks after first evidence of objective response.

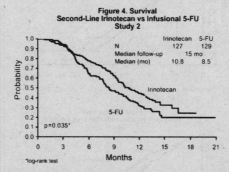

Figure 4. Survival
Second-Line Irinotecan vs Infusional 5-FU
Study 2

	Irinotecan	5-FU
N	127	129
Median follow-up	15 mo	
Median (mo)	10.8	8.5

p=0.035*
*log-rank test

that was derived from two questions about the patient's sense of general well being in the past week. In addition to the global health status subscale, there were five functional (i.e., cognitive, emotional, social, physical, role) and nine symptom (i.e., fatigue, appetite loss, pain assessment, insomnia, constipation, dyspnea, nausea/vomiting, financial impact, diarrhea) subscales. The results as summarized in Table 5 are based on patients' worst post-baseline scores. In Study 1, a multivariate analysis and univariate analyses of the individual subscales were performed and corrected for multivariate testing. Patients receiving irinotecan reported significantly better results for the global health status, on two of five functional subscales, and on four of nine symptom subscales. As expected, patients receiving irinotecan noted significantly more diarrhea than those receiving best supportive care. In Study 2, the multivariate analysis on all 15 subscales did not indicate a statistically significant difference between irinotecan and infusional 5-FU.

[See table 4 on next page]
[See table 5 at bottom of next page]

INDICATIONS AND USAGE

CAMPTOSAR Injection is indicated as a component of first-line therapy in combination with 5-fluorouracil and leucovo-rin for patients with metastatic carcinoma of the colon or rectum. CAMPTOSAR is also indicated for patients with metastatic carcinoma of the colon or rectum whose disease has recurred or progressed following initial fluorouracil-based therapy.

CONTRAINDICATIONS

CAMPTOSAR Injection is contraindicated in patients with a known hypersensitivity to the drug.

WARNINGS
General

Outside of a well-designed clinical study, CAMPTOSAR Injection should not be used in combination with the "Mayo Clinic" regimen of 5-FU/LV (administration for 4-5 consecutive days every 4 weeks) because of reports of increased toxicity, including toxic deaths. CAMPTOSAR should be used as recommended (see DOSAGE AND ADMINISTRATION, Table 10).

In patients receiving either irinotecan/5-FU/LV or 5-FU/LV in the clinical trials, higher rates of hospitalization, neutropenic fever, thromboembolism, first-cycle treatment discontinuation, and early deaths were observed in patients with a baseline performance status of 2 than in patients with a baseline performance status of 0 or 1.

Diarrhea

CAMPTOSAR can induce both early and late forms of diarrhea that appear to be mediated by different mechanisms. Early diarrhea (occurring during or shortly after infusion of CAMPTOSAR) is cholinergic in nature. It is usually transient and only infrequently is severe. It may be accompanied by symptoms of rhinitis, increased salivation, miosis, lacrimation, diaphoresis, flushing, and intestinal hyperperistalsis that can cause abdominal cramping. Early diarrhea and other cholinergic symptoms may be prevented or ameliorated by administration of atropine (see PRECAUTIONS, General, for dosing recommendations for atropine).

Late diarrhea (generally occurring more than 24 hours after administration of CAMPTOSAR) can be life threatening since it may be prolonged and may lead to dehydration, electrolyte imbalance, or sepsis. Late diarrhea should be treated promptly with loperamide (see PRECAUTIONS, Information for Patients, for dosing recommendations for loperamide). Patients with diarrhea should be carefully monitored, should be given fluid and electrolyte replacement if they become dehydrated, and should be given antibiotic support if they develop ileus, fever, or severe neutropenia. After the first treatment, subsequent weekly chemotherapy treatments should be delayed in patients until return of pretreatment bowel function for at least 24 hours without need for antidiarrhea medication. If grade 2, 3, or 4 late diarrhea occurs subsequent doses of CAMPTOSAR should be decreased within the current cycle (see DOSAGE AND ADMINISTRATION).

Neutropenia

Deaths due to sepsis following severe neutropenia have been reported in patients treated with CAMPTOSAR. Neutropenic complications should be managed promptly with antibiotic support (see PRECAUTIONS). Therapy with CAMPTOSAR should be temporarily omitted during a cycle of therapy if neutropenic fever occurs or if the absolute neu-

trophil count drops $<1000/mm^3$. After the patient recovers to an absolute neutrophil count $\geq 1000/mm^3$, subsequent doses of CAMPTOSAR should be reduced depending upon the level of neutropenia observed (see DOSAGE AND ADMINISTRATION).

Routine administration of a colony-stimulating factor (CSF) is not necessary, but physicians may wish to consider CSF use in individual patients experiencing significant neutropenia.

Patients with Reduced UGT1A1 Activity

Individuals who are homozygous for the UGT1A1*28 allele are at increased risk for neutropenia following initiation of CAMPTOSAR treatment. A reduced initial dose should be considered for patients known to be homozygous for the UGT1A1*28 allele (see DOSAGE AND ADMINISTRATION). Heterozygous patients (carriers of one variant allele and one wild-type allele which results in intermediate UGT1A1 activity) may be at increased risk for neutropenia; however, clinical results have been variable and such patients have been shown to tolerate normal starting doses.

Hypersensitivity

Hypersensitivity reactions including severe anaphylactic or anaphylactoid reactions have been observed.

Colitis/Ileus

Cases of colitis complicated by ulceration, bleeding, ileus, and infection have been observed. Patients experiencing ileus should receive prompt antibiotic support (see PRECAUTIONS).

Renal Impairment/Renal Failure

Rare cases of renal impairment and acute renal failure have been identified, usually in patients who became volume depleted from severe vomiting and/or diarrhea.

Thromboembolism

Thromboembolic events have been observed in patients receiving irinotecan-containing regimens; the specific cause of these events has not been determined.

Pregnancy

CAMPTOSAR may cause fetal harm when administered to a pregnant woman. Radioactivity related to ^{14}C-irinotecan crosses the placenta of rats following intravenous administration of 10 mg/kg (which in separate studies produced an irinotecan C_{max} and AUC about 3 and 0.5 times, respectively, the corresponding values in patients administered 125 mg/m^2). Administration of 6 mg/kg/day intravenous irinotecan to rats (which in separate studies produced an irinotecan C_{max} and AUC about 2 and 0.2 times, respectively, the corresponding values in patients administered 125 mg/m^2) and rabbits (about one-half the recommended human weekly starting dose on a mg/m^2 basis) during the period of organogenesis, is embryotoxic as characterized by increased post-implantation loss and decreased numbers of live fetuses. Irinotecan was teratogenic in rats at doses greater than 1.2 mg/kg/day (which in separate studies produced an irinotecan C_{max} and AUC about 2/3 and 1/40th, respectively, of the corresponding values in patients administered 125 mg/m^2) and in rabbits at 6.0 mg/kg/day (about one-half the recommended human weekly starting dose on a mg/m^2 basis). Teratogenic effects included a variety of external, visceral, and skeletal abnormalities. Irinotecan administered to rat dams for the period following organogenesis through weaning at doses of 6 mg/kg/day caused decreased learning ability and decreased female body weights in the offspring. There are no adequate and well-controlled studies of irinotecan in pregnant women. If the drug is used during pregnancy, or if the patient becomes pregnant while receiving this drug, the patient should be apprised of the potential hazard to the fetus. Women of childbearing potential should be advised to avoid becoming pregnant while receiving treatment with CAMPTOSAR.

PRECAUTIONS

General

Care of Intravenous Site: CAMPTOSAR Injection is administered by intravenous infusion. Care should be taken to avoid extravasation, and the infusion site should be monitored for signs of inflammation. Should extravasation occur, flushing the site with sterile water and applications of ice are recommended.

Premedication with Antiemetics: Irinotecan is emetigenic. It is recommended that patients receive premedication with antiemetic agents. In clinical studies of the weekly dosage schedule, the majority of patients received 10 mg of dexamethasone given in conjunction with another type of antiemetic agent, such as a 5-HT^3 blocker (e.g., ondansetron or granisetron). Antiemetic agents should be given on the day of treatment, starting at least 30 minutes before administration of CAMPTOSAR. Physicians should also consider providing patients with an antiemetic regimen (e.g., prochlorperazine) for subsequent use as needed.

Treatment of Cholinergic Symptoms: Prophylactic or therapeutic administration of 0.25 to 1 mg of intravenous or subcutaneous atropine should be considered (unless clinically contraindicated) in patients experiencing rhinitis, increased salivation, miosis, lacrimation, diaphoresis, flushing, abdominal cramping, or diarrhea (occurring during or shortly after infusion of CAMPTOSAR). These symptoms are expected to occur more frequently with higher irinotecan doses.

Patients at Particular Risk: In patients receiving either irinotecan/5-FU/LV or 5-FU/LV in the clinical trials, higher rates of hospitalization, neutropenic fever, thromboembolism, first-cycle treatment discontinuation, and early deaths were observed in patients with a baseline performance status of 2 than in patients with a baseline performance status of 0 or 1. Patients who had previously received pelvic/abdominal radiation and elderly patients with comorbid conditions should be closely monitored.

The use of CAMPTOSAR in patients with significant hepatic dysfunction has not been established. In clinical trials of either dosing schedule, irinotecan was not administered to patients with serum bilirubin >2.0 mg/dL, or transaminase >3 times the upper limit of normal if no liver metastasis, or transaminase >5 times the upper limit of normal with liver metastasis. However in clinical trials of the weekly dosage schedule, it has been noted that patients with modestly elevated baseline serum total bilirubin levels (1.0 to 2.0 mg/dL) have had a significantly greater likelihood of experiencing first-cycle grade 3 or 4 neutropenia than those with bilirubin levels that were less than 1.0 mg/dL (50.0% [19/38] versus 17.7% [47/226]; p<0.001). Patients with abnormal glucuronidation of bilirubin, such as those with Gilbert's syndrome, may also be at greater risk of myelosuppression when receiving therapy with CAMPTOSAR.

Table 4. Once-Every-3-Week Dosage Schedule: Study Results

	Study 1		Study 2	
	Irinotecan	BSC[a]	Irinotecan	5-FU
Number of Patients	189	90	127	129
Demographics and Treatment Administration				
Female/Male (%)	32/68	42/58	43/57	35/65
Median Age in years (range)	59 (22-75)	62 (34-75)	58 (30-75)	58 (25-75)
Performance Status (%)				
0	47	31	58	54
1	39	46	35	43
2	14	23	8	3
Primary Tumor (%)				
Colon	55	52	57	62
Rectum	45	48	43	38
Prior 5-FU Therapy (%)				
For Metastatic Disease	70	63	58	68
As Adjuvant Treatment	30	37	42	32
Prior Irradiation (%)	26	27	18	20
Duration of Study Treatment (median, months) (Log-rank test)	4.1	—	4.2 (p=0.02)	2.8
Relative Dose Intensity (median %)[b]	94	—	95	81-99
Survival				
Survival (median, months) (Log-rank test)	9.2 (p=0.0001)	6.5	10.8 (p=0.035)	8.5

[a]BSC = best supportive care
[b]Relative dose intensity for irinotecan based on planned dose intensity of 116.7 and 100 mg/m^2/wk corresponding with 350 and 300 mg/m^2 starting doses, respectively.

Table 5. EORTC QLQ-C30: Mean Worst Post-Baseline Score[a]

QLQ-C30 Subscale	Study 1			Study 2		
	Irinotecan	BSC	p-value	Irinotecan	5-FU	p-value
Global Health Status	47	37	0.03	53	52	0.9
Functional Scales						
Cognitive	77	68	0.07	79	83	0.9
Emotional	68	64	0.4	64	68	0.9
Social	58	47	0.06	65	67	0.9
Physical	60	40	0.0003	66	66	0.9
Role	53	35	0.02	54	57	0.9
Symptom Scales						
Fatigue	51	63	0.03	47	46	0.9
Appetite Loss	37	57	0.0007	35	38	0.9
Pain Assessment	41	56	0.009	38	34	0.9
Insomnia	39	47	0.3	39	33	0.9
Constipation	28	41	0.03	25	19	0.9
Dyspnea	31	40	0.2	25	24	0.9
Nausea/Vomiting	27	29	0.5	25	16	0.09
Financial Impact	22	26	0.5	24	15	0.3
Diarrhea	32	19	0.01	32	22	0.2

[a]For the five functional subscales and global health status subscale, higher scores imply better functioning, whereas, on the nine symptom subscales, higher scores imply more severe symptoms. The subscale scores of each patient were collected at each visit until the patient dropped out of the study.

Continued on next page

Camptosar—Cont.

An association between baseline bilirubin elevations and an increased risk of late diarrhea has not been observed in studies of the weekly dosage schedule.

Ketoconazole, enzyme-inducing anticonvulsants and St. John's Wort are known to have drug-drug interactions with irinotecan therapy. (See Drug-Drug Interactions sub-section under CLINICAL PHARMACOLOGY)

Information for Patients

Patients and patients' caregivers should be informed of the expected toxic effects of CAMPTOSAR, particularly of its gastrointestinal complications, such as nausea, vomiting, abdominal cramping, diarrhea, and infection. Each patient should be instructed to have loperamide readily available and to begin treatment for late diarrhea (generally occurring more than 24 hours after administration of CAMPTOSAR) at the first episode of poorly formed or loose stools or the earliest onset of bowel movements more frequent than normally expected for the patient. One dosage regimen for loperamide used in clinical trials consisted of the following (Note: This dosage regimen exceeds the usual dosage recommendations for loperamide.): 4 mg at the first onset of late diarrhea and then 2 mg every 2 hours until the patient is diarrhea-free for at least 12 hours. During the night, the patient may take 4 mg of loperamide every 4 hours. Premedication with loperamide is not recommended. The use of drugs with laxative properties should be avoided because of the potential for exacerbation of diarrhea. Patients should be advised to contact their physician to discuss any laxative use.

Patients should be instructed to contact their physician or nurse if any of the following occur: diarrhea for the first time during treatment; black or bloody stools; symptoms of dehydration such as lightheadedness, dizziness, or faintness; inability to take fluids by mouth due to nausea or vomiting; inability to get diarrhea under control within 24 hours; or fever or evidence of infection.

Patients should be alerted to the possibility of alopecia.

Laboratory Tests

Careful monitoring of the white blood cell count with differential, hemoglobin, and platelet count is recommended before each dose of CAMPTOSAR.

Drug Interactions

The adverse effects of CAMPTOSAR, such as myelosuppression and diarrhea, would be expected to be exacerbated by other antineoplastic agents having similar adverse effects. Patients who have previously received pelvic/abdominal irradiation are at increased risk of severe myelosuppression following the administration of CAMPTOSAR. The concurrent administration of CAMPTOSAR with irradiation has not been adequately studied and is not recommended.

Lymphocytopenia has been reported in patients receiving CAMPTOSAR, and it is possible that the administration of dexamethasone as antiemetic prophylaxis may have enhanced the likelihood of this effect. However, serious opportunistic infections have not been observed, and no complications have specifically been attributed to lymphocytopenia.

Hyperglycemia has also been reported in patients receiving CAMPTOSAR. Usually, this has been observed in patients with a history of diabetes mellitus or evidence of glucose intolerance prior to administration of CAMPTOSAR. It is probable that dexamethasone, given as antiemetic prophylaxis, contributed to hyperglycemia in some patients.

The incidence of akathisia in clinical trials of the weekly dosage schedule was greater (8.5%, 4/47 patients) when prochlorperazine was administered on the same day as CAMPTOSAR than when these drugs were given on separate days (1.3%, 1/80 patients). The 8.5% incidence of akathisia, however, is within the range reported for use of prochlorperazine when given as a premedication for other chemotherapies.

It would be expected that laxative use during therapy with CAMPTOSAR would worsen the incidence or severity of diarrhea, but this has not been studied.

In view of the potential risk of dehydration secondary to vomiting and/or diarrhea induced by CAMPTOSAR, the physician may wish to withhold diuretics during dosing with CAMPTOSAR and, certainly, during periods of active vomiting or diarrhea.

Drug-Laboratory Test Interactions

There are no known interactions between CAMPTOSAR and laboratory tests.

Carcinogenesis, Mutagenesis & Impairment of Fertility

Long-term carcinogenicity studies with irinotecan were not conducted. Rats were, however, administered intravenous doses of 2 mg/kg or 25 mg/kg irinotecan once per week for 13 weeks (in separate studies, the 25 mg/kg dose produced an irinotecan C_{max} and AUC that were about 7.0 times and 1.3 times the respective values in patients administered 125 mg/m² weekly) and were then allowed to recover for 91 weeks. Under these conditions, there was a significant linear trend with dose for the incidence of combined uterine horn endometrial stromal polyps and endometrial stromal sarcomas. Neither irinotecan nor SN-38 was mutagenic in the in vitro Ames assay. Irinotecan was clastogenic both in vitro (chromosome aberrations in Chinese hamster ovary cells) and in vivo (micronucleus test in mice). No significant adverse effects on fertility and general reproductive performance were observed after intravenous administration of irinotecan in doses of up to 6 mg/kg/day to rats and rabbits. However, atrophy of male reproductive organs was observed after multiple daily irinotecan doses both in rodents at

---

Table 6. Study 1: Percent (%) of Patients Experiencing Clinically Relevant Adverse Events in Combination Therapies[a]

| Adverse Event | Study 1 | | | | | |
| | Irinotecan + Bolus 5-FU/LV weekly × 4 q 6 weeks N=225 | | Bolus 5-FU/LV daily × 5 q 4 weeks N=219 | | Irinotecan weekly × 4 q 6 weeks N=223 | |
	Grade 1-4	Grade 3&4	Grade 1-4	Grade 3&4	Grade 1-4	Grade 3&4
TOTAL Adverse Events	100	53.3	100	45.7	99.6	45.7
GASTROINTESTINAL						
Diarrhea						
late	84.9	22.7	69.4	13.2	83.0	31.0
grade 3	—	15.1	—	5.9	—	18.4
grade 4	—	7.6	—	7.3	—	12.6
early	45.8	4.9	31.5	1.4	43.0	6.7
Nausea	79.1	15.6	67.6	8.2	81.6	16.1
Abdominal pain	63.1	14.6	50.2	11.5	67.7	13.0
Vomiting	60.4	9.7	46.1	4.1	62.8	12.1
Anorexia	34.2	5.8	42.0	3.7	43.9	7.2
Constipation	41.3	3.1	31.5	1.8	32.3	0.4
Mucositis	32.4	2.2	76.3	16.9	29.6	2.2
HEMATOLOGIC						
Neutropenia	96.9	53.8	98.6	66.7	96.4	31.4
grade 3	—	29.8	—	23.7	—	19.3
grade 4	—	24.0	—	42.5	—	12.1
Leukopenia	96.9	37.8	98.6	23.3	96.4	21.5
Anemia	96.9	8.4	98.6	5.5	96.9	4.5
Neutropenic fever	—	7.1	—	14.6	—	5.8
Thrombocytopenia	96.0	2.6	98.6	2.7	96.0	1.7
Neutropenic infection	—	1.8	—	0	—	2.2
BODY AS A WHOLE						
Asthenia	70.2	19.5	64.4	11.9	69.1	13.9
Pain	30.7	3.1	26.9	3.6	22.9	2.2
Fever	42.2	1.7	32.4	3.6	43.5	0.4
Infection	22.2	0	16.0	1.4	13.9	0.4
METABOLIC & NUTRITIONAL						
↑ Bilirubin	87.6	7.1	92.2	8.2	83.9	7.2
DERMATOLOGIC						
Exfoliative dermatitis	0.9	0	3.2	0.5	0	0
Rash	19.1	0	26.5	0.9	14.3	0.4
Alopecia[b]	43.1	—	26.5	—	46.1	—
RESPIRATORY						
Dyspnea	27.6	6.3	16.0	0.5	22.0	2.2
Cough	26.7	1.3	18.3	0	20.2	0.4
Pneumonia	6.2	2.7	1.4	1.0	3.6	1.3
NEUROLOGIC						
Dizziness	23.1	1.3	16.4	0	21.1	1.8
Somnolence	12.4	1.8	4.6	1.8	9.4	1.3
Confusion	7.1	1.8	4.1	0	2.7	0
CARDIOVASCULAR						
Vasodilatation	9.3	0.9	5.0	0	9.0	0
Hypotension	5.8	1.3	2.3	0.5	5.8	1.7
Thromboembolic events[c]	9.3	—	11.4	—	5.4	—

[a]Severity of adverse events based on NCI CTC (version 1.0)
[b]Complete hair loss = Grade 2
[c]Includes angina pectoris, arterial thrombosis, cerebral infarct, cerebrovascular accident, deep thrombophlebitis, embolus lower extremity, heart arrest, myocardial infarct, myocardial ischemia, peripheral vascular disorder, pulmonary embolus, sudden death, thrombophlebitis, thrombosis, vascular disorder.

---

20 mg/kg (which in separate studies produced an irinotecan C_{max} and AUC about 5 and 1 times, respectively, the corresponding values in patients administered 125 mg/m² weekly) and dogs at 0.4 mg/kg (which in separate studies produced an irinotecan C_{max} and AUC about one-half and 1/15th, respectively, the corresponding values in patients administered 125 mg/m² weekly).

Pregnancy

Pregnancy Category D—see WARNINGS.

Nursing Mothers

Radioactivity appeared in rat milk within 5 minutes of intravenous administration of radiolabeled irinotecan and was concentrated up to 65-fold at 4 hours after administration relative to plasma concentrations. Because many drugs are excreted in human milk and because of the potential for serious adverse reactions in nursing infants, it is recommended that nursing be discontinued when receiving therapy with CAMPTOSAR.

Pediatric Use

The effectiveness of irinotecan in pediatric patients has not been established. Results from two open-label, single arm studies were evaluated. One hundred and seventy children with refractory solid tumors were enrolled in one phase 2 trial in which 50 mg/m² of irinotecan was infused for 5 consecutive days every 3 weeks. Grade 3-4 neutropenia was experienced by 54 (31.8%) patients. Neutropenia was complicated by fever in 15 (8.8%) patients. Grade 3-4 diarrhea was observed in 35 (20.6%) patients. This adverse event profile was comparable to that observed in adults. In the second phase 2 trial of 21 children with previously untreated rhabdomyosarcoma, 20 mg/m² of irinotecan was infused for 5 consecutive days on weeks 0, 1, 3 and 4. This single agent therapy was followed by multimodal therapy. Accrual to the single agent irinotecan phase was halted due to the high

rate (28.6%) of progressive disease and the early deaths (14%). The adverse event profile was different in this study from that observed in adults; the most significant grade 3 or 4 adverse events were dehydration experienced by 6 patients (28.6%) associated with severe hypokalemia in 5 patients (23.8%) and hyponatremia in 3 patients (14.3%); in addition Grade 3-4 infection was reported in 5 patients (23.8%) (across all courses of therapy and irrespective of causal relationship).

Pharmacokinetic parameters for irinotecan and SN-38 were determined in 2 pediatric solid-tumor trials at dose levels of 50 mg/m² (60-min infusion, n=48) and 125 mg/m² (90-min infusion, n=6). Irinotecan clearance (mean ± S.D.) was 17.3 ± 6.7 L/h/m² for the 50mg/m² dose and 16.2 ± 4.6 L/h/m² for the 125 mg/m² dose, which is comparable to that in adults. Dose-normalized SN-38 AUC values were comparable between adults and children. Minimal accumulation of irinotecan and SN-38 was observed in children on daily dosing regimens [daily × 5 every 3 weeks or (daily × 5) × 2 weeks every 3 weeks].

Geriatric Use

Patients greater than 65 years of age should be closely monitored because of a greater risk of late diarrhea in this population (see CLINICAL PHARMACOLOGY, Pharmacokinetics in Special Populations and ADVERSE REACTIONS, Overview of Adverse Events). The starting dose of CAMPTOSAR in patients 70 years and older for the once-every-3-week-dosage schedule should be 300 mg/m² (see DOSAGE AND ADMINISTRATION).

ADVERSE REACTIONS

First-Line Combination Therapy

A total of 955 patients with metastatic colorectal cancer received the recommended regimens of irinotecan in combina-

Table 7. Study 2: Percent (%) of Patients Experiencing Clinically Relevant Adverse Events in Combination Therapies[a]

Adverse Event	Irinotecan + 5-FU/LV infusional d 1&2 q 2 weeks N=145		5-FU/LV infusional d 1&2 q 2 weeks N=143	
	Grade 1-4	Grade 3 & 4	Grade 1-4	Grade 3 & 4
TOTAL Adverse Events	100	72.4	100	39.2
GASTROINTESTINAL				
Diarrhea				
late	72.4	14.4	44.8	6.3
grade 3	—	10.3	—	4.2
grade 4	—	4.1	—	2.1
Cholinergic syndrome[b]	28.3	1.4	0.7	0
Nausea	66.9	2.1	55.2	3.5
Abdominal pain	17.2	2.1	16.8	0.7
Vomiting	44.8	3.5	32.2	2.8
Anorexia	35.2	2.1	18.9	0.7
Constipation	30.3	0.7	25.2	1.4
Mucositis	40.0	4.1	28.7	2.8
HEMATOLOGIC				
Neutropenia	82.5	46.2	47.9	13.4
grade 3	—	36.4	—	12.7
grade 4	—	9.8	—	0.7
Leukopenia	81.3	17.4	42.0	3.5
Anemia	97.2	2.1	90.9	2.1
Neutropenic fever	—	3.4	—	0.7
Thrombocytopenia	32.6	0	32.2	0
Neutropenic infection	—	2.1	—	0
BODY AS A WHOLE				
Asthenia	57.9	9.0	48.3	4.2
Pain	64.1	9.7	61.5	8.4
Fever	22.1	0.7	25.9	0.7
Infection	35.9	7.6	33.6	3.5
METABOLIC & NUTRITIONAL				
↑ Bilirubin	19.1	3.5	35.9	10.6
DERMATOLOGIC				
Hand & foot syndrome	10.3	0.7	12.6	0.7
Cutaneous signs	17.2	0.7	20.3	0
Alopecia[c]	56.6	—	16.8	—
RESPIRATORY				
Dyspnea	9.7	1.4	4.9	0
CARDIOVASCULAR				
Hypotension	3.4	1.4	0.7	0
Thromboembolic events[d]	11.7	—	5.6	—

[a]Severity of adverse events based on NCI CTC (version 1.0)
[b]Includes rhinitis, increased salivation, miosis, lacrimation, diaphoresis, flushing, abdominal cramping or diarrhea (occurring during or shortly after infusion of irinotecan)
[c]Complete hair loss = Grade 2
[d]Includes angina pectoris, arterial thrombosis, cerebral infarct, cerebrovascular accident, deep thrombophlebitis, embolus lower extremity, heart arrest, myocardial infarct, myocardial ischemia, peripheral vascular disorder, pulmonary embolus, sudden death, thrombophlebitis, thrombosis, vascular disorder.

tion with 5-FU/LV, 5-FU/LV alone, or irinotecan alone. In the two phase 3 studies, 370 patients received irinotecan in combination with 5-FU/LV, 362 patients received 5-FU/LV alone, and 223 patients received irinotecan alone. (See Table 10 in DOSAGE AND ADMINISTRATION for recommended combination-agent regimens.)

In Study 1, 49 (7.3%) patients died within 30 days of last study treatment: 21 (9.3%) received irinotecan in combination with 5-FU/LV, 15 (6.8%) received 5-FU/LV alone, and 13 (5.8%) received irinotecan alone. Deaths potentially related to treatment occurred in 2 (0.9%) patients who received irinotecan in combination with 5-FU/LV (2 neutropenic fever/sepsis), 3 (1.4%) patients who received 5-FU/LV alone (1 neutropenic fever/sepsis, 1 CNS bleeding during thrombocytopenia, 1 unknown) and 2 (0.9%) patients who received irinotecan alone (2 neutropenic fever). Deaths from any cause within 60 days of first study treatment were reported for 15 (6.7%) patients who received irinotecan in combination with 5-FU/LV, 16 (7.3%) patients who received 5-FU/LV alone, and 15 (6.7%) patients who received irinotecan alone. Discontinuations due to adverse events were reported for 17 (7.6%) patients who received irinotecan in combination with 5-FU/LV, 14 (6.4%) patients who received 5-FU/LV alone, and 26 (11.7%) patients who received irinotecan alone.

In Study 2, 10 (3.5%) patients died within 30 days of last study treatment: 6 (4.1%) received irinotecan in combination with 5-FU/LV and 4 (2.8%) received 5-FU/LV alone. There was one potentially treatment-related death, which occurred in a patient who received irinotecan in combination with 5-FU/LV (0.7%, neutropenic sepsis). Deaths from any cause within 60 days of first study treatment were reported for 3 (2.1%) patients who received irinotecan in combination with 5-FU/LV and 2 (1.4%) patients who received 5-FU/LV alone. Discontinuations due to adverse events were reported for 9 (6.2%) patients who received irinotecan in combination with 5-FU/LV and 1 (0.7%) patient who received 5-FU/LV alone.

The most clinically significant adverse events for patients receiving irinotecan-based therapy were diarrhea, nausea, vomiting, neutropenia, and alopecia. The most clinically significant adverse events for patients receiving 5-FU/LV therapy were diarrhea, neutropenia, neutropenic fever, and mucositis. In Study 1, grade 4 neutropenia, neutropenic fever (defined as grade 2 fever and grade 4 neutropenia), and mucositis were observed less often with weekly irinotecan/5-FU/LV than with monthly administration of 5-FU/LV.

Tables 6 and 7 list the clinically relevant adverse events reported in Studies 1 and 2, respectively.
[See table 6 at top of previous page]
[See table 7 above]

Second-Line Single-Agent Therapy
Weekly Dosage Schedule
In three clinical studies evaluating the weekly dosage schedule, 304 patients with metastatic carcinoma of the colon or rectum that had recurred or progressed following 5-FU-based therapy were treated with CAMPTOSAR. Seventeen of the patients died within 30 days of the administration of CAMPTOSAR; in five cases (1.6%, 5/304), the deaths were potentially drug-related. These five patients experienced a constellation of medical events that included known effects of CAMPTOSAR. One of these patients died of neutropenic sepsis without fever. Neutropenic fever occurred in nine (3.0%) other patients; these patients recovered with supportive care.

One hundred nineteen (39.1%) of the 304 patients were hospitalized a total of 156 times because of adverse events: 81 (26.6%) patients were hospitalized for events judged to be related to administration of CAMPTOSAR. The primary reasons for drug-related hospitalization were diarrhea, with or without nausea and/or vomiting (18.4%); neutropenia/leukopenia, with or without diarrhea and/or fever (8.2%); and nausea and/or vomiting (4.9%).

Adjustments in the dose of CAMPTOSAR were made during the cycle of treatment and for subsequent cycles based on individual patient tolerance. The first dose of at least one cycle of CAMPTOSAR was reduced for 67% of patients who began the studies at the 125-mg/m² starting dose. Within-cycle dose reductions were required for 32% of the cycles ini-

tiated at the 125-mg/m² dose level. The most common reasons for dose reduction were late diarrhea, neutropenia, and leukopenia. Thirteen (4.3%) patients discontinued treatment with CAMPTOSAR because of adverse events. The adverse events in Table 8 are based on the experience of the 304 patients enrolled in the three studies described in the CLINICAL STUDIES, Studies Evaluating the Weekly Dosage Schedule, section.

Table 8. Adverse Events Occurring in >10% of 304 Previously Treated Patients with Metastatic Carcinoma of the Colon or Rectum[a]

Body System & Event	% of Patients Reporting	
	NCI Grades 1-4	NCI Grades 3 & 4
GASTROINTESTINAL		
Diarrhea (late)[b]	88	31
7-9 stools/day (grade 3)	—	(16)
≥10 stools/day (grade 4)	—	(14)
Nausea	86	17
Vomiting	67	12
Anorexia	55	6
Diarrhea (early)[c]	51	8
Constipation	30	2
Flatulence	12	0
Stomatitis	12	1
Dyspepsia	10	0
HEMATOLOGIC		
Leukopenia	63	28
Anemia	60	7
Neutropenia	54	26
500 to <1000/mm³ (grade 3)	—	(15)
<500/mm³ (grade 4)	—	(12)
BODY AS A WHOLE		
Asthenia	76	12
Abdominal cramping/pain	57	16
Fever	45	1
Pain	24	2
Headache	17	1
Back pain	14	2
Chills	14	0
Minor infection[d]	14	0
Edema	10	1
Abdominal enlargement	10	0
METABOLIC & NUTRITIONAL		
↓ Body weight	30	1
Dehydration	15	4
↑ Alkaline phosphatase	13	4
↑ SGOT	10	1
DERMATOLOGIC		
Alopecia	60	NA[e]
Sweating	16	0
Rash	13	1
RESPIRATORY		
Dyspnea	22	4
↑ Coughing	17	0
Rhinitis	16	0
NEUROLOGIC		
Insomnia	19	0
Dizziness	15	0
CARDIOVASCULAR		
Vasodilation (flushing)	11	0

[a] Severity of adverse events based on NCI CTC (version 1.0)
[b] Occurring >24 hours after administration of CAMPTOSAR
[c] Occurring ≤24 hours after administration of CAMPTOSAR
[d] Primarily upper respiratory infections
[e] Not applicable; complete hair loss = NCI grade 2

Once-Every-3-Week Dosage Schedule
A total of 535 patients with metastatic colorectal cancer whose disease had recurred or progressed following prior 5-FU therapy participated in the two phase 3 studies: 316 received irinotecan, 129 received 5-FU, and 90 received best supportive care. Eleven (3.5%) patients treated with irinotecan died within 30 days of treatment. In three cases (1%, 3/316), the deaths were potentially related to irinotecan treatment and were attributed to neutropenic infection, grade 4 diarrhea, and asthenia, respectively. One (0.8%, 1/129) patient treated with 5-FU died within 30 days of treatment; this death was attributed to grade 4 diarrhea. Hospitalizations due to serious adverse events (whether or not related to study treatment) occurred at least once in 60% (188/316) of patients who received irinotecan, 63% (57/90) who received best supportive care, and 39% (50/129) who received 5-FU-based therapy. Eight percent of patients treated with irinotecan and 7% treated with 5-FU-based therapy discontinued treatment due to adverse events.

Of the 316 patients treated with irinotecan, the most clinically significant adverse events (all grades, 1-4) were diarrhea (84%), alopecia (72%), nausea (70%), vomiting (62%),

Continued on next page

Camptosar—Cont.

cholinergic symptoms (47%), and neutropenia (30%). Table 9 lists the grade 3 and 4 adverse events reported in the patients enrolled to all treatment arms of the two studies described in the CLINICAL STUDIES, Studies Evaluating the Once-Every-3-Week Dosage Schedule, section.

Table 9. Percent Of Patients Experiencing Grade 3 & 4 Adverse Events In Comparative Studies Of Once-Every-3-Week Irinotecan Therapy[a]

Adverse Event	Study 1 Irinotecan N=189	Study 1 BSC[b] N=90	Study 2 Irinotecan N=127	Study 2 5-FU N=129
TOTAL Grade 3/4 Adverse Events	79	67	69	54
GASTROINTESTINAL				
Diarrhea	22	6	22	11
Vomiting	14	8	14	5
Nausea	14	3	11	4
Abdominal pain	14	16	9	8
Constipation	10	8	8	6
Anorexia	5	7	6	4
Mucositis	2	1	2	5
HEMATOLOGIC				
Leukopenia/ Neutropenia	22	0	14	2
Anemia	7	6	6	3
Hemorrhage	5	3	1	3
Thrombocytopenia	1	0	4	2
Infection without grade 3/4 neutropenia	8	3	1	4
with grade 3/4 neutropenia	1	0	2	0
Fever without grade 3/4 neutropenia	2	1	2	0
with grade 3/4 neutropenia	2	0	4	2
BODY AS A WHOLE				
Pain	19	22	17	13
Asthenia	15	19	13	12
METABOLIC & NUTRITIONAL				
Hepatic[c]	9	7	9	6
DERMATOLOGIC				
Hand & foot syndrome	0	0	0	5
Cutaneous signs[d]	2	0	1	3
RESPIRATORY[e]	10	8	5	7
NEUROLOGIC[f]	12	13	9	4
CARDIOVASCULAR[g]	9	3	4	2
OTHER[h]	32	28	12	14

[a] Severity of adverse events based on NCI CTC (version 1.0)
[b] BSC = best supportive care
[c] Hepatic includes events such as ascites and jaundice
[d] Cutaneous signs include events such as rash
[e] Respiratory includes events such as dyspnea and cough
[f] Neurologic includes events such as somnolence
[g] Cardiovascular includes events such as dysrhythmias, ischemia, and mechanical cardiac dysfunction
[h] Other includes events such as accidental injury, hepatomegaly, syncope, vertigo, and weight loss

Overview of Adverse Events
Gastrointestinal: Nausea, vomiting, and diarrhea are common adverse events following treatment with CAMPTOSAR and can be severe. When observed, nausea and vomiting usually occur during or shortly after infusion of CAMPTOSAR. In the clinical studies testing the every 3-week-dosage schedule, the median time to the onset of late diarrhea was 5 days after irinotecan infusion. In the clinical studies evaluating the weekly dosage schedule, the median time to onset of late diarrhea was 11 days following administration of CAMPTOSAR. For patients starting treatment at the 125-mg/m² weekly dose, the median duration of any grade of late diarrhea was 3 days. Among those patients treated at the 125-mg/m² weekly dose who experienced grade 3 or 4 late diarrhea, the median duration of the entire episode of diarrhea was 7 days. The frequency of grade 3 or 4 late diarrhea was somewhat greater in patients starting treatment at 125 mg/m² than in patients given a 100-mg/m² weekly starting dose (34% [65/193] versus 23% [24/102]; p=0.08). The frequency of grade 3 and 4 late diarrhea by age was significantly greater in patients ≥65 years than in patients <65 years (40% [53/133] versus 23% [40/171]; p=0.002). In one study of the weekly dosage treatment, the frequency of grade 3 and 4 late diarrhea was significantly greater in male than in female patients (43% [25/58] versus 16% [5/32]; p=0.01), but there were no gender differences in the frequency of grade 3 and 4 late diarrhea in the other two studies of the weekly dosage treatment schedule.

Table 10. Combination-Agent Dosage Regimens & Dose Modifications[a]

Regimen 1 6-wk cycle with bolus 5-FU/LV (next cycle begins on day 43)	CAMPTOSAR LV 5-FU	125 mg/m² IV over 90 min, d 1,8,15,22 20 mg/m² IV bolus, d 1,8,15,22 500 mg/m² IV bolus, d 1,8,15,22

Starting Dose & Modified Dose Levels (mg/m²)

	Starting Dose	Dose Level -1	Dose Level -2
CAMPTOSAR	125	100	75
LV	20	20	20
5-FU	500	400	300

Regimen 2 6-wk cycle with infusional 5-FU/LV (next cycle begins on day 43)	CAMPTOSAR LV 5-FU Bolus 5-FU Infusion[b]	180 mg/m² IV over 90 min, d 1,15,29 200 mg/m² IV over 2 h, d 1,2,15,16,29,30 400 mg/m² IV bolus, d 1,2,15,16,29,30 600 mg/m² IV over 22 h, d 1,2,15,16,29,30

Starting Dose & Modified Dose Levels (mg/m²)

	Starting Dose	Dose Level -1	Dose Level -2
CAMPTOSAR	180	150	120
LV	200	200	200
5-FU Bolus	400	320	240
5-FU Infusion[b]	600	480	360

[a] Dose reductions beyond dose level −2 by decrements of ≈20% may be warranted for patients continuing to experience toxicity. Provided intolerable toxicity does not develop, treatment with additional cycles may be continued indefinitely as long as patients continue to experience clinical benefit.
[b] Infusion follows bolus administration.

Table 11. Recommended Dose Modifications for CAMPTOSAR/5-Fluorouracil (5-FU)/Leucovorin (LV) Combination Schedules

Patients should return to pre-treatment bowel function without requiring antidiarrhea medications for at least 24 hours before the next chemotherapy administration. A new cycle of therapy should not begin until the granulocyte count has recovered to ≥1500/mm³, and the platelet count has recovered to ≥100,000/mm³, and treatment-related diarrhea is fully resolved. Treatment should be delayed 1 to 2 weeks to allow for recovery from treatment-related toxicities. If the patient has not recovered after a 2-week delay, consideration should be given to discontinuing therapy.

Toxicity NCI CTC Grade[a] (Value)	During a Cycle of Therapy	At the Start of Subsequent Cycles of Therapy[b]
No toxicity	Maintain dose level	Maintain dose level
Neutropenia		
1 (1500 to 1999/mm³)	Maintain dose level	Maintain dose level
2 (1000 to 1499/mm³)	↓ 1 dose level	Maintain dose level
3 (500 to 999/mm³)	Omit dose until resolved to ≤ grade 2, then ↓ 1 dose level	↓ 1 dose level
4 (<500/mm³)	Omit dose until resolved to ≤ grade 2, then ↓ 2 dose levels	↓ 2 dose levels
Neutropenic fever	Omit dose until resolved, then ↓ 2 dose levels	
Other hematologic toxicities	Dose modifications for leukopenia or thrombocytopenia during a cycle of therapy and at the start of subsequent cycles of therapy are also based on NCI toxicity criteria and are the same as recommended for neutropenia above.	
Diarrhea		
1 (2-3 stools/day > pretx[c])	Delay dose until resolved to baseline, then give same dose	Maintain dose level
2 (4-6 stools/day > pretx)	Omit dose until resolved to baseline, then ↓ 1 dose level	Maintain dose level
3 (7-9 stools/day > pretx)	Omit dose until resolved to baseline, then ↓ 1 dose level	↓ 1 dose level
4 (≥10 stools/day > pretx)	Omit dose until resolved to baseline, then ↓ 2 dose levels	↓ 2 dose levels
Other nonhematologic toxicities[d]		
1	Maintain dose level	Maintain dose level
2	Omit dose until resolved to ≤ grade 1, then ↓ 1 dose level	Maintain dose level
3	Omit dose until resolved to ≤ grade 2, then ↓ 1 dose level	↓ 1 dose level
4	Omit dose until resolved to ≤ grade 2, then ↓ 2 dose levels *For mucositis/stomatitis decrease only 5-FU, not CAMPTOSAR*	↓ 2 dose levels *For mucositis/stomatitis decrease only 5-FU, not CAMPTOSAR*

[a] National Cancer Institute Common Toxicity Criteria (version 1.0)
[b] Relative to the starting dose used in the previous cycle
[c] Pretreatment
[d] Excludes alopecia, anorexia, asthenia

Colonic ulceration, sometimes with gastrointestinal bleeding, has been observed in association with administration of CAMPTOSAR.
Hematology: CAMPTOSAR commonly causes neutropenia, leukopenia (including lymphocytopenia), and anemia. Serious thrombocytopenia is uncommon. When evaluated in the trials of weekly administration, the frequency of grade 3 and 4 neutropenia was significantly higher in patients who received previous pelvic/abdominal irradiation than in those who had not received such irradiation (48% [13/27] versus 24% [67/277]; p=0.04). In these same studies, patients with baseline serum total bilirubin levels of 1.0 mg/dL or more also had a significantly greater likelihood of experiencing first-cycle grade 3 or 4 neutropenia than those with bilirubin levels that were less than 1.0 mg/dL (50% [19/38] versus 18% [47/266]; p<0.001). There were no significant differences in the frequency of grade 3 and 4 neutropenia by age or gender. In the clinical studies evaluating the weekly dosage schedule, neutropenic fever (concurrent NCI grade 4 neutropenia and fever of grade 2 or greater) occurred in 3% of the patients; 6% of patients received G-CSF for the treatment of neutropenia. NCI grade 3 or 4 anemia was noted in 7% of the patients receiving weekly treatment; blood transfusions were given to 10% of the patients in these trials.
Body as a Whole: Asthenia, fever, and abdominal pain are generally the most common events of this type.
Cholinergic Symptoms: Patients may have cholinergic symptoms of rhinitis, increased salivation, miosis, lacrimation, diaphoresis, flushing, and intestinal hyperperistalsis that can cause abdominal cramping and early diarrhea. If these symptoms occur, they manifest during or shortly after drug infusion. They are thought to be related to the anticholinesterase activity of the irinotecan parent compound and are expected to occur more frequently with higher irinotecan doses.
Hepatic: In the clinical studies evaluating the weekly dosage schedule, NCI grade 3 or 4 liver enzyme abnormalities were observed in fewer than 10% of patients. These events typically occur in patients with known hepatic metastases.

Dermatologic: Alopecia has been reported during treatment with CAMPTOSAR. Rashes have also been reported but did not result in discontinuation of treatment.
Respiratory: Severe pulmonary events are infrequent. In the clinical studies evaluating the weekly dosage schedule, NCI grade 3 or 4 dyspnea was reported in 4% of patients. Over half the patients with dyspnea had lung metastases; the extent to which malignant pulmonary involvement or other preexisting lung disease may have contributed to dyspnea in these patients is unknown.
Neurologic: Insomnia and dizziness can occur, but are not usually considered to be directly related to the administration of CAMPTOSAR. Dizziness may sometimes represent symptomatic evidence of orthostatic hypotension in patients with dehydration.
Cardiovascular: Vasodilation (flushing) may occur during administration of CAMPTOSAR. Bradycardia may also occur, but has not required intervention. These effects have been attributed to the cholinergic syndrome sometimes observed during or shortly after infusion of CAMPTOSAR. Thromboembolic events have been observed in patients receiving CAMPTOSAR; the specific cause of these events has not been determined.

Other Non-U.S. Clinical Trials

Irinotecan has been studied in over 1100 patients in Japan. Patients in these studies had a variety of tumor types, including cancer of the colon or rectum, and were treated with several different doses and schedules. In general, the types of toxicities observed were similar to those seen in U.S. trials with CAMPTOSAR. There is some information from Japanese trials that patients with considerable ascites or pleural effusions were at increased risk for neutropenia or diarrhea. A potentially life-threatening pulmonary syndrome, consisting of dyspnea, fever, and a reticulonodular pattern on chest x-ray, was observed in a small percentage of patients in early Japanese studies. The contribution of irinotecan to these preliminary events was difficult to assess because these patients also had lung tumors and some had preexisting nonmalignant pulmonary disease. As a result of these observations, however, clinical studies in the United States have enrolled few patients with compromised pulmonary function, significant ascites, or pleural effusions.

Post-Marketing Experience

The following events have been identified during post-marketing use of CAMPTOSAR in clinical practice. Cases of colitis complicated by ulceration, bleeding, ileus, or infection have been observed. There have been rare cases of renal impairment and acute renal failure, generally in patients who became infected and/or volume depleted from severe gastrointestinal toxicities (see WARNINGS).
Hypersensitivity reactions including severe anaphylactic or anaphylactoid reactions have also been observed (see WARNINGS).

OVERDOSAGE

In U.S. phase 1 trials, single doses of up to 345 mg/m^2 of irinotecan were administered to patients with various cancers. Single doses of up to 750 mg/m^2 of irinotecan have been given in non-U.S. trials. The adverse events in these patients were similar to those reported with the recommended dosage and regimen. There is no known antidote for overdosage of CAMPTOSAR. Maximum supportive care should be instituted to prevent dehydration due to diarrhea and to treat any infectious complications.

DOSAGE AND ADMINISTRATION

Combination-Agent Dosage

Dosage Regimens

CAMPTOSAR Injection in Combination with 5-Fluorouracil (5-FU) and Leucovorin (LV)

CAMPTOSAR should be administered as an intravenous infusion over 90 minutes (see Preparation of Infusion Solution). For all regimens, the dose of LV should be administered immediately after CAMPTOSAR, with the administration of 5-FU to occur immediately after receipt of LV. CAMPTOSAR should be used as recommended; the currently recommended regimens are shown in Table 10.
[See table 10 at top of previous page]
Dosing for patients with bilirubin >2 mg/dL cannot be recommended since such patients were not included in clinical studies. It is recommended that patients receive premedication with antiemetic agents. Prophylactic or therapeutic administration of atropine should be considered in patients experiencing cholinergic symptoms. See PRECAUTIONS, General.

Dose Modifications

Patients should be carefully monitored for toxicity and assessed prior to each treatment. Doses of CAMPTOSAR and 5-FU should be modified as necessary to accommodate individual patient tolerance to treatment. Based on the recommended dose-levels described in Table 10, Combination-Agent Dosage Regimens & Dose Modifications, subsequent doses should be adjusted as suggested in Table 11, Recommended Dose Modifications for Combination Schedules. All dose modifications should be based on the worst preceding toxicity. After the first treatment, patients with active diarrhea should return to pre-treatment bowel function without requiring anti-diarrhea medications for at least 24 hours before the next chemotherapy administration.
A new cycle of therapy should not begin until the toxicity has recovered to NCI grade 1 or less. Treatment may be delayed 1 to 2 weeks to allow for recovery from treatment-related toxicity. If the patient has not recovered, consideration should be given to discontinuing therapy. Provided intolerable toxicity does not develop, treatment with additional cycles of CAMPTOSAR/5-FU/LV may be continued indefinitely as long as patients continue to experience clinical benefit.
[See table 11 on previous page]

Single-Agent Dosage Schedules

Dosage Regimens

CAMPTOSAR should be administered as an intravenous infusion over 90 minutes for both the weekly and once-every-3-week dosage schedules (see Preparation of Infusion Solution). Single-agent dosage regimens are shown in Table 12.

Table 12. Single-Agent Regimens of CAMPTOSAR and Dose Modifications

Weekly Regimen[a]	125 mg/m^2 IV over 90 min, d 1,8,15,22 then 2-wk rest		
	Starting Dose & Modified Dose Levels[c] **(mg/m^2)**		
	Starting Dose	Dose Level -1	Dose Level -2
	125	100	75
Once-Every-3-Week Regimen[b]	350 mg/m^2 IV over 90 min, once every 3 wks[c]		
	Starting Dose & Modified Dose Levels (mg/m^2)		
	Starting Dose	Dose Level -1	Dose Level -2
	350	300	250

[a] Subsequent doses may be adjusted as high as 150 mg/m^2 or to as low as 50 mg/m^2 in 25 to 50 mg/m^2 decrements depending upon individual patient tolerance.
[b] Subsequent doses may be adjusted as low as 200 mg/m^2 in 50 mg/m^2 decrements depending upon individual patient tolerance.
[c] Provided intolerable toxicity does not develop, treatment with additional cycles may be continued indefinitely as long as patients continue to experience clinical benefit.

A reduction in the starting dose by one dose level of CAMPTOSAR may be considered for patients with any of the following conditions: age ≥65 years, prior pelvic/abdominal radiotherapy, performance status of 2, or increased bilirubin levels. Dosing for patients with bilirubin >2 mg/dL cannot be recommended since such patients were not included in clinical studies.
A reduction in the starting dose by at least one level of CAMPTOSAR should be considered for patients known to be homozygous for the UGT1A1*28 allele (See CLINICAL PHARMACOLOGY and WARNINGS). The appropriate dose reduction in this patient population is not known.
It is recommended that patients receive premedication with antiemetic agents. Prophylactic or therapeutic administration of atropine should be considered in patients experiencing cholinergic symptoms. See PRECAUTIONS, General.

Dose Modifications

Patients should be carefully monitored for toxicity and doses of CAMPTOSAR should be modified as necessary to accommodate individual patient tolerance to treatment. Based on recommended dose-levels described in Table 12, Single-Agent Regimens of CAMPTOSAR and Dose Modifications, subsequent doses should be adjusted as suggested in Table 13, Recommended Dose Modifications for Single-Agent Schedules. All dose modifications should be based on the worst preceding toxicity.
A new cycle of therapy should not begin until the toxicity has recovered to NCI grade 1 or less. Treatment may be delayed 1 to 2 weeks to allow for recovery from treatment-related toxicity. If the patient has not recovered, consideration should be given to discontinuing this combination therapy. Provided intolerable toxicity does not develop, treatment with additional cycles of CAMPTOSAR may be continued indefinitely as long as patients continue to experience clinical benefit.
[See table 13 above]

Table 13. Recommended Dose Modifications for Single-Agent Schedules[a]

A new cycle of therapy should not begin until the granulocyte count has recovered to ≥1500/mm^3, and the platelet count has recovered to ≥100,000/mm^3, and treatment-related diarrhea is fully resolved. Treatment should be delayed 1 to 2 weeks to allow for recovery from treatment-related toxicities. If the patient has not recovered after a 2-week delay, consideration should be given to discontinuing CAMPTOSAR.

Worst Toxicity NCI Grade[b] (Value)	During a Cycle of Therapy	At the Start of the Next Cycles of Therapy (After Adequate Recovery), Compared with the Starting Dose in the Previous Cycle[a]	
	Weekly	Weekly	Once Every 3 Weeks
No toxicity	Maintain dose level	↑ 25 mg/m^2 up to a maximum dose of 150 mg/m^2	Maintain dose level
Neutropenia			
1 (1500 to 1999/mm^3)	Maintain dose level	Maintain dose level	Maintain dose level
2 (1000 to 1499/mm^3)	↓ 25 mg/m^2	Maintain dose level	Maintain dose level
3 (500 to 999/mm^3)	Omit dose until resolved to ≤ grade 2, then ↓ 25 mg/m^2	↓ 25 mg/m^2	↓ 50 mg/m^2
4 (<500/mm^3)	Omit dose until resolved to ≤ grade 2, then ↓ 50 mg/m^2	↓ 50 mg/m^2	↓ 50 mg/m^2
Neutropenic fever	Omit dose until resolved, then ↓ 50 mg/m^2 when resolved	↓ 50 mg/m^2	↓ 50 mg/m^2
Other hematologic toxicities	Dose modifications for leukopenia, thrombocytopenia, and anemia during a cycle of therapy and at the start of subsequent cycles of therapy are also based on NCI toxicity criteria and are the same as recommended for neutropenia above.		
Diarrhea			
1 (2-3 stools/day > pretx[c])	Maintain dose level	Maintain dose level	Maintain dose level
2 (4-6 stools/day > pretx)	↓ 25 mg/m^2	Maintain dose level	Maintain dose level
3 (7-9 stools/day > pretx)	Omit dose until resolved to ≤ grade 2, then ↓ 25 mg/m^2	↓ 25 mg/m^2	↓ 50 mg/m^2
4 (≥10 stools/day > pretx)	Omit dose until resolved to ≤ grade 2, then ↓ 50 mg/m^2	↓ 50 mg/m^2	↓ 50 mg/m^2
Other nonhematologic toxicities[d]			
1	Maintain dose level	Maintain dose level	Maintain dose level
2	↓ 25 mg/m^2	↓ 25 mg/m^2	↓ 50 mg/m^2
3	Omit dose until resolved to ≤ grade 2, then ↓ 25 mg/m^2	↓ 25 mg/m^2	↓ 50 mg/m^2
4	Omit dose until resolved to ≤ grade 2, then ↓ 50 mg/m^2	↓ 50 mg/m^2	↓ 50 mg/m^2

[a] All dose modifications should be based on the worst preceding toxicity
[b] National Cancer Institute Common Toxicity Criteria (version 1.0)
[c] Pretreatment
[d] Excludes alopecia, anorexia, asthenia

Preparation & Administration Precautions

As with other potentially toxic anticancer agents, care should be exercised in the handling and preparation of infusion solutions prepared from CAMPTOSAR Injection. The use of gloves is recommended. If a solution of CAMPTOSAR contacts the skin, wash the skin immediately and thoroughly with soap and water. If CAMPTOSAR contacts the mucous membranes, flush thoroughly with water.
Several published guidelines for handling and disposal of anticancer agents are available.[1-7]

Preparation of Infusion Solution

Inspect vial contents for particulate matter and repeat inspection when drug product is withdrawn from vial into syringe.

Continued on next page

Camptosar—Cont.

CAMPTOSAR Injection must be diluted prior to infusion. CAMPTOSAR should be diluted in 5% Dextrose Injection, USP, (preferred) or 0.9% Sodium Chloride Injection, USP, to a final concentration range of 0.12 to 2.8 mg/mL. In most clinical trials, CAMPTOSAR was administered in 250 mL to 500 mL of 5% Dextrose Injection, USP.
The solution is physically and chemically stable for up to 24 hours at room temperature (approximately 25°C) and in ambient fluorescent lighting. Solutions diluted in 5% Dextrose Injection, USP, and stored at refrigerated temperatures (approximately 2° to 8°C), and protected from light are physically and chemically stable for 48 hours. Refrigeration of admixtures using 0.9% Sodium Chloride Injection, USP, is not recommended due to a low and sporadic incidence of visible particulates. Freezing CAMPTOSAR and admixtures of CAMPTOSAR may result in precipitation of the drug and should be avoided. Because of possible microbial contamination during dilution, it is advisable to use the admixture prepared with 5% Dextrose Injection, USP, within 24 hours if refrigerated (2° to 8°C, 36° to 46°F). In the case of admixtures prepared with 5% Dextrose Injection, USP, or Sodium Chloride Injection, USP, the solutions should be used within 6 hours if kept at room temperature (15° to 30°C, 59° to 86°F).
Other drugs should not be added to the infusion solution. Parenteral drug products should be inspected visually for particulate matter and discoloration prior to administration whenever solution and container permit.

HOW SUPPLIED

Each mL of CAMPTOSAR Injection contains 20 mg irinotecan (on the basis of the trihydrate salt); 45 mg sorbitol; and 0.9 mg lactic acid. When necessary, pH has been adjusted to 3.5 (range, 3.0 to 3.8) with sodium hydroxide or hydrochloric acid.
CAMPTOSAR Injection is available in single-dose amber glass vials in the following package sizes:

2 mL	NDC 0009-7529-02
5 mL	NDC 0009-7529-01

This is packaged in a backing/plastic blister to protect against inadvertent breakage and leakage. The vial should be inspected for damage and visible signs of leaks before removing the backing/plastic blister. If damaged, incinerate the unopened package.
Store at controlled room temperature 15° to 30°C (59° to 86°F). Protect from light. It is recommended that the vial (and backing/plastic blister) should remain in the carton until the time of use.
Rx only

REFERENCES

1. ONS Clinical Practice Committee. Cancer Chemotherapy Guidelines and Recommendations for Practice. Pittsburgh, Pa: Oncology Nursing Society; 1999:32-41.
2. Recommendations for the safe handling of parenteral antineoplastic drugs. Washington, DC: Division of Safety, National Institutes of Health; 1983. US Dept of Health and Human Services, Public Health Service publication NIH 83-2621.
3. AMA Council on Scientific Affairs. Guidelines for handling parenteral antineoplastics. *JAMA.* 1985;253:1590-1592.
4. National Study Commission on Cytotoxic Exposure. Recommendations for handling cytotoxic agents. 1987. Available from Louis P. Jeffrey, Chairman, National Study Commission on Cytotoxic Exposure. Massachusetts College of Pharmacy and Allied Health Sciences, 179 Longwood Avenue, Boston, MA 02115.
5. Clinical Oncological Society of Australia. Guidelines and recommendations for safe handling of antineoplastic agents. *Med J Australia.* 1983;1:426-428.
6. Jones RB, Frank R, Mass T. Safe handling of chemotherapeutic agents: a report from the Mount Sinai Medical Center. *CA-A Cancer J for Clin.* 1983;33:258-263.
7. American Society of Hospital Pharmacists. ASHP technical assistance bulletin on handling cytotoxic and hazardous drugs. *Am J Hosp Pharm.* 1990;47:1033-1049.
8. Controlling Occupational Exposure to Hazardous Drugs. (OSHA Work-Practice Guidelines). *Am J Health-Syst Pharm.* 1996;53;1669-1685.

Camptosar brand of irinotecan hydrochloride injection
Distributed by
Pfizer
Pharmacia & Upjohn Co
Division of Pfizer Inc, NY, NY 10017
Licensed from Yakult Honsha Co., LTD, Japan, and Daiichi Pharmaceutical Co., LTD, Japan
Revised March 2005

LAB-0134-7.0

DEPO-PROVERA®
CONTRACEPTIVE INJECTION ℞

[*dĕ-pō prō-vĕ-ră*]

medroxyprogesterone acetate injectable suspension, USP

Prescribing information for this product, which appears on pages 2716–2720 of the 2005 PDR, has been completely revised as follows. Please write "See Supplement A" next to the product heading.

Physician Information

Women who use Depo-Provera Contraceptive Injection may lose significant bone mineral density. Bone loss is greater with increasing duration of use and may not be completely reversible.
It is unknown if use of Depo-Provera Contraceptive Injection during adolescence or early adulthood, a critical period of bone accretion, will reduce peak bone mass and increase the risk for osteoporotic fracture in later life.
Depo-Provera Contraceptive Injection should be used as a long-term birth control method (e.g. longer than 2 years) only if other birth control methods are inadequate. (See WARNINGS.)

Patients should be counseled that this product does not protect against HIV infection (AIDS) and other sexually transmitted diseases.

DESCRIPTION

DEPO-PROVERA Contraceptive Injection (CI) contains medroxyprogesterone acetate, a derivative of progesterone, as its active ingredient. Medroxyprogesterone acetate is active by the parenteral and oral routes of administration. It is a white to off-white, odorless crystalline powder that is stable in air and that melts between 200°C and 210°C. It is freely soluble in chloroform, soluble in acetone and dioxane, sparingly soluble in alcohol and methanol, slightly soluble in ether, and insoluble in water.
The chemical name for medroxyprogesterone acetate is pregn-4-ene-3,20-dione, 17-(acetyloxy)-6-methyl-, (6α-). The structural formula is as follows:

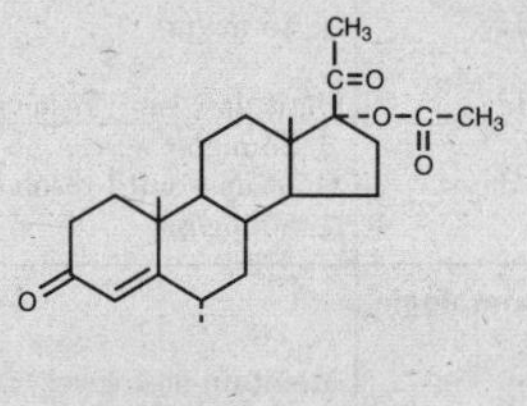

medroxyprogesterone acetate

DEPO-PROVERA CI for intramuscular (IM) injection is available in vials and prefilled syringes, each containing 1 mL of medroxyprogesterone acetate sterile aqueous suspension 150 mg/mL.
Each mL contains:

Medroxyprogesterone acetate	150 mg
Polyethylene glycol 3350	28.9 mg
Polysorbate 80	2.41 mg
Sodium chloride	8.68 mg
Methylparaben	1.37 mg
Propylparaben	0.150 mg
Water for injection	qs

When necessary, pH is adjusted with sodium hydroxide or hydrochloric acid, or both.

CLINICAL PHARMACOLOGY

DEPO-PROVERA CI (medroxyprogesterone acetate), when administered at the recommended dose to women every 3 months, inhibits the secretion of gonadotropins which, in turn, prevents follicular maturation and ovulation and results in endometrial thinning. These actions produce its contraceptive effect.
Following a single 150 mg IM dose of DEPO-PROVERA Contraceptive Injection, medroxyprogesterone acetate concentrations, measured by an extracted radioimmunoassay procedure, increase for approximately 3 weeks to reach peak plasma concentrations of 1 to 7 ng/mL. The levels then decrease exponentially until they become undetectable (<100 pg/mL) between 120 to 200 days following injection. Using an unextracted radioimmunoassay procedure for the assay of medroxyprogesterone acetate in serum, the apparent half-life for medroxyprogesterone acetate following IM administration of DEPO-PROVERA Contraceptive Injection is approximately 50 days.
Women with lower body weights conceive sooner than women with higher body weights after discontinuing DEPO-PROVERA Contraceptive Injection.
The effect of hepatic and/or renal disease on the pharmacokinetics of DEPO-PROVERA Contraceptive Injection is unknown.

INDICATIONS AND USAGE

DEPO-PROVERA CI is indicated only for the prevention of pregnancy. The loss of bone mineral density (BMD) in women of all ages and the impact on peak bone mass in adolescents should be considered, along with the decrease in BMD that occurs during pregnancy and/or lactation, in the risk/benefit assessment for women who use Depo-Provera CI long-term (see WARNINGS.) It is a long-term injectable contraceptive in women when administered at 3-month (13-week) intervals. Dosage does not need to be adjusted for body weight.
In five clinical studies using DEPO-PROVERA CI, the 12-month failure rate for the group of women treated with DEPO-PROVERA CI was zero (no pregnancies reported) to 0.7 by Life-Table method. Pregnancy rates with contraceptive measures are typically reported for only the first year of use as shown in Table 1. Except for intrauterine devices (IUD), implants, sterilization, and DEPO-PROVERA CI, the efficacy of these contraceptive measures depends in part on the reliability of use. The effectiveness of DEPO-PROVERA CI is dependent on the patient returning every 3 months (13 weeks) for reinjection.

Table 1
Lowest Expected and Typical Failure Rates*
Expressed as Percent of Women Experiencing
an Accidental Pregnancy
in the First Year of Continuous Use

Method	Lowest Expected	Typical
Injectable progestogen		
DEPO-PROVERA	0.3	0.3
Implants		
Norplant (6 capsules)	0.2†	0.2†
Female sterilization	0.2	0.4
Male sterilization	0.1	0.15
Pill		3
Combined	0.1	
Progestogen only	0.5	
IUD		3
Progestasert	2	
Copper T 380A	0.8	
Condom	2	12
Diaphragm	6	18
Cap	6	18
Spermicides	3	21
Sponge		
Parous women	9	28
Nulliparous women	6	18
Periodic abstinence	1-9	20
Withdrawal	4	18
No method	85	85

Source: Trussell et al[1]
*Lowest expected - when used exactly as directed.
Typical - includes those not following directions exactly.
†from Norplant® package insert.

CONTRAINDICATIONS

1. Known or suspected pregnancy or as a diagnostic test for pregnancy.
2. Undiagnosed vaginal bleeding.
3. Known or suspected malignancy of breast.
4. Active thrombophlebitis, or current or past history of thromboembolic disorders, or cerebral vascular disease.
5. Significant liver disease.
6. Known hypersensitivity to DEPO-PROVERA CI (medroxyprogesterone acetate or any of its other ingredients).

WARNINGS

1. Loss of Bone Mineral Density

Use of Depo-Provera CI reduces serum estrogen levels and is associated with significant loss of bone mineral density (BMD) as bone metabolism accommodates to a lower estrogen level. This loss of BMD is of particular concern during adolescence and early adulthood, a critical period of bone accretion. It is unknown if use of Depo-Provera CI by younger women will reduce peak bone mass and increase the risk for osteoporotic fracture in later life. In both adults and adolescents, the decrease in BMD appears to be at least partially reversible after Depo-Provera CI is discontinued and ovarian estrogen production increases. A study to assess the reversibility of loss of BMD in adolescents is ongoing.
Depo-Provera CI should be used as a long-term birth control method (e.g. longer than 2 years) only if other birth control methods are inadequate. BMD should be evaluated when a woman needs to continue to use Depo-Provera CI long term. In adolescents, interpretation of BMD results should take into account patient age and skeletal maturity. Other birth control methods should be considered in the risk/benefit analysis for the use of Depo-Provera CI in women with osteoporosis risk factors. Depo-Provera CI can pose an additional risk in patients with risk factors for osteoporosis (e.g., metabolic bone disease, chronic alcohol and/or tobacco use, anorexia nervosa, strong family history of osteoporosis or chronic use of drugs that can reduce bone mass such as anticonvulsants or corticosteroids). Although there are no studies addressing whether calcium and Vitamin D may lessen BMD loss in women using Depo-Provera CI, all patients should have adequate calcium and Vitamin D intake.

BMD Changes in Adult Women

In a controlled, clinical study, adult women using Depo-Provera CI for up to 5 years showed spine and hip BMD mean decreases of 5-6%, compared to no significant change in BMD in the control group. The decline in BMD was more pronounced during the first two years of use, with smaller declines in subsequent years. Mean changes

in lumbar spine BMD of –2.86%, -4.11%, -4.89%, -4.93% and –5.38% after 1, 2, 3, 4, and 5 years, respectively, were observed. Mean decreases in BMD of the total hip and femoral neck were similar.

After stopping use of Depo-Provera CI (150 mg), there was partial recovery of BMD toward baseline values during the 2-year post-therapy period. Longer duration of treatment was associated with less complete recovery during this 2-year period following the last injection. Table 2 shows the extent of recovery of BMD for women who completed 5 years of treatment.

[See table 2 at right]

Table 2. Mean Percent Change from Baseline in BMD in Adults by Skeletal Site and Cohort

Time in Study	Spine		Total Hip		Femoral Neck	
	Depo-Provera*	Control**	Depo-Provera*	Control**	Depo-Provera*	Control**
5 years	n=33 -5.38%	n=105 0.43%	n=21 -5.16%	n=65 0.19%	n=34 -6.12%	n=106 -0.27%
7 years	n=12 -3.13%	n=60 0.53%	n=7 -1.34%	n=39 0.94%	n=13 -5.38%	n=63 -0.11%

***The treatment group consisted of women who received Depo-Provera Contraceptive Injection for 5 years and were then followed for 2 years post-use.**
****The control group consisted of women who did not use hormonal contraception and were followed for 7 years.**

BMD Changes in Adolescent Females (12-18 years of age)

Preliminary results from an ongoing, open-label, self-selected, non-randomized clinical study of adolescent females (12-18 years) also showed that Depo-Provera CI use was associated with a significant decline in BMD from baseline (Table 3). In general, adolescents increase bone density during the period of growth following menarche, as seen in the untreated cohort. However, the two cohorts were not matched at baseline for age, gynecologic age, race, BMD and other factors that influence the rate of acquisition of bone mineral density, with the result that they differed with respect to these demographic factors.

Preliminary data from the small number of adolescents participating in the 2-year post-use observation period demonstrated partial recovery of BMD.

[See table 3 at right]

Table 3. Mean Percent Change from Baseline in BMD in Adolescents by Skeletal Site and Cohort

Duration of Treatment	Depo-Provera CI (150 mg IM)		Unmatched, Untreated Cohort	
	N	Mean % Change	N	Mean % Change
Total Hip BMD				
Week 60 (1.2 years)	103	-2.82	171	1.32
Week 144 (2.8 years)	45	-6.16	111	1.74
Week 240 (4.6 years)	9	-6.92	69	1.12
Femoral Neck BMD				
Week 60	103	-3.05	171	1.87
Week 144	45	-6.01	111	2.54
Week 240	9	-6.06	69	1.45
Lumbar Spine BMD				
Week 60	104	-2.42	171	3.47
Week 144	46	-2.78	111	5.41
Week 240	9	-4.17	70	5.12

2. Bleeding Irregularities

Most women using DEPO-PROVERA CI experience disruption of menstrual bleeding patterns. Altered menstrual bleeding patterns include irregular or unpredictable bleeding or spotting, or rarely, heavy or continuous bleeding. If abnormal bleeding persists or is severe, appropriate investigation should be instituted to rule out the possibility of organic pathology, and appropriate treatment should be instituted when necessary.

As women continue using DEPO-PROVERA CI, fewer experience irregular bleeding and more experience amenorrhea. By month 12 amenorrhea was reported by 55% of women, and by month 24 amenorrhea was reported by 68% of women using DEPO-PROVERA CI.[2]

3. Cancer Risks

Long-term case-controlled surveillance of users of DEPO-PROVERA CI found slight or no increased overall risk of breast cancer[3] and no overall increased risk of ovarian,[4] liver,[5] or cervical[6] cancer and a prolonged, protective effect of reducing the risk of endometrial[7] cancer in the population of users.

A pooled analysis[14] from two case-control studies, the World Health Organization Study[3] and the New Zealand Study[13], reported the relative risk (RR) of breast cancer for women who had ever used DEPO-PROVERA CI as 1.1 (95% confidence interval (CI) 0.97 to 1.4). Overall, there was no increase in risk with increasing duration of use of DEPO-PROVERA CI. The RR of breast cancer for women of all ages who had initiated use of DEPO-PROVERA CI within the previous 5 years was estimated to be 2.0 (95% CI 1.5 to 2.8).

The World Health Organization Study[3], a component of the pooled analysis[14] described above, showed an increased RR of 2.19 (95% CI 1.23 to 3.89) of breast cancer associated with use of DEPO-PROVERA CI in women whose first exposure to drug was within the previous 4 years and who were under 35 years of age. However, the overall RR for ever-users of DEPO-PROVERA CI was only 1.2 (95% CI 0.96 to 1.52). [**NOTE:** A RR of 1.0 indicates neither an increased nor a decreased risk of cancer associated with the use of the drug, relative to no use of the drug. In the case of the subpopulation with a RR of 2.19, the 95% CI is fairly wide and does not include the value of 1.0, thus inferring an increased risk of breast cancer in the defined subgroup relative to nonusers. The value of 2.19 means that women whose first exposure to drug was within the previous 4 years and who are under 35 years of age have a 2.19 fold (95% CI 1.23 to 3.89-fold) increased risk of breast cancer relative to nonusers. The National Cancer Institute[8] reports an average annual incidence rate for breast cancer for US women, all races, age 30 to 34 years of 26.7 per 100,000. A RR of 2.19, thus, increases the possible risk from 26.7 to 58.5 cases per 100,000 women. The attributable risk, thus, is 31.8 per 100,000 women per year.]

A statistically insignificant increase in RR estimates of invasive squamous-cell cervical cancer has been associated with the use of DEPO-PROVERA CI in women who were first exposed before the age of 35 years (RR 1.22 to 1.28 and 95% CI 0.93 to 1.70). The overall, nonsignificant relative rate of invasive squamous-cell cervical cancer in women who ever used DEPO-PROVERA CI was estimated to be 1.11 (95% CI 0.96 to 1.29). No trends in risk with duration of use or times since initial or most recent exposure were observed.

4. Thromboembolic Disorders

The physician should be alert to the earliest manifestations of thrombotic disorders (thrombophlebitis, pulmonary embolism, cerebrovascular disorders, and retinal thrombosis). Should any of these occur or be suspected, the drug should not be readministered.

5. Ocular Disorders

Medication should not be readministered pending examination if there is a sudden partial or complete loss of vision or if there is a sudden onset of proptosis, diplopia, or migraine. If examination reveals papilledema or retinal vascular lesions, medication should not be readministered.

6. Unexpected Pregnancies

To ensure that DEPO-PROVERA CI is not administered inadvertently to a pregnant woman, the first injection must be given **ONLY** during the first 5 days of a normal menstrual period; **ONLY** within the first 5-days postpartum if not breast-feeding, and if exclusively breast-feeding, **ONLY** at the sixth postpartum week (see DOSAGE AND ADMINISTRATION).

Neonates from unexpected pregnancies that occur 1 to 2 months after injection of DEPO-PROVERA CI may be at an increased risk of low birth weight, which, in turn, is associated with an increased risk of neonatal death. The attributable risk is low because such pregnancies are uncommon.[9,10]

A significant increase in incidence of polysyndactyly and chromosomal anomalies was observed among infants of users of DEPO-PROVERA CI, the former being most pronounced in women under 30 years of age. The unrelated nature of these defects, the lack of confirmation from other studies, the distant preconceptual exposure to DEPO-PROVERA CI, and the chance effects due to multiple statistical comparisons, make a causal association unlikely.[11]

Neonates exposed to medroxyprogesterone acetate *in utero* and followed to adolescence, showed no evidence of any adverse effects on their health including their physical, intellectual, sexual, or social development.

Several reports suggest an association between intrauterine exposure to progestational drugs in the first trimester of pregnancy and genital abnormalities in male and female fetuses. The risk of hypospadias (five to eight per 1,000 male births in the general population) may be approximately doubled with exposure to these drugs. There are insufficient data to quantify the risk to exposed female fetuses, but because some of these drugs induce mild virilization of the external genitalia of the female fetus and because of the increased association of hypospadias in the male fetus, it is prudent to avoid the use of these drugs during the first trimester of pregnancy.

To ensure that DEPO-PROVERA CI is not administered inadvertently to a pregnant woman, it is important that the first injection be given only during the first 5 days after the onset of a normal menstrual period within 5 days postpartum if not breast-feeding and if breast-feeding, at the sixth week postpartum (see DOSAGE AND ADMINISTRATION).

7. Ectopic Pregnancy

Health-care providers should be alert to the possibility of an ectopic pregnancy among women using DEPO-PROVERA CI who become pregnant or complain of severe abdominal pain.

8. Lactation

Detectable amounts of drug have been identified in the milk of mothers receiving DEPO-PROVERA CI. In nursing mothers treated with DEPO-PROVERA CI, milk composition, quality, and amount are not adversely affected. Neonates and infants exposed to medroxyprogesterone from breast milk have been studied for developmental and behavioral effects through puberty. No adverse effects have been noted.

9. Anaphylaxis and Anaphylactoid Reaction

Anaphylaxis and anaphylactoid reaction have been reported with the use of DEPO-PROVERA CI. If an anaphylactic reaction occurs appropriate therapy should be instituted. Serious anaphylactic reactions require emergency medical treatment.

PRECAUTIONS

GENERAL

1. Physical Examination

It is good medical practice for all women to have annual history and physical examinations, including women using DEPO-PROVERA CI. The physical examination, however, may be deferred until after initiation of DEPO PROVERA CI if requested by the woman and judged appropriate by the clinician. The physical examination should include special reference to blood pressure, breasts, abdomen and pelvic organs, including cervical cytology and relevant laboratory tests. In case of undiagnosed, persistent or recurrent abnormal vaginal bleeding, appropriate measures should be conducted to rule out malignancy. Women with a strong family history of breast cancer or who have breast nodules should be monitored with particular care.

2. Fluid Retention

Because progestational drugs may cause some degree of fluid retention, conditions that might be influenced by this condition, such as epilepsy, migraine, asthma, and cardiac or renal dysfunction, require careful observation.

3. Weight Changes

There is a tendency for women to gain weight while on therapy with DEPO-PROVERA CI. From an initial average body weight of 136 lb, women who completed 1 year of therapy with DEPO-PROVERA CI gained an average of 5.4 lb. Women who completed 2 years of therapy gained an average of 8.1 lb.

Women who completed 4 years gained an average of 13.8 lb. Women who completed 6 years gained an average of 16.5 lb. Two percent of women withdrew from a large-scale clinical trial because of excessive weight gain.

4. Return of Fertility

DEPO-PROVERA CI has a prolonged contraceptive effect. In a large US study of women who discontinued use of DEPO-PROVERA CI to become pregnant, data are available for 61% of them. Based on Life-Table analysis of these data, it is expected that 68% of women who do become pregnant may conceive within 12 months, 83% may conceive within 15 months, and 93% may conceive within 18 months from the last injection. The median time to conception for those who do conceive is 10 months following the last injection with a range of 4 to 31 months, and is unrelated to the duration of use. No data are available for 39% of the patients who discontinued DEPO-PROVERA CI to become pregnant and who were lost to follow-up or changed their mind.

5. CNS Disorders and Convulsions

Patients who have a history of psychic depression should be carefully observed and the drug not be readministered if the depression recurs.

There have been a few reported cases of convulsions in patients who were treated with DEPO-PROVERA CI. Association with drug use or pre-existing conditions is not clear.

6. Carbohydrate Metabolism

A decrease in glucose tolerance has been observed in some patients on DEPO-PROVERA CI treatment. The mechanism of this decrease is obscure. For this reason, diabetic patients should be carefully observed while receiving such therapy.

7. Liver Function

If jaundice develops, consideration should be given to not readministering the drug.

Continued on next page

Depo-Provera—Cont.

8. Protection Against Sexually Transmitted Diseases
Patients should be counseled that this product does not protect against HIV infection (AIDS) and other sexually transmitted diseases.

DRUG INTERACTIONS
Aminoglutethimide administered concomitantly with the DEPO-PROVERA CI may significantly depress the serum concentrations of medroxyprogesterone acetate.[12] Users of DEPO-PROVERA CI should be warned of the possibility of decreased efficacy with the use of this or any related drugs.

LABORATORY TEST INTERACTIONS
The pathologist should be advised of progestin therapy when relevant specimens are submitted.
The following laboratory tests may be affected by progestins including DEPO-PROVERA CI:
(a) Plasma and urinary steroid levels are decreased (eg, progesterone, estradiol, pregnanediol, testosterone, cortisol).
(b) Gonadotropin levels are decreased.
(c) Sex-hormone-binding-globulin concentrations are decreased.
(d) Protein-bound iodine and butanol extractable protein-bound iodine may increase.
T_3-uptake values may decrease.
(e) Coagulation test values for prothrombin (Factor II), and Factors VII, VIII, IX, and X may increase.
(f) Sulfobromophthalein and other liver function test values may be increased.
(g) The effects of medroxyprogesterone acetate on lipid metabolism are inconsistent. Both increases and decreases in total cholesterol, triglycerides, low-density lipoprotein (LDL) cholesterol, and high-density lipoprotein (HDL) cholesterol have been observed in studies.

CARCINOGENESIS
See "WARNINGS" section 3.

PREGNANCY
Pregnancy Category X. See "WARNINGS" section 6.

NURSING MOTHERS
See "WARNINGS" section 8.

PEDIATRIC USE
Depo-Provera CI is not indicated before menarche. Use of Depo-Provera CI is associated with significant loss of BMD. This loss of BMD is of particular concern during adolescence and early adulthood, a critical period of bone accretion. **In adolescents, interpretation of BMD results should take into account patient age and skeletal maturity.** It is unknown if use of Depo-Provera CI by younger women will reduce peak bone mass and increase the risk of osteoporotic fractures in later life. Other than concerns about loss of BMD, the safety and effectiveness are expected to be the same for postmenarchal adolescents and adult women.

INFORMATION FOR THE PATIENT
See Patient Labeling.
Patient labeling is included with each single-dose vial and prefilled syringe of DEPO-PROVERA CI to help describe its characteristics to the patient. It is recommended that prospective users be given this labeling and be informed about the risks and benefits associated with the use of DEPO-PROVERA CI, as compared with other forms of contraception or with no contraception at all. It is recommended that physicians or other health-care providers responsible for those patients advise them at the beginning of treatment that their menstrual cycle may be disrupted and that irregular and unpredictable bleeding or spotting results, and that this usually decreases to the point of amenorrhea as treatment with DEPO-PROVERA CI continues, without other therapy being required.

ADVERSE REACTIONS
In the largest clinical trial with DEPO-PROVERA CI, over 3,900 women, who were treated for up to 7 years, reported the following adverse reactions, which may or may not be related to the use of DEPO-PROVERA CI.
The following adverse reactions were reported by more than 5% of subjects:
Menstrual irregularities (bleeding or amenorrhea, or both)
Abdominal pain or discomfort
Weight changes
Dizziness
Headache
Asthenia (weakness or fatigue)
Nervousness
Adverse reactions reported by 1% to 5% of subjects using DEPO-PROVERA Contraceptive Injection were:
Decreased libido or anorgasmia
Pelvic pain
Backache
Breast pain
Leg cramps
No hair growth or alopecia
Depression
Bloating
Nausea
Rash
Insomnia
Edema
Leukorrhea
Hot flashes
Acne
Arthralgia
Vaginitis

Events reported by fewer than 1% of subjects included: galactorrhea, melasma, chloasma, convulsions, changes in appetite, gastrointestinal disturbances, jaundice, genitourinary infections, vaginal cysts, dyspareunia, paresthesia, chest pain, pulmonary embolus, allergic reactions, anemia, drowsiness, syncope, dyspnea and asthma, tachycardia, fever, excessive sweating and body odor, dry skin, chills, increased libido, excessive thirst, hoarseness, pain at injection site, blood dyscrasia, rectal bleeding, changes in breast size, breast lumps or nipple bleeding, axillary swelling, breast cancer, prevention of lactation, sensation of pregnancy, lack of return to fertility, paralysis, facial palsy, scleroderma, osteoporosis, uterine hyperplasia, cervical cancer, varicose veins, dysmenorrhea, hirsutism, unexpected pregnancy, thrombophlebitis, deep vein thrombosis.

Postmarketing Experience
There have been rare cases of osteoporosis including osteoporotic fractures reported postmarketing in patients taking Depo-Provera CI. In addition, there have been voluntary reports of anaphylaxis and anaphylactoid reaction associated with the use of Depo-Provera CI.

DOSAGE AND ADMINISTRATION
Both the 1 mL vial and the 1 mL prefilled syringe of DEPO-PROVERA CI should be vigorously shaken just before use to ensure that the dose being administered represents a uniform suspension.
The recommended dose is 150 mg of DEPO-PROVERA CI every 3 months (13 weeks) administered by deep, IM injection in the gluteal or deltoid muscle. To ensure the patient is not pregnant at the time of the first injection, the first injection **MUST** be given **ONLY** during the first 5 days of a normal menstrual period; **ONLY** within the first 5-days postpartum if not breast-feeding; and if exclusively breast-feeding, **ONLY** at the sixth postpartum week. If the time interval between injections is greater than 13 weeks, the physician should determine that the patient is not pregnant before administering the drug. The efficacy of DEPO-PROVERA CI depends on adherence to the dosage schedule of administration.

HOW SUPPLIED
DEPO-PROVERA CI (medroxyprogesterone acetate sterile aqueous suspension 150 mg/mL) is available as:

NDC 0009-0746-30	1 mL vial
NDC 0009-0746-35	25 × 1 mL vials
NDC 0009-7376-01	1 mL prefilled syringe
NDC 0009-7376-02	6 × 1 mL prefilled syringes
NDC 0009-7376-03	24 × 1 mL prefilled syringes

DEPO-PROVERA CI prefilled syringes are available packaged with 22-gauge × 1 1/2 inch BD SafetyGlide™ Needles in the following presentations:

NDC 0009-7376-04	1 mL prefilled syringe
NDC 0009-7376-05	6 × 1 mL prefilled syringes
NDC 0009-7376-06	24 × 1 mL prefilled syringes

Store at controlled room temperature 20° to 25°C (68° to 77°F) [see USP].

REFERENCES

1. Trussell J, Hatcher RA, Cates W Jr, Stewart FH, Kost K. A guide to interpreting contraceptive efficacy studies. Obstet Gynecol. 1990; *76*:558-567.
2. Schwallie PC, Assenzo JR. Contraceptive use-efficacy study utilizing medroxyprogesterone acetate administered as an intramuscular injection once every 90 days. Fertil Steril. 1973; *24*:331-339.
3. WHO Collaborative Study of Neoplasia and Steroid Contraceptives. Breast cancer and depot-medroxyprogesterone acetate: a multi-national study. Lancet. 1991; *338*:833-838.
4. WHO Collaborative Study of Neoplasia and Steroid Contraceptives. Depot-medroxyprogesterone acetate (DMPA) and risk of epithelial ovarian cancer. Int J Cancer. 1991; *49*:191-195.
5. WHO Collaborative Study of Neoplasia and Steroid Contraceptives. Depot-medroxyprogesterone acetate (DMPA) and risk of liver cancer. Int J Cancer. 1991; *49*:182185.
6. WHO Collaborative Study of Neoplasia and Steroid Contraceptives. Depot-medroxyprogesterone acetate (DMPA) and risk of invasive squamous-cell cervical cancer. Contraception. 1992; *45*:299-312.
7. WHO Collaborative Study of Neoplasia and Steroid Contraceptives. Depot-medroxyprogesterone acetate (DMPA) and risk of endometrial cancer. Int J Cancer. 1991; *49*:186-190.
8. Surveillance, Epidemiology, and End Results: Incidence and Mortality Data, 1973-1977. National Cancer Institute Monograph, 57: June 1981. (NIH publication No. 81-2330).
9. Gray RH, Pardthaisong T. *In Utero* exposure to steroid contraceptives and survival during infancy. Am J Epidemiol. 1991; *134*:804-811.
10. Pardthaisong T, Gray RH. *In Utero* exposure to steroid contraceptives and outcome of pregnancy. Am J Epidemiol. 1991; *134*:795-803.
11. Pardthaisong T, Gray RH, McDaniel EB, Chandacham A. Steroid contraceptive use and pregnancy outcome. Teratology. 1988; *38*:51-58.
12. Van Deijk WA, Biljham GH, Mellink WAM, Meulenberg PMM. Influence of aminoglutethimide on plasma levels of medroxyprogesterone acetate: its correlation with serum cortisol. Cancer Treatment Reports. 1985; *69*:1, 85-90.
13. Paul C, Skegg DCG, Spears GFS. Depot medroxyprogesterone (Depo-Provera) and risk of breast cancer. Br Med J. 1989; *299*:759-762.
14. Skegg DCG, Noonan EA, Paul C, Spears GFS, Meirik O, Thomas DB. Depot Medroxyprogesterone Acetate and Breast Cancer: A Pooled Analysis from the World Health Organization and New Zealand Studies. JAMA. 1995; *273(10)*:799-804.

Rx only
DEPO-PROVERA Contraceptive Injection 1 mL vials are manufactured by:
Pharmacia & Upjohn Company
Kalamazoo, MI 49001, USA
Division of Pfizer Inc, NY, NY 10017
DEPO-PROVERA Contraceptive Injection 1 mL prefilled syringes are manufactured by:
Pharmacia & Upjohn, N.V./S.A.
Puurs, Belgium
Division of Pfizer Inc, NY, NY 10017
LAB-0149-4.0 Revised November 2004

DOSTINEX® ℞
[*dŏ-stĭ-nĕks*]
cabergoline tablets

Prescribing information for this product, which appears on pages 2724–2726 of the 2005 PDR, has been completely revised as follows. Please write "See Supplement A" next to the product heading.

DESCRIPTION
DOSTINEX Tablets contain cabergoline, a dopamine receptor agonist. The chemical name for cabergoline is 1-[(6-allylergolin-8β-yl)-carbonyl]-1-[3-(dimethylamino)propyl]-3-ethylurea. Its empirical formula is $C_{26}H_{37}N_5O_2$, and its molecular weight is 451.62. The structural formula is as follows:

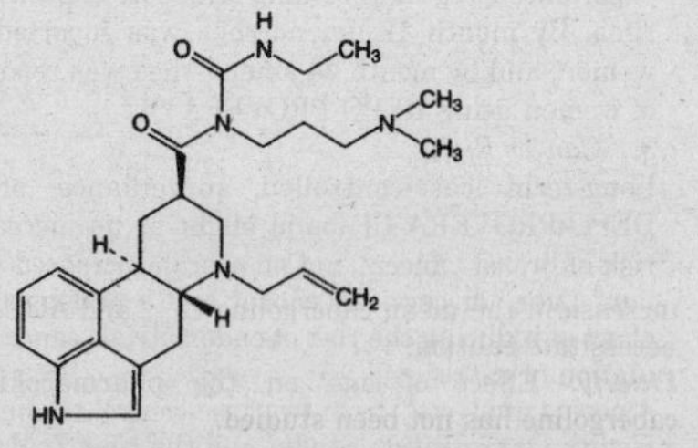

Cabergoline is a white powder soluble in ethyl alcohol, chloroform, and N, N-dimethylformamide (DMF); slightly soluble in 0.1N hydrochloric acid; very slightly soluble in n-hexane; and insoluble in water.
DOSTINEX Tablets, for oral administration, contain 0.5 mg of cabergoline. Inactive ingredients consist of leucine, USP, and lactose, NF.

CLINICAL PHARMACOLOGY
Mechanism of Action: The secretion of prolactin by the anterior pituitary is mainly under hypothalamic inhibitory control, likely exerted through release of dopamine by tuberoinfundibular neurons. Cabergoline is a long-acting dopamine receptor agonist with a high affinity for D_2 receptors. Results of in vitro studies demonstrate that cabergoline exerts a direct inhibitory effect on the secretion of prolactin by rat pituitary lactotrophs. Cabergoline decreased serum prolactin levels in reserpinized rats. Receptor-binding studies indicate that cabergoline has low affinity for dopamine D_1, α_1- and α_2-adrenergic, and 5-HT_1- and 5-HT_2-serotonin receptors.
Clinical Studies: The prolactin-lowering efficacy of DOSTINEX was demonstrated in hyperprolactinemic women in two randomized, double-blind, comparative studies, one with placebo and the other with bromocriptine. In the placebo-controlled study (placebo n=20; cabergoline n=168), DOSTINEX produced a dose-related decrease in serum prolactin levels with prolactin normalized after 4 weeks of treatment in 29%, 76%, 74% and 95% of the patients receiving 0.125, 0.5, 0.75, and 1.0 mg twice weekly respectively.
In the 8-week, double-blind period of the comparative trial with bromocriptine (cabergoline n=223; bromocriptine n=236 in the intent-to-treat analysis), prolactin was normalized in 77% of the patients treated with DOSTINEX at 0.5 mg twice weekly compared with 59% of those treated with bromocriptine at 2.5 mg twice daily. Restoration of menses occurred in 77% of the women treated with DOSTINEX, compared with 70% of those treated with bromocriptine. Among patients with galactorrhea, this symptom disappeared in 73% of those treated with DOSTINEX compared with 56% of those treated with bromocriptine.
Pharmacokinetics
Absorption: Following single oral doses of 0.5 mg to 1.5 mg given to 12 healthy adult volunteers, mean peak plasma levels of 30 to 70 picograms (pg)/mL of cabergoline were observed within 2 to 3 hours. Over the 0.5-to-7 mg dose range, cabergoline plasma levels appeared to be dose-proportional in 12 healthy adult volunteers and nine adult parkinsonian patients. A repeat-dose study in 12 healthy volunteers suggests that steady-state levels following a

once-weekly dosing schedule are expected to be twofold to threefold higher than after a single dose. The absolute bioavailability of cabergoline is unknown. A significant fraction of the administered dose undergoes a first-pass effect. The elimination half-life of cabergoline estimated from urinary data of 12 healthy subjects ranged between 63 to 69 hours. The prolonged prolactin-lowering effect of cabergoline may be related to its slow elimination and long half-life.

Distribution: In animals, based on total radioactivity, cabergoline (and/or its metabolites) has shown extensive tissue distribution. Radioactivity in the pituitary exceeded that in plasma by >100-fold and was eliminated with a half-life of approximately 60 hours. This finding is consistent with the long-lasting prolactin-lowering effect of the drug. Whole body autoradiography studies in pregnant rats showed no fetal uptake but high levels in the uterine wall. Significant radioactivity (parent plus metabolites) detected in the milk of lactating rats suggests a potential for exposure to nursing infants. The drug is extensively distributed throughout the body. Cabergoline is moderately bound (40% to 42%) to human plasma proteins in a concentration-independent manner. Concomitant dosing of highly protein-bound drugs is unlikely to affect its disposition.

Metabolism: In both animals and humans, cabergoline is extensively metabolized, predominately via hydrolysis of the acylurea bond or the urea moiety. Cytochrome P-450 mediated metabolism appears to be minimal. Cabergoline does not cause enzyme induction and/or inhibition in the rat. Hydrolysis of the acylurea or urea moiety abolishes the prolactin-lowering effect of cabergoline, and major metabolites identified thus far do not contribute to the therapeutic effect.

Excretion: After oral dosing of radioactive cabergoline to five healthy volunteers, approximately 22% and 60% of the dose was excreted within 20 days in the urine and feces, respectively. Less than 4% of the dose was excreted unchanged in the urine. Nonrenal and renal clearances for cabergoline are about 3.2 L/min and 0.08 L/min, respectively. Urinary excretion in hyperprolactinemic patients was similar.

Special Populations

Renal Insufficiency: The pharmacokinetics of cabergoline were not altered in 12 patients with moderate-to-severe renal insufficiency as assessed by creatinine clearance.

Hepatic Insufficiency: In 12 patients with mild-to-moderate hepatic dysfunction (Child-Pugh score ≤10), no effect on mean cabergoline C_{max} or area under the plasma concentration curve (AUC) was observed. However, patients with severe insufficiency (Child-Pugh score >10) show a substantial increase in the mean cabergoline C_{max} and AUC, and thus necessitate caution.

Elderly: Effect of age on the pharmacokinetics of cabergoline has not been studied.

Food-Drug Interaction

In 12 healthy adult volunteers, food did not alter cabergoline kinetics.

Pharmacodynamics

Dose response with inhibition of plasma prolactin, onset of maximal effect, and duration of effect has been documented following single cabergoline doses to healthy volunteers (0.05 to 1.5 mg) and hyperprolactinemic patients (0.3 to 1 mg). In volunteers, prolactin inhibition was evident at doses >0.2 mg, while doses ≥0.5 mg caused maximal suppression in most subjects. Higher doses produce prolactin suppression in a greater proportion of subjects and with an earlier onset and longer duration of action. In 12 healthy volunteers, 0.5, 1, and 1.5 mg doses resulted in complete prolactin inhibition, with a maximum effect within 3 hours in 92% to 100% of subjects after the 1 and 1.5 mg doses compared with 50% of subjects after the 0.5 mg dose.

In hyperprolactinemic patients (N=51), the maximal prolactin decrease after a 0.6 mg single dose of cabergoline was comparable to 2.5 mg bromocriptine; however, the duration of effect was markedly longer (14 days vs 24 hours). The time to maximal effect was shorter for bromocriptine than cabergoline (6 hours vs 48 hours).

In 72 healthy volunteers, single or multiple doses (up to 2 mg) of cabergoline resulted in selective inhibition of prolactin with no apparent effect on other anterior pituitary hormones (GH, FSH, LH, ACTH, and TSH) or cortisol.

INDICATIONS AND USAGE

DOSTINEX Tablets are indicated for the treatment of hyperprolactinemic disorders, either idiopathic or due to pituitary adenomas.

CONTRAINDICATIONS

DOSTINEX Tablets are contraindicated in patients with uncontrolled hypertension or known hypersensitivity to ergot derivatives.

WARNINGS

Dopamine agonists in general should not be used in patients with pregnancy-induced hypertension, for example, preeclampsia and eclampsia, unless the potential benefit is judged to outweigh the possible risk.

PRECAUTIONS

General: Initial doses higher than 1.0 mg may produce orthostatic hypotension. Care should be exercised when administering DOSTINEX with other medications known to lower blood pressure.

Postpartum Lactation Inhibition or Suppression: DOSTINEX is not indicated for the inhibition or suppression of physiologic lactation. Use of bromocriptine, another dopamine agonist for this purpose, has been associated with cases of hypertension, stroke, and seizures.

Hepatic Impairment: Since cabergoline is extensively metabolized by the liver, caution should be used, and careful monitoring exercised, when administering DOSTINEX to patients with hepatic impairment.

Information for Patients: A patient should be instructed to notify her physician if she suspects she is pregnant, becomes pregnant, or intends to become pregnant during therapy. A pregnancy test should be done if there is any suspicion of pregnancy and continuation of treatment should be discussed with her physician.

Drug Interactions: DOSTINEX should not be administered concurrently with D_2-antagonists, such as phenothiazines, butyrophenones, thioxanthenes, or metoclopramide.

Carcinogenesis, Mutagenesis, Impairment of Fertility: Carcinogenicity studies were conducted in mice and rats with cabergoline given by gavage at doses up to 0.98 mg/kg/day and 0.32 mg/kg/day, respectively. These doses are 7 times and 4 times the maximum recommended human dose calculated on a body surface area basis using total mg/m^2/week in rodents and mg/m^2/week for a 50 kg human.

There was a slight increase in the incidence of cervical and uterine leiomyomas and uterine leiomyosarcomas in mice. In rats, there was a slight increase in malignant tumors of the cervix and uterus and interstitial cell adenomas. The occurrence of tumors in female rodents may be related to the prolonged suppression of prolactin secretion because prolactin is needed in rodents for the maintenance of the corpus luteum. In the absence of prolactin, the estrogen/progesterone ratio is increased, thereby increasing the risk for uterine tumors. In male rodents, the decrease in serum prolactin levels was associated with an increase in serum luteinizing hormone, which is thought to be a compensatory effect to maintain testicular steroid synthesis. Since these hormonal mechanisms are thought to be species-specific, the relevance of these tumors to humans is not known.

The mutagenic potential of cabergoline was evaluated and found to be negative in a battery of in vitro tests. These tests included the bacterial mutation (Ames) test with *Salmonella typhimurium*, the gene mutation assay with *Schizosaccharomyces pombe* P_1 and V79 Chinese hamster cells, DNA damage and repair in *Saccharomyces cerevisiae* D_4, and chromosomal aberrations in human lymphocytes. Cabergoline was also negative in the bone marrow micronucleus test in the mouse.

In female rats, a daily dose of 0.003 mg/kg for 2 weeks prior to mating and throughout the mating period inhibited conception. This dose represents approximately 1/28 the maximum recommended human dose calculated on a body surface area basis using total mg/m^2/week in rats and mg/m^2/week for a 50 kg human.

Pregnancy: Teratogenic Effects: Category B. Reproduction studies have been performed with cabergoline in mice, rats, and rabbits administered by gavage.

(Multiples of the maximum recommended human dose in this section are calculated on a body surface area basis using total mg/m^2/week for animals and mg/m^2/week for a 50 kg human.)

There were maternotoxic effects but no teratogenic effects in mice given cabergoline at doses up to 8 mg/kg/day (approximately 55 times the maximum recommended human dose) during the period of organogenesis.

A dose of 0.012 mg/kg/day (approximately 1/7 the maximum recommended human dose) during the period of organogenesis in rats caused an increase in post-implantation embryofetal losses. These losses could be due to the prolactin inhibitory properties of cabergoline in rats. At daily doses of 0.5 mg/kg/day (approximately 19 times the maximum recommended human dose) during the period of organogenesis in the rabbit, cabergoline caused maternotoxicity characterized by a loss of body weight and decreased food consumption. Doses of 4 mg/kg/day (approximately 150 times the maximum recommended human dose) during the period of organogenesis in the rabbit caused an increased occurrence of various malformations. However, in another study in rabbits, no treatment-related malformations or embryofetotoxicity were observed at doses up to 8 mg/kg/day (approximately 300 times the maximum recommended human dose).

In rats, doses higher than 0.003 mg/kg/day (approximately 1/28 the maximum recommended human dose) from 6 days before parturition and throughout the lactation period inhibited growth and caused death of offspring due to decreased milk secretion.

There are, however, no adequate and well-controlled studies in pregnant women. Because animal reproduction studies are not always predictive of human response, this drug should be used during pregnancy only if clearly needed.

Nursing Mothers: It is not known whether this drug is excreted in human milk. Because many drugs are excreted in human milk and because of the potential for serious adverse reactions in nursing infants from cabergoline, a decision should be made whether to discontinue nursing or to discontinue the drug, taking into account the importance of the drug to the mother. Use of DOSTINEX for the inhibition or suppression of physiologic lactation is not recommended (see PRECAUTIONS section).

The prolactin-lowering action of cabergoline suggests that it will interfere with lactation. Due to this interference with lactation, DOSTINEX should not be given to women postpartum who are breastfeeding or who are planning to breastfeed.

Pediatric Use: Safety and effectiveness of DOSTINEX in pediatric patients have not been established.

Geriatric Use: Clinical studies of DOSTINEX did not include sufficient numbers of subjects aged 65 and over to determine whether they respond differently from younger patients. Other reported clinical experience has not identified differences in responses between the elderly and younger patients. In general, dose selection for an elderly patient should be cautious, usually starting at the low end of the dosing range, reflecting the greater frequency of decreased hepatic, renal, or cardiac function, and of concomitant disease or other drug therapy.

ADVERSE REACTIONS

The safety of DOSTINEX Tablets has been evaluated in more than 900 patients with hyperprolactinemic disorders. Most adverse events were mild or moderate in severity.

In a 4-week, double-blind, placebo-controlled study, treatment consisted of placebo or cabergoline at fixed doses of 0.125, 0.5, 0.75, or 1.0 mg twice weekly. Doses were halved during the first week. Since a possible dose-related effect was observed for nausea only, the four cabergoline treatment groups have been combined. The incidence of the most common adverse events during the placebo-controlled study is presented in the following table.

Incidence of Reported Adverse Events During the 4-Week, Double-Blind, Placebo-Controlled Trial

Adverse Event*	Cabergoline (n=168) 0.125 to 1 mg two times a week	Placebo (n=20)
	Number (percent)	
Gastrointestinal		
Nausea	45 (27)	4 (20)
Constipation	16 (10)	0
Abdominal pain	9 (5)	1 (5)
Dyspepsia	4 (2)	0
Vomiting	4 (2)	0
Central and Peripheral Nervous System		
Headache	43 (26)	5 (25)
Dizziness	25 (15)	1 (5)
Paresthesia	2 (1)	0
Vertigo	2 (1)	0
Body As a Whole		
Asthenia	15 (9)	2 (10)
Fatigue	12 (7)	0
Hot flashes	2 (1)	1 (5)
Psychiatric		
Somnolence	9 (5)	1 (5)
Depression	5 (3)	1 (5)
Nervousness	4 (2)	0
Autonomic Nervous System		
Postural hypotension	6 (4)	0
Reproductive—Female		
Breast pain	2 (1)	0
Dysmenorrhea	2 (1)	0
Vision		
Abnormal vision	2 (1)	0

*Reported at ≥1% for cabergoline

In the 8-week, double-blind period of the comparative trial with bromocriptine, DOSTINEX (at a dose of 0.5 mg twice weekly) was discontinued because of an adverse event in 4 of 221 patients (2%) while bromocriptine (at a dose of 2.5 mg two times a day) was discontinued in 14 of 231 patients (6%). The most common reasons for discontinuation from DOSTINEX were headache, nausea and vomiting (3, 2 and 2 patients respectively); the most common reasons for discontinuation from bromocriptine were nausea, vomiting, headache, and dizziness or vertigo (10, 3, 3, and 3 patients respectively). The incidence of the most common adverse events during the double-blind portion of the comparative trial with bromocriptine is presented in the following table.

Incidence of Reported Adverse Events During the 8-week, Double-Blind Period of the Comparative Trial With Bromocriptine

Adverse Event*	Cabergoline (n=221)	Bromocriptine (n=231)
	Number (percent)	
Gastrointestinal		
Nausea	63 (29)	100 (43)
Constipation	15 (7)	21 (9)
Abdominal pain	12 (5)	19 (8)
Dyspepsia	11 (5)	16 (7)
Vomiting	9 (4)	16 (7)
Dry mouth	5 (2)	2 (1)
Diarrhea	4 (2)	7 (3)
Flatulence	4 (2)	3 (1)
Throat irritation	2 (1)	0

Continued on next page

Dostinex—Cont.

Toothache	2 (1)	0
Central and Peripheral Nervous System		
Headache	58 (26)	62 (27)
Dizziness	38 (17)	42 (18)
Vertigo	9 (4)	10 (4)
Paresthesia	5 (2)	6 (3)
Body As a Whole		
Asthenia	13 (6)	15 (6)
Fatigue	10 (5)	18 (8)
Syncope	3 (1)	3 (1)
Influenza-like symptoms	2 (1)	0
Malaise	2 (1)	0
Periorbital edema	2 (1)	2 (1)
Peripheral edema	2 (1)	1
Psychiatric		
Depression	7 (3)	5 (2)
Somnolence	5 (2)	5 (2)
Anorexia	3 (1)	3 (1)
Anxiety	3 (1)	3 (1)
Insomnia	3 (1)	2 (1)
Impaired concentration	2 (1)	1
Nervousness	2 (1)	5 (2)
Cardiovascular		
Hot flashes	6 (3)	3 (1)
Hypotension	3 (1)	4 (2)
Dependent edema	2 (1)	1
Palpitation	2 (1)	5 (2)
Reproductive—Female		
Breast pain	5 (2)	8 (3)
Dysmenorrhea	2 (1)	1
Skin and Appendages		
Acne	3 (1)	0
Pruritus	2 (1)	1
Musculoskeletal		
Pain	4 (2)	6 (3)
Arthralgia	2 (1)	0
Respiratory		
Rhinitis	2 (1)	9 (4)
Vision		
Abnormal vision	2 (1)	2 (1)

*Reported at ≥1% for cabergoline

Other adverse events that were reported at an incidence of <1.0% in the overall clinical studies follow.

Body As a Whole: facial edema, influenza-like symptoms, malaise

Cardiovascular System: hypotension, syncope, palpitations

Digestive System: dry mouth, flatulence, diarrhea, anorexia

Metabolic and Nutritional System: weight loss, weight gain

Nervous System: somnolence, nervousness, paresthesia, insomnia, anxiety

Respiratory System: nasal stuffiness, epistaxis

Skin and Appendages: acne, pruritus

Special Senses: abnormal vision

Urogenital System: dysmenorrhea, increased libido

The safety of cabergoline has been evaluated in approximately 1,200 patients with Parkinson's disease in controlled and uncontrolled studies at dosages of up to 11.5 mg/day which greatly exceeds the maximum recommended dosage of cabergoline for hyperprolactinemic disorders. In addition to the adverse events that occurred in the patients with hyperprolactinemic disorders, the most common adverse events in patients with Parkinson's disease were dyskinesia, hallucinations, confusion, and peripheral edema. Heart failure, pleural effusion, pulmonary fibrosis, and gastric or duodenal ulcer occurred rarely. One case of constrictive pericarditis has been reported.

OVERDOSAGE

Overdosage might be expected to produce nasal congestion, syncope, or hallucinations. Measures to support blood pressure should be taken if necessary.

DOSAGE AND ADMINISTRATION

The recommended dosage of DOSTINEX Tablets for initiation of therapy is 0.25 mg twice a week. Dosage may be increased by 0.25 mg twice weekly up to a dosage of 1 mg twice a week according to the patient's serum prolactin level.

Dosage increases should not occur more rapidly than every 4 weeks, so that the physician can assess the patient's response to each dosage level. If the patient does not respond adequately, and no additional benefit is observed with higher doses, the lowest dose that achieved maximal response should be used and other therapeutic approaches considered.

After a normal serum prolactin level has been maintained for 6 months, DOSTINEX may be discontinued, with periodic monitoring of the serum prolactin level to determine whether or when treatment with DOSTINEX should be reinstituted. The durability of efficacy beyond 24 months of therapy with DOSTINEX has not been established.

HOW SUPPLIED

DOSTINEX Tablets are white, scored, capsule-shaped tablets containing 0.5 mg cabergoline. Each tablet is scored on one side and has the letter P and the letter U on either side of the breakline. The other side of the tablet is engraved with the number 700.

DOSTINEX is available as follows:

Bottles of 8 tablets NDC 0013-7001-12

STORAGE

Store at controlled room temperature 20° to 25°C (68° to 77°F) [see USP].

℞ only

U.S. Patent No. 4,526,892.

MADE IN ITALY

Distributed by

Pharmacia & Upjohn Co

Division of Pfizer Inc, NY, NY 10017

816 989 204 Revised September 2004

ELLENCE® ℞

[ĕl-ĕns]

epirubicin hydrochloride injection

Prescribing information for this product, which appears on pages 2726–2730 of the 2005 PDR, has been completely revised as follows. Please write "See Supplement A" next to the product heading.

WARNING

1. Severe local tissue necrosis will occur if there is extravasation during administration (See PRECAUTIONS). Epirubicin must not be given by the intramuscular or subcutaneous route.
2. Myocardial toxicity, manifested in its most severe form by potentially fatal congestive heart failure (CHF), may occur either during therapy with epirubicin or months to years after termination of therapy. The probability of developing clinically evident CHF is estimated as approximately 0.9% at a cumulative dose of 550 mg/m^2, 1.6% at 700 mg/m^2, and 3.3% at 900 mg/m^2. In the adjuvant treatment of breast cancer, the maximum cumulative dose used in clinical trials was 720 mg/m^2. The risk of developing CHF increases rapidly with increasing total cumulative doses of epirubicin in excess of 900 mg/m^2; this cumulative dose should only be exceeded with extreme caution. Active or dormant cardiovascular disease, prior or concomitant radiotherapy to the mediastinal/pericardial area, previous therapy with other anthracyclines or anthracenediones, or concomitant use of other cardiotoxic drugs may increase the risk of cardiac toxicity. Cardiac toxicity with ELLENCE may occur at lower cumulative doses whether or not cardiac risk factors are present.
3. Secondary acute myelogenous leukemia (AML) has been reported in patients with breast cancer treated with anthracyclines, including epirubicin. The occurrence of refractory secondary leukemia is more common when such drugs are given in combination with DNA-damaging antineoplastic agents, when patients have been heavily pretreated with cytotoxic drugs, or when doses of anthracyclines have been escalated. The cumulative risk of developing treatment-related AML or myelodysplastic syndrome (MDS), in 7110 patients with breast cancer who received adjuvant treatment with epirubicin-containing regimens, was estimated as 0.27% at 3 years, 0.46% at 5 years and 0.55% at 8 years.
4. Dosage should be reduced in patients with impaired hepatic function (see DOSAGE AND ADMINISTRATION).
5. Severe myelosuppression may occur.
6. Epirubicin should be administered only under the supervision of a physician who is experienced in the use of cancer chemotherapeutic agents.

DESCRIPTION

ELLENCE Injection (epirubicin hydrochloride injection) is an anthracycline cytotoxic agent, intended for intravenous administration. ELLENCE is supplied as a sterile, clear, red solution and is available in polypropylene vials containing 50 and 200 mg of epirubicin hydrochloride as a preservative-free, ready-to-use solution. Each milliliter of solution contains 2 mg of epirubicin hydrochloride. Inactive ingredients include sodium chloride, USP, and water for injection, USP. The pH of the solution has been adjusted to 3.0 with hydrochloric acid, NF.

Epirubicin hydrochloride is the 4-epimer of doxorubicin and is a semi-synthetic derivative of daunorubicin. The chemical name is (8S-***cis***)-10-[(3-amino-2,3,6-trideoxy-α-L-***arabino***-hexopyranosyl)oxy]-7,8,9,10-tetrahydro-6,8,11-trihydroxy-8-(hydroxyacetyl)-1-methoxy-5,12-naphthacenedione hydrochloride. The active ingredient is a red-orange hygroscopic powder, with the empirical formula $C_{27}H_{29}NO_{11}$ HCl and a molecular weight of 579.95. The structural formula is as follows:

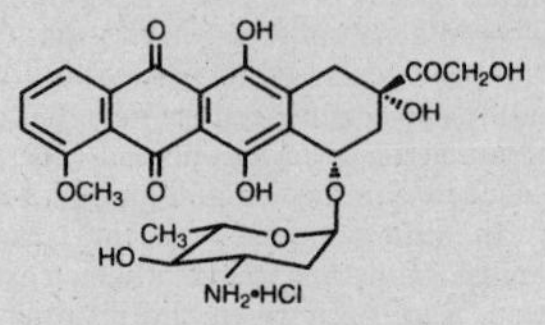

CLINICAL PHARMACOLOGY

Epirubicin is an anthracycline cytotoxic agent. Although it is known that anthracyclines can interfere with a number of biochemical and biological functions within eukaryotic cells, the precise mechanisms of epirubicin's cytotoxic and/or antiproliferative properties have not been completely elucidated.

Epirubicin forms a complex with DNA by intercalation of its planar rings between nucleotide base pairs, with consequent inhibition of nucleic acid (DNA and RNA) and protein synthesis.

Such intercalation triggers DNA cleavage by topoisomerase II, resulting in cytocidal activity. Epirubicin also inhibits DNA helicase activity, preventing the enzymatic separation of double-stranded DNA and interfering with replication and transcription. Epirubicin is also involved in oxidation/reduction reactions by generating cytotoxic free radicals. The antiproliferative and cytotoxic activity of epirubicin is thought to result from these or other possible mechanisms.

Epirubicin is cytotoxic in vitro to a variety of established murine and human cell lines and primary cultures of human tumors. It is also active in vivo against a variety of murine tumors and human xenografts in athymic mice, including breast tumors.

Pharmacokinetics

Epirubicin pharmacokinetics are linear over the dose range of 60 to 150 mg/m^2 and plasma clearance is not affected by the duration of infusion or administration schedule. Pharmacokinetic parameters for epirubicin following 6- to 10-minute, single-dose intravenous infusions of epirubicin at doses of 60 to 150 mg/m^2 in patients with solid tumors are shown in Table 1. The plasma concentration declined in a triphasic manner with mean half-lives for the alpha, beta, and gamma phases of about 3 minutes, 2.5 hours, and 33 hours, respectively.

[See table 1 at top of next page]

Distribution. Following intravenous administration, epirubicin is rapidly and widely distributed into the tissues. Binding of epirubicin to plasma proteins, predominantly albumin, is about 77% and is not affected by drug concentration. Epirubicin also appears to concentrate in red blood cells; whole blood concentrations are approximately twice those of plasma.

Metabolism. Epirubicin is extensively and rapidly metabolized by the liver and is also metabolized by other organs and cells, including red blood cells. Four main metabolic routes have been identified:

(1) reduction of the C-13 keto-group with the formation of the 13(S)-dihydro derivative, epirubicinol; (2) conjugation of both the unchanged drug and epirubicinol with glucuronic acid; (3) loss of the amino sugar moiety through a hydrolytic process with the formation of the doxorubicin and doxorubicinol aglycones; and (4) loss of the amino sugar moiety through a redox process with the formation of the 7-deoxy-doxorubicin aglycone and 7-deoxy-doxorubicinol aglycone. Epirubicinol has in vitro cytotoxic activity one-tenth that of epirubicin. As plasma levels of epirubicinol are lower than those of the unchanged drug, they are unlikely to reach in vivo concentrations sufficient for cytotoxicity. No significant activity or toxicity has been reported for the other metabolites.

Excretion. Epirubicin and its major metabolites are eliminated through biliary excretion and, to a lesser extent, by urinary excretion. Mass-balance data from 1 patient found about 60% of the total radioactive dose in feces (34%) and urine (27%). These data are consistent with those from 3 patients with extrahepatic obstruction and percutaneous drainage, in whom approximately 35% and 20% of the administered dose were recovered as epirubicin or its major metabolites in bile and urine, respectively, in the 4 days after treatment.

Pharmacokinetics in Special Populations

Age. A population analysis of plasma data from 36 cancer patients (13 males and 23 females, 20 to 73 years) showed that age affects plasma clearance of epirubicin in female patients. The predicted plasma clearance for a female patient of 70 years of age was about 35% lower than that for a female patient of 25 years of age. An insufficient number of males > 50 years of age were included in the study to draw conclusions about age-related alterations in clearance in males. Although a lower epirubicin starting dose does not appear necessary in elderly female patients, and was not used in clinical trials, particular care should be taken in monitoring toxicity when epirubicin is administered to female patients > 70 years of age. (See PRECAUTIONS.)

Gender. In patients ≤ 50 years of age, mean clearance values in adult male and female patients were similar. The clearance of epirubicin is decreased in elderly women (see Pharmacokinetics in Special Populations - Age).

Pediatric. The pharmacokinetics of epirubicin in pediatric patients have not been evaluated.

Race. The influence of race on the pharmacokinetics of epirubicin has not been evaluated.

Hepatic Impairment. Epirubicin is eliminated by both hepatic metabolism and biliary excretion and clearance is reduced in patients with hepatic dysfunction. In a study of the effect of hepatic dysfunction, patients with solid tumors were classified into 3 groups. Patients in Group 1 (n=22) had serum AST (SGOT) levels above the upper limit of normal (median: 93 IU/L) and normal serum bilirubin levels (median: 0.5 mg/dL) and were given epirubicin doses of 12.5 to 90 mg/m². Patients in Group 2 had alterations in both serum AST (median: 175 IU/L) and bilirubin levels (median: 2.7 mg/dL) and were treated with an epirubicin dose of 25 mg/m² (n=8). Their pharmacokinetics were compared to those of patients with normal serum AST and bilirubin values, who received epirubicin doses of 12.5 to 120 mg/m². The median plasma clearance of epirubicin was decreased compared to patients with normal hepatic function by about 30% in patients in Group 1 and by 50% in patients in Group 2. Patients with more severe hepatic impairment have not been evaluated. (See WARNINGS and DOSAGE AND ADMINISTRATION.)

Renal Impairment. No significant alterations in the pharmacokinetics of epirubicin or its major metabolite, epirubicinol, have been observed in patients with serum creatinine < 5 mg/dL. A 50% reduction in plasma clearance was reported in four patients with serum creatinine ≥ 5 mg/dL (see WARNINGS and DOSAGE AND ADMINISTRATION). Patients on dialysis have not been studied.

Drug-Drug Interactions

Taxanes. Coadministration of paclitaxel or docetaxel did not affect the pharmacokinetics of epirubicin when given immediately following the taxane.

Cimetidine. Coadministration of cimetidine (400 mg twice daily for 7 days starting 5 days before chemotherapy) increased the mean AUC of epirubicin (100 mg/m²) by 50% and decreased its plasma clearance by 30% (see PRECAUTIONS).

Drugs metabolized by cytochrome P-450 enzymes. No systematic in vitro or in vivo evaluation has been performed to examine the potential for inhibition or induction by epirubicin of oxidative cytochrome P-450 isoenzymes.

CLINICAL STUDIES

Two randomized, open-label, multicenter studies evaluated the use of ELLENCE Injection 100 to 120 mg/m² in combination with cyclophosphamide and fluorouracil for the adjuvant treatment of patients with axillary-node positive breast cancer and no evidence of distant metastatic disease (Stage II or III). Study MA-5 evaluated 120 mg/m² of epirubicin per course in combination with cyclophosphamide and fluorouracil (CEF-120 regimen). This study randomized premenopausal and perimenopausal women with one or more positive lymph nodes to an epirubicin-containing CEF-120 regimen or to a CMF regimen. Study GFEA-05 evaluated the use of 100 mg/m² of epirubicin per course in combination with fluorouracil and cyclophosphamide (FEC-100). This study randomized pre- and postmenopausal women to the FEC-100 regimen or to a lower-dose FEC-50 regimen. In the GFEA-05 study, eligible patients were either required to have ≥ 4 nodes involved with tumor or, if only 1 to 3 nodes were positive, to have negative estrogen- and progesterone-receptors and a histologic tumor grade of 2 or 3. A total of 1281 women participated in these studies. Patients with T4 tumors were not eligible for either study. Table 2 shows the treatment regimens that the patients received. The primary endpoint of the trials was relapse-free survival, ie, time to occurrence of a local, regional, or distant recurrence, or disease-related death. Patients with contralateral breast cancer, second primary malignancy or death from causes other than breast cancer were censored at the time of the last visit prior to these events.

[See table 2 above]

In the MA-5 trial, the median age of the study population was 45 years. Approximately 60% of patients had 1 to 3 involved nodes and approximately 40% had ≥ 4 nodes involved with tumor. In the GFEA-05 study, the median age was 51 years and approximately half of the patients were postmenopausal. About 17% of the study population had 1 to 3 positive nodes and 80% of patients had ≥ 4 involved lymph nodes. Demographic and tumor characteristics were well-balanced between treatment arms in each study.

The efficacy endpoints of relapse-free survival (RFS) and overall survival (OS) were analyzed using Kaplan-Meier methods in the intent-to-treat (ITT) patient populations in each study. Results for endpoints were initially analyzed after up to 5 years of follow-up and these results are presented in the text below and in Table 3. Results after up to 10 years of follow-up are presented in Table 3. In Study MA-5, epirubicin-containing combination therapy (CEF-120) showed significantly longer RFS than CMF (5-year estimates were 62% versus 53%, stratified logrank for the overall RFS p=0.013). The estimated reduction in the risk of relapse was 24% at 5 years. The OS was also greater for the epirubicin-containing CEF-120 regimen than for the CMF regimen (5-year estimate 77% versus 70%; stratified logrank for overall survival p=0.043; non-stratified logrank p=0.13). The estimated reduction in the risk of death was 29% at 5 years.

In Study GFEA-05, patients treated with the higher-dose epirubicin regimen (FEC-100) had a significantly longer 5-year RFS (estimated 65% versus 52%, logrank for the overall RFS p=0.007) and OS (estimated 76% versus 65%, logrank for the overall survival p=0.007) than patients given the lower dose regimen (FEC-50). The estimated reduction in risk of relapse was 32% at 5 years. The estimated reduction in the risk of death was 31% at 5 years. Results of

Table 1. Summary of Mean (± SD) Pharmacokinetic Parameters in Patients[1] with Solid Tumors Receiving Intravenous Epirubicin 60 to 150 mg/m²

Dose[2] (mg/m²)	C_{max}[3] (µg/mL)	AUC[4] (µg • h/mL)	t½[5] (hours)	CL[6] (L/hour)	Vss[7] (L/kg)
60	5.7 ± 1.6	1.6 ± 0.2	35.3 ± 9	65 ± 8	21 ± 2
75	5.3 ± 1.5	1.7 ± 0.3	32.1 ± 5	83 ± 14	27 ± 11
120	9.0 ± 3.5	3.4 ± 0.7	33.7 ± 4	65 ± 13	23 ± 7
150	9.3 ± 2.9	4.2 ± 0.8	31.1 ± 6	69 ± 13	21 ± 7

[1] Advanced solid tumor cancers, primarily of the lung
[2] N=6 patients per dose level
[3] Plasma concentration at the end of 6 to 10 minute infusion
[4] Area under the plasma concentration curve
[5] Half-life of terminal phase
[6] Plasma clearance
[7] Steady state volume of distribution

Table 2. Treatment Regimens Used in Phase 3 Studies of Patients with Early Breast Cancer

	Treatment Groups	Agent	Regimen
MA-5[1] N=716	**CEF-120** (total, 6 cycles)[2] N=356	Cyclophosphamide ELLENCE Fluorouracil	75 mg/m² PO, d 1-14, q 28 days 60 mg/m² IV, d 1 & 8, q 28 days 500 mg/m² IV, d 1 & 8, q 28 days
	CMF (total, 6 cycles) N=360	Cyclophosphamide Methotrexate Fluorouracil	100 mg/m² PO, d 1-14, q 28 days 40 mg/m² IV, d 1 & 8, q 28 days 600 mg/m² IV, d 1 & 8, q 28 days
GFEA-05[3] N=565	**FEC-100** (total, 6 cycles) N=276	Fluorouracil ELLENCE Cyclophosphamide	500 mg/m² IV, d 1, q 21 days 100 mg/m² IV, d 1, q 21 days 500 mg/m² IV, d 1, q 21 days
	FEC-50 (total, 6 cycles) N=289 Tamoxifen 30 mg daily × 3 years, postmenopausal women, any receptor status	Fluorouracil ELLENCE Cyclophosphamide	500 mg/m² IV, d 1, q 21 days 50 mg/m² IV, d 1, q 21 days 500 mg/m² IV, d 1, q 21 days

[1] In women who underwent lumpectomy, breast irradiation was to be administered after completion of study chemotherapy.
[2] Patients also received prophylactic antibiotic therapy with trimethoprim-sulfamethoxazole or fluoroquinolone for the duration of their chemotherapy.
[3] All women were to receive breast irradiation after the completion of chemotherapy.

follow-up up to 10 years (median follow-up = 8.8 years and 8.3 years, respectively for Study MA-5 and Study GFEA-05) are presented in Table 3.

Although the trials were not powered for subgroup analyses, in the MA-5 study improvements in favor of CEF-120 vs. CMF were observed, in RFS and OS both in patients with 1-3 node positive and in those with ≥4 node positive tumor involvement. In the GFEA-05 study improvements in RFS and OS were observed in both pre- and postmenopausal women treated with FEC-100 compared to FEC-50.

[See table 3 at top of next page]

The Kaplan-Meier curves for RFS and OS from Study MA-5 are shown in Figures 1 and 2 and those for Study GFEA-05 are shown in Figure 3 and 4.

Figure 1. Relapse-Free Survival in Study MA-5

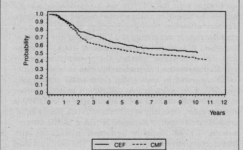

Epirubicin – CTN 068103–999 – 10–years FU
Relapse–Free Survival – Kaplan–Meier Curves by Treatment
(ITT Population)

CEF ---- CMF

Figure 2. Overall Survival in Study MA-5

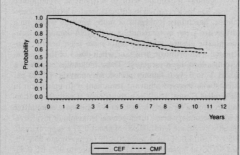

Epirubicin – CTN 068103–999 – 10–years FU
Overall Survival – Kaplan–Meier Curves by Treatment
(ITT Population)

CEF ---- CMF

Figure 3. Relapse-Free Survival in Study GFEA-05

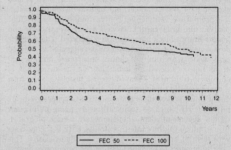

Epirubicin – GFEA 05 – 10–years FU
Relapse–Free Survival – Kaplan–Meier Curves by Treatment
(ITT Population)

FEC 50 ---- FEC 100

Figure 4. Overall Survival in Study GFEA-05

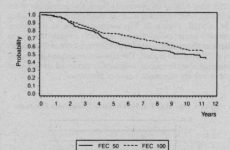

Epirubicin – GFEA 05 – 10–years FU
Overall Survival – Kaplan–Meier Curves by Treatment
(ITT Population)

FEC 50 ---- FEC 100

See Table 3 for statistics on 5 and 10 year analyses.

INDICATIONS AND USAGE

ELLENCE Injection is indicated as a component of adjuvant therapy in patients with evidence of axillary node tumor involvement following resection of primary breast cancer.

CONTRAINDICATIONS

Patients should not be treated with ELLENCE Injection if they have any of the following conditions: baseline neutrophil count < 1500 cells/mm³; severe myocardial insuffi-

Continued on next page

Ellence—Cont.

ciency, recent myocardial infarction, severe arrhythmias; previous treatment with anthracyclines up to the maximum cumulative dose; hypersensitivity to epirubicin, other anthracyclines, or anthracenediones; or severe hepatic dysfunction (see WARNINGS and DOSAGE AND ADMINISTRATION).

WARNINGS

ELLENCE Injection should be administered only under the supervision of qualified physicians experienced in the use of cytotoxic therapy. Before beginning treatment with epirubicin, patients should recover from acute toxicities (such as stomatitis, neutropenia, thrombocytopenia, and generalized infections) of prior cytotoxic treatment. Also, initial treatment with ELLENCE should be preceded by a careful baseline assessment of blood counts; serum levels of total bilirubin, AST, and creatinine; and cardiac function as measured by left ventricular ejection function (LVEF). Patients should be carefully monitored during treatment for possible clinical complications due to myelosuppression. Supportive care may be necessary for the treatment of severe neutropenia and severe infectious complications. Monitoring for potential cardiotoxicity is also important, especially with greater cumulative exposure to epirubicin.

Hematologic Toxicity. A dose-dependent, reversible leukopenia and/or neutropenia is the predominant manifestation of hematologic toxicity associated with epirubicin and represents the most common acute dose-limiting toxicity of this drug. In most cases, the white blood cell (WBC) nadir is reached 10 to 14 days from drug administration. Leukopenia/neutropenia is usually transient, with WBC and neutrophil counts generally returning to normal values by Day 21 after drug administration. As with other cytotoxic agents, ELLENCE at the recommended dose in combination with cyclophosphamide and fluorouracil can produce severe leukopenia and neutropenia. Severe thrombocytopenia and anemia may also occur. Clinical consequences of severe myelosuppression include fever, infection, septicemia, septic shock, hemorrhage, tissue hypoxia, symptomatic anemia, or death. If myelosuppressive complications occur, appropriate supportive measures (e.g., intravenous antibiotics, colony stimulating factors, transfusions) may be required. Myelosuppression requires careful monitoring. Total and differential WBC, red blood cell (RBC), and platelet counts should be assessed before and during each cycle of therapy with ELLENCE.

Cardiac Function. Cardiotoxicity is a known risk of anthracycline treatment. Anthracycline-induced cardiac toxicity may be manifested by early (or acute) or late (delayed) events. Early cardiac toxicity of epirubicin consists mainly of sinus tachycardia and/or ECG abnormalities such as nonspecific ST-T wave changes, but tachyarrhythmias, including premature ventricular contractions and ventricular tachycardia, bradycardia, as well as atrioventricular and bundle-branch block have also been reported. These effects do not usually predict subsequent development of delayed cardiotoxicity, are rarely of clinical importance, and are generally not considered an indication for the suspension of epirubicin treatment. Delayed cardiac toxicity results from a characteristic cardiomyopathy that is manifested by reduced LVEF and/or signs and symptoms of congestive heart failure (CHF) such as tachycardia, dyspnea, pulmonary edema, dependent edema, hepatomegaly, ascites, pleural effusion, gallop rhythm. Life-threatening CHF is the most severe form of anthracycline-induced cardiomyopathy. This toxicity appears to be dependent on the cumulative dose of ELLENCE and represents the cumulative dose-limiting toxicity of the drug. If it occurs, delayed cardiotoxicity usually develops late in the course of therapy with ELLENCE or within 2 to 3 months after completion of treatment, but later events (several months to years after treatment termination) have been reported.

In a retrospective survey, including 9144 patients, mostly with solid tumors in advanced stages, the probability of developing CHF increased with increasing cumulative doses of ELLENCE (Figure 5). The estimated risk of epirubicin-treated patients developing clinically evident CHF was 0.9% at a cumulative dose of 550 mg/m^2, 1.6% at 700 mg/m^2, and 3.3% at 900 mg/m^2. The risk of developing CHF in the absence of other cardiac risk factors increased steeply after an epirubicin cumulative dose of 900 mg/m^2.

Figure 5. Risk of CHF in 9144 Patients Treated with Epirubicin

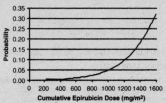

In another retrospective survey of 469 epirubicin-treated patients with metastatic or early breast cancer, the reported risk of CHF was comparable to that observed in the larger study of over 9000 patients.

Given the risk of cardiomyopathy, a cumulative dose of 900 mg/m^2 ELLENCE should be exceeded only with ex-

treme caution. Risk factors (active or dormant cardiovascular disease, prior or concomitant radiotherapy to the mediastinal/pericardial area, previous therapy with other anthracyclines or anthracenediones, concomitant use of other drugs with the ability to suppress cardiac contractility) may increase the risk of cardiac toxicity. Although not formally tested, it is probable that the toxicity of epirubicin and other anthracyclines or anthracenediones is additive. Cardiac toxicity with ELLENCE may occur at lower cumulative doses whether or not cardiac risk factors are present. Although endomyocardial biopsy is recognized as the most sensitive diagnostic tool to detect anthracycline-induced cardiomyopathy, this invasive examination is not practically performed on a routine basis. Electrocardiogram (ECG) changes such as dysrhythmias, a reduction of the QRS voltage, or a prolongation beyond normal limits of the systolic time interval may be indicative of anthracycline-induced cardiomyopathy, but ECG is not a sensitive or specific method for following anthracycline-related cardiotoxicity. The risk of serious cardiac impairment may be decreased through regular monitoring of LVEF during the course of treatment with prompt discontinuation of ELLENCE at the first sign of impaired function. The preferred method for repeated assessment of cardiac function is evaluation of LVEF measured by multi-gated radionuclide angiography (MUGA) or echocardiography (ECHO). A baseline cardiac evaluation with an ECG and a MUGA scan or an ECHO is recommended, especially in patients with risk factors for increased cardiac toxicity. Repeated MUGA or ECHO determinations of LVEF should be performed, particularly with higher, cumulative anthracycline doses. The technique used for assessment should be consistent through follow-up. In patients with risk factors, particularly prior anthracycline or anthracenedione use, the monitoring of cardiac function must be particularly strict and the risk-benefit of continuing treatment with ELLENCE in patients with impaired cardiac function must be carefully evaluated.

Secondary Leukemia. The occurrence of secondary acute myelogenous leukemia, with or without a preleukemic phase, has been reported in patients treated with anthracyclines. Secondary leukemia is more common when such drugs are given in combination with DNA-damaging antineoplastic agents, when patients have been heavily pretreated with cytotoxic drugs, or when doses of the anthracyclines have been escalated. These leukemias can have a short 1- to 3- year latency period. An analysis of 7110 patients who received adjuvant treatment with epirubicin in controlled clinical trials as a component of poly-chemotherapy regimens for early breast cancer, showed a cumulative risk of secondary acute myelogenous leukemia or myelodysplastic syndrome (AML/MDS) of about 0.27% (approximate 95% CI, 0.14-0.40) at 3 years, 0.46% (approximate 95% CI, 0.28-0.65) at 5 years and 0.55% (approximate 95% CI, 0.33-0.78) at 8 years. The risk of developing AML/MDS increased

with increasing epirubicin cumulative doses as shown in Figure 6.

Figure 6. Risk of AML/MDS in 7110 Patients Treated with Epirubicin

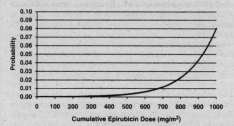

The cumulative probability of developing AML/MDS was found to be particularly increased in patients who received more than the maximum recommended cumulative dose of epirubicin (720 mg/m^2) or cyclophosphamide (6,300 mg/m^2), as shown in Table 4.

[See table 4 at bottom of next page]

ELLENCE is mutagenic, clastogenic, and carcinogenic in animals (see next section, Carcinogenesis, Mutagenesis and Impairment of Fertility).

Carcinogenesis, Mutagenesis & Impairment of Fertility. Treatment-related acute myelogenous leukemia has been reported in women treated with epirubicin-based adjuvant chemotherapy regimens (see above section, WARNINGS, Secondary Leukemia). Conventional long-term animal studies to evaluate the carcinogenic potential of epirubicin have not been conducted, but intravenous administration of a single 3.6 mg/kg epirubicin dose to female rats (about 0.2 times the maximum recommended human dose on a body surface area basis) approximately doubled the incidence of mammary tumors (primarily fibroadenomas) observed at 1 year. Administration of 0.5 mg/kg epirubicin intravenously to rats (about 0.025 times the maximum recommended human dose on a body surface area basis) every 3 weeks for ten doses increased the incidence of subcutaneous fibromas in males over an 18-month observation period. In addition, subcutaneous administration of 0.75 or 1.0 mg/kg/day (about 0.015 times the maximum recommended human dose on a body surface area basis) to newborn rats for 4 days on both the first and tenth day after birth for a total of eight doses increased the incidence of animals with tumors compared to controls during a 24-month observation period.

Epirubicin was mutagenic in vitro to bacteria (Ames test) either in the presence or absence of metabolic activation and to mammalian cells (HGPRT assay in V79 Chinese hamster lung fibroblasts) in the absence but not in the presence of metabolic activation. Epirubicin was clastogenic in vitro (chromosome aberrations in human lymphocytes) both in the presence and absence of metabolic activation and was also clastogenic in vivo (chromosome aberration in mouse bone marrow).

Table 3. Efficacy Results from Phase 3 Studies of Patients with Early Breast Cancer*

	MA-5 Study		GFEA-05 Study	
	CEF-120 N=356	CMF N=360	FEC-100 N=276	FEC-50 N=289
RFS at 5 yrs (%)	62	53	65	52
Hazard ratio[†]	0.76		0.68	
2-sided 95% CI	(0.60, 0.96)		(0.52, 0.89)	
Log-rank Test stratified**	(p = 0.013)		(p = 0.007)	
OS at 5 yrs (%)	77	70	76	65
Hazard ratio[†]	0.71		0.69	
2-sided 95% CI	(0.52, 0.98)		(0.51, 0.92)	
Log-rank Test stratified**	(p = 0.043) (unstratified p = 0.13)		(p = 0.007)	
RFS at 10 yrs (%)	51	44	49	43
Hazard ratio[†]	0.78		0.78	
2-sided 95% CI	(0.63, 0.95)		(0.62, 0.99)	
Log-rank Test stratified**	(p = 0.017) (unstratified p = 0.023)		(p = 0.040) (unstratified p = 0.09)	
OS at 10 yrs (%)	61	57	56	50
Hazard ratio[†]	0.82		0.75	
2-sided 95% CI	(0.65, 1.04)		(0.58, 0.96)	
Log-rank Test stratified**	(p = 0.100) (unstratified p = 0.18)		(p = 0.023) (unstratified p = 0.039)	

*Based on Kaplan-Meier estimates
**Patients in MA-5 were stratified by nodal status (1-3, 4-10, and >10 positive nodes), type of initial surgery (lumpectomy versus mastectomy), and by hormone receptor status (ER or PR positive (≥10 fmol), both negative (<10 fmol), or unknown status). Patients in GFEA-05 were stratified by nodal status (1-3, 4-10, and >10 positive nodes).
[†]Hazard ratio: CMF:CEF-120 in MA-5, FEC-50:FEC-100 in GFEA-05

In fertility studies in rats, males were given epirubicin daily for 9 weeks and mated with females that were given epirubicin daily for 2 weeks prior to mating and through Day 7 of gestation. When 0.3 mg/kg/day (about 0.015 times the maximum recommended human single dose on a body surface area basis) was administered to both sexes, no pregnancies resulted. No effects on mating behavior or fertility were observed at 0.1 mg/kg/day, but male rats had atrophy of the testes and epididymis, and reduced spermatogenesis. The 0.1 mg/kg/day dose also caused embryolethality. An increased incidence of fetal growth retardation was observed in these studies at 0.03 mg/kg/day (about 0.0015 times the maximum recommended human single dose on a body surface area basis). Multiple daily doses of epirubicin to rabbits and dogs also caused atrophy of male reproductive organs. Single 20.5 and 12 mg/kg doses of intravenous epirubicin caused testicular atrophy in mice and rats, respectively (both approximately 0.5 times the maximum recommended human dose on a body surface area basis). A single dose of 16.7 mg/kg epirubicin caused uterine atrophy in rats.
Although experimental data are not available, ELLENCE could induce chromosomal damage in human spermatozoa due to its genotoxic potential. Men undergoing treatment with ELLENCE should use effective contraceptive methods. ELLENCE may cause irreversible amenorrhea (premature menopause) in premenopausal women.

Liver Function. The major route of elimination of epirubicin is the hepatobiliary system (see CLINICAL PHARMACOLOGY, Pharmacokinetics in Special Populations). Serum total bilirubin and AST levels should be evaluated before and during treatment with ELLENCE. Patients with elevated bilirubin or AST may experience slower clearance of drug with an increase in overall toxicity. Lower doses are recommended in these patients (see DOSAGE AND ADMINISTRATION). Patients with severe hepatic impairment have not been evaluated; therefore, epirubicin should not be used in this patient population.

Renal Function. Serum creatinine should be assessed before and during therapy. Dosage adjustment is necessary in patients with serum creatinine >5 mg/dL (see DOSAGE AND ADMINISTRATION). Patients undergoing dialysis have not been studied.

Tumor-Lysis Syndrome. As with other cytotoxic agents, ELLENCE may induce hyperuricemia as a consequence of the extensive purine catabolism that accompanies drug-induced rapid lysis of highly chemosensitive neoplastic cells (tumor lysis syndrome). Other metabolic abnormalities may also occur. While not generally a problem in patients with breast cancer, physicians should consider the potential for tumor-lysis syndrome in potentially susceptible patients and should consider monitoring serum uric acid, potassium, calcium, phosphate, and creatinine immediately after initial chemotherapy administration. Hydration, urine alkalinization, and prophylaxis with allopurinol to prevent hyperuricemia may minimize potential complications of tumor-lysis syndrome.

Pregnancy - Category D. ELLENCE may cause fetal harm when administered to a pregnant woman. Administration of 0.8 mg/kg/day intravenously of epirubicin to rats (about 0.04 times the maximum recommended single human dose on a body surface area basis) during Days 5 to 15 of gestation was embryotoxic (increased resorptions and post-implantation loss) and caused fetal growth retardation (decreased body weight), but was not teratogenic up to this dose. Administration of 2 mg/kg/day intravenously of epirubicin to rats (about 0.1 times the maximum recommended single human dose on a body surface area basis) on Days 9 and 10 of gestation was embryotoxic (increased late resorptions, post-implantation losses, and dead fetuses; and decreased live fetuses), retarded fetal growth (decreased body weight), and caused decreased placental weight. This dose was also teratogenic, causing numerous external (anal atresia, misshapen tail, abnormal genital tubercle), visceral (primarily gastrointestinal, urinary, and cardiovascular systems), and skeletal (deformed long bones and girdles, rib abnormalities, irregular spinal ossification) malformations. Administration of intravenous epirubicin to rabbits at doses up to 0.2 mg/kg/day (about 0.02 times the maximum recommended single human dose on a body surface area basis) during Days 6 to 18 of gestation was not embryotoxic or teratogenic, but a maternally toxic dose of 0.32 mg/kg/day increased abortions and delayed ossification. Administration of a maternally toxic intravenous dose of 1 mg/kg/day epirubicin to rabbits (about 0.1 times the maximum recommended single human dose on a body surface area basis) on Days 10 to 12 of gestation induced abortion, but no other signs of embryofetal toxicity or teratogenicity were observed. When doses up to 0.5 mg/kg/day epirubicin were administered to rat dams from Day 17 of gestation to Day 21 after delivery (about 0.025 times the maximum recommended single human dose on a body surface area basis), no permanent changes were observed in the development, functional activity, behavior, or reproductive performance of the offspring.
There are no adequate and well-controlled studies in pregnant women. Two pregnancies have been reported in women taking epirubicin. A 34-year-old woman, 28 weeks pregnant at her diagnosis of breast cancer, was treated with cyclophosphamide and epirubicin every 3 weeks for 3 cycles. She received the last dose at 34 weeks of pregnancy and delivered a healthy baby at 35 weeks. A second 34-year-old woman with breast cancer metastatic to the liver was randomized to FEC-50 but was removed from study because of pregnancy. She experienced a spontaneous abortion. If epirubicin is used during pregnancy, or if the patient becomes pregnant while taking this drug, the patient should be apprised of the potential hazard to the fetus. Women of childbearing potential should be advised to avoid becoming pregnant.

PRECAUTIONS

General

ELLENCE Injection is administered by intravenous infusion. Venous sclerosis may result from an injection into a small vessel or from repeated injections into the same vein. Extravasation of epirubicin during the infusion may cause local pain, severe tissue lesions (vesication, severe cellulitis) and necrosis. It is recommended that ELLENCE be slowly administered into the tubing of a freely running intravenous infusion. Patients receiving initial therapy at the recommended starting doses of 100-120 mg/m^2 should generally have epirubicin infused over 15-20 minutes. For patients who require lower epirubicin starting doses due to organ dysfunction or who require modification of epirubicin doses during therapy, the epirubicin infusion time may be proportionally decreased, but should not be less than 3 minutes. (see DOSAGE AND ADMINISTRATION, Preparation of Infusion Solution). If possible, veins over joints or in extremities with compromised venous or lymphatic drainage should be avoided. A burning or stinging sensation may be indicative of perivenous infiltration, and the infusion should be immediately terminated and restarted in another vein. Perivenous infiltration may occur without causing pain.
Facial flushing, as well as local erythematous streaking along the vein, may be indicative of excessively rapid administration. It may precede local phlebitis or thrombophlebitis.
Patients administered the 120-mg/m^2 regimen of ELLENCE as a component of combination chemotherapy should also receive prophylactic antibiotic therapy with trimethoprim-sulfamethoxazole (e.g., Septra®, Bactrim®) or a fluoroquinolone (see CLINICAL STUDIES, Early Breast Cancer, and DOSAGE AND ADMINISTRATION).
Epirubicin is emetigenic. Antiemetics may reduce nausea and vomiting; prophylactic use of antiemetics should be considered before administration of ELLENCE, particularly when given in conjunction with other emetigenic drugs.
As with other anthracyclines, administration of ELLENCE after previous radiation therapy may induce an inflammatory recall reaction at the site of the irradiation.
As with other cytotoxic agents, thrombophlebitis and thromboembolic phenomena, including pulmonary embolism (in some cases fatal) have been coincidentally reported with the use of epirubicin.

Information for Patients

Patients should be informed of the expected adverse effects of epirubicin, including gastrointestinal symptoms (nausea, vomiting, diarrhea, and stomatitis) and potential neutropenic complications. Patients should consult their physician if vomiting, dehydration, fever, evidence of infection, symptoms of CHF, or injection-site pain occurs following therapy with ELLENCE. Patients should be informed that they will almost certainly develop alopecia. Patients should be advised that their urine may appear red for 1 to 2 days after administration of ELLENCE and that they should not be alarmed. Patients should understand that there is a risk of irreversible myocardial damage associated with treatment with ELLENCE, as well as a risk of treatment-related leukemia. Because epirubicin may induce chromosomal damage in sperm, men undergoing treatment with ELLENCE should use effective contraceptive methods. Women treated with ELLENCE may develop irreversible amenorrhea, or premature menopause.

Laboratory Testing

See WARNINGS. Blood counts, including absolute neutrophil counts, and liver function should be assessed before and during each cycle of therapy with epirubicin. Repeated evaluations of LVEF should be performed during therapy.

Drug Interactions

ELLENCE when used in combination with other cytotoxic drugs may show on-treatment additive toxicity, especially hematologic and gastrointestinal effects.
Concomitant use of ELLENCE with other cardioactive compounds that could cause heart failure (e.g., calcium channel blockers), requires close monitoring of cardiac function throughout treatment.
There are few data regarding the coadministration of radiation therapy and epirubicin. In adjuvant trials of epirubicin-containing CEF-120 or FEC-100 chemotherapies, breast irradiation was delayed until after chemotherapy was completed. This practice resulted in no apparent increase in local breast cancer recurrence relative to published accounts in the literature. A small number of patients received epirubicin-based chemotherapy concomitantly with radiation therapy but had chemotherapy interrupted in order to avoid potential overlapping toxicities. It is likely that use of epirubicin with radiotherapy may sensitize tissues to the cytotoxic actions of irradiation. Administration of ELLENCE after previous radiation therapy may induce an inflammatory recall reaction at the site of the irradiation.
Epirubicin is extensively metabolized by the liver. Changes in hepatic function induced by concomitant therapies may affect epirubicin metabolism, pharmacokinetics, therapeutic efficacy, and/or toxicity.
Cimetidine increased the AUC of epirubicin by 50%. Cimetidine treatment should be stopped during treatment with ELLENCE (see CLINICAL PHARMACOLOGY).

Drug-Laboratory Test Interactions

There are no known interactions between ELLENCE and laboratory tests.

Carcinogenesis, Mutagenesis & Impairment of Fertility

See WARNINGS.

Pregnancy

Pregnancy Category D - see WARNINGS.

Nursing Mothers

Epirubicin was excreted into the milk of rats treated with 0.50 mg/kg/day of epirubicin during peri- and postnatal periods. It is not known whether epirubicin is excreted in human milk. Because many drugs, including other anthracyclines, are excreted in human milk and because of the potential for serious adverse reactions in nursing infants from epirubicin, mothers should discontinue nursing prior to taking this drug.

Geriatric Use

Although a lower starting dose of ELLENCE was not used in trials in elderly female patients, particular care should be taken in monitoring toxicity when ELLENCE is administered to female patients ≥ 70 years of age. (See CLINICAL PHARMACOLOGY, Pharmacokinetics in Special Populations.)

Pediatric Use

The safety and effectiveness of epirubicin in pediatric patients have not been established in adequate and well-controlled clinical trials. Pediatric patients may be at greater risk for anthracycline-induced acute manifestations of cardiotoxicity and for chronic CHF.

ADVERSE REACTIONS

On-Study Events

Integrated safety data are available from two studies (Studies MA-5 and GFEA-05, see CLINICAL STUDIES) evaluating epirubicin-containing combination regimens in patients with early breast cancer. Of the 1260 patients treated in these studies, 620 patients received the higher-dose epirubicin regimen (FEC-100/CEF-120), 280 patients received the lowerdose epirubicin regimen (FEC-50), and 360 patients received CMF. Serotonin-specific antiemetic therapy and colony-stimulating factors were not used in these trials. Clinically relevant acute adverse events are summarized in Table 5.
[See table 5 at top of next page]
Grade 1 or 2 changes in transaminase levels were observed but were more frequently seen with CMF than with CEF.

Delayed Events

Table 6 describes the incidence of delayed adverse events in patients participating in the MA-5 and GFEA-05 trials.
[See table 6 on next page]
Two cases of acute lymphoid leukemia (ALL) were also observed in patients receiving epirubicin. However, an association between anthracyclines such as epirubicin and ALL has not been clearly established.

Overview of Acute and Delayed Toxicities

Hematologic - See WARNINGS.

Gastrointestinal. A dose-dependent mucositis (mainly oral stomatitis, less often esophagitis) may occur in patients treated with epirubicin. Clinical manifestations of mucositis may include a pain or burning sensation, erythema, erosions, ulcerations, bleeding, or infections. Mucositis generally appears early after drug administration and, if severe, may progress over a few days to mucosal ulcerations; most patients recover from this adverse event by the third week of therapy. Hyperpigmentation of the oral mucosa may also occur.
Nausea, vomiting, and occasionally diarrhea and abdominal pain can also occur. Severe vomiting and diarrhea may pro-

Continued on next page

Table 4. Cumulative probability of AML/MDS in relation to cumulative doses of epirubicin and cyclophosphamide

Years from Treatment Start	Cumulative Probability of Developing AML/MDS % (95% CI)			
	Cyclophosphamide Cumulative Dose ≤6,300 mg/m^2		Cyclophosphamide Cumulative Dose >6,300 mg/m^2	
	Epirubicin Cumulative Dose ≤720 mg/m^2 N=4760	Epirubicin Cumulative Dose >720 mg/m^2 N=111	Epirubicin Cumulative Dose ≤720 mg/m^2 N=890	Epirubicin Cumulative Dose >720 mg/m^2 N=261
3	0.12 (0.01-0.22)	0.00 (0.00-0.00)	0.12 (0.00-0.37)	4.37 (1.69-7.05)
5	0.25 (0.08-0.42)	2.38 (0.00-6.99)	0.31 (0.00-0.75)	4.97 (2.06-7.87)
8	0.37 (0.13-0.61)	2.38 (0.00-6.99)	0.31 (0.00-0.75)	4.97 (2.06-7.87)

Ellence—Cont.

duce dehydration. Antiemetics may reduce nausea and vomiting; prophylactic use of antiemetics should be considered before therapy (see PRECAUTIONS).

Cutaneous and Hypersensitivity Reactions. Alopecia occurs frequently, but is usually reversible, with hair regrowth occurring within 2 to 3 months from the termination of therapy. Flushes, skin and nail hyperpigmentation, photosensitivity and hypersensitivity to irradiated skin (radiation-recall reaction) have been observed. Urticaria and anaphylaxis have been reported in patients treated with epirubicin; signs and symptoms of these reactions may vary from skin rash and pruritus to fever, chills, and shock.

Cardiovascular - See WARNINGS.

Secondary Leukemia - See WARNINGS.

Injection-Site Reactions - See PRECAUTIONS.

OVERDOSAGE

A 36-year-old man with non-Hodgkin's lymphoma received a daily 95 mg/m^2 dose of ELLENCE Injection for 5 consecutive days. Five days later, he developed bone marrow aplasia, grade 4 mucositis, and gastrointestinal bleeding. No signs of acute cardiac toxicity were observed. He was treated with antibiotics, colony-stimulating factors, and antifungal agents, and recovered completely. A 63-year-old woman with breast cancer and liver metastasis received a single 320 mg/m^2 dose of ELLENCE. She was hospitalized with hyperthermia and developed multiple organ failure (respiratory and renal), with lactic acidosis, increased lactate dehydrogenase, and anuria. Death occurred within 24 hours after administration of ELLENCE. Additional instances of administration of doses higher than recommended have been reported at doses ranging from 150 to 250 mg/m^2. The observed adverse events in these patients were qualitatively similar to known toxicities of epirubicin. Most of the patients recovered with appropriate supportive care.

If an overdose occurs, supportive treatment (including antibiotic therapy, blood and platelet transfusions, colony-stimulating factors, and intensive care as needed) should be provided until the recovery of toxicities. Delayed CHF has been observed months after anthracycline administration. Patients must be observed carefully over time for signs of CHF and provided with appropriate supportive therapy.

DOSAGE AND ADMINISTRATION

ELLENCE Injection is administered to patients by intravenous infusion. ELLENCE is given in repeated 3- to 4-week cycles. The total dose of ELLENCE may be given on Day 1 of each cycle or divided equally and given on Days 1 and 8 of each cycle. The recommended dosages of ELLENCE are as follows:

Starting Doses

The recommended starting dose of ELLENCE is 100 to 120 mg/m^2. The following regimens were used in the trials supporting use of ELLENCE as a component of adjuvant therapy in patients with axillary-node positive breast cancer:

[See third table at right]

Patients administered the 120-mg/m^2 regimen of ELLENCE also received prophylactic antibiotic therapy with trimethoprim-sulfamethoxazole (e.g., Septra®, Bactrim®) or a fluoroquinolone.

Bone Marrow Dysfunction. Consideration should be given to administration of lower starting doses (75-90 mg/m^2) for heavily pretreated patients, patients with pre-existing bone marrow depression, or in the presence of neoplastic bone marrow infiltration (see WARNINGS and PRECAUTIONS).

Hepatic Dysfunction. Definitive recommendations regarding use of ELLENCE in patients with hepatic dysfunction are not available because patients with hepatic abnormalities were excluded from participation in adjuvant trials of FEC-100/CEF-120 therapy. In patients with elevated serum AST or serum total bilirubin concentrations, the following dose reductions were recommended in clinical trials, although few patients experienced hepatic impairment:

- Bilirubin 1.2 to 3 mg/dL or AST 2 to 4 times upper limit of normal 1/2 of recommended starting dose
- Bilirubin > 3 mg/dL or AST > 4 times upper limit of normal 1/4 of recommended starting dose

Information regarding experience in patients with hepatic dysfunction is provided in CLINICAL PHARMACOLOGY, Pharmacokinetics In Special Populations.

Renal Dysfunction. While no specific dose recommendation can be made based on the limited available data in patients with renal impairment, lower doses should be considered in patients with severe renal impairment (serum creatinine > 5 mg/dL).

Dose Modifications

Dosage adjustments after the first treatment cycle should be made based on hematologic and nonhematologic toxicities. Patients experiencing during treatment cycle nadir platelet counts <50,000/mm^3, absolute neutrophil counts (ANC) <250/mm^3, neutropenic fever, or Grades 3/4 nonhematologic toxicity should have the Day 1 dose in subsequent cycles reduced to 75% of the Day 1 dose given in the current cycle. Day 1 chemotherapy in subsequent courses of treatment should be delayed until platelet counts are ≥100,000/mm^3, ANC≥1500/mm^3, and nonhematologic toxicities have recovered to ≤ Grade 1.

For patients receiving a divided dose of ELLENCE (Day 1 and Day 8), the Day 8 dose should be 75% of Day 1 if platelet counts are 75,000-100,000/mm^3 and ANC is 1000 to

Table 5. Clinically Relevant Acute Adverse Events in Patients with Early Breast Cancer

Event	% of Patients					
	FEC-100/CEF-120 (N=620)		FEC-50 (N=280)		CMF (N=360)	
	Grades 1-4	Grades 3/4	Grades 1-4	Grades 3/4	Grades 1-4	Grades 3/4
Hematologic						
Leukopenia	80.3	58.6	49.6	1.5	98.1	60.3
Neutropenia	80.3	67.2	53.9	10.5	95.8	78.1
Anemia	72.2	5.8	12.9	0	70.9	0.9
Thrombocytopenia	48.8	5.4	4.6	0	51.4	3.6
Endocrine						
Amenorrhea	71.8	0	69.3	0	67.7	0
Hot flashes	38.9	4.0	5.4	0	69.1	6.4
Body as a Whole						
Lethargy	45.8	1.9	1.1	0	72.7	0.3
Fever	5.2	0	1.4	0	4.5	0
Gastrointestinal						
Nausea/vomiting	92.4	25.0	83.2	22.1	85.0	6.4
Mucositis	58.5	8.9	9.3	0	52.9	1.9
Diarrhea	24.8	0.8	7.1	0	50.7	2.8
Anorexia	2.9	0	1.8	0	5.8	0.3
Infection						
Infection	21.5	1.6	15.0	0	25.9	0.6
Febrile neutropenia	NA	6.1	0	0	NA	1.1
Ocular						
Conjunctivitis/keratitis	14.8	0	1.1	0	38.4	0
Skin						
Alopecia	95.5	56.6	69.6	19.3	84.4	6.7
Local toxicity	19.5	0.3	2.5	0.4	8.1	0
Rash/itch	8.9	0.3	1.4	0	14.2	0
Skin changes	4.7	0	0.7	0	7.2	0

FEC & CEF = cyclophosphamide + epirubicin + fluorouracil; CMF = cyclophosphamide + methotrexate + fluorouracil
NA = not available

Table 6. Long-Term Adverse Events in Patients with Early Breast Cancer

Event	% of Patients		
	FEC-100/CEF-120 (N=620)	FEC-50 (N=280)	CMF (N=360)
Cardiac events			
Asymptomatic drops in LVEF	2.1*	1.4	0.8*
CHF	1.5	0.4	0.3
Leukemia			
AML	0.8	0	0.3

*In study MA-5 cardiac function was not monitored after 5 years.

CEF-120:	Cyclophosphamide	75 mg/m^2 PO D 1-14
	ELLENCE	60 mg/m^2 IV D 1, 8
	5-Fluorouracil	500 mg/m^2 IV D 1, 8
	Repeated every 28 days for 6 cycles	
FEC-100:	5-Fluorouracil	500 mg/m^2
	ELLENCE	100 mg/m^2
	Cyclophosphamide	500 mg/m^2
	All drugs administered intravenously on Day 1 and repeated every 21 days for 6 cycles	

1499/mm^3. If Day 8 platelet counts are <75,000/mm^3, ANC <1000/mm^3, or Grade 3/4 nonhematologic toxicity has occurred, the Day 8 dose should be omitted.

Preparation & Administration Precautions

Parenteral drug products should be inspected visually for particulate matter and discoloration prior to administration, whenever solution and container permit. Procedures normally used for proper handling and disposal of anticancer drugs should be considered for use with ELLENCE. Several guidelines on this subject have been published.[1-8]

Protective measures. The following protective measures should be taken when handling ELLENCE:

- Personnel should be trained in appropriate techniques for reconstitution and handling.
- Pregnant staff should be excluded from working with this drug.
- Personnel handling ELLENCE should wear protective clothing: goggles, gowns and disposable gloves and masks.
- A designated area should be defined for syringe preparation (preferably under a laminar flow system), with the work surface protected by disposable, plastic-backed, absorbent paper.
- All items used for reconstitution, administration or cleaning (including gloves) should be placed in high-risk, waste-disposal bags for high temperature incineration.

Spillage or leakage should be treated with dilute sodium hypochlorite (1% available chlorine) solution, preferably by soaking, and then water. All contaminated and cleaning materials should be placed in high-risk, waste-disposal bags for incineration. Accidental contact with the skin or eyes should be treated immediately by copious lavage with water, or soap and water, or sodium bicarbonate solution. However,

do not abrade the skin by using a scrub brush. Medical attention should be sought. Always wash hands after removing gloves.

Incompatibilities. Prolonged contact with any solution of an alkaline pH should be avoided as it will result in hydrolysis of the drug. ELLENCE should not be mixed with heparin or fluorouracil due to chemical incompatibility that may lead to precipitation.

ELLENCE can be used in combination with other antitumor agents, but it is not recommended that it be mixed with other drugs in the same syringe.

Preparation of Infusion Solution

ELLENCE is provided as a preservative-free, ready-to-use solution.

ELLENCE should be administered into the tubing of a freely flowing intravenous infusion (0.9% sodium chloride or 5% glucose solution). Patients receiving initial therapy at the recommended starting doses of 100-120 mg/m^2 should generally have epirubicin infused over 15-20 minutes. For patients who require lower epirubicin starting doses due to organ dysfunction or who require modification of epirubicin doses during therapy, the epirubicin infusion time may be proportionally decreased, but should not be less than 3 minutes. This technique is intended to minimize the risk of thrombosis or perivenous extravasation, which could lead to severe cellulitis, vesication, or tissue necrosis. A direct push injection is not recommended due to the risk of extravasation, which may occur even in the presence of adequate blood return upon needle aspiration. Venous sclerosis may result from injection into small vessels or repeated injections into the same vein (see PRECAUTIONS). ELLENCE should be used within 24 hours of first penetration of the rubber stopper. Discard any unused solution.

HOW SUPPLIED

ELLENCE Injection is available in polypropylene single-use vials containing 2 mg epirubicin hydrochloride per mL as a sterile, preservative-free, ready-to-use solution in the following strengths:

50 mg/25 mL single-use vial NDC 0009-5091-01
200 mg/100 mL single-use vial NDC 0009-5093-01

Store refrigerated between 2°C and 8°C (36°F and 46°F). Do not freeze. Protect from light. Discard unused portion.

Rx only

US Patent No. 5,977,082

Manufactured for: Pharmacia & Upjohn Company, A subsidiary of Pharmacia Corporation, Kalamazoo, MI 49001 USA
By: Pharmacia (Perth) Pty Limited, Bentley WA 6102 Australia

March 2005 LAB-0078-4.0

REFERENCES

1. ONS Clinical Practice Committee. Cancer Chemotherapy Guidelines and Recommendations for Practice. Pittsburgh, PA: Oncology Nursing Society; 1999: 32-41.
2. Recommendations for the Safe Handling of Parenteral Antineoplastic Drugs. Washington, DC: Division of Safety, Clinical Center Pharmacy Department and Cancer Nursing Services, National Institutes of Health; 1992 US Dept of Health and Human Services. Public Health Service Publication NIH 92-2621.
3. AMA Council on Scientific Affairs. Guidelines for Handling Parenteral Antineoplastics. JAMA 1985; 253(11):1590-1592.
4. National Study Commission on Cytotoxic Exposure – Recommendations for Handling of Cytotoxic Agents. 1987. Available from Louis P. Jeffrey, ScD., Chairman, National Study Commission on Cytotoxic Exposure, Massachusetts College of Pharmacy and Allied Health Sciences, 179 Longwood Avenue, Boston, MA 02115.
5. Clinical Oncology Society of Australia, Guidelines and Recommendations for Safe Handling of Antineoplastic Agents. Med J Australia 1983; 1:426-428.
6. Jones RB, Frank R, Mass T. Safe Handling of Chemotherapeutic Agents: A Report from the Mount Sinai Medical Center. CA-A Cancer J for Clin 1983; 33:258-263.
7. American Society of Hospital Pharmacists. ASHP Technical Assistance Bulletin on Handling Cytotoxic and Hazardous Drugs. AM J Hosp Pharm 1990; 47:1033-1049.
8. Controlling Occupational Exposure to Hazardous Drugs (OSHA Work-Practice Guidelines). Am J Health-Syst Pharm 1996; 53:1669-1685.

ZYVOX®

℞

[zī-vŏks]

linezolid injection
linezolid tablets
linezolid for oral suspension

Prescribing information for this product, which appears on pages 2773–2781 of the 2005 PDR, has been completely revised as follows. Please write "See Supplement A" next to the product heading.

To reduce the development of drug-resistant bacteria and maintain the effectiveness of ZYVOX formulations and other antibacterial drugs, ZYVOX should be used only to treat or prevent infections that are proven or strongly suspected to be caused by bacteria.

DESCRIPTION

ZYVOX I.V. Injection, ZYVOX Tablets, and ZYVOX for Oral Suspension contain linezolid, which is a synthetic antibacterial agent of the oxazolidinone class. The chemical name for linezolid is (S)-N-[[3-[3-Fluoro-4-(4-morpholinyl)phenyl]-2-oxo-5-oxazolidinyl]methyl]-acetamide.

The empirical formula is $C_{16}H_{20}FN_3O_4$. Its molecular weight is 337.35, and its chemical structure is represented below:

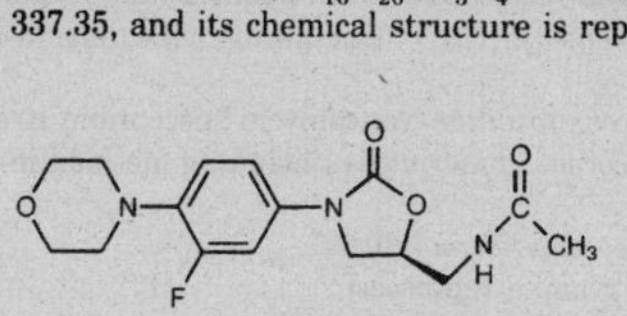

ZYVOX I.V. Injection is supplied as a ready-to-use sterile isotonic solution for intravenous infusion. Each mL contains 2 mg of linezolid. Inactive ingredients are sodium citrate, citric acid, and dextrose in an aqueous vehicle for intravenous administration. The sodium (Na^+) content is 0.38 mg/mL (5 mEq per 300-mL bag; 3.3 mEq per 200-mL bag; and 1.7 mEq per 100-mL bag).

ZYVOX Tablets for oral administration contain 400 mg or 600 mg linezolid as film-coated compressed tablets. Inactive ingredients are corn starch, microcrystalline cellulose, hydroxypropylcellulose, sodium starch glycolate, magnesium stearate, hypromellose, polyethylene glycol, titanium dioxide, and carnauba wax. The sodium (Na^+) content is 1.95 mg per 400-mg tablet and 2.92 mg per 600-mg tablet (0.1 mEq per tablet, regardless of strength).

ZYVOX for Oral Suspension is supplied as an orange-flavored granule/powder for constitution into a suspension for oral administration. Following constitution, each 5 mL contains 100 mg of linezolid. Inactive ingredients are sucrose, citric acid, sodium citrate, microcrystalline cellulose and carboxymethylcellulose sodium, aspartame, xanthan gum, mannitol, sodium benzoate, colloidal silicon dioxide, sodium chloride, and flavors (see **PRECAUTIONS, Information for Patients**). The sodium (Na^+) content is 8.52 mg per 5 mL (0.4 mEq per 5 mL).

Table 1. Mean (Standard Deviation) Pharmacokinetic Parameters of Linezolid in Adults

Dose of Linezolid	C_{max} µg/mL	C_{min} µg/mL	T_{max} hrs	AUC* µg • h/mL	$t_{1/2}$ hrs	CL mL/min
400 mg tablet						
single dose†	8.10 (1.83)	—	1.52 (1.01)	55.10 (25.00)	5.20 (1.50)	146 (67)
every 12 hours	11.00 (4.37)	3.08 (2.25)	1.12 (0.47)	73.40 (33.50)	4.69 (1.70)	110 (49)
600 mg tablet						
single dose	12.70 (3.96)	—	1.28 (0.66)	91.40 (39.30)	4.26 (1.65)	127 (48)
every 12 hours	21.20 (5.78)	6.15 (2.94)	1.03 (0.62)	138.00 (42.10)	5.40 (2.06)	80 (29)
600 mg IV injection‡						
single dose	12.90 (1.60)	—	0.50 (0.10)	80.20 (33.30)	4.40 (2.40)	138 (39)
every 12 hours	15.10 (2.52)	3.68 (2.36)	0.51 (0.03)	89.70 (31.00)	4.80 (1.70)	123 (40)
600 mg oral suspension						
single dose	11.00 (2.76)	—	0.97 (0.88)	80.80 (35.10)	4.60 (1.71)	141 (45)

*AUC for single dose = $AUC_{0-\infty}$; for multiple-dose = $AUC_{0-\tau}$
† Data dose-normalized from 375 mg
‡ Data dose-normalized from 625 mg, IV dose was given as 0.5-hour infusion.
C_{max} = Maximum plasma concentration; C_{min} = Minimum plasma concentration; T_{max} = Time to C_{max};
AUC = Area under concentration-time curve; $t_{1/2}$ = Elimination half-life; CL = Systemic clearance

CLINICAL PHARMACOLOGY

Pharmacokinetics

The mean pharmacokinetic parameters of linezolid in adults after single and multiple oral and intravenous (IV) doses are summarized in Table 1. Plasma concentrations of linezolid at steady-state after oral doses of 600 mg given every 12 hours (q12h) are shown in Figure 1.

[See table 1 above]

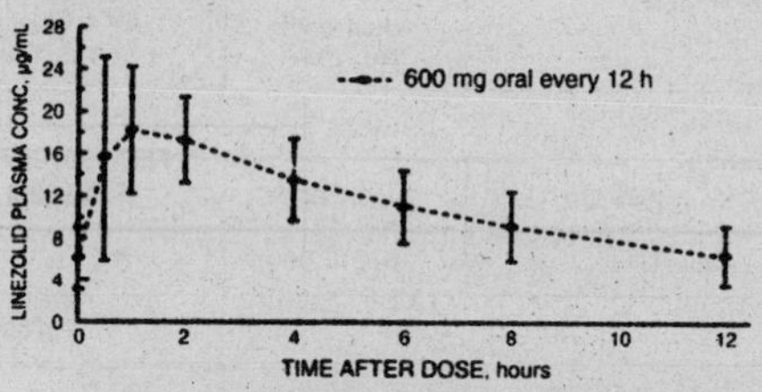

Figure 1. Plasma Concentrations of Linezolid in Adults at Steady-State Following Oral Dosing Every 12 Hours (Mean ± Standard Deviation, n=16)

Absorption: Linezolid is rapidly and extensively absorbed after oral dosing. Maximum plasma concentrations are reached approximately 1 to 2 hours after dosing, and the absolute bioavailability is approximately 100%. Therefore, linezolid may be given orally or intravenously without dose adjustment.

Linezolid may be administered without regard to the timing of meals. The time to reach the maximum concentration is delayed from 1.5 hours to 2.2 hours and C_{max} is decreased by about 17% when high fat food is given with linezolid. However, the total exposure measured as $AUC_{0-\infty}$ values is similar under both conditions.

Distribution: Animal and human pharmacokinetic studies have demonstrated that linezolid readily distributes to well-perfused tissues. The plasma protein binding of linezolid is approximately 31% and is concentration-independent. The volume of distribution of linezolid at steady-state averaged 40 to 50 liters in healthy adult volunteers.

Linezolid concentrations have been determined in various fluids from a limited number of subjects in Phase 1 volunteer studies following multiple dosing of linezolid. The ratio of linezolid in saliva relative to plasma was 1.2 to 1 and for sweat relative to plasma was 0.55 to 1.

Metabolism: Linezolid is primarily metabolized by oxidation of the morpholine ring, which results in two inactive ring-opened carboxylic acid metabolites: the aminoethoxyacetic acid metabolite (A), and the hydroxyethyl glycine metabolite (B). Formation of metabolite B is mediated by a non-enzymatic chemical oxidation mechanism in vitro. Linezolid is not an inducer of cytochrome P450 (CYP) in rats, and it has been demonstrated from in vitro studies that linezolid is not detectably metabolized by human cytochrome P450 and it does not inhibit the activities of clinically significant human CYP isoforms (1A2, 2C9, 2C19, 2D6, 2E1, 3A4).

Excretion: Nonrenal clearance accounts for approximately 65% of the total clearance of linezolid. Under steady-state conditions, approximately 30% of the dose appears in the urine as linezolid, 40% as metabolite B, and 10% as metabolite A. The renal clearance of linezolid is low (average 40 mL/min) and suggests net tubular reabsorption. Virtually no linezolid appears in the feces, while approximately 6% of the dose appears in the feces as metabolite B, and 3% as metabolite A.

A small degree of nonlinearity in clearance was observed with increasing doses of linezolid, which appears to be due to lower renal and nonrenal clearance of linezolid at higher concentrations. However, the difference in clearance was small and was not reflected in the apparent elimination half-life.

Special Populations

Geriatric: The pharmacokinetics of linezolid are not significantly altered in elderly patients (65 years or older). Therefore, dose adjustment for geriatric patients is not necessary.

Pediatric: The pharmacokinetics of linezolid following a single IV dose were investigated in pediatric patients ranging in age from birth through 17 years (including premature and full-term neonates), in healthy adolescent subjects ranging in age from 12 through 17 years, and in pediatric patients ranging in age from 1 week through 12 years. The pharmacokinetic parameters of linezolid are summarized in Table 2 for the pediatric populations studied and healthy adult subjects after administration of single IV doses.

The C_{max} and the volume of distribution (V_{ss}) of linezolid are similar regardless of age in pediatric patients. However, clearance of linezolid varies as a function of age. With the exclusion of pre-term neonates less than one week of age, clearance is most rapid in the youngest age groups ranging from >1 week old to 11 years, resulting in lower single-dose systemic exposure (AUC) and shorter half-life as compared with adults. As age of pediatric patients increases, the clearance of linezolid gradually decreases, and by adolescence mean clearance values approach those observed for the adult population. There is wider inter-subject variability in linezolid clearance and systemic drug exposure (AUC) across all pediatric age groups as compared with adults.

Similar mean daily AUC values were observed in pediatric patients from birth to 11 years of age dosed every 8 hours (q8h) relative to adolescents or adults dosed every 12 hours (q12h). Therefore, the dosage for pediatric patients up to 11 years of age should be 10 mg/kg q8h. Pediatric patients 12 years and older should receive 600 mg q12h (see **DOSAGE AND ADMINISTRATION**).

[See table 2 at top of next page]

Gender: Females have a slightly lower volume of distribution of linezolid than males. Plasma concentrations are higher in females than in males, which is partly due to body weight differences. After a 600-mg dose, mean oral clearance is approximately 38% lower in females than in males. However, there are no significant gender differences in mean apparent elimination-rate constant or half-life. Thus, drug exposure in females is not expected to substantially increase beyond levels known to be well tolerated. Therefore, dose adjustment by gender does not appear to be necessary.

Renal Insufficiency: The pharmacokinetics of the parent drug, linezolid, are not altered in patients with any degree of renal insufficiency; however, the two primary metabolites of linezolid may accumulate in patients with renal insufficiency, with the amount of accumulation increasing with the severity of renal dysfunction (see Table 3). The clinical significance of accumulation of these two metabolites has not been determined in patients with severe renal insufficiency. Because similar plasma concentrations of linezolid are achieved regardless of renal function, no dose adjustment is recommended for patients with renal insufficiency. However, given the absence of information on the clinical significance of accumulation of the primary metabolites, use of linezolid in patients with renal insufficiency should be weighed against the potential risks of accumulation of these metabolites. Both linezolid and the two metabolites are eliminated by dialysis. No information is available on the effect of peritoneal dialysis on the pharmacokinetics of linezolid. Approximately 30% of a dose was eliminated in a

Continued on next page

Zyvox—Cont.

3-hour dialysis session beginning 3 hours after the dose of linezolid was administered; therefore, linezolid should be given after hemodialysis.

[See table 3 at right]

Hepatic Insufficiency: The pharmacokinetics of linezolid are not altered in patients (n=7) with mild-to-moderate hepatic insufficiency (Child-Pugh class A or B). On the basis of the available information, no dose adjustment is recommended for patients with mild-to-moderate hepatic insufficiency. The pharmacokinetics of linezolid in patients with severe hepatic insufficiency have not been evaluated.

Drug-Drug Interactions

Drugs Metabolized by Cytochrome P450: Linezolid is not an inducer of cytochrome P450 (CYP) in rats. It is not detectably metabolized by human cytochrome P450 and it does not inhibit the activities of clinically significant human CYP isoforms (1A2, 2C9, 2C19, 2D6, 2E1, 3A4). Therefore, no CYP450-induced drug interactions are expected with linezolid. Concurrent administration of linezolid does not substantially alter the pharmacokinetic characteristics of (S)-warfarin, which is extensively metabolized by CYP2C9. Drugs such as warfarin and phenytoin, which are CYP2C9 substrates, may be given with linezolid without changes in dosage regimen.

Antibiotics:

Aztreonam: The pharmacokinetics of linezolid or aztreonam are not altered when administered together.

Gentamicin: The pharmacokinetics of linezolid or gentamicin are not altered when administered together.

Monoamine Oxidase Inhibition: Linezolid is a reversible, nonselective inhibitor of monoamine oxidase. Therefore, linezolid has the potential for interaction with adrenergic and serotonergic agents.

Adrenergic Agents: A significant pressor response has been observed in normal adult subjects receiving linezolid and tyramine doses of more than 100 mg. Therefore, patients receiving linezolid need to avoid consuming large amounts of foods or beverages with high tyramine content (see **PRECAUTIONS, Information for Patients**).

A reversible enhancement of the pressor response of either pseudoephedrine HCl (PSE) or phenylpropanolamine HCl (PPA) is observed when linezolid is administered to healthy normotensive subjects (see **PRECAUTIONS, Drug Interactions**). A similar study has not been conducted in hypertensive patients. The interaction studies conducted in normotensive subjects evaluated the blood pressure and heart rate effects of placebo, PPA or PSE alone, linezolid alone, and the combination of steady-state linezolid (600 mg q12h for 3 days) with two doses of PPA (25 mg) or PSE (60 mg) given 4 hours apart. Heart rate was not affected by any of the treatments. Blood pressure was increased with both combination treatments. Maximum blood pressure levels were seen 2 to 3 hours after the second dose of PPA or PSE, and returned to baseline 2 to 3 hours after peak. The results of the PPA study follow, showing the mean (and range) maximum systolic blood pressure in mm Hg: placebo = 121 (103 to 158); linezolid alone = 120 (107 to 135); PPA alone = 125 (106 to 139); PPA with linezolid = 147 (129 to 176). The results from the PSE study were similar to those in the PPA study. The mean maximum increase in systolic blood pressure over baseline was 32 mm Hg (range: 20-52 mm Hg) and 38 mm Hg (range: 18-79 mm Hg) during co-administration of linezolid with pseudoephedrine or phenylpropanolamine, respectively.

Serotonergic Agents: The potential drug-drug interaction with dextromethorphan was studied in healthy volunteers. Subjects were administered dextromethorphan (two 20-mg doses given 4 hours apart) with or without linezolid. No serotonin syndrome effects (confusion, delirium, restlessness, tremors, blushing, diaphoresis, hyperpyrexia) have been observed in normal subjects receiving linezolid and dextromethorphan.

Table 2. Pharmacokinetic Parameters of Linezolid in Pediatrics and Adults Following a Single Intravenous Infusion of 10 mg/kg or 600 mg Linezolid (Mean: (%CV); [Min, Max Values])

Age Group	C_{max} µg/mL	V_{ss} L/kg	AUC* µg•h/mL	$t_{1/2}$ hrs	CL mL/min/kg
Neonatal Patients					
Pre-term** <1 week (N = 9)†	12.7 (30%) [9.6, 22.2]	0.81 (24%) [0.43, 1.05]	108 (47%) [41, 191]	5.6 (46%) [2.4, 9.8]	2.0 (52%) [0.9, 4.0]
Full-term*** <1 week (N = 10)†	11.5 (24%) [8.0, 18.3]	0.78 (20%) [0.45, 0.96]	55 (47%) [19, 103]	3.0 (55%) [1.3, 6.1]	3.8 (55%) [1.5, 8.8]
Full-term*** ≥1 week to -28 days (N = 10)†	12.9 (28%) [7.7, 21.6]	0.66 (29%) [0.35, 1.06]	34 (21%) [23, 50]	1.5 (17%) [1.2, 1.9]	5.1 (22%) [3.3, 7.2]
Infant Patients > 28 days to < 3 Months (N = 12)†	11.0 (27%) [7.2, 18.0]	0.79 (26%) [0.42, 1.08]	33 (26%) [17, 48]	1.8 (28%) [1.2, 2.8]	5.4 (32%) [3.5, 9.9]
Pediatric Patients 3 months through 11 years† (N = 59)	15.1 (30%) [6.8, 36.7]	0.69 (28%) [0.31, 1.50]	58 (54%) [19, 153]	2.9 (53%) [0.9, 8.0]	3.8 (53%) [1.0, 8.5]
Adolescent Subjects and Patients 12 through 17 years‡ (N = 36)	16.7 (24%) [9.9, 28.9]	0.61 (15%) [0.44, 0.79]	95 (44%) [32, 178]	4.1 (46%) [1.3, 8.1]	2.1 (53%) [0.9, 5.2]
Adult Subjects§ (N = 29)	12.5 (21%) [8.2, 19.3]	0.65 (16%) [0.45, 0.84]	91 (33%) [53, 155]	4.9 (35%) [1.8, 8.3]	1.7 (34%) [0.9, 3.3]

* AUC = Single dose $AUC_{0-\infty}$
** In this data set, "pre-term" is defined as <34 weeks gestational age (Note: Only 1 patient enrolled was pre-term with a postnatal age between 1 week and 28 days)
*** In this data set, "full-term" is defined as ≥34 weeks gestational age
† Dose of 10 mg/kg
‡ Dose of 600 mg or 10 mg/kg up to a maximum of 600 mg
§ Dose normalized to 600 mg
C_{max} = Maximum plasma concentration; V_{ss}=Volume of distribution; AUC = Area under concentration-time curve; $t_{1/2}$ = Apparent elimination half-life; CL = Systemic clearance normalized for body weight

Table 3. Mean (Standard Deviation) AUCs and Elimination Half-lives of Linezolid and Metabolites A and B in Patients with Varying Degrees of Renal Insufficiency After a Single 600-mg Oral Dose of Linezolid

Parameter	Healthy Subjects CL_{CR} > 80 mL/min	Moderate Renal Impairment 30 < CL_{CR} < 80 mL/min	Severe Renal Impairment 10 < CL_{CR} < 30 mL/min	Hemodialysis-Dependent	
				Off Dialysis*	On Dialysis
Linezolid					
$AUC_{0-\infty}$, µg h/mL	110 (22)	128 (53)	127 (66)	141 (45)	83 (23)
$t_{1/2}$, hours	6.4 (2.2)	6.1 (1.7)	7.1 (3.7)	8.4 (2.7)	7.0 (1.8)
Metabolite A					
AUC_{0-48}, µg h/mL	7.6 (1.9)	11.7 (4.3)	56.5 (30.6)	185 (124)	68.8 (23.9)
$t_{1/2}$, hours	6.3 (2.1)	6.6 (2.3)	9.0 (4.6)	NA	NA
Metabolite B					
AUC_{0-48}, µg h/mL	30.5 (6.2)	51.1 (38.5)	203 (92)	467 (102)	239 (44)
$t_{1/2}$, hours	6.6 (2.7)	9.9 (7.4)	11.0 (3.9)	NA	NA

* between hemodialysis sessions
NA = Not applicable

MICROBIOLOGY

Linezolid is a synthetic antibacterial agent of a new class of antibiotics, the oxazolidinones, which has clinical utility in the treatment of infections caused by aerobic Gram-positive bacteria. The in vitro spectrum of activity of linezolid also includes certain Gram-negative bacteria and anaerobic bacteria. Linezolid inhibits bacterial protein synthesis through a mechanism of action different from that of other antibacterial agents; therefore, cross-resistance between linezolid and other classes of antibiotics is unlikely. Linezolid binds to a site on the bacterial 23S ribosomal RNA of the 50S subunit and prevents the formation of a functional 70S initiation complex, which is an essential component of the bacterial translation process. The results of time-kill studies have shown linezolid to be bacteriostatic against enterococci and staphylococci. For streptococci, linezolid was found to be bactericidal for the majority of strains.

In clinical trials, resistance to linezolid developed in 6 patients infected with *Enterococcus faecium* (4 patients received 200 mg q12h, lower than the recommended dose, and 2 patients received 600 mg q12h). In a compassionate use program, resistance to linezolid developed in 8 patients with *E. faecium* and in 1 patient with *Enterococcus faecalis*. All patients had either unremoved prosthetic devices or undrained abscesses. Resistance to linezolid occurs in vitro at a frequency of 1×10^{-9} to 1×10^{-11}. In vitro studies have shown that point mutations in the 23S rRNA are associated with linezolid resistance. Reports of vancomycin-resistant *E. faecium* becoming resistant to linezolid during its clinical use have been published.[1] In one report nosocomial spread of vancomycin- and linezolid-resistant *E. faecium* occurred[2]. There has been a report of *Staphylococcus aureus* (methicillin-resistant) developing resistance to linezolid during its clinical use.[3] The linezolid resistance in these organisms was associated with a point mutation in the 23S rRNA (substitution of thymine for guanine at position 2576) of the organism. When antibiotic-resistant organisms are encountered in the hospital, it is important to emphasize infection control policies.[4,5] Resistance to linezolid has not been reported in *Streptococcus* spp., including *Streptococcus pneumoniae*.

In vitro studies have demonstrated additivity or indifference between linezolid and vancomycin, gentamicin, rifampin, imipenem-cilastatin, aztreonam, ampicillin, or streptomycin.

Linezolid has been shown to be active against most isolates of the following microorganisms, both in vitro and in clinical infections, as described in the **INDICATIONS AND USAGE** section.

Aerobic and facultative Gram-positive microorganisms

Enterococcus faecium (vancomycin-resistant strains only)
Staphylococcus aureus (including methicillin-resistant strains)
Streptococcus agalactiae
Streptococcus pneumoniae (including multi-drug resistant isolates [MDRSP]*)
Streptococcus pyogenes

*MDRSP refers to isolates resistant to two or more of the following antibiotics: penicillin, second-generation cephalosporins, macrolides, tetracycline, and trimethoprim/sulfamethoxazole.

The following in vitro data are available, but their clinical significance is unknown. At least 90% of the following microorganisms exhibit an in vitro minimum inhibitory concentration (MIC) less than or equal to the susceptible breakpoint for linezolid. However, the safety and effectiveness of linezolid in treating clinical infections due to these microorganisms have not been established in adequate and well-controlled clinical trials.

Aerobic and facultative Gram-positive microorganisms

Enterococcus faecalis (including vancomycin-resistant strains)
Enterococcus faecium (vancomycin-susceptible strains)
Staphylococcus epidermidis (including methicillin-resistant strains)
Staphylococcus haemolyticus
Viridans group streptococci

Aerobic and facultative Gram-negative microorganisms

Pasteurella multocida

Susceptibility Testing Methods

NOTE: Susceptibility testing by dilution methods requires the use of linezolid susceptibility powder.

When available, the results of in vitro susceptibility tests should be provided to the physician as periodic reports which describe the susceptibility profile of nosocomial and community-acquired pathogens. These reports should aid the physician in selecting the most effective antimicrobial.

Dilution Techniques: Quantitative methods are used to determine antimicrobial minimum inhibitory concentrations (MICs). These MICs provide estimates of the susceptibility of bacteria to antimicrobial compounds. The MICs should be determined using a standardized procedure. Standardized procedures are based on a dilution method[6,7] (broth or agar) or equivalent with standardized inoculum concentrations and standardized concentrations of linezolid powder. The MIC values should be interpreted according to criteria provided in Table 4.

Diffusion Techniques: Quantitative methods that require measurement of zone diameters also provide reproducible estimates of the susceptibility of bacteria to antimicrobial compounds. One such standardized procedure[7,8] requires the use of standardized inoculum concentrations. This procedure uses paper disks impregnated with 30 µg of linezolid to test the susceptibility of microorganisms to linezolid. The disk diffusion interpretive criteria are provided in Table 4.

Table 4. Susceptibility Interpretive Criteria for Linezolid

Pathogen	Susceptibility Interpretive Criteria					
	Minimal Inhibitory Concentrations (MIC in µg/mL)			Disk Diffusion (Zone Diameters in mm)		
	S	I	R	S	I	R
Enterococcus spp	≤ 2	4	≥8	≥ 23	21-22	≤20
Staphylococcus spp[a]	≤4	—	—	≥ 21	—	—
Streptococcus pneumoniae[a]	≤2[b]	—	—	≥ 21[c]	—	—
Streptococcus spp other than S pneumoniae[a]	≤2[b]	—	—	≥ 21[c]	—	—

[a] The current absence of data on resistant strains precludes defining any categories other than "Susceptible." Strains yielding test results suggestive of a "nonsusceptible" category should be retested, and if the result is confirmed, the isolate should be submitted to a reference laboratory for further testing.

[b] These interpretive standards for S. pneumoniae and Streptococcus spp. other than S. pneumoniae are applicable only to tests performed by broth microdilution using cation-adjusted Mueller-Hinton broth with 2 to 5% lysed horse blood inoculated with a direct colony suspension and incubated in ambient air at 35°C for 20 to 24 hours.

[c] These zone diameter interpretive standards are applicable only to tests performed using Mueller-Hinton agar supplemented with 5% defibrinated sheep blood inoculated with a direct colony suspension and incubated in 5% CO_2 at 35°C for 20 to 24 hours.

A report of "Susceptible" indicates that the pathogen is likely to be inhibited if the antimicrobial compound in the blood reaches the concentrations usually achievable. A report of "Intermediate" indicates that the result should be considered equivocal, and, if the microorganism is not fully susceptible to alternative, clinically feasible drugs, the test should be repeated. This category implies possible clinical applicability in body sites where the drug is physiologically concentrated or in situations where high dosage of drug can be used. This category also provides a buffer zone which prevents small uncontrolled technical factors from causing major discrepancies in interpretation. A report of "Resistant" indicates that the pathogen is not likely to be inhibited if the antimicrobial compound in the blood reaches the concentrations usually achievable; other therapy should be selected.

Quality Control
Standardized susceptibility test procedures require the use of quality control microorganisms to control the technical aspects of the test procedures. Standard linezolid powder should provide the following range of values noted in Table 5. **NOTE:** Quality control microorganisms are specific strains of organisms with intrinsic biological properties relating to resistance mechanisms and their genetic expression within bacteria; the specific strains used for microbiological quality control are not clinically significant.

Table 5. Acceptable Quality Control Ranges for Linezolid to be Used in Validation of Susceptibility Test Results

QC Strain	Acceptable Quality Control Ranges	
	Minimum Inhibitory Concentration (MIC in µg/mL)	Disk Diffusion (Zone Diameters in mm)
Enterococcus faecalis ATCC 29212	1 - 4	Not applicable
Staphylococcus aureus ATCC 29213	1 - 4	Not applicable
Staphylococcus aureus ATCC 25923	Not applicable	25 - 32
Streptococcus pneumoniae ATCC 49619[d]	0.50 - 2[e]	25 - 34[f]

[d] This organism may be used for validation of susceptibility test results when testing Streptococcus spp. other than S. pneumoniae.

[e] This quality control range for S. pneumoniae is applicable only to tests performed by broth microdilution using cation-adjusted Mueller-Hinton broth with 2 to 5% lysed horse blood inoculated with a direct colony suspension and incubated in ambient air at 35°C for 20 to 24 hours.

[f] This quality control zone diameter range is applicable only to tests performed using Mueller-Hinton agar supplemented with 5% defibrinated sheep blood inoculated with a direct colony suspension and incubated in 5% CO_2 at 35°C for 20 to 24 hours.

INDICATIONS AND USAGE

ZYVOX formulations are indicated in the treatment of the following infections caused by susceptible strains of the designated microorganisms (see **PRECAUTIONS, Pediatric Use** and **DOSAGE AND ADMINISTRATION**).
Vancomycin-Resistant *Enterococcus faecium* **infections**, including cases with concurrent bacteremia (see **CLINICAL STUDIES**).
Nosocomial pneumonia caused by *Staphylococcus aureus* (methicillin-susceptible and -resistant strains), or *Streptococcus pneumoniae* (including multi-drug resistant strains [MDRSP]). Combination therapy may be clinically indicated if the documented or presumptive pathogens include Gram-negative organisms (see **CLINICAL STUDIES**).
Complicated skin and skin structure infections, including diabetic foot infections, without concomitant osteomyelitis, caused by *Staphylococcus aureus* (methicillin-susceptible and -resistant strains), *Streptococcus pyogenes*, or *Streptococcus agalactiae*. ZYVOX has not been studied in the treatment of decubitus ulcers. Combination therapy may be clinically indicated if the documented or presumptive pathogens include Gram-negative organisms (see **CLINICAL STUDIES**).
Uncomplicated skin and skin structure infections caused by *Staphylococcus aureus* (methicillin-susceptible only) or *Streptococcus pyogenes*.
Community-acquired pneumonia caused by *Streptococcus pneumoniae* (including multi-drug resistant strains [MDRSP]*), including cases with concurrent bacteremia, or *Staphylococcus aureus* (methicillin-susceptible strains only).
To reduce the development of drug-resistant bacteria and maintain the effectiveness of ZYVOX and other antibacterial drugs, ZYVOX should be used only to treat or prevent infections that are proven or strongly suspected to be caused by susceptible bacteria. When culture and susceptibility information are available, they should be considered in selecting or modifying antibacterial therapy. In the absence of such data, local epidemiology and susceptibility patterns may contribute to the empiric selection of therapy.

---

*MDRSP refers to isolates resistant to two or more of the following antibiotics: penicillin, second-generation cephalosporins, macrolides, tetracycline, and trimethoprim/sulfamethoxazole.

CONTRAINDICATIONS

ZYVOX formulations are contraindicated for use in patients who have known hypersensitivity to linezolid or any of the other product components.

WARNINGS

Myelosuppression (including anemia, leukopenia, pancytopenia, and thrombocytopenia) has been reported in patients receiving linezolid. In cases where the outcome is known, when linezolid was discontinued, the affected hematologic parameters have risen toward pretreatment levels. Complete blood counts should be monitored weekly in patients who receive linezolid, particularly in those who receive linezolid for longer than two weeks, those with preexisting myelosuppression, those receiving concomitant drugs that produce bone marrow suppression, or those with a chronic infection who have received previous or concomitant antibiotic therapy. Discontinuation of therapy with linezolid should be considered in patients who develop or have worsening myelosuppression.
In adult and juvenile dogs and rats, myelosuppression, reduced extramedullary hematopoiesis in spleen and liver, and lymphoid depletion of thymus, lymph nodes, and spleen were observed (see **ANIMAL PHARMACOLOGY**).
Pseudomembranous colitis has been reported with nearly all antibacterial agents, including ZYVOX, and may range in severity from mild to life-threatening. Therefore, it is important to consider this diagnosis in patients who present with diarrhea subsequent to the administration of any antibacterial agent.
Treatment with antibacterial agents alters the normal flora of the colon and may permit overgrowth of clostridia. Studies indicated that a toxin produced by *Clostridium difficile* is a primary cause of "antibiotic-associated colitis."
After the diagnosis of pseudomembranous colitis has been established, appropriate therapeutic measures should be initiated. Mild cases of pseudomembranous colitis usually respond to drug discontinuation alone. In moderate to severe cases, consideration should be given to management with fluids and electrolytes, protein supplementation, and treatment with an antibacterial agent clinically effective against *Clostridium difficile*.

PRECAUTIONS

General
Lactic acidosis has been reported with the use of ZYVOX. In reported cases, patients experienced repeated episodes of nausea and vomiting. Patients who develop recurrent nausea or vomiting, unexplained acidosis, or a low bicarbonate level while receiving ZYVOX should receive immediate medical evaluation.

Spontaneous reports of serotonin syndrome associated with the co-administration of ZYVOX and serotonergic agents, including antidepressants such as selective serotonin reuptake inhibitors (SSRIs), have been reported (see **PRECAUTIONS, Drug Interactions**).
The use of antibiotics may promote the overgrowth of non-susceptible organisms. Should superinfection occur during therapy, appropriate measures should be taken.
ZYVOX has not been studied in patients with uncontrolled hypertension, pheochromocytoma, carcinoid syndrome, or untreated hyperthyroidism.
The safety and efficacy of ZYVOX formulations given for longer than 28 days have not been evaluated in controlled clinical trials.
Peripheral and optic neuropathy have been reported in patients treated with ZYVOX, primarily those patients treated for longer than the maximum recommended duration of 28 days. In cases of optic neuropathy that progressed to loss of vision, patients were treated for extended periods beyond the maximum recommended duration.
If symptoms of visual impairment appear, such as changes in visual acuity, changes in color vision, blurred vision, or visual field defect, prompt ophthalmic evaluation is recommended. If peripheral or optic neuropathy occurs, the continued use of ZYVOX in these patients should be weighed against the potential risks.
Prescribing ZYVOX in the absence of a proven or strongly suspected bacterial infection or a prophylactic indication is unlikely to provide benefit to the patient and increases the risk of the development of drug-resistant bacteria.

Information for Patients
Patients should be advised that:
• ZYVOX may be taken with or without food.
• They should inform their physician if they have a history of hypertension.
• Large quantities of foods or beverages with high tyramine content should be avoided while taking ZYVOX. Quantities of tyramine consumed should be less than 100 mg per meal. Foods high in tyramine content include those that may have undergone protein changes by aging, fermentation, pickling, or smoking to improve flavor, such as aged cheeses (0 to 15 mg tyramine per ounce); fermented or air-dried meats (0.1 to 8 mg tyramine per ounce); sauerkraut (8 mg tyramine per 8 ounces); soy sauce (5 mg tyramine per 1 teaspoon); tap beers (4 mg tyramine per 12 ounces); red wines (0 to 6 mg tyramine per 8 ounces). The tyramine content of any protein-rich food may be increased if stored for long periods or improperly refrigerated.[9,10]
• They should inform their physician if taking medications containing pseudoephedrine HCl or phenylpropanolamine HCl, such as cold remedies and decongestants.
• They should inform their physician if taking serotonin reuptake inhibitors or other antidepressants.
• *Phenylketonurics:* Each 5 mL of the 100 mg/5 mL ZYVOX for Oral Suspension contains 20 mg phenylalanine. The other ZYVOX formulations do not contain phenylalanine. Contact your physician or pharmacist.

Patients should be counseled that antibacterial drugs including ZYVOX should only be used to treat bacterial infections. They do not treat viral infections (e.g., the common cold). When ZYVOX is prescribed to treat a bacterial infection, patients should be told that although it is common to feel better early in the course of therapy, the medication should be taken exactly as directed. Skipping doses or not completing the full course of therapy may (1) decrease the effectiveness of the immediate treatment and (2) increase the likelihood that bacteria will develop resistance and will not be treatable by ZYVOX or other antibacterial drugs in the future.

Drug Interactions (see also CLINICAL PHARMACOLOGY, Drug-Drug Interactions)
Monoamine Oxidase Inhibition: Linezolid is a reversible, nonselective inhibitor of monoamine oxidase. Therefore, linezolid has the potential for interaction with adrenergic and serotonergic agents.
Adrenergic Agents: Some individuals receiving ZYVOX may experience a reversible enhancement of the pressor response to indirect-acting sympathomimetic agents, vasopressor or dopaminergic agents. Commonly used drugs such as phenylpropanolamine and pseudoephedrine have been specifically studied. Initial doses of adrenergic agents, such as dopamine or epinephrine, should be reduced and titrated to achieve the desired response.
Serotonergic Agents: Co-administration of linezolid and serotonergic agents was not associated with serotonin syndrome in Phase 1, 2 or 3 studies. Spontaneous reports of serotonin syndrome associated with co-administration of ZYVOX and serotonergic agents, including antidepressants such as selective serotonin reuptake inhibitors (SSRIs), have been reported. Patients who are treated with ZYVOX and concomitant serotonergic agents should be closely observed for signs and symptoms of serotonin syndrome (e.g., cognitive dysfunction, hyperpyrexia, hyperreflexia, incoordination). If any signs or symptoms occur physicians should consider discontinuation of either one or both agents (ZYVOX or concomitant serotonergic agents).

Drug-Laboratory Test Interactions
There are no reported drug-laboratory test interactions.
Carcinogenesis, Mutagenesis, Impairment of Fertility
Lifetime studies in animals have not been conducted to evaluate the carcinogenic potential of linezolid. Neither mutagenic nor clastogenic potential was found in a battery of

Continued on next page

Zyvox—Cont.

tests including: assays for mutagenicity (Ames bacterial reversion and CHO cell mutation), an in vitro unscheduled DNA synthesis (UDS) assay, an in vitro chromosome aberration assay in human lymphocytes, and an in vivo mouse micronucleus assay.

Linezolid did not affect the fertility or reproductive performance of adult female rats. It reversibly decreased fertility and reproductive performance in adult male rats when given at doses ≥ 50 mg/kg/day, with exposures approximately equal to or greater than the expected human exposure level (exposure comparisons are based on AUCs). The reversible fertility effects were mediated through altered spermatogenesis. Affected spermatids contained abnormally formed and oriented mitochondria and were non-viable. Epithelial cell hypertrophy and hyperplasia in the epididymis was observed in conjunction with decreased fertility. Similar epididymal changes were not seen in dogs.

In sexually mature male rats exposed to drug as juveniles, mildly decreased fertility was observed following treatment with linezolid through most of their period of sexual development (50 mg/kg/day from days 7 to 36 of age, and 100 mg/kg/day from days 37 to 55 of age), with exposures up to 1.7-fold greater than mean AUCs observed in pediatric patients aged 3 months to 11 years. Decreased fertility was not observed with shorter treatment periods, corresponding to exposure in utero through the early neonatal period (gestation day 6 through postnatal day 5), neonatal exposure (postnatal days 5 to 21), or to juvenile exposure (postnatal days 22 to 35). Reversible reductions in sperm motility and altered sperm morphology were observed in rats treated from postnatal day 22 to 35.

Pregnancy

Teratogenic Effects. Pregnancy Category C: Linezolid was not teratogenic in mice or rats at exposure levels 6.5-fold (in mice) or equivalent to (in rats) the expected human exposure level, based on AUCs. However, embryo and fetal toxicities were seen (see **Non-teratogenic Effects**). There are no adequate and well-controlled studies in pregnant women. ZYVOX should be used during pregnancy only if the potential benefit justifies the potential risk to the fetus.

Non-teratogenic Effects

In mice, embryo and fetal toxicities were seen only at doses that caused maternal toxicity (clinical signs and reduced body weight gain). A dose of 450 mg/kg/day (6.5-fold the estimated human exposure level based on AUCs) correlated with increased postimplantational embryo death, including total litter loss, decreased fetal body weights, and an increased incidence of costal cartilage fusion.

In rats, mild fetal toxicity was observed at 15 and 50 mg/kg/day (exposure levels 0.22-fold to approximately equivalent to the estimated human exposure, respectively based on AUCs). The effects consisted of decreased fetal body weights and reduced ossification of sternebrae, a finding often seen in association with decreased fetal body weights. Slight maternal toxicity, in the form of reduced body weight gain, was seen at 50 mg/kg/day.

When female rats were treated with 50 mg/kg/day (approximately equivalent to the estimated human exposure based on AUCs) of linezolid during pregnancy and lactation, survival of pups was decreased on postnatal days 1 to 4. Male and female pups permitted to mature to reproductive age, when mated, showed an increase in preimplantation loss.

Nursing Mothers

Linezolid and its metabolites are excreted in the milk of lactating rats. Concentrations in milk were similar to those in maternal plasma. It is not known whether linezolid is excreted in human milk. Because many drugs are excreted in human milk, caution should be exercised when ZYVOX is administered to a nursing woman.

Pediatric Use

The safety and effectiveness of ZYVOX for the treatment of pediatric patients with the following infections are supported by evidence from adequate and well-controlled studies in adults, pharmacokinetic data in pediatric patients, and additional data from a comparator-controlled study of Gram-positive infections in pediatric patients ranging in age from birth through 11 years (see **INDICATIONS AND USAGE** and **CLINICAL STUDIES**):

- nosocomial pneumonia
- complicated skin and skin structure infections
- community-acquired pneumonia (also supported by evidence from an uncontrolled study in patients ranging in age from 8 months through 12 years)
- vancomycin-resistant *Enterococcus faecium* infections

The safety and effectiveness of ZYVOX for the treatment of pediatric patients with the following infection have been established in a comparator-controlled study in pediatric patients ranging in age from 5 through 17 years (see **CLINICAL STUDIES**):

- uncomplicated skin and skin structure infections caused by *Staphylococcus aureus* (methicillin-susceptible strains only) or *Streptococcus pyogenes*

The C_{max} and the volume of distribution (V_{ss}) of linezolid are similar regardless of age in pediatric patients. However, linezolid clearance is a function of age. Excluding neonates less than a week of age, clearance is most rapid in the youngest age groups ranging from >1 week old to 11 years, resulting in lower single-dose systemic exposure (AUC) and shorter half-life as compared with adults. As age of pediatric patients increases, the clearance of linezolid gradually decreases, and by adolescence, mean clearance values approach those observed for the adult population. There is wider inter-subject variability in linezolid clearance and in systemic drug exposure (AUC) across all pediatric age groups as compared with adults.

Similar mean daily AUC values were observed in pediatric patients from birth to 11 years of age dosed q8h relative to adolescents or adults dosed q12h. Therefore, the dosage for pediatric patients up to 11 years of age should be 10 mg/kg q8h. Pediatric patients 12 years and older should receive 600 mg q12h.

Recommendations for the dosage regimen for pre-term neonates less than 7 days of age (gestational age less than 34 weeks) are based on pharmacokinetic data from 9 pre-term neonates. Most of these pre-term neonates have lower systemic linezolid clearance values and larger AUC values than many full-term neonates and older infants. Therefore, these pre-term neonates should be initiated with a dosing regimen of 10 mg/kg q12h. Consideration may be given to the use of a 10 mg/kg q8h regimen in neonates with a sub-optimal clinical response. All neonatal patients should receive 10 mg/kg q8h by 7 days of life (see **CLINICAL PHARMACOLOGY, Special Populations, Pediatric** and **DOSAGE AND ADMINISTRATION**).

In limited clinical experience, 5 out of 6 (83%) pediatric patients with infections due to Gram-positive pathogens with MICs of 4 µg/mL treated with ZYVOX had clinical cures. However, pediatric patients exhibit wider variability in linezolid clearance and systemic exposure (AUC) compared with adults. In pediatric patients with a sub-optimal clinical response, particularly those with pathogens with MIC of 4 µg/mL, lower systemic exposure, site and severity of infection, and the underlying medical condition should be considered when assessing clinical response (see **CLINICAL PHARMACOLOGY, Special Populations, Pediatric** and **DOSAGE AND ADMINISTRATION**).

Geriatric Use

Of the 2046 patients treated with ZYVOX in Phase 3 comparator-controlled clinical trials, 589 (29%) were 65 years or older and 253 (12%) were 75 years or older. No overall differences in safety or effectiveness were observed between these patients and younger patients.

ANIMAL PHARMACOLOGY

Target organs of linezolid toxicity were similar in juvenile and adult rats and dogs. Dose- and time-dependent myelosuppression, as evidenced by bone marrow hypocellularity/decreased hematopoiesis, decreased extramedullary hematopoiesis in spleen and liver, and decreased levels of circulating erythrocytes, leukocytes, and platelets have been seen in animal studies. Lymphoid depletion occurred in thymus, lymph nodes, and spleen. Generally, the lymphoid findings were associated with anorexia, weight loss, and suppression of body weight gain, which may have contributed to the observed effects. These effects were observed at exposure levels that are comparable to those observed in some human subjects. The hematopoietic and lymphoid effects were reversible, although in some studies, reversal was incomplete within the duration of the recovery period.

ADVERSE REACTIONS

Adult Patients

The safety of ZYVOX formulations was evaluated in 2046 adult patients enrolled in seven Phase 3 comparator-controlled clinical trials, who were treated for up to 28 days. In these studies, 85% of the adverse events reported with ZYVOX were described as mild to moderate in intensity. Table 6 shows the incidence of adverse events reported in at least 2% of patients in these trials. The most common adverse events in patients treated with ZYVOX were diarrhea (incidence across studies: 2.8% to 11.0%), headache (incidence across studies: 0.5% to 11.3%), and nausea (incidence across studies: 3.4% to 9.6%).

Table 6. Incidence (%) of Adverse Events Reported in ≥2% of Adult Patients in Comparator-Controlled Clinical Trials with ZYVOX

Event	ZYVOX (n=2046)	All Comparators* (n=2001)
Diarrhea	8.3	6.3
Headache	6.5	5.5
Nausea	6.2	4.6
Vomiting	3.7	2.0
Insomnia	2.5	1.7
Constipation	2.2	2.1
Rash	2.0	2.2
Dizziness	2.0	1.9
Fever	1.6	2.1

*Comparators included cefpodoxime proxetil 200 mg PO q12h; ceftriaxone 1 g IV q12h; clarithromycin 250 mg PO q12h; dicloxacillin 500 mg PO q6h; oxacillin 2 g IV q6h; vancomycin 1 g IV q12h.

Other adverse events reported in Phase 2 and Phase 3 studies included oral moniliasis, vaginal moniliasis, hypertension, dyspepsia, localized abdominal pain, pruritus, and tongue discoloration.

Table 7 shows the incidence of drug-related adverse events reported in at least 1% of adult patients in these trials by dose of ZYVOX.

[See table 7 at left]

Table 7. Incidence (%) of Drug-Related Adverse Events Occurring in >1% of Adult Patients Treated with ZYVOX in Comparator-Controlled Clinical Trials

Adverse Event	Uncomplicated Skin and Skin Structure Infections		All Other Indications	
	ZYVOX 400 mg PO q12h (n=548)	Clarithromycin 250 mg PO q12h (n=537)	ZYVOX 600 mg q12h (n=1498)	All Other Comparators* (n=1464)
% of patients with 1 drug-related adverse event	25.4	19.6	20.4	14.3
% of patients discontinuing due to drug-related adverse events†	3.5	2.4	2.1	1.7
Diarrhea	5.3	4.8	4.0	2.7
Nausea	3.5	3.5	3.3	1.8
Headache	2.7	2.2	1.9	1.0
Taste alteration	1.8	2.0	0.9	0.2
Vaginal moniliasis	1.6	1.3	1.0	0.4
Fungal infection	1.5	0.2	0.1	<0.1
Abnormal liver function tests	0.4	0	1.3	0.5
Vomiting	0.9	0.4	1.2	0.4
Tongue discoloration	1.1	0	0.2	0
Dizziness	1.1	1.5	0.4	0.3
Oral moniliasis	0.4	0	1.1	0.4

*Comparators included cefpodoxime proxetil 200 mg PO q12h; ceftriaxone 1 g IV q12h; dicloxacillin 500 mg PO q6h; oxacillin 2 g IV q6h; vancomycin 1 g IV q12h.

† The most commonly reported drug-related adverse events leading to discontinuation in patients treated with ZYVOX were nausea, headache, diarrhea, and vomiting.

Pediatric Patients

The safety of ZYVOX formulations was evaluated in 215 pediatric patients ranging in age from birth through 11 years, and in 248 pediatric patients aged 5 through 17 years (146 of these 248 were age 5 through 11 and 102 were age 12 to 17). These patients were enrolled in two Phase 3 comparator-controlled clinical trials and were treated for up to 28 days. In these studies, 83% and 99%, respectively, of the adverse events reported with ZYVOX were described as mild to moderate in intensity. In the study of hospitalized pediatric patients (birth through 11 years) with Gram-positive infections, who were randomized 2 to 1 (linezolid:vancomycin), mortality was 6.0% (13/215) in the linezolid arm and 3.0% (3/101) in the vancomycin arm. However, given the severe underlying illness in the patient population, no causality could be established. Table 8 shows the incidence of adverse events reported in at least 2% of pediatric patients treated with ZYVOX in these trials.

[See table 8 at right]

Table 9 shows the incidence of drug-related adverse events reported in more than 1% of pediatric patients (and more than 1 patient) in either treatment group in the comparator-controlled Phase 3 trials.

[See table 9 below and on next page]

Laboratory Changes

ZYVOX has been associated with thrombocytopenia when used in doses up to and including 600 mg every 12 hours for up to 28 days. In Phase 3 comparator-controlled trials, the percentage of adult patients who developed a substantially low platelet count (defined as less than 75% of lower limit of normal and/or baseline) was 2.4% (range among studies: 0.3 to 10.0%) with ZYVOX and 1.5% (range among studies: 0.4 to 7.0%) with a comparator. In a study of hospitalized pediatric patients ranging in age from birth through 11 years, the percentage of patients who developed a substantially low platelet count (defined as less than 75% of lower limit of normal and/or baseline) was 12.9% with ZYVOX and 13.4% with vancomycin. In an outpatient study of pediatric patients aged from 5 through 17 years, the percentage of patients who developed a substantially low platelet count was 0% with ZYVOX and 0.4% with cefadroxil. Thrombocytopenia associated with the use of ZYVOX appears to be dependent on duration of therapy, (generally greater than 2 weeks of treatment). The platelet counts for most patients returned to the normal range/baseline during the follow-up period. No related clinical adverse events were identified in Phase 3 clinical trials in patients developing thrombocytopenia. Bleeding events were identified in thrombocytopenic patients in a compassionate use program for ZYVOX; the role of linezolid in these events cannot be determined (see **WARNINGS**).

Changes seen in other laboratory parameters, without regard to drug relationship, revealed no substantial differences between ZYVOX and the comparators. These changes were generally not clinically significant, did not lead to discontinuation of therapy, and were reversible. The incidence of adult and pediatric patients with at least one substantially abnormal hematologic or serum chemistry value is presented in Tables 10, 11, 12, and 13.

[See table 10 on next page]

[See table 11 on next page]

[See table 12 at top of page 343]

[See table 13 at top of page 343]

Postmarketing Experience

Myelosuppression (including anemia, leukopenia, pancytopenia, and thrombocytopenia) has been reported during postmarketing use of ZYVOX (see **WARNINGS**). Peripheral neuropathy, and optic neuropathy sometimes progressing to loss of vision, have been reported in patients treated with ZYVOX. Lactic acidosis has been reported with the use of ZYVOX (see **PRECAUTIONS**). Although these reports have primarily been in patients treated for longer than the maximum recommended duration of 28 days, these events have also been reported in patients receiving shorter courses of therapy. Serotonin syndrome has been reported in patients receiving concomitant serotonergic agents, including antidepressants such as selective serotonin reuptake inhibitors (SSRIs) and ZYVOX (see **PRECAUTIONS**). These events have been chosen for inclusion due to either their seriousness, frequency of reporting, possible causal connection to ZYVOX, or a combination of these factors. Because they are reported voluntarily from a population of unknown size, estimates of frequency cannot be made and causal relationship cannot be precisely established.

OVERDOSAGE

In the event of overdosage, supportive care is advised, with maintenance of glomerular filtration. Hemodialysis may facilitate more rapid elimination of linezolid. In a Phase 1 clinical trial, approximately 30% of a dose of linezolid was removed during a 3-hour hemodialysis session beginning 3 hours after the dose of linezolid was administered. Data are not available for removal of linezolid with peritoneal dialysis or hemoperfusion. Clinical signs of acute toxicity in animals were decreased activity and ataxia in rats and vomiting and tremors in dogs treated with 3000 mg/kg/day and 2000 mg/kg/day, respectively.

DOSAGE AND ADMINISTRATION

The recommended dosage for ZYVOX formulations for the treatment of infections is described in Table 14.

[See table 14 on page 343]

Adult patients with infection due to MRSA should be treated with ZYVOX 600 mg q12h.

In limited clinical experience, 5 out of 6 (83%) pediatric patients with infections due to Gram-positive pathogens with MICs of 4 µg/mL treated with ZYVOX had clinical cures. However, pediatric patients exhibit wider variability in linezolid clearance and systemic exposure (AUC) compared with adults. In pediatric patients with a sub-optimal clinical response, particularly those with pathogens with MIC of 4 µg/mL, lower systemic exposure, site and severity of infection, and the underlying medical condition should be considered when assessing clinical response (see **CLINICAL PHARMACOLOGY, Special Populations, Pediatric** and **PRECAUTIONS, Pediatric Use**).

In controlled clinical trials, the protocol-defined duration of treatment for all infections ranged from 7 to 28 days. Total treatment duration was determined by the treating physician based on site and severity of the infection, and on the patient's clinical response.

Table 8. Incidence (%) of Adverse Events Reported in ≥2% of Pediatric Patients Treated with ZYVOX in Comparator-Controlled Clinical Trials

Event	Uncomplicated Skin and Skin Structure Infections*		All Other Indications[†]	
	ZYVOX (n=248)	Cefadroxil (n = 251)	ZYVOX (n = 215)	Vancomycin (n=101)
Fever	2.9	3.6	14.1	14.1
Diarrhea	7.8	8.0	10.8	12.1
Vomiting	2.9	6.4	9.4	9.1
Sepsis	0	0	8.0	7.1
Rash	1.6	1.2	7.0	15.2
Headache	6.5	4.0	0.9	0
Anemia	0	0	5.6	7.1
Thrombocytopenia	0	0	4.7	2.0
Upper respiratory infection	3.7	5.2	4.2	1.0
Nausea	3.7	3.2	1.9	0
Dyspnea	0	0	3.3	1.0
Reaction at site of injection or of vascular catheter	0	0	3.3	5.1
Trauma	3.3	4.8	2.8	2.0
Pharyngitis	2.9	1.6	0.5	1.0
Convulsion	0	0	2.8	2.0
Hypokalemia	0	0	2.8	3.0
Pneumonia	0	0	2.8	2.0
Thrombocythemia	0	0	2.8	2.0
Cough	2.4	4.0	0.9	0
Generalized abdominal pain	2.4	2.8	0.9	2.0
Localized abdominal pain	2.4	2.8	0.5	1.0
Apnea	0	0	2.3	2.0
Gastrointestinal bleeding	0	0	2.3	1.0
Generalized edema	0	0	2.3	1.0
Loose stools	1.6	0.8	2.3	3.0
Localized pain	2.0	1.6	0.9	0
Skin disorder	2.0	0	0.9	1.0

* Patients 5 through 11 years of age received ZYVOX 10 mg/kg PO q12h or cefadroxil 15 mg/kg PO q12h. Patients 12 years or older received ZYVOX 600 mg PO q12h or cefadroxil 500 mg PO q12h.
[†] Patients from birth through 11 years of age received ZYVOX 10 mg/kg IV/PO q8h or vancomycin 10 to 15 mg/kg IV q6-24h, depending on age and renal clearance.

Table 9. Incidence (%) of Drug-related Adverse Events Occurring in >1% of Pediatric Patients (and >1 Patient) in Either Treatment Group in Comparator-Controlled Clinical Trials

Event	Uncomplicated Skin and Skin Structure Infections*		All Other Indications[†]	
	ZYVOX (n=248)	Cefadroxil (n=251)	ZYVOX (n=215)	Vancomycin (n=101)
% of patients with ≥1 drug-related adverse event	19.2	14.1	18.8	34.3
% of patients discontinuing due to a drug-related adverse event	1.6	2.4	0.9	6.1
Diarrhea	5.7	5.2	3.8	6.1
Nausea	3.3	2.0	1.4	0
Headache	2.4	0.8	0	0
Loose stools	1.2	0.8	1.9	0
Thrombocytopenia	0	0	1.9	0
Vomiting	1.2	2.4	1.9	1.0

(Table continued on next page)

No dose adjustment is necessary when switching from intravenous to oral administration. Patients whose therapy is started with ZYVOX I.V. Injection may be switched to either ZYVOX Tablets or Oral Suspension at the discretion of the physician, when clinically indicated.

Intravenous Administration

ZYVOX I.V. Injection is supplied in single-use, ready-to-use infusion bags (see **HOW SUPPLIED** for container sizes).

Parenteral drug products should be inspected visually for particulate matter prior to administration. Check for minute leaks by firmly squeezing the bag. If leaks are detected, discard the solution, as sterility may be impaired.

ZYVOX I.V. Injection should be administered by intravenous infusion over a period of 30 to 120 minutes. **Do not use**

Continued on next page

Table 9 (cont.): Incidence (%) of Drug-related Adverse Events Occurring in >1% of Pediatric Patients (and >1 Patient) in Either Treatment Group in Comparator-Controlled Clinical Trials

Event	Uncomplicated Skin and Skin Structure Infections*		All Other Indications[†]	
	ZYVOX (n=248)	Cefadroxil (n=251)	ZYVOX (n=215)	Vancomycin (n=101)
Generalized abdominal pain	1.6	1.2	0	0
Localized abdominal pain	1.6	1.2	0	0
Anemia	0	0	1.4	1.0
Eosinophilia	0.4	0.4	1.4	0
Rash	0.4	1.2	1.4	7.1
Vertigo	1.2	0.4	0	0
Oral moniliasis	0	0	0.9	4.0
Fever	0	0	0.5	3.0
Pruritus at non-application site	0.4	0	0	2.0
Anaphylaxis	0	0	0	10.1[‡]

*Patients 5 through 11 years of age received ZYVOX 10 mg/kg PO q12h or cefadroxil 15 mg/kg PO q12h. Patients 12 years or older received ZYVOX 600 mg PO q12h or cefadroxil 500 mg PO q12h.
[†] Patients from birth through 11 years of age received ZYVOX 10 mg/kg IV/PO q8h or vancomycin 10 to 15 mg/kg IV q6-24h, depending on age and renal clearance.
[‡] These reports were of 'red-man syndrome', which were coded as anaphylaxis.

Table 10. Percent of Adult Patients who Experienced at Least One Substantially Abnormal* Hematology Laboratory Value in Comparator-Controlled Clinical Trials with ZYVOX

Laboratory Assay	Uncomplicated Skin and Skin Structure Infections		All Other Indications	
	ZYVOX 400 mg q12h	Clarithromycin 250 mg q12h	ZYVOX 600 mg q12h	All Other Comparators[†]
Hemoglobin (g/dL)	0.9	0.0	7.1	6.6
Platelet count ($\times 10^3/mm^3$)	0.7	0.8	3.0	1.8
WBC ($\times 10^3/mm^3$)	0.2	0.6	2.2	1.3
Neutrophils ($\times 10^3/mm^3$)	0.0	0.2	1.1	1.2

*<75% (<50% for neutrophils) of Lower Limit of Normal (LLN) for values normal at baseline;
<75% (<50% for neutrophils) of LLN and of baseline for values abnormal at baseline.
[†] Comparators included cefpodoxime proxetil 200 mg PO q12h; ceftriaxone 1 g IV q12h; dicloxacillin 500 mg PO q6h; oxacillin 2 g IV q6h; vancomycin 1 g IV q12h.

Table 11. Percent of Adult Patients who Experienced at Least One Substantially Abnormal* Serum Chemistry Laboratory Value in Comparator-Controlled Clinical Trials with ZYVOX

Laboratory Assay	Uncomplicated Skin and Skin Structure Infections		All Other Indications	
	ZYVOX 400 mg q12h	Clarithromycin 250 mg q12h	ZYVOX 600 mg q12h	All Other Comparators[†]
AST (U/L)	1.7	1.3	5.0	6.8
ALT (U/L)	1.7	1.7	9.6	9.3
LDH (U/L)	0.2	0.2	1.8	1.5
Alkaline phosphatase (U/L)	0.2	0.2	3.5	3.1
Lipase (U/L)	2.8	2.6	4.3	4.2
Amylase (U/L)	0.2	0.2	2.4	2.0
Total bilirubin (mg/dL)	0.2	0.0	0.9	1.1
BUN (mg/dL)	0.2	0.0	2.1	1.5
Creatinine (mg/dL)	0.2	0.0	0.2	0.6

*>2 × Upper Limit of Normal (ULN) for values normal at baseline;
>2 × ULN and >2 × baseline for values abnormal at baseline.
[†] Comparators included cefpodoxime proxetil 200 mg PO q12h; ceftriaxone 1 g IV q12h; dicloxacillin 500 mg PO q6h; oxacillin 2 g IV q6h; vancomycin 1 g IV q12h.

Zyvox—Cont.

this intravenous infusion bag in series connections. Additives should not be introduced into this solution. If ZYVOX I.V. Injection is to be given concomitantly with another drug, each drug should be given separately in accordance with the recommended dosage and route of administration for each product. In particular, physical incompatibilities resulted when ZYVOX I.V. Injection was combined with the following drugs during simulated Y-site administration: amphotericin B, chlorpromazine HCl, diazepam, pentamidine isothionate, erythromycin lactobionate, phenytoin sodium, and trimethoprim-sulfamethoxazole. Additionally, chemical incompatibility resulted when ZYVOX I.V. Injection was combined with ceftriaxone sodium.

If the same intravenous line is used for sequential infusion of several drugs, the line should be flushed before and after infusion of ZYVOX I.V. Injection with an infusion solution compatible with ZYVOX I.V. Injection and with any other drug(s) administered via this common line (see **Compatible Intravenous Solutions**).

Compatible Intravenous Solutions
5% Dextrose Injection, USP
0.9% Sodium Chloride Injection, USP
Lactated Ringer's Injection, USP
Keep the infusion bags in the overwrap until ready to use. Store at room temperature. Protect from freezing. ZYVOX I.V. Injection may exhibit a yellow color that can intensify over time without adversely affecting potency.

Constitution of Oral Suspension
ZYVOX for Oral Suspension is supplied as a powder/granule for constitution. Gently tap bottle to loosen powder. Add a total of 123 mL distilled water in two portions. After adding the first half, shake vigorously to wet all of the powder. Then add the second half of the water and shake vigorously to obtain a uniform suspension. After constitution, each 5 mL of the suspension contains 100 mg of linezolid. Before using, gently mix by inverting the bottle 3 to 5 times. **DO NOT SHAKE.** Store constituted suspension at room temperature. Use within 21 days after constitution.

HOW SUPPLIED
Injection
ZYVOX I.V. Injection is available in single-use, ready-to-use flexible plastic infusion bags in a foil laminate overwrap. The infusion bags and ports are latex-free. The infusion bags are available in the following package sizes:

100 mL bag (200 mg linezolid)	NDC 0009-5137-01
200 mL bag (400 mg linezolid)	NDC 0009-5139-01
300 mL bag (600 mg linezolid)	NDC 0009-5140-01

Tablets
ZYVOX Tablets are available as follows:
400 mg (white, oblong, film-coated tablets printed with "ZYVOX 400mg")

100 tablets in HDPE bottle	NDC 0009-5134-01
20 tablets in HDPE bottle	NDC 0009-5134-02
Unit dose packages of 30 tablets	NDC 0009-5134-03

600 mg (white, capsule-shaped, film-coated tablets printed with "ZYVOX 600 mg")

100 tablets in HDPE bottle	NDC 0009-5135-01
20 tablets in HDPE bottle	NDC 0009-5135-02
Unit dose packages of 30 tablets	NDC 0009-5135-03

Oral Suspension
ZYVOX for Oral Suspension is available as a dry, white to off-white, orange-flavored granule/powder. When constituted as directed, each bottle will contain 150 mL of a suspension providing the equivalent of 100 mg of linezolid per each 5 mL. ZYVOX for Oral Suspension is supplied as follows:
100 mg/5 mL in 240-mL glass bottles   NDC 0009-5136-01
Storage of ZYVOX Formulations
Store at 25°C (77°F); excursions permitted to 15-30°C (59-86°F) [see USP Controlled Room Temperature]. Protect from light. Keep bottles tightly closed to protect from moisture. It is recommended that the infusion bags be kept in the overwrap until ready to use. Protect infusion bags from freezing.

CLINICAL STUDIES
Adults
Vancomycin-Resistant Enterococcal Infections
Adult patients with documented or suspected vancomycin-resistant enterococcal infection were enrolled in a randomized, multi-center, double-blind trial comparing a high dose of ZYVOX (600 mg) with a low dose of ZYVOX (200 mg) given every 12 hours (q12h) either intravenously (IV) or orally for 7 to 28 days. Patients could receive concomitant aztreonam or aminoglycosides. There were 79 patients randomized to high-dose linezolid and 66 to low-dose linezolid. The intent-to-treat (ITT) population with documented vancomycin-resistant enterococcal infection at baseline consisted of 65 patients in the high-dose arm and 52 in the low-dose arm.
The cure rates for the ITT population with documented vancomycin-resistant enterococcal infection at baseline are presented in Table 15 by source of infection. These cure rates do not include patients with missing or indeterminate outcomes. The cure rate was higher in the high-dose arm than in the low-dose arm, although the difference was not statistically significant at the 0.05 level.

Table 15. Cure Rates at the Test-of-Cure Visit for ITT Adult Patients with Documented Vancomycin-Resistant Enterococcal Infections at Baseline

Source of Infection	Cured	
	ZYVOX 600 mg q12h n/N (%)	ZYVOX 200 mg q12h n/N (%)
Any site	39/58 (67)	24/46 (52)
Any site with associated bacteremia	10/17 (59)	4/14 (29)
Bacteremia of unknown origin	5/10 (50)	2/7 (29)
Skin and skin structure	9/13 (69)	5/5 (100)
Urinary tract	12/19 (63)	12/20 (60)
Pneumonia	2/3 (67)	0/1 (0)
Other*	11/13 (85)	5/13 (39)

*Includes sources of infection such as hepatic abscess, biliary sepsis, necrotic gall bladder, pericolonic abscess, pancreatitis, and catheter-related infection.

Nosocomial Pneumonia
Adult patients with clinically and radiologically documented nosocomial pneumonia were enrolled in a randomized, multi-center, double-blind trial. Patients were treated for 7 to 21 days. One group received ZYVOX 600 mg q12h, and the other group received vancomycin 1 g q12h IV. Both groups received concomitant aztreonam (1 to 2 g every 8 hours IV), which could be continued if clinically

indicated. There were 203 linezolid-treated and 193 vancomycin-treated patients enrolled in the study. One hundred twenty-two (60%) linezolid-treated patients and 103 (53%) vancomycin-treated patients were clinically evaluable. The cure rates in clinically evaluable patients were 57% for linezolid-treated patients and 60% for vancomycin-treated patients. The cure rates in clinically evaluable patients with ventilator-associated pneumonia were 47% for linezolid-treated patients and 40% for vancomycin-treated patients. A modified intent-to-treat (MITT) analysis of 94 linezolid-treated patients and 83 vancomycin-treated patients included subjects who had a pathogen isolated before treatment. The cure rates in the MITT analysis were 57% in linezolid-treated patients and 46% in vancomycin-treated patients. The cure rates by pathogen for microbiologically evaluable patients are presented in Table 16.

Table 16. Cure Rates at the Test-of-Cure Visit for Microbiologically Evaluable Adult Patients with Nosocomial Pneumonia

| Pathogen | Cured | |
	ZYVOX n/N (%)	Vancomycin n/N (%)
Staphylococcus aureus	23/38 (61)	14/23 (61)
Methicillin-resistant *S. aureus*	13/22 (59)	7/10 (70)
Streptococcus pneumoniae	9/9 (100)	9/10 (90)

Pneumonia caused by multi-drug resistant *S.pneumoniae* (MDRSP*)

ZYVOX was studied for the treatment of community-acquired (CAP) and hospital-acquired (HAP) pneumonia due to MDRSP by pooling clinical data from seven comparative and non-comparative Phase 2 and Phase 3 studies involving adult and pediatric patients. The pooled MITT population consisted of all patients with *S. pneumoniae* isolated at baseline; the pooled ME population consisted of patients satisfying criteria for microbiologic evaluability. The pooled MITT population with CAP included 15 patients (41%) with severe illness (risk classes IV and V) as assessed by a prediction rule[11]. The pooled clinical cure rates for patients with CAP due to MDRSP were 35/48 (73%) in the MITT and 33/36 (92%) in the ME populations respectively. The pooled clinical cure rates for patients with HAP due to MDRSP were 12/18 (67%) in the MITT and 10/12 (83%) in the ME populations respectively.

* MDRSP refers to isolates resistant to two or more of the following antibiotics: penicillin, second-generation cephalosporins, macrolides, tetracycline, and trimethoprim/sulfamethoxazole.

Table 17. Clinical cure rates for 36 microbiologically-evaluable patients with CAP due to MDRSP* who were treated with ZYVOX (stratified by antibiotic susceptibility)

| Susceptibility Screening | Clinical Cure | |
	n/N[a]	(%)
Penicillin-resistant	14/16	88
2nd generation cephalosporin-resistant[b]	19/22	86
Macrolide-resistant[c]	29/30	97
Tetracycline-resistant	22/24	92
Trimethoprim/sulfamethoxazole-resistant	18/21	86

a) n= pooled number of patients treated successfully; N= pooled number of patients having MDRSP isolates that exhibited resistance to the listed antibiotic
b) 2nd-generation cephalosporin tested was cefuroxime
c) macrolide tested was erythromycin

Complicated Skin and Skin Structure Infections

Adult patients with clinically documented complicated skin and skin structure infections were enrolled in a randomized, multi-center, double-blind, double-dummy trial comparing study medications administered IV followed by medications given orally for a total of 10 to 21 days of treatment. One group of patients received ZYVOX I.V. Injection 600 mg q12h followed by ZYVOX Tablets 600 mg q12h; the other group received oxacillin 2 g every 6 hours (q6h) IV followed by dicloxacillin 500 mg q6h orally. Patients could receive concomitant aztreonam if clinically indicated. There were 400 linezolid-treated and 419 oxacillin-treated patients enrolled in the study. Two hundred forty-five (61%) linezolid-treated patients and 242 (58%) oxacillin-treated patients were clinically evaluable. The cure rates in clinically evaluable patients were 90% in linezolid-treated patients and 85% in oxacillin-treated patients. A modified intent-to-treat (MITT) analysis of 316 linezolid-treated patients and 313 oxacillin-treated patients included subjects who met all criteria for study entry. The cure rates in the MITT analysis were 86% in linezolid-treated patients

Table 12. Percent of Pediatric Patients who Experienced at Least One Substantially Abnormal* Hematology Laboratory Value in Comparator-Controlled Clinical Trials with ZYVOX

| Laboratory Assay | Uncomplicated Skin and Skin Structure Infections[†] | | All Other Indications[‡] | |
	ZYVOX	Cefadroxil	ZYVOX	Vancomycin
Hemoglobin (g/dL)	0.0	0.0	15.7	12.4
Platelet count ($\times 10^3/mm^3$)	0.0	0.4	12.9	13.4
WBC ($\times 10^3/mm^3$)	0.8	0.8	12.4	10.3
Neutrophils ($\times 10^3/mm^3$)	1.2	0.8	5.9	4.3

* <75% (<50% for neutrophils) of Lower Limit of Normal (LLN) for values normal at baseline; <75% (<50% for neutrophils) of LLN and <75% (<50% for neutrophils, <90% for hemoglobin if baseline <LLN) of baseline for values abnormal at baseline.
† Patients 5 through 11 years of age received ZYVOX 10 mg/kg PO q12h or cefadroxil 15 mg/kg PO q12h. Patients 12 years or older received ZYVOX 600 mg PO q12h or cefadroxil 500 mg PO q12h.
‡ Patients from birth through 11 years of age received ZYVOX 10 mg/kg IV/PO q8h or vancomycin 10 to 15 mg/kg IV q6-24h, depending on age and renal clearance.

Table 13. Percent of Pediatric Patients who Experienced at Least One Substantially Abnormal* Serum Chemistry Laboratory Value in Comparator-Controlled Clinical Trials with ZYVOX

| Laboratory Assay | Uncomplicated Skin and Skin Structure Infections[†] | | All Other Indications[‡] | |
	ZYVOX	Cefadroxil	ZYVOX	Vancomycin
ALT (U/L)	0.0	0.0	10.1	12.5
Lipase (U/L)	0.4	1.2	—	—
Amylase (U/L)	—	—	0.6	1.3
Total bilirubin (mg/dL)	—	—	6.3	5.2
Creatinine (mg/dL)	0.4	0.0	2.4	1.0

* >2 × Upper Limit of Normal (ULN) for values normal at baseline; >2 × ULN and >2 (>1.5 for total bilirubin) × baseline for values abnormal at baseline.
† Patients 5 through 11 years of age received ZYVOX 10 mg/kg PO q12h or cefadroxil 15 mg/kg PO q12h. Patients 12 years or older received ZYVOX 600 mg PO q12h or cefadroxil 500 mg PO q12h.
‡ Patients from birth through 11 years of age received ZYVOX 10 mg/kg IV/PO q8h or vancomycjn 10 to 15 mg/kg IV q6-24h, depending on age and renal clearance.

Table 14. Dosage Guidelines for ZYVOX

| Infection* | Dosage and Route of Administration | | Recommended Duration of Treatment (consecutive days) |
	Pediatric Patients[†] (Birth through 11 Years of Age)	Adults and Adolescents (12 Years and Older)	
Complicated skin and skin structure infections	10 mg/kg IV or oral[‡] q8h	600 mg IV or oral[‡] q12h	10 to 14
Community-acquired pneumonia, including concurrent bacteremia			
Nosocomial pneumonia			
Vancomycin-resistant *Enterococcus faecium* infections, including concurrent bacteremia	10 mg/kg IV or oral[‡] q8h	600 mg IV or oral[‡] q12h	14 to 28
Uncomplicated skin and skin structure infections	<5 yrs: 10 mg/kg oral[‡] q8h 5-11 yrs: 10 mg/kg oral[‡] q12h	Adults: 400 mg oral[‡] q12h Adolescents: 600 mg oral[‡] q12h	10 to 14

* Due to the designated pathogens (see **INDICATIONS AND USAGE**)
† **Neonates <7 days:** Most pre-term neonates <7 days of age (gestational age <34 weeks) have lower systemic linezolid clearance values and larger AUC values than many full-term neonates and older infants. These neonates should be initiated with a dosing regimen of 10 mg/kg q12h. Consideration may be given to the use of 10 mg/kg q8h regimen in neonates with a sub-optimal clinical response. All neonatal patients should receive 10 mg/kg q8h by 7 days of life (see **CLINICAL PHARMACOLOGY, Special Populations, Pediatric**).
‡ Oral dosing using either ZYVOX Tablets or ZYVOX for Oral Suspension

and 82% in oxacillin-treated patients. The cure rates by pathogen for microbiologically evaluable patients are presented in Table 18.

Table 18. Cure Rates at the Test-of-Cure Visit for Microbiologically Evaluable Adult Patients with Complicated Skin and Skin Structure Infections

| Pathogen | Cured | |
	ZYVOX n/N (%)	Oxacillin/ Dicloxacillin n/N (%)
Staphylococcus aureus	73/83 (88)	72/84 (86)
Methicillin-resistant *S. aureus*	2/3 (67)	0/0 (-)
Streptococcus agalactiae	6/6 (100)	3/6 (50)
Streptococcus pyogenes	18/26 (69)	21/28 (75)

A separate study provided additional experience with the use of ZYVOX in the treatment of methicillin-resistant *Staphylococcus aureus* (MRSA) infections. This was a randomized, open-label trial in hospitalized adult patients with documented or suspected MRSA infection.

One group of patients received ZYVOX I.V. Injection 600 mg q12h followed by ZYVOX Tablets 600 mg q12h. The other group of patients received vancomycin 1 g q12h IV. Both groups were treated for 7 to 28 days, and could receive concomitant aztreonam or gentamicin if clinically indicated. The cure rates in microbiologically evaluable patients with MRSA skin and skin structure infection were 26/33 (79%) for linezolid-treated patients and 24/33 (73%) for vancomycin-treated patients.

Diabetic Foot Infections

Adult diabetic patients with clinically documented complicated skin and skin structure infections ("diabetic foot infections") were enrolled in a randomized (2:1 ratio), multi-center, open-label trial comparing study medications administered IV or orally for a total of 14 to 28 days of treatment. One group of patients received ZYVOX 600 mg q12h IV or orally; the other group received ampicillin/sulbactam 1.5 to 3 g IV or amoxicillin/clavulanate 500 to 875 mg every 8 to 12 hours (q8-12h) orally. In countries where ampicillin/sulbactam is not marketed, amoxicillin/clavulanate 500 mg to 2 g every 6 hours (q6h) was used for the intravenous regimen. Patients in the comparator group could also be treated with vancomycin 1 g q12h IV if MRSA was isolated from the foot infection. Patients in either treatment group

Continued on next page

Zyvox—Cont.

who had Gram-negative bacilli isolated from the infection site could also receive aztreonam 1 to 2 g q8-12h IV. All patients were eligible to receive appropriate adjunctive treatment methods, such as debridement and off-loading, as typically required in the treatment of diabetic foot infections, and most patients received these treatments. There were 241 linezolid-treated and 120 comparator-treated patients in the intent-to-treat (ITT) study population. Two hundred twelve (86%) linezolid-treated patients and 105 (85%) comparator-treated patients were clinically evaluable. In the ITT population, the cure rates were 68.5% (165/241) in linezolid-treated patients and 64% (77/120) in comparator-treated patients, where those with indeterminate and missing outcomes were considered failures. The cure rates in the clinically evaluable patients (excluding those with indeterminate and missing outcomes) were 83% (159/192) and 73% (74/101) in the linezolid- and comparator-treated patients, respectively. A critical post-hoc analysis focused on 121 linezolid-treated and 60 comparator-treated patients who had a Gram-positive pathogen isolated from the site of infection or from blood, who had less evidence of underlying osteomyelitis than the overall study population, and who did not receive prohibited antimicrobials. Based upon that analysis, the cure rates were 71% (86/121) in the linezolid-treated patients and 63% (38/60) in the comparator-treated patients. None of the above analyses were adjusted for the use of adjunctive therapies. The cure rates by pathogen for microbiologically evaluable patients are presented in Table 19.

Table 19. Cure Rates at the Test-of-Cure Visit for Microbiologically Evaluable Adult Patients with Diabetic Foot Infections

Pathogen	Cured	
	ZYVOX n/N (%)	Comparator n/N (%)
Staphylococcus aureus	49/63 (78)	20/29 (69)
Methicillin-resistant *S. aureus*	12/17 (71)	2/3 (67)
Streptococcus agalactiae	25/29 (86)	9/16 (56)

Pediatric Patients
Infections Due to Gram-positive Organisms
A safety and efficacy study provided experience on the use of ZYVOX in pediatric patients for the treatment of nosocomial pneumonia, complicated skin and skin structure infections, catheter-related bacteremia, bacteremia of unidentified source, and other infections due to Gram-positive bacterial pathogens, including methicillin-resistant and -susceptible *Staphylococcus aureus* and vancomycin-resistant *Enterococcus faecium*. Pediatric patients ranging in age from birth through 11 years with infections caused by the documented or suspected Gram-positive organisms were enrolled in a randomized, open-label, comparator-controlled trial. One group of patients received ZYVOX I.V. Injection 10 mg/kg every 8 hours (q8h) followed by ZYVOX for Oral Suspension 10 mg/kg q8h. A second group received vancomycin 10 to 15 mg/kg IV every 6 to 24 hours, depending on age and renal clearance. Patients who had confirmed VRE infections were placed in a third arm of the study and received ZYVOX 10 mg/kg q8h IV and/or orally. All patients were treated for a total of 10 to 28 days and could receive concomitant Gram-negative antibiotics if clinically indicated. In the intent-to-treat (ITT) population, there were 206 patients randomized to linezolid and 102 patients randomized to vancomycin. One hundred seventeen (57%) linezolid-treated patients and 55 (54%) vancomycin-treated patients were clinically evaluable. The cure rates in ITT patients were 81% in patients randomized to linezolid and 83% in patients randomized to vancomycin (95% Confidence Interval of the treatment difference; -13%, 8%). The cure rates in clinically evaluable patients were 91% in linezolid-treated patients and 91% in vancomycin-treated patients (95% CI; -11%, 11%). Modified intent-to-treat (MITT) patients included ITT patients who, at baseline, had a Gram-positive pathogen isolated from the site of infection or from blood. The cure rates in MITT patients were 80% in patients randomized to linezolid and 90% in patients randomized to vancomycin (95% CI; -23%, 3%). The cure rates for ITT, MITT, and clinically evaluable patients are presented in Table 20, and cure rates by pathogen for microbiologically evaluable patients are provided in Table 21.
[See table 20 below]

Table 21. Cure Rates at the Test-of-Cure Visit for Microbiologically Evaluable Pediatric Patients with Infections due to Gram-positive Pathogens

Pathogen	Microbiologically Evaluable	
	ZYVOX n/N (%)	Vancomycin n/N (%)
Vancomycin-resistant *Enterococcus faecium*	1/1 (100)	0/0 (-)
Staphylococcus aureus	36/38 (95)	23/24 (96)
Methicillin-resistant *S. aureus*	16/17 (94)	9/9 (100)
Streptococcus pyogenes	2/2 (100)	1/2 (50)

REFERENCES

1. Gonzales RD, PC Schreckenberger, MB Graham, et al. Infections due to vancomycin-resistant *Enterococcus faecium* resistant to linezolid. The Lancet 2001;357:1179.
2. Herrero IA, NC Issa, R Patel. Nosocomial spread of linezolid-resistant, vancomycin-resistant *Enterococcus faecium*. The New England Journal of Medicine 2002;346:867-869.
3. Tsiodras S, HS Gold, G Sakoulas, et al. Linezolid resistance in a clinical isolate of *Staphylococcus aureus*. The Lancet 2001;358:207-208.
4. Goldman DA, RA Weinstein, RP Wenzel, et al. Strategies to prevent and control the emergence and spread of antimicrobial-resistant microorganisms in hospitals. A challenge to hospital leadership. The Journal of the American Medical Association 1996;275:234-240.
5. Centers for Disease Control and Prevention. Guideline for hand hygiene in health-care settings: Recommendations of the Healthcare Infection Control Practices Advisory Committee and the HIPAC/SHEA/APIC/IDSA Hand Hygiene Task Force. Morbidity and Mortality Weekly Report 2002;51 (RR-16).
6. National Committee for Clinical Laboratory Standards. Methods for Dilution Antimicrobial Susceptibility Tests for Bacteria that Grow Aerobically. Fifth Edition. Approved Standard NCCLS Document M7-A5, Vol. 20, No. 2, NCCLS, Wayne, PA, January 2000.
7. National Committee for Clinical Laboratory Standards. Twelfth Informational Supplement. Approved NCCLS Document M100-S12, Vol. 21, No. 1, NCCLS, Wayne, PA, January 2002.
8. National Committee for Clinical Laboratory Standards. Performance Standards for Antimicrobial Disk Susceptibility Tests. Seventh Edition. Approved Standard NCCLS Document M2-A7, Vol. 20, No. 1, NCCLS, Wayne, PA, January 2000.
9. Walker SE et al. Tyramine content of previously restricted foods in monoamine oxidase inhibitor diets. Journal of Clinical Psychopharmacology 1996;16(5):383-388.
10. DaPrada M et al. On tyramine, food, beverages and the reversible MAO inhibitor moclobemide. Journal of Neural Transmission 1988; [Supplement] 26:31-56.
11. Fine MJ, Auble TE, Yealy DM, et al. A Prediction Rule to Identify Low-Risk Patients with Community-Acquired Pneumonia. The New England Journal of Medicine. 1997;336 (4):243-250.

Table 20. Cure Rates at the Test-of-Cure Visit for Intent to Treat, Modified Intent to Treat, and Clinically Evaluable Pediatric Patients by Baseline Diagnosis

Population	ITT		MITT*		Clinically Evaluable	
	ZYVOX n/N (%)	Vancomycin n/N (%)	ZYVOX n/N (%)	Vancomycin n/N (%)	ZYVOX n/N (%)	Vancomycin n/N (%)
Any diagnosis	150/186 (81)	69/83 (83)	86/108 (80)	44/49 (90)	106/117 (91)	49/54 (91)
Bacteremia of unidentified source	22/29 (76)	11/16 (69)	8/12 (67)	7/8 (88)	14/17 (82)	7/9 (78)
Catheter-related bacteremia	30/41 (73)	8/12 (67)	25/35 (71)	7/10 (70)	21/25 (84)	7/9 (78)
Complicated skin and skin structure infections	61/72 (85)	31/34 (91)	37/43 (86)	22/23 (96)	46/49 (94)	26/27 (96)
Nosocomial pneumonia	13/18 (72)	11/12 (92)	5/6 (83)	4/4 (100)	7/7 (100)	5/5 (100)
Other infections	24/26 (92)	8/9 (89)	11/12 (92)	4/4 (100)	18/19 (95)	4/4 (100)

* MITT = ITT patients with an isolated Gram-positive pathogen at baseline

Rx only
US Patent Nos. 5,688,792, 6,559,305
Distributed by:
Pfizer
Pharmacia & Upjohn
Division of Pfizer Inc, NY, NY 10017
Revised January 2005 LAB-0139-9.0

Roche Pharmaceuticals

Roche Laboratories Inc.
340 Kingsland Street
Nutley, NJ 07110-1199

For Medical Information:
Call: 1-800-526-6367
Fax: 1-800-532-3931
Write: Professional Product Information
For Patient Assistance Program:
Call: 1-877-75-ROCHE (1-877-757-6243)
Write: Patient Assistance Program

ACCUTANE® ℞
[*acc' u tane*]
(isotretinoin)
Capsules

Prescribing information for this product, which appears on pages 2848–2855 of the 2005 PDR, has been revised as follows. Please write "See Supplement A" next to the product heading.
The **PRECAUTIONS: Information for Patients and Prescribers:** Drug Interactions *section was revised to:*
- *Vitamin A:* Because of the relationship of Accutane to vitamin A, patients should be advised against taking vitamin supplements containing vitamin A to avoid additive toxic effects.
- *Tetracyclines:* Concomitant treatment with Accutane and tetracyclines should be avoided because Accutane use has been associated with a number of cases of pseudotumor cerebri (benign intracranial hypertension), some of which involved concomitant use of tetracyclines.
- *Micro-dosed Progesterone Preparations:* Micro-dosed progesterone preparations ("minipills" that do not contain an estrogen) may be an inadequate method of contraception during Accutane therapy. Although other hormonal contraceptives are highly effective, there have been reports of pregnancy from women who have used combined oral contraceptives, as well as topical/injectable/implantable/insertable hormonal birth control products. These reports are more frequent for women who use only a single method of contraception. It is not known if hormonal contraceptives differ in their effectiveness when used with Accutane. Therefore, it is critically important for women of childbearing potential to select and commit to use 2 forms of effective contraception simultaneously, at least 1 of which must be a primary form, unless absolute abstinence is the chosen method, or the patient has undergone a hysterectomy (see boxed CONTRAINDICATIONS AND WARNINGS).
- *Norethindrone/ethinyl estradiol:* In a study of 31 premenopausal women with severe recalcitrant nodular acne receiving OrthoNovum® 7/7/7 Tablets as an oral contraceptive agent, Accutane at the recommended dose of 1 mg/kg/day, did not induce clinically relevant changes in the pharmacokinetics of ethinyl estradiol and norethindrone and in the serum levels of progesterone, follicle-stimulating hormone (FSH) and luteinizing hormone (LH).
- *Phenytoin:* Accutane has not been shown to alter the pharmacokinetics of phenytoin in a study in seven healthy volunteers. These results are consistent with the in vitro finding that neither isotretinoin nor its metabolites induce or inhibit the activity of the CYP 2C9 human hepatic P450 enzyme. Phenytoin is known to cause osteomalacia. No formal clinical studies have been conducted to assess if there is an interactive effect on bone loss between phenytoin and Accutane. Therefore, caution should be exercised when using these drugs together.
- *Systemic Corticosteroids:* Systemic corticosteroids are known to cause osteoporosis. No formal clinical studies have been conducted to assess if there is an interactive effect on bone loss between systemic corticosteroids and Accutane. Therefore, caution should be exercised when using these drugs together.

Prescribers are advised to consult the package insert of medication administered concomitantly with hormonal contraceptives, since some medications may decrease the effectiveness of these birth control products. **Accutane use is associated with depression in some patients (see WARNINGS: Psychiatric Disorders and ADVERSE REACTIONS: Psychiatric).** Patients should be prospectively cautioned not to self-medicate with the herbal supplement St. John's Wort because a possible interaction has been suggested with hormonal contraceptives based on reports of breakthrough bleeding on oral contraceptives shortly after starting St. John's Wort. Pregnancies have been reported by users of combined hormonal contraceptives who also used some form of St. John's Wort.

Revised: August 2004*

INVIRASE® ℞

[ĭn-vər-ās]

(saquinavir mesylate)

CAPSULES and TABLETS

Prescribing information for this product, which appears on pages 2890–2895 of the 2005 PDR, has been completely revised as follows. Please write "See Supplement A" next to the product heading.

The **DOSAGE AND ADMINISTRATION** *section was revised to:*

INVIRASE (saquinavir mesylate) capsules and FORTOVASE (saquinavir) soft gelatin capsules are not bioequivalent and cannot be used interchangeably. INVIRASE may be used only if it is combined with ritonavir, because it significantly inhibits saquinavir's metabolism to provide plasma saquinavir levels at least equal to those achieved with FORTOVASE at the recommended dose of 1200 mg tid. When using saquinavir as the sole protease inhibitor in an antiretroviral regimen, FORTOVASE is the recommended formulation (see CLINICAL PHARMACOLOGY: Drug Interactions).

Adults (Over the Age of 16 Years)

- INVIRASE 1000-mg bid (5 x 200-mg capsules or 2 x 500-mg tablets) in combination with ritonavir 100-mg bid.
- Ritonavir should be taken at the same time as INVIRASE.
- INVIRASE and ritonavir should be taken within 2 hours after a meal.

Monitoring of Patients

Clinical chemistry tests, viral load, and CD4 count should be performed prior to initiating INVIRASE therapy and at appropriate intervals thereafter. For comprehensive patient monitoring recommendations for other nucleoside analogues, physicians should refer to the complete product information for these drugs.

Dose Adjustment for Combination Therapy with INVIRASE

For serious toxicities that may be associated with INVIRASE, the drug should be interrupted. INVIRASE at doses less than 1000 mg with 100 mg ritonavir bid are not recommended since lower doses have not shown antiviral activity. For recipients of combination therapy with INVIRASE and ritonavir, dose adjustments may be necessary. These adjustments should be based on the known toxicity profile of the individual agent and the pharmacokinetic interaction between saquinavir and the coadministered drug (see **PRECAUTIONS: Drug Interactions**). Physicians should refer to the complete product information for these drugs for comprehensive dose adjustment recommendations and drug-associated adverse reactions of nucleoside analogues.

The **HOW SUPPLIED** *section was revised to:*

INVIRASE 200-mg capsules are light brown and green opaque capsules with ROCHE and 0245 imprinted on the capsule shell—bottles of 270 (NDC 0004-0245-15).

INVIRASE 500-mg film coated tablets are light orange to greyish- or brownish-orange, oval cylindrical, biconvex tablets with ROCHE and SQV 500 imprinted on the tablet face—bottles of 120 (NDC 0004-0244-51).

The capsules and tablets should be stored at 25°C (77°F); excursions permitted to 15° to 30°C (59° to 86°F) [see USP Controlled Room Temperature] in tightly closed bottles.

Manufactured by:

F. Hoffmann-La Roche Ltd., Basel, Switzerland
or Hoffmann-La Roche Inc., Nutley, New Jersey

Revised: December 2004*

KYTRIL® ℞

[*ki-tril*]

(granisetron hydrochloride)

injection

Prescribing information for this product, which appears on pages 2898–2901 of the 2005 PDR, has been revised as follows. Please write "See Supplement A" next to the product heading.

The following paragraphs were revised in **DESCRIPTION:**

KYTRIL 1 mg/1 mL is available in 1 mL single-use and 4 mL multi-use vials. KYTRIL 0.1 mg/1 mL is available in a 1 mL single-use vial.

1 mg/1 mL: Each 1 mL contains 1.12 mg granisetron hydrochloride equivalent to granisetron, 1 mg; sodium chloride, 9 mg; citric acid, 2 mg; and benzyl alcohol, 10 mg, as a preservative. The solution's pH ranges from 4.0 to 6.0.

0.1 mg/1 mL: Each 1 mL contains 0.112 mg granisetron hydrochloride equivalent to granisetron, 0.1 mg; sodium chloride, 9 mg; citric acid, 2 mg. Contains no preservative. The solution's pH ranges from 4.0 to 6.0.

The following sentence was added to **PRECAUTIONS:**

Pregnancy:

Benzyl alcohol may cross the placenta. KYTRIL Injection 1 mg/1 mL is preserved with benzyl alcohol and should be used in pregnancy only if the benefit outweighs the potential risk.

The following paragraph was added to **PRECAUTIONS:**

Pediatric Use:

Benzyl alcohol, a component of KYTRIL 1 mg/1 mL, has been associated with serious adverse events and death, particularly in neonates. The "gasping syndrome," characterized by central nervous system depression, metabolic acidosis, gasping respirations, and high levels of benzyl alcohol and metabolites in blood and urine, has been associated with benzyl alcohol dosages >99 mg/kg/day in neonates and low birth-weight neonates. Additional symptoms may include gradual neurological deterioration, seizures, intracranial hemorrhage, hematologic abnormalities, skin breakdown, hepatic and renal failure, hypotension, bradycardia, and cardiovascular collapse. Although normal therapeutic doses of this product deliver amounts of benzyl alcohol that are substantially lower than those reported in association with the "gasping syndrome," the minimum amount of benzyl alcohol at which toxicity may occur is not known. Premature and low birth-weight infants, as well as patients receiving high dosages, may be more likely to develop toxicity. Practitioners administering this and other medications containing benzyl alcohol should consider the combined daily metabolic load of benzyl alcohol from all sources.

The following was added to **DOSAGE AND ADMINISTRATION:**

NOTE: KYTRIL 1 MG/1 ML CONTAINS BENZYL ALCOHOL (see **PRECAUTIONS**).

The **HOW SUPPLIED** section was revised to:

KYTRIL Injection, 1 mg/1 mL (free base), is supplied in 1 mL Single-Use Vials and 4 mL Multi-Use Vials. CONTAINS BENZYL ALCOHOL.

NDC 0004-0239-09 (package of 1 Single-Use Vial)
NDC 0004-0240-09 (package of 1 Multi-Use Vial)

KYTRIL Injection, 0.1 mg/1 mL (free base), is supplied in 1 mL Single-Use Vials. CONTAINS NO PRESERVATIVE.

NDC 0004-0242-08 (package of 5 Single-Use Vials)

Revised: September 2004*

The sanofi-aventis Group

300 SOMERSET CORPORATE BOULEVARD
BRIDGEWATER, NJ 08807-0977

Direct Inquiries to:
Customer Service
300 Somerset Corporate Boulevard
Bridgewater, NJ 08807-0977
(800) 207-8049

For Medical Information Contact:
Generally:
Medical Information Services
300 Somerset Corporate Boulevard
Bridgewater, NJ 08807-0977
(800) 633-1610
For Oncology Medical Information
call (866) 662-6411

APIDRA™ ℞

[a'pĭ-dră]

insulin glulisine (rDNA origin) injection

Rx only

Rev. April 2004a

Prescribing information for this product, which appears on pages 688–693 of the 2005 PDR, has been completely revised as follows. Please write "See Supplement A" next to the product heading.

DESCRIPTION

APIDRA™ (insulin glulisine [rDNA origin]) is a human insulin analog that is a rapid-acting, parenteral blood glucose lowering agent. Insulin glulisine is produced by recombinant DNA technology utilizing a non-pathogenic laboratory strain of *Escherichia coli* (K12). Insulin glulisine differs from human insulin in that the amino acid asparagine at position B3 is replaced by lysine and the lysine in position B29 is replaced by glutamic acid. Chemically, it is 3^B-lysine-29^B-glutamic acid-human insulin, has the empirical formula $C_{258}H_{384}N_{64}O_{78}S_6$ and a molecular weight of 5823. It has the following structural formula:

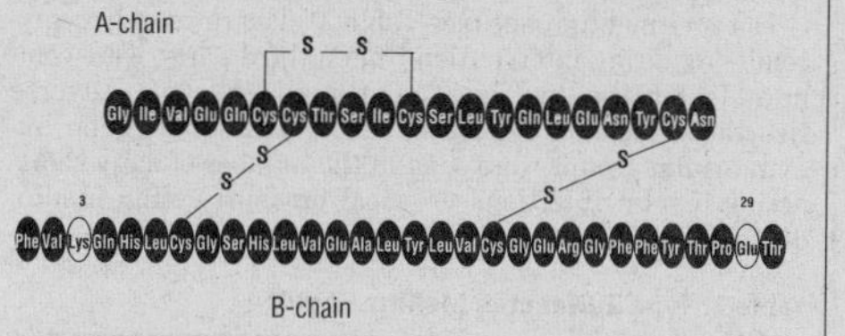

APIDRA is a sterile, aqueous, clear, and colorless solution. Each milliliter of APIDRA (insulin glulisine injection) contains 100 IU (3.49 mg) insulin glulisine, 3.15 mg m-cresol, 6 mg tromethamine, 5 mg sodium chloride, 0.01 mg polysorbate 20, and water for injection. APIDRA has a pH of approximately 7.3. The pH is adjusted by addition of aqueous solutions of hydrochloric acid and/or sodium hydroxide.

CLINICAL PHARMACOLOGY

Mechanism of Action

The primary activity of insulins and insulin analogs, including insulin glulisine, is regulation of glucose metabolism. Insulins lower blood glucose levels by stimulating peripheral glucose uptake by skeletal muscle and fat, and by inhibiting hepatic glucose production. Insulins inhibit lipolysis in the adipocyte, inhibit proteolysis, and enhance protein synthesis.

The glucose lowering activities of APIDRA and of regular human insulin are equipotent when administered by the intravenous route. After subcutaneous administration, the effect of APIDRA is more rapid in onset and of shorter duration compared to regular human insulin.

Pharmacokinetics

Absorption and Bioavailability

Pharmacokinetic profiles in healthy volunteers and patients with diabetes (type 1 or type 2) demonstrated that absorption of insulin glulisine was faster than regular human insulin.

In a study in patients with type 1 diabetes (n=20) after subcutaneous administration of 0.15 IU/kg, the median time to maximum concentration (T_{max}) was 55 minutes (range 34 to 91 minutes) and the peak concentration (C_{max}) was 82 µIU/mL (range 42 to 134 µIU/mL) for insulin glulisine compared to a median T_{max} of 82 minutes (range 52 to 308 minutes) and a C_{max} of 46 µIU/mL (range 32 to 70 µIU/mL) for regular human insulin. The mean residence time of insulin glulisine was shorter (median: 98 minutes, range 55 to 149 minutes) than for regular human insulin (median: 161 minutes, range 133 to 193 minutes). (See Figure 1.)

Figure 1. Pharmacokinetic profile of insulin glulisine and regular human insulin in patients with type 1 diabetes after a dose of 0.15 IU/kg.

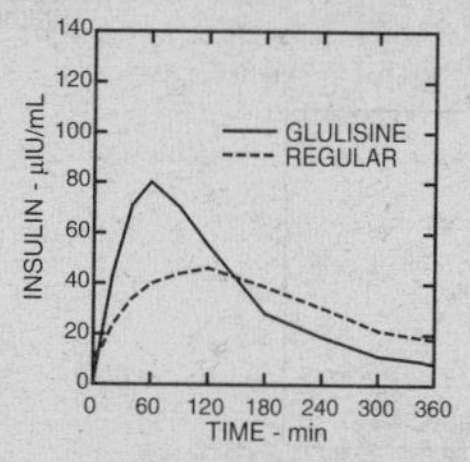

In a euglycemic clamp study in patients with type 2 diabetes (n=24) with a body mass index (BMI) between 20 to 36 kg/m^2 after subcutaneous administration of 0.2 IU/kg, the median time to maximum concentration (T_{max}) was 89 minutes (range 74 to 103 minutes) and the median peak concentration (C_{max}) was 81 µIU/mL (range 75 to 112 µIU/mL) for insulin glulisine compared to a median T_{max} of 94 minutes (range 55 to 140 minutes) and a median C_{max} of 39 µIU/mL (range 30 to 56 µIU/mL) for regular human insulin. The mean residence time of insulin glulisine was shorter (median: 154 minutes, range 122 to 174 minutes) than for regular human insulin (median: 280 minutes, range 227 to 294 minutes).

Figure 2. Pharmacokinetic profile of insulin glulisine and regular human insulin in patients with type 2 diabetes after a dose of 0.2 IU/kg.

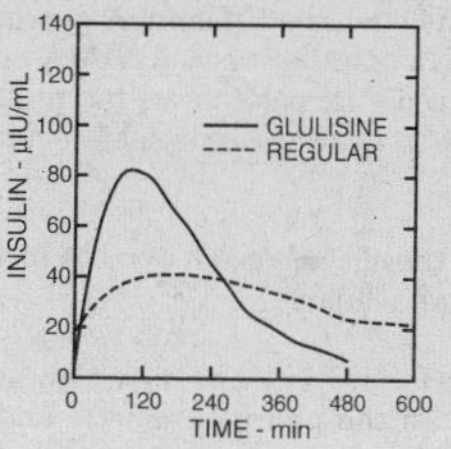

In a euglycemic clamp study in obese, non-diabetic subjects (n=18) with a body mass index (BMI) between 30 to 40 kg/m^2 after subcutaneous administration of 0.3 IU/kg, the median time to maximum concentration (T_{max}) was 76 minutes (range 51 to 118 minutes) and the median peak concentration (C_{max}) was 199 µIU/mL (range 99 to 387 µIU/mL) for insulin glulisine compared to a median T_{max} of 144 minutes (range 110 to 207 minutes) and a median C_{max} of 79 µIU/mL (range 39 to 166 µIU/mL) for regular human insulin. The mean residence time of insulin glulisine was shorter (median: 141 minutes, range 105 to 210 minutes) than for regular human insulin (median: 226 minutes, range 188 to 293 minutes).

When APIDRA was injected subcutaneously into different areas of the body, the time-concentration profiles were similar. The absolute bioavailability of insulin glulisine after subcutaneous administration is about 70%, regardless of injection area (abdomen 73%, deltoid 71%, thigh 68%).

Distribution and Elimination

The distribution and elimination of insulin glulisine and regular human insulin after intravenous administration are similar with volumes of distribution of 13 L and 21 L and half-lives of 13 and 17 minutes, respectively. After subcutaneous administration, insulin glulisine is eliminated more rapidly than regular human insulin with an apparent half-life of 42 minutes compared to 86 minutes.

Pharmacodynamics

Studies in healthy volunteers and patients with diabetes demonstrated that APIDRA has a more rapid onset of action and a shorter duration of activity than regular human insulin when given subcutaneously.

In a study in patients with type 1 diabetes (n= 20), the glucose-lowering profiles of APIDRA and regular human insulin were assessed at various times in relation to a standard meal at a dose of 0.15 IU/kg. (See Figure 3.)

[See figure at top of next column]

The maximum blood glucose excursion (ΔGLU_{max}; baseline subtracted glucose concentration) for APIDRA injected 2 minutes before meal was 65 mg/dL compared to 64 mg/dL for regular human insulin injected 30 minutes before meal (see Figure 3A), and 84 mg.h/dL for regular human insulin

Continued on next page

Apidra—Cont.

Figure 3. Serial mean blood glucose collected up to 6 hours following single dose of APIDRA and regular human insulin. APIDRA given 2 minutes (APIDRA - pre) before the start of a meal compared to regular human insulin given 30 minutes (Regular - 30 min) before start of the meal (Figure 3A) and compared to regular human insulin (Regular - pre) given 2 minutes before a meal (Figure 3B). APIDRA given 15 minutes (APIDRA - post) after start of a meal compared to regular human insulin (Regular - pre) given 2 minutes before a meal (Figure 3C). On the x-axis zero (0) is the start of a 15-minute meal.

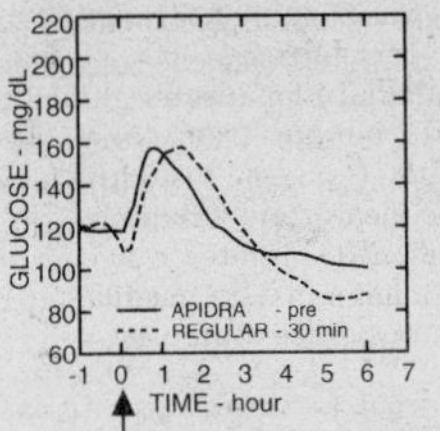

Figure 3A

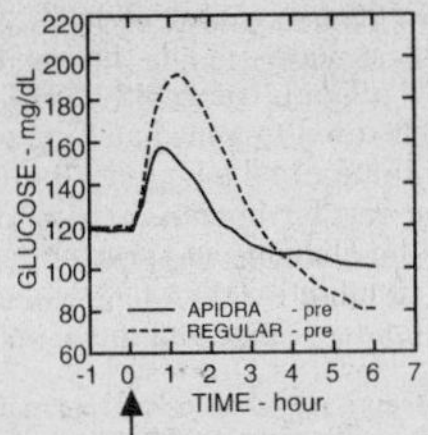

Figure 3B

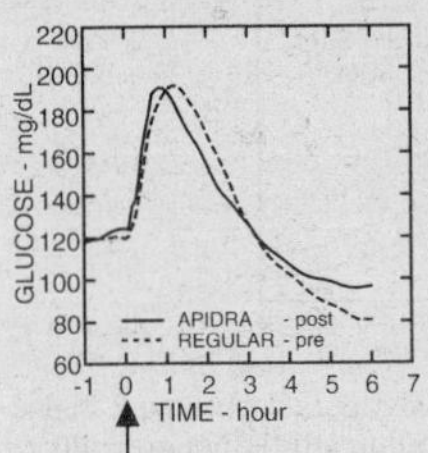

Figure 3C

Start of a 15-minute meal

injected 2 minutes before meal (see Figure 3B). The maximum blood glucose excursion for APIDRA injected 15 minutes after the start of a meal was 85 mg/dL compared to 84 mg.h/dL for regular human insulin injected 2 minutes before meal (see Figure 3C).

Special Populations

Pediatric Patients

The pharmacokinetic and pharmacodynamic properties of APIDRA and regular human insulin were assessed in a study conducted in pediatric patients with type 1 diabetes (children [7 to 11 years, n = 10] and adolescents [12 to 16 years, n = 10]). The relative differences in pharmacokinetics and pharmacodynamics between APIDRA and regular human insulin in pediatric patients with type 1 diabetes were similar to those in healthy adult subjects and adults with type 1 diabetes.

Gender

Information on the effect of gender on the pharmacokinetics of APIDRA is not available.

Race

A study was performed in 24 healthy Caucasians and Japanese to compare the pharmacokinetic and pharmacodynamic parameters after subcutaneous injection of insulin glulisine, insulin lispro, and regular human insulin. With subcutaneous injection of insulin glulisine, Japanese subjects had a greater initial exposure (33%) for the ratio of AUC(0-1hr) to AUC (0-clamp end) than that in Caucasians (21%) though the total exposures were similar. Similar findings were observed with insulin lispro and regular human insulin for the racial difference.

Obesity

The more rapid onset of action and shorter duration of activity of APIDRA and insulin lispro compared to regular human insulin were maintained in an obese non-diabetic population (n= 18). (See Figure 4.)

Figure 4. Glucose infusion rates (GIR) in a euglycemic clamp study after subcutaneous injection of 0.3 IU/kg of APIDRA, insulin lispro or regular human insulin in an obese population.

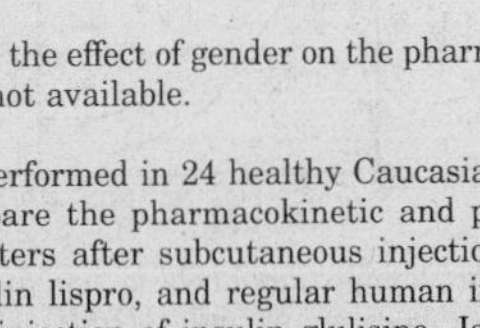

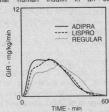

Renal Impairment

Studies with human insulin have shown increased circulating levels of insulin in patients with renal failure. In a study performed in 24 non-diabetic subjects covering a wide range of renal function (Cl_{Cr} >80 mL/min; 30-50 mL/min; <30 mL/min), the subjects with moderate and severe renal impairment showed increased exposure of insulin glulisine by 29% to 40% and reduced clearance of insulin glulisine by 20 to 25% compared to normal subjects. Careful glucose monitoring and dose adjustments of insulin, including APIDRA, may be necessary in patients with renal dysfunction. (See PRECAUTIONS, Renal Impairment.)

Hepatic Impairment

The effect of hepatic impairment on the pharmacokinetics of APIDRA has not been studied. Some studies with human insulin have shown increased circulating levels of insulin in patients with liver failure. Careful glucose monitoring and dose adjustments of insulin, including APIDRA, may be necessary in patients with hepatic dysfunction. (See PRECAUTIONS, Hepatic Impairment.)

Pregnancy

The effect of pregnancy on the pharmacokinetics and pharmacodynamics of APIDRA has not been studied. (See PRECAUTIONS, Pregnancy.)

Smoking

The effect of smoking on the pharmacokinetics and pharmacodynamics of APIDRA has not been studied.

CLINICAL STUDIES

The safety and efficacy of APIDRA was studied in adult patients with type 1 and type 2 diabetes (n=1833). The primary efficacy parameter was glycemic control, as measured by glycated hemoglobin (GHb), and expressed as hemoglobin A1c equivalents (HbA1c).

Type 1 Diabetes:

A 26-week, randomized, open-label, active-control study was conducted in patients with type 1 diabetes to assess the safety and efficacy of APIDRA (n= 339) compared to insulin lispro (n= 333) when administered subcutaneously within 15 minutes before a meal. Lantus® (insulin glargine)† was administered once daily in the evening as the basal insulin. There was a 4-week run-in period combining insulin lispro and Lantus followed by randomization. Most patients were Caucasian (97%). Fifty eight percent of the patients were male. The mean age was 38.5 years (range 18 to 74 years). Glycemic control (see Table 1) and the rates of hypoglycemia requiring intervention from a third party (see Adverse Reactions), were comparable for the two treatment regimens. The number of daily short-acting insulin injections and the total daily doses of APIDRA and insulin lispro were similar. (See Table 1.)

Table 1: Type 1 Diabetes Mellitus–Adult

Treatment duration Treatment in combination with:	26 weeks Lantus®	
	APIDRA	Insulin Lispro
HbA1c (%)		
Number of patients	331	322
Baseline mean	7.60	7.58
Adj. mean change from baseline	-0.14	-0.14
APIDRA – Insulin Lispro	0.00	
95% CI for treatment difference	(-0.09; 0.10)	
Basal insulin dose (IU/day)		
Endstudy mean	24.16	26.43
Adj. mean change from baseline	0.12	1.82
Short-acting insulin dose (IU/day)		
Endstudy mean	29.03	30.12
Adj. mean change from baseline	-1.07	-0.81
Mean number of short-acting insulin injections per day	3.36	3.42

Type 2 Diabetes:

A 26-week, randomized, open-label, active-control study was conducted in insulin-treated patients with type 2 diabetes to assess the safety and efficacy of APIDRA (n= 435) given within 15 minutes before a meal compared to regular human insulin (n=441) administered 30 to 45 minutes prior to a meal. NPH human insulin was given twice a day as the basal insulin. All patients participated in a 4-week run-in period combining regular human insulin and NPH human insulin. Eighty-five percent of patients were Caucasian and 11% were Black. The mean age was 58.3 years (range 26 to 84 years). The average body mass index (BMI) was 34.55 kg/m². At randomization, 58% of the patients were on an oral antidiabetic agent and were instructed to continue use of their oral antidiabetic agent at the same dose. The majority of patients (79%) mixed their short-acting insulin with NPH human insulin immediately prior to injection. The reductions from baseline in HbA1c were similar between treatment groups (see Table 2). The rates of hypoglycemia, requiring intervention from a third party, were comparable for the two treatment regimens (see Adverse Reactions). No differences between APIDRA and regular human insulin groups were seen in the number of daily short-acting insulin injections or basal or short-acting insulin doses. (See Table 2.)

Table 2: Type 2 Diabetes Mellitus–Adult

Treatment duration Treatment in combination with:	26 weeks NPH human insulin	
	APIDRA	Regular Human Insulin
HbA1c (%)		
Number of patients	404	403
Baseline mean	7.57	7.50
Adj. mean change from baseline	-0.46	-0.30
APIDRA – Regular Human Insulin	-0.16	
95% CI for treatment difference	(-0.26; -0.05)	
Basal insulin dose (IU/day)		
Endstudy mean	65.34	63.05
Adj. mean change from baseline	5.73	6.03
Short-acting insulin dose (IU/day)		
Endstudy mean	35.99	36.16
Adj. mean change from baseline	3.69	5.00
Mean number of short-acting insulin injections per day	2.27	2.24

Pre- and Post-Meal Administration (Type 1 Diabetes):

A 12-week, randomized, open-label, active-control study was conducted in patients with type 1 diabetes to assess the safety and efficacy of APIDRA administered at different times with respect to a meal. APIDRA was administered subcutaneously either within 15 minutes before a meal (n=286) or immediately after a meal (n=296) and regular human insulin (n= 278) was administered subcutaneously 30 to 45 minutes prior to a meal. Lantus® was administered once daily at bedtime as the basal insulin. There was a 4-week run-in period combining regular human insulin and Lantus followed by randomization. Most patients were Caucasian (94%). The mean age was 40.3 years (range 18 to 73 years). Glycemic control (see Table 3) and the rates of hypoglycemia requiring intervention from a third party (see Adverse Reactions) were comparable for the treatment regimens. No changes from baseline between the treatments were seen in the total daily number of short-acting insulin injections. (See Table 3.)

Table 3: Type 1 Diabetes Mellitus–Adult

Treatment duration Treatment in combination with:	12 weeks Lantus® APIDRA pre meal	12 weeks Lantus® APIDRA post meal	12 weeks Lantus® Regular Human Insulin
HbA1c (%)			
Number of patients	268	276	257
Baseline mean	7.73	7.70	7.64
Adj. mean change from baseline*	-0.26	-0.11	-0.13
Basal insulin dose (IU/day)			
Endstudy mean	29.49	28.77	28.46
Adj. mean change from baseline	0.99	0.24	0.65
Short-acting insulin dose (IU/day)			
Endstudy mean	28.44	28.06	29.23
Adj. mean change from baseline	-0.88	-0.47	1.75
Mean number of short-acting insulin injections per day	3.15	3.13	3.03

*Adj. mean change from baseline treatment difference (98.33% CI for treatment difference): APIDRA pre meal vs. Regular Human Insulin - 0.13 (-0.26; 0.01); APIDRA post meal vs. Regular Human Insulin 0.02 (-0.11; 0.16); APIDRA post meal vs. pre meal 0.15 (0.02; 0.29).

Continuous Subcutaneous Insulin Infusion (CSII) (Type 1 Diabetes):

To evaluate the use of APIDRA for administration using an external pump, a 12-week randomized, active control study (APIDRA versus insulin aspart) was conducted in patients with type 1 diabetes (APIDRA n=29, insulin aspart n=30). All patients were Caucasian. The mean age was 45.8 (range 21-73 years). Glycemic control (mean HbA1c value at endpoint 6.98% with APIDRA and 7.18% with insulin aspart) and the rates of hypoglycemia requiring intervention from a third party were comparable for the two treatment regimens.

INDICATIONS AND USAGE

APIDRA is indicated for the treatment of adult patients with diabetes mellitus for the control of hyperglycemia.

APIDRA has a more rapid onset of action and a shorter duration of action than regular human insulin. APIDRA should normally be used in regimens that include a longer-acting insulin or basal insulin analog. (See WARNINGS and DOSAGE AND ADMINISTRATION.)

APIDRA may also be infused subcutaneously by external insulin infusion pumps. (See WARNINGS, PRECAUTIONS, Usage in Pumps, Information for Patients, Mixing of Insulins, DOSAGE AND ADMINISTRATION, RECOMMENDED STORAGE.)

CONTRAINDICATIONS

APIDRA is contraindicated during episodes of hypoglycemia and in patients hypersensitive to APIDRA or one of its excipients.

WARNINGS

APIDRA differs from regular human insulin by its rapid onset of action and shorter duration of action. When used as a meal time insulin, the dose of APIDRA should be given within 15 minutes before or immediately after a meal.

Because of the short duration of action of APIDRA, patients with diabetes also require a longer-acting insulin or insulin infusion pump therapy to maintain adequate glucose control.

Any change of insulin should be made cautiously and only under medical supervision. Changes in insulin strength, manufacturer, type (e.g., regular, NPH, analogs), or species (animal, human) may result in the need for a change in dose. Concomitant oral antidiabetic treatment may need to be adjusted.

Glucose monitoring is recommended for all patients with diabetes.

Hypoglycemia is the most common adverse effect of insulin therapy, including APIDRA. The timing of hypoglycemia may differ among various insulin formulations.

Insulin Pumps: When used in an external insulin pump for subcutaneous infusion, APIDRA should not be diluted or mixed with any other insulin. Physicians and patients should carefully evaluate information on pump use in the APIDRA prescribing information, Patient Information Leaflet, and the pump manufacturer's manual. APIDRA-specific information should be followed for in-use time, frequency of changing infusion sets, or other details specific to APIDRA usage, because APIDRA-specific information may differ from general pump manual instructions. Pump or infusion set malfunctions or insulin degradation can lead to hyperglycemia and ketosis in a short time. This is especially pertinent for rapid-acting insulin analogs that are more rapidly absorbed through skin and have a shorter duration of action. Prompt identification and correction of the cause of hyperglycemia or ketosis is necessary. Interim therapy with subcutaneous injection may be required. (See PRECAUTIONS, Usage in Pumps, Information for Patients, Mixing of Insulins, DOSAGE AND ADMINISTRATION, and RECOMMENDED STORAGE.)

PRECAUTIONS

General

As with all insulin preparations, the time course of APIDRA action may vary in different individuals or at different times in the same individual and is dependent on site of injection, blood supply, temperature, and physical activity.

Adjustment of dosage of any insulin may be necessary if patients change their physical activity or their usual meal plan.

Insulin requirements may be altered during intercurrent conditions such as illness, emotional disturbances, or stress.

Hypoglycemia

As with all insulin preparations, hypoglycemic reactions may be associated with the administration of APIDRA. Rapid changes in serum glucose levels may induce symptoms similar to hypoglycemia in persons with diabetes, regardless of the glucose value. Early warning symptoms of hypoglycemia may be different or less pronounced under certain conditions, such as long duration of diabetes, diabetic nerve disease, use of medications such as beta-blockers, or intensified diabetes control. (See PRECAUTIONS, Drug Interactions.)

Such situations may result in severe hypoglycemia (and, possibly, loss of consciousness) prior to patients' awareness of hypoglycemia.

Renal Impairment

The requirements for APIDRA may be reduced in patients with renal impairment. (See CLINICAL PHARMACOLOGY, Special Populations.)

Hepatic Impairment

Studies have not been performed in patients with hepatic impairment. APIDRA requirements may be diminished due to reduced capacity for gluconeogenesis and reduced insulin metabolism, similar to observations found with other insulins. (See CLINICAL PHARMACOLOGY, Special Populations.)

Allergy

Local Allergy

As with other insulin therapy, patients may experience redness, swelling, or itching at the site of injection. These minor reactions usually resolve in a few days to a few weeks. In some instances, these reactions may be related to factors other than insulin, such as irritants in a skin cleansing agent or poor injection technique.

Systemic Allergy

Less common, but potentially more serious, is generalized allergy to insulin, which may cause rash (including pruritus) over the whole body, shortness of breath, wheezing, reduction in blood pressure, rapid pulse, or sweating. Severe cases of generalized allergy, including anaphylactic reactions, may be life threatening.

In controlled clinical trials up to 12 months, potential systemic allergic reactions were reported in 79 of 1833 patients (4.3%) who received APIDRA and 58 of 1524 patients (3.8%) who received the comparator short-acting insulins. During these trials treatment with APIDRA was permanently discontinued in 1 of 1833 patients due to a potential systemic allergic reaction.

Localized reactions and generalized myalgias have been reported with the use of cresol as an injectable excipient.

As with any insulin therapy, lipodystrophy may occur at the injection site and delay insulin absorption.

Antibody Production

In a study in patients with type 1 diabetes (n=333), the concentrations of insulin antibodies that react with both human insulin and insulin glulisine (cross-reactive insulin antibodies) remained near baseline during the first 6 months of the study in the patients treated with APIDRA. A decrease in antibody concentration was observed during the following 6 months of the study. In a study in patients with type 2 diabetes (n=411), a similar increase in cross-reactive insulin antibody concentration was observed in the patients treated with APIDRA and in the patients treated with human insulin during the first 9 months of the study. Thereafter the concentration of antibodies decreased in the APIDRA patients and remained stable in the human insulin patients. There was no correlation between cross-reactive insulin antibody concentration and changes in HbA1c, insulin doses, or incidences of hypoglycemia.

Usage in Pumps

APIDRA has been studied in the following pumps and infusion sets: Disetronic® H-Tron® plus V100 and D-Tron® with Disetronic catheters (Rapid™, Rapid C™, Rapid D™, and Tender™); MiniMed® Models 506, 507, 507c and 508 with MiniMed catheters (Sof-set Ultimate QR™, and Quick-set™)‡.

Based on in vitro studies which have shown loss of m-cresol and insulin degradation, APIDRA should not be used beyond 48 hours at 98.6°F (37°C) in infusion sets and reservoirs. APIDRA in clinical use should not be exposed to temperatures greater than 98.6°F (37°C). **APIDRA should not be mixed with other insulins or with a diluent when used in the pump.** (See WARNINGS, PRECAUTIONS, Information for Patients, Mixing of Insulins, DOSAGE AND ADMINISTRATION, and RECOMMENDED STORAGE.)

Information for Patients

For all patients

Patients should be instructed on self-management procedures including glucose monitoring, proper injection technique, and hypoglycemia and hyperglycemia management. Patients must be instructed on handling of special situations such as intercurrent conditions (illness, stress, or emotional disturbances), an inadequate or skipped insulin dose, inadvertent administration of an increased insulin dose, inadequate food intake, or skipped meals.

Refer patients to the APIDRA Patient Information Leaflet for additional information.

Women with diabetes should be advised to inform their doctor if they are pregnant or are contemplating pregnancy.

For patients using pumps

Patients using external pump infusion therapy should be trained appropriately. APIDRA has been studied in the following pumps and infusion sets: Disetronic H-Tron plus V100 and D-Tron with Disetronic catheters (Rapid, Rapid C, Rapid D, and Tender); MiniMed Models 506, 507, 507c and 508 with MiniMed catheters (Sof-set Ultimate QR, and Quick-set).

To minimize insulin degradation, infusion set occlusion, and loss of the preservative (m-cresol), the infusion sets (reservoir, tubing, and catheter) and the APIDRA in the reservoir should be replaced every 48 hours or less and a new infusion site should be selected. The temperature of the insulin may exceed ambient temperature when the pump housing, cover, tubing or sport case is exposed to sunlight or radiant heat. **Insulin exposed to temperatures higher than 98.6°F (37°C) should be discarded.** Infusion sites that are erythematous, pruritic, or thickened should be reported to the healthcare professional, and a new site selected because continued infusion may increase the skin reaction and/or alter the absorption of APIDRA.

Pump or infusion set malfunctions or insulin degradation can lead to hyperglycemia and ketosis in a short time. This is especially pertinent for rapid-acting insulin analogs that are more rapidly absorbed through skin and have a shorter duration of action. Prompt identification and correction of the cause of hyperglycemia or ketosis is necessary. Problems include pump malfunction, infusion set occlusion, leakage, disconnection or kinking, and degraded insulin. Less commonly, hypoglycemia from pump malfunction may occur. If these problems cannot be promptly corrected, patients should resume therapy with subcutaneous insulin injection and contact their healthcare professional. (See WARNINGS, PRECAUTIONS, Usage in Pumps, Mixing of Insulins, DOSAGE AND ADMINISTRATION, and RECOMMENDED STORAGE.)

Drug Interactions

A number of substances affect glucose metabolism and may require insulin dose adjustment and particularly close monitoring.

The following are examples of substances that may reduce the blood-glucose-lowering effect of insulin: corticosteroids, danazol, diazoxide, diuretics, sympathomimetic agents (e.g., epinephrine, albuterol, terbutaline), glucagon, isoniazid, phenothiazine derivatives, somatropin, thyroid hormones, estrogens, progestogens (e.g., in oral contraceptives), protease inhibitors, and atypical antipsychotic medications (e.g., olanzepine and clozapine).

The following are examples of substances that may increase the blood-glucose-lowering effect and susceptibility to hypoglycemia: oral antidiabetic products, ACE inhibitors, disopyramide, fibrates, fluoxetine, MAO inhibitors, pentoxifylline, propoxyphene, salicylates, sulfonamide antibiotics.

Beta-blockers, clonidine, lithium salts, and alcohol may either potentiate or weaken the blood-glucose-lowering effect of insulin. Pentamidine may cause hypoglycemia, which may sometimes be followed by hyperglycemia.

In addition, under the influence of sympatholytic medicinal products such as beta-blockers, clonidine, guanethidine, and reserpine, the signs of hypoglycemia may be reduced or absent.

Mixing of Insulins

In a clinical study in healthy volunteers (n=32) the total insulin glulisine bioavailability was similar after subcutaneous injection of insulin glulisine and NPH insulin (premixed in the syringe) and following separate simultaneous subcutaneous injections. There was some attenuation (27%) of the maximum concentration (C_{max}) after premixing, however the time to maximum concentration (T_{max}) was not affected. If APIDRA is mixed with NPH human insulin, APIDRA should be drawn into the syringe first. Injection should be made immediately after mixing.

No data are available on mixing APIDRA with insulin preparations other than NPH. (See CLINICAL STUDIES.) APIDRA should not be mixed with insulin preparations other than NPH.

Mixtures should not be administered intravenously.

The effects of mixing APIDRA with diluents or other insulins when used in external subcutaneous infusion pumps for insulin have not been studied. Therefore, APIDRA should not be mixed in these instances.

Carcinogenesis, Mutagenesis, Impairment of Fertility

Standard 2-year carcinogenicity studies in animals have not been performed. In Sprague Dawley rats, a 12-month repeat dose toxicity study was conducted with insulin glulisine at subcutaneous doses of 2.5, 5, 20 or 50 IU/kg twice daily (dose resulting in an exposure 1, 2, 8, and 20 times the average human dose, based on body surface area comparison). There was a non-dose dependent higher incidence of mammary gland tumors in female rats administered insulin glulisine compared to untreated controls. The incidence of mammary tumors for insulin glulisine and regular human insulin was similar. The relevance of these findings to humans is not known.

Insulin glulisine was not mutagenic in the following tests: Ames test, in vitro mammalian chromosome aberration test in V79 Chinese hamster cells, and in vivo mammalian erythrocyte micronucleus test in rats.

In fertility studies in male and female rats at subcutaneous doses up to 10 IU/kg once daily (dose resulting in an exposure 2 times the average human dose, based on body surface area comparison), no clear adverse effects on male and female fertility, or general reproductive performance of animals were observed.

Pregnancy - Teratogenic Effects - Pregnancy Category C

Reproduction and teratology studies have been performed with insulin glulisine in rats and rabbits using regular human insulin as a comparator.

The drug was given to female rats throughout pregnancy at subcutaneous doses up to 10 IU/kg once daily (dose resulting in an exposure 2 times the average human dose, based on body surface area comparison). Insulin glulisine did not have any remarkable toxic effects on the embryo-fetal development in rats.

The drug was given to female rabbits throughout pregnancy at subcutaneous doses up to 1.5 IU/kg/day (dose resulting in an exposure 0.5 times the average human dose, based on body surface area comparison). Adverse effects on embryo-fetal development were only seen at maternal toxic dose levels inducing hypoglycemia. Increased incidence of post-implantation losses and skeletal defects were observed at a dose level of 1.5 IU/kg once daily (dose resulting in an exposure 0.5 times the average human dose, based on body surface area comparison) that also caused mortality in dams. A slight increased incidence of post-implantation losses was seen at the next lower dose level of 0.5 IU/kg once daily (dose resulting in an exposure 0.2 times the average human dose, based on body surface area comparison) which was also associated with severe hypoglycemia but there were no defects at that dose. No effects were observed in rabbits at a dose of 0.25 IU/kg once daily (dose resulting in an exposure 0.1 times the average human dose, based on body surface area comparison). The effects of insulin glulisine did not differ from those observed with subcutaneous regular human insulin at the same doses and were attributed to secondary effects of maternal hypoglycemia.

There are no well-controlled clinical studies of the use of insulin glulisine in pregnant women. Because animal reproduction studies are not always predictive of human response, this drug should be used during pregnancy only if the potential benefit justifies the potential risk to the fetus. It is essential for patients with diabetes or a history of gestational diabetes to maintain good metabolic control before conception and throughout pregnancy. Insulin requirements may decrease during the first trimester, generally increase during the second and third trimesters, and rapidly decline after delivery. Careful monitoring of glucose control is essential in such patients.

Nursing Mothers

It is unknown whether insulin glulisine is excreted in human milk. Many drugs, including human insulin, are excreted in human milk. For this reason, caution should be exercised when APIDRA is administered to a nursing woman. Patients with diabetes who are lactating may require adjustments in APIDRA dose, meal plan, or both.

Pediatric Use

Safety and effectiveness of APIDRA in pediatric patients have not been established.

Geriatric Use

In Phase III clinical trials (n=2408), APIDRA was administered to 147 patients ≥65 years of age and 27 patients ≥75 years of age. The majority of these were patients with type 2 diabetes. The change in HbA1c values and hypoglycemia frequencies did not differ by age, but greater sensitivity of some older individuals cannot be ruled out.

ADVERSE REACTIONS

Overall, clinical studies comparing APIDRA with short-acting insulins did not demonstrate a difference in frequency of adverse events.

Adverse events commonly associated with human insulin therapy include the following:

Body as a whole: allergic reactions. (See PRECAUTIONS.)

Skin and appendages: injection site reaction, lipodystrophy, pruritus, rash. (See PRECAUTIONS.)

Other: hypoglycemia. (See WARNINGS and PRECAUTIONS.)

Continued on next page

Apidra—Cont.

The rates and incidence of severe symptomatic hypoglycemia, defined as hypoglycemia requiring intervention from a third party, were comparable for all treatment regimens (see Table 4).
[See table 4 below]

Continuous Subcutaneous Insulin Infusion (CSII) (Type 1 Diabetes): The rates of catheter occlusions and infusion site reactions were similar for APIDRA and insulin aspart (see Table 5).

Table 5: Catheter Occlusions and Infusion Site Reactions.

	APIDRA	Insulin aspart
Catheter occlusions/ month	0.08	0.15
Infusion site reactions	10.3% (3/29)	13.3% (4/30)

OVERDOSAGE

Hypoglycemia may occur as a result of an excess of insulin relative to food intake, energy expenditure, or both.
Mild/Moderate episodes of hypoglycemia usually can be treated with oral glucose. Adjustments in drug dosage, meal patterns, or exercise may be needed.
Severe episodes with coma, seizure, or neurologic impairment may be treated with intramuscular/subcutaneous glucagon or concentrated intravenous glucose. Sustained carbohydrate intake and observation may be necessary because hypoglycemia may recur after apparent clinical recovery.

DOSAGE AND ADMINISTRATION

APIDRA is a recombinant insulin analog that has been shown to be equipotent to human insulin. One unit of APIDRA has the same glucose-lowering effect as one unit of regular human insulin. After subcutaneous administration, it has a more rapid onset and shorter duration of action.
APIDRA should be given within 15 minutes before a meal or within 20 minutes after starting a meal.
APIDRA is intended for subcutaneous administration and for use by external infusion pump.
The dosage of APIDRA should be individualized and determined based on the physician's advice in accordance with the needs of the patient. APIDRA should normally be used in regimens that include a longer-acting insulin or basal insulin analog.
APIDRA should be administered by subcutaneous injection in the abdominal wall, the thigh or the deltoid or by continuous subcutaneous infusion in the abdominal wall. As with all insulins, injection sites and infusion sites within an injection area (abdomen, thigh or deltoid) should be rotated from one injection to the next.
As for all insulins, the rate of absorption, and consequently the onset and duration of action, may be affected by injection site, exercise and other variables. Blood glucose monitoring is recommended for all patients with diabetes.

Preparation and Handling

Parenteral drug products should be inspected visually prior to administration whenever the solution and the container permit. APIDRA must only be used if the solution is clear and colorless with no particles visible.
When it is used in a pump, APIDRA should not be mixed with other insulins or with a diluent.

HOW SUPPLIED

APIDRA 100 units per mL (U-100) is available in the following package size:
10 mL vials   NDC 0088-2500-33
Storage:
Unopened Vial:
Unopened APIDRA vials should be stored in a refrigerator, 36°F to 46°F (2°C to 8°C). Protect from light. APIDRA should not be stored in the freezer and it should not be allowed to freeze. Discard vial if frozen.
Open (In-Use) Vial:
Opened vials, whether or not refrigerated, must be used within 28 days. They must be discarded if not used within 28 days. If refrigeration is not possible, the open vial in use

can be kept unrefrigerated for up to 28 days away from direct heat and light, as long as the temperature is not greater than 77°F (25°C).

	Not in-use (unopened) Refrigerated	Not in-use (unopened) Room Temperature, below 77°F (25°C)	In-use (opened) Room Temperature, below 77°F (25°C)
10 mL Vial	Until expiration date	28 days	28 days, refrigerated/ room temperature

Infusion sets:
Infusion sets (reservoirs, tubing, and catheters) and the APIDRA in the reservoir should be discarded after no more than 48 hours of use or after exposure to temperatures that exceed 98.6°F (37°C).
Rx only
Rev. April 2004a
Manufactured by:
Aventis Pharma Deutschland GmbH
D-65926 Frankfurt am Main
Frankfurt, Germany
Manufactured for:
Aventis Pharmaceuticals Inc.
Kansas City, MO 64137 USA
US Patent Number 6,221,633
www.aventis-us.com
©2004 Aventis Pharmaceuticals Inc.

†Lantus® is a registered trademark of Aventis Pharmaceuticals Inc.
‡The brands listed are the registered trademarks of their respective owners and are not trademarks of Aventis Pharmaceuticals Inc.

Patient Information

APIDRA™ 10 mL vial (1000 units per vial) 100 units per mL (U-100) (insulin glulisine [recombinant DNA origin] injection)

Read the Patient Information that comes with APIDRA (uh-PEE-druh) before you start using it and each time you get a refill. There may be new information. This leaflet does not take the place of talking with your healthcare provider about your condition or treatment. If you have questions about APIDRA or about diabetes, talk with your healthcare provider.

What is the most important information I should know about APIDRA?

Do not change the insulin you are using without talking to your healthcare provider. Any change in insulin strength, manufacturer, type (regular, NPH, analogs), or species (animal, human) may need a change in the dose. This dose change may be needed right away or later on during the first several weeks or months on the new insulin. Doses of oral antidiabetic medicines may also need to change, if your insulin is changed.

You must test your blood sugar levels while using an insulin such as APIDRA. Your healthcare provider will tell you how often you should test your blood sugar level, and what to do if it is high or low.

When used in a pump do not mix APIDRA with any other insulin or liquid.

APIDRA comes as U-100 insulin and contains 100 units of APIDRA. One milliliter (mL) of U-100 insulin contains 100 units of insulin. (1 mL = 1 cc).

What is APIDRA?

APIDRA is a rapid-acting man-made insulin that is like insulin made by your body. APIDRA is used to treat adults with diabetes for the control of high blood sugar. APIDRA starts working faster than regular insulin and does not work as long. APIDRA is used with a longer-acting insulin or by itself as insulin pump therapy to maintain proper blood sugar control.

Your body needs insulin to turn sugar (glucose) into energy. If your body does not make enough insulin, you need to take more insulin so you will not have too much sugar in your blood.

Insulin injections are important in keeping your diabetes under control. But the way you live, your diet, careful checking of your blood sugar levels, exercise, and planned physical activity, all work with your insulin to help you control your diabetes.
You need a prescription to get APIDRA. Always be sure you receive the right insulin from the pharmacy.

Who should not take APIDRA?

Do not take APIDRA if you are allergic to insulin glulisine or any of the inactive ingredients in APIDRA. See the end of this leaflet for a list of the inactive ingredients.

Before starting APIDRA, tell your healthcare provider
• **about all your medical problems including if you:**
  • **have liver or kidney problems.** Your dose may need to be adjusted.
  • **are pregnant or plan to become pregnant.** It is not known if APIDRA may harm your unborn baby. It is very important to maintain control of your blood sugar levels during pregnancy. Your healthcare provider will decide which insulin is best for you during your pregnancy.
  • **are breast-feeding or plan to breast-feed.** It is not known whether APIDRA passes into your milk. Many medicines, including insulin, pass into human milk, and could affect your baby. Talk to your healthcare provider about the best way to feed your baby.
• **about all the medicines you take including** prescription and non-prescription medicines, vitamins and herbal supplements.

How should I use APIDRA?

See the end of this leaflet for the "**Instructions for Use**" including the sections "**How do I draw the insulin into the syringe?**" and "**How should I infuse APIDRA with an external subcutaneous insulin infusion pump?**"
• Follow the instructions given by your healthcare provider about the type or types of insulin you are using. Do not make any changes with your insulin unless you have talked to your healthcare provider. Your insulin needs may change because of illness, stress, other medicines, or changes in diet or activity level. Talk to your healthcare provider about how to adjust your insulin dose.
• You should take APIDRA within 15 minutes before a meal or within 20 minutes after starting the meal. Only use APIDRA that is clear and colorless. If your APIDRA is cloudy or colored, return it to your pharmacy for a replacement.
• Follow your healthcare provider's instructions for testing your blood sugar.
• Inject APIDRA under your skin (subcutaneously) in your upper arm, abdomen (stomach area), or thigh (upper leg). Never inject it into a vein or muscle. If you use a pump, infuse APIDRA through the skin of your abdomen.
• Change (rotate) injection sites within the same body area.

What kind of syringe should I use?
• Always use a syringe that is marked for U-100 insulin. If you use the wrong syringe, you may get the wrong dose. You could get a blood sugar level that is too low or too high.

Mixing with APIDRA
• If you are mixing APIDRA with NPH human insulin, draw APIDRA into the syringe first. Inject the mixture right away. **Do not mix APIDRA with any other type of insulin than NPH.**
• **Do not mix APIDRA with any other insulin when used in a pump.**

What can affect how much insulin I need?

Illness. Illness may change how much insulin you need. It is a good idea to think ahead and make a "sick day" plan with your healthcare provider in advance so you will be ready when this happens. Be sure to test your blood sugar more often and call your healthcare provider if you are sick.

Medicines. Many medicines can affect your insulin needs. Other medicines, including prescription and non-prescription medicines, vitamins and herbal supplements, can change the way insulin works. You may need a different dose of insulin when you are taking certain other medicines.

Know all the medicines you take, including prescription and non-prescription medicines, vitamins and herbal supplements. You may want to keep a list of the medicines you take. You can show this list to all your healthcare providers and pharmacists anytime you get a new medicine or refill. They will tell you if your insulin dose needs to be changed.

Meals. The amount of food you eat can affect your insulin needs. If you eat less food, skip meals, or eat more food than usual, you may need a different dose of insulin. Talk to your healthcare provider if you change your diet so that you know how to adjust your APIDRA and other insulin doses.

Alcohol. Alcohol, including beer and wine, may affect the way APIDRA works and affect your blood sugar levels. Talk to your healthcare provider about drinking alcohol.

Exercise or Activity level. Exercise or activity level may change the way your body uses insulin. Check with your healthcare provider before you start an exercise program because your dose may need to be changed.

Travel. If you travel across time zones, talk with your healthcare professional about how to time your injections. When you travel, wear your medical alert identification. Take extra insulin and supplies with you.

Table 4: Severe Symptomatic Hypoglycemia

	Type 1 Diabetes Mellitus– Adult 12 weeks in combination with Lantus®*		Type 1 Diabetes Mellitus– Adult 26 weeks in combination with Lantus®***			Type 2 Diabetes Mellitus– Adult 26 weeks in combination with NPH human insulin**	
	APIDRA Pre-meal	APIDRA Post-meal	Regular Human Insulin	APIDRA	Insulin Lispro	APIDRA	Regular Human Insulin
Severe symptomatic hypoglycemia (events/month/patient)	0.05	0.05	0.13	0.02	0.02	0.00	0.00
Severe symptomatic hypoglycemia Percent of patients (n/total N)	8.4% (24/286)	8.4% (25/296)	10.1% (28/278)	4.8% (16/335)	4.0% (13/326)	1.4% (6/416)	1.2% (5/420)

*Entire treatment phase (3 months) has been included.
**Last three months of treatment have been considered.

What are the possible side effects of APIDRA and other insulins?

Hypoglycemia (low blood glucose):

Hypoglycemia is often called an "insulin reaction" or "low blood sugar". It may happen when you do not have enough sugar in your blood. Common causes of hypoglycemia are illness, emotional or physical stress, too much insulin, too little food or missed meals, and too much exercise or activity.

Early warning signs of hypoglycemia may be different, less noticeable or not noticeable at all in some people. That is why it is important to check your blood sugar as you have been advised by your healthcare provider.

Hypoglycemia can happen with:

- **The wrong insulin dose.** This can happen when too much insulin is injected. For pump users it could happen if the pump dose is too high.
- **Not enough carbohydrate (sugar or starch) intake.** This can happen if: a meal or snack is missed or delayed.
- **Vomiting or diarrhea** that decreases the amount of sugar absorbed by your body.
- **Intake of alcohol.**
- **Medicines that affect insulin.** Be sure to discuss all your medicines with your healthcare provider. **Do not start any new medicines until you know how they may affect your insulin dose.**
- **Medical conditions that can affect your blood sugar levels or insulin.** These conditions include diseases of the adrenal glands, the pituitary, the thyroid gland, the liver, and the kidney.
- **Too much glucose use by the body.** This can happen if you exercise too much or have a fever.
- **Injecting insulin the wrong way or in the wrong injection area.**

Hypoglycemia can be mild to severe. Its onset may be rapid. Some patients have few or no warning symptoms, including:

- patients with diabetes for a long time
- patients with diabetic neuropathy (nerve problems)
- or patients using certain medicines for high blood pressure or heart problems.

Hypoglycemia may reduce your ability to drive a car or use mechanical equipment and you may risk injury to yourself or others.

Severe hypoglycemia can be dangerous and can cause temporary or permanent harm to your heart or brain. **It may cause unconsciousness, seizures, or death.**

Symptoms of hypoglycemia may include:

- anxiety, irritability, restlessness, trouble concentrating, personality changes, mood changes, or other abnormal behavior
- tingling in your hands, feet, lips, or tongue
- dizziness, light-headedness, or drowsiness
- nightmares or trouble sleeping
- headache
- blurred vision
- slurred speech
- palpitations (fast heart beat)
- sweating
- tremor (shaking)
- unsteady gait (walking).

If you have hypoglycemia often or it is hard for you to know if you have the symptoms of hypoglycemia, talk to your healthcare provider.

Mild to moderate hypoglycemia can be treated by eating or drinking carbohydrates such as fruit juice, raisins, sugar candies, milk or glucose tablets. Talk to your healthcare provider about the amount of carbohydrates you should eat to treat mild to moderate hypoglycemia.

Severe hypoglycemia may require the help of another person or emergency medical people. Someone with hypoglycemia who cannot take foods or liquids with sugar by mouth needs medical help fast and will need treatment with a glucagon injection or glucose given intravenously (IV). Without medical help right away, serious reactions or even death could happen.

Hyperglycemia (high blood glucose):

Hyperglycemia occurs when you have too much sugar in your blood. Usually, it means there is not enough insulin to break down the food you eat into energy your body can use. Hyperglycemia can be caused by a fever, an infection, stress, eating more than you should, taking less insulin than prescribed, or it can mean your diabetes is getting worse.

Hyperglycemia can happen with:

- **The wrong insulin dose.** This can happen from:
  - injecting too little or no insulin
  - incorrect storage (freezing, excessive heat)
  - use after the expiration date.

For pump users this can also be caused when the bolus dose of APIDRA infusion or the basal infusion is set too low or the pump is delivering too little insulin.

- **Too much carbohydrate intake.** This can happen if you eat larger meals, eat more often or increase the amount of carbohydrate in your meals.
- **Medicines that affect insulin.** Be sure to discuss all your medicines with your healthcare provider. **Do not start any new medicines until you know how they may affect your insulin dose.**
- **Medical conditions that affect insulin.** These medical conditions include fevers, infections, heart attacks, and stress.
- **Injecting insulin the wrong way or in the wrong injection area.**

Testing your blood or urine often will let you know if you have hyperglycemia. If your tests are often high, tell your healthcare provider so your dose of medicine can be changed.

Hyperglycemia can be mild or severe. It can **progress to diabetic acidosis (DKA) (ketoacidosis) or very high glucose levels (hyperosmolar coma) and result in unconsciousness and death.**

Diabetic ketoacidosis occurs most often in patients with type 1 diabetes. It can also happen in patients with type 2 diabetes who become very sick. Because some patients get few symptoms of hyperglycemia, it is important to check your blood sugar regularly.

Symptoms of hyperglycemia include:

- confusion or drowsiness
- increased thirst
- decreased appetite, nausea, or vomiting
- rapid heart rate
- increased urination and dehydration (too little fluid in your body).

Symptoms of DKA also include:

- fruity smelling breath
- fast, deep breathing
- stomach area (abdominal) pain.

Severe or continuing hyperglycemia or DKA needs evaluation and treatment right away by your healthcare provider.

Other possible side effects of APIDRA include:

Serious allergic reactions:

Some times severe, life-threatening allergic reactions can happen with insulin. If you think you are having a severe allergic reaction, get medical help right away. Signs of insulin allergy include:

- a rash all over your body
- shortness of breath
- wheezing (trouble breathing)
- a fast pulse
- sweating
- low blood pressure.

Reactions at the injection site:

Injecting insulin can cause the following reactions on the skin at the injection site:

- a little depression in the skin (lipoatrophy)
- skin thickening (lipohypertrophy)
- red, swelling, itchy skin (injection site reaction).

You can reduce the chance of getting an injection site reaction if you change (rotate) the injection site each time. An injection site reaction should clear up in a few days or a few weeks. If injection site reactions do not go away or keep happening call your healthcare provider.

Tell your healthcare provider if you have any side effects that bother you.

These are not all the side effects of APIDRA. Ask your healthcare provider or pharmacist for more information.

How should I store APIDRA?

- **Unopened vial:**
  Store new unopened APIDRA vials in the refrigerator (not the freezer) between 36°F to 46°F (2°C to 8°C). Do not freeze APIDRA. Keep APIDRA out of direct heat and light. If a vial freezes or overheats, throw it away.
- **Open (In-Use) vial:**
  Once a vial is opened, you can keep it in the refrigerator or as cool as possible (below 77°F [25°C]), but the opened vial must be used within 28 days. If refrigeration is not possible, the open vial in use can be kept unrefrigerated for up to 28 days away from direct heat and light, as long as the temperature is not greater than 77°F (25°C). For example, do not leave it in a car on a summer day.

	Not in-use (unopened) Refrigerated	Not in-use (unopened) Room Temperature, below 77°F (25°C)	In-use (opened) Room Temperature, below 77°F (25°C)
10 mL Vial	Until expiration date	28 days	28 days, refrigerated/ room temperature

- **Insulin pump infusion sets:** Infusion sets (reservoirs, tubing, and catheters) and the APIDRA in the reservoir should be thrown away:
  - after no more than 48 hours of use or
  - after exposure to temperatures higher than 98.6°F (37°C).
- Do not use a vial of APIDRA after the expiration date stamped on the label.
- Do not use APIDRA if it is cloudy or if you see particles.

General Information about APIDRA

Use APIDRA only to treat your diabetes. **Do not** give or share APIDRA with another person, even if they have diabetes also. It may harm them.

This leaflet summarizes the most important information about APIDRA. If you would like more information, talk with your healthcare provider. You can ask your healthcare provider or pharmacist for information about APIDRA that is written for health professionals. For more information about APIDRA call 1-800-633-1610 or go to website www.aventis-us.com.

What are the ingredients in APIDRA?

Active Ingredient: insulin glulisine

Inactive Ingredients: m-cresol, tromethamine, sodium chloride, polysorbate 20, and water for injection.

Instructions for Use

How do I draw the insulin into the syringe?

- **The syringe must be new and not contain any other medicine.**
- **Do not mix APIDRA with any other type of insulin than NPH.** If you are mixing APIDRA with NPH human insulin, draw APIDRA into the syringe first. Inject the mixture right away.

Follow these steps:

1. Wash your hands.
2. Check the insulin to make sure it is clear and colorless. Do not use it after the expiration date or if it is cloudy or if you see particles.
3. If you are using a new vial, remove the protective cap. **Do not** remove the stopper.
4. Wipe the top of the vial with an alcohol swab. You do not have to shake the vial of APIDRA before use.
5. Use a new needle and syringe every time you take a dose. Use disposable syringes and needles only once. Throw them away properly. **Never** share needles and syringes.
6. Draw air into the syringe equal to your insulin dose. Put the needle through the rubber top of the vial and push the plunger to inject the air into the vial.
7. Leave the syringe in the vial and turn both upside down. Hold the syringe and vial firmly in one hand.
8. Make sure the tip of the needle is in the insulin. With your free hand, pull the plunger to withdraw the correct dose into the syringe.
9. Before you take the needle out of the vial, check the syringe for air bubbles. If bubbles are in the syringe, hold the syringe straight up and tap the side of the syringe until the bubbles float to the top. Push the bubbles out with the plunger and draw insulin back in until you have the correct dose. If you are mixing APIDRA with NPH insulin check with your healthcare professional on how to mix.
10. Remove the needle from the vial. Do not let the needle touch anything. You are now ready to inject.

How do I inject APIDRA?

Inject APIDRA under your skin. Take APIDRA as prescribed by your healthcare provider.

You should look at the medicine in the vial. If the medicine is cloudy or has particles in it, do not use it. Contact your healthcare provider. Use a new vial.

Follow these steps:

1. Decide on an injection area - either upper arm, thigh or abdomen. Injection sites within an injection area must be different from one injection to the next.
2. Use alcohol or soap and water to clean the skin where you are going to inject. The injection site should be dry before you inject.
3. Pinch the skin. Stick the needle in the way your healthcare provider showed you. Release the skin.
4. Slowly push in the plunger of the syringe all the way, making sure you have injected all the insulin. Leave the needle in the skin for about 10 seconds.
   Pull the needle straight out and gently press on the spot where you injected yourself for several seconds. **Do not rub the area.**
5. Follow your healthcare provider's instructions for throwing away the needle and syringe. Do not recap the syringe. Used needle and syringe should be placed in sharps containers (such as red biohazard containers), hard plastic containers (such as detergent bottles), or metal containers (such as an empty coffee can). Such containers should be sealed and disposed of properly.

How should I infuse APIDRA with an external subcutaneous insulin infusion pump?

Do not mix APIDRA with any other insulin or liquid when used in a pump.

- APIDRA is recommended for use in the following pumps and infusion sets: Disetronic® H-Tron® plus V100 and D-Tron® with Disetronic catheters (Rapid™, Rapid C™, Rapid D™, and Tender™); MiniMed® Models 506, 507, 507c and 508 with MiniMed catheters (Sof-set Ultimate QR™, and Quick-set™)‡. Refer to the instruction manual of your specific pump on proper use of insulin in a pump. Call your healthcare provider if you have questions about using the pump.
- If the pump or infusion set does not work right you may not receive the right dose of insulin. Hypoglycemia, hyperglycemia or ketosis can happen. Problems should be identified and corrected as quickly as possible, see instruction manual for your pump. Because APIDRA starts working faster and does not work as long, you may have less time to identify and correct the problem than with regular insulin.
- If you start using APIDRA by pump infusion, you may need to adjust your insulin doses. Check with your healthcare provider.
- You must use insulin from a new vial of APIDRA if unexplained hyperglycemia happens, or if pump alarms do not respond to all of the following:
- a repeat dose (injection or bolus) of APIDRA
- a change in the infusion set, including the reservoir with APIDRA
- a change in the infusion site.

Continued on next page

Apidra—Cont.

If these actions do not work, you may need to restart your injections with syringes and you must call your healthcare provider. Continue to check your blood sugar often.

The infusion set, reservoir with insulin, and infusion site should be changed:

- every 48 hours or less
- when unexpected hyperglycemia or ketosis occurs
- when alarms sound, as specified by your pump manual
- if the insulin has been exposed to temperatures over 98.6°F (37°C). If the insulin or pump could have absorbed radiant heat, for example from sunlight, that would heat the insulin to over 98.6°F (37°C). Dark colored pump cases or sport covers can increase this type of heat. The location where the pump is worn may affect the temperature.
- Patients who get skin reactions at the infusion site may need to change infusion sites more often.

ADDITIONAL INFORMATION

DIABETES FORECAST is a national magazine designed especially for patients with diabetes and their families and is available by subscription from the American Diabetes Association, National Service Center, 1701 N. Beauregard Street, Alexandria, Virginia 22311, 1-800-DIABETES (1-800-342-2383). You may also visit the ADA website at www.diabetes.org.

Another publication, **DIABETES COUNTDOWN**, is available from the Juvenile Diabetes Research Foundation International (JDRF), 120 Wall Street, 19th Floor, New York, New York 10005, 1-800-JDF-CURE (1-800-533-2873). You may also visit the JDRF website at www.jdf.org.

To get more information about diabetes, check with your healthcare professional or diabetes educator or visit www.DiabetesWatch.com.

Rev. April 2004a
Aventis Pharmaceuticals Inc.
Kansas City, MO 64137 USA

† Lantus® is a registered trademark of Aventis Pharmaceuticals Inc.

‡ The brands listed are the registered trademarks of their respective owners and are not trademarks of Aventis Pharmaceuticals Inc.

ARAVA® Tablets ℞

[ă-ră-vă]
(leflunomide)
10 mg, 20 mg, 100 mg
Rev. November 2004
Rx only

Prescribing information for this product, which appears on pages 693–699 of the 2005 PDR, has been completely revised as follows. Please write "See Supplement A" next to the product heading.

CONTRAINDICATIONS AND WARNINGS

PREGNANCY MUST BE EXCLUDED BEFORE THE START OF TREATMENT WITH ARAVA. ARAVA IS CONTRAINDICATED IN PREGNANT WOMEN, OR WOMEN OF CHILDBEARING POTENTIAL WHO ARE NOT USING RELIABLE CONTRACEPTION. (SEE CONTRAINDICATIONS AND WARNINGS.) PREGNANCY MUST BE AVOIDED DURING ARAVA TREATMENT OR PRIOR TO THE COMPLETION OF THE DRUG ELIMINATION PROCEDURE AFTER ARAVA TREATMENT.

DESCRIPTION

ARAVA® (leflunomide) is a pyrimidine synthesis inhibitor. The chemical name for leflunomide is N-(4′-trifluoromethylphenyl)-5-methylisoxazole-4-carboxamide. It has an empirical formula $C_{12}H_9F_3N_2O_2$, a molecular weight of 270.2 and the following structural formula:

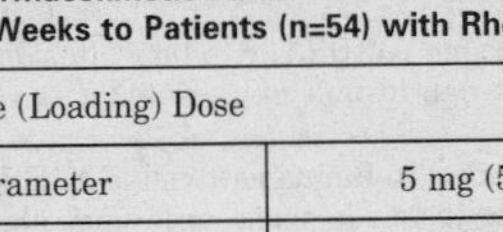

ARAVA is available for oral administration as tablets containing 10, 20, or 100 mg of active drug. Combined with leflunomide are the following inactive ingredients: colloidal silicon dioxide, crospovidone, hypromellose, lactose monohydrate, magnesium stearate, polyethylene glycol, povidone, starch, talc, titanium dioxide, and yellow ferric oxide (20 mg tablet only).

CLINICAL PHARMACOLOGY

Mechanism of Action

Leflunomide is an isoxazole immunomodulatory agent which inhibits dihydroorotate dehydrogenase (an enzyme involved in de novo pyrimidine synthesis) and has antiproliferative activity. Several *in vivo* and *in vitro* experimental models have demonstrated an anti-inflammatory effect.

Pharmacokinetics

Following oral administration, leflunomide is metabolized to an active metabolite A77 1726 (hereafter referred to as M1) which is responsible for essentially all of its activity *in vivo*. Plasma levels of leflunomide are occasionally seen, at very low levels. Studies of the pharmacokinetics of leflunomide have primarily examined the plasma concentrations of this active metabolite.

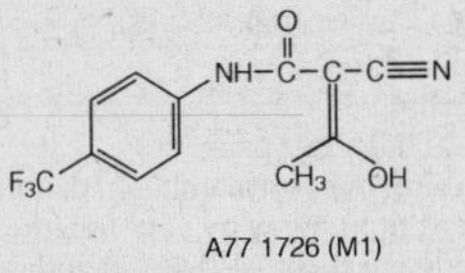

A77 1726 (M1)

Absorption

Following oral administration, peak levels of the active metabolite, M1, occurred between 6-12 hours after dosing. Due to the very long half-life of M1 (~2 weeks), a loading dose of 100 mg for 3 days was used in clinical studies to facilitate the rapid attainment of steady-state levels of M1. Without a loading dose, it is estimated that attainment of steady-state plasma concentrations would require nearly two months of dosing. The resulting plasma concentrations following both loading doses and continued clinical dosing indicate that M1 plasma levels are dose proportional.

[See table 1 below]

Relative to an oral solution, ARAVA tablets are 80% bioavailable. Co-administration of leflunomide tablets with a high fat meal did not have a significant impact on M1 plasma levels.

Distribution

M1 has a low volume of distribution (Vss = 0.13 L/kg) and is extensively bound (>99.3%) to albumin in healthy subjects. Protein binding has been shown to be linear at therapeutic concentrations. The free fraction of M1 is slightly higher in patients with rheumatoid arthritis and approximately doubled in patients with chronic renal failure; the mechanism and significance of these increases are unknown.

Metabolism

Leflunomide is metabolized to one primary (M1) and many minor metabolites. Of these minor metabolites, only 4-trifluoromethylaniline (TFMA) is quantifiable, occurring at low levels in the plasma of some patients. The parent compound is rarely detectable in plasma. At the present time the specific site of leflunomide metabolism is unknown. *In vivo* and *in vitro* studies suggest a role for both the GI wall and the liver in drug metabolism. No specific enzyme has been identified as the primary route of metabolism for leflunomide; however, hepatic cytosolic and microsomal cellular fractions have been identified as sites of drug metabolism.

Elimination

The active metabolite M1 is eliminated by further metabolism and subsequent renal excretion as well as by direct biliary excretion. In a 28 day study of drug elimination (n=3) using a single dose of radiolabeled compound, approximately 43% of the total radioactivity was eliminated in the urine and 48% was eliminated in the feces. Subsequent analysis of the samples revealed the primary urinary metabolites to be leflunomide glucuronides and an oxanilic acid derivative of M1. The primary fecal metabolite was M1. Of these two routes of elimination, renal elimination is more significant over the first 96 hours after which fecal elimination begins to predominate. In a study involving the intravenous administration of M1, the clearance was estimated to be 31 mL/hr.

In small studies using activated charcoal (n=1) or cholestyramine (n=3) to facilitate drug elimination, the *in vivo* plasma half-life of M1 was reduced from >1 week to approximately 1 day. (See **PRECAUTIONS – General – Need for Drug Elimination**). Similar reductions in plasma half-life were observed for a series of volunteers (n=96) enrolled in pharmacokinetic trials who were given cholestyramine. This suggests that biliary recycling is a major contributor to the long elimination half-life of M1. Studies with both hemodialysis and CAPD (chronic ambulatory peritoneal dialysis) indicate that M1 is not dialyzable.

Special Populations

Gender. Gender has not been shown to cause a consistent change in the *in vivo* pharmacokinetics of M1.

Age. Age has been shown to cause a change in the *in vivo* pharmacokinetics of M1 (see **CLINICAL PHARMACOLOGY – Special Populations – *Pediatrics***).

Smoking. A population based pharmacokinetic analysis of the phase III data indicates that smokers have a 38% increase in clearance over nonsmokers; however, no difference in clinical efficacy was seen between smokers and nonsmokers.

Chronic Renal Insufficiency. In single dose studies in patients (n=6) with chronic renal insufficiency requiring either chronic ambulatory peritoneal dialysis (CAPD) or hemodialysis, neither had a significant impact on circulating levels of M1. The free fraction of M1 was almost doubled, but the mechanism of this increase is not known. In light of the fact that the kidney plays a role in drug elimination, and without adequate studies of leflunomide use in subjects with renal insufficiency, caution should be used when ARAVA is administered to these patients.

Hepatic Insufficiency. Studies of the effect of hepatic insufficiency on M1 pharmacokinetics have not been done. Given the need to metabolize leflunomide into the active species, the role of the liver in drug elimination/recycling, and the possible risk of increased hepatic toxicity, the use of leflunomide in patients with hepatic insufficiency is not recommended.

Pediatrics

The pharmacokinetics of M1 following oral administration of leflunomide have been investigated in 73 pediatric patients with polyarticular course Juvenile Rheumatoid Arthritis (JRA) who ranged in age from 3 to 17 years. The results of a population pharmacokinetic analysis of these trials have demonstrated that pediatric patients with body weights ≤40 kg have a reduced clearance of M1 (see Table 2) relative to adult rheumatoid arthritis patients.

Table 2: Population Pharmacokinetic Estimate of M1 Clearance Following Oral Administration of Leflunomide in Pediatric Patients with Polyarticular Course JRA Mean ± SD [Range]

N	Body Weight (kg)	CL (mL/h)
10	<20	18 ± 9.8 [6.8-37]
30	20-40	18 ± 9.5 [4.2-43]
33	>40	26 ± 16 [9.7-93.6]

Drug Interactions

In vivo drug interaction studies have demonstrated a lack of a significant drug interaction between leflunomide and tri-phasic oral contraceptives, and cimetidine.

In vitro studies of protein binding indicated that warfarin did not affect M1 protein binding. At the same time M1 was shown to cause increases ranging from 13-50% in the free fraction of diclofenac, ibuprofen and tolbutamide at concentrations in the clinical range. *In vitro* studies of drug metabolism indicate that M1 inhibits CYP 450 2C9, which is responsible for the metabolism of phenytoin, tolbutamide, warfarin and many NSAIDs. M1 has been shown to inhibit the formation of 4-hydroxydiclofenac from diclofenac *in vitro*. The clinical significance of these findings with regard to phenytoin and tolbutamide is unknown, however, there was extensive concomitant use of NSAIDs in the clinical studies and no differential effect was observed. (See **PRECAUTIONS – Drug Interactions**).

Methotrexate. Coadministration, in 30 patients, of ARAVA (100 mg/day × 2 days followed by 10-20 mg/day) with methotrexate (10 - 25 mg/week, with folate) demonstrated no pharmacokinetic interaction between the two drugs. However, co-administration increased risk of hepatotoxicity (see **PRECAUTIONS – Drug Interactions – Hepatotoxic Drugs**).

Rifampin. Following concomitant administration of a single dose of ARAVA to subjects receiving multiple doses of rifampin, M1 peak levels were increased (~40%) over those seen when ARAVA was given alone. Because of the potential for ARAVA levels to continue to increase with multiple dosing, caution should be used if patients are to receive both ARAVA and rifampin.

CLINICAL STUDIES

A. ADULTS

The efficacy of ARAVA in the treatment of rheumatoid arthritis (RA) was demonstrated in three controlled trials showing reduction in signs and symptoms, and inhibition of structural damage. In two placebo controlled trials, efficacy was demonstrated for improvement in physical function.

1. Reduction of signs and symptoms

Relief of signs and symptoms was assessed using the American College of Rheumatology (ACR)20 Responder Index, a composite of clinical, laboratory, and functional measures in rheumatoid arthritis. An "ACR20 Responder" is a patient who had ≥ 20% improvement in both tender and swollen joint counts and in 3 of the following 5 criteria: physician global assessment, patient global assessment, functional ability measure [Modified Health Assessment Questionnaire (MHAQ)], visual analog pain scale, and erythrocyte sedimentation rate or C-reactive protein. An "ACR20 Re-

Table 1. Pharmacokinetic Parameters for M1 after Administration of Leflunomide at Doses of 5, 10, and 25 mg/day for 24 Weeks to Patients (n=54) with Rheumatoid Arthritis (Mean ± SD) (Study YU204)

Maintenance (Loading) Dose

Parameter	5 mg (50 mg)	10 mg (100 mg)	25 mg (100 mg)
C_{24} (Day 1) (μg/mL)[1]	4.0 ± 0.6	8.4 ± 2.1	8.5 ± 2.2
C_{24} (ss) (μg/mL)[2]	8.8 ± 2.9	18 ± 9.6	63 ± 36
$t_{1/2}$ (DAYS)	15 ± 3	14 ± 5	18 ± 9

[1] Concentration at 24 hours after loading dose
[2] Concentration at 24 hours after maintenance doses at steady state

Table 3: Withdrawals in US301

	n(%) patients		
	Leflunomide 190	Placebo 128	Methotrexate 190
Withdrawals in Year-1			
Lack of efficacy	33 (17.4)	70 (54.7)	50 (26.3)
Safety	44 (23.2)	12 (9.4)	22 (11.6)
Other[1]	15 (7.9)	10 (7.8)	17 (9.0)
Total	92 (48.4)	92 (71.9)	89 (46.8)
Patients entering Year 2	98	36	101
Withdrawals in Year-2			
Lack of efficacy	4 (4.1)	1 (2.8)	4 (4.0)
Safety	8 (8.2)	0 (0.0)	10 (9.9)
Other[1]	3 (3.1)	8 (22.2)	7 (6.9)
Total	15 (15.3)	9 (25.0)	21 (20.8)

[1]Includes: lost to follow up, protocol violation, noncompliance, voluntary withdrawal, investigator discretion.

Table 4: Withdrawals in study MN301/303/305

	n(%) patients		
	Leflunomide 133	Placebo 92	Sulfasalazine 133
Withdrawals in MN301 (Mo 0-6)			
Lack of efficacy	10 (7.5)	29 (31.5)	14 (10.5)
Safety	19 (14.3)	6 (6.5)	25 (18.8)
Other[1]	8 (6.0)	6 (6.5)	11 (8.3)
Total	37 (27.8)	41 (44.6)	50 (37.6)
Patients entering MN303	80		76
Withdrawals in MN303 (Mo 7-12)			
Lack of efficacy	4 (5.0)		2 (2.6)
Safety	2 (2.5)		5 (6.6)
Other[1]	3 (3.8)		1 (1.3)
Total	9 (11.3)		8 (10.5)
Patients entering MN305	60		60
Withdrawals in MN305 (Mo 13-24)			
Lack of efficacy	0 (0.0)		3 (5.0)
Safety	6 (10.0)		8 (13.3)
Other[1]	1 (1.7)		2 (3.3)
Total	7 (11.7)		13 (21.7)

[1]Includes: lost to follow up, protocol violation, noncompliance, voluntary withdrawal, investigator discretion.

Table 5: Withdrawals in MN302/304

	n(%) patients	
	Leflunomide 501	Methotrexate 498
Withdrawals in MN302 (Year-1)		
Lack of efficacy	37 (7.4)	15 (3.0)
Safety	98 (19.6)	79 (15.9)
Other[1]	17 (3.4)	17 (3.4)
Total	152 (30.3)	111 (22.3)
Patients entering MN304	292	320
Withdrawals in MN304 (Year-2)		
Lack of efficacy	13 (4.5)	9 (2.8)
Safety	11 (3.8)	22 (6.9)
Other[1]	12 (4.1)	12 (3.8)
Total	36 (12.3)	43 (13.4)

[1] Includes: lost to follow up, protocol violation, noncompliance, voluntary withdrawal, investigator discretion.

sponder at Endpoint" is a patient who completed the study and was an ACR20 Responder at the completion of the study.

2. Inhibition of structural damage
Inhibition of structural damage compared to control was assessed using the Sharp Score (Sharp, JT. Scoring Radiographic Abnormalities in Rheumatoid Arthritis, Radiologic Clinics of North America, 1996; vol. 34, pp. 233-241), a composite score of X-ray erosions and joint space narrowing in hands/wrists and forefeet.

3. Improvement in physical function
Improvement in physical function was assessed using the Health Assessment Questionnaire (HAQ) and the Medical Outcomes Survey Short Form (SF-36). In all Arava monotherapy studies, an initial loading dose of 100 mg per day for three days only was used followed by 20 mg per day thereafter.

US301 Clinical Trial in Adults
Study US301, a 2 year study, randomized 482 patients with active RA of at least 6 months duration to leflunomide 20 mg/day (n=182), methotrexate 7.5 mg/week increasing to 15 mg/week (n=182), or placebo (n=118). All patients received folate 1 mg BID. Primary analysis was at 52 weeks with blinded treatment to 104 weeks.
Overall, 235 of the 508 randomized treated patients (482 in primary data analysis and an additional 26 patients), continued into a second 12 months of double-blind treatment (98 leflunomide, 101 methotrexate, 36 placebo). Leflunomide dose continued at 20 mg/day and the methotrexate dose could be increased to a maximum of 20 mg/

week. In total, 190 patients (83 leflunomide, 80 methotrexate, 27 placebo) completed 2 years of double-blind treatment.
The rate and reason for withdrawal is summarized in Table 3.
[See table 3 above]

MN301/303/305 Clinical Trial in Adults
Study MN301 randomized 358 patients with active RA to leflunomide 20 mg/day (n=133), sulfasalazine 2.0 g/day (n=133), or placebo (n=92). Treatment duration was 24 weeks. An extension of the study was an optional 6-month blinded continuation of MN301 without the placebo arm, resulting in a 12-month comparison of leflunomide and sulfasalazine (study MN303).
Of the 168 patients who completed 12 months of treatment in MN301 and MN303, 146 patients (87%) entered a 1-year extension study of double blind active treatment (MN305; 60 leflunomide, 60 sulfasalazine, 26 placebo/sulfasalazine). Patients continued on the same daily dosage of leflunomide or sulfasalazine that they had been taking at the completion of MN301/303. A total of 121 patients (53 leflunomide, 47 sulfasalazine, 21 placebo/sulfasalazine) completed the 2 years of double-blind treatment.
Patient withdrawal data in MN301/303/305 is summarized in Table 4.
[See table 4 above]

MN302/304 Clinical Trial in Adults
Study MN302 randomized 999 patients with active RA to leflunomide 20 mg/day (n=501) or methotrexate at 7.5 mg/

week increasing to 15 mg/week (n=498). Folate supplementation was used in 10% of patients. Treatment duration was 52 weeks.
Of the 736 patients who completed 52 weeks of treatment in study MN302, 612 (83%) entered the double-blind, 1-year extension study MN304 (292 leflunomide; 320 methotrexate). Patients continued on the same daily dosage of leflunomide or methotrexate that they had been taking at the completion of MN302. There were 533 patients (256 leflunomide, 277 methotrexate) who completed 2 years of double-blind treatment.
Patient withdrawal data in MN302/304 is summarized in Table 5.
[See table 5 at left]

Clinical Trial Data
1. Signs and symptoms Rheumatoid Arthritis
The ACR20 Responder at Endpoint rates are shown in Figure 1. ARAVA was statistically significantly superior to placebo in reducing the signs and symptoms of RA by the primary efficacy analysis, ACR20 Responder at Endpoint, in study US301 (at the primary 12 months endpoint) and MN301 (at 6 month endpoint). ACR20 Responder at Endpoint rates with ARAVA treatment were consistent across the 6 and 12 month studies (41-49%). No consistent differences were demonstrated between leflunomide and methotrexate or between leflunomide and sulfasalazine. ARAVA treatment effect was evident by 1 month, stabilized by 3 - 6 months, and continued throughout the course of treatment as shown in Figure 2.

Figure 1

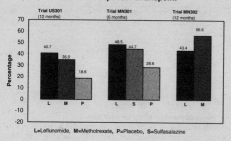

% ACR 20 Responder at Endpoint

L=Leflunomide, M=Methotrexate, P=Placebo, S=Sulfasalazine

	Comparisons	95% Confidence Interval	p Value
US301	Leflunomide vs. Placebo	(12, 32)	<0.0001
	Methotrexate vs. Placebo	(8, 30)	<0.0001
	Leflunomide vs. Methotrexate	(-4, 16)	NS
MN301	Leflunomide vs. Placebo	(7, 33)	0.0026
	Sulfasalazine vs. Placebo	(4, 29)	0.0121
	Leflunomide vs. Sulfasalazine	(-8, 16)	NS
MN302	Leflunomide vs. Methotrexate	(-19, -7)	<0.0001

Figure 2

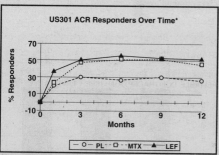

US301 ACR Responders Over Time*

PL --- MTX --- LEF

*Last Observation Carried Forward.

ACR50 and ACR70 Responders are defined in an analogous manner to the ACR 20 Responder, but use improvements of 50% or 70%, respectively (Table 6). Mean change for the individual components of the ACR Responder Index are shown in Table 7.
[See table 6 at top of next page]
Table 7 shows the results of the components of the ACR response criteria for US301, MN301, and MN302. ARAVA was significantly superior to placebo in all components of the ACR Response criteria in study US301 and MN301. In addition, Arava was significantly superior to placebo in improving morning stiffness, a measure of RA disease activity, not included in the ACR Response criteria. No consistent differences were demonstrated between ARAVA and the active comparators.
[See table 7 at top of next page]

Maintenance of effect
After completing 12 months of treatment, patients continuing on study treatment were evaluated for an additional 12 months of double-blind treatment (total treatment period of 2 years) in studies US301, MN305, and MN304. ACR Responder rates at 12 months were maintained over 2 years in most patients continuing a second year of treatment.
Improvement from baseline in the individual components of the ACR responder criteria was also sustained in most patients during the second year of Arava treatment in all three trials.

Continued on next page

Arava—Cont.

2. Inhibition of structural damage

The change from baseline to endpoint in progression of structural disease, as measured by the Sharp X-ray score, is displayed in Figure 3. ARAVA was statistically significantly superior to placebo in inhibiting the progression of disease by the Sharp Score. No consistent differences were demonstrated between leflunomide and methotrexate or between leflunomide and sulfasalazine.

Figure 3

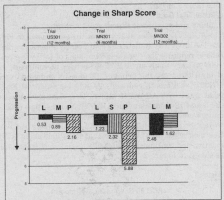

Change in Sharp Score

L= Leflunomide; M=methotrexate; S=sulfasalazine; P=placebo

	Comparisons	95% Confidence Interval	p Value
US301	Leflunomide vs. Placebo	(-4.0, -1.1)	0.0007
	Methotrexate vs. Placebo	(-2.6, -0.2)	0.0196
	Leflunomide vs. Methotrexate	(-2.3, 0.0)	0.0499
MN301	Leflunomide vs. Placebo	(-6.2, -1.8)	0.0004
	Sulfasalazine vs. Placebo	(-6.9, 0.0)	0.0484
	Leflunomide vs. Sulfasalazine	(-3.3, 1.2)	NS
MN302	Leflunomide vs. Methotrexate	(-2.2, 7.4)	NS

3. Improvement in physical function

The Health Assessment Questionnaire (HAQ) assesses a patient's physical function and degree of disability. The mean change from baseline in functional ability as measured by the HAQ Disability Index (HAQ DI) in the 6 and 12 month placebo and active controlled trials is shown in Figure 4. ARAVA was statistically significantly superior to placebo in improving physical function. Superiority to placebo was demonstrated consistently across all eight HAQ DI subscales (dressing, arising, eating, walking, hygiene, reach, grip and activities) in both placebo controlled studies.

The Medical Outcomes Survey Short Form 36 (SF-36), a generic health-related quality of life questionnaire, further addresses physical function. In US301, at 12 months, ARAVA provided statistically significant improvements compared to placebo in the Physical Component Summary (PCS) Score.

Figure 4

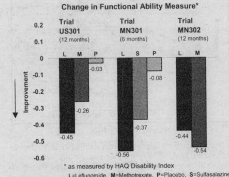

Change in Functional Ability Measure*

* as measured by HAQ Disability Index
L=Leflunomide, M=Methotrexate, P=Placebo, S=Sulfasalazine

	Comparison	95% Confidence Interval	p Value
US301	Leflunomide vs. Placebo	(-0.58, -0.29)	0.0001
	Leflunomide vs. Methotrexate	(-0.34, -0.07)	0.0026
MN301	Leflunomide vs. Placebo	(-0.67, -0.36)	<0.0001
	Leflunomide vs. Sulfasalazine	(-0.33, -0.03)	0.0163
MN302	Leflunomide vs. Methotrexate	(0.01, 0.16)	0.0221

Maintenance of effect

The improvement in physical function demonstrated at 6 and 12 months was maintained over two years. In those patients continuing therapy for a second year, this improvement in physical function as measured by HAQ and SF-36 (PCS) was maintained.

B. PEDIATRICS

Clinical Trials in Pediatrics

ARAVA was studied in a single multicenter, double-blind, active-controlled trial in 94 patients (1:1 randomization) with polyarticular course juvenile rheumatoid arthritis (JRA) as defined by the American College of Rheumatology (ACR). Approximately 68% of pediatric patients receiving ARAVA, versus 89% of pediatric patients receiving the active comparator, improved by Week 16 (end-of-study) employing the JRA Definition of Improvement (DOI) ≥ 30 % responder endpoint. In this trial, the loading dose and maintenance dose of ARAVA was based on three weight categories: <20 kg, 20-40kg, and ≥40 kg. The response rate

Table 6. Summary of ACR Response Rates*

Study and Treatment Group	ACR20	ACR50	ACR70
Placebo-Controlled Studies			
US301 (12 months)			
Leflunomide (n=178)[†]	52.2[‡]	34.3[‡]	20.2[‡]
Placebo (n=118)[†]	26.3	7.6	4.2
Methotrexate (n=180)[†]	45.6	22.8	9.4
MN301 (6 months)			
Leflunomide (n=130)[†]	54.6[‡]	33.1[‡]	10.0[§]
Placebo (n=91)[†]	28.6	14.3	2.2
Sulfasalazine (n=132)[†]	56.8	30.3	7.6
Non-Placebo Active-Controlled Studies			
MN302 (12 months)			
Leflunomide (n=495)[†]	51.1	31.1	9.9
Methotrexate (n=489)[†]	65.2	43.8	16.4

* Intent to treat (ITT) analysis using last observation carried forward (LOCF) technique for patients who discontinued early.
[†] N is the number of ITT patients for whom adequate data were available to calculate the indicated rates.
[‡] p<0.001 leflunomide vs placebo
[§] p<0.02 leflunomide vs placebo

Table 7. Mean Change in the Components of the ACR Responder Index*

Components	Placebo-Controlled Studies						Non-placebo Controlled Study	
	US301 (12 months)			MN301 Non-US (6 months)			MN302 Non-US (12 months)	
	Leflunomide	Methotrexate	Placebo	Leflunomide	Sulfasalazine	Placebo	Leflunomide	Methotrexate
Tender joint count[1]	-7.7	-6.6	-3.0	-9.7	-8.1	-4.3	-8.3	-9.7
Swollen joint count[1]	-5.7	-5.4	-2.9	-7.2	-6.2	-3.4	-6.8	-9.0
Patient global assessment[2]	-2.1	-1.5	0.1	-2.8	-2.6	-0.9	-2.3	-3.0
Physician global assessment[2]	-2.8	-2.4	-1.0	-2.7	-2.5	-0.8	-2.3	-3.1
Physical function/ disability (MHAQ/ HAQ)	-0.29	-0.15	0.07	-0.50	-0.29	-0.04	-0.37	-0.44
Pain intensity[2]	-2.2	-1.7	-0.5	-2.7	-2.0	-0.9	-2.1	-2.9
Erythrocyte Sedimentation rate	-6.26	-6.48	2.56	-7.48	-16.56	3.44	-10.12	-22.18
C-reactive protein	-0.62	-0.50	0.47	-2.26	-1.19	0.16	-1.86	-2.45
Not included in the ACR Responder Index								
Morning Stiffness (min)	-101.4	-88.7	14.7	-93.0	-42.4	-6.8	-63.7	-86.6

* Last Observation Carried Forward; Negative Change Indicates Improvement
[1] Based on 28 joint count
[2] Visual Analog Scale - 0=Best; 10=Worst

to ARAVA in pediatric patients ≤40 kg was less robust than in pediatric patients >40 kg suggesting suboptimal dosing in smaller weight pediatric patients, as studied, resulting in less than efficacious plasma concentrations, despite reduced clearance of M1. (See **PHARMACOKINETICS – Pediatrics**).

INDICATIONS AND USAGE

ARAVA is indicated in adults for the treatment of active rheumatoid arthritis (RA):
1. to reduce signs and symptoms
2. to inhibit structural damage as evidenced by X-ray erosions and joint space narrowing
3. to improve physical function.
(see **CLINICAL STUDIES**)

Aspirin, nonsteroidal anti-inflammatory agents and/or low dose corticosteroids may be continued during treatment with ARAVA (see **PRECAUTIONS – Drug Interactions – NSAIDs**). The combined use of ARAVA with antimalarials, intramuscular or oral gold, D penicillamine, azathioprine, or methotrexate has not been adequately studied. (See **WARNINGS – Immunosuppression Potential/Bone Marrow Suppression**)

CONTRAINDICATIONS

ARAVA is contraindicated in patients with known hypersensitivity to leflunomide or any of the other components of ARAVA.

ARAVA can cause fetal harm when administered to a pregnant woman. Leflunomide, when administered orally to rats during organogenesis at a dose of 15 mg/kg, was teratogenic (most notably anophthalmia or microophthalmia and inter-

nal hydrocephalus). The systemic exposure of rats at this dose was approximately 1/10 the human exposure level based on AUC. Under these exposure conditions, leflunomide also caused a decrease in the maternal body weight and an increase in embryolethality with a decrease in fetal body weight for surviving fetuses. In rabbits, oral treatment with 10 mg/kg of leflunomide during organogenesis resulted in fused, dysplastic sternebrae. The exposure level at this dose was essentially equivalent to the maximum human exposure level based on AUC. At a 1 mg/kg dose, leflunomide was not teratogenic in rats and rabbits. When female rats were treated with 1.25 mg/kg of leflunomide beginning 14 days before mating and continuing until the end of lactation, the offspring exhibited marked (greater than 90%) decreases in postnatal survival. The systemic exposure level at 1.25 mg/kg was approximately 1/100 the human exposure level based on AUC.

ARAVA is contraindicated in women who are or may become pregnant. If this drug is used during pregnancy, or if the patient becomes pregnant while taking this drug, the patient should be apprised of the potential hazard to the fetus.

WARNINGS

Immunosuppression Potential/Bone Marrow Suppression

ARAVA is not recommended for patients with severe immunodeficiency, bone marrow dysplasia, or severe, uncontrolled infections. In the event that a serious infection occurs, it may be necessary to interrupt therapy with ARAVA and administer cholestyramine or charcoal (see **PRECAUTIONS – General – Need for Drug Elimination**). Medications like leflunomide that have immunosuppression potential may cause patients to be more susceptible to infections, including opportunistic infections. Rarely, severe infections including sepsis, which may be fatal, have been reported in patients receiving ARAVA. Most of the reports were confounded by concomitant immunosuppressant therapy and/or comorbid illness which, in addition to rheumatoid disease, may predispose patients to infection.

There have been rare reports of pancytopenia, agranulocytosis and thrombocytopenia in patients receiving ARAVA alone. These events have been reported most frequently in patients who received concomitant treatment with methotrexate or other immunosuppressive agents, or who had recently discontinued these therapies; in some cases, patients had a prior history of a significant hematologic abnormality.

Patients taking ARAVA should have platelet, white blood cell count and hemoglobin or hematocrit monitored at baseline and monthly for six months following initiation of therapy and every 6 to 8 weeks thereafter. If used with concomitant methotrexate and/or other potential immunosuppressive agents, chronic monitoring should be monthly. If evidence of bone marrow suppression occurs in a patient taking ARAVA, treatment with ARAVA should be stopped, and cholestyramine or charcoal should be used to reduce the plasma concentration of leflunomide active metabolite (see **PRECAUTIONS – General – Need for Drug Elimination**).

In any situation in which the decision is made to switch from ARAVA to another anti-rheumatic agent with a known potential for hematologic suppression, it would be prudent to monitor for hematologic toxicity, because there will be overlap of systemic exposure to both compounds. ARAVA washout with cholestyramine or charcoal may decrease this risk, but also may induce disease worsening if the patient had been responding to ARAVA treatment.

Hepatotoxicity

RARE CASES OF SEVERE LIVER INJURY, INCLUDING CASES WITH FATAL OUTCOME, HAVE BEEN REPORTED DURING TREATMENT WITH LEFLUNOMIDE. MOST CASES OF SEVERE LIVER INJURY OCCUR WITHIN 6 MONTHS OF THERAPY AND IN A SETTING OF MULTIPLE RISK FACTORS FOR HEPATOTOXICITY (liver disease, other hepatotoxins). (See PRECAUTIONS).

At minimum, ALT (SGPT) must be performed at baseline and monitored initially at monthly intervals during the first six months then, if stable, every 6 to 8 weeks thereafter. In addition, if ARAVA and methotrexate are given concomitantly, ACR guidelines for monitoring methotrexate liver toxicity must be followed with ALT, AST, and serum albumin testing monthly.

Guidelines for dose adjustment or discontinuation based on the severity and persistence of ALT elevation are recommended as follows: For confirmed ALT elevations between 2- and 3-fold ULN, dose reduction to 10 mg/day may allow continued administration of ARAVA under close monitoring. If elevations between 2- and 3-fold ULN persist despite dose reduction or if ALT elevations of >3-fold ULN are present, ARAVA should be discontinued and cholestyramine or charcoal should be administered (see **PRECAUTIONS – General – Need for Drug Elimination**) with close monitoring, including retreatment with cholestyramine or charcoal as indicated.

In clinical trials, ARAVA treatment as monotherapy or in combination with methotrexate was associated with elevations of liver enzymes, primarily ALT and AST, in a significant number of patients; these effects were generally reversible. Most transaminase elevations were mild (≤ 2-fold ULN) and usually resolved while continuing treatment. Marked elevations (>3-fold ULN) occurred infrequently and reversed with dose reduction or discontinuation of treatment. Table 8 shows liver enzyme elevations seen with monthly monitoring in clinical trials US301 and MN301. It was notable that the absence of folate use in MN302 was associated with a considerably greater incidence of liver enzyme elevation on methotrexate.

[See table 8 above]

Table 8. Liver Enzyme Elevations >3-fold Upper Limits of Normal (ULN)

	US301			MN301			MN302*	
	LEF	**PL**	**MTX**	**LEF**	**PL**	**SSZ**	**LEF**	**MTX**
ALT (SGPT)								
>3-fold ULN	8	3	5	2	1	2	13	83
(n %)	(4.4)	(2.5)	(2.7)	(1.5)	(1.1)	(1.5)	(2.6)	(16.7)
Reversed to ≤2-fold ULN:	8	3	5	2	1	2	12	82
Timing of Elevation								
0-3 Months	6	1	1	2	1	2	7	27
4-6 Months	1	1	3	—	—	—	1	34
7-9 Months	1	1	1	—	—	—	—	16
10-12 Months	—	—	—	—	—	—	5	6

*Only 10% of patients in MN302 received folate. All patients in US301 received folate.

In a 6 month study of 263 patients with persistent active rheumatoid arthritis despite methotrexate therapy, and with normal LFTs, leflunomide was added to a group of 133 patients starting at 10 mg per day and increased to 20 mg as needed. An increase in ALT greater than or equal to three times the ULN was observed in 3.8% of patients compared to 0.8% in 130 patients continued on methotrexate with placebo added.

Pre-existing Hepatic Disease

Given the possible risk of increased hepatotoxicity, and the role of the liver in drug activation, elimination and recycling, the use of ARAVA is not recommended in patients with significant hepatic impairment or evidence of infection with hepatitis B or C viruses. (See **Warnings – Hepatotoxicity**).

Skin Reactions

Rare cases of Stevens-Johnson syndrome and toxic epidermal necrolysis have been reported in patients receiving ARAVA. If a patient taking ARAVA develops any of these conditions, ARAVA therapy should be stopped, and a drug elimination procedure is recommended. (See **PRECAUTIONS – General – Need for Drug Elimination**).

Malignancy

The risk of malignancy, particularly lymphoproliferative disorders, is increased with the use of some immunosuppression medications. There is a potential for immunosuppression with ARAVA. No apparent increase in the incidence of malignancies and lymphoproliferative disorders was reported in the clinical trials of ARAVA, but larger and longer-term studies would be needed to determine whether there is an increased risk of malignancy or lymphoproliferative disorders with ARAVA.

Use in Women of Childbearing Potential

There are no adequate and well-controlled studies evaluating ARAVA in pregnant women. However, based on animal studies, leflunomide may increase the risk of fetal death or teratogenic effects when administered to a pregnant woman (see **CONTRAINDICATIONS**). Women of childbearing potential must not be started on ARAVA until pregnancy is excluded and it has been confirmed that they are using reliable contraception. Before starting treatment with ARAVA, patients must be fully counseled on the potential for serious risk to the fetus.

The patient must be advised that if there is any delay in onset of menses or any other reason to suspect pregnancy, they must notify the physician immediately for pregnancy testing and, if positive, the physician and patient must discuss the risk to the pregnancy. It is possible that rapidly lowering the blood level of the active metabolite by instituting the drug elimination procedure described below at the first delay of menses may decrease the risk to the fetus from ARAVA.

Upon discontinuing ARAVA, it is recommended that all women of childbearing potential undergo the drug elimination procedure described below. Women receiving ARAVA treatment who wish to become pregnant must discontinue ARAVA and undergo the drug elimination procedure described below which includes verification of M1 metabolite plasma levels less than 0.02 mg/L (0.02 µg/mL). Human plasma levels of the active metabolite (M1) less than 0.02 mg/L (0.02 µg/mL) are expected to have minimal risk based on available animal data.

Drug Elimination Procedure

The following drug elimination procedure is recommended to achieve non-detectable plasma levels (less than 0.02 mg/L or 0.02 µg/mL) after stopping treatment with ARAVA:

1) Administer cholestyramine 8 grams 3 times daily for 11 days. (The 11 days do not need to be consecutive unless there is a need to lower the plasma level rapidly.)
2) Verify plasma levels less than 0.02 mg/L (0.02 µg/mL) by two separate tests at least 14 days apart. If plasma levels are higher than 0.02 mg/L, additional cholestyramine treatment should be considered.

Without the drug elimination procedure, it may take up to 2 years to reach plasma M1 metabolite levels less than 0.02 mg/L due to individual variation in drug clearance.

PRECAUTIONS

General

Need for Drug Elimination

The active metabolite of leflunomide is eliminated slowly from the plasma. In instances of any serious toxicity from ARAVA, including hypersensitivity, use of a drug elimination procedure as described in this section is highly recommended to reduce the drug concentration more rapidly after stopping ARAVA therapy. If hypersensitivity is the suspected clinical mechanism, more prolonged cholestyramine or charcoal administration may be necessary to achieve rapid and sufficient clearance. The duration may be modified based on the clinical status of the patient.

Cholestyramine given orally at a dose of 8 g three times a day for 24 hours to three healthy volunteers decreased plasma levels of M1 by approximately 40% in 24 hours and by 49 to 65% in 48 hours.

Administration of activated charcoal (powder made into a suspension) orally or via nasogastric tube (50 g every 6 hours for 24 hours) has been shown to reduce plasma concentrations of the active metabolite, M1, by 37% in 24 hours and by 48% in 48 hours.

These drug elimination procedures may be repeated if clinically necessary.

Respiratory

Interstitial lung disease has been reported during treatment with leflunomide and has been associated with fatal outcomes (see **ADVERSE REACTIONS**). Interstitial lung disease is a potentially fatal disorder, which may occur acutely at any time during therapy and has a variable clinical presentation. New onset or worsening pulmonary symptoms, such as cough and dyspnea, with or without associated fever, may be a reason for discontinuation of the therapy and for further investigation as appropriate. If discontinuation of the drug is necessary, initiation of wash-out procedures should be considered. (See **WARNINGS – Drug Elimination Procedure**).

Renal Insufficiency

Single dose studies in dialysis patients show a doubling of the free fraction of M1 in plasma. There is no clinical experience in the use of ARAVA in patients with renal impairment. Caution should be used when administering this drug in this population.

Vaccinations

No clinical data are available on the efficacy and safety of vaccinations during ARAVA treatment. Vaccination with live vaccines is, however, not recommended. The long half-life of ARAVA should be considered when contemplating administration of a live vaccine after stopping ARAVA.

Information for Patients

- The potential for increased risk of birth defects should be discussed with female patients of childbearing potential. It is recommended that physicians advise women that they may be at increased risk of having a child with birth defects if they are pregnant when taking ARAVA, become pregnant while taking ARAVA, or do not wait to become pregnant until they have stopped taking ARAVA and followed the drug elimination procedure (as described in **WARNINGS – Use In Women of Childbearing Potential – Drug Elimination Procedure**).
- Patients should be advised of the possibility of rare, serious skin reactions. Patients should be instructed to inform their physicians promptly if they develop a skin rash or mucous membrane lesions.
- Patients should be advised of the potential hepatotoxic effects of ARAVA and of the need for monitoring liver enzymes. Patients should be instructed to notify their physicians if they develop symptoms such as unusual tiredness, abdominal pain or jaundice.
- Patients should be advised that they may develop a lowering of their blood counts and should have frequent hematologic monitoring. This is particularly important for patients who are receiving other immunosuppressive therapy concurrently with ARAVA, who have recently discontinued such therapy before starting treatment with ARAVA, or who have had a history of a significant hematologic abnormality. Patients should be instructed to notify their physicians promptly if they notice symptoms of pancytopenia (such as easy bruising or bleeding, recurrent infections, fever, paleness or unusual tiredness).
- Patients should be informed about the early warning signs of interstitial lung disease and asked to contact their physician as soon as possible if these symptoms appear or worsen during therapy.

Laboratory Tests

Hematologic Monitoring

At minimum, patients taking ARAVA should have platelet, white blood cell count and hemoglobin or hematocrit monitored at baseline and monthly for six months following initiation of therapy and every 6 to 8 weeks thereafter.

Bone Marrow Suppression Monitoring

If used with concomitantly with immunosuppressants such as methotrexate, chronic monitoring should be monthly. (See **WARNINGS – Immunosuppression Potential/Bone Marrow Suppression**).

Liver Enzyme Monitoring

ALT (SGPT) must be performed at baseline and monitored at monthly intervals during the first six months then, if stable, every 6 to 8 weeks thereafter. In addition, if ARAVA and methotrexate are given concomitantly, ACR guidelines for monitoring methotrexate liver toxicity must be followed with ALT, AST, and serum albumin testing every month. (See **WARNINGS – Hepatotoxicity**.)

Due to a specific effect on the brush border of the renal proximal tubule, ARAVA has a uricosuric effect. A separate effect of hypophosphaturia is seen in some patients. These effects have not been seen together, nor have there been alterations in renal function.

Drug Interactions

Cholestyramine and Charcoal

Administration of cholestyramine or activated charcoal in patients (n=13) and volunteers (n=96) resulted in a rapid and significant decrease in plasma M1 (the active metabolite of leflunomide) concentration (see **PRECAUTIONS – General – Need for Drug Elimination**).

Hepatotoxic Drugs

Increased side effects may occur when leflunomide is given concomitantly with hepatotoxic substances. This is also to be considered when leflunomide treatment is followed by such drugs without a drug elimination procedure. In a small (n=30) combination study of ARAVA with methotrexate, a 2- to 3-fold elevation in liver enzymes was seen in 5 of 30 patients. All elevations resolved, 2 with continuation of both drugs and 3 after discontinuation of leflunomide. A >3-fold increase was seen in another 5 patients. All of these also resolved, 2 with continuation of both drugs and 3 after discontinuation of leflunomide. Three patients met "ACR crite-

Continued on next page

Arava—Cont.

ria" for liver biopsy (1: Roegnik Grade I, 2: Roegnik Grade IIIa). No pharmacokinetic interaction was identified (see **CLINICAL PHARMACOLOGY**).

NSAIDs
In *in vitro* studies, M1 was shown to cause increases ranging from 13-50% in the free fraction of diclofenac and ibuprofen at concentrations in the clinical range. The clinical significance of this finding is unknown; however, there was extensive concomitant use of NSAIDs in clinical studies and no differential effect was observed.

Tolbutamide
In *in vitro* studies, M1 was shown to cause increases ranging from 13-50% in the free fraction of tolbutamide at concentrations in the clinical range. The clinical significance of this finding is unknown.

Rifampin
Following concomitant administration of a single dose of ARAVA to subjects receiving multiple doses of rifampin, M1 peak levels were increased (~40%) over those seen when ARAVA was given alone. Because of the potential for ARAVA levels to continue to increase with multiple dosing, caution should be used if patients are to be receiving both ARAVA and rifampin.

Warfarin
Increased INR (International Normalized Ratio) when ARAVA and warfarin were co-administered has been rarely reported.

Carcinogenesis, Mutagenesis, and Impairment of Fertility
No evidence of carcinogenicity was observed in a 2-year bioassay in rats at oral doses of leflunomide up to the maximally tolerated dose of 6 mg/kg (approximately 1/40 the maximum human M1 systemic exposure based on AUC). However, male mice in a 2-year bioassay exhibited an increased incidence in lymphoma at an oral dose of 15 mg/kg, the highest dose studied (1.7 times the human M1 exposure based on AUC). Female mice, in the same study, exhibited a dose-related increased incidence of bronchoalveolar adenomas and carcinomas combined beginning at 1.5 mg/kg (approximately 1/10 the human M1 exposure based on AUC). The significance of the findings in mice relative to the clinical use of ARAVA is not known.

Leflunomide was not mutagenic in the Ames Assay, the Unscheduled DNA Synthesis Assay, or in the HGPRT Gene Mutation Assay. In addition, leflunomide was not clastogenic in the *in vivo* Mouse Micronucleus Assay nor in the *in vivo* Cytogenetic Test in Chinese Hamster Bone Marrow Cells. However, 4-trifluoromethylaniline (TFMA), a minor metabolite of leflunomide, was mutagenic in the Ames Assay and in the HGPRT Gene Mutation Assay, and was clastogenic in the *in vitro* Assay for Chromosome Aberrations in the Chinese Hamster Cells. TFMA was not clastogenic in the *in vivo* Mouse Micronucleus Assay nor in the *in vivo* Cytogenetic Test in Chinese Hamster Bone Marrow Cells. Leflunomide had no effect on fertility in either male or female rats at oral doses up to 4.0 mg/kg (approximately 1/30 the human M1 exposure based on AUC).

Pregnancy
Pregnancy Category X. (See **CONTRAINDICATIONS** section). Pregnancy Registry: To monitor fetal outcomes of pregnant women exposed to leflunomide, health care providers are encouraged to register such patients by calling 1-877-311-8972.

Nursing Mothers
ARAVA should not be used by nursing mothers. It is not known whether ARAVA is excreted in human milk. Many drugs are excreted in human milk, and there is a potential for serious adverse reactions in nursing infants from ARAVA. Therefore, a decision should be made whether to proceed with nursing or to initiate treatment with ARAVA, taking into account the importance of the drug to the mother.

Use in Males
Available information does not suggest that ARAVA would be associated with an increased risk of male-mediated fetal toxicity. However, animal studies to evaluate this specific risk have not been conducted. To minimize any possible risk, men wishing to father a child should consider discontinuing use of ARAVA and taking cholestyramine 8 grams 3 times daily for 11 days.

Pediatric Use
The safety and effectiveness of ARAVA in pediatric patients with polyarticular course juvenile rheumatoid arthritis (JRA) have not been fully evaluated. (See **CLINICAL STUDIES** and **ADVERSE REACTIONS**).

Geriatric Use
Of the total number of subjects in controlled clinical (Phase III) studies of ARAVA, 234 subjects were 65 years and over. No overall differences in safety or effectiveness were observed between these subjects and younger subjects, other reported clinical experience has not identified differences in responses between the elderly and younger patients, but greater sensitivity of some older individuals cannot be ruled out. No dosage adjustment is needed in patients over 65.

ADVERSE REACTIONS
Adverse reactions associated with the use of leflunomide in RA include diarrhea, elevated liver enzymes (ALT and AST), alopecia and rash. In the controlled studies at one year, the following adverse events were reported, regardless of causality. (See Table 9.)
[See table 9 at left and on next page]
Adverse events during a second year of treatment with leflunomide in clinical trials were consistent with those observed during the first year of treatment and occurred at a similar or lower incidence.
In addition, the following adverse events have been reported in 1% to <3% of the RA patients in the leflunomide treatment group in controlled clinical trials.
Body as a Whole: abscess, cyst, fever, hernia, malaise, pain, neck pain, pelvic pain;
Cardiovascular: angina pectoris, migraine, palpitation, tachycardia, varicose vein, vasculitis, vasodilatation;
Gastrointestinal: cholelithiasis, colitis, constipation, esophagitis, flatulence, gastritis, gingivitis, melena, oral moniliasis, pharyngitis, salivary gland enlarged, stomatitis (or aphthous stomatitis), tooth disorder;
Endocrine: diabetes mellitus, hyperthyroidism;
Hemic and Lymphatic System: anemia (including iron deficiency anemia), ecchymosis;
Metabolic and Nutritional: creatine phosphokinase increased, hyperglycemia, hyperlipidemia, peripheral edema;
Musculo-Skeletal System: arthrosis, bone necrosis, bone pain, bursitis, muscle cramps, myalgia, tendon rupture;
Nervous System: anxiety, depression, dry mouth, insomnia, neuralgia, neuritis, sleep disorder, sweating increased, vertigo;
Respiratory System: asthma, dyspnea, epistaxis, lung disorder;
Skin and Appendages: acne, contact dermatitis, fungal dermatitis, hair discoloration, hematoma, herpes simplex, herpes zoster, maculopapular rash, nail disorder, skin discoloration, skin disorder, skin nodule, subcutaneous nodule, ulcer skin;
Special Senses: blurred vision, cataract, conjunctivitis, eye disorder, taste perversion;
Urogenital System: albuminuria, cystitis, dysuria, hematuria, menstrual disorder, prostate disorder, urinary frequency, vaginal moniliasis.
Other less common adverse events seen in clinical trials include: 1 case of anaphylactic reaction occurred in Phase 2 following rechallenge of drug after withdrawal due to rash (rare); urticaria; eosinophilia; transient thrombocytopenia (rare); and leukopenia <2000 WBC/mm[3] (rare).
Adverse events during a second year of treatment with leflunomide in clinical trials were consistent with those observed during the first year of treatment and occurred at a similar or lower incidence.

Table 9. Percentage Of Patients With Adverse Events ≥3% In Any Leflunomide Treated Group

	All RA Studies	Placebo-Controlled Trials				Active-Controlled Trials	
		MN 301 and US 301				MN 302*	
	LEF (N=1339)[1]	LEF (N=315)	PBO (N=210)	SSZ (N=133)	MTX (N=182)	LEF (N=501)	MTX (N=498)
BODY AS A WHOLE							
Allergic Reaction	2%	5%	2%	0%	6%	1%	2%
Asthenia	3%	6%	4%	5%	6%	3%	3%
Flu Syndrome	2%	4%	2%	0%	7%	0%	0%
Infection, upper respiratory	4%	0%	0%	0%	0%	0%	0%
Injury Accident	5%	7%	5%	3%	11%	6%	7%
Pain	2%	4%	2%	2%	5%	1%	<1%
Abdominal Pain	6%	5%	4%	4%	8%	6%	4%
Back Pain	5%	6%	3%	4%	9%	8%	7%
CARDIOVASCULAR							
Hypertension[2]	10%	9%	4%	4%	3%	10%	4%
- New onset of hypertension		1%	<1%	0%	2%	2%	<1%
Chest Pain	2%	4%	2%	2%	4%	1%	2%
GASTROINTESTINAL							
Anorexia	3%	3%	2%	5%	2%	3%	3%
Diarrhea	17%	27%	12%	10%	20%	22%	10%
Dyspepsia	5%	10%	10%	9%	13%	6%	7%
Gastroenteritis	3%	1%	1%	0%	6%	3%	3%
Abnormal Liver Enzymes	5%	10%	2%	4%	10%	6%	17%
Nausea	9%	13%	11%	19%	18%	13%	18%
GI/Abdominal Pain	5%	6%	4%	7%	8%	8%	8%
Mouth Ulcer	3%	5%	4%	3%	10%	3%	6%
Vomiting	3%	5%	4%	4%	3%	3%	3%
METABOLIC AND NUTRITIONAL							
Hypokalemia	1%	3%	1%	1%	1%	1%	<1%
Weight Loss[3]	4%	2%	1%	2%	0%	2%	2%
MUSCULO-SKELETAL SYSTEM							
Arthralgia	1%	4%	3%	0%	9%	<1%	1%
Leg Cramps	1%	4%	2%	2%	6%	0%	0%
Joint Disorder	4%	2%	2%	2%	2%	8%	6%
Synovitis	2%	<1%	1%	0%	2%	4%	2%
Tenosynovitis	3%	2%	0%	1%	2%	5%	1%
NERVOUS SYSTEM							
Dizziness	4%	5%	3%	6%	5%	7%	6%
Headache	7%	13%	11%	12%	21%	10%	8%
Paresthesia	2%	3%	1%	1%	2%	4%	3%

(Table continued on next page)

Table 9 *(cont.)*: Percentage Of Patients With Adverse Events ≥3% In Any Leflunomide Treated Group

	All RA Studies	Placebo-Controlled Trials				Active-Controlled Trials	
		MN 301 and US 301				MN 302*	
	LEF (N=1339)[1]	LEF (N=315)	PBO (N=210)	SSZ (N=133)	MTX (N=182)	LEF (N=501)	MTX (N=498)
RESPIRATORY SYSTEM							
Bronchitis	7%	5%	2%	4%	7%	8%	7%
Increased Cough	3%	4%	5%	3%	6%	5%	7%
Respiratory Infection	15%	21%	21%	20%	32%	27%	25%
Pharyngitis	3%	2%	1%	2%	1%	3%	3%
Pneumonia	2%	3%	0%	0%	1%	2%	2%
Rhinitis	2%	5%	2%	4%	3%	2%	2%
Sinusitis	2%	5%	5%	0%	10%	1%	1%
SKIN AND APPENDAGES							
Alopecia	10%	9%	1%	6%	6%	17%	10%
Eczema	2%	1%	1%	1%	1%	3%	2%
Pruritus	4%	5%	2%	3%	2%	6%	2%
Rash	10%	12%	7%	11%	9%	11%	10%
Dry Skin	2%	3%	2%	2%	0%	3%	1%
UROGENITAL SYSTEM							
Urinary Tract Infection	5%	5%	7%	4%	2%	5%	6%

* Only 10% of patients in MN302 received folate. All patients in US301 received folate; none in MN301 received folate.
[1] Includes all controlled and uncontrolled trials with leflunomide (duration up to 12 months).
[2] Hypertension as a preexisting condition was overrepresented in all leflunomide treatment groups in phase III trials.
[3] In a meta-analysis of all phase II and III studies, during the first 6 months in patients receiving leflunomide, 10% lost 10-19 lbs (24 cases per 100 patient years) and 2% lost at least 20 lbs (4 cases/100 patient years). Of patients receiving leflunomide 4% lost 10% of their baseline weight during the first 6 months of treatment.

ARAVA® (leflunomide) Tablets

Strength	Quantity	NDC Number	Description
10 mg	30 count bottle	0088-2160-30	White, round film-coated tablet embossed with "ZBN" on one side.
20 mg	30 count bottle	0088-2161-30	Light yellow, triangular film-coated tablet embossed with "ZBO" on one side.
100 mg	3 count blister pack	0088-2162-03	White, round film-coated tablet embossed with "ZBP" on one side.

In post-marketing experience, the following have been reported rarely:
Body as a whole: opportunistic infections, severe infections including sepsis that may be fatal;
Gastrointestinal: pancreatitis;
Hematologic: agranulocytosis, leukopenia, neutropenia, pancytopenia, thrombocytopenia;
Hypersensitivity: angioedema;
Hepatic: hepatitis, jaundice/cholestasis, severe liver injury such as hepatic failure and acute hepatic necrosis that may be fatal;
Respiratory: interstitial lung disease, including interstitial pneumonitis and pulmonary fibrosis, which may be fatal;
Nervous system: peripheral neuropathy;
Skin and Appendages: erythema multiforme, Stevens-Johnson syndrome, toxic epidermal necrolysis.

Adverse Reactions (Pediatric Patients)
The safety of ARAVA was studied in 74 patients with polyarticular course juvenile rheumatoid arthritis ranging in age from 3-17 years (47 patients from the active-controlled study and 27 from the open-label safety and pharmacokinetic study). The most common adverse events included abdominal pain, diarrhea, nausea, vomiting, oral ulcers, upper respiratory tract infections, alopecia, rash, headache, and dizziness. Less common adverse events included anemia, hypertension, and weight loss. Fourteen pediatric patients experienced ALT and/or AST elevations, nine between 1.2 and 3-fold the upper limit of normal, five between 3 and 8-fold the upper limit of normal.

DRUG ABUSE AND DEPENDENCE
ARAVA has no known potential for abuse or dependence.

OVERDOSAGE
In mouse and rat acute toxicology studies, the minimally toxic dose for oral leflunomide was 200-500 mg/kg and 100 mg/kg, respectively (approximately >350 times the maximum recommended human dose, respectively).
There have been reports of chronic overdose in patients taking ARAVA at daily dose up to five times the recommended daily dose and reports of acute overdose in adults or children. There were no adverse events reported in the majority of case reports of overdose. Adverse events were consistent with the safety profile for ARAVA (see **ADVERSE REACTIONS**). The most frequent adverse events observed were diarrhea, abdominal pain, leukopenia, anemia and elevated liver function tests.
In the event of a significant overdose or toxicity, cholestyramine or charcoal administration is recommended to accelerate elimination (see **PRECAUTIONS – General – Need for Drug Elimination**).
Studies with both hemodialysis and CAPD (chronic ambulatory peritoneal dialysis) indicate that M1, the primary metabolite of leflunomide, is not dialyzable. (See **CLINICAL PHARMACOLOGY – Elimination**).

DOSAGE AND ADMINISTRATION
Loading Dose
Due to the long half-life in patients with RA and recommended dosing interval (24 hours), a loading dose is needed to provide steady-state concentrations more rapidly. It is recommended that ARAVA therapy be initiated with a loading dose of one 100 mg tablet per day for 3 days.
Elimination of the loading dose regimen may decrease the risk of adverse events. This could be especially important for patients at increased risk of hematologic or hepatic toxicity, such as those receiving concomitant treatment with methotrexate or other immunosuppressive agents or on such medications in the recent past. (See **WARNINGS – Hepatotoxicity**).

Maintenance Therapy
Daily dosing of 20 mg is recommended for treatment of patients with RA. A small cohort of patients (n=104), treated with 25 mg/day, experienced a greater incidence of side effects; alopecia, weight loss, liver enzyme elevations. Doses higher than 20 mg/day are not recommended. If dosing at 20 mg/day is not well tolerated clinically, the dose may be decreased to 10 mg daily. Liver enzymes must be monitored and dose adjustments may be necessary (see **WARNINGS – Hepatotoxicity**). Due to the prolonged half-life of the active metabolite of leflunomide, patients should be carefully observed after dose reduction, since it may take several weeks for metabolite levels to decline.

HOW SUPPLIED
ARAVA Tablets in 10 and 20 mg strengths are packaged in bottles. ARAVA Tablets 100 mg strength are packaged in blister packs.

[See second table at left]
Store at 25°C (77°F); excursions permitted to 15-30°C (59-86°F) [see USP Controlled Room Temperature]. Protect from light.
Rx only.
Rev. November 2004
Manufactured by
Aventis Pharma Specialites, 60200 Compiegne, France
for
Aventis Pharmaceuticals Inc.
Kansas City, MO 64137
Made in France
©2004 Aventis Pharmaceuticals Inc.

LANTUS® ℞

[lăn' tus]

(insulin glargine [rDNA origin] injection)
Rev. August 2004
Rx Only

Prescribing information for this product, which appears on pages 715-719 of the 2005 PDR, has been completely revised as follows. Please write "See Supplement A" next to the product heading.

LANTUS® must NOT be diluted or mixed with any other insulin or solution.

DESCRIPTION
LANTUS® (insulin glargine [rDNA origin] injection) is a sterile solution of insulin glargine for use as an injection. Insulin glargine is a recombinant human insulin analog that is a long-acting (up to 24-hour duration of action), parenteral blood-glucose-lowering agent. (See CLINICAL PHARMACOLOGY). LANTUS is produced by recombinant DNA technology utilizing a non-pathogenic laboratory strain of *Escherichia coli* (K12) as the production organism. Insulin glargine differs from human insulin in that the amino acid asparagine at position A21 is replaced by glycine and two arginines are added to the C-terminus of the B-chain. Chemically, it is 21^A-Gly-30^{B}a-L-Arg-30^{B}b-L-Arg-human insulin and has the empirical formula $C_{267}H_{404}N_{72}O_{78}S_6$ and a molecular weight of 6063. It has the following structural formula:

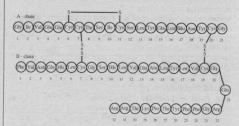

LANTUS consists of insulin glargine dissolved in a clear aqueous fluid. Each milliliter of LANTUS (insulin glargine injection) contains 100 IU (3.6378 mg) insulin glargine, 30 mcg zinc, 2.7 mg m-cresol, 20 mg glycerol 85%, and water for injection. The pH is adjusted by addition of aqueous solutions of hydrochloric acid and sodium hydroxide. LANTUS has a pH of approximately 4.

CLINICAL PHARMACOLOGY
Mechanism of Action:
The primary activity of insulin, including insulin glargine, is regulation of glucose metabolism. Insulin and its analogs lower blood glucose levels by stimulating peripheral glucose uptake, especially by skeletal muscle and fat, and by inhibiting hepatic glucose production. Insulin inhibits lipolysis in the adipocyte, inhibits proteolysis, and enhances protein synthesis.

Pharmacodynamics:
Insulin glargine is a human insulin analog that has been designed to have low aqueous solubility at neutral pH. At pH 4, as in the LANTUS injection solution, it is completely soluble. After injection into the subcutaneous tissue, the acidic solution is neutralized, leading to formation of microprecipitates from which small amounts of insulin glargine are slowly released, resulting in a relatively constant concentration/time profile over 24 hours with no pronounced peak. This profile allows once-daily dosing as a patient's basal insulin.
In clinical studies, the glucose-lowering effect on a molar basis (i.e., when given at the same doses) of intravenous insulin glargine is approximately the same as human insulin. In euglycemic clamp studies in healthy subjects or in patients with type 1 diabetes, the onset of action of subcutaneous insulin glargine was slower than NPH human insulin. The effect profile of insulin glargine was relatively constant with no pronounced peak and the duration of its effect was prolonged compared to NPH human insulin. *Figure 1* shows results from a study in patients with type 1 diabetes conducted for a maximum of 24 hours after the injection. The median time between injection and the end of pharmacological effect was 14.5 hours (range: 9.5 to 19.3 hours) for NPH human insulin, and 24 hours (range: 10.8 to >24.0 hours) (24 hours was the end of the observation period) for insulin glargine.

Continued on next page

Lantus—Cont.

Figure 1. Activity Profile in Patients with Type 1 Diabetes†

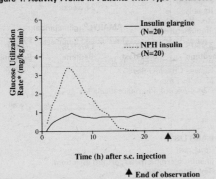

Insulin glargine
(N=20)

NPH insulin
(N=20)

Glucose Utilization Rate* (mg/kg/min)

Time (h) after s.c. injection

▲ End of observation
period

* Determined as amount of glucose infused to maintain constant plasma glucose levels (hourly mean values); indicative of insulin activity.
† Between-patient variability (CV, coefficient of variation); insulin glargine, 84% and NPH, 78%.

The longer duration of action (up to 24 hours) of LANTUS is directly related to its slower rate of absorption and supports once-daily subcutaneous administration. The time course of action of insulins, including LANTUS, may vary between individuals and/or within the same individual.

Pharmacokinetics:

Absorption and Bioavailability. After subcutaneous injection of insulin glargine in healthy subjects and in patients with diabetes, the insulin serum concentrations indicated a slower, more prolonged absorption and a relatively constant concentration/time profile over 24 hours with no pronounced peak in comparison to NPH human insulin. Serum insulin concentrations were thus consistent with the time profile of the pharmacodynamic activity of insulin glargine.

After subcutaneous injection of 0.3 IU/kg insulin glargine in patients with type 1 diabetes, a relatively constant concentration/time profile has been demonstrated. The duration of action after abdominal, deltoid, or thigh subcutaneous administration was similar.

Metabolism. A metabolism study in humans indicates that insulin glargine is partly metabolized at the carboxyl terminus of the B chain in the subcutaneous depot to form two active metabolites with in vitro activity similar to that of insulin, M1 (21^A-Gly-insulin) and M2 (21^A-Gly-des-30^B-Thr-insulin). Unchanged drug and these degradation products are also present in the circulation.

Special Populations:

Age, Race, and Gender. Information on the effect of age, race, and gender on the pharmacokinetics of LANTUS is not available. However, in controlled clinical trials in adults (n=3890) and a controlled clinical trial in pediatric patients (n=349), subgroup analyses based on age, race, and gender did not show differences in safety and efficacy between insulin glargine and NPH human insulin.

Smoking. The effect of smoking on the pharmacokinetics/pharmacodynamics of LANTUS has not been studied.

Pregnancy. The effect of pregnancy on the pharmacokinetics and pharmacodynamics of LANTUS has not been studied (see PRECAUTIONS, Pregnancy).

Obesity. In controlled clinical trials, which included patients with Body Mass Index (BMI) up to and including 49.6 kg/m², subgroup analyses based on BMI did not show any differences in safety and efficacy between insulin glargine and NPH human insulin.

Renal Impairment. The effect of renal impairment on the pharmacokinetics of LANTUS has not been studied. However, some studies with human insulin have shown increased circulating levels of insulin in patients with renal failure. Careful glucose monitoring and dose adjustments of insulin, including LANTUS, may be necessary in patients with renal dysfunction (see PRECAUTIONS, Renal Impairment).

Hepatic Impairment. The effect of hepatic impairment on the pharmacokinetics of LANTUS has not been studied. However, some studies with human insulin have shown increased circulating levels of insulin in patients with liver failure. Careful glucose monitoring and dose adjustments of insulin, including LANTUS, may be necessary in patients with hepatic dysfunction (see PRECAUTIONS, Hepatic Impairment).

Clinical Studies

The safety and effectiveness of insulin glargine given once-daily at bedtime was compared to that of once-daily and twice-daily NPH human insulin in open-label, randomized, active-control, parallel studies of 2327 adult patients and 349 pediatric patients with type 1 diabetes mellitus and 1563 adult patients with type 2 diabetes mellitus (see Tables 1-3). In general, the reduction in glycated hemoglobin (HbA1c) with LANTUS was similar to that with NPH human insulin. The overall rates of hypoglycemia did not differ between patients with diabetes treated to LANTUS compared with NPH human insulin.

Type 1 Diabetes—Adult (see Table 1). In two large, randomized, controlled clinical studies (Studies A and B), patients with type 1 diabetes (Study A; n=585, Study B; n=534) were randomized to basal-bolus treatment with

Table 1: Type 1 Diabetes Mellitus—Adult

	Study A 28 weeks Regular insulin		Study B 28 weeks Regular insulin		Study C 16 weeks Insulin lispro	
Treatment duration Treatment in combination with						
	LANTUS	NPH	LANTUS	NPH	LANTUS	NPH
Number of subjects treated	292	293	264	270	310	309
HbA1c						
Endstudy mean	8.13	8.07	7.55	7.49	7.53	7.60
Adj. mean change from baseline	+0.21	+0.10	-0.16	-0.21	-0.07	-0.08
LANTUS—NPH	+0.11		+0.05		+0.01	
95% CI for Treatment difference	(-0.03; +0.24)		(-0.08; +0.19)		(-0.11; +0.13)	
Basal insulin dose						
Endstudy mean	19.2	22.8	24.8	31.3	23.9	29.2
Mean change from baseline	-1.7	-0.3	-4.1	+1.8	-4.5	+0.9
Total insulin dose						
Endstudy mean	46.7	51.7	50.3	54.8	47.4	50.7
Mean change from baseline	-1.1	-0.1	+0.3	+3.7	-2.9	+0.3
Fasting blood glucose (mg/dL)						
Endstudy mean	146.3	150.8	147.8	154.4	144.4	161.3
Adj. mean change from baseline	-21.1	-16.0	-20.2	-16.9	-29.3	-11.9

Table 2: Type 1 Diabetes Mellitus—Pediatric

	Study D 28 weeks Regular insulin	
Treatment duration Treatment in combination with		
	LANTUS	NPH
Number of subjects treated	174	175
HbA1c		
Endstudy mean	8.91	9.18
Adj. mean change from baseline	+0.28	+0.27
LANTUS—NPH	+0.01	
95% CI for Treatment difference	(-0.24; +0.26)	
Basal insulin dose		
Endstudy mean	18.2	21.1
Mean change from baseline	-1.3	+2.4
Total insulin dose		
Endstudy mean	45.0	46.0
Mean change from baseline	+1.9	+3.4
Fasting blood glucose (mg/dL)		
Endstudy mean	171.9	182.7
Adj. mean change from baseline	-23.2	-12.2

Table 3: Type 2 Diabetes Mellitus—Adult

	Study E 52 weeks Oral agents		Study F 28 weeks Regular insulin	
Treatment duration Treatment in combination with				
	LANTUS	NPH	LANTUS	NPH
Number of subjects treated	289	281	259	259
HbA1c				
Endstudy mean	8.51	8.47	8.14	7.96
Adj. mean change from baseline	-0.46	-0.38	-0.41	-0.59
LANTUS—NPH	-0.08		+0.17	
95% CI for Treatment difference	(-0.28; +0.12)		(-0.00; +0.35)	
Basal insulin dose				
Endstudy mean	25.9	23.6	42.9	52.5
Mean change from baseline	+11.5	+9.0	-1.2	+7.0
Total insulin dose				
Endstudy mean	25.9	23.6	74.3	80.0
Mean change from baseline	+11.5	+9.0	+10.0	+13.1
Fasting blood glucose (mg/dL)				
Endstudy mean	126.9	129.4	141.5	144.5
Adj. mean change from baseline	-49.0	-46.3	-23.8	-21.6

LANTUS once daily at bedtime or to NPH human insulin once or twice daily and treated for 28 weeks. Regular human insulin was administered before each meal. LANTUS was administered at bedtime. NPH human insulin was administered once daily at bedtime or in the morning and at bedtime when used twice daily. In one large, randomized, controlled clinical study (Study C), patients with type 1 diabetes (n=619) were treated for 16 weeks with a basal-bolus insulin regimen where insulin lispro was used before each meal. LANTUS was administered once daily at bedtime and NPH human insulin was administered once or twice daily. In these studies, LANTUS and NPH human insulin had a similar effect on glycohemoglobin with a similar overall rate of hypoglycemia.
[See table 1 above]

Type 1 Diabetes—Pediatric (see Table 2). In a randomized, controlled clinical study (Study D), pediatric patients (age range 6 to 15 years) with type 1 diabetes (n=349) were treated for 28 weeks with a basal-bolus insulin regimen where regular human insulin was used before each meal. LANTUS was administered once daily at bedtime and NPH human insulin was administered once or twice daily. Similar effects on glycohemoglobin and the incidence of hypoglycemia were observed in both treatment groups.
[See table 2 above]

Type 2 Diabetes—Adult (see Table 3). In a large, randomized, controlled clinical study (Study E) (n=570), LANTUS was evaluated for 52 weeks as part of a regimen of combination therapy with insulin and oral antidiabetes agents (a sulfonylurea, metformin, acarbose, or combinations of these drugs). LANTUS administered once daily at bedtime was as

effective as NPH human insulin administered once daily at bedtime in reducing glycohemoglobin and fasting glucose. There was a low rate of hypoglycemia that was similar in LANTUS and NPH human insulin treated patients. In a large, randomized, controlled clinical study (Study F), in patients with type 2 diabetes not using oral antidiabetes agents (n=518), a basal-bolus regimen of LANTUS once daily at bedtime or NPH human insulin administered once or twice daily was evaluated for 28 weeks. Regular human insulin was used before meals as needed. LANTUS had similar effectiveness as either once- or twice-daily NPH human insulin in reducing glycohemoglobin and fasting glucose with a similar incidence of hypoglycemia.
[See table 3 above]

LANTUS Flexible Daily Dosing

The safety and efficacy of LANTUS administered pre-breakfast, pre-dinner, or at bedtime were evaluated in a large, randomized, controlled clinical study, in patients with type 1 diabetes (study G, n=378). Patients were also treated with insulin lispro at mealtime. LANTUS administered at different times of the day resulted in similar reductions in glycated hemoglobin compared to that with bedtime administration (see Table 4). In these patients, data are available from 8-point home glucose monitoring. The maximum mean blood glucose level was observed just prior to injection of LANTUS regardless of time of administration, i.e. pre-breakfast, pre-dinner, or bedtime.

In this study, 5% of patients in the LANTUS-breakfast arm discontinued treatment because of lack of efficacy. No patients in the other two arms discontinued for this reason. Routine monitoring during this trial revealed the following mean changes in systolic blood pressure: pre-breakfast group, 1.9 mm Hg; pre-dinner group, 0.7 mm Hg; pre-bedtime group, -2.0 mm Hg.

The safety and efficacy of LANTUS administered pre-breakfast or at bedtime were also evaluated in a large, randomized, active-controlled clinical study (Study H, n=697) in type 2 diabetes patients no longer adequately controlled on oral agent therapy. All patients in this study also received AMARYL® (glimepiride) 3 mg daily. LANTUS given before breakfast was at least as effective in lowering glycated hemoglobin A1c (HbA1c) as LANTUS given at bedtime or NPH human insulin given at bedtime (see Table 4).

[See table 4 at right]

Table 4: Flexible LANTUS Daily Dosing in Type 1 (Study G) and Type 2 (Study H) Diabetes Mellitus

Treatment duration Treatment in combination with:	Study G 24 weeks Insulin lispro			Study H 24 weeks AMARYL® (glimepiride)		
	LANTUS Breakfast	LANTUS Dinner	LANTUS Bedtime	LANTUS Breakfast	LANTUS Bedtime	NPH Bedtime
Number of subjects treated*	112	124	128	234	226	227
HbA1c						
Baseline mean	7.56	7.53	7.61	9.13	9.07	9.09
Endstudy mean	7.39	7.42	7.57	7.87	8.12	8.27
Mean change from baseline	-0.17	-0.11	-0.04	-1.26	-0.95	-0.83
Basal insulin dose (IU)						
Endstudy mean	27.3	24.6	22.8	40.4	38.5	36.8
Mean change from baseline	5.0	1.8	1.5			
Total insulin dose (IU)				NA**	NA	NA
Endstudy mean	53.3	54.7	51.5			
Mean change from baseline	1.6	3.0	2.3			

*Intent to treat
**Not applicable

INDICATIONS AND USAGE

LANTUS is indicated for once-daily subcutaneous administration for the treatment of adult and pediatric patients with type 1 diabetes mellitus or adult patients with type 2 diabetes mellitus who require basal (long-acting) insulin for the control of hyperglycemia.

CONTRAINDICATIONS

LANTUS is contraindicated in patients hypersensitive to insulin glargine or the excipients.

WARNINGS

Hypoglycemia is the most common adverse effect of insulin, including LANTUS. As with all insulins, the timing of hypoglycemia may differ among various insulin formulations. Glucose monitoring is recommended for all patients with diabetes.

Any change of insulin should be made cautiously and only under medical supervision. Changes in insulin strength, timing of dosing, manufacturer, type (e.g., regular, NPH, or insulin analogs), species (animal, human), or method of manufacture (recombinant DNA versus animal-source insulin) may result in the need for a change in dosage. Concomitant oral antidiabetes treatment may need to be adjusted.

PRECAUTIONS

General:

LANTUS is not intended for intravenous administration. The prolonged duration of activity of insulin glargine is dependent on injection into subcutaneous tissue. Intravenous administration of the usual subcutaneous dose could result in severe hypoglycemia.

LANTUS must NOT be diluted or mixed with any other insulin or solution. If LANTUS is diluted or mixed, the solution may become cloudy, and the pharmacokinetic/pharmacodynamic profile (e.g., onset of action, time to peak effect) of LANTUS and/or the mixed insulin may be altered in an unpredictable manner. When LANTUS and regular human insulin were mixed immediately before injection in dogs, a delayed onset of action and time to maximum effect for regular human insulin was observed. The total bioavailability of the mixture was also slightly decreased compared to separate injections of LANTUS and regular human insulin. The relevance of these observations in dogs to humans is not known.

As with all insulin preparations, the time course of LANTUS action may vary in different individuals or at different times in the same individual and the rate of absorption is dependent on blood supply, temperature, and physical activity.

Insulin may cause sodium retention and edema, particularly if previously poor metabolic control is improved by intensified insulin therapy.

Hypoglycemia:

As with all insulin preparations, hypoglycemic reactions may be associated with the administration of LANTUS. Hypoglycemia is the most common adverse effect of insulins. Early warning symptoms of hypoglycemia may be different or less pronounced under certain conditions, such as long duration of diabetes, diabetes nerve disease, use of medications such as beta-blockers, or intensified diabetes control (see PRECAUTIONS, Drug Interactions). Such situations may result in severe hypoglycemia (and, possibly, loss of consciousness) prior to patients' awareness of hypoglycemia.

The time of occurrence of hypoglycemia depends on the action profile of the insulins used and may, therefore, change when the treatment regimen or timing of dosing is changed. Patients being switched from twice daily NPH insulin to once-daily LANTUS should have their initial LANTUS dose reduced by 20% from the previous total daily NPH dose to reduce the risk of hypoglycemia (see DOSAGE AND ADMINISTRATION, Changeover to LANTUS).

The prolonged effect of subcutaneous LANTUS may delay recovery from hypoglycemia.

In a clinical study, symptoms of hypoglycemia or counterregulatory hormone responses were similar after intravenous insulin glargine and regular human insulin both in healthy subjects and patients with type 1 diabetes.

Renal Impairment:

Although studies have not been performed in patients with diabetes and renal impairment, LANTUS requirements may be diminished because of reduced insulin metabolism, similar to observations found with other insulins (see CLINICAL PHARMACOLOGY, Special Populations).

Hepatic Impairment:

Although studies have not been performed in patients with diabetes and hepatic impairment, LANTUS requirements may be diminished due to reduced capacity for gluconeogenesis and reduced insulin metabolism, similar to observations found with other insulins (see CLINICAL PHARMACOLOGY, Special Populations).

Injection Site and Allergic Reactions:

As with any insulin therapy, lipodystrophy may occur at the injection site and delay insulin absorption. Other injection site reactions with insulin therapy include redness, pain, itching, hives, swelling, and inflammation. Continuous rotation of the injection site within a given area may help to reduce or prevent these reactions. Most minor reactions to insulins usually resolve in a few days to a few weeks.

Reports of injection site pain were more frequent with LANTUS than NPH human insulin (2.7% insulin glargine versus 0.7% NPH). The reports of pain at the injection site were usually mild and did not result in discontinuation of therapy.

Immediate-type allergic reactions are rare. Such reactions to insulin (including insulin glargine) or the excipients may, for example, be associated with generalized skin reactions, angioedema, bronchospasm, hypotension, or shock and may be life threatening.

Intercurrent Conditions:

Insulin requirements may be altered during intercurrent conditions such as illness, emotional disturbances, or stress.

Information for Patients:

LANTUS must only be used if the solution is clear and colorless with no particles visible (see DOSAGE AND ADMINISTRATION, Preparation and Handling).

Patients must be advised that LANTUS must NOT be diluted or mixed with any other insulin or solution (see PRECAUTIONS, General).

Patients should be instructed on self-management procedures including glucose monitoring, proper injection technique, and hypoglycemia and hyperglycemia management. Patients must be instructed on handling of special situations such as intercurrent conditions (illness, stress, or emotional disturbances), an inadequate or skipped insulin dose, inadvertent administration of an increased insulin dose, inadequate food intake, or skipped meals. Refer patients to the LANTUS "Patient Information" circular for additional information.

As with all patients who have diabetes, the ability to concentrate and/or react may be impaired as a result of hypoglycemia or hyperglycemia.

Patients with diabetes should be advised to inform their health care professional if they are pregnant or are contemplating pregnancy.

Drug Interactions:

A number of substances affect glucose metabolism and may require insulin dose adjustment and particularly close monitoring.

The following are examples of substances that may increase the blood-glucose-lowering effect and susceptibility to hypoglycemia: oral antidiabetes products, ACE inhibitors, disopyramide, fibrates, fluoxetine, MAO inhibitors, propoxyphene, salicylates, somatostatin analog (e.g., octreotide), sulfonamide antibiotics.

The following are examples of substances that may reduce the blood-glucose-lowering effect of insulin: corticosteroids, danazol, diuretics, sympathomimetic agents (e.g., epinephrine, albuterol, terbutaline), isoniazid, phenothiazine derivatives, somatropin, thyroid hormones, estrogens, progestogens (e.g., in oral contraceptives).

Beta-blockers, clonidine, lithium salts, and alcohol may either potentiate or weaken the blood-glucose-lowering effect of insulin. Pentamidine may cause hypoglycemia, which may sometimes be followed by hyperglycemia.

In addition, under the influence of sympatholytic medicinal products such as beta-blockers, clonidine, guanethidine, and reserpine, the signs of hypoglycemia may be reduced or absent.

Carcinogenesis, Mutagenesis, Impairment of Fertility:

In mice and rats, standard two-year carcinogenicity studies with insulin glargine were performed at doses up to 0.455 mg/kg, which is for the rat approximately 10 times and for the mouse approximately 5 times the recommended human subcutaneous starting dose of 10 IU (0.008 mg/kg/day), based on mg/m^2. The findings in female mice were not conclusive due to excessive mortality in all dose groups during the study. Histiocytomas were found at injection sites in male rats (statistically significant) and male mice (not statistically significant) in acid vehicle containing groups. These tumors were not found in female animals, in saline control, or insulin comparator groups using a different vehicle. The relevance of these findings to humans is unknown.

Insulin glargine was not mutagenic in tests for detection of gene mutations in bacteria and mammalian cells (Ames- and HGPRT-test) and in tests for detection of chromosomal aberrations (cytogenetics in vitro in V79 cells and in vivo in Chinese hamsters).

In a combined fertility and prenatal and postnatal study in male and female rats at subcutaneous doses up to 0.36 mg/kg/day, which is approximately 7 times the recommended human subcutaneous starting dose of 10 IU (0.008 mg/kg/day), based on mg/m^2, maternal toxicity due to dose-dependent hypoglycemia, including some deaths, was observed. Consequently, a reduction of the rearing rate occurred in the high-dose group only. Similar effects were observed with NPH human insulin.

Pregnancy:

Teratogenic Effects: Pregnancy Category C. Subcutaneous reproduction and teratology studies have been performed with insulin glargine and regular human insulin in rats and Himalayan rabbits. The drug was given to female rats before mating, during mating, and throughout pregnancy at doses up to 0.36 mg/kg/day, which is approximately 7 times the recommended human subcutaneous starting dose of 10 IU (0.008 mg/kg/day), based on mg/m^2. In rabbits, doses of 0.072 mg/kg/day, which is approximately 2 times the recommended human subcutaneous starting dose of 10 IU (0.008 mg/kg/day), based on mg/m^2, were administered during organogenesis. The effects of insulin glargine did not generally differ from those observed with regular human insulin in rats or rabbits. However, in rabbits, five fetuses from two litters of the high-dose group exhibited dilation of the cerebral ventricles. Fertility and early embryonic development appeared normal.

There are no well-controlled clinical studies of the use of insulin glargine in pregnant women. It is essential for patients with diabetes or a history of gestational diabetes to maintain good metabolic control before conception and throughout pregnancy. Insulin requirements may decrease during the first trimester, generally increase during the second and third trimesters, and rapidly decline after delivery. Careful monitoring of glucose control is essential in such patients. Because animal reproduction studies are not always predictive of human response, this drug should be used during pregnancy only if clearly needed.

Nursing Mothers:

It is unknown whether insulin glargine is excreted in significant amounts in human milk. Many drugs, including human insulin, are excreted in human milk. For this reason, caution should be exercised when LANTUS is administered to a nursing woman. Lactating women may require adjustments in insulin dose and diet.

Pediatric Use:

Safety and effectiveness of LANTUS have been established in the age group 6 to 15 years with type 1 diabetes.

Geriatric Use:

In controlled clinical studies comparing insulin glargine to NPH human insulin, 593 of 3890 patients with type 1 and type 2 diabetes were 65 years and older. The only difference in safety or effectiveness in this subpopulation compared to the entire study population was an expected higher incidence of cardiovascular events in both insulin glargine and NPH human insulin-treated patients.

In elderly patients with diabetes, the initial dosing, dose increments, and maintenance dosage should be conservative to avoid hypoglycemic reactions. Hypoglycemia may be difficult to recognize in the elderly (see PRECAUTIONS, Hypoglycemia).

ADVERSE REACTIONS

The adverse events commonly associated with LANTUS include the following:

Continued on next page

Lantus—Cont.

Body as a whole: allergic reactions (see PRECAUTIONS).
Skin and appendages: injection site reaction, lipodystrophy, pruritus, rash (see PRECAUTIONS).
Other: hypoglycemia (see WARNINGS and PRECAUTIONS).
In clinical studies in adult patients, there was a higher incidence of treatment-emergent injection site pain in LANTUS-treated patients (2.7%) compared to NPH insulin-treated patients (0.7%). The reports of pain at the injection site were usually mild and did not result in discontinuation of therapy. Other treatment-emergent injection site reactions occurred at similar incidences with both insulin glargine and NPH human insulin.
Retinopathy was evaluated in the clinical studies by means of retinal adverse events reported and fundus photography. The numbers of retinal adverse events reported for LANTUS and NPH treatment groups were similar for patients with type 1 and type 2 diabetes. Progression of retinopathy was investigated by fundus photography using a grading protocol derived from the Early Treatment Diabetic Retinopathy Study (ETDRS). In one clinical study involving patients with type 2 diabetes, a difference in the number of subjects with ≥3-step progression in ETDRS scale over a 6-month period was noted by fundus photography (7.5% in LANTUS group versus 2.7% in NPH treated group). The overall relevance of this isolated finding cannot be determined due to the small number of patients involved, the short follow-up period, and the fact that this finding was not observed in other clinical studies.

OVERDOSAGE

An excess of insulin relative to food intake, energy expenditure, or both may lead to severe and sometimes long-term and life-threatening hypoglycemia. Mild episodes of hypoglycemia can usually be treated with oral carbohydrates. Adjustments in drug dosage, meal patterns, or exercise may be needed.
More severe episodes with coma, seizure, or neurologic impairment may be treated with intramuscular/subcutaneous glucagon or concentrated intravenous glucose. After apparent clinical recovery from hypoglycemia, continued observation and additional carbohydrate intake may be necessary to avoid reoccurrence of hypoglycemia.

DOSAGE AND ADMINISTRATION

LANTUS is a recombinant human insulin analog. Its potency is approximately the same as human insulin. It exhibits a relatively constant glucose-lowering profile over 24 hours that permits once-daily dosing.
LANTUS may be administered at any time during the day. LANTUS should be administered subcutaneously once a day at the same time every day. For patients adjusting timing of dosing with LANTUS, see **WARNINGS** and **PRECAUTIONS, Hypoglycemia**. LANTUS is not intended for intravenous administration (see PRECAUTIONS). Intravenous administration of the usual subcutaneous dose could result in severe hypoglycemia. The desired blood glucose levels as well as the doses and timing of antidiabetes medications must be determined individually. Blood glucose monitoring is recommended for all patients with diabetes. The prolonged duration of activity of LANTUS is dependent on injection into subcutaneous space.
As with all insulins, injection sites within an injection area (abdomen, thigh, or deltoid) must be rotated from one injection to the next.
In clinical studies, there was no relevant difference in insulin glargine absorption after abdominal, deltoid, or thigh subcutaneous administration. As for all insulins, the rate of absorption, and consequently the onset and duration of action, may be affected by exercise and other variables.
LANTUS is not the insulin of choice for the treatment of diabetes ketoacidosis. Intravenous short-acting insulin is the preferred treatment.

Pediatric Use:
LANTUS can be safely administered to pediatric patients ≥6 years of age. Administration to pediatric patients <6 years has not been studied. Based on the results of a study in pediatric patients, the dose recommendation for changeover to LANTUS is the same as described for adults in DOSAGE AND ADMINISTRATION, Changeover to LANTUS.

Initiation of LANTUS Therapy:
In a clinical study with insulin naïve patients with type 2 diabetes already treated with oral antidiabetes drugs, LANTUS was started at an average dose of 10 IU once daily, and subsequently adjusted according to the patient's need to a total daily dose ranging from 2 to 100 IU.

Changeover to LANTUS:
If changing from a treatment regimen with an intermediate- or long-acting insulin to a regimen with LANTUS, the amount and timing of short-acting insulin or fast-acting insulin analog or the dose of any oral antidiabetes drug may need to be adjusted. In clinical studies, when patients were transferred from once-daily NPH human insulin or ultralente human insulin to once-daily LANTUS, the initial dose was usually not changed. However, when patients were transferred from twice-daily NPH human insulin to LANTUS once daily, to reduce the risk of hypoglycemia, the initial dose (IU) was usually reduced by approximately 20% (compared to total daily IU of NPH human insulin) and then adjusted based on patient response (see PRECAUTIONS, Hypoglycemia).

	Not in-use (unopened) Refrigerated	Not in-use (unopened) Room Temperature	In-use (opened) (See Temperature Below)
10 mL Vial	Until expiration date	28 days	28 days Refrigerated or room temperature
3 mL Cartridge system	Until expiration date	28 days	28 days Refrigerated or room temperature
3 mL Cartridge system inserted into OptiClik™			28 days Room temperature only (Do not refrigerate)

A program of close metabolic monitoring under medical supervision is recommended during transfer and in the initial weeks thereafter. The amount and timing of short-acting insulin or fast-acting insulin analog may need to be adjusted. This is particularly true for patients with acquired antibodies to human insulin needing high-insulin doses and occurs with all insulin analogs. Dose adjustment of LANTUS and other insulins or oral antidiabetes drugs may be required; for example, if the patient's timing of dosing, weight or lifestyle changes, or other circumstances arise that increase susceptibility to hypoglycemia or hyperglycemia (see PRECAUTIONS, Hypoglycemia).
The dose may also have to be adjusted during intercurrent illness (see PRECAUTIONS, Intercurrent Conditions).

Preparation and Handling:
Parenteral drug products should be inspected visually prior to administration whenever the solution and the container permit. LANTUS must only be used if the solution is clear and colorless with no particles visible.

Mixing and diluting: LANTUS must NOT be diluted or mixed with any other insulin or solution (see PRECAUTIONS, General).

Vial: **The syringes must not contain any other medicinal product or residue.**

Cartridge system: If OptiClik™, the Insulin Delivery Device for LANTUS, malfunctions, LANTUS may be drawn from the cartridge system into a U-100 syringe and injected.

HOW SUPPLIED

LANTUS 100 units per mL (U-100) is available in the following package size:
10 mL vials (NDC 0088-2220-33)
3 mL cartridge system*, package of 5 (NDC 0088-2220-52)
*Cartridge systems are for use only in OptiClik™ (Insulin Delivery Device)

Storage:

Unopened Vial/Cartridge system:
Unopened LANTUS vials and cartridge systems should be stored in a refrigerator, 36°F-46°F (2°C-8°C). LANTUS should not be stored in the freezer and it should not be allowed to freeze. Discard if it has been frozen.

Open (In-Use) Vial/Cartridge system:
Opened vials, whether or not refrigerated, must be used within 28 days after the first use. They must be discarded if not used within 28 days. If refrigeration is not possible, the open vial can be kept unrefrigerated for up to 28 days away from direct heat and light, as long as the temperature is not greater than 86°F (30°C).
The opened (in-use) cartridge system in OptiClik™ should **NOT** be refrigerated but should be kept at room temperature (below 86°F [30°C]) away from direct heat and light. The opened (in-use) cartridge system in OptiClik™ kept at room temperature must be discarded after 28 days. Do not store OptiClik™, with or without cartridge system, in a refrigerator at any time.
LANTUS should not be stored in the freezer and it should not be allowed to freeze. Discard if it has been frozen.
These storage conditions are summarized in the table:
[See table above]
Rev. August 2004
Manufactured by:
Aventis Pharma Deutschland GmbH
D-65926 Frankfurt am Main
Frankfurt, Germany
Manufactured for:
Aventis Pharmaceuticals Inc.
Kansas City, MO 64137 USA
US Patents 5,656,722, 5,370,629, and 5,509,905
Made in Germany
www.lantus.com

LANTUS®

(insulin glargine [Recombinant DNA origin] injection)

Patient Information

LANTUS® 10 mL vial (1000 units per vial) 100 units per mL (U-100)
(insulin glargine [recombinant DNA origin] injection)

- What is the most important information I should know about LANTUS?
- What is LANTUS?
- Who should NOT take LANTUS?
- How should I use LANTUS?
- What kind of syringe should I use?
- Mixing with LANTUS
- Instructions for Use
  - How do I draw the insulin into the syringe?
  - How do I inject LANTUS?
- What can affect how much insulin I need?
- What are the possible side effects of LANTUS and other insulins?
- How should I store LANTUS?
- General Information about LANTUS

Read this "Patient Information" that comes with LANTUS (LAN-tus) before you start using it and each time you get a refill because there may be new information. This leaflet does not take the place of talking with your healthcare provider about your condition or treatment. If you have questions about LANTUS or about diabetes, talk with your healthcare provider.

What is the most important information I should know about LANTUS?

- **Do not change the insulin you are using without talking to your healthcare provider.** Any change of insulin should be made cautiously and only under medical supervision. Changes in insulin strength, manufacturer, type (for example: Regular, NPH, analogs), species (beef, pork, beef-pork, human) or method of manufacture (recombinant DNA versus animal-source insulin) may need a change in the dose. This dose change may be needed right away or later on during the first several weeks or months on the new insulin. Doses of oral anti-diabetic medicines may also need to change, if your insulin is changed.
- **You must test your blood sugar levels while using an insulin, such as LANTUS.** Your healthcare provider will tell you how often you should test your blood sugar level, and what to do if it is high or low.
- **Do NOT dilute or mix LANTUS with any other insulin or solution.** It will not work and you may lose blood sugar control, which could be serious.
- **LANTUS** comes as U-100 insulin and contains 100 units of LANTUS per milliliter (mL). One milliliter of U-100 insulin contains 100 units of insulin. (1 mL = 1 cc).

What is Diabetes?

- Your body needs insulin to turn sugar (glucose) into energy. If your body does not make enough insulin, you need to take more insulin so you will not have too much sugar in your blood.
- Insulin injections are important in keeping your diabetes under control. But the way you live, your diet, careful checking of your blood sugar levels, exercise, and planned physical activity, all work with your insulin to help you control your diabetes.

What is LANTUS?

- LANTUS (insulin glargine [recombinant DNA origin]) is a long-acting insulin. Because Lantus is made by recombinant DNA technology (rDNA) and is chemically different from the insulin made by the human body, it is called an insulin analog. LANTUS is used to treat patients with diabetes for the control of high blood sugar. It is used once a day to lower blood sugar.
- LANTUS is a clear, colorless, sterile solution for injection under the skin (subcutaneously).
- The active ingredient in LANTUS is insulin glargine. The concentration of insulin glargine is 100 units per milliliter (mL), or U-100. LANTUS also contains zinc, metacresol, glycerol, and water for injection as inactive ingredients. Hydrochloric acid and/or sodium hydroxide may be added to adjust the pH.
- You need a prescription to get LANTUS. Always be sure you receive the right insulin from the pharmacy. The carton and vial should look like the ones in this picture.

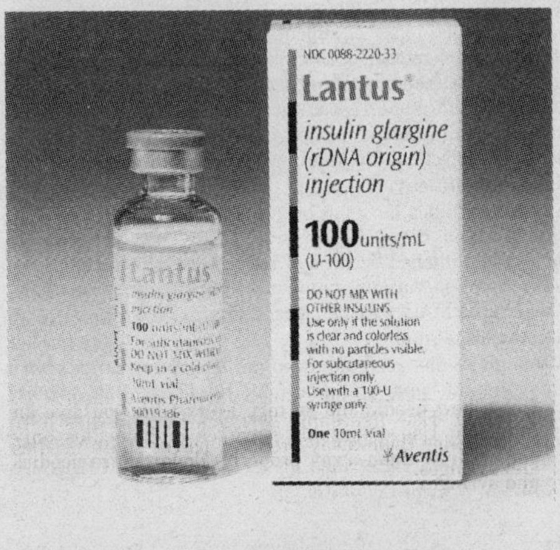

Who should NOT take LANTUS?

Do not take LANTUS if you are allergic to insulin glargine or any of the inactive ingredients in LANTUS. Check with your healthcare provider if you are not sure.

Before starting LANTUS, tell your healthcare provider about all your medical conditions including if you:

- **have liver or kidney problems.** Your dose may need to be adjusted.
- **are pregnant or plan to become pregnant.** It is not known if LANTUS may harm your unborn baby. It is very important to maintain control of your blood sugar levels during pregnancy. Your healthcare provider will decide which insulin is best for you during your pregnancy.
- **are breast-feeding or plan to breast-feed.** It is not known whether LANTUS passes into your milk. Many medicines, including insulin, pass into human milk, and could affect your baby. Talk to your healthcare provider about the best way to feed your baby.
- **about all the medicines you take including** prescription and non-prescription medicines, vitamins, and herbal supplements.

How should I use LANTUS?

See the "**Instructions for Use**" including the "**How do I draw the insulin into the syringe?**" **section for additional information.**

- Follow the instructions given by your healthcare provider about the type or types of insulin you are using. Do not make any changes with your insulin unless you have talked to your healthcare provider. Your insulin needs may change because of illness, stress, other medicines, or changes in diet or activity level. Talk to your healthcare provider about how to adjust your insulin dose.
- You may take LANTUS at any time during the day but you must take it at the same time every day.
- Only use LANTUS that is clear and colorless. If your LANTUS is cloudy or slightly colored, return it to your pharmacy for a replacement.
- Follow your healthcare provider's instructions for testing your blood sugar.
- Inject LANTUS under your skin (subcutaneously) in your upper arm, abdomen (stomach area), or thigh (upper leg). Never inject it into a vein or muscle.
- Change (rotate) injection sites within the same body area.

What kind of syringe should I use?

- Always use a syringe that is marked for U-100 insulin. If you use other than U-100 insulin syringe, you may get the wrong dose of insulin causing serious problems for you, such as a blood sugar level that is too low or too high. Always use a new needle and syringe each time you give LANTUS injection.
- **NEEDLES AND SYRINGES MUST NOT BE SHARED.**
- Disposable syringes and needles should be used only once. Used syringe and needle should be placed in sharps containers (such as red biohazard containers), hard plastic containers (such as detergent bottles), or metal containers (such as an empty coffee can). Such containers should be sealed and disposed of properly.

Mixing with LANTUS

- **Do NOT dilute or mix LANTUS with any other insulin or solution.** It will not work as intended and you may lose blood sugar control, which could be serious.

Instructions for Use

How do I draw the insulin into the syringe?

- **The syringe must be new and does not contain any other medicine.**
- **Do not mix LANTUS with any other type of insulin.**

Follow these steps:

1. Wash your hands with soap and water or with alcohol.
2. Check the insulin to make sure it is clear and colorless. Do not use the insulin after the expiration date stamped on the label, if it is colored or cloudy, or if you see particles in the solution.
3. If you are using a new vial, remove the protective cap. **Do not** remove the stopper.

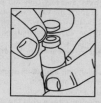

4. Wipe the top of the vial with an alcohol swab. You do not have to shake the vial of LANTUS before use.

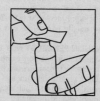

5. Use a new needle and syringe every time you give an injection. Use disposable syringes and needles only once. Throw them away properly. **Never** share needles and syringes.

6. Draw air into the syringe equal to your insulin dose. Put the needle through the rubber top of the vial and push the plunger to inject the air into the vial.

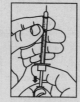 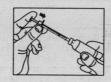

7. Leave the syringe in the vial and turn both upside down. Hold the syringe and vial firmly in one hand.
8. Make sure the tip of the needle is in the insulin. With your free hand, pull the plunger to withdraw the correct dose into the syringe.

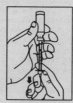

9. Before you take the needle out of the vial, check the syringe for air bubbles. If bubbles are in the syringe, hold the syringe straight up and tap the side of the syringe until the bubbles float to the top. Push the bubbles out with the plunger and draw insulin back in until you have the correct dose.

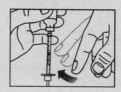

10. Remove the needle from the vial. Do not let the needle touch anything. You are now ready to inject.

How do I inject LANTUS?

Inject LANTUS under your skin. Take LANTUS as prescribed by your healthcare provider.

Follow these steps:

1. Decide on an injection area - either upper arm, thigh or abdomen. Injection sites within an injection area must be different from one injection to the next.
2. Use alcohol or soap and water to clean the injection site. The injection site should be dry before you inject.

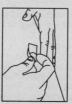

3. Pinch the skin. Stick the needle in the way your healthcare provider showed you. Release the skin.
4. Slowly push in the plunger of the syringe all the way, making sure you have injected all the insulin. Leave the needle in the skin for about 10 seconds.

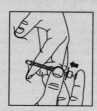

5. Pull the needle straight out and gently press on the spot where you injected yourself for several seconds. **Do not rub the area.**
6. Follow your healthcare provider's instructions for throwing away the used needle and syringe. Do not recap the used needle. Used needle and syringe should be placed in sharps containers (such as red biohazard containers), hard plastic containers (such as detergent bottles), or metal containers (such as an empty coffee can). Such containers should be sealed and disposed of properly.

What can affect how much insulin I need?

Illness. Illness may change how much insulin you need. It is a good idea to think ahead and make a "sick day" plan with your healthcare provider in advance so you will be ready when this happens. Be sure to test your blood sugar more often and call your healthcare provider if you are sick.

Medicines. Many medicines can affect your insulin needs. Other medicines, including prescription and non-prescription medicines, vitamins, and herbal supplements, can change the way insulin works. You may need a different dose of insulin when you are taking certain other medicines.

Know all the medicines you take, including prescription and non-prescription medicines, vitamins, and herbal supplements. You may want to keep a list of the medicines you take. You can show this list to your healthcare provider anytime you get a new medicine or refill. Your healthcare provider will tell you if your insulin dose needs to be changed.

Meals. The amount of food you eat can affect your insulin needs. If you eat less food, skip meals, or eat more food than usual, you may need a different dose of insulin. Talk to your healthcare provider if you change your diet so that you know how to adjust your LANTUS and other insulin doses.

Alcohol. Alcohol, including beer and wine, may affect the way LANTUS works and affect your blood sugar levels. Talk to your healthcare provider about drinking alcohol.

Exercise or Activity level. Exercise or activity level may change the way your body uses insulin. Check with your healthcare provider before you start an exercise program because your dose may need to be changed.

Travel. If you travel across time zones, talk with your healthcare provider about how to time your injections. When you travel, wear your medical alert identification. Take extra insulin and supplies with you.

Pregnancy or nursing. The effects of LANTUS on an unborn child or on a nursing baby are unknown. Therefore, tell your healthcare provider if you planning to have a baby, are pregnant, or nursing a baby. Good control of diabetes is especially important during pregnancy and nursing.

What are the possible side effects of LANTUS and other insulins?

Insulins, including LANTUS, can cause hypoglycemia (low blood sugar), hyperglycemia (high blood sugar), allergy, and skin reactions.

Hypoglycemia (low blood sugar):

Hypoglycemia is often called an "insulin reaction" or "low blood sugar". It may happen when you do not have enough sugar in your blood. Common causes of hypoglycemia are illness, emotional or physical stress, too much insulin, too little food or missed meals, and too much exercise or activity.

Early warning signs of hypoglycemia may be different, less noticeable or not noticeable at all in some people. That is why it is important to check your blood sugar as you have been advised by your healthcare provider.

Hypoglycemia can happen with:

- **Taking too much insulin.** This can happen when too much insulin is injected.
- **Not enough carbohydrate (sugar or starch) intake.** This can happen if a meal or snack is missed or delayed.
- **Vomiting or diarrhea** that decreases the amount of sugar absorbed by your body.
- **Intake of alcohol.**
- **Medicines that affect insulin.** Be sure to discuss all your medicines with your healthcare provider. **Do not start any new medicines until you know how they may affect your insulin dose.**
- **Medical conditions that can affect your blood sugar levels or insulin.** These conditions include diseases of the adrenal glands, the pituitary, the thyroid gland, the liver, and the kidney.
- **Too much glucose use by the body.** This can happen if you exercise too much or have a fever.
- **Injecting insulin the wrong way or in the wrong injection area.**

Hypoglycemia can be mild to severe. Its onset may be rapid. Some patients have few or no warning symptoms, including:

- patients with diabetes for a long time
- patients with diabetic neuropathy (nerve problems)
- or patients using certain medicines for high blood pressure or heart problems.

Hypoglycemia may reduce your ability to drive a car or use mechanical equipment and you may risk injury to yourself or others.

Severe hypoglycemia can be dangerous and can cause temporary or permanent harm to your heart or brain. **It may cause unconsciousness, seizures, or death.**

Symptoms of hypoglycemia may include:

- anxiety, irritability, restlessness, trouble concentrating, personality changes, mood changes, or other abnormal behavior
- tingling in your hands, feet, lips, or tongue
- dizziness, light-headedness, or drowsiness
- nightmares or trouble sleeping
- headache
- blurred vision
- slurred speech
- palpitations (fast heart beat)
- sweating
- tremor (shaking)
- unsteady gait (walking).

If you have hypoglycemia often or it is hard for you to know if you have the symptoms of hypoglycemia, talk to your healthcare provider.

Mild to moderate hypoglycemia is treated by eating or drinking carbohydrates, such as fruit juice, raisins, sugar candies, milk or glucose tablets. Talk to your healthcare provider about the amount of carbohydrates you should eat to treat mild to moderate hypoglycemia.

Severe hypoglycemia may require the help of another person or emergency medical people. A person with hypoglycemia who is unable to take foods or liquids with sugar by mouth, or is unconscious needs medical help fast and will

Continued on next page

Lantus—Cont.

need treatment with a glucagon injection or glucose given intravenously (IV). Without medical help right away, serious reactions or even death could happen.

Hyperglycemia (high blood sugar):

Hyperglycemia happens when you have too much sugar in your blood. Usually, it means there is not enough insulin to break down the food you eat into energy your body can use. Hyperglycemia can be caused by a fever, an infection, stress, eating more than you should, taking less insulin than prescribed, or it can mean your diabetes is getting worse.

Hyperglycemia can happen with:

- **Insufficient (too little) insulin.** This can happen from:
  - injecting too little or no insulin
  - incorrect storage (freezing, excessive heat)
  - use after the expiration date.
- **Too much carbohydrate intake.** This can happen if you eat larger meals, eat more often, or increase the amount of carbohydrate in your meals.
- **Medicines that affect insulin.** Be sure to discuss all your medicines with your healthcare provider. **Do not start any new medicines until you know how they may affect your insulin dose.**
- **Medical conditions that affect insulin.** These medical conditions include fevers, infections, heart attacks, and stress.
- **Injecting insulin the wrong way or in the wrong injection area.**

Testing your blood or urine often will let you know if you have hyperglycemia. If your tests are often high, tell your healthcare provider so your dose of insulin can be changed. Hyperglycemia can be mild or severe. Hyperglycemia can **progress to diabetic ketoacidosis (DKA) or very high glucose levels (hyperosmolar coma) and result in unconsciousness and death.**

Although diabetic ketoacidosis occurs most often in patients with type 1 diabetes, it can also happen in patients with type 2 diabetes who become very sick. Because some patients get few symptoms of hyperglycemia, it is important to check your blood sugar/urine sugar and ketones regularly.

Symptoms of hyperglycemia include:

- confusion or drowsiness
- increased thirst
- decreased appetite, nausea, or vomiting
- rapid heart rate
- increased urination and dehydration (too little fluid in your body).

Symptoms of DKA also include:

- fruity smelling breath
- fast, deep breathing
- stomach area (abdominal) pain.

Severe or continuing hyperglycemia or DKA needs evaluation and treatment right away by your healthcare provider. Do not use LANTUS to treat diabetic ketoacidosis.

Other possible side effects of LANTUS include:

Serious allergic reactions:

Some times severe, life-threatening allergic reactions can happen with insulin. If you think you are having a severe allergic reaction, get medical help right away. Signs of insulin allergy include:

- rash all over your body
- shortness of breath
- wheezing (trouble breathing)
- fast pulse
- sweating
- low blood pressure.

Reactions at the injection site:

Injecting insulin can cause the following reactions on the skin at the injection site:

- little depression in the skin (lipoatrophy)
- skin thickening (lipohypertrophy)
- red, swelling, itchy skin (injection site reaction).

You can reduce the chance of getting an injection site reaction if you change (rotate) the injection site each time. An injection site reaction should clear up in a few days or a few weeks. If injection site reactions do not go away or keep happening, call your healthcare provider.

Tell your healthcare provider if you have any side effects that bother you.

These are not all the side effects of LANTUS. Ask your healthcare provider or pharmacist for more information.

How should I store LANTUS?

- **Unopened vial:**
  Store new (unopened) LANTUS vials in a refrigerator (not the freezer) between 36°F to 46°F (2°C to 8°C). Do not freeze LANTUS. Keep LANTUS out of direct heat and light. If a vial has been frozen or overheated, throw it away.
- **Open (In-Use) vial:**
  Once a vial is opened, you can keep it in a refrigerator or at room temperature (below 86°F [30°C]) but away from direct heat and light. Opened vial, either kept in a refrigerator or at room temperature, should be discarded 28 days after the first use even if it still contains LANTUS. Do not leave your insulin in a car on a summer day.

These storage conditions are summarized in the following table:
[See table below]

- Do not use a vial of LANTUS after the expiration date stamped on the label.
- Do not use LANTUS if it is cloudy, colored, or if you see particles.

General Information about LANTUS

- Use LANTUS only to treat your diabetes. **Do not** give or share LANTUS with another person, even if they have diabetes also. It may harm them.
- This leaflet summarizes the most important information about LANTUS. If you would like more information, talk with your healthcare provider. You can ask your doctor or pharmacist for information about LANTUS that is written for healthcare professionals. For more information about LANTUS call 1-800-633-1610 or go to website www.lantus.com.

ADDITIONAL INFORMATION

DIABETES FORECAST is a national magazine designed especially for patients with diabetes and their families and is available by subscription from the American Diabetes Association (ADA), P.O. Box 363, Mt. Morris, IL 61054-0363, 1-800-DIABETES (1-800-342-2383). You may also visit the ADA website at www.diabetes.org.

Another publication, **COUNTDOWN**, is available from the Juvenile Diabetes Research Foundation International (JDRF), 120 Wall Street, 19th Floor, New York, New York 10005, 1-800-JDF-CURE (1-800-533-2873). You may also visit the JDRF website at www.jdf.org.

To get more information about diabetes, check with your healthcare professional or diabetes educator or visit www.DiabetesWatch.com.

Additional information about LANTUS can be obtained by calling 1-800-633-1610 or by visiting www.lantus.com.

Rev. August 2004

Aventis Pharmaceuticals Inc.
Kansas City, MO 64137 USA
©2004 Aventis Pharmaceuticals Inc.
† Lantus® is a registered trademark of Aventis Pharmaceuticals Inc.

LANTUS®

(insulin glargine [Recombinant DNA origin] injection)

Patient Information

LANTUS® 3 mL cartridge system (300 units per cartridge system)
100 units per mL (U-100)
(insulin glargine [recombinant DNA origin] injection)

- What is the most important information I should know about LANTUS?
- What is LANTUS?
- Who should NOT take LANTUS?
- How should I use LANTUS?
- What kind of insulin Pen should I use?
- Mixing with LANTUS
- Instructions for Use
- What can affect how much insulin I need?
- What are the possible side effects of LANTUS and other insulins?
- How should I store LANTUS?
- General Information about LANTUS

Read this "Patient Information" that comes with LANTUS (LAN-tus) before you start using it and each time you get a refill because there may be new information. This leaflet does not take the place of talking with your healthcare provider about your condition or treatment. If you have questions about LANTUS or about diabetes, talk with your healthcare provider.

What is the most important information I should know about LANTUS?

- **Do not change the insulin you are using without talking to your healthcare provider.** Any change of insulin should be made cautiously and only under medical supervision. Changes in insulin strength, manufacturer, type (for example: Regular, NPH, analogs), species (beef, pork, beef-pork, human) or method of manufacture (recombinant DNA versus animal-source insulin) may need a change in the dose. This dose change may be needed right away or later on during the first several weeks or months on the new insulin. Doses of oral anti-diabetic medicines may also need to change, if your insulin is changed.
- **You must test your blood sugar levels while using an insulin, such as LANTUS.** Your healthcare provider will tell you how often you should test your blood sugar level, and what to do if it is high or low.
- **Do NOT dilute or mix LANTUS with any other insulin or solution.** It will not work and you may lose blood sugar control, which could be serious.
- **LANTUS** comes as U-100 insulin and contains 100 units of LANTUS per milliliter (mL). One milliliter of U-100 insulin contains 100 units of insulin. (1 mL = 1 cc).

What is Diabetes?

- Your body needs insulin to turn sugar (glucose) into energy. If your body does not make enough insulin, you need

to take more insulin so you will not have too much sugar in your blood.

- Insulin injections are important in keeping your diabetes under control. But the way you live, your diet, careful checking of your blood sugar levels, exercise, and planned physical activity, all work with your insulin to help you control your diabetes.

What is LANTUS?

- LANTUS (insulin glargine [recombinant DNA origin]) is a long-acting insulin. Because Lantus is made by recombinant DNA technology (rDNA) and is chemically different from the insulin made by the human body, it is called an insulin analog. LANTUS is used to treat patients with diabetes for the control of high blood sugar. It is used once a day to lower blood glucose.
- LANTUS is a clear, colorless, sterile solution for injection under the skin (subcutaneously).
- The active ingredient in LANTUS is insulin glargine. The concentration of insulin glargine is 100 units per milliliter (mL), or U-100. LANTUS also contains zinc, metacresol, glycerol, and water for injection as inactive ingredients. Hydrochloric acid and/or sodium hydroxide may be added to adjust the pH.
- You need a prescription to get LANTUS. Always be sure you receive the right insulin from the pharmacy. The carton and cartridge system should look like the ones in this picture.

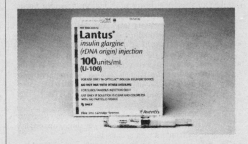

Who should NOT take LANTUS?

Do not take LANTUS if you are allergic to insulin glargine or any of the inactive ingredients in LANTUS. Check with your healthcare provider if you are not sure.

- **Before starting LANTUS, tell your healthcare provider about all your medical conditions including if you:**
  - **have liver or kidney problems.** Your dose may need to be adjusted.
  - **are pregnant or plan to become pregnant.** It is not known if LANTUS may harm your unborn baby. It is very important to maintain control of your blood sugar levels during pregnancy. Your healthcare provider will decide which insulin is best for you during your pregnancy.
  - **are breast-feeding or plan to breast-feed.** It is not known whether LANTUS passes into your milk. Many medicines, including insulin, pass into human milk, and could affect your baby. Talk to your healthcare provider about the best way to feed your baby.
  - **about all the medicines you take including** prescription and non-prescription medicines, vitamins and herbal supplements.

How should I use LANTUS?

See the "Instructions for OptiClik™ Use" section for additional information.

- Follow the instructions given by your healthcare provider about the type or types of insulin you are using. Do not make any changes with your insulin unless you have talked to your healthcare provider. Your insulin needs may change because of illness, stress, other medicines, or changes in diet or activity level. Talk to your healthcare provider about how to adjust your insulin dose.
- You may take LANTUS at any time during the day but you must take it at the same time every day.
- Only use LANTUS that is clear and colorless. If your LANTUS is cloudy or slightly colored, return it to your pharmacy for a replacement.
- Follow your healthcare provider's instructions for testing your blood sugar.
- Inject LANTUS under your skin (subcutaneously) in your upper arm, abdomen (stomach area), or thigh (upper leg). Never inject it into a vein or muscle.
- Change (rotate) injection sites within the same body area.

What kind of insulin Pen should I use?

- Always use the OptiClik™ device distributed by Aventis Pharmaceuticals. If you use any other device than OptiClik™ insulin Pen with this cartridge, you may get the wrong dose of insulin causing serious problems for you, such as a blood sugar level that is too low or too high. Always use a new needle each time you give LANTUS injection.
- **NEEDLES AND INSULIN PEN MUST NOT BE SHARED.**
- Disposable needle should be used only once. Used needle should be placed in sharps containers (such as red biohazard containers), hard plastic containers (such as detergent bottles), or metal containers (such as an empty coffee can). Such containers should be sealed and disposed of properly.

Mixing with LANTUS

- **Do NOT dilute or mix LANTUS with any other insulin or solution.** It will not work as intended and you may lose blood sugar control, which could be serious.

	Not in-use (unopened) Refrigerated	Not in-use (unopened) Room Temperature	In-use (opened) (See Temperature Below)
10 mL Vial	Until expiration date	28 days	28 days Refrigerated or room temperature

Instructions for OptiClik™ Use

It is important to read, understand, and follow the step-by-step instructions in the "OptiClik™ Instruction Leaflet" before using OptiClik™ insulin Pen. Failure to follow the instructions may result in getting too much or too little insulin. If you have lost your leaflet or have a question, go to www.opticlik.com or call 1-800-633-1610.

The following general notes should be taken into consideration before injecting Lantus:

- Always wash your hands before handling the cartridge system and/or the OptiClik™ insulin Pen.
- Always attach a new needle before use.
- Always perform the safety test before use.
- Check the insulin solution in the cartridge system to make sure it is clear, colorless, and free of particles. If it is not, throw it away.
- Do NOT mix or dilute LANTUS with any other insulin or solution. LANTUS will not work if it is mixed or diluted and you may lose blood sugar control, which could be serious.
- Decide on an injection area - either upper arm, thigh, or abdomen. Do not use the same injection site as your last injection.
- After injecting LANTUS, leave the needle in the skin for an additional 10 seconds. Then pull the needle straight out. Gently press on the spot where you injected yourself for a few seconds. **Do not rub the area.**
- Do not drop the OptiClik™ insulin Pen.

If your blood glucose reading is high or low, tell your healthcare provider so the dose can be adjusted.

What can affect how much insulin I need?

Illness. Illness may change how much insulin you need. It is a good idea to think ahead and make a "sick day" plan with your healthcare provider in advance so you will be ready when this happens. Be sure to test your blood sugar more often and call your healthcare provider if you are sick.

Medicines. Many medicines can affect your insulin needs. Other medicines, including prescription and non-prescription medicines, vitamins, and herbal supplements, can change the way insulin works. You may need a different dose of insulin when you are taking certain other medicines. **Know all the medicines you take,** including prescription and non-prescription medicines, vitamins, and herbal supplements. You may want to keep a list of the medicines you take. You can show this list to your healthcare provider and pharmacists anytime you get a new medicine or refill. Your healthcare provider will tell you if your insulin dose needs to be changed.

Meals. The amount of food you eat can affect your insulin needs. If you eat less food, skip meals, or eat more food than usual, you may need a different dose of insulin. Talk to your healthcare provider if you change your diet so that you know how to adjust your LANTUS and other insulin doses.

Alcohol. Alcohol, including beer and wine, may affect the way LANTUS works and affect your blood sugar levels. Talk to your healthcare provider about drinking alcohol.

Exercise or Activity level. Exercise or activity level may change the way your body uses insulin. Check with your healthcare provider before you start an exercise program because your dose may need to be changed.

Travel. If you travel across time zones, talk with your healthcare provider about how to time your injections. When you travel, wear your medical alert identification. Take extra insulin and supplies with you.

Pregnancy or nursing. The effects of LANTUS on an unborn child or on a nursing baby are unknown. Therefore, tell your healthcare provider if you planning to have a baby, are pregnant, or nursing a baby. Good control of diabetes is especially important during pregnancy and nursing.

What are the possible side effects of LANTUS and other insulins?

Insulins, including LANTUS, can cause hypoglycemia (low blood sugar), hyperglycemia (high blood sugar), allergy, and skin reactions.

Hypoglycemia (low blood sugar):

Hypoglycemia is often called an "insulin reaction" or "low blood sugar". It may happen when you do not have enough sugar in your blood. Common causes of hypoglycemia are illness, emotional or physical stress, too much insulin, too little food or missed meals, and too much exercise or activity.

Early warning signs of hypoglycemia may be different, less noticeable or not noticeable at all in some people. That is why it is important to check your blood sugar as you have been advised by your healthcare provider.

Hypoglycemia can happen with:

- **Taking too much insulin.** This can happen when too much insulin is injected.
- **Not enough carbohydrate (sugar or starch) intake.** This can happen if a meal or snack is missed or delayed.
- **Vomiting or diarrhea** that decreases the amount of sugar absorbed by your body.
- **Intake of alcohol.**
- **Medicines that affect insulin.** Be sure to discuss all your medicines with your healthcare provider. **Do not start any new medicines until you know how they may affect your insulin dose.**
- **Medical conditions that can affect your blood sugar levels or insulin.** These conditions include diseases of the adrenal glands, the pituitary, the thyroid gland, the liver, and the kidney.

- **Too much glucose use by the body.** This can happen if you exercise too much or have a fever.
- **Injecting insulin the wrong way or in the wrong injection area.**

Hypoglycemia can be mild to severe. Its onset may be rapid. Some patients have few or no warning symptoms, including:

- patients with diabetes for a long time
- patients with diabetic neuropathy (nerve problems)
- or patients using certain medicines for high blood pressure or heart problems.

Hypoglycemia may reduce your ability to drive a car or use mechanical equipment and you may risk injury to yourself or others.

Severe hypoglycemia can be dangerous and can cause temporary or permanent harm to your heart or brain. **It may cause unconsciousness, seizures, or death.**

Symptoms of hypoglycemia may include:

- anxiety, irritability, restlessness, trouble concentrating, personality changes, mood changes, or other abnormal behavior
- tingling in your hands, feet, lips, or tongue
- dizziness, light-headedness, or drowsiness
- nightmares or trouble sleeping
- headache
- blurred vision
- slurred speech
- palpitations (fast heart beat)
- sweating
- tremor (shaking)
- unsteady gait (walking).

If you have hypoglycemia often or it is hard for you to know if you have the symptoms of hypoglycemia, talk to your healthcare provider.

Mild to moderate hypoglycemia is treated by eating or drinking carbohydrates, such as fruit juice, raisins, sugar candies, milk or glucose tablets. Talk to your healthcare provider about the amount of carbohydrates you should eat to treat mild to moderate hypoglycemia.

Severe hypoglycemia may require the help of another person or emergency medical people. A person with hypoglycemia who is unable to take foods or liquids with sugar by mouth, or is unconscious needs medical help fast and will need treatment with a glucagon injection or glucose given intravenously (IV). Without medical help right away, serious reactions or even death could happen.

Hyperglycemia (high blood sugar):

Hyperglycemia happens when you have too much sugar in your blood. Usually, it means there is not enough insulin to break down the food you eat into energy your body can use. Hyperglycemia can be caused by a fever, an infection, stress, eating more than you should, taking less insulin than prescribed, or it can mean your diabetes is getting worse.

Hyperglycemia can happen with:

- **Insufficient (too little) insulin.** This can happen from:
  - injecting too little or no insulin
  - incorrect storage (freezing, excessive heat)
  - use after the expiration date.
- **Too much carbohydrate intake.** This can happen if you eat larger meals, eat more often, or increase the amount of carbohydrate in your meals.
- **Medicines that affect insulin.** Be sure to discuss all your medicines with your healthcare provider. **Do not start any new medicines until you know how they may affect your insulin dose.**
- **Medical conditions that affect insulin.** These medical conditions include fevers, infections, heart attacks, and stress.
- **Injecting insulin the wrong way or in the wrong injection area.**

Testing your blood or urine often will let you know if you have hyperglycemia. If your tests are often high, tell your healthcare provider so your dose of insulin can be changed. Hyperglycemia can be mild or severe. It can **progress to diabetic ketoacidosis (DKA) or very high glucose levels (hyperosmolar coma) and result in unconsciousness and death.**

Although diabetic ketoacidosis occurs most often in patients with type 1 diabetes, it can also happen in patients with type 2 diabetes who become very sick. Because some patients get few symptoms of hyperglycemia, it is important to check your blood sugar/urine sugar and ketones regularly.

Symptoms of hyperglycemia include:

- confusion or drowsiness
- increased thirst
- decreased appetite, nausea, or vomiting
- rapid heart rate
- increased urination and dehydration (too little fluid in your body).

Symptoms of DKA also include:

- fruity smelling breath
- fast, deep breathing
- stomach area (abdominal) pain.

Severe or continuing hyperglycemia or DKA needs evaluation and treatment right away by your healthcare provider.

	Not in-use (unopened) Refrigerated	Not in-use (unopened) Room Temperature	In-use (opened) (See Temperature Below)
3 mL Cartridge System	Until expiration date	28 days	28 days Refrigerated or room temperature
3 mL cartridge system inserted in OptiClik™ insulin Pen			28 days Room temperature only (Do not refrigerate)

Do not use LANTUS to treat diabetic ketoacidosis.

Other possible side effects of LANTUS include:

Serious allergic reactions:

Some times severe, life-threatening allergic reactions can happen with insulin. If you think you are having a severe allergic reaction, get medical help right away. Signs of insulin allergy include:

- rash all over your body
- shortness of breath
- wheezing (trouble breathing)
- fast pulse
- sweating
- low blood pressure.

Reactions at the injection site:

Injecting insulin can cause the following reactions on the skin at the injection site:

- little depression in the skin (lipoatrophy)
- skin thickening (lipohypertrophy)
- red, swelling, itchy skin (injection site reaction).

You can reduce the chance of getting an injection site reaction if you change (rotate) the injection site each time. An injection site reaction should clear up in a few days or a few weeks. If injection site reactions do not go away or keep happening, call your healthcare provider.

Tell your healthcare provider if you have any side effects that bother you.

These are not all the side effects of LANTUS. Ask your healthcare provider or pharmacist for more information.

How should I store LANTUS?

- **Unopened cartridge system:**
  Store new unopened LANTUS cartridge systems in a refrigerator (not the freezer) between 36°F to 46°F (2°C to 8°C). Do not freeze LANTUS. Keep LANTUS out of direct heat and light. If a cartridge system has been frozen or overheated, throw it away.
- **Open (In-Use) cartridge system:**
  Once a cartridge system is opened, you can keep it at room temperature (below 86°F [30°C]) but away from direct heat and light for 28 days. Cartridge system in OptiClik™ insulin Pen must be discarded 28 days after the first use even if it still contains LANTUS. The opened cartridge system in OptiClik™ insulin Pen should be kept at room temperature (below 86°F [30°C]) and away from direct heat and light for up to 28 days. For example, do not leave it in a car on a summer day. Do not store OptiClik™, with or without cartridge system, in a refrigerator at any time.

These storage conditions are summarized in the following table:

[See table above]

- Do not use a cartridge system of LANTUS after the expiration date stamped on the label.
- Do not use LANTUS if it is cloudy, colored, or if you see particles.

General Information about LANTUS

- Use LANTUS only to treat your diabetes. **Do not** give or share LANTUS with another person, even if they have diabetes also. It may harm them.
- This leaflet summarizes the most important information about LANTUS. If you would like more information, talk with your healthcare provider. You can ask your healthcare provider or pharmacist for information about LANTUS that is written for healthcare professionals. For more information about LANTUS call 1-800-633-1610 or go to website www.lantus.com.

ADDITIONAL INFORMATION

DIABETES FORECAST is a national magazine designed especially for patients with diabetes and their families and is available by subscription from the American Diabetes Association (ADA), P.O. Box 363, Mt. Morris, IL 61054-0363, 1-800-DIABETES (1-800-342-2383). You may also visit the ADA website at www.diabetes.org.

Another publication, **COUNTDOWN**, is available from the Juvenile Diabetes Research Foundation International (JDRF), 120 Wall Street, 19th Floor, New York, New York 10005, 1-800-JDF-CURE (1-800-533-2873). You may also visit the JDRF website at www.jdf.org.

To get more information about diabetes, check with your healthcare professional or diabetes educator or visit www.DiabetesWatch.com.

Additional information about LANTUS can be obtained by calling 1-800-633-1610 or by visiting www.lantus.com.

Rev. August 2004a

Aventis Pharmaceuticals Inc.
Kansas City, MO 64137 USA

©2004 Aventis Pharmaceuticals Inc.

† Lantus® is a registered trademark of Aventis Pharmaceuticals Inc.

Continued on next page

LOVENOX® ℞

[lō'və-nŏks]

(enoxaparin sodium injection)

Rx only

Rev. July 2004

Prescribing information for this product, which appears on pages 719–725 of the 2005 PDR, has been completely revised as follows. Please write "See Supplement A" next to the product heading.

SPINAL / EPIDURAL HEMATOMAS

When neuraxial anesthesia (epidural/spinal anesthesia) or spinal puncture is employed, patients anticoagulated or scheduled to be anticoagulated with low molecular weight heparins or heparinoids for prevention of thromboembolic complications are at risk of developing an epidural or spinal hematoma which can result in long-term or permanent paralysis.

The risk of these events is increased by the use of indwelling epidural catheters for administration of analgesia or by the concomitant use of drugs affecting hemostasis such as non steroidal anti-inflammatory drugs (NSAIDs), platelet inhibitors, or other anticoagulants. The risk also appears to be increased by traumatic or repeated epidural or spinal puncture.

Patients should be frequently monitored for signs and symptoms of neurological impairment. If neurologic compromise is noted, urgent treatment is necessary.

The physician should consider the potential benefit versus risk before neuraxial intervention in patients anticoagulated or to be anticoagulated for thromboprophylaxis (see also **WARNINGS, Hemorrhage,** and **PRECAUTIONS, Drug Interactions**).

DESCRIPTION

Lovenox Injection is a sterile aqueous solution containing enoxaparin sodium, a low molecular weight heparin.

Lovenox Injection is available in two concentrations:

1. 100 mg per mL

-Prefilled Syringes	30 mg / 0.3 mL, 40 mg / 0.4 mL
-Graduated Prefilled Syringes	60 mg / 0.6 mL, 80 mg / 0.8 mL, 100 mg / 1 mL
-Multiple-Dose Vials	300 mg / 3.0 mL

Lovenox Injection 100 mg/mL Concentration contains 10 mg enoxaparin sodium (approximate anti-Factor Xa activity of 1000 IU [with reference to the W.H.O. First International Low Molecular Weight Heparin Reference Standard]) per 0.1 mL Water for Injection.

2. 150 mg per mL

-Graduated Prefilled Syringes	120 mg / 0.8 mL, 150 mg / 1 mL

Lovenox Injection 150 mg/mL Concentration contains 15 mg enoxaparin sodium (approximate anti-Factor Xa activity of 1500 IU [with reference to the W.H.O. First International Low Molecular Weight Heparin Reference Standard]) per 0.1 mL Water for Injection.

The Lovenox prefilled syringes and graduated prefilled syringes are preservative-free and intended for use only as a single-dose injection. The multiple-dose vial contains 15 mg/1.0 mL benzyl alcohol as a preservative. (See **DOSAGE AND ADMINISTRATION** and **HOW SUPPLIED** for dosage unit descriptions.) The pH of the injection is 5.5 to 7.5.

Enoxaparin sodium is obtained by alkaline depolymerization of heparin benzyl ester derived from porcine intestinal mucosa. Its structure is characterized by a 2-O-sulfo-4-enepyranosuronic acid group at the non-reducing end and a 2-N,6-O-disulfo-D-glucosamine at the reducing end of the chain. About 20% (ranging between 15% and 25%) of the enoxaparin structure contains an 1,6 anhydro derivative on the reducing end of the polysaccharide chain. The drug substance is the sodium salt. The average molecular weight is about 4500 daltons. The molecular weight distribution is:

<2000 daltons	≤20%
2000 to 8000 daltons	≥68%
>8000 daltons	≤18%

STRUCTURAL FORMULA

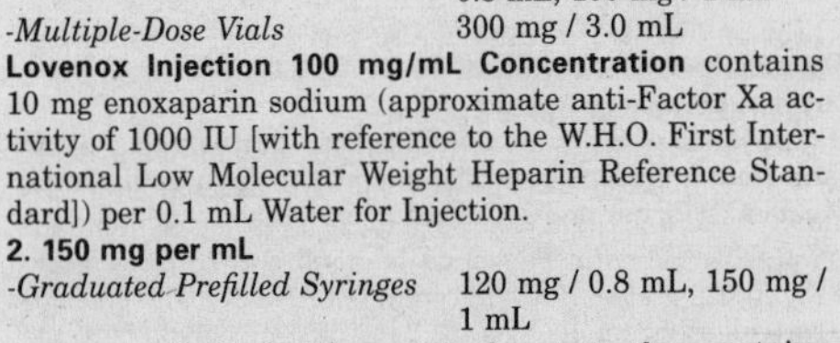
COONa
OR1
OH
NHR2
OR1
R
n

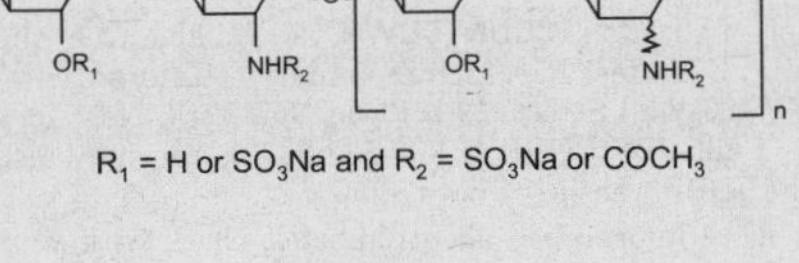

R_1 = H or SO_3Na and R_2 = SO_3Na or $COCH_3$

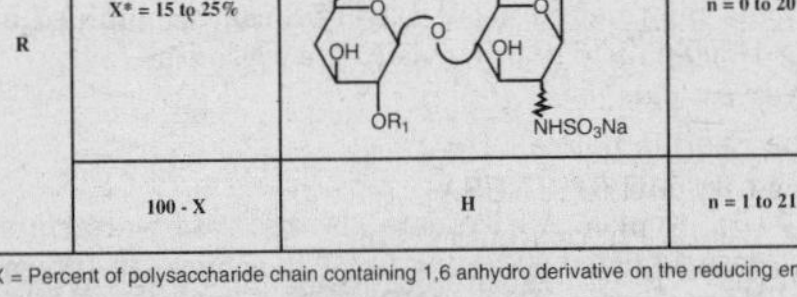

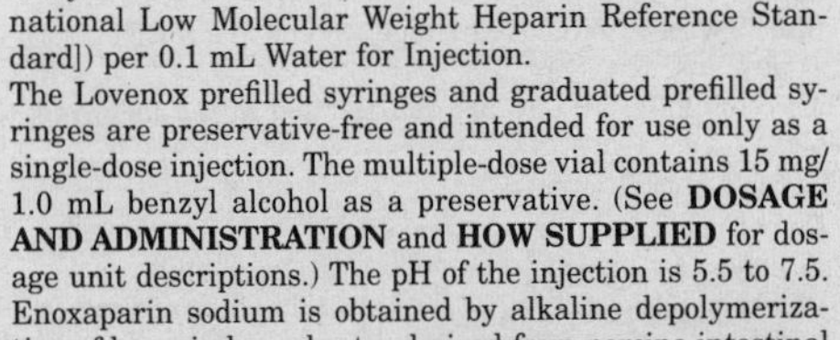
R
X* = 15 to 25%
COONa
OH
OR1
NHSO3Na
n = 0 to 20
100 - X
H
n = 1 to 21

*X = Percent of polysaccharide chain containing 1,6 anhydro derivative on the reducing end.

CLINICAL PHARMACOLOGY

Enoxaparin is a low molecular weight heparin which has antithrombotic properties. In humans, enoxaparin given at a dose of 1.5 mg/kg subcutaneously (SC) is characterized by a higher ratio of anti-Factor Xa to anti-Factor IIa activity (mean±SD, 14.0±3.1) (based on areas under anti-Factor activity versus time curves) compared to the ratios observed for heparin (mean±SD, 1.22±0.13). Increases of up to 1.8 times the control values were seen in the thrombin time (TT) and the activated partial thromboplastin time (aPTT). Enoxaparin at a 1 mg/kg dose (100 mg / mL concentration), administered SC every 12 hours to patients in a large clinical trial resulted in aPTT values of 45 seconds or less in the majority of patients (n = 1607).

Pharmacokinetics (conducted using 100 mg / mL concentration):

Absorption. Maximum anti-Factor Xa and anti-thrombin (anti-Factor IIa) activities occur 3 to 5 hours after SC injection of enoxaparin. Mean peak anti-Factor Xa activity was 0.16 IU/mL (1.58 µg/mL) and 0.38 IU/mL (3.83 µg/mL) after the 20 mg and the 40 mg clinically tested SC doses, respectively. Mean (n = 46) peak anti-Factor Xa activity was 1.1 IU/mL at steady state in patients with unstable angina receiving 1mg/kg SC every 12 hours for 14 days. Mean absolute bioavailability of enoxaparin, after 1.5 mg/kg given SC, based on anti-Factor Xa activity is approximately 100% in healthy volunteers.

Enoxaparin pharmacokinetics appear to be linear over the recommended dosage ranges (see **Dosage and Administration**). After repeated subcutaneous administration of 40 mg once daily and 1.5 mg/kg once-daily regimens in healthy volunteers, the steady state is reached on day 2 with an average exposure ratio about 15% higher than after a single dose. Steady-state enoxaparin activity levels are well predicted by single-dose pharmacokinetics. After repeated subcutaneous administration of the 1 mg/kg twice daily regimen, the steady state is reached from day 4 with mean exposure about 65% higher than after a single dose and mean peak and trough levels of about 1.2 and 0.52 IU/mL, respectively. Based on enoxaparin sodium pharmacokinetics, this difference in steady state is expected and within the therapeutic range.

Although not studied clinically, the 150 mg/mL concentration of enoxaparin sodium is projected to result in anticoagulant activities similar to those of 100 mg/mL and 200 mg/mL concentrations at the same enoxaparin dose. When a daily 1.5 mg/kg SC injection of enoxaparin sodium was given to 25 healthy male and female subjects using a 100 mg/mL or a 200 mg/mL concentration the following pharmacokinetic profiles were obtained (see table below):

[See table above]

Pharmacokinetic Parameters* After 5 Days of 1.5 mg/kg SC Once Daily Doses of Enoxaparin Sodium Using 100 mg/mL *or* 200 mg/mL Concentrations

	Concentration	Anti-Xa	Anti-IIa	Heptest	aPTT
Amax (IU/mL or Δ sec)	100 mg/mL	1.37 (±0.23)	0.23 (±0.05)	104.5 (±16.6)	19.3 (±4.7)
	200 mg/mL	1.45 (±0.22)	0.26 (±0.05)	110.9 (±17.1)	22 (±6.7)
	90% CI	102-110%		102-111%	
tmax** (h)	100 mg/mL	3 (2-6)	4 (2-5)	2.5 (2-4.5)	3 (2-4.5)
	200 mg/mL	3.5 (2-6)	4.5 (2.5-6)	3.3 (2-5)	3 (2-5)
AUC (ss) (h*IU/mL or h*Δ sec)	100 mg/mL	14.26 (±2.93)	1.54 (±0.61)	1321 (±219)	
	200 mg/mL	15.43 (±2.96)	1.77 (±0.67)	1401 (±227)	
	90% CI	105-112%		103-109%	

*Means ± SD at Day 5 and 90% Confidence Interval (CI) of the ratio

**Median (range)

Distribution. The volume of distribution of anti-Factor Xa activity is about 4.3 L.

Elimination. Following intravenous (i.v.) dosing, the total body clearance of enoxaparin is 26 mL/min. After i.v. dosing of enoxaparin labeled with the gamma-emitter, ^{99m}Tc, 40% of radioactivity and 8 to 20% of anti-Factor Xa activity were recovered in urine in 24 hours. Elimination half-life based on anti-Factor Xa activity was 4.5 hours after a single SC dose to about 7 hours after repeated dosing. Following a 40 mg SC once a day dose, significant anti-Factor Xa activity persists in plasma for about 12 hours.

Following SC dosing, the apparent clearance (CL/F) of enoxaparin is approximately 15 mL/min.

Metabolism. Enoxaparin sodium is primarily metabolized in the liver by desulfation and/or depolymerization to lower molecular weight species with much reduced biological potency. Renal clearance of active fragments represents about 10% of the administered dose and total renal excretion of active and non-active fragments 40% of the dose.

Special Populations

Gender: Apparent clearance and A_{max} derived from anti-Factor Xa values following single SC dosing (40 mg and 60 mg) were slightly higher in males than in females. The source of the gender difference in these parameters has not been conclusively identified, however, body weight may be a contributing factor.

Geriatric: Apparent clearance and A_{max} derived from anti-Factor Xa values following single and multiple SC dosing in elderly subjects were close to those observed in young subjects. Following once a day SC dosing of 40 mg enoxaparin, the Day 10 mean area under anti-Factor Xa activity versus time curve (AUC) was approximately 15% greater than the mean Day 1 AUC value. (See **PRECAUTIONS**.)

Renal Impairment: A linear relationship between anti-Factor Xa plasma clearance and creatinine clearance at steady-state has been observed, which indicates decreased clearance of enoxaparin sodium in patients with reduced renal function. Anti-Factor Xa exposure represented by AUC, at steady-state, is marginally increased in mild (creatinine clearance 50-80 mL/min) and moderate (creatinine clearance 30-50 mL/min) renal impairment after repeated subcutaneous 40 mg once daily doses. In patients with severe renal impairment (creatinine clearance <30 mL/min), the AUC at steady state is significantly increased on average by 65% after repeated subcutaneous 40-mg once-daily doses (see **PRECAUTIONS** and **DOSAGE AND ADMINISTRATION**).

Weight: After repeated subcutaneous 1.5 mg/kg once daily dosing, mean AUC of anti-Factor Xa activity is marginally higher at steady-state in obese healthy volunteers (BMI 30-48 kg/m^2) compared to non-obese control subjects, while Amax is not increased.

When non-weight adjusted dosing was administered, it was found after a single-subcutaneous 40-mg dose, that anti-Factor Xa exposure is 52% higher in low-weight women (<45 kg) and 27% higher in low-weight men (<57 kg) when compared to normal weight control subjects (see **PRECAUTIONS**).

Hemodialysis: In a single study, elimination rate appeared similar but AUC was two-fold higher than control population, after a single 0.25 or 0.50 mg/kg intravenous dose.

CLINICAL TRIALS

Prophylaxis of Deep Vein Thrombosis Following Abdominal Surgery in Patients at Risk for Thromboembolic Complications: Abdominal surgery patients at risk include those who are over 40 years of age, obese, undergoing surgery under general anesthesia lasting longer than 30 minutes or who have additional risk factors such as malignancy or a history of deep vein thrombosis or pulmonary embolism.

In a double-blind, parallel group study of patients undergoing elective cancer surgery of the gastrointestinal, urological, or gynecological tract, a total of 1116 patients were enrolled in the study, and 1115 patients were treated. Patients ranged in age from 32 to 97 years (mean age 67 years) with 52.7% men and 47.3% women. Patients were 98% Caucasian, 1.1% Black, 0.4% Oriental, and 0.4% others. Lovenox Injection 40 mg SC, administered once a day, beginning 2 hours prior to surgery and continuing for a maximum of 12 days after surgery, was comparable to heparin 5000 U every 8 hours SC in reducing the risk of deep vein thrombosis (DVT). The efficacy data are provided below.

Efficacy of Lovenox Injection in the Prophylaxis of Deep Vein Thrombosis Following Abdominal Surgery

	Dosing Regimen	
Indication	**Lovenox Inj.** 40 mg q.d. SC n (%)	**Heparin** 5000 U q8h SC n (%)
All Treated Abdominal Surgery Patients	555 (100)	560 (100)
Treatment Failures		
Total VTE[1] (%)	56 (10.1) (95% CI[2]: 8 to 13)	63 (11.3) (95% CI: 9 to 14)
DVT Only (%)	54 (9.7) (95% CI: 7 to 12)	61 (10.9) (95% CI: 8 to 13)

[1] VTE = Venous thromboembolic events which included DVT, PE, and death considered to be thromboembolic in origin.

[2] CI = Confidence Interval

Efficacy of Lovenox Injection in the Prophylaxis of Deep Vein Thrombosis Following Hip Replacement Surgery

	Dosing Regimen		
Indication	**10 mg q.d. SC** n (%)	**30 mg q12h SC** n (%)	**40 mg q.d. SC** n (%)
All Treated Hip Replacement Patients	161 (100)	208 (100)	199 (100)
Treatment Failures Total DVT (%)	40 (25)	22 (11)[1]	27 (14)
Proximal DVT (%)	17 (11)	8 (4)[2]	9 (5)

[1] p value versus Lovenox 10 mg once a day = 0.0008
[2] p value versus Lovenox 10 mg once a day = 0.0168

In a second double-blind, parallel group study, Lovenox Injection 40 mg SC once a day was compared to heparin 5000 U every 8 hours SC in patients undergoing colorectal surgery (one-third with cancer). A total of 1347 patients were randomized in the study and all patients were treated. Patients ranged in age from 18 to 92 years (mean age 50.1 years) with 54.2% men and 45.8% women. Treatment was initiated approximately 2 hours prior to surgery and continued for approximately 7 to 10 days after surgery. The efficacy data are provided below.

Efficacy of Lovenox Injection in the Prophylaxis of Deep Vein Thrombosis Following Colorectal Surgery

	Dosing Regimen	
Indication	**Lovenox Inj.** 40 mg q.d. SC n (%)	**Heparin** 5000 U q8h SC n (%)
All Treated Colorectal Surgery Patients	673 (100)	674 (100)
Treatment Failures Total VTE[1] (%)	48 (7.1) (95% CI[2]: 5 to 9)	45 (6.7) (95% CI: 5 to 9)
DVT Only (%)	47 (7.0) (95% CI: 5 to 9)	44 (6.5) (95% CI: 5 to 8)

[1] VTE = Venous thromboembolic events which included DVT, PE, and death considered to be thromboembolic in origin.
[2] CI = Confidence Interval

Prophylaxis of Deep Vein Thrombosis Following Hip or Knee Replacement Surgery: Lovenox Injection has been shown to reduce the risk of post-operative deep vein thrombosis (DVT) following hip or knee replacement surgery.

In a double-blind study, Lovenox Injection 30 mg every 12 hours SC was compared to placebo in patients with hip replacement. A total of 100 patients were randomized in the study and all patients were treated. Patients ranged in age from 41 to 84 years (mean age 67.1 years) with 45% men and 55% women. After hemostasis was established, treatment was initiated 12 to 24 hours after surgery and was continued for 10 to 14 days after surgery. The efficacy data are provided below.

Efficacy of Lovenox Injection in the Prophylaxis of Deep Vein Thrombosis Following Hip Replacement Surgery

	Dosing Regimen	
Indication	**Lovenox Inj.** 30 mg q12h SC n (%)	**Placebo** q12h SC n (%)
All Treated Hip Replacement Patients	50 (100)	50 (100)
Treatment Failures Total DVT (%)	5 (10)[1]	23 (46)
Proximal DVT (%)	1 (2)[2]	11 (22)

[1] p value versus placebo = 0.0002
[2] p value versus placebo = 0.0134

A double-blind, multicenter study compared three dosing regimens of Lovenox Injection in patients with hip replacement. A total of 572 patients were randomized in the study and 568 patients were treated. Patients ranged in age from 31 to 88 years (mean age 64.7 years) with 63% men and 37% women. Patients were 93% Caucasian, 6% Black, <1% Oriental, and 1% others. Treatment was initiated within two days after surgery and was continued for 7 to 11 days after surgery. The efficacy data are provided below.

[See table above]

There was no significant difference between the 30 mg every 12 hours and 40 mg once a day regimens. In a double-blind study, Lovenox Injection 30 mg every 12 hours SC was compared to placebo in patients undergoing knee replacement surgery. A total of 132 patients were randomized in the study and 131 patients were treated, of which 99 had total knee replacement and 32 had either unicompartmental knee replacement or tibial osteotomy. The 99 patients with total knee replacement ranged in age from 42 to 85 years (mean age 70.2 years) with 36.4% men and 63.6% women. After hemostasis was established, treatment was initiated 12 to 24 hours after surgery and was continued up to 15 days after surgery. The incidence of proximal and total DVT after surgery was significantly lower for Lovenox Injection compared to placebo. The efficacy data are provided below.

Efficacy of Lovenox Injection in the Prophylaxis of Deep Vein Thrombosis Following Total Knee Replacement Surgery

	Dosing Regimen	
Indication	**Lovenox Inj.** 30 mg q12h SC n (%)	**Placebo** q12h SC n (%)
All Treated Total Knee Replacement Patients	47 (100)	52 (100)
Treatment Failures Total DVT (%)	5 (11)[1] (95% CI[2]: 1 to 21)	32 (62) (95% CI: 47 to 76)
Proximal DVT (%)	0 (0)[3] (95% Upper CL[4]: 5)	7 (13) (95% CI: 3 to 24)

[1] p value versus placebo = 0.0001
[2] CI = Confidence Interval
[3] p value versus placebo = 0.013
[4] CL = Confidence Limit

Additionally, in an open-label, parallel group, randomized clinical study, Lovenox Injection 30 mg every 12 hours SC in patients undergoing elective knee replacement surgery was compared to heparin 5000 U every 8 hours SC. A total of 453 patients were randomized in the study and all were treated. Patients ranged in age from 38 to 90 years (mean age 68.5 years) with 43.7% men and 56.3% women. Patients were 92.5% Caucasian, 5.3% Black, 0.2% Oriental, and 0.4% others. Treatment was initiated after surgery and continued up to 14 days. The incidence of deep vein thrombosis was significantly lower for Lovenox Injection compared to heparin.

Extended Prophylaxis of Deep Vein Thrombosis Following Hip Replacement Surgery: In a study of extended prophylaxis for patients undergoing hip replacement surgery, patients were treated, while hospitalized, with Lovenox Injection 40 mg SC, initiated up to 12 hours prior to surgery for the prophylaxis of post-operative DVT. At the end of the peri-operative period, all patients underwent bilateral venography. In a double-blind design, those patients with no venous thromboembolic disease were randomized to a post-discharge regimen of either Lovenox Injection 40 mg (n = 90) once a day SC or to placebo (n = 89) for 3 weeks. A total of 179 patients were randomized in the double-blind phase of the study and all patients were treated. Patients ranged in age from 47 to 87 years (mean age 69.4 years) with 57% men and 43% women. In this population of patients, the incidence of DVT during extended prophylaxis was significantly lower for Lovenox Injection compared to placebo. The efficacy data are provided below.

Efficacy of Lovenox Injection in the Extended Prophylaxis of Deep Vein Thrombosis Following Hip Replacement Surgery

	Post-Discharge Dosing Regimen	
Indication (Post-Discharge)	**Lovenox Inj.** 40 mg q.d. SC n (%)	**Placebo** q.d. SC n (%)
All Treated Extended Prophylaxis Patients	90 (100)	89 (100)
Treatment Failures Total DVT (%)	6 (7)[1] (95% CI[2]: 3 to 14)	18 (20) (95% CI: 12 to 30)
Proximal DVT (%)	5 (6)[3] (95% CI: 2 to 13)	7 (8) (95% CI: 3 to 16)

[1] p value versus placebo = 0.008
[2] CI= Confidence Interval
[3] p value versus placebo = 0.537

In a second study, patients undergoing hip replacement surgery were treated, while hospitalized, with Lovenox Injection 40 mg SC, initiated up to 12 hours prior to surgery. All patients were examined for clinical signs and symptoms of venous thromboembolic (VTE) disease. In a double-blind design, patients without clinical signs and symptoms of VTE disease were randomized to a post-discharge regimen of either Lovenox Injection 40 mg (n = 131) once a day SC or to placebo (n = 131) for 3 weeks. A total of 262 patients were randomized in the study double-blind phase and all patients were treated. Patients ranged in age from 44 to 87 years (mean age 68.5 years) with 43.1% men and 56.9% women. Similar to the first study the incidence of DVT during extended prophylaxis was significantly lower for Lovenox Injection compared to placebo, with a statistically significant difference in both total DVT (Lovenox Injection 21 [16%] versus placebo 45 [34%]; p = 0.001) and proximal DVT (Lovenox Injection 8 [6%] versus placebo 28 [21%]; p = <0.001).

Prophylaxis of Deep Vein Thrombosis (DVT) In Medical Patients with Severely Restricted Mobility During Acute Illness: In a double blind multicenter, parallel group study, Lovenox Injection 20 mg or 40 mg once a day SC was compared to placebo in the prophylaxis of DVT in medical patients with severely restricted mobility during acute illness (defined as walking distance of <10 meters for ≤3 days). This study included patients with heart failure (NYHA Class III or IV); acute respiratory failure or complicated chronic respiratory insufficiency (not requiring ventilatory support): acute infection (excluding septic shock); or acute rheumatic disorder [acute lumbar or sciatic pain, vertebral compression (due to osteoporosis or tumor), acute arthritic episodes of the lower extremities]. A total of 1102 patients were enrolled in the study, and 1073 patients were treated. Patients ranged in age from 40 to 97 years (mean age 73 years) with equal proportions of men and women. Treatment continued for a maximum of 14 days (median duration 7 days). When given at a dose of 40 mg once a day SC, Lovenox Injection significantly reduced the incidence of DVT as compared to placebo. The efficacy data are provided below.

[See first table at top of next page]

At approximately 3 months following enrollment, the incidence of venous thromboembolism remained significantly lower in the Lovenox Injection 40 mg treatment group versus the placebo treatment group.

Prophylaxis of Ischemic Complications in Unstable Angina and Non-Q-Wave Myocardial Infarction: In a multicenter, double-blind, parallel group study, patients who recently experienced unstable angina or non-Q-wave myocardial infarction were randomized to either Lovenox Injection 1 mg/kg every 12 hours SC or heparin i.v. bolus (5000 U) followed by a continuous infusion (adjusted to achieve an aPTT of 55 to 85 seconds). A total of 3171 patients were enrolled in the study, and 3107 patients were treated. Patients ranged in age from 25-94 years (median age 64 years), with 33.4% of patients female and 66.6% male. Race was distributed as follows: 89.8% Caucasian, 4.8% Black, 2.0% Oriental, and 3.5% other. All patients were also treated with aspirin 100 to 325 mg per day. Treatment was initiated within 24 hours of the event and continued until clinical stabilization, revascularization procedures, or hospital discharge, with a maximal duration of 8 days of therapy. The combined incidence of the triple endpoint of death, myocardial infarction, or recurrent angina was lower for Lovenox Injection compared with heparin therapy at 14 days after initiation of treatment. The lower incidence of the triple endpoint was sustained up to 30 days after initiation of treatment. These results were observed in an analysis of both all-randomized and all-treated patients. The efficacy data are provided below.

[See second table at top of next page]

The combined incidence of death or myocardial infarction at all time points was lower for Lovenox Injection compared to standard heparin therapy, but did not achieve statistical significance. The efficacy data are provided below.

[See third table on next page]

In a survey one year following treatment, with information available for 92% of enrolled patients, the combined incidence of death, myocardial infarction, or recurrent angina remained lower for Lovenox Injection versus heparin (32.0% vs 35.7%).

Urgent revascularization procedures were performed less frequently in the Lovenox Injection group as compared to the heparin group, 6.3% compared to 8.2% at 30 days (p = 0.047).

Treatment of Deep Vein Thrombosis (DVT) with or without Pulmonary Embolism (PE): In a multicenter, parallel group study, 900 patients with acute lower extremity DVT with or without PE were randomized to an inpatient (hospital) treatment of either (i) Lovenox Injection 1.5 mg/kg once a day SC, (ii) Lovenox Injection 1 mg/kg every 12 hours SC, or (iii) heparin i.v. bolus (5000 IU) followed by a continuous infusion (administered to achieve an aPTT of 55 to 85 seconds). A total of 900 patients were randomized in the study and all patients were treated. Patients ranged in age from 18 to 92 years (mean age 60.7 years) with 54.7% men and 45.3% women. All patients also received warfarin sodium (dose adjusted according to PT to achieve an International Normalization Ratio [INR] of 2.0 to 3.0), commencing

Continued on next page

Lovenox—Cont.

within 72 hours of initiation of Lovenox Injection or standard heparin therapy, and continuing for 90 days. Lovenox Injection or standard heparin therapy was administered for a minimum of 5 days and until the targeted warfarin sodium INR was achieved. Both Lovenox Injection regimens were equivalent to standard heparin therapy in reducing the risk of recurrent venous thromboembolism (DVT and/or PE). The efficacy data are provided below.
[See fourth table at right]

Similarly, in a multicenter, open-label, parallel group study, patients with acute proximal DVT were randomized to Lovenox Injection or heparin. Patients who could not receive outpatient therapy were excluded from entering the study. Outpatient exclusion criteria included the following: inability to receive outpatient heparin therapy because of associated comorbid conditions or potential for non-compliance and inability to attend follow-up visits as an outpatient because of geographic inaccessibility. Eligible patients could be treated in the hospital, but ONLY Lovenox Injection patients were permitted to go home on therapy (72%). A total of 501 patients were randomized in the study and all patients were treated. Patients ranged in age from 19 to 96 years (mean age 57.8 years) with 60.5% men and 39.5% women. Patients were randomized to either Lovenox Injection 1 mg/kg every 12 hours SC or heparin i.v. bolus (5000 IU) followed by a continuous infusion administered to achieve an aPTT of 60 to 85 seconds (in-patient treatment). All patients also received warfarin sodium as described in the previous study. Lovenox Injection or standard heparin therapy was administered for a minimum of 5 days. Lovenox Injection was equivalent to standard heparin therapy in reducing the risk of recurrent venous thromboembolism. The efficacy data are provided below.

Efficacy of Lovenox Injection in Treatment of Deep Vein Thrombosis

| Indication | Dosing Regimen[1] | |
	Lovenox Inj. 1 mg/kg q12h SC n (%)	Heparin aPTT Adjusted i.v. Therapy n (%)
All Treated DVT Patients	247 (100)	254 (100)
Patient Outcome Total VTE[2] (%)	13 (5.3)[3]	17 (6.7)
DVT Only (%)	11 (4.5)	14 (5.5)
Proximal DVT (%)	10 (4.0)	12 (4.7)
PE (%)	2 (0.8)	3 (1.2)

[1] All patients were also treated with warfarin sodium commencing on the evening of the second day of Lovenox Injection or standard heparin therapy.
[2] VTE = venous thromboembolic event (deep vein thrombosis [DVT] and/or pulmonary embolism [PE]).
[3] The 95% Confidence Intervals for the treatment difference for total VTE was: Lovenox Injection versus heparin (-5.6 to 2.7).

INDICATIONS AND USAGE

- Lovenox Injection is indicated for the prophylaxis of deep vein thrombosis, which may lead to pulmonary embolism:
  - in patients undergoing abdominal surgery who are at risk for thromboembolic complications;
  - in patients undergoing hip replacement surgery, during and following hospitalization;
  - in patients undergoing knee replacement surgery;
  - in medical patients who are at risk for thromboembolic complications due to severely restricted mobility during acute illness.
- Lovenox Injection is indicated for the prophylaxis of ischemic complications of unstable angina and non-Q-wave myocardial infarction, when concurrently administered with aspirin.
- Lovenox Injection is indicated for:
  - the **inpatient treatment** of acute deep vein thrombosis **with or without pulmonary embolism,** when administered in conjunction with warfarin sodium;
  - the **outpatient treatment** of acute deep vein thrombosis **without pulmonary embolism** when administered in conjunction with warfarin sodium.

See **DOSAGE AND ADMINISTRATION: Adult Dosage** for appropriate dosage regimens.

CONTRAINDICATIONS

Lovenox Injection is contraindicated in patients with active major bleeding, in patients with thrombocytopenia associated with a positive *in vitro* test for anti-platelet antibody in the presence of enoxaparin sodium, or in patients with hypersensitivity to enoxaparin sodium.
Patients with known hypersensitivity to heparin or pork products should not be treated with Lovenox Injection or any of its constituents.

WARNINGS

Lovenox Injection is not intended for intramuscular administration.

Efficacy of Lovenox Injection in the Prophylaxis of Deep Vein Thrombosis in Medical Patients With Severely Restricted Mobility During Acute Illness

| Indication | Dosing Regimen | | |
	Lovenox Inj. 20 mg q.d. SC n (%)	Lovenox Inj. 40 mg q.d. SC n (%)	Placebo n (%)
All Treated Medical Patients During Acute Illness	351 (100)	360 (100)	362 (100)
Treatment Failure[1] Total VTE[2] (%)	43 (12.3)	16 (4.4)	43 (11.9)
Total DVT (%)	43 (12.3) (95% CI[3] 8.8 to 15.7)	16 (4.4) (95% CI[3] 2.3 to 6.6)	41 (11.3) (95% CI[3] 8.1 to 14.6)
Proximal DVT (%)	13 (3.7)	5 (1.4)	14 (3.9)

[1] Treatment failures during therapy, between Days 1 and 14.
[2] VTE = Venous thromboembolic events which included DVT, PE, and death considered to be thromboembolic in origin.
[3] CI = Confidence Interval

Efficacy of Lovenox Injection in the Prophylaxis of Ischemic Complications in Unstable Angina and Non-Q-Wave Myocardial Infarction (Combined Endpoint of Death, Myocardial Infarction, or Recurrent Angina)

| Indication | Dosing Regimen[1] | | Reduction (%) | p Value |
	Lovenox Inj. 1 mg/kg q12h SC n (%)	Heparin aPTT Adjusted i.v. Therapy n (%)		
All Treated Unstable Angina and Non-Q-Wave MI Patients	1578 (100)	1529 (100)		
Timepoint[2] 48 Hours	96 (6.1)	112 (7.3)	1.2	0.120
14 Days	261 (16.5)	303 (19.8)	3.3	0.017
30 Days	313 (19.8)	358 (23.4)	3.6	0.014

[1] All patients were also treated with aspirin 100 to 325 mg per day.
[2] Evaluation timepoints are after initiation of treatment. Therapy continued for up to 8 days (median duration of 2.6 days).

Efficacy of Lovenox Injection in the Prophylaxis of Ischemic Complications in Unstable Angina and Non-Q-Wave Myocardial Infarction (Combined Endpoint of Death or Myocardial Infarction)

| Indication | Dosing Regimen[1] | | Reduction (%) | p Value |
	Lovenox Inj. 1 mg/kg q12h SC n (%)	Heparin aPTT Adjusted i.v. Therapy n (%)		
All Treated Unstable Angina and Non-Q-Wave MI Patients	1578 (100)	1529 (100)		
Timepoint[2] 48 Hours	16 (1.0)	20 (1.3)	0.3	0.126
14 Days	76 (4.8)	93 (6.1)	1.3	0.115
30 Days	96 (6.1)	118 (7.7)	1.6	0.069

[1] All patients were also treated with aspirin 100 to 325 mg per day.
[2] Evaluation timepoints are after initiation of treatment. Therapy continued for up to 8 days (median duration of 2.6 days).

Efficacy of Lovenox Injection in Treatment of Deep Vein Thrombosis With or Without Pulmonary Embolism

| Indication | Dosing Regimen[1] | | |
	Lovenox Inj. 1.5 mg/kg q.d. SC n (%)	Lovenox Inj. 1 mg/kg q12h SC n (%)	Heparin aPTT Adjusted i.v. Therapy n (%)
All Treated DVT Patients with or without PE	298 (100)	312 (100)	290 (100)
Patient Outcome Total VTE[2] (%)	13 (4.4)[3]	9 (2.9)[3]	12 (4.1)
DVT Only (%)	11 (3.7)	7 (2.2)	8 (2.8)
Proximal DVT (%)	9 (3.0)	6 (1.9)	7 (2.4)
PE (%)	2 (0.7)	2 (0.6)	4 (1.4)

[1] All patients were also treated with warfarin sodium commencing within 72 hours of Lovenox Injection or standard heparin therapy.
[2] VTE = venous thromboembolic event (DVT and/or PE).
[3] The 95% Confidence Intervals for the treatment differences for total VTE were:
Lovenox Injection once a day versus heparin (-3.0 to 3.5)
Lovenox Injection every 12 hours versus heparin (-4.2 to 1.7).

Lovenox Injection cannot be used interchangeably (unit for unit) with heparin or other low molecular weight heparins as they differ in manufacturing process, molecular weight distribution, anti-Xa and anti-IIa activities, units, and dosage. Each of these medicines has its own instructions for use.

Lovenox Injection should be used with extreme caution in patients with a history of heparin-induced thrombocytopenia.

Hemorrhage: Lovenox Injection, like other anticoagulants, should be used with extreme caution in conditions with increased risk of hemorrhage, such as bacterial endocarditis, congenital or acquired bleeding disorders, active ulcerative and angiodysplastic gastrointestinal disease, hemorrhagic stroke, or shortly after brain, spinal, or ophthalmological surgery, or in patients treated concomitantly with platelet inhibitors.

Cases of epidural or spinal hematomas have been reported with the associated use of Lovenox Injection and spinal/epidural anesthesia or spinal puncture resulting in long-term or permanent paralysis. The risk of these events is higher with the use of post-operative indwelling epidural catheters or by the concomitant use of additional drugs affecting hemostasis such as NSAIDs (see boxed WARNING; ADVERSE REACTIONS, Ongoing Safety Surveillance; and PRECAUTIONS, Drug Interactions).

Major hemorrhages including retroperitoneal and intracranial bleeding have been reported. Some of these cases have been fatal.

Bleeding can occur at any site during therapy with Lovenox Injection. An unexplained fall in hematocrit or blood pressure should lead to a search for a bleeding site.

Thrombocytopenia: Thrombocytopenia can occur with the administration of Lovenox Injection.

Moderate thrombocytopenia (platelet counts between 100,000/mm^3 and 50,000/mm^3) occurred at a rate of 1.3% in patients given Lovenox Injection, 1.2% in patients given heparin, and 0.7% in patients given placebo in clinical trials.

Platelet counts less than 50,000/mm^3 occurred at a rate of 0.1% in patients given Lovenox Injection, in 0.2% of patients given heparin, and 0.4% of patients given placebo in the same trials.

Thrombocytopenia of any degree should be monitored closely. If the platelet count falls below 100,000/mm^3, Lovenox Injection should be discontinued. Cases of heparin-induced thrombocytopenia with thrombosis have also been observed in clinical practice. Some of these cases were complicated by organ infarction, limb ischemia, or death.

Pregnant Women with Mechanical Prosthetic Heart Valves: The use of Lovenox Injection for thromboprophylaxis in pregnant women with mechanical prosthetic heart valves has not been adequately studied. In a clinical study of pregnant women with mechanical prosthetic heart valves given enoxaparin (1 mg/kg bid) to reduce the risk of thromboembolism, 2 of 8 women developed clots resulting in blockage of the valve and leading to maternal and fetal death. Although a causal relationship has not been established these deaths may have been due to therapeutic failure or inadequate anticoagulation. No patients in the heparin/warfarin group (0 of 4 women) died. There also have been isolated postmarketing reports of valve thrombosis in pregnant women with mechanical prosthetic heart valves while receiving enoxaparin for thromboprophylaxis. Women with mechanical prosthetic heart valves may be at higher risk for thromboembolism during pregnancy, and, when pregnant, have a higher rate of fetal loss from stillbirth, spontaneous abortion and premature delivery. Therefore, frequent monitoring of peak and trough anti-Factor Xa levels, and adjusting of dosage may be needed.

Miscellaneous: Lovenox multiple-dose vials contain benzyl alcohol as a preservative. The administration of medications containing benzyl alcohol as a preservative to premature neonates has been associated with a fatal "Gasping Syndrome". Because benzyl alcohol may cross the placenta, Lovenox multiple-dose vials, preserved with benzyl alcohol, should be used with caution in pregnant women and only if clearly needed (see **PRECAUTIONS, Pregnancy**).

PRECAUTIONS

General: Lovenox Injection should not be mixed with other injections or infusions.

Lovenox Injection should be used with care in patients with a bleeding diathesis, uncontrolled arterial hypertension or a history of recent gastrointestinal ulceration, diabetic retinopathy, and hemorrhage. Lovenox Injection should be used with care in elderly patients who may show delayed elimination of enoxaparin.

If thromboembolic events occur despite Lovenox Injection prophylaxis, appropriate therapy should be initiated.

Mechanical Prosthetic Heart Valves: The use of Lovenox Injection has not been adequately studied for thromboprophylaxis in patients with mechanical prosthetic heart valves and has not been adequately studied for long-term use in this patient population. Isolated cases of prosthetic heart valve thrombosis have been reported in patients with mechanical prosthetic heart valves who have received enoxaparin for thromboprophylaxis. Some of these cases were pregnant women in whom thrombosis led to maternal and fetal deaths. Insufficient data, the underlying disease and the possibility of inadequate anticoagulation complicate the evaluation of these cases. Pregnant women with mechanical prosthetic heart valves may be at higher risk for thromboembolism (see **WARNINGS, Pregnant Women with Mechanical Prosthetic Heart Valves**).

Renal Impairment: In patients with renal impairment, there is an increase in exposure of enoxaparin sodium. All such patients should be observed carefully for signs and symptoms of bleeding. Because exposure of enoxaparin sodium is significantly increased in patients with severe renal impairment (creatinine clearance <30 mL/min), a dosage adjustment is recommended for therapeutic and prophylactic dosage ranges. No dosage adjustment is recommended in patients with moderate (creatinine clearance 30–50 mL/min) and mild (creatinine clearance 50–80 mL/min) renal impairment. (see **DOSAGE AND ADMINISTRATION** and **CLINICAL PHARMACOLOGY, Pharmacokinetics, Special Populations**).

Low-Weight Patients: An increase in exposure of enoxaparin sodium with prophylactic dosages (non-weight adjusted) has been observed in low-weight women (<45 kg) and low-weight men (<57 kg). All such patients should be observed carefully for signs and symptoms of bleeding (see **CLINICAL PHARMACOLOGY, Pharmacokinetics, Special Populations**).

Laboratory Tests: Periodic complete blood counts, including platelet count, and stool occult blood tests are recommended during the course of treatment with Lovenox Injection. When administered at recommended prophylaxis doses, routine coagulation tests such as Prothrombin Time (PT) and Activated Partial Thromboplastin Time (aPTT) are relatively insensitive measures of Lovenox Injection activity and, therefore, unsuitable for monitoring. Anti-Factor Xa may be used to monitor the anticoagulant effect of Lovenox Injection in patients with significant renal impairment. If during Lovenox Injection therapy abnormal coagulation parameters or bleeding should occur, anti-Factor Xa levels may be used to monitor the anticoagulant effects of Lovenox Injection (see **CLINICAL PHARMACOLOGY: Pharmacokinetics**).

Drug Interactions: Unless really needed, agents which may enhance the risk of hemorrhage should be discontinued prior to initiation of Lovenox Injection therapy. These agents include medications such as: anticoagulants, platelet inhibitors including acetylsalicylic acid, salicylates, NSAIDs (including ketorolac tromethamine), dipyridamole, or sulfinpyrazone. If co-administration is essential, conduct close clinical and laboratory monitoring (see **PRECAUTIONS: Laboratory Tests**).

Carcinogenesis, Mutagenesis, Impairment of Fertility: No long-term studies in animals have been performed to evaluate the carcinogenic potential of enoxaparin. Enoxaparin was not mutagenic in *in vitro* tests, including the Ames test, mouse lymphoma cell forward mutation test, and human lymphocyte chromosomal aberration test, and the *in vivo* rat bone marrow chromosomal aberration test. Enoxaparin was found to have no effect on fertility or reproductive performance of male and female rats at SC doses up to 20 mg/kg/day or 141 mg/m^2/day. The maximum human dose in clinical trials was 2.0 mg/kg/day or 78 mg/m^2/day (for an average body weight of 70 kg, height of 170 cm, and body surface area of 1.8 m^2).

Pregnancy: Pregnancy Category B:

All pregnancies have a background risk of birth defects, loss, or other adverse outcome regardless of drug exposure. The fetal risk summary below describes Lovenox's potential to increase the risk of developmental abnormalities above background risk.

Fetal Risk Summary

Lovenox is not predicted to increase the risk of developmental abnormalities. Lovenox does not cross the placenta, based on human and animal studies, and shows no evidence of teratogenic effects or fetotoxicity.

Clinical Considerations

It is not known if dose adjustment or monitoring of anti-Xa activity of enoxaparin are necessary during pregnancy.

Pregnancy alone confers an increased risk for thromboembolism, that is even higher for women with thromboembolic disease and certain high risk pregnancy conditions. While not adequately studied, pregnant women with mechanical prosthetic heart valves may be at even higher risk for thrombosis (See **WARNINGS, Pregnant Women with Mechanical Prosthetic Heart Valves** and **PRECAUTIONS, Mechanical Prosthetic Heart Valves**.) Pregnant women with thromboembolic disease, including those with mechanical prosthetic heart valves, and those with inherited or acquired thrombophilias, also have an increased risk of other maternal complications and fetal loss regardless of the type of anticoagulant used.

All patients receiving anticoagulants such as enoxaparin, including pregnant women, are at risk for bleeding. Pregnant women receiving enoxaparin should be carefully monitored for evidence of bleeding or excessive anticoagulation. Consideration for use of a shorter acting anticoagulant should be specifically addressed as delivery approaches (see **BOXED WARNING, SPINAL/EPIDURAL HEMATOMAS**).

Hemorrhage can occur at any site and may lead to death of mother and/or fetus. Pregnant women should be apprised of the potential hazard to the fetus and the mother if enoxaparin is administered during pregnancy.

Data

- Human Data - There are no adequate and well-controlled studies in pregnant women.

  A retrospective study reviewed the records of 604 women who used enoxaparin during pregnancy. A total of 624 pregnancies resulted in 693 live births. There were 72 hemorrhagic events (11 serious) in 63 women. There were 14 cases of neonatal hemorrhage. Major congenital anomalies in live births occurred at rates (2.5%) similar to background rates.[1]

  There have been postmarketing reports of fetal death when pregnant women received Lovenox Injection. Causality for these cases has not been determined. Insufficient data, the underlying disease, and the possibility of inadequate anticoagulation complicate the evaluation of these cases.

  See **WARNINGS: Pregnant Women with Mechanical Prosthetic Heart Valves** for a clinical study of pregnant women with mechanical prosthetic heart valves.

- Animal Data - Teratology studies have been conducted in pregnant rats and rabbits at SC doses of enoxaparin up to 30 mg/kg/day or 211 mg/m^2/day and 410 mg/m^2/day, respectively. There was no evidence of teratogenic effects or fetotoxicity due to enoxaparin. Because animal reproduction studies are not always predictive of human response, this drug should be used during pregnancy only if clearly needed.

Cases of "Gasping Syndrome" have occurred in premature infants when large amounts of benzyl alcohol have been administered (99-405 mg/kg/day). The multiple-dose vial of Lovenox solution contains 15 mg/1.0 mL benzyl alcohol as a preservative (see **WARNINGS, Miscellaneous**).

Nursing Mothers: It is not known whether this drug is excreted in human milk. Because many drugs are excreted in human milk, caution should be exercised when Lovenox Injection is administered to nursing women.

Pediatric Use: Safety and effectiveness of Lovenox Injection in pediatric patients have not been established.

Geriatric Use: Over 2800 patients, 65 years and older, have received Lovenox Injection in pivotal clinical trials. The efficacy of Lovenox Injection in the elderly (≥65 years) was similar to that seen in younger patients (<65 years). The incidence of bleeding complications was similar between elderly and younger patients when 30 mg every 12 hours or 40 mg once a day doses of Lovenox Injection were employed. The incidence of bleeding complications was higher in elderly patients as compared to younger patients when Lovenox Injection was administered at doses of 1.5 mg/kg once a day or 1 mg/kg every 12 hours. The risk of Lovenox Injection-associated bleeding increased with age. Serious adverse events increased with age for patients receiving Lovenox Injection. Other clinical experience (including postmarketing surveillance and literature reports) has not revealed additional differences in the safety of Lovenox Injection between elderly and younger patients. Careful attention to dosing intervals and concomitant medications (especially antiplatelet medications) is advised. Monitoring of geriatric patients with low body weight (<45 kg) and those predisposed to decreased renal function should be considered (see **CLINICAL PHARMACOLOGY** and **General** and **Laboratory Tests** subsections of **PRECAUTIONS**).

ADVERSE REACTIONS

Hemorrhage: The incidence of major hemorrhagic complications during Lovenox Injection treatment has been low. The following rates of major bleeding events have been reported during clinical trials with Lovenox Injection.

Major Bleeding Episodes Following Abdominal and Colorectal Surgery[1]

	Dosing Regimen	
Indications	**Lovenox Inj.** 40 mg q.d. SC	**Heparin** 5000 U q8h SC
Abdominal Surgery	n = 555 23 (4%)	n = 560 16 (3%)
Colorectal Surgery	n = 673 28 (4%)	n = 674 21 (3%)

[1] Bleeding complications were considered major: (1) if the hemorrhage caused a significant clinical event, or (2) if accompanied by a hemoglobin decrease ≥2 g/dL or transfusion of 2 or more units of blood products. Retroperitoneal, intraocular, and intracranial hemorrhages were always considered major.

Major Bleeding Episodes Following Hip or Knee Replacement Surgery[1]

	Dosing Regimen		
Indications	**Lovenox Inj.** 40 mg q.d. SC	**Lovenox Inj.** 30 mg q12h SC	**Heparin** 15,000 U/24h SC
Hip Replacement Surgery Without Extended Prophylaxis[2]		n = 786 31 (4%)	n = 541 32 (6%)
Hip Replacement Surgery With Extended Prophylaxis			
Peri-operative Period[3]	n = 288 4 (2%)		
Extended Prophylaxis Period[4]	n = 221 0 (0%)		
Knee Replacement Surgery Without Extended Prophylaxis[2]		n = 294 3 (1%)	n = 225 3 (1%)

[1] Bleeding complications were considered major: (1) if the hemorrhage caused a significant clinical event, or (2) if ac-

Continued on next page

Lovenox—Cont.

companied by a hemoglobin decrease ≥ 2 g/dL or transfusion of 2 or more units of blood products. Retroperitoneal and intracranial hemorrhages were always considered major. In the knee replacement AST surgery trials, intraocular hemorrhages were also considered major hemorrhages.
[2] Lovenox Injection 30 mg every 12 hours SC initiated 12 to 24 hours after surgery and continued for up to 14 days after surgery.
[3] Lovenox Injection 40 mg SC once a day initiated up to 12 hours prior to surgery and continued for up to 7 days after surgery.
[4] Lovenox Injection 40 mg SC once a day for up to 21 days after discharge.
NOTE: At no time point were the 40 mg once a day preoperative and the 30 mg every 12 hours post-operative hip replacement surgery prophylactic regimens compared in clinical trials.
Injection site hematomas during the extended prophylaxis period after hip replacement surgery occurred in 9% of the Lovenox Injection patients versus 1.8% of the placebo patients.

Major Bleeding Episodes in Medical Patients With Severely Restricted Mobility During Acute Illness[1]

Indications	Dosing Regimen		
	Lovenox Inj.[2] 20 mg q.d. SC	Lovenox Inj.[2] 40 mg q.d. SC	Placebo[2]
Medical Patients During Acute Illness	n = 351 1 (<1%)	n = 360 3 (<1%)	n = 362 2 (<1%)

[1] Bleeding complications were considered major: (1) if the hemorrhage caused a significant clinical event, (2) if the hemorrhage caused a decrease in hemoglobin of ≥ 2 g/dL or transfusion of 2 or more units of blood products. Retroperitoneal and intracranial hemorrhages were always considered major although none were reported during the trial.
[2] The rates represent major bleeding on study medication up to 24 hours after last dose.

Major Bleeding Episodes in Unstable Angina and Non-Q-Wave Myocardial Infarction

Indication	Dosing Regimen	
	Lovenox Inj.[1] 1 mg/kg q12h SC	Heparin[1] aPTT Adjusted i.v. Therapy
Unstable Angina and Non-Q-Wave MI[2,3]	n = 1578 17 (1%)	n = 1529 18 (1%)

[1] The rates represent major bleeding on study medication up to 12 hours after dose.
[2] Aspirin therapy was administered concurrently (100 to 325 mg per day).
[3] Bleeding complications were considered major: (1) if the hemorrhage caused a significant clinical event, or (2) if accompanied by a hemoglobin decrease by ≥ 3 g/dL or transfusion of 2 or more units of blood products. Intraocular, retroperitoneal, and intracranial hemorrhages were always considered major.

Major Bleeding Episodes in Deep Vein Thrombosis With or Without Pulmonary Embolism Treatment[1]

Indication	Dosing Regimen[2]		
	Lovenox Inj. 1.5 mg/kg q.d. SC	Lovenox Inj. 1 mg/kg q12h SC	Heparin aPTT Adjusted i.v. Therapy
Treatment of DVT and PE	n = 298 5 (2%)	n = 559 9 (2%)	n = 554 9 (2%)

[1] Bleeding complications were considered major: (1) if the hemorrhage caused a significant clinical event, or (2) if accompanied by a hemoglobin decrease ≥2 g/dL or transfusion of 2 or more units of blood products. Retroperitoneal, intraocular, and intracranial hemorrhages were always considered major.
[2] All patients also received warfarin sodium (dose-adjusted according to PT to achieve an INR of 2.0 to 3.0) commencing within 72 hours of Lovenox Injection or standard heparin therapy and continuing for up to 90 days.

Thrombocytopenia: see **WARNINGS: Thrombocytopenia.**
Elevations of Serum Aminotransferases: Asymptomatic increases in aspartate (AST [SGOT]) and alanine (ALT [SGPT]) aminotransferase levels greater than three times the upper limit of normal of the laboratory reference range have been reported in up to 6.1% and 5.9% of patients, respectively, during treatment with Lovenox Injection. Similar significant increases in aminotransferase levels have also been observed in patients and healthy volunteers

Adverse Events Occurring at ≥2% Incidence in Lovenox Injection Treated Patients[1] Undergoing Abdominal or Colorectal Surgery

Adverse Event	Dosing Regimen			
	Lovenox Inj. 40 mg q.d. SC n = 1228		Heparin 5000 U q8h SC n = 1234	
	Severe	Total	Severe	Total
Hemorrhage	<1%	7%	<1%	6%
Anemia	<1%	3%	<1%	3%
Ecchymosis	0%	3%	0%	3%

[1] Excluding unrelated adverse events.

Adverse Events Occurring at ≥2% Incidence in Lovenox Injection Treated Patients[1] Undergoing Hip or Knee Replacement Surgery

Adverse Event	Dosing Regimen									
	Lovenox Inj. 40 mg q.d. SC				Lovenox Inj. 30 mg q12h SC		Heparin 15,000 U/24h SC		Placebo q12h SC	
	Peri-operative Period n = 288[2]		Extended Prophylaxis Period n = 131[3]		n = 1080		n = 766		n = 115	
	Severe	Total	Severe	Total	Severe	Total	Severe	Total	Severe	Total
Fever	0%	8%	0%	0%	<1%	5%	<1%	4%	0%	3%
Hemorrhage	<1%	13%	0%	5%	<1%	4%	1%	4%	0%	3%
Nausea					<1%	3%	<1%	2%	0%	2%
Anemia	0%	16%	0%	<2%	<1%	2%	2%	5%	<1%	7%
Edema					<1%	2%	<1%	2%	0%	2%
Peripheral edema	0%	6%	0%	0%	<1%	3%	<1%	4%	0%	3%

[1] Excluding unrelated adverse events.
[2] Data represents Lovenox Injection 40 mg SC once a day initiated up to 12 hours prior to surgery in 288 hip replacement surgery patients who received Lovenox Injection peri-operatively in an unblinded fashion in one clinical trial.
[3] Data represents Lovenox Injection 40 mg SC once a day given in a blinded fashion as extended prophylaxis at the end of the peri-operative period in 131 of the original 288 hip replacement surgery patients for up to 21 days in one clinical trial.

treated with heparin and other low molecular weight heparins. Such elevations are fully reversible and are rarely associated with increases in bilirubin.
Since aminotransferase determinations are important in the differential diagnosis of myocardial infarction, liver disease, and pulmonary emboli, elevations that might be caused by drugs like Lovenox Injection should be interpreted with caution.
Local Reactions: Mild local irritation, pain, hematoma, ecchymosis, and erythema may follow SC injection of Lovenox Injection.
Other: Other adverse effects that were thought to be possibly or probably related to treatment with Lovenox Injection, heparin, or placebo in clinical trials with patients undergoing hip or knee replacement surgery, abdominal or colorectal surgery, or treatment for DVT and that occurred at a rate of at least 2% in the Lovenox Injection group, are provided below.
[See first table above]
[See second table above]

Adverse Events Occurring at ≥2% Incidence in Lovenox Injection Treated Medical Patients[1] With Severely Restricted Mobility During Acute Illness

Adverse Event	Dosing Regimen	
	Lovenox Inj. 40 mg q.d. SC n = 360 (%)	Placebo q.d. SC n = 362 (%)
Dyspnea	3.3	5.2
Thrombocytopenia	2.8	2.8
Confusion	2.2	1.1
Diarrhea	2.2	1.7
Nausea	2.5	1.7

[1] Excluding unrelated and unlikely adverse events.

Adverse Events in Lovenox Injection Treated Patients With Unstable Angina or Non-Q-Wave Myocardial Infarction: Non-hemorrhagic clinical events reported to be related to Lovenox Injection therapy occurred at an incidence of ≤1%. Non-major hemorrhagic episodes, primarily injection site ecchymoses and hematomas, were more frequently reported in patients treated with SC Lovenox Injection than in patients treated with i.v. heparin.
Serious adverse events with Lovenox Injection or heparin in a clinical trial in patients with unstable angina or non-Q-wave myocardial infarction that occurred at a rate of at least 0.5% in the Lovenox Injection group, are provided below (irrespective of relationship to drug therapy).

Serious Adverse Events Occurring at ≥0.5% Incidence in Lovenox Injection Treated Patients With Unstable Angina or Non-Q-Wave Myocardial Infarction

Adverse Event	Dosing Regimen	
	Lovenox Inj. 1 mg/kg q12h SC n = 1578 n (%)	Heparin aPTT Adjusted i.v. Therapy n = 1529 n (%)
Atrial fibrillation	11 (0.70)	3 (0.20)
Heart failure	15 (0.95)	11 (0.72)
Lung edema	11 (0.70)	11 (0.72)
Pneumonia	13 (0.82)	9 (0.59)

[See first table at top of next page]
Ongoing Safety Surveillance: Since 1993, there have been over 80 reports of epidural or spinal hematoma formation with concurrent use of Lovenox Injection and spinal/epidural anesthesia or spinal puncture. The majority of patients had a post-operative indwelling epidural catheter placed for analgesia or received additional drugs affecting hemostasis such as NSAIDs. Many of the epidural or spinal hematomas caused neurologic injury, including long-term or permanent paralysis. Because these events were reported voluntarily from a population of unknown size, estimates of frequency cannot be made.
Other Ongoing Safety Surveillance Reports: local reactions at the injection site (i.e., skin necrosis, nodules, inflammation, oozing), systemic allergic reactions (i.e., pruritus, urticaria, anaphylactoid reactions), vesiculobullous rash, rare cases of hypersensitivity cutaneous vasculitis, purpura, thrombocytosis, and thrombocytopenia with thrombosis (see **WARNINGS, Thrombocytopenia**). Very rare cases of hyperlipidemia have been reported, with one case of hyperlipidemia, with marked hypertriglyceridemia, reported in a diabetic pregnant woman; causality has not been determined.

OVERDOSAGE

Symptoms/Treatment: Accidental overdosage following administration of Lovenox Injection may lead to hemorrhagic complications. Injected Lovenox Injection may be largely neutralized by the slow i.v. injection of protamine sulfate (1% solution). The dose of protamine sulfate should be equal to the dose of Lovenox Injection injected: 1 mg protamine sulfate should be administered to neutralize 1 mg Lovenox Injection, if enoxaparin sodium was administered in the previous 8 hours. An infusion of 0.5 mg protamine per 1 mg of enoxaparin sodium may be administered if enoxaparin sodium was administered greater than 8 hours previous to the protamine administration, or if it has been de-

Adverse Events Occurring at ≥2% Incidence in Lovenox Injection Treated Patients[1] Undergoing Treatment of Deep Vein Thrombosis With or Without Pulmonary Embolism

Adverse Event	Dosing Regimen					
	Lovenox Inj. 1.5 mg/kg q.d. SC n = 298		Lovenox Inj. 1 mg/kg q12h SC n = 559		Heparin aPTT Adjusted i.v. Therapy n = 544	
	Severe	Total	Severe	Total	Severe	Total
Injection Site Hemorrhage	0%	5%	0%	3%	<1%	<1%
Injection Site Pain	0%	2%	0%	2%	0%	0%
Hematuria	0%	2%	0%	<1%	<1%	2%

[1] Excluding unrelated adverse events.

100 mg/mL Concentration

Dosage Unit/Strength[1]	Anti-Xa Activity[2]	Package Size (per carton)	Label Color	NDC # 0075-
Prefilled Syringes[3] 30 mg / 0.3 mL	3000 IU	10 syringes	Medium Blue	0624-30
40 mg / 0.4 mL	4000 IU	10 syringes	Yellow	0620-40
Graduated Prefilled Syringes[3] 60 mg / 0.6 mL	6000 IU	10 syringes	Orange	0621-60
80 mg / 0.8 mL	8000 IU	10 syringes	Brown	0622-80
100 mg / 1 mL	10,000 IU	10 syringes	Black	0623-00
Multiple-Dose Vial[4] 300 mg / 3.0 mL	30,000 IU	1 vial	Red	0626-03

[1] Strength represents the number of milligrams of enoxaparin sodium in Water for Injection. **Lovenox Injection** 30 and 40 mg prefilled syringes, and 60, 80, and 100 mg graduated prefilled syringes each contain **10 mg enoxaparin sodium per 0.1 mL Water for Injection.**
[2] Approximate anti-Factor Xa activity based on reference to the W.H.O. First International Low Molecular Weight Heparin Reference Standard.
[3] Each **Lovenox Injection** syringe is affixed with a 27 gauge × 1/2 inch needle.
[4] Each Lovenox multiple-dose vial contains 15 mg / 1.0 mL of benzyl alcohol as a preservative.

150 mg/mL Concentration

Dosage Unit/Strength[1]	Anti-Xa Activity[2]	Package Size (per carton)	Syringe Label Color	NDC # 0075-
Graduated Prefilled Syringes[3] 120 mg / 0.8 mL	12,000 IU	10 syringes	Purple	2912-01
150 mg / 1 mL	15,000 IU	10 syringes	Navy Blue	2915-01

[1] Strength represents the number of milligrams of enoxaparin sodium in Water for Injection. **Lovenox Injection** 120 and 150 mg graduated prefilled syringes contain **15 mg enoxaparin sodium per 0.1 mL** Water for Injection.
[2] Approximate anti-Factor Xa activity based on reference to the W.H.O. First International Low Molecular Weight Heparin Reference Standard.
[3] Each **Lovenox Injection** graduated prefilled syringe is affixed with a 27 gauge × 1/2 inch needle.

termined that a second dose of protamine is required. The second infusion of 0.5 mg protamine sulfate per 1 mg of Lovenox Injection may be administered if the aPTT measured 2 to 4 hours after the first infusion remains prolonged.

After 12 hours of the enoxaparin sodium injection, protamine administration may not be required. However, even with higher doses of protamine, the aPTT may remain more prolonged than under normal conditions found following administration of heparin. In all cases, the anti-Factor Xa activity is never completely neutralized (maximum about 60%). Particular care should be taken to avoid overdosage with protamine sulfate. Administration of protamine sulfate can cause severe hypotensive and anaphylactoid reactions. Because fatal reactions, often resembling anaphylaxis, have been reported with protamine sulfate, it should be given only when resuscitation techniques and treatment of anaphylactic shock are readily available. For additional information consult the labeling of Protamine Sulfate Injection, USP, products.

A single SC dose of 46.4 mg/kg enoxaparin was lethal to rats. The symptoms of acute toxicity were ataxia, decreased motility, dyspnea, cyanosis, and coma.

DOSAGE AND ADMINISTRATION

All patients should be evaluated for a bleeding disorder before administration of Lovenox Injection, unless the medication is needed urgently. Since coagulation parameters are unsuitable for monitoring Lovenox Injection activity, routine monitoring of coagulation parameters is not required (see **PRECAUTIONS, Laboratory Tests**).

Note: Lovenox Injection is available in two concentrations:
1. 100 mg/mL Concentration: 30 mg / 0.3 mL and 40 mg / 0.4 mL prefilled single-dose syringes, 60 mg / 0.6 mL, 80 mg / 0.8 mL, and 100 mg / 1 mL prefilled, graduated, single-dose syringes, 300 mg / 3.0 mL multiple-dose vials.
2. 150 mg/mL Concentration: 120 mg / 0.8 mL and 150 mg / 1 mL prefilled, graduated, single-dose syringes.

Adult Dosage:

Abdominal Surgery: In patients undergoing abdominal surgery who are at risk for thromboembolic complications, the recommended dose of Lovenox Injection is **40 mg once a day** administered by SC injection with the initial dose given 2 hours prior to surgery. The usual duration of administration is 7 to 10 days; up to 12 days administration has been well tolerated in clinical trials.

Hip or Knee Replacement Surgery: In patients undergoing hip or knee replacement surgery, the recommended dose of Lovenox Injection is **30 mg every 12 hours** administered by SC injection. Provided that hemostasis has been established, the initial dose should be given 12 to 24 hours after surgery. For hip replacement surgery, a dose of **40 mg once a day** SC, given initially 12 (±3) hours prior to surgery, may be considered. Following the initial phase of thromboprophylaxis in hip replacement surgery patients, continued prophylaxis with Lovenox Injection 40 mg once a day administered by SC injection for 3 weeks is recommended. The usual duration of administration is 7 to 10 days; up to 14 days administration has been well tolerated in clinical trials.

Medical Patients During Acute Illness: In medical patients at risk for thromboembolic complications due to severely restricted mobility during acute illness, the recommended dose of Lovenox Injection is **40 mg once a day** administered by SC injection. The usual duration of administration is 6 to 11 days; up to 14 days of Lovenox Injection has been well tolerated in the controlled clinical trial.

Unstable Angina and Non-Q-Wave Myocardial Infarction: In patients with unstable angina or non-Q-wave myocardial infarction, the recommended dose of Lovenox Injection is **1 mg/kg** administered SC **every 12 hours** in conjunction with oral aspirin therapy (100 to 325 mg once daily). Treatment with Lovenox Injection should be prescribed for a minimum of 2 days and continued until clinical stabilization. To minimize the risk of bleeding following vascular instrumentation during the treatment of unstable angina, adhere pre-

cisely to the intervals recommended between Lovenox Injection doses. The vascular access sheath for instrumentation should remain in place for 6 to 8 hours following a dose of Lovenox Injection. The next scheduled dose should be given no sooner than 6 to 8 hours after sheath removal. The site of the procedure should be observed for signs of bleeding or hematoma formation. The usual duration of treatment is 2 to 8 days; up to 12.5 days of Lovenox Injection has been well tolerated in clinical trials.

Treatment of Deep Vein Thrombosis With or Without Pulmonary Embolism: In **outpatient treatment**, patients with acute deep vein thrombosis without pulmonary embolism who can be treated at home, the recommended dose of Lovenox Injection is **1 mg/kg every 12 hours** administered SC. In **inpatient (hospital) treatment**, patients with acute deep vein thrombosis with pulmonary embolism or patients with acute deep vein thrombosis without pulmonary embolism (who are not candidates for outpatient treatment), the recommended dose of Lovenox Injection is **1 mg/kg every 12 hours** administered SC **or 1.5 mg/kg once a day** administered SC at the same time every day. In both outpatient and inpatient (hospital) treatments, warfarin sodium therapy should be initiated when appropriate (usually within 72 hours of Lovenox Injection). Lovenox Injection should be continued for a minimum of 5 days and until a therapeutic oral anticoagulant effect has been achieved (International Normalization Ratio 2.0 to 3.0). The average duration of administration is 7 days; up to 17 days of Lovenox Injection administration has been well tolerated in controlled clinical trials.

Renal Impairment: Although no dose adjustment is recommended in patients with moderate (creatinine clearance 30-50 mL/min) and mild (creatinine clearance 50-80 mL/min) renal impairment, all such patients should be observed carefully for signs and symptoms of bleeding.

The recommended prophylaxis and treatment dosage regimens for patients with severe renal impairment (creatinine clearance <30 mL/min) are described in the following table (see **CLINICAL PHARMACOLOGY, Pharmacokinetics, Special Populations** and **PRECAUTIONS, Renal Impairment**).

Dosage Regimens for Patients with Severe Renal Impairment (creatinine clearance <30mL/minute)

Indication	Dosage Regimen
Prophylaxis in abdominal surgery	30 mg administered SC once daily
Prophylaxis in hip or knee replacement surgery	30 mg administered SC once daily
Prophylaxis in medical patients during acute illness	30 mg administered SC once daily
Prophylaxis of ischemic complications of unstable angina and non-Q-wave myocardial infarction, when concurrently administered with aspirin	1 mg/kg administered SC once daily
Inpatient treatment of acute deep vein thrombosis with or without pulmonary embolism, when administered in conjunction with warfarin sodium	1 mg/kg administered SC once daily
Outpatient treatment of acute deep vein thrombosis without pulmonary embolism, when administered in conjunction with warfarin sodium	1 mg/kg administered SC once daily

Administration: Lovenox Injection is a clear, colorless to pale yellow sterile solution, and as with other parenteral drug products, should be inspected visually for particulate matter and discoloration prior to administration.

The use of a tuberculin syringe or equivalent is recommended when using Lovenox multiple-dose vials to assure withdrawal of the appropriate volume of drug.

Lovenox Injection is administered by SC injection. It must not be administered by intramuscular injection. Lovenox Injection is intended for use under the guidance of a physician. Patients may self-inject only if their physician determines that it is appropriate and with medical follow-up, as necessary. Proper training in subcutaneous injection technique (with or without the assistance of an injection device) should be provided.

Subcutaneous Injection Technique: Patients should be lying down and Lovenox Injection administered by deep SC injection. To avoid the loss of drug when using the 30 and 40 mg prefilled syringes, do not expel the air bubble from the syringe before the injection. Administration should be alternated between the left and right anterolateral and left and right posterolateral abdominal wall. The whole length of the needle should be introduced into a skin fold held between the thumb and forefinger; the skin fold should be held throughout the injection. To minimize bruising, do not rub the injection site after completion of the injection.

Continued on next page

Lovenox—Cont.

Lovenox Injection prefilled syringes and graduated prefilled syringes are available with a system that shields the needle after injection.
- Remove the needle shield by pulling it straight off the syringe. If adjusting the dose is required, the dose adjustment must be done prior to injecting the prescribed dose to the patient.

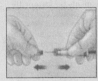

- Inject using standard technique, pushing the plunger to the bottom of the syringe.

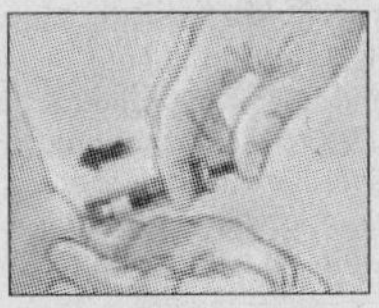

- Remove the syringe from the injection site keeping your finger on the plunger rod.

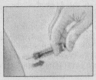

- Orienting the needle away from you and others, activate the safety system by firmly pushing the plunger rod. The protective sleeve will automatically cover the needle and an audible "click" will be heard to confirm shield activation.

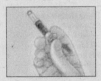

- Immediately dispose of the syringe in the nearest sharps container.

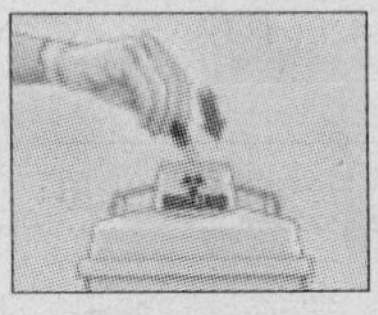

NOTE:
- The safety system can only be activated once the syringe has been emptied.
- Activation of the safety system must be done only after removing the needle from the patient's skin.
- Do not replace the needle shield after injection.
- The safety system should not be sterilized.
- Activation of the safety system may cause minimal splatter of fluid. For optimal safety activate the system while orienting it downwards away from yourself and others.

HOW SUPPLIED

Lovenox® (enoxaparin sodium injection) is available in two concentrations:
[See second table at top of previous page]
[See third table on previous page]
Store at 25°C (77°F); excursions permitted to 15-30°C (59-86°F) [see USP Controlled Room Temperature].
Keep out of the reach of children.

[1]Lepercq J, Conard J, Borel-Derlon A, et al. Venous thromboembolism during pregnancy: a retrospective study of enoxaparin safety in 624 pregnancies. *Br J Obstet Gynec* 2001; 108 (11): 1134-40.
Lovenox Injection prefilled and graduated prefilled syringes manufactured by:
Aventis Pharma Specialties
94700 Maisons-Alfort
France
And
Aventis Pharma
Boulevard Industriel
76580 Le Trait
France
Lovenox multiple-dose vials manufactured by:
DSM Pharmaceuticals, Inc.
Greenville, NC 27835

Manufactured for:
Aventis Pharmaceuticals Inc.
Bridgewater, NJ 08807
©2004 Aventis Pharmaceuticals Inc.
Rev. July 2004

PLAVIX® ℞
[plă-vĭcks]
clopidogrel bisulfate tablets

Prescribing information for this product, which appears on pages 3009–3012 of the 2005 PDR, has been completely revised as follows. Please write "See Supplement A" next to the product heading.

DESCRIPTION

PLAVIX (clopidogrel bisulfate) is an inhibitor of ADP-induced platelet aggregation acting by direct inhibition of adenosine diphosphate (ADP) binding to its receptor and of the subsequent ADP-mediated activation of the glycoprotein GPIIb/IIIa complex. Chemically it is methyl (+)-(S)-α-(2-chlorophenyl)-6,7-dihydrothieno[3,2-c]pyridine-5(4H)-acetate sulfate (1:1). The empirical formula of clopidogrel bisulfate is $C_{16}H_{16}ClNO_2S \bullet H_2SO_4$ and its molecular weight is 419.9.
The structural formula is as follows:

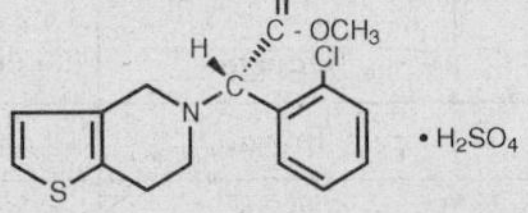

$$\bullet H_2SO_4$$

Clopidogrel bisulfate is a white to off-white powder. It is practically insoluble in water at neutral pH but freely soluble at pH 1. It also dissolves freely in methanol, dissolves sparingly in methylene chloride, and is practically insoluble in ethyl ether. It has a specific optical rotation of about +56°.
PLAVIX for oral administration is provided as pink, round, biconvex, debossed film-coated tablets containing 97.875 mg of clopidogrel bisulfate which is the molar equivalent of 75 mg of clopidogrel base.
Each tablet contains hydrogenated castor oil, hydroxypropylcellulose, mannitol, microcrystalline cellulose and polyethylene glycol 6000 as inactive ingredients. The pink film coating contains ferric oxide, hypromellose 2910, lactose monohydrate, titanium dioxide and triacetin. The tablets are polished with Carnauba wax.

CLINICAL PHARMACOLOGY
Mechanism of Action

Clopidogrel is an inhibitor of platelet aggregation. A variety of drugs that inhibit platelet function have been shown to decrease morbid events in people with established cardiovascular atherosclerotic disease as evidenced by stroke or transient ischemic attacks, myocardial infarction, unstable angina or the need for vascular bypass or angioplasty. This indicates that platelets participate in the initiation and/or evolution of these events and that inhibiting them can reduce the event rate.

Pharmacodynamic Properties

Clopidogrel selectively inhibits the binding of adenosine diphosphate (ADP) to its platelet receptor and the subsequent ADP-mediated activation of the glycoprotein GPIIb/IIIa complex, thereby inhibiting platelet aggregation. Biotransformation of clopidogrel is necessary to produce inhibition of platelet aggregation, but an active metabolite responsible for the activity of the drug has not been isolated. Clopidogrel also inhibits platelet aggregation induced by agonists other than ADP by blocking the amplification of platelet activation by released ADP. Clopidogrel does not inhibit phosphodiesterase activity.
Clopidogrel acts by irreversibly modifying the platelet ADP receptor. Consequently, platelets exposed to clopidogrel are affected for the remainder of their lifespan.
Dose dependent inhibition of platelet aggregation can be seen 2 hours after single oral doses of PLAVIX. Repeated doses of 75 mg PLAVIX per day inhibit ADP-induced platelet aggregation on the first day, and inhibition reaches steady state between Day 3 and Day 7. At steady state, the average inhibition level observed with a dose of 75 mg PLAVIX per day was between 40% and 60%. Platelet aggregation and bleeding time gradually return to baseline values after treatment is discontinued, generally in about 5 days.

Pharmacokinetics and Metabolism

After repeated 75-mg oral doses of clopidogrel (base), plasma concentrations of the parent compound, which has no platelet inhibiting effect, are very low and are generally below the quantification limit (0.00025 mg/L) beyond 2 hours after dosing. Clopidogrel is extensively metabolized by the liver. The main circulating metabolite is the carboxylic acid derivative, and it has no effect on platelet aggregation. It represents about 85% of the circulating drug-related compounds in plasma.
Following an oral dose of ^{14}C-labeled clopidogrel in humans, approximately 50% was excreted in the urine and approximately 46% in the feces in the 5 days after dosing. The elimination half-life of the main circulating metabolite was 8 hours after single and repeated administration. Covalent binding to platelets accounted for 2% of radiolabel with a half-life of 11 days.
Effect of Food: Administration of PLAVIX (clopidogrel bisulfate) with meals did not significantly modify the bioavail-

---

ability of clopidogrel as assessed by the pharmacokinetics of the main circulating metabolite.
Absorption and Distribution: Clopidogrel is rapidly absorbed after oral administration of repeated doses of 75 mg clopidogrel (base), with peak plasma levels (≅3 mg/L) of the main circulating metabolite occurring approximately 1 hour after dosing. The pharmacokinetics of the main circulating metabolite are linear (plasma concentrations increased in proportion to dose) in the dose range of 50 to 150 mg of clopidogrel. Absorption is at least 50% based on urinary excretion of clopidogrel-related metabolites.
Clopidogrel and the main circulating metabolite bind reversibly *in vitro* to human plasma proteins (98% and 94%, respectively). The binding is nonsaturable *in vitro* up to a concentration of 100 μg/mL.
Metabolism and Elimination: In vitro and in vivo, clopidogrel undergoes rapid hydrolysis into its carboxylic acid derivative. In plasma and urine, the glucuronide of the carboxylic acid derivative is also observed.
Special Populations
Geriatric Patients: Plasma concentrations of the main circulating metabolite are significantly higher in elderly (≥75 years) compared to young healthy volunteers but these higher plasma levels were not associated with differences in platelet aggregation and bleeding time. No dosage adjustment is needed for the elderly.
Renally Impaired Patients: After repeated doses of 75 mg PLAVIX per day, plasma levels of the main circulating metabolite were lower in patients with severe renal impairment (creatinine clearance from 5 to 15 mL/min) compared to subjects with moderate renal impairment (creatinine clearance 30 to 60 mL/min) or healthy subjects. Although inhibition of ADP-induced platelet aggregation was lower (25%) than that observed in healthy volunteers, the prolongation of bleeding time was similar to healthy volunteers receiving 75 mg of PLAVIX per day.
Gender: No significant difference was observed in the plasma levels of the main circulating metabolite between males and females. In a small study comparing men and women, less inhibition of ADP-induced platelet aggregation was observed in women, but there was no difference in prolongation of bleeding time. In the large, controlled clinical study (Clopidogrel vs. Aspirin in Patients at Risk of Ischemic Events; CAPRIE), the incidence of clinical outcome events, other adverse clinical events, and abnormal clinical laboratory parameters was similar in men and women.
Race: Pharmacokinetic differences due to race have not been studied.

CLINICAL STUDIES

The clinical evidence for the efficacy of PLAVIX is derived from two double-blind trials: the CAPRIE study (Clopidogrel vs. Aspirin in Patients at Risk of Ischemic Events), a comparison of Plavix to aspirin, and the CURE study (Clopidogrel in Unstable Angina to Prevent Recurrent Ischemic Events), a comparison of Plavix to placebo, both given in combination with aspirin and other standard therapy.
The CAPRIE trial was a 19,185-patient, 304-center, international, randomized, double-blind, parallel-group study comparing PLAVIX (75 mg daily) to aspirin (325 mg daily). The patients randomized had: 1) recent histories of myocardial infarction (within 35 days); 2) recent histories of ischemic stroke (within 6 months) with at least a week of residual neurological signs; or 3) objectively established peripheral arterial disease. Patients received randomized treatment for an average of 1.6 years (maximum of 3 years). The trial's primary outcome was the time to first occurrence of new ischemic stroke (fatal or not), new myocardial infarction (fatal or not), or other vascular death. Deaths not easily attributable to nonvascular causes were all classified as vascular.

Table 1: Outcome Events in the CAPRIE Primary Analysis

Patients	PLAVIX 9599		aspirin 9586	
IS (fatal or not)	438	(4.6%)	461	(4.8%)
MI (fatal or not)	275	(2.9%)	333	(3.5%)
Other vascular death	226	(2.4%)	226	(2.4%)
Total	939	(9.8%)	1020	(10.6%)

As shown in the table, PLAVIX (clopidogrel bisulfate) was associated with a lower incidence of outcome events of every kind. The overall risk reduction (9.8% vs. 10.6%) was 8.7%, P=0.045. Similar results were obtained when all-cause mortality and all-cause strokes were counted instead of vascular mortality and ischemic strokes (risk reduction 6.9%). In patients who survived an on-study stroke or myocardial infarction, the incidence of subsequent events was again lower in the PLAVIX group.
The curves showing the overall event rate are shown in Figure 1. The event curves separated early and continued to diverge over the 3-year follow-up period.
[See figure 1 at top of next column]
Although the statistical significance favoring PLAVIX over aspirin was marginal (P=0.045), and represents the result of a single trial that has not been replicated, the comparator drug, aspirin, is itself effective (vs. placebo) in reducing cardiovascular events in patients with recent myocardial infarction or stroke. Thus, the difference between PLAVIX and placebo, although not measured directly, is substantial. The CAPRIE trial included a population that was randomized on the basis of 3 entry criteria. The efficacy of PLAVIX relative to aspirin was heterogeneous across these randomized subgroups (P=0.043). It is not clear whether this difference is real or a chance occurrence. Although the CAPRIE

Figure 1: Fatal or Non-Fatal Vascular Events in the CAPRIE Study

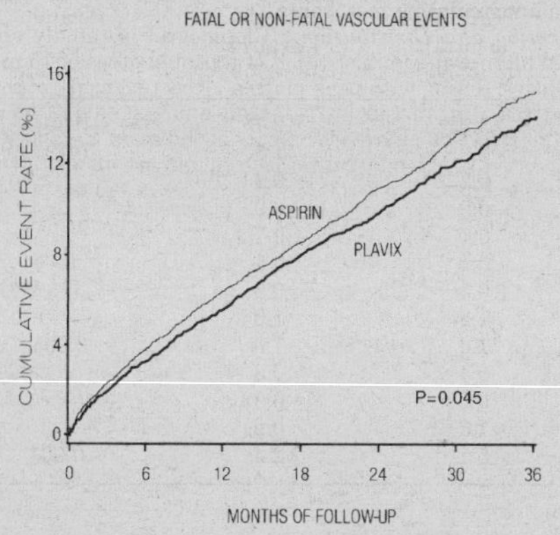
FATAL OR NON-FATAL VASCULAR EVENTS
CUMULATIVE EVENT RATE (%)
ASPIRIN
PLAVIX
P=0.045
MONTHS OF FOLLOW-UP

trial was not designed to evaluate the relative benefit of PLAVIX over aspirin in the individual patient subgroups, the benefit appeared to be strongest in patients who were enrolled because of peripheral vascular disease (especially those who also had a history of myocardial infarction) and weaker in stroke patients. In patients who were enrolled in the trial on the sole basis of a recent myocardial infarction, PLAVIX was not numerically superior to aspirin.

In the meta-analyses of studies of aspirin vs. placebo in patients similar to those in CAPRIE, aspirin was associated with a reduced incidence of thrombotic events. There was a suggestion of heterogeneity in these studies too, with the effect strongest in patients with a history of myocardial infarction, weaker in patients with a history of stroke, and not discernible in patients with a history of peripheral vascular disease. With respect to the inferred comparison of PLAVIX to placebo, there is no indication of heterogeneity.

The CURE study included 12,562 patients with acute coronary syndrome without ST segment elevation (unstable angina or non-Q-wave myocardial infarction) and presenting within 24 hours of onset of the most recent episode of chest pain or symptoms consistent with ischemia. Patients were required to have either ECG changes compatible with new ischemia (without ST segment elevation) or elevated cardiac enzymes or troponin I or T to at least twice the upper limit of normal. The patient population was largely Caucasian (82%) and included 38% women, and 52% patients ≥65 years of age.

Patients were randomized to receive PLAVIX (300 mg loading dose followed by 75 mg/day) or placebo, and were treated for up to one year. Patients also received aspirin (75–325 mg once daily) and other standard therapies such as heparin. The use of GPIIb/IIIa inhibitors was not permitted for three days prior to randomization.

The number of patients experiencing the primary outcome (CV death, MI, or stroke) was 582 (9.30%) in the PLAVIX-treated group and 719 (11.41%) in the placebo-treated group, a 20% relative risk reduction (95% CI of 10%-28%; P=0.00009) for the PLAVIX-treated group (see Table 2).

At the end of 12 months, the number of patients experiencing the co-primary outcome (CV death, MI, stroke or refractory ischemia) was 1035 (16.54%) in the PLAVIX-treated group and 1187 (18.83%) in the placebo-treated group, a 14% relative risk reduction (95% CI of 6%-21%, P=0.0005) for the PLAVIX-treated group (see Table 2).

In the PLAVIX-treated group, each component of the two primary endpoints (CV death, MI, stroke, refractory ischemia) occurred less frequently than in the placebo-treated group.

[See table 2 above]

The benefits of PLAVIX (clopidogrel bisulfate) were maintained throughout the course of the trial (up to 12 months).

Figure 2: Cardiovascular Death, Myocardial Infarction, and Stroke in the CURE Study

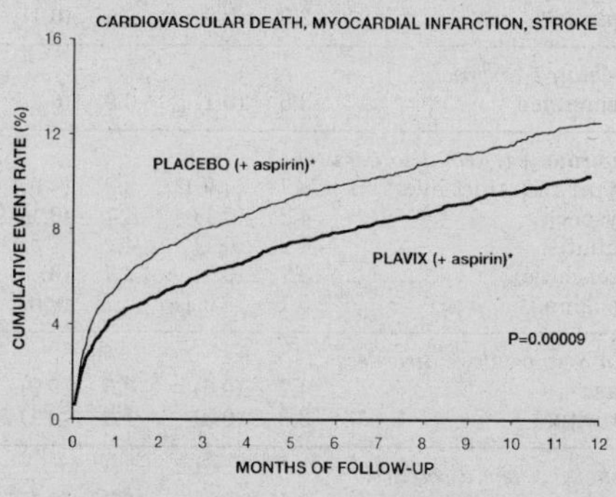
CARDIOVASCULAR DEATH, MYOCARDIAL INFARCTION, STROKE
CUMULATIVE EVENT RATE (%)
PLACEBO (+ aspirin)*
PLAVIX (+ aspirin)*
P=0.00009
MONTHS OF FOLLOW-UP

*Other standard therapies were used as appropriate

In CURE, the use of PLAVIX was associated with a lower incidence of CV death, MI or stroke in patient populations with different characteristics, as shown in Figure 3. The benefits associated with PLAVIX were independent of the

Table 2: Outcome Events in the CURE Primary Analysis

Outcome	PLAVIX (+ aspirin)* (n=6259)		Placebo (+ aspirin)* (n=6303)		Relative Risk Reduction (%) (95% CI)
Primary outcome (Cardiovascular death, MI, Stroke)	582	(9.3%)	719	(11.4%)	20% (10.3, 27.9) P=0.00009
Co-primary outcome (Cardiovascular death, MI, Stroke, Refractory Ischemia)	1035	(16.5%)	1187	(18.8%)	14% (6.2, 20.6) P=0.00052
All Individual Outcome Events:†					
CV death	318	(5.1%)	345	(5.5%)	7% (-7.7, 20.6)
MI	324	(5.2%)	419	(6.6%)	23% (11.0, 33.4)
Stroke	75	(1.2%)	87	(1.4%)	14% (-17.7, 36.6)
Refractory ischemia	544	(8.7%)	587	(9.3%)	7% (-4.0, 18.0)

*Other standard therapies were used as appropriate.
†The individual components do not represent a breakdown of the primary and co-primary outcomes, but rather the total number of subjects experiencing an event during the course of the study.

use of other acute and long-term cardiovascular therapies, including heparin/LMWH (low molecular weight heparin), IV glycoprotein IIb/IIIa (GPIIb/IIIa) inhibitors, lipid-lowering drugs, beta-blockers, and ACE-inhibitors. The efficacy of PLAVIX was observed independently of the dose of aspirin (75-325 mg once daily). The use of oral anticoagulants, nonstudy anti-platelet drugs and chronic NSAIDs was not allowed in CURE.

Figure 3. Hazard Ratio for Patient Baseline Characteristics and On-Study Concomitant Medications/Interventions for the CURE Study

Baseline Characteristics		N	Percent Events PLAVIX (+aspirin)*	Percent Events Placebo (+aspirin)*
Overall		12562	9.3	11.4
Diagnosis	Non-Q-W	3295	12.7	15.5
	Unst Ang	8298	7.3	8.7
	Other	968	15.1	19.7
Age	< 65	5996	5.2	7.6
	65-74	4136	10.2	12.4
	≥ 75	2430	17.8	19.2
Gender	Male	7725	9.1	11.9
	Female	4836	9.5	10.7
Race	Caucas	10308	9.1	11.0
	Non-Cauc	2250	10.1	13.2
Elev Card Enzy	No	9381	8.8	10.9
	Yes	3176	10.7	13.0
ST Depr >1.0mm	No	7273	7.5	8.9
	Yes	5288	11.8	14.8
Diabetes	No	9721	7.9	9.9
	Yes	2840	14.2	16.7
Previous MI	No	8517	7.8	9.5
	Yes	4044	12.5	15.4
Previous Stroke	No	12055	8.9	11.0
	Yes	506	17.9	22.4
Concomitant Medication / Therapy				
Heparin/LMWH	No	951	4.9	7.7
	Yes	11611	9.7	11.7
Aspirin	<100mg	1927	8.5	9.7
	100-200mg	7428	9.2	10.9
	>200mg	3201	9.9	13.7
GPIIb/IIIa Antag	No	11739	8.9	10.8
	Yes	823	15.7	19.2
Beta-Blocker	No	2032	9.9	12.0
	Yes	10530	9.2	11.3
ACEI	No	4813	6.3	8.1
	Yes	7749	11.2	13.5
Lipid-Lowering	No	4461	10.9	13.1
	Yes	8101	8.4	10.5
PTCA/CABG	No	7977	8.1	10.0
	Yes	4585	11.4	13.8

*Other standard therapies were used as appropriate

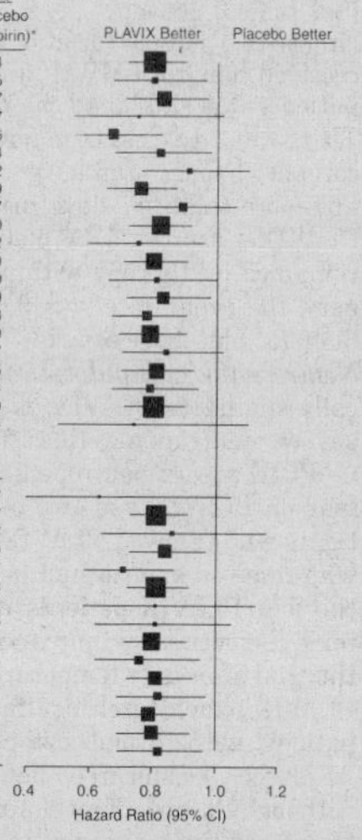
PLAVIX Better
Placebo Better
0.4
0.6
0.8
1.0
1.2
Hazard Ratio (95% CI)

The use of PLAVIX in CURE was associated with a decrease in the use of thrombolytic therapy (71 patients [1.1%] in the PLAVIX group, 126 patients [2.0%] in the placebo group; relative risk reduction of 43%, P=0.0001), and GPIIb/IIIa inhibitors (369 patients [5.9%] in the PLAVIX group, 454 patients [7.2%] in the placebo group, relative risk reduction of 18%, P=0.003). The use of PLAVIX in CURE did not impact the number of patients treated with CABG or PCI (with or without stenting), (2253 patients [36.0%] in the PLAVIX group, 2324 patients [36.9%] in the placebo group; relative risk reduction of 4.0%, P=0.1658).

INDICATIONS AND USAGE

PLAVIX (clopidogrel bisulfate) is indicated for the reduction of thrombotic events as follows:

- **Recent MI, Recent Stroke or Established Peripheral Arterial Disease**
  For patients with a history of recent myocardial infarction (MI), recent stroke, or established peripheral arterial disease, PLAVIX has been shown to reduce the rate of a combined endpoint of new ischemic stroke (fatal or not), new MI (fatal or not), and other vascular death.
- **Acute Coronary Syndrome**
  For patients with acute coronary syndrome (unstable angina/non-Q-wave MI) including patients who are to be managed medically and those who are to be managed with percutaneous coronary intervention (with or without stent) or CABG, PLAVIX has been shown to decrease the rate of a combined endpoint of cardiovascular death, MI, or stroke as well as the rate of a combined endpoint of cardiovascular death, MI, stroke, or refractory ischemia.

CONTRAINDICATIONS

The use of PLAVIX is contraindicated in the following conditions:

- Hypersensitivity to the drug substance or any component of the product.
- Active pathological bleeding such as peptic ulcer or intracranial hemorrhage.

WARNINGS

Thrombotic thrombocytopenic purpura (TTP): TTP has been reported rarely following use of PLAVIX, sometimes after a short exposure (<2 weeks). TTP is a serious condition and requires urgent referral to a hematologist for prompt treatment. It is characterized by thrombocytopenia, microangiopathic hemolytic anemia (schistocytes [fragmented RBCs] seen on peripheral smear), neurological findings, renal dysfunction, and fever. TTP was not seen during clopidogrel's clinical trials, which included over 17,500 clopidogrel-treated patients. In world-wide postmarketing experience, however, TTP has been reported at a rate of about four cases per million patients exposed, or about 11 cases per million patient-years. The background rate is thought to be about four cases per million person-years. (See **ADVERSE REACTIONS**.)

PRECAUTIONS

General

As with other antiplatelet agents,PLAVIX prolongs the bleeding time and therefore should be used with caution in patients who may be at risk of increased bleeding from trauma, surgery, or other pathological conditions (particularly gastrointestinal and intraocular). If a patient is to undergo elective surgery and an antiplatelet effect is not desired, PLAVIX should be discontinued 5 days prior to surgery.

Due to the risk of bleeding and undesirable hematological effects, blood cell count determination and/or other appropriate testing should be promptly considered, whenever such suspected clinical symptoms arise during the course of treatment (see **ADVERSE REACTIONS**).

GI Bleeding: In CAPRIE, PLAVIX was associated with a rate of gastrointestinal bleeding of 2.0%, vs. 2.7% on aspirin. In CURE, the incidence of major gastrointestinal bleeding was 1.3% vs. 0.7% (PLAVIX + aspirin vs. placebo + aspirin, respectively). PLAVIX should be used with caution in patients who have lesions with a propensity to bleed (such as ulcers). Drugs that might induce such lesions should be used with caution in patients taking PLAVIX.

Use in Hepatically Impaired Patients: Experience is limited in patients with severe hepatic disease, who may have bleeding diatheses. PLAVIX should be used with caution in this population.

Use in Renally-impaired Patients: Experience is limited in patients with severe renal impairment. PLAVIX should be used with caution in this population.

Information for Patients

Patients should be told that they may bleed more easily and it may take them longer than usual to stop bleeding when they take PLAVIX or PLAVIX combined with aspirin, and that they should report any unusual bleeding to their physician. Patients should inform physicians and dentists that they are taking PLAVIX and/or any other product known to affect bleeding before any surgery is scheduled and before any new drug is taken.

Drug Interactions

Study of specific drug interactions yielded the following results:

Aspirin: Aspirin did not modify the clopidogrel-mediated inhibition of ADP-induced platelet aggregation. Concomitant administration of 500 mg of aspirin twice a day for 1 day did not significantly increase the prolongation of bleeding time induced by PLAVIX. PLAVIX potentiated the effect of aspirin on collagen-induced platelet aggregation. PLAVIX and aspirin have been administered together for up to one year.

Heparin: In a study in healthy volunteers, PLAVIX did not necessitate modification of the heparin dose or alter the effect of heparin on coagulation. Coadministration of heparin had no effect on inhibition of platelet aggregation induced by PLAVIX.

Continued on next page

Plavix—Cont.

Nonsteroidal Anti-Inflammatory Drugs (NSAIDs): In healthy volunteers receiving naproxen, concomitant administration of PLAVIX was associated with increased occult gastrointestinal blood loss. NSAIDs and PLAVIX should be coadministered with caution.

Warfarin: Because of the increased risk of bleeding, the concomitant administration of warfarin with PLAVIX should be undertaken with caution. (See **PRECAUTIONS–General**.)

Other Concomitant Therapy: No clinically significant pharmacodynamic interactions were observed when PLAVIX was coadministered with **atenolol, nifedipine,** or both atenolol and nifedipine. The pharmacodynamic activity of PLAVIX was also not significantly influenced by the coadministration of **phenobarbital, cimetidine** or **estrogen**.

The pharmacokinetics of **digoxin** or **theophylline** were not modified by the coadministration of PLAVIX (clopidogrel bisulfate).

At high concentrations *in vitro*, clopidogrel inhibits P_{450} (2C9). Accordingly, PLAVIX may interfere with the metabolism of **phenytoin, tamoxifen, tolbutamide, warfarin, torsemide, fluvastatin,** and many **non-steroidal anti-inflammatory agents,** but there are no data with which to predict the magnitude of these interactions. Caution should be used when any of these drugs is coadministered with PLAVIX.

In addition to the above specific interaction studies, patients entered into clinical trials with PLAVIX received a variety of concomitant medications including **diuretics, beta-blocking agents, angiotensin converting enzyme inhibitors, calcium antagonists, cholesterol lowering agents, coronary vasodilators, antidiabetic agents** (including **insulin**), **antiepileptic agents, hormone replacement therapy, heparins** (unfractionated and LMWH) and **GPIIb/IIIa antagonists** without evidence of clinically significant adverse interactions. The use of oral anticoagulants, non-study antiplatelet drug and chronic NSAIDs was not allowed in CURE and there are no data on their concomitant use with clopidogrel.

Drug/Laboratory Test Interactions

None known.

Carcinogenesis, Mutagenesis, Impairment of Fertility

There was no evidence of tumorigenicity when clopidogrel was administered for 78 weeks to mice and 104 weeks to rats at dosages up to 77 mg/kg per day, which afforded plasma exposures >25 times that in humans at the recommended daily dose of 75 mg.

Clopidogrel was not genotoxic in four *in vitro* tests (Ames test, DNA-repair test in rat hepatocytes, gene mutation assay in Chinese hamster fibroblasts, and metaphase chromosome analysis of human lymphocytes) and in one *in vivo* test (micronucleus test by oral route in mice).

Clopidogrel was found to have no effect on fertility of male and female rats at oral doses up to 400 mg/kg per day (52 times the recommended human dose on a mg/m^2 basis).

Pregnancy

Pregnancy Category B. Reproduction studies performed in rats and rabbits at doses up to 500 and 300 mg/kg/day (respectively, 65 and 78 times the recommended daily human dose on a mg/m^2 basis), revealed no evidence of impaired fertility or fetotoxicity due to clopidogrel. There are, however, no adequate and well-controlled studies in pregnant women. Because animal reproduction studies are not always predictive of a human response, PLAVIX should be used during pregnancy only if clearly needed.

Nursing Mothers

Studies in rats have shown that clopidogrel and/or its metabolites are excreted in the milk. It is not known whether this drug is excreted in human milk. Because many drugs are excreted in human milk and because of the potential for serious adverse reactions in nursing infants, a decision should be made whether to discontinue nursing or to discontinue the drug, taking into account the importance of the drug to the nursing woman.

Pediatric Use

Safety and effectiveness in the pediatric population have not been established.

Geriatric Use

Of the total number of subjects in controlled clinical studies, approximately 50% of patients treated with PLAVIX were 65 years of age and over. Approximately 16% of patients treated with PLAVIX were 75 years of age and over.

The observed difference in risk of thrombotic events with clopidogrel plus aspirin versus placebo plus aspirin by age category is provided in Figure 3 (see **CLINICAL STUDIES**). The observed difference in risk of bleeding events with clopidogrel plus aspirin versus placebo plus aspirin by age category is provided in Table 3 (see **ADVERSE REACTIONS**).

ADVERSE REACTIONS

PLAVIX has been evaluated for safety in more than 17,500 patients, including over 9,000 patients treated for 1 year or more. The overall tolerability of PLAVIX in CAPRIE was similar to that of aspirin regardless of age, gender and race, with an approximately equal incidence (13%) of patients withdrawing from treatment because of adverse reactions. The clinically important adverse events observed in CAPRIE and CURE are discussed below.

Hemorrhagic: In CAPRIE patients receiving PLAVIX, gastrointestinal hemorrhage occurred at a rate of 2.0%, and required hospitalization in 0.7%. In patients receiving aspirin, the corresponding rates were 2.7% and 1.1%, respectively.

Table 3: CURE Incidence of bleeding complications (% patients)

Event	PLAVIX (+ aspirin)* (n=6259)	Placebo (+ aspirin)* (n=6303)	*P*-value
Major bleeding†	3.7‡	2.7§	0.001
Life-threatening bleeding	2.2	1.8	0.13
Fatal	0.2	0.2	
5 g/dL hemoglobin drop	0.9	0.9	
Requiring surgical intervention	0.7	0.7	
Hemorrhagic strokes	0.1	0.1	
Requiring inotropes	0.5	0.5	
Requiring transfusion (≥4 units)	1.2	1.0	
Other major bleeding	1.6	1.0	0.005
Significantly disabling	0.4	0.3	
Intraocular bleeding with significant loss of vision	0.05	0.03	
Requiring 2–3 units of blood	1.3	0.9	
Minor bleeding¶	5.1	2.4	<0.001

* Other standard therapies were used as appropriate.
† Life threatening and other major bleeding.
‡ Major bleeding event rate for PLAVIX + aspirin was dose-dependent on aspirin: <100 mg=2.6%; 100-200 mg=3.5%; >200 mg=4.9%
Major bleeding event rates for PLAVIX + aspirin by age were: <65 years = 2.5%, ≥65 to <75 years = 4.1%, ≥75 years 5.9%
§ Major bleeding event rate for placebo + aspirin was dose-dependent on aspirin: <100 mg=2.0%; 100-200 mg=2.3%; >200 mg=4.0%
Major bleeding event rates for placebo + aspirin by age were: <65 years = 2.1%, ≥65 to <75 years = 3.1%, ≥75 years 3.6%
¶ Led to interruption of study medication.

The incidence of intracranial hemorrhage was 0.4% for PLAVIX compared to 0.5% for aspirin.

In CURE, PLAVIX use with aspirin was associated with an increase in bleeding compared to placebo with aspirin (see Table 3). There was an excess in major bleeding in patients receiving PLAVIX plus aspirin compared with placebo plus aspirin, primarily gastrointestinal and at puncture sites. The incidence of intracranial hemorrhage (0.1%), and fatal bleeding (0.2%), were the same in both groups.

The overall incidence of bleeding is described in Table 3 for patients receiving both PLAVIX and aspirin in CURE.

[See table 3 above]

Ninety-two percent (92%) of the patients in the CURE study received heparin/LMWH, and the rate of bleeding in these patients was similar to the overall results.

There was no excess in major bleeds within seven days after coronary bypass graft surgery in patients who stopped therapy more than five days prior to surgery (event rate 4.4% PLAVIX + aspirin; 5.3% placebo + aspirin). In patients who remained on therapy within five days of bypass graft surgery, the event rate was 9.6% for PLAVIX + aspirin, and 6.3% for placebo + aspirin.

Neutropenia/agranulocytosis: Ticlopidine, a drug chemically similar to PLAVIX, is associated with a 0.8% rate of severe neutropenia (less than 450 neutrophils/μL). In CAPRIE severe neutropenia was observed in six patients, four on PLAVIX and two on aspirin. Two of the 9599 patients who received PLAVIX and none of the 9586 patients who received aspirin had neutrophil counts of zero. One of the four PLAVIX patients in CAPRIE was receiving cytotoxic chemotherapy, and another recovered and returned to the trial after only temporarily interrupting treatment with PLAVIX (clopidogrel bisulfate). In CURE, the numbers of patients with thrombocytopenia (19 PLAVIX + aspirin vs. 24 placebo + aspirin) or neutropenia (3 vs. 3) were similar. Although the risk of myelotoxicity with PLAVIX (clopidogrel bisulfate) thus appears to be quite low, this possibility should be considered when a patient receiving PLAVIX demonstrates fever or other sign of infection.

Gastrointestinal: Overall, the incidence of gastrointestinal events (e.g. abdominal pain, dyspepsia, gastritis and constipation) in patients receiving PLAVIX (clopidogrel bisulfate) was 27.1%, compared to 29.8% in those receiving aspirin in the CAPRIE trial. In the CURE trial the incidence of these gastrointestinal events for patients receiving PLAVIX + aspirin was 11.7% compared to 12.5% for those receiving placebo + aspirin.

In the CAPRIE trial, the incidence of peptic, gastric or duodenal ulcers was 0.7% for PLAVIX and 1.2% for aspirin. In the CURE trial the incidence of peptic, gastric or duodenal ulcers was 0.4% for PLAVIX + aspirin and 0.3% for placebo + aspirin.

Cases of diarrhea were reported in the CAPRIE trial in 4.5% of patients in the PLAVIX group compared to 3.4% in the aspirin group. However, these were rarely severe (PLAVIX=0.2% and aspirin=0.1%). In the CURE trial, the incidence of diarrhea for patients receiving PLAVIX + aspirin was 2.1% compared to 2.2% for those receiving placebo + aspirin.

In the CAPRIE trial, the incidence of patients withdrawing from treatment because of gastrointestinal adverse reactions was 3.2% for PLAVIX (clopidogrel bisulfate) and 4.0% for aspirin. In the CURE trial, the incidence of patients withdrawing from treatment because of gastrointestinal adverse reactions was 0.9% for PLAVIX + aspirin compared with 0.8% for placebo + aspirin.

Rash and Other Skin Disorders: In the CAPRIE trial, the incidence of skin and appendage disorders in patients receiving PLAVIX was 15.8% (0.7% serious); the corresponding rate in aspirin patients was 13.1% (0.5% serious). In the CURE trial the incidence of rash or other skin disorders in patients receiving PLAVIX + aspirin was 4.0% compared to 3.5% for those receiving placebo + aspirin.

In the CAPRIE trial, the overall incidence of patients withdrawing from treatment because of skin and appendage disorders adverse reactions was 1.5% for PLAVIX and 0.8% for aspirin. In the CURE trial, the incidence of patients withdrawing because of skin and appendage disorders adverse reactions was 0.7% for PLAVIX + aspirin compared with 0.3% for placebo + aspirin.

Adverse events occurring in ≥2.5% of patients on PLAVIX in the CAPRIE controlled clinical trial are shown below regardless of relationship to PLAVIX. The median duration of therapy was 20 months, with a maximum of 3 years.

Table 4: Adverse Events Occurring in ≥2.5% of PLAVIX Patients in CAPRIE

	% Incidence (% Discontinuation)			
Body System **Event**	**PLAVIX [n=9599]**		**Aspirin [n=9586]**	
Body as a Whole-general disorders				
Chest Pain	8.3	(0.2)	8.3	(0.3)
Accidental/Inflicted Injury	7.9	(0.1)	7.3	(0.1)
Influenza-like symptoms	7.5	(<0.1)	7.0	(<0.1)
Pain	6.4	(0.1)	6.3	(0.1)
Fatigue	3.3	(0.1)	3.4	(0.1)
Cardiovascular disorders, general				
Edema	4.1	(<0.1)	4.5	(<0.1)
Hypertension	4.3	(<0.1)	5.1	(<0.1)
Central & peripheral nervous system disorders				
Headache	7.6	(0.3)	7.2	(0.2)
Dizziness	6.2	(0.2)	6.7	(0.3)
Gastrointestinal system disorders				
Abdominal pain	5.6	(0.7)	7.1	(1.0)
Dyspepsia	5.2	(0.6)	6.1	(0.7)
Diarrhea	4.5	(0.4)	3.4	(0.3)
Nausea	3.4	(0.5)	3.8	(0.4)
Metabolic & nutritional disorders				
Hypercholesterolemia	4.0	(0)	4.4	(<0.1)
Musculo-skeletal system disorders				
Arthralgia	6.3	(0.1)	6.2	(0.1)
Back Pain	5.8	(0.1)	5.3	(<0.1)
Platelet, bleeding, & clotting disorders				
Purpura/Bruise	5.3	(0.3)	3.7	(0.1)
Epistaxis	2.9	(0.2)	2.5	(0.1)
Psychiatric disorders				
Depression	3.6	(0.1)	3.9	(0.2)
Respiratory system disorders				
Upper resp tract infection	8.7	(<0.1)	8.3	(<0.1)
Dyspnea	4.5	(0.1)	4.7	(0.1)
Rhinitis	4.2	(0.1)	4.2	(<0.1)
Bronchitis	3.7	(0.1)	3.7	(0)
Coughing	3.1	(<0.1)	2.7	(<0.1)
Skin & appendage disorders				
Rash	4.2	(0.5)	3.5	(0.2)
Pruritus	3.3	(0.3)	1.6	(0.1)
Urinary system disorders				
Urinary tract infection	3.1	(0)	3.5	(0.1)

Incidence of discontinuation, regardless of relationship to therapy, is shown in parentheses.

Adverse events occurring in ≥2.0% of patients on PLAVIX in the CURE controlled clinical trial are shown below regardless of relationship to PLAVIX.

Table 5: Adverse Events Occurring in ≥2.0% of PLAVIX Patients in CURE

Body System / Event	PLAVIX (+ aspirin)* [n=6259] % Incidence	(% Discontinuation)	Placebo (+ aspirin)* [n=6303] % Incidence	(% Discontinuation)
Body as a Whole-general disorders				
Chest Pain	2.7	(<0.1)	2.8	(0.0)
Central & peripheral nervous system disorders				
Headache	3.1	(0.1)	3.2	(0.1)
Dizziness	2.4	(0.1)	2.0	(<0.1)
Gastrointestinal system disorders				
Abdominal pain	2.3	(0.3)	2.8	(0.3)
Dyspepsia	2.0	(0.1)	1.9	(<0.1)
Diarrhea	2.1	(0.1)	2.2	(0.1)

*Other standard therapies were used as appropriate.

Other adverse experiences of potential importance occurring in 1% to 2.5% of patients receiving PLAVIX (clopidogrel bisulfate) in the CAPRIE or CURE controlled clinical trials are listed below regardless of relationship to PLAVIX. In general, the incidence of these events was similar to that in patients receiving aspirin (in CAPRIE) or placebo + aspirin (in CURE).

Autonomic Nervous System Disorders: Syncope, Palpitation. *Body as a Whole-general disorders:* Asthenia, Fever, Hernia. *Cardiovascular disorders:* Cardiac failure. *Central and peripheral nervous system disorders:* Cramps legs, Hypoaesthesia, Neuralgia, Paraesthesia, Vertigo. *Gastrointestinal system disorders:* Constipation, Vomiting. *Heart rate and rhythm disorders:* Fibrillation atrial. *Liver and biliary system disorders:* Hepatic enzymes increased. *Metabolic and nutritional disorders:* Gout, hyperuricemia, non-protein nitrogen (NPN) increased. *Musculo-skeletal system disorders:* Arthritis, Arthrosis. *Platelet, bleeding & clotting disorders:* GI hemorrhage, hematoma, platelets decreased. *Psychiatric disorders:* Anxiety, Insomnia. *Red blood cell disorders:* Anemia. *Respiratory system disorders:* Pneumonia, Sinusitis. *Skin and appendage disorders:* Eczema, Skin ulceration. *Urinary system disorders:* Cystitis. *Vision disorders:* Cataract, Conjunctivitis.

Other potentially serious adverse events which may be of clinical interest but were rarely reported (<1%) in patients who received PLAVIX in the CAPRIE or CURE controlled clinical trials are listed below regardless of relationship to PLAVIX. In general, the incidence of these events was similar to that in patients receiving aspirin (in CAPRIE) or placebo + aspirin (in CURE).

Body as a whole: Allergic reaction, necrosis ischemic. *Cardiovascular disorders:* Edema generalized. *Gastrointestinal system disorders:* Gastric ulcer perforated, gastritis hemorrhagic, upper GI ulcer hemorrhagic. *Liver and Biliary system disorders:* Bilirubinemia, hepatitis infectious, liver fatty. *Platelet, bleeding and clotting disorders:* hemarthrosis, hematuria, hemoptysis, hemorrhage intracranial, hemorrhage retroperitoneal, hemorrhage of operative wound, ocular hemorrhage, pulmonary hemorrhage, purpura allergic, thrombocytopenia. *Red blood cell disorders:* Anemia aplastic, anemia hypochromic. *Reproductive disorders, female:* Menorrhagia. *Respiratory system disorders:* Hemothorax. *Skin and appendage disorders:* Bullous eruption, rash erythematous, rash maculopapular, urticaria. *Urinary system disorders:* Abnormal renal function, acute renal failure. *White cell and reticuloendothelial system disorders:* Agranulocytosis, granulocytopenia, leukemia, leukopenia, neutrophils decreased.

Postmarketing Experience

The following events have been reported spontaneously from worldwide postmarketing experience:

- *Body as a whole:*
  - hypersensitivity reactions, anaphylactoid reactions
- *Central and Peripheral Nervous System disorders:*
  - confusion, hallucinations, taste disorders
- *Hepato-biliary disorders:*
  - abnormal liver function test, hepatitis (non-infectious)
- *Platelet, Bleeding and Clotting disorders:*
  - cases of bleeding with fatal outcome (especially intracranial, gastrointestinal and retroperitoneal hemorrhage)
  - agranulocytosis, aplastic anemia/pancytopenia, thrombotic thrombocytopenic purpura (TTP) – some cases with fatal outcome – (see **WARNINGS**).
  - conjunctival, ocular and retinal bleeding
- *Respiratory, thoracic and mediastinal disorders:*
  - bronchospasm
- *Skin and subcutaneous tissue disorders:*
  - angioedema, erythema multiforme, Stevens-Johnson syndrome, lichen planus
- *Renal and urinary disorders:*
  - glomerulopathy, increased creatinine levels
- *Vascular disorders:*
  - vasculitis, hypotension
- *Gastrointestinal disorders:*
  - colitis (including ulcerative or lymphocytic colitis), pancreatitis
- *Musculoskeletal, connective tissue and bone disorders:*
  - myalgia

OVERDOSAGE

Overdose following clopidogrel administration may lead to prolonged bleeding time and subsequent bleeding complications. Appropriate therapy should be considered if bleeding is observed. A single oral dose of clopidogrel at 1500 or 2000 mg/kg was lethal to mice and to rats and at 3000 mg/kg to baboons. Symptoms of acute toxicity were vomiting (in baboons), prostration, difficult breathing, and gastrointestinal hemorrhage in all species.

Recommendations About Specific Treatment:

Based on biological plausibility, platelet transfusion may be appropriate to reverse the pharmacological effects of PLAVIX if quick reversal is required.

DOSAGE AND ADMINISTRATION

Recent MI, Recent Stroke, or Established Peripheral Arterial Disease

The recommended daily dose of PLAVIX is 75 mg once daily.

Acute Coronary Syndrome

For patients with acute coronary syndrome (unstable angina/non-Q-wave MI), PLAVIX should be initiated with a single 300 mg loading dose and then continued at 75 mg once daily. Aspirin (75 mg-325 mg once daily) should be initiated and continued in combination with PLAVIX. In CURE, most patients with Acute Coronary Syndrome also received heparin acutely (see **CLINICAL STUDIES**).

PLAVIX can be administered with or without food.

No dosage adjustment is necessary for elderly patients or patients with renal disease. (See **Clinical Pharmacology: Special Populations.**)

HOW SUPPLIED

PLAVIX (clopidogrel bisulfate) is available as a pink, round, biconvex, film-coated tablet debossed with "75" on one side and "1171" on the other. Tablets are provided as follows:

NDC 63653-1171-6 bottles of 30
NDC 63653-1171-1 bottles of 90
NDC 63653-1171-5 bottles of 500
NDC 63653-1171-3 blisters of 100

Storage

Store at 25° C (77° F); excursions permitted to 15°-30° C (59°-86° F) [See USP Controlled Room Temperature].

Distributed by:
Bristol-Myers Squibb/Sanofi Pharmaceuticals Partnership
New York, NY 10016

sanofi~synthelabo **Bristol-Myers-Squibb Company**

PLAVIX® is a registered trademark of Sanofi-Synthelabo.

51-021345-05 Revised November 2004

TAXOTERE® ℞

[*tax-ō-tĕr*]
(docetaxel)
Injection Concentrate

Prescribing Information as of February 2005
℞ only

Prescribing information for this product, which appears on pages 746–754 of the 2005 PDR, has been completely revised as follows. Please write "See Supplement A" next to the product heading.

WARNING

TAXOTERE® (docetaxel) Injection Concentrate should be administered under the supervision of a qualified physician experienced in the use of antineoplastic agents. Appropriate management of complications is possible only when adequate diagnostic and treatment facilities are readily available.

The incidence of treatment-related mortality associated with TAXOTERE therapy is increased in patients with abnormal liver function, in patients receiving higher doses, and in patients with non-small cell lung carcinoma and a history of prior treatment with platinum-based chemotherapy who receive TAXOTERE as a single agent at a dose of 100 mg/m^2 (see **WARNINGS**).

TAXOTERE should generally not be given to patients with bilirubin > upper limit of normal (ULN), or to patients with SGOT and/or SGPT >1.5 × ULN concomitant with alkaline phosphatase > 2.5 × ULN. Patients with elevations of bilirubin or abnormalities of transaminase concurrent with alkaline phosphatase are at increased risk for the development of grade 4 neutropenia, febrile neutropenia, infections, severe thrombocytopenia, severe stomatitis, severe skin toxicity, and toxic death. Patients with isolated elevations of transaminase > 1.5 × ULN also had a higher rate of febrile neutropenia grade 4 but did not have an increased incidence of toxic death. Bilirubin, SGOT or SGPT, and alkaline phosphatase values should be obtained prior to each cycle of TAXOTERE therapy and reviewed by the treating physician.

TAXOTERE therapy should not be given to patients with neutrophil counts of < 1500 cells/mm^3. In order to monitor the occurrence of neutropenia, which may be severe and result in infection, frequent blood cell counts should be performed on all patients receiving TAXOTERE.

Severe hypersensitivity reactions characterized by hypotension and/or bronchospasm, or generalized rash/erythema occurred in 2.2% (2/92) of patients who received the recommended 3-day dexamethasone premedication. Hypersensitivity reactions requiring discontinuation of the TAXOTERE infusion were reported in five patients who did not receive premedication. These reactions resolved after discontinuation of the infusion and the administration of appropriate therapy. TAXOTERE must not be given to patients who have a history of severe hypersensitivity reactions to TAXOTERE or to other drugs formulated with polysorbate 80 (see **WARNINGS**).

Severe fluid retention occurred in 6.5% (6/92) of patients despite use of a 3-day dexamethasone premedication regimen. It was characterized by one or more of the following events: poorly tolerated peripheral edema, generalized edema, pleural effusion requiring urgent drainage, dyspnea at rest, cardiac tamponade, or pronounced abdominal distention (due to ascites) (see **PRECAUTIONS**).

DESCRIPTION

Docetaxel is an antineoplastic agent belonging to the taxoid family. It is prepared by semisynthesis beginning with a precursor extracted from the renewable needle biomass of yew plants. The chemical name for docetaxel is (2R,3S)-N-carboxy-3-phenylisoserine,N-*tert*-butyl ester, 13-ester with 5β-20-epoxy-1,2α,4,7β,10β,13α-hexahydroxytax-11-en-9-one 4-acetate 2-benzoate, trihydrate. Docetaxel has the following structural formula:

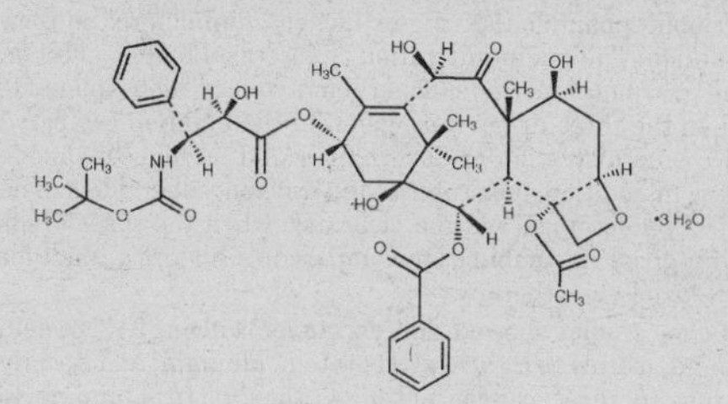

Docetaxel is a white to almost-white powder with an empirical formula of $C_{43}H_{53}NO_{14} \cdot 3H_2O$, and a molecular weight of 861.9. It is highly lipophilic and practically insoluble in water. TAXOTERE (docetaxel) Injection Concentrate is a clear yellow to brownish-yellow viscous solution. TAXOTERE is sterile, non-pyrogenic, and is available in single-dose vials containing 20 mg (0.5 mL) or 80 mg (2 mL) docetaxel (anhydrous). Each mL contains 40 mg docetaxel (anhydrous) and 1040 mg polysorbate 80.

TAXOTERE Injection Concentrate requires dilution prior to use. A sterile, non-pyrogenic, single-dose diluent is supplied for that purpose. The diluent for TAXOTERE contains 13% ethanol in water for injection, and is supplied in vials.

CLINICAL PHARMACOLOGY

Docetaxel is an antineoplastic agent that acts by disrupting the microtubular network in cells that is essential for mitotic and interphase cellular functions. Docetaxel binds to free tubulin and promotes the assembly of tubulin into stable microtubules while simultaneously inhibiting their disassembly. This leads to the production of microtubule bundles without normal function and to the stabilization of microtubules, which results in the inhibition of mitosis in cells. Docetaxel's binding to microtubules does not alter the number of protofilaments in the bound microtubules, a feature which differs from most spindle poisons currently in clinical use.

HUMAN PHARMACOKINETICS

The pharmacokinetics of docetaxel have been evaluated in cancer patients after administration of 20-115 mg/m^2 in phase I studies. The area under the curve (AUC) was dose proportional following doses of 70-115 mg/m^2 with infusion times of 1 to 2 hours. Docetaxel's pharmacokinetic profile is consistent with a three-compartment pharmacokinetic model, with half-lives for the α, β, and γ phases of 4 min, 36 min, and 11.1 hr, respectively. The initial rapid decline represents distribution to the peripheral compartments and the late (terminal) phase is due, in part, to a relatively slow efflux of docetaxel from the peripheral compartment. Mean values for total body clearance and steady state volume of distribution were 21 L/h/m^2 and 113 L, respectively. Mean total body clearance for Japanese patients dosed at the range of 10-90 mg/m^2 was similar to that of European/American populations dosed at 100 mg/m^2, suggesting no significant difference in the elimination of docetaxel in the two populations.

A study of ^{14}C-docetaxel was conducted in three cancer patients. Docetaxel was eliminated in both the urine and feces following oxidative metabolism of the *tert*-butyl ester group, but fecal excretion was the main elimination route. Within 7 days, urinary and fecal excretion accounted for approximately 6% and 75% of the administered radioactivity, respectively. About 80% of the radioactivity recovered in feces is excreted during the first 48 hours as 1 major and 3 minor metabolites with very small amounts (less than 8%) of unchanged drug.

A population pharmacokinetic analysis was carried out after TAXOTERE treatment of 535 patients dosed at 100 mg/m^2. Pharmacokinetic parameters estimated by this analysis were very close to those estimated from phase I studies. The pharmacokinetics of docetaxel were not influenced by age or gender and docetaxel total body clearance was not modified by pretreatment with dexamethasone. In patients with clin-

Continued on next page

Taxotere—Cont.

ical chemistry data suggestive of mild to moderate liver function impairment (SGOT and/or SGPT >1.5 times the upper limit of normal [ULN] concomitant with alkaline phosphatase >2.5 times ULN), total body clearance was lowered by an average of 27%, resulting in a 38% increase in systemic exposure (AUC). This average, however, includes a substantial range and there is, at present, no measurement that would allow recommendation for dose adjustment in such patients. Patients with combined abnormalities of transaminase and alkaline phosphatase should, in general, not be treated with TAXOTERE.

Clearance of docetaxel in combination therapy with cisplatin was similar to that previously observed following monotherapy with docetaxel. The pharmacokinetic profile of cisplatin in combination therapy with docetaxel was similar to that observed with cisplatin alone.

A population pharmacokinetic analysis of plasma data from 40 patients with hormone-refractory metastatic prostate cancer indicated that docetaxel systemic clearance in combination with prednisone is similar to that observed following administration of docetaxel alone.

A study was conducted in 30 patients with advanced breast cancer to determine the potential for drug-drug interactions between docetaxel (75 mg/m^2), doxorubicin (50 mg/m^2), and cyclophosphamide (500 mg/m^2) when administered in combination. The coadministration of docetaxel had no effect on the pharmacokinetics of doxorubicin and cyclophosphamide when the three drugs were given in combination compared to coadministration of doxorubicin and cyclophosphamide only. In addition, doxorubicin and cyclophosphamide had no effect on docetaxel plasma clearance when the three drugs were given in combination compared to historical data for docetaxel monotherapy.

In vitro studies showed that docetaxel is about 94% protein bound, mainly to α_1-acid glycoprotein, albumin, and lipoproteins. In three cancer patients, the *in vitro* binding to plasma proteins was found to be approximately 97%. Dexamethasone does not affect the protein binding of docetaxel.

In vitro drug interaction studies revealed that docetaxel is metabolized by the CYP3A4 isoenzyme, and its metabolism can be inhibited by CYP3A4 inhibitors, such as ketoconazole, erythromycin, troleandomycin, and nifedipine. Based on *in vitro* findings, it is likely that CYP3A4 inhibitors and/or substrates may lead to substantial increases in docetaxel blood concentrations. No clinical studies have been performed to evaluate this finding (see **PRECAUTIONS**).

CLINICAL STUDIES
Breast Cancer
The efficacy and safety of TAXOTERE have been evaluated in locally advanced or metastatic breast cancer after failure of previous chemotherapy (alkylating agent-containing regimens or anthracycline-containing regimens).

Randomized Trials

In one randomized trial, patients with a history of prior treatment with an anthracycline-containing regimen were assigned to treatment with TAXOTERE (100 mg/m^2 every 3 weeks) or the combination of mitomycin (12 mg/m^2 every 6 weeks) and vinblastine (6 mg/m^2 every 3 weeks). 203 patients were randomized to TAXOTERE and 189 to the comparator arm. Most patients had received prior chemotherapy for metastatic disease; only 27 patients on the TAXOTERE arm and 33 patients on the comparator arm entered the study following relapse after adjuvant therapy. Three-quarters of patients had measurable, visceral metastases. The primary endpoint was time to progression. The following table summarizes the study results:

[See first table above]

In a second randomized trial, patients previously treated with an alkylating-containing regimen were assigned to treatment with TAXOTERE (100 mg/m^2) or doxorubicin (75 mg/m^2) every 3 weeks. 161 patients were randomized to TAXOTERE and 165 patients to doxorubicin. Approximately one-half of patients had received prior chemotherapy for metastatic disease, and one-half entered the study following relapse after adjuvant therapy. Three-quarters of patients had measurable, visceral metastases. The primary endpoint was time to progression. The study results are summarized below:

[See second table above]

In another multicenter open-label, randomized trial (TAX313), in the treatment of patients with advanced breast cancer who progressed or relapsed after one prior chemotherapy regimen, 527 patients were randomized to receive TAXOTERE monotherapy 60 mg/m^2 (n=151), 75 mg/m^2 (n=188) or 100 mg/m^2 (n=188). In this trial, 94% of patients had metastatic disease and 79% had received prior anthracycline therapy. Response rate was the primary endpoint. Response rates increased with TAXOTERE dose: 19.9% for the 60 mg/m^2 group compared to 22.3% for the 75 mg/m^2 and 29.8% for the 100 mg/m^2 group; pair-wise comparison between the 60 mg/m^2 and 100 mg/m^2 groups was statistically significant, (p=0.037).

Single Arm Studies

TAXOTERE at a dose of 100 mg/m^2 was studied in six single arm studies involving a total of 309 patients with metastatic breast cancer in whom previous chemotherapy had failed. Among these, 190 patients had anthracycline-resistant breast cancer, defined as progression during an anthracycline-containing chemotherapy regimen for metastatic disease, or relapse during an anthracycline-containing ad-

Efficacy of TAXOTERE in the Treatment of Breast Cancer Patients Previously Treated with an Anthracycline-Containing Regimen (Intent-to-Treat Analysis)

Efficacy Parameter	Docetaxel (n=203)	Mitomycin/ Vinblastine (n=189)	p-value
Median Survival	11.4 months	8.7 months	
Risk Ratio*, Mortality (Docetaxel: Control)	.73		p=0.01 Log Rank
95% CI (Risk Ratio)	0.58-0.93		
Median Time to Progression	4.3 months	2.5 months	
Risk Ratio*, Progression (Docetaxel: Control)	0.75		p=0.01 Log Rank
95% CI (Risk Ratio)	0.61-0.94		
Overall Response Rate	28.1%	9.5%	p<0.0001
Complete Response Rate	3.4%	1.6%	Chi Square

*For the risk ratio, a value less than 1.00 favors docetaxel.

Efficacy of TAXOTERE in the Treatment of Breast Cancer Patients Previously Treated with an Alkylating-Containing Regimen (Intent-to-Treat Analysis)

Efficacy Parameter	Docetaxel (n=161)	Doxorubicin (n=165)	p-value
Median Survival	14.7 months	14.3 months	
Risk Ratio*, Mortality (Docetaxel: Control)	0.89		p=0.39 Log Rank
95% CI (Risk Ratio)	0.68-1.16		
Median Time to Progression	6.5 months	5.3 months	
Risk Ratio*, Progression (Docetaxel: Control)	0.93		p=0.45 Log Rank
95% CI (Risk Ratio)	0.71-1.16		
Overall Response Rate	45.3%	29.7%	p=0.004
Complete Response Rate	6.8%	4.2%	Chi Square

*For the risk ratio, a value less than 1.00 favors docetaxel.

Subset Analyses-Adjuvant Breast Cancer Study

Patient subset	Number of patients	Disease Free Survival		Overall Survival	
		Hazard ratio*	95% CI	Hazard ratio*	95% CI
No. of positive nodes					
Overall	744	0.74	(0.60, 0.92)	0.69	(0.53, 0.90)
1-3	467	0.64	(0.47, 0.87)	0.45	(0.29, 0.70)
4+	277	0.84	(0.63, 1.12)	0.93	(0.66, 1.32)
Receptor status					
Positive	566	0.76	(0.59, 0.98)	0.69	(0.48, 0.99)
Negative	178	0.68	(0.48, 0.97)	0.66	(0.44, 0.98)

*a hazard ratio of less than 1 indicates that TAC is associated with a longer disease free survival or overall survival compared to FAC.

juvant regimen. In anthracycline-resistant patients, the overall response rate was 37.9% (72/190; 95% C.I.: 31.0–44.8) and the complete response rate was 2.1%.

TAXOTERE was also studied in three single arm Japanese studies at a dose of 60 mg/m^2, in 174 patients who had received prior chemotherapy for locally advanced or metastatic breast cancer. Among 26 patients whose best response to an anthracycline had been progression, the response rate was 34.6% (95% C.I.: 17.2-55.7), similar to the response rate in single arm studies of 100 mg/m^2.

Adjuvant Treatment of Breast Cancer
A multicenter, open-label, randomized trial (TAX316) evaluated the efficacy and safety of TAXOTERE for the adjuvant treatment of patients with axillary-node-positive breast cancer and no evidence of distant metastatic disease. After stratification according to the number of positive lymph nodes (1-3, 4+), 1491 patients were randomized to receive either TAXOTERE 75 mg/m^2 administered 1-hour after doxorubicin 50 mg/m^2 and cyclophosphamide 500 mg/m^2 (TAC arm), or doxorubicin 50 mg/m^2 followed by fluorouracil 500 mg/m^2 and cyclosphosphamide 500 mg/m^2 (FAC arm). Both regimens were administered every 3 weeks for 6 cycles. TAXOTERE was administered as a 1-hour infusion; all other drugs were given as IV bolus on day 1. In both arms, after the last cycle of chemotherapy, patients with positive estrogen and/or progesterone receptors received tamoxifen 20 mg daily for up to 5 years. Adjuvant radiation therapy was prescribed according to guidelines in place at

participating institutions and was given to 69% of patients who received TAC and 72% of patients who received FAC. Results from a second interim analysis (median follow-up 55 months) are as follows: In study TAX 316, the docetaxel-containing combination regimen TAC showed significantly longer disease-free survival (DFS) than FAC (hazard ratio=0.74; 2-sided 95% CI=0.60, 0.92, stratified log rank p=0.0047). The primary endpoint, disease-free survival, included local and distant recurrences, contralateral breast cancer and deaths from any cause. The overall reduction in risk of relapse was 25.7% for TAC-treated patients. (See Figure 1).

At the time of this interim analysis, based on 219 deaths, overall survival was longer for TAC than FAC (hazard ratio=0.69, 2-sided 95% CI=0.53, 0.90). (See Figure 2). There will be further analysis at the time survival data mature.

[See figure 1 in next column]
[See figure 2 in next column]
The following table describes the results of subgroup analyses for DFS and OS.
[See third table above]

Non-Small Cell Lung Cancer (NSCLC)
The efficacy and safety of TAXOTERE has been evaluated in patients with unresectable, locally advanced or metastatic non-small cell lung cancer whose disease has failed prior platinum-based chemotherapy or in patients who are chemotherapy-naïve.

Monotherapy with TAXOTERE for NSCLC Previously Treated with Platinum-Based Chemotherapy

Efficacy of TAXOTERE in the Treatment of Non-Small Cell Lung Cancer Patients Previously Treated with a Platinum-Based Chemotherapy Regimen (Intent-to-Treat Analysis)

	TAX317		TAX320	
	Docetaxel 75 mg/m² n=55	Best Supportive Care/75 n=49	Docetaxel 75 mg/m² n=125	Control (V/I) n=123
Overall Survival Log-rank Test	p=0.01		p=0.13	
Risk Ratio[††], Mortality (Docetaxel: Control) 95% CI (Risk Ratio)	0.56 (0.35, 0.88)		0.82 (0.63, 1.06)	
Median Survival 95% CI	7.5 months* (5.5, 12.8)	4.6 months (3.7, 6.1)	5.7 months (5.1, 7.1)	5.6 months (4.4, 7.9)
% 1-year Survival 95% CI	37%*[†] (24, 50)	12% (2, 23)	30%*[†] (22, 39)	20% (13, 27)
Time to Progression 95% CI	12.3 weeks* (9.0, 18.3)	7.0 weeks (6.0, 9.3)	8.3 weeks (7.0, 11.7)	7.6 weeks (6.7, 10.1)
Response Rate 95% CI	5.5% (1.1, 15.1)	Not Applicable	5.7% (2.3, 11.3)	0.8% (0.0, 4.5)

* $p \leq 0.05$; [†] uncorrected for multiple comparisons; [††] a value less than 1.00 favors docetaxel.

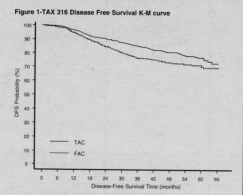

Figure 1-TAX 316 Disease Free Survival K-M curve

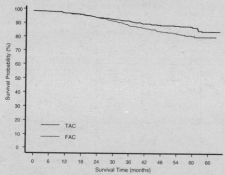

Figure 2-TAX 316 Overall Survival K-M Curve

Two randomized, controlled trials established that a TAXOTERE dose of 75 mg/m² was tolerable and yielded a favorable outcome in patients previously treated with platinum-based chemotherapy (see below). TAXOTERE at a dose of 100 mg/m², however, was associated with unacceptable hematologic toxicity, infections, and treatment-related mortality and this dose should not be used (see **BOXED WARNING, WARNINGS,** and **DOSAGE AND ADMINISTRATION** sections).

One trial (TAX317), randomized patients with locally advanced or metastatic non-small cell lung cancer, a history of prior platinum-based chemotherapy, no history of taxane exposure, and an ECOG performance status ≤2 to TAXOTERE or best supportive care. The primary endpoint of the study was survival. Patients were initially randomized to TAXOTERE 100 mg/m² or best supportive care, but early toxic deaths at this dose led to a dose reduction to TAXOTERE 75 mg/m². A total of 104 patients were randomized in this amended study to either TAXOTERE 75 mg/m² or best supportive care.

In a second randomized trial (TAX320), 373 patients with locally advanced or metastatic non-small cell lung cancer, a history of prior platinum-based chemotherapy, and an ECOG performance status ≤2 were randomized to TAXOTERE 75 mg/m², TAXOTERE 100 mg/m² and a treatment in which the investigator chose either vinorelbine 30 mg/m² days 1, 8, and 15 repeated every 3 weeks **or** ifosfamide 2 g/m² days 1-3 repeated every 3 weeks. Forty percent of the patients in this study had a history of prior paclitaxel exposure. The primary endpoint was survival in both trials. The efficacy data for the TAXOTERE 75 mg/m² arm and the comparator arms are summarized in the table below and in figures 3 and 4 showing the survival curves for the two studies.
[See table above]

Only one of the two trials (TAX317) showed a clear effect on survival, the primary endpoint; that trial also showed an increased rate of survival to one year. In the second study (TAX320) the rate of survival at one year favored TAXOTERE 75 mg/m².

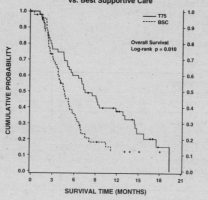

Figure 3: TAX317 Survival K-M Curves - TAXOTERE 75 mg/m² vs. Best Supportive Care

Patients treated with TAXOTERE at a dose of 75 mg/m² experienced no deterioration in performance status and body weight relative to the comparator arms used in these trials.
Combination Therapy with TAXOTERE for Chemotherapy-Naïve NSCLC
In a randomized controlled trial (TAX326), 1218 patients with unresectable stage IIIB or IV NSCLC and no prior chemotherapy were randomized to receive one of three treatments: TAXOTERE 75 mg/m² as a 1 hour infusion immediately followed by cisplatin 75 mg/m² over 30-60 minutes every 3 weeks; vinorelbine 25 mg/m² administered over 6-10 minutes on days 1, 8, 15, 22 followed by cisplatin 100 mg/m² administered on day 1 of cycles repeated every 4 weeks; or a combination of TAXOTERE and carboplatin. The primary efficacy endpoint was overall survival. Treatment with TAXOTERE+cisplatin did not result in a statistically significantly superior survival compared to

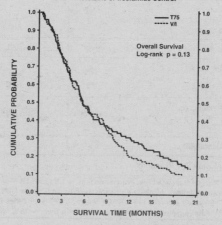

Figure 4: TAX320 Survival K-M Curves - TAXOTERE 75 mg/m² vs. Vinorelbine or Ifosfamide Control

vinorelbine+cisplatin (see table below). The 95% confidence interval of the hazard ratio (adjusted for interim analysis and multiple comparisons) shows that the addition of TAXOTERE to cisplatin results in an outcome ranging from a 6% inferior to a 26% superior survival compared to the addition of vinorelbine to cisplatin. The results of a further statistical analysis showed that at least (the lower bound of the 95% confidence interval) 62% of the known survival effect of vinorelbine when added to cisplatin (about a 2-month increase in median survival; Wozniak et al. JCO, 1998) was maintained. The efficacy data for the TAXOTERE+cisplatin arm and the comparator arm are summarized in the table below.

Survival Analysis of TAXOTERE in Combination Therapy for Chemotherapy-Naïve NSCLC

Comparison	Taxotere +Cisplatin n=408	Vinorelbine +Cisplatin n=405
Kaplan-Meier Estimate of Median Survival	10.9 months	10.0 months
p-value[a]	0.122	
Estimated Hazard Ratio[b]	0.88	
Adjusted 95% CI[c]	(0.74, 1.06)	

[a]From the superiority test (stratified log rank) comparing TAXOTERE+cisplatin to vinorelbine+cisplatin
[b]Hazard ratio of TAXOTERE+cisplatin vs. vinorelbine+cisplatin. A hazard ratio of less than 1 indicates that TAXOTERE+cisplatin is associated with a longer survival.
[c]Adjusted for interim analysis and multiple comparisons.

The second comparison in the study, vinorelbine+cisplatin versus TAXOTERE+carboplatin, did not demonstrate superior survival associated with the TAXOTERE arm (Kaplan-Meier estimate of median survival was 9.1 months for TAXOTERE+carboplatin compared to 10.0 months on the vinorelbine+cisplatin arm) and the TAXOTERE+carboplatin arm did not demonstrate preservation of at least 50% of the survival effect of vinorelbine added to cisplatin. Secondary endpoints evaluated in the trial included objective response and time to progression. There was no statistically significant difference between TAXOTERE+cisplatin and vinorelbine+cisplatin with respect to objective response and time to progression (see table below).

Response and TTP Analysis of TAXOTERE in Combination Therapy for Chemotherapy-Naïve NSCLC

Endpoint	TAXOTERE +Cisplatin	Vinorelbine +Cisplatin	p-value
Objective Response Rate (95% CI)[a]	31.6% (26.5%, 36.8%)	24.4% (19.8%, 29.2%)	Not Significant
Median Time to Progression[b] (95% CI)[a]	21.4 weeks (19.3, 24.6)	22.1 weeks (18.1, 25.6)	Not Significant

[a]Adjusted for multiple comparisons.
[b]Kaplan-Meier estimates.

Prostate Cancer
The safety and efficacy of TAXOTERE in combination with prednisone in patients with androgen independent (hormone refractory) metastatic prostate cancer were evaluated in a randomized multicenter active control trial. A total of 1006 patients with Karnofsky Performance Status (KPS) ≥60 were randomized to the following treatment groups:
• TAXOTERE 75 mg/m² every 3 weeks for 10 cycles.
• TAXOTERE 30 mg/m² administered weekly for the first 5 weeks in a 6-week cycle for 5 cycles.
• Mitoxantrone 12 mg/m² every 3 weeks for 10 cycles.
All 3 regimens were administered in combination with prednisone 5 mg twice daily, continuously.
In the TAXOTERE every three week arm, a statistically significant overall survival advantage was demonstrated compared to mitoxantrone. In the TAXOTERE weekly arm, no overall survival advantage was demonstrated compared to the mitoxantrone control arm. Efficacy results for the TAXOTERE every 3 week arm versus the control arm are summarized in the following table and figure 5:

Efficacy of TAXOTERE in the Treatment of Patients with Androgen Independent (Hormone Refractory) Metastatic Prostate Cancer (Intent-to-Treat Analysis)

	TAXOTERE every 3 weeks	Mitoxantrone every 3 weeks
Number of patients	335	337
Median survival (months)	18.9	16.5

Continued on next page

Taxotere—Cont.

95% CI	(17.0-21.2)	(14.4-18.6)
Hazard ratio	0.761	–
95% CI	(0.619-0.936)	–
p-value*	0.0094	–

*Stratified log rank test. Threshold for statistical significance = 0.0175 because of 3 arms.

Figure 5 - TAX327 Survival K-M Curves

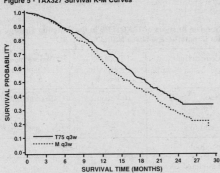

INDICATIONS AND USAGE

Breast Cancer

TAXOTERE is indicated for the treatment of patients with locally advanced or metastatic breast cancer after failure of prior chemotherapy.

TAXOTERE in combination with doxorubicin and cyclophosphamide is indicated for the adjuvant treatment of patients with operable node-positive breast cancer.

Non-Small Cell Lung Cancer

TAXOTERE as a single agent is indicated for the treatment of patients with locally advanced or metastatic non-small cell lung cancer after failure of prior platinum-based chemotherapy.

TAXOTERE in combination with cisplatin is indicated for the treatment of patients with unresectable, locally advanced or metastatic non-small cell lung cancer who have not previously received chemotherapy for this condition.

Prostate Cancer

TAXOTERE in combination with prednisone is indicated for the treatment of patients with androgen independent (hormone refractory) metastatic prostate cancer.

CONTRAINDICATIONS

TAXOTERE is contraindicated in patients who have a history of severe hypersensitivity reactions to docetaxel or to other drugs formulated with polysorbate 80.

TAXOTERE should not be used in patients with neutrophil counts of <1500 cells/mm³.

WARNINGS

TAXOTERE should be administered under the supervision of a qualified physician experienced in the use of antineoplastic agents. Appropriate management of complications is possible only when adequate diagnostic and treatment facilities are readily available.

Toxic Deaths

Breast Cancer

TAXOTERE administered at 100 mg/m² was associated with deaths considered possibly or probably related to treatment in 2.0% (19/965) of metastatic breast cancer patients, both previously treated and untreated, with normal baseline liver function and in 11.5% (7/61) of patients with various tumor types who had abnormal baseline liver function (SGOT and/or SGPT > 1.5 times ULN together with AP > 2.5 times ULN). Among patients dosed at 60 mg/m², mortality related to treatment occurred in 0.6% (3/481) of patients with normal liver function, and in 3 of 7 patients with abnormal liver function. Approximately half of these deaths occurred during the first cycle. Sepsis accounted for the majority of the deaths.

Non-Small Cell Lung Cancer

TAXOTERE administered at a dose of 100 mg/m² in patients with locally advanced or metastatic non-small cell lung cancer who had a history of prior platinum-based chemotherapy was associated with increased treatment-related mortality (14% and 5% in two randomized, controlled studies). There were 2.8% treatment-related deaths among the 176 patients treated at the 75 mg/m² dose in the randomized trials. Among patients who experienced treatment-related mortality at the 75 mg/m² dose level, 3 of 5 patients had a PS of 2 at study entry (see **BOXED WARNING, CLINICAL STUDIES**, and **DOSAGE AND ADMINISTRATION** sections).

Premedication Regimen

All patients should be premedicated with oral corticosteroids (see below for prostate cancer) such as dexamethasone 16 mg per day (e.g., 8 mg BID) for 3 days starting 1 day prior to TAXOTERE to reduce the severity of fluid retention and hypersensitivity reactions (see **DOSAGE AND ADMINISTRATION** section). This regimen was evaluated in 92 patients with metastatic breast cancer previously treated with chemotherapy given TAXOTERE at a dose of 100 mg/m² every 3 weeks.

The pretreatment regimen for hormone-refractory metastatic prostate cancer is oral dexamethasone 8 mg, at 12 hours, 3 hours and 1 hour before the TAXOTERE infusion (see **DOSAGE AND ADMINISTRATION** section).

Summary of Adverse Events in Patients Receiving TAXOTERE at 100 mg/m²

Adverse Event	All Tumor Types Normal LFTs* n=2045 %	All Tumor Types Elevated LFTs** n=61 %	Breast Cancer Normal LFTs* n=965 %
Hematologic			
Neutropenia			
<2000 cells/mm³	95.5	96.4	98.5
<500 cells/mm³	75.4	87.5	85.9
Leukopenia			
<4000 cells/mm³	95.6	98.3	98.6
<1000 cells/mm³	31.6	46.6	43.7
Thrombocytopenia			
<100,000 cells/mm³	8.0	24.6	9.2
Anemia			
<11 g/dL	90.4	91.8	93.6
<8 g/dL	8.8	31.1	7.7
Febrile Neutropenia***	11.0	26.2	12.3
Septic Death	1.6	4.9	1.4
Non-Septic Death	0.6	6.6	0.6
Infections			
Any	21.6	32.8	22.2
Severe	6.1	16.4	6.4
Fever in Absence of Infection			
Any	31.2	41.0	35.1
Severe	2.1	8.2	2.2
Hypersensitivity Reactions			
Regardless of Premedication			
Any	21.0	19.7	17.6
Severe	4.2	9.8	2.6
With 3-day Premedication	n=92	n=3	n=92
Any	15.2	33.3	15.2
Severe	2.2	0	2.2
Fluid Retention			
Regardless of Premedication			
Any	47.0	39.3	59.7
Severe	6.9	8.2	8.9
With 3-day Premedication	n=92	n=3	n=92
Any	64.1	66.7	64.1
Severe	6.5	33.3	6.5
Neurosensory			
Any	49.3	34.4	58.3
Severe	4.3	0	5.5
Cutaneous			
Any	47.6	54.1	47.0
Severe	4.8	9.8	5.2
Nail Changes			
Any	30.6	23.0	40.5
Severe	2.5	4.9	3.7
Gastrointestinal			
Nausea	38.8	37.7	42.1
Vomiting	22.3	23.0	23.4
Diarrhea	38.7	32.8	42.6
Severe	4.7	4.9	5.5
Stomatitis			
Any	41.7	49.2	51.7
Severe	5.5	13.0	7.4
Alopecia	75.8	62.3	74.2
Asthenia			
Any	61.8	52.5	66.3
Severe	12.8	24.6	14.9
Myalgia			
Any	18.9	16.4	21.1
Severe	1.5	1.6	1.8
Arthralgia	9.2	6.6	8.2
Infusion Site Reactions	4.4	3.3	4.0

*Normal Baseline LFTs: Transaminases ≤ 1.5 times ULN or alkaline phosphatase ≤ 2.5 times ULN or isolated elevations of transaminases or alkaline phosphatase up to 5 times ULN
**Elevated Baseline LFTs: SGOT and/or SGPT >1.5 times ULN concurrent with alkaline phosphatase >2.5 times ULN
***Febrile Neutropenia: ANC grade 4 with fever > 38°C with IV antibiotics and/or hospitalization

Hypersensitivity Reactions

Patients should be observed closely for hypersensitivity reactions, especially during the first and second infusions. Severe hypersensitivity reactions characterized by hypotension and/or bronchospasm, or generalized rash/erythema occurred in 2.2% of the 92 patients premedicated with 3-day corticosteroids. Hypersensitivity reactions requiring discontinuation of the TAXOTERE infusion were reported in 5 out of 1260 patients with various tumor types who did not receive premedication, but in 0/92 patients premedicated with 3-day corticosteroids. Patients with a history of severe hypersensitivity reactions should not be rechallenged with TAXOTERE.

Hematologic Effects

Neutropenia (< 2000 neutrophils/mm³) occurs in virtually all patients given 60-100 mg/m² of TAXOTERE and grade 4 neutropenia (<500 cells/mm³) occurs in 85% of patients given 100 mg/m² and 75% of patients given 60 mg/m². Fre-

quent monitoring of blood counts is, therefore, essential so that dose can be adjusted. TAXOTERE should not be administered to patients with neutrophils < 1500 cells/mm³. Febrile neutropenia occurred in about 12% of patients given 100 mg/m² but was very uncommon in patients given 60 mg/m². Hematologic responses, febrile reactions and infections, and rates of septic death for different regimens are dose related and are described in **CLINICAL STUDIES**.

Three breast cancer patients with severe liver impairment (bilirubin > 1.7 times ULN) developed fatal gastrointestinal bleeding associated with severe drug-induced thrombocytopenia.

Hepatic Impairment
(see **BOXED WARNING**).

Fluid Retention
(see **BOXED WARNING**).

Acute Myeloid Leukemia

Treatment-related acute myeloid leukemia (AML) has occurred in patients given anthracyclines and/or cyclophosphamide, including use in adjuvant therapy for breast cancer. In the adjuvant breast cancer trial (TAX316, see CLINICAL STUDIES) AML occurred in 3 of 744 patients who received TAXOTERE, doxorubicin and cyclophosphamide and in 1 of 736 patients who received fluorouracil, doxorubicin and cyclophosphamide (see ADVERSE REACTIONS).

Pregnancy

TAXOTERE can cause fetal harm when administered to pregnant women. Studies in both rats and rabbits at doses ≥ 0.3 and 0.03 mg/kg/day, respectively (about 1/50 and 1/300 the daily maximum recommended human dose on a mg/m^2 basis), administered during the period of organogenesis, have shown that TAXOTERE is embryotoxic and fetotoxic (characterized by intrauterine mortality, increased resorption, reduced fetal weight, and fetal ossification delay). The doses indicated above also caused maternal toxicity.

There are no adequate and well-controlled studies in pregnant women using TAXOTERE. If TAXOTERE is used during pregnancy, or if the patient becomes pregnant while receiving this drug, the patient should be apprised of the potential hazard to the fetus or potential risk for loss of the pregnancy. Women of childbearing potential should be advised to avoid becoming pregnant during therapy with TAXOTERE.

PRECAUTIONS

General

Responding patients may not experience an improvement in performance status on therapy and may experience worsening. The relationship between changes in performance status, response to therapy, and treatment-related side effects has not been established.

Hematologic Effects

In order to monitor the occurrence of myelotoxicity, it is recommended that frequent peripheral blood cell counts be performed on all patients receiving TAXOTERE. Patients should not be retreated with subsequent cycles of TAXOTERE until neutrophils recover to a level > 1500 cells/mm^3 and platelets recover to a level > 100,000 cells/mm^3. A 25% reduction in the dose of TAXOTERE is recommended during subsequent cycles following severe neutropenia (<500 cells/mm^3) lasting 7 days or more, febrile neutropenia, or a grade 4 infection in a TAXOTERE cycle (see DOSAGE AND ADMINISTRATION section).

Hypersensitivity Reactions

Hypersensitivity reactions may occur within a few minutes following initiation of a TAXOTERE infusion. If minor reactions such as flushing or localized skin reactions occur, interruption of therapy is not required. More severe reactions, however, require the immediate discontinuation of TAXOTERE and aggressive therapy. All patients should be premedicated with an oral corticosteroid prior to the initiation of the infusion of TAXOTERE (see BOXED WARNING and WARNINGS: Premedication Regimen).

Cutaneous

Localized erythema of the extremities with edema followed by desquamation has been observed. In case of severe skin toxicity, an adjustment in dosage is recommended (see DOSAGE AND ADMINISTRATION section). The discontinuation rate due to skin toxicity was 1.6% (15/965) for metastatic breast cancer patients. Among 92 breast cancer patients premedicated with 3-day corticosteroids, there were no cases of severe skin toxicity reported and no patient discontinued TAXOTERE due to skin toxicity.

Fluid Retention

Severe fluid retention has been reported following TAXOTERE therapy (see BOXED WARNING and WARNINGS: Premedication Regimen). Patients should be premedicated with oral corticosteroids prior to each TAXOTERE administration to reduce the incidence and severity of fluid retention (see DOSAGE AND ADMINISTRATION section). Patients with pre-existing effusions should be closely monitored from the first dose for the possible exacerbation of the effusions.

When fluid retention occurs, peripheral edema usually starts in the lower extremities and may become generalized with a median weight gain of 2 kg.

Among 92 breast cancer patients premedicated with 3-day corticosteroids, moderate fluid retention occurred in 27.2% and severe fluid retention in 6.5%. The median cumulative dose to onset of moderate or severe fluid retention was 819 mg/m^2. 9.8% (9/92) of patients discontinued treatment due to fluid retention: 4 patients discontinued with severe fluid retention; the remaining 5 had mild or moderate fluid retention. The median cumulative dose to treatment discontinuation due to fluid retention was 1021 mg/m^2. Fluid retention was completely, but sometimes slowly, reversible with a median of 16 weeks from the last infusion of TAXOTERE to resolution (range: 0 to 42+ weeks). Patients developing peripheral edema may be treated with standard measures, e.g., salt restriction, oral diuretic(s).

Neurologic

Severe neurosensory symptoms (paresthesia, dysesthesia, pain) were observed in 5.5% (53/965) of metastatic breast cancer patients, and resulted in treatment discontinuation in 6.1%. When these symptoms occur, dosage must be adjusted. If symptoms persist, treatment should be discontinued (see DOSAGE AND ADMINISTRATION section). Patients who experienced neurotoxicity in clinical trials and for whom follow-up information on the complete resolution of the event was available had spontaneous reversal of symptoms with a median of 9 weeks from onset (range: 0 to 106 weeks). Severe peripheral motor neuropathy mainly manifested as distal extremity weakness occurred in 4.4% (42/965).

Hematologic Adverse Events in Breast Cancer Patients Previously Treated with Chemotherapy Treated at TAXOTERE 100 mg/m² with Normal or Elevated Liver Function Tests or 60 mg/m² with Normal Liver Function Tests

Adverse Event		TAXOTERE 100 mg/m²		TAXOTERE 60 mg/m²
		Normal LFTs* n=730 %	Elevated LFTs** n=18 %	Normal LFTs* n=174 %
Neutropenia				
Any	<2000 cells/mm³	98.4	100	95.4
Grade 4	<500 cells/mm³	84.4	93.8	74.9
Thrombocytopenia				
Any	<100,000 cells/mm³	10.8	44.4	14.4
Grade 4	<20,000 cells/mm³	0.6	16.7	1.1
Anemia <11 g/dL		94.6	94.4	64.9
Infection*				
Any		22.5	38.9	1.1
Grade 3 and 4		7.1	33.3	0
Febrile Neutropenia**				
By Patient		11.8	33.3	0
By Course		2.4	8.6	0
Septic Death		1.5	5.6	1.1
Non-Septic Death		1.1	11.1	0

*Normal Baseline LFTs: Transaminases ≤ 1.5 times ULN or alkaline phosphatase ≤ 2.5 times ULN or isolated elevations of transaminases or alkaline phosphatase up to 5 times ULN
**Elevated Baseline LFTs: SGOT and/or SGPT >1.5 times ULN concurrent with alkaline phosphatase >2.5 times ULN
***Incidence of infection requiring hospitalization and/or intravenous antibiotics was 8.5% (n=62) among the 730 patients with normal LFTs at baseline; 7 patients had concurrent grade 3 neutropenia, and 46 patients had grade 4 neutropenia.
****Febrile Neutropenia: For 100 mg/m², ANC grade 4 and fever > 38°C with IV antibiotics and/or hospitalization; for 60 mg/m², ANC grade 3/4 and fever > 38.1°C

Non-Hematologic Adverse Events in Breast Cancer Patients Previously Treated with Chemotherapy Treated at TAXOTERE 100 mg/m² with Normal or Elevated Liver Function Tests or 60 mg/m² with Normal Liver Function Tests

Adverse Event	TAXOTERE 100 mg/m²		TAXOTERE 60 mg/m²
	Normal LFTs* n=730 %	Elevated LFTs** n=18 %	Normal LFTs* n=174 %
Acute Hypersensitivity Reaction Regardless of Premedication			
Any	13.0	5.6	0.6
Severe	1.2	0	0
Fluid Retention* Regardless of Premedication**			
Any	56.2	61.1	12.6
Severe	7.9	16.7	0
Neurosensory			
Any	56.8	50	19.5
Severe	5.8	0	0
Myalgia	22.7	33.3	3.4
Cutaneous			
Any	44.8	61.1	30.5
Severe	4.8	16.7	0
Asthenia			
Any	65.2	44.4	65.5
Severe	16.6	22.2	0
Diarrhea			
Any	42.2	27.8	NA
Severe	6.3	11.1	
Stomatitis			
Any	53.3	66.7	19.0
Severe	7.8	38.9	0.6

*Normal Baseline LFTs: Transaminases ≤ 1.5 times ULN or alkaline phosphatase ≤ 2.5 times ULN or isolated elevations of transaminases or alkaline phosphatase up to 5 times ULN
** Elevated Baseline Liver Function: SGOT and/or SGPT >1.5 times ULN concurrent with alkaline phosphatase >2.5 times ULN
***Fluid Retention includes (by COSTART): edema (peripheral, localized, generalized, lymphedema, pulmonary edema, and edema otherwise not specified) and effusion (pleural, pericardial, and ascites); no premedication given with the 60 mg/m² dose
NA = not available

Asthenia

Severe asthenia has been reported in 14.9% (144/965) of metastatic breast cancer patients but has led to treatment discontinuation in only 1.8%. Symptoms of fatigue and weakness may last a few days up to several weeks and may be associated with deterioration of performance status in patients with progressive disease.

Information for Patients

For additional information, see the accompanying Patient Information Leaflet.

Drug Interactions

There have been no formal clinical studies to evaluate the drug interactions of TAXOTERE with other medications. In vitro studies have shown that the metabolism of docetaxel may be modified by the concomitant administration of compounds that induce, inhibit, or are metabolized by cytochrome P450 3A4, such as cyclosporine, terfenadine, ketoconazole, erythromycin, and troleandomycin. Caution

Continued on next page

Taxotere—Cont.

should be exercised with these drugs when treating patients receiving TAXOTERE as there is a potential for a significant interaction.

Carcinogenicity, Mutagenicity, Impairment of Fertility

No studies have been conducted to assess the carcinogenic potential of TAXOTERE. TAXOTERE has been shown to be clastogenic in the *in vitro* chromosome aberration test in CHO-K$_1$ cells and in the *in vivo* micronucleus test in the mouse, but it did not induce mutagenicity in the Ames test or the CHO/HGPRT gene mutation assays. TAXOTERE produced no impairment of fertility in rats when administered in multiple IV doses of up to 0.3 mg/kg (about 1/50 the recommended human dose on a mg/m^2 basis), but decreased testicular weights were reported. This correlates with findings of a 10-cycle toxicity study (dosing once every 21 days for 6 months) in rats and dogs in which testicular atrophy or degeneration was observed at IV doses of 5 mg/kg in rats and 0.375 mg/kg in dogs (about 1/3 and 1/15 the recommended human dose on a mg/m^2 basis, respectively). An increased frequency of dosing in rats produced similar effects at lower dose levels.

Pregnancy

Pregnancy Category D (see **WARNINGS** section).

Nursing Mothers

It is not known whether TAXOTERE is excreted in human milk. Because many drugs are excreted in human milk, and because of the potential for serious adverse reactions in nursing infants from TAXOTERE, mothers should discontinue nursing prior to taking the drug.

Pediatric Use

The safety and effectiveness of TAXOTERE in pediatric patients have not been established.

Geriatric Use

In a study conducted in chemotherapy-naïve patients with NSCLC (TAX326), 148 patients (36%) in the TAXOTERE+cisplatin group were 65 years of age or greater. There were 128 patients (32%) in the vinorelbine+cisplatin group 65 years of age or greater. In the TAXOTERE+ cisplatin group, patients less than 65 years of age had a median survival of 10.3 months (95% CI : 9.1 months, 11.8 months) and patients 65 years or older had a median survival of 12.1 months (95% CI : 9.3 months, 14 months). In patients 65 years of age or greater treated with TAXOTERE+cisplatin, diarrhea (55%), peripheral edema (39%) and stomatitis (28%) were observed more frequently than in the vinorelbine+cisplatin group (diarrhea 24%, peripheral edema 20%, stomatitis 20%). Patients treated with TAXOTERE+cisplatin who were 65 years of age or greater were more likely to experience diarrhea (55%), infections (42%), peripheral edema (39%) and stomatitis (28%) compared to patients less than the age of 65 administered the same treatment (43%, 31%, 31% and 21%, respectively).

When TAXOTERE was combined with carboplatin for the treatment of chemotherapy-naïve, advanced non-small cell lung carcinoma, patients 65 years of age or greater (28%) experienced higher frequency of infection compared to similar patients treated with TAXOTERE+cisplatin; and a higher frequency of diarrhea, infection and peripheral edema than elderly patients treated with vinorelbine+ cisplatin.

Of the 333 patients treated with TAXOTERE every three weeks plus prednisone in the prostate cancer study (TAX327), 209 patients were 65 years of age or greater and 68 patients were older than 75 years. In patients treated with TAXOTERE every three weeks, the following TEAEs occurred at rates $\geq$ 10% higher in patients 65 years of age or greater compared to younger patients: anemia (71% vs. 59%), infection (37% vs. 24%), nail changes (34% vs. 23%), anorexia (21% vs. 10%), weight loss (15% vs. 5%) respectively.

In the adjuvant breast cancer trial (TAX316), TAXOTERE in combination with doxorubicin and cyclophosphamide was administered to 744 patients of whom 48 (6%) were 65 years of age or greater. The number of elderly patients who received this regimen was not sufficient to determine whether there were differences in safety and efficacy between elderly and younger patients.

ADVERSE REACTIONS

Adverse reactions are described for TAXOTERE according to indication:

— in the treatment of breast cancer, at the maximum dose of 100 mg/m^2
— in the treatment of advanced breast cancer at doses of 60, 75 and 100 mg/m^2
— in the adjuvant therapy of breast cancer at a dose of 75 mg/m^2, in combination with doxorubicin and cyclophosphamide
— in the treatment of advanced non-small cell lung cancer after prior platinum-based chemotherapy, at a dose of 75 mg/m^2
— in the treatment of non-small cell lung cancer in patients who have not previously received chemotherapy for this condition, at a dose of 75 mg/m^2, in combination with cisplatin
— in the treatment of androgen independent (hormone refractory) metastatic prostate cancer, at a dose of 75 mg/m^2 every three weeks in combination with prednisone

Monotherapy with TAXOTERE for Locally Advanced or Metastatic Breast Cancer After Failure of Prior Chemotherapy

Clinically Important Treatment Emergent Adverse Events Regardless of Causal Relationship in Patients Receiving TAXOTERE in Combination with Doxorubicin and Cyclophosphamide (TAX 316).				
	TAXOTERE 75 mg/m^2+ Doxorubicin 50 mg/m^2+ Cyclophosphamide 500 mg/m^2 (TAC) n=744 %		Fluorouracil 500 mg/m^2+ Doxorubicin 50 mg/m^2+ Cyclophosphamide 500 mg/m^2 (FAC) n=736 %	
Adverse Event	Any	G 3/4	Any	G 3/4
Anemia	91.5	4.3	71.7	1.6
Neutropenia	71.4	65.5	82.0	49.3
Fever in absence of infection	46.5	1.3	17.1	0.0
Infection	39.4	3.9	36.3	2.2
Thrombocytopenia	39.4	2.0	27.7	1.2
Febrile neutropenia	24.7	N/A	2.5	N/A
Neutropenic infection	12.1	N/A	6.3	N/A
Hypersensitivity reactions	13.4	1.3	3.7	0.1
Lymphedema	4.4	0.0	1.2	0.0
Fluid Retention*	35.1	0.9	14.7	0.1
Peripheral edema	26.9	0.4	7.3	0.0
Weight gain	12.9	0.3	8.6	0.3
Neuropathy sensory	25.5	0.0	10.2	0.0
Neuro-cortical	5.1	0.5	6.4	0.7
Neuropathy motor	3.8	0.1	2.2	0.0
Neuro-cerebellar	2.4	0.1	2.0	0.0
Syncope	1.6	0.5	1.2	0.3
Alopecia	97.8	N/A	97.1	N/A
Skin toxicity	26.5	0.8	17.7	0.4
Nail disorders	18.5	0.4	14.4	0.1
Nausea	80.5	5.1	88.0	9.5
Stomatitis	69.4	7.1	52.9	2.0
Vomiting	44.5	4.3	59.2	7.3
Diarrhea	35.2	3.8	27.9	1.8
Constipation	33.9	1.1	31.8	1.4
Taste perversion	27.8	0.7	15.1	0.0
Anorexia	21.6	2.2	17.7	1.2
Abdominal Pain	10.9	0.7	5.3	0.0
Amenorrhea	61.7	N/A	52.4	N/A
Cough	13.7	0.0	9.8	0.1
Cardiac dysrhythmias	7.9	0.3	6.0	0.3
Vasodilatation	27.0	1.1	21.2	0.5
Hypotension	2.6	0.0	1.1	0.1
Phlebitis	1.2	0.0	0.8	0.0
Asthenia	80.8	11.2	71.2	5.6
Myalgia	26.7	0.8	9.9	0.0
Arthralgia	19.4	0.5	9.0	0.3
Lacrimation disorder	11.3	0.1	7.1	0.0
Conjunctivitis	5.1	0.3	6.9	0.1

* COSTART term and grading system for events related to treatment.

TAXOTERE 100 mg/m^2: Adverse drug reactions occurring in at least 5% of patients are compared for three populations who received TAXOTERE administered at 100 mg/m^2 as a 1-hour infusion every 3 weeks: 2045 patients with various tumor types and normal baseline liver function tests; the subset of 965 patients with locally advanced or metastatic breast cancer, both previously treated and untreated with chemotherapy, who had normal baseline liver function tests; and an additional 61 patients with various tumor types who had abnormal liver function tests at baseline. These reactions were described using COSTART terms and were considered possibly or probably related to TAXOTERE. At least 95% of these patients did not receive hematopoietic support. The safety profile is generally similar in patients receiving TAXOTERE for the treatment of breast cancer and in patients with other tumor types.

[See table at top of page 374] .

Hematologic: (see **WARNINGS**).

Reversible marrow suppression was the major dose-limiting toxicity of TAXOTERE. The median time to nadir was 7 days, while the median duration of severe neutropenia (<500 cells/mm^3) was 7 days. Among 2045 patients with solid tumors and normal baseline LFTs, severe neutropenia occurred in 75.4% and lasted for more than 7 days in 2.9% of cycles.

Febrile neutropenia (<500 cells/mm^3 with fever > 38°C with IV antibiotics and/or hospitalization) occurred in 11% of patients with solid tumors, in 12.3% of patients with metastatic breast cancer, and in 9.8% of 92 breast cancer patients premedicated with 3-day corticosteroids.

Severe infectious episodes occurred in 6.1% of patients with solid tumors, in 6.4% of patients with metastatic breast cancer, and in 5.4% of 92 breast cancer patients premedicated with 3-day corticosteroids.

Thrombocytopenia (<100,000 cells/mm^3) associated with fatal gastrointestinal hemorrhage has been reported.

Hypersensitivity Reactions

Severe hypersensitivity reactions are discussed in the **BOXED WARNING, WARNINGS,** and **PRECAUTIONS** sections. Minor events, including flushing, rash with or without pruritus, chest tightness, back pain, dyspnea, drug fever, or chills, have been reported and resolved after discontinuing the infusion and appropriate therapy.

Fluid Retention: (see **BOXED WARNING, WARNINGS: Premedication Regimen,** and **PRECAUTIONS** sections).

Cutaneous

Severe skin toxicity is discussed in **PRECAUTIONS**. Reversible cutaneous reactions characterized by a rash including localized eruptions, mainly on the feet and/or hands, but also on the arms, face, or thorax, usually associated with pruritus, have been observed. Eruptions generally occurred within 1 week after TAXOTERE infusion, recovered before the next infusion, and were not disabling.

Severe nail disorders were characterized by hypo- or hyperpigmentation, and occasionally by onycholysis (in 0.8% of patients with solid tumors) and pain.

Neurologic: (see **PRECAUTIONS**).

Gastrointestinal

Gastrointestinal reactions (nausea and/or vomiting and/or diarrhea) were generally mild to moderate. Severe reactions occurred in 3-5% of patients with solid tumors and to a similar extent among metastatic breast cancer patients. The incidence of severe reactions was 1% or less for the 92 breast cancer patients premedicated with 3-day corticosteroids.

Severe stomatitis occurred in 5.5% of patients with solid tumors, in 7.4% of patients with metastatic breast cancer, and in 1.1% of the 92 breast cancer patients premedicated with 3-day corticosteroids.

Cardiovascular

Hypotension occurred in 2.8% of patients with solid tumors; 1.2% required treatment. Clinically meaningful events such as heart failure, sinus tachycardia, atrial flutter, dysrhythmia, unstable angina, pulmonary edema, and hypertension occurred rarely. 8.1% (7/86) of metastatic breast cancer patients receiving TAXOTERE 100 mg/m^2 in a randomized trial and who had serial left ventricular ejection fractions assessed developed deterioration of LVEF by ≥ 10% associated with a drop below the institutional lower limit of normal.

Infusion Site Reactions

Infusion site reactions were generally mild and consisted of hyperpigmentation, inflammation, redness or dryness of the skin, phlebitis, extravasation, or swelling of the vein.

Hepatic

In patients with normal LFTs at baseline, bilirubin values greater than the ULN occurred in 8.9% of patients. Increases in SGOT or SGPT > 1.5 times the ULN, or alkaline phosphatase > 2.5 times ULN, were observed in 18.9% and 7.3% of patients, respectively. While on TAXOTERE, increases in SGOT and/or SGPT > 1.5 times ULN concomitant with alkaline phosphatase > 2.5 times ULN occurred in 4.3% of patients with normal LFTs at baseline. (Whether these changes were related to the drug or underlying disease has not been established.)

Hematologic and Other Toxicity: Relation to dose and baseline liver chemistry abnormalities.

Hematologic and other toxicity is increased at higher doses and in patients with elevated baseline liver function tests (LFTs). In the following tables, adverse drug reactions are compared for three populations: 730 patients with normal LFTs given TAXOTERE at 100 mg/m^2 in the randomized and single arm studies of metastatic breast cancer after failure of previous chemotherapy; 18 patients in these studies who had abnormal baseline LFTs (defined as SGOT and/or SGPT > 1.5 times ULN concurrent with alkaline phosphatase > 2.5 times ULN); and 174 patients in Japanese studies given TAXOTERE at 60 mg/m^2 who had normal LFTs.

[See first table at top of page 375]

[See second table on page 375]

In the three-arm monotherapy trial, TAX313, which compared TAXOTERE 60, 75 and 100 mg/m^2 in advanced breast cancer, the overall safety profile was consistent with the safety profile observed in previous TAXOTERE trials. Grade 3/4 or severe adverse events occurred in 49.0% of patients treated with TAXOTERE 60 mg/m^2 compared to 55.3% and 65.9% treated with 75 and 100 mg/m^2 respectively. Discontinuation due to adverse events was reported in 5.3% of patients treated with 60 mg/m^2 vs. 6.9% and 16.5% for patients treated at 75 and 100 mg/m^2 respectively. Deaths within 30 days of last treatment occurred in 4.0% of patients treated with 60 mg/m^2 compared to 5.3% and 1.6% for patients treated at 75 and 100 mg/m^2 respectively.

The following adverse events were associated with increasing docetaxel doses: fluid retention (26%, 38%, and 46% at 60, 75, and 100 mg/m^2 respectively), thrombocytopenia (7%, 11% and 12% respectively), neutropenia (92%, 94%, and 97% respectively), febrile neutropenia (5%, 7%, and 14% respectively), treatment-related grade 3/4 infection (2%, 3%, and 7% respectively) and anemia (87%, 94%, and 97% respectively).

Treatment Emergent Adverse Events Regardless of Relationship to Treatment in Patients Receiving TAXOTERE as Monotherapy for Non-Small Cell Lung Cancer Previously Treated with Platinum-Based Chemotherapy*

Adverse Event	TAXOTERE 75 mg/m^2 n=176 %	Best Supportive Care n=49 %	Vinorelbine/ Ifosfamide n=119 %
Neutropenia			
Any	84.1	14.3	83.2
Grade 3/4	65.3	12.2	57.1
Leukopenia			
Any	83.5	6.1	89.1
Grade 3/4	49.4	0	42.9
Thrombocytopenia			
Any	8.0	0	7.6
Grade 3/4	2.8	0	1.7
Anemia			
Any	91.0	55.1	90.8
Grade 3/4	9.1	12.2	14.3
Febrile Neutropenia**	6.3	NA†	0.8
Infection			
Any	33.5	28.6	30.3
Grade 3/4	10.2	6.1	9.2
Treatment Related Mortality	2.8	NA†	3.4
Hypersensitivity Reactions			
Any	5.7	0	0.8
Grade 3/4	2.8	0	0
Fluid Retention			
Any	33.5	ND††	22.7
Severe	2.8		3.4
Neurosensory			
Any	23.3	14.3	28.6
Grade 3/4	1.7	6.1	5.0
Neuromotor			
Any	15.9	8.2	10.1
Grade 3/4	4.5	6.1	3.4
Skin			
Any	19.9	6.1	16.8
Grade 3/4	0.6	2.0	0.8
Gastrointestinal			
Nausea			
Any	33.5	30.6	31.1
Grade 3/4	5.1	4.1	7.6
Vomiting			
Any	21.6	26.5	21.8
Grade 3/4	2.8	2.0	5.9
Diarrhea			
Any	22.7	6.1	11.8
Grade 3/4	2.8	0	4.2
Alopecia	56.3	34.7	49.6
Asthenia			
Any	52.8	57.1	53.8
Severe***	18.2	38.8	22.7
Stomatitis			
Any	26.1	6.1	7.6
Grade 3/4	1.7	0	0.8
Pulmonary			
Any	40.9	49.0	45.4
Grade 3/4	21.0	28.6	18.5
Nail Disorder			
Any	11.4	0	1.7
Severe***	1.1	0	0
Myalgia			
Any	6.3	0	2.5
Severe***	0	0	0
Arthralgia			
Any	3.4	2.0	1.7
Severe***	0	0	0.8
Taste Perversion			
Any	5.7	0	0
Severe***	0.6	0	0

*Normal Baseline LFTs: Transaminases ≤ 1.5 times ULN or alkaline phosphatase ≤ 2.5 times ULN or isolated elevations of transaminases or alkaline phosphatase up to 5 times ULN

** Febrile Neutropenia: ANC grade 4 with fever > 38°C with IV antibiotics and/or hospitalization

*** COSTART term and grading system

† Not Applicable; †† Not Done

Combination Therapy with TAXOTERE in the Adjuvant Treatment of Breast Cancer

The following table presents treatment emergent adverse events (TEAEs) observed in 744 patients, who were treated with TAXOTERE 75 mg/m^2 every 3 weeks in combination with doxorubicin and cyclophosphamide.

[See table at top of previous page]

Of the 744 patients treated with TAC, 36.3% experienced severe TEAEs compared to 26.6% of the 736 patients treated with FAC. Dose reductions due to hematologic toxicity occurred in 1% of cycles in the TAC arm versus 0.1% of cycles in the FAC arm. Six percent of patients treated with

Continued on next page

Taxotere—Cont.

TAC discontinued treatment due to adverse events, compared to 1.1% treated with FAC; fever in the absence of infection and allergy being the most common reasons for withdrawal among TAC-treated patients. Two patients died in each arm within 30 days of their last study treatment; 1 death per arm was attributed to study drugs.

Fever and Infection

Fever in the absence of infection was seen in 46.5% of TAC-treated patients and in 17.1% of FAC-treated patients. Grade 3/4 fever in the absence of infection was seen in 1.3% and 0% of TAC- and FAC-treated patients respectively. Infection was seen in 39.4% of TAC-treated patients compared to 36.3% of FAC-treated patients. Grade 3/4 infection was seen in 3.9% and 2.2% of TAC-treated and FAC-treated patients respectively. There were no septic deaths in either treatment arm.

Gastrointestinal events

In addition to gastrointestinal events reflected in the table above, 7 patients in the TAC arm were reported to have colitis/enteritis/large intestine perforation vs. one patient in the FAC arm. Five of the 7 TAC-treated patients required treatment discontinuation; no deaths due to these events occurred.

Cardiovascular events

More cardiovascular events were reported in the TAC arm vs. the FAC arm; dysrhythmias, all grades (7.9% vs. 6.0%), hypotension, all grades (2.6% vs. 1.1%) and CHF (1.6% vs. 0.5%). One patient in each arm died due to heart failure.

Acute Myeloid Leukemia

Treatment-related acute myeloid leukemia (AML) is known to occur in patients treated with anthracyclines and/or cyclophosphamide, including use in adjuvant therapy for breast cancer. AML occurs at a higher frequency when these agents are given in combination with radiation therapy. AML occurred in the adjuvant breast cancer trial (TAX316). The cumulative risk of developing treatment-related AML at 5 years in TAX316 was 0.4% for TAC-treated patients and 0.1% for FAC-treated patients. This risk of AML is comparable to the risk observed for other anthracyclines/cyclophosphamide containing adjuvant breast chemotherapy regimens.

Monotherapy with TAXOTERE for Unresectable, Locally Advanced or Metastatic NSCLC Previously Treated with Platinum-Based Chemotherapy

TAXOTERE 75 mg/m^2: Treatment emergent adverse drug reactions are shown below. Included in this table are safety data for a total of 176 patients with non-small cell lung carcinoma and a history of prior treatment with platinum-based chemotherapy who were treated in two randomized, controlled trials. These reactions were described using NCI Common Toxicity Criteria regardless of relationship to study treatment, except for the hematologic toxicities or otherwise noted.

[See table at top of previous page]

Combination Therapy with TAXOTERE in Chemotherapy-Naïve Advanced Unresectable or Metastatic NSCLC

The table below presents safety data from two arms of an open label, randomized controlled trial (TAX326) that enrolled patients with unresectable stage IIIB or IV non-small cell lung cancer and no history of prior chemotherapy. Adverse reactions were described using the NCI Common Toxicity Criteria except where otherwise noted.

Adverse Events Regardless of Relationship to Treatment in Chemotherapy-Naïve Advanced Non-Small Cell Lung Cancer Patients Receiving TAXOTERE in Combination with Cisplatin

Adverse Event	TAXOTERE 75 mg/m^2 + Cisplatin 75 mg/m^2 n=406 %	Vinorelbine 25 mg/m^2 + Cisplatin 100 mg/m^2 n=396 %
Neutropenia		
Any	91	90
Grade 3/4	74	78
Febrile Neutropenia	5	5
Thrombocytopenia		
Any	15	15
Grade 3/4	3	4
Anemia		
Any	89	94
Grade 3/4	7	25
Infection		
Any	35	37
Grade 3/4	8	8
Fever in absence of infection		
Any	33	29
Grade 3/4	< 1	1
Hypersensitivity Reaction*		
Any	12	4
Grade 3/4	3	< 1

Fluid Retention**		
Any	54	42
All severe or life-threatening events	2	2
Pleural effusion		
Any	23	22
All severe or life-threatening events	2	2
Peripheral edema		
Any	34	18
All severe or life-threatening events	< 1	< 1
Weight gain		
Any	15	9
All severe or life-threatening events	< 1	< 1
Neurosensory		
Any	47	42
Grade 3/4	4	4
Neuromotor		
Any	19	17
Grade 3/4	3	6
Skin		
Any	16	14
Grade 3/4	< 1	1
Nausea		
Any	72	76
Grade 3/4	10	17
Vomiting		
Any	55	61
Grade 3/4	8	16
Diarrhea		
Any	47	25
Grade 3/4	7	3
Anorexia**		
Any	42	40
All severe or life-threatening events	5	5
Stomatitis		
Any	24	21
Grade 3/4	2	1
Alopecia		
Any	75	42
Grade 3/4	< 1	0
Asthenia**		
Any	74	75
All severe or life-threatening events	12	14
Nail Disorder**		
Any	14	< 1
All severe events	< 1	0
Myalgia**		
Any	18	12
All severe events	< 1	< 1

* Replaces NCI term "Allergy"
** COSTART term and grading system

Deaths within 30 days of last study treatment occurred in 31 patients (7.6%) in the docetaxel+cisplatin arm and 37 patients (9.3%) in the vinorelbine+cisplatin arm. Deaths within 30 days of last study treatment attributed to study drug occurred in 9 patients (2.2%) in the docetaxel+cisplatin arm and 8 patients (2.0%) in the vinorelbine+cisplatin arm. The second comparison in the study, vinorelbine+cisplatin versus TAXOTERE+carboplatin (which did not demonstrate a superior survival associated with TAXOTERE, see **CLINICAL STUDIES** section) demonstrated a higher incidence of thrombocytopenia, diarrhea, fluid retention, hypersensitivity reactions, skin toxicity, alopecia and nail changes on the TAXOTERE+carboplatin arm, while a higher incidence of anemia, neurosensory toxicity, nausea, vomiting, anorexia and asthenia was observed on the vinorelbine+cisplatin arm.

Combination Therapy with TAXOTERE in Patients with Prostate Cancer

The following data are based on the experience of 332 patients, who were treated with TAXOTERE 75 mg/m^2 every 3 weeks in combination with prednisone 5 mg orally twice daily.

[See table at bottom of next page]

Post-marketing Experiences

The following adverse events have been identified from clinical trials and/or post-marketing surveillance. Because they are reported from a population of unknown size, precise estimates of frequency cannot be made.

Body as a whole: diffuse pain, chest pain, radiation recall phenomenon

Cardiovascular: atrial fibrillation, deep vein thrombosis, ECG abnormalities, thrombophlebitis, pulmonary embolism, syncope, tachycardia, myocardial infarction

Cutaneous: rare cases of bullous eruption such as erythema multiforme, Stevens-Johnson syndrome, toxic epidermal necrolysis. Multiple factors may have contributed to the development of these effects. Severe hand and foot syndrome has been reported.

Gastrointestinal: abdominal pain, anorexia, constipation, duodenal ulcer, esophagitis, gastrointestinal hemorrhage, gastrointestinal perforation, ischemic colitis, colitis, intestinal obstruction, ileus, neutropenic enterocolitis and dehydration as a consequence to gastrointestinal events have been reported.

Hematologic: bleeding episodes

Hepatic: rare cases of hepatitis, sometimes fatal primarily in patients with pre-existing liver disorders, have been reported.

Neurologic: confusion, rare cases of seizures or transient loss of consciousness have been observed, sometimes appearing during the infusion of the drug.

Ophthalmologic: conjunctivitis, lacrimation or lacrimation with or without conjunctivitis. Excessive tearing which may be attributable to lacrimal duct obstruction has been reported. Rare cases of transient visual disturbances (flashes, flashing lights, scotomata) typically occurring during drug infusion and in association with hypersensitivity reactions have been reported. These were reversible upon discontinuation of the infusion.

Respiratory: dyspnea, acute pulmonary edema, acute respiratory distress syndrome, interstitial pneumonia. Pulmonary fibrosis has been rarely reported.

Urogenital: renal insufficiency

OVERDOSAGE

There is no known antidote for TAXOTERE overdosage. In case of overdosage, the patient should be kept in a specialized unit where vital functions can be closely monitored. Anticipated complications of overdosage include: bone marrow suppression, peripheral neurotoxicity, and mucositis. Patients should receive therapeutic G-CSF as soon as possible after discovery of overdose. Other appropriate symptomatic measures should be taken, as needed.

In two reports of overdose, one patient received 150 mg/m^2 and the other received 200 mg/m^2 as 1-hour infusions. Both patients experienced severe neutropenia, mild asthenia, cutaneous reactions, and mild paresthesia, and recovered without incident.

In mice, lethality was observed following single IV doses that were ≥154 mg/kg (about 4.5 times the recommended human dose on a mg/m^2 basis); neurotoxicity associated with paralysis, non-extension of hind limbs, and myelin degeneration was observed in mice at 48 mg/kg (about 1.5 times the recommended human dose on a mg/m^2 basis). In male and female rats, lethality was observed at a dose of 20 mg/kg (comparable to the recommended human dose on a mg/m^2 basis) and was associated with abnormal mitosis and necrosis of multiple organs.

DOSAGE AND ADMINISTRATION

Breast Cancer

The recommended dose of TAXOTERE is 60-100 mg/m^2 administered intravenously over 1 hour every 3 weeks.

In the adjuvant treatment of operable node-positive breast cancer, the recommended TAXOTERE dose is 75 mg/m^2 administered 1-hour after doxorubicin 50 mg/m^2 and cyclophosphamide 500 mg/m^2 every 3 weeks for 6 courses. Prophylactic G-CSF may be used to mitigate the risk of hematological toxicities (see also **Dosage Adjustments**).

Non-Small Cell Lung Cancer

For treatment after failure of prior platinum-based chemotherapy, TAXOTERE was evaluated as monotherapy, and the recommended dose is 75 mg/m^2 administered intravenously over 1 hour every 3 weeks. A dose of 100 mg/m^2 in patients previously treated with chemotherapy was associated with increased hematologic toxicity, infection, and treatment-related mortality in randomized, controlled trials (see **BOXED WARNING, WARNINGS** and **CLINICAL STUDIES** sections).

For chemotherapy-naïve patients, TAXOTERE was evaluated in combination with cisplatin. The recommended dose of TAXOTERE is 75 mg/m^2 administered intravenously over 1 hour immediately followed by cisplatin 75 mg/m^2 over 30-60 minutes every 3 weeks.

Prostate cancer

For hormone-refractory metastatic prostate cancer, the recommended dose of TAXOTERE is 75 mg/m^2 every 3 weeks as a 1 hour infusion. Prednisone 5 mg orally twice daily is administered continuously.

Premedication Regimen

All patients should be premedicated with oral corticosteroids (see below for prostate cancer) such as dexamethasone 16 mg per day (e.g., 8 mg BID) for 3 days starting 1 day prior to TAXOTERE administration in order to reduce the incidence and severity of fluid retention as well as the severity of hypersensitivity reactions (see **BOXED WARNING, WARNINGS,** and **PRECAUTIONS** sections).

For hormone-refractory metastatic prostate cancer, given the concurrent use of prednisone, the recommended premedication regimen is oral dexamethasone 8 mg, at 12 hours, 3 hours and 1 hour before the TAXOTERE infusion (see **WARNINGS,** and **PRECAUTIONS** sections).

Dosage Adjustments During Treatment

Breast Cancer

Patients who are dosed initially at 100 mg/m^2 and who experience either febrile neutropenia, neutrophils < 500 cells/mm^3 for more than 1 week, or severe or cumulative cutaneous reactions during TAXOTERE therapy should have the dosage adjusted from 100 mg/m^2 to 75 mg/

m². If the patient continues to experience these reactions, the dosage should either be decreased from 75 mg/m² to 55 mg/m² or the treatment should be discontinued. Conversely, patients who are dosed initially at 60 mg/m² and who do not experience febrile neutropenia, neutrophils <500 cells/mm³ for more than 1 week, severe or cumulative cutaneous reactions, or severe peripheral neuropathy during TAXOTERE therapy may tolerate higher doses. Patients who develop ≥ grade 3 peripheral neuropathy should have TAXOTERE treatment discontinued entirely.

Combination Therapy with TAXOTERE in the Adjuvant Treatment of Breast Cancer

TAXOTERE in combination with doxorubicin and cyclophosphamide should be administered when the neutrophil count is ≥ 1,500 cells/mm³. Patients who experience febrile neutropenia should receive G-CSF in all subsequent cycles. Patients who continue to experience this reaction should remain on G-CSF and have their TAXOTERE dose reduced to 60 mg/m². Patients who experience Grade 3 or 4 stomatitis should have their TAXOTERE dose decreased to 60 mg/m². Patients who experience severe or cumulative cutaneous reactions or moderate neurosensory signs and/or symptoms during TAXOTERE therapy should have their dosage of TAXOTERE reduced from 75 to 60 mg/m². If the patient continues to experience these reactions at 60 mg/m², treatment should be discontinued.

Non-Small Cell Lung Cancer

Monotherapy with TAXOTERE for NSCLC Treatment After Failure of Prior Platinum-Based Chemotherapy

Patients who are dosed initially at 75 mg/m² and who experience either febrile neutropenia, neutrophils <500 cells/mm³ for more than one week, severe or cumulative cutaneous reactions, or other grade 3/4 non-hematological toxicities during TAXOTERE treatment should have treatment withheld until resolution of the toxicity and then resumed at 55 mg/m². Patients who develop ≥ grade 3 peripheral neuropathy should have TAXOTERE treatment discontinued entirely.

Combination Therapy with TAXOTERE for Chemotherapy-Naïve NSCLC

For patients who are dosed initially at TAXOTERE 75 mg/m² in combination with cisplatin, and whose nadir of platelet count during the previous course of therapy is <25,000 cells/mm³, in patients who experience febrile neutropenia, and in patients with serious non-hematologic toxicities, the TAXOTERE dosage in subsequent cycles should be reduced to 65 mg/m². In patients who require a further dose reduction, a dose of 50 mg/m² is recommended. For cisplatin dosage adjustments, see manufacturers' prescribing information.

Combination Therapy with TAXOTERE for Hormone-Refractory Metastatic Prostate Cancer

TAXOTERE should be administered when the neutrophil count is ≥ 1,500 cells/mm³. Patients who experience either febrile neutropenia, neutrophils < 500 cells/mm³ for more than one week, severe or cumulative cutaneous reactions or moderate neurosensory signs and/or symptoms during TAXOTERE therapy should have the dosage of TAXOTERE reduced from 75 to 60 mg/m². If the patient continues to experience these reactions at 60 mg/m², the treatment should be discontinued.

Special Populations

Hepatic Impairment: Patients with bilirubin > ULN should generally not receive TAXOTERE. Also, patients with SGOT and/or SGPT > 1.5 × ULN concomitant with alkaline phosphatase > 2.5 × ULN should generally not receive TAXOTERE.

Children: The safety and effectiveness of docetaxel in pediatric patients below the age of 16 years have not been established.

Elderly: See **Precautions, Geriatric Use.** In general, dose selection for an elderly patient should be cautious, reflecting the greater frequency of decreased hepatic, renal, or cardiac function and of concomitant disease or other drug therapy in elderly patients.

PREPARATION AND ADMINISTRATION
Administration Precautions

TAXOTERE is a cytotoxic anticancer drug and, as with other potentially toxic compounds, caution should be exercised when handling and preparing TAXOTERE solutions. The use of gloves is recommended. Please refer to **Handling and Disposal** section.

If TAXOTERE Injection Concentrate, initial diluted solution, or final dilution for infusion should come into contact with the skin, immediately and thoroughly wash with soap and water.

If TAXOTERE Injection Concentrate, initial diluted solution, or final dilution for infusion should come into contact with mucosa, immediately and thoroughly wash with water.

Contact of the TAXOTERE concentrate with plasticized PVC equipment or devices used to prepare solutions for infusion is not recommended. In order to minimize patient exposure to the plasticizer DEHP (di-2-ethylhexyl phthalate), which may be leached from PVC infusion bags or sets, the final TAXOTERE dilution for infusion should be stored in bottles (glass, polypropylene) or plastic bags (polypropylene, polyolefin) and administered through polyethylene-lined administration sets.

TAXOTERE Injection Concentrate requires two dilutions prior to administration. Please follow the preparation instructions provided below. **Note:** Both the TAXOTERE Injection Concentrate and the diluent vials contain an overfill to compensate for liquid loss during preparation. This overfill ensures that after dilution with the **entire** contents of the accompanying diluent, there is an initial diluted solution containing 10 mg/mL docetaxel.

The table below provides the fill range of the diluent, the approximate extractable volume of diluent when the entire contents of the diluent vial are withdrawn, and the concentration of the initial diluted solution for TAXOTERE 20 mg and TAXOTERE 80 mg.

Product	Diluent 13% (w/w) ethanol in water for injection Fill Range (mL)	Approximate extractable volume of diluent when entire contents are withdrawn (mL)	Concentration of the initial diluted solution (mg/mL docetaxel)
Taxotere® 20 mg/0.5 mL	1.88 - 2.08 mL	1.8 mL	10 mg/mL
Taxotere® 80 mg/2 mL	6.96 - 7.70 mL	7.1 mL	10 mg/mL

Preparation and Administration

A. Initial Diluted Solution
1. TAXOTERE vials should be stored between 2 and 25°C (36 and 77°F). If the vials are stored under refrigeration, allow the appropriate number of vials of TAXOTERE Injection Concentrate and diluent (13% ethanol in water for injection) vials to stand at room temperature for approximately 5 minutes.
2. Aseptically withdraw the **entire** contents of the appropriate diluent vial (approximately 1.8 mL for TAXOTERE 20 mg and approximately 7.1 mL for TAXOTERE 80 mg) into a syringe by partially inverting the vial, and transfer it to the appropriate vial of TAXOTERE Injection Concentrate. **If the procedure is followed as described, an initial diluted solution of 10mg docetaxel/mL will result.**
3. Mix the initial diluted solution by repeated inversions for at least 45 seconds to assure full mixture of the concentrate and diluent. Do not shake.
4. The initial diluted TAXOTERE solution (10 mg docetaxel/mL) should be clear; however, there may be some foam on top of the solution due to the polysorbate 80. Allow the solution to stand for a few minutes to allow any foam to dissipate. It is not required that all foam dissipate prior to continuing the preparation process.

The initial diluted solution may be used immediately or stored either in the refrigerator or at room temperature for a maximum of 8 hours.

B. Final Dilution for Infusion
1. Aseptically withdraw the required amount of initial diluted TAXOTERE solution (10 mg docetaxel/mL) with a calibrated syringe and inject into a 250 mL infusion bag or bottle of either 0.9% Sodium Chloride solution or 5% Dextrose solution to produce a final concentration of 0.3 to 0.74 mg/mL.

If a dose greater than 200 mg of TAXOTERE is required, use a larger volume of the infusion vehicle so that a concentration of 0.74 mg/mL TAXOTERE is not exceeded.
2. Thoroughly mix the infusion by manual rotation.
3. As with all parenteral products, TAXOTERE should be inspected visually for particulate matter or discoloration prior to administration whenever the solution and container permit. If the TAXOTERE initial diluted solution or final dilution for infusion is not clear or appears to have precipitation, these should be discarded.

The final TAXOTERE dilution for infusion should be administered intravenously as a 1-hour infusion under ambient room temperature and lighting conditions.

Stability

TAXOTERE infusion solution, if stored between 2 and 25°C (36 and 77°F) is stable for 4 hours. Fully prepared

---

Clinically Important Treatment Emergent Adverse Events (Regardless of Relationship) in Patients with Prostate Cancer who Received TAXOTERE in Combination with Prednisone (TAX 327)

Adverse Event	TAXOTERE 75 mg/m² every 3 weeks + prednisone 5 mg twice daily n=332 %		Mitoxantrone 12 mg/m² every 3 weeks + prednisone 5 mg twice daily n=335 %	
	Any	G 3/4	Any	G 3/4
Anemia	66.5	4.9	57.8	1.8
Neutropenia	40.9	32.0	48.2	21.7
Thrombocytopenia	3.4	0.6	7.8	1.2
Febrile neutropenia	2.7	N/A	1.8	N/A
Infection	32.2	5.7	20.3	4.2
Epistaxis	5.7	0.3	1.8	0.0
Allergic Reactions	8.4	0.6	0.6	0.0
Fluid Retention*	24.4	0.6	4.5	0.3
Weight Gain*	7.5	0.3	3.0	0.0
Peripheral Edema*	18.1	0.3	1.5	0.0
Neuropathy Sensory	30.4	1.8	7.2	0.3
Neuropathy Motor	7.2	1.5	3.0	0.9
Rash/Desquamation	6.0	0.3	3.3	0.6
Alopecia	65.1	N/A	12.8	N/A
Nail Changes	29.5	0.0	7.5	0.0
Nausea	41.0	2.7	35.5	1.5
Diarrhea	31.6	2.1	9.6	1.2
Stomatitis/Pharyngitis	19.6	0.9	8.4	0.0
Taste Disturbance	18.4	0.0	6.6	0.0
Vomiting	16.9	1.5	14.0	1.5
Anorexia	16.6	1.2	14.3	0.3
Cough	12.3	0.0	7.8	0.0
Dyspnea	15.1	2.7	8.7	0.9
Cardiac left ventricular function	9.6	0.3	22.1	1.2
Fatigue	53.3	4.5	34.6	5.1
Myalgia	14.5	0.3	12.8	0.9
Tearing	9.9	0.6	1.5	0.0
Arthralgia	8.1	0.6	5.1	1.2

*Related to treatment

Continued on next page

Taxotere—Cont.

TAXOTERE infusion solution (in either 0.9% Sodium Chloride solution or 5% Dextrose solution) should be used within 4 hours (including the 1 hour i.v. administration).

HOW SUPPLIED

TAXOTERE Injection Concentrate is supplied in a single-dose vial as a sterile, pyrogen-free, non-aqueous, viscous solution with an accompanying sterile, non-pyrogenic, Diluent (13% ethanol in water for injection) vial. The following strengths are available:

TAXOTERE 80 MG/2 ML   (NDC 0075-8001-80)

TAXOTERE (docetaxel) Injection Concentrate 80 mg/2 mL: 80 mg docetaxel in 2 mL polysorbate 80 and Diluent for TAXOTERE 80 mg (13% (w/w) ethanol in water for injection). Both items are in a blister pack in one carton.

TAXOTERE 20 MG/0.5 ML   (NDC 0075-8001-20)

TAXOTERE (docetaxel) Injection Concentrate 20 mg/0.5 mL: 20 mg docetaxel in 0.5 mL polysorbate 80 and diluent for TAXOTERE 20 mg (13% (w/w) ethanol in water for injection). Both items are in a blister pack in one carton.

Storage

Store between 2 and 25°C (36 and 77°F). Retain in the original package to protect from bright light. Freezing does not adversely affect the product.

Handling and Disposal

Procedures for proper handling and disposal of anticancer drugs should be considered. Several guidelines on this subject have been published[1-7]. There is no general agreement that all of the procedures recommended in the guidelines are necessary or appropriate.

REFERENCES

1. OSHA Work-Practice Guidelines for Controlling Occupational Exposure to Hazardous Drugs. *Am J Health-Syst Pharm.* 1996; 53: 1669-1685.
2. American Society of Hospital Pharmacists Technical Assistance Bulletin on Handling Cytotoxic and Hazardous Drugs. *Am J Hosp Pharm.* 1990; 47(95): 1033-1049.
3. AMA Council Report. Guidelines for Handling Parenteral Antineoplastics. *JAMA.* 1985; 253(11): 1590-1592.
4. Recommendations for the Safe Handling of Parenteral Antineoplastic Drugs. NIH Publication No. 83-2621. For sale by the Superintendent of Documents, US Government Printing Office, Washington, DC 20402.
5. National Study Commission on Cytotoxic Exposure - Recommendations for Handling Cytotoxic Agents. Available from Louis P. Jeffry, Chairman, National Study Commission on Cytotoxic Exposure. Massachusetts College of Pharmacy and Allied Health Sciences, 179 Longwood Avenue, Boston, MA 02115.
6. Clinical Oncological Society of Australia. Guidelines and Recommendations for Safe Handling of Antineoplastic Agents. *Med J Austr.* 1983; 426-428.
7. Jones, RB, et al. Safe Handling of Chemotherapeutic Agents: A Report from the Mt. Sinai Medical Center. *CA-A Cancer Journal for Clinicians.* 1983; Sept/Oct: 258-263.

Prescribing Information as of February 2005
Manufactured by Aventis Pharma Ltd.
Dagenham, Essex RM10 7XS
United Kingdom
Manufactured for
Aventis Pharmaceuticals Inc.
Bridgewater, NJ 08807 USA
www.aventis-us.com
©2005 Aventis Pharmaceuticals

Patient Information Leaflet

Questions and Answers About Taxotere® Injection Concentrate

(generic name = docetaxel)
(pronounced as TAX-O-TEER)

What is Taxotere?

Taxotere is a medication to treat breast cancer, non-small cell lung cancer and prostate cancer. It has severe side effects in some patients. This leaflet is designed to help you understand how to use Taxotere and avoid its side effects to the fullest extent possible. The more you understand your treatment, the better you will be able to participate in your care. If you have questions or concerns, be sure to ask your doctor or nurse. They are always your best source of information about your condition and treatment.

What is the most important information about Taxotere?

- Since this drug, like many other cancer drugs, affects your blood cells, your doctor will ask for routine blood tests. These will include regular checks of your white blood cell counts. People with low blood counts can develop life-threatening infections. The earliest sign of infection may be fever, so if you experience a fever, tell your doctor right away.
- Occasionally, serious allergic reactions have occurred with this medicine. If you have any allergies, tell your doctor before receiving this medicine.
- A small number of people who take Taxotere have severe fluid retention, which can be life-threatening. To help avoid this problem, you must take another medication such as dexamethasone (DECKS-A-METH-A-SONE) prior to each Taxotere treatment. You must follow the schedule and take the exact dose of dexamethasone prescribed (see schedule at end of brochure). If you forget to take a dose or do not take it on schedule you must tell the doctor or nurse prior to your Taxotere treatment.

- If you are using any other medicines, tell your doctor before receiving your infusions of Taxotere.

How does Taxotere work?

Taxotere works by attacking cancer cells in your body. Different cancer medications attack cancer cells in different ways.

Here's how Taxotere works: Every cell in your body contains a supporting structure (like a skeleton). Damage to this "skeleton" can stop cell growth or reproduction. Taxotere makes the "skeleton" in some cancer cells very stiff, so that the cells can no longer grow.

How will I receive Taxotere?

Taxotere is given by an infusion directly into your vein. Your treatment will take about 1 hour. Generally, people receive Taxotere every 3 weeks. The amount of Taxotere and the frequency of your infusions will be determined by your doctor.

As part of your treatment, to reduce side effects your doctor will prescribe another medicine called dexamethasone. Your doctor will tell you how and when to take this medicine. It is important that you take the dexamethasone on the schedule set by your doctor. If you forget to take your medication, or do not take it on schedule, make sure to tell your doctor or nurse **BEFORE** you receive your Taxotere treatment. **Included with this information leaflet is a chart to help you remember when to take your dexamethasone.**

What should be avoided while receiving Taxotere?

Taxotere can interact with other medicines. Use only medicines that are prescribed for you by your doctor and **be sure** to tell your doctor all the medicines that you use, including nonprescription drugs.

What are the possible side effects of Taxotere?

Low Blood Cell Count—Many cancer medications, including Taxotere, cause a temporary drop in the number of white blood cells. These cells help protect your body from infection. Your doctor will routinely check your blood count and tell you if it is too low. Although most people receiving Taxotere do not have an infection even if they have a low white blood cell count, the risk of infection is increased. **Fever is often one of the most common and earliest signs of infection. Your doctor will recommend that you take your temperature frequently, especially during the days after treatment with Taxotere. If you have a fever, tell your doctor or nurse immediately.**

Allergic Reactions—This type of reaction, which occurs during the infusion of Taxotere, is infrequent. If you feel a warm sensation, a tightness in your chest, or itching during or shortly after your treatment, tell your doctor or nurse immediately.

Fluid Retention—This means that your body is holding extra water. If this fluid retention is in the chest or around the heart it can be life-threatening. If you notice swelling in the feet and legs or a slight weight gain, this may be the first warning sign. Fluid retention usually does not start immediately; but, if it occurs, it may start around your 5th treatment. Generally, fluid retention will go away within weeks or months after your treatments are completed.

Dexamethasone tablets may protect patients from significant fluid retention. It is important that you take this medicine on schedule. If you have not taken dexamethasone on schedule, you must tell your doctor or nurse before receiving your next Taxotere treatment.

Gastrointestinal—Diarrhea has been associated with TAXOTERE use and can be severe in some patients. Nausea and/or vomiting are common in patients receiving TAXOTERE. Severe inflammation of the bowel can also occur in some patients and may be life threatening.

Hair Loss—Loss of hair occurs in most patients taking Taxotere (including the hair on your head, underarm hair, pubic hair, eyebrows, and eyelashes). Hair loss will begin after the first few treatments and varies from patient to patient. Once you have completed all your treatments, hair generally grows back.

Your doctor or nurse can refer you to a store that carries wigs, hairpieces, and turbans for patients with cancer.

Fatigue—A number of patients (about 10%) receiving Taxotere feel very tired following their treatments. If you feel tired or weak, allow yourself extra rest before your next treatment. If it is bothersome or lasts for longer than 1 week, inform your doctor or nurse.

Muscle Pain—This happens about 20% of the time, but is rarely severe. You may feel pain in your muscles or joints. Tell your doctor or nurse if this happens. They may suggest ways to make you more comfortable.

Rash—This side effect occurs commonly but is severe in about 5%. You may develop a rash that looks like a blotchy, hive-like reaction. This usually occurs on the hands and feet but may also appear on the arms, face, or body. Generally, it will appear between treatments and will go away before the next treatment. Inform your doctor or nurse if you experience a rash. They can help you avoid discomfort.

Odd Sensations—About half of patients getting Taxotere will feel numbness, tingling, or burning sensations in their hands and feet. If you do experience this, tell your doctor or nurse. Generally, these go away within a few weeks or months after your treatments are completed. About 14% of patients may also develop weakness in their hands and feet.

Nail Changes—Color changes to your fingernails or toenails may occur while taking Taxotere. In extreme, but rare, cases nails may fall off. After you have finished Taxotere treatments, your nails will generally grow back.

Eye Changes—Excessive tearing, which can be related to conjunctivitis or blockage of the tear ducts, may occur.

If you are interested in learning more about this drug, ask your doctor for a copy of the package insert.
Aventis Pharmaceuticals Inc.
Bridgewater, NJ 08807 USA
www.aventis-us.com
Rev. February 2005

Every three-week injection of TAXOTERE for breast and non-small cell lung cancers Take dexamethasone tablets, 8 mg twice daily Dexamethasone dosing:				
Day 1 Date:	Time:		AM	PM
Day 2 Date:	Time:		AM	PM
(Taxotere Treatment Day)				
Day 3 Date:	Time:		AM	PM

Every three-week injection of TAXOTERE for prostate cancer Take dexamethasone 8 mg, at 12 hours, 3 hours and 1 hour before TAXOTERE infusion. Dexamethasone dosing:	
Date:	Time:
Date:	Time:
(Taxotere Treatment Day)	
	Time:

Schering Corporation

a wholly-owned subsidiary of Schering-Plough Corporation
GALLOPING HILL ROAD
KENILWORTH, NJ 07033

Direct Inquiries to:
(908) 298-4000
CUSTOMER SERVICE:
(800) 222-7579
FAX: (908) 595-3729

For Medical Information Contact:
Schering Laboratories
Drug Information Services
2000 Galloping Hill Road
Kenilworth, NJ 07033
(800) 526-4099
FAX: (973) 921-7228

CLARINEX®   ℞

[*klă-rĭ-nĕks*]
(desloratadine)
TABLETS, SYRUP, REDITABS® TABLETS

Prescribing information for this product, which appears on page(s) 3021–3023 of the 2005 PDR, has been completely revised as follows. Please write "See Supplement A" next to the product heading.

DESCRIPTION

CLARINEX (desloratadine) Tablets are light blue, round, film coated tablets containing 5 mg desloratadine, an antihistamine, to be administered orally. It also contains the following excipients: dibasic calcium phosphate dihydrate USP, microcrystalline cellulose NF, corn starch NF, talc USP, carnauba wax NF, white wax NF, coating material consisting of lactose monohydrate, hydroxypropyl methylcellulose, titanium dioxide, polyethylene glycol, and FD&C Blue #2 Aluminum Lake.

CLARINEX Syrup is a clear orange colored liquid containing 0.5 mg/1mL desloratadine. The syrup contains the following inactive ingredients: propylene glycol USP, sorbitol solution USP, citric acid (anhydrous) USP, sodium citrate dihydrate USP, sodium benzoate NF, disodium edetate USP, purified water USP. It also contains granulated sugar, natural and artificial flavor for bubble gum and FDC Yellow #6 dye.

The CLARINEX RediTabs® brand of desloratadine orally-disintegrating tablets is a pink colored round tablet shaped units with a "C" debossed on one side. Each RediTabs unit contains 5 mg of desloratadine. It also contains the following inactive ingredients: gelatin Type B NF, mannitol USP, aspartame NF, polarcrillin potassium NF, citric acid USP, red dye and tutti frutti flavoring.

Desloratadine is a white to off-white powder that is slightly soluble in water, but very soluble in ethanol and propylene glycol. It has an empirical formula: $C_{19}H_{19}ClN_2$ and a molecular weight of 310.8. The chemical name is 8-chloro-6,11-dihydro-11-(4-piperidinylidene)-5H-benzo[5,6]cyclohepta[1,2-b]pyridine and has the following structure:
[See chemical structure at top of next column]

CLINICAL PHARMACOLOGY

Mechanism of Action: Desloratadine is a long-acting tricyclic histamine antagonist with selective H_1-receptor histamine antagonist activity. Receptor binding data indicates that at a concentration of 2-3 ng/mL (7 nanomolar), desloratadine shows significant interaction with the human

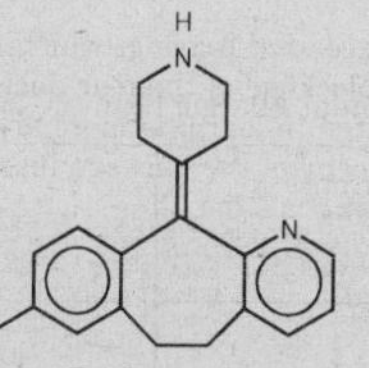

histamine H_1-receptor. Desloratadine inhibited histamine release from human mast cells *in vitro*.

Results of a radiolabeled tissue distribution study in rats and a radioligand H_1-receptor binding study in guinea pigs showed that desloratadine did not readily cross the blood brain barrier.

Pharmacokinetics: Absorption: Following oral administration of desloratadine 5 mg once daily for 10 days to normal healthy volunteers, the mean time to maximum plasma concentrations (T_{max}) occurred at approximately 3 hours post dose and mean steady state peak plasma concentrations (C_{max}) and area under the concentration-time curve (AUC) of 4 ng/mL and 56.9 ng.hr/mL were observed, respectively. Neither food nor grapefruit juice had an effect on the bioavailability (C_{max} and AUC) of desloratadine.

The pharmacokinetic profile of CLARINEX Syrup was evaluated in a three-way crossover study in 30 adult volunteers. A single dose of 10 mL of CLARINEX Syrup containing 5 mg of desloratadine was bioequivalent to a single dose of 5 mg CLARINEX Tablet. Food had no effect on the bioavailability (AUC and C_{max}) of CLARINEX Syrup.

The pharmacokinetic profile of CLARINEX RediTabs Tablets was evaluated in a three-way crossover study in 30 adult volunteers. A single CLARINEX RediTabs Tablet containing 5 mg of desloratadine was bioequivalent to a single 5 mg CLARINEX Tablet and was bioequivalent to 10 mL of CLARINEX Syrup containing 5 mg of desloratadine for both desloratadine and 3-hydroxydesloratadine. In a separate study with 30 adult volunteers, food or water had no effect on the bioavailability (AUC and C_{max}) of CLARINEX RediTabs Tablets, however, food shifted the desloratadine median T_{max} value from 2.5 to 4 hr.

Distribution: Desloratadine and 3-hydroxydesloratadine are approximately 82% to 87% and 85% to 89%, bound to plasma proteins, respectively. Protein binding of desloratadine and 3-hydroxydesloratadine was unaltered in subjects with impaired renal function.

Metabolism: Desloratadine (a major metabolite of loratadine) is extensively metabolized to 3-hydroxydesloratadine, an active metabolite, which is subsequently glucuronidated. The enzyme(s) responsible for the formation of 3-hydroxydesloratadine have not been identified. Data from clinical trials indicate that a subset of the general population has a decreased ability to form 3-hydroxydesloratadine, and are poor metabolizers of desloratadine. In pharmacokinetic studies (n= 3748), approximately 6% of subjects were poor metabolizers of desloratadine (defined as a subject with an AUC ratio of 3-hydroxydesloratadine to desloratadine less than 0.1, or a subject with a desloratadine half-life exceeding 50 hours). These pharmacokinetic studies included subjects between the ages of 2 and 70 years, including 977 subjects aged 2-5 years, 1575 subjects aged 6-11 years, and 1196 subjects aged 12-70 years. There was no difference in the prevalence of poor metabolizers across age groups. The frequency of poor metabolizers was higher in Blacks (17%, n=988) as compared to Caucasians (2%, n=1462) and Hispanics (2%, n=1063). The median exposure (AUC) to desloratadine in the poor metabolizers was approximately 6-fold greater than in the subjects who are not poor metabolizers. Subjects who are poor metabolizers of desloratadine cannot be prospectively identified and will be exposed to higher levels of desloratadine following dosing with the recommended dose of desloratadine. In multidose clinical safety studies, where metabolizer status was identified, a total of 94 poor metabolizers and 123 normal metabolizers were enrolled and treated with CLARINEX for 15-35 days. In these studies, no overall differences in safety were observed between poor metabolizers and normal metabolizers. Although not seen in these studies, an increased risk of exposure-related adverse events in patients who are poor metabolizers cannot be ruled out.

Elimination: The mean elimination half-life of desloratadine was 27 hours. C_{max} and AUC values increased in a dose proportional manner following single oral doses between 5 and 20 mg. The degree of accumulation after 14 days of dosing was consistent with the half-life and dosing frequency. A human mass balance study documented a recovery of approximately 87% of the ^{14}C-desloratadine dose, which was equally distributed in urine and feces as metabolic products. Analysis of plasma 3-hydroxydesloratadine showed similar T_{max} and half-life values compared to desloratadine.

Special Populations: Geriatric: In older subjects ($\geq$ 65 years old; n=17) following multiple-dose administration of CLARINEX Tablets, the mean C_{max} and AUC values for desloratadine were 20% greater than in younger subjects (< 65 years old). The oral total body clearance (CL/F) when normalized for body weight was similar between the two age groups. The mean plasma elimination half-life of desloratadine was 33.7 hr in subjects $\geq$ 65 years old. The pharmacokinetics for 3-hydroxydesloratadine appeared unchanged in older versus younger subjects. These age-related differences are unlikely to be clinically relevant and no dosage adjustment is recommended in elderly subjects.

Pediatric Subjects: In subjects 6 to 11 years old, a single dose of 5 mL of CLARINEX Syrup containing 2.5 mg of desloratadine, resulted in desloratadine plasma concentrations similar to those achieved in adults administered a single 5 mg CLARINEX Tablet. In subjects 2 to 5 years old, a single dose of 2.5 mL of CLARINEX Syrup containing 1.25 mg of desloratadine, resulted in desloratadine plasma concentrations similar to those achieved in adults administered a single 5 mg CLARINEX Tablet. However, the C_{max} and AUC of the metabolite (3-OH desloratadine) were 1.27 and 1.61 times higher for the 5 mg dose of syrup administered in adults compared to the C_{max} and AUC obtained in children 2-11 years of age receiving 1.25-2.5 mg of CLARINEX Syrup.

A single dose of either 2.5 mL or 1.25 mL of CLARINEX Syrup containing 1.25 mg or 0.625 mg, respectively, of desloratadine was administered to subjects 6 to 11 months of age and 12 to 23 months of age. The results of a population pharmacokinetic analysis indicated that a dose of 1 mg for subjects aged 6 to 11 months and 1.25 mg for subjects 12 to 23 months of age is required to obtain desloratadine plasma concentrations similar to those achieved in adults administered a single 5 mg dose of CLARINEX Syrup.

Renally Impaired: Desloratadine pharmacokinetics following a single dose of 7.5 mg were characterized in patients with mild (n=7; creatinine clearance 51-69 mL/min/1.73 m^2), moderate (n=6; creatinine clearance 34-43 mL/min/1.73 m^2), and severe (n=6; creatinine clearance 5-29 mL/min/1.73 m^2) renal impairment or hemodialysis dependent (n=6) patients. In patients with mild and moderate renal impairment, median C_{max} and AUC values increased by approximately 1.2- and 1.9-fold, respectively, relative to subjects with normal renal function. In patients with severe renal impairment or who were hemodialysis dependent, C_{max} and AUC values increased by approximately 1.7- and 2.5-fold, respectively. Minimal changes in 3-hydroxydesloratadine concentrations were observed. Desloratadine and 3-hydroxydesloratadine were poorly removed by hemodialysis. Plasma protein binding of desloratadine and 3-hydroxydesloratadine was unaltered by renal impairment. Dosage adjustment for patients with renal impairment is recommended (see **DOSAGE AND ADMINISTRATION** section).

Hepatically Impaired: Desloratadine pharmacokinetics were characterized following a single oral dose in patients with mild (n=4), moderate (n=4), and severe (n=4) hepatic impairment as defined by the Child-Pugh classification of hepatic function and 8 subjects with normal hepatic function. Patients with hepatic impairment, regardless of severity, had approximately a 2.4-fold increase in AUC as compared with normal subjects. The apparent oral clearance of desloratadine in patients with mild, moderate, and severe hepatic impairment was 37%, 36%, and 28% of that in normal subjects, respectively. An increase in the mean elimination half-life of desloratadine in patients with hepatic impairment was observed. For 3-hydroxydesloratadine, the mean C_{max} and AUC values for patients with hepatic impairment were not statistically significantly different from subjects with normal hepatic function. Dosage adjustment for patients with hepatic impairment is recommended (see **DOSAGE AND ADMINISTRATION** section).

Gender: Female subjects treated for 14 days with CLARINEX Tablets had 10% and 3% higher desloratadine C_{max} and AUC values, respectively, compared with male subjects. The 3-hydroxydesloratadine C_{max} and AUC values were also increased by 45% and 48%, respectively, in females compared with males. However, these apparent differences are not likely to be clinically relevant and therefore no dosage adjustment is recommended.

Race: Following 14 days of treatment with CLARINEX Tablets, the C_{max} and AUC values for desloratadine were 18% and 32% higher, respectively, in Blacks compared with Caucasians. For 3-hydroxydesloratadine there was a corresponding 10% reduction in C_{max} and AUC values in Blacks compared to Caucasians. These differences are not likely to be clinically relevant and therefore no dose adjustment is recommended.

Drug Interactions: In two controlled crossover clinical pharmacology studies in healthy male (n=12 in each study) and female (n=12 in each study) volunteers, desloratadine 7.5 mg (1.5 times the daily dose) once daily was coadministered with erythromycin 500 mg every 8 hours or ketoconazole 200 mg every 12 hours for 10 days. In three separate controlled, parallel group clinical pharmacology studies, desloratadine at the clinical dose of 5 mg has been coadministered with azithromycin 500 mg followed by 250 mg once daily for 4 days (n=18) or with fluoxetine 20 mg once daily for 7 days after a 23 day pretreatment period with fluoxetine (n=18) or with cimetidine 600 mg every 12 hours for 14 days (n=18) under steady state conditions to normal healthy male and female volunteers. Although increased plasma concentrations (C_{max} and AUC 0-24 hrs) of desloratadine and 3-hydroxydesloratadine were observed (see Table 1), there were no clinically relevant changes in the safety profile of desloratadine, as assessed by electrocardiographic parameters (including the corrected QT interval), clinical laboratory tests, vital signs, and adverse events.

[See table 1 above]

Table 1

Changes in Desloratadine and 3-Hydroxydesloratadine Pharmacokinetics in Healthy Male and Female Volunteers

	Desloratadine		3-Hydroxydesloratadine	
	C_{max}	AUC 0-24 hrs	C_{max}	AUC 0-24 hrs
Erythromycin (500 mg Q8h)	+24%	+14%	+43%	+40%
Ketoconazole (200 mg Q12h)	+45%	+39%	+43%	+72%
Azithromycin (500 mg day 1, 250 mg QD × 4 days)	+15%	+5%	+15%	+4%
Fluoxetine (20 mg QD)	+15%	+0%	+17%	+13%
Cimetidine (600 mg Q12h)	+12%	+19%	-11%	-3%

Pharmacodynamics: Wheal and Flare: Human histamine skin wheal studies following single and repeated 5 mg doses of desloratadine have shown that the drug exhibits an antihistaminic effect by 1 hour; this activity may persist for as long as 24 hours. There was no evidence of histamine-induced skin wheal tachyphylaxis within the desloratadine 5 mg group over the 28 day treatment period. The clinical relevance of histamine wheal skin testing is unknown.

Effects on QT_c: Single dose administration of desloratadine did not alter the corrected QT interval (QT_c) in rats (up to 12 mg/kg, oral), or guinea pigs (25 mg/kg, intravenous). Repeated oral administration at doses up to 24 mg/kg for durations up to 3 months in monkeys did not alter the QT_c at an estimated desloratadine exposure (AUC) that was approximately 955 times the mean AUC in humans at the recommended daily oral dose. See **OVERDOSAGE** section for information on human QT_c experience.

Clinical Trials: Seasonal Allergic Rhinitis: The clinical efficacy and safety of CLARINEX Tablets were evaluated in over 2,300 patients 12 to 75 years of age with seasonal allergic rhinitis. A total of 1,838 patients received 2.5-20 mg/day of CLARINEX in four double-blind, randomized, placebo-controlled clinical trials of 2 to 4 weeks' duration conducted in the United States. The results of these studies demonstrated the efficacy and safety of CLARINEX 5 mg in the treatment of adult and adolescent patients with seasonal allergic rhinitis. In a dose ranging trial, CLARINEX 2.5-20 mg/day was studied. Doses of 5, 7.5, 10, and 20 mg/day were superior to placebo; and no additional benefit was seen at doses above 5.0 mg. In the same study, an increase in the incidence of somnolence was observed at doses of 10 mg/day and 20 mg/day (5.2% and 7.6%, respectively), compared to placebo (2.3%).

Table 2

TOTAL SYMPTOM SCORE (TSS)

Changes in a 2-Week Clinical Trial in Patients with Seasonal Allergic Rhinitis

Treatment Group (n)	Mean Baseline* (sem)	Change from Baseline** (sem)	Placebo Comparison (*P*-value)
CLARINEX 5.0 mg (171)	14.2 (0.3)	-4.3 (0.3)	*P*<0.01
Placebo (173)	13.7 (0.3)	-2.5 (0.3)	

* At baseline, a total nasal symptom score (sum of 4 individual symptoms) of at least 6 and a total non-nasal symptom score (sum of 4 individual symptoms) of at least 5 (each symptom scored 0 to 3 where 0=no symptom and 3=severe symptoms) was required for trial eligibility. TSS ranges from 0=no symptoms to 24=maximal symptoms.

**Mean reduction in TSS averaged over the 2-week treatment period.

In two 4-week studies of 924 patients (aged 15 to 75 years) with seasonal allergic rhinitis and concomitant asthma, CLARINEX Tablets 5 mg once daily improved rhinitis symptoms, with no decrease in pulmonary function. This supports the safety of administering CLARINEX Tablets to adult patients with seasonal allergic rhinitis with mild to moderate asthma.

Continued on next page

Clarinex—Cont.

CLARINEX Tablets 5 mg once daily significantly reduced the Total Symptom Scores (the sum of individual scores of nasal and non-nasal symptoms) in patients with seasonal allergic rhinitis. See Table 2.

[See table 2 at top of previous page]

There were no significant differences in the effectiveness of CLARINEX Tablets 5 mg across subgroups of patients defined by gender, age, or race.

Perennial Allergic Rhinitis: The clinical efficacy and safety of CLARINEX Tablets 5 mg were evaluated in over 1,300 patients 12 to 80 years of age with perennial allergic rhinitis. A total of 685 patients received 5 mg/day of CLARINEX in two double-blind, randomized, placebo-controlled clinical trials of 4 weeks' duration conducted in the United States and internationally. In one of these studies CLARINEX Tablets 5 mg once daily was shown to significantly reduce symptoms of perennial allergic rhinitis (Table 3).

[See table 3 at right]

Table 3
TOTAL SYMPTOM SCORE (TSS)
Changes in a 4-Week Clinical Trial in Patients with Perennial Allergic Rhinitis

Treatment Group (n)	Mean Baseline* (sem)	Change from Baseline** (sem)	Placebo Comparison (*P*-value)
CLARINEX 5.0 mg (337)	12.37 (0.18)	-4.06 (0.21)	*P*=0.01
Placebo (337)	12.30 (0.18)	-3.27 (0.21)	

* At baseline, average of total symptom score (sum of 5 individual nasal symptoms and 3 non-nasal symptoms, each symptom scored 0 to 3 where 0=no symptom and 3=severe symptoms) of at least 10 was required for trial eligibility. TSS ranges from 0=no symptoms to 24=maximal symptoms.
**Mean reduction in TSS averaged over the 4-week treatment period.

Chronic Idiopathic Urticaria: The efficacy and safety of CLARINEX Tablets 5 mg once daily was studied in 416 chronic idiopathic urticaria patients 12 to 84 years of age, of whom 211 received CLARINEX. In two double-blind, placebo-controlled, randomized clinical trials of six weeks' duration, at the pre-specified one-week primary time point evaluation, CLARINEX Tablets significantly reduced the severity of pruritus when compared to placebo (Table 4). Secondary endpoints were also evaluated and during the first week of therapy CLARINEX Tablets 5 mg reduced the secondary endpoints, "Number of Hives" and the "Size of the Largest Hive," when compared to placebo.

[See table 4 at right]

Table 4
PRURITUS SYMPTOM SCORE (TSS)
Changes in the First Week of a Clinical Trial in Patients with Chronic Idiopathic Urticaria

Treatment Group (n)	Mean Baseline (sem)	Change from Baseline* (sem)	Placebo Comparison (*P*-value)
CLARINEX 5.0 mg (115)	2.19 (0.04)	-1.05 (0.07)	*P*<0.01
Placebo (110)	2.21 (0.04)	-0.52 (0.07)	

Pruritus scored 0 to 3 where 0=no symptom to 3=maximal symptom
*Mean reduction in pruritus averaged over the first week of treatment.

The clinical safety of CLARINEX Syrup was documented in three, 15-day, double-blind, placebo-controlled safety studies in pediatric subjects with a documented history of allergic rhinitis, chronic idiopathic urticaria, or subjects who were candidates for antihistamine therapy. In the first study, 2.5 mg of CLARINEX Syrup was administered to 60 pediatric subjects 6 to 11 years of age. The second study evaluated 1.25 mg of CLARINEX Syrup administered to 55 pediatric subjects 2 to 5 years of age. In the third study, 1.25 mg of CLARINEX Syrup was administered to 65 pediatric subjects 12 to 23 months of age and 1.0 mg of CLARINEX Syrup was administered to 66 pediatric subjects 6 to 11 months of age. The results of these studies demonstrated the safety of CLARINEX Syrup in pediatric subjects 6 months to 11 years of age.

INDICATIONS AND USAGE

Seasonal Allergic Rhinitis: CLARINEX indicated for the relief of the nasal and non-nasal symptoms of seasonal allergic rhinitis in patients 2 years of age and older.

Perennial Allergic Rhinitis: CLARINEX is indicated for the relief of the nasal and non-nasal symptoms of perennial allergic rhinitis in patients 6 months of age and older.

Chronic Idiopathic Urticaria: CLARINEX is indicated for the symptomatic relief of pruritus, reduction in the number of hives, and size of hives, in patients with chronic idiopathic urticaria 6 months of age and older.

CONTRAINDICATIONS

CLARINEX Tablets 5 mg are contraindicated in patients who are hypersensitive to this medication or to any of its ingredients, or to loratadine.

PRECAUTIONS

Carcinogenesis, Mutagenesis, Impairment of Fertility: The carcinogenic potential of desloratadine was assessed using loratadine studies. In an 18-month study in mice and a 2-year study in rats, loratadine was administered in the diet at doses up to 40 mg/kg/day in mice (estimated desloratadine and desloratadine metabolite exposures were approximately 3 times the AUC in humans at the recommended daily oral dose) and 25 mg/kg/day in rats (estimated desloratadine and desloratadine metabolite exposures were approximately 30 times the AUC in humans at the recommended daily oral dose). Male mice given 40 mg/kg/day loratadine had a significantly higher incidence of hepatocellular tumors (combined adenomas and carcinomas) than concurrent controls. In rats, a significantly higher incidence of hepatocellular tumors (combined adenomas and carcinomas) was observed in males given 10 mg/kg/day and in males and females given 25 mg/kg/day. The estimated desloratadine and desloratadine metabolite exposures of rats given 10 mg/kg of loratadine were approximately 7 times the AUC in humans at the recommended daily oral dose. The clinical significance of these findings during long-term use of desloratadine is not known.

In genotoxicity studies with desloratadine, there was no evidence of genotoxic potential in a reverse mutation assay (*Salmonella*/*E. coli* mammalian microsome bacterial mutagenicity assay) or in two assays for chromosomal aberrations (human peripheral blood lymphocyte clastogenicity assay and mouse bone marrow micronucleus assay).

There was no effect on female fertility in rats at desloratadine doses up to 24 mg/kg/day (estimated desloratadine and desloratadine metabolite exposures were approximately 130 times the AUC in humans at the recommended daily oral dose). A male specific decrease in fertility, demonstrated by reduced female conception rates, decreased sperm numbers and motility, and histopathologic testicular changes, occurred at an oral desloratadine dose of 12 mg/kg in rats (estimated desloratadine exposures were approximately 45 times the AUC in humans at the recommended daily oral dose). Desloratadine had no effect on fertility in rats at an oral dose of 3 mg/kg/day (estimated desloratadine and desloratadine metabolite exposures were approximately 8 times the AUC in humans at the recommended daily oral dose).

Pregnancy Category C: Desloratadine was not teratogenic in rats at doses up to 48 mg/kg/day (estimated desloratadine and desloratadine metabolite exposures were approximately 210 times the AUC in humans at the recommended daily oral dose) or in rabbits at doses up to 60 mg/kg/day (estimated desloratadine exposures were approximately 230 times the AUC in humans at the recommended daily oral dose). In a separate study, an increase in pre-implantation loss and a decreased number of implantations and fetuses were noted in female rats at 24 mg/kg (estimated desloratadine and desloratadine metabolite exposures were approximately 120 times the AUC in humans at the recommended daily oral dose). Reduced body weight and slow righting reflex were reported in pups at doses of 9 mg/kg/day or greater (estimated desloratadine and desloratadine metabolite exposures were approximately 50 times or greater than the AUC in humans at the recommended daily oral dose). Desloratadine had no effect on pup development at an oral dose of 3 mg/kg/day (estimated desloratadine and desloratadine metabolite exposures were approximately 7 times the AUC in humans at the recommended daily oral dose). There are, however, no adequate and well-controlled studies in pregnant women. Because animal reproduction studies are not always predictive of human response, desloratadine should be used during pregnancy only if clearly needed.

Nursing Mothers: Desloratadine passes into breast milk, therefore a decision should be made whether to discontinue nursing or to discontinue desloratadine, taking into account the importance of the drug to the mother.

Pediatric Use: The recommended dose of CLARINEX Syrup in the pediatric population is based on cross-study comparison of the plasma concentration of CLARINEX in adults and pediatric subjects. The safety of CLARINEX Syrup has been established in 246 pediatric subjects aged 6 months to 11 years in three placebo-controlled clinical studies. Since the course of seasonal and perennial allergic rhinitis and chronic idiopathic urticaria and the effects of CLARINEX are sufficiently similar in the pediatric and adult populations, it allows extrapolation from the adult efficacy data to pediatric patients. The effectiveness of CLARINEX Syrup in these age groups is supported by evidence from adequate and well-controlled studies of CLARINEX Tablets in adults. The safety and effectiveness of CLARINEX Tablets or CLARINEX Syrup have not been demonstrated in pediatric patients less than 6 months of age.

Geriatric Use: Clinical studies of desloratadine did not include sufficient numbers of subjects aged 65 and over to determine whether they respond differently from younger subjects. Other reported clinical experience has not identified differences between the elderly and younger patients. In general, dose selection for an elderly patient should be cautious, reflecting the greater frequency of decreased hepatic, renal, or cardiac function, and of concomitant disease or other drug therapy (see **CLINICAL PHARMACOLOGY – Special Populations**).

Information for Patients: Patients should be instructed to use CLARINEX Tablets as directed. As there are no food effects on bioavailability, patients can be instructed that CLARINEX Tablets may be taken without regard to meals. Patients should be advised not to increase the dose or dosing frequency as studies have not demonstrated increased effectiveness at higher doses and somnolence may occur. Phenylketonurics: CLARINEX RediTabs Tablets contain phenylalanine 1.75 mg per tablet.

ADVERSE REACTIONS

Adults and Adolescents

Allergic Rhinitis: In multiple-dose placebo-controlled trials, 2,834 patients ages 12 years or older received CLARINEX Tablets at doses of 2.5 mg to 20 mg daily, of whom 1,655 patients received the recommended daily dose of 5 mg. In patients receiving 5 mg daily, the rate of adverse events was similar between CLARINEX and placebo-treated patients. The percent of patients who withdrew prematurely due to adverse events was 2.4% in the CLARINEX group and 2.6% in the placebo group. There were no serious adverse events in these trials in patients receiving desloratadine. All adverse events that were reported by greater than or equal to 2% of patients who received the recommended daily dose of CLARINEX Tablets (5.0 mg once-daily), and that were more common with CLARINEX Tablets than placebo, are listed in Table 5.

Table 5
Incidence of Adverse Events Reported by 2% or More of Adult and Adolescent Allergic Rhinitis Patients in Placebo-Controlled, Multiple-Dose Clinical Trials with the Tablet Formulation of CLARINEX

Adverse Experience	CLARINEX Tablets 5 mg (n=1,655)	Placebo (n=1,652)
Pharyngitis	4.1%	2.0%
Dry Mouth	3.0%	1.9%
Myalgia	2.1%	1.8%
Fatigue	2.1%	1.2%
Somnolence	2.1%	1.8%
Dysmenorrhea	2.1%	1.6%

The frequency and magnitude of laboratory and electrocardiographic abnormalities were similar in CLARINEX and placebo-treated patients.

There were no differences in adverse events for subgroups of patients as defined by gender, age, or race.

Chronic Idiopathic Urticaria: In multiple-dose, placebo-controlled trials of chronic idiopathic urticaria, 211 patients ages 12 years or older received CLARINEX Tablets and 205 received placebo. Adverse events that were reported by greater than or equal to 2% of patients who received CLARINEX Tablets and that were more common with CLARINEX than placebo were (rates for CLARINEX and placebo, respectively): headache (14%, 13%), nausea (5%, 2%), fatigue (5%, 1%), dizziness (4%, 3%), pharyngitis (3%, 2%), dyspepsia (3%, 1%), and myalgia (3%, 1%).

Pediatrics: Two hundred and forty-six pediatric subjects 6 months to 11 years of age received CLARINEX Syrup for 15 days in three placebo-controlled clinical trials. Pediatric subjects aged 6 to 11 years received 2.5 mg once a day, subjects aged 1 to 5 years received 1.25 mg once a day, and subjects 6 to 11 months of age received 1.0 mg once a day. In subjects 6 to 11 years of age, no individual adverse event was reported by 2 percent or more of the subjects. In subjects 2 to 5 years of age, adverse events reported for CLARINEX and placebo in at least 2 percent of subjects receiving CLARINEX Syrup and at frequency greater than placebo were fever (5.5%, 5.4%), urinary tract infection (3.6%, 0%) and varicella (3.6%, 0%). In subjects 12 months to 23 months of age, adverse events reported for the CLARINEX product and placebo in at least 2 percent of subjects receiving CLARINEX Syrup and at a frequency greater than placebo were fever (16.9%, 12.9%), diarrhea (15.4% 11.3%), upper respiratory tract infections (10.8%, 9.7%), coughing (10.8%, 6.5%), appetite increased (3.1%, 1.6%), emotional lability (3.1%, 0%), epistaxis (3.1%, 0%), parasitic infection, (3.1%, 0%) pharyngitis (3.1%, 0%), rash maculopapular (3.1%, 0%). In subjects 6 months to 11 months of age, adverse events reported for CLARINEX and placebo in at least 2 percent of subjects receiving CLARINEX Syrup and at a frequency greater than placebo were upper respiratory tract infections (21.2%, 12.9%), diarrhea (19.7% 8.1%), fever (12.1%, 1.6%), irritability (12.1%, 11.3%) coughing (10.6%, 9.7%), somnolence (9.1%, 8.1%), bronchitis (6.1%, 0%), otitis media (6.1%, 1.6%), vomiting (6.1%, 3.2%), anorexia (4.5%, 1.6%), pharyngitis (4.5%, 1.6%), insomnia (4.5%, 0%), rhinorrhea (4.5%, 3.2%), erythema (3.0%, 1.6%), and nausea (3.0%, 0%). There were no clinically meaningful changes in any electrocardiographic parameter, including the QTc interval. Only one of the 246 pediatric subjects receiving CLARINEX Syrup in the clinical trials discontinued treatment because of an adverse event.

Observed During Clinical Practice: The following spontaneous adverse events have been reported during the marketing of desloratadine: tachycardia, palpitations and rarely hypersensitivity reactions (such as rash, pruritus, urticaria, edema, dyspnea, and anaphylaxis), and elevated liver enzymes including bilirubin.

DRUG ABUSE AND DEPENDENCE

There is no information to indicate that abuse or dependency occurs with CLARINEX Tablets.

OVERDOSAGE

Information regarding acute overdosage is limited to experience from clinical trials conducted during the development of the CLARINEX product. In a dose ranging trial, at doses of 10 mg and 20 mg/day somnolence was reported.

Single daily doses of 45 mg were given to normal male and female volunteers for 10 days. All ECGs obtained in this study were manually read in a blinded fashion by a cardiologist. In CLARINEX-treated subjects, there was an increase in mean heart rate of 9.2 bpm relative to placebo. The QT interval was corrected for heart rate (QTc) by both the Bazett and Fridericia methods. Using the QTc (Bazett) there was a mean increase of 8.1 msec in CLARINEX-treated subjects relative to placebo. Using QTc (Fridericia) there was a mean increase of 0.4 msec in CLARINEX-treated subjects relative to placebo. No clinically relevant adverse events were reported.

In the event of overdose, consider standard measures to remove any unabsorbed drug. Symptomatic and supportive treatment is recommended. Desloratadine and 3-hydroxy-desloratadine are not eliminated by hemodialysis.

Lethality occurred in rats at oral doses of 250 mg/kg or greater (estimated desloratadine and desloratadine metabolite exposures were approximately 120 times the AUC in humans at the recommended daily oral dose). The oral median lethal dose in mice was 353 mg/kg (estimated desloratadine exposures were approximately 290 times the human daily oral dose on a mg/m^2 basis). No deaths occurred at oral doses up to 250 mg/kg in monkeys (estimated desloratadine exposures were approximately 810 times the human daily oral dose on a mg/m^2 basis).

DOSAGE AND ADMINISTRATION

Adults and children 12 years of age and over: the recommended dose of CLARINEX Tablets or CLARINEX RediTabs Tablets is one 5 mg tablet once daily or the recommended dose of CLARINEX Syrup is 2 teaspoonfuls (5 mg in 10 mL) once daily.

Children 6 to 11 years of age: The recommended dose of CLARINEX Syrup is 1 teaspoonful (2.5 mg in 5 mL) once daily.

Children 12 months to 5 years of age: The recommended dose of CLARINEX Syrup is ½ teaspoonful (1.25 mg in 2.5 mL) once daily.

Children 6 to 11 months of age: The recommended dose of CLARINEX Syrup is 2 mL (1.0 mg) once daily.

The age-appropriate dose of CLARINEX Syrup should be administered with a commercially available measuring dropper or syringe that is calibrated to deliver 2 mL and 2.5 mL (½ teaspoon).

In adult patients with liver or renal impairment, a starting dose of one 5 mg tablet every other day is recommended based on pharmacokinetic data. Dosing recommendation for children with liver or renal impairment cannot be made due to lack of data.

Administration of CLARINEX RediTabs Tablets: Place CLARINEX (desloratadine) RediTabs Tablets on the tongue. Tablet disintegration occurs rapidly. Administer with or without water. Take tablet immediately after opening the blister.

HOW SUPPLIED

CLARINEX Tablets: Embossed "C5", light blue film coated tablets; that are packaged in high-density polyethylene plastic bottles of 100 (NDC 0085-1264-01) and 500 (NDC 0085-1264-02). Also available, CLARINEX Unit-of-Use package of 30 tablets (3 × 10; 10 blisters per card) (NDC 0085-1264-04); and Unit Dose-Hospital Pack of 100 Tablets (10 × 10; 10 blisters per card) (NDC 0085-1264-03).

Protect Unit-of-Use packaging and Unit Dose-Hospital Pack from excessive moisture.

Store at 25°C (77°F); excursions permitted to 15-30°C (59-86°F) [see USP Controlled Room Temperature]

Heat Sensitive. Avoid exposure at or above 30°C (86°F).

CLARINEX Syrup: clear orange colored liquid containing 0.5 mg/1mL desloratadine in a 16-ounce Amber glass bottle (NDC 0085-1334-01).

Store syrup at 25°C (77°F); excursions permitted between 15-30°C (59-86°F) [see USP Controlled Room Temperature] Protect from light.

CLARINEX REDITABS (desloratadine orally-disintegrating tablets) 5 mg: "C" debossed, pink tablets in foil/foil blisters. Packs of 30 tablets (containing 3 × 10's) NDC 0085-1280-01.

Store at 25°C (77°F); excursions permitted to 15-30°C (59-86°F) [see USP Controlled Room Temperature]

Schering
Schering Corporation
Kenilworth, NJ 07033 USA
Rev. 8/04   23882167T
CLARINEX REDITABS brand of desloratadine orally-disintegrating tablets are manufactured for Schering Corporation by Cardinal Health UK. 416 Limited, England.
U.S. Patent Nos. 4,659,716; 4,804,666; 4,863,931; 5,595,997; and 6,100,274

INTRON® A ℞

[ĭn'trŏn]
Interferon alfa-2b, recombinant
For Injection

Prescribing information for this product, which appears on pages 3035–3044 of the 2005 PDR, has been completely revised as follows. Please write "See Supplement A" next to the product heading.

> **WARNING**
>
> Alpha interferons, including INTRON® A, cause or aggravate fatal or life-threatening neuropsychiatric, autoimmune, ischemic, and infectious disorders. Patients should be monitored closely with periodic clinical and laboratory evaluations. Patients with persistently severe or worsening signs or symptoms of these conditions should be withdrawn from therapy. In many but not all cases these disorders resolve after stopping INTRON A therapy. See **WARNINGS** and **ADVERSE REACTIONS**.

DESCRIPTION

INTRON A Interferon alfa-2b, recombinant for intramuscular, subcutaneous, intralesional, or intravenous Injection is a purified sterile recombinant interferon product.

Interferon alfa-2b, recombinant for Injection has been classified as an alfa interferon and is a water-soluble protein with a molecular weight of 19,271 daltons produced by recombinant DNA techniques. It is obtained from the bacterial fermentation of a strain of *Escherichia coli* bearing a genetically engineered plasmid containing an interferon alfa-2b gene from human leukocytes. The fermentation is carried out in a defined nutrient medium containing the antibiotic tetracycline hydrochloride at a concentration of 5 to 10 mg/L; the presence of this antibiotic is not detectable in the final product. The specific activity of Interferon alfa-2b, recombinant is approximately 2.6×10^8 IU/mg protein as measured by the HPLC assay.
[See first table below]

Prior to administration, the INTRON A Powder for Injection is to be with the provided Diluent for INTRON A Interferon alfa-2b, recombinant for Injection (Sterile Water for Injec-

tion, USP) (see **DOSAGE AND ADMINISTRATION**)
INTRON A Powder for Injection is a white to cream-colored powder.
[See second table below]
[See table at top of next page]

CLINICAL PHARMACOLOGY

General The interferons are a family of naturally occurring small proteins and glycoproteins with molecular weights of approximately 15,000 to 27,600 daltons produced and secreted by cells in response to viral infections and to synthetic or biological inducers.

Preclinical Pharmacology Interferons exert their cellular activities by binding to specific membrane receptors on the cell surface. Once bound to the cell membrane, interferons initiate a complex sequence of intracellular events. *In vitro* studies demonstrated that these include the induction of certain enzymes, suppression of cell proliferation, immunomodulating activities such as enhancement of the phagocytic activity of macrophages and augmentation of the specific cytotoxicity of lymphocytes for target cells, and inhibition of virus replication in virus-infected cells.

In a study using human hepatoblastoma cell line, HB 611, the *in vitro* antiviral activity of alfa interferon was demonstrated by its inhibition of hepatitis B virus (HBV) replication.

The correlation between these *in vitro* data and the clinical results is unknown. Any of these activities might contribute to interferon's therapeutic effects.

Pharmacokinetics The pharmacokinetics of INTRON A Interferon alfa-2b, recombinant for Injection were studied in 12 healthy male volunteers following single doses of 5 million IU/m^2 administered intramuscularly, subcutaneously, and as a 30-minute intravenous infusion in a crossover design.

The mean serum INTRON A concentrations following intramuscular and subcutaneous injections were comparable. The maximum serum concentrations obtained via these routes were approximately 18 to 116 IU/mL and occurred 3 to 12 hours after administration. The elimination half-life of INTRON A Interferon alfa-2b, recombinant for Injection following both intramuscular and subcutaneous injections was approximately 2 to 3 hours. Serum concentrations were undetectable by 16 hours after the injections.

After intravenous administration, serum INTRON A concentrations peaked (135 to 273 IU/mL) by the end of the 30-minute infusion, then declined at a slightly more rapid rate than after intramuscular or subcutaneous drug administration, becoming undetectable 4 hours after the infusion. The elimination half-life was approximately 2 hours.

Urine INTRON A concentrations following a single dose (5 million IU/m^2) were not detectable after any of the parenteral routes of administration. This result was expected since preliminary studies with isolated and perfused rabbit kidneys have shown that the kidney may be the main site of interferon catabolism.

There are no pharmacokinetic data available for the intralesional route of administration.

Serum Neutralizing Antibodies In INTRON A treated patients tested for antibody activity in clinical trials, serum anti-interferon neutralizing antibodies were detected in 0% (0/90) of patients with hairy cell leukemia, 0.8% (2/260) of patients treated intralesionally for condylomata acuminata, and 4% (1/24) of patients with AIDS-Related Kaposi's Sarcoma. Serum neutralizing antibodies have been detected in

Continued on next page

Powder for Injection

Vial Strength Million IU	mL Diluent	Final Concentration after Reconstitution million IU/mL*	mg INTRON A[†] Interferon alfa-2b, recombinant per vial	Route of Administration
10	1	10	0.038	IM, SC, IV, IL
18	1	18	0.069	IM, SC, IV
50	1	50	0.192	IM, SC, IV

*Each mL also contains 20 mg glycine, 2.3 mg sodium phosphate dibasic, 0.55 mg sodium phosphate monobasic, and 1.0 mg human albumin.
[†]Based on the specific activity of approximately 2.6×10^8 IU/mg protein, as measured by HPLC assay.

Solution Vials for Injection

Vial Strength	Concentration*	mg INTRON A[†] Interferon alfa-2b, recombinant per vial	Route of Administration
10 MIU single dose	10 million IU/1.0 mL	0.038	SC, IL
18[‡] MIU multidose	3 million IU/0.5 mL	0.088	IM, SC
25[¶] MIU multidose	5 million IU/0.5 mL	0.123	IM, SC, IL

*Each mL contains 7.5 mg sodium chloride, 1.8 mg sodium phosphate dibasic, 1.3 mg sodium phosphate monobasic, 0.1 mg edetate disodium, 0.1 mg polysorbate 80, and 1.5 mg m-cresol as a preservative.
[†] Based on the specific activity of approximately 2.6×10^8 IU/mg protein as measured by HPLC assay.
[‡] This is a multidose vial which contains a total of 22.8 million IU of interferon alfa-2b, recombinant per 3.8 mL in order to provide the delivery of six 0.5-mL doses, each containing 3 million IU of INTRON A Interferon alfa-2b, recombinant for Injection (for a label strength of 18 million IU).
[¶] This is a multidose vial which contains a total of 32.0 million IU of interferon alfa-2b, recombinant per 3.2 mL in order to provide the delivery of five 0.5-mL doses, each containing 5 million IU of INTRON A Interferon alfa-2b, recombinant for Injection (for a label strength of 25 million IU).

Intron A—Cont.

<3% of patients treated with higher INTRON A doses in malignancies other than hairy cell leukemia or AIDS-Related Kaposi's Sarcoma. The clinical significance of the appearance of serum anti-interferon neutralizing activity in these indications is not known.

Serum anti-interferon neutralizing antibodies were detected in 7% (12/168) of patients either during treatment or after completing 12 to 48 weeks of treatment with 3 million IU TIW of INTRON A therapy for chronic hepatitis C and in 13% (6/48) of patients who received INTRON A therapy for chronic hepatitis B at 5 million IU QD for 4 months, and in 3% (1/33) of patients treated at 10 million IU TIW. Serum anti-interferon neutralizing antibodies were detected in 9% (5/53) of pediatric patients who received INTRON A therapy for chronic hepatitis B at 6 million IU/m² TIW. Among all chronic hepatitis B or C patients, pediatric and adults with detectable serum neutralizing antibodies, the titers detected were low (22/24 with titers ≤1:40 and 2/24 with titers ≤1:160). The appearance of serum anti-interferon neutralizing activity did not appear to affect safety or efficacy.

Hairy Cell Leukemia In clinical trials in patients with hairy cell leukemia, there was depression of hematopoiesis during the first 1 to 2 months of INTRON A treatment, resulting in reduced numbers of circulating red and white blood cells, and platelets. Subsequently, both splenectomized and nonsplenectomized patients achieved substantial and sustained improvements in granulocytes, platelets, and hemoglobin levels in 75% of treated patients and at least some improvement (minor responses) occurred in 90%. INTRON A treatment resulted in a decrease in bone marrow hypercellularity and hairy cell infiltrates. The hairy cell index (HCI), which represents the percent of bone marrow cellularity times the percent of hairy cell infiltrate, was ≥50% at the beginning of the study in 87% of patients. The percentage of patients with such an HCI decreased to 25% after 6 months and to 14% after 1 year. These results indicate that even though hematologic improvement had occurred earlier, prolonged INTRON A treatment may be required to obtain maximal reduction in tumor cell infiltrates in the bone marrow.

The percentage of patients with hairy cell leukemia who required red blood cell or platelet transfusions decreased significantly during treatment and the percentage of patients with confirmed and serious infections declined as granulocyte counts improved. Reversal of splenomegaly and of clinically significant hypersplenism was demonstrated in some patients.

A study was conducted to assess the effects of extended INTRON A treatment on duration of response for patients who responded to initial therapy. In this study, 126 responding patients were randomized to receive additional INTRON A treatment for 6 months or observation for a comparable period, after 12 months of initial INTRON A therapy. During this 6-month period, 3% (2/66) of INTRON A treated patients relapsed compared with 18% (11/60) who were not treated. This represents a significant difference in time to relapse in favor of continued INTRON A treatment (p=0.006/0.01, Log Rank/Wilcoxon). Since a small proportion of the total population had relapsed, median time to relapse could not be estimated in either group. A similar pattern in relapses was seen when all randomized treatment, including that beyond 6 months, and available follow-up data were assessed. The 15% (10/66) relapses among INTRON A patients occurred over a significantly longer period of time than the 40% (24/60) with observation (p=0.0002/0.0001, Log Rank/Wilcoxon). Median time to relapse was estimated, using the Kaplan-Meier method, to be 6.8 months in the observation group but could not be estimated in the INTRON A group.

Subsequent follow-up with a median time of approximately 40 months demonstrated an overall survival of 87.8%. In a comparable historical control group followed for 24 months, overall median survival was approximately 40%.

Malignant Melanoma The safety and efficacy of INTRON A Interferon alfa-2b, recombinant for Injection was evaluated as adjuvant to surgical treatment in patients with melanoma who were free of disease (post surgery) but at high risk for systemic recurrence. These included patients with lesions of Breslow thickness >4 mm, or patients with lesions of any Breslow thickness with primary or recurrent nodal involvement. In a randomized, controlled trial in 280 patients, 143 patients received INTRON A therapy at 20 million IU/m² intravenously five times per week for 4 weeks (induction phase) followed by 10 million IU/m² subcutaneously three times per week for 48 weeks (maintenance phase). In the clinical trial, the median daily INTRON A dose administered to patients was 19.1 million IU/m² during the induction phase and 9.1 million IU/m² during the maintenance phase. INTRON A therapy was begun ≤56 days after surgical resection. The remaining 137 patients were observed.

INTRON A therapy produced a significant increase in relapse-free and overall survival. Median time to relapse for the INTRON A treated patients vs observation patients was 1.72 years vs 0.98 years (p<0.01, stratified Log Rank). The estimated 5-year relapse-free survival rate, using the Kaplan-Meier method, was 37% for INTRON A treated patients vs 26% for observation patients. Median overall survival time for INTRON A treated patients vs observation patients was 3.82 years vs 2.78 years (p=0.047, stratified Log Rank). The estimated 5-year overall survival rate, using the Kaplan-Meier method, was 46% for INTRON A treated patients vs 37% for observation patients.

Solution in Multidose Pens for Injection

Pen Strength	Concentration* million IU/1.5 mL	INTRON A Dose Delivered (6 doses, 0.2 mL each)	mg INTRON A† Interferon alfa-2b, recombinant per 1.5 mL	Route of Administration
3 MIU	22.5	3 MIU/0.2 mL	0.087	SC
5 MIU	37.5	5 MIU/0.2 mL	0.144	SC
10 MIU	75	10 MIU/0.2 mL	0.288	SC

*Each mL also contains 7.5 mg sodium chloride, 1.8 mg sodium phosphate dibasic, 1.3 mg sodium phosphate monobasic, 0.1 mg edetate disodium, 0.1 mg polysorbate 80, and 1.5 mg m-cresol as a preservative.

† Based on the specific activity of approximately 2.6×10^8 IU/mg protein as measured by HPLC assay. These packages do not require reconstitution prior to administration (see **DOSAGE AND ADMINISTRATION**) INTRON A Solution for Injection is a clear, colorless solution.

In a second study of 642 resected high-risk melanoma patients, subjects were randomized equally to one of three groups: high-dose INTRON A therapy for 1 year (same schedule as above), low-dose INTRON A therapy for 2 years (3 MU/d TIW SC), and observation. Consistent with the earlier trial, high-dose INTRON A therapy demonstrated an improvement in relapse-free survival (3-year estimated RFS 48% vs 41%; median RFS 2.4 vs 1.6 years, p=not significant). Relapse-free survival in the low-dose INTRON A arm was similar to that seen in the observation arm. Neither high-dose nor low-dose INTRON A therapy showed a benefit in overall survival as compared to observation in this study.

Follicular Lymphoma The safety and efficacy of INTRON A in conjunction with CHVP, a combination chemotherapy regimen, was evaluated as initial treatment in patients with clinically aggressive, large tumor burden, Stage III/IV follicular Non-Hodgkin's Lymphoma. Large tumor burden was defined by the presence of any one of the following: a nodal or extranodal tumor mass with a diameter of >7 cm; involvement of at least three nodal sites (each with a diameter of >3 cm); systemic symptoms; splenomegaly; serous effusion, orbital or epidural involvement; ureteral compression; or leukemia.

In a randomized, controlled trial, 130 patients received CHVP therapy and 135 patients received CHVP therapy plus INTRON A therapy at 5 million IU subcutaneously three times weekly for the duration of 18 months. CHVP chemotherapy consisted of cyclophosphamide 600 mg/m², doxorubicin 25 mg/m², and teniposide (VM-26) 60 mg/m², administered intravenously on Day 1 and prednisone at a daily dose of 40 mg/m² given orally on Days 1 to 5. Treatment consisted of six CHVP cycles administered monthly, followed by an additional six cycles administered every 2 months for 1 year. Patients in both treatment groups received a total of 12 CHVP cycles over 18 months.

The group receiving the combination of INTRON A therapy plus CHVP had a significantly longer progression-free survival (2.9 years vs 1.5 years, p=0.0001, Log Rank test). After a median follow-up of 6.1 years, the median survival for patients treated with CHVP alone was 5.5 years while median survival for patients treated with CHVP plus INTRON A therapy had not been reached (p=0.004, Log Rank test). In three additional published, randomized, controlled studies of the addition of interferon alfa to anthracycline-containing combination chemotherapy regimens,[1-3] the addition of interferon alfa was associated with significantly prolonged progression-free survival. Differences in overall survival were not consistently observed.

Condylomata Acuminata Condylomata acuminata (venereal or genital warts) are associated with infections of the human papilloma virus (HPV). The safety and efficacy of INTRON A Interferon alfa-2b, recombinant for Injection in the treatment of condylomata acuminata were evaluated in three controlled double-blind clinical trials. In these studies, INTRON A doses of 1 million IU per lesion were administered intralesionally three times a week (TIW), in ≤5 lesions per patient for 3 weeks. The patients were observed for up to 16 weeks after completion of the full treatment course.

INTRON A treatment of condylomata was significantly more effective than placebo, as measured by disappearance of lesions, decreases in lesion size, and by an overall change in disease status. Of 192 INTRON A treated patients and 206 placebo treated patients who were evaluable for efficacy at the time of best response during the course of the study, 42% of INTRON A patients vs 17% of placebo patients experienced clearing of all treated lesions. Likewise, 24% of INTRON A patients vs 8% of placebo patients experienced marked (≥75% to <100%) reduction in lesion size, 18% vs 9% experienced moderate (≥50% to ≤75%) reduction in lesion size, 10% vs 42% had a slight (<50%) reduction in lesion size, 5% vs 24% had no change in lesion size, and 0% vs 1% experienced exacerbation (p<0.001).

In one of these studies, 43% (54/125) of patients in whom multiple (≤3) lesions were treated, experienced complete clearing of all treated lesions during the course of the study. Of these patients, 81% remained cleared 16 weeks after treatment was initiated.

Patients who did not achieve total clearing of all their treated lesions had these same lesions treated with a second course of therapy. During this second course of treatment, 38% to 67% of patients had clearing of all treated lesions. The overall percentage of patients who had cleared all their treated lesions after two courses of treatment ranged from 57% to 85%.

INTRON A treated lesions showed improvement within 2 to 4 weeks after the start of treatment in the above study; maximal response to INTRON A therapy was noted 4 to 8 weeks after initiation of treatment.

The response to INTRON A therapy was better in patients who had condylomata for shorter durations than in patients with lesions for a longer duration.

Another study involved 97 patients in whom three lesions were treated with either an intralesional injection of 1.5 million IU of INTRON A Interferon alfa-2b, recombinant for Injection per lesion followed by a topical application of 25% podophyllin, or a topical application of 25% podophyllin alone. Treatment was given once a week for 3 weeks. The combined treatment of INTRON A Interferon alfa-2b, recombinant for Injection and podophyllin was shown to be significantly more effective than podophyllin alone, as determined by the number of patients whose lesions cleared. This significant difference in response was evident after the second treatment (Week 3) and continued through 8 weeks posttreatment. At the time of the patient's best response, 67% (33/49) of the INTRON A Interferon alfa-2b, recombinant for Injection and podophyllin treated patients had all three treated lesions clear while 42% (20/48) of the podophyllin treated patients had all three clear (p=0.003).

AIDS-Related Kaposi's Sarcoma The safety and efficacy of INTRON A Interferon alfa-2b, recombinant for Injection in the treatment of Kaposi's Sarcoma (KS), a common manifestation of the Acquired Immune Deficiency Syndrome (AIDS), were evaluated in clinical trials in 144 patients.

In one study, INTRON A doses of 30 million IU/m² were administered subcutaneously three times per week (TIW), to patients with AIDS-Related KS. Doses were adjusted for patient tolerance. The average weekly dose delivered in the first 4 weeks was 150 million IU; at the end of 12 weeks this averaged 110 million IU/week; and by 24 weeks averaged 75 million IU/week.

Forty-four percent of asymptomatic patients responded vs 7% of symptomatic patients. The median time to response was approximately 2 months and 1 month, respectively, for asymptomatic and symptomatic patients. The median duration of response was approximately 3 months and 1 month, respectively, for the asymptomatic and symptomatic patients. Baseline T4/T8 ratios were 0.46 for responders vs 0.33 for nonresponders.

In another study, INTRON A doses of 35 million IU were administered subcutaneously, daily (QD), for 12 weeks. Maintenance treatment, with every other day dosing (QOD), was continued for up to 1 year in patients achieving antitumor and antiviral responses. The median time to response was 2 months and the median duration of response was 5 months in the asymptomatic patients.

In all studies, the likelihood of response was greatest in patients with relatively intact immune systems as assessed by baseline CD4 counts (interchangeable with T4 counts). Results at doses of 30 million IU/m² TIW and 35 million IU/QD were subcutaneously similar and are provided together in TABLE 1. This table demonstrates the relationship of response to baseline CD4 count in both asymptomatic and symptomatic patients in the 30 million IU/m² TIW and the 35 million IU/QD treatment groups.

In the 30 million IU study group, 7% (5/72) of patients were complete responders and 22% (16/72) of the patients were partial responders. The 35 million IU study had 13% (3/23 patients) complete responders and 17% (4/23) partial responders.

For patients who received 30 million IU TIW, the median survival time was longer in patients with CD4 >200 (30.7 months) than in patients with CD4 ≤200 (8.9 months). Among responders, the median survival time was 22.6 months vs 9.7 months in nonresponders.

TABLE 1
*RESPONSE BY BASELINE CD4 COUNT**
IN AIDS-RELATED KS PATIENTS
30 million IU/m²
TIW, SC and 35 million IU QD, SC

	Asymptomatic			Symptomatic	
CD4<200	4/14	(29%)		0/19	(0%)
200≤CD4≤400	6/12	(50%)	} 58%	0/5	(0%)
CD4>400	5/7	(71%)		0/0	(0%)

*Data for CD4, and asymptomatic and symptomatic classification were not available for all patients.

Chronic Hepatitis C The safety and efficacy of INTRON A Interferon alfa-2b, recombinant for Injection in the treatment of chronic hepatitis C was evaluated in 5 randomized clinical studies in which an INTRON A dose of 3 million IU three times a week (TIW) was assessed. The initial three studies were placebo-controlled trials that evaluated a 6-month (24 week) course of therapy. In each of the three studies, INTRON A therapy resulted in a reduction in serum alanine aminotransferase (ALT) in a greater proportion of patients vs control patients at the end of 6 months of dosing. During the 6 months of follow-up, approximately 50% of the patients who responded maintained their ALT response. A combined analysis comparing pretreatment and posttreatment liver biopsies revealed histological improvement in a statistically significantly greater proportion of INTRON A treated patients compared to controls.

Two additional studies have investigated longer treatment durations (up to 24 months).[5,6] Patients in the two studies to evaluate longer duration of treatment had hepatitis with or without cirrhosis in the absence of decompensated liver disease. Complete response to treatment was defined as normalization of the final two serum ALT levels during the treatment period. A sustained response was defined as a complete response at the end of the treatment period with sustained normal ALT values lasting at least 6 months following discontinuation of therapy.

In Study 1, all patients were initially treated with INTRON A 3 million IU TIW subcutaneously for 24 weeks (run-in-period). Patients who completed the initial 24-week treatment period were then randomly assigned to receive no further treatment, or to receive 3 million IU TIW for an additional 48 weeks. In Study 2, patients who met the entry criteria were randomly assigned to receive INTRON A 3 million IU TIW subcutaneously for 24 weeks or to receive INTRON A 3 million IU TIW subcutaneously for 96 weeks. In both studies, patient follow-up was variable and some data collection was retrospective.

Results show that longer durations of INTRON A therapy improved the sustained response rate (see TABLE 2). In patients with complete responses (CR) to INTRON A therapy after 6 months of treatment (149/352 [42%]), responses were less often sustained if drug was discontinued (21/70 [30%]) than if it was continued for 18 to 24 months (44/79 [56%]). Of all patients randomized, the sustained response rate in the patients receiving 18 or 24 months of therapy was 22% and 26%, respectively, in the two trials. In patients who did not have a CR by 6 months, additional therapy did not result in significantly more responses, since almost all patients who responded to therapy did so within the first 16 weeks of treatment.

A subset (<50%) of patients from the combined extended dosing studies had liver biopsies performed both before and after INTRON A treatment. Improvement in necroinflammatory activity as assessed retrospectively by the Knodell (Study 1) and Scheuer (Study 2) Histology Activity Indices was observed in both studies. A higher number of patients (58%, 45/78) improved with extended therapy than with shorter (6 months) therapy (38%, 34/89) in this subset.

REBETRON® Combination Therapy containing INTRON A and REBETOL® (ribavirin, USP) Capsules has been shown to provide a significant reduction in virologic load and improved histologic response in patients with compensated liver disease who have relapsed following therapy with alfa interferon alone and in patients previously untreated with alfa interferon. See REBETRON Combination Therapy package insert for additional information.

[See table 2 above]

Chronic Hepatitis B ***Adults*** The safety and efficacy of INTRON A Interferon alfa-2b, recombinant for Injection in the treatment of chronic hepatitis B were evaluated in three clinical trials in which INTRON A doses of 30 to 35 million IU per week were administered subcutaneously (SC), as either 5 million IU daily (QD), or 10 million IU three times a week (TIW) for 16 weeks vs no treatment. All patients were 18 years of age or older with compensated liver disease, and had chronic hepatitis B virus (HBV) infection (serum HBsAg positive for at least 6 months) and HBV replication (serum HBeAg positive). Patients were also serum HBV-DNA positive, an additional indicator of HBV replication, as measured by a research assay.[7,8] All patients had elevated serum alanine aminotransferase (ALT) and liver biopsy findings compatible with the diagnosis of chronic hepatitis. Patients with the presence of antibody to human immunodeficiency virus (anti-HIV) or antibody to hepatitis delta virus (anti-HDV) in the serum were excluded from the studies.

Virologic response to treatment was defined in these studies as a loss of serum markers of HBV replication (HBeAg and HBV DNA). Secondary parameters of response included loss of serum HBsAg, decreases in serum ALT, and improvement in liver histology.

In each of two randomized controlled studies, a significantly greater proportion of INTRON A treated patients exhibited a virologic response compared with untreated control patients (see TABLE 3). In a third study without a concurrent control group, a similar response rate to INTRON A therapy was observed. Pretreatment with prednisone, evaluated in two of the studies, did not improve the response rate and provided no additional benefit.

The response to INTRON A therapy was durable. No patient responding to INTRON A therapy at a dose of 5 million IU QD or 10 million IU TIW, relapsed during the follow-up period which ranged from 2 to 6 months after treatment ended. The loss of serum HBeAg and HBV DNA was maintained in 100% of 19 responding patients followed for 3.5 to 36 months after the end of therapy.

TABLE 2
SUSTAINED ALT RESPONSE RATE VS DURATION OF THERAPY
IN **CHRONIC HEPATITIS C** *PATIENTS*
INTRON A 3 Million IU TIW
Treatment Group—Number of Patients (%)*

Study Number	*INTRON A 3 million IU 24 weeks of treatment*		*INTRON A 3 million IU 72 or 96 weeks of treatment*†		*Difference (Extended– 24 weeks) (95% CI)*‡	
			ALT response at the end of follow-up			
1	12/101	(12%)	23/104	(22%)	10%	(-3, 24)
2	9/67	(13%)	21/80	(26%)	13%	(-4, 30)
Combined Studies	**21/168**	**(12.5%)**	**44/184**	**(24%)**	**11.4%**	**(2, 21)**
			ALT response at the end of treatment			
1	40/101	(40%)	51/104	(49%)	—	
2	32/67	(48%)	35/80	(44%)	—	

*Intent to treat groups.
† Study 1: 72 weeks of treatment; Study 2: 96 weeks of treatment.
‡ Confidence intervals adjusted for multiple comparisons due to 3 treatment arms in the study.

TABLE 3
*VIROLOGIC RESPONSE**
IN **CHRONIC HEPATITIS B** *PATIENTS*
Treatment Group†—Number of Patients (%)

Study Number	*INTRON A 5 million IU QD*		*INTRON A 10 million IU TIW*		*Untreated Controls*		*P‡ Value*
1[7]	15/38	(39%)	—	—	3/42	(7%)	0.0009
2	—	—	10/24	(42%)	1/22	(5%)	0.005
3[8]	—	—	13/24§	(54%)	2/27	(7%)§	NA§
All Studies	**15/38**	**(39%)**	**23/48**	**(48%)**	**6/91**	**(7%)**	—

*Loss of HBeAg and HBV DNA by 6 months posttherapy.
† Patients pretreated with prednisone not shown.
‡ INTRON A treatment group vs untreated control.
§ Untreated control patients evaluated after 24-week observation period. A subgroup subsequently received INTRON A therapy. A direct comparison is not applicable (NA).

TABLE 4
*ALT RESPONSES**
IN **CHRONIC HEPATITIS B** *PATIENTS*
Treatment Group—Number of Patients (%)

Study Number	*INTRON A 5 million IU QD*		*INTRON A 10 million IU TIW*		*Untreated Controls*		*P† Value*
1	16/38	(42%)	—	—	8/42	(19%)	0.03
2	—	—	10/24	(42%)	1/22	(5%)	0.0034
3	—	—	12/24‡	(50%)	2/27	(7%)‡	NA‡
All Studies	**16/38**	**(42%)**	**22/48**	**(46%)**	**11/91**	**(12%)**	—

*Reduction in serum ALT to normal by 6 months posttherapy.
† INTRON A treatment group vs untreated control.
‡ Untreated control patients evaluated after 24-week observation period. A subgroup subsequently received INTRON A therapy. A direct comparison is not applicable (NA).

In a proportion of responding patients, loss of HBeAg was followed by the loss of HBsAg. HBsAg was lost in 27% (4/15) of patients who responded to INTRON A therapy at a dose of 5 million IU QD, and 35% (8/23) of patients who responded to 10 million IU TIW. No untreated control patient lost HBsAg in these studies.

[See table 3 above]

In an ongoing study to assess the long-term durability of virologic response, 64 patients responding to INTRON A therapy have been followed for 1.1 to 6.6 years after treatment; 95% (61/64) remain serum HBeAg negative and 49% (30/61) lost serum HBsAg.

INTRON A therapy resulted in normalization of serum ALT in a significantly greater proportion of treated patients compared to untreated patients in each of two controlled studies (see TABLE 4). In a third study without a concurrent control group, normalization of serum ALT was observed in 50% (12/24) of patients receiving INTRON A therapy.

Virologic response was associated with a reduction in serum ALT to normal or near normal ($\leq 1.5 \times$ the upper limit of normal) in 87% (13/15) of patients responding to INTRON A therapy at 5 million IU QD, and 100% (23/23) of patients responding to 10 million IU TIW.

Improvement in liver histology was evaluated in Studies 1 and 3 by comparison of pretreatment and 6-month posttreatment liver biopsies using the semiquantitative Knodell Histology Activity Index.[9] No statistically significant difference in liver histology was observed in treated patients compared to control patients in Study 1. Although statistically significant histological improvement from baseline was observed in treated patients in Study 3 ($p \leq 0.01$), there was no control group for comparison. Of those patients exhibiting a virologic response following treatment with 5 million IU QD or 10 million IU TIW, histological improvement was observed in 85% (17/20) compared to 36% (9/25) of patients who were not virologic responders. The histological improvement was due primarily to decreases in severity of necrosis, degeneration, and inflammation in the periportal, lobular, and portal regions of the liver (Knodell Categories I + II + III). Continued histological improvement was observed in four responding patients who lost serum HBsAg and were followed 2 to 4 years after the end of INTRON A therapy.[10]

Pediatrics The safety and efficacy of INTRON A Interferon alfa-2b, recombinant for Injection in the treatment of chronic hepatitis B was evaluated in one randomized controlled trial of 149 patients ranging from 1 year to 17 years of age. Seventy-two patients were treated with 3 million IU/m^2 of INTRON A therapy administered subcutaneously three times a week (TIW) for 1 week: the dose was then escalated to 6 million IU/m^2 TIW for a minimum of 16 weeks up to 24 weeks. The maxiumum weekly dosage was 10 million IU TIW. Seventy-seven patients were untreated controls. Study entry and response criteria were identical to those described in the adult patient population.

Patients treated with INTRON A therapy had a better response (loss of HBV DNA and HBeAg at 24 weeks of follow-up) compared to the untreated controls (24% [17/72] vs 10% [8/77] p=0.05). Sixteen of the 17 responders treated with INTRON A therapy remained HBV DNA and HBeAg negative and had a normal serum ALT 12 to 24 months after completion of treatment. Serum HBsAg became negative in 7 out of 17 patients who responded to INTRON A therapy. None of the control patients who had an HBV DNA and HBeAg response became HBsAg negative. At 24 weeks of follow-up, normalization of serum ALT was similar in patients treated with INTRON A therapy (17%, 12/72) and in untreated control patients (16%, 12/77). Patients with a baseline HBV DNA <100 pg/mL were more likely to respond to INTRON A therapy than were patients with a baseline HBV DNA >100 pg/mL (35% vs 9%, respectively). Patients who contracted hepatitis B through maternal vertical transmission had lower response rates than those who contracted the disease by other means (5% vs 31%, respectively). There was no evidence that the effects on HBV DNA and HBeAg were limited to specific subpopulations based on age, gender, or race.

[See table 4 above]

INDICATIONS AND USAGE

Hairy Cell Leukemia INTRON A Interferon alfa-2b, recombinant for Injection is indicated for the treatment of patients 18 years of age or older with hairy cell leukemia.

Malignant Melanoma INTRON A Interferon alfa-2b, recombinant for Injection is indicated as adjuvant to surgical treatment in patients 18 years of age or older with malignant melanoma who are free of disease but at high risk for systemic recurrence, within 56 days of surgery.

Follicular Lymphoma INTRON A Interferon alfa-2b, recombinant for Injection is indicated for the initial treatment of clinically aggressive (see **Clinical Experience**) follicular Non-Hodgkin's Lymphoma in conjunction with anthracycline-containing combination chemotherapy in patients 18 years of age or older. Efficacy of INTRON A therapy in pa-

Continued on next page

Intron A—Cont.

tients with low-grade, low-tumor burden follicular Non-Hodgkin's Lymphoma has not been demonstrated.

Condylomata Acuminata INTRON A Interferon alfa-2b, recombinant for Injection is indicated for intralesional treatment of selected patients 18 years of age or older with condylomata acuminata involving external surfaces of the genital and perianal areas (see **DOSAGE AND ADMINISTRATION**).

The use of this product in adolescents has not been studied.

AIDS-Related Kaposi's Sarcoma INTRON A Interferon alfa-2b, recombinant for Injection is indicated for the treatment of selected patients 18 years of age or older with AIDS-Related Kaposi's Sarcoma. The likelihood of response to INTRON A therapy is greater in patients who are without systemic symptoms, who have limited lymphadenopathy and who have a relatively intact immune as indicated by total CD4 count.

Chronic Hepatitis C INTRON A Interferon alfa-2b, recombinant for Injection is indicated for the treatment of chronic hepatitis C in patients 18 years of age or older with compensated liver disease who have a history of blood or blood-product exposure and/or are HCV antibody positive. Studies in these patients demonstrated that INTRON A therapy can produce clinically meaningful effects on this disease, manifested by normalization of serum alanine aminotransferase (ALT) and reduction in liver necrosis and degeneration.

A liver biopsy should be performed to establish the diagnosis of chronic hepatitis. Patients should be tested for the presence of antibody to HCV. Patients with other causes of chronic hepatitis, including autoimmune hepatitis, should be excluded. Prior to initiation of INTRON A therapy, the physician should establish that the patient has compensated liver disease. The following patient entrance criteria for compensated liver disease were used in the clinical studies and should be considered before INTRON A treatment of patients with chronic hepatitis C:

- No history of hepatic encephalopathy, variceal bleeding, ascites, or other clinical signs of decompensation
- Bilirubin $\leq$2 mg/dL
- Albumin Stable and within normal limits
- Prothrombin Time <3 seconds prolonged
- WBC $\geq$3000/mm^3
- Platelets $\geq$70,000/mm^3

Serum creatinine should be normal or near normal.

Prior to initiation of INTRON A therapy, CBC and platelet counts should be evaluated in order to establish baselines for monitoring potential toxicity. These tests should be repeated at Weeks 1 and 2 following initiation of INTRON A therapy, and monthly thereafter. Serum ALT should be evaluated at approximately 3-month intervals to assess response to treatment (see **DOSAGE AND ADMINISTRATION**).

Patients with preexisting thyroid abnormalities may be treated if thyroid-stimulating hormone (TSH) levels can be maintained in the normal range by medication. TSH levels must be within normal limits upon initiation of INTRON A treatment and TSH testing should be repeated at 3 and 6 months (see **PRECAUTIONS – Laboratory Tests**).

INTRON A in combination with REBETOL (ribavirin, USP) Capsules is indicated for the treatment of chronic hepatitis C in patients with compensated liver disease previously untreated with alfa interferon therapy or who have relapsed following alfa interferon therapy. See REBETRON Combination Therapy package insert for additional information.

Chronic Hepatitis B INTRON A Interferon alfa-2b, recombinant for Injection is indicated for the treatment of chronic hepatitis B in patients 1 year of age or older with compensated liver disease. Patients who have been serum HBsAg positive for at least 6 months and have evidence of HBV replication (serum HBeAg positive) with elevated serum ALT are candidates for treatment. Studies in these patients demonstrated that INTRON A therapy can produce virologic remission of this disease (loss of serum HBeAg), and normalization of serum aminotransferases. INTRON A therapy resulted in the loss of serum HBsAg in some responding patients.

Prior to initiation of INTRON A therapy, it is recommended that a liver biopsy be performed to establish the presence of chronic hepatitis and the extent of liver damage. The physician should establish that the patient has compensated liver disease. The following patient entrance criteria for compensated liver disease were used in the clinical studies and should be considered before INTRON A treatment of patients with chronic hepatitis B:

- No history of hepatic encephalopathy, variceal bleeding, ascites, or other signs of clinical decompensation

• Bilirubin	Normal	
• Albumin	Stable and within normal limits	
• Prothrombin Time	*Adults* <3 seconds prolonged	*Pediatrics* $\leq$2 seconds prolonged
• WBC	$\geq$4000/mm^3	
• Platelets	*Adults* $\geq$100,000/mm^3	*Pediatrics* $\geq$150,000/mm^3

Patients with causes of chronic hepatitis other than chronic hepatitis B or chronic hepatitis C should not be treated with INTRON A Interferon alfa-2b, recombinant for Injection. CBC and platelet counts should be evaluated prior to initiation of INTRON A therapy in order to establish baselines for monitoring potential toxicity. These tests should be repeated at treatment Weeks 1, 2, 4, 8, 12, and 16. Liver function tests, including serum ALT, albumin, and bilirubin, should be evaluated at treatment Weeks 1, 2, 4, 8, 12, and 16. HBeAg, HBsAg, and ALT should be evaluated at the end of therapy, as well as 3- and 6-months posttherapy, since patients may become virologic responders during the 6-month period following the end of treatment. In clinical studies in adults, 39% (15/38) of responding patients lost HBeAg 1 to 6 months following end of INTRON A therapy. Of responding patients who lost HBsAg, 58% (7/12) did so 1- to 6-months posttreatment.

A transient increase in ALT $\geq$2 × baseline value (flare) can occur during INTRON A therapy for chronic hepatitis B. In clinical trials in adults and pediatrics, this flare generally occurred 8 to 12 weeks after initiation of therapy and was more frequent in INTRON A responders (*adults* 63%, 24/38; *pediatrics* 59%, 10/17) than in nonresponders (*adults* 27%, 13/48; *pediatrics* 35%, 19/55). However, in adults and pediatrics, elevations in bilirubin $\geq$3 mg/dL ($\geq$2 times ULN) occurred infrequently (*adults* 2%, 2/86; *pediatrics* 3%, 2/72) during therapy. When ALT flare occurs, in general, INTRON A therapy should be continued unless signs and symptoms of liver failure are observed. During ALT flare, clinical symptomatology and liver function tests including ALT, prothrombin time, alkaline phosphatase, albumin, and bilirubin, should be monitored at approximately 2-week intervals (see **WARNINGS**).

CONTRAINDICATIONS

INTRON A Interferon alfa-2b, recombinant for Injection is contraindicated in patients with a history of hypersensitivity to interferon alfa or any component of the injection. REBETRON Combination Therapy containing INTRON A and REBETOL (ribavirin, USP) Capsules must not be used by women who are pregnant or by men whose female partners are pregnant. Extreme care must be taken to avoid pregnancy in female patients and in female partners of patients taking combination INTRON A/REBETOL therapy. Patients with autoimmune hepatitis must not be treated with combination INTRON A/REBETOL therapy. See REBETRON Combination Therapy package insert for additional information.

WARNINGS

General Moderate to severe adverse experiences may require modification of the patient's dosage regimen, or in some cases termination of INTRON A therapy. Because of the fever and other "flu-like" symptoms associated with INTRON A administration, it should be used cautiously in patients with debilitating medical conditions, such as those with a history of pulmonary disease (eg, chronic obstructive pulmonary disease), or diabetes mellitus prone to ketoacidosis. Caution should also be observed in patients with coagulation disorders (eg, thrombophlebitis, pulmonary embolism) or severe myelosuppression.

INTRON A therapy should be used cautiously in patients with a history of cardiovascular disease. Those patients with a history of myocardial infarction and/or previous or current arrhythmic disorder who require INTRON A therapy should be closely monitored (see **Laboratory Tests**). Cardiovascular adverse experiences, which include hypotension, arrhythmia, or tachycardia of 150 beats per minute or greater, and rarely, cardiomyopathy and myocardial infarction have been observed in some INTRON A treated patients. Some patients with these adverse events had no history of cardiovascular disease. Transient cardiomyopathy was reported in approximately 2% of the AIDS-Related Kaposi's Sarcoma patients treated with INTRON A Interferon alfa-2b, recombinant for Injection. Hypotension may occur during INTRON A administration, or up to 2 days post-therapy, and may require supportive therapy including fluid replacement to maintain intravascular volume.

Supraventricular arrhythmias occurred rarely and appeared to be correlated with preexisting conditions and prior therapy with cardiotoxic agents. These adverse experiences were controlled by modifying the dose or discontinuing treatment, but may require specific additional therapy. DEPRESSION AND SUICIDAL BEHAVIOR INCLUDING SUICIDAL IDEATION, SUICIDAL ATTEMPTS, AND COMPLETED SUICIDES HAVE BEEN REPORTED IN ASSOCIATION WITH TREATMENT WITH ALFA INTERFERONS, INCLUDING INTRON A THERAPY. Patients with a preexisting psychiatric condition, especially depression, or a history of severe psychiatric disorder should not be treated with INTRON A Interferon alfa-2b, recombinant for Injection.[11] INTRON A therapy should be discontinued for any patient developing severe depression or other psychiatric disorder during treatment. Obtundation and coma have also been observed in some patients, usually elderly, treated at higher doses. While these effects are usually rapidly reversible upon discontinuation of therapy, full resolution of symptoms has taken up to 3 weeks in a few severe episodes. Narcotics, hypnotics, or sedatives may be used concurrently with caution and patients should be closely monitored until the adverse effects have resolved.

Bone marrow toxicity INTRON A therapy suppresses bone marrow function and may result in severe cytopenias including very rare events of aplastic anemia. It is advised that complete blood counts (CBC) be obtained pretreatment and monitored routinely during therapy (see **PRECAUTIONS: Laboratory Tests**). INTRON A therapy should be discontinued in patients who develop severe decreases in neutrophil (<0.5 × 10^9/L) or platelet counts (<25 × 10^9/L) (see **DOSAGE AND ADMINISTRATION**: Guidelines for Dose Modification).

Ophthalmologic Disorders Decrease or loss of vision, retinopathy including macular edema, retinal artery or vein thrombosis, retinal hemorrhages and cotton wool spots; optic neuritis and papilledema may be induced or aggravated by treatment with Interferon alfa-2b or other alpha interferons. All patients should receive an eye examination at baseline. Patients with preexisting ophthalmologic disorders (eg, diabetic or hypertensive retinopathy) should receive periodic ophthalmologic exams during interferon alpha treatment. Any patient who develops ocular symptoms should receive a prompt and complete eye examination. Interferon alfa-2b treatment should be discontinued in patients who develop new or worsening ophthalmologic disorders.

Infrequently, patients receiving INTRON A therapy developed thyroid abnormalities, either hypothyroid or hyperthyroid. The mechanism by which INTRON A Interferon alfa-2b, recombinant for Injection may alter thyroid status is unknown. Patients with preexisting thyroid abnormalities whose thyroid function cannot be maintained in the normal range by medication should not be treated with INTRON A Interferon alfa-2b, recombinant for Injection. Prior to initiation of INTRON A therapy, serum TSH should be evaluated. Patients developing symptoms consistent with possible thyroid dysfunction during the course of INTRON A therapy should have their thyroid function evaluated and appropriate treatment instituted. Therapy should be discontinued for patients developing thyroid abnormalities during treatment whose thyroid function cannot be normalized by medication. Discontinuation of INTRON A therapy has not always reversed thyroid dysfunction occurring during treatment.

Hepatotoxicity, including fatality, has been observed in interferon alfa treated patients, including those treated with INTRON A Interferon alfa-2b, recombinant for Injection. Any patient developing liver function abnormalities during treatment should be monitored closely and if appropriate, treatment should be discontinued.

Pulmonary infiltrates, pneumonitis and pneumonia, including fatality, have been observed in interferon alfa treated patients, including those treated with INTRON A Interferon alfa-2b, recombinant for Injection. The etiologic explanation for these pulmonary findings has yet to be established. Any patient developing fever, cough, dyspnea, or other respiratory symptoms should have a chest x-ray taken. If the chest x-ray shows pulmonary infiltrates or there is evidence of pulmonary function impairment, the patient should be closely monitored, and, if appropriate, interferon alfa treatment should be discontinued. While this has been reported more often in patients with chronic hepatitis C treated with interferon alfa, it has also been reported in patients with oncologic diseases treated with interferon alfa.

Rare cases of autoimmune diseases including thrombocytopenia, vasculitis, Raynaud's phenomenon, rheumatoid arthritis, lupus erythematosus, and rhabdomyolysis have been observed in patients treated with alfa interferons, including patients treated with INTRON A Interferon alfa-2b, recombinant for Injection. In very rare cases the event resulted in fatality. The mechanism by which these events develop and their relationship to interferon alfa therapy is not clear. Any patient developing an autoimmune disorder during treatment should be closely monitored and, if appropriate, treatment should be discontinued.

Diabetes mellitus and hyperglycemia have been observed rarely in patients treated with INTRON A Interferon alfa-2b, recombinant for Injection. Symptomatic patients should have their blood glucose measured and followed up accordingly. Patients with diabetes mellitus may require adjustment of their antidiabetic regimen.

The powder formulations of this product contain albumin, a derivative of human blood. Based on effective donor screening and product manufacturing processes, it carries an extremely remote risk for transmission of viral diseases. A theoretical risk for transmission of Creutzfeldt-Jakob disease (CJD) also is considered extremely remote. No cases of transmission of viral diseases or CJD have ever been identified for albumin.

AIDS-Related Kaposi's Sarcoma INTRON A therapy should not be used for patients with rapidly progressive visceral disease (see **CLINICAL PHARMACOLOGY**). Also of note, there may be synergistic adverse effects between INTRON A Interferon alfa-2b, recombinant for Injection and zidovudine. Patients receiving concomitant zidovudine have had a higher incidence of neutropenia than that expected with zidovudine alone. Careful monitoring of the WBC count is indicated in all patients who are myelosuppressed and in all patients receiving other myelosuppressive medications. The effects of INTRON A Interferon alfa-2b, recombinant for Injection when combined with other drugs used in the treatment of AIDS-Related disease are unknown.

Chronic Hepatitis C and Chronic Hepatitis B Patients with decompensated liver disease, autoimmune hepatitis or a history of autoimmune disease, and patients who are immunosuppressed transplant recipients should not be treated with INTRON A Interferon alfa-2b, recombinant for Injection. There are reports of worsening liver disease, including jaundice, hepatic encephalopathy, hepatic failure, and death following INTRON A therapy in such patients. Therapy should be discontinued for any patient developing signs and symptoms of liver failure.

Chronic hepatitis B patients with evidence of decreasing hepatic synthetic functions, such as decreasing albumin levels or prolongation of prothrombin time, who nevertheless meet the entry criteria to start therapy, may be at increased risk of clinical decompensation if a flare of aminotransferases occurs during INTRON A treatment. In such patients, if increases in ALT occur during INTRON A therapy for chronic hepatitis B, they should be followed carefully including

TREATMENT-RELATED ADVERSE EXPERIENCES BY INDICATION
Dosing Regimens
Percentage (%) of Patients*

ADVERSE EXPERIENCE	MALIGNANT MELANOMA 20 MIU/m² Induction (IV) / 10 MIU/m² Maintenance (SC)	FOLLICULAR LYMPHOMA 5 MIU TIW/SC	HAIRY CELL LEUKEMIA 2 MIU/m² TIW/SC	CONDYLOMATA ACUMINATA 1 MIU/lesion	AIDS-RELATED KAPOSI'S SARCOMA 30 MIU/m² TIW/SC	AIDS-RELATED KAPOSI'S SARCOMA 35 MIU QD/SC	CHRONIC HEPATITIS C‖ 3 MIU TIW	CHRONIC HEPATITIS B Adults 5 MIU QD	CHRONIC HEPATITIS B Adults 10 MIU TIW	CHRONIC HEPATITIS B Pediatrics 6 MIU/m² TIW
	N=143	N=135	N=145	N=352	N=74	N=29	N=183	N=101	N=78	N=116
Application-Site Disorders										
injection site inflammation	—	1	20	—	—	—	5	3	—	—
other (≤5%)	burning, injection site bleeding, injection site pain, injection site reaction (5% in chronic hepatitis B pediatrics), itching									
Blood Disorders (<5%)	anemia, anemia hypochromic, granulocytopenia, hemolytic anemia, leukopenia, lymphocytosis, neutropenia (9% in chronic hepatitis C, 14% in chronic hepatitis B pediatrics), thrombocytopenia (10% in chronic hepatitis C) (bleeding 8% in malignant melanoma), thrombocytopenic purpura									
Body as a Whole										
facial edema	—	1	—	<1	—	10	<1	3	1	<1
weight decrease	3	13	<1	<1	—	5	3	2	5	3
other (≤5%)	allergic reaction, cachexia, dehydration, earache, hernia, edema, hypercalcemia, hyperglycemia, hypothermia, inflammation nonspecific, lymphadenitis, lymphadenopathy, mastitis, periorbital edema, poor peripheral circulation, peripheral edema (6% in follicular lymphoma), phlebitis superficial, scrotal/penile edema, thirst, weakness, weight increase									
Cardiovascular System Disorders (<5%)	angina, arrhythmia, atrial fibrillation, bradycardia, cardiac failure, cardiomegaly, cardiomyopathy, coronary artery disorder, extrasystoles, heart valve disorder, hematoma, hypertension (9% in chronic hepatitis C), hypotension, palpitations, phlebitis, postural hypotension, pulmonary embolism, Raynaud's disease, tachycardia, thrombosis, varicose vein									
Endocrine System Disorders (<5%)	aggravation of diabetes mellitus, goiter, gynecomastia, hyperglycemia, hyperthyroidism, hypertriglyceridemia, hypothyroidism, virilism									
Flu-like Symptoms										
fever	81	56	68	56	47	55	34	66	86	94
headache	62	21	39	47	36	21	43	61	44	57
chills	54	—	46	45	—	—	43	61	44	57
myalgia	75	16	39	44	34	28	43	59	40	27
fatigue	96	8	61	18	84	48	23	75	69	71
increased sweating	6	13	8	2	4	21	4	1	1	3
asthenia	—	63	7	—	11	—	40	5	15	5
rigors	2	7	—	—	30	14	16	38	42	30
arthralgia	6	8	8	9	—	3	16	19	8	15
dizziness	23	—	12	9	7	24	9	13	10	8
influenza-like symptoms	10	18	37	—	45	79	26	5	—	<1
back pain	—	15	19	—	6	3	—	—	—	—
dry mouth	1	2	19	—	22	28	5	6	5	—
chest pain	2	8	<1	<1	1	28	4	4	—	—
malaise	6	—	—	14	5	—	13	9	6	3
pain (unspecified)	15	9	18	3	3	3	—	—	—	—
other (<5%)	chest pain substernal, hyperthermia, rhinitis, rhinorrhea									
Gastrointestinal System Disorders										
diarrhea	35	19	18	2	18	45	13	19	8	12
anorexia	69	21	19	1	38	41	14	43	53	43
nausea	66	24	21	17	28	21	19	50	33	18
taste alteration	24	2	13	<1	5	7	2	10	—	—
abdominal pain	2	20	<5	1	5	21	16	5	4	23
loose stools	—	1	—	<1	—	10	2	2	—	2
vomiting	†	32	6	2	11	14	8	7	10	27
constipation	1	14	<1	—	1	10	4	5	—	2
gingivitis	2‡	7‡	—	—	—	14	—	1	—	—
dyspepsia	—	2	—	2	4	—	7	3	8	3
other (<5%)	abdominal ascites, abdominal distension, colitis, dysphagia, eructation, esophagitis, flatulence, gallstones, gastric ulcer, gastritis, gastroenteritis, gastrointestinal disorder (7% in follicular lymphoma), gastrointestinal hemorrhage, gastrointestinal mucosal discoloration, gingival bleeding, gum hyperplasia, halitosis, hemorrhoids, increased appetite, increased saliva, intestinal disorder, melena, mouth ulceration, mucositis, oral hemorrhage, oral leukoplakia, rectal bleeding after stool, rectal hemorrhage, stomatitis, stomatitis ulcerative, taste loss, tongue disorder, tooth disorder									
Liver and Biliary System Disorders (<5%)	abnormal hepatic function tests, biliary pain, bilirubinemia, hepatitis, increased lactate dehydrogenase, increased transaminases (SGOT/SGPT) (elevated SGOT 63% in malignant melanoma and 24% in follicular lymphoma), jaundice, right upper quadrant pain (15% in chronic hepatitis C), and very rarely, hepatic encephalopathy, hepatic failure, and death									

(Table continued on next page)

---

close monitoring of clinical symptomatology and liver function tests, including ALT, prothrombin time, alkaline phosphatase, albumin, and bilirubin. In considering these patients for INTRON A therapy, the potential risks must be evaluated against the potential benefits of treatment.

REBETRON Combination Therapy containing INTRON A and REBETOL (ribavirin, USP) Capsules was associated with hemolytic anemia. Hemoglobin <10 g/dL was observed in approximately 10% of patients in clinical trials. Anemia occurred within 1 to 2 weeks of initiation of ribavirin therapy. REBETRON Combination Therapy containing INTRON A and REBETOL is not recommended in patients with severe renal impairment and should be used with caution in patients with moderate renal impairment. See REBETRON Combination Therapy package insert for additional information.

PRECAUTIONS
General Acute serious hypersensitivity reactions (eg, urticaria, angioedema, bronchoconstriction, anaphylaxis) have been observed rarely in INTRON A treated patients; if such an acute reaction develops, the drug should be discontinued immediately and appropriate medical therapy instituted. Transient rashes have occurred in some patients following injection, but have not necessitated treatment interruption. While fever may be related to the flu-like syndrome reported commonly in patients treated with interferon, other causes of persistent fever should be ruled out.

There have been reports of interferon, including INTRON A Interferon alfa-2b, recombinant for Injection, exacerbating preexisting psoriasis and sarcoidosis as well as development of new sarcoidosis. Therefore, INTRON A therapy should be used in these patients only if the potential benefit justifies the potential risk.

Variations in dosage, routes of administration, and adverse reactions exist among different brands of interferon. Therefore, do not use different brands of interferon in any single treatment regimen.

Triglycerides Elevated triglyceride levels have been observed in patients treated with interferons including INTRON A therapy. Elevated triglyceride levels should be managed as clinically appropriate. Hypertriglyceridemia may result in pancreatitis. Discontinuation of INTRON A therapy should be considered for patients with persistently elevated triglycerides (eg, triglycerides >1000 mg/dL) associated with symptoms of potential pancreatitis, such as abdominal pain, nausea, or vomiting.

Drug Interactions Interactions between INTRON A Interferon alfa-2b, recombinant for Injection and other drugs have not been fully evaluated. Caution should be exercised when administering INTRON A therapy in combination with other potentially myelosuppressive agents such as zidovudine. Concomitant use of alfa interferon and theophylline decreases theophylline clearance, resulting in a 100% increase in serum theophylline levels.

Information for Patients Patients receiving INTRON A alone or in combination with REBETOL should be informed of the risks and benefits associated with treatment and should be instructed on proper use of the product. To supplement your discussion with a patient, you may wish to provide patients with a copy of the **MEDICATION GUIDE**.

Patients should be informed of, and advised to seek medical attention for symptoms indicative of serious adverse reactions associated with this product. Such adverse reactions may include depression (suicidal ideation), cardiovascular (chest pain), ophthalmologic toxicity (decrease in/or loss of vision), pancreatitis or colitis (severe abdominal pain) and cytopenias (high persistent fevers, bruising, dypsnea). Patients should be advised that some side effects such as fatigue and decreased concentration might interfere with the ability to perform certain tasks. Patients who are taking INTRON A in combination with REBETOL must be thoroughly informed of the risks to a fetus. Female patients and female partners of male patients must be told to use two forms of birth control during treatment and for six months after therapy is discontinued (see **MEDICATION GUIDE**).

Patients should be advised to remain well hydrated during the initial stages of treatment and that use of an antipyretic may ameliorate some of the flu-like symptoms.

If a decision is made to allow a patient to self-administer INTRON A, a puncture resistant container for the disposal of needles and syringes should be supplied. Patients self-

Continued on next page

TREATMENT-RELATED ADVERSE EXPERIENCES BY INDICATION (cont.)
Dosing Regimens
Percentage (%) of Patients*

ADVERSE EXPERIENCE	Malignant Melanoma 20 MIU/m² Induction (IV) 10 MIU/m² Maintenance (SC)	Follicular Lymphoma 5 MIU TIW/SC	Hairy Cell Leukemia 2 MIU/m² TIW/SC	Condylomata Acuminata 1 MIU/lesion	AIDS-Related Kaposi's Sarcoma 30 MIU/m² TIW/SC	AIDS-Related Kaposi's Sarcoma 35 MIU QD/SC	Chronic Hepatitis C[||] 3 MIU TIW	Chronic Hepatitis B Adults 5 MIU QD	Chronic Hepatitis B Adults 10 MIU TIW	Chronic Hepatitis B Pediatrics 6 MIU/m² TIW
	N=143	N=135	N=145	N=352	N=74	N=29	N=183	N=101	N=78	N=116
Musculoskeletal System Disorders										
musculoskeletal pain	—	18	—	—	—	—	21	9	1	10
other (<5%)	arteritis, arthritis, arthritis aggravated, arthrosis, bone disorder, bone pain, carpal tunnel syndrome, hyporeflexia, leg cramps, muscle atrophy, muscle weakness, polyarteritis nodosa, tendinitis, rheumatoid arthritis, spondylitis									
Nervous System and Psychiatric Disorders										
depression	40	9	6	3	9	28	19	17	6	4
paresthesia	13	13	6	1	3	21	5	6	3	<1
impaired concentration	—	1	—	<1	3	14	3	8	5	3
amnesia	§	1	<5	—	—	14	—	—	—	2
confusion	8	2	<5	4	12	10	1	—	—	—
hypoesthesia	—	1	<5	1	—	10	—	—	—	—
irritability	1	1	—	—	—	—	13	16	12	22
somnolence	1	2	<5	3	3	—	33¶	14	9	5
anxiety	1	9	5	<1	1	3	5	2	—	3
insomnia	5	4	—	<1	3	3	12	11	6	8
nervousness	1	1	—	1	—	3	2	3	—	3
decreased libido	1	1	<5	—	—	—	1	5	1	—
other (<5%)	abnormal coordination, abnormal dreaming, abnormal gait, abnormal thinking, aggravated depression, aggressive reaction, agitation (7% in chronic hepatitis B pediatrics) alcohol intolerance, apathy, aphasia, ataxia, Bell's palsy, CNS dysfunction, coma, convulsions, delirium, dysphonia, emotional lability, extrapyramidal disorder, feeling of ebriety, flushing, hearing disorder, hearing impairment, hot flashes, hyperesthesia, hyperkinesia, hypertonia, hypokinesia, impaired consciousness, labyrinthine disorder, loss of consciousness, manic depression, manic reaction, migraine, neuralgia, neuritis, neuropathy, neurosis, paresis, paroniria, parosmia, personality disorder, polyneuropathy, psychosis, speech disorder, stroke, suicidal ideation, suicide attempt, syncope, tinnitus, tremor, twitching, vertigo (8% in follicular lymphoma)									
Reproduction System Disorders (<5%)	amenorrhea (12% in follicular lymphoma), dysmenorrhea, impotence, leukorrhea, menorrhagia, menstrual irregularity, pelvic pain, penis disorder, sexual dysfunction, uterine bleeding, vaginal dryness									
Resistance Mechanism Disorders										
moniliasis	—	1	—	<1	—	17	—	—	—	—
herpes simplex	1	2	—	3	—	3	1	5	—	—
other (<5%)	abscess, conjunctivitis, fungal infection, hemophilus, herpes zoster, infection, infection bacterial, infection nonspecific (7% in follicular lymphoma), infection parasitic, otitis media, sepsis, stye, trichomonas, upper respiratory tract infection, viral infection (7% in chronic hepatitis C)									
Respiratory System Disorders										
dyspnea	15	14	<1	—	1	34	3	5	—	—
coughing	6	13	<1	—	—	31	1	4	—	5
pharyngitis	2	8	<5	1	1	31	3	7	1	7
sinusitis	1	4	—	—	—	21	2	—	—	—
nonproductive coughing	2	7	—	—	—	14	0	1	—	—
nasal congestion	1	7	—	—	1	10	<1	4	—	—
other (≤5%)	asthma, bronchitis (10% in follicular lymphoma), bronchospasm, cyanosis, epistaxis (7% in chronic hepatitis B pediatrics), hemoptysis, hypoventilation, laryngitis, lung fibrosis, pleural effusion, orthopnea, pleural pain, pneumonia, pneumonitis, pneumothorax, rales, respiratory disorder, respiratory insufficiency, sneezing, tonsillitis, tracheitis, wheezing									
Skin and Appendages Disorders										
dermatitis	1	—	8	—	—	—	2	1	—	—
alopecia	29	23	8	—	12	31	28	26	38	17
pruritus	—	10	11	1	7	—	9	6	4	3
rash	19	13	25	—	9	10	5	8	1	5
dry skin	1	3	9	—	9	10	4	3	—	<1
other (<5%)	abnormal hair texture, acne, cellulitis, cyanosis of the hand, cold and clammy skin, dermatitis lichenoides, eczema, epidermal necrolysis, erythema, erythema nodosum, folliculitis, furunculosis, increased hair growth, lacrimal gland disorder, lacrimation, lipoma, maculopapular rash, melanosis, nail disorders, nonherpetic cold sores, pallor, peripheral ischemia, photosensitivity, pruritus genital, psoriasis, psoriasis aggravated, purpura (5% in chronic hepatitis C), rash erythematous, sebaceous cyst, skin depigmentation, skin discoloration, skin nodule, urticaria, vitiligo									
Urinary System Disorders (<5%)	albumin/protein in urine, cystitis, dysuria, hematuria, incontinence, increased BUN, micturition disorder, micturition frequency, nocturia, polyuria (10% in follicular lymphoma), renal insufficiency, urinary tract infection (5% in chronic hepatitis C)									
Vision Disorders (<5%)	abnormal vision, blurred vision, diplopia, dry eyes, eye pain, nystagmus, photophobia									

* Dash (—) indicates not reported
[†] Vomiting was reported with nausea as a single term
[‡] Includes stomatitis/mucositis
[§] Amnesia was reported with confusion as a single term
[||] Percentages based upon a summary of all adverse events during 18 to 24 months of treatment
[¶] Predominantly lethargy

Intron A—Cont.

administering INTRON A should be instructed on the proper disposal of needles and syringes and cautioned against reuse.

Laboratory Tests In addition to those tests normally required for monitoring patients, the following laboratory tests are recommended for all patients on INTRON A therapy, prior to beginning treatment and then periodically thereafter.

- Standard hematologic tests – including hemoglobin, complete and differential white blood cell counts, and platelet count.
- Blood chemistries – electrolytes, liver function tests, and TSH.

Those patients who have preexisting cardiac abnormalities and/or are in advanced stages of cancer should have electrocardiograms taken prior to and during the course of treatment.

Mild-to-moderate leukopenia and elevated serum liver enzyme (SGOT) levels have been reported with intralesional administration of INTRON A Interferon alfa-2b, recombinant for Injection (see **ADVERSE REACTIONS**); therefore, the monitoring of these laboratory parameters should be considered.

Baseline chest x-rays are suggested and should be repeated if clinically indicated.

For malignant melanoma patients, differential WBC count and liver function tests should be monitored weekly during the induction phase of therapy and monthly during the maintenance phase of therapy.

For specific recommendations in chronic hepatitis C and chronic hepatitis B, see **INDICATIONS AND USAGE**.

Carcinogenesis, Mutagenesis, Impairment of Fertility Studies with INTRON A Interferon alfa-2b, recombinant for Injection have not been performed to determine carcinogenicity.

Interferon may impair fertility. In studies of interferon administration in nonhuman primates, menstrual cycle abnormalities have been observed. Decreases in serum estradiol and progesterone concentrations have been reported in women treated with human leukocyte interferon.[12] Therefore, fertile women should not receive INTRON A therapy unless they are using effective contraception during the therapy period. INTRON A therapy should be used with caution in fertile men.

Mutagenicity studies have demonstrated that INTRON A Interferon alfa-2b, recombinant for Injection is not mutagenic.

Studies in mice (0.1, 1.0 million IU/day), rats (4, 20, 100 million IU/kg/day), and cynomolgus monkeys (1.1 million IU/kg/day; 0.25, 0.75, 2.5 million IU/kg/day) injected with INTRON A Interferon alfa-2b, recombinant for Injection for up to 9 days, 3 months, and 1 month, respectively, have revealed no evidence of toxicity. However, in cynomolgus monkeys (4, 20, 100 million IU/kg/day) injected daily for 3 months with INTRON A Interferon alfa-2b, recombinant for Injection toxicity was observed at the mid and high doses and mortality was observed at the high dose.

However, due to the known species-specificity of interferon, the effects in animals are unlikely to be predictive of those in man.

INTRON A in combination with REBETOL (ribavirin, USP) Capsules should be used with caution in fertile men. See the REBETRON Combination Therapy package insert for additional information.

Pregnancy Category C INTRON A Interferon alfa-2b, recombinant for Injection has been shown to have abortifacient effects in *Macaca mulatta* (rhesus monkeys) at 15 and

ABNORMAL LABORATORY TEST VALUES BY INDICATION
Dosing Regimens
Percentage (%) of Patients

	Malignant Melanoma	Follicular Lymphoma	Hairy Cell Leukemia	Condylomata Acuminata	AIDS-Related Kaposi's Sarcoma		Chronic Hepatitis C	Chronic Hepatitis B		
								Adults		Pediatrics
	20 MIU/m² Induction (IV) 10 MIU/m² Maintenance (SC)	*5 MIU TIW/SC*	*2 MIU/m² TIW/SC*	*1 MIU/ lesion*	*30 MIU/m² TIW/SC*	*35 MIU QD/SC*	*3 MIU TIW*	*5 MIU QD*	*10 MIU TIW*	*6 MIU/m² TIW*
Laboratory Tests	N=143	N=135	N=145	N=352	N=69–73	N=26–28	N=140–171	N=96–101	N=75–103	N=113–115
Hemoglobin	22	8	NA	—	1	15	26¶	32*	23*	17**
White Blood Cell Count	‖	—	NA	17	10	22	26†	68†	34†	9†
Platelet Count	15	13	NA	—	0	8	15‡	12‡	5‡	1‡
Serum Creatinine	3	2	0	—	—	—	6	3	0	3
Alkaline Phosphatase	13	—	4	—	—	—	—	8	4	0
Lactate Dehydrogenase	1	—	0	—	—	—	—	—	—	—
Serum Urea Nitrogen	12	4	0	—	—	—	—	2	0	2
SGOT	63	24	4	12	11	41	—	—	—	—
SGPT	2	—	13	—	10	15	—	—	—	—
Granulocyte Count										
• Total	92	36	NA	—	31	39	45§	75§	61§	70§
• 1000 –<1500/mm³	66	—	—	—	—	—	32	30	32	43
• 750 –<1000/mm³	—	21	—	—	—	—	10	24	18	18
• 500 –<750/mm³	25	—	—	—	—	—	1	17	9	7
• <500/mm³	1	13	—	—	—	—	2	4	2	2

NA—Not Applicable—Patients' initial hematologic laboratory test values were abnormal due to their condition.
* Decrease of ≥2 g/dL
**Decrease of ≥2 g/dL; 14% 2–<3 g/dL; 3%≥3g/dL
† Decrease to <3000/mm³
‡ Decrease to <70,000/mm³
§ Neutrophils plus bands
‖ White Blood Cell Count was reported as neutropenia
¶ Decrease of ≥2 g/dL; 20% 2–<3 g/dL; 6% ≥3 g/dL

30 million IU/kg (estimated human equivalent of 5 and 10 million IU/kg, based on body surface area adjustment for a 60-kg adult). There are no adequate and well-controlled studies in pregnant women. INTRON A therapy should be used during pregnancy only if the potential benefit justifies the potential risk to the fetus.

Pregnancy Category X applies to REBETRON Combination Therapy containing INTRON A and REBETOL (ribavirin, USP) Capsules (see **CONTRAINDICATIONS**). See REBETRON Combination Therapy package insert for additional information.

Nursing Mothers It is not known whether this drug is excreted in human milk. However, studies in mice have shown that mouse interferons are excreted into the milk. Because of the potential for serious adverse reactions from the drug in nursing infants, a decision should be made whether to discontinue nursing or to discontinue INTRON A therapy, taking into account the importance of the drug to the mother.

Pediatric Use *General* Safety and effectiveness in pediatric patients below the age of 18 years have not been established for indications other than chronic hepatitis B.

Chronic Hepatitis B Safety and effectiveness in pediatric patients ranging in age from 1 to 17 years have been established based upon one controlled clinical trial (see **CLINICAL PHARMACOLOGY, INDICATIONS AND USAGE, DOSAGE AND ADMINISTRATION; Chronic Hepatitis B**). Safety and effectiveness in pediatric patients below the age of 1 year have not been established.

Geriatric Use In all clinical studies of INTRON A (Interferon alfa-2b, recombinant), including studies as monotherapy and in combination with REBETOL (ribavirin, USP) Capsules, only a small percentage of the subjects were aged 65 and over. These numbers were too few to determine if they respond differently from younger subjects except for the clinical trials of INTRON A in combination with REBETOL, where elderly subjects had a higher frequency of anemia (67%) than did younger patients (28%).

In a database consisting of clinical study and postmarketing reports for various indications, cardiovascular adverse events and confusion were reported more frequently in elderly patients receiving INTRON A therapy compared to younger patients.

In general, INTRON A therapy should be administered to elderly patients cautiously, reflecting the greater frequency of decreased hepatic, renal, bone marrow, and/or cardiac function and concomitant disease or other drug therapy. INTRON A is known to be substantially excreted by the kidney, and the risk of adverse reactions to INTRON A may be greater in patients with impaired renal function. Because elderly patients often have decreased renal function, patients should be carefully monitored during treatment, and dose adjustments made based on symptoms and/or laboratory abnormalities (see **CLINICAL PHARMACOLOGY**, and **DOSAGE AND ADMINISTRATION**).

ADVERSE REACTIONS

General The adverse experiences listed below were reported to be possibly or probably related to INTRON A therapy during clinical trials. Most of these adverse reactions were mild to moderate in severity and were manageable. Some were transient and most diminished with continued therapy.

The most frequently reported adverse reactions were "flu-like" symptoms, particularly fever, headache, chills, myalgia, and fatigue. More severe toxicities are observed generally at higher doses and may be difficult for patients to tolerate.

In addition, the following spontaneous adverse experiences have been reported during the marketing surveillance of INTRON A Interferon alfa-2b, recombinant for Injection: nephrotic syndrome, pancreatitis, psychosis, including hallucinations, renal failure, and renal insufficiency. Very rarely, INTRON A used alone or in combination with REBETOL (ribavirin, USP) Capsules may be associated with aplastic anemia. Rarely sarcoidosis or exacerbation of sarcoidosis has been reported.

[See table on pages 387 and 388]

Hairy Cell Leukemia The adverse reactions most frequently reported during clinical trials in 145 patients with hairy cell leukemia were the "flu-like" symptoms of fever (68%), fatigue (61%), and chills (46%).

Malignant Melanoma The INTRON A dose was modified because of adverse events in 65% (n=93) of the patients. INTRON A therapy was discontinued because of adverse events in 8% of the patients during induction and 18% of the patients during maintenance. The most frequently reported adverse reaction was fatigue which was observed in 96% of patients. Other adverse reactions that were recorded in >20% of INTRON A treated patients included neutropenia (92%), fever (81%), myalgia (75%), anorexia (69%), vomiting/nausea (66%), increased SGOT (63%), headache (62%), chills (54%), depression (40%), diarrhea (35%), alopecia (29%), altered taste sensation (24%), dizziness/vertigo (23%), and anemia (22%).

Adverse reactions classified as severe or life threatening (ECOG Toxicity Criteria grade 3 or 4) were recorded in 66% and 14% of INTRON A treated patients, respectively. Severe adverse reactions recorded in >10% of INTRON A treated patients included neutropenia/leukopenia (26%), fatigue (23%), fever (18%), myalgia (17%), headache (17%), chills (16%), and increased SGOT (14%). Grade 4 fatigue was recorded in 4% and grade 4 depression was recorded in 2% of INTRON A treated patients. No other grade 4 AE was reported in more than 2 INTRON A treated patients. Lethal hepatotoxicity occurred in 2 INTRON A treated patients early in the clinical trial. No subsequent lethal hepatotoxicities were observed with adequate monitoring of liver function tests (see **PRECAUTIONS – Laboratory Tests**).

Follicular Lymphoma Ninety-six percent of patients treated with CHVP plus INTRON A therapy and 91% of patients treated with CHVP alone reported an adverse event of any severity. Asthenia, fever, neutropenia, increased hepatic enzymes, alopecia, headache, anorexia, "flu-like" symptoms, myalgia, dyspnea, thrombocytopenia, paresthesia, and polyuria occurred more frequently in the CHVP plus INTRON A treated patients than in patients treated with CHVP alone. Adverse reactions classified as severe or life threatening (World Health Organization grade 3 or 4) recorded in >5% of CHVP plus INTRON A treated patients included neutropenia (34%), asthenia (10%), and vomiting (10%). The incidence of neutropenic infection was 6% in CHVP plus INTRON A vs 2% in CHVP alone. One patient in each treatment group required hospitalization.

Twenty-eight percent of CHVP plus INTRON A treated patients had a temporary modification/interruption of their INTRON A therapy, but only 13 patients (10%) permanently stopped INTRON A therapy because of toxicity. There were four deaths on study; two patients committed suicide in the CHVP plus INTRON A arm and two patients in the CHVP arm had unwitnessed sudden death. Three patients with hepatitis B (one of whom also had alcoholic cirrhosis) developed hepatotoxicity leading to discontinuation of INTRON A. Other reasons for discontinuation included intolerable asthenia (5/135), severe flu symptoms (2/135), and one patient each with exacerbation of ankylosing spondylitis, psychosis, and decreased ejection fraction.

Condylomata Acuminata Eighty-eight percent (311/352) of patients treated with INTRON A Interferon alfa-2b, recombinant for injection for condylomata acuminata who were evaluable for safety, reported an adverse reaction during treatment. The incidence of the adverse reactions reported increased when the number of treated lesions increased from one to five. All 40 patients who had five warts treated, reported some type of adverse reaction during treatment.

Adverse reactions and abnormal laboratory test values reported by patients who were retreated were qualitatively and quantitatively similar to those reported during the initial INTRON A treatment period.

AIDS-Related Kaposi's Sarcoma In patients with AIDS-Related Kaposi's Sarcoma, some type of adverse reaction occurred in 100% of the 74 patients treated with 30 million IU/m² three times a week and in 97% of the 29 patients treated with 35 million IU per day.

Of these adverse reactions, those classified as severe (World Health Organization grade 3 or 4) were reported in 27% to 55% of patients. Severe adverse reactions in the 30 million IU/m² TIW study included: fatigue (20%), influenza-like symptoms (15%), anorexia (12%), dry mouth (4%), headache (4%), confusion (3%), fever (3%), myalgia (3%), and nausea and vomiting (1% each). Severe adverse reactions for patients who received the 35 million IU QD included: fever (24%), fatigue (17%), influenza-like symptoms (14%), dyspnea (14%), headache (10%), pharyngitis (7%), and ataxia, confusion, dysphagia, GI hemorrhage, abnormal hepatic function, increased SGOT, myalgia, cardiomyopathy, face edema, depression, emotional lability, suicide attempt, chest pain, and coughing (1 patient each). Overall, the incidence of severe toxicity was higher among patients who received the 35 million IU per day dose.

Chronic Hepatitis C Two studies of extended treatment (18 to 24 months) with INTRON A Interferon alfa-2b, recombinant for Injection show that approximately 95% of all patients treated experience some type of adverse event and that patients treated for extended duration continue to experience adverse events throughout treatment. Most adverse events reported are mild to moderate in severity. However, 29/152 (19%) of patients treated for 18 to 24 months experienced a serious adverse event compared to 11/163 (7%) of those treated for 6 months. Adverse events which occur or persist during extended treatment are similar in type and severity to those occurring during short-course therapy.

Of the patients achieving a complete response after 6 months of therapy, 12/79 (15%) subsequently discontinued INTRON A treatment during extended therapy because of adverse events, and 23/79 (29%) experienced severe adverse events (WHO grade 3 or 4) during extended therapy.

In patients using REBETRON Combination Therapy containing INTRON A and REBETOL (ribavirin, USP) Capsules, the primary toxicity observed was hemolytic anemia. Reductions in hemoglobin levels occurred within the first 1

Continued on next page

Intron A—Cont.

to 2 weeks of therapy. Cardiac and pulmonary events associated with anemia occurred in approximately 10% of patients treated with INTRON A/REBETOL therapy. See REBETRON Combination Therapy package insert for additional information.

Chronic Hepatitis B *Adults* In patients with chronic hepatitis B, some type of adverse reaction occurred in 98% of the 101 patients treated at 5 million IU QD and 90% of the 78 patients treated at 10 million IU TIW. Most of these adverse reactions were mild to moderate in severity, were manageable, and were reversible following the end of therapy.

Adverse reactions classified as severe (causing a significant interference with normal daily activities or clinical state) were reported in 21% to 44% of patients. The severe adverse reactions reported most frequently were the "flu-like" symptoms of fever (28%), fatigue (15%), headache (5%), myalgia (4%), rigors (4%), and other severe "flu-like" symptoms which occurred in 1% to 3% of patients. Other severe adverse reactions occurring in more than one patient were alopecia (8%), anorexia (6%), depression (3%), nausea (3%), and vomiting (2%).

To manage side effects, the dose was reduced, or INTRON A therapy was interrupted in 25% to 38% of patients. Five percent of patients discontinued treatment due to adverse experiences.

Pediatrics In pediatric patients, the most frequently reported adverse events were those commonly associated with interferon treatment; flu-like symptoms (100%), gastrointestinal system disorders (46%), and nausea and vomiting (40%). Neutropenia (13%) and thrombocytopenia (3%) were also reported. None of the adverse events were life threatening. The majority were moderate to severe and resolved upon dose reduction or drug discontinuation.

[See table at top of previous page]

OVERDOSAGE

There is limited experience with overdosage. Postmarketing surveillance includes reports of patients receiving a single dose as great as 10 times the recommended dose. In general, the primary effects of an overdose are consistent with the effects seen with therapeutic doses of interferon alfa-2b. Hepatic enzyme abnormalities, renal failure, hemorrhage, and myocardial infarction have been reported with single administration overdoses and/or with longer durations of treatment than prescribed (see **ADVERSE REACTIONS**). Toxic effects after ingestion of interferon alfa-2b are not expected because interferons are poorly absorbed orally. Consultation with a poison center is recommended.

Treatment. There is no specific antidote for interferon alfa-2b. Hemodialysis and peritoneal dialysis are not considered effective for treatment of overdose.

DOSAGE AND ADMINISTRATION
General

IMPORTANT: INTRON A Interferon alfa-2b, is supplied as 1) Powder for Injection/Reconstitution; 2) Solution for Injection in vials; 3) Solution for Injection in multidose pens. **Not all dosage forms and strengths are appropriate for some indications.** It is important that you carefully read the instructions below for the indication you are treating to ensure you are using an appropriate dosage form and strength.

To enhance the tolerability of INTRON A, injections should be administered in the evening when possible.

To reduce the incidence of certain adverse reactions, acetaminophen may be administered at the time of injection.

Hairy Cell Leukemia (see DOSAGE AND ADMINISTRATION, General)

Dose: The recommended dose for the treatment of hairy cell leukemia is 2 million IU/m^2 administered intramuscularly or subcutaneously 3 times a week for up to 6 months. Patients with platelet counts of less than 50,000/mm^3 should not be administered INTRON A Interferon alfa-2b, recombinant for Injection intramuscularly, but instead by subcutaneous administration. Patients who are responding to therapy may benefit from continued treatment.

[See first table above]

NOTE: INTRON A Powder for Injection does not contain a preservative. The vial must be discarded after reconstitution and withdrawal of a single dose.

Dose adjustment:
- If severe adverse reactions develop, the dosage should be modified (50% reduction) or therapy should be temporarily withheld until the adverse reactions abate and then resume at 50% (1 MIU/m^2 TIW).
- If severe adverse reactions persist or recur following dosage adjustment, INTRON A should be permanently discontinued.
- INTRON A should be discontinued for progressive disease or failure to respond after six months of treatment.

Malignant Melanoma (see DOSAGE AND ADMINISTRATION, General)

INTRON A adjuvant treatment of malignant melanoma is given in two phases, induction and maintenance.

Induction Recommended Dose:

The recommended daily dose of INTRON A in induction is 20 million IU/m^2 as an intravenous infusion, over 20 minutes, 5 consecutive days per week, for 4 weeks (see Dose adjustment below).

Dosage Forms for This Indication

Dosage Form	Concentration	Route	Fixed Doses
Powder 10 MIU (single dose)	10 MIU/mL	IM, SC	N/A
Solution 10 MIU (single dose)	10 MIU/mL	SC	N/A
Solution 18 MIU multidose	6 MIU/mL	IM, SC	N/A
Solution 25 MIU multidose	10 MIU/mL	IM, SC	N/A
Pen 3 MIU/dose multidose	15 MIU/mL	SC	1.5, 3.0, 4.5
Pen 5 MIU/dose multidose	25 MIU/mL	SC	2.5, 5.0

Dosage Forms for This Indication

Dosage Form	Concentration	Route	Fixed Doses
Powder 10 MIU (single dose)*	10 MIU/mL	SC	N/A
Powder 18 MIU (single dose)**	18 MIU/mL	SC	N/A
Solution 10 MIU	10 MIU/mL	SC	N/A
Solution 18 MIU multidose	6 MIU/mL	SC	N/A
Solution 25 MIU multidose	10 MIU/mL	SC	N/A
Pen 3 MIU/dose multidose*	15 MIU/mL	SC	4.5, 6.0
Pen 5 MIU/dose multidose	25 MIU/mL	SC	7.5, 10.0
Pen 10 MIU/dose multidose	50 MIU/mL	SC	10.0, 15.0, 20.0

*Patients receiving 50% dose reduction only
**Patients receiving full dose only

Dosage Forms for This Indication

Dosage Form	Concentration	Route	Fixed Doses
Powder 10 MIU (single dose)	10 MIU/mL	SC	N/A
Solution 10 MIU (single dose)	10 MIU/mL	SC	N/A
Solution 18 MIU multidose	6 MIU/mL	SC	N/A
Solution 25 MIU multidose	10 MIU/mL	SC	N/A
Pen 5 MIU/dose multidose	25 MIU/mL	SC	2.5, 5.0
Pen 10 MIU/dose multidose	50 MIU/mL	SC	5.0

Dosage Forms for This Indication

Dosage Form	Concentration	Route
Powder 10 MIU	10 MIU/mL	IV
Powder 18 MIU	18 MIU/mL	IV
Powder 50 MIU	50 MIU/mL	IV

NOTE: INTRON A Solution for Injection in vials or multidose pens is NOT recommended for intravenous administration and should not be used for the induction phase of malignant melanoma.

NOTE: INTRON A Powder for Injection does not contain a preservative. The vial must be discarded after reconstitution and withdrawal of a single dose.

Dose adjustment:
NOTE: Regular laboratory testing should be performed to monitor laboratory abnormalities for the purpose of dose modifications (see **PRECAUTIONS-Laboratory Tests**).
- INTRON A should be withheld for severe adverse reactions, including granulocyte counts >250mm^3 but <500mm^3 or SGPT/SGOT >5-10x upper limit of normal, until adverse reactions abate. INTRON A treatment should be restarted at 50% of the previous dose.
- INTRON A should be permanently discontinued for:
  - Toxicity that does not abate after withholding INTRON A
  - Severe adverse reactions which recur in patients receiving reduced doses of INTRON A
  - Granulocyte count <250mm^3 or SGPT/SGOT of >10x upper limit of normal

Maintenance Recommended Dose:
The recommended dose of INTRON A for maintenance is 10 million IU/m^2 as a subcutaneous injection three times per week for 48 weeks (see Dose adjustment below).
[See second table above]
NOTE: INTRON A Powder for Injection does not contain a preservative. The vial must be discarded after reconstitution and withdrawal of a single dose.

Dose adjustment:
NOTE: Regular laboratory testing should be performed to monitor laboratory abnormalities for the purpose of dose modifications (see **PRECAUTIONS-Laboratory Tests**).
- INTRON A should be withheld for severe adverse reactions, including granulocyte counts >250mm^3 but <500mm^3 or SGPT/SGOT >5-10x upper limit of normal, until adverse reactions abate. INTRON A treatment should be restarted at 50% of the previous dose.

- INTRON A should be permanently discontinued for:
  - Toxicity that does not abate after withholding INTRON A
  - Severe adverse reactions which recur in patients receiving reduced doses of INTRON A
  - Granulocyte count <250mm^3 or SGPT/SGOT of >10x upper limit of normal

Follicular Lymphoma (see DOSAGE and ADMINISTRATION, General)

Dose: The recommended dose of INTRON A for the treatment of follicular lymphoma is 5 million IU subcutaneously three times per week for up to 18 months in conjunction with anthracycline-containing chemotherapy regimen and following completion of the chemotherapy regimen.
[See third table above]
NOTE: INTRON A Powder for Injection does not contain a preservative. The vial must be discarded after reconstitution and withdrawal of a single dose.

Dose adjustment:
- Doses of myelosuppressive drugs were reduced by 25% from a full-dose CHOP regimen, and cycle length increased by 33% (eg, from 21 to 28 days) when alfa interferon was added to the regimen.
- Delay chemotherapy cycle if neutrophil count was <1500/mm^3 or platelet count was <75,000/mm^3
- INTRON A should be permanently discontinued if SGOT exceeds >5x the upper limit of normal or serum creatinine >2.0 mg/dL (see **WARNINGS**).
- Administration of INTRON A therapy should be withheld for a neutrophil count <1000/mm^3, or a platelet count <50,000/mm^3.
- INTRON A dose should be reduced by 50% (2.5 MIU TIW) for a neutrophil count >1000/mm^3, but <1500/mm^3. The INTRON A dose may be re-escalated to the starting dose (5 million IU TIW) after resolution of hematologic toxicity (ANC >1500/mm^3).

Condylomata Acuminata (see DOSAGE and ADMINISTRATION, General)

Dose: The recommended dose is 1.0 million IU per lesion in a maximum of 5 lesions in a single course. The lesions should be injected three times weekly on alternate days for 3 weeks. An additional course may be administered at 12-16 weeks.

Dosage Forms for This Indication

Dosage Form	Concentration	Route
Powder 10 MIU (single dose)	10 MIU/mL	IL

Solution 10 MIU (single dose)	10 MIU/mL	IL
Solution 25 MIU multidose	10 MIU/mL	IL

NOTE: INTRON A Powder for Injection does not contain a preservative. The vial must be discarded after reconstitution and withdrawal of a single dose.

NOTE: Do not use the following formulations for this indication:
• the 18 million or 50 million IU Powder for Injection
• the 18 million IU multidose INTRON A Solution for Injection
• the multidose pens

Dose adjustment: None

Technique for Injection:

The injection should be administered intralesionally using a Tuberculin or similar syringe and a 25-to-30 gauge needle. The needle should be directed at the center of the base of the wart and at an angle almost parallel to the plane of the skin (approximately that in the commonly used PPD test). This will deliver the interferon to the dermal core of the lesion, infiltrating the lesion and causing a small wheal. Care should be taken not to go beneath the lesion too deeply; subcutaneous injection should be avoided, since this area is below the base of the lesion. Do not inject too superficially since this will result in possible leakage, infiltrating only the keratinized layer and not the dermal core.

AIDS-Related Kaposi's Sarcoma (see DOSAGE and ADMINISTRATION, General)

Dose: The recommended dose of INTRON A for Kaposi's Sarcoma is 30 million IU/m² /dose administered subcutaneously or intramuscularly three times a week until disease progression or maximal response has been achieved after 16 weeks of treatment. Dose reduction is frequently required (see Dose adjustment below).

Dosage Forms for This Indication

Dosage Form	Concentration	Route
Powder 50 MIU	50 MIU/mL	IM, SC

NOTE: INTRON A Solution for Injection either in vials or in multidose pens should NOT be used for AIDS-Related Kaposi's Sarcoma.

NOTE: INTRON A Powder for Injection does not contain a preservative. The vial must be discarded after reconstitution and withdrawal of a single dose.

Dose adjustment:
• INTRON A dose should be reduced by 50% or withheld for severe adverse reactions.
• INTRON A may be resumed reduced dose if severe adverse reactions abate with interruption of dosing.
• INTRON A should be permanently discontinued if severe adverse reactions persist or if they recur in patients receiving a reduced dose.

Chronic Hepatitis C (see DOSAGE and ADMINISTRATION, General)

Dose: The recommended dose of INTRON A for the treatment of chronic hepatitis C is 3 million IU three times a week (TIW) administered subcutaneously or intramuscularly. In patients tolerating therapy with normalization of ALT at 16 weeks of treatment, INTRON A therapy should be extended to 18 to 24 months (72 to 96 weeks) at 3 million IU TIW to improve the sustained response rate (see **CLINICAL PHARMACOLOGY - Chronic Hepatitis C**). Patients who do not normalize their ALTs after 16 weeks of therapy rarely achieve a sustained response with extension of treatment. Consideration should be given to discontinuing these patients from therapy.

See REBETRON Combination Therapy package insert for dosing when used in combination with REBETOL (ribavirin, USP) Capsules.

[See first table above]

Dose adjustment: If severe adverse reactions develop during INTRON A treatment, the dose should be modified (50% reduction) or therapy should be temporarily discontinued until the adverse reactions abate. If intolerance persists after dose adjustment, INTRON A therapy should be discontinued.

Chronic Hepatitis B Adults (see DOSAGE and ADMINISTRATION, General)

Dose: The recommended dose of INTRON A for the treatment of chronic hepatitis B is 30 to 35 million IU per week, administered subcutaneously or intramuscularly, either as 5 million IU daily (QD) or as 10 million IU three times a week (TIW) for 16 weeks.

[See second table above]

NOTE: INTRON A Powder for Injection does not contain a preservative. The vial must be discarded after reconstitution and withdrawal of a single dose.

Chronic Hepatitis B Pediatrics (see DOSAGE and ADMINISTRATION, General)

Dose: The recommended dose of INTRON A Interferon alfa-2b, recombinant for Injection for the treatment of chronic hepatitis B is 3 million IU/m² three times a week (TIW) for the first week of therapy followed by dose escalation to 6 million IU/m² TIW (maximum of 10 million IU TIW) administered subcutaneously for a total duration of 16 to 24 weeks.

[See third table above]

NOTE: INTRON A Powder for Injection does not contain a preservative. The vial must be discarded after reconstitution and withdrawal of a single dose.

Dosage Forms for This Indication

Dosage Form	Concentration	Route	Fixed Doses
Solution 18 MIU multidose	6 MIU/mL	IM, SC	N/A
Pen 3 MIU/dose multidose	15 MIU/mL	SC	1.5, 3.0

Dosage Forms for This Indication

Dosage Form	Concentration	Route	Fixed Doses
Powder 10 MIU (single dose)	10 MIU/mL	IM, SC	N/A
Solution 10 MIU (single dose)	10 MIU/mL	SC	N/A
Solution 25 MIU multidose	10 MIU/mL	IM, SC	N/A
Pen 5 MIU/dose multidose	25 MIU/mL	SC	2.5, 5.0, 10.0
Pen 10 MIU/dose multidose	50 MIU/mL	SC	5.0, 10.0

Dosage Forms for This Indication

Dosage Form	Concentration	Route	Fixed Doses
Powder 10 MIU (single dose)	10 MIU/mL	SC	N/A
Solution 10 MIU (single dose)	10 MIU/mL	SC	N/A
Solution 25 MIU multidose	10 MIU/mL	SC	N/A
Pen 3 MIU/dose multidose	15 MIU/mL	SC	1.5, 3.0, 4.5, 6.0
Pen 5 MIU/dose multidose	25 MIU/mL	SC	2.5, 5.0, 7.5, 10.0
Pen 10 MIU/dose multidose	50 MIU/mL	SC	5.0, 10.0, 15.0, 20.0

INTRON A Dose	White Blood Cell Count	Granulocyte Count	Platelet Count
Reduce 50%	$<1.5 \times 10^9/L$	$<0.75 \times 10^9/L$	$<50 \times 10^9/L$
Permanently Discontinue	$<1.0 \times 10^9/L$	$<0.5 \times 10^9/L$	$<25 \times 10^9/L$

Dose adjustment: If severe adverse reactions or laboratory abnormalities develop during INTRON A therapy, the dose should be modified (50% reduction) or discontinued if appropriate, until the adverse reactions abate. If intolerance persists after dose adjustment, INTRON A therapy should be discontinued.

For patients with decreases in white blood cell, granulocyte or platelet counts, the following guidelines for dose modification should be followed:

[See fourth table above]

INTRON A therapy was resumed at up to 100% of the initial dose when white blood cell, granulocyte, and/or platelet counts returned to normal or baseline values.

PREPARATION AND ADMINISTRATION

Reconstitution of INTRON A Powder for Injection

The INTRON A powder reconstituted with Sterile Water for Injection, USP is a single-use vial and does not contain a preservative. The reconstituted solution is clear and colorless to light yellow. **DO NOT RE-ENTER VIAL AFTER WITHDRAWING THE DOSE. DISCARD UNUSED PORTION** (see **DOSAGE and ADMINISTRATION**). Once the dose from the single-dose vial has been withdrawn, the sterility of any remaining product can no longer be guaranteed. Pooling of unused portions of some medications has been linked to bacterial contamination and morbidity.

• Intramuscular, Subcutaneous, or Intralesional Administration

Inject 1 mL Diluent (Sterile Water for Injection, USP) for INTRON A into the INTRON A vial. Swirl gently to hasten complete dissolution of the powder. The appropriate INTRON A dose should then be withdrawn and injected intramuscularly, subcutaneously, or intralesionally (see **MEDICATION GUIDE** for detailed instructions).

Please refer to the **Medication Guide** for detailed, step-by-step instructions on how to inject the INTRON A dose. After preparation and administration of the INTRON A injection, it is essential to follow the procedure for proper disposal of syringes and needles (see **MEDICATION GUIDE** for detailed instructions).

Parenteral drug products should be inspected visually for particulate matter and discoloration prior to administration.

• Intravenous Infusion

The infusion solution should be prepared immediately prior to use. Based on the desired dose, the appropriate vial strength(s) of INTRON A Interferon alfa-2b, recombinant Powder for Injection should be reconstituted with the diluent provided. Inject 1 mL Diluent (Sterile Water for Injection, USP) for INTRON A Interferon alfa-2b, into the INTRON A vial. Swirl gently to hasten complete dissolution of the powder. The appropriate INTRON A dose should then be withdrawn and injected into a 100-mL bag of 0.9% Sodium Chloride Injection, USP. The final concentration of INTRON A Interferon alfa-2b, recombinant for Injection should not be less than 10 million IU/100 mL.

Please refer to the **Medication Guide** for detailed, step-by-step instructions on how to inject the INTRON A dose. After

preparation and administration of INTRON A, it is essential to follow the procedure for proper disposal of syringes and needles.

INTRON A Solution for Injection in Vials

INTRON A Solution for Injection is supplied in a single-use vial and two multidose vials. The solutions for injection do not require reconstitution prior to administration; the solution is clear and colorless.

The appropriate dose should be withdrawn from the vial and injected intramuscularly, subcutaneously, or intralesionally.

The single-use 10 million IU vial is supplied with B-D Safety-Lok* syringes. The Safety-Lok* syringe contains a plastic safety sleeve to be pulled over the needle after use. The syringe locks with an audible click when the green stripe on the safety sleeve covers the red stripe on the needle. The B-D Safety-Lok* syringes provided with the 10 MIU Solution for Injection cannot be used for IM injections.

INTRON A Solution for Injection is not recommended for intravenous administration.

Solution for Injection in Multidose Pens

The INTRON A Solution for Injection multidose pens are designed to deliver 3-12 doses depending on the individual dose using a simple dial mechanism and are for subcutaneous injections only. Only the needles provided in the packaging should be used for the INTRON A Solution for Injection multidose pen. A new needle is to be used each time a dose is delivered using the pen. To avoid the possible transmission of disease, each INTRON A Solution for Injection multidose pen is for single patient use only.

Please refer to the **Medication Guide** for detailed, step-by-step instructions on how to inject the INTRON A dose. After preparation and administration of INTRON A, it is essential to follow the procedure for proper disposal of syringes and needles.

HOW SUPPLIED

INTRON A Powder for Injection INTRON A Interferon alfa-2b, recombinant Powder for Injection, 10 million IU per vial and Diluent for Injection INTRON A Interferon alfa-2b, recombinant for Injection (Sterile Water for Injection, USP) 1 mL per vial; boxes containing 1 INTRON A vial and 1 vial of INTRON A Diluent (NDC 0085-0571-02).

INTRON A Interferon alfa-2b, recombinant Powder for Injection, 18 million IU per vial and Diluent for INTRON A Interferon alfa-2b, recombinant for Injection (Sterile Water for Injection, USP) 1 mL per vial; boxes containing 1 vial of INTRON A and 1 vial of INTRON A Diluent (NDC 0085-1110-01).

INTRON A Interferon alfa-2b, recombinant Powder for Injection, 50 million IU per vial and Diluent for INTRON A Interferon alfa-2b, recombinant for Injection (Sterile Water for Injection, USP) 1 mL per vial; boxes containing 1 INTRON A vial and 1 vial of INTRON A Diluent (NDC 0085-0539-01).

Continued on next page

Intron A—Cont.

INTRON A Solution for Injection in Multidose Pens

INTRON A Interferon alfa-2b, recombinant Solution for Injection, 6 doses of 3 million IU (18 million IU) multidose pen (22.5 million IU per 1.5 mL per pen); boxes containing 1 INTRON A multidose pen, six disposable needles and alcohol swabs (NDC 0085-1242-01).

INTRON A Interferon alfa-2b, recombinant Solution for Injection, 6 doses of 5 million IU (30 million IU) multidose pen (37.5 million IU per 1.5 mL per pen); boxes containing 1 INTRON A multidose pen, six disposable needles and alcohol swabs (NDC 0085-1235-01).

INTRON A Interferon alfa-2b, recombinant Solution for Injection, 6 doses of 10 million IU (60 million IU) multidose pen (75 million IU per 1.5 mL per pen); boxes containing 1 INTRON A multidose pen, six disposable needles and alcohol swabs (NDC 0085-1254-01).

INTRON A Solution for Injection in Vials

INTRON A Interferon alfa-2b, recombinant Solution for Injection INTRON A, Pak-10, containing 6 INTRON A vials, 10 million IU per vial; and 6 B-D Safety-Lok* syringes with a safety sleeve (NDC 0085-1179-02).

INTRON A Interferon alfa-2b, recombinant Solution for Injection, 18 million IU multidose vial (22.8 million IU per 3.8 mL per vial); boxes containing 1 vial of INTRON A Solution Injection (NDC 0085-1168-01).

INTRON A Interferon alfa-2b, recombinant Solution for Injection, 25 million IU multidose vial (32 million IU per 3.2 mL per vial); boxes containing 1 vial of INTRON A Solution for Injection (NDC 0085-1133-01).

Storage

- **INTRON A Powder for Injection/Reconstitution**

INTRON A Powder for Injection should be stored at 2° to 8°C (36° to 46°F). After reconstitution, the solution should be used immediately, but may be stored up to 24 hours at 2° to 8°C (36° to 46°F).

- **INTRON A Solution for Injection in Vials**

INTRON A Solution for Injection in vials should be stored at 2° to 8°C (36° to 46°F).

- **INTRON A Solution for Injection in Multidose Pens**

INTRON A Solution for Injection in multidose pens should be stored at 2° to 8°C (36° to 46°F).

REFERENCES

1. Smalley R, et al. *N Engl J Med.* 1992;327:1336–1341.
2. Aviles A, et al. *Leukemia and Lymphoma.* 1996;20:495–499.
3. Unterhalt M, et al. *Blood.* 1996;88 (10 Suppl 1):1744A.
4. Schiller J, et al. *J Biol Response Mod.* 1989;8:252–261.
5. Poynard T, et al. *N Engl J Med.* 1995;332:(22)1457–1462.
6. Lin R, et al. *J Hepatol.* 1995;23:487–496.
7. Perrillo R, et al. *N Engl J Med.* 1990;323:295–301.
8. Perez V, et al. *J Hepatol.* 1990;11:S113–S117.
9. Knodell R, et al. *Hepatology.* 1981;1:431–435.
10. Perrillo R, et al. *Ann Intern Med.* 1991;115:113–115.
11. Renault P, et al. *Arch Intern Med.* 1987;147:1577–1580.
12. Kauppila A, et al. *Int J Cancer.* 1982;29:291–294.

Schering Corporation
Kenilworth, NJ 07033 USA B-27783503T
Rev. 3/04

*Safety-Lok is a trademark of Becton, Dickinson and Company

NASONEX® ℞

[*nā-sō-nĕks*]

(mometasone furoate monohydrate)
Nasal Spray, 50 mcg*
FOR INTRANASAL USE ONLY

*calculated on the anhydrous basis

Prescribing information for this product, which appears on pages 3044–3046 of the 2005 PDR, has been completely revised as follows. Please write "See Supplement A" next to the product heading.

DESCRIPTION

Mometasone furoate monohydrate, the active component of NASONEX Nasal Spray, 50 mcg, is an anti-inflammatory corticosteroid having the chemical name, 9,21-Dichloro-11β,17-dihydroxy-16α-methylpregna-1,4-diene-3,20-dione 17-(2 furoate) monohydrate, and the following chemical structure:

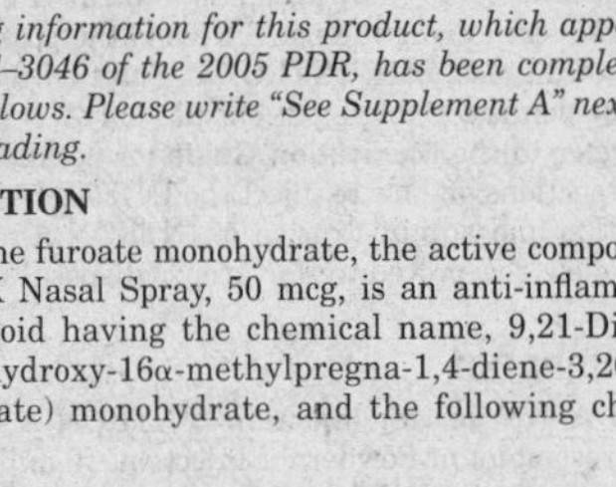

Mometasone furoate monohydrate is a white powder, with an empirical formula of $C_{27}H_{30}Cl_2O_6 \cdot H_2O$, and a molecular weight of 539.45. It is practically insoluble in water; slightly soluble in methanol, ethanol, and isopropanol; soluble in acetone and chloroform; and freely soluble in tetrahydrofuran. Its partition coefficient between octanol and water is greater than 5000.

NASONEX Nasal Spray, 50 mcg is a metered-dose, manual pump spray unit containing an aqueous suspension of mometasone furoate monohydrate equivalent to 0.05% w/w mometasone furoate calculated on the anhydrous basis; in an aqueous medium containing glycerin, microcrystalline cellulose and carboxymethylcellulose sodium, sodium citrate, citric acid, benzalkonium chloride, and polysorbate 80. The pH is between 4.3 and 4.9.

After initial priming (10 actuations), each actuation of the pump delivers a metered spray containing 100 mg of suspension containing mometasone furoate monohydrate equivalent to 50 mcg of mometasone furoate calculated on the anhydrous basis. Each bottle of NASONEX Nasal Spray, 50 mcg provides 120 sprays.

CLINICAL PHARMACOLOGY

NASONEX Nasal Spray, 50 mcg is a corticosteroid demonstrating anti-inflammatory properties. The precise mechanism of corticosteroid action on allergic rhinitis is not known. Corticosteroids have been shown to have a wide range of effects on multiple cell types (eg, mast cells, eosinophils, neutrophils, macrophages, and lymphocytes) and mediators (eg, histamine, eicosanoids, leukotrienes, and cytokines) involved in inflammation.

In two clinical studies utilizing nasal antigen challenge, NASONEX Nasal Spray, 50 mcg decreased some markers of the early- and late-phase allergic response. These observations included decreases (vs placebo) in histamine and eosinophil cationic protein levels, and reductions (vs baseline) in eosinophils, neutrophils, and epithelial cell adhesion proteins. The clinical significance of these findings is not known.

The effect of NASONEX Nasal Spray, 50 mcg on nasal mucosa following 12 months of treatment was examined in 46 patients with allergic rhinitis. There was no evidence of atrophy and there was a marked reduction in intraepithelial eosinophilia and inflammatory cell infiltration (eg, eosinophils, lymphocytes, monocytes, neutrophils, and plasma cells).

Pharmacokinetics: ***Absorption:*** Mometasone furoate monohydrate administered as a nasal spray is virtually undetectable in plasma from adult and pediatric subjects despite the use of a sensitive assay with a lower quantitation limit (LOQ) of 50 pcg/mL.

Distribution: The *in vitro* protein binding for mometasone furoate was reported to be 98% to 99% in concentration range of 5 to 500 ng/mL.

Metabolism: Studies have shown that any portion of a mometasone furoate dose which is swallowed and absorbed undergoes extensive metabolism to multiple metabolites. There are no major metabolites detectable in plasma. Upon *in vitro* incubation, one of the minor metabolites formed is 6β-hydroxy-mometasone furoate. In human liver microsomes, the formation of the metabolite is regulated by cytochrome P-450 3A4 (CYP3A4).

Elimination: Following intravenous administration, the effective plasma elimination half-life of mometasone furoate is 5.8 hours. Any absorbed drug is excreted as metabolites mostly via the bile, and to a limited extent, into the urine.

Special Populations: The effects of renal impairment, hepatic impairment, age, or gender on mometasone furoate pharmacokinetics have not been adequately investigated.

Pharmacodynamics: Four clinical pharmacology studies have been conducted in humans to assess the effect of NASONEX Nasal Spray, 50 mcg at various doses on adrenal function. In one study, daily doses of 200 and 400 mcg of NASONEX Nasal Spray, 50 mcg and 10 mg of prednisone were compared to placebo in 64 patients with allergic rhinitis. Adrenal function before and after 36 consecutive days of treatment was assessed by measuring plasma cortisol levels following a 6-hour Cortrosyn (ACTH) infusion and by measuring 24-hour urinary-free cortisol levels. NASONEX Nasal Spray, 50 mcg, at both the 200- and 400-mcg dose, was not associated with a statistically significant decrease in mean plasma cortisol levels post-Cortrosyn infusion or a statistically significant decrease in the 24-hour urinary-free cortisol levels compared to placebo. A statistically significant decrease in the mean plasma cortisol levels post-Cortrosyn infusion and 24-hour urinary-free cortisol levels was detected in the prednisone treatment group compared to placebo.

A second study assessed adrenal response to NASONEX Nasal Spray, 50 mcg (400 and 1600 mcg/day), prednisone (10 mg/day), and placebo, administered for 29 days in 48 male volunteers. The 24-hour plasma cortisol area under the curve (AUC_{0-24}), during and after an 8-hour Cortrosyn infusion and 24-hour urinary-free cortisol levels were determined at baseline and after 29 days of treatment. No statistically significant differences of adrenal function were observed with NASONEX Nasal Spray, 50 mcg compared to placebo.

A third study evaluated single, rising doses of NASONEX Nasal Spray, 50 mcg (1000, 2000, and 4000 mcg/day), orally administered mometasone furoate (2000, 4000, and 8000 mcg/day), orally administered dexamethasone (200, 400, and 800 mcg/day), and placebo (administered at the end of each series of doses) in 24 male volunteers. Dose administrations were separated by at least 72 hours. Determination of serial plasma cortisol levels at 8 AM and for the 24-hour period following each treatment were used to calculate the plasma cortisol area under the curve (AUC_{0-24}). In addition, 24-hour urinary-free cortisol levels were collected prior to initial treatment administration and during the period immediately following each dose. No statistically significant decreases in the plasma cortisol AUC, 8 AM cortisol levels, or 24-hour urinary-free cortisol levels were observed in volunteers treated with either NASONEX Nasal Spray, 50 mcg or oral mometasone, as compared with placebo treatment. Conversely, nearly all volunteers treated with the three doses of dexamethasone demonstrated abnormal 8 AM cortisol levels (defined as a cortisol level <10 mcg/dL), reduced 24-hour plasma AUC values, and decreased 24-hour urinary-free cortisol levels, as compared to placebo treatment.

In a fourth study, adrenal function was assessed in 213 patients with nasal polyps before and after 4 months of treatment with either NASONEX Nasal Spray, 50 mcg, (200 mcg once or twice daily) or placebo by measuring 24-hour urinary-free cortisol levels. NASONEX Nasal Spray, 50 mcg, at both doses (200 and 400 mcg/day), was not associated with statistically significant decreases in the 24-hour urinary-free cortisol levels compared to placebo.

Three clinical pharmacology studies have been conducted in pediatric patients to assess the effect of mometasone furoate nasal spray on the adrenal function at daily doses of 50, 100, and 200 mcg vs placebo. In one study, adrenal function before and after 7 consecutive days of treatment was assessed in 48 pediatric patients with allergic rhinitis (ages 6 to 11 years) by measuring morning plasma cortisol and 24-hour urinary-free cortisol levels. Mometasone furoate nasal spray, at all three doses, was not associated with a statistically significant decrease in mean plasma cortisol levels or a statistically significant decrease in the 24-hour urinary-free cortisol levels compared to placebo. In the second study, adrenal function before and after 14 consecutive days of treatment was assessed in 48 pediatric patients (ages 3 to 5 years) with allergic rhinitis by measuring plasma cortisol levels following a 30-minute Cortrosyn infusion. Mometasone furoate nasal spray, 50 mcg, at all three doses (50, 100, and 200 mcg/day), was not associated with a statistically significant decrease in mean plasma cortisol levels post-Cortrosyn infusion compared to placebo. All patients had a normal response to Cortrosyn. In the third study, adrenal function before and after up to 42 consecutive days of once-daily treatment was assessed in 52 patients with allergic rhinitis (ages 2 to 5 years), 28 of whom received mometasone furoate nasal spray, 50 mcg per nostril (total daily dose 100 mcg), by measuring morning plasma cortisol and 24-hour urinary-free cortisol levels. Mometasone furoate nasal spray was not associated with a statistically significant decrease in mean plasma cortisol levels or a statistically significant decrease in the 24-hour urinary-free cortisol levels compared to placebo.

CLINICAL STUDIES

Allergic Rhinitis. The efficacy and safety of NASONEX Nasal Spray, 50 mcg in the prophylaxis and treatment of seasonal allergic rhinitis and the treatment of perennial allergic rhinitis have been evaluated in 18 controlled trials, and one uncontrolled clinical trial, in approximately 3000 adults (ages 17 to 85 years) and adolescents (ages 12 to 16 years). This included 1757 males and 1453 females, including a total of 283 adolescents (182 boys and 101 girls) with seasonal allergic or perennial allergic rhinitis, treated with NASONEX Nasal Spray, 50 mcg at doses ranging from 50 to 800 mcg/day. The majority of patients were treated with 200 mcg/day. These trials evaluated the total nasal symptom scores that included stuffiness, rhinorrhea, itching, and sneezing. Patients treated with NASONEX Nasal Spray, 50 mcg, 200 mcg/day had a significant decrease in total nasal symptom scores compared to placebo-treated patients. No additional benefit was observed for mometasone furoate doses greater than 200 mcg/day. A total of 350 patients have been treated with NASONEX Nasal Spray, 50 mcg for 1 year or longer.

The efficacy and safety of NASONEX Nasal Spray, 50 mcg in the treatment of seasonal allergic and perennial allergic rhinitis in pediatric patients (ages 3 to 11 years) have been evaluated in four controlled trials. This included approximately 990 pediatric patients ages 3 to 11 years (606 males and 384 females) with seasonal allergic or perennial allergic rhinitis treated with mometasone furoate nasal spray at doses ranging from 25 to 200 mcg/day. Pediatric patients treated with NASONEX Nasal Spray, 50 mcg (100 mcg total daily dose, 374 patients) had a significant decrease in total nasal symptom (congestion, rhinorrhea, itching, and sneezing) scores, compared to placebo-treated patients. No additional benefit was observed for the 200-mcg mometasone furoate total daily dose in pediatric patients (ages 3 to 11 years). A total of 163 pediatric patients have been treated for 1 year.

In patients with seasonal allergic rhinitis, NASONEX Nasal Spray, 50 mcg, demonstrated improvement in nasal symptoms (vs placebo) within 11 hours after the first dose based on one single-dose, parallel-group study of patients in an outdoor "park" setting (park study) and one environmental exposure unit (EEU) study, and within 2 days in two randomized, double-blind, placebo-controlled, parallel-group seasonal allergic rhinitis studies. Maximum benefit is usually achieved within 1 to 2 weeks after initiation of dosing.

Prophylaxis of seasonal allergic rhinitis for patients 12 years of age and older with NASONEX Nasal Spray, 50 mcg, given at a dose of 200 mcg/day, was evaluated in two clinical studies in 284 patients. These studies were designed such that patients received 4 weeks of prophylaxis with NASONEX Nasal Spray, 50 mcg prior to the anticipated onset of the pollen season; however, some patients received only 2 to 3 weeks of prophylaxis. Patients receiving 2 to 4 weeks of prophylaxis with NASONEX Nasal Spray, 50 mcg demonstrated a statistically significantly smaller mean increase in total nasal symptom scores with onset of the pollen season as compared to placebo patients.

Nasal Polyps. Two studies were performed to evaluate the efficacy and safety of NASONEX Nasal Spray in the treatment of nasal polyps. These studies involved 664 patients with nasal polyps, 441 of whom received NASONEX Nasal Spray. These studies were randomized, double-blind, placebo-controlled, parallel group, multicenter studies in patients 18 to 86 years of age with bilateral nasal polyps. Patients were randomized to receive NASONEX Nasal Spray 200 mcg once daily, 200 mcg twice daily or placebo for a period of 4 months. The co-primary efficacy endpoints were 1) change from baseline in nasal congestion/obstruction averaged over the first month of treatment; and 2) change from baseline to last assessment in bilateral polyp grade during the entire 4 months of treatment as assessed by endoscopy. Efficacy was demonstrated in both studies at a dose of 200 mcg twice daily and in one study at a dose of 200 mcg once a day (see table below).

[See table above]

EFFECT OF NASONEX NASAL SPRAY IN TWO RANDOMIZED, PLACEBO-CONTROLLED TRIALS IN PATIENTS WITH NASAL POLYPS

	NASONEX 200 mcg qd	NASONEX 200 mcg bid	Placebo	*P* value for NASONEX 200 mcg qd vs placebo	*P* value for NASONEX 200 mcg bid vs placebo
Study 1	N = 115	N = 122	N = 117		
Baseline bilateral polyp grade*	4.21	4.27	4.25		
Mean change from baseline in bilateral polyp grade	-1.15	-0.96	-0.50	<0.001	0.01
Baseline nasal congestion**	2.29	2.35	2.28		
Mean change from baseline in nasal congestion	-0.47	-0.61	-0.24	0.001	<0.001
Study 2	N = 102	N = 102	N = 106		
Baseline bilateral polyp grade*	4.00	4.10	4.17		
Mean change from baseline in bilateral polyp grade	-0.78	-0.96	-0.62	0.33	0.04
Baseline nasal congestion**	2.23	2.20	2.18		
Mean change from baseline in nasal congestion	-0.42	-0.66	-0.23	0.01	<0.001

*polyps in each nasal fossa were graded by the investigator based on endoscopic visualization, using a scale of 0-3 where 0 = no polyps; 1 = polyps in the middle meatus, not reaching below the inferior border of the middle turbinate; 2 = polyps reaching below the inferior border of the middle turbinate but not the inferior border of the inferior turbinate; 3 = polyps reaching to or below the border of the inferior turbinate, or polyps medial to the middle turbinate (score reflects sum of left and right nasal fossa grades).
**nasal congestion/obstruction was scored daily by the patient using a 0-3 categorical scale where 0 = no symptoms, 1 = mild symptoms, 2 = moderate symptoms and 3 = severe symptoms.

There were no clinically relevant differences in the effectiveness of NASONEX Nasal Spray, 50 mcg, in the studies evaluating treatment of nasal polyps across subgroups of patients defined by gender, age, or race.

INDICATIONS AND USAGE

NASONEX Nasal Spray, 50 mcg is indicated for the treatment of the nasal symptoms of seasonal allergic and perennial allergic rhinitis, in adults and pediatric patients 2 years of age and older. NASONEX Nasal Spray, 50 mcg is indicated for the prophylaxis of the nasal symptoms of seasonal allergic rhinitis in adult and adolescent patients 12 years and older. In patients with a known seasonal allergen that precipitates nasal symptoms of seasonal allergic rhinitis, initiation of prophylaxis with NASONEX Nasal Spray, 50 mcg is recommended 2 to 4 weeks prior to the anticipated start of the pollen season. Safety and effectiveness of NASONEX Nasal Spray, 50 mcg in pediatric patients less than 2 years of age have not been established.

NASONEX Nasal Spray, 50 mcg, is indicated for the treatment of nasal polyps in patients 18 years of age and older. Safety and effectiveness of NASONEX Nasal Spray, 50 mcg, for the treatment of nasal polyps in pediatric patients less than 18 years of age have not been established.

CONTRAINDICATIONS

Hypersensitivity to any of the ingredients of this preparation contraindicates its use.

WARNINGS

The replacement of a systemic corticosteroid with a topical corticosteroid can be accompanied by signs of adrenal insufficiency and, in addition, some patients may experience symptoms of withdrawal; ie, joint and/or muscular pain, lassitude, and depression. Careful attention must be given when patients previously treated for prolonged periods with systemic corticosteroids are transferred to topical corticosteroids, with careful monitoring for acute adrenal insufficiency in response to stress. This is particularly important in those patients who have associated asthma or other clinical conditions where too rapid a decrease in systemic corticosteroid dosing may cause a severe exacerbation of their symptoms.

If recommended doses of intranasal corticosteroids are exceeded or if individuals are particularly sensitive or predisposed by virtue of recent systemic steroid therapy, symptoms of hypercorticism may occur, including very rare cases of menstrual irregularities, acneiform lesions, and cushingoid features. If such changes occur, topical corticosteroids should be discontinued slowly, consistent with accepted procedures for discontinuing oral steroid therapy.

Persons who are on drugs which suppress the immune system are more susceptible to infections than healthy individuals. Chickenpox and measles, for example, can have a more serious or even fatal course in nonimmune children or adults on corticosteroids. In such children or adults who have not had these diseases, particular care should be taken to avoid exposure. How the dose, route, and duration of corticosteroid administration affects the risk of developing a disseminated infection is not known. The contribution of the underlying disease and/or prior corticosteroid treatment to the risk is also not known. If exposed to chickenpox, prophylaxis with varicella zoster immune globin (VZIG) may be indicated. If exposed to measles, prophylaxis with pooled intramuscular immunoglobulin (IG) may be indicated. (See the respective package inserts for complete VZIG and IG prescribing information.) If chickenpox develops, treatment with antiviral agents may be considered.

PRECAUTIONS

General: Intranasal corticosteroids may cause a reduction in growth velocity when administered to pediatric patients (see **PRECAUTIONS, Pediatric Use** section). In clinical studies with NASONEX Nasal Spray, 50 mcg, the development of localized infections of the nose and pharynx with *Candida albicans* has occurred only rarely. When such an infection develops, use of NASONEX Nasal Spray, 50 mcg should be discontinued and appropriate local or systemic therapy instituted, if needed.

Nasal corticosteroids should be used with caution, if at all, in patients with active or quiescent tuberculous infection of the respiratory tract, or in untreated fungal, bacterial, systemic viral infections, or ocular herpes simplex.

Rarely, immediate hypersensitivity reactions may occur after the intranasal administration of mometasone furoate monohydrate. Extremely rare instances of wheezing have been reported.

Rare instances of nasal septum perforation and increased intraocular pressure have also been reported following the intranasal application of aerosolized corticosteroids. As with any long-term topical treatment of the nasal cavity, patients using NASONEX Nasal Spray, 50 mcg over several months or longer should be examined periodically for possible changes in the nasal mucosa.

Because of the inhibitory effect of corticosteroids on wound healing, patients who have experienced recent nasal septum ulcers, nasal surgery, or nasal trauma should not use a nasal corticosteroid until healing has occurred.

Glaucoma and cataract formation was evaluated in one controlled study of 12 weeks' duration and one uncontrolled study of 12 months' duration in patients treated with NASONEX Nasal Spray, 50 mcg at 200 mcg/day, using intraocular pressure measurements and slit lamp examination. No significant change from baseline was noted in the mean intraocular pressure measurements for the 141 NASONEX-treated patients in the 12-week study, as compared with 141 placebo-treated patients. No individual NASONEX-treated patient was noted to have developed a significant elevation in intraocular pressure or cataracts in this 12-week study. Likewise, no significant change from baseline was noted in the mean intraocular pressure measurements for the 139 NASONEX-treated patients in the 12-month study and again, no cataracts were detected in these patients. Nonetheless, nasal and inhaled corticosteroids have been associated with the development of glaucoma and/or cataracts. Therefore, close follow-up is warranted in patients with a change in vision and with a history of glaucoma and/or cataracts.

When nasal corticosteroids are used at excessive doses, systemic corticosteroid effects such as hypercorticism and adrenal suppression may appear. If such changes occur, NASONEX Nasal Spray, 50 mcg should be discontinued slowly, consistent with accepted procedures for discontinuing oral steroid therapy.

Information for Patients: Patients being treated with NASONEX Nasal Spray, 50 mcg should be given the following information and instructions. This information is intended to aid in the safe and effective use of this medication. It is not a disclosure of all intended or possible adverse effects. Patients should use NASONEX Nasal Spray, 50 mcg at regular intervals (see **DOSAGE AND ADMINISTRATION**) since its effectiveness depends on regular use. Improvement in nasal symptoms of allergic rhinitis has been shown to occur within 11 hours after the first dose based on one single-dose, parallel-group study of patients in an outdoor "park" setting (park study) and one environmental exposure unit (EEU) study and within 2 days after the first dose in two randomized, double-blind, placebo-controlled, parallel-group seasonal allergic rhinitis studies. Maximum benefit is usually achieved within 1 to 2 weeks after initiation of dosing. Patients should take the medication as directed and should not increase the prescribed dosage in an attempt to increase its effectiveness. Patients should contact their physician if symptoms do not improve, or if the condition worsens. To assure proper use of this nasal spray, and to attain maximum benefit, patients should read and follow the accompanying Patient's Instructions for Use carefully. Administration to young children should be aided by an adult.

Patients should be cautioned not to spray NASONEX Nasal Spray, 50 mcg into the eyes or directly onto the nasal septum.

Persons who are on immunosuppressant doses of corticosteroids should be warned to avoid exposure to chickenpox or measles, and patients should also be advised that if they are exposed, medical advice should be sought without delay.

Carcinogenesis, Mutagenesis, Impairment of Fertility: In a 2-year carcinogenicity study in Sprague Dawley rats, mometasone furoate demonstrated no statistically significant increase in the incidence of tumors at inhalation doses up to 67 mcg/kg (approximately 1 and 2 times the maximum recommended daily intranasal dose [MRDID] in adults [400 mcg] and children [100 mcg], respectively, on a mcg/m^2 basis). In a 19-month carcinogenicity study in Swiss CD-1 mice, mometasone furoate demonstrated no statistically significant increase in the incidence of tumors at inhalation doses up to 160 mcg/kg (approximately 2 times the MRDID in adults and children, respectively, on a mcg/m^2 basis).

Mometasone furoate increased chromosomal aberrations in an *in vitro* Chinese hamster ovary-cell assay, but did not increase chromosomal aberrations in an *in vitro* Chinese hamster lung cell assay. Mometasone furoate was not mutagenic in the Ames test or mouse-lymphoma assay, and was not clastogenic in an *in vivo* mouse micronucleus assay and a rat bone marrow chromosomal aberration assay or a mouse male germ-cell chromosomal aberration assay. Mometasone furoate also did not induce unscheduled DNA synthesis *in vivo* in rat hepatocytes.

In reproductive studies in rats, impairment of fertility was not produced by subcutaneous doses up to 15 mcg/kg (less than the MRDID in adults on a mcg/m^2 basis).

Pregnancy: *Teratogenic Effects: Pregnancy Category C:* When administered to pregnant mice, rats, and rabbits, mometasone furoate increased fetal malformations. The doses that produced malformations also decreased fetal growth, as measured by lower fetal weights and/or delayed ossification. Mometasone furoate also caused dystocia and related complications when administered to rats during the end of pregnancy.

In mice, mometasone furoate caused cleft palate at subcutaneous doses of 60 mcg/kg and above (less than the MRDID in adults on a mcg/m^2 basis). Fetal survival was reduced at 180 mcg/kg (approximately 2 times the MRDID in adults on a mcg/m^2 basis). No toxicity was observed at 20 mcg/kg (less than the MRDID in adults on a mcg/m^2 basis).

In rats, mometasone furoate produced umbilical hernia at topical dermal doses of 600 mcg/kg and above (approximately 10 times the MRDID in adults on a mcg/m^2 basis). A dose of 300 mcg/kg (approximately 6 times the MRDID in adults on a mcg/m^2 basis) produced delays in ossification, but no malformations.

In rabbits, mometasone furoate caused multiple malformations (eg, flexed front paws, gallbladder agenesis, umbilical hernia, hydrocephaly) at topical dermal doses of 150 mcg/kg and above (approximately 6 times the MRDID in adults on a mcg/m^2 basis). In an oral study, mometasone furoate increased resorptions and caused cleft palate and/or head malformations (hydrocephaly or domed head) at 700 mcg/kg (approximately 30 times the MRDID in adults on a mcg/m^2 basis). At 2800 mcg/kg (approximately 110 times the MRDID in adults on a mcg/m^2 basis), most litters were aborted or resorbed. No toxicity was observed at 140 mcg/kg (approximately 6 times the MRDID in adults on a mcg/m^2 basis).

Continued on next page

Nasonex—Cont.

When rats received subcutaneous doses of mometasone furoate throughout pregnancy or during the later stages of pregnancy, 15 mcg/kg (less than the MRDID in adults on a mcg/m^2 basis) caused prolonged and difficult labor and reduced the number of live births, birth weight, and early pup survival. Similar effects were not observed at 7.5 mcg/kg (less than the MRDID in adults on a mcg/m^2 basis).

There are no adequate and well-controlled studies in pregnant women. NASONEX Nasal Spray, 50 mcg, like other corticosteroids, should be used during pregnancy only if the potential benefits justify the potential risk to the fetus. Experience with oral corticosteroids since their introduction in pharmacologic, as opposed to physiologic, doses suggests that rodents are more prone to teratogenic effects from corticosteroids than humans. In addition, because there is a natural increase in corticosteroid production during pregnancy, most women will require a lower exogenous corticosteroid dose and many will not need corticosteroid treatment during pregnancy.

Nonteratogenic Effects: Hypoadrenalism may occur in infants born to women receiving corticosteroids during pregnancy. Such infants should be carefully monitored.

Nursing Mothers: It is not known if mometasone furoate is excreted in human milk. Because other corticosteroids are excreted in human milk, caution should be used when NASONEX Nasal Spray, 50 mcg is administered to nursing women.

Pediatric Use: Controlled clinical studies have shown intranasal corticosteroids may cause a reduction in growth velocity in pediatric patients. This effect has been observed in the absence of laboratory evidence of hypothalamic-pituitary-adrenal (HPA) axis suppression, suggesting that growth velocity is a more sensitive indicator of systemic corticosteroid exposure in pediatric patients than some commonly used tests of HPA axis function. The long-term effects of this reduction in growth velocity associated with intranasal corticosteroids, including the impact on final adult height, are unknown. The potential for "catch up" growth following discontinuation of treatment with intranasal corticosteroids has not been adequately studied. The growth of pediatric patients receiving intranasal corticosteroids, including NASONEX Nasal Spray, 50 mcg, should be monitored routinely (eg, via stadiometry). The potential growth effects of prolonged treatment should be weighed against clinical benefits obtained and the availability of safe and effective noncorticosteroid treatment alternatives. To minimize the systemic effects of intranasal corticosteroids, including NASONEX Nasal Spray, 50 mcg, each patient should be titrated to his/her lowest effective dose.

Seven hundred and twenty (720) patients 3 to 11 years of age with allergic rhinitis were treated with mometasone furoate nasal spray, 50 mcg (100 mcg total daily dose) in controlled clinical trials (see **CLINICAL PHARMACOLOGY, Clinical Studies** section). Twenty-eight (28) patients 2 to 5 years of age with allergic rhinitis were treated with mometasone furoate nasal spray, 50 mcg (100 mcg total daily dose) in a controlled trial to evaluate safety (see **CLINICAL PHARMACOLOGY, Pharmacokinetics** section). Safety and effectiveness in children less than 2 years of age with allergic rhinitis and in children less than 18 years of age with nasal polyps have not been established.

A clinical study has been conducted for 1 year in pediatric patients with allergic rhinitis (ages 3 to 9 years) to assess the effect of NASONEX Nasal Spray, 50 mcg (100 mcg total daily dose) on growth velocity. No statistically significant effect on growth velocity was observed for NASONEX Nasal Spray, 50 mcg compared to placebo. No evidence of clinically relevant HPA axis suppression was observed following a 30-minute cosyntropin infusion.

The potential of NASONEX Nasal Spray, 50 mcg to cause growth suppression in susceptible patients or when given at higher doses cannot be ruled out.

Geriatric Use: A total of 280 patients above 64 years of age with allergic rhinitis or nasal polyps (age range 64 to 86 years) have been treated with NASONEX Nasal Spray, 50 mcg for up to 3 or 4 months, respectively. The adverse reactions reported in this population were similar in type and incidence to those reported by younger patients.

ADVERSE REACTIONS

Allergic Rhinitis. In controlled US and international clinical studies, a total of 3210 adult and adolescent patients ages 12 years and older with allergic rhinitis received treatment with NASONEX Nasal Spray, 50 mcg at doses of 50 to 800 mcg/day. The majority of patients (n = 2103) were treated with 200 mcg/day. In controlled US and international studies, a total of 990 pediatric patients (ages 3 to 11 years) with allergic rhinitis received treatment with NASONEX Nasal Spray, 50 mcg, at doses of 25 to 200 mcg/day. The majority of pediatric patients (720) were treated with 100 mcg/day. A total of 513 adult, adolescent, and pediatric patients have been treated for 1 year or longer. The overall incidence of adverse events for patients treated with NASONEX Nasal Spray, 50 mcg was comparable to patients treated with the vehicle placebo. Also, adverse events did not differ significantly based on age, sex, or race. Three percent or less of patients in clinical trials discontinued treatment because of adverse events; this rate was similar for the vehicle and active comparators.

All adverse events (regardless of relationship to treatment) reported by 5% or more of adult and adolescent patients ages 12 years and older who received NASONEX Nasal Spray, 50 mcg, 200 mcg/day and by pediatric patients ages 3 to 11 years who received NASONEX Nasal Spray, 50 mcg, 100 mcg/day in clinical trials vs placebo and that were more common with NASONEX Nasal Spray, 50 mcg than placebo, are displayed in the table below.

[See table below]

Other adverse events which occurred in less than 5% but greater than or equal to 2% of mometasone furoate adult and adolescent patients (ages 12 years and older) treated with 200-mcg doses (regardless of relationship to treatment), and more frequently than in the placebo group included: arthralgia, asthma, bronchitis, chest pain, conjunctivitis, diarrhea, dyspepsia, earache, flu-like symptoms, myalgia, nausea, and rhinitis.

Other adverse events which occurred in less than 5% but greater than or equal to 2% of mometasone furoate pediatric patients ages 3 to 11 years treated with 100-mcg doses vs placebo (regardless of relationship to treatment) and more frequently than in the placebo group included: diarrhea, nasal irritation, otitis media, and wheezing.

The adverse event (regardless of relationship to treatment) reported by 5% of pediatric patients ages 2 to 5 years who received NASONEX Nasal Spray, 50 mcg, 100 mcg/day in a clinical trial vs placebo including 56 subjects (28 each NASONEX Nasal Spray, 50 mcg and placebo) and that was more common with NASONEX Nasal Spray, 50 mcg than placebo, included: upper respiratory tract infection (7% vs 0%, respectively). The other adverse event which occurred in less than 5% but greater than or equal to 2% of mometasone furoate pediatric patients ages 2 to 5 years treated with 100-mcg doses vs placebo (regardless of relationship to treatment) and more frequently than in the placebo group included: skin trauma.

Nasal Polyps. In controlled clinical studies, the types of adverse events observed in patients with nasal polyps were similar to those observed for patients with allergic rhinitis. A total of 594 adult patients (ages 18 to 86 years) received NASONEX Nasal Spray, 50 mcg, at doses of 200 mcg once or twice daily for up to 4 months for treatment of nasal polyps. The overall incidence of adverse events for patients treated with NASONEX Nasal Spray, 50 mcg was comparable to patients treated with the placebo except for epistaxis, which was 9% for 200 mcg once daily, 13% for 200 mcg twice daily, and 5% for placebo.

Rare cases of nasal ulcers and nasal and oral candidiasis were also reported in patients treated with NASONEX Nasal Spray, 50 mcg, primarily in patients treated for longer than 4 weeks.

In postmarketing surveillance of this product, cases of nasal burning and irritation, anaphylaxis and angioedema, and rare cases of nasal septal perforation have been reported. Disturbances of taste and smell have been reported very rarely.

ADVERSE EVENTS FROM CONTROLLED CLINICAL TRIALS IN SEASONAL ALLERGIC AND PERENNIAL ALLERGIC RHINITIS (PERCENT OF PATIENTS REPORTING)

	Adult and Adolescent Patients 12 years and older		Pediatric Patients Ages 3 to 11 years	
	NASONEX 200 mcg (n = 2103)	VEHICLE PLACEBO (n = 1671)	NASONEX 100 mcg (n = 374)	VEHICLE PLACEBO (n = 376)
Headache	26	22	17	18
Viral Infection	14	11	8	9
Pharyngitis	12	10	10	10
Epistaxis/Blood-Tinged Mucus	11	6	8	9
Coughing	7	6	13	15
Upper Respiratory Tract Infection	6	2	5	4
Dysmenorrhea	5	3	1	0
Musculoskeletal Pain	5	3	1	1
Sinusitis	5	3	4	4
Vomiting	1	1	5	4

OVERDOSAGE

There are no data available on the effects of acute or chronic overdosage with NASONEX Nasal Spray, 50 mcg. Because of low systemic bioavailability, and an absence of acute drug-related systemic findings in clinical studies, overdose is unlikely to require any therapy other than observation. Intranasal administration of 1600 mcg (4 times the recommended dose of NASONEX Nasal Spray, 50 mcg) daily for 29 days, to healthy human volunteers, was well tolerated with no increased incidence of adverse events. Single intranasal doses up to 4000 mcg have been studied in human volunteers with no adverse effects reported. Single oral doses up to 8000 mcg have been studied in human volunteers with no adverse effects reported. Chronic overdosage with any corticosteroid may result in signs or symptoms of hypercorticism (see **PRECAUTIONS**). Acute overdosage with this dosage form is unlikely since one bottle of NASONEX Nasal Spray, 50 mcg contains approximately 8500 mcg of mometasone furoate.

DOSAGE AND ADMINISTRATION

Allergic Rhinitis: Adults and Children 12 Years of Age and Older: The recommended dose for prophylaxis and treatment of the nasal symptoms of seasonal allergic rhinitis and treatment of the nasal symptoms of perennial allergic rhinitis is two sprays (50 mcg of mometasone furoate in each spray) in each nostril once daily (total daily dose of 200 mcg).

In patients with a known seasonal allergen that precipitates nasal symptoms of seasonal allergic rhinitis, prophylaxis with NASONEX Nasal Spray, 50 mcg (200 mcg/day) is recommended 2 to 4 weeks prior to the anticipated start of the pollen season.

Children 2 to 11 Years of Age: The recommended dose for treatment of the nasal symptoms of seasonal allergic and perennial allergic rhinitis is one spray (50 mcg of mometasone furoate in each spray) in each nostril once daily (total daily dose of 100 mcg).

Improvement in nasal symptoms of allergic rhinitis has been shown to occur within 11 hours after the first dose based on one single-dose, parallel-group study of patients in an outdoor "park" setting (park study) and one environmental exposure unit (EEU) study and within 2 days after the first dose in two randomized, double-blind, placebo-controlled, parallel-group seasonal allergic rhinitis studies. Maximum benefit is usually achieved within 1 to 2 weeks. Patients should use NASONEX Nasal Spray, 50 mcg only once daily for allergic rhinitis at a regular interval.

Nasal Polyps: Adults 18 years of Age and Older: The recommended dose for nasal polyps is two sprays (50 mcg of mometasone furoate in each spray) in each nostril twice daily (total daily dose of 400 mcg). A dose of two sprays (50 mcg of mometasone furoate in each spray) in each nostril once daily (total daily dose of 200 mcg) is also effective in some patients.

Prior to initial use of NASONEX Nasal Spray, 50 mcg, the pump must be primed by actuating ten times or until a fine spray appears. The pump may be stored unused for up to 1 week without repriming. If unused for more than 1 week, reprime by actuating two times, or until a fine spray appears.

Directions for Use: Illustrated **Patient's Instructions for Use** accompany each package of NASONEX Nasal Spray, 50 mcg.

Directions for Cleaning: Illustrated **Applicator Cleaning Instructions** accompany each package of NASONEX Nasal Spray, 50 mcg.

HOW SUPPLIED

NASONEX (mometasone furoate monohydrate) Nasal Spray, 50 mcg is supplied in a white, high-density, polyethylene bottle fitted with a white metered-dose, manual spray pump, and blue cap. It contains 17 g of product formulation, 120 sprays, each delivering 50 mcg of mometasone furoate per actuation. Supplied with **Patient's Instructions for Use** (NDC 0085-1288-01).

Store at 25°C (77°F); excursions permitted to 15–30°C (59–86°F) [see USP Controlled Room Temperature]. Protect from light.

When NASONEX Nasal Spray, 50 mcg is removed from its cardboard container, prolonged exposure of the product to direct light should be avoided. Brief exposure to light, as with normal use, is acceptable.

SHAKE WELL BEFORE EACH USE.

Schering®
Schering Corporation
Kenilworth, NJ 07033 USA

Copyright © 1997, 2003, 2005, Schering Corporation.
All rights reserved.

Rev. 12/04
26405262T

PEG-INTRON® ℞

[pĕg ĭn-trŏn]
(Peginterferon alfa-2b)
Powder for Injection

Prescribing information for this product, which appears on pages 3046–3053 of the 2005 PDR, has been completely revised as follows. Please write "See Supplement A" next to the product heading.

Alpha interferons, including PEG-Intron, may cause or aggravate fatal or life-threatening neuropsychiatric, autoimmune, ischemic, and infectious disorders. Patients should be monitored closely with periodic clinical and laboratory evaluations. Patients with persistently severe or worsening signs or symptoms of these conditions should be withdrawn from therapy. In many but not all cases these disorders resolve after stopping PEG-Intron therapy. See WARNINGS, ADVERSE REACTIONS.

Use with Ribavirin. Ribavirin may cause birth defects and/or death of the unborn child. Extreme care must be taken to avoid pregnancy in female patients and in female partners of male patients. Ribavirin causes hemolytic anemia. The anemia associated with REBETOL therapy may result in a worsening of cardiac disease. Ribavirin is genotoxic and mutagenic and should be considered a potential carcinogen. (See REBETOL package insert for additional information and other warnings.)

DESCRIPTION

PEG-Intron®, peginterferon alfa-2b, Powder for Injection is a covalent conjugate of recombinant alfa-2b interferon with monomethoxy polyethylene glycol (PEG). The average molecular weight of the PEG portion of the molecule is 12,000 daltons. The average molecular weight of the PEG-Intron molecule is approximately 31,000 daltons. The specific activity of peginterferon alfa-2b is approximately 0.7×10^8 IU/mg protein.

Interferon alfa-2b, is a water-soluble protein with a molecular weight of 19,271 daltons produced by recombinant DNA techniques. It is obtained from the bacterial fermentation of a strain of *Escherichia coli* bearing a genetically engineered plasmid containing an interferon gene from human leukocytes.

PEG-Intron is supplied in both vials and the Redipen® for subcutaneous use.

Vials

Each vial contains either 74 µg, 118.4 µg, 177.6 µg, or 222 µg of PEG-Intron as a white to off-white tablet-like solid, that is whole/in pieces or as a loose powder, and 1.11 mg dibasic sodium phosphate anhydrous, 1.11 mg monobasic sodium phosphate dihydrate, 59.2 mg sucrose and 0.074 mg polysorbate 80. Following reconstitution with 0.7 mL of the supplied Sterile Water for Injection, USP, each vial contains PEG-Intron at strengths of either 50 µg per 0.5 mL, 80 µg per 0.5 mL, 120 µg per 0.5 mL, or 150 µg per 0.5 mL.

Redipen®

Redipen® is a dual-chamber glass cartridge containing lyophilized PEG-Intron as a white to off-white tablet or powder that is whole or in pieces in the sterile active chamber and a second chamber containing Sterile Water for Injection, USP. Each PEG-Intron Redipen® contains either 67.5 µg, 108 µg, 162 µg, or 202.5 µg of PEG-Intron, and 1.013 mg dibasic sodium phosphate anhydrous, 1.013 mg monobasic sodium phosphate dihydrate, 54 mg sucrose and 0.0675 mg polysorbate 80. Each cartridge is reconstituted to allow for the administration of up to 0.5 mL of solution. Following reconstitution, each Redipen® contains PEG-Intron at strengths of either 50 µg per 0.5 mL, 80 µg per 0.5 mL, 120 µg per 0.5 mL, or 150 µg per 0.5 mL for a single use. Because a small volume of reconstituted solution is lost during preparation of PEG-Intron, each Redipen® contains an excess amount of PEG-Intron powder and diluent to ensure delivery of the labeled dose.

CLINICAL PHARMACOLOGY

General: The biological activity of PEG-Intron is derived from its interferon alfa-2b moiety. Interferons exert their cellular activities by binding to specific membrane receptors on the cell surface and initiate a complex sequence of intracellular events. These include the induction of certain enzymes, suppression of cell proliferation, immunomodulating activities such as enhancement of the phagocytic activity of macrophages and augmentation of the specific cytotoxicity of lymphocytes for target cells, and inhibition of virus replication in virus-infected cells. Interferon alfa upregulates the Th1 T-helper cell subset in *in vitro* studies. The clinical relevance of these findings is not known.

Pharmacodynamics: PEG-Intron raises concentrations of effector proteins such as serum neopterin and 2′5′ oligoadenylate synthetase, raises body temperature, and causes reversible decreases in leukocyte and platelet counts. The correlation between the *in vitro* and *in vivo* pharmacologic and pharmacodynamic and clinical effects is unknown.

Pharmacokinetics: Following a single subcutaneous (SC) dose of PEG-Intron, the mean absorption half-life (t ½ k_a) was 4.6 hours. Maximal serum concentrations (C_{max}) occur between 15–44 hours post-dose, and are sustained for up to 48–72 hours. The C_{max} and AUC measurements of PEG-Intron increase in a dose-related manner. After multiple dosing, there is an increase in bioavailability of PEG-Intron. Week 48 mean trough concentrations (320 pg/mL; range 0, 2960) are approximately 3-fold higher than Week 4 mean trough concentrations (94 pg/mL; range 0, 416). The mean PEG-Intron elimination half-life is approximately 40 hours (range 22 to 60 hours) in patients with HCV infection. The apparent clearance of PEG-Intron is estimated to be approximately 22.0 mL/hr•kg. Renal elimination accounts for 30% of the clearance.

Pegylation of interferon alfa-2b produces a product (PEG-Intron) whose clearance is lower than that of non-pegylated interferon alfa-2b. When compared to INTRON A, PEG-Intron (1.0 µ/kg) has approximately a seven-fold lower mean apparent clearance and a five-fold greater mean half-life permitting a reduced dosing frequency. At effective therapeutic doses, PEG-Intron has approximately ten-fold greater C_{max} and 50-fold greater AUC than interferon alfa-2b.

Special Populations

Renal Dysfunction

Following multiple dosing of PEG-Intron (1 mcg/kg SC given every week for four weeks) the clearance of PEG-Intron is reduced by a mean of 17% in patients with moderate renal impairment (creatinine clearance 30–49 mL/min) and by a mean of 44% in patients with severe renal impairment (creatinine clearance 10–29 mL/min) compared to subjects with normal renal function. Clearance was similar in patients with severe renal impairment not on dialysis and patients who are receiving hemodialysis. The dose of PEG-Intron for monotherapy should be reduced in patients with moderate or severe renal impairment (See **DOSAGE AND ADMINISTRATION: DOSE REDUCTION**). REBETOL should not be used in patients with creatinine clearance < 50 mL/min (See **REBETOL Package Insert, WARNINGS**).

Gender

During the 48 week treatment period with PEG-Intron, no differences in the pharmacokinetic profiles were observed between male and female patients with chronic hepatitis C infection.

Geriatric Patients

The pharmacokinetics of geriatric subjects (> 65 years of age) treated with a single subcutaneous dose of 1.0 µg/kg of PEG-Intron were similar in C_{max}, AUC, clearance, or elimination half-life as compared to younger subjects (28 to 44 years of age).

Effect of Food on Absorption of Ribavirin Both AUC_{tf} and C_{max} increased by 70% when REBETOL Capsules were administered with a high-fat meal (841 kcal, 53.8 g fat, 31.6 g protein, and 57.4 g carbohydrate) in a single-dose pharmacokinetic study. (See **DOSAGE AND ADMINISTRATION**).

Drug Interactions: It is not known if PEG-Intron therapy causes clinically significant drug-drug interactions with drugs metabolized by the liver in patients with hepatitis C. In 12 healthy subjects known to be CYP2D6 extensive metabolizers, a single subcutaneous dose of 1 µg/kg PEG-Intron did not inhibit CYP1A2, 2C8/9, 2D6, hepatic 3A4 or N-acetyltransferase; the effects of PEG-Intron on CYP2C19 were not assessed.

Methadone

The pharmacokinetics of concomitant administration of methadone and PEG-Intron were evaluated in 18 PEG-Intron naïve chronic hepatitis C patients receiving 1.5 µg/kg/week PEG-Intron SC weekly. All patients were on stable methadone maintenance therapy receiving ≥40 mg/day prior to initiating PEG-Intron. Mean methadone AUC was approximately 16% higher after 4 weeks of PEG-Intron treatment as compared to baseline. In 2 patients, methadone AUC was approximately double after 4 weeks of PEG-Intron treatment as compared to baseline (see **PRECAUTIONS: Drug Interactions**).

CLINICAL STUDIES

PEG-Intron Monotherapy-Study 1

A randomized study compared treatment with PEG-Intron (0.5, 1.0, or 1.5 µg/kg once weekly SC) to treatment with INTRON A, (3 million units three times weekly SC) in 1219 adults with chronic hepatitis from HCV infection. The patients were not previously treated with interferon alfa, had compensated liver disease, detectable HCV RNA, elevated ALT, and liver histopathology consistent with chronic hepatitis. Patients were treated for 48 weeks and were followed for 24 weeks post-treatment. Seventy percent of all patients were infected with HCV genotype 1, and 74 percent of all patients had high baseline levels of HCV RNA (more than 2 million copies per mL of serum), two factors known to predict poor response to treatment.

Response to treatment was defined as undetectable HCV RNA and normalization of ALT at 24 weeks post-treatment. The response rates to the 1.0 and 1.5 µg/kg PEG-Intron doses were similar (approximately 24%) to each other and were both higher than the response rate to INTRON A (12%). (See **Table 1**.)

[See table 1 above]

TABLE 1. Rates of Response to Treatment-Study 1

	A PEG-Intron 0.5 µg/kg (N=315)	B PEG-Intron 1.0 µg/kg (N=298)	C INTRON A 3 MIU TIW (N=307)	B-C (95% CI) Difference between PEG-Intron 1.0 µg/kg and INTRON A
Treatment Response (Combined Virologic Response and ALT Normalization)	17%	24%	12%	11 (5, 18)
Virologic Response[a]	18%	25%	12%	12 (6, 19)
ALT Normalization	24%	29%	18%	11 (5, 18)

[a]Serum HCV is measured by a research-based quantitative polymerase chain reaction assay by a central laboratory.

Patients with both viral genotype 1 and high serum levels of HCV RNA at baseline were less likely to respond to treatment with PEG-Intron. Among patients with the two unfavorable prognostic variables, 8% (12/157) responded to PEG-Intron treatment and 2% (4/169) responded to INTRON A. Doses of PEG-Intron higher than the recommended dose did not result in higher response rates in these patients.

Patients receiving PEG-Intron with viral genotype 1 had a response rate of 14% (28/199) while patients with other viral genotypes had a 45% (43/96) response rate.

Ninety-six percent of the responders in the PEG-Intron groups and 100% of responders in the INTRON A group first cleared their viral RNA by week 24 of treatment. (See **DOSAGE AND ADMINISTRATION**.)

The treatment response rates were similar in men and women. Response rates were lower in African American and Hispanic patients and higher in Asians compared to Caucasians. Although African Americans had a higher proportion of poor prognostic factors compared to Caucasians the number of non-Caucasians studied (9% of the total) was insufficient to allow meaningful conclusions about differences in response rates after adjusting for prognostic factors.

Liver biopsies were obtained before and after treatment in 60% of patients. A modest reduction in inflammation compared to baseline that was similar in all four treatment groups was observed.

PEG-Intron/REBETOL Combination Therapy-Study 2

A randomized study compared treatment with two PEG-Intron/REBETOL regimens [PEG-Intron 1.5 µg/kg SC once weekly (QW)/REBETOL 800 mg PO daily (in divided doses); PEG-Intron 1.5 µg/kg SC QW for 4 weeks then 0.5 µg/kg SC QW for 44 weeks/REBETOL 1000/1200 mg PO daily (in divided doses)] with INTRON A [3 MIU SC thrice weekly (TIW)/REBETOL 1000/1200 mg PO daily (in divided doses)] in 1530 adults with chronic hepatitis C. Interferon naïve patients were treated for 48 weeks and followed for 24 weeks posttreatment. Eligible patients had compensated liver disease, detectable HCV RNA, elevated ALT, and liver histopathology consistent with chronic hepatitis.

Response to treatment was defined as undetectable HCV RNA at 24 weeks posttreatment. The response rate to the PEG-Intron 1.5 µg/kg plus ribavirin 800 mg dose was higher than the response rate to INTRON A/REBETOL (see **Table 2**). The response rate to PEG-Intron 1.5 >0.5 µg/kg/REBETOL was essentially the same as the response to INTRON A/REBETOL (data not shown).

[See table 2 at top of next page]

Patients with viral genotype 1, regardless of viral load, had a lower response rate to PEG-Intron (1.5 µg/kg)/REBETOL compared to patients with other viral genotypes. Patients with both poor prognostic factors (genotype 1 and high viral load) had a response rate of 30% (78/256) compared to a response rate of 29% (71/247) with INTRON A/REBETOL.

Patients with lower body weight tended to have higher adverse event rates (see **ADVERSE REACTIONS**) and higher response rates than patients with higher body weights. Differences in response rates between treatment arms did not substantially vary with body weight.

Treatment response rates with PEG-Intron/REBETOL were 49% in men and 56% in women. Response rates were lower in African American and Hispanic patients and higher in Asians compared to Caucasians. Although African Americans had a higher proportion of poor prognostic factors compared to Caucasians the number of non-Caucasians studied (11% of the total) was insufficient to allow meaningful conclusions about differences in response rates after adjusting for prognostic factors.

Liver biopsies were obtained before and after treatment in 68% of patients. Compared to baseline approximately 2/3 of patients in all treatment groups were observed to have a modest reduction in inflammation.

INDICATIONS AND USAGE

PEG-Intron, peginterferon alfa-2b, is indicated for use alone or in combination with REBETOL (ribavirin, USP) for the treatment of chronic hepatitis C in patients with compensated liver disease who have not been previously treated with interferon alpha and are at least 18 years of age.

CONTRAINDICATIONS

PEG-Intron is contraindicated in patients with:

- hypersensitivity to PEG-Intron or any other component of the product
- autoimmune hepatitis
- decompensated liver disease

PEG-Intron/REBETOL combination therapy is additionally contraindicated in:

- patients with hypersensitivity to ribavirin or any other component of the product

Continued on next page

Peg-Intron—Cont.

- women who are pregnant
- men whose female partners are pregnant
- patients with hemoglobinopathies (e.g., thalassemia major, sickle-cell anemia)
- patients with creatinine clearance < 50 mL/min

WARNINGS

Patients should be monitored for the following serious conditions, some of which may become life threatening. Patients with persistently severe or worsening signs or symptoms should be withdrawn from therapy.

Neuropsychiatric events
Life-threatening or fatal neuropsychiatric events, including suicide, suicidal and homicidal ideation, depression, relapse of drug addiction/overdose, and aggressive behavior have occurred in patients with and without a previous psychiatric disorder during PEG-Intron treatment and follow-up. Psychoses, hallucinations, bipolar disorders, and mania have been observed in patients treated with alpha interferons. PEG-Intron should be used with extreme caution in patients with a history of psychiatric disorders. Patients should be advised to report immediately any symptoms of depression and/or suicidal ideation to their prescribing physicians. Physicians should monitor all patients for evidence of depression and other psychiatric symptoms. In severe cases, PEG-Intron should be stopped immediately and psychiatric intervention instituted. (See **DOSAGE AND ADMINISTRATION: Dose Reduction.**)

Bone marrow toxicity
PEG-Intron suppresses bone marrow function, sometimes resulting in severe cytopenias. PEG-Intron should be discontinued in patients who develop severe decreases in neutrophil or platelet counts. (See **DOSAGE AND ADMINISTRATION: Dose Reduction.**) Ribavirin may potentiate the neutropenia induced by interferon alpha. Very rarely alpha interferons may be associated with aplastic anemia.

Endocrine disorders
PEG-Intron causes or aggravates hypothyroidism and hyperthyroidism. Hyperglycemia has been observed in patients treated with PEG-Intron. Diabetes mellitus has been observed in patients treated with alpha interferons. Patients with these conditions who cannot be effectively treated by medication should not begin PEG-Intron therapy. Patients who develop these conditions during treatment and cannot be controlled with medication should not continue PEG-Intron therapy.

Cardiovascular events
Cardiovascular events, which include hypotension, arrhythmia, tachycardia, cardiomyopathy, angina pectoris, and myocardial infarction, have been observed in patients treated with PEG-Intron. PEG-Intron should be used cautiously in patients with cardiovascular disease. Patients with a history of myocardial infarction and arrhythmic disorder who require PEG-Intron therapy should be closely monitored (see **Laboratory Tests**). Patients with a history of significant or unstable cardiac disease should not be treated with PEG-Intron/REBETOL combination therapy. (See **REBETOL package insert.**)

Pulmonary disorders
Dyspnea, pulmonary infiltrates, pneumonia, bronchiolitis obliterans, interstitial pneumonitis and sarcoidosis, some resulting in respiratory failure and/or patient deaths, may be induced or aggravated by PEG-Intron or alpha interferon therapy. Recurrence of respiratory failure has been observed with interferon rechallenge. PEG-Intron combination treatment should be suspended in patients who develop pulmonary infiltrates or pulmonary function impairment. Patients who resume interferon treatment should be closely monitored.

Colitis
Fatal and nonfatal ulcerative or hemorrhagic/ischemic colitis have been observed within 12 weeks of the start of alpha interferon treatment. Abdominal pain, bloody diarrhea, and fever are the typical manifestations. PEG-Intron treatment should be discontinued immediately in patients who develop these symptoms and signs. The colitis usually resolves within 1–3 weeks of discontinuation of alpha interferons.

Pancreatitis
Fatal and nonfatal pancreatitis have been observed in patients treated with alpha interferon. PEG-Intron therapy should be suspended in patients with signs and symptoms suggestive of pancreatitis and discontinued in patients diagnosed with pancreatitis.

Autoimmune disorders
Development or exacerbation of autoimmune disorders (eg, thyroiditis, thrombocytopenia, rheumatoid arthritis, interstitial nephritis, systemic lupus erythematosus, psoriasis) have been observed in patients receiving PEG-Intron. PEG-Intron should be used with caution in patients with autoimmune disorders.

Ophthalmologic disorders
Decrease or loss of vision, retinopathy including macular edema, retinal artery or vein thrombosis, retinal hemorrhages and cotton wool spots, optic neuritis, and papilledema may be induced or aggravated by treatment with peginterferon alfa-2b or other alpha interferons. All patients should receive an eye examination at baseline. Patients with preexisting ophthalmologic disorders (eg, diabetic or hypertensive retinopathy) should receive periodic ophthalmologic exams during interferon alpha treatment. Any patient who develops ocular symptoms should receive a prompt and complete eye examination. Peginterferon alfa-2b treatment should be discontinued in patients who develop new or worsening ophthalmologic disorders.

TABLE 2. Rates of Response to Treatment-Study 2

	PEG-Intron 1.5 µg/kg QW REBETOL 800 mg QD	INTRON A 3 MIU TIW REBETOL 1000/1200 mg QD
Overall response[1,2]	52% (264/511)	46% (231/505)
Genotype 1	41% (141/348)	33% (112/343)
Genotype 2-6	75% (123/163)	73% (119/162)

[1]Serum HCV RNA is measured with a research-based quantitative polymerase chain reaction assay by a central laboratory.
[2]Difference in overall treatment response (PEG-Intron/REBETOL vs. INTRON A/REBETOL) is 6% with 95% confidence interval of 0.18, 11.63 adjusted for viral genotype and presence of cirrhosis at baseline.

Hypersensitivity
Serious, acute hypersensitivity reactions (eg, urticaria, angioedema, bronchoconstriction, anaphylaxis) and cutaneous eruptions (Stevens Johnson syndrome, toxic epidermal necrolysis) have been rarely observed during alpha interferon therapy. If such a reaction develops during treatment with PEG-Intron, discontinue treatment and institute appropriate medical therapy immediately. Transient rashes do not necessitate interruption of treatment.

Use with Ribavirin–(See also REBETOL Package Insert.)
REBETOL may cause birth defects and/or death of the unborn child. REBETOL therapy should not be started until a report of a negative pregnancy test has been obtained immediately prior to planned initiation of therapy. Patients should use at least two forms of contraception and have monthly pregnancy tests (see BOXED WARNING, CONTRAINDICATIONS and PRECAUTIONS: Information for Patients and REBETOL package insert).

Anemia
Ribavirin caused hemolytic anemia in 10% of PEG-Intron/REBETOL treated patients within 1–4 weeks of initiation of therapy. Complete blood counts should be obtained pretreatment and at week 2 and week 4 of therapy or more frequently if clinically indicated. Anemia associated with REBETOL therapy may result in a worsening of cardiac disease. Decrease in dosage or discontinuation of REBETOL may be necessary. (See **DOSAGE AND ADMINISTRATION: Dose Reduction.**)

PRECAUTIONS

- PEG-Intron alone or in combination with REBETOL has not been studied in patients who have failed other alpha interferon treatments.
- The safety and efficacy of PEG-Intron alone or in combination with REBETOL for the treatment of hepatitis C in liver or other organ transplant recipients have not been studied. In a small (n=16) single-center, uncontrolled case experience, renal failure in renal allograft recipients receiving interferon alpha and ribavirin combination therapy was more frequent than expected from the center's previous experience with renal allograft recipients not receiving combination therapy. The relationship of the renal failure to renal allograft rejection is not clear.
- The safety and efficacy of PEG-Intron/REBETOL for the treatment of patients with HCV co-infected with HIV or HBV have not been established.

Triglycerides: Elevated triglyceride levels have been observed in patients treated with interferon-alfa including PEG-Intron therapy. Hypertriglyceridemia may result in pancreatitis (see **WARNINGS: Pancreatitis**). Elevated triglyceride levels should be managed as clinically appropriate. Discontinuation of PEG-Intron therapy should be considered for patients with symptoms of potential pancreatitis, such as abdominal pain, nausea, or vomiting and persistently elevated triglycerides (eg. triglycerides >1000 mg/dL).

Patients with renal insufficiency: Increases in serum creatinine levels have been observed in patients with renal insufficiency receiving interferon alfa products, including PEG-Intron. Patients with impaired renal function should be closely monitored for signs and symptoms of interferon toxicity, including increases in serum creatinine, and PEG-Intron dosing should be adjusted accordingly or discontinued (see **CLINICAL PHARMACOLOGY: Pharmacokinetics** and **DOSAGE AND ADMINISTRATION: Dose Reduction**). PEG-Intron monotherapy should be used with caution in patients with creatinine clearance <50 mL/min; the potential risks should be weighed against the potential benefits in these patients. Combination therapy with REBETOL must not be used in patients with creatinine clearance < 50 mL/min (see **REBETOL Package Insert WARNINGS**).

Information for Patients: Patients receiving PEG-Intron alone or in combination with REBETOL should be directed in its appropriate use, informed of the benefits and risks associated with treatment, and referred to the **MEDICATION GUIDES for PEG-Intron and, if applicable, REBETOL (ribavirin, USP).**

Patients must be informed that REBETOL may cause birth defects and/or death of the unborn child. Extreme care must be taken to avoid pregnancy in female patients and in female partners of male patients during treatment with combination PEG-Intron/REBETOL therapy and for 6 months post-therapy. Combination PEG-Intron/REBETOL therapy should not be initiated until a report of a negative pregnancy test has been obtained immediately prior to initiation of therapy. It is recommended that patients undergo monthly pregnancy tests during therapy and for 6 months post-therapy. **(See CONTRAINDICATIONS and REBETOL package insert.)**

Patients should be informed that there are no data regarding whether PEG-Intron therapy will prevent transmission of HCV infection to others. Also, it is not known if treatment with PEG-Intron will cure hepatitis C or prevent cirrhosis, liver failure, or liver cancer that may be the result of infection with the hepatitis C virus.

Patients should be advised that laboratory evaluations are required before starting therapy and periodically thereafter (see **Laboratory Tests**). It is advised that patients be well hydrated, especially during the initial stages of treatment. "Flu-like" symptoms associated with administration of PEG-Intron may be minimized by bedtime administration of PEG-Intron or by use of antipyretics.

Patients should be advised to use a puncture-resistant container for the disposal of used syringes, needles, and the Redipen®. The full container should be disposed of in accordance with state and local laws. Patients should be thoroughly instructed in the importance of proper disposal. Patients should also be cautioned against reusing or sharing needles, syringes, or the Redipen®.

Laboratory Tests: PEG-Intron alone or in combination with ribavirin may cause severe decreases in neutrophil and platelet counts, and hematologic, endocrine (eg, TSH) and hepatic abnormalities. Transient elevations in ALT (2–5 fold above baseline) were observed in 10% of patients treated with PEG-Intron, and was not associated with deterioration of other liver functions. Triglyceride levels are frequently elevated in patients receiving alpha interferon therapy including PEG-Intron and should be periodically monitored.

Patients on PEG-Intron or PEG-Intron/REBETOL combination therapy should have hematology and blood chemistry testing before the start of treatment and then periodically thereafter. In the clinical trial CBC (including hemoglobin, neutrophil and platelet counts) and chemistries (including AST, ALT, bilirubin, and uric acid) were measured during the treatment period at weeks 2, 4, 8, 12, and then at 6-week intervals or more frequently if abnormalities developed. TSH levels were measured every 12 weeks during the treatment period.

HCV RNA should be measured at 6 months of treatment. PEG-Intron or PEG-Intron/REBETOL combination therapy should be discontinued in patients with persistent high viral levels.

Patients who have pre-existing cardiac abnormalities should have electrocardiograms administered before treatment with PEG-Intron/REBETOL.

Drug Interactions
In a pharmacokinetic study of 18 chronic hepatitis C patients concomitantly receiving methadone, treatment with PEG-Intron once weekly for 4 weeks was associated with a mean increase of 16% in methadone AUC; in 2 out of 18 patients, methadone AUC doubled (see **CLINICAL PHARMACOLOGY: Drug Interactions**). The clinical significance of this finding is unknown; however, patients should be monitored for the signs and symptoms of increased narcotic effect.

Carcinogenesis, Mutagenesis, and Impairment of Fertility
Carcinogenesis and Mutagenesis: PEG-Intron has not been tested for its carcinogenic potential. Neither PEG-Intron, nor its components interferon or methoxy polyethylene glycol caused damage to DNA when tested in the standard battery of mutagenesis assays, in the presence and absence of metabolic activation.

Use with Ribavirin: Ribavirin is genotoxic and mutagenic and should be considered a potential carcinogen. See REBETOL package insert for additional warnings relevant to PEG-Intron therapy in combination with ribavirin.

Impairment of Fertility: PEG-Intron may impair human fertility. Irregular menstrual cycles were observed in female cynomolgus monkeys given subcutaneous injections of 4239 µg/m^2 PEG-Intron alone every other day for 1 month (approximately 345 times the recommended weekly human dose based upon body surface area). These effects included transiently decreased serum levels of estradiol and progesterone, suggestive of anovulation. Normal menstrual cycles and serum hormone levels resumed in these animals 2 to 3 months following cessation of PEG-Intron treatment. Every other day dosing with 262 µg/m^2 (approximately 21 times the weekly human dose) had no effects on cycle duration or reproductive hormone status. The effects of PEG-Intron on male fertility have not been studied.

Pregnancy Category C: PEG-Intron monotherapy: Nonpegylated Interferon alfa-2b, has been shown to have abortifacient effects in *Macaca mulatta* (rhesus monkeys) at 15 and 30 million IU/kg (estimated human equivalent of 5 and 10 million IU/kg, based on body surface area adjustment for a 60 kg adult). PEG-Intron should be assumed to also have

TABLE 3. Adverse Events Occurring in >5% of Patients

Percentage of Patients Reporting Adverse Events*

Adverse Events	Study 1		Study 2	
	PEG-Intron 1.0 µg/kg (n=297)	INTRON A 3 MIU (n=303)	PEG-Intron 1.5 µg/kg/ REBETOL (n=511)	INTRON A/ REBETOL (n=505)
Application Site				
Injection Site Inflammation/Reaction	47	20	75	49
Autonomic Nervous Sys.				
Mouth Dry	6	7	12	8
Sweating Increased	6	7	11	7
Flushing	6	3	4	3
Body as a Whole				
Fatigue/Asthenia	52	54	66	63
Headache	56	52	62	58
Rigors	23	19	48	41
Fever	22	12	46	33
Weight Decrease	11	13	29	20
RUQ Pain	8	8	12	6
Chest Pain	6	4	8	7
Malaise	7	6	4	6
Central/Periph. Nerv. Sys.				
Dizziness	12	10	21	17
Endocrine				
Hypothyroidism	5	3	5	4
Gastrointestinal				
Nausea	26	20	43	33
Anorexia	20	17	32	27
Diarrhea	18	16	22	17
Vomiting	7	6	14	12
Abdominal Pain	15	11	13	13
Dyspepsia	6	7	9	8
Constipation	1	3	5	5
Hematologic Disorders				
Neutropenia	6	2	26	14
Anemia	0	0	12	17
Leukopenia	<1	0	6	5
Thrombocytopenia	7	<1	5	2
Liver and Biliary System				
Hepatomegaly	6	5	4	4
Musculoskeletal				
Myalgia	54	53	56	50
Arthralgia	23	27	34	28
Musculoskeletal Pain	28	22	21	19
Psychiatric				
Insomnia	23	23	40	41
Depression	29	25	31	34
Anxiety/Emotional Lability/Irritability	28	34	47	47
Concentration Impaired	10	8	17	21
Agitation	2	2	8	5
Nervousness	4	3	6	6
Reproductive, Female				
Menstrual Disorder	4	3	7	6
Resistance Mechanism				
Infection Viral	11	10	12	12
Infection Fungal	<1	3	6	1
Respiratory System				
Dyspnea	4	2	26	24
Coughing	8	5	23	16
Pharyngitis	10	7	12	13
Rhinitis	2	2	8	6
Sinusitis	7	7	6	5
Skin and Appendages				
Alopecia	22	22	36	32
Pruritus	12	8	29	28
Rash	6	7	24	23
Skin Dry	11	9	24	23
Special Senses Other				
Taste Perversion	<1	2	9	4
Vision Disorders				
Vision Blurred	2	3	5	6
Conjunctivitis	4	2	4	5

* Patients reporting one or more adverse events. A patient may have reported more than one adverse event within a body system/organ class category.

abortifacient potential. There are no adequate and well-controlled studies in pregnant women. PEG-Intron therapy is to be used during pregnancy only if the potential benefit justifies the potential risk to the fetus. Therefore, PEG-Intron is recommended for use in fertile women only when they are using effective contraception during the treatment period.

Pregnancy Category X: Use with Ribavirin
Significant teratogenic and/or embryocidal effects have been demonstrated in all animal species exposed to ribavirin. REBETOL therapy is contraindicated in women who are

pregnant and in the male partners of women who are pregnant. See CONTRAINDICATIONS and the REBETOL Package Insert.

If pregnancy occurs in a patient or partner of a patient during treatment with PEG-Intron and REBETOL or during the 6 months after treatment cessation, physicians should report such cases by calling (800) 727-7064.

Nursing Mothers: It is not known whether the components of PEG-Intron and/or REBETOL are excreted in human milk. Studies in mice have shown that mouse interferons are excreted in breast milk. Because of the potential for ad-

verse reactions from the drug in nursing infants, a decision must be made whether to discontinue nursing or discontinue the PEG-Intron and REBETOL treatment, taking into account the importance of the therapy to the mother.

Pediatric: Safety and effectiveness in pediatric patients below the age of 18 years have not been established.

Geriatric: In general, younger patients tend to respond better than older patients to interferon-based therapies. Clinical studies of PEG-Intron alone or in combination with REBETOL did not include sufficient numbers of subjects aged 65 and over, however, to determine whether they respond differently than younger subjects. Treatment with alpha interferons, including PEG-Intron, is associated with neuropsychiatric, cardiac, pulmonary, GI and systemic (flu-like) adverse effects. Because these adverse reactions may be more severe in the elderly, caution should be exercised in the use of PEG-Intron in this population. This drug is known to be substantially excreted by the kidney. Because elderly patients are more likely to have decreased renal function, the risk of toxic reactions to this drug may be greater in patients with impaired renal function (see **CLINICAL PHARMACOLOGY: Special Populations: Renal dysfunction**). REBETOL should not be used in patients with creatinine clearance <50 mL/min. When using PEG-Intron/REBETOL therapy, refer also to the REBETOL Package Insert.

ADVERSE REACTIONS

Nearly all study patients in clinical trials experienced one or more adverse events. In the PEG monotherapy trial the incidence of serious adverse events was similar (about 12%) in all treatment groups. In the PEG-Intron/REBETOL combination trial the incidence of serious adverse events was 17% in the PEG-Intron/REBETOL groups compared to 14% in the INTRON A/REBETOL group.

In many but not all cases, adverse events resolved after dose reduction or discontinuation of therapy. Some patients experienced ongoing or new serious adverse events during the 6-month follow-up period. In the PEG-Intron/REBETOL trial 13 patients experienced life-threatening psychiatric events (suicidal ideation or attempt) and one patient accomplished suicide.

There have been five patient deaths which occurred in clinical trials: one suicide in a patient receiving PEG-Intron monotherapy and one suicide in a patient receiving PEG-Intron/REBETOL combination therapy; two deaths among patients receiving INTRON A monotherapy (1 murder/suicide and 1 sudden death) and one patient death in the INTRON A/REBETOL group (motor vehicle accident).

Overall, 10–14% of patients receiving PEG-Intron, alone or in combination with REBETOL, discontinued therapy compared with 6% treated with INTRON A alone and 13% treated with INTRON A in combination with REBETOL. The most common reasons for discontinuation of therapy were related to psychiatric, systemic (eg, fatigue, headache), or gastrointestinal adverse events.

In the combination therapy trial, dose reductions due to adverse reactions occurred in 42% of patients receiving PEG-Intron (1.5 µg/kg)/REBETOL and in 34% of those receiving INTRON A/REBETOL. The majority of patients (57%) weighing 60 kg or less receiving PEG-Intron (1.5 µg/kg)/REBETOL required dose reduction. Reduction of interferon was dose related (PEG-Intron 1.5 µg/kg >PEG-Intron 0.5 µg/kg or INTRON A), 40%, 27%, 28%, respectively. Dose reduction for REBETOL was similar across all three groups, 33–35%. The most common reasons for dose modifications were neutropenia (18%), or anemia (9%) (see **Laboratory Values**). Other common reasons included depression, fatigue, nausea, and thrombocytopenia.

In the PEG-Intron/REBETOL combination trial the most common adverse events were psychiatric which occurred among 77% of patients and included most commonly depression, irritability, and insomnia, each reported by approximately 30-40% of subjects in all treatment groups. Suicidal behavior (ideation, attempts, and suicides) occurred in 2% of all patients during treatment or during follow-up after treatment cessation (see **WARNINGS**).

PEG-Intron induced fatigue or headache in approximately two-thirds of patients, and induced fever or rigors in approximately half of the patients. The severity of some of these systemic symptoms (eg, fever and headache) tended to decrease as treatment continues. The incidence tends to be higher with PEG-Intron than with INTRON A therapy alone or in combination with REBETOL.

Application site inflammation and reaction (eg, bruise, itchiness, irritation) occurred at approximately twice the incidence with PEG-Intron therapies (in up to 75% of patients) compared with INTRON A. However injection site pain was infrequent (2–3%) in all groups.

Other common adverse events in the PEG-Intron/REBETOL group included myalgia (56%), arthralgia (34%), nausea (43%), anorexia (32%), weight loss (29%), alopecia (36%), and pruritus (29%).

In the PEG-Intron monotherapy trial the incidence of severe adverse events was 13% in the INTRON A group and 17% in the PEG-Intron groups. In the PEG-Intron/REBETOL combination therapy trial the incidence of severe adverse events was 23% in the INTRON A/REBETOL group and 31–34% in the PEG-Intron/REBETOL groups. The incidence of life-threatening adverse events was ≤1% across all groups in the monotherapy and combination therapy trials.

Adverse events that occurred in the clinical trial at >5% incidence are provided in **Table 3** by treatment group. Due to potential differences in ascertainment procedures, adverse event rate comparisons across studies should not be made. [See table 3 above]

Continued on next page

Peg-Intron—Cont.

Many patients continued to experience adverse events several months after discontinuation of therapy. By the end of the 6-month follow-up period the incidence of ongoing adverse events by body class in the PEG-Intron 1.5/REBETOL group was 33% (psychiatric), 20% (musculoskeletal), and 10% (for endocrine and for GI). In approximately 10–15% of patients weight loss, fatigue, and headache had not resolved.

Individual serious adverse events occurred at a frequency ≤1% and included suicide attempt, suicidal ideation, severe depression; psychosis, aggressive reaction, relapse of drug addiction/overdose; nerve palsy (facial, oculomotor); cardiomyopathy, myocardial infarction, angina, pericardial effusion, retinal ischemia, retinal artery or vein thrombosis, blindness, decreased visual acuity, optic neuritis, transient ischemic attack, supraventricular arrhythmias, loss of consciousness; neutropenia, infection (sepsis, pneumonia, abscess, cellulitis); emphysema, bronchiolitis obliterans, pleural effusion, gastroenteritis, pancreatitis, gout, hyperglycemia, hyperthyroidism and hypothyroidism, autoimmune thrombocytopenia with or without purpura, rheumatoid arthritis, interstitial nephritis, lupus-like syndrome, sarcoidosis, aggravated psoriasis; urticaria, injection-site necrosis, vasculitis, phototoxicity.

Laboratory Values
Changes in selected laboratory values during treatment with PEG-Intron alone or in combination with REBETOL treatment are described below. **Decreases in hemoglobin, neutrophils, and platelets may require dose reduction or permanent discontinuation from therapy. (See DOSAGE AND ADMINISTRATION: Dose Reduction.)**

Hemoglobin. REBETOL induced a decrease in hemoglobin levels in approximately two thirds of patients. Hemoglobin levels decreased to <11 g/dL in about 30% of patients. Severe anemia (<8 g/dL) occurred in <1% of patients. Dose modification was required in 9% and 13% of patients in the PEG-Intron/REBETOL and INTRON A/REBETOL groups. Hemoglobin levels become stable by treatment week 4–6 on average. Hemoglobin levels return to baseline between 4 and 12 weeks posttreatment. In the PEG-Intron monotherapy trial hemoglobin decreases were generally mild and dose modifications were rarely necessary. (See **DOSAGE AND ADMINISTRATION: Dose Reduction.**)

Neutrophils. Decreases in neutrophil counts were observed in a majority of patients treated with PEG-Intron alone (70%) or as combination therapy with REBETOL (85%) and INTRON A/REBETOL (60%). Severe potentially life-threatening neutropenia (<0.5 × 10^9/L) occurred in 1% of patients treated with PEG-Intron monotherapy, 2% of patients treated with INTRON A/REBETOL and in 4% of patients treated with PEG-Intron/REBETOL. Two percent of patients receiving PEG-Intron monotherapy and 18% of patients receiving PEG-Intron/REBETOL required modification of interferon dosage. Few patients (≤1%) required permanent discontinuation of treatment. Neutrophil counts generally return to pretreatment levels within 4 weeks of cessation of therapy. (See **DOSAGE AND ADMINISTRATION: Dose Reduction.**)

Platelets. Platelet counts decrease in approximately 20% of patients treated with PEG-Intron alone or with REBETOL and in 6% of patients treated with INTRON A/REBETOL. Severe decreases in platelet counts (<50,000/mm³) occur in <1% of patients. Patients may require discontinuation or dose modification as a result of platelet decreases. (See **DOSAGE AND ADMINISTRATION: Dose Reduction.**) In the PEG-Intron/REBETOL combination therapy trial 1% or 3% of patients required dose modification of INTRON A or PEG-Intron respectively. Platelet counts generally returned to pretreatment levels within 4 weeks of the cessation of therapy.

Triglycerides. Elevated triglyceride levels have been observed in patients treated with interferon alfas including PEG-Intron.

Thyroid Function. Development of TSH abnormalities, with and without clinical manifestations, are associated with interferon therapies. Clinically apparent thyroid disorders occur among patients treated with either INTRON A or PEG-Intron (with or without REBETOL) at a similar incidence (5% for hypothyroidism and 3% for hyperthyroidism). Subjects developed new onset TSH abnormalities while on treatment and during the follow-up period. At the end of the follow-up period 7% of subjects still had abnormal TSH values.

Bilirubin and uric acid. In the PEG-Intron/REBETOL trial 10–14% of patients developed hyperbilirubinemia and 33–38% developed hyperuricemia in association with hemolysis. Six patients developed mild to moderate gout.

Postmarketing Experience
The following adverse reactions have been identified and reported during post-approval use of PEG-Intron therapy: seizures, hearing impairment, hearing loss, peripheral neuropathy, rhabdomyolysis, myositis, aphthous stomatitis, vertigo, renal insufficiency, renal failure, Stevens Johnson syndrome, toxic epidermal necrolysis, and erythema multiforme. Because the reports of these reactions are voluntary and the population of uncertain size, it is not always possible to reliably estimate the frequency of the reaction or establish a causal relationship to drug exposure.

TABLE 4. Recommended PEG-Intron Monotherapy Dosing

Body weight (kg)	PEG-Intron Redipen® or Vial Strength to Use	Amount of PEG-Intron (µg) to Administer	Volume (mL)* of PEG-Intron to Administer
≤45	50 µg per 0.5 mL	40	0.4
46–56		50	0.5
57–72	80 µg per 0.5 mL	64	0.4
73–88		80	0.5
89–106	120 µg per 0.5 mL	96	0.4
107–136		120	0.5
137–160	150 µg per 0.5 mL	150	0.5

* When reconstituted as directed

TABLE 5. Recommended PEG-Intron Combination Therapy Dosing

Body weight (kg)	PEG-Intron Redipen® or Vial Strength to Use	Amount of PEG-Intron (µg) to Administer	Volume (mL)* of PEG-Intron to Administer
<40	50 µg per 0.5 mL	50	0.5
40–50	80 µg per 0.5 mL	64	0.4
51–60		80	0.5
61–75	120 µg per 0.5 mL	96	0.4
76–85		120	0.5
>85	150 µg per 0.5 mL	150	0.5

* When reconstituted as directed

TABLE 6. Guidelines for Modification or Discontinuation of PEG-Intron or PEG-Intron/REBETOL and for Scheduling Visits for Patients with Depression

Depression Severity[1]	Initial Management (4–8 wks)			Depression	
	Dose modification	Visit schedule	Remains stable	Improves	Worsens
Mild	No change	Evaluate once weekly by visit and/or phone.	Continue weekly visit schedule.	Resume normal visit schedule.	(See moderate or severe depression)
Moderate	Decrease IFN dose 50%	Evaluate once weekly (office visit at least every other week).	Consider psychiatric consultation. Continue reduced dosing.	If symptoms improve and are stable for 4 wks, may resume normal visit schedule. Continue reducing dosing or return to normal dose.	(See severe depression)
Severe	Discontinue IFN/R permanently.	Obtain immediate psychiatric consultation.	Psychiatric therapy necessary		

[1]See DSM-IV for definitions

Immunogenicity: Approximately 2% of patients receiving PEG-Intron (32/1759) or INTRON A (11/728) with or without REBETOL developed low-titer (≤160) neutralizing antibodies to PEG-Intron or INTRON A. The clinical and pathological significance of the appearance of serum neutralizing antibodies is unknown. No apparent correlation of antibody development to clinical response or adverse events was observed. The incidence of posttreatment binding antibody ranged from 8 to 15 percent. The data reflect the percentage of patients whose test results were considered positive for antibodies to PEG-Intron in a Biacore assay that is used to measure binding antibodies, and in an antiviral neutralization assay, which measures serum-neutralizing antibodies. The percentage of patients whose test results were considered positive for antibodies is highly dependent on the sensitivity and specificity of the assays. Additionally the observed incidence of antibody positivity in these assays may be influenced by several factors including sample timing and handling, concomitant medications, and underlying disease. For these reasons, comparison of the incidence of antibodies to PEG-Intron with the incidence of antibodies to other products may be misleading.

OVERDOSAGE
There is limited experience with overdosage. In the clinical studies, a few patients accidentally received a dose greater than that prescribed. There were no instances in which a participant in the monotherapy or combination therapy trials received more than 10.5 times the intended dose of PEG-Intron. The maximum dose received by any patient was 3.45 µg/kg weekly over a period of approximately 12 weeks. The maximum known overdosage of REBETOL was an intentional ingestion of 10 g (fifty 200-mg capsules). There were no serious reactions attributed to these overdosages. In cases of overdosing, symptomatic treatment and close observation of the patient are recommended.

DOSAGE AND ADMINISTRATION
There are no safety and efficacy data on treatment for longer than 1 year. A patient should self-inject PEG-Intron only if it has been determined that it is appropriate and the patient agrees to medical follow-up as necessary and training in proper injection technique has been given to him/her.

It is recommended that patients receiving PEG-Intron, alone or in combination with ribavirin, be discontinued from therapy if HCV viral levels remain high after 6 months of therapy.

PEG-Intron Monotherapy
The recommended dose of PEG-Intron regimen is 1.0 µg/kg/week subcutaneously for 1 year. The dose should be administered on the same day of the week.

The volume of PEG-Intron to be injected depends on the patient weight (see **Table 4** below).

[See table 4 above]

PEG-Intron/REBETOL Combination Therapy
When administered in combination with REBETOL, the recommended dose of PEG-Intron is 1.5 micrograms/kg/week. The volume of PEG-Intron to be injected depends on the strength of PEG-Intron and patient's body weight. (See **Table 5.**)

[See table 5 above]

The recommended dose of REBETOL is 800 mg/day in 2 divided doses: two capsules (400 mg) with breakfast and two capsules (400 mg) with dinner. REBETOL should not be used in patients with creatinine clearance <50 mL/min.

Dose Reduction
If a serious adverse reaction develops during the course of treatment (see **WARNINGS**) discontinue or modify the dosage of PEG-Intron and/or REBETOL until the adverse event abates or decreases in severity. If persistent or recurrent serious adverse events develop despite adequate dosage adjustment, discontinue treatment. For guidelines for dose modifications and discontinuation based on laboratory parameters, see **Tables 6** and **7**. Dose reduction of PEG-Intron may be accomplished by utilizing a lower dose strength as shown in **Table 8** or **9**. For vials, 50% dose reduction may also be accomplished by reducing the volume administered by one-half without changing the dose

strength. In the combination therapy trial dose reductions occurred among 42% of patients receiving PEG-Intron 1.5 µg/kg/REBETOL 800 mg daily including 57% of those patients weighing 60 kg or less (see **ADVERSE REACTIONS**).

[See table 6 on previous page]
[See table 7 at right]
[See table 8 at right]
[See table 9 at right]

Renal Function

In patients with moderate renal dysfunction (creatinine clearance 30–50 mL/min), the PEG-Intron dose should be reduced by 25%. Patients with severe renal dysfunction (creatinine clearance 10–29 mL/min) including those on hemodialysis, should have the PEG-Intron dose reduced by 50%. If renal function decreases during treatment, PEG-Intron therapy should be discontinued.

Preparation and Administration

PEG-Intron Redipen®

PEG-Intron Redipen® consists of a dual-chamber glass cartridge with sterile, lyophilized peginterferon alfa-2b in the active chamber and Sterile Water for Injection, USP in the diluent chamber. The PEG-Intron in the glass cartridge should appear as a white to off-white tablet-shaped solid that is whole or in pieces, or powder. To reconstitute the lyophilized peginterferon alfa-2b in the Redipen®, hold the Redipen® upright (dose button down) and press the two halves of the pen together until there is an audible click. Gently invert the pen to mix the solution. **DO NOT SHAKE**. The reconstituted solution has a concentration of either 50 µg per 0.5 mL, 80 µg per 0.5 mL, 120 µg per 0.5 mL, or 150 µg per 0.5 mL for a single subcutaneous injection. Visually inspect the solution for particulate matter and discoloration prior to administration. The reconstituted solution should be clear and colorless. Do not use if the solution is discolored or cloudy, or if particulates are present.

Keeping the pen upright, attach the supplied needle and select the appropriate PEG-Intron dose by pulling back on the dosing button until the dark bands are visible and turning the button until the dark band is aligned with the correct dose. The prepared PEG-Intron solution is to be injected subcutaneously.

The PEG-Intron Redipen® is a single-use pen and does not contain a preservative. The reconstituted solution should be used immediately and cannot be stored for more than 24 hours at 2°-8°C (see **Storage**). **DO NOT REUSE THE REDIPEN®**. The sterility of any remaining product can no longer be guaranteed. **DISCARD THE UNUSED PORTION**. Pooling of unused portions of some medications has been linked to bacterial contamination and morbidity.

PEG-Intron Vials

Two B-D Safety-Lok™ syringes are provided in the package; one syringe is for the reconstitution steps and one for the patient injection. There is a plastic safety sleeve to be pulled over the needle after use. The syringe locks with an audible click when the green stripe on the safety sleeve covers the red stripe on the needle. Instructions for the preparation and administration of PEG-Intron Powder for Injection are provided below.

Reconstitute the PEG-Intron lyophilized product with only 0.7 mL of 1.25 mL of supplied diluent (Sterile Water for Injection, USP).**The diluent vial is for single use only.The remaining diluent should be discarded.** No other medications should be added to solutions containing PEG-Intron, and PEG-Intron should not be reconstituted with other diluents. Swirl gently to hasten complete dissolution of the powder. The reconstituted solution should be clear and colorless. Visually inspect the solution for particulate matter and discoloration prior to administration. The solution should not be used if discolored or cloudy, or if particulates are present. The appropriate PEG-Intron dose should be withdrawn and injected subcutaneously. PEG-Intron vials are for single use only and do not contain a preservative. The reconstituted solution should be used immediately and cannot be stored for more than 24 hours at 2°–8°C (see **Storage**). **DO NOT REUSE THE VIAL**. The sterility of any remaining product can no longer be guaranteed. **DISCARD THE UNUSED PORTION**. Pooling of unused portions of some medications has been linked to bacterial contamination and morbidity.

After preparation and administration of the PEG-Intron for injection, it is essential to follow the state and/or local procedures for proper disposal of syringes, needles, and the Redipen®. A puncture-resistant container should be used for disposal. Patients should be instructed in how to properly dispose of used syringes, needles, or the Redipen® and be cautioned against the reuse of these items.

Storage

PEG-Intron Redipen®

PEG-Intron Redipen® should be stored at 2° to 8°C (36° to 46°F). After reconstitution, the solution should be used immediately, but may be stored up to 24 hours at 2° to 8°C (36° to 46°F). The reconstituted solution contains no preservative, and is clear and colorless. **DO NOT FREEZE**.

PEG-Intron Vials

PEG-Intron should be stored at 25°C (77°F); excursions permitted to 15°–30°C (59°–86°F) [see USP Controlled Room Temperature]. After reconstitution with supplied Diluent the solution should be used immediately, but may be stored up to 24 hours at 2° to 8°C (36° to 46°F). The reconstituted solution contains no preservative, is clear and colorless. **DO NOT FREEZE**.

TABLE 7. Guidelines for Dose Modification and Discontinuation of PEG-Intron or PEG-Intron/REBETOL for Hematologic Toxicity

Laboratory Values		PEG-Intron	REBETOL
Hgb*	<10.0 g/dL	--------------------------	Decrease by 200 mg/day
	<8.5 g/dL	Permanently discontinue	Permanently discontinue
WBC	<1.5 × 10⁹/L	Reduce dose by 50%	--------------------------
	<1.0 × 10⁹/L	Permanently discontinue	Permanently discontinue
Neutrophil	<0.75 × 10⁹/L	Reduce dose by 50%	--------------------------
	<0.5 × 10⁹/L	Permanently discontinue	Permanently discontinue
Platelets	<80 × 10⁹/L	Reduce dose by 50%	--------------------------
	<50 × 10⁹/L	Permanently discontinue	Permanently discontinue

* For patients with a history of stable cardiac disease receiving PEG-Intron in combination with ribavirin, the PEG-Intron dose should be reduced by half and the ribavirin dose by 200 mg/day if a >2g/dL decrease in hemoglobin is observed during any 4-week period. Both PEG-Intron and ribavirin should be permanently discontinued if patients have hemoglobin levels <12 g/dL after this ribavirin dose reduction.

TABLE 8. Reduced PEG-Intron Dose (0.5 µg/kg) for (1.0 µg/kg) Monotherapy

Body weight (kg)	PEG-Intron Redipen® or Vial Strength to Use	Amount of PEG-Intron (µg) to Administer	Volume (mL)** of PEG-Intron to Administer
≤ 45	50 µg per 0.5 mL*	20	0.2
46–56		25	0.25
57–72	50 µg per 0.5 mL	30	0.3
73–88		40	0.4
89–106	50 µg per 0.5 mL	50	0.5
107–136	80 µg per 0.5 mL	64	0.4
137–160		80	0.5

* Must use vial. Minimum delivery for Redipen® 0.3 mL
** When reconstituted as directed

TABLE 9. Reduced PEG-Intron Dose (0.75 µg/kg) for (1.5 µg/kg) Combination Therapy

Body weight (kg)	PEG-Intron Redipen® or Vial Strength to Use	Amount of PEG-Intron (µg) to Administer	Volume (mL)** of PEG-Intron to Administer
≤ 40	50 µg per 0.5 mL*	25	0.25
40–50	50 µg per 0.5 mL	30	0.3
51–60		40	0.4
61–75	50 µg per 0.5 mL	50	0.5
76–85	80 µg per 0.5 mL	64	0.4
> 85		80	0.5

* Must use vial. Minimum delivery for Redipen® 0.3 mL
** When reconstituted as directed

HOW SUPPLIED

PEG-Intron Redipen®

Each PEG-Intron Redipen® Package Contains:	
A box containing one 50 µg per 0.5 mL PEG-Intron Redipen® and 1 B-D needle and 2 alcohol swabs.	(NDC 0085-1323-01)
A box containing one 80 µg per 0.5 mL PEG-Intron Redipen® and 1 B-D needle and 2 alcohol swabs.	(NDC 0085-1316-01)
A box containing one 120 µg per 0.5 mL PEG-Intron Redipen® and 1 B-D needle and 2 alcohol swabs.	(NDC 0085-1297-01)
A box containing one 150 µg per 0.5 mL PEG-Intron Redipen® and 1 B-D needle and 2 alcohol swabs.	(NDC 0085-1370-01)

Each PEG-Intron Redipen® PAK 4 Contains:	
A box containing four 50 µg per 0.5 mL PEG-Intron Redipen® Units, each containing 1 B-D needle and 2 alcohol swabs.	(NDC 0085-1323-02)
A box containing four 80 µg per 0.5 mL PEG-Intron Redipen® Units, each containing 1 B-D needle and 2 alcohol swabs.	(NDC 0085-1316-02)
A box containing four 120 µg per 0.5 mL PEG-Intron Redipen® Units, each containing 1 B-D needle and 2 alcohol swabs.	(NDC 0085-1297-02)
A box containing four 150 µg per 0.5 mL PEG-Intron Redipen® Units, each containing 1 B-D needle and 2 alcohol swabs.	(NDC 0085-1370-02)

PEG-Intron Vials

Each PEG-Intron Package Contains:	
A box containing one 50 µg per 0.5 mL vial of PEG-Intron Powder for Injection and one 1.25 mL vial of Diluent (Sterile Water for Injection, USP), 2 B-D Safety-Lok™* syringes with a safety sleeve and 2 alcohol swabs.	(NDC 0085-1368-01)
A box containing one 80 µg per 0.5 mL vial of PEG-Intron Powder for Injection and one 1.25 mL vial of Diluent (Sterile Water for Injection, USP), 2 B-D Safety-Lok™* syringes with a safety sleeve and 2 alcohol swabs.	(NDC 0085-1291-01)
A box containing one 120 µg per 0.5 mL vial of PEG-Intron Powder for Injection and one 1.25 mL vial of Diluent (Sterile Water for Injection, USP), 2 B-D Safety-Lok™* syringes with a safety sleeve and 2 alcohol swabs.	(NDC 0085-1304-01)
A box containing one 150 µg per 0.5 mL vial of PEG-Intron Powder for Injection and one 1.25 mL vial of Diluent (Sterile Water for Injection, USP), 2 B-D Safety-Lok™* syringes with a safety sleeve and 2 alcohol swabs.	(NDC 0085-1279-01)

Schering®
Schering Corporation
Kenilworth, NJ 07033 USA

Continued on next page

Peg-Intron—Cont.

 Rev. 2/05

*Safety-Lok is a trademark of Becton Dickinson and Company.

27664431T

TEMODAR® ℞

[*tĕm-ō-dăr*]
(temozolomide)
CAPSULES

PRODUCT INFORMATION

Prescribing information for this product, which appears on pages 3067–3070 of the 2005 PDR, has been completely revised as follows. Please write "See Supplement A" next to the product heading.

DESCRIPTION

TEMODAR Capsules for oral administration contain temozolomide, an imidazotetrazine derivative. The chemical name of temozolomide is 3,4-dihydro-3-methyl-4-oxoimidazo[5,1-d]-*as*-tetrazine-8-carboxamide. The structural formula is:

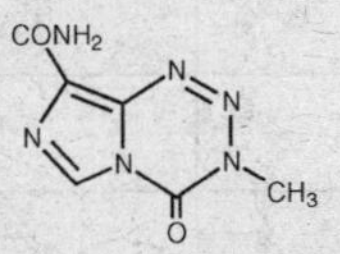
CONH2
N
N
N
N
N
CH3
O

The material is a white to light tan/light pink powder with a molecular formula of $C_6H_6N_6O_2$ and a molecular weight of 194.15. The molecule is stable at acidic pH (<5), and labile at pH >7, hence TEMODAR can be administered orally. The prodrug, temozolomide, is rapidly hydrolyzed to the active 5-(3-methyltriazen-1-yl)imidazole-4-carboxamide (MTIC) at neutral and alkaline pH values, with hydrolysis taking place even faster at alkaline pH.

Each capsule contains either 5 mg, 20 mg, 100 mg, or 250 mg of temozolomide. The inactive ingredients for TEMODAR Capsules are lactose anhydrous, colloidal silicon dioxide, sodium starch glycolate, tartaric acid, and stearic acid. Gelatin capsule shells contain titanium dioxide. The capsules are white and imprinted with pharmaceutical ink.

TEMODAR 5 mg: green imprint contains pharmaceutical grade shellac, anhydrous ethyl alcohol, isopropyl alcohol, n-butyl alcohol, propylene glycol, ammonium hydroxide, titanium dioxide, yellow iron oxide, and FD&C Blue #2 aluminum lake.

TEMODAR 20 mg: brown imprint contains pharmaceutical grade shellac, anhydrous ethyl alcohol, isopropyl alcohol, n-butyl alcohol, propylene glycol, purified water, ammonium hydroxide, potassium hydroxide, titanium dioxide, black iron oxide, yellow iron oxide, brown iron oxide, and red iron oxide.

TEMODAR 100 mg: blue imprint contains pharmaceutical glaze (modified) in an ethanol/shellac mixture, isopropyl alcohol, n-butyl alcohol, propylene glycol, titanium dioxide, and FD&C Blue #2 aluminum lake.

TEMODAR 250 mg: black imprint contains pharmaceutical grade shellac, anhydrous ethyl alcohol, isopropyl alcohol, n-butyl alcohol, propylene glycol, purified water, ammonium hydroxide, potassium hydroxide, and black iron oxide.

CLINICAL PHARMACOLOGY

Mechanism of Action: Temozolomide is not directly active but undergoes rapid nonenzymatic conversion at physiologic pH to the reactive compound MTIC. The cytotoxicity of MTIC is thought to be primarily due to alkylation of DNA. Alkylation (methylation) occurs mainly at the O^6 and N^7 positions of guanine.

Pharmacokinetics: Temozolomide is rapidly and completely absorbed after oral administration; peak plasma concentrations occur in 1 hour. Food reduces the rate and extent of temozolomide absorption. Mean peak plasma concentration and AUC decreased by 32% and 9%, respectively, and T_{max} increased 2-fold (from 1.1 to 2.25 hours) when temozolomide was administered after a modified high-fat breakfast. Temozolomide is rapidly eliminated with a mean elimination half-life of 1.8 hours and exhibits linear kinetics over the therapeutic dosing range. Temozolomide has a mean apparent volume of distribution of 0.4 L/kg (%CV=13%). It is weakly bound to human plasma proteins; the mean percent bound of drug-related total radioactivity is 15%.

Metabolism and Elimination: Temozolomide is spontaneously hydrolyzed at physiologic pH to the active species, 3-methyl-(triazen-1-yl)imidazole-4-carboxamide (MTIC) and to temozolomide acid metabolite. MTIC is further hydrolyzed to 5-amino-imidazole-4-carboxamide (AIC) which is known to be an intermediate in purine and nucleic acid biosynthesis and to methylhydrazine, which is believed to be the active alkylating species. Cytochrome P450 enzymes play only a minor role in the metabolism of temozolomide and MTIC. Relative to the AUC of temozolomide, the exposure to MTIC and AIC is 2.4% and 23%, respectively. About 38% of the administered temozolomide total radioactive dose is recovered over 7 days; 37.7% in urine and 0.8% in feces. The majority of the recovery of radioactivity in urine is as unchanged temozolomide (5.6%), AIC (12%), temozolomide acid metabolite (2.3%), and unidentified polar metabolite(s) (17%). Overall clearance of temozolomide is about 5.5 L/hr/m^2.

Special Populations: *Age* Population pharmacokinetic analysis indicates that age (range 19 to 78 years) has no influence on the pharmacokinetics of temozolomide. In the anaplastic astrocytoma study population, patients 70 years of age or older had a higher incidence of Grade 4 neutropenia and Grade 4 thrombocytopenia in the first cycle of therapy than patients under 70 years of age (see **PRECAUTIONS**).

Gender Population pharmacokinetic analysis indicates that women have an approximately 5% lower clearance (adjusted for body surface area) for temozolomide than men. Women have higher incidences of Grade 4 neutropenia and thrombocytopenia in the first cycle of therapy than men (see **ADVERSE REACTIONS**).

Race The effect of race on the pharmacokinetics of temozolomide has not been studied.

Tobacco Use Population pharmacokinetic analysis indicates that the oral clearance of temozolomide is similar in smokers and nonsmokers.

Creatinine Clearance Population pharmacokinetic analysis indicates that creatinine clearance over the range of 36-130 mL/min/m^2 has no effect on the clearance of temozolomide after oral administration. The pharmacokinetics of temozolomide have not been studied in patients with severely impaired renal function (CLcr < 36 mL/min/m^2). Caution should be exercised when TEMODAR Capsules are administered to patients with severe renal impairment. TEMODAR has not been studied in patients on dialysis.

Hepatically Impaired Patients In a pharmacokinetic study, the pharmacokinetics of temozolomide in patients with mild-to-moderate hepatic impairment (Child's-Pugh Class I - II) were similar to those observed in patients with normal hepatic function. Caution should be exercised when temozolomide is administered to patients with severe hepatic impairment.

Drug-Drug Interactions In a multiple-dose study, administration of TEMODAR Capsules with ranitidine did not change the C_{max} or AUC values for temozolomide or MTIC. Population analysis indicates that administration of valproic acid decreases the clearance of temozolomide by about 5% (see **PRECAUTIONS**).

Population analysis failed to demonstrate any influence of coadministered dexamethasone, prochlorperazine, phenytoin, carbamazepine, ondansetron, H_2-receptor antagonists, or phenobarbital on the clearance of orally administered temozolomide.

CLINICAL STUDIES

Newly Diagnosed Glioblastoma Multiforme Five hundred and seventy-three patients were randomized to receive either TEMODAR (TMZ) + Radiotherapy (RT) (n=287) or RT alone (n=286). Patients in the TEMODAR + RT arm received concomitant TEMODAR (75 mg/m^2) once daily, starting the first day of RT until the last day of RT, for 42 days (with a maximum of 49 days). This was followed by 6 cycles of TEMODAR alone (150 or 200 mg/m^2) on Day 1-5 of every 28-day cycle, starting 4 weeks after the end of RT. Patients in the control arm received RT only. In both arms, focal radiation therapy was delivered as 60 Gy/30 fractions. Focal RT includes the tumor bed or resection site with a 2-3 cm margin. *Pneumocystis carinii* pneumonia (PCP) prophylaxis was required during the TMZ + radiotherapy treatment, regardless of lymphocyte count, and was to continue until recovery of lymphocyte count to less than or equal to Grade 1. At the time of disease progression, TEMODAR was administered as salvage therapy in 161 patients of the 282 (57%) in the RT alone arm, and 62 patients of the 277 (22%) in the TEMODAR + RT arm.

The addition of concomitant and maintenance TEMODAR to radiotherapy in the treatment of patients with newly diagnosed GBM showed a statistically significant improvement in overall survival compared to radiotherapy alone (Figure 1). The hazard ratio (HR) for overall survival was 0.63 (95% CI for HR=0.52-0.75) with a log-rank p<0.0001 in favor of the TEMODAR arm. The median survival was increased by 2 months in the TEMODAR arm.

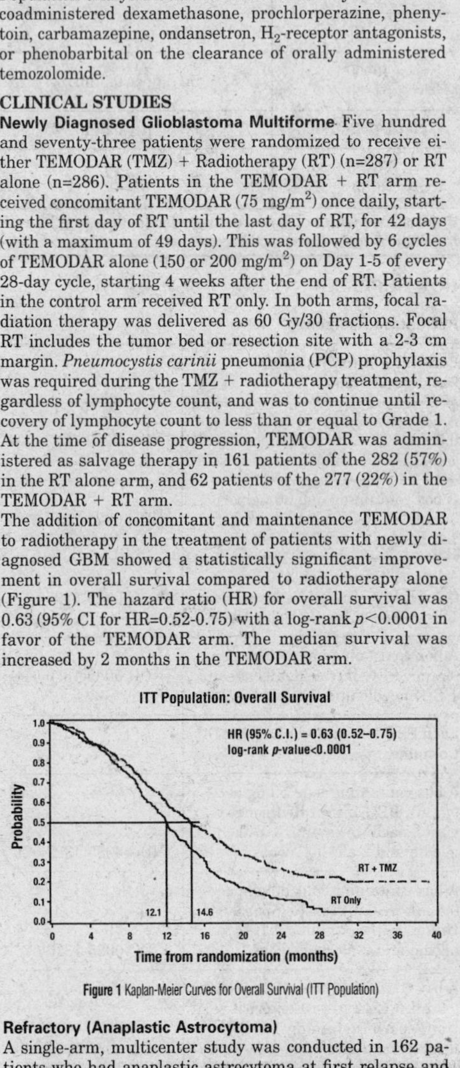
ITT Population: Overall Survival
HR (95% C.I.) = 0.63 (0.52–0.75)
log-rank p-value<0.0001
Probability
1.0
0.9
0.8
0.7
0.6
0.5
0.4
0.3
0.2
0.1
0.0
RT + TMZ
RT Only
12.1
14.6
0
4
8
12
16
20
24
28
32
36
40
Time from randomization (months)

Figure 1 Kaplan-Meier Curves for Overall Survival (ITT Population)

Refractory (Anaplastic Astrocytoma)

A single-arm, multicenter study was conducted in 162 patients who had anaplastic astrocytoma at first relapse and who had a baseline Karnofsky performance status of 70 or greater. Patients had previously received radiation therapy and may also have previously received a nitrosourea with or without other chemotherapy. Fifty-four patients had disease progression on prior therapy with both a nitrosourea and procarbazine and their malignancy was considered refractory to chemotherapy (refractory anaplastic astrocytoma population). Median age of this subgroup of 54 patients was 42 years (19 to 76). Sixty-five percent were male. Seventy-two percent of patients had a KPS of >80. Sixty-three percent of patients had surgery other than a biopsy at the time of initial diagnosis. Of those patients undergoing resection, 73% underwent a subtotal resection and 27% underwent a gross total resection. Eighteen percent of patients had surgery at the time of first relapse. The median time from initial diagnosis to first relapse was 13.8 months (4.2 to 75.4). TEMODAR Capsules were given for the first 5 consecutive days of a 28-day cycle at a starting dose of 150 mg/m^2/day. If the nadir and day of dosing (Day 29, Day 1 of next cycle) absolute neutrophil count was ≥1.5 × 10^9/L (1,500/μL) and the nadir and Day 29, Day 1 of next cycle, platelet count was ≥100 × 10^9/L (100,000/μL), the TEMODAR dose was increased to 200 mg/m^2/day for the first 5 consecutive days of a 28-day cycle.

In the refractory anaplastic astrocytoma population, the overall tumor response rate (CR + PR) was 22% (12/54 patients) and the complete response rate was 9% (5/54 patients). The median duration of all responses was 50 weeks (range of 16 to 114 weeks) and the median duration of complete responses was 64 weeks (range of 52 to 114 weeks). In this population, progression-free survival at 6 months was 45% (95% confidence interval 31% to 58%) and progression-free survival at 12 months was 29% (95% confidence interval 16% to 42%). Median progression-free survival was 4.4 months. Overall survival at 6 months was 74% (95% confidence interval 62% to 86%) and 12-month overall survival was 65% (95% confidence interval 52% to 78%). Median overall survival was 15.9 months.

INDICATIONS AND USAGE

TEMODAR (temozolomide) Capsules are indicated for the treatment of adult patients with newly diagnosed glioblastoma multiforme concomitantly with radiotherapy and then as maintenance treatment.

TEMODAR Capsules are indicated for the treatment of adult patients with refractory anaplastic astrocytoma, ie, patients who have experienced disease progression on a drug regimen containing nitrosourea and procarbazine.

CONTRAINDICATIONS

TEMODAR (temozolomide) Capsules are contraindicated in patients who have a history of hypersensitivity reaction to any of its components. TEMODAR is also contraindicated in patients who have a history of hypersensitivity to DTIC, since both drugs are metabolized to MTIC.

WARNINGS

Patients treated with TEMODAR Capsules may experience myelosuppression. Prior to dosing, patients must have an absolute neutrophil count (ANC) ≥1.5 × 10^9/L and a platelet count ≥100 × 10^9/L. A complete blood count should be obtained on Day 22 (21 days after the first dose) or within 48 hours of that day, and weekly until the ANC is above 1.5 × 10^9/L and platelet count exceeds 100 × 10^9/L. Geriatric patients and women have been shown in clinical trials to have a higher risk of developing myelosuppression.

Very rare cases of myelodysplastic syndrome and secondary malignancies, including myeloid leukemia, have also been observed.

For treatment of newly diagnosed glioblastoma multiforme: Prophylaxis against *Pneumocystis carinii* pneumonia is required for all patients receiving concomitant TEMODAR and radiotherapy for the 42 day regimen.

There may be a higher occurrence of PCP when temozolomide is administered during a longer dosing regimen. However, all patients receiving temozolomide, particularly patients receiving steroids, should be observed closely for the development of PCP regardless of the regimen.

Pregnancy: Temozolomide may cause fetal harm when administered to a pregnant woman. Five consecutive days of oral administration of 75 mg/m^2/day in rats and 150 mg/m^2/day in rabbits during the period of organogenesis (3/8 and 3/4 the maximum recommended human dose, respectively) caused numerous malformations of the external organs, soft tissues, and skeleton in both species. Doses of 150 mg/m^2/day in rats and rabbits also caused embryolethality as indicated by increased resorptions. There are no adequate and well-controlled studies in pregnant women. If this drug is used during pregnancy, or if the patient becomes pregnant while taking this drug, the patient should be apprised of the potential hazard to the fetus. Women of childbearing potential should be advised to avoid becoming pregnant during therapy with TEMODAR Capsules.

PRECAUTIONS

Information for Patients: Nausea and vomiting were among the most frequently occurring adverse events. These were usually either self-limiting or readily controlled with standard antiemetic therapy. Capsules should not be opened. If capsules are accidentally opened or damaged, rigorous precautions should be taken with the capsule contents to avoid inhalation or contact with the skin or mucous membranes. The medication should be kept away from children and pets.

Drug Interaction: Administration of valproic acid decreases oral clearance of temozolomide by about 5%. The clinical implication of this effect is not known.

Patients with Severe Hepatic or Renal Impairment: Caution should be exercised when TEMODAR Capsules are administered to patients with severe hepatic or renal impairment (see **Special Populations**).

Geriatrics: Clinical studies of temozolomide did not include sufficient numbers of subjects aged 65 and over to determine whether they responded differently from younger subjects. Other reported clinical experience has not identified differences in responses between the elderly and younger patients. Caution should be exercised when treating elderly patients.

In the anaplastic astrocytoma study population, patients 70 years of age or older had a higher incidence of Grade 4 neutropenia and Grade 4 thrombocytopenia (2/8; 25%, p=0.31 and 2/10; 20%, p=0.09, respectively) in the first cycle of therapy than patients under 70 years of age (see **ADVERSE REACTIONS**).

In newly diagnosed patients with glioblastoma multiforme, the adverse event profile was similar in younger patients (<65 years) vs older (≥65 years).

Laboratory Tests: For the concomitant treatment phase with RT, a complete blood count should be obtained weekly. For the 28 day treatment cycles, a complete blood count should be obtained on Day 22 (21 days after the first dose). Blood counts should be performed weekly until recovery if the ANC falls below 1.5×10^9/L and the platelet count falls below 100×10^9/L.

Carcinogenesis, Mutagenesis, and Impairment of Fertility: Standard carcinogenicity studies were not conducted with temozolomide. In rats treated with 200 mg/m² temozolomide (equivalent to the maximum recommended daily human dose) on 5 consecutive days every 28 days for 3 cycles, mammary carcinomas were found in both males and females. With 6 cycles of treatment at 25, 50, and 125 mg/m² (about 1/8 to 1/2 the maximum recommended daily human dose), mammary carcinomas were observed at all doses and fibrosarcomas of the heart, eye, seminal vesicles, salivary glands, abdominal cavity, uterus, and prostate; carcinoma of the seminal vesicles, schwannoma of the heart, optic nerve, and harderian gland; and adenomas of the skin, lung, pituitary, and thyroid were observed at the high dose.

Temozolomide was mutagenic *in vitro* in bacteria (Ames assay) and clastogenic in mammalian cells (human peripheral blood lymphocyte assays).

Reproductive function studies have not been conducted with temozolomide. However, multicycle toxicology studies in rats and dogs have demonstrated testicular toxicity (syncytial cells/immature sperm, testicular atrophy) at doses of 50 mg/m² in rats and 125 mg/m² in dogs (1/4 and 5/8, respectively, of the maximum recommended human dose on a body surface area basis).

Pregnancy Category D: See **WARNINGS** section.

Nursing Mothers: It is not known whether this drug is excreted in human milk. Because many drugs are excreted in human milk and because of the potential for serious adverse reactions in nursing infants from TEMODAR Capsules, patients receiving TEMODAR should discontinue nursing.

Pediatric Use: TEMODOR effectiveness in children has not been demonstrated. TEMODAR Capsules have been studied in 2 open label Phase 2 studies in pediatric patients (age 3-18 years) at a dose of 160-200 mg/m² daily for 5 days every 28 days. In one trial conducted by the Schering Corporation, 29 patients with recurrent brain stem glioma and 34 patients with recurrent high grade astrocytoma were enrolled. All patients had failed surgery and radiation therapy, while 31% also failed chemotherapy. In a second Phase 2 open label study conducted by the Children's Oncology Group (COG), 122 patients were enrolled, including medulloblastoma/PNET (29), high grade astrocytoma (23), low grade astrocytoma (22), brain stem glioma (16), ependymoma (14), other CNS tumors (9) and non-CNS tumors (9). The TEMODAR toxicity profile in children is similar to adults. Table 1 shows the adverse events in 122 children in the COG Phase 2 study.

[See table 1 above]

ADVERSE REACTIONS IN ADULTS

Newly Diagnosed Glioblastoma Multiforme

During the concomitant phase (TEMODAR + radiotherapy), adverse events including thrombocytopenia, nausea, vomiting, anorexia and constipation, were more frequent in the TEMODAR + RT arm. The incidence of other adverse events was comparable in the two arms. The most common adverse events across the cumulative TEMODAR experience were alopecia, nausea, vomiting, anorexia, headache, and constipation (see **Table 2**). Forty-nine percent (49%) of patients treated with TEMODAR reported one or more severe or life-threatening events, most commonly fatigue (13%), convulsions (6%), headache (5%), and thrombocytopenia (5%). Overall, the pattern of events during the maintenance phase was consistent with the known safety profile of TEMODAR.

[See table 2 at right]

Myelosuppression, (neutropenia and thrombocytopenia), which are known dose limiting toxicities for most cytotoxic agents, including TEMODAR, were observed. When laboratory abnormalities and adverse events were combined, Grade 3 or Grade 4 neutrophil abnormalities including neutropenic events were observed in 8% of the patients and Grade 3 or Grade 4 platelet abnormalities, including thrombocytopenic events were observed in 14% of the patients treated with TEMODAR.

Refractory Anaplastic Astrocytoma

Tables 3 and 4 show the incidence of adverse events in the 158 patients in the anaplastic astrocytoma study for whom data are available. In the absence of a control group, it is not clear in many cases whether these events should be attributed to temozolomide or the patients' underlying conditions, but nausea, vomiting, fatigue, and hematologic effects appear to be clearly drug related. The most frequently occurring side effects were nausea, vomiting, headache, and fatigue. The adverse events were usually NCI Common Toxicity Criteria (CTC) Grade 1 or 2 (mild to moderate in severity) and were self-limiting, with nausea and vomiting

Table 1
Adverse Events Reported in Pediatric Cooperative Group Trial (≥10%)

Body System/Organ Class Adverse Event	No. (%) of TEMODAR Patients (N=122)[a]	
	All Events	Gr 3/4
Subjects Reporting an AE	107 (88)	69 (57)
Body as a Whole		
Central and Peripheral Nervous System		
Central cerebral CNS cortex	22 (18)	13 (11)
Gastrointestinal System		
Nausea	56 (46)	5 (4)
Vomiting	62 (51)	4 (3)
Platelet, Bleeding and Clotting		
Thrombocytopenia	71 (58)	31 (25)
Red Blood Cell Disorders		
Decreased Hemoglobin	62 (51)	7 (6)
White Cell and RES Disorders		
Decreased WBC	71 (58)	21 (17)
Lymphopenia	73 (60)	48 (39)
Neutropenia	62 (51)	24 (20)

[a] These various tumors included the following: PNET-medulloblastoma, glioblastoma, low grade astrocytoma, brain stem tumor, ependymona, mixed glioma, oligodendroglioma, neuroblastoma, Ewing's sarcoma, pineoblastoma, alveolar soft part sarcoma, neurofibrosarcoma, optic glioma, and osteosarcoma.

Table 2

Number (%) of Patients with Adverse Events: All and Severe/Life Threatening (Incidence of 5% or Greater)

	Concomitant Phase RT Alone (n=285)		Concomitant Phase RT+TMZ (n=288)*		Maintenance Phase TMZ (n=224)	
	All	Grade ≥ 3	All	Grade ≥ 3	All	Grade ≥ 3
Subjects Reporting any Adverse Event	258 (91)	74 (26)	266 (92)	80 (28)	206 (92)	82 (37)
Body as a Whole - General Disorders						
Anorexia	25 (9)	1 (<1)	56 (19)	2 (1)	61 (27)	3 (1)
Dizziness	10 (4)	0	12 (4)	2 (1)	12 (5)	0
Fatigue	139 (49)	15 (5)	156 (54)	19 (7)	137 (61)	20 (9)
Headache	49 (17)	11 (4)	56 (19)	5 (2)	51 (23)	9 (4)
Weakness	9 (3)	3 (1)	10 (3)	5 (2)	16 (7)	4 (2)
Central and Peripheral Nervous System Disorders						
Confusion	12 (4)	6 (2)	11 (4)	4 (1)	12 (5)	4 (2)
Convulsions	20 (7)	9 (3)	17 (6)	10 (3)	25 (11)	7 (3)
Memory Impairment	12 (4)	1 (<1)	8 (3)	1 (<1)	16 (7)	2 (1)
Disorders of the Eye						
Vision Blurred	25 (9)	4 (1)	26 (9)	2 (1)	17 (8)	0
Disorders of the Immume System						
Allergic Reaction	7 (2)	1 (<1)	13 (5)	0	6 (3)	0
Gastrointestinal System Disorders						
Abdominal Pain	2 (1)	0	7 (2)	1 (<1)	11 (5)	1 (<1)
Constipation	18 (6)	0	53 (18)	3 (1)	49 (22)	0
Diarrhea	9 (3)	0	18 (6)	0	23 (10)	2 (1)
Nausea	45 (16)	1 (<1)	105 (36)	2 (1)	110 (49)	3 (1)
Stomatitis	14 (5)	1 (<1)	19 (7)	0	20 (9)	3 (1)
Vomiting	16 (6)	1 (<1)	57 (20)	1 (<1)	66 (29)	4 (2)
Injury and Poisoning						
Radiation Injury NOS	11 (4)	1 (<1)	20 (7)	0	5 (2)	0
Musculoskeletal System Disorders						
Arthralgia	2 (1)	0	7 (2)	1 (<1)	14 (6)	0
Platelet, Bleeding and Clotting Disorders						
Thrombocytopenia	3 (1)	0	11 (4)	8 (3)	19 (8)	8 (4)
Psychiatric Disorders						
Insomnia	9 (3)	1 (<1)	14 (5)	0	9 (4)	0
Respiratory System Disorders						
Coughing	3 (1)	0	15 (5)	2 (1)	19 (8)	1 (<1)
Dyspnea	9 (3)	4 (1)	11 (4)	5 (2)	12 (5)	1 (<1)
Skin and Subcutaneous Tissue Disorders						
Alopecia	179 (63)	0	199 (69)	0	124 (55)	0
Dry Skin	6 (2)	0	7 (2)	0	11 (5)	1 (<1)
Erythema	15 (5)	0	14 (5)	0	2 (1)	0
Pruritus	4 (1)	0	11 (4)	0	11 (5)	0
Rash	42 (15)	0	56 (19)	3 (1)	29 (13)	3 (1)
Special Senses Other, Disorders						
Taste Perversion	6 (2)	0	18 (6)	0	11 (5)	0

*One patient who was randomized to RT only arm received RT + temozolomide

RT+TMZ = radiotherapy plus temozolomide; LT = life threatening; SGPT = serum glutamic pyruvic transaminase (= alanine aminotransferase [ALT]); NOS = not otherwise specified.

Note: Grade 5 (fatal) adverse events are included in the Grade ≥ 3 column.

Continued on next page

Temodar—Cont.

readily controlled with antiemetics. The incidence of severe nausea and vomiting (CTC Grade 3 or 4) was 10% and 6%, respectively. Myelosuppression (thrombocytopenia and neutropenia) was the dose-limiting adverse event. It usually occurred within the first few cycles of therapy and was not cumulative.

Myelosuppression occurred late in the treatment cycle and returned to normal, on average, within 14 days of nadir counts. The median nadirs occurred at 26 days for platelets (range 21 to 40 days) and 28 days for neutrophils (range 1 to 44 days). Only 14% (22/158) of patients had a neutrophil nadir and 20% (32/158) of patients had a platelet nadir which may have delayed the start of the next cycle. Less than 10% of patients required hospitalization, blood transfusion, or discontinuation of therapy due to myelosuppression.

In clinical trial experience with 110 to 111 women and 169 to 174 men (depending on measurements), there were higher rates of Grade 4 neutropenia (ANC < 500 cells/μL) and thrombocytopenia (< 20,000 cells/μL) in women than men in the first cycle of therapy: (12% versus 5% and 9% versus 3%, respectively).

In the entire safety database for which hematologic data exist (N=932), 7% (4/61) and 9.5% (6/63) of patients over age 70 experienced Grade 4 neutropenia or thrombocytopenia in the first cycle, respectively. For patients less than or equal to age 70, 7% (62/871) and 5.5% (48/879) experienced Grade 4 neutropenia or thrombocytopenia in the first cycle, respectively. Pancytopenia, leukopenia, and anemia have also been reported.

Table 3

Adverse Events in the Anaplastic Astrocytoma Trial in Adults (≥5%)

Any Adverse Event	No. (%) of TEMODAR Patients (N=158)	
	All Events 153 (97)	Grade 3/4 79 (50)
Body as a Whole		
Headache	65 (41)	10 (6)
Fatigue	54 (34)	7 (4)
Asthenia	20 (13)	9 (6)
Fever	21 (13)	3 (2)
Back pain	12 (8)	4 (3)
Cardiovascular		
Edema peripheral	17 (11)	1 (1)
Central and Peripheral Nervous System		
Convulsions	36 (23)	8 (5)
Hemiparesis	29 (18)	10 (6)
Dizziness	19 (12)	1 (1)
Coordination abnormal	17 (11)	2 (1)
Amnesia	16 (10)	6 (4)
Insomnia	16 (10)	0
Paresthesia	15 (9)	1 (1)
Somnolence	15 (9)	5 (3)
Paresis	13 (8)	4 (3)
Urinary incontinence	13 (8)	3 (2)
Ataxia	12 (8)	3 (2)
Dysphasia	11 (7)	1 (1)
Convulsions local	9 (6)	0
Gait abnormal	9 (6)	1 (1)
Confusion	8 (5)	0
Endocrine		
Adrenal hypercorticism	13 (8)	0
Gastrointestinal System		
Nausea	84 (53)	16 (10)
Vomiting	66 (42)	10 (6)
Constipation	52 (33)	1 (1)
Diarrhea	25 (16)	3 (2)
Abdominal pain	14 (9)	2 (1)
Anorexia	14 (9)	1 (1)
Metabolic		
Weight increase	8 (5)	0
Musculoskeletal System		
Myalgia	8 (5)	
Psychiatric Disorders		
Anxiety	11 (7)	1 (1)
Depression	10 (6)	0
Reproductive Disorders		
Breast pain, female	4 (6)	
Resistance Mechanism Disorders		
Infection viral	17 (11)	0
Respiratory System		
Upper respiratory tract infection	13 (8)	0
Pharyngitis	12 (8)	0
Sinusitis	10 (6)	0
Coughing	8 (5)	0
Skin and Appendages		
Rash	13 (8)	0

Pruritus	12 (8)	2 (1)
Urinary System		
Urinary tract infection	12 (8)	0
Micturition increased frequency	9 (6)	0
Vision		
Diplopia	8 (5)	0
Vision Abnormal*	8 (5)	

*Blurred vision, visual deficit, vision changes, vision troubles.

Table 4

Adverse Hematologic Effects (Grade 3 to 4) in the Anaplastic Astrocytoma Trial in Adults

	TEMODAR[a]
Hemoglobin	7/158 (4%)
Lymphopenia	83/152 (55%)
Neutrophils	20/142 (14%)
Platelets	29/156 (19%)
WBC	18/158 (11%)

[a]Change from Grade 0 to 2 at baseline to Grade 3 or 4 during treatment.

In addition, the following spontaneous adverse experiences have been reported during the marketing surveillance of TEMODAR Capsules: allergic reactions, including rare cases of anaphylaxis. Rare cases of erythema multiforme have been reported which resolved after discontinuation of TEMODAR and, in some cases, recurred upon rechallenge. Rare cases of opportunistic infections including *Pneumocystis carinii* pneumonia (PCP) have also been reported.

OVERDOSAGE

Doses of 500, 750, 1000, and 1250 mg/m² (total dose per cycle over 5 days) have been evaluated clinically in patients. Dose-limiting toxicity was hematologic and was reported with any dose but is expected to be more severe at higher doses. An overdose of 2000 mg per day for 5 days was taken by one patient and the adverse events reported were pancytopenia, pyrexia, multi-organ failure and death. There are reports of patients who have taken more than 5 days of treatment (up to 64 days) with adverse events reported including bone marrow suppression, which in some cases was severe and prolonged, and infections and resulted in death. In the event of an overdose, hematologic evaluation is needed. Supportive measures should be provided as necessary.

DOSAGE AND ADMINISTRATION

Dosage of TEMODAR Capsules must be adjusted according to nadir neutrophil and platelet counts in the previous cycle and the neutrophil and platelet counts at the time of initiating the next cycle.

For TEMODAR dosage calculations based on body surface area (BSA) see **Table 9**. For suggested capsule combinations on a daily dose see **Table 10**.

Patients with Newly Diagnosed High Grade Glioma: Concomitant Phase

TEMODAR is administered orally at 75 mg/m² daily for 42 days concomitant with focal radiotherapy (60 Gy administered in 30 fractions) followed by maintenance TEMODAR for 6 cycles. Focal RT includes the tumor bed or resection site with a 2-3 cm margin. No dose reductions are recommended during the concomitant phase; however, dose interruptions or discontinuation may occur based on toxicity. The TEMODAR dose should be continued throughout the 42 day concomitant period up to 49 days if all of the following conditions are met: absolute neutrophil count ≥ 1.5 × 10⁹/L; platelet count ≥ 100 × 10⁹/L common toxicity criteria (CTC) non-hematological toxicity ≤ Grade 1 (except for alopecia, nausea and vomiting). During treatment a complete blood count should be obtained weekly. Temozolomide dosing should be interrupted or discontinued during concomitant phase according to the hematological and non-hematological toxicity criteria as noted in **Table 5**. PCP prophylaxis is required during the concomitant administration of TEMODAR and radiotherapy and should be continued in patients who develop lymphocytopenia until recovery from lymphocytopenia (CTC grade ≤ 1).

Table 5

Temozolomide Dosing Interruption or Discontinuation During Concomitant Radiotherapy and Temozolomide

Toxicity	TMZ Interruption[a]	TMZ Discontinuation
Absolute Neutrophil Count	≥0.5 and <1.5 × 10⁹/L	<0.5 × 10⁹/L
Platelet Count	≥10 and <100 × 10⁹/L	<10 × 10⁹/L

Toxicity		
CTC Non-hematological Toxicity (except for alopecia, nausea, vomiting)	CTC Grade 2	CTC Grade 3 or 4

[a]Treatment with concomitant TMZ could be continued when all of the following conditions were met: absolute neutrophil count ≥ 1.5 × 10⁹/L; platelet count ≥ 100 × 10⁹/L; CTC non-hematological toxicity ≤ Grade 1 (except for alopecia, nausea, vomiting).

TMZ = temozolomide; CTC = Common Toxicity Criteria.

Maintenance Phase Cycle 1:

Four weeks after completing the TEMODAR + RT phase, TEMODAR is administered for an additional 6 cycles of maintenance treatment. Dosage in Cycle 1 (maintenance) is 150 mg/m² once daily for 5 days followed by 23 days without treatment.

Cycles 2-6:

At the start of Cycle 2, the dose is escalated to 200 mg/m², if the CTC non-hematologic toxicity for Cycle 1 is Grade ≤ 2 (except for alopecia, nausea and vomiting), absolute neutrophil count (ANC) is ≥ 1.5 × 10⁹/L, and the platelet count is ≥ 100 × 10⁹/L. The dose remains at 200 mg/m² per day for the first 5 days of each subsequent cycle except if toxicity occurs. If the dose was not escalated at Cycle 2, escalation should not be done in subsequent cycles.

Dose reduction or discontinuation during maintenance:

Dose reductions during the maintenance phase should be applied according to **Tables 6** and **7**.

During treatment a complete blood count should be obtained on Day 22 (21 days after the first dose of TEMODAR) or within 48 hours of that day, and weekly until the ANC is above 1.5 × 10⁹/L (1500/μL) and the platelet count exceeds 100 × 10⁹/L (100,000/μL). The next cycle of TEMODAR should not be started until the ANC and platelet count exceed these levels. Dose reductions during the next cycle should be based on the lowest blood counts and worst non-hematologic toxicity during the previous cycle. Dose reductions or discontinuations during the maintenance phase should be applied according to **Tables 6** and **7**.

Table 6

Temozolomide Dose Levels for Maintenance Treatment

Dose Level	Dose (mg/m²/day)	Remarks
−1	100	Reduction for prior toxicity
0	150	Dose during Cycle 1
1	200	Dose during Cycles 2-6 in absence of toxicity

Table 7

Temozolomide Dose Reduction or Discontinuation During Maintenance Treatment

Toxicity	Reduce TMZ by 1 Dose Level[a]	Discontinue TMZ
Absolute Neutrophil Count	<1.0 × 10⁹/L	See footnote b
Platelet Count	<50 × 10⁹/L	See footnote b
CTC Non-hematological Toxicity (except for alopecia, nausea, vomiting)	CTC Grade 3	CTC Grade 4[b]

[a]TMZ dose levels are listed in **Table 6**.
[b]TMZ is to be discontinued if dose reduction to <100 mg/m² is required or if the same Grade 3 non-hematological toxicity (except for alopecia, nausea, vomiting) recurs after dose reduction.

TMZ = temozolomide; CTC = Common Toxicity Criteria.

Patients with Refractory Anaplastic Astrocytoma

For adults the initial dose is 150 mg/m² orally once daily for 5 consecutive days per 28-day treatment cycle. For adult patients, if both the nadir and day of dosing (Day 29, Day 1 of next cycle) ANC are ≥1.5 × 10⁹/L (1500/μL) and both the nadir and Day 29, Day 1 of next cycle platelet counts are ≥100 × 10⁹/L (100,000/μL); the TEMODAR dose may be increased to 200 mg/m²/day for 5 consecutive days per 28-day treatment cycle. During treatment, a complete blood count should be obtained on Day 22 (21 days after the first dose) or within 48 hours of that day, and weekly until the ANC is above 1.5 × 10⁹/L (1500/μL) and the platelet count exceeds 100 × 10⁹/L (100,000/μL). The next cycle of TEMODAR should not be started until the ANC and platelet count exceed these levels. If the ANC falls to <1.0 × 10⁹/L (1000/μL) or the platelet count is <50 × 10⁹/L (50,000/μL) during any cycle, the next cycle should be reduced by 50 mg/m², but not below 100 mg/m², the lowest recommended dose (see **Table 8**). TEMODAR therapy can be continued until disease progression. In the clinical trial, treatment could be continued for a maximum of 2 years; but the optimum duration of therapy is not known.

Table 8 Dosing Modification Table

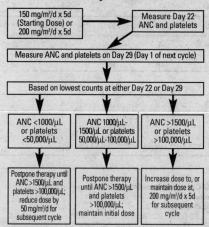

Table 9

Daily Dose Calculations by Body Surface Area (BSA)

Total BSA (m^2)	75 mg/m^2 (mg daily)	150 mg/m^2 (mg daily)	200 mg/m^2 (mg daily)
1.0	75	150	200
1.1	82.5	165	220
1.2	90	180	240
1.3	97.5	195	260
1.4	105	210	280
1.5	112.5	225	300
1.6	120	240	320
1.7	127.5	255	340
1.8	135	270	360
1.9	142.5	285	380
2.0	150	300	400
2.1	157.5	315	420
2.2	165	330	440
2.3	172.5	345	460
2.4	180	360	480
2.5	187.5	375	500

Table 10

Suggested Capsule Combinations Based on Daily Dose in Adults

Total Daily Dose (mg)	Number of Daily Capsules by Strength (mg)			
	250	100	20	5
75	0	0	3	3
82.5	0	0	4	0
90	0	0	4	2
97.5	0	1	0	0
105	0	1	0	1
112.5	0	1	0	2
120	0	1	1	0
127.5	0	1	1	1
135	0	1	1	3
142.5	0	1	2	0
150	0	1	2	2
157.5	0	1	3	0
165	0	1	3	1
172.5	0	1	3	2
180	0	1	4	0
187.5	0	1	4	1
195	0	1	4	3
200	0	2	0	0
210	0	2	0	2
220	0	2	1	0
225	0	2	1	1
240	0	2	2	0
255	1	0	0	1
260	1	0	0	2
270	1	0	1	0
280	1	0	1	2
285	1	0	1	3
300	0	3	0	0
315	0	3	0	3
320	0	3	1	0
330	1	0	4	0
340	0	3	2	0
345	0	3	2	1
360	0	3	3	0
375	1	1	1	1
380	1	1	1	2
400	0	4	0	0
420	0	4	1	0
440	0	4	2	0
460	1	2	0	2
480	1	2	1	2
500	2	0	0	0

In clinical trials, TEMODAR was administered under both fasting and non-fasting conditions; however, absorption is affected by food (see **CLINICAL PHARMACOLOGY**) and consistency of administration with respect to food is recommended. There are no dietary restrictions with TEMODAR. To reduce nausea and vomiting, TEMODAR should be taken on an empty stomach. Bedtime administration may be advised. Antiemetic therapy may be administered prior to and/or following administration of TEMODAR Capsules.
TEMODAR (temozolomide) Capsules should not be opened or chewed. They should be swallowed whole with a glass of water.

Handling and Disposal: TEMODAR causes the rapid appearance of malignant tumors in rats. Capsules should not be opened. If capsules are accidentally opened or damaged, rigorous precautions should be taken with the capsule contents to avoid inhalation or contact with the skin or mucous membranes. Procedures for proper handling and disposal of anticancer drugs should be considered.[1-7] Several guidelines on this subject have been published. There is no general agreement that all of the procedures recommended in the guidelines are necessary or appropriate.

HOW SUPPLIED

TEMODAR (temozolomide) Capsules are supplied in amber glass bottles with child-resistant polypropylene caps containing the following capsule strengths:
TEMODAR (temozolomide) Capsules 5 mg: 5 and 20 capsule bottles.
5 count - NDC 0085-1248-01
20 count - NDC 0085-1248-02
TEMODAR (temozolomide) Capsules 20 mg: 5 and 20 capsule bottles.
5 count - NDC 0085-1244-01
20 count - NDC 0085-1244-02
TEMODAR (temozolomide) Capsules 100 mg: 5 and 20 capsule bottles.
5 count - NDC 0085-1259-01
20 count - NDC 0085-1259-02
TEMODAR (temozolomide) Capsules 250 mg: 5 and 20 capsule bottles.
5 count - NDC 0085-1252-01
20 count - NDC 0085-1252-02
Store at 25°C (77°F); excursions permitted to 15-30°C (59-86°F).
[see USP Controlled Room Temperature]

REFERENCES

1. Recommendations for the Safe Handling of Parenteral Antineoplastic Drugs, NIH Publication No. 83-2621. For sale by the Superintendent of Documents, U.S. Government Printing Office, Washington, DC 20402.
2. AMA Council Report, Guidelines for Handling Parenteral Antineoplastics. *JAMA.* 1985;2.53(11):1590-1592.
3. National Study Commission on Cytotoxic Exposure— Recommendations for Handling Cytotoxic Agents. Available from Louis P. Jeffrey, ScD., Chairman, National Study Commission on Cytotoxic Exposure, Massachusetts College of Pharmacy and Allied Health Sciences, 179 Longwood Avenue, Boston, Massachusetts 02115.
4. Clinical Oncological Society of Australia, Guidelines and Recommendations for Safe Handling of Antineoplastic Agents. *Med J Australia.* 1983;1:426-428.
5. Jones RB, et al. Safe Handling Of Chemotherapeutic Agents: A Report from the Mount Sinai Medical Center. CA - *A Cancer Journal for Clinicians.* 1983;(Sept/Oct):258-263.
6. American Society of Hospital Pharmacists Technical Assistance Bulletin on Handling Cytotoxic and Hazardous Drugs. *Am J Hosp Pharm.* 1990;47:1033-1049.
7. Controlling Occupational Exposure to Hazardous Drugs. (OSHA Work-Practice Guidelines), *Am J Health-Syst Pharm.* 1996;53:1669-1685.

Schering®
Schering Corporation
Kenilworth, NJ 07033 USA
Rev. 11/04   22487876
U.S. Patent No. 5,260,291.

ZETIA®   ℞
[zĕt' ē ă]
(EZETIMIBE)
TABLETS

Prescribing information for this product, which appears on pages 3075–3080 of the 2005 PDR, has been completely revised as follows. Please write "See Supplement A" next to the product heading.

DESCRIPTION

ZETIA (ezetimibe) is in a class of lipid-lowering compounds that selectively inhibits the intestinal absorption of cholesterol and related phytosterols. The chemical name of ezetimibe is 1-(4-fluorophenyl)-3(R)-[3-(4-fluorophenyl)-3(S)-hydroxypropyl]-4(S)-(4-hydroxyphenyl)-2-azetidinone.

The empirical formula is $C_{24}H_{21}F_2NO_3$. Its molecular weight is 409.4 and its structural formula is:

Ezetimibe is a white, crystalline powder that is freely to very soluble in ethanol, methanol, and acetone and practically insoluble in water. Ezetimibe has a melting point of about 163°C and is stable at ambient temperature. ZETIA is available as a tablet for oral administration containing 10 mg of ezetimibe and the following inactive ingredients: croscarmellose sodium NF, lactose monohydrate NF, magnesium stearate NF, microcrystalline cellulose NF, povidone USP, and sodium lauryl sulfate NF.

CLINICAL PHARMACOLOGY

Background
Clinical studies have demonstrated that elevated levels of total cholesterol (total-C), low density lipoprotein cholesterol (LDL-C) and apolipoprotein B (Apo B), the major protein constituent of LDL, promote human atherosclerosis. In addition, decreased levels of high density lipoprotein cholesterol (HDL-C) are associated with the development of atherosclerosis. Epidemiologic studies have established that cardiovascular morbidity and mortality vary directly with the level of total-C and LDL-C and inversely with the level of HDL-C. Like LDL, cholesterol-enriched triglyceride-rich lipoproteins, including very-low-density lipoproteins (VLDL), intermediate-density lipoproteins (IDL), and remnants, can also promote atherosclerosis. The independent effect of raising HDL-C or lowering triglycerides (TG) on the risk of coronary and cardiovascular morbidity and mortality has not been determined.
ZETIA reduces total-C, LDL-C, Apo B, and TG, and increases HDL-C in patients with hypercholesterolemia. Administration of ZETIA with an HMG-CoA reductase inhibitor is effective in improving serum total-C, LDL-C, Apo B, TG, and HDL-C beyond either treatment alone. The effects of ezetimibe given either alone or in addition to an HMG-CoA reductase inhibitor on cardiovascular morbidity and mortality have not been established.
Mode of Action
Ezetimibe reduces blood cholesterol by inhibiting the absorption of cholesterol by the small intestine. In a 2-week clinical study in 18 hypercholesterolemic patients, ZETIA inhibited intestinal cholesterol absorption by 54%, compared with placebo. ZETIA had no clinically meaningful effect on the plasma concentrations of the fat-soluble vitamins A, D, and E (in a study of 113 patients), and did not impair adrenocortical steroid hormone production (in a study of 118 patients).
The cholesterol content of the liver is derived predominantly from three sources. The liver can synthesize cholesterol, take up cholesterol from the blood from circulating lipoproteins, or take up cholesterol absorbed by the small intestine. Intestinal cholesterol is derived primarily from cholesterol secreted in the bile and from dietary cholesterol. Ezetimibe has a mechanism of action that differs from those of other classes of cholesterol-reducing compounds (HMG-CoA reductase inhibitors, bile acid sequestrants [resins], fibric acid derivatives, and plant stanols).
Ezetimibe does not inhibit cholesterol synthesis in the liver, or increase bile acid excretion. Instead, ezetimibe localizes and appears to act at the brush border of the small intestine and inhibits the absorption of cholesterol, leading to a decrease in the delivery of intestinal cholesterol to the liver. This causes a reduction of hepatic cholesterol stores and an increase in clearance of cholesterol from the blood; this distinct mechanism is complementary to that of HMG-CoA reductase inhibitors (see CLINICAL STUDIES).
Pharmacokinetics
Absorption
After oral administration, ezetimibe is absorbed and extensively conjugated to a pharmacologically active phenolic glucuronide (ezetimibe-glucuronide). After a single 10-mg dose of ZETIA to fasted adults, mean ezetimibe peak plasma concentrations (C_{max}) of 3.4 to 5.5 ng/mL were attained within 4 to 12 hours (T_{max}). Ezetimibe-glucuronide mean C_{max} values of 45 to 71 ng/mL were achieved between 1 and 2 hours (T_{max}). There was no substantial deviation from dose proportionality between 5 and 20 mg. The absolute bioavailability of ezetimibe cannot be determined, as the compound is virtually insoluble in aqueous media suitable for injection. Ezetimibe has variable bioavailability; the coefficient of variation, based on inter-subject variability, was 35 to 60% for AUC values.
Effect of Food on Oral Absorption
Concomitant food administration (high fat or non-fat meals) had no effect on the extent of absorption of ezetimibe when administered as ZETIA 10-mg tablets. The C_{max} value of ezetimibe was increased by 38% with consumption of high fat meals. ZETIA can be administered with or without food.
Distribution
Ezetimibe and ezetimibe-glucuronide are highly bound (>90%) to human plasma proteins.
Metabolism and Excretion
Ezetimibe is primarily metabolized in the small intestine and liver via glucuronide conjugation (a phase II reaction)

Continued on next page

Zetia—Cont.

with subsequent biliary and renal excretion. Minimal oxidative metabolism (a phase I reaction) has been observed in all species evaluated.

In humans, ezetimibe is rapidly metabolized to ezetimibe-glucuronide. Ezetimibe and ezetimibe-glucuronide are the major drug-derived compounds detected in plasma, constituting approximately 10 to 20% and 80 to 90% of the total drug in plasma, respectively. Both ezetimibe and ezetimibe-glucuronide are slowly eliminated from plasma with a half-life of approximately 22 hours for both ezetimibe and ezetimibe-glucuronide. Plasma concentration-time profiles exhibit multiple peaks, suggesting enterohepatic recycling. Following oral administration of ^{14}C-ezetimibe (20 mg) to human subjects, total ezetimibe (ezetimibe + ezetimibe-glucuronide) accounted for approximately 93% of the total radioactivity in plasma. After 48 hours, there were no detectable levels of radioactivity in the plasma.

Approximately 78% and 11% of the administered radioactivity were recovered in the feces and urine, respectively, over a 10-day collection period. Ezetimibe was the major component in feces and accounted for 69% of the administered dose, while ezetimibe-glucuronide was the major component in urine and accounted for 9% of the administered dose.

Special Populations
Geriatric Patients
In a multiple dose study with ezetimibe given 10 mg once daily for 10 days, plasma concentrations for total ezetimibe were about 2-fold higher in older (≥65 years) healthy subjects compared to younger subjects.

Pediatric Patients
In a multiple dose study with ezetimibe given 10 mg once daily for 7 days, the absorption and metabolism of ezetimibe were similar in adolescents (10 to 18 years) and adults. Based on total ezetimibe, there are no pharmacokinetic differences between adolescents and adults. Pharmacokinetic data in the pediatric population <10 years of age are not available.

Gender
In a multiple dose study with ezetimibe given 10 mg once daily for 10 days, plasma concentrations for total ezetimibe were slightly higher (<20%) in women than in men.

Race
Based on a meta-analysis of multiple-dose pharmacokinetic studies, there were no pharmacokinetic differences between Blacks and Caucasians. There were too few patients in other racial or ethnic groups to permit further pharmacokinetic comparisons.

Hepatic Insufficiency
After a single 10-mg dose of ezetimibe, the mean area under the curve (AUC) for total ezetimibe was increased approximately 1.7-fold in patients with mild hepatic insufficiency (Child-Pugh score 5 to 6), compared to healthy subjects. The mean AUC values for total ezetimibe and ezetimibe were increased approximately 3- to 4-fold and 5- to 6- fold, respectively, in patients with moderate (Child-Pugh score 7 to 9) or severe hepatic impairment (Child-Pugh score 10 to 15). In a 14-day, multiple-dose study (10 mg daily) in patients with moderate hepatic insufficiency, the mean AUC values for total ezetimibe and ezetimibe were increased approximately 4-fold on Day 1 and Day 14 compared to healthy subjects. Due to the unknown effects of the increased exposure to ezetimibe in patients with moderate or severe hepatic insufficiency, ZETIA is not recommended in these patients (see CONTRAINDICATIONS and PRECAUTIONS, *Hepatic Insufficiency*).

Renal Insufficiency
After a single 10-mg dose of ezetimibe in patients with severe renal disease (n=8; mean CrCl ≤30 mL/min/1.73 m²), the mean AUC values for total ezetimibe, ezetimibe-glucuronide, and ezetimibe were increased approximately 1.5-fold, compared to healthy subjects (n=9).

Drug Interactions (See also PRECAUTIONS, *Drug Interactions*)
ZETIA had no significant effect on a series of probe drugs (caffeine, dextromethorphan, tolbutamide, and IV midazolam) known to be metabolized by cytochrome P450 (1A2, 2D6, 2C8/9 and 3A4) in a "cocktail" study of twelve healthy adult males. This indicates that ezetimibe is neither an inhibitor nor an inducer of these cytochrome P450 isozymes, and it is unlikely that ezetimibe will affect the metabolism of drugs that are metabolized by these enzymes.

Warfarin: Concomitant administration of ezetimibe (10 mg once daily) had no significant effect on bioavailability of warfarin and prothrombin time in a study of twelve healthy adult males.

Digoxin: Concomitant administration of ezetimibe (10 mg once daily) had no significant effect on the bioavailability of digoxin and the ECG parameters (HR, PR, QT, and QTc intervals) in a study of twelve healthy adult males.

Gemfibrozil: In a study of twelve healthy adult males, concomitant administration of gemfibrozil (600 mg twice daily) significantly increased the oral bioavailability of total ezetimibe by a factor of 1.7. Ezetimibe (10 mg once daily) did not significantly affect the bioavailability of gemfibrozil.

Oral Contraceptives: Co-administration of ezetimibe (10 mg once daily) with oral contraceptives had no significant effect on the bioavailability of ethinyl estradiol or levonorgestrel in a study of eighteen healthy adult females.

Cimetidine: Multiple doses of cimetidine (400 mg twice daily) had no significant effect on the oral bioavailability of ezetimibe and total ezetimibe in a study of twelve healthy adults.

Table 1
Response to ZETIA in Patients with Primary Hypercholesterolemia
(Mean[a] % Change from Untreated Baseline[b])

	Treatment group	N	Total-C	LDL-C	Apo B	TG[a]	HDL-C
Study 1[c]	Placebo	205	+1	+1	-1	-1	-1
	Ezetimibe	622	-12	-18	-15	-7	+1
Study 2[c]	Placebo	226	+1	+1	-1	+2	-2
	Ezetimibe	666	-12	-18	-16	-9	+1
Pooled Data[c] (Studies 1 & 2)	Placebo	431	0	+1	-2	0	-2
	Ezetimibe	1288	-13	-18	-16	-8	+1

[a] For triglycerides, median % change from baseline
[b] Baseline - on no lipid-lowering drug
[c] ZETIA significantly reduced total-C, LDL-C, Apo B, and TG, and increased HDL-C compared to placebo.

Table 2
Response to Addition of ZETIA to On-going HMG-CoA Reductase Inhibitor Therapy[a] in Patients with Hypercholesterolemia
(Mean[b] % Change from Treated Baseline[c])

Treatment (Daily Dose)	N	Total-C	LDL-C	Apo B	TG[b]	HDL-C
On-going HMG-CoA reductase inhibitor + Placebo[d]	390	-2	-4	-3	-3	+1
On-going HMG-CoA reductase inhibitor + ZETIA[d]	379	-17	-25	-19	-14	+3

[a] Patients receiving each HMG-CoA reductase inhibitor: 40% atorvastatin, 31% simvastatin, 29% others (pravastatin, fluvastatin, cerivastatin, lovastatin)
[b] For triglycerides, median % change from baseline
[c] Baseline - on an HMG-CoA reductase inhibitor alone.
[d] ZETIA + HMG-CoA reductase inhibitor significantly reduced total-C, LDL-C, Apo B, and TG, and increased HDL-C compared to HMG-CoA reductase inhibitor alone.

Antacids: In a study of twelve healthy adults, a single dose of antacid (Supralox™ 20 mL) administration had no significant effect on the oral bioavailability of total ezetimibe, ezetimibe-glucuronide, or ezetimibe based on AUC values. The C_{max} value of total ezetimibe was decreased by 30%.

Glipizide: In a study of twelve healthy adult males, steady-state levels of ezetimibe (10 mg once daily) had no significant effect on the pharmacokinetics and pharmacodynamics of glipizide. A single dose of glipizide (10 mg) had no significant effect on the exposure to total ezetimibe or ezetimibe.

HMG-CoA Reductase Inhibitors: In studies of healthy hypercholesterolemic (LDL-C ≥130 mg/dL) adult subjects, concomitant administration of ezetimibe (10 mg once daily) had no significant effect on the bioavailability of either lovastatin, simvastatin, pravastatin, atorvastatin, or fluvastatin. No significant effect on the bioavailability of total ezetimibe and ezetimibe was demonstrated by either lovastatin (20 mg once daily), pravastatin (20 mg once daily), atorvastatin (10 mg once daily), or fluvastatin (20 mg once daily).

Fenofibrate: In a study of thirty-two healthy hypercholesterolemic (LDL-C ≥130 mg/dL) adult subjects, concomitant fenofibrate (200 mg once daily) administration increased the mean C_{max} and AUC values of total ezetimibe approximately 64% and 48%, respectively. Pharmacokinetics of fenofibrate were not significantly affected by ezetimibe (10 mg once daily).

Cholestyramine: In a study of forty healthy hypercholesterolemic (LDL-C ≥130 mg/dL) adult subjects, concomitant cholestyramine (4 g twice daily) administration decreased the mean AUC values of total ezetimibe and ezetimibe approximately 55% and 80%, respectively.

Cyclosporine: In a study of eight post-renal transplant patients with mildly impaired or normal renal function (creatinine clearance of >50 mL/min), stable doses of cyclosporine (75 to 150 mg twice daily) increased the mean AUC and C_{max} values of total ezetimibe 3.4-fold (range 2.3- to 7.9-fold) and 3.9-fold (range 3.0- to 4.4-fold), respectively, compared to a historical healthy control population (n=17). In a different study, a renal transplant patient with severe renal insufficiency (creatinine clearance of 13.2 mL/min/1.73 m²) who was receiving multiple medications, including cyclosporine, demonstrated a 12-fold greater exposure to total ezetimibe compared to healthy subjects.

ANIMAL PHARMACOLOGY

The hypocholesterolemic effect of ezetimibe was evaluated in cholesterol-fed Rhesus monkeys, dogs, rats, and mouse models of human cholesterol metabolism. Ezetimibe was found to have an ED$_{50}$ value of 0.5 µg/kg/day for inhibiting the rise in plasma cholesterol levels in monkeys. The ED$_{50}$ values in dogs, rats, and mice were 7, 30, and 700 µg/kg/day, respectively. These results are consistent with ZETIA being a potent cholesterol absorption inhibitor.

In a rat model, where the glucuronide metabolite of ezetimibe (SCH 60663) was administered intraduodenally, the metabolite was as potent as the parent compound (SCH 58235) in inhibiting the absorption of cholesterol, suggesting that the glucuronide metabolite had activity similar to the parent drug.

In 1-month studies in dogs given ezetimibe (0.03-300 mg/kg/day), the concentration of cholesterol in gallbladder bile increased ~2- to 4-fold. However, a dose of 300 mg/kg/day administered to dogs for one year did not result in gallstone

formation or any other adverse hepatobiliary effects. In a 14-day study in mice given ezetimibe (0.3-5 mg/kg/day) and fed a low-fat or cholesterol-rich diet, the concentration of cholesterol in gallbladder bile was either unaffected or reduced to normal levels, respectively.

A series of acute preclinical studies was performed to determine the selectivity of ZETIA for inhibiting cholesterol absorption. Ezetimibe inhibited the absorption of ^{14}C-cholesterol with no effect on the absorption of triglycerides, fatty acids, bile acids, progesterone, ethyl estradiol, or the fat-soluble vitamins A and D.

In 4- to 12-week toxicity studies in mice, ezetimibe did not induce cytochrome P450 drug metabolizing enzymes. In toxicity studies, a pharmacokinetic interaction of ezetimibe with HMG-CoA reductase inhibitors (parents or their active hydroxy acid metabolites) was seen in rats, dogs, and rabbits.

CLINICAL STUDIES
Primary Hypercholesterolemia
ZETIA reduces total-C, LDL-C, Apo B, and TG, and increases HDL-C in patients with hypercholesterolemia. Maximal to near maximal response is generally achieved within 2 weeks and maintained during chronic therapy.

ZETIA is effective in patients with hypercholesterolemia, in men and women, in younger and older patients, alone or administered with an HMG-CoA reductase inhibitor. Experience in pediatric and adolescent patients (ages 9 to 17) has been limited to patients with homozygous familial hypercholesterolemia (HoFH) or sitosterolemia.

Experience in non-Caucasians is limited and does not permit a precise estimate of the magnitude of the effects of ZETIA.

Monotherapy
In two, multicenter, double-blind, placebo-controlled, 12-week studies in 1719 patients with primary hypercholesterolemia, ZETIA significantly lowered total-C, LDL-C, Apo B, and TG, and increased HDL-C compared to placebo (see Table 1). Reduction in LDL-C was consistent across age, sex, and baseline LDL-C.

[See table 1 above]
Combination with HMG-CoA Reductase Inhibitors
ZETIA Added to On-going HMG-CoA Reductase Inhibitor Therapy
In a multicenter, double-blind, placebo-controlled, 8-week study, 769 patients with primary hypercholesterolemia, known coronary heart disease or multiple cardiovascular risk factors who were already receiving HMG-CoA reductase inhibitor monotherapy, but who had not met their NCEP ATP II target LDL-C goal were randomized to receive either ZETIA or placebo in addition to their on-going HMG-CoA reductase inhibitor therapy.

ZETIA, added to on-going HMG-CoA reductase inhibitor therapy, significantly lowered total-C, LDL-C, Apo B, and TG, and increased HDL-C compared with an HMG-CoA reductase inhibitor administered alone (see Table 2). LDL-C reductions induced by ZETIA were generally consistent across all HMG-CoA reductase inhibitors.

[See table 2 above]
ZETIA Initiated Concurrently with an HMG-CoA Reductase Inhibitor
In four, multicenter, double-blind, placebo-controlled, 12-week trials, in 2382 hypercholesterolemic patients, ZETIA or placebo was administered alone or with various doses of atorvastatin, simvastatin, pravastatin, or lovastatin.

When all patients receiving ZETIA with an HMG-CoA reductase inhibitor were compared to all those receiving the corresponding HMG-CoA reductase inhibitor alone, ZETIA significantly lowered total-C, LDL-C, Apo B, and TG, and, with the exception of pravastatin, increased HDL-C compared to the HMG-CoA reductase inhibitor administered alone. LDL-C reductions induced by ZETIA were generally consistent across all HMG-CoA reductase inhibitors. (See footnote c, Tables 3 to 6.)

[See table 3 at right]
[See table 4 at right]
[See table 5 on next page]
[See table 6 at top of next page]

Homozygous Familial Hypercholesterolemia (HoFH)
A study was conducted to assess the efficacy of ZETIA in the treatment of HoFH. This double-blind, randomized, 12-week study enrolled 50 patients with a clinical and/or genotypic diagnosis of HoFH, with or without concomitant LDL apheresis, already receiving atorvastatin or simvastatin (40 mg). Patients were randomized to one of three treatment groups, atorvastatin or simvastatin (80 mg), ZETIA administered with atorvastatin or simvastatin (40 mg), or ZETIA administered with atorvastatin or simvastatin (80 mg). Due to decreased bioavailability of ezetimibe in patients concomitantly receiving cholestyramine (see PRECAUTIONS), ezetimibe was dosed at least 4 hours before or after administration of resins. Mean baseline LDL-C was 341 mg/dL in those patients randomized to atorvastatin 80 mg or simvastatin 80 mg alone and 316 mg/dL in the group randomized to ZETIA plus atorvastatin 40 or 80 mg or simvastatin 40 or 80 mg. ZETIA, administered with atorvastatin or simvastatin (40 and 80 mg statin groups, pooled), significantly reduced LDL-C (21%) compared with increasing the dose of simvastatin or atorvastatin monotherapy from 40 to 80 mg (7%). In those treated with ZETIA plus 80 mg atorvastatin or with ZETIA plus 80 mg simvastatin, LDL-C was reduced by 27%.

Homozygous Sitosterolemia (Phytosterolemia)
A study was conducted to assess the efficacy of ZETIA in the treatment of homozygous sitosterolemia. In this multicenter double-blind, placebo-controlled, 8-week trial, 37 patients with homozygous sitosterolemia with elevated plasma sitosterol levels (>5 mg/dL) on their current therapeutic regimen (diet, bile-acid-binding resins, HMG-CoA reductase inhibitors, ileal bypass surgery and/or LDL apheresis), were randomized to receive ZETIA (n=30) or placebo (n=7). Due to decreased bioavailability of ezetimibe in patients concomitantly receiving cholestyramine (see PRECAUTIONS), ezetimibe was dosed at least 2 hours before or 4 hours after resins were administered. Excluding the one subject receiving LDL apheresis, ZETIA significantly lowered plasma sitosterol and campesterol, by 21% and 24% from baseline, respectively. In contrast, patients who received placebo had increases in sitosterol and campesterol of 4% and 3% from baseline, respectively. For patients treated with ZETIA, mean plasma levels of plant sterols were reduced progressively over the course of the study. The effects of reducing plasma sitosterol and campesterol on reducing the risks of cardiovascular morbidity and mortality have not been established.
Reductions in sitosterol and campesterol were consistent between patients taking ZETIA concomitantly with bile acid sequestrants (n=8) and patients not on concomitant bile acid sequestrant therapy (n=21).

INDICATIONS AND USAGE
Primary Hypercholesterolemia
Monotherapy
ZETIA, administered alone, is indicated as adjunctive therapy to diet for the reduction of elevated total-C, LDL-C, and Apo B in patients with primary (heterozygous familial and non-familial) hypercholesterolemia.
Combination therapy with HMG-CoA reductase inhibitors
ZETIA, administered in combination with an HMG-CoA reductase inhibitor, is indicated as adjunctive therapy to diet for the reduction of elevated total-C, LDL-C, and Apo B in patients with primary (heterozygous familial and non-familial) hypercholesterolemia.
Homozygous Familial Hypercholesterolemia (HoFH)
The combination of ZETIA and atorvastatin or simvastatin, is indicated for the reduction of elevated total-C and LDL-C levels in patients with HoFH, as an adjunct to other lipid-lowering treatments (e.g., LDL apheresis) or if such treatments are unavailable.
Homozygous Sitosterolemia
ZETIA is indicated as adjunctive therapy to diet for the reduction of elevated sitosterol and campesterol levels in patients with homozygous familial sitosterolemia.
Therapy with lipid-altering agents should be a component of multiple risk-factor intervention in individuals at increased risk for atherosclerotic vascular disease due to hypercholesterolemia. Lipid-altering agents should be used in addition to an appropriate diet (including restriction of saturated fat and cholesterol) and when the response to diet and other non-pharmacological measures has been inadequate. (See NCEP Adult Treatment Panel (ATP) III Guidelines, summarized in Table 7.)
[See table 7 at top of page 407]
Prior to initiating therapy with ZETIA, secondary causes for dyslipidemia (i.e., diabetes, hypothyroidism, obstructive liver disease, chronic renal failure, and drugs that increase LDL-C and decrease HDL-C [progestins, anabolic steroids, and corticosteroids]), should be excluded or, if appropriate, treated. A lipid profile should be performed to measure

Table 3
Response to ZETIA and Atorvastatin Initiated Concurrently in Patients with Primary Hypercholesterolemia (Mean[a] % Change from Untreated Baseline[b])

Treatment (Daily Dose)	N	Total-C	LDL-C	Apo B	TG[a]	HDL-C
Placebo	60	+4	+4	+3	-6	+4
ZETIA	65	-14	-20	-15	-5	+4
Atorvastatin 10 mg	60	-26	-37	-28	-21	+6
ZETIA + Atorvastatin 10 mg	65	-38	-53	-43	-31	+9
Atorvastatin 20 mg	60	-30	-42	-34	-23	+4
ZETIA + Atorvastatin 20 mg	62	-39	-54	-44	-30	+9
Atorvastatin 40 mg	66	-32	-45	-37	-24	+4
ZETIA + Atorvastatin 40 mg	65	-42	-56	-45	-34	+5
Atorvastatin 80 mg	62	-40	-54	-46	-31	+3
ZETIA + Atorvastatin 80 mg	63	-46	-61	-50	-40	+7
Pooled data (All Atorvastatin Doses)[c]	248	-32	-44	-36	-24	+4
Pooled data (All ZETIA + Atorvastatin Doses)[c]	255	-41	-56	-45	-33	+7

[a] For triglycerides, median % change from baseline
[b] Baseline - on no lipid-lowering drug
[c] ZETIA + all doses of atorvastatin pooled (10-80 mg) significantly reduced total-C, LDL-C, Apo B, and TG, and increased HDL-C compared to all doses of atorvastatin pooled (10-80 mg).

Table 4
Response to ZETIA and Simvastatin Initiated Concurrently in Patients with Primary Hypercholesterolemia (Mean[a] % Change from Untreated Baseline[b])

Treatment (Daily Dose)	N	Total-C	LDL-C	Apo B	TG[a]	HDL-C
Placebo	70	-1	-1	0	+2	+1
ZETIA	61	-13	-19	-14	-11	+5
Simvastatin 10 mg	70	-18	-27	-21	-14	+8
ZETIA + Simvastatin 10 mg	67	-32	-46	-35	-26	+9
Simvastatin 20 mg	61	-26	-36	-29	-18	+6
ZETIA + Simvastatin 20 mg	69	-33	-46	-36	-25	+9
Simvastatin 40 mg	65	-27	-38	-32	-24	+6
ZETIA + Simvastatin 40 mg	73	-40	-56	-45	-32	+11
Simvastatin 80 mg	67	-32	-45	-37	-23	+8
ZETIA + Simvastatin 80 mg	65	-41	-58	-47	-31	+8
Pooled data (All Simvastatin Doses)[c]	263	-26	-36	-30	-20	+7
Pooled data (All ZETIA + Simvastatin Doses)[c]	274	-37	-51	-41	-29	+9

[a] For triglycerides, median % change from baseline
[b] Baseline - on no lipid-lowering drug
[c] ZETIA + all doses of simvastatin pooled (10-80 mg) significantly reduced total-C, LDL-C, Apo B, and TG, and increased HDL-C compared to all doses of simvastatin pooled (10-80 mg).

total-C, LDL-C, HDL-C and TG. For TG levels >400 mg/dL (>4.5 mmol/L), LDL-C concentrations should be determined by ultracentrifugation.
At the time of hospitalization for an acute coronary event, lipid measures should be taken on admission or within 24 hours. These values can guide the physician on initiation of LDL-lowering therapy before or at discharge.

CONTRAINDICATIONS
Hypersensitivity to any component of this medication.
The combination of ZETIA with an HMG-CoA reductase inhibitor is contraindicated in patients with active liver disease or unexplained persistent elevations in serum transaminases.
All HMG-CoA reductase inhibitors are contraindicated in pregnant and nursing women. When ZETIA is administered with an HMG-CoA reductase inhibitor in a woman of childbearing potential, refer to the pregnancy category and product labeling for the HMG-CoA reductase inhibitor. (See PRECAUTIONS, *Pregnancy*.)

PRECAUTIONS
Concurrent administration of ZETIA with a specific HMG-CoA reductase inhibitor should be in accordance with the product labeling for that HMG-CoA reductase inhibitor.
Liver Enzymes
In controlled clinical monotherapy studies, the incidence of consecutive elevations ($\geq 3 \times$ the upper limit of normal [ULN]) in serum transaminases was similar between ZETIA (0.5%) and placebo (0.3%).

Continued on next page

Zetia—Cont.

In controlled clinical combination studies of ZETIA initiated concurrently with an HMG-CoA reductase inhibitor, the incidence of consecutive elevations ($\geq 3 \times$ ULN) in serum transaminases was 1.3% for patients treated with ZETIA administered with HMG-CoA reductase inhibitors and 0.4% for patients treated with HMG-CoA reductase inhibitors alone. These elevations in transaminases were generally asymptomatic, not associated with cholestasis, and returned to baseline after discontinuation of therapy or with continued treatment. When ZETIA is co-administered with an HMG-CoA reductase inhibitor, liver function tests should be performed at initiation of therapy and according to the recommendations of the HMG-CoA reductase inhibitor.

Skeletal Muscle
In clinical trials, there was no excess of myopathy or rhabdomyolysis associated with ZETIA compared with the relevant control arm (placebo or HMG-CoA reductase inhibitor alone). However, myopathy and rhabdomyolysis are known adverse reactions to HMG-CoA reductase inhibitors and other lipid-lowering drugs. In clinical trials, the incidence of CPK >10 × ULN was 0.2% for ZETIA vs 0.1% for placebo, and 0.1% for ZETIA co-administered with an HMG-CoA reductase inhibitor vs 0.4% for HMG-CoA reductase inhibitors alone.

Hepatic Insufficiency
Due to the unknown effects of the increased exposure to ezetimibe in patients with moderate or severe hepatic insufficiency, ZETIA is not recommended in these patients. (See CLINICAL PHARMACOLOGY, *Special Populations.*)

Drug Interactions (See also CLINICAL PHARMACOLOGY, *Drug Interactions*)
Cholestyramine: Concomitant cholestyramine administration decreased the mean AUC of total ezetimibe approximately 55%. The incremental LDL-C reduction due to adding ezetimibe to cholestyramine may be reduced by this interaction.
Fibrates: The safety and effectiveness of ezetimibe administered with fibrates have not been established.
Fibrates may increase cholesterol excretion into the bile, leading to cholelithiasis. In a preclinical study in dogs, ezetimibe increased cholesterol in the gallbladder bile (see ANIMAL PHARMACOLOGY). Co-administration of ZETIA with fibrates is not recommended until use in patients is studied.
Fenofibrate: In a pharmacokinetic study, concomitant fenofibrate administration increased total ezetimibe concentrations approximately 1.5-fold.
Gemfibrozil: In a pharmacokinetic study, concomitant gemfibrozil administration increased total ezetimibe concentrations approximately 1.7-fold.
HMG-CoA Reductase Inhibitors: No clinically significant pharmacokinetic interactions were seen when ezetimibe was co-administered with atorvastatin, simvastatin, pravastatin, lovastatin, or fluvastatin.
Cyclosporine: Caution should be exercised when initiating ezetimibe in patients treated with cyclosporine due to increased exposure to ezetimibe. This exposure may be greater in patients with severe renal insufficiency. In patients treated with cyclosporine, the potential effects of the increased exposure to ezetimibe from concomitant use should be carefully weighed against the benefits of alterations in lipid levels provided by ezetimibe. In a pharmacokinetic study in post-renal transplant patients with mildly impaired or normal renal function (creatinine clearance >50 mL/min), concomitant cyclosporine administration increased the mean AUC and C_{max} of total ezetimibe 3.4-fold (range 2.3- to 7.9-fold) and 3.9-fold (range 3.0- to 4.4-fold), respectively. In a separate study, the total ezetimibe exposure increased 12-fold in one renal transplant patient with severe renal insufficiency receiving multiple medications, including cyclosporine (see CLINICAL PHARMACOLOGY, *Drug Interactions*).

Carcinogenesis, Mutagenesis, Impairment of Fertility
A 104-week dietary carcinogenicity study with ezetimibe was conducted in rats at doses up to 1500 mg/kg/day (males) and 500 mg/kg/day (females) ($\sim$20 times the human exposure at 10 mg daily based on AUC_{0-24hr} for total ezetimibe). A 104-week dietary carcinogenicity study with ezetimibe was also conducted in mice at doses up to 500 mg/kg/day (>150 times the human exposure at 10 mg daily based on AUC_{0-24hr} for total ezetimibe). There were no statistically significant increases in tumor incidences in drug-treated rats or mice.
No evidence of mutagenicity was observed *in vitro* in a microbial mutagenicity (Ames) test with *Salmonella typhimurium* and *Escherichia coli* with or without metabolic activation. No evidence of clastogenicity was observed *in vitro* in a chromosomal aberration assay in human peripheral blood lymphocytes with or without metabolic activation. In addition, there was no evidence of genotoxicity in the *in vivo* mouse micronucleus test.
In oral (gavage) fertility studies of ezetimibe conducted in rats, there was no evidence of reproductive toxicity at doses up to 1000 mg/kg/day in male or female rats ($\sim$7 times the human exposure at 10 mg daily based on AUC_{0-24hr} for total ezetimibe).

Pregnancy
Pregnancy Category: C
There are no adequate and well-controlled studies of ezetimibe in pregnant women. Ezetimibe should be used during pregnancy only if the potential benefit justifies the risk to the fetus.

Table 5
Response to ZETIA and Pravastatin Initiated Concurrently in Patients with Primary Hypercholesterolemia
(Mean[a] % Change from Untreated Baseline[b])

Treatment (Daily Dose)	N	Total-C	LDL-C	Apo B	TG[a]	HDL-C
Placebo	65	0	-1	-2	-1	+2
ZETIA	64	-13	-20	-15	-5	+4
Pravastatin 10 mg	66	-15	-21	-16	-14	+6
ZETIA + Pravastatin 10 mg	71	-24	-34	-27	-23	+8
Pravastatin 20 mg	69	-15	-23	-18	-8	+8
ZETIA + Pravastatin 20 mg	66	-27	-40	-31	-21	+8
Pravastatin 40 mg	70	-22	-31	-26	-19	+6
ZETIA + Pravastatin 40 mg	67	-30	-42	-32	-21	+8
Pooled data (All Pravastatin Doses)[c]	205	-17	-25	-20	-14	+7
Pooled data (All ZETIA + Pravastatin Doses)[c]	204	-27	-39	-30	-21	+8

[a] For triglycerides, median % change from baseline
[b] Baseline - on no lipid-lowering drug
[c] ZETIA + all doses of pravastatin pooled (10-40 mg) significantly reduced total-C, LDL-C, Apo B, and TG compared to all doses of pravastatin pooled (10-40 mg).

Table 6
Response to ZETIA and Lovastatin Initiated Concurrently in Patients with Primary Hypercholesterolemia
(Mean[a] % Change from Untreated Baseline[b])

Treatment (Daily Dose)	N	Total-C	LDL-C	Apo B	TG[a]	HDL-C
Placebo	64	+1	0	+1	+6	0
ZETIA	72	-13	-19	-14	-5	+3
Lovastatin 10 mg	73	-15	-20	-17	-11	+5
ZETIA + Lovastatin 10 mg	65	-24	-34	-27	-19	+8
Lovastatin 20 mg	74	-19	-26	-21	-12	+3
ZETIA + Lovastatin 20 mg	62	-29	-41	-34	-27	+9
Lovastatin 40 mg	73	-21	-30	-25	-15	+5
ZETIA + Lovastatin 40 mg	65	-33	-46	-38	-27	+9
Pooled data (All Lovastatin Doses)[c]	220	-18	-25	-21	-12	+4
Pooled data (All ZETIA + Lovastatin Doses)[c]	192	-29	-40	-33	-25	+9

[a] For triglycerides, median % change from baseline
[b] Baseline - on no lipid-lowering drug
[c] ZETIA + all doses of lovastatin pooled (10-40 mg) significantly reduced total-C, LDL-C, Apo B, and TG, and increased HDL-C compared to all doses of lovastatin pooled (10-40 mg).

In oral (gavage) embryo-fetal development studies of ezetimibe conducted in rats and rabbits during organogenesis, there was no evidence of embryolethal effects at the doses tested (250, 500, 1000 mg/kg/day). In rats, increased incidences of common fetal skeletal findings (extra pair of thoracic ribs, unossified cervical vertebral centra, shortened ribs) were observed at 1000 mg/kg/day ($\sim$10 times the human exposure at 10 mg daily based on AUC_{0-24hr} for total ezetimibe). In rabbits treated with ezetimibe, an increased incidence of extra thoracic ribs was observed at 1000 mg/kg/day (150 times the human exposure at 10 mg daily based on AUC_{0-24hr} for total ezetimibe). Ezetimibe crossed the placenta when pregnant rats and rabbits were given multiple oral doses.
Multiple dose studies of ezetimibe given in combination with HMG-CoA reductase inhibitors (statins) in rats and rabbits during organogenesis result in higher ezetimibe and statin exposures. Reproductive findings occur at lower doses in combination therapy compared to monotherapy.
All HMG-CoA reductase inhibitors are contraindicated in pregnant and nursing women. When ZETIA is administered with an HMG-CoA reductase inhibitor in a woman of childbearing potential, refer to the pregnancy category and product labeling for the HMG-CoA reductase inhibitor. (See CONTRAINDICATIONS.)

Labor and Delivery
The effects of ZETIA on labor and delivery in pregnant women are unknown.
Nursing Mothers
In rat studies, exposure to total ezetimibe in nursing pups was up to half of that observed in maternal plasma. It is not known whether ezetimibe is excreted into human breast milk; therefore, ZETIA should not be used in nursing mothers unless the potential benefit justifies the potential risk to the infant.
Pediatric Use
The pharmacokinetics of ZETIA in adolescents (10 to 18 years) have been shown to be similar to that in adults. Treatment experience with ZETIA in the pediatric population is limited to 4 patients (9 to 17 years) in the sitosterolemia study and 5 patients (11 to 17 years) in the HoFH study. Treatment with ZETIA in children (<10 years) is not recommended. (See CLINICAL PHARMACOLOGY, *Special Populations.*)
Geriatric Use
Of the patients who received ZETIA in clinical studies, 948 were 65 and older (this included 206 who were 75 and older). The effectiveness and safety of ZETIA were similar between these patients and younger subjects. Greater sen-

Table 7
Summary of NCEP ATP III Guidelines

Risk Category	LDL Goal (mg/dL)	LDL Level at Which to Initiate Therapeutic Lifestyle Changes[a] (mg/dL)	LDL level at Which to Consider Drug Therapy (mg/dL)
CHD or CHD risk equivalents[b] (10-year risk >20%)[c]	<100	≥100	≥130 (100-129: drug optional)[d]
2+ Risk factors[e] (10-year risk ≤20%)[c]	<130	≥130	10-year risk 10-20%: ≥130[c] 10-year risk <10%: ≥160[c]
0-1 Risk factor[f]	<160	≥160	≥190 (160-189: LDL-lowering drug optional)

[a] Therapeutic lifestyle changes include: 1) dietary changes: reduced intake of saturated fats (<7% of total calories) and cholesterol (<200 mg per day), and enhancing LDL lowering with plant stanols/sterols (2 g/d) and increased viscous (soluble) fiber (10-25 g/d), 2) weight reduction, and 3) increased physical activity.

[b] CHD risk equivalents comprise: diabetes, multiple risk factors that confer a 10-year risk for CHD >20%, and other clinical forms of atherosclerotic disease (peripheral arterial disease, abdominal aortic aneurysm and symptomatic carotid artery disease).

[c] Risk assessment for determining the 10-year risk for developing CHD is carried out using the Framingham risk scoring. Refer to JAMA, May 16, 2001; 285 (19): 2486-2497, or the NCEP website (http://www.nhlbi.nih.gov) for more details.

[d] Some authorities recommend use of LDL-lowering drugs in this category if an LDL cholesterol <100 mg/dL cannot be achieved by therapeutic lifestyle changes. Others prefer use of drugs that primarily modify triglycerides and HDL, e.g., nicotinic acid or fibrate. Clinical judgment also may call for deferring drug therapy in this subcategory.

[e] Major risk factors (exclusive of LDL cholesterol) that modify LDL goals include cigarette smoking, hypertension (BP ≥140/90 mm Hg or on anti-hypertensive medication), low HDL cholesterol (<40 mg/dL), family history of premature CHD (CHD in male first-degree relative <55 years; CHD in female first-degree relative <65 years), age (men ≥45 years; women ≥55 years). HDL cholesterol ≥60 mg/dL counts as a "negative" risk factor; its presence removes one risk factor from the total count.

[f] Almost all people with 0-1 risk factor have a 10-year risk <10%; thus, 10-year risk assessment in people with 0-1 risk factor is not necessary.

Table 9*
Clinical Adverse Events Occurring in ≥2% of Patients and at an Incidence Greater than Placebo, Regardless of Causality, in ZETIA/Statin Combination Studies

Body System/Organ Class Adverse Event	Placebo (%) n=259	ZETIA 10 mg (%) n=262	All Statins** (%) n=936	ZETIA + All Statins** (%) n=925
Body as a whole – general disorders				
Chest pain	1.2	3.4	2.0	1.8
Dizziness	1.2	2.7	1.4	1.8
Fatigue	1.9	1.9	1.4	2.8
Headache	5.4	8.0	7.3	6.3
Gastro-intestinal system disorders				
Abdominal pain	2.3	2.7	3.1	3.5
Diarrhea	1.5	3.4	2.9	2.8
Infection and infestations				
Pharyngitis	1.9	3.1	2.5	2.3
Sinusitis	1.9	4.6	3.6	3.5
Upper respiratory tract infection	10.8	13.0	13.6	11.8
Musculo-skeletal system disorders				
Arthralgia	2.3	3.8	4.3	3.4
Back pain	3.5	3.4	3.7	4.3
Myalgia	4.6	5.0	4.1	4.5

*Includes four placebo-controlled combination studies in which ZETIA was initiated concurrently with an HMG-CoA reductase inhibitor.

**All Statins = all doses of all HMG-CoA reductase inhibitors.

sitivity of some older individuals cannot be ruled out. (See CLINICAL PHARMACOLOGY, *Special Populations*, and ADVERSE REACTIONS.)

ADVERSE REACTIONS

ZETIA has been evaluated for safety in more than 4700 patients in clinical trials. Clinical studies of ZETIA (administered alone or with an HMG-CoA reductase inhibitor) demonstrated that ZETIA was generally well tolerated. The overall incidence of adverse events reported with ZETIA was similar to that reported with placebo, and the discontinuation rate due to adverse events was also similar for ZETIA and placebo.

Monotherapy
Adverse experiences reported in ≥2% of patients treated with ZETIA and at an incidence greater than placebo in placebo-controlled studies of ZETIA, regardless of causality assessment, are shown in Table 8.

Table 8*
Clinical Adverse Events Occurring in ≥2% of Patients Treated with ZETIA and at an Incidence Greater than Placebo, Regardless of Causality

Body System/Organ Class Adverse Event	Placebo (%) n = 795	ZETIA 10 mg (%) n = 1691
Body as a whole – general disorders		
Fatigue	1.8	2.2
Gastro-intestinal system disorders		
Abdominal pain	2.8	3.0
Diarrhea	3.0	3.7
Infection and infestations		
Infection viral	1.8	2.2
Pharyngitis	2.1	2.3
Sinusitis	2.8	3.6
Musculo-skeletal system disorders		
Arthralgia	3.4	3.8
Back pain	3.9	4.1
Respiratory system disorders		
Coughing	2.1	2.3

*Includes patients who received placebo or ZETIA alone reported in Table 9.

The frequency of less common adverse events was comparable between ZETIA and placebo.

Combination with an HMG-CoA Reductase Inhibitor
ZETIA has been evaluated for safety in combination studies in more than 2000 patients.
In general, adverse experiences were similar between ZETIA administered with HMG-CoA reductase inhibitors and HMG-CoA reductase inhibitors alone. However, the frequency of increased transaminases was slightly higher in patients receiving ZETIA administered with HMG-CoA reductase inhibitors than in patients treated with HMG-CoA reductase inhibitors alone. (See PRECAUTIONS, *Liver Enzymes*.)
Clinical adverse experiences reported in ≥2% of patients and at an incidence greater than placebo in four placebo-controlled trials where ZETIA was administered alone or initiated concurrently with various HMG-CoA reductase inhibitors, regardless of causality assessment, are shown in Table 9.
[See table 9 above]

Post-marketing Experience
The following adverse reactions have been reported in post-marketing experience, regardless of causality assessment: Hypersensitivity reactions, including angioedema and rash; myalgia; increased CPK; elevations in liver transaminases; hepatitis; thrombocytopenia; pancreatitis; nausea; cholelithiasis; cholecystitis; and, very rarely in patients taking an HMG-CoA reductase inhibitor with ZETIA, rhabdomyolysis (see PRECAUTIONS, *Skeletal Muscle*).

OVERDOSAGE

In clinical studies, administration of ezetimibe, 50 mg/day to 15 healthy subjects for up to 14 days, or 40 mg/day to 18 patients with primary hypercholesterolemia for up to 56 days, was generally well tolerated.
A few cases of overdosage with ZETIA have been reported; most have not been associated with adverse experiences. Reported adverse experiences have not been serious. In the event of an overdose, symptomatic and supportive measures should be employed.

DOSAGE AND ADMINISTRATION

The patient should be placed on a standard cholesterol-lowering diet before receiving ZETIA and should continue on this diet during treatment with ZETIA.
The recommended dose of ZETIA is 10 mg once daily. ZETIA can be administered with or without food.
ZETIA may be administered with an HMG-CoA reductase inhibitor for incremental effect. For convenience, the daily dose of ZETIA may be taken at the same time as the HMG-CoA reductase inhibitor, according to the dosing recommendations for the HMG-CoA reductase inhibitor.
Patients with Hepatic Insufficiency
No dosage adjustment is necessary in patients with mild hepatic insufficiency (see PRECAUTIONS, *Hepatic Insufficiency*).
Patients with Renal Insufficiency
No dosage adjustment is necessary in patients with renal insufficiency (see CLINICAL PHARMACOLOGY, *Special Populations*).
Geriatric Patients
No dosage adjustment is necessary in geriatric patients (see CLINICAL PHARMACOLOGY, *Special Populations*).
Co-administration with Bile Acid Sequestrants
Dosing of ZETIA should occur either ≥2 hours before or ≥4 hours after administration of a bile acid sequestrant (see PRECAUTIONS, *Drug Interactions*).

HOW SUPPLIED

No. 3861-Tablets ZETIA, 10 mg, are white to off-white, capsule-shaped tablets debossed with "414" on one side. They are supplied as follows:
NDC 66582-414-31 bottles of 30
NDC 66582-414-54 bottles of 90
NDC 66582-414-74 bottles of 500
NDC 66582-414-28 unit dose packages of 100.
Storage
Store at 25°C (77°F); excursions permitted to 15-30°C (59-86°F). [See USP Controlled Room Temperature.] Protect from moisture.
MERCK/Schering-Plough Pharmaceuticals
Manufactured for: Merck/Schering-Plough Pharmaceuticals, North Wales, PA 19454, USA
By: Schering Corporation, Kenilworth, NJ 07033, USA or Merck & Co., Inc., Whitehouse Station, NJ 08889, USA
Issued November 2004
REV 05   25751876T
COPYRIGHT © Merck/Schering-Plough Pharmaceuticals, 2001, 2002. All rights reserved. Printed in USA.

G.D. Searle & Co.
A division of Pfizer
235 EAST 42ND STREET
NEW YORK, NY 10017-5755

For updates to the product information listed below, please check the Pfizer Web site, http://www.pfizer.com, or call (800) 438-1985. For complete product listing, please see the Manufacturers' Index.
For Medical Information, Contact:
(800) 438-1985
24 hours a day, seven days a week

Distribution:
1855 Shelby Oaks Drive North
Memphis, TN 38134
(901) 387-5200

Customer Service:
(800) 533-4535

CELEBREX®   ℞
[sĕ-lĕ-brĕks]
celecoxib capsules

Prescribing information for this product, which appears on pages 3095–3099 of the 2005 PDR, has been completely revised as follows. Please write "See Supplement A" next to the product heading.

DESCRIPTION

CELEBREX (celecoxib) is chemically designated as 4-[5-(4-methylphenyl)-3-(trifluoromethyl)-1H-pyrazol-1-yl] benzenesulfonamide and is a diaryl-substituted pyrazole. It has the following chemical structure:
[See chemical structure at top of next column]
The empirical formula for celecoxib is $C_{17}H_{14}F_3N_3O_2S$, and the molecular weight is 381.38.
CELEBREX oral capsules contain either 100 mg, 200 mg or 400 mg of celecoxib.

Continued on next page

Celebrex—Cont.

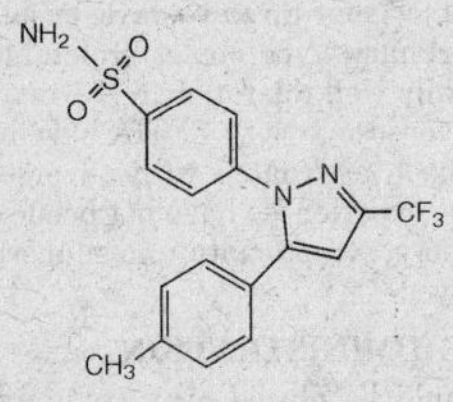

The inactive ingredients in CELEBREX capsules include: croscarmellose sodium, edible inks, gelatin, lactose monohydrate, magnesium stearate, povidone, sodium lauryl sulfate and titanium dioxide.

CLINICAL PHARMACOLOGY

Mechanism of Action: CELEBREX is a nonsteroidal anti-inflammatory drug that exhibits anti-inflammatory, analgesic, and antipyretic activities in animal models. The mechanism of action of CELEBREX is believed to be due to inhibition of prostaglandin synthesis, primarily via inhibition of cyclooxygenase-2 (COX-2), and at therapeutic concentrations in humans, CELEBREX does not inhibit the cyclooxygenase-1 (COX-1) isoenzyme. In animal colon tumor models, celecoxib reduced the incidence and multiplicity of tumors.

Pharmacokinetics:

Absorption

Peak plasma levels of celecoxib occur approximately 3 hrs after an oral dose. Under fasting conditions, both peak plasma levels (C_{max}) and area under the curve (AUC) are roughly dose proportional up to 200 mg BID; at higher doses there are less than proportional increases in C_{max} and AUC (see Food Effects). Absolute bioavailability studies have not been conducted. With multiple dosing, steady state conditions are reached on or before day 5.

The pharmacokinetic parameters of celecoxib in a group of healthy subjects are shown in Table 1.

[See table 1 above]

Table 1
Summary of Single Dose (200 mg) Disposition Kinetics of Celecoxib in Healthy Subjects[1]

Mean (%CV) PK Parameter Values				
C_{max}, ng/mL	T_{max}, hr	Effective $t_{1/2}$, hr	V_{ss}/F, L	CL/F, L/hr
705 (38)	2.8 (37)	11.2 (31)	429 (34)	27.7 (28)

[1]Subjects under fasting conditions (n=36, 19–52 yrs.)

Food Effects

When CELEBREX capsules were taken with a high fat meal, peak plasma levels were delayed for about 1 to 2 hours with an increase in total absorption (AUC) of 10% to 20%. Under fasting conditions, at doses above 200 mg, there is less than a proportional increase in C_{max} and AUC, which is thought to be due to the low solubility of the drug in aqueous media. Coadministration of CELEBREX with an aluminum- and magnesium-containing antacid resulted in a reduction in plasma celecoxib concentrations with a decrease of 37% in C_{max} and 10% in AUC. CELEBREX, at doses up to 200 mg BID can be administered without regard to timing of meals. Higher doses (400 mg BID) should be administered with food to improve absorption.

Distribution

In healthy subjects, celecoxib is highly protein bound (~97%) within the clinical dose range. *In vitro* studies indicate that celecoxib binds primarily to albumin and, to a lesser extent, α_1-acid glycoprotein. The apparent volume of distribution at steady state (V_{ss}/F) is approximately 400 L, suggesting extensive distribution into the tissues. Celecoxib is not preferentially bound to red blood cells.

Metabolism

Celecoxib metabolism is primarily mediated via cytochrome P450 2C9. Three metabolites, a primary alcohol, the corresponding carboxylic acid and its glucuronide conjugate, have been identified in human plasma. These metabolites are inactive as COX-1 or COX-2 inhibitors. Patients who are known or suspected to be P450 2C9 poor metabolizers based on a previous history should be administered celecoxib with caution as they may have abnormally high plasma levels due to reduced metabolic clearance.

Excretion

Celecoxib is eliminated predominantly by hepatic metabolism with little (<3%) unchanged drug recovered in the urine and feces. Following a single oral dose of radiolabeled drug, approximately 57% of the dose was excreted in the feces and 27% was excreted into the urine. The primary metabolite in both urine and feces was the carboxylic acid metabolite (73% of dose) with low amounts of the glucuronide also appearing in the urine. It appears that the low solubility of the drug prolongs the absorption process making terminal half-life ($t_{1/2}$) determinations more variable. The effective half-life is approximately 11 hours under fasted conditions. The apparent plasma clearance (CL/F) is about 500 mL/min.

Special Populations

Geriatric: At steady state, elderly subjects (over 65 years old) had a 40% higher C_{max} and a 50% higher AUC compared to the young subjects. In elderly females, celecoxib C_{max} and AUC are higher than those for elderly males, but these increases are predominantly due to lower body weight in elderly females. Dose adjustment in the elderly is not generally necessary. However, for patients of less than 50 kg in body weight, initiate therapy at the lowest recommended dose.

Pediatric: CELEBREX capsules have not been investigated in pediatric patients below 18 years of age.

Race: Meta-analysis of pharmacokinetic studies has suggested an approximately 40% higher AUC of celecoxib in Blacks compared to Caucasians. The cause and clinical significance of this finding is unknown.

Hepatic Insufficiency: A pharmacokinetic study in subjects with mild (Child-Pugh Class A) and moderate (Child-Pugh Class B) hepatic impairment has shown that steady-state celecoxib AUC is increased about 40% and 180%, respectively, above that seen in healthy control subjects. Therefore, the daily recommended dose of CELEBREX capsules should be reduced by approximately 50% in patients with moderate (Child-Pugh Class B) hepatic impairment. Patients with severe hepatic impairment (Child-Pugh Class C) have not been studied. The use of CELEBREX in patients with severe hepatic impairment is not recommended.

Renal Insufficiency: In a cross-study comparison, celecoxib AUC was approximately 40% lower in patients with chronic renal insufficiency (GFR 35-60 mL/min) than that seen in subjects with normal renal function. No significant relationship was found between GFR and celecoxib clearance. Patients with severe renal insufficiency have not been studied. Similar to other NSAIDs, CELEBREX is not recommended in patients with severe renal insufficiency (see WARNINGS – Advanced Renal Disease).

Drug Interactions

Also see **PRECAUTIONS – Drug Interactions.**

General: Significant interactions may occur when celecoxib is administered together with drugs that inhibit P450 2C9. *In vitro* studies indicate that celecoxib is not an inhibitor of cytochrome P450 2C9, 2C19 or 3A4.

Clinical studies with celecoxib have identified potentially significant interactions with fluconazole and lithium. Experience with nonsteroidal anti-inflammatory drugs (NSAIDs) suggests the potential for interactions with furosemide and ACE inhibitors. The effects of celecoxib on the pharmacokinetics and/or pharmacodynamics of glyburide, ketoconazole, methotrexate, phenytoin, and tolbutamide have been studied *in vivo* and clinically important interactions have not been found.

CLINICAL STUDIES

Osteoarthritis (OA): CELEBREX has demonstrated significant reduction in joint pain compared to placebo. CELEBREX was evaluated for treatment of the signs and the symptoms of OA of the knee and hip in approximately 4,200 patients in placebo- and active-controlled clinical trials of up to 12 weeks duration. In patients with OA, treatment with CELEBREX 100 mg BID or 200 mg QD resulted in improvement in WOMAC (Western Ontario and McMaster Universities) osteoarthritis index, a composite of pain, stiffness, and functional measures in OA. In three 12-week studies of pain accompanying OA flare, CELEBREX doses of 100 mg BID and 200 mg BID provided significant reduction of pain within 24-48 hours of initiation of dosing. At doses of 100 mg BID or 200 mg BID the effectiveness of CELEBREX was shown to be similar to that of naproxen 500 mg BID. Doses of 200 mg BID provided no additional benefit above that seen with 100 mg BID. A total daily dose of 200 mg has been shown to be equally effective whether administered as 100 mg BID or 200 mg QD.

Rheumatoid Arthritis (RA): CELEBREX has demonstrated significant reduction in joint tenderness/pain and joint swelling compared to placebo. CELEBREX was evaluated for treatment of the signs and symptoms of RA in approximately 2,100 patients in placebo- and active-controlled clinical trials of up to 24 weeks in duration. CELEBREX was shown to be superior to placebo in these studies, using the ACR20 Responder Index, a composite of clinical, laboratory, and functional measures in RA. CELEBREX doses of 100 mg BID and 200 mg BID were similar in effectiveness and both were comparable to naproxen 500 mg BID.

Although CELEBREX 100 mg BID and 200 mg BID provided similar overall effectiveness, some patients derived additional benefit from the 200 mg BID dose. Doses of 400 mg BID provided no additional benefit above that seen with 100–200 mg BID.

Analgesia, including primary dysmenorrhea: In acute analgesic models of post-oral surgery pain, post-orthopedic surgical pain, and primary dysmenorrhea, CELEBREX relieved pain that was rated by patients as moderate to severe. Single doses (see DOSAGE AND ADMINISTRATION) of CELEBREX provided pain relief within 60 minutes.

Familial Adenomatous Polyposis (FAP): CELEBREX was evaluated to reduce the number of adenomatous colorectal polyps. A randomized double-blind placebo-controlled study was conducted in 83 patients with FAP. The study population included 58 patients with a prior subtotal or total colectomy and 25 patients with an intact colon. Thirteen patients had the attenuated FAP phenotype.

One area in the rectum and up to four areas in the colon were identified at baseline for specific follow-up, and polyps were counted at baseline and following six months of treatment. The mean reduction in the number of colorectal polyps was 28% for CELEBREX 400 mg BID, 12% for CELEBREX 100 mg BID and 5% for placebo. The reduction in polyps observed with CELEBREX 400 mg BID was statistically superior to placebo at the six-month timepoint (p=0.003). (See Figure 1.)

Figure 1
Percent Change from Baseline in Number of Colorectal Polyps (FAP Patients)

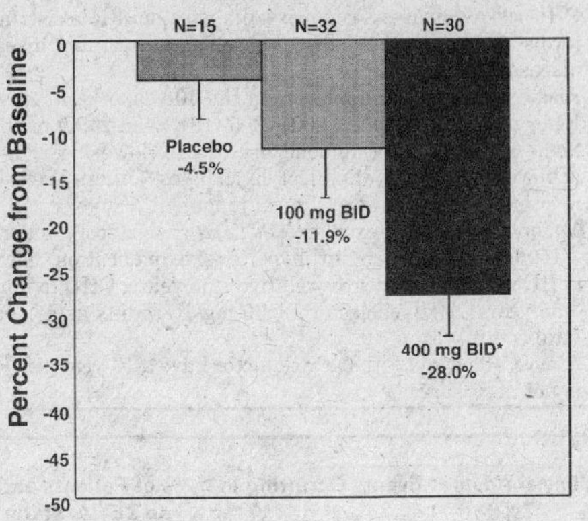

*p=0.003 versus placebo

Special Studies

Endoscopic Studies: Scheduled upper GI endoscopic evaluations were performed in over 4,500 arthritis patients who were enrolled in five controlled randomized 12-24 week trials using active comparators, two of which also included placebo controls. There was no consistent relationship between the incidence of gastroduodenal ulcers and the dose of CELEBREX over the range studied.

Table 2 summarizes the incidence of endoscopic ulcers in two 12-week studies that enrolled patients in whom baseline endoscopies revealed no ulcers.

Table 2
Incidence of Gastroduodenal Ulcers from Endoscopic Studies in OA and RA Patients

	3 Month Studies	
	Study 1 (n = 1108)	Study 2 (n = 1049)
Placebo	2.3% (5/217)	2.0% (4/200)
Celebrex 50 mg BID	3.4% (8/233)	—
Celebrex 100 mg BID	3.1% (7/227)	4.0% (9/223)
Celebrex 200 mg BID	5.9% (13/221)	2.7% (6/219)
Celebrex 400 mg BID	—	4.1% (8/197)
Naproxen 500 mg BID	16.2% (34/210)*	17.6% (37/210)*

*p≤0.05 vs all other treatments

Table 3 summarizes data from two 12-week studies that enrolled patients in whom baseline endoscopies revealed no ulcers. Patients underwent interval endoscopies every 4 weeks to give information on ulcer risk over time.

[See table 3 at top of next page]

One randomized and double-blind 6-month study in 430 RA patients was conducted in which an endoscopic examination was performed at 6 months. The incidence of endoscopic ulcers in patients taking CELEBREX 200 mg BID was 4% vs 15% for patients taking diclofenac SR 75 mg BID (p<0.001).

In 4 of the 5 endoscopic studies, approximately 11% of patients (440/4,000) were taking aspirin (≤325 mg/day). In the CELEBREX groups, the endoscopic ulcer rate appeared to be higher in aspirin users than in non-users. However, the increased rate of ulcers in these aspirin users was less than the endoscopic ulcer rates observed in the active comparator groups, with or without aspirin.

The correlation between findings of endoscopic studies, and the relative incidence of clinically significant serious upper GI events has not been established. Serious clinically significant upper GI bleeding has been observed in patients receiving CELEBREX in controlled and open-labeled trials, albeit infrequently (see *Use with Aspirin* and WARNINGS — Gastrointestinal (GI) Effects).

Use with Aspirin: The Celecoxib Long-Term Arthritis Safety Study (CLASS) was a prospective long-term safety outcome study conducted postmarketing in approximately 5,800 OA patients and 2,200 RA patients. Patients received CELEBREX 400 mg BID (4-fold and 2-fold the recommended OA and RA doses, respectively, and the approved dose for FAP), ibuprofen 800 mg TID or diclofenac 75 mg BID (common therapeutic doses). Median exposures for CELEBREX (n = 3,987) and diclofenac (n = 1,996) were 9 months while ibuprofen (n = 1,985) was 6 months. The Kaplan-Meier cumulative rates at 9 months are provided for all analyses. The primary endpoint of this outcome study was the incidence of *complicated ulcers* (gastrointestinal bleeding, perforation or obstruction). Patients were allowed to take concomitant low-dose (≤ 325 mg/day) aspirin (ASA) for cardiovascular prophylaxis (ASA subgroups: CELEBREX, n = 882; diclofenac, n = 445; ibuprofen, n = 412). Differences in the incidence of *complicated ulcers* between CELEBREX and the combined group of ibuprofen and diclofenac were not statistically significant. Those patients on CELEBREX and concomitant low-dose ASA experienced 4-fold higher rates of *complicated ulcers* compared to those not on ASA (see WARNINGS — Gastrointestinal (GI) Effects). The results for CELEBREX are displayed in Table 4. For *complicated and symptomatic ulcer* rates, see WARNINGS — Gastrointestinal (GI) Effects - Risk of GI Ulceration, Bleeding, and Perforation.

Table 4
Effects of Co-Administration of Low-Dose Aspirin on *Complicated Ulcer* Rates with CELEBREX 400 mg BID (Kaplan-Meier Rates at 9 months [%])

	Non-Aspirin Users n=3105	Aspirin Users n=882
Complicated Ulcers	0.32	1.12

Platelets: In clinical trials, CELEBREX at single doses up to 800 mg and multiple doses of 600 mg BID for up to 7 days duration (higher than recommended therapeutic doses) had no effect on platelet aggregation and bleeding time. Comparators (naproxen 500 mg BID, ibuprofen 800 mg TID, diclofenac 75 mg BID) significantly reduced platelet aggregation and prolonged bleeding time.

Because of its lack of platelet effects, CELEBREX is not a substitute for aspirin for cardiovascular prophylaxis.

INDICATIONS AND USAGE

CELEBREX is indicated:

1) For relief of the signs and symptoms of osteoarthritis.
2) For relief of the signs and symptoms of rheumatoid arthritis in adults.
3) For the management of acute pain in adults (see CLINICAL STUDIES).
4) For the treatment of primary dysmenorrhea.
5) To reduce the number of adenomatous colorectal polyps in familial adenomatous polyposis (FAP), as an adjunct to usual care (e.g., endoscopic surveillance, surgery). It is not known whether there is a clinical benefit from a reduction in the number of colorectal polyps in FAP patients. It is also not known whether the effects of CELEBREX treatment will persist after CELEBREX is discontinued. The efficacy and safety of CELEBREX treatment in patients with FAP beyond six months have not been studied (see CLINICAL STUDIES, WARNINGS and PRECAUTIONS sections).

CONTRAINDICATIONS

CELEBREX is contraindicated in patients with known hypersensitivity to celecoxib.

CELEBREX should not be given to patients who have demonstrated allergic-type reactions to sulfonamides.

CELEBREX should not be given to patients who have experienced asthma, urticaria, or allergic-type reactions after taking aspirin or other NSAIDs. Severe, rarely fatal, anaphylactic-like reactions to NSAIDs have been reported in such patients (see WARNINGS — Anaphylactoid Reactions, and PRECAUTIONS — Preexisting Asthma).

WARNINGS

Gastrointestinal (GI) Effects—Risk of GI Ulceration, Bleeding, and Perforation

Serious gastrointestinal toxicity such as bleeding, ulceration, and perforation of the stomach, small intestine or large intestine, can occur at any time, with or without warning symptoms, in patients treated with nonsteroidal anti-inflammatory drugs (NSAIDs). Minor upper gastrointestinal problems, such as dyspepsia, are common and may also occur at any time during NSAID therapy. Therefore, physicians and patients should remain alert for ulceration and bleeding, even in the absence of previous GI tract symptoms (see PRECAUTIONS - Hematological Effects). Patients should be informed about the signs and/or symptoms of serious GI toxicity and the steps to take if they occur. The utility of periodic laboratory monitoring has not been demonstrated, nor has it been adequately assessed. Only one in five patients who develop a serious upper GI adverse event on NSAID therapy is symptomatic. It has been demonstrated that upper GI ulcers, gross bleeding or perforation, caused by NSAIDs, appear to occur in approximately 1% of patients treated for 3–6 months, and in about 2–4% of patients treated for one year. These trends continue thus, increasing the likelihood of developing a serious GI event at some time during the course of therapy. However, even short-term therapy is not without risk.

NSAIDs should be prescribed with extreme caution in patients with a prior history of ulcer disease or gastrointestinal bleeding. Most spontaneous reports of fatal GI events are in elderly or debilitated patients and therefore special care should be taken in treating this population. **To minimize the potential risk for an adverse GI event, the lowest effective dose should be used for the shortest possible duration.** For high risk patients, alternate therapies that do not involve NSAIDs should be considered.

Studies have shown that patients with a *prior history of peptic ulcer disease and/or gastrointestinal bleeding* and who use NSAIDs, have a greater than 10-fold higher risk for developing a GI bleed than patients with neither of these risk factors. In addition to a past history of ulcer disease, pharmacoepidemiological studies have identified several other co-therapies or co-morbid conditions that may increase the risk for GI bleeding such as: treatment with oral corticosteroids, treatment with anticoagulants, longer duration of NSAID therapy, smoking, alcoholism, older age, and poor general health status.

Table 3
Incidence of Gastroduodenal Ulcers from 3-Month Serial Endoscopy Studies in OA and RA Patients

	Week 4	Week 8	Week 12	Final
Study 3 (n=523)				
Celebrex 200 mg BID	4.0% (10/252)*	2.2% (5/227)*	1.5% (3/196)*	7.5% (20/266)*
Naproxen 500 mg BID	19.0% (47/247)	14.2% (26/182)	9.9% (14/141)	34.6% (89/257)
Study 4 (n=1062)				
Celebrex **200 mg BID**	3.9% (13/337)†	2.4% (7/296)†	1.8% (5/274)†	7.0% (25/356)†
Diclofenac 75 mg BID	5.1% (18/350)	3.3% (10/306)	2.9% (8/278)	9.7% (36/372)
Ibuprofen 800 mg TID	13.0% (42/323)	6.2% (15/241)	9.6% (21/219)	23.3% (78/334)

*p ≤0.05 Celebrex vs. naproxen based on interval and cumulative analyses
†p ≤0.05 Celebrex vs. ibuprofen based on interval and cumulative analyses

CLASS Study: The estimated cumulative rates at 9 months of *complicated and symptomatic ulcers* (an adverse event similar but not identical to the "upper GI ulcers, gross bleeding or perforation" described in the preceding paragraphs) for patients treated with CELEBREX 400 mg BID (see Special Studies – *Use with Aspirin*) are described in Table 5. Table 5 also displays results for patients less than or greater than or equal to the age of 65 years. The differences in rates between CELEBREX alone and CELEBREX with ASA groups may be due to the higher risk for GI events in ASA users.

Table 5
***Complicated and Symptomatic Ulcer* Rates in Patients Taking CELEBREX 400 mg BID (Kaplan-Meier Rates at 9 months [%]) Based on Risk Factors**

	Complicated and Symptomatic Ulcer Rates
All Patients	
Celebrex alone (n=3105)	0.78
Celebrex with ASA (n=882)	2.19
Patients <65 Years	
Celebrex alone (n=2025)	0.47
Celebrex with ASA (n=403)	1.26
Patients ≥65 Years	
Celebrex alone (n=1080)	1.40
Celebrex with ASA (n=479)	3.06

In a small number of patients with a history of ulcer disease, the *complicated and symptomatic ulcer* rates in patients taking CELEBREX alone or CELEBREX with ASA were, respectively, 2.56% (n=243) and 6.85% (n=91) at 48 weeks. These results are to be expected in patients with a prior history of ulcer disease (see WARNINGS – Gastrointestinal (GI) Effects – Risk of GI Ulceration, Bleeding, and Perforation).

Anaphylactoid Reactions

As with NSAIDs in general, anaphylactoid reactions have occurred in patients without known prior exposure to CELEBREX. In post-marketing experience, rare cases of anaphylactic reactions and angioedema have been reported in patients receiving CELEBREX. CELEBREX should not be given to patients with the aspirin triad. This symptom complex typically occurs in asthmatic patients who experience rhinitis with or without nasal polyps, or who exhibit severe, potentially fatal bronchospasm after taking aspirin or other NSAIDs (see CONTRAINDICATIONS and PRECAUTIONS — Preexisting Asthma). Emergency help should be sought in cases where an anaphylactoid reaction occurs.

Advanced Renal Disease

No information is available from controlled clinical studies regarding the use of CELEBREX in patients with advanced kidney disease. Therefore, treatment with CELEBREX is not recommended in these patients with advanced kidney disease. If CELEBREX therapy must be initiated, close monitoring of the patient's kidney function is advisable (see PRECAUTIONS — Renal Effects).

Pregnancy

In late pregnancy CELEBREX should be avoided because it may cause premature closure of the ductus arteriosus (see PRECAUTIONS – Pregnancy).

Familial Adenomatous Polyposis (FAP): Treatment with CELEBREX in FAP has not been shown to reduce the risk of gastrointestinal cancer or the need for prophylactic colectomy or other FAP-related surgeries. Therefore, the usual care of FAP patients should not be altered because of the concurrent administration of CELEBREX. In particular, the frequency of routine endoscopic surveillance should not be decreased and prophylactic colectomy or other FAP-related surgeries should not be delayed.

PRECAUTIONS

General: CELEBREX cannot be expected to substitute for corticosteroids or to treat corticosteroid insufficiency. Abrupt discontinuation of corticosteroids may lead to exacerbation of corticosteroid-responsive illness. Patients on prolonged corticosteroid therapy should have their therapy tapered slowly if a decision is made to discontinue corticosteroids.

The pharmacological activity of CELEBREX in reducing inflammation, and possibly fever, may diminish the utility of these diagnostic signs in detecting infectious complications of presumed noninfectious, painful conditions.

Hepatic Effects: Borderline elevations of one or more liver associated enzymes may occur in up to 15% of patients taking NSAIDs, and notable elevations of ALT or AST (approximately 3 or more times the upper limit of normal) have been reported in approximately 1% of patients in clinical trials with NSAIDs. These laboratory abnormalities may progress, may remain unchanged, or may be transient with continuing therapy. Rare cases of severe hepatic reactions, including jaundice and fatal fulminant hepatitis, liver necrosis and hepatic failure (some with fatal outcome) have been reported with NSAIDs, including CELEBREX (see ADVERSE REACTIONS – post-marketing experience). In controlled clinical trials of CELEBREX, the incidence of borderline elevations (greater than or equal to 1.2 times and less than 3 times the upper limit of normal) of liver associated enzymes was 6% for CELEBREX and 5% for placebo, and approximately 0.2% of patients taking CELEBREX and 0.3% of patients taking placebo had notable elevations of ALT and AST.

A patient with symptoms and/or signs suggesting liver dysfunction, or in whom an abnormal liver test has occurred, should be monitored carefully for evidence of the development of a more severe hepatic reaction while on therapy with CELEBREX. If clinical signs and symptoms consistent with liver disease develop, or if systemic manifestations occur (e.g., eosinophilia, rash, etc.), CELEBREX should be discontinued.

Renal Effects: Long-term administration of NSAIDs has resulted in renal papillary necrosis and other renal injury. Renal toxicity has also been seen in patients in whom renal prostaglandins have a compensatory role in the maintenance of renal perfusion. In these patients, administration of a nonsteroidal anti-inflammatory drug may cause a dose-dependent reduction in prostaglandin formation and, secondarily, in renal blood flow, which may precipitate overt renal decompensation. Patients at greatest risk of this reaction are those with impaired renal function, heart failure, liver dysfunction, those taking diuretics and ACE inhibitors, and the elderly. Discontinuation of NSAID therapy is usually followed by recovery to the pretreatment state. Clinical trials with CELEBREX have shown renal effects similar to those observed with comparator NSAIDs.

Caution should be used when initiating treatment with CELEBREX in patients with considerable dehydration. It is advisable to rehydrate patients first and then start therapy with CELEBREX. Caution is also recommended in patients with preexisting kidney disease (see WARNINGS—Advanced Renal Disease).

Hematological Effects: Anemia is sometimes seen in patients receiving CELEBREX. In controlled clinical trials the incidence of anemia was 0.6% with CELEBREX and 0.4% with placebo. Patients on long-term treatment with CELEBREX should have their hemoglobin or hematocrit checked if they exhibit any signs or symptoms of anemia or blood loss. CELEBREX does not generally affect platelet counts, prothrombin time (PT), or partial thromboplastin time (PTT), and does not inhibit platelet aggregation at indicated dosages (see CLINICAL STUDIES—Special Studies—Platelets).

Fluid Retention, Edema, and Hypertension: Fluid retention and edema have been observed in some patients taking CELEBREX (see ADVERSE REACTIONS). In the CLASS study (see Special Studies – *Use with Aspirin*), the Kaplan-Meier cumulative rates at 9 months of peripheral edema in patients on CELEBREX 400 mg BID (4-fold and 2-fold the recommended OA and RA doses, respectively, and the approved dose for FAP), ibuprofen 800 mg TID and diclofenac 75 mg BID were 4.5%, 6.9% and 4.7%, respectively. The rates of hypertension in the CELEBREX, ibuprofen and diclofenac

Continued on next page

Celebrex—Cont.

treated patients were 2.4%, 4.2% and 2.5%, respectively. As with other NSAIDs, CELEBREX should be used with caution in patients with fluid retention, hypertension, or heart failure.

Preexisting Asthma: Patients with asthma may have aspirin-sensitive asthma. The use of aspirin in patients with aspirin-sensitive asthma has been associated with severe bronchospasm which can be fatal. Since cross reactivity, including bronchospasm, between aspirin and other nonsteroidal anti-inflammatory drugs has been reported in such aspirin-sensitive patients, CELEBREX should not be administered to patients with this form of aspirin sensitivity and should be used with caution in patients with preexisting asthma.

Information for Patients: CELEBREX can cause discomfort and, rarely, more serious side effects, such as gastrointestinal bleeding, which may result in hospitalization and even fatal outcomes. Although serious GI tract ulcerations and bleeding can occur without warning symptoms, patients should be alert for the signs and symptoms of ulcerations and bleeding, and should ask for medical advice when observing any indicative signs or symptoms. Patients should be apprised of the importance of this follow-up (see WARNINGS — Gastrointestinal (GI) Effects – Risk of Gastrointestinal Ulceration, Bleeding, and Perforation).

Patients should promptly report signs or symptoms of gastrointestinal ulceration or bleeding, skin rash, unexplained weight gain, or edema to their physicians.

Patients should be informed of the warning signs and symptoms of hepatotoxicity (e.g., nausea, fatigue, lethargy, pruritus, jaundice, right upper quadrant tenderness, and "flu-like" symptoms). If these occur, patients should be instructed to stop therapy and seek immediate medical therapy.

Patients should also be instructed to seek immediate emergency help in the case of an anaphylactoid reaction (see WARNINGS).

In late pregnancy CELEBREX should be avoided because it may cause premature closure of the ductus arteriosus.

Patients with familial adenomatous polyposis (FAP) should be informed that CELEBREX has not been shown to reduce colorectal, duodenal or other FAP-related cancers, or the need for endoscopic surveillance, prophylactic or other FAP-related surgery. Therefore, all patients with FAP should be instructed to continue their usual care while receiving CELEBREX.

Laboratory Tests: Because serious GI tract ulcerations and bleeding can occur without warning symptoms, physicians should monitor for signs or symptoms of GI bleeding. In controlled clinical trials, elevated BUN occurred more frequently in patients receiving CELEBREX compared with patients on placebo. This laboratory abnormality was also seen in patients who received comparator NSAIDs in these studies. The clinical significance of this abnormality has not been established.

Drug Interactions

General: Celecoxib metabolism is predominantly mediated via cytochrome P450 2C9 in the liver. Co-administration of celecoxib with drugs that are known to inhibit 2C9 should be done with caution.

In vitro studies indicate that celecoxib, although not a substrate, is an inhibitor of cytochrome P450 2D6. Therefore, there is a potential for an *in vivo* drug interaction with drugs that are metabolized by P450 2D6.

ACE-inhibitors: Reports suggest that NSAIDs may diminish the antihypertensive effect of Angiotensin Converting Enzyme (ACE) inhibitors. This interaction should be given consideration in patients taking CELEBREX concomitantly with ACE-inhibitors.

Furosemide: Clinical studies, as well as post marketing observations, have shown that NSAIDs can reduce the natriuretic effect of furosemide and thiazides in some patients. This response has been attributed to inhibition of renal prostaglandin synthesis.

Aspirin: CELEBREX can be used with low-dose aspirin. However, concomitant administration of aspirin with CELEBREX increases the rate of GI ulceration or other complications, compared to use of CELEBREX alone (see CLINICAL STUDIES — Special Studies — *Use with Aspirin* and WARNINGS – Gastrointestinal (GI) Effects – Risk of GI Ulceration, Bleeding, and Perforation – CLASS Study).

Because of its lack of platelet effects, CELEBREX is not a substitute for aspirin for cardiovascular prophylaxis.

Fluconazole: Concomitant administration of fluconazole at 200 mg QD resulted in a two-fold increase in celecoxib plasma concentration. This increase is due to the inhibition of celecoxib metabolism via P450 2C9 by fluconazole (see Pharmacokinetics — Metabolism). CELEBREX should be introduced at the lowest recommended dose in patients receiving fluconazole.

Lithium: In a study conducted in healthy subjects, mean steady-state lithium plasma levels increased approximately 17% in subjects receiving lithium 450 mg BID with CELEBREX 200 mg BID as compared to subjects receiving lithium alone. Patients on lithium treatment should be closely monitored when CELEBREX is introduced or withdrawn.

Methotrexate: In an interaction study of rheumatoid arthritis patients taking methotrexate, CELEBREX did not have a significant effect on the pharmacokinetics of methotrexate.

Warfarin: Anticoagulant activity should be monitored, particularly in the first few days, after initiating or changing CELEBREX therapy in patients receiving warfarin or similar agents, since these patients are at an increased risk of bleeding complications. The effect of celecoxib on the anticoagulant effect of warfarin was studied in a group of healthy subjects receiving daily doses of 2-5 mg of warfarin. In these subjects, celecoxib did not alter the anticoagulant effect of warfarin as determined by prothrombin time. However, in post-marketing experience, serious bleeding events, some of which were fatal, have been reported, predominantly in the elderly, in association with increases in prothrombin time in patients receiving CELEBREX concurrently with warfarin.

Table 6
Adverse Events Occurring in ≥2% of CELEBREX Patients From CELEBREX Premarketing Controlled Arthritis Trials

	CELEBREX (100-200 mg BID or 200 mg QD) (n=4146)	Placebo (n=1864)	Naproxen 500 mg BID (n=1366)	Diclofenac 75 mg BID (n=387)	Ibuprofen 800 mg TID (n=345)
Gastrointestinal					
Abdominal pain	4.1%	2.8%	7.7%	9.0%	9.0%
Diarrhea	5.6%	3.8%	5.3%	9.3%	5.8%
Dyspepsia	8.8%	6.2%	12.2%	10.9%	12.8%
Flatulence	2.2%	1.0%	3.6%	4.1%	3.5%
Nausea	3.5%	4.2%	6.0%	3.4%	6.7%
Body as a whole					
Back pain	2.8%	3.6%	2.2%	2.6%	0.9%
Peripheral edema	2.1%	1.1%	2.1%	1.0%	3.5%
Injury-accidental	2.9%	2.3%	3.0%	2.6%	3.2%
Central and peripheral nervous system					
Dizziness	2.0%	1.7%	2.6%	1.3%	2.3%
Headache	15.8%	20.2%	14.5%	15.5%	15.4%
Psychiatric					
Insomnia	2.3%	2.3%	2.9%	1.3%	1.4%
Respiratory					
Pharyngitis	2.3%	1.1%	1.7%	1.6%	2.6%
Rhinitis	2.0%	1.3%	2.4%	2.3%	0.6%
Sinusitis	5.0%	4.3%	4.0%	5.4%	5.8%
Upper respiratory tract infection	8.1%	6.7%	9.9%	9.8%	9.9%
Skin					
Rash	2.2%	2.1%	2.1%	1.3%	1.2%

Carcinogenesis, mutagenesis, impairment of fertility: Celecoxib was not carcinogenic in rats given oral doses up to 200 mg/kg for males and 10 mg/kg for females (approximately 2- to 4-fold the human exposure as measured by the AUC_{0-24} at 200 mg BID) or in mice given oral doses up to 25 mg/kg for males and 50 mg/kg for females (approximately equal to human exposure as measured by the AUC_{0-24} at 200 mg BID) for two years.

Celecoxib was not mutagenic in an Ames test and a mutation assay in Chinese hamster ovary (CHO) cells, nor clastogenic in a chromosome aberration assay in CHO cells and an *in vivo* micronucleus test in rat bone marrow.

Celecoxib did not impair male and female fertility in rats at oral doses up to 600 mg/kg/day (approximately 11-fold human exposure at 200 mg BID based on the AUC_{0-24}).

Pregnancy

Teratogenic effects: Pregnancy Category C. Celecoxib at oral doses ≥150 mg/kg/day (approximately 2-fold human exposure at 200 mg BID as measured by AUC_{0-24}), caused an increased incidence of ventricular septal defects, a rare event, and fetal alterations, such as ribs fused, sternebrae fused and sternebrae misshapen when rabbits were treated throughout organogenesis. A dose-dependent increase in diaphragmatic hernias was observed when rats were given celecoxib at oral doses ≥30 mg/kg/day (approximately 6-fold human exposure based on the AUC_{0-24} at 200 mg BID) throughout organogenesis. There are no studies in pregnant women. CELEBREX should be used during pregnancy only if the potential benefit justifies the potential risk to the fetus.

Nonteratogenic effects: Celecoxib produced pre-implantation and post-implantation losses and reduced embryo/fetal survival in rats at oral dosages ≥50 mg/kg/day (approximately 6-fold human exposure based on the AUC_{0-24} at 200 mg BID). These changes are expected with inhibition of prostaglandin synthesis and are not the result of permanent alteration of female reproductive function, nor are they expected at clinical exposures. No studies have been conducted to evaluate the effect of celecoxib on the closure of the ductus arteriosus in humans. Therefore, use of CELEBREX during the third trimester of pregnancy should be avoided.

Labor and delivery: Celecoxib produced no evidence of delayed labor or parturition at oral doses up to 100 mg/kg in rats (approximately 7-fold human exposure as measured by the AUC_{0-24} at 200 mg BID). The effects of CELEBREX on labor and delivery in pregnant women are unknown.

Nursing mothers: Celecoxib is excreted in the milk of lactating rats at concentrations similar to those in plasma. Limited data from one subject indicate that celecoxib is also excreted in human milk. Because many drugs are excreted in human milk and because of the potential for serious adverse reactions in nursing infants from CELEBREX, a decision should be made whether to discontinue nursing or to discontinue the drug, taking into account the importance of the drug to the mother.

Pediatric Use

Safety and effectiveness in pediatric patients below the age of 18 years have not been evaluated.

Geriatric Use

Of the total number of patients who received CELEBREX in clinical trials, more than 3,300 were 65-74 years of age, while approximately 1,300 additional patients were 75 years and over. No substantial differences in effectiveness were observed between these subjects and younger subjects. In clinical studies comparing renal function as measured by the GFR, BUN and creatinine, and platelet function as measured by bleeding time and platelet aggregation, the results were not different between elderly and young volunteers. However, as with other NSAIDs, including those that selectively inhibit COX-2, there have been more spontaneous post-marketing reports of fatal GI events and acute renal failure in the elderly than in younger patients (see WARNINGS – Gastrointestinal (GI) Effects – Risk of GI Ulceration, Bleeding, and Perforation).

ADVERSE REACTIONS

Of the CELEBREX treated patients in the premarketing controlled clinical trials, approximately 4,250 were patients with OA, approximately 2,100 were patients with RA, and approximately 1,050 were patients with post-surgical pain. More than 8,500 patients have received a total daily dose of CELEBREX of 200 mg (100 mg BID or 200 mg QD) or more, including more than 400 treated at 800 mg (400 mg BID). Approximately 3,900 patients have received CELEBREX at these doses for 6 months or more; approximately 2,300 of these have received it for 1 year or more and 124 of these have received it for 2 years or more.

Adverse events from CELEBREX premarketing controlled arthritis trials: Table 6 lists all adverse events, regardless of causality, occurring in ≥2% of patients receiving CELEBREX from 12 controlled studies conducted in patients with OA or RA that included a placebo and/or a positive control group.

[See table 6 above]

In placebo- or active-controlled clinical trials, the discontinuation rate due to adverse events was 7.1% for patients receiving CELEBREX and 6.1% for patients receiving placebo. Among the most common reasons for discontinuation due to adverse events in the CELEBREX treatment groups were dyspepsia and abdominal pain (cited as reasons for discontinuation in 0.8% and 0.7% of CELEBREX patients, respectively). Among patients receiving placebo, 0.6% discontinued due to dyspepsia and 0.6% withdrew due to abdominal pain.

The following adverse events occurred in 0.1 - 1.9% of patients regardless of causality.

[See first table at bottom of next page]

Other serious adverse reactions which occur rarely (estimated <0.1%), regardless of causality: The following serious adverse events have occurred rarely in patients taking CELEBREX. Cases reported only in the post-marketing experience are indicated in italics.

[See second table at bottom of next page]

Safety Data from CLASS Study:

Hematological Events:

During this study (see Special Studies – *Use with Aspirin*), the incidence of clinically significant decreases in hemoglobin (>2 g/dL) confirmed by repeat testing was lower in patients on CELEBREX 400 mg BID (4-fold and 2-fold the recommended OA and RA doses, respectively, and the approved dose for FAP) compared to patients on either diclofenac 75 mg BID or ibuprofen 800 mg TID: 0.5%, 1.3% and 1.9%, respectively. The lower incidence of events with CELEBREX was maintained with or without ASA use (see CLINICAL STUDIES – Special Studies – Platelets).

Withdrawals/Serious Adverse Events:

Kaplan-Meier cumulative rates at 9 months for withdrawals due to adverse events for CELEBREX, diclofenac and ibuprofen were 24%, 29%, and 26%, respectively. Rates for serious adverse events (i.e. those causing hospitalization or felt to be life threatening or otherwise medically significant) regardless of causality were not different across treatment groups, respectively, 8%, 7%, and 8%.

Based on Kaplan-Meier cumulative rates for investigator-reported serious cardiovascular thromboembolic adverse events*, there were no differences between the CELEBREX, diclofenac, or ibuprofen treatment groups. The rates in all patients at 9 months for CELEBREX, diclofenac, and ibuprofen were 1.2%, 1.4%, and 1.1%, respectively. The rates for non-

ASA users in each of the three treatment groups were less than 1%. The rates for myocardial infarction in each of the three non-ASA treatment groups were less than 0.2%.

---

*includes myocardial infarction, pulmonary embolism, deep venous thrombosis, unstable angina, transient ischemic attacks or ischemic cerebrovascular accidents.

Adverse events from analgesia and dysmenorrhea studies: Approximately 1,700 patients were treated with Celebrex in analgesia and dysmenorrhea studies. All patients in post-oral surgery pain studies received a single dose of study medication. Doses up to 600 mg/day of Celebrex were studied in primary dysmenorrhea and post-orthopedic surgery pain studies. The types of adverse events in the analgesia and dysmenorrhea studies were similar to those reported in arthritis studies. The only additional adverse event reported was post-dental extraction alveolar osteitis (dry socket) in the post-oral surgery pain studies.

Adverse events from the controlled trial in familial adenomatous polyposis: The adverse event profile reported for the 83 patients with familial adenomatous polyposis enrolled in the randomized, controlled clinical trial was similar to that reported for patients in the arthritis controlled trials. Intestinal anastomotic ulceration was the only new adverse event reported in the FAP trial, regardless of causality, and was observed in 3 of 58 patients (one at 100 mg BID, and two at 400 mg BID) who had prior intestinal surgery.

OVERDOSAGE

No overdoses of Celebrex were reported during clinical trials. Doses up to 2400 mg/day for up to 10 days in 12 patients did not result in serious toxicity. Symptoms following acute NSAID overdoses are usually limited to lethargy, drowsiness, nausea, vomiting, and epigastric pain, which are generally reversible with supportive care. Gastrointestinal bleeding can occur. Hypertension, acute renal failure, respiratory depression and coma may occur, but are rare. Anaphylactoid reactions have been reported with therapeutic ingestion of NSAIDs, and may occur following an overdose. Patients should be managed by symptomatic and supportive care following an NSAID overdose. There are no specific antidotes. No information is available regarding the removal of celecoxib by hemodialysis, but based on its high degree of plasma protein binding (>97%) dialysis is unlikely to be useful in overdose. Emesis and/or activated charcoal (60 to 100 g in adults, 1 to 2 g/kg in children) and/or osmotic cathartic may be indicated in patients seen within 4 hours of ingestion with symptoms or following a large overdose. Forced diuresis, alkalinization of urine, hemodialysis, or hemoperfusion may not be useful due to high protein binding.

DOSAGE AND ADMINISTRATION

For osteoarthritis and rheumatoid arthritis, the lowest dose of Celebrex should be sought for each patient. These doses can be given without regard to timing of meals.

Osteoarthritis: For relief of the signs and symptoms of osteoarthritis the recommended oral dose is 200 mg per day administered as a single dose or as 100 mg twice per day.

Rheumatoid arthritis: For relief of the signs and symptoms of rheumatoid arthritis the recommended oral dose is 100 to 200 mg twice per day.

Management of Acute Pain and Treatment of Primary Dysmenorrhea: The recommended dose of Celebrex is 400 mg initially, followed by an additional 200 mg dose if needed on the first day. On subsequent days, the recommended dose is 200 mg twice daily as needed.

Familial adenomatous polyposis (FAP): Usual medical care for FAP patients should be continued while on Celebrex. To reduce the number of adenomatous colorectal polyps in patients with FAP, the recommended oral dose is 400 mg twice per day to be taken with food.

Special Populations

Hepatic insufficiency: The daily recommended dose of Celebrex capsules in patients with moderate hepatic impairment (Child-Pugh Class B) should be reduced by approximately 50% (see CLINICAL PHARMACOLOGY – Special Populations).

HOW SUPPLIED

Celebrex 100-mg capsules are white, reverse printed white on blue band of body and cap with markings of 7767 on the cap and 100 on the body, supplied as:

NDC Number	Size
0025-1520-31	bottle of 100
0025-1520-51	bottle of 500
0025-1520-34	carton of 100 unit dose

Celebrex 200-mg capsules are white, with reverse printed white on gold band with markings of 7767 on the cap and 200 on the body, supplied as:

NDC Number	Size
0025-1525-31	bottle of 100
0025-1525-51	bottle of 500
0025-1525-34	carton of 100 unit dose

Celebrex 400-mg capsules are white, with reverse printed white on green band with markings of 7767 on the cap and 400 on the body, supplied as:

NDC Number	Size
0025-1530-02	bottle of 60
0025-1530-01	carton of 100 unit dose

Store at 25°C (77°F); excursions permitted to 15-30°C (59-86°F) [see USP Controlled Room Temperature].

Rx only Revised: February 2005

Distributed by
Pfizer
G.D. Searle LLC
Division of Pfizer Inc, NY, NY 10017
CELEBREX ®
celecoxib capsules
LAB-0036-7.0

COVERA-HS® ℞

[cō-vər′ ə]
(verapamil hydrochloride)
Extended-Release Tablets
Controlled-Onset

Prescribing information for this product, which appears on pages 3099–3102 of the 2005 PDR, has been completely revised as follows. Please write "See Supplement A" next to the product heading.

DESCRIPTION

Covera-HS (verapamil hydrochloride) is a calcium ion influx inhibitor (slow-channel blocker or calcium ion antagonist). Covera-HS is available for oral administration as pale yellow, round, film-coated tablets containing 240 mg of verapamil hydrochloride and as lavender, round, film-coated tablets containing 180 mg of verapamil hydrochloride. Verapamil is administered as a racemic mixture of the R and S enantiomers. The structural formulae of the verapamil HCl enantiomers are:

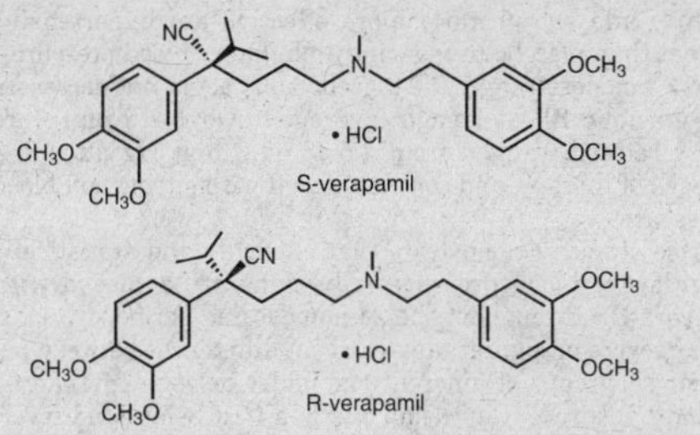

$C_{27}H_{38}N_2O_4 \cdot HCl$ M.W. = 491.07

Benzeneacetonitrile, (±)-α-[3[[2-(3,4-dimethoxyphenyl) ethyl]methylamino]propyl]-3,4-dimethoxy-α-(1-methylethyl) hydrochloride

Verapamil HCl is an almost white, crystalline powder, practically free of odor, with a bitter taste. It is soluble in water, chloroform, and methanol. Verapamil HCl is not chemically related to other cardioactive drugs.

Inactive ingredients are black ferric oxide, BHT, cellulose acetate, hydroxyethyl cellulose, hydroxypropyl cellulose, hypromellose, magnesium stearate, polyethylene glycol, polyethylene oxide, polysorbate 80, povidone, sodium chloride, titanium dioxide, and coloring agents: 240-mg—FD&C Blue No. 2 Lake and D&C Yellow No. 10 Lake; 180-mg—FD&C Blue No. 2 Lake and D&C Red No. 30 Lake.

System components and performance: The Covera-HS formulation has been designed to initiate the release of verapamil 4–5 hours after ingestion. This delay is introduced by a layer between the active drug core and outer semipermeable membrane. As water from the gastrointestinal tract enters the tablet, this delay coating is solubilized and released. As tablet hydration continues, the osmotic layer expands and pushes against the drug layer, releasing drug through precision laser-drilled orifices in the outer membrane at a constant rate. This controlled rate of drug delivery in the gastrointestinal lumen is independent of posture, pH, gastrointestinal motility, and fed or fasting conditions.

The biologically inert components of the delivery system remain intact during GI transit and are eliminated in the feces as an insoluble shell.

CLINICAL PHARMACOLOGY

Covera-HS has a unique delivery system, designed for bedtime dosing, incorporating a 4 to 5-hour delay in drug delivery. The unique controlled-onset, extended-release (COER) delivery system, which is designed for bedtime dosing, results in a maximum plasma concentration (C_{max}) of verapamil in the morning hours.

Verapamil is a calcium ion influx inhibitor (L-type calcium channel blocker or calcium channel antagonist). Verapamil exerts its pharmacologic effects by selectively inhibiting the transmembrane influx of ionic calcium into arterial smooth muscle as well as in conductile and contractile myocardial cells without altering serum calcium concentrations.

Mechanism of action

In vitro: Verapamil binding is voltage-dependent with affinity increasing as the vascular smooth muscle membrane potential is reduced. In addition, verapamil binding is frequency dependent and apparent affinity increases with increased frequency of depolarizing stimulus.

The L-type calcium channel is an oligomeric structure consisting of five putative subunits designated alpha-1, alpha-2, beta, tau, and epsilon. Biochemical evidence points to separate binding sites for 1,4-dihydropyridines, phenylalkylamines, and the benzothiazepines (all located on the alpha-1 subunit). Although they share a similar mechanism

Continued on next page

Celebrex (100 - 200 mg BID or 200 mg QD)	
Gastrointestinal:	Constipation, diverticulitis, dysphagia, eructation, esophagitis, gastritis, gastroenteritis, gastroesophageal reflux, hemorrhoids, hiatal hernia, melena, dry mouth, stomatitis, tenesmus, tooth disorder, vomiting
Cardiovascular:	Aggravated hypertension, angina pectoris, coronary artery disorder, myocardial infarction
General:	Allergy aggravated, allergic reaction, asthenia, chest pain, cyst NOS, edema generalized, face edema, fatigue, fever, hot flushes, influenza-like symptoms, pain, peripheral pain
Resistance mechanism disorders:	Herpes simplex, herpes zoster, infection bacterial, infection fungal, infection soft tissue, infection viral, moniliasis, moniliasis genital, otitis media
Central, peripheral nervous system:	Leg cramps, hypertonia, hypoesthesia, migraine, neuralgia, neuropathy, paresthesia, vertigo
Female reproductive:	Breast fibroadenosis, breast neoplasm, breast pain, dysmenorrhea, menstrual disorder, vaginal hemorrhage, vaginitis
Male reproductive:	Prostatic disorder
Hearing and vestibular:	Deafness, ear abnormality, earache, tinnitus
Heart rate and rhythm:	Palpitation, tachycardia
Liver and biliary system:	Hepatic function abnormal, SGOT increased, SGPT increased
Metabolic and nutritional:	BUN increased, CPK increased, diabetes mellitus, hypercholesterolemia, hyperglycemia, hypokalemia, NPN increase, creatinine increased, alkaline phosphatase increased, weight increase
Musculoskeletal:	Arthralgia, arthrosis, bone disorder, fracture accidental, myalgia, neck stiffness, synovitis, tendinitis
Platelets (bleeding or clotting):	Ecchymosis, epistaxis, thrombocythemia
Psychiatric:	Anorexia, anxiety, appetite increased, depression, nervousness, somnolence
Hemic:	Anemia
Respiratory:	Bronchitis, bronchospasm, bronchospasm aggravated, coughing, dyspnea, laryngitis, pneumonia
Skin and appendages:	Alopecia, dermatitis, nail disorder, photosensitivity reaction, pruritus, rash erythematous, rash maculopapular, skin disorder, skin dry, sweating increased, urticaria
Application site disorders:	Cellulitis, dermatitis contact, injection site reaction, skin nodule
Special senses:	Taste perversion
Urinary system:	Albuminuria, cystitis, dysuria, hematuria, micturition frequency, renal calculus, urinary incontinence, urinary tract infection
Vision:	Blurred vision, cataract, conjunctivitis, eye pain, glaucoma

Cardiovascular:	Syncope, congestive heart failure, ventricular fibrillation, pulmonary embolism, cerebrovascular accident, peripheral gangrene, thrombophlebitis, *vasculitis*
Gastrointestinal:	Intestinal obstruction, intestinal perforation, gastrointestinal bleeding, colitis with bleeding, esophageal perforation, pancreatitis, ileus
Liver and biliary system:	Cholelithiasis, *hepatitis, jaundice, liver failure*
Hemic and lymphatic:	Thrombocytopenia, *agranulocytosis, aplastic anemia, pancytopenia, leukopenia*
Metabolic:	*Hypoglycemia, hyponatremia*
Nervous system:	*Aseptic meningitis,* ataxia, suicide, *ageusia, anosmia, fatal intracranial hemorrhage* (see PRECAUTIONS – Drug Interactions – *Warfarin*)
Renal:	Acute renal failure, *interstitial nephritis*
Skin:	*Erythema multiforme, exfoliative dermatitis, Stevens-Johnson syndrome, toxic epidermal necrolysis*
General:	Sepsis, sudden death, *anaphylactoid reaction, angioedema*

Covera-HS—Cont.

of action, calcium channel blockers represent three heterogeneous categories of drugs with differing vascular-cardiac selectivity ratios.

Essential hypertension: Verapamil produces its antihypertensive effect by a combination of vascular and cardiac effects. It acts as a vasodilator with selectivity for the arterial portion of the peripheral vasculature. As a result the systemic vascular resistance is reduced and usually without orthostatic hypotension or reflex tachycardia. Bradycardia (rate less than 50 beats/min) is uncommon (<1% with Covera-HS as assessed by ECG). During isometric or dynamic exercise Covera-HS does not alter systolic cardiac function in patients with normal ventricular function.

Covera-HS does not alter total serum calcium levels. However, one report has suggested that calcium levels above the normal range may alter the therapeutic effect of verapamil. Covera-HS regularly reduces the total systemic resistance (afterload) against which the heart works both at rest and at a given level of exercise by dilating peripheral arterioles.

Effects in hypertension: Covera-HS was evaluated in two placebo-controlled, parallel design, double-blind studies of 382 patients with mild to moderate hypertension.

In a clinical trial, 287 patients were randomized to placebo, 120 mg, 180 mg, 360 mg, or 540 mg and treated for 8 weeks (the two higher doses were titrated from low doses and maintained for 6 and 4 weeks, respectively). Covera-HS or placebo was given once daily at 10 pm and blood pressure changes were measured with 36-hour ambulatory blood pressure monitoring (ABPM). The results of these studies demonstrate that Covera-HS, at 180–540 mg, is a consistently and significantly more effective antihypertensive agent than placebo in reducing ambulatory blood pressures. Over this dose range, the placebo-subtracted net decreases in diastolic BP at trough (averaged over 6–10 pm) were dose-related, ranged from 4.5 to 11.2 mm Hg after 4–8 weeks of therapy, and correlated well with sitting cuff blood pressures.

These studies demonstrate that clinically and statistically significant blood pressure reductions are achieved with Covera-HS throughout the 24-hour dosing period.

There were no significant treatment differences between patient subgroups of different age (older or younger than 65 years), sex, race (Caucasian and non-Caucasian) and severity of hypertension at baseline (cuff BP below and above 105 mm Hg).

Angina: Verapamil dilates the main coronary arteries and coronary arterioles, both in normal and ischemic regions, and is a potent inhibitor of coronary artery spasm, whether spontaneous or ergonovine-induced. This property increases myocardial oxygen delivery in patients with coronary artery spasm and is responsible for the effectiveness of verapamil in vasospastic (Prinzmetal's or variant) as well as unstable angina at rest. Whether this effect plays any role in classical effort angina is not clear, but studies of exercise tolerance have not shown an increase in the maximum exercise rate-pressure product, a widely accepted measure of oxygen utilization. This suggests that, in general, relief of spasm or dilation of coronary arteries is not an important factor in classical angina.

Verapamil regularly reduces the total systemic resistance (afterload) against which the heart works both at rest and at a given level of exercise by dilating peripheral arterioles.

Effect in chronic stable angina: Covera-HS was evaluated in two placebo-controlled, parallel design, double-blind studies of 453 patients with chronic stable angina.

In the first clinical trial 277 patients were randomized to placebo, 180 mg, 360 mg, or 540 mg and treated for 4 weeks (the two higher doses were titrated from low doses and maintained for 3 and 2 weeks, respectively). A single dose of 240 mg was compared to placebo in a separate study of 176 patients. In these studies Covera-HS was significantly more effective than placebo in improvement of exercise tolerance. Placebo-adjusted net increases in median exercise times at the end of the dosing interval were 0.1 to 1.0 minute for symptom limited duration, 0.3 to 1.4 minutes for time to angina, and 0.1 to 1.1 minutes for time to ST change. Increases in exercise tolerance were in general greater at higher doses, but dose-response relationship was not well defined due to shorter treatment duration for high doses.

In addition, in the first study, 24 to 34% of patients treated with Covera-HS did not experience exercise-limiting angina on exercise treadmill testing (ETT) versus 12% of patients on placebo.

Electrophysiologic effects: Electrical activity through the AV node depends, to a significant degree, upon the transmembrane influx of extracellular calcium through the L-type (slow) channel. By decreasing the influx of calcium, verapamil prolongs the effective refractory period within the AV node and slows AV conduction in a rate-related manner.

Normal sinus rhythm is usually not affected, but in patients with sick sinus syndrome, verapamil may interfere with sinus-node impulse generation and may induce sinus arrest or sinoatrial block. Atrioventricular block can occur in patients without preexisting conduction defects (see Warnings).

Covera-HS does not alter the normal atrial action potential or intraventricular conduction time, but depresses amplitude, velocity of depolarization, and conduction in depressed atrial fibers. Verapamil may shorten the antegrade effective refractory period of the accessory bypass tract. Acceleration of ventricular rate and/or ventricular fibrillation has been

reported in patients with atrial flutter or atrial fibrillation and a coexisting accessory AV pathway following administration of verapamil (see Warnings).

Verapamil has a local anesthetic action that is 1.6 times that of procaine on an equimolar basis. It is not known whether this action is important at the doses used in man.

Pharmacokinetics and metabolism: Verapamil is administered as a racemic mixture of the R and S enantiomers. The systemic concentrations of R and S enantiomers, as well as overall bioavailability, are dependent upon the route of administration and the rate and extent of release from the dosage forms. Upon oral administration, there is rapid stereoselective biotransformation during the first pass of verapamil through the portal circulation. In a study in 5 subjects with oral immediate-release verapamil, the systemic bioavailability was from 33% to 65% for the R enantiomer and from 13% to 34% for the S enantiomer. The R and S enantiomers have differing levels of pharmacologic activity. In studies in animals and humans, the S enantiomer has 8 to 20 times the activity of the R enantiomer in slowing AV conduction. In animal studies, the S enantiomer has 15 and 50 times the activity of the R enantiomer in reducing myocardial contractility in isolated blood-perfused dog papillary muscle and isolated rabbit papillary muscle, respectively, and twice the effect in reducing peripheral resistance. In isolated septal strip preparations from 5 patients, the S enantiomer was 8 times more potent than the R in reducing myocardial contractility. Dose escalation study data indicate that verapamil concentrations increase disproportionally to dose as measured by relative peak plasma concentrations (C_{max}) or areas under the plasma concentration vs time curves (AUC).

Pharmacokinetic Characteristics of Verapamil Enantiomers After Administration of Escalating Doses

		Total Dose of Racemic Verapamil (mg)			
	Isomer	120	180	360	540
Dose Ratio	—	1	1.5	3	4.5
Relative C_{max}	R	1	1.55	4.47	7.06
	S	1	1.62	5.17	9.21
Relative AUC	R	1	1.59	6.14	11.1
	S	1	1.89	8.17	15.9

Pharmacokinetic Characteristics of Verapamil Enantiomers After Administration of a Single 180 mg Dose and at Steady State

	Isomer	First Dose (Verapamil-naive subject)	Steady State (Current verapamil exposure)
C_{max} (ng/ml)	R	59.4	90.5
	S	11.7	21.2
AUC (0-24h) (ng·hr/ml)	R	644	1,223
	S	111	266

Racemic verapamil is released from Covera-HS at a constant rate following solubilization and release of the delay coat through the tablet orifices. This delay coat produces a lag period in drug release for approximately 4–5 hours. The drug release phase is prolonged with the peak plasma concentration (C_{max}) occurring approximately 11 hours after administration. Trough concentrations occur approximately 4 hours after bedtime dosing while the patient is sleeping. Steady-state pharmacokinetics were determined in healthy volunteers. Steady-state concentration is reached by the third or fourth day of dosing.

Steady-State Pharmacokinetics of Verapamil Enantiomers in Healthy Humans

	Isomer	Verapamil Dose (mg)	
		180	240
Mean C_{max} (ng/ml)	R	90.5	120
	S	21.2	28.7
AUC (0-24h) (ng·hr/ml)	R	1,223	1,470
	S	266	322

Consumption of a high fat meal just prior to dosing at night had no effect on the pharmacokinetics of Covera-HS. The pharmacokinetics were also not affected by whether the volunteers were supine or ambulatory for the 8 hours following dosing. Administering Covera-HS in the morning led to a slower rate of absorption and/or elimination, but did not affect the extent of absorption or extent of metabolism to norverapamil.

Orally administered verapamil undergoes extensive metabolism in the liver. Thirteen metabolites have been identified in urine. Norverapamil enantiomers can reach steady-state plasma concentrations approximately equal to those of the enantiomers of the parent drug. The cardiovascular activity of norverapamil appears to be approximately 20% that of verapamil. Approximately 70% of an administered dose is

excreted as metabolites in the urine and 16% or more in the feces within 5 days. About 3% to 4% is excreted in the urine as unchanged drug. R-verapamil is 94% bound to plasma albumin, while S-verapamil is 88% bound. In addition, R-verapamil is 92% and S-verapamil 86% bound to alpha-1 acid glycoprotein. In patients with hepatic insufficiency, metabolism of immediate-release verapamil is delayed and elimination half-life prolonged up to 14 to 16 hours because of the extensive hepatic metabolism (see Precautions). In addition, in these patients there is a reduced first pass effect, and verapamil is more bioavailable. Verapamil clearance values suggest that patients with liver dysfunction may attain therapeutic verapamil plasma concentrations with one third of the oral daily dose required for patients with normal liver function.

After four weeks of oral dosing of immediate release verapamil (120 mg q.i.d.), verapamil and norverapamil levels were noted in the cerebrospinal fluid with estimated partition coefficient of 0.06 for verapamil and 0.04 for norverapamil.

Geriatric use: The pharmacokinetics of Covera-HS were studied after 5 consecutive nights of dosing 180 mg in 30 healthy young (19-43 years) versus 30 healthy elderly (65-80 years) male and female subjects. Older subjects had significantly higher mean verapamil C_{max}, C_{min}, and $AUC_{(0-24h)}$ compared to younger subjects. Older subjects had mean AUCs that were approximately 1.7-2.0 times higher than those of younger subjects as well as a longer average verapamil $t_{1/2}$ (approximately 20 hr vs 13 hr). These results were typical of the age-related differences seen with many drug products in clinical medicine. Lean body mass was inversely related to AUC, but no gender difference was observed in the clinical trials of Covera-HS. However, there are conflicting data in the literature suggesting that verapamil clearance may decrease with age in women to a greater degree than in men. Mean T_{max} was similar in young and elderly subjects.

Hemodynamics: Verapamil reduces afterload and myocardial contractility. In most patients, including those with organic cardiac disease, the negative inotropic action of verapamil is countered by reduction of afterload and cardiac index remains unchanged. During isometric or dynamic exercise, verapamil does not alter systolic cardiac function in patients with normal ventricular function. Improved left ventricular diastolic function in patients with IHSS and those with coronary heart disease has also been observed with verapamil. In patients with severe left ventricular dysfunction (eg, pulmonary wedge pressure above 20 mm Hg or ejection fraction less than 30%), or in patients taking beta-adrenergic blocking agents or other cardiodepressant drugs, deterioration of ventricular function may occur (see Drug interactions).

Pulmonary function: Verapamil does not induce bronchoconstriction and, hence, does not impair ventilatory function.

Verapamil has been shown to have either a neutral or relaxant effect on bronchial smooth muscle.

INDICATIONS AND USAGE

Covera-HS is indicated for the management of hypertension and angina.

CONTRAINDICATIONS

Covera-HS is contraindicated in:
1. Severe left ventricular dysfunction (see Warnings)
2. Hypotension (systolic pressure less than 90 mm Hg) or cardiogenic shock
3. Sick sinus syndrome (except in patients with a functioning artificial ventricular pacemaker)
4. Second- or third-degree AV block (except in patients with a functioning artificial ventricular pacemaker)
5. Patients with atrial flutter or atrial fibrillation and an accessory bypass tract (eg, Wolff-Parkinson-White, Lown-Ganong-Levine syndromes). (See Warnings.)
6. Patients with known hypersensitivity to verapamil hydrochloride.

WARNINGS

Heart failure: Verapamil has a negative inotropic effect, which in most patients is compensated by its afterload reduction (decreased systemic vascular resistance) properties without a net impairment of ventricular performance. In previous clinical experience with 4,954 patients primarily with immediate-release verapamil, 1.8% developed congestive heart failure or pulmonary edema. Verapamil should be avoided in patients with severe left ventricular dysfunction (eg, ejection fraction less than 30%) or moderate to severe symptoms of cardiac failure and in patients with any degree of ventricular dysfunction if they are receiving a beta-adrenergic blocker (see Drug interactions). Patients with milder ventricular dysfunction should, if possible, be controlled with optimum doses of digitalis and/or diuretics before verapamil treatment is started. (**Note interactions with digoxin under Precautions.**)

Hypotension: Occasionally, the pharmacologic action of verapamil may produce a decrease in blood pressure below normal levels, which may result in dizziness or symptomatic hypotension. In previous verapamil clinical trials the incidence observed in 4,954 patients was 2.5%. In clinical studies of Covera-HS, 0.4% of hypertensive patients and 1.0% of angina patients developed significant hypotension. In hypertensive patients, decreases in blood pressure below normal are unusual. Tilt-table testing (60 degrees) was not able to induce orthostatic hypotension.

Elevated liver enzymes: Elevations of transaminases with and without concomitant elevations in alkaline phosphatase and bilirubin have been reported. Such elevations have sometimes been transient and may disappear even in the face of continued verapamil treatment. Several cases of hepatocellular injury related to verapamil have been proven by rechallenge; half of these had clinical symptoms (malaise, fever, and/or right upper quadrant pain) in addition to elevation of SGOT, SGPT, and alkaline phosphatase. Periodic monitoring of liver function in patients receiving verapamil is therefore prudent.

Accessory bypass tract (Wolff-Parkinson-White or Lown-Ganong-Levine): Some patients with paroxysmal and/or chronic atrial fibrillation or atrial flutter and a coexisting accessory AV pathway have developed increased antegrade conduction across the accessory pathway bypassing the AV node, producing a very rapid ventricular response or ventricular fibrillation after receiving intravenous verapamil (or digitalis). Although a risk of this occurring with oral verapamil has not been established, such patients receiving oral verapamil may be at risk and its use in these patients is contraindicated (see *Contraindications*). Treatment is usually DC-cardioversion. Cardioversion has been used safely and effectively after oral verapamil.

Atrioventricular block: The effect of verapamil on AV conduction and the SA node may cause asymptomatic first-degree AV block and transient bradycardia, sometimes accompanied by nodal escape rhythms. PR-interval prolongation is correlated with verapamil plasma concentrations, especially during the early titration phase of therapy. Higher degrees of AV block, however, were infrequently (0.8%) observed in previous verapamil clinical trials. Marked first-degree block or progressive development to second- or third-degree AV block requires a reduction in dosage or, in rare instances, discontinuation of verapamil HCl and institution of appropriate therapy, depending upon the clinical situation.

Patients with hypertrophic cardiomyopathy (IHSS): In 120 patients with hypertrophic cardiomyopathy (most of them refractory or intolerant to propranolol) who received therapy with verapamil at doses up to 720 mg/day, a variety of serious adverse effects were seen. Three patients died in pulmonary edema; all had severe left ventricular outflow obstruction and a past history of left ventricular dysfunction. Eight other patients had pulmonary edema and/or severe hypotension; abnormally high (greater than 20 mm Hg) pulmonary wedge pressure and a marked left ventricular outflow obstruction were present in most of these patients. Concomitant administration of quinidine (see *Drug interactions*) preceded the severe hypotension in 3 of the 8 patients (2 of whom developed pulmonary edema). Sinus bradycardia occurred in 11% of the patients, second-degree AV block in 4%, and sinus arrest in 2%. It must be appreciated that this group of patients had a serious disease with a high mortality rate. Most adverse effects responded well to dose reduction, and only rarely did verapamil use have to be discontinued.

PRECAUTIONS

General

Formulation specific: As with any other non-deformable dosage form caution should be used when administering Covera-HS in patients with preexisting severe gastrointestinal narrowing (pathologic or iatrogenic). In patients with extremely short GI transit time (<7 hrs), pharmacokinetic data are not available and dosage adjustment may be required.

Use in patients with impaired hepatic function: Since verapamil is highly metabolized by the liver, it should be administered cautiously to patients with impaired hepatic function. Severe liver dysfunction prolongs the elimination half-life of immediate-release verapamil to about 14 to 16 hours; hence, approximately 30% of the dose given to patients with normal liver function should be administered to these patients. Careful monitoring for abnormal prolongation of the PR interval or other signs of excessive pharmacologic effects (see *Overdosage*) should be carried out.

Use in patients with attenuated (decreased) neuromuscular transmission: It has been reported that verapamil decreases neuromuscular transmission in patients with Duchenne's muscular dystrophy, prolongs recovery from the neuromuscular blocking agent vecuronium, and causes a worsening of myasthenia gravis. It may be necessary to decrease the dosage of verapamil when it is administered to patients with attenuated neuromuscular transmission.

Use in patients with impaired renal function: About 70% of an administered dose of verapamil is excreted as metabolites in the urine. Verapamil is not removed by hemodialysis. Until further data are available, verapamil should be administered cautiously to patients with impaired renal function. These patients should be carefully monitored for abnormal prolongation of the PR interval or other signs of overdosage (see *Overdosage*).

Information for patients: Covera-HS tablets should be swallowed whole; do not break, crush, or chew. The medication in the Covera-HS tablet is released slowly through an outer shell that does not dissolve. The patient should not be concerned if they occasionally observe this outer shell in their stool as it passes from the body.

Drug-Drug Interactions

Drug interactions: Effects of other drugs on verapamil pharmacokinetics: In vitro metabolic studies indicate that verapamil is metabolized by cytochrome P450 CYP3A4, CYP1A2, and CYP2C. Clinically significant interactions have been reported with inhibitors of CYP3A4 (eg, erythromycin, ritonavir) causing elevation of plasma levels of vera-

pamil while inducers of CYP3A4 (eg, rifampin) have caused a lowering of plasma levels of verapamil.

Alcohol: Verapamil may increase blood alcohol concentrations and prolong its effects.

Aspirin: In a few reported cases, coadministration of verapamil with aspirin has led to increased bleeding times greater than observed with aspirin alone.

Grapefruit juice: Grapefruit juice may significantly increase concentrations of verapamil. Grapefruit juice given to nine healthy volunteers increased S- and R-verapamil AUC_{0-12} by 36% and 28%, respectively. Steady state C_{max} and C_{min} of S-verapamil increased by 57% and 16.7%, respectively, with grapefruit juice compared to control. Similarly, C_{max} and C_{min} of R-verapamil increased by 40% and 13%, respectively. Grapefruit juice did not affect half-life, nor was there a significant change in AUC_{0-12} ratio R/S compared to control. Grapefruit juice did not cause a significant difference in the PK of norverapamil. This increase in verapamil plasma concentration is not expected to have any clinical consequences.

Beta-blockers: Concomitant therapy with beta-adrenergic blockers and verapamil may result in additive negative effects on heart rate, atrioventricular conduction and/or cardiac contractility. The combination of sustained-release verapamil and beta-adrenergic blocking agents has not been studied. However, there have been reports of excessive bradycardia and AV block, including complete heart block, when the combination has been used for the treatment of hypertension. For hypertensive patients, the risks of combined therapy may outweigh the potential benefits. The combination should be used only with caution and close monitoring.

Asymptomatic bradycardia (36 beats/min) with a wandering atrial pacemaker has been observed in a patient receiving concomitant timolol (a beta-adrenergic blocker) eyedrops and oral verapamil.

A decrease in metoprolol and propranolol clearance has been observed when either drug is administered concomitantly with verapamil. A variable effect has been seen when verapamil and atenolol were given together.

Digitalis: Clinical use of verapamil in digitalized patients has shown the combination to be well tolerated if digoxin doses are properly adjusted. However, chronic verapamil treatment can increase serum digoxin levels by 50% to 75% during the first week of therapy, and this can result in digitalis toxicity. In patients with hepatic cirrhosis the influence of verapamil on digoxin kinetics is magnified. Verapamil may reduce total body clearance and extrarenal clearance of digitoxin by 27% and 29%, respectively. Maintenance and digitalization doses should be reduced when verapamil is administered, and the patient should be reassessed to avoid over- to underdigitalization. Whenever overdigitalization is suspected, the daily dose of digitalis should be reduced or temporarily discontinued. On discontinuation of verapamil use, the patient should be reassessed to avoid underdigitalization. In previous clinical trials with other verapamil formulations related to the control of ventricular response in digitalized patients who had atrial fibrillation or atrial flutter, ventricular rates below 50/min at rest occurred in 15% of patients, and asymptomatic hypotension occurred in 5% of patients.

Antihypertensive agents: Verapamil administered concomitantly with oral antihypertensive agents (eg, vasodilators, angiotensin-converting enzyme inhibitors, diuretics, beta-blockers) will usually have an additive effect on lowering blood pressure. Patients receiving these combinations should be appropriately monitored. Concomitant use of agents that attenuate alpha-adrenergic function with verapamil may result in a reduction in blood pressure that is excessive in some patients. Such an effect was observed in one study following the concomitant administration of verapamil and prazosin.

Antiarrhythmic agents:

Disopyramide: Until data on possible interactions between verapamil and disopyramide are obtained, disopyramide should not be administered within 48 hours before or 24 hours after verapamil administration.

Flecainide: A study in healthy volunteers showed that the concomitant administration of flecainide and verapamil may have additive effects on myocardial contractility, AV conduction, and repolarization. Concomitant therapy with flecainide and verapamil may result in additive negative inotropic effect and prolongation of atrioventricular conduction.

Quinidine: In a small number of patients with hypertrophic cardiomyopathy (IHSS), concomitant use of verapamil and quinidine resulted in significant hypotension. Until further data are obtained, combined therapy of verapamil and quinidine in patients with hypertrophic cardiomyopathy should probably be avoided.

The electrophysiologic effects of quinidine and verapamil on AV conduction were studied in 8 patients. Verapamil significantly counteracted the effects of quinidine on AV conduction. There has been a report of increased quinidine levels during verapamil therapy.

Other:

Nitrates: Verapamil has been given concomitantly with short- and long-acting nitrates without any undesirable drug interactions. The pharmacologic profile of both drugs and clinical experience suggest beneficial interactions.

Cimetidine: The interaction between cimetidine and chronically administered verapamil has not been studied. Variable results on clearance have been obtained in acute studies of healthy volunteers; clearance of verapamil was either reduced or unchanged.

Lithium: Increased sensitivity to the effects of lithium (neurotoxicity) has been reported during concomitant verapamil-lithium therapy; lithium levels have been observed sometimes to increase, sometimes to decrease, and sometimes to be unchanged. Patients receiving both drugs must be monitored carefully.

Carbamazepine: Verapamil therapy may increase carbamazepine concentrations during combined therapy. This may produce carbamazepine side effects such as diplopia, headache, ataxia, or dizziness.

Rifampin: Therapy with rifampin may markedly reduce oral verapamil bioavailability.

Phenobarbital: Phenobarbital therapy may increase verapamil clearance.

Cyclosporin: Verapamil therapy may increase serum levels of cyclosporin.

Theophylline: Verapamil may inhibit the clearance and increase the plasma levels of theophylline.

Inhalation anesthetics: Animal experiments have shown that inhalation anesthetics depress cardiovascular activity by decreasing the inward movement of calcium ions. When used concomitantly, inhalation anesthetics and calcium channel blocking agents, such as verapamil, should each be titrated carefully to avoid excessive cardiovascular depression.

Neuromuscular blocking agents: Clinical data and animal studies suggest that verapamil may potentiate the activity of neuromuscular blocking agents (curare-like and depolarizing). It may be necessary to decrease the dose of verapamil and/or the dose of the neuromuscular blocking agent when the drugs are used concomitantly.

Carcinogenesis, mutagenesis, impairment of fertility: An 18-month toxicity study in rats, at a low multiple (6-fold) of the maximum recommended human dose, not the maximum tolerated dose, did not suggest a tumorigenic potential. There was no evidence of a carcinogenic potential of verapamil administered in the diet of rats for two years at doses of 10, 35, and 120 mg/kg/day or approximately 1, 3.5, and 12 times, respectively, the maximum recommended human daily dose (480 mg/day or 9.6 mg/kg/day).

Verapamil was not mutagenic in the Ames test in 5 test strains at 3 mg per plate with or without metabolic activation.

Studies in female rats at daily dietary doses up to 5.5 times (55 mg/kg/day) the maximum recommended human dose did not show impaired fertility. Effects on male fertility have not been determined.

Pregnancy: Pregnancy Category C. Reproduction studies have been performed in rabbits and rats at oral doses up to 1.5 (15 mg/kg/day) and 6 (60 mg/kg/day) times the human oral daily dose, respectively, and have revealed no evidence of teratogenicity. In the rat, however, this multiple of the human dose was embryocidal and retarded fetal growth and development, probably because of adverse maternal effects reflected in reduced weight gains of the dams. This oral dose has also been shown to cause hypotension in rats. There are no adequate and well-controlled studies in pregnant women. Because animal reproduction studies are not always predictive of human response, this drug should be used during pregnancy only if clearly needed. Verapamil crosses the placental barrier and can be detected in umbilical vein blood at delivery.

Labor and delivery: It is not known whether the use of verapamil during labor or delivery has immediate or delayed adverse effects on the fetus, or whether it prolongs the duration of labor or increases the need for forceps delivery or other obstetric intervention. Such adverse experiences have not been reported in the literature, despite a long history of use of verapamil in Europe in the treatment of cardiac side effects of beta-adrenergic agonist agents used to treat premature labor.

Nursing mothers: Verapamil is excreted in human milk. Because of the potential for adverse reactions in nursing infants from verapamil, nursing should be discontinued while verapamil is administered.

Pediatric use: Safety and effectiveness in pediatric patients have not been established.

Geriatric use: Clinical studies of Covera-HS did not include sufficient numbers of subjects aged under 65 to determine whether they responded differently from older subjects. Other reported clinical experience has not identified differences in responses between the elderly and younger patients. In general, dose selection for an elderly patient should be cautious, usually starting at the low end of the dosing range, reflecting the greater frequency of decreased hepatic, renal, or cardiac function, and of concomitant disease or other drug therapy.

Animal pharmacology and/or animal toxicology: In chronic animal toxicology studies verapamil caused lenticular and/or suture line changes at 30 mg/kg/day or greater, and frank cataracts at 62.5 mg/kg/day or greater in the beagle dog but not in the rat. Development of cataracts due to verapamil has not been reported in man.

ADVERSE REACTIONS

Serious adverse reactions are uncommon when verapamil therapy is initiated with upward dose titration within the recommended single and total daily dose. See *Warnings* for discussion of heart failure, hypotension, elevated liver enzymes, AV block, and rapid ventricular response. Reversible (upon discontinuation of verapamil) non-obstructive, paralytic ileus has been infrequently reported in association with the use of verapamil. The following reactions to orally

Continued on next page

Covera-HS—Cont.

administered Covera-HS occurred at rates greater than 2.0% or occurred at lower rates but appeared drug-related in clinical trials in hypertension and angina:

	Placebo n=261 %	All doses studied n=572 %
Constipation	2.7	11.7*
Headache	7.3	6.6
Upper respiratory infection	4.6	5.4
Dizziness	2.7	4.7
Fatigue	3.8	4.5
Edema	3.1	3.0
Nausea	1.9	2.1
AV block (1°)	0.0	1.7
Elevated liver enzymes (see *Warnings*)	0.8	1.4
Bradycardia	0.4	1.4
Paresthesia	0.0	1.0
Flushing	0.3	0.8
Hypotension	0.0	0.7
Postural hypotension	0.3	0.4

*Constipation was typically mild, easily manageable, and the incidence usually diminished within about one week. At a typical once-daily dose of 240 mg, the observed incidence was 7.2%.

In previous experience with other formulations of verapamil, the following reactions occurred at rates greater than 1.0% or occurred at lower rates but appeared clearly drug related in clinical trials in 4,954 patients.

Constipation	7.3%
Dizziness	3.3%
Nausea	2.7%
Hypotension	2.5%
Headache	2.2%
Edema	1.9%
CHF/Pulmonary Edema	1.8%
Fatigue	1.7%
Dyspnea	1.4%
Bradycardia (HR < 50/min)	1.4%
AV Block total (1°,2°,3°)	1.2%
AV Block 2° and 3°	0.8%
Rash	1.2%
Flushing	0.6%
Elevated liver enzymes (see *Warnings*)	

The following reactions, reported with orally administered verapamil in 2% or less of patients, occurred under conditions (open trials, marketing experience) where a causal relationship is uncertain; they are listed to alert the physician to a possible relationship:
Cardiovascular: angina pectoris, AV block (2° & 3°), atrioventricular dissociation, CHF, pulmonary edema, chest pain, claudication, myocardial infarction, palpitations, purpura (vasculitis), syncope.
Digestive system: diarrhea, dry mouth, gastrointestinal distress, gingival hyperplasia.
Hemic and lymphatic: ecchymosis or bruising.
Nervous system: cerebrovascular accident, confusion, equilibrium disorders, insomnia, muscle cramps, psychotic symptoms, shakiness, somnolence, extrapyramidal symptoms.
Skin: arthralgia and rash, exanthema, hair loss, hyperkeratosis, macules, sweating, urticaria, Stevens-Johnson syndrome, erythema multiforme.
Special senses: blurred vision, tinnitus.
Urogenital: gynecomastia, galactorrhea/hyperprolactinemia, increased urination, spotty menstruation, impotence.
Other: allergy aggravated, dyspnea.
Treatment of acute cardiovascular adverse reactions: The frequency of cardiovascular adverse reactions that require therapy is rare; hence, experience with their treatment is limited. Whenever severe hypotension or complete AV block occurs following oral administration of verapamil, the appropriate emergency measures should be applied immediately; eg, intravenously administered norepinephrine bitartrate, atropine sulfate, isoproterenol HCl (all in usual doses), or calcium gluconate (10% solution). In patients with hypertrophic cardiomyopathy (IHSS), alpha-adrenergic agents (phenylephrine HCl, metaraminol bitartrate, or methoxamine HCl) should be used to maintain blood pressure, and isoproterenol and norepinephrine should be avoided. If further support is necessary, dopamine HCl or dobutamine HCl may be administered. Actual treatment and dosage should depend on the severity of the clinical situation and the judgement and experience of the treating physician.

OVERDOSAGE

Treat all verapamil overdoses as serious and maintain observation for at least 48 hours (especially sustained-release verapamil products), preferably under continuous hospital care. Delayed pharmacodynamic consequences may occur with the sustained-release formulations. Verapamil is known to decrease gastrointestinal transit time.
Treatment of overdosage should be supportive. Beta-adrenergic stimulation or parenteral administration of calcium solutions may increase calcium ion flux across the slow channel and have been used effectively in treatment of deliberate overdosage with verapamil. In a few reported cases, overdose with calcium channel blockers has been associated with hypotension and bradycardia, initially refractory to atropine but becoming more responsive to this treatment when the patients received large doses (close to 1 gram/hour for more than 24 hours) of calcium chloride. Verapamil cannot be removed by hemodialysis. Clinically significant hypotensive reactions or high degree AV block should be treated with vasopressor agents or cardiac pacing, respectively. Asystole should be handled by the usual measures including cardiopulmonary resuscitation.

DOSAGE AND ADMINISTRATION

Covera-HS should be administered once daily at bedtime. Clinical trials explored dose ranges between 180 mg and 540 mg given at bedtime and found effects to persist throughout the dosing interval.
Covera-HS tablets should be swallowed whole and not chewed, broken, or crushed.
For both hypertension and angina the dose of Covera-HS should be individualized by titration. Initiate therapy with 180 mg of Covera-HS.
If an adequate response is not obtained with 180 mg of Covera-HS, the dose may be titrated upward in the following manner:
a) 240 mg each evening
b) 360 mg each evening (2 × 180 mg)
c) 480 mg each evening (2 × 240 mg)
When Covera-HS is administered at bedtime, office evaluation of blood pressure during morning and early afternoon hours is essentially a measure of peak effect. The usual evaluation of trough effect, which sometimes might be needed to evaluate the appropriateness of any given dose of Covera-HS, would be just prior to bedtime.

HOW SUPPLIED

Covera-HS 240-mg tablets are pale yellow, round, film coated with COVERA–HS 2021 printed on one side, supplied as:

NDC Number	Size
0025-2021-31	bottle of 100
0025-2021-34	carton of 100 unit dose

Covera-HS 180-mg tablets are lavender, round, film coated, with COVERA–HS 2011 printed on one side, supplied as:

NDC Number	Size
0025-2011-31	bottle of 100
0025-2011-34	carton of 100 unit dose

Store at controlled room temperature 20°–25°C (68°–77°F) [see USP]. Dispense in tight, light-resistant containers.
Rx only Revised: May 2004
Distributed by
G.D. Searle LLC
Division of Pfizer Inc, NY, NY 10017
Covera-HS®
(verapamil hydrochloride)
Extended-Release Tablets
Controlled-Onset
818 875 103 P04027-4

Shire US Inc.
725 CHESTERBROOK BLVD.
WAYNE, PA 19087

Direct Inquiries to:
Customer Service
(800) 828-2088

For Medical Information Contact:
(800) 828-2088

ADDERALL® Ⓒ℞
[*ăd-dĕr-ăll*]
5mg, 7.5mg, 10mg, 12.5mg, 15mg, 20mg & 30mg
Rx ONLY

Prescribing information for this product, which appears on pages 3131–3132 of the 2005 PDR, has been completely revised as follows. Please write "See Supplement A" next to the product heading.

AMPHETAMINES HAVE A HIGH POTENTIAL FOR ABUSE. ADMINISTRATION OF AMPHETAMINES FOR PROLONGED PERIODS OF TIME MAY LEAD TO DRUG DEPENDENCE AND MUST BE AVOIDED. PARTICULAR ATTENTION SHOULD BE PAID TO THE POSSIBILITY OF SUBJECTS OBTAINING AMPHETAMINES FOR NON-THERAPEUTIC USE OR DISTRIBUTION TO OTHERS, AND THE DRUGS SHOULD BE PRESCRIBED OR DISPENSED SPARINGLY.
MISUSE OF AMPHETAMINE MAY CAUSE SUDDEN DEATH AND SERIOUS CARDIOVASCULAR ADVERSE EVENTS.

DESCRIPTION

A single entity amphetamine product combining the neutral sulfate salts of dextroamphetamine and amphetamine, with the dextro isomer of amphetamine saccharate and d, l-amphetamine aspartate monohydrate.
[See table at top of next page]
Inactive Ingredients: microcrystalline cellulose, colloidal silicon dioxide, and magnesium stearate, and other ingredients.
Colors: ADDERALL® 5 mg is a white to off-white tablet, which contains no color additives.
ADDERALL® 7.5 mg and 10 mg contain FD & C Blue #1.
ADDERALL® 12.5 mg, 15 mg, 20 mg and 30 mg contain FD & C Yellow #6 as a color additive.

CLINICAL PHARMACOLOGY

Amphetamines are non-catecholamine sympathomimetic amines with CNS stimulant activity. Peripheral actions include elevation of systolic and diastolic blood pressures and weak bronchodilator and respiratory stimulant action.
There is neither specific evidence which clearly establishes the mechanism whereby amphetamine produces mental and behavioral effects in children, nor conclusive evidence regarding how these effects relate to the condition of the central nervous system.
Pharmacokinetics
ADDERALL® tablets contain d-amphetamine and l-amphetamine salts in the ratio of 3:1. Following administration of a single dose 10 or 30 mg of ADDERALL® to healthy volunteers under fasted conditions, peak plasma concentrations occurred approximately 3 hours post-dose for both d-amphetamine and l-amphetamine. The mean elimination half-life ($t_{1/2}$) for d-amphetamine was shorter than the $t_{1/2}$ of the l-isomer (9.77–11 hours vs. 11.5–13.8 hours). The PK parameters (C_{max}, $AUC_{0\text{-}inf}$) of d-and l-amphetamine increased approximately three-fold from 10 mg to 30 mg indicating dose-proportional pharmacokinetics.
The effect of food on the bioavailability of ADDERALL® has not been studied.

INDICATIONS

Attention Deficit Disorder with Hyperactivity: ADDERALL® is indicated as an integral part of a total treatment program which typically includes other remedial measures (psychological, educational, social) for a stabilizing effect in children with behavioral syndrome characterized by the following group of developmentally inappropriate symptoms: moderate to severe distractibility, short attention span, hyperactivity, emotional lability, and impulsivity. The diagnosis of this syndrome should not be made with finality when these symptoms are only of comparatively recent origin. Nonlocalizing (soft) neurological signs, learning disability and abnormal EEG may or may not be present, and a diagnosis of central nervous system dysfunction may or may not be warranted.
In Narcolepsy

CONTRAINDICATIONS

Advanced arteriosclerosis, symptomatic cardiovascular disease, moderate to severe hypertension, hyperthyroidism, known hypersensitivity or idiosyncrasy to the sympathomimetic amines, glaucoma.
Agitated states.
Patients with a history of drug abuse.
During or within 14 days following the administration of monoamine oxidase inhibitors (hypertensive crises may result).

WARNINGS

Psychosis: Clinical experience suggests that in psychotic children, administration of amphetamine may exacerbate symptoms of behavior disturbance and thought disorder.
Long-Term Suppression of Growth: Data are inadequate to determine whether chronic administration of amphetamine may be associated with growth inhibition; therefore, growth should be monitored during treatment.
Sudden Death and Pre-existing Structural Cardiac Abnormalities: Sudden death has been reported in association with amphetamine treatment at usual doses in children with structural cardiac abnormalities. Adderall generally should not be used in children or adults with structural cardiac abnormalities.
Usage in Nursing Mothers: Amphetamines are excreted in human milk. Mothers taking amphetamines should be advised to refrain from nursing.

PRECAUTIONS

General: The least amount feasible should be prescribed or dispensed at one time in order to minimize the possibility of overdosage.
Hypertension: Caution is to be exercised in prescribing amphetamines for patients with even mild hypertension. Blood pressure and pulse should be monitored at appropriate intervals in patients taking Adderall, especially patients with hypertension.
Information for Patients: Amphetamines may impair the ability of the patient to engage in potentially hazardous activities such as operating machinery or vehicles; the patient should therefore be cautioned accordingly.
Drug Interactions: *Acidifying agents*—Gastrointestinal acidifying agents (guanethidine, reserpine, glutamic acid HCl, ascorbic acid, fruit juices, etc.) lower absorption of amphetamines.
Urinary acidifying agents—(ammonium chloride, sodium acid phosphate, etc.) Increase the concentration of the ionized species of the amphetamine molecule, thereby increasing urinary excretion. Both groups of agents lower blood levels and efficacy of amphetamines.
Adrenergic blocker—Adrenergic blockers are inhibited by amphetamines.
Alkalinizing agents—Gastrointestinal alkalinizing agents (sodium bicarbonate, etc.) increase absorption of amphetamines. Urinary alkalinizing agents (acetazolamide, some

thiazides) increase the concentration of the non-ionized species of the amphetamine molecule, thereby decreasing urinary excretion. Both groups of agents increase blood levels and therefore potentiate the actions of amphetamines.

Antidepressants, tricyclic—Amphetamines may enhance the activity of tricyclic or sympathomimetic agents; d-amphetamine with desipramine or protriptyline and possibly other tricyclics cause striking and sustained increases in the concentration of d-amphetamine in the brain; cardiovascular effects can be potentiated.

MAO inhibitors—MAOI antidepressants, as well as a metabolite of furazolidone, slow amphetamine metabolism. This slowing potentiates amphetamines, increasing their effect on the release of norepinephrine and other monoamines from adrenergic nerve endings; this can cause headaches and other signs of hypertensive crisis. A variety of neurological toxic effects and malignant hyperpyrexia can occur, sometimes with fatal results.

Antihistamines—Amphetamines may counteract the sedative effect of antihistamines.

Antihypertensives—Amphetamines may antagonize the hypotensive effects of antihypertensives.

Chlorpromazine—Chlorpromazine blocks dopamine and norepinephrine receptors, thus inhibiting the central stimulant effects of amphetamines, and can be used to treat amphetamine poisoning.

Ethosuximide—Amphetamines may delay intestinal absorption of ethosuximide.

Haloperidol—Haloperidol blocks dopamine receptors, thus inhibiting the central stimulant effects of amphetamines.

Lithium carbonate—The anorectic and stimulatory effects of amphetamines may be inhibited by lithium carbonate.

Meperidine—Amphetamines potentiate the analgesic effect of meperidine.

Methenamine therapy—Urinary excretion of amphetamines is increased, and efficacy is reduced, by acidifying agents used in methenamine therapy.

Norepinephrine—Amphetamines enhance the adrenergic effect of norepinephrine.

Phenobarbital—Amphetamines may delay intestinal absorption of phenobarbital; co-administration of phenobarbital may produce a synergistic anticonvulsant action.

Phenytoin—Amphetamines may delay intestinal absorption of phenytoin; co-administration of phenytoin may produce a synergistic anticonvulsant action.

Propoxyphene—In cases of propoxyphene overdosage, amphetamine CNS stimulation is potentiated and fatal convulsions can occur.

Veratrum alkaloids—Amphetamines inhibit the hypotensive effect of veratrum alkaloids.

Drug/Laboratory Test Interactions:
• Amphetamines can cause a significant elevation in plasma corticosteroid levels. This increase is greatest in the evening.
• Amphetamines may interfere with urinary steroid determinations.

Carcinogenesis/Mutagenesis: Mutagenicity studies and long-term studies in animals to determine the carcinogenic potential of amphetamine, have not been performed.

Pregnancy—Teratogenic Effects: Pregnancy Category C. Amphetamine has been shown to have embryotoxic and teratogenic effects when administered to A/Jax mice and C57BL mice in doses approximately 41 times the maximum human dose. Embryotoxic effects were not seen in New Zealand white rabbits given the drug in doses 7 times the human dose nor in rats given 12.5 times the maximum human dose. While there are no adequate and well-controlled studies in pregnant women, there has been one report of severe congenital bony deformity, tracheoesophageal fistula, and anal atresia (vater association) in a baby born to a woman who took dextroamphetamine sulfate with lovastatin during the first trimester of pregnancy. Amphetamines should be used during pregnancy only if the potential benefit justifies the potential risk to the fetus.

Nonteratogenic Effects: Infants born to mothers dependent on amphetamines have an increased risk of premature delivery and low birth weight. Also, these infants may experience symptoms of withdrawal as demonstrated by dysphoria, including agitation, and significant lassitude.

Pediatric Use: Long-term effects of amphetamines in children have not been well established. Amphetamines are not recommended for use in children under 3 years of age with Attention Deficit Disorder with Hyperactivity described under INDICATIONS AND USAGE.

Amphetamines have been reported to exacerbate motor and phonic tics and Tourette's syndrome. Therefore, clinical evaluation for tics and Tourette's syndrome in children and their families should precede use of stimulant medications.

Drug treatment is not indicated in all cases of Attention Deficit Disorder with Hyperactivity and should be considered only in light of the complete history and evaluation of the child. The decision to prescribe amphetamines should depend on the physician's assessment of the chronicity and severity of the child's symptoms and their appropriateness for his/her age. Prescription should not depend solely on the presence of one or more of the behavioral characteristics. When these symptoms are associated with acute stress reactions, treatment with amphetamines is usually not indicated.

ADVERSE REACTIONS

Cardiovascular: Palpitations, tachycardia, elevation of blood pressure, sudden death, myocardial infarction. There have been isolated reports of cardiomyopathy associated with chronic amphetamine use.

EACH TABLET CONTAINS:	5 mg	7.5 mg	10 mg	12.5 mg	15 mg	20 mg	30 mg
Dextroamphetamine Saccharate	1.25 mg	1.875 mg	2.5 mg	3.125 mg	3.75 mg	5 mg	7.5 mg
Amphetamine Aspartate Monohydrate	1.25 mg	1.875 mg	2.5 mg	3.125 mg	3.75 mg	5 mg	7.5 mg
Dextroamphetamine Sulfate USP	1.25 mg	1.875 mg	2.5 mg	3.125 mg	3.75 mg	5 mg	7.5 mg
Amphetamine Sulfate USP	1.25 mg	1.875 mg	2.5 mg	3.125 mg	3.75 mg	5 mg	7.5 mg
Total amphetamine base equivalence	3.13 mg	4.7 mg	6.3 mg	7.8 mg	9.4 mg	12.6 mg	18.8 mg

Central Nervous System: Psychotic episodes at recommended doses (rare), overstimulation, restlessness, dizziness, insomnia, euphoria, dyskinesia, dysphoria, depression, tremor, headache, exacerbation of motor and phonic tics and Tourette's syndrome, seizures, stroke.

Gastrointestinal: Dryness of the mouth, unpleasant taste, diarrhea, constipation, other gastrointestinal disturbances. Anorexia and weight loss may occur as undesirable effects when amphetamines are used for other than the anorectic effect.

Allergic: Urticaria.

Endocrine: Impotence, changes in libido.

DRUG ABUSE AND DEPENDENCE

Dextroamphetamine Sulfate, Amphetamine Sulfate, Amphetamine Aspartate Monohydrate, and Dextroamphetamine Saccharate are Schedule II controlled substance. Amphetamines have been extensively abused. Tolerance, extreme psychological dependence, and severe social disability have occurred. There are reports of patients who have increased the dosage to many times than recommended. Abrupt cessation following prolonged high dosage administration results in extreme fatigue and mental depression; changes are also noted on the sleep EEG. Manifestations of chronic intoxication with amphetamines include severe dermatoses, marked insomnia, irritability, hyperactivity, and personality changes. The most severe manifestation of chronic intoxication is psychosis, often clinically indistinguishable from schizophrenia. This is rare with oral amphetamines.

OVERDOSAGE

Individual patient response to amphetamines varies widely. While toxic symptoms occasionally occur as an idiosyncrasy at doses as low as 2 mg, they are rare with doses of less than 15 mg; 30 mg can produce severe reactions, yet doses of 400 to 500 mg are not necessarily fatal.

In rats, the oral LD_{50} of dextroamphetamine sulfate is 96.8 mg/kg.

Symptoms: Manifestations of acute overdosage with amphetamines include restlessness, tremor, hyperreflexia, rapid respiration, confusion, assaultiveness, hallucinations, panic states, hyperpyrexia and rhabdomyolysis.

Fatigue and depression usually follow the central stimulation.

Cardiovascular effects include arrhythmias, hypertension or hypotension and circulatory collapse.

Gastrointestinal symptoms include nausea, vomiting, diarrhea, and abdominal cramps. Fatal poisoning is usually preceded by convulsions and coma.

Treatment: Consult with a Certified Poison Control Center for up to date guidance and advice. Management of acute amphetamine intoxication is largely symptomatic and includes gastric lavage, administration of activated charcoal, administration of a cathartic and sedation. Experience with hemodialysis or peritoneal dialysis is inadequate to permit recommendation in this regard. Acidification of the urine increases amphetamine excretion, but is believed to increase risk of acute renal failure if myoglobinuria is present. If acute, severe hypertension complicates amphetamine overdosage, administration of intravenous phentolamine has been suggested. However, a gradual drop in blood pressure will usually result when sufficient sedation has been achieved. Chlorpromazine antagonizes the central stimulant effects of amphetamines and can be used to treat amphetamine intoxication.

DOSAGE AND ADMINISTRATION

Regardless of indication, amphetamines should be administered at the lowest effective dosage and dosage should be individually adjusted. Late evening doses should be avoided because of the resulting insomnia.

Attention Deficit Disorder with Hyperactivity: Not recommended for children under 3 years of age. In children from 3 to 5 years of age, start with 2.5 mg daily; daily dosage may be raised in increments of 2.5 mg at weekly intervals until optimal response is obtained.

In children 6 years of age and older, start with 5 mg once or twice daily; daily dosage may be raised in increments of 5 mg at weekly intervals until optimal response is obtained. Only in rare cases will it be necessary to exceed a total of 40 mg per day. Give first dose on awakening; additional doses (1 or 2) at intervals of 4 to 6 hours.

Where possible, drug administration should be interrupted occasionally to determine if there is a recurrence of behavioral symptoms sufficient to require continued therapy.

Narcolepsy: Usual dose 5 mg to 60 mg per day in divided doses, depending on the individual patient response.

Narcolepsy seldom occurs in children under 12 years of age; however, when it does, dextroamphetamine sulfate may be used. The suggested initial dose for patients aged 6–12 is 5 mg daily; daily dose may be raised in increments of 5 mg at weekly intervals until optimal response is obtained. In patients 12 years of age and older, start with 10 mg daily; daily dosage may be raised in increments of 10 mg at weekly intervals until optimal response is obtained. If bothersome adverse reactions appear (e.g., insomnia or anorexia), dosage should be reduced. Give first dose on awakening; additional doses (1 or 2) at intervals of 4 to 6 hours.

HOW SUPPLIED

ADDERALL® 5 mg: A round, flat-faced beveled edge, white to off-white tablet, "5" embossed on one side with partial bisect and "AD" embossed on the other side (NDC 54092-371-01)

ADDERALL® 7.5 mg: An oval, convex, blue tablet, "7.5" embossed on one side with a partial bisect and "AD" embossed on the other side with a full and partial bisect (NDC 54092-372-01)

ADDERALL® 10 mg: A round, convex, blue tablet, "10" embossed on one side with a full and partial bisect and "AD" embossed on the other side (NDC 54092-373-01)

ADDERALL® 12.5 mg: A round, flat-faced beveled edge, orange tablet, "12.5" embossed on one side and "AD" embossed on the other side with a full and partial bisect (NDC 54092-374-01)

ADDERALL® 15 mg: An oval, convex, orange tablet, "15" embossed on one side with a partial bisect and "AD" embossed on the other side with a full and partial bisect (NDC 54092-375-01)

ADDERALL® 20 mg: A round, convex, orange tablet, "20" embossed on one side with a full and partial bisect and "AD" embossed on the other side (NDC 54092-376-01)

ADDERALL® 30 mg: A round, flat-faced beveled edge, orange tablet, "30" embossed on one side with a full and partial bisect and "AD" embossed on the other side (NDC 54092-377-01)

In bottles of 100 tablets.

Dispense in a tight, light-resistant container as defined in the USP.

Store at 25°C (77°F), excursions permitted to 15°–30°C (59–86°F) [see USP Controlled Room Temperature]

Rx only.

001375

Revised: 03/05
371 0107 003

Manufactured for: Shire US Inc.
725 Chesterbrook Blvd.
Wayne, PA 19087

Manufactured by: DSM Pharmaceuticals Inc.
5900 NW Greenville Blvd.
Greenville, NC 27834

Made in USA
1-800-828-2088
©2005 Shire US Inc.

ADDERALL XR®

5 mg, 10 mg, 15 mg, 20 mg, 25 mg, 30 mg Capsules
(mixed salts of a single-entity Amphetamine Product)
Dextroamphetamine Sulfate Dextromphetamine
Saccharate Amphetomine Asparate Monohydrate
Amphetamine Sulfate
CAPSULES

Prescribing information for this product, which appears on pages 3132–3134 of the 2005 PDR, has been completely revised as follows. Please write "See Supplement A" next to the product heading.

> AMPHETAMINES HAVE A HIGH POTENTIAL FOR ABUSE. ADMINISTRATION OF AMPHETAMINES FOR PROLONGED PERIODS OF TIME MAY LEAD TO DRUG DEPENDENCE. PARTICULAR ATTENTION SHOULD BE PAID TO THE POSSIBILITY OF SUBJECTS OBTAINING AMPHETAMINES FOR NON-THERAPEUTIC USE OR DISTRIBUTION TO OTHERS AND THE DRUGS SHOULD BE PRESCRIBED OR DISPENSED SPARINGLY.
>
> MISUSE OF AMPHETAMINE MAY CAUSE SUDDEN DEATH AND SERIOUS CARDIOVASCULAR ADVERSE EVENTS.

DESCRIPTION

ADDERALL XR® is a once daily extended-release, single-entity amphetamine product. ADDERALL XR® combines the neutral sulfate salts of dextroamphetamine and amphetamine, with the dextro isomer of amphetamine saccharate and d,l-amphetamine aspartate monohydrate. The ADDERALL XR® capsule contains two types of drug-containing beads designed to give a double-pulsed delivery of amphetamines, which prolongs the release of amphetamine from ADDERALL XR® compared to the conventional ADDERALL® (immediate-release) tablet formulation.
[See table at top of next page]

Inactive Ingredients and Colors: The inactive ingredients in ADDERALL XR® capsules include: gelatin capsules, hydroxypropyl methylcellulose, methacrylic acid copolymer, opadry beige, sugar spheres, talc, and triethyl citrate. Gelatin capsules contain edible inks, kosher gelatin, and titanium dioxide. The 5 mg, 10 mg, and 15 mg capsules also contain FD&C Blue #2. The 20 mg, 25 mg, and 30 mg capsules also contain red iron oxide and yellow iron oxide.

CLINICAL PHARMACOLOGY

Pharmacodynamics

Amphetamines are non-catecholamine sympathomimetic amines with CNS stimulant activity. The mode of therapeu-

Continued on next page

Adderall XR—Cont.

EACH CAPSULE CONTAINS:	5 mg	10 mg	15 mg	20 mg	25 mg	30 mg
Dextroamphetamine Saccharate	1.25 mg	2.5 mg	3.75 mg	5.0 mg	6.25 mg	7.5 mg
Amphetamine Aspartate Monohydrate	1.25 mg	2.5 mg	3.75 mg	5.0 mg	6.25 mg	7.5 mg
Dextroamphetamine Sulfate USP	1.25 mg	2.5 mg	3.75 mg	5.0 mg	6.25 mg	7.5 mg
Amphetamine Sulfate USP	1.25 mg	2.5 mg	3.75 mg	5.0 mg	6.25 mg	7.5 mg
Total amphetamine base equivalent	3.1 mg	6.3 mg	9.4 mg	12.5 mg	15.6 mg	18.8 mg

tic action in Attention Deficit Hyperactivity Disorder (ADHD) is not known. Amphetamines are thought to block the reuptake of norepinephrine and dopamine into the presynaptic neuron and increase the release of these monoamines into the extraneuronal space.

Pharmacokinetics

Pharmacokinetic studies of ADDERALL XR® have been conducted in healthy adult and pediatric (6–12 yrs) subjects, and pediatric patients with ADHD. Both ADDERALL® (immediate-release) tablets and ADDERALL XR® capsules contain d-amphetamine and l-amphetamine salts in the ratio of 3:1. Following administration of ADDERALL® (immediate-release), the peak plasma concentrations occurred in about 3 hours for both d-amphetamine and l-amphetamine.

The time to reach maximum plasma concentration (T_{max}) for ADDERALL XR® is about 7 hours, which is about 4 hours longer compared to ADDERALL® (immediate-release). This is consistent with the extended-release nature of the product.

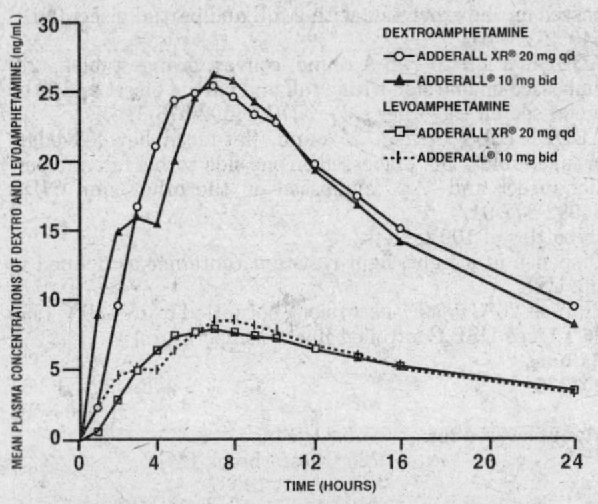

Figure 1 Mean d-amphetamine and l-amphetamine plasma concentrations following administration of ADDERALL XR® 20 mg (8 am) and ADDERALL® (immediate-release) 10 mg bid (8 am 12 noon) in the fed state.

A single dose of ADDERALL XR® 20 mg capsules provided comparable plasma concentration profiles of both d-amphetamine and l-amphetamine to ADDERALL® (immediate-release) 10 mg bid administered 4 hours apart.

The mean elimination half-lives for d-amphetamine and l-amphetamine in adults are 10 hours and 13 hours, respectively. In children aged 6 to 12 years, the mean elimination half-life is 1 hour shorter for d-amphetamine (9 hours) and 2 hours shorter for l-amphetamine (11 hours). Children had higher systemic exposure to amphetamine (C_{max} and AUC) than adults for a given dose of ADDERALL®, which was attributed to the higher dose administered to children on a mg/kg body weight basis compared to adults. Upon dose normalization on a mg/kg basis, children showed 30% less systemic exposure compared to adults.

ADDERALL XR® demonstrates linear pharmacokinetics over the dose range of 20 to 60 mg in adults and 5 to 30 mg in children aged 6 to 12 years. There is no unexpected accumulation at steady state in children.

Food does not affect the extent of absorption of d-amphetamine and l-amphetamine, but prolongs T_{max} by 2.5 hours (from 5.2 hrs at fasted state 7.7 hrs after a high-fat meal) for d-amphetamine and 2.1 hours (from 5.6 hrs at fasted state to 7.7 hrs after a high fat meal) for l-amphetamine after administration of ADDERALL XR® 30 mg. Opening the capsule and sprinkling the contents on applesauce results in comparable absorption to the intact capsule taken in the fasted state. Equal doses of ADDERALL XR® strengths are bioequivalent.

Special Populations

Pediatric Patients

Children eliminated amphetamine faster than adults. The elimination half-life ($t_{1/2}$) is approximately 1 hour shorter for d-amphetamine and 2 hours shorter for l-amphetamine in children than in adults. However, children had higher systemic exposure to amphetamine (C_{max} and AUC) than adults for a given dose of ADDERALL XR®, which was attributed to the higher dose administered to children on a mg/kg body weight basis compared to adults. Upon dose normalization on a mg/kg basis, children showed 30% less systemic exposure compared to adults.

Gender

Systemic exposure to amphetamine was 20-30% higher in women (N=20) than in men (N=20) due to the higher dose administered to women on a mg/kg body weight basis. When the exposure parameters (C_{max} and AUC) were normalized by dose (mg/kg), these differences diminished.

Race

Formal pharmacokinetic studies for race have not been conducted. However, amphetamine pharmacokinetics appeared to be comparable among Caucasians (N=33), Blacks (N=8) and Hispanics (N=10).

Clinical Trials

Children

A double-blind, randomized, placebo-controlled, parallel-group study was conducted in children aged 6-12 (N=584) who met DSM-IV criteria for ADHD (either the combined type or the hyperactive-impulsive type). Patients were randomized to fixed dose treatment groups receiving final doses of 10, 20, or 30 mg of ADDERALL XR® or placebo once daily in the morning for three weeks. Significant improvements in patient behavior, based upon teacher ratings of attention and hyperactivity, were observed for all ADDERALL XR® doses compared to patients who received placebo, for all three weeks, including the first week of treatment, when all ADDERALL XR® subjects were receiving a dose of 10 mg/day. Patients who received ADDERALL XR® showed behavioral improvements in both morning and afternoon assessments compared to patients on placebo.

In a classroom analogue study, patients (N=51) receiving fixed doses of 10 mg, 20 mg or 30 mg ADDERALL XR® demonstrated statistically significant improvements in teacher-rated behavior and performance measures, compared to patients treated with placebo.

Adults

A double-blind, randomized, placebo-controlled, parallel-group study was conducted in adults (N=255) who met DSM-IV-TR criteria for ADHD. Patients were randomized to fixed dose treatment groups receiving final doses of 20, 40, or 60 mg of ADDERALL XR® or placebo once daily in the morning for four weeks. Significant improvements, measured with the Attention Deficit Hyperactivity Disorder-Rating Scale (ADHD-RS), an 18-item scale that measures the core symptoms of ADHD, were observed at endpoint for all ADDERALL XR® doses compared to patients who received placebo for all four weeks. There was not adequate evidence that doses greater than 20 mg/day conferred additional benefit.

INDICATIONS

ADDERALL XR® is indicated for the treatment of Attention Deficit Hyperactivity Disorder (ADHD).

The efficacy of ADDERALL XR® in the treatment of ADHD was established on the basis of two controlled trials in children aged 6 to 12 and one controlled trial in adults who met DSM-IV criteria for ADHD (see CLINICAL PHARMACOLOGY), along with extrapolation from the known efficacy of ADDERALL®, the immediate-release formulation of this substance.

A diagnosis of Attention Deficit Hyperactivity Disorder (ADHD; DSM-IV) implies the presence of hyperactive-impulsive or inattentive symptoms that caused impairment and were present before age 7 years. The symptoms must cause clinically significant impairment, e.g., in social, academic, or occupational functioning, and be present in two or more settings, e.g., school (or work) and at home. The symptoms must not be better accounted for by another mental disorder. For the Inattentive Type, at least six of the following symptoms must have persisted for at least 6 months: lack of attention to details/careless mistakes; lack of sustained attention; poor listener; failure to follow through on tasks; poor organization; avoids tasks requiring sustained mental effort; loses things; easily distracted; forgetful. For the Hyperactive-Impulsive Type, at least six of the following symptoms must have persisted for at least 6 months: fidgeting/squirming; leaving seat; inappropriate running/climbing; difficulty with quiet activities; "on the go;" excessive talking; blurting answers; can't wait turn; intrusive. The Combined Type requires both inattentive and hyperactive-impulsive criteria to be met.

Special Diagnostic Considerations: Specific etiology of this syndrome is unknown, and there is no single diagnostic test. Adequate diagnosis requires the use not only of medical but of special psychological, educational, and social resources. Learning may or may not be impaired. The diagnosis must be based upon a complete history and evaluation of the child and not solely on the presence of the required number of DSM-IV characteristics.

Need for Comprehensive Treatment Program: ADDERALL XR® is indicated as an integral part of a total treatment program for ADHD that may include other measures (psychological, educational, social) for patients with this syndrome. Drug treatment may not be indicated for all children with this syndrome. Stimulants are not intended for use in the child who exhibits symptoms secondary to environmental factors and/or other primary psychiatric disorders, including psychosis. Appropriate educational placement is essential and psychosocial intervention is often helpful. When remedial measures alone are insufficient, the decision to prescribe stimulant medication will depend upon the physician's assessment of the chronicity and severity of the child's symptoms.

Long-Term Use: The effectiveness of ADDERALL XR® for long-term use, i.e., for more than 3 weeks in children and 4 weeks in adults, has not been systematically evaluated in controlled trials. Therefore, the physician who elects to use ADDERALL XR® for extended periods should periodically re-evaluate the long-term usefulness of the drug for the individual patient.

CONTRAINDICATIONS

Advanced arteriosclerosis, symptomatic cardiovascular disease, moderate to severe hypertension, hyperthyroidism, known hypersensitivity or idiosyncrasy to the sympathomimetic amines, glaucoma.

Agitated states.

Patients with a history of drug abuse.

During or within 14 days following the administration of monoamine oxidase inhibitors (hypertensive crises may result).

WARNINGS

Psychosis: Clinical experience suggests that, in psychotic patients, administration of amphetamine may exacerbate symptoms of behavior disturbance and thought disorder.

Long-Term Suppression of Growth: Data are inadequate to determine whether chronic use of stimulants in children, including amphetamine, may be causally associated with suppression of growth. Therefore, growth should be monitored during treatment, and patients who are not growing or gaining weight as expected should have their treatment interrupted.

Sudden Death and Pre-existing Structural Cardiac Abnormalities: Sudden death has been reported in association with amphetamine treatment at usual doses in children with structural cardiac abnormalities. Adderall XR® generally should not be used in children or adults with structural cardiac abnormalities.

PRECAUTIONS

General: The least amount of amphetamine feasible should be prescribed or dispensed at one time in order to minimize the possibility of overdosage.

Hypertension: Caution is to be exercised in prescribing amphetamines for patients with even mild hypertension (see CONTRAINDICATIONS). Blood pressure and pulse should be monitored at appropriate intervals in patients taking ADDERALL XR®, especially patients with hypertension.

Tics: Amphetamines have been reported to exacerbate motor and phonic tics and Tourette's syndrome. Therefore, clinical evaluation for tics and Tourette's syndrome in children and their families should precede use of stimulant medications.

Information for Patients: Amphetamines may impair the ability of the patient to engage in potentially hazardous activities such as operating machinery or vehicles; the patient should therefore be cautioned accordingly.

Drug Interactions: *Acidifying agents*—Gastrointestinal acidifying agents (guanethidine, reserpine, glutamic acid HCl, ascorbic acid, etc.) lower absorption of amphetamines.

Urinary acidifying agents—These agents (ammonium chloride, sodium acid phosphate, etc.) increase the concentration of the ionized species of the amphetamine molecule, thereby increasing urinary excretion. Both groups of agents lower blood levels and efficacy of amphetamines.

Adrenergic blockers—Adrenergic blockers are inhibited by amphetamines.

Alkalinizing agents—Gastrointestinal alkalinizing agents (sodium bicarbonate, etc.) increase absorption of amphetamines. Co-administration of ADDERALL XR® and gastrointestinal alkalinizing agents, such as antacids, should be avoided. Urinary alkalinizing agents (acetazolamide, some thiazides) increase the concentration of the non-ionized species of the amphetamine molecule, thereby decreasing urinary excretion. Both groups of agents increase blood levels and therefore potentiate the actions of amphetamines.

Antidepressants, tricyclic—Amphetamines may enhance the activity of tricyclic antidepressants or sympathomimetic agents; d-amphetamine with desipramine or protriptyline and possibly other tricyclics cause striking and sustained increases in the concentration of d-amphetamine in the brain; cardiovascular effects can be potentiated.

MAO inhibitors—MAOI antidepressants, as well as a metabolite of furazolidone, slow amphetamine metabolism. This slowing potentiates amphetamines, increasing their effect on the release of norepinephrine and other monoamines from adrenergic nerve endings; this can cause headaches and other signs of hypertensive crisis. A variety of toxic neurological effects and malignant hyperpyrexia can occur, sometimes with fatal results.

Antihistamines—Amphetamines may counteract the sedative effect of antihistamines.

Antihypertensives—Amphetamines may antagonize the hypotensive effects of antihypertensives.

Chlorpromazine—Chlorpromazine blocks dopamine and norepinephrine receptors, thus inhibiting the central stimulant effects of amphetamines, and can be used to treat amphetamine poisoning.

Ethosuximide—Amphetamines may delay intestinal absorption of ethosuximide.

Haloperidol—Haloperidol blocks dopamine receptors, thus inhibiting the central stimulant effects of amphetamines.

Lithium carbonate—The anorectic and stimulatory effects of amphetamines may be inhibited by lithium carbonate.

Meperidine—Amphetamines potentiate the analgesic effect of meperidine.

Methenamine therapy—Urinary excretion of amphetamines is increased, and efficacy is reduced, by acidifying agents used in methenamine therapy.

Norepinephrine—Amphetamines enhance the adrenergic effect of norepinephrine.

Phenobarbital—Amphetamines may delay intestinal absorption of phenobarbital; co-administration of phenobarbital may produce a synergistic anticonvulsant action.

Phenytoin—Amphetamines may delay intestinal absorption of phenytoin; co-administration of phenytoin may produce a synergistic anticonvulsant action.

Propoxyphene—In cases of propoxyphene overdosage, amphetamine CNS stimulation is potentiated and fatal convulsions can occur.

Veratrum alkaloids—Amphetamines inhibit the hypotensive effect of veratrum alkaloids.

Drug/Laboratory Test Interactions: Amphetamines can cause a significant elevation in plasma corticosteroid levels. This increase is greatest in the evening. Amphetamines may interfere with urinary steroid determinations.

Carcinogenesis/Mutagenesis and Impairment of Fertility: No evidence of carcinogenicity was found in studies in which d,l-amphetamine (enantiomer ratio of 1:1) was administered to mice and rats in the diet for 2 years at doses of up to 30 mg/kg/day in male mice, 19 mg/kg/day in female mice, and 5 mg/kg/day in male and female rats. These doses are approximately 2.4, 1.5, and 0.8 times, respectively, the maximum recommended human dose of 30 mg/day [child] on a mg/m^2 body surface area basis.

Amphetamine, in the enantiomer ratio present in ADDERALL® (immediate-release)(d- to l- ratio of 3:1), was not clastogenic in the mouse bone marrow micronucleus test *in vivo* and was negative when tested in the E. coli component of the Ames test *in vitro*. d,l-Amphetamine (1:1 enantiomer ratio) has been reported to produce a positive response in the mouse bone marrow micronucleus test, an equivocal response in the Ames test, and negative responses in the *in vitro* sister chromatid exchange and chromosomal aberration assays.

Amphetamine, in the enantiomer ratio present in ADDERALL® (immediate-release)(d- to l- ratio of 3:1), did not adversely affect fertility or early embryonic development in the rat at doses of up to 20 mg/kg/day (approximately 5 times the maximum recommended human dose of 30 mg/day on a mg/m^2 body surface area basis).

Pregnancy: Pregnancy Category C. Amphetamine, in the enantiomer ratio present in ADDERALL® (d- to l- ratio of 3:1), had no apparent effects on embryofetal morphological development or survival when orally administered to pregnant rats and rabbits throughout the period of organogenesis at doses of up to 6 and 16 mg/kg/day, respectively. These doses are approximately 1.5 and 8 times, respectively, the maximum recommended human dose of 30 mg/day [child] on a mg/m^2 body surface area basis. Fetal malformations and death have been reported in mice following parenteral administration of d-amphetamine doses of 50 mg/kg/day (approximately 6 times that of a human dose of 30 mg/day [child] on a mg/m^2 basis) or greater to pregnant animals. Administration of these doses was also associated with severe maternal toxicity.

A number of studies in rodents indicate that prenatal or early postnatal exposure to amphetamine (d- or d,l-), at doses similar to those used clinically, can result in long-term neurochemical and behavioral alterations. Reported behavioral effects include learning and memory deficits, altered locomotor activity, and changes in sexual function.

There are no adequate and well-controlled studies in pregnant women. There has been one report of severe congenital bony deformity, tracheo-esophageal fistula, and anal atresia (vater association) in a baby born to a woman who took dextroamphetamine sulfate with lovastatin during the first trimester of pregnancy. Amphetamines should be used during pregnancy only if the potential benefit justifies the potential risk to the fetus.

Nonteratogenic Effects: Infants born to mothers dependent on amphetamines have an increased risk of premature delivery and low birth weight. Also, these infants may experience symptoms of withdrawal as demonstrated by dysphoria, including agitation, and significant lassitude.

Usage in Nursing Mothers: Amphetamines are excreted in human milk. Mothers taking amphetamines should be advised to refrain from nursing.

Pediatric Use: ADDERALL XR® is indicated for use in children 6 years of age and older.

Use in Children Under Six Years of Age: Effects of ADDERALL XR® in 3-5 year olds have not been studied. Long-term effects of amphetamines in children have not been well established. Amphetamines are not recommended for use in children under 3 years of age.

Geriatric Use: ADDERALL XR® has not been studied in the geriatric population.

ADVERSE EVENTS

The premarketing development program for ADDERALL XR® included exposures in a total of 965 participants in clinical trials (635 pediatric patients, 248 adult patients, and 82 healthy adult subjects). Of these, 635 patients (ages 6 to 12) were evaluated in two controlled clinical studies, and one open-label clinical study, and two single-dose clinical pharmacology studies (N= 40). Safety data on all patients are included in the discussion that follows. Adverse reactions were assessed by collecting adverse events, results of physical examinations, vital signs, weights, laboratory analyses, and ECGs.

Adverse events during exposure were obtained primarily by general inquiry and recorded by clinical investigators using terminology of their own choosing. Consequently, it is not possible to provide a meaningful estimate of the proportion of individuals experiencing adverse events without first grouping similar types of events into a smaller number of standardized event categories. In the tables and listings that follow, COSTART terminology has been used to classify reported adverse events.

Table 1 Adverse Events Reported by More Than 1% of Pediatric Patients Receiving ADDERALL XR® with Higher Incidence Than on Placebo in a 584 Patient Clinical Study

Body System	Preferred Term	ADDERALL XR® (n=374)	Placebo (n=210)
General	Abdominal Pain (stomachache)	14%	10%
	Accidental injury	3%	2%
	Asthenia (fatigue)	2%	0%
	Fever	5%	2%
	Infection	4%	2%
	Viral Infection	2%	0%
Digestive System	Loss of Appetite	22%	2%
	Diarrhea	2%	1%
	Dyspepsia	2%	1%
	Nausea	5%	3%
	Vomiting	7%	4%
Nervous System	Dizziness	2%	0%
	Emotional Lability	9%	2%
	Insomnia	17%	2%
	Nervousness	6%	2%
Metabolic/Nutritional	Weight Loss	4%	0%

Table 2 Adverse Events Reported by 5% or More of Adults Receiving ADDERALL XR® with Higher Incidence Than on Placebo in a 255 Patient Clinical Forced Weekly-Dose Titration Study*

Body System	Preferred Term	ADDERALL XR® (n=191)	Placebo (n=64)
General	Asthenia	6%	5%
	Headache	26%	13%
Digestive System	Loss of Appetite	33%	3%
	Diarrhea	6%	0%
	Dry Mouth	35%	5%
	Nausea	8%	3%
Nervous System	Agitation	8%	5%
	Anxiety	8%	5%
	Dizziness	7%	0%
	Insomnia	27%	13%
Cardiovascular System	Tachycardia	6%	3%
Metabolic/Nutritional	Weight Loss	11%	0%
Urogenital System	Urinary Tract Infection	5%	0%

Note: The following events did not meet the criterion for inclusion in Table 2 but were reported by 2% to 4% of adult patients receiving ADDERALL XR® with a higher incidence than patients receiving placebo in this study: infection, photosensitivity reaction, constipation, tooth disorder, emotional lability, libdo decreased, somnolence, speech disorder, palpitation, twitching, dyspnea, sweating, dysmenorrhea, and impotence.

*included doses up to 60 mg.

The stated frequencies of adverse events represent the proportion of individuals who experienced, at least once, a treatment-emergent adverse event of the type listed.

Adverse events associated with discontinuation of treatment: In two placebo-controlled studies of up to 5 weeks duration among children with ADHD, 2.4% (10/425) of ADDERALL XR® treated patients discontinued due to adverse events (including 3 patients with loss of appetite, one of whom also reported insomnia) compared to 2.7% (7/259) receiving placebo. The most frequent adverse events associated with discontinuation of ADDERALL XR® in controlled and uncontrolled, multiple-dose clinical trials of pediatric patients (N=595) are presented below. Over half of these patients were exposed to ADDERALL XR® for 12 months or more.

Adverse event	% of patients discontinuing (N=595)
Anorexia (loss of appetite)	2.9
Insomnia	1.5
Weight loss	1.2
Emotional lability	1.0
Depression	0.7

In one placebo-controlled 4-week study among adults with ADHD, patients who discontinued treatment due to adverse events among ADDERALL XR®-treated patients (N=191) were 3.1% (n=6) for nervousness including anxiety and irritability, 2.6% (n=5) for insomnia, 1% (n=2) each for headache, palpitation, and somnolence; and, 0.5% (n=1) each for ALT increase, agitation, chest pain, cocaine craving, elevated blood pressure, and weight loss.

Adverse events occurring in a controlled trial: Adverse events reported in a 3-week clinical trial of pediatric patients and a 4-week clinical trial in adults treated with ADDERALL XR® or placebo are presented in the tables below.

The prescriber should be aware that these figures cannot be used to predict the incidence of adverse events in the course of usual medical practice where patient characteristics and other factors differ from those which prevailed in the clinical trials. Similarly, the cited frequencies cannot be compared with figures obtained from other clinical investigations involving different treatments, uses, and investigators. The cited figures, however, do provide the prescribing physician with some basis for estimating the relative contribution of drug and non-drug factors to the adverse event incidence rate in the population studied.

[See table 1 above]
[See table 2 above]

The following adverse reactions adverse reactions have been associated with amphetamine use:

Cardiovascular: Palpitations, tachycardia, elevation of blood pressure, sudden death, myocardial infarction. There have been isolated reports of cardiomyopathy associated with chronic amphetamine use.

Central Nervous System: Psychotic episodes at recommended doses, overstimulation, restlessness, dizziness, insomnia, euphoria, dyskinesia, dysphoria, depression, tremor, headache, exacerbation of motor and phonic tics and Tourette's syndrome, seizures, stroke.

Gastrointestinal: Dryness of the mouth, unpleasant taste, diarrhea, constipation, other gastrointestinal disturbances. Anorexia and weight loss may occur as undesirable effects.

Allergic: Urticaria.

Endocrine: Impotence, changes in libido.

DRUG ABUSE AND DEPENDENCE

ADDERALL XR® is a Schedule II controlled substance. Amphetamines have been extensively abused. Tolerance, extreme psychological dependence, and severe social disability have occurred. There are reports of patients who have increased the dosage to many times that recommended. Abrupt cessation following prolonged high dosage administration results in extreme fatigue and mental depression; changes are also noted on the sleep EEG. Manifestations of chronic intoxication with amphetamines may include severe dermatoses, marked insomnia, irritability, hyperactivity, and personality changes. The most severe manifestation of chronic intoxication is psychosis, often clinically indistinguishable from schizophrenia.

OVERDOSAGE

Individual patient response to amphetamines varies widely. Toxic symptoms may occur idiosyncratically at low doses.

Symptoms: Manifestations of acute overdosage with amphetamines include restlessness, tremor, hyperreflexia, rapid respiration, confusion, assaultiveness, hallucinations,

Continued on next page

Adderall XR—Cont.

panic states, hyperpyrexia and rhabdomyolysis. Fatigue and depression usually follow the central nervous system stimulation. Cardiovascular effects include arrhythmias, hypertension or hypotension and circulatory collapse. Gastrointestinal symptoms include nausea, vomiting, diarrhea, and abdominal cramps. Fatal poisoning is usually preceded by convulsions and coma.

Treatment: Consult with a Certified Poison Control Center for up to date guidance and advice. Management of acute amphetamine intoxication is largely symptomatic and includes gastric lavage, administration of activated charcoal, administration of a cathartic and sedation. Experience with hemodialysis or peritoneal dialysis is inadequate to permit recommendation in this regard. Acidification of the urine increases amphetamine excretion, but is believed to increase risk of acute renal failure if myoglobinuria is present. If acute severe hypertension complicates amphetamine overdosage, administration of intravenous phentolamine has been suggested. However, a gradual drop in blood pressure will usually result when sufficient sedation has been achieved. Chlorpromazine antagonizes the central stimulant effects of amphetamines and can be used to treat amphetamine intoxication.

The prolonged release of mixed amphetamine salts from ADDERALL XR® should be considered when treating patients with overdose.

DOSAGE AND ADMINISTRATION

Dosage should be individualized according to the therapeutic needs and response of the patient. ADDERALL XR® should be administered at the lowest effective dosage.

Children

In children with ADHD who are 6 years of age and older and are either starting treatment for the first time or switching from another medication, start with 10 mg once daily in the morning; daily dosage may be adjusted in increments of 5 mg or 10 mg at weekly intervals. When in the judgment of the clinician a lower initial dose is appropriate, patients may begin treatment with 5 mg once daily in the morning. The maximum recommended dose for children is 30 mg/day; doses greater than 30 mg/day of ADDERALL XR® have not been studied in children. Amphetamines are not recommended for children under 3 years of age. ADDERALL XR® has not been studied in children under 6 years of age.

Adults

In adults with ADHD who are either starting treatment for the first time or switching from medication, the recommended dose is 20 mg/day.

Patients Currently Using ADDERALL®—Based on bioequivalence data, patients taking divided doses of immediate-release for example twice a day, may be switched to ADDERALL XR® at the same total daily dose taken once daily. Titrate at weekly intervals to appropriate efficacy and tolerability as indicated.

ADDERALL XR® capsules may be taken whole, or the capsule may be opened and the entire contents sprinkled on applesauce. If the patient is using the sprinkle administration method, the sprinkled applesauce should be consumed immediately; it should not be stored. Patients should take the applesauce with sprinkled beads in its entirety without chewing. The dose of a single capsule should not be divided. The contents of the entire capsule should be taken, and patients should not take anything less than one capsule per day.

ADDERALL XR® may be taken with or without food.

ADDERALL XR® should be given upon awakening. Afternoon doses should be avoided because of the potential for insomnia.

Where possible, drug administration should be interrupted occasionally to determine if there is a recurrence of behavioral symptoms sufficient to require continued therapy.

HOW SUPPLIED

ADDERALL XR® 5 mg Capsules: Clear/blue (imprinted ADDERALL XR 5 mg), bottles of 100, NDC 54092-381-01

ADDERALL XR® 10 mg Capsules: Blue/blue (imprinted ADDERALL XR 10 mg), bottles of 100, NDC 54092-383-01

ADDERALL XR® 15 mg Capsules: Blue/white (imprinted ADDERALL XR 15 mg), bottles of 100, NDC 54092-385-01

ADDERALL XR® 20 mg Capsules: Orange/orange (imprinted ADDERALL XR 20 mg), bottles of 100, NDC 54092-387-01

ADDERALL XR® 25 mg Capsules: Orange/white (imprinted ADDERALL XR 25 mg), bottles of 100, NDC 54092-389-01

ADDERALL XR® 30 mg Capsules: Natural/orange (imprinted ADDERALL XR 30 mg), bottles of 100, NDC 54092-391-01

Dispense in a tight, light-resistant container as defined in the USP.

Store at 25° C (77° F). Excursions permitted to 15-30°C (59-86° F) [see USP Controlled Room Temperature]

ANIMAL TOXICOLOGY

Acute administration of high doses of amphetamine (d- or d,l-) has been shown to produce long-lasting neurotoxic effects, including irreversible nerve fiber damage, in rodents. The significance of these findings to humans is unknown.

Manufactured for Shire US Inc., Newport, KY 41071

For more information call 1-800-828-2088 or visit www.adderallxr.com

Made in USA

001268
381 0107 005 Rev. 11/04

AGRYLIN® ℞

[ă-grĭ-lĭn]
(anagrelide hydrochloride)
Capsules
Rx only

Prescribing information for this product, which appears on pages 3134–3136 of the 2005 PDR, has been completely revised as follows. Please write "See Supplement A" next to the product heading.

DESCRIPTION

Name: AGRYLIN® (anagrelide hydrochloride)
Dosage Form: 0.5 mg and 1 mg capsules for oral administration
Active Ingredient: AGRYLIN® Capsules contain either 0.5 mg or 1 mg of anagrelide base (as anagrelide hydrochloride).
Inactive Ingredients: Anhydrous Lactose NF, Crospovidone NF, Lactose Monohydrate NF, Magnesium stearate NF, Microcrystalline cellulose NF, Povidone USP.
Pharmacological Classification: Platelet-reducing agent.
Chemical Name: 6,7-dichloro-1,5-dihydroimidazo[2,1-b]quinazolin-2(3H)-one monohydrochloride monohydrate.
Molecular formula: $C_{10}H_7Cl_2N_3O \bullet HCl \bullet H_2O$
Molecular weight: 310.55
Structural formula:

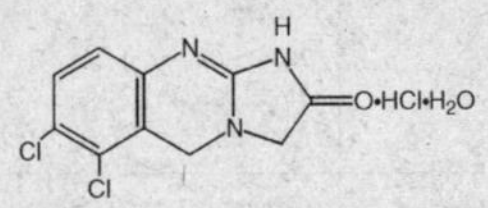

Appearance: Off-white powder.
Solubility: Water .... Very slightly soluble
Dimethyl Sulfoxide .... Sparingly soluble
Dimethylformamide .... Sparingly soluble

CLINICAL PHARMACOLOGY

The mechanism by which anagrelide reduces blood platelet count is still under investigation. Studies in patients support a hypothesis of dose-related reduction in platelet production resulting from a decrease in megakaryocyte hypermaturation. In blood withdrawn from normal volunteers treated with anagrelide, a disruption was found in the postmitotic phase of megakaryocyte development and a reduction in megakaryocyte size and ploidy. At therapeutic doses, anagrelide does not produce significant changes in white cell counts or coagulation parameters, and may have a small, but clinically insignificant effect on red cell parameters. Anagrelide inhibits cyclic AMP phosphodiesterase III (PDEIII). PDEIII inhibitors can also inhibit platelet aggregation. However, significant inhibition of platelet aggregation is observed only at doses of anagrelide higher than those required to reduce platelet count.

Following oral administration of ^{14}C-anagrelide in people, more than 70% of radioactivity was recovered in urine. Based on limited data, there appears to be a trend toward dose linearity between doses of 0.5 mg and 2.0 mg. At fasting and at a dose of 0.5 mg of anagrelide, the plasma half-life is 1.3 hours. The available plasma concentration time data at steady state in patients showed that anagrelide does not accumulate in plasma after repeated administration. Two major metabolites have been identified (RL603 and 3-hydroxy anagrelide).

There were no apparent differences between patient groups (pediatric versus adult patients) for t_{max} and $t_{1/2}$ for anagrelide, 3-hydroxy anagrelide, or RL603.

Pharmacokinetic data obtained from healthy volunteers comparing the pharmacokinetics of anagrelide in the fed and fasted states showed that administration of a 1 mg dose of anagrelide with food decreased the C_{max} by 14%, but increased the AUC by 20%.

Pharmacokinetic (PK) data from pediatric (age range 7-14 years) and adult (age range 16-86 years) patients with thrombocythemia secondary to a myeloproliferative disorder (MPD), indicate that dose and body weight-normalized exposure, C_{max} and AUC_t, of anagrelide were lower in the pediatric patients compared to the adult patients (C_{max} 48%, AUC_t 55%).

A pharmacokinetic study at a single dose of 1 mg anagrelide in subjects with severe renal impairment (creatinine clearance <30ml/min) showed no significant effects on the pharmacokinetics of anagrelide.

A pharmacokinetic study at a single dose of 1 mg anagrelide in subjects with moderate hepatic impairment showed an 8-fold increase in total exposure (AUC) to anagrelide.

CLINICAL STUDIES

A total of 942 patients with myeloproliferative disorders including 551 patients with Essential Thrombocythemia (ET), 117 patients with Polycythemia Vera (PV), 178 patients with Chronic Myelogenous Leukemia (CML), and 96 patients with other myeloproliferative disorders (OMPD), were treated with anagrelide in three clinical trials. Patients with OMPD included 87 patients who had Myeloid Metaplasia with Myelofibrosis (MMM), and 9 patients who had unknown myeloproliferative disorders.

Clinical Studies

Patients with ET, PV, CML, or MMM were diagnosed based on the following criteria:

[See table below]

Patients were enrolled in clinical trials if their platelet count was ≥ 900,000/µL on two occasions or ≥ 650,000/µL on two occasions with documentation of symptoms associated with thrombocythemia. The mean duration of anagrelide therapy for ET, PV, CML, and OMPD patients was 65, 67, 40, and 44 weeks, respectively; 23% of patients received treatment for 2 years. Patients were treated with anagrelide starting at doses of 0.5-2.0 mg every 6 hours. The dose was increased if the platelet count was still high, but to no more than 12 mg each day. Efficacy was defined as reduction of platelet count to or near physiologic levels (150,000-400,000/µL). The criteria for defining subjects as "responders" were reduction in platelets for at least 4 weeks to ≤600,000/µL, or by at least 50% from baseline value. Subjects treated for less than 4 weeks were not considered evaluable. The results are depicted graphically below:

Patients with Thrombocytosis Secondary to Myeloproliferative Disorders: Mean Platelet Count During Anagrelide Therapy

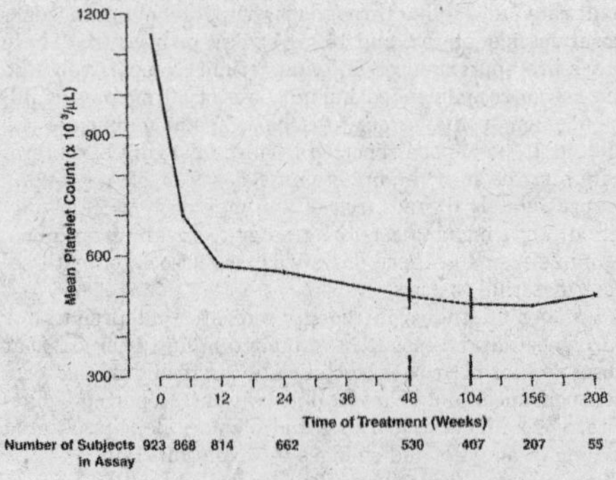

	Time on Treatment						
	Weeks				Years		
Baseline	4	12	24	48	2	3	4
Mean* 1131	683	575	526	484	460	437	457
N 923†	868	814	662	530	407	207	55

*x 10³/µL

† Nine hundred and forty-two subjects with myeloproliferative disorders were enrolled in three research studies. Of these, 923 had platelet counts over the duration of the studies.

AGRYLIN® was effective in phlebotomized patients as well as in patients treated with other concomitant therapies including hydroxyurea, aspirin, interferon, radioactive phosphorus, and alkylating agents.

INDICATIONS AND USAGE

AGRYLIN® Capsules are indicated for the treatment of patients with thrombocythemia, secondary to myeloproliferative disorders, to reduce the elevated platelet count and the risk of thrombosis and to ameliorate associated symptoms including thrombo-hemorrhagic events (see CLINICAL STUDIES, DOSAGE and ADMINISTRATION).

ET

- Platelet count ≥ 900,000/µL on two determinations
- Profound megakaryocytic hyperplasia in bone marrow
- Absence of Philadelphia chromosome
- Normal red cell mass
- Normal serum iron and ferritin and normal marrow iron stores

CML

- Persistent granulocyte count ≥ 50,000/µL without evidence of infection
- Absolute basophil count ≥ 100/µL
- Evidence for hyperplasia of the granulocytic line in the bone marrow
- Philadelphia chromosome is present
- Leucocyte alkaline phophatase ≤ lower limit of the laboratory normal range

PV†

- A1 Increased red cell mass
- A2 Normal arterial oxygen saturation
- A3 Splenomegaly
- B1 Platelet count ≥ 400,000/µL, in absence of iron deficiency or bleeding
- B2 Leucocytosis (≥ 12,000/µL, in the absence of infection)
- B3 Elevated leucocyte alkaline phosphatase
- B4 Elevated Serum B_{12}

†Diagnosis positive if A1, A2, and A3 present; or, if no splenomegaly, diagnosis is positive if A1 and A2 are present with any two of B1, B2, or B3.

MMM

- Myelofibrotic (hypocellular, fibrotic) bone marrow
- Prominent megakaryocytic metaplasia in bone marrow
- Splenomegaly
- Moderate to severe normochromic normocytic anemia
- White cell count may be variable; (80,000-100,000/µL)
- Increased platelet count
- Variable red cell mass; teardrop poikilocytes
- Normal to high leucocyte alkaline phosphatase
- Absence of Philadelphia chromosome

CONTRAINDICATIONS

Anagrelide is contraindicated in patients with severe hepatic impairment. Exposure to anagrelide is increased 8-fold in patients with moderate hepatic impairment (See CLINICAL PHARMACOLOGY). Use of anagrelide in patients with severe hepatic impairment has not been studied. (See also WARNINGS: Hepatic Impairment).

WARNINGS

Cardiovascular

Anagrelide should be used with caution in patients with known or suspected heart disease, and only if the potential benefits of therapy outweigh the potential risks. Because of the positive inotropic effects and side-effects of anagrelide, a pre-treatment cardiovascular examination is recommended along with careful monitoring during treatment. In humans, therapeutic doses of anagrelide may cause cardiovascular effects, including vasodilation, tachycardia, palpitations, and congestive heart failure.

Hepatic

Exposure to anagrelide is increased 8-fold in patients with moderate hepatic impairment (See CLINICAL PHARMACOLOGY). Use of anagrelide in patients with severe hepatic impairment has not been studied. The potential risks and benefits of anagrelide therapy in a patient with mild and moderate impairment of hepatic function should be assessed before treatment is commenced. In patients with moderate hepatic impairment, dose reduction is required and patients should be carefully monitored for cardiovascular effects (See DOSAGE AND ADMINISTRATION for specific dosing recommendations).

PRECAUTIONS

Laboratory Tests: Anagrelide therapy requires close clinical supervision of the patient. While the platelet count is being lowered (usually during the first two weeks of treatment), blood counts (hemoglobin, white blood cells), liver function (SGOT, SGPT) and renal function (serum creatinine, BUN) should be monitored. In 9 subjects receiving a single 5 mg dose of anagrelide, standing blood pressure fell an average of 22/15 mm Hg, usually accompanied by dizziness. Only minimal changes in blood pressure were observed following a dose of 2 mg.

Cessation of AGRYLIN® Treatment: In general, interruption of anagrelide treatment is followed by an increase in platelet count. After sudden stoppage of anagrelide therapy, the increase in platelet count can be observed within four days.

Drug Interactions: Limited PK and/or PD studies investigating possible interactions between anagrelide and other medicinal products have been conducted. *In vivo* interaction studies in humans have demonstrated that digoxin and warfarin do not affect the PK properties of anagrelide, nor does anagrelide affect the PK properties of digoxin or warfarin.

Although additional drug interaction studies have not been conducted, the most common medications used concomitantly with anagrelide in clinical trials were aspirin, acetaminophen, furosemide, iron, ranitidine, hydroxyurea, and allopurinol. There is no clinical evidence to suggest that anagrelide interacts with any of these compounds.

An *in vivo* interaction study in humans demonstrated that a single 1mg dose of anagrelide administered concomitantly with a single 900 mg dose of aspirin was generally well tolerated. There was no effect on bleeding time, PT or aPTT. No clinically relevant pharmacokinetic interactions between anagrelide and acetylsalicylic acid were observed. In that same study, aspirin alone produced a marked inhibition in platelet aggregation *ex vivo*. Anagrelide alone had no effect on platelet aggregation, but did slightly enhance the inhibition of platelet aggregation by aspirin.

Anagrelide is metabolized at least in part by CYP1A2. It is known that CYP1A2 is inhibited by several medicinal products, including fluvoxamine, and such medicinal products could theoretically adversely influence the clearance of anagrelide. Anagrelide demonstrates some limited inhibitory activity towards CYP1A2 which may present a theoretical potential for interaction with other co-administered medicinal products sharing that clearance mechanism e.g. theophylline.

Anagrelide is an inhibitor of cyclic AMP PDE III. The effects of medicinal products with similar properties such as inotropes milrinone, enoximone, amrinone, olprinone and cilostazol may be exacerbated by anagrelide.

There is a single case report which suggests that sucralfate may interfere with anagrelide absorption.

Food has no clinically significant effect on the bioavailability of anagrelide.

Carcinogenesis, Mutagenesis, Impairment of Fertility: No long-term studies in animals have been performed to evaluate carcinogenic potential of anagrelide hydrochloride. Anagrelide hydrochloride was not genotoxic in the Ames test, the mouse lymphoma cell (L5178Y, $TK^{+/-}$) forward mutation test, the human lymphocyte chromosome aberration test, or the mouse micronucleus test. Anagrelide hydrochloride at oral doses up to 240 mg/kg/day (1,440 mg/m^2/day, 195 times the recommended maximum human dose based on body surface area) was found to have no effect on fertility and reproductive performance of male rats. However, in female rats, at oral doses of 60 mg/kg/day (360 mg/m^2/day, 49 times the recommended maximum human dose based on body surface area) or higher, it disrupted implantation when administered in early pregnancy and retarded or blocked parturition when administered in late pregnancy.

Pregnancy: Pregnancy Category C.

(i) Teratogenic Effects

Teratology studies have been performed in pregnant rats at oral doses up to 900 mg/kg/day (5,400 mg/m^2/day, 730 times the recommended maximum human dose based on body surface area) and in pregnant rabbits at oral doses up to 20 mg/kg/day (240 mg/m^2/day, 32 times the recommended maximum human dose based on body surface area) and have revealed no evidence of impaired fertility or harm to the fetus due to anagrelide hydrochloride.

(ii) Nonteratogenic Effects

A fertility and reproductive performance study performed in female rats revealed that anagrelide hydrochloride at oral doses of 60 mg/kg/day (360 mg/m^2/day, 49 times the recommended maximum human dose based on body surface area) or higher disrupted implantation and exerted adverse effect on embryo/fetal survival.

A perinatal and postnatal study performed in female rats revealed that anagrelide hydrochloride at oral doses of 60 mg/kg/day (360 mg/m^2/day, 49 times the recommended maximum human dose based on body surface area) or higher produced delay or blockage of parturition, deaths of nondelivering pregnant dams and their fully developed fetuses, and increased mortality in the pups born.

Five women became pregnant while on anagrelide treatment at doses of 1 to 4 mg/day. Treatment was stopped as soon as it was realized that they were pregnant. All delivered normal, healthy babies. There are no adequate and well-controlled studies in pregnant women.

Anagrelide hydrochloride should be used during pregnancy only if the potential benefit justifies the potential risk to the fetus.

Anagrelide is not recommended in women who are or may become pregnant. If this drug is used during pregnancy, or if the patient becomes pregnant while taking this drug, the patient should be apprised of the potential harm to the fetus. Women of child-bearing potential should be instructed that they must not be pregnant and that they should use contraception while taking anagrelide. Anagrelide may cause fetal harm when administered to a pregnant woman.

Nursing Mothers: It is not known whether this drug is excreted in human milk. Because many drugs are excreted in human milk and because of the potential for serious adverse reaction in nursing infants from anagrelide hydrochloride, a decision should be made whether to discontinue nursing or to discontinue the drug, taking into account the importance of the drug to the mother.

Pediatric Use: Myeloproliferative disorders are uncommon in pediatric patients and limited data are available in this population. An open label safety and PK/PD study (See Clinical Pharmacology section) was conducted in 17 pediatric patients 7-14 years of age (8 patients 7-11 years of age and 9 patients 11-14 years of age, mean age of 11 years; 8 males and 9 females) with thrombocythemia secondary to ET as compared to 18 adult patients (mean age of 63 years, 9 males and 9 females). Prior to entry on to the study, 16 of 17 pediatric patients and 13 of 18 adult patients had received anagrelide treatment for an average of 2 years. The median starting total daily dose, determined by retrospective chart review, for pediatric and adult ET patients who had received anagrelide prior to study entry was 1mg for each of the three age groups (7-11 and 11-14 year old patients and adults). The starting dose for 6 anagrelide-naive patients at study entry was 0.5mg once daily. At study completion, the median total daily maintenance doses were similar across age groups, median of 1.75mg for patients of 7-11 years of age, 2mg in patients 11-14 years of age, and 1.5mg for adults.

The study evaluated the pharmacokinetic (PK) and pharmacodynamic (PD) profile of anagrelide, including platelet counts (See Clinical Pharmacology section).

The frequency of adverse events observed in pediatric patients was similar to adult patients. The most common adverse events observed in pediatric patients were fever, epistaxis, headache, and fatigue during a 3-months treatment of anagrelide in the study. Adverse events that had been reported in these pediatric patients prior to the study and were considered to be related to anagrelide treatment based on retrospective review were palpitation, headache, nausea, vomiting, abdominal pain, back pain, anorexia, fatigue, and muscle cramps. Episodes of increased pulse rate and decreased systolic or diastolic blood pressure beyond the normal ranges in the absence of clinical symptoms were observed in some patients. Reported AEs were consistent with the known pharmacological profile of anagrelide and the underlying disease. There were no apparent trends or differences in the types of adverse events observed between the pediatric patients compared with those of the adult patients. No overall difference in dosing and safety were observed between pediatric and adult patients.

In another open-label study, anagrelide had been used successfully in 12 pediatric patients (age range 6.8 to 17.4 years; 6 male and 6 female), including 8 patients with ET, 2 patients with CML, 1 patient with PV, and 1 patient with OMPD. Patients were started on therapy with 0.5 mg qid up to a maximum daily dose of 10 mg. The median duration of treatment was 18.1 months with a range of 3.1 to 92 months. Three patients received treatment for greater than three years. Other adverse events reported in spontaneous reports and literature reviews include anemia, cutaneous photosensitivity and elevated leukocyte count.

Geriatric Use: Of the total number of subjects in clinical studies of **AGRYLIN®**, 42.1% were 65 years and over, while 14.9% were 75 years and over. No overall differences in safety or effectiveness were observed between these subjects and younger subjects, and other reported clinical experience has not identified differences in response between the elderly and younger patients, but greater sensitivity of some older individuals cannot be ruled out.

ADVERSE REACTIONS

Analysis of the adverse events in a population consisting of 942 patients in 3 clinical studies diagnosed with myeloproliferataive diseases of varying etiology (ET: 551; PV: 117; OMPD: 274) has shown that all disease groups have the same adverse event profile. While most reported adverse events during anagrelide therapy have been mild in intensity and have decreased in frequency with continued therapy, serious adverse events were reported in these patients. These include the following: congestive heart failure, myocardial infarction, cardiomyopathy, cardiomegaly, complete heart block, atrial fibrillation, cerebrovascular accident, pericarditis, pericardial effusion, pleural effusion, pulmonary infiltrates, pulmonary fibrosis, pulmonary hypertension, pancreatitis, gastric/duodenal ulceration, and seizure.

Of the 942 patients treated with anagrelide for a mean duration of approximately 65 weeks, 161 (17%) were discontinued from the study because of adverse events or abnormal laboratory test results. The most common adverse events for treatment discontinuation were headache, diarrhea, edema, palpitation, and abdominal pain. Overall, the occurrence rate of all adverse events was 17.9 per 1,000 treatment days. The occurrence rate of adverse events increased at higher dosages of anagrelide.

The most frequently reported adverse reactions to anagrelide (in 5% or greater of 942 patients with myeloproliferative disease) in clinical trials were:

Headache	43.5%
Palpitations	26.1%
Diarrhea	25.7%
Asthenia	23.1%
Edema, other	20.6%
Nausea	17.1%
Abdominal Pain	16.4%
Dizziness	15.4%
Pain, other	15.0%
Dyspnea	11.9%
Flatulence	10.2%
Vomiting	9.7%
Fever	8.9%
Peripheral Edema	8.5%
Rash, including urticaria	8.3%
Chest Pain	7.8%
Anorexia	7.7%
Tachycardia	7.5%
Pharyngitis	6.8%
Malaise	6.4%
Cough	6.3%
Paresthesia	5.9%
Back Pain	5.9%
Pruritus	5.5%
Dyspepsia	5.2%

Adverse events with an incidence of 1% to < 5% included:

Body as a Whole System: Flu symptoms, chills, photosensitivity.

Cardiovascular System: Arrhythmia, hemorrhage, hypertension, cardiovascular disease, angina pectoris, heart failure, postural hypotension, thrombosis, vasodilatation, migraine, syncope.

Digestive System: Constipation, GI distress, GI hemorrhage, gastritis, melena, aphthous stomatitis, eructation.

Hemic & Lymphatic System: Anemia, thrombocytopenia, ecchymosis, lymphadenopathy.

Platelet counts below 100,000/µL occurred in 84 patients (ET: 35; PV: 9; OMPD: 40), reduction below 50,000/µL occurred in 44 patients (ET: 7; PV: 6; OMPD: 31) while on anagrelide therapy. Thrombocytopenia promptly recovered upon discontinuation of anagrelide.

Hepatic System: Elevated liver enzymes were observed in 3 patients (ET: 2; OMPD: 1) during anagrelide therapy.

Musculoskeletal System: Arthralgia, myalgia, leg cramps.

Nervous System: Depression, somnolence, confusion, insomnia, nervousness, amnesia.

Nutritional Disorders: Dehydration.

Respiratory System: Rhinitis, epistaxis, respiratory disease, sinusitis, pneumonia, bronchitis, asthma.

Skin and Appendages System: Skin disease, alopecia.

Special Senses: Amblyopia, abnormal vision, tinnitus, visual field abnormality, diplopia.

Urogenital System: Dysuria, hematuria.

Renal abnormalities occurred in 15 patients (ET: 10; PV: 4; OMPD: 1). Six ET, 4 PV and 1 with OMPD experienced renal failure (approximately 1%) while on anagrelide treatment; in 4 cases, the renal failure was considered to be possibly related to anagrelide treatment. The remaining 11 were found to have pre-existing renal impairment. Doses ranged from 1.5-6.0 mg/day, with exposure periods of 2 to 12 months. No dose adjustment was required because of renal insufficiency.

The adverse event profile for patients in three clinical trials on anagrelide therapy (in 5% or greater of 942 patients with

Continued on next page

Agrylin—Cont.

myeloproliferative diseases) is shown in the following bar graph:

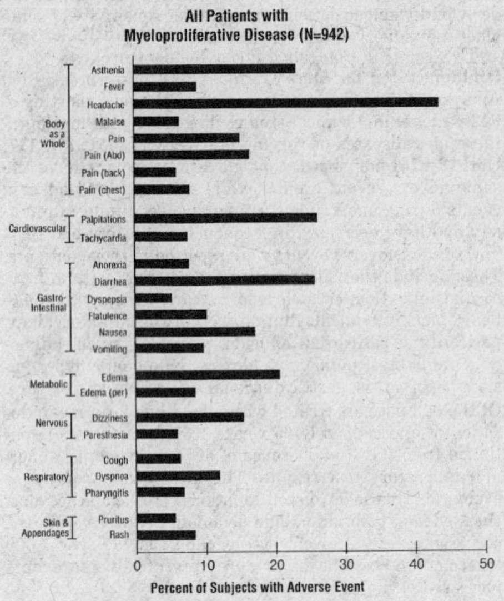
All Patients with
Myeloproliferative Disease (N=942)
Body as a Whole
Asthenia
Fever
Headache
Malaise
Pain
Pain (Abd)
Pain (back)
Pain (chest)
Cardiovascular
Palpitations
Tachycardia
Gastro-Intestinal
Anorexia
Diarrhea
Dyspepsia
Flatulence
Nausea
Vomiting
Metabolic
Edema
Edema (per)
Nervous
Dizziness
Paresthesia
Respiratory
Cough
Dyspnea
Pharyngitis
Skin & Appendages
Pruritus
Rash
0
10
20
30
40
50
Percent of Subjects with Adverse Event

OVERDOSAGE

Acute Toxicity and Symptoms

Single oral doses of anagrelide hydrochloride at 2,500, 1,500 and 200 mg/kg in mice, rats and monkeys, respectively, were not lethal. Symptoms of acute toxicity were: decreased motor activity in mice and rats and softened stools and decreased appetite in monkeys.

There are no reports of overdosage with anagrelide hydrochloride. Platelet reduction from anagrelide therapy is dose-related; therefore, thrombocytopenia, which can potentially cause bleeding, is expected from overdosage. Should overdosage occur, cardiac and central nervous system toxicity can also be expected.

Management and Treatment

In case of overdosage, close clinical supervision of the patient is required; this especially includes monitoring of the platelet count for thrombocytopenia. Dosage should be decreased or stopped, as appropriate, until the platelet count returns to within the normal range.

DOSAGE AND ADMINISTRATION

Treatment with **AGRYLIN®** Capsules should be initiated under close medical supervision. The recommended starting dosage of **AGRYLIN®** for adult patients is 0.5 mg qid or 1 mg bid, which should be maintained for at least one week. Starting doses in pediatric patients have ranged from 0.5 mg per day to 0.5 mg qid. As there are limited data on the appropriate starting dose for pediatric patients, an initial dose of 0.5 mg per day is recommended. In both adult and pediatric patients, dosage should then be adjusted to the lowest effective dosage required to reduce and maintain platelet count below 600,000/µL, and ideally to the normal range. The dosage should be increased by not more than 0.5 mg/day in any one week. Maintenance dosing is not expected to be different between adult and pediatric patients. Dosage should not exceed 10 mg/day or 2.5 mg in a single dose (see PRECAUTIONS).

There are no special requirements for dosing the geriatric population.

It is recommended that patients with moderate hepatic impairment start anagrelide therapy at a dose of 0.5mg/day and be maintained for a minimum of one week with careful monitoring of cardiovascular effects. The dosage increment must not exceed more than 0.5mg/day in any one-week. The potential risks and benefits of anagrelide therapy in a patient with mild and moderate impairment of hepatic function should be assessed before treatment is commenced. Use of anagrelide in patients with severe hepatic impairment has not been studied. Use of anagrelide in patients with severe hepatic impairment is contraindicated (See CONTRAINDICATIONS).

To monitor the effect of anagrelide and prevent the occurrence of thrombocytopenia, platelet counts should be performed every two days during the first week of treatment and at least weekly thereafter until the maintenance dosage is reached.

Typically, platelet count begins to respond within 7 to 14 days at the proper dosage. The time to complete response, defined as platelet count ≤ 600,000/µL, ranged from 4 to 12 weeks. Most patients will experience an adequate response at a dose of 1.5 to 3.0 mg/day. Patients with known or suspected heart disease, renal insufficiency, or hepatic dysfunction should be monitored closely.

HOW SUPPLIED

AGRYLIN® is available as:

0.5 mg, opaque, white capsules imprinted "S 063" in black ink: NDC 54092-063-01 = bottle of 100

1 mg, opaque, gray capsules imprinted "S 064" in black ink: NDC 54092-064-01 = bottle of 100

Store at 25°C (77°F) excursions permitted to 15-30°C (59-86°F), [See USP Controlled Room Temperature]. Store in a light resistant container.

Manufactured for **Shire US Inc.**, 725 Chesterbrook Blvd., Wayne, PA 19087-5637 USA
By MALLINCKRODT INC., Hobart, NY 13788

Rev. 12/04 063 0117 013
Printed in USA
MG #12610

PENTASA® ℞

[*pĕn-tă-să*]
(mesalamine)
Controlled-Release Capsules 250 mg and 500 mg

Prescribing information for this product, which appears on pages 3141–3142 of the 2005 PDR, has been completely revised as follows. Please write "See Supplement A" next to the product heading.

Prescribing Information as of July 2004
Rx only

DESCRIPTION

PENTASA (mesalamine) for oral administration is a controlled-release formulation of mesalamine, an aminosalicylate anti-inflammatory agent for gastrointestinal use. Chemically, mesalamine is 5-amino-2-hydroxybenzoic acid. It has a molecular weight of 153.14.

The structural formula is:

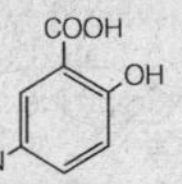
COOH
OH
H2N

Each 250 mg capsule contains 250 mg of mesalamine. It also contains the following inactive ingredients: acetylated monoglyceride, castor oil, colloidal silicon dioxide, ethylcellulose, hydroxypropyl methylcellulose, starch, stearic acid, sugar, talc, and white wax. The capsule shell contains D&C Yellow #10, FD&C Blue #1, FD&C Green #3, gelatin, titanium dioxide, and other ingredients.

Each 500 mg capsule contains 500 mg of mesalamine. It also contains the following inactive ingredients: acetylated monoglyceride, castor oil, colloidal silicon dioxide, ethylcellulose, hydroxypropyl methylcellulose, starch, stearic acid, sugar, talc, and white wax. The capsule shell contains FD&C Blue #1, gelatin, titanium dioxide, and other ingredients.

CLINICAL PHARMACOLOGY

Sulfasalazine is split by bacterial action in the colon into sulfapyridine (SP) and mesalamine (5-ASA). It is thought that the mesalamine component is therapeutically active in ulcerative colitis. The usual oral dose of sulfasalazine for active ulcerative colitis in adults is 2 to 4 g per day in divided doses. Four grams of sulfasalazine provide 1.6 g of free mesalamine to the colon.

The mechanism of action of mesalamine (and sulfasalazine) is unknown, but appears to be topical rather than systemic. Mucosal production of arachidonic acid (AA) metabolites, both through the cyclooxygenase pathways, ie, prostanoids, and through the lipoxygenase pathways, ie, leukotrienes (LTs) and hydroxyeicosatetraenoic acids (HETEs), is increased in patients with chronic inflammatory bowel disease, and it is possible that mesalamine diminishes inflammation by blocking cyclooxygenase and inhibiting prostaglandin (PG) production in the colon.

Human Pharmacokinetics and Metabolism

Absorption. PENTASA is an ethylcellulose-coated, controlled-release formulation of mesalamine designed to release therapeutic quantities of mesalamine throughout the gastrointestinal tract. Based on urinary excretion data, 20% to 30% of the mesalamine in PENTASA is absorbed. In contrast, when mesalamine is administered orally as an unformulated 1-g aqueous suspension, mesalamine is approximately 80% absorbed.

Plasma mesalamine concentration peaked at approximately 1 µg/mL 3 hours following a 1-g PENTASA dose and declined in a biphasic manner. The literature describes a mean terminal half-life of 42 minutes for mesalamine following intravenous administration. Because of the continuous release and absorption of mesalamine from PENTASA throughout the gastrointestinal tract, the true elimination half-life cannot be determined after oral administration. N-acetylmesalamine, the major metabolite of mesalamine, peaked at approximately 3 hours at 1.8 µg/mL, and its concentration followed a biphasic decline. Pharmacological activities of N-acetylmesalamine are unknown, and other metabolites have not been identified.

Oral mesalamine pharmacokinetics were nonlinear when PENTASA capsules were dosed from 250 mg to 1 g four times daily, with steady-state mesalamine plasma concentrations increasing about nine times, from 0.14 µg/mL to 1.21 µg/mL, suggesting saturable first-pass metabolism. N-acetylmesalamine pharmacokinetics were linear.

Elimination. About 130 mg free mesalamine was recovered in the feces following a single 1-g PENTASA dose, which was comparable to the 140 mg of mesalamine recovered from the molar equivalent sulfasalazine tablet dose of 2.5 g. Elimination of free mesalamine and salicylates in feces increased proportionately with PENTASA dose. N-acetylmesalamine was the primary compound excreted in the urine (19% to 30%) following PENTASA dosing.

CLINICAL TRIALS

In two randomized, double-blind, placebo-controlled, dose-response trials (UC-1 and UC-2) of 625 patients with active mild to moderate ulcerative colitis, PENTASA, at an oral dose of 4 g/day given 1 g four times daily, produced consistent improvement in prospectively identified primary efficacy parameters, PGA, Tx F, and SI as shown in the table below.

The 4-g dose of PENTASA also gave consistent improvement in secondary efficacy parameters, namely the frequency of trips to the toilet, stool consistency, rectal bleeding, abdominal/rectal pain, and urgency. The 4-g dose of PENTASA induced remission as assessed by endoscopic and symptomatic endpoints.

In some patients, the 2-g dose of PENTASA was observed to improve efficacy parameters measured. However, the 2-g dose gave inconsistent results in primary efficacy parameters across the two adequate and well-controlled trials.

[See table below]

INDICATIONS AND USAGE

PENTASA is indicated for the induction of remission and for the treatment of patients with mildly to moderately active ulcerative colitis.

CONTRAINDICATIONS

PENTASA is contraindicated in patients who have demonstrated hypersensitivity to mesalamine, any other components of this medication, or salicylates.

PRECAUTIONS

General

Caution should be exercised if PENTASA is administered to patients with impaired hepatic function.

Mesalamine has been associated with an acute intolerance syndrome that may be difficult to distinguish from a flare of inflammatory bowel disease. Although the exact frequency of occurrence cannot be ascertained, it has occurred in 3% of patients in controlled clinical trials of mesalamine or sulfasalazine. Symptoms include cramping, acute abdominal pain and bloody diarrhea, sometimes fever, headache, and rash. If acute intolerance syndrome is suspected, prompt withdrawal is required. If a rechallenge is performed later in order to validate the hypersensitivity, it should be carried out under close medical supervision at reduced dose and only if clearly needed.

Renal

Caution should be exercised if PENTASA is administered to patients with impaired renal function. Single reports of nephrotic syndrome and interstitial nephritis associated with mesalamine therapy have been described in the foreign literature. There have been rare reports of interstitial nephritis in patients receiving PENTASA. In animal studies, a 13-week oral toxicity study in mice and 13-week and 52-week oral toxicity studies in rats and cynomolgus monkeys have shown the kidney to be the major target organ of mesalamine toxicity. Oral daily doses of 2400 mg/kg in mice and 1150 mg/kg in rats produced renal lesions including granular and hyaline casts, tubular degeneration, tubular dilation, renal infarct, papillary necrosis, tubular necrosis,

	Clinical Trial UC-1			Clinical Trial UC-2		
		PENTASA			PENTASA	
Parameter Evaluated	PL (n=90)	4 g/day (n=95)	2 g/day (n=97)	PL (n=83)	4 g/day (n=85)	2 g/day (n=83)
PGA	36%	59%*	57%*	31%	55%*	41%
Tx F	22%	9%*	18%	31%	9%*	17%*
SI	−2.5	−5.0*	−4.3*	−1.6	−3.8*	−2.6
Remission†	12%	26%*	24%*	12%	27%*	12%

* $p < 0.05$ vs placebo.

PGA: Physician Global Assessment: proportion of patients with complete or marked improvement.

Tx F: Treatment Failure: proportion of patients developing severe or fulminant UC requiring steroid therapy or hospitalization or worsening of the disease at 7 days of therapy, or lack of significant improvement by 14 days of therapy.

SI: Sigmoidoscopic Index: an objective measure of disease activity rated by a standard (15-point) scale that includes mucosal vascular pattern, erythema, friability, granularity/ulcerations, and mucopus: improvement over baseline.

† Defined as complete resolution of symptoms plus improvement of endoscopic endpoints. To be considered in remission, patients had a "1" score for one of the endoscopic components (mucosal vascular pattern, erythema, granularity, or friability) and "0" for the others.

Table 1. Adverse Events Occurring in More Than 1% of Either Placebo or PENTASA Patients in Domestic Placebo-controlled Ulcerative Colitis Trials. (PENTASA Comparison to Placebo)

Event	PENTASA n=451	Placebo n=173
Diarrhea	16 (3.5%)	13 (7.5%)
Headache	10 (2.2%)	6 (3.5%)
Nausea	14 (3.1%)	—
Abdominal Pain	5 (1.1%)	7 (4.0%)
Melena (Bloody Diarrhea)	4 (0.9%)	6 (3.5%)
Rash	6 (1.3%)	2 (1.2%)
Anorexia	5 (1.1%)	2 (1.2%)
Fever	4 (0.9%)	2 (1.2%)
Rectal Urgency	1 (0.2%)	4 (2.3%)
Nausea and Vomiting	5 (1.1%)	—
Worsening of Ulcerative Colitis	2 (0.4%)	2 (1.2%)
Acne	1 (0.2%)	2 (1.2%)

and interstitial nephritis. In cynomolgus monkeys, oral daily doses of 250 mg/kg or higher produced nephrosis, papillary edema, and interstitial fibrosis. Patients with pre-existing renal disease, increased BUN or serum creatinine, or proteinuria should be carefully monitored.

Carcinogenesis, Mutagenesis, Impairment of Fertility

In a 104-week dietary carcinogenicity study of mesalamine, CD-1 mice were treated with doses up to 2500 mg/kg/day and it was not tumorigenic. For a 50 kg person of average height (1.46 m^2 body surface area), this represents 2.5 times the recommended human dose on a body surface area basis (2960 mg/m^2/day). In a 104-week dietary carcinogenicity study in Wistar rats, mesalamine up to a dose of 800 mg/kg/day was not tumorigenic. This dose represents 1.5 times the recommended human dose on a body surface area basis.

No evidence of mutagenicity was observed in an in vitro Ames test and an in vivo mouse micronucleus test.

No effects on fertility or reproductive performance were observed in male or female rats at oral doses of mesalamine up to 400 mg/kg/day (0.8 times the recommended human dose based on body surface area).

Semen abnormalities and infertility in men, which have been reported in association with sulfasalazine, have not been seen with PENTASA capsules during controlled clinical trials.

Pregnancy

Category B. Reproduction studies have been performed in rats at doses up to 1000 mg/kg/day (5900 mg/M^2) and rabbits at doses of 800 mg/kg/day (6856 mg/M^2) and have revealed no evidence of teratogenic effects or harm to the fetus due to mesalamine. There are, however, no adequate and well-controlled studies in pregnant women. Because animal reproduction studies are not always predictive of human response, PENTASA should be used during pregnancy only if clearly needed.

Mesalamine is known to cross the placental barrier.

Nursing Mothers

Minute quantities of mesalamine were distributed to breast milk and amniotic fluid of pregnant women following sulfasalazine therapy. When treated with sulfasalazine at a dose equivalent to 1.25 g/day of mesalamine, 0.02 µg/mL to 0.08 µg/mL and trace amounts of mesalamine were measured in amniotic fluid and breast milk, respectively. N-acetylmesalamine, in quantities of 0.07 µg/mL to 0.77 µg/mL and 1.13 µg/mL to 3.44 µg/mL, was identified in the same fluids, respectively.

Caution should be exercised when PENTASA is administered to a nursing woman.

Pediatric Use

Safety and efficacy of PENTASA in pediatric patients have not been established.

ADVERSE REACTIONS

In combined domestic and foreign clinical trials, more than 2100 patients with ulcerative colitis or Crohn's disease received PENTASA therapy. Generally, PENTASA therapy was well tolerated. The most common events (ie, greater than or equal to 1%) were diarrhea (3.4%), headache (2.0%), nausea (1.8%), abdominal pain (1.7%), dyspepsia (1.6%), vomiting (1.5%), and rash (1.0%).

In two domestic placebo-controlled trials involving over 600 ulcerative colitis patients, adverse events were fewer in PENTASA-treated patients than in the placebo group (PENTASA 14% vs placebo 18%) and were not dose-related. Events occurring at 1% or more are shown in the table below. Of these, only nausea and vomiting were more frequent in the PENTASA group. Withdrawal from therapy due to adverse events was more common on placebo than PENTASA (7% vs 4%).

[See table 1 above]

Clinical laboratory measurements showed no significant abnormal trends for any test, including measurement of hematologic, liver, and kidney function.

The following adverse events, presented by body system, were reported infrequently (ie, less than 1%) during domestic ulcerative colitis and Crohn's disease trials. In many cases, the relationship to PENTASA has not been established.

Gastrointestinal: abdominal distention, anorexia, constipation, duodenal ulcer, dysphagia, eructation, esophageal ulcer, fecal incontinence, GGTP increase, GI bleeding, increased alkaline phosphatase, LDH increase, mouth ulcer, oral moniliases, pancreatitis, rectal bleeding, SGOT increase, SGPT increase, stool abnormalities (color or texture change), thirst

Dermatological: acne, alopecia, dry skin, eczema, erythema nodosum, nail disorder, photosensitivity, pruritus, sweating, urticaria

Nervous System: depression, dizziness, insomnia, somnolence, paresthesia

Cardiovascular: palpitations, pericarditis, vasodilation

Other: albuminuria, amenorrhea, amylase increase, arthralgia, asthenia, breast pain, conjunctivitis, ecchymosis, edema, fever, hematuria, hypomenorrhea, Kawasaki-like syndrome, leg cramps, lichen planus, lipase increase, malaise, menorrhagia, metrorrhagia, myalgia, pulmonary infiltrates, thrombocythemia, thrombocytopenia, urinary frequency

One week after completion of an 8-week ulcerative colitis study, a 72-year-old male, with no previous history of pulmonary problems, developed dyspnea. The patient was subsequently diagnosed with interstitial pulmonary fibrosis without eosinophilia by one physician and bronchiolitis obliterans with organizing pneumonitis by a second physician. A causal relationship between this event and mesalamine therapy has not been established.

Published case reports and/or spontaneous postmarketing surveillance have described infrequent instances of pericarditis, fatal myocarditis, chest pain and T-wave abnormalities, hypersensitivity pneumonitis, pancreatitis, nephrotic syndrome, interstitial nephritis, hepatitis, aplastic anemia, pancytopenia, leukopenia, agranulocytosis, or anemia while receiving mesalamine therapy. Anemia can be a part of the clinical presentation of inflammatory bowel disease. Allergic reactions, which could involve eosinophilia, can be seen in connection with PENTASA therapy.

Postmarketing Reports

The following events have been identified during post-approval use of products which contain (or are metabolized to) mesalamine in clinical practice. Because they are reported voluntarily from a population of unknown size, estimates of frequency cannot be made. These events have been chosen for inclusion due to a combination of seriousness, frequency of reporting, or potential causal connection to mesalamine:

Gastrointestinal: Reports of hepatotoxicity, including elevated liver function tests (SGOT/AST, SGPT/ALT, GGT, LDH, alkaline phosphatase, bilirubin), jaundice, cholestatic jaundice, cirrhosis, and possible hepatocellular damage including liver necrosis and liver failure. Some of these cases were fatal. One case of Kawasaki-like syndrome which included hepatic function changes was also reported.

OVERDOSAGE

Single oral doses of mesalamine up to 5 g/kg in pigs or a single intravenous dose of mesalamine at 920 mg/kg in rats were not lethal.

There is no clinical experience with PENTASA overdosage. PENTASA is an aminosalicylate, and symptoms of salicylate toxicity may be possible, such as: tinnitus, vertigo, headache, confusion, drowsiness, sweating, hyperventilation, vomiting, and diarrhea. Severe intoxication with salicylates can lead to disruption of electrolyte balance and blood pH, hyperthermia, and dehydration.

Treatment of Overdosage. Since PENTASA is an aminosalicylate, conventional therapy for salicylate toxicity may be beneficial in the event of acute overdosage. This includes prevention of further gastrointestinal tract absorption by emesis and, if necessary, by gastric lavage. Fluid and electrolyte imbalance should be corrected by the administration of appropriate intravenous therapy. Adequate renal function should be maintained.

DOSAGE AND ADMINISTRATION

The recommended dosage for the induction of remission and the symptomatic treatment of mildly to moderately active ulcerative colitis is 1g (4 PENTASA 250 mg capsules or 2 PENTASA 500 mg capsules) 4 times a day for a total daily dosage of 4g. Treatment duration in controlled trials was up to 8 weeks.

HOW SUPPLIED

PENTASA controlled-release 250 mg capsules are supplied in bottles of 240 capsules (NDC 54092-189-81); and blister packs of 80 capsules (NDC 54092-189-80). Each green and blue capsule contains 250 mg of mesalamine in controlled-release beads. PENTASA controlled-release capsules are identified with a pentagonal starburst logo and the number 2010 on the green portion and PENTASA 250 mg on the blue portion of the capsules.

PENTASA controlled-release 500 mg capsules are supplied in bottles of 120 capsules (NDC 54092-191-12); and blister packs of 80 capsules (NDC 54092-191-80). Each blue capsule contains 500 mg of mesalamine in controlled-release beads. PENTASA controlled-release capsules are identified with a pentagonal starburst logo and PENTASA 500 mg on the capsules.

Store at 25°C (77°F) excursions permitted to 15-30°C (59-86°F) [see USP Controlled Room Temperature].

Manufactured for **Shire US Inc.**, 725 Chesterbrook Blvd., Wayne, PA 19087, USA

©2004 Shire US Inc.   189 0107 007A

Licensed U.S. Patent Nos. B1 4,496,553 and 4,980,173.

Licensed from Ferring A/S, Denmark   Rev. 07/2004

Wyeth Pharmaceuticals

Division of Wyeth
P.O. BOX 8299
PHILADELPHIA, PA 19101

For Product Information Contact:
(800) 934-5556
For Product Quality Contact:
(800) 999-9384
For Sales Representative Information Contact:
(800) 395-9938
For Customer Service and Ordering Information Contact:
Pharmaceuticals and Vaccines: (800) 666-7248
For Patient Assistance Program Contact:
(800) 568-9938
For All Other Inquiries:
(610) 688-4400
www.wyeth.com

Since the publication of this reference book, there may have been revisions to the labeling of the Wyeth Pharmaceuticals products listed below. For further product information and current package inserts please visit www.wyeth.com or call our Global Medical Communications Department toll-free at 1-800-934-5556.

BENEFIX®   ℞

[bĕně-fĭks]

Coagulation Factor IX (Recombinant)

USA: ℞ only

Prescribing information for this product, which appears on pages 3318–3321 of the 2005 PDR, has been revised as follows. Please write "See Supplement A" next to the product heading.

This product's label may have been revised after this insert was used in production. For further product information and current package insert, please visit www.wyeth.com or call our medical communications department toll-free at 1-800-934-5556.

In the **Instructions For Use** section, the following paragraph was added at the end of the "Reconstitution" subsection.

BeneFix, when reconstituted, contains polysorbate-80, which is known to increase the rate of di-(2-ethylhexyl)-phthalate (DEHP) extraction from polyvinyl chloride (PVC). This should be considered during the preparation and administration of BeneFix, including storage time elapsed in a PVC container following reconstitution. It is important that the recommendations in **DOSAGE AND ADMINISTRATION** be followed closely.

Manufactured by:
Wyeth Pharmaceuticals Inc.
Philadelphia, PA 19101
US Govt. License No. 3
Imported and Distributed in Canada by:
Wyeth Canada
Montreal, Canada
W10483C006
ET01
Rev 10/04

EFFEXOR®   ℞

[ĕ-fĕks-ōr]

(venlafaxine hydrochloride)

Tablets

℞ only

Prescribing information for this product, which appears on pages 3321–3326 of the 2005 PDR, has been completely revised as follows. Please write "See Supplement A" next to the product heading.

This product's label may have been revised after this insert was used in production. For further product information

Continued on next page

Effexor—Cont.

and current package insert, please visit www.wyeth.com or call our medical communications department toll-free at 1-800-934-5556.

Suicidality in Children and Adolescents
Antidepressants increased the risk of suicidal thinking and behavior (suicidality) in short-term studies in children and adolescents with Major Depressive Disorder (MDD) and other psychiatric disorders. Anyone considering the use of Effexor or any other antidepressant in a child or adolescent must balance this risk with the clinical need. Patients who are started on therapy should be observed closely for clinical worsening, suicidality, or unusual changes in behavior. Families and caregivers should be advised of the need for close observation and communication with the prescriber. Effexor is not approved for use in pediatric patients. (See WARNINGS and PRECAUTIONS, Pediatric Use.)
Pooled analyses of short-term (4 to 16 weeks) placebo-controlled trials of 9 antidepressant drugs (SSRIs and others) in children and adolescents with major depressive disorder (MDD), obsessive compulsive disorder (OCD), or other psychiatric disorders (a total of 24 trials involving over 4400 patients) have revealed a greater risk of adverse events representing suicidal thinking or behavior (suicidality) during the first few months of treatment in those receiving antidepressants. The average risk of such events in patients receiving antidepressants was 4%, twice the placebo risk of 2%. No suicides occurred in these trials.

DESCRIPTION

Effexor (venlafaxine hydrochloride) is a structurally novel antidepressant for oral administration. It is designated (R/S)-1-[2-(dimethylamino)-1-(4-methoxyphenyl)ethyl] cyclohexanol hydrochloride or (±)-1-[α-[(dimethyl-amino)-methyl]-p-methoxybenzyl] cyclohexanol hydrochloride and has the empirical formula of $C_{17}H_{27}NO_2$ HCl. Its molecular weight is 313.87. The structural formula is shown below.

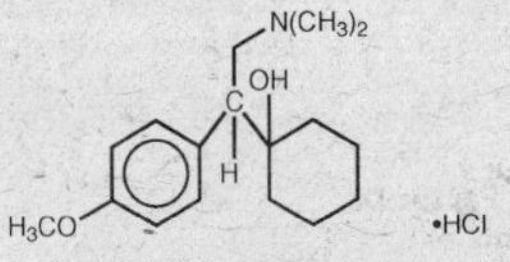

venlafaxine hydrochloride

Venlafaxine hydrochloride is a white to off-white crystalline solid with a solubility of 572 mg/mL in water (adjusted to ionic strength of 0.2 M with sodium chloride). Its octanol:water (0.2 M sodium chloride) partition coefficient is 0.43.
Compressed tablets contain venlafaxine hydrochloride equivalent to 25 mg, 37.5 mg, 50 mg, 75 mg, or 100 mg venlafaxine. Inactive ingredients consist of cellulose, iron oxides, lactose, magnesium stearate, and sodium starch glycolate.

CLINICAL PHARMACOLOGY

Pharmacodynamics

The mechanism of the antidepressant action of venlafaxine in humans is believed to be associated with its potentiation of neurotransmitter activity in the CNS. Preclinical studies have shown that venlafaxine and its active metabolite, O-desmethylvenlafaxine (ODV), are potent inhibitors of neuronal serotonin and norepinephrine reuptake and weak inhibitors of dopamine reuptake. Venlafaxine and ODV have no significant affinity for muscarinic, histaminergic, or α-1 adrenergic receptors in vitro. Pharmacologic activity at these receptors is hypothesized to be associated with the various anticholinergic, sedative, and cardiovascular effects seen with other psychotropic drugs. Venlafaxine and ODV do not possess monoamine oxidase (MAO) inhibitory activity.

Pharmacokinetics

Venlafaxine is well absorbed and extensively metabolized in the liver. O-desmethylvenlafaxine (ODV) is the only major active metabolite. On the basis of mass balance studies, at least 92% of a single dose of venlafaxine is absorbed. Approximately 87% of a venlafaxine dose is recovered in the urine within 48 hours as either unchanged venlafaxine (5%), unconjugated ODV (29%), conjugated ODV (26%), or other minor inactive metabolites (27%). Renal elimination of venlafaxine and its metabolites is the primary route of excretion. The relative bioavailability of venlafaxine from a tablet was 100% when compared to an oral solution. Food has no significant effect on the absorption of venlafaxine or on the formation of ODV.
The degree of binding of venlafaxine to human plasma is 27% ± 2% at concentrations ranging from 2.5 to 2215 ng/mL. The degree of ODV binding to human plasma is 30% ± 12% at concentrations ranging from 100 to 500 ng/mL. Protein-binding-induced drug interactions with venlafaxine are not expected.
Steady-state concentrations of both venlafaxine and ODV in plasma were attained within 3 days of multiple-dose therapy. Venlafaxine and ODV exhibited linear kinetics over the dose range of 75 to 450 mg total dose per day (administered on a q8h schedule). Plasma clearance, elimination half-life and steady-state volume of distribution were unaltered for both venlafaxine and ODV after multiple-dosing. Mean ± SD steady-state plasma clearance of venlafaxine and ODV is 1.3 ± 0.6 and 0.4 ± 0.2 L/h/kg, respectively; elimination half-life is 5 ± 2 and 11 ± 2 hours, respectively; and steady-state volume of distribution is 7.5 ± 3.7 L/kg and 5.7 ± 1.8 L/kg, respectively. When equal daily doses of venlafaxine were administered as either b.i.d. or t.i.d. regimens, the drug exposure (AUC) and fluctuation in plasma levels of venlafaxine and ODV were comparable following both regimens.

Age and Gender

A pharmacokinetic analysis of 404 venlafaxine-treated patients from two studies involving both b.i.d. and t.i.d. regimens showed that dose-normalized trough plasma levels of either venlafaxine or ODV were unaltered due to age or gender differences. Dosage adjustment based upon the age or gender of a patient is generally not necessary (see **DOSAGE AND ADMINISTRATION**).

Liver Disease

In 9 patients with hepatic cirrhosis, the pharmacokinetic disposition of both venlafaxine and ODV was significantly altered after oral administration of venlafaxine. Venlafaxine elimination half-life was prolonged by about 30%, and clearance decreased by about 50% in cirrhotic patients compared to normal subjects. ODV elimination half-life was prolonged by about 60% and clearance decreased by about 30% in cirrhotic patients compared to normal subjects. A large degree of intersubject variability was noted. Three patients with more severe cirrhosis had a more substantial decrease in venlafaxine clearance (about 90%) compared to normal subjects.
Dosage adjustment is necessary in these patients (see **DOSAGE AND ADMINISTRATION**).

Renal Disease

In a renal impairment study, venlafaxine elimination half-life after oral administration was prolonged by about 50% and clearance was reduced by about 24% in renally impaired patients (GFR = 10-70 mL/min), compared to normal subjects. In dialysis patients, venlafaxine elimination half-life was prolonged by about 180% and clearance was reduced by about 57% compared to normal subjects. Similarly, ODV elimination half-life was prolonged by about 40% although clearance was unchanged in patients with renal impairment (GFR = 10-70 mL/min) compared to normal subjects. In dialysis patients, ODV elimination half-life was prolonged by about 142% and clearance was reduced by about 56%, compared to normal subjects. A large degree of intersubject variability was noted.
Dosage adjustment is necessary in these patients (see **DOSAGE AND ADMINISTRATION**).

CLINICAL TRIALS

The efficacy of Effexor (venlafaxine hydrochloride) as a treatment for major depressive disorder was established in 5 placebo-controlled, short-term trials. Four of these were 6-week trials in adult outpatients meeting DSM-III or DSM-III-R criteria for major depression: two involving dose titration with Effexor in a range of 75 to 225 mg/day (t.i.d. schedule), the third involving fixed Effexor doses of 75, 225, and 375 mg/day (t.i.d. schedule), and the fourth involving doses of 25, 75, and 200 mg/day (b.i.d. schedule). The fifth was a 4-week study of adult inpatients meeting DSM-III-R criteria for major depression with melancholia whose Effexor doses were titrated in a range of 150 to 375 mg/day (t.i.d. schedule). In these 5 studies, Effexor was shown to be significantly superior to placebo on at least 2 of the following 3 measures: Hamilton Depression Rating Scale (total score), Hamilton depressed mood item, and Clinical Global Impression-Severity of Illness rating. Doses from 75 to 225 mg/day were superior to placebo in outpatient studies and a mean dose of about 350 mg/day was effective in inpatients. Data from the 2 fixed-dose outpatient studies were suggestive of a dose-response relationship in the range of 75 to 225 mg/day. There was no suggestion of increased response with doses greater than 225 mg/day.
While there were no efficacy studies focusing specifically on an elderly population, elderly patients were included among the patients studied. Overall, approximately 2/3 of all patients in these trials were women. Exploratory analyses for age and gender effects on outcome did not suggest any differential responsiveness on the basis of age or sex.
In one longer-term study, adult outpatients meeting DSM-IV criteria for major depressive disorder who had responded during an 8-week open trial on Effexor XR (75, 150, or 225 mg, qAM) were randomized to continuation of their same Effexor XR dose or to placebo, for up to 26 weeks of observation for relapse. Response during the open phase was defined as a CGI Severity of Illness item score of ≤3 and a HAM-D-21 total score of ≤10 at the day 56 evaluation. Relapse during the double-blind phase was defined as follows: (1) a reappearance of major depressive disorder as defined by DSM-IV criteria and a CGI Severity of Illness item score of ≥4 (moderately ill), (2) 2 consecutive CGI Severity of Illness item scores of ≥4, or (3) a final CGI Severity of Illness item score of ≥4 for any patient who withdrew from the study for any reason. Patients receiving continued Effexor XR treatment experienced significantly lower relapse rates over the subsequent 26 weeks compared with those receiving placebo.
In a second longer-term trial, adult outpatients meeting DSM-III-R criteria for major depression, recurrent type, who had responded (HAM-D-21 total score ≤12 at the day 56 evaluation) and continued to be improved [defined as the following criteria being met for days 56 through 180: (1) no HAM-D-21 total score ≥20; (2) no more than 2 HAM-D-21 total scores >10; and (3) no single CGI Severity of Illness item score ≥4 (moderately ill)] during an initial 26 weeks of treatment on Effexor (100 to 200 mg/day, on a b.i.d. schedule) were randomized to continuation of their same Effexor dose or to placebo. The follow-up period to observe patients for relapse, defined as a CGI Severity of Illness item score ≥4, was for up to 52 weeks. Patients receiving continued Effexor treatment experienced significantly lower relapse rates over the subsequent 52 weeks compared with those receiving placebo.

INDICATIONS AND USAGE

Effexor (venlafaxine hydrochloride) is indicated for the treatment of major depressive disorder.
The efficacy of Effexor in the treatment of major depressive disorder was established in 6-week controlled trials of adult outpatients whose diagnoses corresponded most closely to the DSM-III or DSM-III-R category of major depression and in a 4-week controlled trial of inpatients meeting diagnostic criteria for major depression with melancholia (see **CLINICAL TRIALS**).
A major depressive episode implies a prominent and relatively persistent depressed or dysphoric mood that usually interferes with daily functioning (nearly every day for at least 2 weeks); it should include at least 4 of the following 8 symptoms: change in appetite, change in sleep, psychomotor agitation or retardation, loss of interest in usual activities or decrease in sexual drive, increased fatigue, feelings of guilt or worthlessness, slowed thinking or impaired concentration, and a suicide attempt or suicidal ideation.
The efficacy of Effexor XR in maintaining an antidepressant response for up to 26 weeks following 8 weeks of acute treatment was demonstrated in a placebo-controlled trial. The efficacy of Effexor in maintaining an antidepressant response in patients with recurrent depression who had responded and continued to be improved during an initial 26 weeks of treatment and were then followed for a period of up to 52 weeks was demonstrated in a second placebo-controlled trial (see **CLINICAL TRIALS**). Nevertheless, the physician who elects to use Effexor/Effexor XR for extended periods should periodically re-evaluate the long-term usefulness of the drug for the individual patient.

CONTRAINDICATIONS

Hypersensitivity to venlafaxine hydrochloride or to any excipients in the formulation.
Concomitant use in patients taking monoamine oxidase inhibitors (MAOIs) is contraindicated (see **WARNINGS**).

WARNINGS

Clinical Worsening and Suicide Risk

Patients with major depressive disorder (MDD), both adult and pediatric, may experience worsening of their depression and/or the emergence of suicidal ideation and behavior (suicidality) or unusual changes in behavior, whether or not they are taking antidepressant medications, and this risk may persist until significant remission occurs. There has been a long-standing concern that antidepressants may have a role in inducing worsening of depression and the emergence of suicidality in certain patients. Antidepressants increased the risk of suicidal thinking and behavior (suicidality) in short-term studies in children and adolescents with Major Depressive Disorder (MDD) and other psychiatric disorders.
Pooled analyses of short-term placebo-controlled trials of 9 antidepressant drugs (SSRIs and others) in children and adolescents with MDD, OCD, or other psychiatric disorders (a total of 24 trials involving over 4400 patients) have revealed a greater risk of adverse events representing suicidal behavior or thinking (suicidality) during the first few months of treatment in those receiving antidepressants. The average risk of such events in patients receiving antidepressants was 4%, twice the placebo risk of 2%. There was considerable variation in risk among drugs, but a tendency toward an increase for almost all drugs studied. The risk of suicidality was most consistently observed in the MDD trials, but there were signals of risk arising from some trials in other psychiatric indications (obsessive compulsive disorder and social anxiety disorder) as well. **No suicides occurred in any of these trials.** It is unknown whether the suicidality risk in pediatric patients extends to longer-term use, i.e., beyond several months. It is also unknown whether the suicidality risk extends to adults.
All pediatric patients being treated with antidepressants for any indication should be observed closely for clinical worsening, suicidality, and unusual changes in behavior, especially during the initial few months of a course of drug therapy, or at times of dose changes, either increases or decreases. Such observation would generally include at least weekly face-to-face contact with patients or their family members or caregivers during the first 4 weeks of treatment, then every other week visits for the next 4 weeks, then at 12 weeks, and as clinically indicated beyond 12 weeks. Additional contact by telephone may be appropriate between face-to-face visits.
Adults with MDD or co-morbid depression in the setting of other psychiatric illness being treated with antidepressants

should be observed similarly for clinical worsening and suicidality, especially during the initial few months of a course of drug therapy, or at times of dose changes, either increases or decreases.

The following symptoms, anxiety, agitation, panic attacks, insomnia, irritability, hostility, aggressiveness, impulsivity, akathisia (psychomotor restlessness), hypomania, and mania, have been reported in adult and pediatric patients being treated with antidepressants for major depressive disorder as well as for other indications, both psychiatric and nonpsychiatric. Although a causal link between the emergence of such symptoms and either the worsening of depression and/or the emergence of suicidal impulses has not been established, there is concern that such symptoms may represent precursors to emerging suicidality.

Consideration should be given to changing the therapeutic regimen, including possibly discontinuing the medication, in patients whose depression is persistently worse, or who are experiencing emergent suicidality or symptoms that might be precursors to worsening depression or suicidality, especially if these symptoms are severe, abrupt in onset, or were not part of the patient's presenting symptoms.

If the decision has been made to discontinue treatment, medication should be tapered, as rapidly as is feasible, but with recognition that abrupt discontinuation can be associated with certain symptoms (see **PRECAUTIONS** and **DOSAGE AND ADMINISTRATION, Discontinuation of Treatment with Effexor,** for a description of the risks of discontinuation of Effexor).

Families and caregivers of pediatric patients being treated with antidepressants for major depressive disorder or other indications, both psychiatric and nonpsychiatric, should be alerted about the need to monitor patients for the emergence of agitation, irritability, unusual changes in behavior, and the other symptoms described above, as well as the emergence of suicidality, and to report such symptoms immediately to health care providers. Such monitoring should include daily observation by families and caregivers. Prescriptions for Effexor should be written for the smallest quantity of tablets consistent with good patient management, in order to reduce the risk of overdose. Families and caregivers of adults being treated for depression should be similarly advised.

Screening Patients for Bipolar Disorder: A major depressive episode may be the initial presentation of bipolar disorder. It is generally believed (though not established in controlled trials) that treating such an episode with an antidepressant alone may increase the likelihood of precipitation of a mixed/manic episode in patients at risk for bipolar disorder. Whether any of the symptoms described above represent such a conversion is unknown. However, prior to initiating treatment with an antidepressant, patients with depressive symptoms should be adequately screened to determine if they are at risk for bipolar disorder; such screening should include a detailed psychiatric history, including a family history of suicide, bipolar disorder, and depression. It should be noted that Effexor is not approved for use in treating bipolar depression.

Potential for Interaction with Monoamine Oxidase Inhibitors

Adverse reactions, some of which were serious, have been reported in patients who have recently been discontinued from a monoamine oxidase inhibitor (MAOI) and started on Effexor, or who have recently had Effexor therapy discontinued prior to initiation of an MAOI. These reactions have included tremor, myoclonus, diaphoresis, nausea, vomiting, flushing, dizziness, hyperthermia with features resembling neuroleptic malignant syndrome, seizures, and death. In patients receiving antidepressants with pharmacological properties similar to venlafaxine in combination with a monoamine oxidase inhibitor, there have also been reports of serious, sometimes fatal, reactions. For a selective serotonin reuptake inhibitor, these reactions have included hyperthermia, rigidity, myoclonus, autonomic instability with possible rapid fluctuations of vital signs, and mental status changes that include extreme agitation progressing to delirium and coma. Some cases presented with features resembling neuroleptic malignant syndrome. Severe hyperthermia and seizures, sometimes fatal, have been reported in association with the combined use of tricyclic antidepressants and MAOIs. These reactions have also been reported in patients who have recently discontinued these drugs and have been started on an MAOI. Therefore, it is recommended that Effexor not be used in combination with an MAOI, or within at least 14 days of discontinuing treatment with an MAOI. Based on the half-life of Effexor, at least 7 days should be allowed after stopping Effexor before starting an MAOI.

Sustained Hypertension

Venlafaxine treatment is associated with sustained increases in blood pressure in some patients. (1) In a premarketing study comparing three fixed doses of venlafaxine (75, 225, and 375 mg/day) and placebo, a mean increase in supine diastolic blood pressure (SDBP) of 7.2 mm Hg was seen in the 375 mg/day group at week 6 compared to essentially no changes in the 75 and 225 mg/day groups and a mean decrease in SDBP of 2.2 mm Hg in the placebo group. (2) An analysis for patients meeting criteria for sustained hypertension (defined as treatment-emergent SDBP ≥ 90 mm Hg *and* ≥ 10 mm Hg above baseline for 3 consecutive visits) revealed a dose-dependent increase in the incidence of sustained hypertension for venlafaxine:

Probability of Sustained Elevation in SDBP
(Pool of Premarketing Venlafaxine Studies)

Treatment Group	Incidence of Sustained Elevation in SDBP
Venlafaxine	
<100 mg/day	3%
101–200 mg/day	5%
201–300 mg/day	7%
>300 mg/day	13%
Placebo	2%

An analysis of the patients with sustained hypertension and the 19 venlafaxine patients who were discontinued from treatment because of hypertension (<1% of total venlafaxine-treated group) revealed that most of the blood pressure increases were in a modest range (10 to 15 mm Hg, SDBP). Nevertheless, sustained increases of this magnitude could have adverse consequences. Therefore, it is recommended that patients receiving venlafaxine have regular monitoring of blood pressure. For patients who experience a sustained increase in blood pressure while receiving venlafaxine, either dose reduction or discontinuation should be considered.

PRECAUTIONS

General

Discontinuation of Treatment with Effexor

Discontinuation symptoms have been systematically evaluated in patients taking venlafaxine, to include prospective analyses of clinical trials in Generalized Anxiety Disorder and retrospective surveys of trials in major depressive disorder. Abrupt discontinuation or dose reduction of venlafaxine at various doses has been found to be associated with the appearance of new symptoms, the frequency of which increased with increased dose level and with longer duration of treatment. Reported symptoms include agitation, anorexia, anxiety, confusion, coordination impaired, diarrhea, dizziness, dry mouth, dysphoric mood, fasciculation, fatigue, headaches, hypomania, insomnia, nausea, nervousness, nightmares, sensory disturbances (including shock-like electrical sensations), somnolence, sweating, tremor, vertigo, and vomiting.

During marketing of Effexor, other SNRIs (Serotonin and Norepinephrine Reuptake Inhibitors), and SSRIs (Selective Serotonin Reuptake Inhibitors), there have been spontaneous reports of adverse events occurring upon discontinuation of these drugs, particularly when abrupt, including the following: dysphoric mood, irritability, agitation, dizziness, sensory disturbances (e.g. paresthesias such as electric shock sensations), anxiety, confusion, headache, lethargy, emotional lability, insomnia, hypomania, tinnitus, and seizures. While these events are generally self-limiting, there have been reports of serious discontinuation symptoms.

Patients should be monitored for these symptoms when discontinuing treatment with Effexor. A gradual reduction in the dose rather than abrupt cessation is recommended whenever possible. If intolerable symptoms occur following a decrease in the dose or upon discontinuation of treatment, then resuming the previously prescribed dose may be considered. Subsequently, the physician may continue decreasing the dose but at a more gradual rate (see **DOSAGE AND ADMINISTRATION**).

Anxiety and Insomnia

Treatment-emergent anxiety, nervousness, and insomnia were more commonly reported for venlafaxine-treated patients compared to placebo-treated patients in a pooled analysis of short-term, double-blind, placebo-controlled depression studies:

Symptom	Venlafaxine n = 1033	Placebo n = 609
Anxiety	6%	3%
Nervousness	13%	6%
Insomnia	18%	10%

Anxiety, nervousness, and insomnia led to drug discontinuation in 2%, 2%, and 3%, respectively, of the patients treated with venlafaxine in the Phase 2 and Phase 3 depression studies.

Changes in Weight

Adult Patients: A dose-dependent weight loss was noted in patients treated with venlafaxine for several weeks. A loss of 5% or more of body weight occurred in 6% of patients treated with venlafaxine compared with 1% of patients treated with placebo and 3% of patients treated with another antidepressant. However, discontinuation for weight loss associated with venlafaxine was uncommon (0.1% of venlafaxine-treated patients in the Phase 2 and Phase 3 depression trials).

The safety and efficacy of venlafaxine therapy in combination with weight loss agents, including phentermine, have not been established. Co-administration of Effexor and weight loss agents is not recommended. Effexor is not indicated for weight loss alone or in combination with other products.

Pediatric Patients: Weight loss has been observed in pediatric patients (ages 6-17) receiving Effexor XR. In a pooled analysis of four eight-week, double-blind, placebo-controlled, flexible dose outpatient trials for major depressive disorder (MDD) and generalized anxiety disorder (GAD), Effexor XR-treated patients lost an average of 0.45 kg (n = 333), while placebo-treated patients gained an average of 0.77 kg (n = 333). More patients treated with Effexor XR than with placebo experienced a weight loss of at least 3.5% in both the MDD and the GAD studies (18% of Effexor XR-treated patients vs. 3.6% of placebo-treated patients; p<0.001). Weight loss was not limited to patients with treatment-emergent anorexia (see **PRECAUTIONS, General,** *Changes in Appetite*).

The risks associated with longer-term Effexor XR use were assessed in an open-label study of children and adolescents who received Effexor XR for up to six months. The children and adolescents in the study had increases in weight that were less than expected based on data from age- and sex-matched peers. The difference between observed weight gain and expected weight gain was larger for children (<12 years old) than for adolescents (>12 years old).

Changes in Height

Pediatric Patients: During the eight-week placebo-controlled GAD studies, Effexor XR-treated patients (ages 6-17) grew an average of 0.3 cm (n = 122), while placebo-treated patients grew an average of 1.0 cm (n = 132); p=0.041. This difference in height increase was most notable in patients younger than twelve. During the eight-week placebo-controlled MDD studies, Effexor XR-treated patients grew an average of 0.8 cm (n = 146), while placebo-treated patients grew an average of 0.7 cm (n = 147). In the six-month open-label study, children and adolescents had height increases that were less than expected based on data from age- and sex-matched peers. The difference between observed growth rates and expected growth rates was larger for children (<12 years old) than for adolescents (>12 years old).

Changes in Appetite

Adult Patients: Treatment-emergent anorexia was more commonly reported for venlafaxine-treated (11%) than placebo-treated patients (2%) in the pool of short-term, double-blind, placebo-controlled depression studies.

Pediatric Patients: Decreased appetite been observed in pediatric patients receiving Effexor XR. In the placebo-controlled trials for GAD and MDD, 10% of patients aged 6-17 treated with Effexor XR for up to eight weeks and 3% of patients treated with placebo reported treatment-emergent anorexia (decreased appetite). None of the patients receiving Effexor XR discontinued for anorexia or weight loss.

Activation of Mania/Hypomania

During Phase 2 and Phase 3 trials, hypomania or mania occurred in 0.5% of patients treated with venlafaxine. Activation of mania/hypomania has also been reported in a small proportion of patients with major affective disorder who were treated with other marketed antidepressants. As with all antidepressants, Effexor (venlafaxine hydrochloride) should be used cautiously in patients with a history of mania.

Hyponatremia

Hyponatremia and/or the syndrome of inappropriate antidiuretic hormone secretion (SIADH) may occur with venlafaxine. This should be taken into consideration in patients who are, for example, volume-depleted, elderly, or taking diuretics.

Mydriasis

Mydriasis has been reported in association with venlafaxine; therefore patients with raised intraocular pressure or at risk of acute narrow-angle glaucoma (angle-closure glaucoma) should be monitored.

Seizures

During premarketing testing, seizures were reported in 0.26% (8/3082) of venlafaxine-treated patients. Most seizures (5 of 8) occurred in patients receiving doses of 150 mg/day or less. Effexor should be used cautiously in patients with a history of seizures. It should be discontinued in any patient who develops seizures.

Abnormal Bleeding

There have been reports of abnormal bleeding (most commonly ecchymosis) associated with venlafaxine treatment. While a causal relationship to venlafaxine is unclear, impaired platelet aggregation may result from platelet serotonin depletion and contribute to such occurrences.

Serum Cholesterol Elevation

Clinically relevant increases in serum cholesterol were recorded in 5.3% of venlafaxine-treated patients and 0.0% of placebo-treated patients treated for at least 3 months in placebo-controlled trials (see **ADVERSE REACTIONS–Laboratory Changes**). Measurement of serum cholesterol levels should be considered during long-term treatment.

Use in Patients with Concomitant Illness

Clinical experience with Effexor in patients with concomitant systemic illness is limited. Caution is advised in administering Effexor to patients with diseases or conditions that could affect hemodynamic responses or metabolism.

Effexor has not been evaluated or used to any appreciable extent in patients with a recent history of myocardial infarction or unstable heart disease. Patients with these diagnoses were systematically excluded from many clinical studies during the product's premarketing testing. Evaluation of the electrocardiograms for 769 patients who received Effexor in 4- to 6-week double-blind placebo-controlled trials, however, showed that the incidence of trial-emergent conduction abnormalities did not differ from that with placebo. The mean heart rate in Effexor-treated patients was increased relative to baseline by about 4 beats per minute. The electrocardiograms for 357 patients who received Effexor XR (the extended-release form of venlafaxine) and

Continued on next page

Effexor—Cont.

285 patients who received placebo in 8- to 12-week double-blind, placebo-controlled trials were analyzed. The mean change from baseline in corrected QT interval (QTc) for Effexor XR-treated patients was increased relative to that for placebo-treated patients (increase of 4.7 msec for Effexor XR and decrease of 1.9 msec for placebo). In these same trials, the mean change from baseline in heart rate for Effexor XR-treated patients was significantly higher than that for placebo (a mean increase of 4 beats per minute for Effexor XR and 1 beat per minute for placebo). In a flexible-dose study, with Effexor doses in the range of 200 to 375 mg/day and mean dose greater than 300 mg/day, Effexor-treated patients had a mean increase in heart rate of 8.5 beats per minute compared with 1.7 beats per minute in the placebo group.

As increases in heart rate were observed, caution should be exercised in patients whose underlying medical conditions might be compromised by increases in heart rate (eg, patients with hyperthyroidism, heart failure, or recent myocardial infarction), particularly when using doses of Effexor above 200 mg/day.

In patients with renal impairment (GFR=10 to 70 mL/min) or cirrhosis of the liver, the clearances of venlafaxine and its active metabolite were decreased, thus prolonging the elimination half-lives of these substances. A lower dose may be necessary (see **DOSAGE AND ADMINISTRATION**).

Effexor (venlafaxine hydrochloride), like all antidepressants, should be used with caution in such patients.

Information for Patients

Prescribers or other health professionals should inform patients, their families, and their caregivers about the benefits and risks associated with treatment with Effexor and should counsel them in its appropriate use. A patient Medication Guide About Using Antidepressants in Children and Teenagers is available for Effexor. The prescriber or health professional should instruct patients, their families, and their caregivers to read the Medication Guide and should assist them in understanding its contents. Patients should be given the opportunity to discuss the contents of the Medication Guide and to obtain answers to any questions they may have. The complete text of the Medication Guide is reprinted at the end of this document.

Patients should be advised of the following issues and asked to alert their prescriber if these occur while taking Effexor.

Clinical Worsening and Suicide Risk: Patients, their families, and their caregivers should be encouraged to be alert to the emergence of anxiety, agitation, panic attacks, insomnia, irritability, hostility, aggressiveness, impulsivity, akathisia (psychomotor restlessness), hypomania, mania, other unusual changes in behavior, worsening of depression, and suicidal ideation, especially early during antidepressant treatment and when the dose is adjusted up or down. Families and caregivers of patients should be advised to observe for the emergence of such symptoms on a day-to-day basis, since changes may be abrupt. Such symptoms should be reported to the patient's prescriber or health professional, especially if they are severe, abrupt in onset, or were not part of the patient's presenting symptoms. Symptoms such as these may be associated with an increased risk for suicidal thinking and behavior and indicate a need for very close monitoring and possibly changes in the medication.

Interference with Cognitive and Motor Performance
Clinical studies were performed to examine the effects of venlafaxine on behavioral performance of healthy individuals. The results revealed no clinically significant impairment of psychomotor, cognitive, or complex behavior performance. However, since any psychoactive drug may impair judgment, thinking, or motor skills, patients should be cautioned about operating hazardous machinery, including automobiles, until they are reasonably certain that Effexor therapy does not adversely affect their ability to engage in such activities.

Pregnancy
Patients should be advised to notify their physician if they become pregnant or intend to become pregnant during therapy.

Nursing
Patients should be advised to notify their physician if they are breast-feeding an infant.

Concomitant Medication
Patients should be advised to inform their physicians if they are taking, or plan to take, any prescription or over-the-counter drugs, including herbal preparations, since there is a potential for interactions.

Alcohol
Although Effexor has not been shown to increase the impairment of mental and motor skills caused by alcohol, patients should be advised to avoid alcohol while taking Effexor.

Allergic Reactions
Patients should be advised to notify their physician if they develop a rash, hives, or a related allergic phenomenon.

Laboratory Tests

There are no specific laboratory tests recommended.

Drug Interactions

As with all drugs, the potential for interaction by a variety of mechanisms is a possibility.

Alcohol
A single dose of ethanol (0.5 g/kg) had no effect on the pharmacokinetics of venlafaxine or ODV when venlafaxine was administered at 150 mg/day in 15 healthy male subjects. Additionally, administration of venlafaxine in a stable regimen did not exaggerate the psychomotor and psychometric effects induced by ethanol in these same subjects when they were not receiving venlafaxine.

Cimetidine
Concomitant administration of cimetidine and venlafaxine in a steady-state study for both drugs resulted in inhibition of first-pass metabolism of venlafaxine in 18 healthy subjects. The oral clearance of venlafaxine was reduced by about 43%, and the exposure (AUC) and maximum concentration (C_{max}) of the drug were increased by about 60%. However, co-administration of cimetidine had no apparent effect on the pharmacokinetics of ODV, which is present in much greater quantity in the circulation than is venlafaxine. The overall pharmacological activity of venlafaxine plus ODV is expected to increase only slightly, and no dosage adjustment should be necessary for most normal adults. However, for patients with pre-existing hypertension, and for elderly patients or patients with hepatic dysfunction, the interaction associated with the concomitant use of venlafaxine and cimetidine is not known and potentially could be more pronounced. Therefore, caution is advised with such patients.

Diazepam
Under steady-state conditions for venlafaxine administered at 150 mg/day, a single 10 mg dose of diazepam did not appear to affect the pharmacokinetics of either venlafaxine or ODV in 18 healthy male subjects. Venlafaxine also did not have any effect on the pharmacokinetics of diazepam or its active metabolite, desmethyldiazepam, or affect the psychomotor and psychometric effects induced by diazepam.

Haloperidol
Venlafaxine administered under steady-state conditions at 150 mg/day in 24 healthy subjects decreased total oral-dose clearance (Cl/F) of a single 2 mg dose of haloperidol by 42%, which resulted in a 70% increase in haloperidol AUC. In addition, the haloperidol C_{max} increased 88% when coadministered with venlafaxine, but the haloperidol elimination half-life ($t_{1/2}$) was unchanged. The mechanism explaining this finding is unknown.

Lithium
The steady-state pharmacokinetics of venlafaxine administered at 150 mg/day were not affected when a single 600 mg oral dose of lithium was administered to 12 healthy male subjects. O-desmethylvenlafaxine (ODV) also was unaffected. Venlafaxine had no effect on the pharmacokinetics of lithium (see also *CNS-Active Drugs*, below).

Drugs Highly Bound to Plasma Protein
Venlafaxine is not highly bound to plasma proteins; therefore, administration of Effexor to a patient taking another drug that is highly protein bound should not cause increased free concentrations of the other drug.

Drugs that Inhibit Cytochrome P450 Isoenzymes
CYP2D6 Inhibitors: In vitro and in vivo studies indicate that venlafaxine is metabolized to its active metabolite, ODV, by CYP2D6, the isoenzyme that is responsible for the genetic polymorphism seen in the metabolism of many antidepressants. Therefore, the potential exists for a drug interaction between drugs that inhibit CYP2D6-mediated metabolism and venlafaxine. However, although imipramine partially inhibited the CYP2D6-mediated metabolism of venlafaxine, resulting in higher plasma concentrations of venlafaxine and lower plasma concentrations of ODV, the total concentration of active compounds (venlafaxine plus ODV) was not affected. Additionally, in a clinical study involving CYP2D6-poor and -extensive metabolizers, the total concentration of active compounds (venlafaxine plus ODV), was similar in the two metabolizer groups. Therefore, no dosage adjustment is required when venlafaxine is coadministered with a CYP2D6 inhibitor.
CYP3A4 Inhibitors: In vitro studies indicate that venlafaxine is likely metabolized to a minor, less active metabolite, N-desmethylvenlafaxine, by CYP3A4. Because CYP3A4 is typically a minor pathway relative to CYP2D6 in the metabolism of venlafaxine, the potential for a clinically significant drug interaction between drugs that inhibit CYP3A4-mediated metabolism and venlafaxine is small.
The concomitant use of venlafaxine with a drug treatment(s) that potently inhibits both CYP2D6 and CYP3A4, the primary metabolizing enzymes for venlafaxine, has not been studied. Therefore, caution is advised should a patient's therapy include venlafaxine and any agent(s) that produce potent simultaneous inhibition of these two enzyme systems.

Drugs Metabolized by Cytochrome P450 Isoenzymes
CYP2D6: In vitro studies indicate that venlafaxine is a relatively weak inhibitor of CYP2D6. These findings have been confirmed in a clinical drug interaction study comparing the effect of venlafaxine to that of fluoxetine on the CYP2D6-mediated metabolism of dextromethorphan to dextrorphan.
Imipramine—Venlafaxine did not affect the pharmacokinetics of imipramine and 2-OH-imipramine. However, desipramine AUC, C_{max}, and C_{min} increased by about 35% in the presence of venlafaxine. The 2-OH-desipramine AUCs increased by at least 2.5 fold (with venlafaxine 37.5 mg q12h) and by 4.5 fold (with venlafaxine 75 mg q12h). Imipramine did not affect the pharmacokinetics of venlafaxine and ODV. The clinical significance of elevated 2-OH-desipramine levels is unknown.
Risperidone—Venlafaxine administered under steady-state conditions at 150 mg/day slightly inhibited the CYP2D6-mediated metabolism of risperidone (administered as a single 1 mg oral dose) to its active metabolite, 9-hydroxyrisperidone, resulting in an approximate 32% increase in risperidone AUC. However, venlafaxine coadministration did not significantly alter the pharmacokinetic profile of the total active moiety (risperidone plus 9-hydroxyrisperidone).
CYP3A4: Venlafaxine did not inhibit CYP3A4 in vitro. This finding was confirmed in vivo by clinical drug interaction studies in which venlafaxine did not inhibit the metabolism of several CYP3A4 substrates, including alprazolam, diazepam, and terfenadine.
Indinavir—In a study of 9 healthy volunteers, venlafaxine administered under steady-state conditions at 150 mg/day resulted in a 28% decrease in the AUC of a single 800 mg oral dose of indinavir and a 36% decrease in indinavir C_{max}. Indinavir did not affect the pharmacokinetics of venlafaxine and ODV. The clinical significance of this finding is unknown.
CYP1A2: Venlafaxine did not inhibit CYP1A2 in vitro. This finding was confirmed in vivo by a clinical drug interaction study in which venlafaxine did not inhibit the metabolism of caffeine, a CYP1A2 substrate.
CYP2C9: Venlafaxine did not inhibit CYP2C9 in vitro. In vivo, venlafaxine 75 mg by mouth every 12 hours did not alter the pharmacokinetics of a single 500 mg dose of tolbutamide or the CYP2C9 mediated formation of 4-hydroxytolbutamide.
CYP2C19: Venlafaxine did not inhibit the metabolism of diazepam which is partially metabolized by CYP2C19 (see *Diazepam* above).

Monoamine Oxidase Inhibitors
See **CONTRAINDICATIONS** and **WARNINGS**.

CNS-Active Drugs
The risk of using venlafaxine in combination with other CNS-active drugs has not been systematically evaluated (except in the case of those CNS-active drugs noted above). Consequently, caution is advised if the concomitant administration of venlafaxine and such drugs is required. Based on the mechanism of action of venlafaxine and the potential for serotonin syndrome, caution is advised when venlafaxine is co-administered with other drugs that may affect the serotonergic neurotransmitter systems, such as triptans, serotonin reuptake inhibitors (SRIs), or lithium.

Electroconvulsive Therapy
There are no clinical data establishing the benefit of electroconvulsive therapy combined with Effexor treatment.

Postmarketing Spontaneous Drug Interaction Reports
See **ADVERSE REACTIONS, Postmarketing Reports.**

Carcinogenesis, Mutagenesis, Impairment of Fertility

Carcinogenesis
Venlafaxine was given by oral gavage to mice for 18 months at doses up to 120 mg/kg per day, which was 16 times, on a mg/kg basis, and 1.7 times on a mg/m² basis, the maximum recommended human dose. Venlafaxine was also given to rats by oral gavage for 24 months at doses up to 120 mg/kg per day. In rats receiving the 120 mg/kg dose, plasma levels of venlafaxine were 1 times (male rats) and 6 times (female rats) the plasma levels of patients receiving the maximum recommended human dose. Plasma levels of the O-desmethyl metabolite were lower in rats than in patients receiving the maximum recommended dose. Tumors were not increased by venlafaxine treatment in mice or rats.

Mutagenicity
Venlafaxine and the major human metabolite, O-desmethylvenlafaxine (ODV), were not mutagenic in the Ames reverse mutation assay in Salmonella bacteria or the CHO/HGPRT mammalian cell forward gene mutation assay. Venlafaxine was also not mutagenic in the in vitro BALB/c-3T3 mouse cell transformation assay, the sister chromatid exchange assay in cultured CHO cells, or the in vivo chromosomal aberration assay in rat bone marrow. ODV was not mutagenic in the in vitro CHO cell chromosomal aberration assay. There was a clastogenic response in the in vivo chromosomal aberration assay in rat bone marrow in male rats receiving 200 times, on a mg/kg basis, or 50 times, on a mg/m² basis, the maximum human daily dose. The no effect dose was 67 times (mg/kg) or 17 times (mg/m²) the human dose.

Impairment of Fertility
Reproduction and fertility studies in rats showed no effects on male or female fertility at oral doses of up to 8 times the maximum recommended human daily dose on a mg/kg basis, or up to 2 times on a mg/m² basis.

Pregnancy

Teratogenic Effects—Pregnancy Category C
Venlafaxine did not cause malformations in offspring of rats or rabbits given doses up to 11 times (rat) or 12 times (rabbit) the maximum recommended human daily dose on a mg/kg basis, or 2.5 times (rat) and 4 times (rabbit) the human daily dose on a mg/m² basis. However, in rats, there was a decrease in pup weight, an increase in stillborn pups, and an increase in pup deaths during the first 5 days of lactation, when dosing began during pregnancy and continued until weaning. The cause of these deaths is not known. These effects occurred at 10 times (mg/kg) or 2.5 times (mg/m²) the maximum human daily dose. The no effect dose for rat pup mortality was 1.4 times the human dose on a mg/kg basis or 0.25 times the human dose on a mg/m² basis. There are no adequate and well-controlled studies in pregnant women. Because animal reproduction studies are not always predictive of human response, this drug should be used during pregnancy only if clearly needed.

Non-teratogenic Effects
Neonates exposed to Effexor, other SNRIs (Serotonin and Norepinephrine Reuptake Inhibitors), or SSRIs (Selective Serotonin Reuptake Inhibitors), late in the third trimester have developed complications requiring prolonged hospitalization, respiratory support, and tube feeding. Such complications can arise immediately upon delivery. Reported clin-

ical findings have included respiratory distress, cyanosis, apnea, seizures, temperature instability, feeding difficulty, vomiting, hypoglycemia, hypotonia, hypertonia, hyperreflexia, tremor, jitteriness, irritability, and constant crying. These features are consistent with either a direct toxic effect of SSRIs and SNRIs or, possibly, a drug discontinuation syndrome. It should be noted that, in some cases, the clinical picture is consistent with serotonin syndrome (see **PRECAUTIONS-Drug Interactions**-*CNS-Active Drugs*). When treating a pregnant woman with Effexor during the third trimester, the physician should carefully consider the potential risks and benefits of treatment (see **DOSAGE AND ADMINISTRATION**).

Labor and Delivery
The effect of Effexor® (venlafaxine hydrochloride) on labor and delivery in humans is unknown.

Nursing Mothers
Venlafaxine and ODV have been reported to be excreted in human milk. Because of the potential for serious adverse reactions in nursing infants from Effexor, a decision should be made whether to discontinue nursing or to discontinue the drug, taking into account the importance of the drug to the mother.

Pediatric Use
Safety and effectiveness in the pediatric population have not been established (see **BOX WARNING** and **WARNINGS, Clinical Worsening and Suicide Risk**). Two placebo-controlled trials in 766 pediatric patients with MDD and two placebo-controlled trials in 793 pediatric patients with GAD have been conducted with Effexor XR, and the data were not sufficient to support a claim for use in pediatric patients.

Anyone considering the use of Effexor in a child or adolescent must balance the potential risks with the clinical need. Although no studies have been designed to primarily assess Effexor XR's impact on the growth, development, and maturation of children and adolescents, the studies that have been done suggest that Effexor XR may adversely affect weight and height (see **PRECAUTIONS, General**, *Changes in Height* and *Changes in Weight*). Should the decision be made to treat a pediatric patient with Effexor, regular monitoring of weight and height is recommended during treatment, particularly if it is to be continued long term. The safety of Effexor XR treatment for pediatric patients has not been systematically assessed for chronic treatment longer than six months in duration.

In the studies conducted in pediatric patients (ages 6-17), the occurrence of blood pressure and cholesterol increases considered to be clinically relevant in pediatric patients was similar to that observed in adult patients. Consequently, the precautions for adults apply to pediatric patients (see **WARNINGS, Sustained Hypertension**, and **PRECAUTIONS, General**, *Serum Cholesterol Elevation*).

Geriatric Use
Of the 2,897 patients in Phase 2 and Phase 3 depression studies with Effexor, 12% (357) were 65 years of age or over. No overall differences in effectiveness or safety were observed between these patients and younger patients, and other reported clinical experience generally has not identified differences in response between the elderly and younger patients. However, greater sensitivity of some older individuals cannot be ruled out. As with other antidepressants, several cases of hyponatremia and syndrome of inappropriate antidiuretic hormone secretion (SIADH) have been reported, usually in the elderly.

The pharmacokinetics of venlafaxine and ODV are not substantially altered in the elderly (see **CLINICAL PHARMACOLOGY**). No dose adjustment is recommended for the elderly on the basis of age alone, although other clinical circumstances, some of which may be more common in the elderly, such as renal or hepatic impairment, may warrant a dose reduction (see **DOSAGE AND ADMINISTRATION**).

ADVERSE REACTIONS
Associated with Discontinuation of Treatment
Nineteen percent (537/2897) of venlafaxine patients in Phase 2 and Phase 3 depression studies discontinued treatment due to an adverse event. The more common events (≥ 1%) associated with discontinuation and considered to be drug-related (ie, those events associated with dropout at a rate approximately twice or greater for venlafaxine compared to placebo) included:

CNS	Venlafaxine	Placebo
Somnolence	3%	1%
Insomnia	3%	1%
Dizziness	3%	—
Nervousness	2%	—
Dry mouth	2%	—
Anxiety	2%	1%
Gastrointestinal		
Nausea	6%	1%
Urogenital		
Abnormal ejaculation*	3%	—
Other		
Headache	3%	1%
Asthenia	2%	—
Sweating	2%	—

* Percentages based on the number of males.
— Less than 1%

Incidence in Controlled Trials
Commonly Observed Adverse Events in Controlled Clinical Trials
The most commonly observed adverse events associated with the use of Effexor® (incidence of 5% or greater) and not

TABLE 1
Treatment-Emergent Adverse Experience Incidence in 4- to 8-Week Placebo-Controlled Clinical Trials[1]

Body System	Preferred Term	Effexor (n=1033)	Placebo (n=609)
Body as a Whole	Headache	25%	24%
	Asthenia	12%	6%
	Infection	6%	5%
	Chills	3%	—
	Chest pain	2%	1%
	Trauma	2%	1%
Cardiovascular	Vasodilatation	4%	3%
	Increased blood pressure/hypertension	2%	—
	Tachycardia	2%	—
	Postural hypotension	1%	—
Dermatological	Sweating	12%	3%
	Rash	3%	2%
	Pruritus	1%	—
Gastrointestinal	Nausea	37%	11%
	Constipation	15%	7%
	Anorexia	11%	2%
	Diarrhea	8%	7%
	Vomiting	6%	2%
	Dyspepsia	5%	4%
	Flatulence	3%	2%
Metabolic	Weight loss	1%	—
Nervous System	Somnolence	23%	9%
	Dry mouth	22%	11%
	Dizziness	19%	7%
	Insomnia	18%	10%
	Nervousness	13%	6%
	Anxiety	6%	3%
	Tremor	5%	1%
	Abnormal dreams	4%	3%
	Hypertonia	3%	2%
	Paresthesia	3%	2%
	Libido decreased	2%	—
	Agitation	2%	—
	Confusion	2%	1%
	Thinking abnormal	2%	1%
	Depersonalization	1%	—
	Depression	1%	—
	Urinary retention	1%	—
	Twitching	1%	—
Respiration	Yawn	3%	—
Special Senses	Blurred vision	6%	2%
	Taste perversion	2%	—
	Tinnitus	2%	—
	Mydriasis	2%	—
Urogenital System	Abnormal ejaculation/orgasm	12%[2]	—[2]
	Impotence	6%[2]	—[2]
	Urinary frequency	3%	2%
	Urination impaired	2%	—
	Orgasm disturbance	2%[3]	—[3]

[1] Events reported by at least 1% of patients treated with Effexor (venlafaxine hydrochloride) are included, and are rounded to the nearest %. Events for which the Effexor incidence was equal to or less than placebo are not listed in the table, but included the following: abdominal pain, pain, back pain, flu syndrome, fever, palpitation, increased appetite, myalgia, arthralgia, amnesia, hypesthesia, rhinitis, pharyngitis, sinusitis, cough increased, and dysmenorrhea[3].
— Incidence less than 1%.
[2] Incidence based on number of male patients.
[3] Incidence based on number of female patients.

seen at an equivalent incidence among placebo-treated patients (ie, incidence for Effexor at least twice that for placebo), derived from the 1% incidence table below, were asthenia, sweating, nausea, constipation, anorexia, vomiting, somnolence, dry mouth, dizziness, nervousness, anxiety, tremor, and blurred vision as well as abnormal ejaculation/orgasm and impotence in men.

Adverse Events Occurring at an Incidence of 1% or More Among Effexor-Treated Patients
The table that follows enumerates adverse events that occurred at an incidence of 1% or more, and were more frequent than in the placebo group, among Effexor-treated patients who participated in short-term (4- to 8-week) placebo-controlled trials in which patients were administered doses in a range of 75 to 375 mg/day. This table shows the percentage of patients in each group who had at least one episode of an event at some time during their treatment. Reported adverse events were classified using a standard COSTART-based Dictionary terminology.

The prescriber should be aware that these figures cannot be used to predict the incidence of side effects in the course of usual medical practice where patient characteristics and other factors differ from those which prevailed in the clinical trials. Similarly, the cited frequencies cannot be compared with figures obtained from other clinical investigations involving different treatments, uses and investigators. The cited figures, however, do provide the prescribing physician with some basis for estimating the relative contribution of drug and nondrug factors to the side effect incidence rate in the population studied.
[See table 1 above]
Dose Dependency of Adverse Events
A comparison of adverse event rates in a fixed-dose study comparing Effexor (venlafaxine hydrochloride) 75, 225, and 375 mg/day with placebo revealed a dose dependency for some of the more common adverse events associated with Effexor use, as shown in the table that follows. The rule for including events was to enumerate those that occurred at an incidence of 5% or more for at least one of the venlafaxine groups and for which the incidence was at least twice the placebo incidence for at least one Effexor group. Tests for potential dose relationships for these events (Cochran-

Armitage Test, with a criterion of exact 2-sided p-value ≤ 0.05) suggested a dose-dependency for several adverse events in this list, including chills, hypertension, anorexia, nausea, agitation, dizziness, somnolence, tremor, yawning, sweating, and abnormal ejaculation.
[See table 2 at top of next page]
Adaptation to Certain Adverse Events
Over a 6-week period, there was evidence of adaptation to some adverse events with continued therapy (eg, dizziness and nausea), but less to other effects (eg, abnormal ejaculation and dry mouth).

Vital Sign Changes
Effexor (venlafaxine hydrochloride) treatment (averaged over all dose groups) in clinical trials was associated with a mean increase in pulse rate of approximately 3 beats per minute, compared to no change for placebo. In a flexible-dose study, with doses in the range of 200 to 375 mg/day and mean dose greater than 300 mg/day, the mean pulse was increased by about 2 beats per minute compared with a decrease of about 1 beat per minute for placebo.

In controlled clinical trials, Effexor was associated with mean increases in diastolic blood pressure ranging from 0.7 to 2.5 mm Hg averaged over all dose groups, compared to mean decreases ranging from 0.9 to 3.8 mm Hg for placebo. However, there is a dose dependency for blood pressure increase (see **WARNINGS**).

Laboratory Changes
Of the serum chemistry and hematology parameters monitored during clinical trials with Effexor, a statistically significant difference with placebo was seen only for serum cholesterol. In premarketing trials, treatment with Effexor tablets was associated with a mean final on-therapy increase in total cholesterol of 3 mg/dL.

Patients treated with Effexor tablets for at least 3 months in placebo-controlled 12-month extension trials had a mean final on-therapy increase in total cholesterol of 9.1 mg/dL compared with a decrease of 7.1 mg/dL among placebo-treated patients. This increase was duration dependent over the study period and tended to be greater with higher

Continued on next page

Effexor—Cont.

doses. Clinically relevant increases in serum cholesterol, defined as 1) a final on-therapy increase in serum cholesterol ≥50 mg/dL from baseline and to a value ≥261 mg/dL or 2) an average on-therapy increase in serum cholesterol ≥50 mg/dL from baseline and to a value ≥261 mg/dL, were recorded in 5.3% of venlafaxine-treated patients and 0.0% of placebo-treated patients (see **PRECAUTIONS-General-** *Serum Cholesterol Elevation*).

ECG Changes

In an analysis of ECGs obtained in 769 patients treated with Effexor and 450 patients treated with placebo in controlled clinical trials, the only statistically significant difference observed was for heart rate, ie, a mean increase from baseline of 4 beats per minute for Effexor. In a flexible-dose study, with doses in the range of 200 to 375 mg/day and mean dose greater than 300 mg/day, the mean change in heart rate was 8.5 beats per minute compared with 1.7 beats per minute for placebo (see **PRECAUTIONS, General,** *Use in Patients with Concomitant Illness*).

Other Events Observed During the Premarketing Evaluation of Venlafaxine

During its premarketing assessment, multiple doses of Effexor were administered to 2897 patients in Phase 2 and Phase 3 studies. In addition, in premarketing assessment of Effexor XR (the extended release form of venlafaxine), multiple doses were administered to 705 patients in Phase 3 major depressive disorder studies and Effexor was administered to 96 patients. During its premarketing assessment, multiple doses of Effexor XR were also administered to 1381 patients in Phase 3 GAD studies and 277 patients in Phase 3 Social Anxiety Disorder studies. The conditions and duration of exposure to venlafaxine in both development programs varied greatly, and included (in overlapping categories) open and double-blind studies, uncontrolled and controlled studies, inpatient (Effexor only) and outpatient studies, fixed-dose and titration studies. Untoward events associated with this exposure were recorded by clinical investigators using terminology of their own choosing. Consequently, it is not possible to provide a meaningful estimate of the proportion of individuals experiencing adverse events without first grouping similar types of untoward events into a smaller number of standardized event categories.

In the tabulations that follow, reported adverse events were classified using a standard COSTART-based Dictionary terminology. The frequencies presented, therefore, represent the proportion of the 5356 patients exposed to multiple doses of either formulation of venlafaxine who experienced an event of the type cited on at least one occasion while receiving venlafaxine. All reported events are included except those already listed in Table 1 and those events for which a drug cause was remote. If the COSTART term for an event was so general as to be uninformative, it was replaced with a more informative term. It is important to emphasize that, although the events reported occurred during treatment with venlafaxine, they were not necessarily caused by it.

Events are further categorized by body system and listed in order of decreasing frequency using the following definitions: **frequent** adverse events are defined as those occurring on one or more occasions in at least 1/100 patients; **infrequent** adverse events are those occurring in 1/100 to 1/1000 patients; **rare** events are those occurring in fewer than 1/1000 patients.

Body as a whole—**Frequent:** accidental injury, chest pain substernal, neck pain; **Infrequent:** face edema, intentional injury, malaise, moniliasis, neck rigidity, pelvic pain, photosensitivity reaction, suicide attempt, withdrawal syndrome; **Rare:** appendicitis, bacteremia, carcinoma, cellulitis.

Cardiovascular system—**Frequent:** migraine; **Infrequent:** angina pectoris, arrhythmia, extrasystoles, hypotension, peripheral vascular disorder (mainly cold feet and/or cold hands), syncope, thrombophlebitis; **Rare:** aortic aneurysm, arteritis, first-degree atrioventricular block, bigeminy, bradycardia, bundle branch block, capillary fragility, cardiovascular disorder (mitral valve and circulatory disturbance), cerebral ischemia, coronary artery disease, congestive heart failure, heart arrest, mucocutaneous hemorrhage, myocardial infarct, pallor.

Digestive system—**Frequent:** eructation; **Infrequent:** bruxism, colitis, dysphagia, tongue edema, esophagitis, gastritis, gastroenteritis, gastrointestinal ulcer, gingivitis, glossitis, rectal hemorrhage, hemorrhoids, melena, oral moniliasis, stomatitis, mouth ulceration; **Rare:** cheilitis, cholecystitis, cholelithiasis, duodenitis, esophageal spasm, hematemesis, gastrointestinal hemorrhage, gum hemorrhage, hepatitis, ileitis, jaundice, intestinal obstruction, parotitis, periodontitis, proctitis, increased salivation, soft stools, tongue discoloration.

Endocrine system—**Rare:** goiter, hyperthyroidism, hypothyroidism, thyroid nodule, thyroiditis.

Hemic and lymphatic system—**Frequent:** ecchymosis; **Infrequent:** anemia, leukocytosis, leukopenia, lymphadenopathy, thrombocythemia, thrombocytopenia; **Rare:** basophilia, bleeding time increased, cyanosis, eosinophilia, lymphocytosis, multiple myeloma, purpura.

Metabolic and nutritional—**Frequent:** edema, weight gain; **Infrequent:** alkaline phosphatase increased, dehydration, hypercholesteremia, hyperglycemia, hyperlipemia, hypokalemia, SGOT (AST) increased, SGPT (ALT) increased, thirst; **Rare:** alcohol intolerance, bilirubinemia, BUN increased, creatinine increased, diabetes mellitus, glycosuria, gout, healing abnormal, hemochromatosis, hypercalcinuria, hyperkalemia, hyperphosphatemia, hyperuricemia, hypocholesteremia, hypoglycemia, hyponatremia, hypophosphatemia, hypoproteinemia, uremia.

TABLE 2
Treatment-Emergent Adverse Experience Incidence in a Dose Comparison Trial

Body System/ Preferred Term	Placebo (n=92)	Effexor (mg/day) 75 (n=89)	225 (n=89)	375 (n=88)
Body as a Whole				
Abdominal pain	3.3%	3.4%	2.2%	8.0%
Asthenia	3.3%	16.9%	14.6%	14.8%
Chills	1.1%	2.2%	5.6%	6.8%
Infection	2.2%	2.2%	5.6%	2.3%
Cardiovascular System				
Hypertension	1.1%	1.1%	2.2%	4.5%
Vasodilatation	0.0%	4.5%	5.6%	2.3%
Digestive System				
Anorexia	2.2%	14.6%	13.5%	17.0%
Dyspepsia	2.2%	6.7%	6.7%	4.5%
Nausea	14.1%	32.6%	38.2%	58.0%
Vomiting	1.1%	7.9%	3.4%	6.8%
Nervous System				
Agitation	0.0%	1.1%	2.2%	4.5%
Anxiety	4.3%	11.2%	4.5%	2.3%
Dizziness	4.3%	19.1%	22.5%	23.9%
Insomnia	9.8%	22.5%	20.2%	13.6%
Libido decreased	1.1%	2.2%	1.1%	5.7%
Nervousness	4.3%	21.3%	13.5%	12.5%
Somnolence	4.3%	16.9%	18.0%	26.1%
Tremor	0.0%	1.1%	2.2%	10.2%
Respiratory System				
Yawn	0.0%	4.5%	5.6%	8.0%
Skin and Appendages				
Sweating	5.4%	6.7%	12.4%	19.3%
Special Senses				
Abnormality of accommodation	0.0%	9.1%	7.9%	5.6%
Urogenital System				
Abnormal ejaculation/orgasm	0.0%	4.5%	2.2%	12.5%
Impotence	0.0%	5.8%	2.1%	3.6%
(Number of men)	(n=63)	(n=52)	(n=48)	(n=56)

Musculoskeletal system—**Infrequent:** arthritis, arthrosis, bone pain, bone spurs, bursitis, leg cramps, myasthenia, tenosynovitis; **Rare:** pathological fracture, myopathy, osteoporosis, osteosclerosis, plantar fasciitis, rheumatoid arthritis, tendon rupture.

Nervous system—**Frequent:** trismus, vertigo; **Infrequent:** akathisia, apathy, ataxia, circumoral paresthesia, CNS stimulation, emotional lability, euphoria, hallucinations, hostility, hyperesthesia, hyperkinesia, hypotonia, incoordination, libido increased, manic reaction, myoclonus, neuralgia, neuropathy, psychosis, seizure, abnormal speech, stupor; **Rare:** akinesia, alcohol abuse, aphasia, bradykinesia, buccoglossal syndrome, cerebrovascular accident, loss of consciousness, delusions, dementia, dystonia, facial paralysis, feeling drunk, abnormal gait, Guillain-Barre Syndrome, hyperchlorhydria, hypokinesia, impulse control difficulties, neuritis, nystagmus, paranoid reaction, paresis, psychotic depression, reflexes decreased, reflexes increased, suicidal ideation, torticollis.

Respiratory system—**Frequent:** bronchitis, dyspnea; **Infrequent:** asthma, chest congestion, epistaxis, hyperventilation, laryngismus, laryngitis, pneumonia, voice alteration; **Rare:** atelectasis, hemoptysis, hypoventilation, hypoxia, larynx edema, pleurisy, pulmonary embolus, sleep apnea.

Skin and appendages—**Infrequent:** acne, alopecia, brittle nails, contact dermatitis, dry skin, eczema, skin hypertrophy, maculopapular rash, psoriasis, urticaria; **Rare:** erythema nodosum, exfoliative dermatitis, lichenoid dermatitis, hair discoloration, skin discoloration, furunculosis, hirsutism, leukoderma, petechial rash, pustular rash, vesiculobullous rash, seborrhea, skin atrophy, skin striae.

Special senses—**Frequent:** abnormality of accommodation, abnormal vision; **Infrequent:** cataract, conjunctivitis, corneal lesion, diplopia, dry eyes, eye pain, hyperacusis, otitis media, parosmia, photophobia, taste loss, visual field defect; **Rare:** blepharitis, chromatopsia, conjunctival edema, deafness, exophthalmos, glaucoma, retinal hemorrhage, subconjunctival hemorrhage, keratitis, labyrinthitis, miosis, papilledema, decreased pupillary reflex, otitis externa, scleritis, uveitis.

Urogenital system—**Frequent:** metrorrhagia*, prostatic disorder (prostatitis and enlarged prostate)*, vaginitis*; **Infrequent:** albuminuria, amenorrhea*, cystitis, dysuria, hematuria, leukorrhea*, menorrhagia*, nocturia, bladder pain, breast pain, polyuria, pyuria, urinary incontinence, urinary urgency, vaginal hemorrhage*; **Rare:** abortion*, anuria, balanitis*, breast discharge, breast engorgement, breast enlargement, endometriosis*, fibrocystic breast, calcium crystalluria, cervicitis*, ovarian cyst*, prolonged erection*, gynecomastia (male)*, hypomenorrhea*, kidney calculus, kidney pain, kidney function abnormal, female lactation*, mastitis, menopause*, oliguria, orchitis*, pyelonephritis, salpingitis*, urolithiasis, uterine hemorrhage*, uterine spasm.* vaginal dryness*.

* Based on the number of men and women as appropriate.

Postmarketing Reports

Voluntary reports of other adverse events temporally associated with the use of venlafaxine that have been received since market introduction and that may have no causal relationship with the use of venlafaxine include the following: agranulocytosis, anaphylaxis, aplastic anemia, catatonia, congenital anomalies, CPK increased, deep vein thrombophlebitis, delirium, EKG abnormalities such as QT prolongation; cardiac arrhythmias including atrial fibrillation, supraventricular tachycardia, ventricular extrasystole, and rare reports of ventricular fibrillation and ventricular tachycardia, including torsade de pointes; epidermal necrosis/Stevens-Johnson Syndrome, erythema multiforme, extrapyramidal symptoms (including dyskinesia and tardive dyskinesia), angle-closure glaucoma, hemorrhage (including eye and gastrointestinal bleeding), hepatic events (including GGT elevation; abnormalities of unspecified liver function tests; liver damage, necrosis, or failure; and fatty liver), involuntary movements, LDH increased, neuroleptic malignant syndrome-like events (including a case of a 10-year-old who may have been taking methylphenidate, was treated and recovered), neutropenia, night sweats, pancreatitis, pancytopenia, panic, prolactin increased, pulmonary eosinophilia, renal failure, rhabdomyolysis, serotonin syndrome, shock-like electrical sensations or tinnitus (in some cases, subsequent to the discontinuation of venlafaxine or tapering of dose), and syndrome of inappropriate antidiuretic hormone secretion (usually in the elderly).

There have been reports of elevated clozapine levels that were temporally associated with adverse events, including seizures, following the addition of venlafaxine. There have been reports of increases in prothrombin time, partial thromboplastin time, or INR when venlafaxine was given to patients receiving warfarin therapy.

DRUG ABUSE AND DEPENDENCE

Controlled Substance Class

Effexor (venlafaxine hydrochloride) is not a controlled substance.

Physical and Psychological Dependence

In vitro studies revealed that venlafaxine has virtually no affinity for opiate, benzodiazepine, phencyclidine (PCP), or N-methyl-D-aspartic acid (NMDA) receptors.

Venlafaxine was not found to have any significant CNS stimulant activity in rodents. In primate drug discrimination studies, venlafaxine showed no significant stimulant or depressant abuse liability.

Discontinuation effects have been reported in patients receiving venlafaxine (see **DOSAGE AND ADMINISTRATION**).

While Effexor has not been systematically studied in clinical trials for its potential for abuse, there was no indication of drug-seeking behavior in the clinical trials. However, it is not possible to predict on the basis of premarketing experience the extent to which a CNS active drug will be misused, diverted, and/or abused once marketed. Consequently, physicians should carefully evaluate patients for history of drug abuse and follow such patients closely, observing them for signs of misuse or abuse of Effexor (eg, development of tolerance, incrementation of dose, drug-seeking behavior).

OVERDOSAGE

Human Experience

There were 14 reports of acute overdose with Effexor (venlafaxine hydrochloride), either alone or in combination with other drugs and/or alcohol, among the patients included in the premarketing evaluation. The majority of the reports involved ingestions in which the total dose of Effexor taken was estimated to be no more than several-fold higher than the usual therapeutic dose. The 3 patients who took the highest doses were estimated to have ingested approximately 6.75 g, 2.75 g, and 2.5 g. The resultant peak plasma levels of venlafaxine for the latter 2 patients were 6.24 and 2.35 µg/mL, respectively, and the peak plasma levels of O-desmethylvenlafaxine were 3.37 and 1.30 µg/mL, respectively. Plasma venlafaxine levels were not obtained for the patient who ingested 6.75 g of venlafaxine. All 14 patients recovered without sequelae. Most patients reported no symptoms. Among the remaining patients, somnolence was the most commonly reported symptom. The patient who ingested 2.75 g of venlafaxine was observed to have 2 generalized convulsions and a prolongation of QTc to 500 msec, compared with 405 msec at baseline. Mild sinus tachycardia was reported in 2 of the other patients.

In postmarketing experience, overdose with venlafaxine has occurred predominantly in combination with alcohol and/or other drugs. Electrocardiogram changes (eg, prolongation of QT interval, bundle branch block, QRS prolongation), sinus and ventricular tachycardia, bradycardia, hypotension, altered level of consciousness (ranging from somnolence to coma), rhabdomyolysis, seizures, vertigo, and death have been reported.

Management of Overdosage
Treatment should consist of those general measures employed in the management of overdosage with any antidepressant.

Ensure an adequate airway, oxygenation, and ventilation. Monitor cardiac rhythm and vital signs. General supportive and symptomatic measures are also recommended. Induction of emesis is not recommended. Gastric lavage with a large-bore orogastric tube with appropriate airway protection, if needed, may be indicated if performed soon after ingestion or in symptomatic patients. Activated charcoal should be administered. Due to the large volume of distribution of this drug, forced diuresis, dialysis, hemoperfusion and exchange transfusion are unlikely to be of benefit. No specific antidotes for venlafaxine are known.

In managing overdosage, consider the possibility of multiple drug involvement. The physician should consider contacting a poison control center for additional information on the treatment of any overdose. Telephone numbers for certified poison control centers are listed in the *Physicians' Desk Reference (PDR)*.

DOSAGE AND ADMINISTRATION
Initial Treatment
The recommended starting dose for Effexor is 75 mg/day, administered in two or three divided doses, taken with food. Depending on tolerability and the need for further clinical effect, the dose may be increased to 150 mg/day. If needed, the dose should be further increased up to 225 mg/day. When increasing the dose, increments of up to 75 mg/day should be made at intervals of no less than 4 days. In outpatient settings there was no evidence of usefulness of doses greater than 225 mg/day for moderately depressed patients, but more severely depressed inpatients responded to a mean dose of 350 mg/day. Certain patients, including more severely depressed patients, may therefore respond more to higher doses, up to a maximum of 375 mg/day, generally in three divided doses (see **PRECAUTIONS, General,** *Use in Patients with Concomitant Illness*).

Special Populations
Treatment of Pregnant Women During the Third Trimester
Neonates exposed to Effexor, other SNRIs, or SSRIs, late in the third trimester have developed complications requiring prolonged hospitalization, respiratory support, and tube feeding (see **PRECAUTIONS**). When treating pregnant women with Effexor during the third trimester, the physician should carefully consider the potential risks and benefits of treatment. The physician may consider tapering Effexor in the third trimester.

Dosage for Patients with Hepatic Impairment
Given the decrease in clearance and increase in elimination half-life for both venlafaxine and ODV that is observed in patients with hepatic cirrhosis compared to normal subjects (see **CLINICAL PHARMACOLOGY**), it is recommended that the total daily dose be reduced by 50% in patients with moderate hepatic impairment. Since there was much individual variability in clearance between patients with cirrhosis, it may be necessary to reduce the dose even more than 50%, and individualization of dosing may be desirable in some patients.

Dosage for Patients with Renal Impairment
Given the decrease in clearance for venlafaxine and the increase in elimination half-life for both venlafaxine and ODV that is observed in patients with renal impairment (GFR = 10 to 70 mL/min) compared to normals (see **CLINICAL PHARMACOLOGY**), it is recommended that the total daily dose be reduced by 25% in patients with mild to moderate renal impairment. It is recommended that the total daily dose be reduced by 50% and the dose be withheld until the dialysis treatment is completed (4 hrs) in patients undergoing hemodialysis. Since there was much individual variability in clearance between patients with renal impairment, individualization of dosing may be desirable in some patients.

Dosage for Elderly Patients
No dose adjustment is recommended for elderly patients on the basis of age. As with any antidepressant, however, caution should be exercised in treating the elderly. When individualizing the dosage, extra care should be taken when increasing the dose.

Maintenance Treatment
It is generally agreed that acute episodes of major depressive disorder require several months or longer of sustained pharmacological therapy beyond response to the acute episode. In one study, in which patients responding during 8 weeks of acute treatment with Effexor XR were assigned randomly to placebo or to the same dose of Effexor XR (75, 150, or 225 mg/day, qAM) during 26 weeks of maintenance treatment as they had received during the acute stabilization phase, longer-term efficacy was demonstrated. A second longer-term study has demonstrated the efficacy of Effexor in maintaining an antidepressant response in patients with recurrent depression who had responded and continued to be improved during an initial 26 weeks of treatment and were then randomly assigned to placebo or Effexor for periods of up to 52 weeks on the same dose (100 to 200 mg/day, on a b.i.d. schedule) (see **CLINICAL TRIALS**). Based on these limited data, it is not known whether or not the dose of Effexor/Effexor XR needed for maintenance treatment is identical to the dose needed to achieve an initial response. Patients should be periodically reassessed to determine the need for maintenance treatment and the appropriate dose for such treatment.

Discontinuing Effexor (venlafaxine hydrochloride)
Symptoms associated with discontinuation of Effexor, other SNRIs, and SSRIs, have been reported (see **PRECAUTIONS**). Patients should be monitored for these symptoms when discontinuing treatment. A gradual reduction in the dose rather than abrupt cessation is recommended whenever possible. If intolerable symptoms occur following a decrease in the dose or upon discontinuation of treatment, then resuming the previously prescribed dose may be considered. Subsequently, the physician may continue decreasing the dose but at a more gradual rate.

SWITCHING PATIENTS TO OR FROM A MONOAMINE OXIDASE INHIBITOR
At least 14 days should elapse between discontinuation of an MAOI and initiation of therapy with Effexor. In addition, at least 7 days should be allowed after stopping Effexor before starting an MAOI (see **CONTRAINDICATIONS** and **WARNINGS**).

HOW SUPPLIED
Effexor® (venlafaxine hydrochloride) Tablets are available as follows: 25 mg, peach, shield-shaped tablet with "25" and a "W" on one side and "701" on scored reverse side.
   NDC 0008-0701-01, bottle of 100 tablets.
   NDC 0008-0701-02, carton of 10 Redipak® blister strips of 10 tablets each.
37.5 mg, peach, shield-shaped tablet with "37.5" and a "W" on one side and "781" on scored reverse side.
   NDC 0008-0781-01, bottle of 100 tablets.
   NDC 0008-0781-02, carton of 10 Redipak® blister strips of 10 tablets each.
50 mg, peach, shield-shaped tablet with "50" and a "W" on one side and "703" on scored reverse side.
   NDC 0008-0703-01, bottle of 100 tablets.
   NDC 0008-0703-02, carton of 10 Redipak® blister strips of 10 tablets each.
75 mg, peach, shield-shaped tablet with "75" and a "W" on one side and "704" on scored reverse side.
   NDC 0008-0704-01, bottle of 100 tablets.
   NDC 0008-0704-02, carton of 10 Redipak® blister strips of 10 tablets each.
100 mg, peach, shield-shaped tablet with "100" and a "W" on one side and "705" on scored reverse side.
   NDC 0008-0705-01, bottle of 100 tablets.
   NDC 0008-0705-02, carton of 10 Redipak® blister strips of 10 tablets each.
The appearance of these tablets is a trademark of Wyeth Pharmaceuticals.
Store at controlled room temperature 20° to 25°C (68° to 77°F) in a dry place.
Dispense in a well-closed container as defined in the USP.

Medication Guide
About Using Antidepressants in Children and Teenagers
What is the most important information I should know if my child is being prescribed an antidepressant?
Parents or guardians need to think about 4 important things when their child is prescribed an antidepressant:
1. There is a risk of suicidal thoughts or actions.
2. How to try to prevent suicidal thoughts or actions in your child.
3. You should watch for certain signs if your child is taking an antidepressant.
4. There are benefits and risks when using antidepressants.

1. There is a Risk of Suicidal Thoughts or Actions
Children and teenagers sometimes think about suicide, and many report trying to kill themselves.

Antidepressants increase suicidal thoughts and actions in some children and teenagers. But suicidal thoughts and actions can also be caused by depression, a serious medical condition that is commonly treated with antidepressants. Thinking about killing yourself or trying to kill yourself is called *suicidality* or *being suicidal*.

A large study combined the results of 24 different studies of children and teenagers with depression or other illnesses. In these studies, patients took either a placebo (sugar pill) or an antidepressant for 1 to 4 months. **No one committed suicide in these studies**, but some patients became suicidal. On sugar pills, 2 out of every 100 became suicidal. On the antidepressants, 4 out of every 100 patients became suicidal.

For some children and teenagers, the risks of suicidal actions may be especially high. These include patients with:
• Bipolar illness (sometimes called manic-depressive illness)
• A family history of bipolar illness
• A personal or family history of attempting suicide
If any of these are present, make sure you tell your healthcare provider before your child takes an antidepressant.
2. How to Try to Prevent Suicidal Thoughts and Actions
To try to prevent suicidal thoughts and actions in your child, pay close attention to changes in her or his moods or actions, especially if the changes occur suddenly. Other important people in your child's life can help by paying attention as well (e.g., your child, brothers and sisters, teachers, and other important people). The changes to look out for are listed in Section 3, on what to watch for.
Whenever an antidepressant is started or its dose is changed, pay close attention to your child.
After starting an antidepressant, your child should generally see his or her healthcare provider:
• Once a week for the first 4 weeks
• Every 2 weeks for the next 4 weeks
• After taking the antidepressant for 12 weeks
• After 12 weeks, follow your healthcare provider's advice about how often to come back
• More often if problems or questions arise (see Section 3)
You should call your child's healthcare provider between visits if needed.
3. You Should Watch for Certain Signs If Your Child is Taking an Antidepressant
Contact your child's healthcare provider *right away* if your child exhibits any of the following signs for the first time, or if they seem worse, or worry you, your child, or your child's teacher:
• Thoughts about suicide or dying
• Attempts to commit suicide
• New or worse depression
• New or worse anxiety
• Feeling very agitated or restless
• Panic attacks
• Difficulty sleeping (insomnia)
• New or worse irritability
• Acting aggressive, being angry, or violent
• Acting on dangerous impulses
• An extreme increase in activity and talking
• Other unusual changes in behavior or mood
Never let your child stop taking an antidepressant without first talking to his or her healthcare provider. Stopping an antidepressant suddenly can cause other symptoms.
4. There are Benefits and Risks When Using Antidepressants
Antidepressants are used to treat depression and other illnesses. Depression and other illnesses can lead to suicide. In some children and teenagers, treatment with an antidepressant increases suicidal thinking or actions. It is important to discuss all the risks of treating depression and also the risks of not treating it. You and your child should discuss all treatment choices with your healthcare provider, not just the use of antidepressants.
Other side effects can occur with antidepressants (see section below).
Of all the antidepressants, only fluoxetine (Prozac®) has been FDA approved to treat pediatric depression.
For obsessive compulsive disorder in children and teenagers, FDA has approved only fluoxetine (Prozac®), sertraline (Zoloft®), fluvoxamine, and clomipramine (Anafranil®).*
Your healthcare provider may suggest other antidepressants based on the past experience of your child or other family members.

Is this all I need to know if my child is being prescribed an antidepressant?
No. This is a warning about the risk for suicidality. Other side effects can occur with antidepressants. Be sure to ask your healthcare provider to explain all the side effects of the particular drug he or she is prescribing. Also ask about drugs to avoid when taking an antidepressant. Ask your healthcare provider or pharmacist where to find more information.

---

*Prozac® is a registered trademark of Eli Lilly and Company
Zoloft® is a registered trademark of Pfizer Pharmaceuticals
Anafranil® is a registered trademark of Mallinckrodt Inc.

This Medication Guide has been approved by the U.S. Food and Drug Administration for all antidepressants.
Wyeth®
Wyeth Pharmaceuticals Inc.
Philadelphia, PA 19101

W10402C011
ET01
Rev 01/05

EFFEXOR® XR ℞
[ĕ-fĕks-ōr]
(venlafaxine hydrochloride)
Extended-Release Capsules
℞ only

Prescribing information for this product, which appears on pages 3326–3333 of the 2005 PDR, has been completely revised as follows. Please write "See Supplement A" next to the product heading.

Continued on next page

Effexor XR—Cont.

This product's label may have been revised after this insert was used in production. For further product information and current package insert, please visit www.wyeth.com or call our medical communications department toll-free at 1-800-934-5556.

Suicidality in Children and Adolescents
Antidepressants increased the risk of suicidal thinking and behavior (suicidality) in short-term studies in children and adolescents with Major Depressive Disorder (MDD) and other psychiatric disorders. Anyone considering the use of Effexor XR or any other antidepressant in a child or adolescent must balance this risk with the clinical need. Patients who are started on therapy should be observed closely for clinical worsening, suicidality, or unusual changes in behavior. Families and caregivers should be advised of the need for close observation and communication with the prescriber. Effexor XR is not approved for use in pediatric patients. (See WARNINGS and PRECAUTIONS, Pediatric Use.)
Pooled analyses of short-term (4 to 16 weeks) placebo-controlled trials of 9 antidepressant drugs (SSRIs and others) in children and adolescents with major depressive disorder (MDD), obsessive compulsive disorder (OCD), or other psychiatric disorders (a total of 24 trials involving over 4400 patients) have revealed a greater risk of adverse events representing suicidal thinking or behavior (suicidality) during the first few months of treatment in those receiving antidepressants. The average risk of such events in patients receiving antidepressants was 4%, twice the placebo risk of 2%. No suicides occurred in these trials.

DESCRIPTION

Effexor XR is an extended-release capsule for oral administration that contains venlafaxine hydrochloride, a structurally novel antidepressant. It is designated (R/S)-1-[2-(dimethylamino)-1-(4-methoxyphenyl)ethyl] cyclohexanol hydrochloride or (±)-1-[α-[(dimethylamino)methyl]-p-methoxybenzyl] cyclohexanol hydrochloride and has the empirical formula of $C_{17}H_{27}NO_2$ HCl. Its molecular weight is 313.87. The structural formula is shown below.

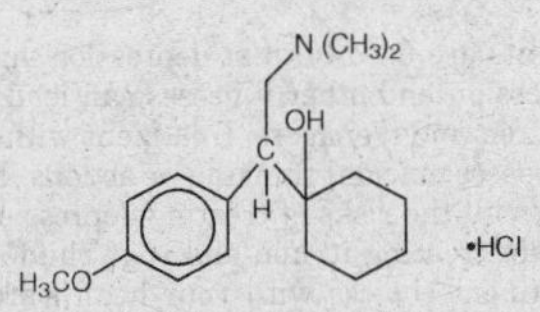

venlafaxine hydrochloride

Venlafaxine hydrochloride is a white to off-white crystalline solid with a solubility of 572 mg/mL in water (adjusted to ionic strength of 0.2 M with sodium chloride). Its octanol: water (0.2 M sodium chloride) partition coefficient is 0.43.
Effexor XR is formulated as an extended-release capsule for once-a-day oral administration. Drug release is controlled by diffusion through the coating membrane on the spheroids and is not pH dependent. Capsules contain venlafaxine hydrochloride equivalent to 37.5 mg, 75 mg, or 150 mg venlafaxine. Inactive ingredients consist of cellulose, ethylcellulose, gelatin, hypromellose, iron oxide, and titanium dioxide.

CLINICAL PHARMACOLOGY

Pharmacodynamics

The mechanism of the antidepressant action of venlafaxine in humans is believed to be associated with its potentiation of neurotransmitter activity in the CNS. Preclinical studies have shown that venlafaxine and its active metabolite, O-desmethylvenlafaxine (ODV), are potent inhibitors of neuronal serotonin and norepinephrine reuptake and weak inhibitors of dopamine reuptake. Venlafaxine and ODV have no significant affinity for muscarinic cholinergic, H_1-histaminergic, or α_1-adrenergic receptors in vitro. Pharmacologic activity at these receptors is hypothesized to be associated with the various anticholinergic, sedative, and cardiovascular effects seen with other psychotropic drugs. Venlafaxine and ODV do not possess monoamine oxidase (MAO) inhibitory activity.

Pharmacokinetics

Steady-state concentrations of venlafaxine and ODV in plasma are attained within 3 days of oral multiple dose therapy. Venlafaxine and ODV exhibited linear kinetics over the dose range of 75 to 450 mg/day. Mean±SD steady-state plasma clearance of venlafaxine and ODV is 1.3±0.6 and 0.4±0.2 L/h/kg, respectively; apparent elimination half-life is 5±2 and 11±2 hours, respectively; and apparent (steady-state) volume of distribution is 7.5±3.7 and 5.7±1.8 L/kg, respectively. Venlafaxine and ODV are minimally bound at therapeutic concentrations to plasma proteins (27% and 30%, respectively).

Absorption

Venlafaxine is well absorbed and extensively metabolized in the liver. O-desmethylvenlafaxine (ODV) is the only major active metabolite. On the basis of mass balance studies, at least 92% of a single oral dose of venlafaxine is absorbed. The absolute bioavailability of venlafaxine is about 45%.
Administration of Effexor XR (150 mg q24 hours) generally resulted in lower C_{max} (150 ng/mL for venlafaxine and 260 ng/mL for ODV) and later T_{max} (5.5 hours for venlafaxine and 9 hours for ODV) than for immediate release venlafaxine tablets (C_{max}'s for immediate release 75 mg q12 hours were 225 ng/mL for venlafaxine and 290 ng/mL for ODV; T_{max}'s were 2 hours for venlafaxine and 3 hours for ODV). When equal daily doses of venlafaxine were administered as either an immediate release tablet or the extended-release capsule, the exposure to both venlafaxine and ODV was similar for the two treatments, and the fluctuation in plasma concentrations was slightly lower with the Effexor XR capsule. Effexor XR, therefore, provides a slower rate of absorption, but the same extent of absorption compared with the immediate release tablet.
Food did not affect the bioavailability of venlafaxine or its active metabolite, ODV. Time of administration (AM vs PM) did not affect the pharmacokinetics of venlafaxine and ODV from the 75 mg Effexor XR capsule.

Metabolism and Excretion

Following absorption, venlafaxine undergoes extensive presystemic metabolism in the liver, primarily to ODV, but also to N-desmethylvenlafaxine, N,O-didesmethylvenlafaxine, and other minor metabolites. In vitro studies indicate that the formation of ODV is catalyzed by CYP2D6; this has been confirmed in a clinical study showing that patients with low CYP2D6 levels ("poor metabolizers") had increased levels of venlafaxine and reduced levels of ODV compared to people with normal CYP2D6 ("extensive metabolizers"). The differences between the CYP2D6 poor and extensive metabolizers, however, are not expected to be clinically important because the sum of venlafaxine and ODV is similar in the two groups and venlafaxine and ODV are pharmacologically approximately equiactive and equipotent.
Approximately 87% of a venlafaxine dose is recovered in the urine within 48 hours as unchanged venlafaxine (5%), unconjugated ODV (29%), conjugated ODV (26%), or other minor inactive metabolites (27%). Renal elimination of venlafaxine and its metabolites is thus the primary route of excretion.

Special Populations

Age and Gender: A population pharmacokinetic analysis of 404 venlafaxine-treated patients from two studies involving both b.i.d. and t.i.d. regimens showed that dose-normalized trough plasma levels of either venlafaxine or ODV were unaltered by age or gender differences. Dosage adjustment based on the age or gender of a patient is generally not necessary (see **DOSAGE AND ADMINISTRATION**).
Extensive/Poor Metabolizers: Plasma concentrations of venlafaxine were higher in CYP2D6 poor metabolizers than extensive metabolizers. Because the total exposure (AUC) of venlafaxine and ODV was similar in poor and extensive metabolizer groups, however, there is no need for different venlafaxine dosing regimens for these two groups.
Liver Disease: In 9 patients with hepatic cirrhosis, the pharmacokinetic disposition of both venlafaxine and ODV was significantly altered after oral administration of venlafaxine. Venlafaxine elimination half-life was prolonged by about 30%, and clearance decreased by about 50% in cirrhotic patients compared to normal subjects. ODV elimination half-life was prolonged by about 60%, and clearance decreased by about 30% in cirrhotic patients compared to normal subjects. A large degree of intersubject variability was noted. Three patients with more severe cirrhosis had a more substantial decrease in venlafaxine clearance (about 90%) compared to normal subjects. Dosage adjustment is necessary in these patients (see **DOSAGE AND ADMINISTRATION**).
Renal Disease: In a renal impairment study, venlafaxine elimination half-life after oral administration was prolonged by about 50% and clearance was reduced by about 24% in renally impaired patients (GFR=10 to 70 mL/min), compared to normal subjects. In dialysis patients, venlafaxine elimination half-life was prolonged by about 180% and clearance was reduced by about 57% compared to normal subjects. Similarly, ODV elimination half-life was prolonged by about 40% although clearance was unchanged in patients with renal impairment (GFR=10 to 70 mL/min) compared to normal subjects. In dialysis patients, ODV elimination half-life was prolonged by about 142% and clearance was reduced by about 56% compared to normal subjects. A large degree of intersubject variability was noted. Dosage adjustment is necessary in these patients (see **DOSAGE AND ADMINISTRATION**).

Clinical Trials

Major Depressive Disorder

The efficacy of Effexor XR (venlafaxine hydrochloride) extended-release capsules as a treatment for major depressive disorder was established in two placebo-controlled, short-term, flexible-dose studies in adult outpatients meeting DSM-III-R or DSM-IV criteria for major depressive disorder.
A 12-week study utilizing Effexor XR doses in a range 75 to 150 mg/day (mean dose for completers was 136 mg/day) and an 8-week study utilizing Effexor XR doses in a range 75 to 225 mg/day (mean dose for completers was 177 mg/day) both demonstrated superiority of Effexor XR over placebo on the HAM-D total score, HAM-D Depressed Mood Item, the MADRS total score, the Clinical Global Impressions (CGI) Severity of Illness item, and the CGI Global Improvement item. In both studies, Effexor XR was also significantly better than placebo for certain factors of the HAM-D, including the anxiety/somatization factor, the cognitive disturbance factor, and the retardation factor, as well as for the psychic anxiety score.
A 4-week study of inpatients meeting DSM-III-R criteria for major depressive disorder with melancholia utilizing Effexor (the immediate release form of venlafaxine) in a range of 150 to 375 mg/day (t.i.d. schedule) demonstrated superiority of Effexor over placebo. The mean dose in completers was 350 mg/day.
Examination of gender subsets of the population studied did not reveal any differential responsiveness on the basis of gender.
In one longer-term study, adult outpatients meeting DSM-IV criteria for major depressive disorder who had responded during an 8-week open trial on Effexor XR (75, 150, or 225 mg, qAM) were randomized to continuation of their same Effexor XR dose or to placebo, for up to 26 weeks of observation for relapse. Response during the open phase was defined as a CGI Severity of Illness item score of ≤3 and a HAM-D-21 total score of ≤10 at the day 56 evaluation. Relapse during the double-blind phase was defined as follows: (1) a reappearance of major depressive disorder as defined by DSM-IV criteria and a CGI Severity of Illness item score of ≥4 (moderately ill), (2) 2 consecutive CGI Severity of Illness item scores of ≥4, or (3) a final CGI Severity of Illness item score of ≥4 for any patient who withdrew from the study for any reason. Patients receiving continued Effexor XR treatment experienced significantly lower relapse rates over the subsequent 26 weeks compared with those receiving placebo.
In a second longer-term trial, adult outpatients meeting DSM-III-R criteria for major depressive disorder, recurrent type, who had responded (HAM-D-21 total score ≤12 at the day 56 evaluation) and continued to be improved [defined as the following criteria being met for days 56 through 180: (1) no HAM-D-21 total score ≥20; (2) no more than 2 HAM-D-21 total scores >10, and (3) no single CGI Severity of Illness item score ≥4 (moderately ill)] during an initial 26 weeks of treatment on Effexor (100 to 200 mg/day, on a b.i.d. schedule) were randomized to continuation of their same Effexor dose or to placebo. The follow-up period to observe patients for relapse, defined as a CGI Severity of Illness item score ≥4, was for up to 52 weeks. Patients receiving continued Effexor treatment experienced significantly lower relapse rates over the subsequent 52 weeks compared with those receiving placebo.

Generalized Anxiety Disorder

The efficacy of Effexor XR capsules as a treatment for Generalized Anxiety Disorder (GAD) was established in two 8-week, placebo-controlled, fixed-dose studies, one 6-month, placebo-controlled, fixed-dose study, and one 6-month, placebo-controlled, flexible-dose study in adult outpatients meeting DSM-IV criteria for GAD.
One 8-week study evaluating Effexor XR doses of 75, 150, and 225 mg/day, and placebo showed that the 225 mg/day dose was more effective than placebo on the Hamilton Rating Scale for Anxiety (HAM-A) total score, both the HAM-A anxiety and tension items, and the Clinical Global Impressions (CGI) scale. While there was also evidence for superiority over placebo for the 75 and 150 mg/day doses, these doses were not as consistently effective as the highest dose.
A second 8-week study evaluating Effexor XR doses of 75 and 150 mg/day and placebo showed that both doses were more effective than placebo on some of these same outcomes; however, the 75 mg/day dose was more consistently effective than the 150 mg/day dose. A dose-response relationship for effectiveness in GAD was not clearly established in the 75 to 225 mg/day dose range utilized in these two studies.
Two 6-month studies, one evaluating Effexor XR doses of 37.5, 75, and 150 mg/day and the other evaluating Effexor XR doses of 75 to 225 mg/day, showed that daily doses of 75 mg or higher were more effective than placebo on the HAM-A total, both the HAM-A anxiety and tension items, and the CGI scale during 6 months of treatment. While there was also evidence for superiority over placebo for the 37.5 mg/day dose, this dose was not as consistently effective as the higher doses.
Examination of gender subsets of the population studied did not reveal any differential responsiveness on the basis of gender.

Social Anxiety Disorder (Social Phobia)

The efficacy of Effexor XR capsules as a treatment for Social Anxiety Disorder (also known as Social Phobia) was established in two double-blind, parallel group, 12-week, multicenter, placebo-controlled, flexible-dose studies in adult outpatients meeting DSM-IV criteria for Social Anxiety Disorder. Patients received doses in a range of 75 to 225 mg/day. Efficacy was assessed with the Liebowitz Social Anxiety Scale (LSAS). In these two trials, Effexor XR was significantly more effective than placebo on change from baseline to endpoint on the LSAS total score.
Examination of subsets of the population studied did not reveal any differential responsiveness on the basis of gender. There was insufficient information to determine the effect of age or race on outcome in these studies.

INDICATIONS AND USAGE

Major Depressive Disorder

Effexor XR (venlafaxine hydrochloride) extended-release capsules is indicated for the treatment of major depressive disorder.
The efficacy of Effexor XR in the treatment of major depressive disorder was established in 8- and 12-week controlled trials of adult outpatients whose diagnoses corresponded most closely to the DSM-III-R or DSM-IV category of major depressive disorder (see **Clinical Trials**).
A major depressive episode (DSM-IV) implies a prominent and relatively persistent (nearly every day for at least 2 weeks) depressed mood or the loss of interest or pleasure in

nearly all activities, representing a change from previous functioning, and includes the presence of at least five of the following nine symptoms during the same two-week period: depressed mood, markedly diminished interest or pleasure in usual activities, significant change in weight and/or appetite, insomnia or hypersomnia, psychomotor agitation or retardation, increased fatigue, feelings of guilt or worthlessness, slowed thinking or impaired concentration, a suicide attempt or suicidal ideation.

The efficacy of Effexor (the immediate release form of venlafaxine) in the treatment of major depressive disorder in adult inpatients meeting diagnostic criteria for major depressive disorder with melancholia was established in a 4-week controlled trial (see **Clinical Trials**). The safety and efficacy of Effexor XR in hospitalized depressed patients have not been adequately studied.

The efficacy of Effexor XR in maintaining a response in major depressive disorder for up to 26 weeks following 8 weeks of acute treatment was demonstrated in a placebo-controlled trial. The efficacy of Effexor in maintaining a response in patients with recurrent major depressive disorder who had responded and continued to be improved during an initial 26 weeks of treatment and were then followed for a period of up to 52 weeks was demonstrated in a second placebo-controlled trial (see **Clinical Trials**). Nevertheless, the physician who elects to use Effexor/Effexor XR for extended periods should periodically re-evaluate the long-term usefulness of the drug for the individual patient (see **DOSAGE AND ADMINISTRATION**).

Generalized Anxiety Disorder

Effexor XR is indicated for the treatment of Generalized Anxiety Disorder (GAD) as defined in DSM-IV. Anxiety or tension associated with the stress of everyday life usually does not require treatment with an anxiolytic.

The efficacy of Effexor XR in the treatment of GAD was established in 8-week and 6-month placebo-controlled trials in adult outpatients diagnosed with GAD according to DSM-IV criteria (see **Clinical Trials**).

Generalized Anxiety Disorder (DSM-IV) is characterized by excessive anxiety and worry (apprehensive expectation) that is persistent for at least 6 months and which the person finds difficult to control. It must be associated with at least 3 of the following 6 symptoms: restlessness or feeling keyed up or on edge, being easily fatigued, difficulty concentrating or mind going blank, irritability, muscle tension, sleep disturbance.

Although the effectiveness of Effexor XR has been demonstrated in 6-month clinical trials in patients with GAD, the physician who elects to use Effexor XR for extended periods should periodically re-evaluate the long-term usefulness of the drug for the individual patient (see **DOSAGE AND ADMINISTRATION**).

Social Anxiety Disorder

Effexor XR is indicated for the treatment of Social Anxiety Disorder, also known as Social Phobia, as defined in DSM-IV (300.23).

Social Anxiety Disorder (DSM-IV) is characterized by a marked and persistent fear of 1 or more social or performance situations in which the person is exposed to unfamiliar people or to possible scrutiny by others. Exposure to the feared situation almost invariably provokes anxiety, which may approach the intensity of a panic attack. The feared situations are avoided or endured with intense anxiety or distress. The avoidance, anxious anticipation, or distress in the feared situation(s) interferes significantly with the person's normal routine, occupational or academic functioning, or social activities or relationships, or there is a marked distress about having the phobias. Lesser degrees of performance anxiety or shyness generally do not require psychopharmacological treatment.

The efficacy of Effexor XR in the treatment of Social Anxiety Disorder was established in two 12-week placebo-controlled trials in adult outpatients with Social Anxiety Disorder (DSM-IV). Effexor XR has not been studied in children or adolescents with Social Anxiety Disorder (see **Clinical Trials**).

The effectiveness of Effexor XR in the long-term treatment of Social Anxiety Disorder, ie, for more than 12 weeks, has not been systematically evaluated in adequate and well-controlled trials. Therefore, the physician who elects to use Effexor XR for extended periods should periodically re-evaluate the long-term usefulness of the drug for the individual patient (see **DOSAGE AND ADMINISTRATION**).

CONTRAINDICATIONS

Hypersensitivity to venlafaxine hydrochloride or to any excipients in the formulation.

Concomitant use in patients taking monoamine oxidase inhibitors (MAOIs) is contraindicated (see **WARNINGS**).

WARNINGS

Clinical Worsening and Suicide Risk

Patients with major depressive disorder (MDD), both adult and pediatric, may experience worsening of their depression and/or the emergence of suicidal ideation and behavior (suicidality) or unusual changes in behavior, whether or not they are taking antidepressant medications, and this risk may persist until significant remission occurs. There has been a long-standing concern that antidepressants may have a role in inducing worsening of depression and the emergence of suicidality in certain patients. Antidepressants increased the risk of suicidal thinking and behavior (suicidality) in short-term studies in children and adolescents with Major Depressive Disorder (MDD) and other psychiatric disorders.

Pooled analyses of short-term placebo-controlled trials of 9 antidepressant drugs (SSRIs and others) in children and adolescents with MDD, OCD, or other psychiatric disorders (a total of 24 trials involving over 4400 patients) have revealed a greater risk of adverse events representing suicidal behavior or thinking (suicidality) during the first few months of treatment in those receiving antidepressants. The average risk of such events in patients receiving antidepressants was 4%, twice the placebo risk of 2%. There was considerable variation in risk among drugs, but a tendency toward an increase for almost all drugs studied. The risk of suicidality was most consistently observed in the MDD trials, but there were signals of risk arising from some trials in other psychiatric indications (obsessive compulsive disorder and social anxiety disorder) as well. **No suicides occurred in any of these trials.** It is unknown whether the suicidality risk in pediatric patients extends to longer-term use, i.e., beyond several months. It is also unknown whether the suicidality risk extends to adults.

All pediatric patients being treated with antidepressants for any indication should be observed closely for clinical worsening, suicidality, and unusual changes in behavior, especially during the initial few months of a course of drug therapy, or at times of dose changes, either increases or decreases. Such observation would generally include at least weekly face-to-face contact with patients or their family members or caregivers during the first 4 weeks of treatment, then every other week visits for the next 4 weeks, then at 12 weeks, and as clinically indicated beyond 12 weeks. Additional contact by telephone may be appropriate between face-to-face visits.

Adults with MDD or co-morbid depression in the setting of other psychiatric illness being treated with antidepressants should be observed similarly for clinical worsening and suicidality, especially during the initial few months of a course of drug therapy, or at times of dose changes, either increases or decreases.

The following symptoms, anxiety, agitation, panic attacks, insomnia, irritability, hostility, aggressiveness, impulsivity, akathisia (psychomotor restlessness), hypomania, and mania, have been reported in adult and pediatric patients being treated with antidepressants for major depressive disorder as well as for other indications, both psychiatric and nonpsychiatric. Although a causal link between the emergence of such symptoms and either the worsening of depression and/or the emergence of suicidal impulses has not been established, there is concern that such symptoms may represent precursors to emerging suicidality.

Consideration should be given to changing the therapeutic regimen, including possibly discontinuing the medication, in patients whose depression is persistently worse, or who are experiencing emergent suicidality or symptoms that might be precursors to worsening depression or suicidality, especially if these symptoms are severe, abrupt in onset, or were not part of the patient's presenting symptoms.

If the decision has been made to discontinue treatment, medication should be tapered, as rapidly as is feasible, but with recognition that abrupt discontinuation can be associated with certain symptoms (see **PRECAUTIONS** and **DOSAGE AND ADMINISTRATION, Discontinuation of Treatment with Effexor XR**, for a description of the risks of discontinuation of Effexor XR).

Families and caregivers of pediatric patients being treated with antidepressants for major depressive disorder or other indications, both psychiatric and nonpsychiatric, should be alerted about the need to monitor patients for the emergence of agitation, irritability, unusual changes in behavior, and the other symptoms described above, as well as the emergence of suicidality, and to report such symptoms immediately to health care providers. Such monitoring should include daily observation by families and caregivers. Prescriptions for Effexor XR should be written for the smallest quantity of capsules consistent with good patient management, in order to reduce the risk of overdose. Families and caregivers of adults being treated for depression should be similarly advised.

Screening Patients for Bipolar Disorder: A major depressive episode may be the initial presentation of bipolar disorder. It is generally believed (though not established in controlled trials) that treating such an episode with an antidepressant alone may increase the likelihood of precipitation of a mixed/manic episode in patients at risk for bipolar disorder. Whether any of the symptoms described above represent such a conversion is unknown. However, prior to initiating treatment with an antidepressant, patients with depressive symptoms should be adequately screened to determine if they are at risk for bipolar disorder; such screening should include a detailed psychiatric history, including a family history of suicide, bipolar disorder, and depression. It should be noted that Effexor XR is not approved for use in treating bipolar depression.

Potential for Interaction with Monoamine Oxidase Inhibitors

Adverse reactions, some of which were serious, have been reported in patients who have recently been discontinued from a monoamine oxidase inhibitor (MAOI) and started on venlafaxine, or who have recently had venlafaxine therapy discontinued prior to initiation of an MAOI. These reactions have included tremor, myoclonus, diaphoresis, nausea, vomiting, flushing, dizziness, hyperthermia with features resembling neuroleptic malignant syndrome, seizures, and death. In patients receiving antidepressants with pharmacological properties similar to venlafaxine in combination with an MAOI, there have also been reports of serious, sometimes fatal, reactions. For a selective serotonin reuptake inhibitor, these reactions have included hyperthermia, rigidity, myoclonus, autonomic instability with possible rapid fluctuations of vital signs, and mental status changes that include extreme agitation progressing to delirium and coma. Some cases presented with features resembling neuroleptic malignant syndrome. Severe hyperthermia and seizures, sometimes fatal, have been reported in association with the combined use of tricyclic antidepressants and MAOIs. These reactions have also been reported in patients who have recently discontinued these drugs and have been started on an MAOI. The effects of combined use of venlafaxine and MAOIs have not been evaluated in humans or animals. Therefore, because venlafaxine is an inhibitor of both norepinephrine and serotonin reuptake, it is recommended that Effexor XR (venlafaxine hydrochloride) extended-release capsules not be used in combination with an MAOI, or within at least 14 days of discontinuing treatment with an MAOI. Based on the half-life of venlafaxine, at least 7 days should be allowed after stopping venlafaxine before starting an MAOI.

Sustained Hypertension

Venlafaxine treatment is associated with sustained increases in blood pressure in some patients. Among patients treated with 75 to 375 mg/day of Effexor XR in premarketing studies in patients with major depressive disorder, 3% (19/705) experienced sustained hypertension [defined as treatment-emergent supine diastolic blood pressure (SDBP) ≥ 90 mm Hg and ≥ 10 mm Hg above baseline for 3 consecutive on-therapy visits]. Among patients treated with 37.5 to 225 mg/day of Effexor XR in premarketing GAD studies, 0.5% (5/1011) experienced sustained hypertension. Among patients treated with 75 to 225 mg/day of Effexor XR in premarketing Social Anxiety Disorder studies, 1.4% (4/277) experienced sustained hypertension. Experience with the immediate-release venlafaxine showed that sustained hypertension was dose-related, increasing from 3% to 7% at 100 to 300 mg/day to 13% at doses above 300 mg/day. An insufficient number of patients received mean doses of Effexor XR over 300 mg/day to fully evaluate the incidence of sustained increases in blood pressure at these higher doses.

In placebo-controlled premarketing studies in patients with major depressive disorder with Effexor XR 75 to 225 mg/day, a final on-drug mean increase in supine diastolic blood pressure (SDBP) of 1.2 mm Hg was observed for Effexor XR-treated patients compared with a mean decrease of 0.2 mm Hg for placebo-treated patients. In placebo-controlled premarketing GAD studies with Effexor XR 37.5 to 225 mg/day, up to 8 weeks or up to 6 months, a final on-drug mean increase in SDBP of 0.3 mm Hg was observed for Effexor XR-treated patients compared with a mean decrease of 0.9 and 0.8 mm Hg, respectively, for placebo-treated patients. In placebo-controlled premarketing Social Anxiety Disorder studies with Effexor XR 75 to 225 mg/day up to 12 weeks, a final on-drug mean increase in SDBP of 1.3 mm Hg was observed for Effexor XR-treated patients compared with a mean decrease of 1.3 mm Hg for placebo-treated patients.

In premarketing major depressive disorder studies, 0.7% (5/705) of the Effexor XR-treated patients discontinued treatment because of elevated blood pressure. Among these patients, most of the blood pressure increases were in a modest range (12 to 16 mm Hg, SDBP). In premarketing GAD studies up to 8 weeks and up to 6 months, 0.7% (10/1381) and 1.3% (7/535) of the Effexor XR-treated patients, respectively, discontinued treatment because of elevated blood pressure. Among these patients, most of the blood pressure increases were in a modest range (12 to 25 mm Hg, SDBP up to 8 weeks; 8 to 28 mm Hg up to 6 months). In premarketing Social Anxiety Disorder studies up to 12 weeks, 0.4% (1/277) of the Effexor XR-treated patients discontinued treatment because of elevated blood pressure. In this patient, the blood pressure increase was modest (13 mm Hg, SDBP).

Sustained increases of SDBP could have adverse consequences. Therefore, it is recommended that patients receiving Effexor XR have regular monitoring of blood pressure. For patients who experience a sustained increase in blood pressure while receiving venlafaxine, either dose reduction or discontinuation should be considered.

PRECAUTIONS

General

Discontinuation of Treatment with Effexor XR

Discontinuation symptoms have been systematically evaluated in patients taking venlafaxine, to include prospective analyses of clinical trials in Generalized Anxiety Disorder and retrospective surveys of trials in major depressive disorder. Abrupt discontinuation or dose reduction of venlafaxine at various doses has been found to be associated with the appearance of new symptoms, the frequency of which increased with increased dose level and with longer duration of treatment. Reported symptoms include agitation, anorexia, anxiety, confusion, coordination impaired, diarrhea, dizziness, dry mouth, dysphoric mood, fasciculation, fatigue, headaches, hypomania, insomnia, nausea, nervousness, nightmares, sensory disturbances (including shock-like electrical sensations), somnolence, sweating, tremor, vertigo, and vomiting.

During marketing of Effexor XR, other SNRIs (Serotonin and Norepinephrine Reuptake Inhibitors), and SSRIs (Selective Serotonin Reuptake Inhibitors), there have been spontaneous reports of adverse events occurring upon discontinuation of these drugs, particularly when abrupt, in-

Continued on next page

Effexor XR—Cont.

cluding the following: dysphoric mood, irritability, agitation, dizziness, sensory disturbances (e.g. paresthesias such as electric shock sensations), anxiety, confusion, headache, lethargy, emotional lability, insomnia, hypomania, tinnitus, and seizures. While these events are generally self-limiting, there have been reports of serious discontinuation symptoms.

Patients should be monitored for these symptoms when discontinuing treatment with Effexor XR. A gradual reduction in the dose rather than abrupt cessation is recommended whenever possible. If intolerable symptoms occur following a decrease in the dose or upon discontinuation of treatment, then resuming the previously prescribed dose may be considered. Subsequently, the physician may continue decreasing the dose but at a more gradual rate (see **DOSAGE AND ADMINISTRATION**).

Insomnia and Nervousness

Treatment-emergent insomnia and nervousness were more commonly reported for patients treated with Effexor XR (venlafaxine hydrochloride) extended-release capsules than with placebo in pooled analyses of short-term major depressive disorder, GAD, and Social Anxiety Disorder studies, as shown in Table 1.

[See table 1 below]

Insomnia and nervousness each led to drug discontinuation in 0.9% of the patients treated with Effexor XR in major depressive disorder studies.

In GAD trials, insomnia and nervousness led to drug discontinuation in 3% and 2%, respectively, of the patients treated with Effexor XR up to 8 weeks and 2% and 0.7%, respectively, of the patients treated with Effexor XR up to 6 months.

In Social Anxiety Disorder trials, insomnia and nervousness led to drug discontinuation in 3% and 0%, respectively, of the patients treated with Effexor XR up to 12 weeks.

Changes in Weight

Adult Patients: A loss of 5% or more of body weight occurred in 7% of Effexor XR-treated and 2% of placebo-treated patients in the short-term placebo-controlled major depressive disorder trials. The discontinuation rate for weight loss associated with Effexor XR was 0.1% in major depressive disorder studies. In placebo-controlled GAD studies, a loss of 7% or more of body weight occurred in 3% of Effexor XR patients and 1% of placebo patients who received treatment for up to 6 months. The discontinuation rate for weight loss was 0.3% for patients receiving Effexor XR in GAD studies for up to eight weeks. In placebo-controlled Social Anxiety Disorder trials, 3% of the Effexor XR-treated and 0.4% of the placebo-treated patients sustained a loss of 7% or more of body weight during up to 12 weeks of treatment. None of the patients receiving Effexor XR in Social Anxiety Disorder studies discontinued for weight loss. The safety and efficacy of venlafaxine therapy in combination with weight loss agents, including phentermine, have not been established. Co-administration of Effexor XR and weight loss agents is not recommended. Effexor XR is not indicated for weight loss alone or in combination with other products.

Pediatric Patients: Weight loss has been observed in pediatric patients (ages 6-17) receiving Effexor XR. In a pooled analysis of four eight-week, double-blind, placebo-controlled, flexible dose outpatient trials for major depressive disorder (MDD) and generalized anxiety disorder (GAD), Effexor XR-treated patients lost an average of 0.45 kg (n = 333), while placebo-treated patients gained an average of 0.77 kg (n = 333). More patients treated with Effexor XR than with placebo experienced a weight loss of at least 3.5% in both the MDD and the GAD studies (18% of Effexor XR-treated patients vs. 3.6% of placebo-treated patients; $p<0.001$). Weight loss was not limited to patients with treatment-emergent anorexia (see **PRECAUTIONS, General**, *Changes in Appetite*).

The risks associated with longer-term Effexor XR use were assessed in an open-label study of children and adolescents who received Effexor XR for up to six months. The children and adolescents in the study had increases in weight that were less than expected based on data from age- and sex-matched peers. The difference between observed weight gain and expected weight gain was larger for children (<12 years old) than for adolescents (>12 years old).

Changes in Height

Pediatric Patients: During the eight-week placebo-controlled GAD studies, Effexor XR-treated patients (ages 6-17) grew an average of 0.3 cm (n = 122), while placebo-treated patients grew an average of 1.0 cm (n = 132); p=0.041. This difference in height increase was most notable in patients younger than twelve. During the eight-week placebo-controlled MDD studies, Effexor XR-treated patients grew an average of 0.8 cm (n = 146), while placebo-treated patients grew an average of 0.7 cm (n = 147). In the six-month open-label study, children and adolescents had height increases that were less than expected based on data from age- and sex-matched peers. The difference between observed growth rates and expected growth rates was larger for children (<12 years old) than for adolescents (>12 years old).

Changes in Appetite

Adult Patients: Treatment-emergent anorexia was more commonly reported for Effexor XR-treated (8%) than placebo-treated patients (4%) in the pool of short-term, double-blind, placebo-controlled major depressive disorder studies. The discontinuation rate for anorexia associated with Effexor XR was 1.0% in major depressive disorder studies. Treatment-emergent anorexia was more commonly reported for Effexor XR-treated (8%) than placebo-treated patients (2%) in the pool of short-term, double-blind, placebo-controlled GAD studies. The discontinuation rate for anorexia was 0.9% for patients receiving Effexor XR for up to 8 weeks in GAD studies. Treatment-emergent anorexia was more commonly reported for Effexor XR-treated (20%) than placebo-treated patients (2%) in the pool of short-term, double-blind, placebo-controlled Social Anxiety Disorder studies. The discontinuation rate for anorexia was 0.4% for patients receiving Effexor XR for up to 12 weeks in Social Anxiety Disorder studies.

Pediatric Patients: Decreased appetite has been observed in pediatric patients receiving Effexor XR. In the placebo-controlled trials for GAD and MDD, 10% of patients aged 6-17 treated with Effexor XR for up to eight weeks and 3% of patients treated with placebo reported treatment-emergent anorexia (decreased appetite). None of the patients receiving Effexor XR discontinued for anorexia or weight loss.

Activation of Mania/Hypomania

During premarketing major depressive disorder studies, mania or hypomania occurred in 0.3% of Effexor XR-treated patients and 0.0% placebo patients. In premarketing GAD studies, 0.0% of Effexor XR-treated patients and 0.2% of placebo-treated patients experienced mania or hypomania. In premarketing Social Anxiety Disorder studies, no Effexor XR-treated patients and no placebo-treated patients experienced mania or hypomania. In all premarketing major depressive disorder trials with Effexor, mania or hypomania occurred in 0.5% of venlafaxine-treated patients compared with 0% of placebo patients. Mania/hypomania has also been reported in a small proportion of patients with mood disorders who were treated with other marketed drugs to treat major depressive disorder. As with all drugs effective in the treatment of major depressive disorder, Effexor XR should be used cautiously in patients with a history of mania.

Hyponatremia

Hyponatremia and/or the syndrome of inappropriate antidiuretic hormone secretion (SIADH) may occur with venlafaxine. This should be taken into consideration in patients who are, for example, volume-depleted, elderly, or taking diuretics.

Mydriasis

Mydriasis has been reported in association with venlafaxine; therefore patients with raised intraocular pressure or those at risk of acute narrow-angle glaucoma (angle-closure glaucoma) should be monitored.

Seizures

During premarketing experience, no seizures occurred among 705 Effexor XR-treated patients in the major depressive disorder studies, among 1381 Effexor XR-treated patients in GAD studies, or among 277 Effexor XR-treated patients in Social Anxiety Disorder studies. In all premarketing major depressive disorder trials with Effexor, seizures were reported at various doses in 0.3% (8/3082) of venlafaxine-treated patients. Effexor XR, like many antidepressants, should be used cautiously in patients with a history of seizures and should be discontinued in any patient who develops seizures.

Abnormal Bleeding

There have been reports of abnormal bleeding (most commonly ecchymosis) associated with venlafaxine treatment. While a causal relationship to venlafaxine is unclear, impaired platelet aggregation may result from platelet serotonin depletion and contribute to such occurrences.

Serum Cholesterol Elevation

Clinically relevant increases in serum cholesterol were recorded in 5.3% of venlafaxine-treated patients and 0.0% of placebo-treated patients treated for at least 3 months in placebo-controlled trials (see **ADVERSE REACTIONS-Laboratory Changes**). Measurement of serum cholesterol levels should be considered during long-term treatment.

Use in Patients With Concomitant Illness

Premarketing experience with venlafaxine in patients with concomitant systemic illness is limited. Caution is advised in administering Effexor XR to patients with diseases or conditions that could affect hemodynamic responses or metabolism.

Venlafaxine has not been evaluated or used to any appreciable extent in patients with a recent history of myocardial infarction or unstable heart disease. Patients with these diagnoses were systematically excluded from many clinical studies during venlafaxine's premarketing testing. The electrocardiograms were analyzed for 275 patients who received Effexor XR and 220 patients who received placebo in 8- to 12-week double-blind, placebo-controlled trials in major depressive disorder, for 610 patients who received Effexor XR and 298 patients who received placebo in 8-week double-blind, placebo-controlled trials in GAD, and for 195 patients who received Effexor XR and 228 patients who received placebo in 12-week double-blind, placebo-controlled trials in Social Anxiety Disorder. The mean change from baseline in corrected QT interval (QTc) for Effexor XR-treated patients in major depressive disorder studies was increased relative to that for placebo-treated patients (increase of 4.7 msec for Effexor XR and decrease of 1.9 msec for placebo). The mean change from baseline in corrected QT interval (QTc) for Effexor XR-treated patients in the GAD studies did not differ significantly from that with placebo. The mean change from baseline in QTc for Effexor XR-treated patients in the Social Anxiety Disorder studies was increased relative to that for placebo-treated patients (increase of 2.8 msec for Effexor XR and decrease of 2.0 msec for placebo).

In these same trials, the mean change from baseline in heart rate for Effexor XR-treated patients in the major depressive disorder studies was significantly higher than that for placebo (a mean increase of 4 beats per minute for Effexor XR and 1 beat per minute for placebo). The mean change from baseline in heart rate for Effexor XR-treated patients in the GAD studies was significantly higher than that for placebo (a mean increase of 3 beats per minute for Effexor XR and no change for placebo). The mean change from baseline in heart rate for Effexor XR-treated patients in the Social Anxiety Disorder studies was significantly higher than that for placebo (a mean increase of 5 beats per minute for Effexor XR and no change for placebo).

In a flexible-dose study, with Effexor doses in the range of 200 to 375 mg/day and mean dose greater than 300 mg/day, Effexor-treated patients had a mean increase in heart rate of 8.5 beats per minute compared with 1.7 beats per minute in the placebo group.

As increases in heart rate were observed, caution should be exercised in patients whose underlying medical conditions might be compromised by increases in heart rate (eg, patients with hyperthyroidism, heart failure, or recent myocardial infarction), particularly when using doses of Effexor above 200 mg/day.

Evaluation of the electrocardiograms for 769 patients who received immediate release Effexor in 4- to 6-week double-blind, placebo-controlled trials showed that the incidence of trial-emergent conduction abnormalities did not differ from that with placebo.

In patients with renal impairment (GFR = 10 to 70 mL/min) or cirrhosis of the liver, the clearances of venlafaxine and its active metabolites were decreased, thus prolonging the elimination half-lives of these substances. A lower dose may be necessary (see **DOSAGE AND ADMINISTRATION**). Effexor XR, like all drugs effective in the treatment of major depressive disorder, should be used with caution in such patients.

Information for Patients

Prescribers or other health professionals should inform patients, their families, and their caregivers about the benefits and risks associated with treatment with Effexor XR and should counsel them in its appropriate use. A patient Medication Guide About Using Antidepressants in Children and Teenagers is available for Effexor XR. The prescriber or health professional should instruct patients, their families, and their caregivers to read the Medication Guide and should assist them in understanding its contents. Patients should be given the opportunity to discuss the contents of the Medication Guide and to obtain answers to any questions they may have. The complete text of the Medication Guide is reprinted at the end of this document.

Patients should be advised of the following issues and asked to alert their prescriber if these occur while taking Effexor XR.

Clinical Worsening and Suicide Risk: Patients, their families, and their caregivers should be encouraged to be alert to the emergence of anxiety, agitation, panic attacks, insomnia, irritability, hostility, aggressiveness, impulsivity, akathisia (psychomotor restlessness), hypomania, mania, other unusual changes in behavior, worsening of depression, and suicidal ideation, especially early during antidepressant treatment and when the dose is adjusted up or down. Families and caregivers of patients should be advised to observe for the emergence of such symptoms on a day-to-day basis, since changes may be abrupt. Such symptoms should be reported to the patient's prescriber or health professional, especially if they are severe, abrupt in onset, or were not part of the patient's presenting symptoms. Symptoms such as these may be associated with an increased risk for suicidal thinking and behavior and indicate a need for very close monitoring and possibly changes in the medication.

Interference with Cognitive and Motor Performance

Clinical studies were performed to examine the effects of venlafaxine on behavioral performance of healthy individuals. The results revealed no clinically significant impairment of psychomotor, cognitive, or complex behavior performance. However, since any psychoactive drug may impair judgment, thinking, or motor skills, patients should be cautioned about operating hazardous machinery, including au-

Table 1
Incidence of Insomnia and Nervousness in Placebo-Controlled Major Depressive Disorder, GAD, and Social Anxiety Disorder Trials

Symptom	Major Depressive Disorder Effexor XR n = 357	Major Depressive Disorder Placebo n = 285	GAD Effexor XR n = 1381	GAD Placebo n = 555	Social Anxiety Disorder Effexor XR n = 277	Social Anxiety Disorder Placebo n = 274
Insomnia	17%	11%	15%	10%	23%	7%
Nervousness	10%	5%	6%	4%	11%	3%

tomobiles, until they are reasonably certain that venlafaxine therapy does not adversely affect their ability to engage in such activities.

Concomitant Medication

Patients should be advised to inform their physicians if they are taking, or plan to take, any prescription or over-the-counter drugs, including herbal preparations, since there is a potential for interactions.

Alcohol

Although venlafaxine has not been shown to increase the impairment of mental and motor skills caused by alcohol, patients should be advised to avoid alcohol while taking venlafaxine.

Allergic Reactions

Patients should be advised to notify their physician if they develop a rash, hives, or a related allergic phenomenon.

Pregnancy

Patients should be advised to notify their physician if they become pregnant or intend to become pregnant during therapy.

Nursing

Patients should be advised to notify their physician if they are breast-feeding an infant.

Laboratory Tests

There are no specific laboratory tests recommended.

Drug Interactions

As with all drugs, the potential for interaction by a variety of mechanisms is a possibility.

Alcohol

A single dose of ethanol (0.5 g/kg) had no effect on the pharmacokinetics of venlafaxine or O-desmethylvenlafaxine (ODV) when venlafaxine was administered at 150 mg/day in 15 healthy male subjects. Additionally, administration of venlafaxine in a stable regimen did not exaggerate the psychomotor and psychometric effects induced by ethanol in these same subjects when they were not receiving venlafaxine.

Cimetidine

Concomitant administration of cimetidine and venlafaxine in a steady-state study for both drugs resulted in inhibition of first-pass metabolism of venlafaxine in 18 healthy subjects. The oral clearance of venlafaxine was reduced by about 43%, and the exposure (AUC) and maximum concentration (C_{max}) of the drug were increased by about 60%. However, coadministration of cimetidine had no apparent effect on the pharmacokinetics of ODV, which is present in much greater quantity in the circulation than venlafaxine. The overall pharmacological activity of venlafaxine plus ODV is expected to increase only slightly, and no dosage adjustment should be necessary for most normal adults. However, for patients with pre-existing hypertension, and for elderly patients or patients with hepatic dysfunction, the interaction associated with the concomitant use of venlafaxine and cimetidine is not known and potentially could be more pronounced. Therefore, caution is advised with such patients.

Diazepam

Under steady-state conditions for venlafaxine administered at 150 mg/day, a single 10 mg dose of diazepam did not appear to affect the pharmacokinetics of either venlafaxine or ODV in 18 healthy male subjects. Venlafaxine also did not have any effect on the pharmacokinetics of diazepam or its active metabolite, desmethyldiazepam, or affect the psychomotor and psychometric effects induced by diazepam.

Haloperidol

Venlafaxine administered under steady-state conditions at 150 mg/day in 24 healthy subjects decreased total oral-dose clearance (Cl/F) of a single 2 mg dose of haloperidol by 42%, which resulted in a 70% increase in haloperidol AUC. In addition, the haloperidol C_{max} increased 88% when coadministered with venlafaxine, but the haloperidol elimination half-life ($t_{1/2}$) was unchanged. The mechanism explaining this finding is unknown.

Lithium

The steady-state pharmacokinetics of venlafaxine administered at 150 mg/day were not affected when a single 600 mg oral dose of lithium was administered to 12 healthy male subjects. ODV also was unaffected. Venlafaxine had no effect on the pharmacokinetics of lithium (see also *CNS-Active Drugs*, below).

Drugs Highly Bound to Plasma Proteins

Venlafaxine is not highly bound to plasma proteins; therefore, administration of Effexor XR to a patient taking another drug that is highly protein bound should not cause increased free concentrations of the other drug.

Drugs that Inhibit Cytochrome P450 Isoenzymes

CYP2D6 Inhibitors: In vitro and in vivo studies indicate that venlafaxine is metabolized to its active metabolite, ODV, by CYP2D6, the isoenzyme that is responsible for the genetic polymorphism seen in the metabolism of many antidepressants. Therefore, the potential exists for a drug interaction between drugs that inhibit CYP2D6-mediated metabolism of venlafaxine, reducing the metabolism of venlafaxine to ODV, resulting in increased plasma concentrations of venlafaxine and decreased concentrations of the active metabolite. CYP2D6 inhibitors such as quinidine would be expected to do this, but the effect would be similar to what is seen in patients who are genetically CYP2D6 poor metabolizers (see *Metabolism and Excretion* under **CLINICAL PHARMACOLOGY**). Therefore, no dosage adjustment is required when venlafaxine is coadministered with a CYP2D6 inhibitor.

The concomitant use of venlafaxine with drug treatment(s) that potentially inhibits both CYP2D6 and CYP3A4, the primary metabolizing enzymes for venlafaxine, has not been studied.

Therefore, caution is advised should a patient's therapy include venlafaxine and any agent(s) that produce simultaneous inhibition of these two enzyme systems.

Drugs Metabolized by Cytochrome P450 Isoenzymes

CYP2D6: In vitro studies indicate that venlafaxine is a relatively weak inhibitor of CYP2D6. These findings have been confirmed in a clinical drug interaction study comparing the effect of venlafaxine with that of fluoxetine on the CYP2D6-mediated metabolism of dextromethorphan to dextrorphan.

Imipramine—Venlafaxine did not affect the pharmacokinetics of imipramine and 2-OH-imipramine. However, desipramine AUC, C_{max}, and C_{min} increased by about 35% in the presence of venlafaxine. The 2-OH-desipramine AUC's increased by at least 2.5 fold (with venlafaxine 37.5 mg q12h) and by 4.5 fold (with venlafaxine 75 mg q12h). Imipramine did not affect the pharmacokinetics of venlafaxine and ODV. The clinical significance of elevated 2-OH-desipramine levels is unknown.

Risperidone—Venlafaxine administered under steady-state conditions at 150 mg/day slightly inhibited the CYP2D6-mediated metabolism of risperidone (administered as a single 1 mg oral dose) to its active metabolite, 9-hydroxyrisperidone, resulting in an approximate 32% increase in risperidone AUC. However, venlafaxine coadministration did not significantly alter the pharmacokinetic profile of the total active moiety (risperidone plus 9-hydroxyrisperidone).

CYP3A4: Venlafaxine did not inhibit CYP3A4 in vitro. This finding was confirmed in vivo by clinical drug interaction studies in which venlafaxine did not inhibit the metabolism of several CYP3A4 substrates, including alprazolam, diazepam, and terfenadine.

Indinavir—In a study of 9 healthy volunteers, venlafaxine administered under steady-state conditions at 150 mg/day resulted in a 28% decrease in the AUC of a single 800 mg oral dose of indinavir and a 36% decrease in indinavir C_{max}. Indinavir did not affect the pharmacokinetics of venlafaxine and ODV. The clinical significance of this finding is unknown.

CYP1A2: Venlafaxine did not inhibit CYP1A2 in vitro. This finding was confirmed in vivo by a clinical drug interaction study in which venlafaxine did not inhibit the metabolism of caffeine, a CYP1A2 substrate.

CYP2C9: Venlafaxine did not inhibit CYP2C9 in vitro. In vivo, venlafaxine 75 mg by mouth every 12 hours did not alter the pharmacokinetics of a single 500 mg dose of tolbutamide or the CYP2C9 mediated formation of 4-hydroxy-tolbutamide.

CYP2C19: Venlafaxine did not inhibit the metabolism of diazepam, which is partially metabolized by CYP2C19 (see *Diazepam* above).

Monoamine Oxidase Inhibitors

See **CONTRAINDICATIONS** and **WARNINGS**.

CNS-Active Drugs

The risk of using venlafaxine in combination with other CNS-active drugs has not been systematically evaluated (except in the case of those CNS-active drugs noted above). Consequently, caution is advised if the concomitant administration of venlafaxine and such drugs is required. Based on the mechanism of action of venlafaxine and the potential for serotonin syndrome, caution is advised when venlafaxine is co-administered with other drugs that may affect the serotonergic neurotransmitter systems, such as triptans, serotonin reuptake inhibitors (SRIs), or lithium.

Electroconvulsive Therapy

There are no clinical data establishing the benefit of electroconvulsive therapy combined with Effexor XR (venlafaxine hydrochloride) extended-release capsules treatment.

Postmarketing Spontaneous Drug Interaction Reports

See **ADVERSE REACTIONS, Postmarketing Reports**.

Carcinogenesis, Mutagenesis, Impairment of Fertility

Carcinogenesis

Venlafaxine was given by oral gavage to mice for 18 months at doses up to 120 mg/kg per day, which was 1.7 times the maximum recommended human dose on a mg/m² basis. Venlafaxine was also given to rats by oral gavage for 24 months at doses up to 120 mg/kg per day. In rats receiving the 120 mg/kg dose, plasma concentrations of venlafaxine at necropsy were 1 times (male rats) and 6 times (female rats) the plasma concentrations of patients receiving the maximum recommended human dose. Plasma levels of the O-desmethyl metabolite were lower in rats than in patients receiving the maximum recommended dose. Tumors were not increased by venlafaxine treatment in mice or rats.

Mutagenesis

Venlafaxine and the major human metabolite, O-desmethylvenlafaxine (ODV), were not mutagenic in the Ames reverse mutation assay in Salmonella bacteria or the Chinese hamster ovary/HGPRT mammalian cell forward gene mutation assay. Venlafaxine was also not mutagenic or clastogenic in the in vitro BALB/c-3T3 mouse cell transformation assay, the sister chromatid exchange assay in cultured Chinese hamster ovary cells, or in the in vivo chromosomal aberration assay in rat bone marrow. ODV was not clastogenic in the in vitro Chinese hamster ovary cell chromosomal aberration assay, but elicited a clastogenic response in the in vivo chromosomal aberration assay in rat bone marrow.

Impairment of Fertility

Reproduction and fertility studies in rats showed no effects on male or female fertility at oral doses of up to 2 times the maximum recommended human dose on a mg/m² basis.

Pregnancy

Teratogenic Effects - Pregnancy Category C

Venlafaxine did not cause malformations in offspring of rats or rabbits given doses up to 2.5 times (rat) or 4 times (rabbit) the maximum recommended human daily dose on a mg/m² basis. However, in rats, there was a decrease in pup weight, an increase in stillborn pups, and an increase in pup deaths during the first 5 days of lactation, when dosing began during pregnancy and continued until weaning. The cause of these deaths is not known. These effects occurred at 2.5 times (mg/m²) the maximum human daily dose. The no effect dose for rat pup mortality was 0.25 times the human dose on a mg/m² basis. There are no adequate and well-controlled studies in pregnant women. Because animal reproduction studies are not always predictive of human response, this drug should be used during pregnancy only if clearly needed.

Non-teratogenic Effects

Neonates exposed to Effexor XR, other SNRIs (Serotonin and Norepinephrine Reuptake Inhibitors), or SSRIs (Selective Serotonin Reuptake Inhibitors), late in the third trimester have developed complications requiring prolonged hospitalization, respiratory support, and tube feeding. Such complications can arise immediately upon delivery. Reported clinical findings have included respiratory distress, cyanosis, apnea, seizures, temperature instability, feeding difficulty, vomiting, hypoglycemia, hypotonia, hypertonia, hyperreflexia, tremor, jitteriness, irritability, and constant crying. These features are consistent with either a direct toxic effect of SSRIs and SNRIs or, possibly, a drug discontinuation syndrome. It should be noted that, in some cases, the clinical picture is consistent with serotonin syndrome (see **PRECAUTIONS-Drug Interactions**-*CNS-Active Drugs*). When treating a pregnant woman with Effexor XR during the third trimester, the physician should carefully consider the potential risks and benefits of treatment (see **DOSAGE AND ADMINISTRATION**).

Labor and Delivery

The effect of venlafaxine on labor and delivery in humans is unknown.

Nursing Mothers

Venlafaxine and ODV have been reported to be excreted in human milk. Because of the potential for serious adverse reactions in nursing infants from Effexor XR, a decision should be made whether to discontinue nursing or to discontinue the drug, taking into account the importance of the drug to the mother.

Pediatric Use

Safety and effectiveness in the pediatric population have not been established (see **BOX WARNING** and **WARNINGS, Clinical Worsening and Suicide Risk**). Two placebo-controlled trials in 766 pediatric patients with MDD and two placebo-controlled trials in 793 pediatric patients with GAD have been conducted with Effexor XR, and the data were not sufficient to support a claim for use in pediatric patients.

Anyone considering use of Effexor XR in a child or adolescent must balance the potential risks with the clinical need. Although no studies have been designed to primarily assess Effexor XR's impact on the growth, development, and maturation of children and adolescents, the studies that have been done suggest that Effexor XR may adversely affect weight and height (see **PRECAUTIONS, General**, *Changes in Height* and *Changes in Weight*). Should the decision be made to treat a pediatric patient with Effexor XR, regular monitoring of weight and height is recommended during treatment, particularly if it is to be continued long term. The safety of Effexor XR treatment for pediatric patients has not been systematically assessed for chronic treatment longer than six months in duration.

In the studies conducted in pediatric patients (ages 6-17), the occurrence of blood pressure and cholesterol increases considered to be clinically relevant in pediatric patients was similar to that observed in adult patients. Consequently, the precautions for adults apply to pediatric patients (see **WARNINGS, Sustained Hypertension**, and **PRECAUTIONS, General**, *Serum Cholesterol Elevation*).

Geriatric Use

Approximately 4% (14/357), 6% (77/1381), and 2% (6/277) of Effexor XR-treated patients in placebo-controlled premarketing major depressive disorder, GAD, and Social Anxiety Disorder trials, respectively, were 65 years of age or over. Of 2,897 Effexor-treated patients in premarketing phase major depressive disorder studies, 12% (357) were 65 years of age or over. No overall differences in effectiveness or safety were observed between geriatric patients and younger patients, and other reported clinical experience generally has not identified differences in response between the elderly and younger patients. However, greater sensitivity of some older individuals cannot be ruled out. As with other antidepressants, several cases of hyponatremia and syndrome of inappropriate antidiuretic hormone secretion (SIADH) have been reported, usually in the elderly.

The pharmacokinetics of venlafaxine and ODV are not substantially altered in the elderly (see **CLINICAL PHARMACOLOGY**). No dose adjustment is recommended for the elderly on the basis of age alone, although other clinical circumstances, some of which may be more common in the elderly, such as renal or hepatic impairment, may warrant a dose reduction (see **DOSAGE AND ADMINISTRATION**).

ADVERSE REACTIONS

The information included in the **Adverse Findings Observed in Short-Term, Placebo-Controlled Studies with Effexor XR**

Continued on next page

Effexor XR—Cont.

subsection is based on data from a pool of three 8- and 12-week controlled clinical trials in major depressive disorder (includes two U.S. trials and one European trial), on data up to 8 weeks from a pool of five controlled clinical trials in GAD with Effexor XR®, and on data up to 12 weeks from a pool of two controlled clinical trials in Social Anxiety Disorder. Information on additional adverse events associated with Effexor XR in the entire development program for the formulation and with Effexor (the immediate release formulation of venlafaxine) is included in the **Other Adverse Events Observed During the Premarketing Evaluation of Effexor and Effexor XR** subsection (see also **WARNINGS** and **PRECAUTIONS**).

Adverse Findings Observed in Short-Term, Placebo-Controlled Studies with Effexor XR

Adverse Events Associated with Discontinuation of Treatment

Approximately 11% of the 357 patients who received Effexor® XR (venlafaxine hydrochloride) extended-release capsules in placebo-controlled clinical trials for major depressive disorder discontinued treatment due to an adverse experience, compared with 6% of the 285 placebo-treated patients in those studies. Approximately 18% of the 1381 patients who received Effexor XR capsules in placebo-controlled clinical trials for GAD discontinued treatment due to an adverse experience, compared with 12% of the 555 placebo-treated patients in those studies. Approximately 17% of the 277 patients who received Effexor XR capsules in placebo-controlled clinical trials for Social Anxiety Disorder discontinued treatment due to an adverse experience, compared with 5% of the 274 placebo-treated patients in those studies. The most common events leading to discontinuation and considered to be drug-related (ie, leading to discontinuation in at least 1% of the Effexor XR-treated patients at a rate at least twice that of placebo for either indication) are shown in Table 2.

[See table 2 below]

Adverse Events Occurring at an Incidence of 2% or More Among Effexor XR-Treated Patients

Tables 3, 4, and 5 enumerate the incidence, rounded to the nearest percent, of treatment-emergent adverse events that occurred during acute therapy of major depressive disorder (up to 12 weeks; dose range of 75 to 225 mg/day), of GAD (up to 8 weeks; dose range of 37.5 to 225 mg/day), and of Social Anxiety Disorder (up to 12 weeks; dose range of 75 to 225 mg/day), respectively, in 2% or more of patients treated with Effexor XR (venlafaxine hydrochloride) where the incidence in patients treated with Effexor XR was greater than the incidence for the respective placebo-treated patients. The table shows the percentage of patients in each group who had at least one episode of an event at some time during their treatment. Reported adverse events were classified using a standard COSTART-based Dictionary terminology. The prescriber should be aware that these figures cannot be used to predict the incidence of side effects in the course of usual medical practice where patient characteristics and other factors differ from those which prevailed in the clinical trials. Similarly, the cited frequencies cannot be compared with figures obtained from other clinical investigations involving different treatments, uses and investigators. The cited figures, however, do provide the prescribing physician with some basis for estimating the relative contribution of drug and nondrug factors to the side effect incidence rate in the population studied.

Commonly Observed Adverse Events from Tables 3, 4, and 5:

Major Depressive Disorder

Note in particular the following adverse events that occurred in at least 5% of the Effexor XR patients and at a rate at least twice that of the placebo group for all placebo-controlled trials for the major depressive disorder (Table 3): Abnormal ejaculation, gastrointestinal complaints (nausea, dry mouth, and anorexia), CNS complaints (dizziness, somnolence, and abnormal dreams), and sweating. In the two U.S. placebo-controlled trials, the following additional events occurred in at least 5% of Effexor XR-treated patients (n = 192) and at a rate at least twice that of the placebo group: Abnormalities of sexual function (impotence in men, anorgasmia in women, and libido decreased), gastrointestinal complaints (constipation and flatulence), CNS complaints (insomnia, nervousness, and tremor), problems of special senses (abnormal vision), cardiovascular effects (hypertension and vasodilatation), and yawning.

Generalized Anxiety Disorder

Note in particular the following adverse events that occurred in at least 5% of the Effexor XR patients and at a rate at least twice that of the placebo group for all placebo-controlled trials for the GAD indication (Table 4): Abnormalities of sexual function (abnormal ejaculation and impotence), gastrointestinal complaints (nausea, dry mouth, anorexia, and constipation), problems of special senses (abnormal vision), and sweating.

Social Anxiety Disorder

Note in particular the following adverse events that occurred in at least 5% of the Effexor XR patients and at a rate at least twice that of the placebo group for the 2 placebo-controlled trials for the Social Anxiety Disorder indication (Table 5): Asthenia, gastrointestinal complaints (anorexia, dry mouth, nausea), CNS complaints (anxiety, insomnia, libido decreased, nervousness, somnolence, dizziness), abnormalities of sexual function (abnormal ejaculation, orgasmic dysfunction, impotence), yawn, sweating, and abnormal vision.

Table 3
Treatment-Emergent Adverse Event Incidence in Short-Term Placebo-Controlled Effexor XR Clinical Trials in Patients with Major Depressive Disorder[1,2]

Body System Preferred Term	% Reporting Event	
	Effexor XR (n=357)	Placebo (n=285)
Body as a Whole		
Asthenia	8%	7%
Cardiovascular System		
Vasodilatation[3]	4%	2%
Hypertension	4%	1%
Digestive System		
Nausea	31%	12%
Constipation	8%	5%
Anorexia	8%	4%
Vomiting	4%	2%
Flatulence	4%	3%
Metabolic/Nutritional		
Weight Loss	3%	0%
Nervous System		
Dizziness	20%	9%
Somnolence	17%	8%
Insomnia	17%	11%
Dry Mouth	12%	6%
Nervousness	10%	5%
Abnormal Dreams[4]	7%	2%
Tremor	5%	2%
Depression	3%	<1%
Paresthesia	3%	1%
Libido Decreased	3%	<1%
Agitation	3%	1%
Respiratory System		
Pharyngitis	7%	6%
Yawn	3%	0%
Skin		
Sweating	14%	3%
Special Senses		
Abnormal Vision[5]	4%	<1%
Urogenital System		
Abnormal Ejaculation (male)[6,7]	16%	<1%
Impotence[7]	4%	<1%
Anorgasmia (female)[8,9]	3%	<1%

[1] Incidence, rounded to the nearest %, for events reported by at least 2% of patients treated with Effexor XR, except the following events which had an incidence equal to or less than placebo: abdominal pain, accidental injury, anxiety, back pain, bronchitis, diarrhea, dysmenorrhea, dyspepsia, flu syndrome, headache, infection, pain, palpitation, rhinitis, and sinusitis.
[2] <1% indicates an incidence greater than zero but less than 1%.
[3] Mostly "hot flashes."
[4] Mostly "vivid dreams," "nightmares," and "increased dreaming."
[5] Mostly "blurred vision" and "difficulty focusing eyes."
[6] Mostly "delayed ejaculation."
[7] Incidence is based on the number of male patients.
[8] Mostly "delayed orgasm" or "anorgasmia."
[9] Incidence is based on the number of female patients.

Table 4
Treatment-Emergent Adverse Event Incidence in Short-Term Placebo-Controlled Effexor XR Clinical Trials in GAD Patients[1,2]

Body System Preferred Term	% Reporting Event	
	Effexor XR (n=1381)	Placebo (n=555)
Body as a Whole		
Asthenia	12%	8%
Cardiovascular System		
Vasodilatation[3]	4%	2%
Digestive System		
Nausea	35%	12%
Constipation	10%	4%
Anorexia	8%	2%
Vomiting	5%	3%
Nervous System		
Dizziness	16%	11%
Dry Mouth	16%	6%
Insomnia	15%	10%
Somnolence	14%	8%
Nervousness	6%	4%
Libido Decreased	4%	2%
Tremor	4%	<1%
Abnormal Dreams[4]	3%	2%
Hypertonia	3%	2%
Paresthesia	2%	1%
Respiratory System		
Yawn	3%	<1%
Skin		
Sweating	10%	3%
Special Senses		
Abnormal Vision[5]	5%	<1%
Urogenital System		
Abnormal Ejaculation[6,7]	11%	<1%
Impotence[7]	5%	<1%
Orgasmic Dysfunction (female)[8,9]	2%	0%

[1] Adverse events for which the Effexor XR reporting rate was less than or equal to the placebo rate are not included. These events are: abdominal pain, accidental injury, anxiety, back pain, diarrhea, dysmenorrhea, dyspepsia, flu syndrome, headache, infection, myalgia, pain, palpitation, pharyngitis, rhinitis, tinnitus, and urinary frequency.
[2] <1% means greater than zero but less than 1%.
[3] Mostly "hot flashes."
[4] Mostly "vivid dreams," "nightmares," and "increased dreaming."
[5] Mostly "blurred vision" and "difficulty focusing eyes."
[6] Includes "delayed ejaculation" and "anorgasmia."
[7] Percentage based on the number of males (Effexor XR = 525, placebo = 220).
[8] Includes "delayed orgasm," "abnormal orgasm," and "anorgasmia."

Table 2
Common Adverse Events Leading to Discontinuation of Treatment in Placebo-Controlled Trials[1]

Adverse Event	Percentage of Patients Discontinuing Due to Adverse Event					
	Major Depressive Disorder Indication[2]		GAD Indication[3,4]		Social Anxiety Disorder Indication	
	Effexor XR n=357	Placebo n=285	Effexor XR n=1381	Placebo n=555	Effexor XR n=277	Placebo n=274
Body as a Whole						
Asthenia	—	—	3%	<1%	1%	<1%
Headache	—	—	—	—	2%	<1%
Digestive System						
Nausea	4%	<1%	8%	<1%	4%	0%
Anorexia	1%	<1%	—	—	—	—
Dry Mouth	1%	0%	2%	<1%	—	—
Vomiting	—	—	1%	<1%	—	—
Nervous System						
Dizziness	2%	1%	—	—	2%	0%
Insomnia	1%	<1%	3%	<1%	3%	<1%
Somnolence	2%	<1%	3%	<1%	2%	<1%
Nervousness	—	—	2%	<1%	—	—
Tremor	—	—	1%	0%	—	—
Anxiety	—	—	—	—	1%	<1%
Skin						
Sweating	—	—	2%	<1%	1%	0%
Urogenital System						
Impotence[5]	—	—	—	—	3%	0%

[1] Two of the major depressive disorder studies were flexible dose and one was fixed dose. Four of the GAD studies were fixed dose and one was flexible dose. Both of the Social Anxiety Disorder studies were flexible dose.
[2] In U.S. placebo-controlled trials for major depressive disorder, the following were also common events leading to discontinuation and were considered to be drug-related for Effexor XR-treated patients (% Effexor XR [n = 192], % Placebo [n = 202]): hypertension (1%, <1%); diarrhea (1%, 0%); paresthesia (1%, 0%); tremor (1%, 0%); abnormal vision, mostly blurred vision (1%, 0%); and abnormal, mostly delayed, ejaculation (1%, 0%).
[3] In two short-term U.S. placebo-controlled trials for GAD, the following were also common events leading to discontinuation and were considered to be drug-related for Effexor XR-treated patients (% Effexor XR [n = 476]), % Placebo [n = 201]): headache (4%, <1%); vasodilatation (1%, 0%); anorexia (2%, <1%); dizziness (4%, 1%); thinking abnormal (1%, 0%); and abnormal vision (1%, 0%).
[4] In long-term placebo-controlled trials for GAD, the following was also a common event leading to discontinuation and was considered to be drug-related for Effexor XR-treated patients (% Effexor XR [n = 535], % Placebo [n = 257]): decreased libido (1%, 0%).
[5] Incidence is based on the number of men (Effexor XR = 158, placebo = 153).

[9]Percentage based on the number of females (Effexor XR = 856, placebo = 335).

Table 5
Treatment-Emergent Adverse Event Incidence in Short-Term Placebo-Controlled Effexor XR Clinical Trials in Social Anxiety Disorder Patients[1,2]

Body System Preferred Term	% Reporting Event	
	Effexor XR (n=277)	Placebo (n=274)
Body as a Whole		
Headache	34%	33%
Asthenia	17%	8%
Flu Syndrome	6%	5%
Accidental Injury	5%	3%
Abdominal Pain	4%	3%
Cardiovascular System		
Hypertension	5%	4%
Vasodilatation[3]	3%	1%
Palpitation	3%	1%
Digestive System		
Nausea	29%	9%
Anorexia[4]	20%	1%
Constipation	8%	4%
Diarrhea	6%	5%
Vomiting	3%	2%
Eructation	2%	0%
Metabolic/Nutritional		
Weight Loss	4%	0%
Nervous System		
Insomnia	23%	7%
Dry Mouth	17%	4%
Dizziness	16%	8%
Somnolence	16%	8%
Nervousness	11%	3%
Libido Decreased	9%	<1%
Anxiety	5%	3%
Agitation	4%	1%
Tremor	4%	<1%
Abnormal Dreams[5]	4%	<1%
Paresthesia	3%	<1%
Twitching	2%	0%
Respiratory System		
Yawn	5%	<1%
Sinusitis	2%	1%
Skin		
Sweating	13%	2%
Special Senses		
Abnormal Vision[6]	6%	3%
Urogenital System		
Abnormal Ejaculation[7,8]	16%	1%
Impotence[8]	10%	1%
Orgasmic Dysfunction[9,10]	8%	0%

[1] Adverse events for which the Effexor XR reporting rate was less than or equal to the placebo rate are not included. These events are: back pain, depression, dysmenorrhea, dyspepsia, infection, myalgia, pain, pharyngitis, rash, rhinitis, and upper respiratory infection.
[2] <1% means greater than zero but less than 1%.
[3] Mostly "hot flashes."
[4] Mostly "decreased appetite" and "loss of appetite."
[5] Mostly "vivid dreams," "nightmares," and "increased dreaming."
[6] Mostly "blurred vision."
[7] Includes "delayed ejaculation" and "anorgasmia."
[8] Percentage based on the number of males (Effexor XR = 158, placebo = 153).
[9] Includes "abnormal orgasm" and "anorgasmia."
[10] Percentage based on the number of females (Effexor XR = 119, placebo = 121).

Vital Sign Changes
Effexor XR (venlafaxine hydrochloride) extended-release capsules treatment for up to 12 weeks in premarketing placebo-controlled major depressive disorder trials was associated with a mean final on-therapy increase in pulse rate of approximately 2 beats per minute, compared with 1 beat per minute for placebo. Effexor XR treatment for up to 8 weeks in premarketing placebo-controlled GAD trials was associated with a mean final on-therapy increase in pulse rate of approximately 2 beats per minute, compared with less than 1 beat per minute for placebo. Effexor XR treatment for up to 12 weeks in premarketing placebo-controlled Social Anxiety Disorder trials was associated with a mean final on-therapy increase in pulse rate of approximately 4 beats per minute, compared with an increase of 1 beat per minute for placebo. (See the **Sustained Hypertension** section of **WARNINGS** for effects on blood pressure.)
In a flexible-dose study, with Effexor doses in the range of 200 to 375 mg/day and mean dose greater than 300 mg/day, the mean pulse was increased by about 2 beats per minute compared with a decrease of about 1 beat per minute for placebo.

Laboratory Changes
Effexor XR (venlafaxine hydrochloride) extended-release capsules treatment for up to 12 weeks in premarketing placebo-controlled trials for major depressive disorder was associated with a mean final on-therapy increase in serum cholesterol concentration of approximately 1.5 mg/dL compared with a mean final decrease of 7.4 mg/dL for placebo. Effexor XR treatment for up to 8 weeks and up to 6 months in premarketing placebo-controlled GAD trials was associ-

ated with mean final on-therapy increases in serum cholesterol concentration of approximately 1.0 mg/dL and 2.3 mg/dL, respectively while placebo subjects experienced mean final decreases of 4.9 mg/dL and 7.7 mg/dL, respectively. Effexor XR treatment for up to 12 weeks in premarketing placebo-controlled Social Anxiety Disorder trials was associated with mean final on-therapy increases in serum cholesterol concentration of approximately 11.4 mg/dL compared with a mean final decrease of 2.2 mg/dL for placebo. Patients treated with Effexor tablets (the immediate-release form of venlafaxine) for at least 3 months in placebo-controlled 12-month extension trials had a mean final on-therapy increase in total cholesterol of 9.1 mg/dL compared with a decrease of 7.1 mg/dL among placebo-treated patients. This increase was duration dependent over the study period and tended to be greater with higher doses. Clinically relevant increases in serum cholesterol, defined as 1) a final on-therapy increase in serum cholesterol ≥50 mg/dL from baseline and to a value ≥261 mg/dL, or 2) an average on-therapy increase in serum cholesterol ≥50 mg/dL from baseline and to a value ≥261 mg/dL, were recorded in 5.3% of venlafaxine-treated patients and 0.0% of placebo-treated patients (see **PRECAUTIONS-General-***Serum Cholesterol Elevation*).

ECG Changes
In a flexible-dose study, with Effexor doses in the range of 200 to 375 mg/day and mean dose greater than 300 mg/day, the mean change in heart rate was 8.5 beats per minute compared with 1.7 beats per minute for placebo.
(See the *Use in Patients with Concomitant Illness* section of **PRECAUTIONS**).

Other Adverse Events Observed During the Premarketing Evaluation of Effexor and Effexor XR
During its premarketing assessment, multiple doses of Effexor XR were administered to 705 patients in Phase 3 major depressive disorder studies and Effexor was administered to 96 patients. During its premarketing assessment, multiple doses of Effexor XR were also administered to 1381 patients in Phase 3 GAD studies and 277 patients in Phase 3 Social Anxiety Disorder studies. In addition, in premarketing assessment of Effexor, multiple doses were administered to 2897 patients in Phase 2 to Phase 3 studies for major depressive disorder. The conditions and duration of exposure to venlafaxine in both development programs varied greatly, and included (in overlapping categories) open and double-blind studies, uncontrolled and controlled studies, inpatient (Effexor only) and outpatient studies, fixed-dose, and titration studies. Untoward events associated with this exposure were recorded by clinical investigators using terminology of their own choosing. Consequently, it is not possible to provide a meaningful estimate of the proportion of individuals experiencing adverse events without first grouping similar types of untoward events into a smaller number of standardized event categories.
In the tabulations that follow, reported adverse events were classified using a standard COSTART-based Dictionary terminology. The frequencies presented, therefore, represent the proportion of the 5356 patients exposed to multiple doses of either formulation of venlafaxine who experienced an event of the type cited on at least one occasion while receiving venlafaxine. All reported events are included except those already listed in Tables 3, 4, and 5 and those events for which a drug cause was remote. If the COSTART term for an event was so general as to be uninformative, it was replaced with a more informative term. It is important to emphasize that, although the events reported occurred during treatment with venlafaxine, they were not necessarily caused by it.
Events are further categorized by body system and listed in order of decreasing frequency using the following definitions: **frequent** adverse events are defined as those occurring on one or more occasions in at least 1/100 patients; **infrequent** adverse events are those occurring in 1/100 to 1/1000 patients; **rare** events are those occurring in fewer than 1/1000 patients.
Body as a whole—**Frequent:** chest pain substernal, chills, fever, neck pain; **Infrequent:** face edema, intentional injury, malaise, moniliasis, neck rigidity, pelvic pain, photosensitivity reaction, suicide attempt, withdrawal syndrome; **Rare:** appendicitis, bacteremia, carcinoma, cellulitis.
Cardiovascular system—**Frequent:** migraine, postural hypotension, tachycardia; **Infrequent:** angina pectoris, arrhythmia, extrasystoles, hypotension, peripheral vascular disorder (mainly cold feet and/or cold hands), syncope, thrombophlebitis; **Rare:** aortic aneurysm, arteritis, first-degree atrioventricular block, bigeminy, bradycardia, bundle branch block, capillary fragility, cerebral ischemia, coronary artery disease, congestive heart failure, heart arrest, cardiovascular disorder (mitral valve and circulatory disturbance), mucocutaneous hemorrhage, myocardial infarct, pallor.
Digestive system—**Frequent:** increased appetite; **Infrequent:** bruxism, colitis, dysphagia, tongue edema, esophagitis, gastritis, gastroenteritis, gastrointestinal ulcer, gingivitis, glossitis, rectal hemorrhage, hemorrhoids, melena, oral moniliasis, stomatitis, mouth ulceration; **Rare:** cheilitis, cholecystitis, cholelithiasis, esophageal spasms, duodenitis, hematemesis, gastrointestinal hemorrhage, gum hemorrhage, hepatitis, ileitis, jaundice, intestinal obstruction, parotitis, periodontitis, proctitis, increased salivation, soft stools, tongue discoloration.
Endocrine system—**Rare:** goiter, hyperthyroidism, hypothyroidism, thyroid nodule, thyroiditis.
Hemic and lymphatic system—**Frequent:** ecchymosis; **Infrequent:** anemia, leukocytosis, leukopenia, lymphadenopathy,

thrombocythemia, thrombocytopenia; **Rare:** basophilia, bleeding time increased, cyanosis, eosinophilia, lymphocytosis, multiple myeloma, purpura.
Metabolic and nutritional—**Frequent:** edema, weight gain; **Infrequent:** alkaline phosphatase increased, dehydration, hypercholesteremia, hyperglycemia, hyperlipemia, hypokalemia, SGOT (AST) increased, SGPT (ALT) increased, thirst; **Rare:** alcohol intolerance, bilirubinemia, BUN increased, creatinine increased, diabetes mellitus, glycosuria, gout, healing abnormal, hemochromatosis, hypercalcinuria, hyperkalemia, hyperphosphatemia, hyperuricemia, hypocholesteremia, hypoglycemia, hyponatremia, hypophosphatemia, hypoproteinemia, uremia.
Musculoskeletal system—**Frequent:** arthralgia; **Infrequent:** arthritis, arthrosis, bone pain, bone spurs, bursitis, leg cramps, myasthenia, tenosynovitis; **Rare:** pathological fracture, myopathy, osteoporosis, osteosclerosis, plantar fasciitis, rheumatoid arthritis, tendon rupture.
Nervous system—**Frequent:** amnesia, confusion, depersonalization, hypesthesia, thinking abnormal, trismus, vertigo; **Infrequent:** akathisia, apathy, ataxia, circumoral paresthesia, CNS stimulation, emotional lability, euphoria, hallucinations, hostility, hyperesthesia, hyperkinesia, hypotonia, incoordination, libido increased, manic reaction, myoclonus, neuralgia, neuropathy, psychosis, seizure, abnormal speech, stupor; **Rare:** akinesia, alcohol abuse, aphasia, bradykinesia, buccoglossal syndrome, cerebrovascular accident, feeling drunk, loss of consciousness, delusions, dementia, dystonia, facial paralysis, abnormal gait, Guillain-Barre Syndrome, hyperchlorhydria, hypokinesia, impulse control difficulties, neuritis, nystagmus, paranoid reaction, paresis, psychotic depression, reflexes decreased, reflexes increased, suicidal ideation, torticollis.
Respiratory system—**Frequent:** cough increased, dyspnea; **Infrequent:** asthma, chest congestion, epistaxis, hyperventilation, laryngismus, laryngitis, pneumonia, voice alteration; **Rare:** atelectasis, hemoptysis, hypoventilation, hypoxia, larynx edema, pleurisy, pulmonary embolus, sleep apnea.
Skin and appendages—**Frequent:** pruritus; **Infrequent:** acne, alopecia, brittle nails, contact dermatitis, dry skin, eczema, skin hypertrophy, maculopapular rash, psoriasis, urticaria; **Rare:** erythema nodosum, exfoliative dermatitis, lichenoid dermatitis, hair discoloration, skin discoloration, furunculosis, hirsutism, leukoderma, petechial rash, pustular rash, vesiculobullous rash, seborrhea, skin atrophy, skin striae.
Special senses—**Frequent:** abnormality of accommodation, mydriasis, taste perversion; **Infrequent:** cataract, conjunctivitis, corneal lesion, diplopia, dry eyes, eye pain, hyperacusis, otitis media, parosmia, photophobia, taste loss, visual field defect; **Rare:** blepharitis, chromatopsia, conjunctival edema, deafness, exophthalmos, glaucoma, retinal hemorrhage, subconjunctival hemorrhage, keratitis, labyrinthitis, miosis, papilledema, decreased pupillary reflex, otitis externa, scleritis, uveitis.
Urogenital system—**Frequent:** metrorrhagia,* prostatic disorder (prostatitis and enlarged prostate),* urination impaired, vaginitis*; **Infrequent:** albuminuria, amenorrhea,* cystitis, dysuria, hematuria, leukorrhea,* menorrhagia,* nocturia, bladder pain, breast pain, polyuria, pyuria, urinary incontinence, urinary retention, urinary urgency, vaginal hemorrhage*; **Rare:** abortion,* anuria, breast discharge, breast engorgement, balanitis,* breast enlargement, endometriosis,* female lactation,* fibrocystic breast, calcium crystalluria, cervicitis,* orchitis,* ovarian cyst,* prolonged erection,* gynecomastia (male),* hypomenorrhea,* kidney calculus, kidney pain, kidney function abnormal, mastitis, menopause,* pyelonephritis, oliguria, salpingitis,* urolithiasis, uterine hemorrhage,* uterine spasm,* vaginal dryness.*

---

*Based on the number of men and women as appropriate.
Postmarketing Reports
Voluntary reports of other adverse events temporally associated with the use of venlafaxine that have been received since market introduction and that may have no causal relationship with the use of venlafaxine include the following: agranulocytosis, anaphylaxis, aplastic anemia, catatonia, congenital anomalies, CPK increased, deep vein thrombophlebitis, delirium, EKG abnormalities such as QT prolongation; cardiac arrhythmias including atrial fibrillation, supraventricular tachycardia, ventricular extrasystoles, and rare reports of ventricular fibrillation and ventricular tachycardia, including torsade de pointes; epidermal necrosis/Stevens-Johnson Syndrome, erythema multiforme, extrapyramidal symptoms (including dyskinesia and tardive dyskinesia), angle-closure glaucoma, hemorrhage (including eye and gastrointestinal bleeding), hepatic events (including GGT elevation; abnormalities of unspecified liver function tests; liver damage, necrosis, or failure; and fatty liver), involuntary movements, LDH increased, neuroleptic malignant syndrome-like events (including a case of a 10-year-old who may have been taking methylphenidate, was treated and recovered), neutropenia, night sweats, pancreatitis, pancytopenia, panic, prolactin increased, pulmonary eosinophilia, renal failure, rhabdomyolysis, serotonin syndrome, shock-like electrical sensations or tinnitus (in some cases, subsequent to the discontinuation of venlafaxine or tapering of dose), and syndrome of inappropriate antidiuretic hormone secretion (usually in the elderly).
There have been reports of elevated clozapine levels that were temporally associated with adverse events, including

Continued on next page

Effexor XR—Cont.

seizures, following the addition of venlafaxine. There have been reports of increases in prothrombin time, partial thromboplastin time, or INR when venlafaxine was given to patients receiving warfarin therapy.

DRUG ABUSE AND DEPENDENCE

Controlled Substance Class

Effexor XR (venlafaxine hydrochloride) extended-release capsules is not a controlled substance.

Physical and Psychological Dependence

In vitro studies revealed that venlafaxine has virtually no affinity for opiate, benzodiazepine, phencyclidine (PCP), or N-methyl-D-aspartic acid (NMDA) receptors.

Venlafaxine was not found to have any significant CNS stimulant activity in rodents. In primate drug discrimination studies, venlafaxine showed no significant stimulant or depressant abuse liability.

Discontinuation effects have been reported in patients receiving venlafaxine (see **DOSAGE AND ADMINISTRATION**).

While venlafaxine has not been systematically studied in clinical trials for its potential for abuse, there was no indication of drug-seeking behavior in the clinical trials. However, it is not possible to predict on the basis of premarketing experience the extent to which a CNS active drug will be misused, diverted, and/or abused once marketed. Consequently, physicians should carefully evaluate patients for history of drug abuse and follow such patients closely, observing them for signs of misuse or abuse of venlafaxine (eg, development of tolerance, incrementation of dose, drug-seeking behavior).

OVERDOSAGE

Human Experience

Among the patients included in the premarketing evaluation of Effexor XR, there were 2 reports of acute overdosage with Effexor XR in major depressive disorder trials, either alone or in combination with other drugs. One patient took a combination of 6 g of Effexor XR and 2.5 mg of lorazepam. This patient was hospitalized, treated symptomatically, and recovered without any untoward effects. The other patient took 2.85 g of Effexor XR. This patient reported paresthesia of all four limbs but recovered without sequelae.

There were 2 reports of acute overdose with Effexor XR in GAD trials. One patient took a combination of 0.75 g of Effexor XR and 200 mg of paroxetine and 50 mg of zolpidem. This patient was described as being alert, able to communicate, and a little sleepy. This patient was hospitalized, treated with activated charcoal, and recovered without any untoward effects. The other patient took 1.2 g of Effexor XR. This patient recovered and no other specific problems were found. The patient had moderate dizziness, nausea, numb hands and feet, and hot-cold spells 5 days after the overdose. These symptoms resolved over the next week.

There were no reports of acute overdose with Effexor XR in Social Anxiety Disorder trials.

Among the patients included in the premarketing evaluation with Effexor, there were 14 reports of acute overdose with venlafaxine, either alone or in combination with other drugs and/or alcohol. The majority of the reports involved ingestion in which the total dose of venlafaxine taken was estimated to be no more than several-fold higher than the usual therapeutic dose. The 3 patients who took the highest doses were estimated to have ingested approximately 6.75 g, 2.75 g, and 2.5 g. The resultant peak plasma levels of venlafaxine for the latter 2 patients were 6.24 and 2.35 µg/mL, respectively, and the peak plasma levels of O-desmethylvenlafaxine were 3.37 and 1.30 µg/mL, respectively. Plasma venlafaxine levels were not obtained for the patient who ingested 6.75 g of venlafaxine. All 14 patients recovered without sequelae. Most patients reported no symptoms. Among the remaining patients, somnolence was the most commonly reported symptom. The patient who ingested 2.75 g of venlafaxine was observed to have 2 generalized convulsions and a prolongation of QTc to 500 msec, compared with 405 msec at baseline. Mild sinus tachycardia was reported in 2 of the other patients.

In postmarketing experience, overdose with venlafaxine has occurred predominantly in combination with alcohol and/or other drugs. Electrocardiogram changes (eg, prolongation of QT interval, bundle branch block, QRS prolongation), sinus and ventricular tachycardia, bradycardia, hypotension, altered level of consciousness (ranging from somnolence to coma), rhabdomyolysis, seizures, vertigo, and death have been reported.

Management of Overdosage

Treatment should consist of those general measures employed in the management of overdosage with any antidepressant.

Ensure an adequate airway, oxygenation, and ventilation. Monitor cardiac rhythm and vital signs. General supportive and symptomatic measures are also recommended. Induction of emesis is not recommended. Gastric lavage with a large bore orogastric tube with appropriate airway protection, if needed, may be indicated if performed soon after ingestion or in symptomatic patients.

Activated charcoal should be administered. Due to the large volume of distribution of this drug, forced diuresis, dialysis, hemoperfusion, and exchange transfusion are unlikely to be of benefit. No specific antidotes for venlafaxine are known. In managing overdosage, consider the possibility of multiple drug involvement. The physician should consider contacting a poison control center for additional information on the treatment of any overdose. Telephone numbers for certified poison control centers are listed in the *Physicians' Desk Reference® (PDR).*

DOSAGE AND ADMINISTRATION

Effexor XR should be administered in a single dose with food either in the morning or in the evening at approximately the same time each day. Each capsule should be swallowed whole with fluid and not divided, crushed, chewed, or placed in water, or it may be administered by carefully opening the capsule and sprinkling the entire contents on a spoonful of applesauce. This drug/food mixture should be swallowed immediately without chewing and followed with a glass of water to ensure complete swallowing of the pellets.

Initial Treatment

Major Depressive Disorder

For most patients, the recommended starting dose for Effexor XR is 75 mg/day, administered in a single dose. In the clinical trials establishing the efficacy of Effexor XR in moderately depressed outpatients, the initial dose of venlafaxine was 75 mg/day. For some patients, it may be desirable to start at 37.5 mg/day for 4 to 7 days, to allow new patients to adjust to the medication before increasing to 75 mg/day. While the relationship between dose and antidepressant response for Effexor XR has not been adequately explored, patients not responding to the initial 75 mg/day dose may benefit from dose increases to a maximum of approximately 225 mg/day. Dose increases should be in increments of up to 75 mg/day, as needed, and should be made at intervals of not less than 4 days, since steady state plasma levels of venlafaxine and its major metabolites are achieved in most patients by day 4. In the clinical trials establishing efficacy, upward titration was permitted at intervals of 2 weeks or more; the average doses were about 140 to 180 mg/day (see **Clinical Trials** under **CLINICAL PHARMACOLOGY**).

It should be noted that, while the maximum recommended dose for moderately depressed outpatients is also 225 mg/day for Effexor (the immediate release form of venlafaxine), more severely depressed inpatients in one study of the development program for that product responded to a mean dose of 350 mg/day (range of 150 to 375 mg/day). Whether or not higher doses of Effexor XR are needed for more severely depressed patients is unknown; however, the experience with Effexor XR doses higher than 225 mg/day is very limited. (See **PRECAUTIONS-General**-*Use in Patients with Concomitant Illness*.)

Generalized Anxiety Disorder

For most patients, the recommended starting dose for Effexor XR is 75 mg/day, administered in a single dose. In clinical trials establishing the efficacy of Effexor XR in outpatients with Generalized Anxiety Disorder (GAD), the initial dose of venlafaxine was 75 mg/day. For some patients, it may be desirable to start at 37.5 mg/day for 4 to 7 days, to allow new patients to adjust to the medication before increasing to 75 mg/day. Although a dose-response relationship for effectiveness in GAD was not clearly established in fixed-dose studies, certain patients not responding to the initial 75 mg/day dose may benefit from dose increases to a maximum of approximately 225 mg/day. Dose increases should be in increments of up to 75 mg/day, as needed, and should be made at intervals of not less than 4 days. (See the *Use in Patients with Concomitant Illness* section of **PRECAUTIONS**.)

Social Anxiety Disorder (Social Phobia)

For most patients, the recommended starting dose for Effexor XR is 75 mg/day, administered in a single dose. In clinical trials establishing the efficacy of Effexor XR in outpatients with Social Anxiety Disorder, the initial dose of Effexor XR was 75 mg/day and the maximum dose was 225 mg/day. For some patients, it may be desirable to start at 37.5 mg/day for 4 to 7 days, to allow new patients to adjust to the medication before increasing to 75 mg/day. Although a dose-response relationship for effectiveness in patients with Social Anxiety Disorder was not clearly established in fixed-dose studies, certain patients not responding to the initial 75 mg/day dose may benefit from dose increases to a maximum of approximately 225 mg/day. Dose increases should be in increments of up to 75 mg/day, as needed, and should be made at intervals of not less than 4 days. (See the *Use in Patients with Concomitant Illness* section of **PRECAUTIONS**.)

Switching Patients from Effexor Tablets

Depressed patients who are currently being treated at a therapeutic dose with Effexor may be switched to Effexor XR at the nearest equivalent dose (mg/day), eg, 37.5 mg venlafaxine two-times-a-day to 75 mg Effexor XR once daily. However, individual dosage adjustments may be necessary.

Special Populations

Treatment of Pregnant Women During the Third Trimester

Neonates exposed to Effexor XR, other SNRIs, or SSRIs, late in the third trimester have developed complications requiring prolonged hospitalization, respiratory support, and tube feeding (see **PRECAUTIONS**). When treating pregnant women with Effexor XR during the third trimester, the physician should carefully consider the potential risks and benefits of treatment. The physician may consider tapering Effexor XR in the third trimester.

Patients with Hepatic Impairment

Given the decrease in clearance and increase in elimination half-life for both venlafaxine and ODV that is observed in patients with hepatic cirrhosis compared with normal subjects (see **CLINICAL PHARMACOLOGY**), it is recommended that the starting dose be reduced by 50% in patients with moderate hepatic impairment. Because there was much individual variability in clearance between patients with cirrhosis, individualization of dosage may be desirable in some patients.

Patients with Renal Impairment

Given the decrease in clearance for venlafaxine and the increase in elimination half-life for both venlafaxine and ODV that is observed in patients with renal impairment (GFR = 10 to 70 mL/min) compared with normal subjects (see **CLINICAL PHARMACOLOGY**), it is recommended that the total daily dose be reduced by 25% to 50%. In patients undergoing hemodialysis, it is recommended that the total daily dose be reduced by 50% and that the dose be withheld until the dialysis treatment is completed (4 hrs). Because there was much individual variability in clearance between patients with renal impairment, individualization of dosage may be desirable in some patients.

Elderly Patients

No dose adjustment is recommended for elderly patients solely on the basis of age. As with any drug for the treatment of major depressive disorder, Generalized Anxiety Disorder, or Social Anxiety Disorder, however, caution should be exercised in treating the elderly. When individualizing the dosage, extra care should be taken when increasing the dose.

Maintenance Treatment

There is no body of evidence available from controlled trials to indicate how long patients with major depressive disorder, Generalized Anxiety Disorder, or Social Anxiety Disorder should be treated with Effexor XR.

It is generally agreed that acute episodes of major depressive disorder require several months or longer of sustained pharmacological therapy beyond response to the acute episode. In one study, in which patients responding during 8 weeks of acute treatment with Effexor XR were assigned randomly to placebo or to the same dose of Effexor XR (75, 150, or 225 mg/day, qAM) during 26 weeks of maintenance treatment as they had received during the acute stabilization phase, longer-term efficacy was demonstrated. A second longer-term study has demonstrated the efficacy of Effexor in maintaining a response in patients with recurrent major depressive disorder who had responded and continued to be improved during an initial 26 weeks of treatment and were then randomly assigned to placebo or Effexor for periods of up to 52 weeks on the same dose (100 to 200 mg/day, on a b.i.d. schedule) (see **Clinical Trials** under **CLINICAL PHARMACOLOGY**). Based on these limited data, it is not known whether or not the dose of Effexor/Effexor XR needed for maintenance treatment is identical to the dose needed to achieve an initial response. Patients should be periodically reassessed to determine the need for maintenance treatment and the appropriate dose for such treatment.

In patients with Generalized Anxiety Disorder, Effexor XR has been shown to be effective in 6-month clinical trials. The need for continuing medication in patients with GAD who improve with Effexor XR treatment should be periodically reassessed.

In patients with Social Anxiety Disorder, there are no efficacy data beyond 12 weeks of treatment with Effexor XR. The need for continuing medication in patients with Social Anxiety Disorder who improve with Effexor XR treatment should be periodically reassessed.

Discontinuing Effexor XR

Symptoms associated with discontinuation of Effexor XR, other SNRIs, and SSRIs, have been reported (see **PRECAUTIONS**). Patients should be monitored for these symptoms when discontinuing treatment. A gradual reduction in the dose rather than abrupt cessation is recommended whenever possible. If intolerable symptoms occur following a decrease in the dose or upon discontinuation of treatment, then resuming the previously prescribed dose may be considered. Subsequently, the physician may continue decreasing the dose but at a more gradual rate. In clinical trials with Effexor XR, tapering was achieved by reducing the daily dose by 75 mg at 1 week intervals. Individualization of tapering may be necessary.

Switching Patients To or From a Monoamine Oxidase Inhibitor

At least 14 days should elapse between discontinuation of an MAOI and initiation of therapy with Effexor XR. In addition, at least 7 days should be allowed after stopping Effexor XR before starting an MAOI (see **CONTRAINDICATIONS** and **WARNINGS**).

HOW SUPPLIED

Effexor® XR (venlafaxine hydrochloride) extended-release capsules are available as follows:

37.5 mg, grey cap/peach body with W and "Effexor XR" on the cap and "37.5" on the body.

NDC 0008-0837-01, bottle of 100 capsules.
NDC 0008-0837-03, carton of 10 Redipak® blister strips of 10 capsules each.

Store at controlled room temperature, 20°C to 25°C (68°F to 77°F).

75 mg, peach cap and body with W and "Effexor XR" on the cap and "75" on the body.

NDC 0008-0833-01, bottle of 100 capsules.
NDC 0008-0833-03, carton of 10 Redipak® blister strips of 10 capsules each.

Store at controlled room temperature, 20°C to 25°C (68°F to 77°F).

150 mg, dark orange cap and body with W and "Effexor XR" on the cap and "150" on the body.

NDC 0008-0836-01, bottle of 100 capsules.
NDC 0008-0836-03, carton of 10 Redipak® blister strips of 10 capsules each.

Store at controlled room temperature, 20°C to 25°C (68°F to 77°F).

The appearance of these capsules is a trademark of Wyeth Pharmaceuticals.

Medication Guide

About Using Antidepressants in Children and Teenagers

What is the most important information I should know if my child is being prescribed an antidepressant?

Parents or guardians need to think about 4 important things when their child is prescribed an antidepressant:

1. There is a risk of suicidal thoughts or actions.
2. How to try to prevent suicidal thoughts or actions in your child.
3. You should watch for certain signs if your child is taking an antidepressant.
4. There are benefits and risks when using antidepressants.

1. There is a Risk of Suicidal Thoughts or Actions

Children and teenagers sometimes think about suicide, and many report trying to kill themselves.

Antidepressants increase suicidal thoughts and actions in some children and teenagers. But suicidal thoughts and actions can also be caused by depression, a serious medical condition that is commonly treated with antidepressants. Thinking about killing yourself or trying to kill yourself is called *suicidality* or *being suicidal*.

A large study combined the results of 24 different studies of children and teenagers with depression or other illnesses. In these studies, patients took either a placebo (sugar pill) or an antidepressant for 1 to 4 months. ***No one committed suicide in these studies***, but some patients became suicidal. On sugar pills, 2 out of every 100 became suicidal. On the antidepressants, 4 out of every 100 patients became suicidal.

For some children and teenagers, the risks of suicidal actions may be especially high. These include patients with:

- Bipolar illness (sometimes called manic-depressive illness)
- A family history of bipolar illness
- A personal or family history of attempting suicide

If any of these are present, make sure you tell your healthcare provider before your child takes an antidepressant.

2. How to Try to Prevent Suicidal Thoughts and Actions

To try to prevent suicidal thoughts and actions in your child, pay close attention to changes in her or his moods or actions, especially if the changes occur suddenly. Other important people in your child's life can help by paying attention as well (e.g., your child, brothers and sisters, teachers, and other important people). The changes to look out for are listed in Section 3, on what to watch for.

Whenever an antidepressant is started or its dose is changed, pay close attention to your child.

After starting an antidepressant, your child should generally see his or her healthcare provider:

- Once a week for the first 4 weeks
- Every 2 weeks for the next 4 weeks
- After taking the antidepressant for 12 weeks
- After 12 weeks, follow your healthcare provider's advice about how often to come back
- More often if problems or questions arise (see Section 3)

You should call your child's healthcare provider between visits if needed.

3. You Should Watch for Certain Signs If Your Child is Taking an Antidepressant

Contact your child's healthcare provider ***right away*** if your child exhibits any of the following signs for the first time, or if they seem worse, or worry you, your child, or your child's teacher:

- Thoughts about suicide or dying
- Attempts to commit suicide
- New or worse depression
- New or worse anxiety
- Feeling very agitated or restless
- Panic attacks
- Difficulty sleeping (insomnia)
- New or worse irritability
- Acting aggressive, being angry, or violent
- Acting on dangerous impulses
- An extreme increase in activity and talking
- Other unusual changes in behavior or mood

Never let your child stop taking an antidepressant without first talking to his or her healthcare provider. Stopping an antidepressant suddenly can cause other symptoms.

4. There are Benefits and Risks When Using Antidepressants

Antidepressants are used to treat depression and other illnesses. Depression and other illnesses can lead to suicide. In some children and teenagers, treatment with an antidepressant increases suicidal thinking or actions. It is important to discuss all the risks of treating depression and also the risks of not treating it. You and your child should discuss all treatment choices with your healthcare provider, not just the use of antidepressants.

Other side effects can occur with antidepressants (see section below).

Of all the antidepressants, only fluoxetine (Prozac®) has been FDA approved to treat pediatric depression.

For obsessive compulsive disorder in children and teenagers, FDA has approved only fluoxetine (Prozac®), sertraline (Zoloft®), fluvoxamine, and clomipramine (Anafranil®).*

Your healthcare provider may suggest other antidepressants based on the past experience of your child or other family members.

Is this all I need to know if my child is being prescribed an antidepressant?

No. This is a warning about the risk for suicidality. Other side effects can occur with antidepressants. Be sure to ask your healthcare provider to explain all the side effects of the particular drug he or she is prescribing. Also ask about drugs to avoid when taking an antidepressant. Ask your healthcare provider or pharmacist where to find more information.

*Prozac® is a registered trademark of Eli Lilly and Company
Zoloft® is a registered trademark of Pfizer Pharmaceuticals
Anafranil® is a registered trademark of Mallinckrodt Inc.

This Medication Guide has been approved by the U.S. Food and Drug Administration for all antidepressants.

Wyeth®
Wyeth Pharmaceuticals Inc.
Philadelphia, PA 19101

W10404C013
ET01
Rev 01/05

HibTITER® ℞

[*hĭb-tī-tər*]

HAEMOPHILUS b CONJUGATE VACCINE
(Diphtheria CRM_{197} Protein Conjugate)
℞ only

Prescribing information for this product, which appears on pages 3333–3336 of the 2005 PDR, has been completely revised as follows. Please write "See Supplement A" next to the product heading.

This product's label may have been revised after this insert was used in production. For further product information and current package insert, please visit www.wyeth.com or call our medical communications department toll-free at 1-800-934-5556.

DESCRIPTION

Haemophilus b Conjugate Vaccine (Diphtheria CRM_{197} Protein Conjugate) HibTITER is a sterile solution of a conjugate of oligosaccharides of the capsular antigen of *Haemophilus influenzae* type b (Haemophilus b) and diphtheria CRM_{197} protein (CRM_{197}) dissolved in 0.9% sodium chloride. The oligosaccharides are derived from highly purified capsular polysaccharide, polyribosylribitol phosphate, isolated from Haemophilus b strain Eagan grown in a chemically defined medium (a mixture of mineral salts, amino acids, and cofactors). The oligosaccharides are purified and sized by diafiltrations through a series of ultrafiltration membranes, and coupled by reductive amination directly to highly purified CRM_{197}.[1,2] CRM_{197} is a nontoxic variant of diphtheria toxin isolated from cultures of *Corynebacterium diphtheriae* C7 (β197) grown in a casamino acids and yeast extract-based medium that is ultrafiltered before use. CRM_{197} is purified through ultrafiltration, ammonium sulfate precipitation, and ion-exchange chromatography to high purity. The conjugate is purified to remove unreacted protein, oligosaccharides, and reagents; sterilized by filtration; and filled into vials. HibTITER is intended for intramuscular use.

The vaccine is a clear, colorless solution. Each single dose of 0.5 mL is formulated to contain 10 µg of purified Haemophilus b saccharide and approximately 25 µg of CRM_{197} protein. The potency of HibTITER is determined by chemical assay for polyribosylribitol.

CLINICAL PHARMACOLOGY

For several decades *Haemophilus influenzae* type b (Haemophilus b) was the most common cause of invasive bacterial disease, including meningitis, in young children in the United States. Although nonencapsulated *H. influenzae* are common and six capsular polysaccharide types are known, strains with the type b capsule caused most of the invasive Haemophilus diseases.[3]

Haemophilus b diseases occurred primarily in children under 5 years of age prior to immunization with *Haemophilus influenzae* type b vaccines. In the US, the cumulative risk of developing invasive Haemophilus b disease during the first 5 years of life was estimated to be about 1 in 200. Approximately 60% of cases were meningitis. Cellulitis, epiglottitis, pericarditis, pneumonia, sepsis, or septic arthritis made up the remaining 40%. An estimated 12,000 cases of Haemophilus b meningitis occurred annually prior to the routine use of conjugate vaccines in toddlers.[3,4] The mortality rate can be 5%, and neurologic sequelae have been observed in up to 38% of survivors.[5]

The incidence of invasive Haemophilus b disease peaks between 6 months and 1 year of age, and approximately 55% of disease occurs between 6 and 18 months of age.[3] Interpersonal transmission of Haemophilus b occurs and risk of invasive disease is increased in children younger than 4 years of age who are exposed in the household to a primary case of disease. Clusters of cases in children in day care have been reported and recent studies suggest that the rate of secondary cases may also be increased among children exposed to a primary case in the daycare setting.[3,6]

The incidence of invasive Haemophilus b disease is increased in certain children, such as those who are native Americans, black, or from lower socioeconomic status, and those with medical conditions such as asplenia, sickle cell disease, malignancies associated with immunosuppression, and antibody deficiency syndromes.[3,4,6]

The protective activity of antibody to Haemophilus b polysaccharide was demonstrated by passive antibody studies in animals and in children with agammaglobulinemia or with Haemophilus b disease[7] and confirmed with the efficacy study of Haemophilus b polysaccharide (HbPs) vaccine.[8] Data from passive antibody studies indicate that a preexisting titer of antibody to HbPs of 0.15 µg/mL correlates with protection.[9] Data from a Finnish field trial in children 18 to 71 months of age indicate that a titer of > 1.0 µg/mL 3 weeks after vaccination is associated with long-term protection.[10,11]

Linkage of Haemophilus b saccharides to a protein such as CRM_{197} converts the saccharide (HbO) to a T-dependent (HbOC) antigen, and results in an enhanced antibody response to the saccharide in young infants that primes for an anamnestic response and is predominantly of the IgG class.[12] Laboratory evidence indicates that the native state of the CRM_{197} protein and the use of oligosaccharides in the formulation of HibTITER enhances its immunogenicity.[13–15]

Prior to licensure, the immunogenicity of HibTITER was evaluated in US infants and children.[15] Infants 1 to 6 months of age at first immunization received three doses at approximately 2-month intervals.[16] Children 7 to 11 and 12 to 14 months of age received 2 doses at the same interval.[15] Children 15 to 23 months of age received a single dose.[17] HibTITER was highly immunogenic in all age groups studied, with 97% to 100% of 1,232 infants attaining titers of ≥ 1 µg/mL and 92% to 100% for bactericidal activity.[15–17]

Long-term persistence of the antibody response was observed. More than 80% of 235 infants who received three doses of vaccine had an anti-HbPs antibody level ≥ 1 µg/mL at 2 years of age.[18]

The vaccine generated an immune response characteristic of a protein antigen. IgG anti-HbPs antibodies of IgG_1 subclass predominated and the immune system was primed for a booster response to HibTITER. There is some evidence suggesting natural increases in antibody levels over time after vaccination, most probably the result of contact with Haemophilus type b organisms or cross-reactive antigens.[18] These studies were carried out at a time when significant levels of Haemophilus b disease were still present in the community.

Antibody generated by HibTITER has been found to have high avidity, a measure of the functional affinity of antibody to bind to antigen. High-avidity antibody is more potent than low-avidity antibody in serum bactericidal assays.[19] The contribution to clinical protection is unknown.

Immunogenicity of HibTITER was evaluated in 26 children 22 months to 5 years of age who had not responded to earlier vaccination with Haemophilus b polysaccharide vaccine. One dose of HibTITER was immunogenic in all 26 children and generated titers of ≥ 1 µg/mL in 25 of the 26 infants.[20] HibTITER has been found to be immunogenic in children with sickle cell disease, a condition that may cause increased susceptibility to Haemophilus b disease.[21] HibTITER has also been shown to be immunogenic in native American infants, such as the group of 50 studied in Alaska who received three doses at 2, 4, and 6 months of age.[20] Antibody levels achieved were comparable to those seen in healthy US infants who received their first dose at 1 to 2 months of age and subsequent doses at 4 to 6 months of age.[15,16,20]

Postlicensure surveillance of immunogenicity was conducted during the distribution of the first 30 million doses of HibTITER and during the time period over which Haemophilus b disease in children has been decreasing significantly in areas of extensive vaccine usage.[20,22–29] After three doses, titers ranged from 2.37 to 8.45 µg/mL with 67% to 94% attaining ≥ 1 µg/mL.[20,24,25]

Persistence of antibody was examined in several cohorts of subjects that received either a selected commercial lot or that were part of the initial efficacy trial in northern California. Geometric mean titers for these cohorts were between 0.51 and 1.96 just prior to boosting at 15 to 18 months. These lots not only induced persistent antibody but also provided effective priming for a booster dose with commercial lots, with postboosting titers greater than 1.0 µg/mL in 80% to 97% of subjects.[20]

HibTITER (HbOC) was shown to be effective in a large-scale controlled clinical trial in a multiethnic population in northern California carried out between February 1988 and June 1990.[30,31] There were no (0) vaccine failures in infants who received three doses of HibTITER and 12 cases of Haemophilus b disease (6 cases of meningitis) in the control group. The estimate of efficacy is 100% (*P*= .0002) with 95% confidence intervals of 68% to 100%. Through the end of 1991, with an additional 49,000 person-years of follow-up, there were still no cases of Haemophilus b disease in fully vaccinated infants less than 2 years of age.[22,23] One case of disease has been reported in a 3 1/2-year-old child who did not receive a booster dose as recommended.

A comparative clinical trial was performed in Finland where approximately 53,000 infants received HibTITER at 4 and 6 months of age and a booster dose at 14 months in a trial conducted from January 1988 through December 1990. Only two children developed Haemophilus b disease after receiving the two-dose primary immunization schedule. One child became ill at 15 months of age and the other at 18 months of age; neither child received the scheduled booster

Continued on next page

HibTITER—Cont.

at 14 months of age. No vaccine failure has been reported in children who received the two-dose primary series and the booster dose at 14 months of age. Based on more than 32,000 person-years of follow-up time, the estimate of efficacy is about 95% when compared to historical control groups followed between 1985 and 1988.[20] Historical controls were used since all infants received one of two Haemophilus b conjugate vaccines during the period of the trial.

Evidence of efficacy postlicensure includes significant reductions in Haemophilus b disease that are closely associated with increases in the net doses of Haemophilus b Conjugate Vaccine distributed in the US.[20,22–29] In the northern California Kaiser Permanente there has been a 94% decrease in Haemophilus disease incidence in 1991 for children younger than 18 months of age, compared to 1984-1988, when HibTITER was not available for this age group.[22,23] Furthermore, active surveillance by the Centers for Disease Control and Prevention (CDC) has shown a 71% decrease in Haemophilus b disease in children less than 15 months old, between 1989 and 1991, which corresponds temporally and geographically with increases in net doses of Haemophilus b conjugate vaccine distributed in the US.[26] As with all vaccines, this conjugate vaccine cannot be expected to be 100% effective. There have been rare reports to the Vaccine Adverse Event Reporting System (VAERS) of Haemophilus b disease following full primary immunization.

INDICATIONS AND USAGE

Haemophilus b Conjugate Vaccine (Diphtheria CRM_{197} Protein Conjugate) HibTITER is indicated for the immunization of children 2 months to 71 months of age against invasive diseases caused by *H. influenza* type b.

As with any vaccine, HibTITER may not protect 100% of individuals receiving the vaccine.

The American Academy of Pediatrics (AAP), the Advisory Committee on Immunization Practices (ACIP) and the American Academy of Family Physicians (AAFP) encourage the routine simultaneous administration of *Haemophilus influenzae* type b vaccines with other currently recommended vaccines, but at different sites (see **DRUG INTERACTIONS**).[32,33,34,35]

CONTRAINDICATIONS

Hypersensitivity to any component of the vaccine, including diphtheria toxoid, is a contraindication to the use of HibTITER.

The occurrence of an allergic or anaphylactic reaction following a prior dose of HibTITER is a contraindication to the use of HibTITER.

WARNINGS

HibTITER WILL NOT PROTECT AGAINST *H. INFLUENZA* OTHER THAN TYPE b STRAINS, NOR WILL HibTITER PROTECT AGAINST OTHER MICROORGANISMS THAT CAUSE MENINGITIS OR SEPTIC DISEASE.

AS WITH ANY INTRAMUSCULAR INJECTION, HibTITER SHOULD BE GIVEN WITH CAUTION TO INFANTS OR CHILDREN WITH THROMBOCYTOPENIA OR ANY COAGULATION DISORDER, OR TO THOSE RECEIVING ANTICOAGULANT THERAPY (SEE **DRUG INTERACTIONS**).

ANTIGENURIA HAS BEEN DETECTED FOLLOWING RECEIPT OF HAEMOPHILUS b CONJUGATE VACCINE[36] AND THEREFORE ANTIGEN DETECTION IN URINE MAY NOT HAVE DIAGNOSTIC VALUE IN SUSPECTED HAEMOPHILUS b DISEASE WITHIN 2 WEEKS OF IMMUNIZATION.

The vial stopper contains dry natural rubber that may cause hypersensitivity reactions when handled by or when the product is injected into persons with known or possible latex sensitivity.

PRECAUTIONS

GENERAL

1. CARE IS TO BE TAKEN BY THE HEALTH CARE PROVIDER FOR SAFE AND EFFECTIVE USE OF THIS PRODUCT.
2. PRIOR TO ADMINISTRATION OF ANY DOSE OF HibTITER, THE PARENT OR GUARDIAN SHOULD BE ASKED ABOUT THE PERSONAL HISTORY, FAMILY HISTORY, AND RECENT HEALTH STATUS OF THE VACCINE RECIPIENT. THE HEALTH CARE PROVIDER SHOULD ASCERTAIN PREVIOUS IMMUNIZATION HISTORY, CURRENT HEALTH STATUS, AND OCCURRENCE OF ANY SYMPTOMS AND/OR SIGNS OF AN ADVERSE EVENT AFTER PREVIOUS IMMUNIZATION IN THE CHILD TO BE IMMUNIZED, IN ORDER TO DETERMINE THE EXISTENCE OF ANY CONTRAINDICATION TO IMMUNIZATION WITH HibTITER AND TO ALLOW AN ASSESSMENT OF BENEFITS AND RISKS.
3. BEFORE THE INJECTION OF ANY BIOLOGICAL, THE HEALTH CARE PROVIDER SHOULD TAKE ALL PRECAUTIONS KNOWN FOR THE PREVENTION OF ALLERGIC OR ANY OTHER SIDE REACTIONS. This should include: a review of the patient's history regarding possible sensitivity; the ready availability of epinephrine 1:1,000 and other appropriate agents used for control of immediate allergic reactions; and a knowledge of the recent literature pertaining to use of the biological concerned, including the nature of side effects and adverse reactions that may follow its use.
4. Children with impaired immune responsiveness, whether due to the use of immunosuppressive therapy (including irradiation, corticosteroids, antimetabolites, alkylating agents, and cytotoxic agents), a genetic defect, human immunodeficiency virus (HIV) infection, or other causes, may have reduced antibody response to active immunization procedures.[37,38] Deferral of administration of vaccine may be considered in individuals receiving immunosuppressive therapy.[37] Other groups should receive this vaccine according to the usual recommended schedule.[37–39] (See **DRUG INTERACTIONS**.)
5. Minor illnesses, such as mild respiratory infection with or without low-grade fever, are not generally contraindications to vaccination. The decision to administer or delay vaccination because of a current or recent febrile illness depends largely on the severity of the symptoms and their etiology. The administration of HibTITER® should be postponed in subjects suffering from acute severe febrile illness.
6. This product is not contraindicated based on the presence of human immunodeficiency virus infection.[40]
7. As reported with Haemophilus b polysaccharide vaccine, cases of Haemophilus b disease may occur prior to the onset of the protective effects of the vaccine.[3,41]
8. The vaccine should not be injected intradermally, subcutaneously, or intravenously since the safety and immunogenicity of these routes have not been evaluated. The vaccine should be given intramuscularly.
9. A separate sterile syringe and needle or a sterile disposable unit should be used for each individual patient to prevent transmission of infectious agents from one person to another. Needles should be disposed of properly and should not be recapped.
10. Special care should be taken to prevent injection into a blood vessel.
11. The vaccine is to be administered immediately after being drawn up into a syringe. Single dose 0.5 mL vial contains no preservative. Use one dose per vial; do not reenter vial. Discard unused portions.
12. As with any vaccine, HibTITER® may not protect 100% of individuals receiving the vaccine.

ALTHOUGH SOME ANTIBODY RESPONSE TO DIPHTHERIA TOXIN OCCURS, IMMUNIZATION WITH HibTITER DOES NOT SUBSTITUTE FOR ROUTINE DIPHTHERIA IMMUNIZATION.

The vial stopper contains dry natural rubber that may cause hypersensitivity reactions when handled by or when the product is injected into persons with known or possible latex sensitivity.

INFORMATION FOR PATIENT

PRIOR TO ADMINISTRATION OF HibTITER, HEALTH CARE PERSONNEL SHOULD INFORM THE PARENT, GUARDIAN OR OTHER RESPONSIBLE ADULT, OF THE RECOMMENDED IMMUNIZATION SCHEDULE FOR PROTECTION AGAINST HAEMOPHILUS b DISEASE AND THE BENEFITS AND RISKS TO THE CHILD RECEIVING THIS VACCINE. GUIDANCE SHOULD BE PROVIDED ON MEASURES TO BE TAKEN SHOULD ADVERSE EVENTS OCCUR, SUCH AS, ANTIPYRETIC MEASURES FOR ELEVATED TEMPERATURES AND THE NEED TO REPORT ADVERSE EVENTS TO THE HEALTH CARE PROVIDER. Parents should be provided with vaccine information pamphlets at the time of each vaccination, as stated in the National Childhood Vaccine Injury Act.[42]

PATIENTS, PARENTS, OR GUARDIANS SHOULD BE INSTRUCTED TO REPORT ANY SERIOUS ADVERSE REACTIONS TO THEIR HEALTH CARE PROVIDER.

TABLE 1

Number of Subjects (Percent) Manifesting Side Effects Associated with HibTITER Administered Independently from DTP* (Infants Vaccinated Initially at 1-6 Months of Age)

	Dose 1 n = 401			Dose 2 n = 383			Dose 3 n = 334		
Symptoms	Same Day As Vacc.	+1 Day	+2 Days	Same Day As Vacc.	+1 Day	+2 Days	Same Day As Vacc.	+1 Day	+2 Days
Temp > 38.3°C	0 -	2 < 1%	2 < 1%	2 < 1%	3 < 1%	2 < 1%	2 < 1%	6 1.8%	5 1.5%
Redness ≥ 2 cm	1 < 1%	0 -	0 -	1 < 1%	6 1.6%	0 -	5 1.5%	4 1.2%	0 -
Warmth ≥ 2 cm	1 < 1%	1 < 1%	0 -	2 < 1%	1 < 1%	0 -	1 < 1%	6 1.8%	0 -
Swelling ≥ 2 cm	5 1.2%	1 < 1%	0 -	2 < 1%	2 < 1%	0 -	1 < 1%	0 -	0 -

*DTP and HibTITER given 2 weeks apart with DTP having been given first.

DRUG INTERACTIONS

Children receiving therapy with immunosuppressive agents (large amounts of corticosteroids, antimetabolites, alkylating agents, cytotoxic agents) may not respond optimally to active immunization.[37,38,39] (See **PRECAUTIONS, GENERAL**.)

As with other intramuscular injections, HibTITER should be given with caution to children on anticoagulant therapy.

No impairment of the antibody response to the individual antigens was demonstrated when HibTITER was given at the same time but at separate sites as diphtheria tetanus pertussis vaccine (DTP) plus oral polio vaccine (OPV) to children 2 to 20 months of age or measles-mumps-rubella (MMR) to children 15 ± 1 month of age.[20,43,44]

There are no clinical studies where a direct comparison of the immune responses to HibTITER was compared with the concurrent administration of diphtheria and tetanus toxoids and acellular pertussis vaccine (DTaP), hepatitis B vaccine (Hep B), inactivated poliovirus vaccine (IPV), 7-valent Conjugate Vaccine-Diphtheria CRM_{197} Protein (Prevnar), or Varicella vaccine. However, in clinical trials where HibTITER and DTaP or HibTITER, DTaP, IPV, and Hep B vaccines were administered concurrently with or without Prevnar in children at 2, 4, and 6 months of age, the percentage of children achieving Hib antibody levels of ≥0.15 or ≥1.0 μg/mL were similar.[45,46] In one study where children 12-15 months of age were administered a booster dose of HibTITER concurrently with DTaP and Prevnar, some suppression of the Hib antibody response was observed, but over 97% of children achieved titers of ≥1.0 μg/mL.[47,48] However, in another study where a booster dose of HibTITER was administered to children at 12-15 months of age concurrently with or without Prevnar the percentage of children achieving Hib antibody levels of ≥0.15 or ≥1.0 μg/mL was found to be similar.[49,50]

HibTITER and DTaP administered concurrently with and without Prevnar at 2, 4, and 6, and 12–15 months of age did not impair immune responses to the seven Pneumococcal vaccine serotypes in Prevnar.[47,48,51,52]

There are no clinical trials where the local and systemic reactogenicity of HibTITER was directly compared with the concurrent administration of DTaP, Hep B, IPV, Prevnar, or Varicella vaccines.

The American Academy of Pediatrics (AAP), the Advisory Committee on Immunization Practices (ACIP) and the American Academy of Family Physicians (AAFP) encourage routine simultaneous administration of DTaP, IPV, *Haemophilus influenzae* type b vaccine, pneumococcal conjugate vaccine, measles-mumps-rubella (MMR), varicella vaccine and hepatitis B vaccine for children who are the recommended age to receive these vaccines and for whom no specific contraindications exist at the time of the visit, unless, in the judgment of the provider, complete vaccination of the child will not be compromised by administering different vaccines at different visits. Simultaneous administration is particularly important if the child might not return for subsequent vaccinations.[32,33,34,35]

CARCINOGENESIS, MUTAGENESIS, IMPAIRMENT OF FERTILITY

HibTITER has not been evaluated for its carcinogenic, mutagenic potential, or impairment of fertility.

PREGNANCY

REPRODUCTIVE STUDIES— PREGNANCY CATEGORY C

Animal reproduction studies have not been conducted with HibTITER. It is also not known whether HibTITER can cause fetal harm when administered to a pregnant woman or can affect reproduction capability. HibTITER is NOT recommended for use in a pregnant woman.

GERIATRIC USE

This vaccine is NOT recommended for use in adult populations.

PEDIATRIC USE

The safety and effectiveness of HibTITER in children below the age of 6 weeks have not been established.

ADVERSE REACTIONS

Adverse reactions associated with HibTITER have been evaluated in 401 infants who were vaccinated initially at 1 to 6 months of age and were given 1,118 doses independent of DTP vaccine. Observations were made during the day of vaccination and days 1 and 2 postvaccination. A temperature > 38.3°C was recorded at least once during the observation period following 2% of the vaccinations. Local erythema, warmth, or swelling (≥ 2 cm) was observed following 3.3% of vaccinations. The incidence of temperature > 38.3°C was greater during the first postvaccination day than during the day of vaccination or the second postvaccination day. The incidence of local erythema, warmth, or swelling was similar during the day of vaccination and the first postvaccination day; it was lower during the second postvaccination day. All side effects have been infrequent, mild, and transient with no serious sequelae (Table 1). No difference in the rates of these complaints was reported after dose 1, 2, or 3.

[See table 1 at left]

The following complaints were also observed after 1,118 vaccinations with HibTITER: irritability (133), sleepiness (91), prolonged crying [≥4 hours] (38), appetite loss (23), vomiting (9), diarrhea (2), and rash (1).

Additional safety data with HibTITER are available from the efficacy studies conducted in young infants.[30] There were 79,483 doses given to 30,844 infants at approximately 2, 4, and 6 months of age in California, usually at the same time as DTP (but at a separate injection site) and OPV; approximately 100,000 doses have been given to 53,000 infants at 4 and 6 months in Finland at the same time as a combined DTP and inactivated polio (IPV) vaccine (but at a separate injection site). The rate and type of reactions associated with the vaccinations were no different from those seen when DTP or DTP-IPV was administered alone. These included fever, local reactions, rash, and one hyporesponsive episode with a single seizure. The safety of HibTITER was also evaluated in the California study by direct phone questioning of the parents or guardians of 6,887 vaccine recipients. The incidence and type of side effects reported within 24 hours of vaccination were similar to those cited in Table 1. In addition, analysis of emergency room (ER) visits within 30 days and hospitalization within 60 days after receipt of 23,800 doses of HibTITER showed no increase in the rates of any type of ER visit or hospitalization.

Table 2 details the side effects associated with a single vaccination of HibTITER given (without DTP) to infants of 15 to 23 months of age.

TABLE 2
Selected Adverse Reactions* in Children of 15-23 Months of Age Following Vaccination with HibTITER

Adverse Reaction	No. of Subjects	Reaction Within 24 h	% Postvaccination At 48 h
Fever >38.3°C	354	1.4	0.6
Erythema	354	2.0	—
Swelling	354	1.7	—
Tenderness	354	3.7	0.3

*The following complaints were reported after vaccination of these 354 children in the indicated number of children: diarrhea (9), vomiting (5), prolonged crying [>4 hours] (4), and rashes (2).

Similar results have been observed in the analysis of 2,285 subjects of 18 to 60 months of age, vaccinated as part of a postmarketing safety study of HibTITER.[20] These data were collected by telephone survey 24 to 48 hours postvaccination. Additional observations included irritability, restless sleep, and GI symptoms (diarrhea, vomiting, and loss of appetite) in the group that received HibTITER alone. A cause and effect relationship between these observations and the vaccinations has not been established.

Post Approval Experience
The following adverse reactions have been identified during post approval use of HibTITER. Because these reactions are reported voluntarily from a population of uncertain size, it is not always possible to reliably estimate their frequency or establish a causal relationship to drug exposure. Decisions to include these reactions in labeling are typically based on one or more of the following factors: (1) seriousness of the reaction, (2) frequency of reporting, or (3) strength of causal connection to the vaccine for post marketing surveillance information.

Injection Site Reactions

Injection site reactions including hypersensitivity (including urticaria), induration, inflammation, mass, and skin discoloration.

Systemic Events

Anaphylactoid/anaphylactic reactions (including shock), angioneurotic edema, convulsions,[53] erythema multiforme, facial edema, febrile seizures, Guillain-Barré syndrome,[54] headache, hives (urticaria), hypersensitivity reaction, lethargy, and malaise. Also reported, hypotonia or hyporesponsive-hypotonic-episodes (in many instances pertussis-containing vaccine was coadministered).

There have been spontaneous reports of apnea in temporal association with the administration of HibTITER. In most cases HibTITER was administered concomitantly with other vaccines including DTP, DTaP, hepatitis B vaccine, IPV, OPV, pneumococcal 7-valent conjugate vaccine, MMR, and/or meningococcal group C conjugate vaccine (not licensed in the US). In addition, in some of the reports existing medical conditions such as prematurity and/or history of apnea were present.

Reporting of Adverse Reactions
Any suspected adverse events following immunization should be reported by the healthcare professional to the US Department of Health and Human Services (DHHS). The National Vaccine Injury Compensation Program requires that the manufacturer and lot number of the vaccine administered be recorded by the healthcare professional in the vaccine recipient's permanent medical record (or in a permanent office log or file), along with the date of administration of the vaccine and the name, address, and title of the person administering the vaccine. The DHHS has established the Vaccine Adverse Event Reporting System (VAERS) to accept all reports of suspected adverse events after the administration of any vaccine, including but not limited to the reporting of events required by the National Childhood Vaccine Injury Act of 1986.[42] The VAERS FDA web site is:

http://www.fda.gov/cber/vaers/vaers.htm

The VAERS toll-free number for VAERS forms and information is 800-822-7967.

OVERDOSAGE
There have been reports of overdose with HibTITER. Many cases were due to inadvertent coadministration with another Haemophilus b conjugate-containing vaccine. Most in-

dividuals were asymptomatic. In general, adverse events reported with overdosage have also been reported with recommended single doses of HibTITER.

DOSAGE AND ADMINISTRATION
HibTITER is for intramuscular use only.

Any parenteral drug product should be inspected visually for particulate matter and/or discoloration prior to administration whenever solution and container permit. If these conditions exist, or if cloudy, HibTITER should not be administered.

Before injection, the skin over the site to be injected should be cleansed with a suitable germicide. After insertion of the needle, aspirate to help avoid inadvertent injection into a blood vessel.

The vaccine should be injected intramuscularly, preferably into the midlateral muscles of the thigh or deltoid, with care to avoid major peripheral nerve trunks. Do not inject in the gluteal area.

The vaccine is to be administered immediately after being drawn up into a syringe. Single dose 0.5 mL vial contains no preservative. Use one dose per vial; do not re-enter vial. Discard unused portions.

HibTITER is indicated for children 2 months to 71 months of age for the prevention of invasive Haemophilus b disease. For infants 2 to 6 months of age, the immunizing dose is three separate injections of 0.5 mL given at approximately 2-month intervals. Previously unvaccinated infants from 7 through 11 months of age should receive two separate injections approximately 2 months apart. Children from 12 through 14 months of age who have not been vaccinated previously receive one injection. All vaccinated children receive a single booster dose at 15 months of age or older, but not less than 2 months after the previous dose. Previously unvaccinated children 15 to 71 months of age receive a single injection of HibTITER.[32,33] Preterm infants should be vaccinated with HibTITER according to their chronological age, from birth.[32]

Recommended Immunization Schedule

Age at First Immunization (Mo)	No. of Doses	Booster
2-6	3	Yes
7-11	2	Yes
12-14	1	Yes
15 and over	1	No

Interruption of the recommended schedules with a delay between doses does not interfere with the final immunity achieved nor does it necessitate starting the series over again, regardless of the length of time elapsed between doses.[32,33]

Data support that HibTITER may be interchanged with other Haemophilus influenzae type b conjugate vaccines for the primary immunization series[55,56]

Each dose of 0.5 mL is formulated to contain 10 µg of purified Haemophilus b saccharide and approximately 25 µg of CRM_{197} protein.

STORAGE
DO NOT FREEZE. Store refrigerated away from freezer compartments at 2°C-8°C (36°F-46°F). Discard if the vaccine has been frozen.

HOW SUPPLIED
Vial, 1 Dose (5 per package) – Product No. 0005-0104-32

REFERENCES
1. United States Patent Number 4,902,506 by Anderson PW, Eby filed May 5, 1986 issued February 20, 1990.
2. Seid RC Jr, Boykins RA, Liu DF, et al. Chemical evidence for covalent linkage of a semi-synthetic glycoconjugate vaccine for Haemophilus influenzae type b disease. Glycoconjugate J 1989;6:489-498.
3. Wenger JD, Ward JL, Broome CV. Prevention of Haemophilus influenzae type b disease: vaccines and passive prophylaxis. In: Remington JS, Swartz MS, eds. Current Clinical Topics in Infectious Diseases. New York, NY: McGraw-Hill Inc; 1989;10: 306-339.
4. Recommendation of the Immunization Practices Advisory Committee (ACIP) – polysaccharide vaccine for prevention of Haemophilus influenzae type b disease. MMWR. 1985;34:201-205.
5. Sell SH. Long term sequelae of bacterial meningitis in children. Pediatr Infect Dis J. 1983;2:90-93.
6. Broome CV. Epidemiology of Haemophilus influenzae type b infections in the United States. Pediatr Infect Dis J. 1987;6:779-782.
7. Alexander HE. The productive or curative element in type b Haemophilus influenzae rabbit serum. Yale J Biol Med. 1944;16:425-434.
8. Peltola H, Kayhty H, Sivonen A. Haemophilus influenzae type b capsular polysaccharide vaccine in children: a double-blind field study of 100,000 vaccinees 3 months to 5 years of age in Finland. Pediatrics. 1977;60:730-737.
9. Robbins JB, Parke JC Jr, Schneerson R. Quantitative measurement of "natural" and immunization-induced Haemophilus influenzae type b capsular polysaccharide antibodies. Pediatr Res. 1973;7:103-110.
10. Kayhty H, Peltola H, Karanko V, et al. The protective level of serum antibodies to the capsular polysaccharide of Haemophilus influenzae type b. J Infect Dis. 1983;147:1100.
11. Kayhty H, Karanko V, Peltola H, et al. Serum antibodies after vaccination with Haemophilus influenzae type b

capsular polysaccharide and responses to reimmunization: no evidence immunologic tolerance or memory. Pediatrics. 1984;74:857-865.
12. Weinberg GA, Granoff DM. Polysaccharide-protein conjugate vaccines for the prevention of Haemophilus influenzae type b disease. J Pediatr. 1988;113:621-631.
13. Makela O, Péterfy F, Outshoorn IG, et al. Immunogenic properties of a (1-6) dextran, its protein conjugates, and conjugates of its breakdown products in mice. Scand J Immunol. 1984;19:541-550.
14. Anderson P, Pichichero ME, Insel RA. Immunogens consisting of oligosaccharides from Haemophilus influenzae type b coupled to diphtheria toxoid or the toxin protein CRM197. J Clin Invest. 1985;76:52-59.
15. Madore DV, Phipps DC, Eby R, et al. Immune response of young children vaccinated with Haemophilus influenzae type b conjugate vaccines. In: Cruse JM, Lewis RE, eds. Contributions to Microbiology and Immunology: Conjugate Vaccines. New York, NY: Karger Medical and Scientific Publishers; 1989;10:125-150.
16. Madore DV, Phipps DC, Eby R, et al. Safety and immunologic response to Haemophilus influenzae type b oligosaccharide-CRM197 conjugate vaccine in 1- to 6-month-old infants. Pediatrics. 1990;85:331-337.
17. Madore DV, Johnson CL, Phipps DC, et al. Safety and immunogenicity of Haemophilus influenzae type b oligosaccharide-CRM197 conjugate vaccine in infants aged 15-23 months. Pediatrics. 1990;86:527-534.
18. Rothstein EP, Madore DV, Long S. Antibody persistence four years after primary immunization of infants and toddlers with Haemophilus influenzae type b CRM197 conjugate vaccine. J Pediatr. 1991; 119:655-657.
19. Schlesinger Y, Granoff DM. Avidity and bactericidal activity of antibodies elicited by different Haemophilus influenzae type b conjugate vaccines. JAMA. 1992;267:1489-1494.
20. Unpublished data available from Lederle Laboratories.
21. Gigliotti F, Feldman S, Wang WC, et al. Immunization of young infants with sickle cell disease with a Haemophilus influenzae type b saccharide-diphtheria CRM197 protein conjugate vaccine. J Pediatr. 1989;114:1006-1010.
22. Black SB, Shinefield HR, The Kaiser Permanente Pediatric Vaccine Study Group. Immunization with oligosaccharide conjugate Haemophilus influenzae type b (HbOC) vaccine on a large health maintenance organization population: extended follow-up and impact on Haemophilus influenzae disease epidemiology. Pediatric Infect Dis J. 1992;11:610-613.
23. Black SB, Shinefield HR, Fireman B, et al. Safety, immunogenicity, and efficacy in infancy of oligosaccharide conjugate Haemophilus influenzae type b vaccine in a United States Population: possible implications for optimal use. J Infect Dis. 1992;165 (suppl 1):S139-S143.
24. Granoff DM, Anderson EL, Osterholm MT, et al. Differences in the immunogenicity of three Haemophilus influenzae type b conjugate vaccines in infants. J Pediatr. 1992;121:187-194.
25. Decker MD, Edwards KM, Bradley R, et al. Comparative trial in infants of four conjugate Haemophilus influenzae type b vaccines. J Pediatr. 1992;120:184-189.
26. Adams WG, Deaver KA, Cochi SL, et al. Decline of childhood Haemophilus influenzae type b (Hib) disease in the Hib vaccine era. JAMA. 1993;269:221-226.
27. Murphy TV, White KE, Pastor P, et al. Declining incidence of Haemophilus influenzae type b disease since introduction of vaccination. JAMA. 1993;269:246-248.
28. Broadhurst LE, Erickson RL, Kelley PW. Decreases in invasive Haemophilus influenzae diseases in US Army children, 1984 through 1991. JAMA. 1993;269:227-231.
29. Shapiro ED. Infections caused by Haemophilus influenzae type b: the beginning of the end? JAMA. 1993;269:264-266.
30. Black SB, Shinefield HR, Lampert D, et al. Safety and immunogenicity of oligosaccharide conjugate Haemophilus influenzae type b (HbOC) vaccine in infancy. Pediatr Infect Dis J. 1991;10:92-96.
31. Black SB, Shinefield HR, Fireman B, et al. Efficacy in infancy of oligosaccharide conjugate Haemophilus influenzae type b (HbOC) vaccine in a United States Population of 61,080 children. Pediatr Infect Dis J. 1991;10:97-104.
32. Recommendations of the AAP: Haemophilus influenzae type b conjugate vaccines: recommendations for immunization of infants and children 2 months of age and older: update. Pediatrics. 1991;88:169-172.
33. Recommendation of the ACIP: Haemophilus b conjugate vaccines for prevention of Haemophilus influenzae type b disease among infants and children two months of age and older. MMWR. 1991;40:1-7.
34. Centers for Disease Control and Prevention. General recommendations on immunization: Recommendations of the Advisory Committee on Immunization Practices (ACIP) and the American Academy of Family Physicians (AAFP). MMWR. 2002;51(No. RR-2);1-36.
35. 2000 Red Book: Report of the Committee on Infectious Diseases. 25th ed. Elk Grove Village, IL: American Academy of Pediatrics; 2000: 26, 266-72.
36. Jones RG, Bass JW, Weisse ME, et al. Antigenuria after immunization with Haemophilus influenzae oligosaccharide CRM197 conjugate (HbOC) vaccine. Pediatr Infect Dis J. 1991;10:557-559.

Continued on next page

HibTITER—Cont.

37. American Academy of Pediatrics: Report of the Committee on Infectious Diseases. 22nd ed. Elk Grove Village, Ill: American Academy of Pediatrics; 1991.
38. Recommendation of the ACIP: Immunization of children infected with human T-lymphotrophic virus type III/lymphadenopathy-associated virus. *MMWR.* 1986; 35(38):595-606.
39. Immunization of children infected with human immunodeficiency virus – supplementary ACIP statement. *MMWR.* 1988;37(12):181-183.
40. General Recommendations on Immunization: Recommendations of the Immunization Practices Advisory Committee (ACIP). *MMWR.* 1989;38(13):221.
41. Spinola SM, Sheaffer CI, Philbrick KB, et al. Antigenuria after *Haemophilus influenzae* type b polysaccharide immunization: a prospective study. *J Pediatr.* 1986;109:835-837.
42. CDC. Vaccine Adverse Event Reporting System – United States. *MMWR.* 1990;39:730-733.
43. Paradiso PR. Combined childhood immunizations. *JAMA.* 1992;268:1685.
44. Paradiso PR, Hogerman DA, Madore DV, et al. Safety and immunogenicity of a combined diphtheria, tetanus, pertussis and *Haemophilus influenzae* type b vaccine in young infants. *Pediatrics.* 1993;92(6):827-32.
45. Wyeth Pharmaceuticals, Data on File: Prevnar Study D118-P12.
46. Wyeth Pharmaceuticals, Data on File: Prevnar Study D118-P16.
47. Wyeth Pharmaceuticals, Data on File: Prevnar Study D118-P7.
48. Shinefield H, Black S, Ray P, et al. Safety and immunogenicity of heptavalent pneumococcal CRM_{197} conjugate vaccine in infants and toddlers. *Pediatr Infect Dis J.* 1999;18:757-63.
49. Wyeth Pharmaceuticals, Data on File: Prevnar Study D118-P3.
50. Rennels MB, Edwards KM, Keyserling HL, et al. Safety and immunogenicity of heptavalent pneumococcal vaccine conjugated to CRM_{197} in United States infants. *Pediatrics.* 1998;101(4):604-11.
51. Wyeth Pharmaceuticals, Data on File: Prevnar Study D118-P8.
52. Black S, Shinefield H, Fireman B, et al. Efficacy, safety and immunogenicity of heptavalent pneumococcal conjugate vaccine in children. *Pediatr Infect Dis J.* 2000;19:187-95.
53. Milstein JB, Gross TP, Kuritsky JN. Adverse reactions reported following receipt of *Haemophilus influenzae* type b vaccine: an analysis after one year of marketing. *Pediatrics.* 1987;80:270-274.
54. D'Cruz DF, Shapiro ED, Spiegelman KN, et al. Acute inflammatory demyelinating polyradiculoneuropathy (Guillain-Barré syndrome) after immunization with *Haemophilus influenzae* type b conjugate vaccine. *J Pediatr.* 1989;115:743-746.
55. Greenberg DP, Lieberman JM, Marcy SM, et al. Enhanced antibody responses in infants given different sequences of heterogenous *Haemophilus influenzae* type b conjugate vaccines. *J Pediatr.* 1995;126:206-11.
56. Anderson EL, Decker MD, Englund JA, et al. Interchangeability of conjugated *Haemophilus influenzae* type b vaccines in infants. *JAMA.* 1995;273:849-53.

Wyeth®

Manufactured by: W10461C004
Wyeth Pharmaceuticals Inc. ET01
Philadelphia, PA 19101 Rev 02/05
US Govt. License No. 3

MYLOTARG® ℞

[mī'lō-tărg]

(gemtuzumab ozogamicin for Injection)
FOR INTRAVENOUS USE ONLY

Prescribing information for this product, which appears on pages 3344–3347 of the 2005 PDR, has been revised as follows. Please write "See Supplement A" next to the product heading.

This product's label may have been revised after this insert was used in production. For further product information and current package insert, please visit www.wyeth.com or call our medical communications department toll-free at 1-800-943-5556.

In the **Dosage and Administration** section, the *"Instructions for Reconstitution," "Instructions for Dilution," "Administration," "Stability and Storage,"* and *"Instructions for Use, Handling and for Disposal,"* subsections were revised as follows:

Instructions for Reconstitution

The drug product is light sensitive and must be protected from direct and indirect sunlight and unshielded fluorescent light during the preparation and administration of the infusion. **All preparation should take place in a biologic safety hood with shielded fluorescent light.** Reconstitute the contents of each vial with 5 mL Sterile Water for Injection, USP, using sterile syringes. Gently swirl each vial. Each vial should be inspected for complete dissolution of the drug. The final concentration of the reconstituted drug solution is 1 mg/mL. See Tables 10 and 11 for storage conditions for reconstituted product.

TABLE 10: REFRIGERATION STORAGE CONDITION TIMES

The following time intervals for reconstitution, dilution, and administration should be followed for refrigeration storage of the reconstituted solution.

Time Intervals			Total Maximum Hours[a]
Reconstitution	Dilution	Administration	
≤ 8 hours at refrigeration	Immediate use	2 hour infusion	10

a: Total maximum storage time from reconstitution of product through completion of infusion.

TABLE 11: ROOM TEMPERATURE STORAGE CONDITION TIMES

The following time intervals for reconstitution, dilution, and administration should be followed for room temperature storage of the reconstituted solution.

Time Intervals			Total Maximum Hours[a]
Reconstitution	Dilution	Administration	
≤ 2 hours at room temperature	≤ 16 hours at room temperature	2 hour infusion	20

a: Total maximum storage time from reconstitution of product through completion of infusion.

Instructions for Dilution

Prepare an admixture corresponding to 9 mg/m^2 dose of Mylotarg by injecting the reconstituted solution into a 100 mL 0.9% sodium chloride injection solution in either a polyvinyl chloride (PVC) or ethylene/polypropylene copolymer (non-PVC) IV bag covered by an ultraviolet (UV) light protector. Mylotarg should only be diluted with 0.9% sodium chloride solution. DO NOT DILUTE WITH ANY OTHER ELECTROLYTE SOLUTIONS or 5% DEXTROSE or MIX WITH OTHER DRUGS. See Tables 10 and 11 for storage conditions for diluted product.

The drug solution in the vial, transfer syringe, or the IV bag may appear hazy due to normal light scattering from the protein.

Administration

DO NOT ADMINISTER AS AN INTRAVENOUS (IV) PUSH OR BOLUS

Once the reconstituted Mylotarg is diluted into the IV bag containing normal saline, the resulting solution should be infused over a 2-hour period. See Tables 10 and 11 for infusion times. Mylotarg may be given peripherally or through a central line. During the infusion, only the IV bag needs to be protected from light. An in-line, low protein binding filter must be used for the infusion of Mylotarg. The following filter membranes are qualified: 0.22 µm or 1.2 µm polyether sulfone (PES) (Supor®); 1.2 µm acrylic copolymer hydrophilic filter (Versapor®); 0.8 µm cellulose mixed ester (acetate and nitrate) membrane; 0.2 µm cellulose acetate membrane. DO NOT CO-ADMINISTER OTHER DRUGS THROUGH THE SAME INFUSION LINE. Premedication, consisting of acetaminophen and diphenhydramine, should be given before each infusion to reduce the incidence of a post-infusion symptom complex (see **ADVERSE REACTIONS, Acute Infusion-Related Events**).

Stability and Storage:

Prior to Reconstitution: Mylotarg should be stored refrigerated 2° to 8° C (36° to 46° F) and protected from light.

After Reconstitution: Follow the instructions for reconstitution, dilution, and administration in the section above. See Tables 10 and 11 below for reconstitution, dilution, and administration storage conditions and time intervals.

[See table 10 above]
[See table 11 above]

Instructions for Use, Handling and for Disposal: Mylotarg should be inspected visually for particulate matter and discoloration, once in the transfer syringe. Additionally, the diluted admixture solution should be inspected visually for particulate matter and discoloration. Protect from light and use an UV protective bag over the IV bag during infusion. Vials are for single use. Aseptic technique must be strictly observed throughout the handling of Mylotarg since no bacteriostatic agent or preservative is present. Institutional procedures for handling and disposal of anticancer drugs should be used. Several guidelines on this subject have been published.[1,2,3]

Wyeth®

Wyeth Pharmaceuticals Inc. W10477C007
Philadelphia, PA 19101 ET01
Rev 11/04

PHENERGAN® ℞

[fĕn-ər-jăn]

(promethazine HCl)
Tablets and Suppositories

Prescribing information for this product, which appears on pages 3362–3363 of the 2005 PDR, has been completely revised as follows. Please write "See Supplement A" next to the product heading.

℞ only

DESCRIPTION

Each tablet of Phenergan contains 12.5 mg, 25 mg, or 50 mg promethazine HCl. The inactive ingredients present are lactose, magnesium stearate, and methylcellulose. Each dosage strength also contains the following:

12.5 mg—FD&C Yellow 6 and saccharin sodium;
25 mg—saccharin sodium;
50 mg—FD&C Red 40.

Each rectal suppository of Phenergan contains 12.5 mg, 25 mg, or 50 mg promethazine HCl with ascorbyl palmitate, silicon dioxide, white wax, and cocoa butter. Phenergan Suppositories are for rectal administration only.

Promethazine HCl is a racemic compound; the empirical formula is $C_{17}H_{20}N_2S \cdot HCl$ and its molecular weight is 320.88.

Promethazine HCl, a phenothiazine derivative, is designated chemically as 10*H*-Phenothiazine-10-ethanamine, *N,N*,α-trimethyl-, monohydrochloride, (±)- with the following structural formula:

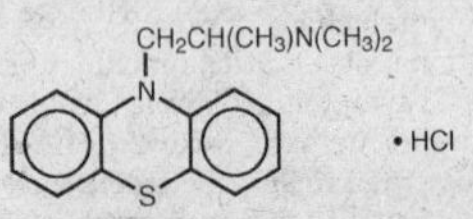

Promethazine HCl occurs as a white to faint yellow, practically odorless, crystalline powder which slowly oxidizes and turns blue on prolonged exposure to air. It is freely soluble in water and soluble in alcohol.

CLINICAL PHARMACOLOGY

Promethazine is a phenothiazine derivative which differs structurally from the antipsychotic phenothiazines by the presence of a branched side chain and no ring substitution. It is thought that this configuration is responsible for its relative lack (1/10 that of chlorpromazine) of dopamine antagonist properties.

Promethazine is an H_1 receptor blocking agent. In addition to its antihistaminic action, it provides clinically useful sedative and antiemetic effects.

Promethazine is well absorbed from the gastrointestinal tract. Clinical effects are apparent within 20 minutes after oral administration and generally last four to six hours, although they may persist as long as 12 hours. Promethazine is metabolized by the liver to a variety of compounds; the sulfoxides of promethazine and N-demethylpromethazine are the predominant metabolites appearing in the urine.

INDICATIONS AND USAGE

Phenergan, either orally or by suppository, is useful for:
Perennial and seasonal allergic rhinitis.
Vasomotor rhinitis.
Allergic conjunctivitis due to inhalant allergens and foods.
Mild, uncomplicated allergic skin manifestations of urticaria and angioedema.
Amelioration of allergic reactions to blood or plasma.
Dermographism.
Anaphylactic reactions, as adjunctive therapy to epinephrine and other standard measures, after the acute manifestations have been controlled.
Preoperative, postoperative, or obstetric sedation.
Prevention and control of nausea and vomiting associated with certain types of anesthesia and surgery.
Therapy adjunctive to meperidine or other analgesics for control of post-operative pain.
Sedation in both children and adults, as well as relief of apprehension and production of light sleep from which the patient can be easily aroused.
Active and prophylactic treatment of motion sickness.
Antiemetic therapy in postoperative patients.

CONTRAINDICATIONS

Phenergan Tablets and Suppositories are contraindicated for use in pediatric patients less than two years of age.

Phenergan Tablets and Suppositories are contraindicated in comatose states, and in individuals known to be hypersensitive or to have had an idiosyncratic reaction to promethazine or to other phenothiazines.

Antihistamines are contraindicated for use in the treatment of lower respiratory tract symptoms including asthma.

WARNINGS

> PHENERGAN SHOULD NOT BE USED IN PEDIATRIC PATIENTS LESS THAN 2 YEARS OF AGE BECAUSE OF THE POTENTIAL FOR FATAL RESPIRATORY DEPRESSION.
>
> POSTMARKETING CASES OF RESPIRATORY DEPRESSION, INCLUDING FATALITIES, HAVE BEEN REPORTED WITH USE OF PHENERGAN IN PEDIATRIC PATIENTS LESS THAN 2 YEARS OF AGE. A WIDE RANGE OF WEIGHT-BASED DOSES OF PHENERGAN HAVE RESULTED IN RESPIRATORY DEPRESSION IN THESE PATIENTS.
>
> CAUTION SHOULD BE EXERCISED WHEN ADMINISTERING PHENERGAN TO PEDIATRIC PATIENTS 2 YEARS OF AGE AND OLDER. IT IS RECOMMENDED THAT THE LOWEST EFFECTIVE DOSE OF PHENERGAN BE USED IN PEDIATRIC PATIENTS 2 YEARS OF AGE AND OLDER AND CONCOMITANT ADMINISTRATION OF OTHER DRUGS WITH RESPIRATORY DEPRESSANT EFFECTS BE AVOIDED.

CNS Depression
Phenergan Tablets and Suppositories may impair the mental and/or physical abilities required for the performance of potentially hazardous tasks, such as driving a vehicle or operating machinery. The impairment may be amplified by concomitant use of other central-nervous-system depressants such as alcohol, sedatives/hypnotics (including barbiturates), narcotics, narcotic analgesics, general anesthetics, tricyclic antidepressants, and tranquilizers; therefore such agents should either be eliminated or given in reduced dosage in the presence of promethazine HCl (see **PRECAUTIONS—Information for Patients** and **Drug Interactions**).

Respiratory Depression
Phenergan Tablets and Suppositories may lead to potentially fatal respiratory depression.
Use of Phenergan Tablets and Suppositories in patients with compromised respiratory function (e.g., COPD, sleep apnea) should be avoided.

Lower Seizure Threshold
Phenergan Tablets and Suppositories may lower seizure threshold. It should be used with caution in persons with seizure disorders or in persons who are using concomitant medications, such as narcotics or local anesthetics, which may also affect seizure threshold.

Bone-Marrow Depression
Phenergan Tablets and Suppositories should be used with caution in patients with bone-marrow depression. Leukopenia and agranulocytosis have been reported, usually when Phenergan (promethazine HCl) has been used in association with other known marrow-toxic agents.

Neuroleptic Malignant Syndrome
A potentially fatal symptom complex sometimes referred to as Neuroleptic Malignant Syndrome (NMS) has been reported in association with promethazine HCl alone or in combination with antipsychotic drugs. Clinical manifestations of NMS are hyperpyrexia, muscle rigidity, altered mental status and evidence of autonomic instability (irregular pulse or blood pressure, tachycardia, diaphoresis and cardiac dysrhythmias).
The diagnostic evaluation of patients with this syndrome is complicated. In arriving at a diagnosis, it is important to identify cases where the clinical presentation includes both serious medical illness (e.g. pneumonia, systemic infection, etc.) and untreated or inadequately treated extrapyramidal signs and symptoms (EPS). Other important considerations in the differential diagnosis include central anticholinergic toxicity, heat stroke, drug fever and primary central nervous system (CNS) pathology.
The management of NMS should include 1) immediate discontinuation of promethazine HCl, antipsychotic drugs, if any, and other drugs not essential to concurrent therapy, 2) intensive symptomatic treatment and medical monitoring, and 3) treatment of any concomitant serious medical problems for which specific treatments are available. There is no general agreement about specific pharmacological treatment regimens for uncomplicated NMS.
Since recurrences of NMS have been reported with phenothiazines, the reintroduction of promethazine HCl should be carefully considered.

Use in Pediatric Patients
PHENERGAN TABLETS AND SUPPOSITORIES ARE CONTRAINDICATED FOR USE IN PEDIATRIC PATIENTS LESS THAN TWO YEARS OF AGE.
CAUTION SHOULD BE EXERCISED WHEN ADMINISTERING PHENERGAN TABLETS AND SUPPOSITORIES TO PEDIATRIC PATIENTS 2 YEARS OF AGE AND OLDER BECAUSE OF THE POTENTIAL FOR FATAL RESPIRATORY DEPRESSION. RESPIRATORY DEPRESSION AND APNEA, SOMETIMES ASSOCIATED WITH DEATH, ARE STRONGLY ASSOCIATED WITH PROMETHAZINE PRODUCTS AND ARE NOT DIRECTLY RELATED TO INDIVIDUALIZED WEIGHT-BASED DOSING, WHICH MIGHT OTHERWISE PERMIT SAFE ADMINISTRATION. CONCOMITANT ADMINISTRATION OF PROMETHAZINE PRODUCTS WITH OTHER RESPIRATORY DEPRESSANTS HAS AN ASSOCIATION WITH RESPIRATORY DEPRESSION, AND SOMETIMES DEATH, IN PEDIATRIC PATIENTS.
ANTIEMETICS ARE NOT RECOMMENDED FOR TREATMENT OF UNCOMPLICATED VOMITING IN PEDIATRIC PATIENTS, AND THEIR USE SHOULD BE LIMITED TO PROLONGED VOMITING OF KNOWN ETIOLOGY. THE EXTRAPYRAMIDAL SYMPTOMS WHICH CAN OCCUR SECONDARY TO PHENERGAN TABLETS AND SUPPOSITORIES ADMINISTRATION MAY BE CONFUSED WITH THE CNS SIGNS OF UNDIAGNOSED PRIMARY DISEASE, e.g., ENCEPHALOPATHY OR REYE'S SYNDROME. THE USE OF PHENERGAN TABLETS AND SUPPOSITORIES SHOULD BE AVOIDED IN PEDIATRIC PATIENTS WHOSE SIGNS AND SYMPTOMS MAY SUGGEST REYE'S SYNDROME OR OTHER HEPATIC DISEASES.
Excessively large dosages of antihistamines, including Phenergan Tablets and Suppositories, in pediatric patients may cause sudden death (see **OVERDOSAGE**). Hallucinations and convulsions have occurred with therapeutic doses and overdoses of Phenergan in pediatric patients. In pediatric patients who are acutely ill associated with dehydration, there is an increased susceptibility to dystonias with the use of promethazine HCl.

Other Considerations
Administration of promethazine HCl has been associated with reported cholestatic jaundice.

PRECAUTIONS
General
Drugs having anticholinergic properties should be used with caution in patients with narrow-angle glaucoma, prostatic hypertrophy, stenosing peptic ulcer, pyloroduodenal obstruction, and bladder-neck obstruction.
Phenergan Tablets and Suppositories should be used cautiously in persons with cardiovascular disease or with impairment of liver function.

Information for Patients
Phenergan Tablets and Suppositories may cause marked drowsiness or impair the mental and/or physical abilities required for the performance of potentially hazardous tasks, such as driving a vehicle or operating machinery. The use of alcohol or other central-nervous-system depressants such as sedatives/hypnotics (including barbiturates), narcotics, narcotic analgesics, general anesthetics, tricyclic antidepressants, and tranquilizers, may enhance impairment (see **WARNINGS—CNS Depression** and **PRECAUTIONS—Drug Interactions**). Pediatric patients should be supervised to avoid potential harm in bike riding or in other hazardous activities.
Patients should be advised to report any involuntary muscle movements.
Avoid prolonged exposure to the sun.

Drug Interactions
CNS Depressants—Phenergan Tablets and Suppositories may increase, prolong, or intensify the sedative action of other central-nervous-system depressants, such as alcohol, sedatives/hypnotics (including barbiturates), narcotics, narcotic analgesics, general anesthetics, tricyclic antidepressants, and tranquilizers; therefore, such agents should be avoided or administered in reduced dosage to patients receiving promethazine HCl. When given concomitantly with Phenergan Tablets and Suppositories, the dose of barbiturates should be reduced by at least one-half, and the dose of narcotics should be reduced by one-quarter to one-half. Dosage must be individualized. Excessive amounts of promethazine HCl relative to a narcotic may lead to restlessness and motor hyperactivity in the patient with pain; these symptoms usually disappear with adequate control of the pain.
Epinephrine—Because of the potential for Phenergan to reverse epinephrine's vasopressor effect, epinephrine should NOT be used to treat hypotension associated with Phenergan Tablets and Suppositories overdose.
Anticholinergics—Concomitant use of other agents with anticholinergic properties should be undertaken with caution.
Monoamine Oxidase Inhibitors (MAOI)—Drug interactions, including an increased incidence of extrapyramidal effects, have been reported when some MAOI and phenothiazines are used concomitantly. This possibility should be considered with Phenergan Tablets and Suppositories.

Drug/Laboratory Test Interactions
The following laboratory tests may be affected in patients who are receiving therapy with promethazine HCl:
Pregnancy Tests
Diagnostic pregnancy tests based on immunological reactions between HCG and anti-HCG may result in false-negative or false-positive interpretations.
Glucose Tolerance Test
An increase in blood glucose has been reported in patients receiving promethazine HCl.

Carcinogenesis, Mutagenesis, Impairment of Fertility
Long-term animal studies have not been performed to assess the carcinogenic potential of promethazine, nor are there other animal or human data concerning carcinogenicity, mutagenicity, or impairment of fertility with this drug. Promethazine was nonmutagenic in the *Salmonella* test system of Ames.

Pregnancy
Teratogenic Effects—Pregnancy Category C
Teratogenic effects have not been demonstrated in rat-feeding studies at doses of 6.25 and 12.5 mg/kg of promethazine HCl. These doses are from approximately 2.1 to 4.2 times the maximum recommended total daily dose of promethazine for a 50-kg subject, depending upon the indication for which the drug is prescribed. Daily doses of 25 mg/kg intraperitoneally have been found to produce fetal mortality in rats.
Specific studies to test the action of the drug on parturition, lactation, and development of the animal neonate were not done, but a general preliminary study in rats indicated no effect on these parameters. Although antihistamines have been found to produce fetal mortality in rodents, the pharmacological effects of histamine in the rodent do not parallel those in man. There are no adequate and well-controlled studies of Phenergan® Tablets and Suppositories in pregnant women.
Phenergan (promethazine HCl) Tablets and Suppositories should be used during pregnancy only if the potential benefit justifies the potential risk to the fetus.
Nonteratogenic Effects
Phenergan Tablets and Suppositories administered to a pregnant woman within two weeks of delivery may inhibit platelet aggregation in the newborn.

Labor and Delivery
Promethazine HCl may be used alone or as an adjunct to narcotic analgesics during labor (see **DOSAGE AND ADMINISTRATION**). Limited data suggest that use of Phenergan during labor and delivery does not have an appreciable effect on the duration of labor or delivery and does not increase the risk of need for intervention in the newborn. The effect on later growth and development of the newborn is unknown. (See also *Nonteratogenic Effects*.)

Nursing Mothers
It is not known whether promethazine HCl is excreted in human milk. Because many drugs are excreted in human milk and because of the potential for serious adverse reactions in nursing infants from Phenergan Tablets and Suppositories, a decision should be made whether to discontinue nursing or to discontinue the drug, taking into account the importance of the drug to the mother.

Pediatric Use
PHENERGAN TABLETS AND SUPPOSITORIES ARE CONTRAINDICATED FOR USE IN PEDIATRIC PATIENTS LESS THAN TWO YEARS OF AGE (see **WARNINGS–Black Box Warning** and **Use in Pediatric Patients**).
Phenergan Tablets and Suppositories should be used with caution in pediatric patients 2 years of age and older (see **WARNINGS—Use in Pediatric Patients**).

Geriatric Use
Clinical studies of Phenergan formulations did not include sufficient numbers of subjects aged 65 and over to determine whether they respond differently from younger subjects. Other reported clinical experience has not identified differences in responses between the elderly and younger patients. In general, dose selection for an elderly patient should be cautious, usually starting at the low end of the dosing range, reflecting the greater frequency of decreased hepatic, renal or cardiac function, and of concomitant disease or other drug therapy.
Sedating drugs may cause confusion and over-sedation in the elderly; elderly patients generally should be started on low doses of Phenergan Tablets and Suppositories and observed closely.

ADVERSE REACTIONS
Central Nervous System
Drowsiness is the most prominent CNS effect of this drug. Sedation, somnolence, blurred vision, dizziness; confusion, disorientation, and extrapyramidal symptoms such as oculogyric crisis, torticollis, and tongue protrusion; lassitude, tinnitus, incoordination, fatigue, euphoria, nervousness, diplopia, insomnia, tremors, convulsive seizures, excitation, catatonic-like states, hysteria. Hallucinations have also been reported.
Cardiovascular—Increased or decreased blood pressure, tachycardia, bradycardia, faintness.
Dermatologic—Dermatitis, photosensitivity, urticaria.
Hematologic—Leukopenia, thrombocytopenia, thrombocytopenic purpura, agranulocytosis.
Gastrointestinal—Dry mouth, nausea, vomiting, jaundice.
Respiratory—Asthma, nasal stuffiness, respiratory depression (potentially fatal) and apnea (potentially fatal). (See **WARNINGS—Respiratory Depression**.)
Other—Angioneurotic edema. Neuroleptic malignant syndrome (potentially fatal) has also been reported. (See **WARNINGS—Neuroleptic Malignant Syndrome**.)

Paradoxical Reactions
Hyperexcitability and abnormal movements have been reported in patients following a single administration of promethazine HCl. Consideration should be given to the discontinuation of promethazine HCl and to the use of other drugs if these reactions occur. Respiratory depression, nightmares, delirium, and agitated behavior have also been reported in some of these patients.

OVERDOSAGE
Signs and symptoms of overdosage with promethazine HCl range from mild depression of the central nervous system and cardiovascular system to profound hypotension, respiratory depression, unconsciousness, and sudden death. Other reported reactions include hyperreflexia, hypertonia, ataxia, athetosis, and extensor-plantar reflexes (Babinski reflex).
Stimulation may be evident, especially in children and geriatric patients. Convulsions may rarely occur. A paradoxical-type reaction has been reported in children receiving single doses of 75 mg to 125 mg orally, characterized by hyperexcitability and nightmares.
Atropine-like signs and symptoms—dry mouth, fixed, dilated pupils, flushing, as well as gastrointestinal symptoms—may occur.

Treatment
Treatment of overdosage is essentially symptomatic and supportive. Only in cases of extreme overdosage or individual sensitivity do vital signs, including respiration, pulse, blood pressure, temperature, and EKG, need to be monitored. Activated charcoal orally or by lavage may be given,

Continued on next page

Phenergan—Cont.

or sodium or magnesium sulfate orally as a cathartic. Attention should be given to the reestablishment of adequate respiratory exchange through provision of a patent airway and institution of assisted or controlled ventilation. Diazepam may be used to control convulsions. Acidosis and electrolyte losses should be corrected. Note that any depressant effects of promethazine HCl are not reversed by naloxone. Avoid analeptics which may cause convulsions.

The treatment of choice for resulting hypotension is administration of intravenous fluids, accompanied by repositioning if indicated. In the event that vasopressors are considered for the management of severe hypotension which does not respond to intravenous fluids and repositioning, the administration of norepinephrine or phenylephrine should be considered. EPINEPHRINE SHOULD NOT BE USED, since its use in patients with partial adrenergic blockade may further lower the blood pressure. Extrapyramidal reactions may be treated with anticholinergic antiparkinsonian agents, diphenhydramine, or barbiturates. Oxygen may also be administered.

Limited experience with dialysis indicates that it is not helpful.

DOSAGE AND ADMINISTRATION

Phenergan Tablets and Phenergan Rectal Suppositories are contraindicated for children under 2 years of age (see WARNINGS—Black Box Warning and Use in Pediatric Patients).

Phenergan Suppositories are for rectal administration only.

Allergy

The average oral dose is 25 mg taken before retiring; however, 12.5 mg may be taken before meals and on retiring, if necessary. Single 25-mg doses at bedtime or 6.25 to 12.5 mg taken three times daily will usually suffice. After initiation of treatment in children or adults, dosage should be adjusted to the smallest amount adequate to relieve symptoms. The administration of promethazine HCl in 25-mg doses will control minor transfusion reactions of an allergic nature.

Motion Sickness

The average adult dose is 25 mg taken twice daily. The initial dose should be taken one-half to one hour before anticipated travel and be repeated 8 to 12 hours later, if necessary. On succeeding days of travel, it is recommended that 25 mg be given on arising and again before the evening meal. For children, Phenergan Tablets, Syrup, or Rectal Suppositories, 12.5 to 25 mg, twice daily, may be administered.

Nausea and Vomiting

Antiemetics should not be used in vomiting of unknown etiology in children and adolescents (see **WARNINGS-Use in Pediatric Patients**).

The average effective dose of Phenergan for the active therapy of nausea and vomiting in children or adults is 25 mg. When oral medication cannot be tolerated, the dose should be given parenterally (cf. Phenergan Injection) or by rectal suppository. 12.5- to 25-mg doses may be repeated, as necessary, at 4- to 6-hour intervals.

For nausea and vomiting in children, the usual dose is 0.5 mg per pound of body weight, and the dose should be adjusted to the age and weight of the patient and the severity of the condition being treated.

For prophylaxis of nausea and vomiting, as during surgery and the postoperative period, the average dose is 25 mg repeated at 4- to 6-hour intervals, as necessary.

Sedation

This product relieves apprehension and induces a quiet sleep from which the patient can be easily aroused. Administration of 12.5 to 25 mg Phenergan by the oral route or by rectal suppository at bedtime will provide sedation in children. Adults usually require 25 to 50 mg for nighttime, presurgical, or obstetrical sedation.

Pre- and Postoperative Use

Phenergan in 12.5- to 25-mg doses for children and 50-mg doses for adults the night before surgery relieves apprehension and produces a quiet sleep.

For preoperative medication, children require doses of 0.5 mg per pound of body weight in combination with an appropriately reduced dose of narcotic or barbiturate and the appropriate dose of an atropine-like drug. Usual adult dosage is 50 mg Phenergan with an appropriately reduced dose of narcotic or barbiturate and the required amount of a belladonna alkaloid.

Postoperative sedation and adjunctive use with analgesics may be obtained by the administration of 12.5 to 25 mg in children and 25- to 50-mg doses in adults.

Phenergan Tablets and Phenergan Rectal Suppositories are contraindicated for children under 2 years of age.

HOW SUPPLIED

Phenergan® (promethazine HCl) Tablets are available as follows:

12.5 mg, orange tablet with "WYETH" on one side and "19" on the scored reverse side.

NDC 0008-0019-01, bottle of 100 tablets.

25 mg, white tablet with "WYETH" and "27" on one side and scored on the reverse side.

NDC 0008-0027-02, bottle of 100 tablets.

NDC 0008-0027-07, Redipak® carton of 100 tablets (10 blister strips of 10).

50 mg, pink tablet with "WYETH" on one side and "227" on the other side.

NDC 0008-0227-01, bottle of 100 tablets.

Keep tightly closed.

Store at controlled room temperature 20° to 25°C (68° to 77°F).

Protect from light.

Dispense in light-resistant, tight container.

Use carton to protect contents from light.

Phenergan® (promethazine HCl) Rectal Suppositories are available in boxes of 12 as follows:

12.5 mg, ivory, torpedo-shaped suppository wrapped in copper-colored foil, NDC 0008-0498-01.

25 mg, ivory, torpedo-shaped suppository wrapped in light-green foil, NDC 0008-0212-01.

50 mg, ivory, torpedo-shaped suppository wrapped in blue foil, NDC 0008-0229-01.

Store refrigerated between 2°–8°C (36°–46°F).

Dispense in well-closed container.

Wyeth®

Wyeth Pharmaceuticals Inc.
Philadelphia, PA 19101

W10448C003
ET01
Rev 12/04

PREMARIN® ℞

[prĕm'ă-rĭn]

Intravenous

(conjugated estrogens, USP) for injection

Specially prepared for Intravenous & Intramuscular use ℞ only

Prescribing information for this product, which appears on pages 3363–3366 of the 2005 PDR, has been completely revised as follows. Please write "See Supplement A" next to the product heading.

> **ESTROGENS INCREASE THE RISK OF ENDOMETRIAL CANCER**
>
> Close clinical surveillance of all women taking estrogens is important. Adequate diagnostic measures, including endometrial sampling when indicated, should be undertaken to rule out malignancy in all cases of undiagnosed persistent or recurring abnormal vaginal bleeding. There is no evidence that the use of "natural" estrogens results in a different endometrial risk profile than synthetic estrogens of equivalent estrogen doses.
>
> **CARDIOVASCULAR AND OTHER RISKS**
>
> Estrogens with or without progestins should not be used for the prevention of cardiovascular disease or dementia.
>
> The Women's Health Initiative (WHI) study reported increased risks of stroke and deep-vein thrombosis in postmenopausal women (50 to 79 years of age) during 6.8 years of treatment with conjugated estrogens (0.625 mg) relative to placebo.
>
> The WHI study reported increased risks of myocardial infarction, stroke, invasive breast cancer, pulmonary emboli, and deep vein thrombosis in postmenopausal women (50 to 79 years of age) during 5 years of treatment with conjugated estrogens (0.625 mg) combined with medroxyprogesterone acetate (2.5 mg) relative to placebo. (See **CLINICAL PHARMACOLOGY, Clinical Studies**.)
>
> The Women's Health Initiative Memory Study (WHIMS), a substudy of WHI, reported increased risk of developing probable dementia in postmenopausal women 65 years of age or older during 4 to 5.2 years of treatment with conjugated estrogens, with or without medroxyprogesterone acetate, relative to placebo. It is unknown whether this finding applies to younger postmenopausal women.
>
> Other doses of conjugated estrogens and medroxyprogesterone acetate, and other combinations and dosage forms of estrogens and progestins were not studied in the WHI clinical trials and, in the absence of comparable data, these risks should be assumed to be similar. Because of these risks, estrogens with or without progestins should be prescribed at the lowest effective doses and for the shortest duration consistent with treatment goals and risks for the individual woman.

DESCRIPTION

Premarin® Intravenous (conjugated estrogens, USP) for injection contains a mixture of conjugated estrogens obtained exclusively from natural sources, occurring as the sodium salts of water-soluble estrogen sulfates blended to represent the average composition of materials derived from pregnant mares' urine. It is a mixture of sodium estrone sulfate and sodium equilin sulfate. It contains as concomitant components, as sodium sulfate conjugates, 17α-dihydroequilin, 17α-estradiol, and 17β-dihydroequilin.

Each Secule® vial contains 25 mg of conjugated estrogens, USP, in a sterile lyophilized cake which also contains lactose 200 mg, sodium citrate 12.2 mg, and simethicone 0.2 mg. The pH is adjusted with sodium hydroxide or hydrochloric acid. A sterile diluent (5 mL) containing 2% benzyl alcohol in sterile water is provided for reconstitution. The reconstituted solution is suitable for intravenous or intramuscular injection.

CLINICAL PHARMACOLOGY

Endogenous estrogens are largely responsible for the development and maintenance of the female reproductive system

---

and secondary sexual characteristics. Although circulating estrogens exist in a dynamic equilibrium of metabolic interconversions, estradiol is the principal intracellular human estrogen and is substantially more potent than its metabolites, estrone and estriol, at the receptor level. The primary source of estrogen in normally cycling adult women is the ovarian follicle, which secretes 70 to 500 mcg of estradiol daily, depending on the phase of the menstrual cycle. After menopause, most endogenous estrogen is produced by conversion of androstenedione, secreted by the adrenal cortex, to estrone by peripheral tissues. Thus, estrone and the sulfate-conjugated form, estrone sulfate, are the most abundant circulating estrogen in postmenopausal women.

Estrogens act through binding to nuclear receptors in estrogen-responsive tissues. To date, two estrogen receptors have been identified. These vary in proportion from tissue to tissue.

Circulating estrogens modulate the pituitary secretion of the gonadotropins, luteinizing hormone (LH) and follicle stimulating hormone (FSH) through a negative feedback mechanism. Estrogens act to reduce the elevated levels of these gonadotropins seen in postmenopausal women.

Pharmacokinetics

Absorption

Conjugated estrogens are soluble in water and are well absorbed through the skin, mucous membranes, and gastrointestinal tract after release from the drug formulation.

Distribution

The distribution of exogenous estrogens is similar to that of endogenous estrogens. Estrogens are widely distributed in the body and are generally found in higher concentration in the sex hormone target organs. Estrogens circulate in the blood largely bound to sex hormone-binding globulin (SHBG) and albumin.

Metabolism

Exogenous estrogens are metabolized in the same manner as endogenous estrogens. Circulating estrogens exist in a dynamic equilibrium of metabolic interconversions. These transformations take place mainly in the liver. Estradiol is converted reversibly to estrone, and both can be converted to estriol, which is the major urinary metabolite. Estrogens also undergo enterohepatic recirculation via sulfate and glucuronide conjugation in the liver, biliary secretion of conjugates into the intestine, and hydrolysis in the gut followed by reabsorption. In postmenopausal women a significant proportion of the circulating estrogens exists as sulfate conjugates, especially estrone sulfate, which serves as a circulating reservoir for the formation of more active estrogens.

Excretion

Estradiol, estrone, and estriol are excreted in the urine along with glucuronide and sulfate conjugates.

Special Populations

No pharmacokinetic studies were conducted in special populations, including patients with renal or hepatic impairment.

Drug Interactions

Data from a single-dose drug-drug interaction study involving oral conjugated estrogens and medroxyprogesterone acetate indicate that the pharmacokinetic dispositions of both drugs are not altered when the drugs are coadministered. No other clinical drug-drug interaction studies have been conducted with conjugated estrogens.

In vitro and in vivo studies have shown that estrogens are metabolized partially by cytochrome P450 3A4 (CYP3A4). Therefore, inducers or inhibitors of CYP3A4 may affect estrogen drug metabolism. Inducers of CYP3A4 such as St. John's Wort preparations (Hypericum perforatum), phenobarbital, carbamazepine, and rifampin may reduce plasma concentrations of estrogens, possibly resulting in a decrease in therapeutic effects and/or changes in the uterine bleeding profile. Inhibitors of CYP3A4 such as erythromycin, clarithromycin, ketoconazole, itraconazole, ritonavir, and grapefruit juice may increase plasma concentrations of estrogens and may result in side effects.

Clinical Studies

Women's Health Initiative Studies.

The Women's Health Initiative (WHI) enrolled a total of 27,000 predominantly healthy postmenopausal women to assess the risks and benefits of either the use of Premarin tablets (0.625 mg conjugated estrogens per day) alone or the use of PREMPRO™ tablets (0.625 mg conjugated estrogens plus 2.5 mg medroxyprogesterone acetate per day) compared to placebo in the prevention of certain chronic diseases. The primary endpoint was the incidence of coronary heart disease (CHD) (nonfatal myocardial infarction and CHD death), with invasive breast cancer as the primary adverse outcome studied. A "global index" included the earliest occurrence of CHD, invasive breast cancer, stroke, pulmonary embolism (PE), endometrial cancer, colorectal cancer, hip fracture, or death due to other cause. The study did not evaluate the effects of Premarin tablets or PREMPRO on menopausal symptoms.

The estrogen plus progestin substudy was stopped early because, according to the predefined stopping rule, the increased risk of breast cancer and cardiovascular events exceeded the specified benefits included in the "global index." Results of the estrogen plus progestin substudy, which included 16,608 women (average age of 63 years, range 50 to 79; 83.9% White, 6.5% Black, 5.5% Hispanic), after an average follow-up of 5.2 years, are presented in Table 1 below:

[See table 1 at bottom of next page]

For those outcomes included in the "global index," the absolute excess risks per 10,000 women-years in the group treated with PREMPRO were 7 more CHD events, 8 more strokes, 8 more PEs, and 8 more invasive breast cancers, while the absolute risk reductions per 10,000 women-years were 6 fewer colorectal cancers and 5 fewer hip fractures. The absolute excess risk of events included in the "global index" was 19 per 10,000 women-years. There was no difference between the groups in terms of all-cause mortality. (See **BOXED WARNINGS, WARNINGS,** and **PRECAUTIONS.**)

INDICATIONS AND USAGE

Premarin Intravenous (conjugated estrogens, USP) for injection is indicated in the treatment of abnormal uterine bleeding due to hormonal imbalance in the absence of organic pathology.

Premarin Intravenous is indicated for short-term use only, to provide a rapid and temporary increase in estrogen levels.

CONTRAINDICATIONS

Premarin Intravenous should not be used in individuals with any of the following conditions:

1. Undiagnosed abnormal genital bleeding.
2. Known, suspected, or history of cancer of the breast.
3. Known or suspected estrogen-dependent neoplasia.
4. Active deep vein thrombosis, pulmonary embolism or a history of these conditions.
5. Active or recent (e.g., within past year) arterial thromboembolic disease (e.g., stroke, myocardial infarction).
6. Liver dysfunction or disease.
7. Premarin Intravenous for injection should not be used in patients with known hypersensitivity to its ingredients.
8. Known or suspected pregnancy. There is no indication for Premarin Intravenous in pregnancy. There appears to be little or no increased risk of birth defects in children born to women who have used estrogen and progestins from oral contraceptives inadvertently during pregnancy. (See **PRECAUTIONS.**)

WARNINGS

See **BOXED WARNINGS.**

Premarin Intravenous is indicated for short-term use. However, warnings, precautions and adverse reactions associated with Premarin tablets should be taken into account.

1. **Cardiovascular disorders.**

Estrogen and estrogen/progestin therapy have been associated with an increased risk of cardiovascular events such as myocardial infarction and stroke, as well as venous thrombosis and pulmonary embolism (venous thromboembolism or VTE). Should any of these occur or be suspected, estrogens should be discontinued immediately.

Risk factors for arterial vascular disease (e.g., hypertension, diabetes mellitus, tobacco use, hypercholesterolemia, and obesity) and/or venous thromboembolism (e.g., personal history or family history of VTE, obesity, and systemic lupus erythematosus) should be managed appropriately.

a. Coronary heart disease and stroke. In the Premarin tablets substudy of the Women's Health Initiative (WHI) study, an increase in the number of myocardial infarctions and strokes has been observed in women receiving Premarin compared to placebo. (See **CLINICAL PHARMACOLOGY, Clinical Studies.**)

In the estrogen plus progestin substudy of WHI, an increased risk of coronary heart disease (CHD) events (defined as nonfatal myocardial infarction and CHD death) was observed in women receiving PREMPRO (0.625 mg conjugated estrogens plus 2.5 mg medroxyprogesterone acetate) per day compared to women receiving placebo (37 vs 30 per 10,000 women-years). The increase in risk was observed in year one and persisted.

In the same substudy of WHI, an increased risk of stroke was observed in women receiving PREMPRO compared to women receiving placebo (29 vs 21 per 10,000 women-years). The increase in risk was observed after the first year and persisted.

In postmenopausal women with documented heart disease (n = 2,763, average age 66.7 years) a controlled clinical trial of secondary prevention of cardiovascular disease (Heart and Estrogen/progestin Replacement Study; HERS) treatment with PREMPRO (0.625 mg conjugated estrogen plus 2.5 mg medroxyprogesterone acetate per day) demonstrated no cardiovascular benefit. During an average follow-up of 4.1 years, treatment with PREMPRO did not reduce the overall rate of CHD events in postmenopausal women with established coronary heart disease. There were more CHD events in the PREMPRO-treated group than in the placebo group in year 1, but not during the subsequent years. Two thousand three hundred and twenty one women from the original HERS trial agreed to participate in an open label extension of HERS, HERS II. Average follow-up in HERS II was an additional 2.7 years, for a total of 6.8 years overall. Rates of CHD events were comparable among women in the PREMPRO group and the placebo group in HERS, HERS II, and overall.

Large doses of estrogen (5 mg conjugated estrogens per day), comparable to those used to treat cancer of the prostate and breast, have been shown in a large prospective clinical trial in men to increase the risks of nonfatal myocardial infarction, pulmonary embolism, and thrombophlebitis.

b. Venous thromboembolism (VTE). In the Premarin tablets substudy of the Women's Health Initiative (WHI), an increase in VTE has been observed in women receiving Premarin compared to placebo. (See **CLINICAL PHARMACOLOGY, Clinical Studies.**)

In the estrogen plus progestin substudy of WHI, a 2-fold greater rate of VTE, including deep venous thrombosis and pulmonary embolism, was observed in women receiving PREMPRO compared to women receiving placebo. The rate of VTE was 34 per 10,000 women-years in the PREMPRO group compared to 16 per 10,000 women-years in the placebo group. The increase in VTE risk was observed during the first year and persisted.

2. **Malignant neoplasms.**

a. Endometrial cancer. The use of unopposed estrogens in women with intact uteri has been associated with an increased risk of endometrial cancer. The reported endometrial cancer risk among unopposed estrogen users is about 2- to 12-fold greater than in non-users, and appears dependent on duration of treatment and on estrogen dose. Most studies show no significant increased risk associated with use of estrogens for less than one year. The greatest risk appears associated with prolonged use, with increased risks of 15- to 24-fold for five to ten years or more and this risk has been shown to persist for at least 8 to 15 years after estrogen therapy is discontinued.

Table 1. RELATIVE AND ABSOLUTE RISK SEEN IN THE ESTROGEN PLUS PROGESTIN SUBSTUDY OF WHI[a]

Event[c]	Relative Risk Prempro vs Placebo at 5.2 Years (95% CI*)	Placebo n = 8102	Prempro n = 8506
		Absolute Risk per 10,000 Women-years	
CHD events	1.29 (1.02-1.63)	30	37
Non-fatal MI	*1.32 (1.02-1.72)*	*23*	*30*
CHD death	*1.18 (0.70-1.97)*	*6*	*7*
Invasive breast cancer[b]	1.26 (1.00-1.59)	30	38
Stroke	1.41 (1.07-185)	21	29
Pulmonary embolism	2.13 (1.39-3.25)	8	16
Colorectal cancer	0.63 (0.43-0.92)	16	10
Endometrial cancer	0.83 (0.47-1.47)	6	5
Hip fracture	0.66 (0.45-0.98)	15	10
Death due to causes other than the events above	0.92 (0.74-1.14)	40	37
Global Index[c]	1.15 (1.03-1.28)	151	170
Deep vein thrombosis[d]	2.07 (1.49-2.87)	13	26
Vertebral fractures[d]	0.66 (0.44-0.98)	15	9
Other osteoporotic fractures[d]	0.77 (0.69-0.86)	170	131

[a] adapted from JAMA, 2002; 288:321–333
[b] includes metastatic and non-metastatic breast cancer with the exception of in situ breast cancer
[c] a subset of the events was combined in a "global index", defined as the earliest occurrence of CHD events, invasive breast cancer, stroke, pulmonary embolism, endometrial cancer, colorectal cancer, hip fracture, or death due to other causes
[d] not included in Global Index
* nominal confidence intervals unadjusted for multiple looks and multiple comparisons

b. Breast cancer. The use of estrogens and progestins by postmenopausal women has been reported to increase the risk of breast cancer. The most important randomized clinical trial providing information about this issue is the Women's Health Initiative (WHI) trial of estrogen plus progestin (see **CLINICAL PHARMACOLOGY, Clinical Studies**). The results from observational studies are generally consistent with those of the WHI clinical trial.

After a mean follow-up of 5.6 years, the WHI trial reported an increased risk of breast cancer in women who took estrogen plus progestin. Observational studies have also reported an increased risk for estrogen/progestin combination therapy, and a smaller increased risk for estrogen alone therapy, after several years of use. For both findings, the excess risk increased with duration of use, and appeared to return to baseline over about five years after stopping treatment (only the observational studies have substantial data on risk after stopping). In these studies, the risk of breast cancer was greater, and became apparent earlier, with estrogen/progestin combination therapy as compared to estrogen alone therapy. However, these studies have not found significant variation in the risk of breast cancer among different estrogens or among different estrogen/progestin combinations, doses, or routes of administration.

In the WHI trial of estrogen plus progestin, 26% of the women reported prior use of estrogen alone and/or estrogen/progestin combination hormone therapy. After a mean follow-up of 5.6 years during the clinical trial, the overall relative risk of invasive breast cancer was 1.24 (95% confidence interval 1.01-1.54), and the overall absolute risk was 41 vs. 33 cases per 10,000 women-years, for estrogen plus progestin compared with placebo. Among women who reported prior use of hormone therapy, the relative risk of invasive breast cancer was 1.86, and the absolute risk was 46 vs. 25 cases per 10,000 women-years, for estrogen plus progestin compared with placebo. Among women who reported no prior use of hormone therapy, the relative risk of invasive breast cancer was 1.09, and the absolute risk was 40 vs. 36 cases per 10,000 women-years for estrogen plus progestin compared with placebo. In the WHI trial, invasive breast cancers were larger and diagnosed at a more advanced stage in the estrogen plus progestin group compared with the placebo group. Metastatic disease was rare with no apparent difference between the two groups. Other prognostic factors such as histologic subtype, grade and hormone receptor status did not differ between the groups.

The observational Million Women Study in Europe reported an increased risk of mortality due to breast cancer among current users of estrogens alone or estrogens plus progestins compared to never users, while the estrogen plus progestin sub-study of WHI showed no effect on breast cancer mortality with a mean follow-up of 5.6 years.

The use of estrogen plus progestin has been reported to result in an increase in abnormal mammograms requiring further evaluation. All women should receive yearly breast examinations by a healthcare provider and perform monthly breast self-examinations. In addition, mammography examinations should be scheduled based on patient age, risk factors, and prior mammogram results.

3. **Gallbladder disease.**

A 2- to 4-fold increase in the risk of gallbladder disease requiring surgery in postmenopausal women receiving postmenopausal estrogens has been reported.

4. **Hypercalcemia.**

Estrogen administration may lead to severe hypercalcemia in patients with breast cancer and bone metastases. If hypercalcemia occurs, use of the drug should be stopped and appropriate measures taken to reduce the serum calcium level.

5. **Visual abnormalities.**

Retinal vascular thrombosis has been reported in patients receiving estrogens. Discontinue medication pending examination if there is sudden partial or complete loss of vision, or a sudden onset of proptosis, diplopia, or migraine. If examination reveals papilledema or retinal vascular lesions, estrogens should be discontinued.

PRECAUTIONS

A. General

Premarin Intravenous is indicated for short-term use. However, warnings, precautions and adverse reactions associated with Premarin tablets should be taken into account.

1. ***Addition of a progestin when a woman has not had a hysterectomy.***

Studies of the addition of a progestin for 10 or more days of a cycle of estrogen administration or daily with estrogen in a continuous regimen have reported a lowered incidence of endometrial hyperplasia than would be induced by estrogen treatment alone. Endometrial hyperplasia may be a precursor to endometrial cancer.

There are, however, possible risks which may be associated with the use of progestins with estrogens compared to estrogen-alone regimens. These include a possible increased risk of breast cancer, adverse effects on lipoprotein metabolism (e.g., lowering HDL, raising LDL) and impairment of glucose tolerance.

2. ***Elevated blood pressure.***

In a small number of case reports, substantial increases in blood pressure have been attributed to idiosyncratic reactions to estrogens. In a large, randomized, placebo-controlled clinical trial, a generalized effect of estrogen therapy on blood pressure was not seen. Blood pressure should be monitored at regular intervals with estrogen use.

Continued on next page

Premarin for Injection—Cont.

3. *Hypertriglyceridemia.*

In patients with pre-existing hypertriglyceridemia, estrogen therapy may be associated with elevations of plasma triglycerides leading to pancreatitis and other complications.

4. *Impaired liver function and past history of cholestatic jaundice.*

Estrogens may be poorly metabolized in patients with impaired liver function. For patients with a history of cholestatic jaundice associated with past estrogen use or with pregnancy, caution should be exercised and in the case of recurrence, medication should be discontinued.

5. *Hypothyroidism.*

Estrogen administration leads to increased thyroid-binding globulin (TBG) levels. Patients with normal thyroid function can compensate for the increased TBG by making more thyroid hormone, thus maintaining free T_4 and T_3 serum concentrations in the normal range. Patients dependent on thyroid hormone replacement therapy who are also receiving estrogens may require increased doses of their thyroid replacement therapy. These patients should have their thyroid function monitored in order to maintain their free thyroid hormone levels in an acceptable range.

6. *Fluid retention.*

Because estrogens may cause some degree of fluid retention, patients with conditions that might be influenced by this factor, such as a cardiac or renal dysfunction, warrant careful observation when estrogens are prescribed.

7. *Hypocalcemia.*

Estrogens should be used with caution in individuals with severe hypocalcemia.

8. *Ovarian cancer.*

The estrogen plus progestin substudy of WHI reported that after an average follow-up of 5.6 years, the relative risk of ovarian cancer for estrogen plus progestin versus placebo was 1.58 (95% confidence interval 0.77 – 3.24) but was not statistically significant. The absolute risk for estrogen plus progestin versus placebo was 4.2 versus 2.7 cases per 10,000 women-years. In some epidemiologic studies, the use of estrogen-only products, in particular for ten or more years, has been associated with an increased risk of ovarian cancer. Other epidemiologic studies have not found these associations.

9. *Exacerbation of endometriosis.*

Endometriosis may be exacerbated with administration of estrogen therapy.

A few cases of malignant transformation of residual endometrial implants have been reported in women treated post-hysterectomy with estrogen alone therapy. For patients known to have residual endometriosis post-hysterectomy, the addition of progestin should be considered.

10. *Exacerbation of other conditions.*

Estrogen therapy may cause an exacerbation of asthma, diabetes mellitus, epilepsy, migraine, porphyria, systemic lupus erythematosus, and hepatic hemangiomas and should be used with caution in women with these conditions.

B. Patient Information

Physicians are advised to discuss the contents of the PATIENT INFORMATION leaflet with patients who are being treated with Premarin Intravenous.

C. Laboratory Tests

Estrogen administration should be guided by clinical response at the lowest dose, rather than laboratory monitoring.

D. Drug/Laboratory Test Interactions

1. Accelerated prothrombin time, partial thromboplastin time, and platelet aggregation time; increased platelet count; increased factors II, VII antigen, VIII antigen, VIII coagulant activity, IX, X, XII, VII-X complex, II-VII-X complex, and beta-thromboglobulin; decreased levels of antifactor Xa and antithrombin III, decreased antithrombin III activity; increased levels of fibrinogen and fibrinogen activity; increased plasminogen antigen and activity.

2. Increased thyroid-binding globulin (TBG) leading to increased circulating total thyroid hormone, as measured by protein-bound iodine (PBI), T_4 levels (by column or by radioimmunoassay) or T_3 levels by radioimmunoassay. T_3 resin uptake is decreased, reflecting the elevated TBG. Free T_4 and free T_3 concentrations are unaltered. Patients on thyroid replacement therapy may require higher doses of thyroid hormone.

3. Other binding proteins may be elevated in serum, i.e., corticosteroid binding globulin (CBG), sex hormone-binding globulin (SHBG), leading to increased total circulating corticosteroids and sex steroids respectively. Free hormone concentrations may be decreased. Other plasma proteins may be increased (angiotensinogen/renin substrate, alpha-1-antitrypsin, ceruloplasmin).

4. Increased plasma HDL and HDL_2 subfraction concentrations, reduced LDL cholesterol concentration, increased triglyceride levels.

5. Impaired glucose tolerance.

6. Reduced response to metyrapone test.

E. Carcinogenesis, Mutagenesis, and Impairment of Fertility

(See **BOXED WARNINGS, WARNINGS,** and **PRECAUTIONS**.)

Long-term continuous administration of natural and synthetic estrogens in certain animal species increases the frequency of carcinomas of the breast, uterus, cervix, vagina, testis, and liver.

F. Pregnancy

Premarin Intravenous should not be used during pregnancy. (See **CONTRAINDICATIONS**.)

G. Nursing Mothers

Estrogen administration to nursing mothers has been shown to decrease the quantity and quality of breast milk. Detectable amounts of estrogens have been identified in the milk of mothers receiving the drug. Caution should be exercised when Premarin Intravenous is administered to a nursing woman.

H. Pediatric Use

Estrogen therapy has been used for the induction of puberty in adolescents with some forms of pubertal delay. Safety and effectiveness in pediatric patients have not otherwise been established.

Large and repeated doses of estrogen over an extended time period have been shown to accelerate epiphyseal closure, which could result in short adult stature if treatment is initiated before the completion of physiologic puberty in normally developing children. If estrogen is administered to patients whose bone growth is not complete, periodic monitoring of bone maturation and effects on epiphyseal centers is recommended during estrogen administration.

Estrogen treatment of prepubertal girls also induces premature breast development and vaginal cornification, and may induce vaginal bleeding. In boys, estrogen treatment may modify the normal pubertal process and induce gynecomastia.

I. Geriatric Use

Of the total number of subjects in the estrogen plus progestin substudy of the Women's Health Initiative study, 44% (n = 7,320) were 65 years and over, while 6.6% (n = 1,095) were 75 years and over (see **CLINICAL PHARMACOLOGY, Clinical Studies**). There was a higher incidence of stroke and invasive breast cancer in women 75 and over compared to women less than 75 years of age.

There have not been sufficient numbers of geriatric patients involved in studies utilizing Premarin to determine whether those over 65 years of age differ from younger subjects in their response to Premarin.

ADVERSE REACTIONS

See **BOXED WARNINGS, WARNINGS,** and **PRECAUTIONS**.

Premarin Intravenous is indicated for short-term use. However, the warnings, precautions and adverse reactions associated with Premarin tablets should be taken into account.

1. *Genitourinary system.*

Changes in vaginal bleeding pattern and abnormal withdrawal bleeding or flow; breakthrough bleeding, spotting.
Increase in size of uterine leiomyomata.
Vaginal candidiasis.
Change in amount of cervical secretion.

2. *Breasts.*

Pain, tenderness, enlargement.

3. *Cardiovascular.*

Venous thrombosis.
Pulmonary embolism.
Superficial thrombophlebitis.
Hypotension.
Myocardial infarction.
Stroke.

4. *Gastrointestinal.*

Nausea, vomiting.
Abdominal cramps, bloating.
Cholestatic jaundice.
Increased incidence of gallbladder disease.
Pancreatitis.
Enlargement of hepatic hemangiomas.

5. *Skin.*

Chloasma or melasma that may persist when drug is discontinued.
Erythema multiforme.
Erythema nodosum.
Hemorrhagic eruption.
Loss of scalp hair.
Hirsutism.
Pruritis.
Rash.

6. *Eyes.*

Retinal vascular thrombosis.
Intolerance to contact lenses.

7. *Central Nervous System.*

Headache.
Migraine.
Dizziness.
Mental depression.
Chorea.
Nervousness.
Exacerbation of epilepsy.
Dementia.

8. *Miscellaneous.*

Increase or decrease in weight.
Reduced carbohydrate tolerance.
Aggravation of porphyria.
Edema.
Changes in libido.
Anaphylactoid/anaphylactic reactions.
Urticaria.
Angioedema.
Injection site pain.
Injection site edema.
Phlebitis (injection site).
Exacerbation of asthma.

OVERDOSAGE

Serious ill effects have not been reported following acute ingestion of large doses of estrogen-containing drug products by young children. Overdosage of estrogen may cause nausea and vomiting, and withdrawal bleeding may occur in females.

DOSAGE AND ADMINISTRATION

For treatment of abnormal uterine bleeding due to hormonal imbalance in the absence of organic pathology:

One 25 mg injection, intravenously or intramuscularly. Intravenous use is preferred since more rapid response can be expected from this mode of administration. Repeat in 6 to 12 hours if necessary. The use of Premarin Intravenous for injection does not preclude the advisability of other appropriate measures.

One should adhere to the usual precautionary measures governing intravenous administration. Injection should be made SLOWLY to obviate the occurrence of flushes.

Infusion of Premarin Intravenous for injection with other agents is not generally recommended. In emergencies, however, when an infusion has already been started it may be expedient to make the injection into the tubing just distal to the infusion needle. If so used, compatibility of solutions must be considered.

COMPATIBILITY OF SOLUTIONS: Premarin Intravenous is compatible with normal saline, dextrose, and invert sugar solutions. **It is not compatible with protein hydrolysate, ascorbic acid, or any solution with an acid pH.**

DIRECTIONS FOR STORAGE AND RECONSTITUTION

STORAGE BEFORE RECONSTITUTION: Store package in refrigerator, 2° to 8°C (36° to 46°F).

TO RECONSTITUTE: First withdraw air from Secule® vial so as to facilitate introduction of sterile diluent. Then, flow the sterile diluent slowly against the side of Secule® vial and agitate gently. **Do not shake violently.**

STORAGE AFTER RECONSTITUTION: It is common practice to utilize the reconstituted solution within a few hours. If it is necessary to keep the reconstituted solution for more than a few hours, store the reconstituted solution under refrigeration (2° to 8°C). Under these conditions, the solution is stable for 60 days, and is suitable for use unless darkening or precipitation occurs.

HOW SUPPLIED

NDC 0046-0749-05–Each package provides: (1) One Secule® vial containing 25 mg of conjugated estrogens, USP, for injection (also lactose 200 mg, sodium citrate 12.2 mg, and simethicone 0.2 mg). The pH is adjusted with sodium hydroxide or hydrochloric acid. (2) One 5 mL ampul of sterile diluent with 2% benzyl alcohol in sterile water.

Premarin Intravenous (conjugated estrogens, USP) for injection is prepared by cryodesiccation.

SECULE®-Registered trademark to designate a vial containing an injectable preparation in dry form.

PATIENT INFORMATION

(Updated January 19, 2005)

Premarin® Intravenous (conjugated estrogens, USP) for injection

Read this PATIENT INFORMATION which describes the benefit and major risks of your treatment, as well as how and when treatment should be used. This information does not take the place of talking to your healthcare provider about your medical condition or your treatment.

What is the most important information I should know about Premarin Intravenous (an estrogen mixture)?

- Estrogens increase the chances of getting cancer of the uterus.

  Report any unusual vaginal bleeding right away while you are taking Premarin. Vaginal bleeding after menopause may be a warning sign of cancer of the uterus (womb). Your healthcare provider should check any unusual vaginal bleeding to find out the cause.

- Do not use estrogens with or without progestins to prevent heart disease, heart attacks, strokes, or dementia.

  Using estrogens with or without progestins may increase your chances of getting heart attacks, strokes, breast cancer, and blood clots. Using estrogens, with or without progestins, may increase your risk of dementia, based on a study of women age 65 years or older. You and your healthcare provider should talk regularly about whether you still need treatment with estrogens.

What is Premarin Intravenous?

Premarin Intravenous is a medicine that contains a mixture of estrogen hormones.

Premarin Intravenous is used to:

- treat certain types of abnormal uterine bleeding due to hormonal imbalance when your doctor has found no other cause of bleeding.

Who should not use Premarin Intravenous?

Premarin Intravenous should not be used if you:

- **have unusual vaginal bleeding that has not been evaluated by your healthcare provider.**

- **currently have or have had certain cancers.**

  Estrogens may increase the chances of getting certain types of cancers, including cancer of the breast or uterus. If you have or have had cancer, talk with your healthcare provider.

- **had a stroke or heart attack in the past year.**
- **currently have or have had blood clots.**
- **currently have liver problems.**
- **are allergic to Premarin Intravenous or any of its ingredients.**
  See the end of this leaflet for a list of all the ingredients in Premarin Intravenous.
- **think you may be pregnant.**

Tell your healthcare provider:

- **if you are breast feeding.** The hormones in Premarin Intravenous can pass into your milk.
- **about all of your medical problems.** Your healthcare provider may need to check you more carefully if you have certain conditions, such as asthma (wheezing), epilepsy (seizures), migraine, endometriosis, lupus, problems with your heart, liver, thyroid, kidneys, or have high calcium levels in your blood.
- **about all the medicines you take,** including prescription and nonprescription medicines, vitamins, and herbal supplements. Some medicines may affect how Premarin Intravenous works.

What are the possible side effects of Premarin Intravenous?

Premarin Intravenous is for short-term use only. However, the risks associated with Premarin tablets should be taken into account.

Less common but serious side effects include:

- Breast cancer
- Cancer of the uterus
- Stroke
- Heart attack
- Blood clots
- Dementia
- Gallbladder disease
- Ovarian cancer

These are some of the warning signs of serious side effects:

- Breast lumps
- Unusual vaginal bleeding
- Dizziness and faintness
- Changes in speech
- Severe headaches
- Chest pain
- Shortness of breath
- Pains in your legs
- Changes in vision
- Vomiting

Call your healthcare provider right away if you get any of these warning signs, or any other unusual symptom that concerns you.

Common side effects include:

- Headache
- Breast tenderness
- Irregular vaginal bleeding or spotting
- Stomach/abdominal cramps, bloating
- Nausea and vomiting
- Hair loss

Other side effects include:

- High blood pressure
- Liver problems
- High blood sugar
- Fluid retention
- Enlargement of benign tumors of the uterus ("fibroids")
- Vaginal yeast infections

These are not all the possible side effects of Premarin. For more information, ask your healthcare provider or pharmacist.

What can I do to lower my chances of getting a serious side effect with Premarin Intravenous?

- If you have high blood pressure, high cholesterol (fat in the blood), diabetes, are overweight, or if you use tobacco, you may have higher chances for getting heart disease. Ask your healthcare provider for ways to lower your chances for getting heart disease.

General information about the safe and effective use of Premarin Intravenous

Medicines are sometimes prescribed for conditions that are not mentioned in patient information leaflets. Do not use Premarin Intravenous for conditions for which it was not prescribed. Do not give Premarin Intravenous to other people, even if they have the same symptoms you have. It may harm them. **Keep Premarin Intravenous out of the reach of children.**

This leaflet provides a summary of the most important information about Premarin Intravenous. If you would like more information, talk with your healthcare provider or pharmacist. You can ask for information about Premarin Intravenous that is written for health professionals. You can get more information by calling the toll free number 1-800-934-5556.

What are the ingredients in Premarin IV?

Premarin Intravenous for injection contains a mixture of conjugated estrogens, which are a mixture of sodium estrone sulfate and sodium equilin sulfate and other components including sodium sulfate conjugates: 17α-dihydroequilin, 17α-estradiol, and 17β-dihydroequilin. Premarin Intravenous for injection also contains lactose, sodium citrate, simethicone, and sodium hydroxide or hydrochloric acid in dry form. A sterile diluent containing benzyl alcohol in sterile water is provided for reconstitution. The reconstituted solution is suitable for intravenous or intramuscular injection.

Each Premarin Intravenous (conjugated estrogens, USP) for injection package provides 25 mg of conjugated estrogens, USP, in dry form and 5 mL of sterile diluent for intravenous or intramuscular use.

This product's label may have been revised after this insert was used in production. For further product information and current package insert, please visit www.wyeth.com or call our medical communications department toll-free at 1-800-934-5556.

Wyeth®
Wyeth Pharmaceuticals Inc.
Philadelphia, PA 19101

W10411C005
ET01
Revised January 19, 2005

PREMARIN® ℞

[prĕm'ă-rĭn]
(conjugated estrogens tablets, USP)
℞ only

Prescribing information for this product, which appears on pages 3366–3371 of the 2005 PDR, has been completely revised as follows. Please write "See Supplement A" next to the product heading.

ESTROGENS INCREASE THE RISK OF ENDOMETRIAL CANCER

Close clinical surveillance of all women taking estrogens is important. Adequate diagnostic measures, including endometrial sampling when indicated, should be undertaken to rule out malignancy in all cases of undiagnosed persistent or recurring abnormal vaginal bleeding. There is no evidence that the use of "natural" estrogens results in a different endometrial risk profile than synthetic estrogens of equivalent estrogen dose. (See **WARNINGS, Malignant neoplasms, *Endometrial cancer*.**)

CARDIOVASCULAR AND OTHER RISKS

Estrogens with or without progestins should not be used for the prevention of cardiovascular disease or dementia. (See **WARNINGS, Cardiovascular disorders** and **Dementia.**)

The Women's Health Initiative (WHI) study reported increased risks of stroke and deep vein thrombosis in postmenopausal women (50 to 79 years of age) during 6.8 years of treatment with conjugated estrogens (0.625 mg) relative to placebo. (See **CLINICAL PHARMACOLOGY, Clinical Studies** and **WARNINGS, Cardiovascular disorders.**)

The WHI study reported increased risks of myocardial infarction, stroke, invasive breast cancer, pulmonary emboli, and deep vein thrombosis in postmenopausal women (50 to 79 years of age) during 5 years of treatment with conjugated estrogens (0.625 mg) combined with medroxyprogesterone acetate (2.5 mg) relative to placebo. (See **CLINICAL PHARMACOLOGY, Clinical Studies** and **WARNINGS, Cardiovascular disorders** and **Malignant neoplasms, *Breast cancer*.**)

The Women's Health Initiative Memory Study (WHIMS), a substudy of WHI, reported increased risk of developing probable dementia in postmenopausal women 65 years of age or older during 5.2 years of treatment with conjugated estrogens alone and during 4 years of treatment with conjugated estrogens combined with medroxyprogesterone acetate, relative to placebo. It is unknown whether this finding applies to younger postmenopausal women. (See **CLINICAL PHARMACOLOGY, Clinical Studies, WARNINGS, Dementia** and **PRECAUTIONS, Geriatric Use.**)

Other doses of conjugated estrogens and medroxyprogesterone acetate, and other combinations and dosage forms of estrogens and progestins were not studied in the WHI clinical trials and, in the absence of comparable data, these risks should be assumed to be similar. Because of these risks, estrogens with or without progestins should be prescribed at the lowest effective doses and for the shortest duration consistent with treatment goals and risks for the individual woman.

DESCRIPTION

Premarin® (conjugated estrogens tablets, USP) for oral administration contains a mixture of conjugated estrogens obtained exclusively from natural sources, occurring as the sodium salts of water-soluble estrogen sulfates blended to represent the average composition of material derived from pregnant mares' urine. It is a mixture of sodium estrone sulfate and sodium equilin sulfate. It contains as concomitant components, as sodium sulfate conjugates, 17α-dihydroequilin, 17α-estradiol, and 17β-dihydroequilin. Tablets for oral administration are available in 0.3 mg, 0.45 mg, 0.625 mg, 0.9 mg, and 1.25 mg strengths of conjugated estrogens.

Premarin 0.3 mg, 0.45 mg, 0.625 mg, and 0.9 mg tablets contain the following inactive ingredients: calcium phosphate tribasic, calcium sulfate, carnauba wax, microcrystalline cellulose, powdered cellulose, glyceryl monooleate, lactose monohydrate, magnesium stearate, methylcellulose, pharmaceutical glaze, polyethylene glycol, stearic acid (not present in 0.45 mg tablet), sucrose, and titanium dioxide.

Premarin 1.25 mg tablets contain the following inactive ingredients: calcium phosphate tribasic, hydroxypropyl cellulose, microcrystalline cellulose, powdered cellulose, hypromellose, lactose monohydrate, magnesium stearate, polyethylene glycol, sucrose, and titanium dioxide.

— 0.3 mg tablets also contain: D&C Yellow No. 10, FD&C Blue No. 1, FD&C Blue No. 2, FD&C Yellow No. 6.
— 0.45 mg tablets also contain: FD&C Blue No. 2.
— 0.625 mg tablets also contain: FD&C Blue No. 2, D&C Red No. 27, FD&C Red No. 40.
— 0.9 mg tablets also contain: D&C Red No. 6, D&C Red No. 7.
— 1.25 mg tablets also contain: black iron oxide, D&C Yellow No. 10, FD&C Yellow No. 6.

Premarin tablets comply with USP Drug Release Test criteria as outlined below:

Premarin 0.3 mg, 0.45 mg, and 0.625 mg tablets	Test 1
Premarin 0.9 mg tablets	Test 2
Premarin 1.25 mg tablets	USP Drug Release Test pending

CLINICAL PHARMACOLOGY

Endogenous estrogens are largely responsible for the development and maintenance of the female reproductive system and secondary sexual characteristics. Although circulating estrogens exist in a dynamic equilibrium of metabolic interconversions, estradiol is the principal intracellular human estrogen and is substantially more potent than its metabolites, estrone and estriol, at the receptor level.

The primary source of estrogen in normally cycling adult women is the ovarian follicle, which secretes 70 to 500 mcg of estradiol daily, depending on the phase of the menstrual cycle. After menopause, most endogenous estrogen is produced by conversion of androstenedione, secreted by the adrenal cortex, to estrone by peripheral tissues. Thus, estrone and the sulfate-conjugated form, estrone sulfate, are the most abundant circulating estrogens in postmenopausal women.

Estrogens act through binding to nuclear receptors in estrogen-responsive tissues. To date, two estrogen receptors have been identified. These vary in proportion from tissue to tissue.

Circulating estrogens modulate the pituitary secretion of the gonadotropins, luteinizing hormone (LH) and follicle stimulating hormone (FSH) through a negative feedback mechanism. Estrogens act to reduce the elevated levels of these gonadotropins seen in postmenopausal women.

Pharmacokinetics

Absorption

Conjugated estrogens are soluble in water and are well absorbed from the gastrointestinal tract after release from the drug formulation. The Premarin tablet releases conjugated estrogens slowly over several hours. Table 1 summarizes the mean pharmacokinetic parameters for unconjugated and conjugated estrogens following administration of 2 × 0.3 mg, 2 × 0.45 mg, and 2 × 0.625 mg tablets to healthy postmenopausal women.

[See table 1 at top of next page]

Distribution

The distribution of exogenous estrogens is similar to that of endogenous estrogens. Estrogens are widely distributed in the body and are generally found in higher concentration in the sex hormone target organs. Estrogens circulate in the blood largely bound to sex hormone binding globulin (SHBG) and albumin.

Metabolism

Exogenous estrogens are metabolized in the same manner as endogenous estrogens. Circulating estrogens exist in a dynamic equilibrium of metabolic interconversions. These transformations take place mainly in the liver. Estradiol is converted reversibly to estrone, and both can be converted to estriol, which is the major urinary metabolite. Estrogens also undergo enterohepatic recirculation via sulfate and glucuronide conjugation in the liver, biliary secretion of conjugates into the intestine, and hydrolysis in the gut followed by reabsorption. In postmenopausal women a significant proportion of the circulating estrogens exists as sulfate conjugates, especially estrone sulfate, which serves as a circulating reservoir for the formation of more active estrogens.

Excretion

Estradiol, estrone, and estriol are excreted in the urine along with glucuronide and sulfate conjugates.

Special Populations

No pharmacokinetic studies were conducted in special populations, including patients with renal or hepatic impairment.

Drug Interactions

Data from a single-dose drug-drug interaction study involving conjugated estrogens and medroxyprogesterone acetate indicate that the pharmacokinetic dispositions of both drugs are not altered when the drugs are coadministered. No other clinical drug-drug interaction studies have been conducted with conjugated estrogens.

In vitro and in vivo studies have shown that estrogens are metabolized partially by cytochrome P450 3A4 (CYP3A4). Therefore, inducers or inhibitors of CYP3A4 may affect estrogen drug metabolism. Inducers of CYP3A4 such as St. John's Wort preparations (Hypericum perforatum), phenobarbital, carbamazepine, and rifampin may reduce plasma concentrations of estrogens, possibly resulting in a decrease in therapeutic effects and/or changes in the uterine bleeding profile. Inhibitors of CYP3A4 such as erythromycin, clarithromycin, ketoconazole, itraconazole, ritonavir and grapefruit juice may increase plasma concentrations of estrogens and may result in side effects.

Clinical Studies

Effects on vasomotor symptoms.

In the first year of the Health and Osteoporosis, Progestin and Estrogen (HOPE) Study, a total of 2805 postmeno-

Continued on next page

Premarin—Cont.

pausal women (average age 53.3 ± 4.9 years) were randomly assigned to one of eight treatment groups, receiving either placebo or conjugated estrogens with or without medroxyprogesterone acetate. Efficacy for vasomotor symptoms was assessed during the first 12 weeks of treatment in a subset of symptomatic women (n = 241) who had at least 7 moderate to severe hot flushes daily or at least 50 moderate to severe hot flushes during the week before randomization. Premarin (0.3 mg, 0.45 mg, and 0.625 mg tablets) was shown to be statistically better than placebo at weeks 4 and 12 for relief of both the frequency and severity of moderate to severe vasomotor symptoms. Table 2 shows the adjusted mean number of hot flushes in the Premarin 0.3 mg, 0.45 mg, and 0.625 mg and placebo treatment groups over the initial 12-week period.
[See table 2 below]

Effects on vulvar and vaginal atrophy.
Results of vaginal maturation indexes at cycles 6 and 13 showed that the differences from placebo were statistically significant (p<0.001) for all treatment groups (conjugated estrogens alone and conjugated estrogens/medroxyprogesterone acetate treatment groups).

Effects on bone mineral density.
Health and Osteoporosis, Progestin and Estrogen (HOPE) Study
The HOPE study was a double-blind, randomized, placebo/active-drug-controlled, multicenter study of healthy post-menopausal women with an intact uterus. Subjects (mean age 53.3 ± 4.9 years) were 2.3 ± 0.9 years, on average, since menopause, and took one 600-mg tablet of elemental calcium (Caltrate) daily. Subjects were not given vitamin D supplements. They were treated with Premarin 0.625 mg, 0.45 mg, 0.3 mg, or placebo. Prevention of bone loss was assessed by measurement of bone mineral density (BMD), primarily at the anteroposterior lumbar spine (L_2 to L_4). Secondarily, BMD measurements of the total body, femoral neck, and trochanter were also analyzed. Serum osteocalcin, urinary calcium, and N-telopeptide were used as bone turnover markers (BTM) at cycles 6, 13, 19, and 26.

Intent-to-treat subjects
All active treatment groups showed significant differences from placebo in each of the 4 BMD endpoints at cycles 6, 13, 19, and 26. The mean percent increases in the primary efficacy measure (L_2 to L_4 BMD) at the final on-therapy evaluation (cycle 26 for those who completed and the last available evaluation for those who discontinued early) were 2.46% with 0.625 mg, 2.26% with 0.45 mg, and 1.13% with 0.3 mg. The placebo group showed a mean percent decrease from baseline at the final evaluation of 2.45%. These results show that the lower dosages of Premarin were effective in increasing L_2 to L_4 BMD compared with placebo and, therefore, support the efficacy of the lower doses.
The analysis for the other 3 BMD endpoints yielded mean percent changes from baseline in femoral trochanter that were generally larger than those seen for L_2 to L_4 and changes in femoral neck and total body that were generally smaller than those seen for L_2 to L_4. Significant differences between groups indicated that each of the Premarin treatments was more effective than placebo for all 3 of these additional BMD endpoints. With regard to femoral neck and total body, the active treatment groups all showed mean percent increases in BMD while placebo treatment was accompanied by mean percent decreases. For femoral trochanter, each of the Premarin dose groups showed a mean percent increase that was significantly greater than the small increase seen in the placebo group. The percent changes from baseline to final evaluation are shown in Table 3.
[See table 3 at top of next page]
Figure 1 shows the cumulative percentage of subjects with changes from baseline equal to or greater than the value shown on the x-axis.

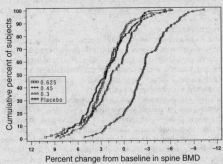

Figure 1. CUMULATIVE PERCENT OF SUBJECTS WITH CHANGES FROM BASELINE IN SPINE BMD OF GIVEN MAGNITUDE OR GREATER IN PREMARIN AND PLACEBO GROUPS

The mean percent changes from baseline in L_2 to L_4 BMD for women who completed the bone density study are shown with standard error bars by treatment group in Figure 2. Significant differences between each of the Premarin dosage groups and placebo were found at cycles 6, 13, 19, and 26.
[See figure 2 at top of next page]
The bone turnover markers serum osteocalcin and urinary N-telopeptide significantly decreased (p<0.001) in all active-treatment groups at cycles 6, 13, 19, and 26 compared with the placebo group. Larger mean decreases from baseline were seen with the active groups than with the placebo group. Significant differences from placebo were seen less frequently in urine calcium.

TABLE 1. PHARMACOKINETIC PARAMETERS FOR PREMARIN

Pharmacokinetic Profile of Unconjugated Estrogens Following a Dose of 2 × 0.3 mg

PK Parameter Arithmetic Mean (%CV)	C_{max} (pg/mL)	t_{max} (h)	$t_{1/2}$ (h)	AUC (pg•h/mL)
Estrone	82 (33)	7.8 (27)	54.7 (42)	5390 (50)
Baseline-adjusted estrone	58 (42)	7.8 (27)	21.1 (45)	1467 (41)
Equilin	31 (47)	7.2 (28)	18.3 (110)	652 (68)

Pharmacokinetic Profile of Conjugated Estrogens Following a Dose of 2 × 0.3 mg

PK Parameter Arithmetic Mean (%CV)	C_{max} (ng/mL)	t_{max} (h)	$t_{1/2}$ (h)	AUC (ng•h/mL)
Estrone	2.5 (32)	6.5 (29)	25.4 (22)	61.0 (43)
Baseline-adjusted total estrone	2.4 (32)	6.5 (29)	16.2 (34)	40.8 (36)
Equilin	1.6 (40)	5.9 (27)	11.8 (21)	22.4 (42)

Pharmacokinetic Profile of Unconjugated Estrogens Following a Dose of 2 × 0.45 mg

PK Parameter Arithmetic Mean (%CV)	C_{max} (pg/mL)	t_{max} (h)	$t_{1/2}$ (h)	AUC (pg•h/mL)
Estrone	92 (32)	8.7 (28)	56.4 (68)	6344 (56)
Baseline-adjusted estrone	65 (40)	8.7 (28)	20.3 (38)	1940 (40)
Equilin	35 (49)	7.6 (33)	21.9 (113)	849 (60)

Pharmacokinetic Profile of Conjugated Estrogens Following a Dose of 2 × 0.45 mg

PK Parameter Arithmetic Mean (%CV)	C_{max} (ng/mL)	t_{max} (h)	$t_{1/2}$ (h)	AUC (ng•h/mL)
Total estrone	2.8 (46)	7.1 (27)	27.6 (35)	77 (34)
Baseline-adjusted total estrone	2.6 (46)	7.1 (27)	14.7 (42)	48 (38)
Total equilin	1.9 (53)	5.9 (32)	11.8 (32)	29 (55)

Pharmacokinetic Profile of Unconjugated Estrogens Following a Dose of 2 × 0.625 mg

PK Parameter Arithmetic Mean (%CV)	C_{max} (pg/mL)	t_{max} (h)	$t_{1/2}$ (h)	AUC (pg•h/mL)
Estrone	139 (37)	8.8 (20)	28.0 (30)	5016 (34)
Baseline-adjusted estrone	120 (41)	8.8 (20)	17.4 (37)	2956 (39)
Equilin	66 (42)	7.9 (19)	13.6 (52)	1210 (37)

Pharmacokinetic Profile of Conjugated Estrogens Following a Dose of 2 × 0.625 mg

PK Parameter Arithmetic Mean (%CV)	C_{max} (ng/mL)	t_{max} (h)	$t_{1/2}$ (h)	AUC (ng•h/mL)
Total estrone	7.3 (41)	7.3 (24)	15.0 (25)	134 (42)
Baseline-adjusted total estrone	7.1 (41)	7.3 (24)	13.6 (23)	122 (38)
Total equilin	5.0 (42)	6.2 (26)	10.1 (26)	65 (44)

Pharmacokinetic Profile of Unconjugated Estrogens Following a Dose of 1 × 1.25 mg

PK Parameter Arithmetic Mean (%CV)	C_{max} (pg/mL)	t_{max} (h)	$t_{1/2}$ (h)	AUC (pg•h/mL)
Estrone	124 (30)	10.0 (32)	38.1 (37)	6332 (44)
Baseline-adjusted estrone	102 (35)	10.0 (32)	19.7 (48)	3159 (53)
Equilin	59 (43)	8.8 (36)	10.9 (47)	1182 (42)

Pharmacokinetic Profile of Conjugated Estrogens Following a Dose of 1 × 1.25 mg

PK Parameter Arithmetic Mean (%CV)	C_{max} (ng/mL)	t_{max} (h)	$t_{1/2}$ (h)	AUC (ng•h/mL)
Total Estrone	4.5 (39)	8.2 (58)	26.5 (40)	109 (46)
Baseline-adjusted total estrone	4.3 (41)	8.2 (58)	17.5 (41)	87 (44)
Total equilin	2.9 (42)	6.8 (49)	12.5 (34)	48 (51)

TABLE 2. SUMMARY TABULATION OF THE NUMBER OF HOT FLUSHES PER DAY– MEAN VALUES AND COMPARISONS BETWEEN THE ACTIVE TREATMENT GROUPS AND THE PLACEBO GROUP: PATIENTS WITH AT LEAST 7 MODERATE TO SEVERE FLUSHES PER DAY OR AT LEAST 50 PER WEEK AT BASELINE, LOCF

Treatment (No. of Patients) Time Period (week)	Baseline Mean ± SD	Observed Mean ± SD	Mean Change± SD	p-Values vs. Placebo[a]
0.625 mg CE (n = 27)				
4	12.29 ± 3.89	1.95 ± 2.77	-10.34 ± 4.73	<0.001
12	12.29 ± 3.89	0.75 ± 1.82	-11.54 ± 4.62	<0.001
0.45 mg CE (n = 32)				
4	12.25 ± 5.04	5.04 ± 5.31	-7.21 ± 4.75	<0.001
12	12.25 ± 5.04	2.32 ± 3.32	-9.93 ± 4.64	<0.001
0.3 mg CE (n = 30)				
4	13.77 ± 4.78	4.65 ± 3.71	-9.12 ± 4.71	<0.001
12	13.77 ± 4.78	2.52 ± 3.23	-11.25 ± 4.60	<0.001
Placebo (n = 28)				
4	11.69 ± 3.87	7.89 ± 5.28	-3.80 ± 4.71	—
12	11.69 ± 3.87	5.71 ± 5.22	-5.98 ± 4.60	—

a: Based on analysis of covariance with treatment as factor and baseline as covariate.

Women's Health Initiative Studies.
The Women's Health Initiative (WHI) enrolled a total of 27,000 predominantly healthy postmenopausal women to

Figure 2. ADJUSTED MEAN (SE) PERCENT CHANGE FROM BASELINE AT EACH CYCLE IN SPINE BMD: SUBJECTS COMPLETING IN PREMARIN GROUPS AND PLACEBO

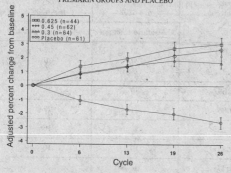

assess the risks and benefits of either the use of Premarin (0.625 mg conjugated estrogens per day) alone or the use of PREMPRO™ (0.625 mg conjugated estrogens plus 2.5 mg medroxyprogesterone acetate per day) compared to placebo in the prevention of certain chronic diseases. The primary endpoint was the incidence of coronary heart disease (CHD) (nonfatal myocardial infarction and CHD death), with invasive breast cancer as the primary adverse outcome studied. A "global index" included the earliest occurrence of CHD, invasive breast cancer, stroke, pulmonary embolism (PE), endometrial cancer, colorectal cancer, hip fracture, or death due to other cause. The study did not evaluate the effects of Premarin or PREMPRO on menopausal symptoms.

The estrogen alone substudy was stopped early because an increased risk of stroke was observed and it was deemed that no further information would be obtained regarding the risks and benefits of estrogen alone in predetermined primary endpoints. Results of the estrogen alone substudy, which included 10,739 women (average age of 63 years, range 50 to 79; 75.3% White, 15% Black, 6.1% Hispanic), after an average follow-up of 6.8 years are presented in Table 4 below.

[See table 4 at right]

For those outcomes included in the WHI "global index" that reached statistical significance, the absolute excess risk per 10,000 women-years in the group treated with Premarin alone were 12 more strokes while the absolute risk reduction per 10,000 women-years was 6 fewer hip fractures. The absolute excess risk of events included in the "global index" was a nonsignificant 2 events per 10,000 women-years. There was no difference between the groups in terms of all-cause mortality. (See **BOXED WARNINGS, WARNINGS,** and **PRECAUTIONS**.)

The estrogen plus progestin substudy was also stopped early because, according to the predefined stopping rule, the increased risk of breast cancer and cardiovascular events exceeded the specified benefits included in the "global index." Results of the estrogen plus progestin substudy, which included 16,608 women (average age of 63 years, range 50 to 79; 83.9% White, 6.5% Black, 5.5% Hispanic), after an average follow-up of 5.2 years are presented in Table 5 below.

[See table 5 at top of next page]

For those outcomes included in the WHI "global index," the absolute excess risks per 10,000 women-years in the group treated with PREMPRO were 7 more CHD events, 8 more strokes, 8 more PEs, and 8 more invasive breast cancers, while the absolute risk reductions per 10,000 women-years were 6 fewer colorectal cancers and 5 fewer hip fractures. The absolute excess risk of events included in the "global index" was 19 per 10,000 women-years. There was no difference between the groups in all-cause mortality. (See **BOXED WARNINGS, WARNINGS,** and **PRECAUTIONS**.)

Women's Health Initiative Memory Study.
The estrogen alone Women's Health Initiative Memory Study (WHIMS), a substudy of WHI, enrolled 2,947 predominantly healthy postmenopausal women 65 years of age and older (45% were age 65 to 69 years, 36% were 70 to 74 years, and 19% were 75 years of age and older) to evaluate the effects of Premarin (0.625 mg conjugated estrogens) on the incidence of probable dementia (primary outcome) compared with placebo.

After an average follow-up of 5.2 years, 28 women in the estrogen alone group (37 per 10,000 women-years) and 19 in the placebo group (25 per 10,000 women-years) were diagnosed with probable dementia. The relative risk of probable dementia in the estrogen alone group was 1.49 (95% CI, 0.83 to 2.66) compared to placebo. It is unknown whether these findings apply to younger postmenopausal women.
(See **BOXED WARNINGS, WARNINGS, Dementia** and **PRECAUTIONS, Geriatric Use**.)
The estrogen plus progestin WHIMS substudy enrolled 4,532 predominantly healthy postmenopausal women 65 years of age and older (47% were age 65 to 69 years, 35% were 70 to 74 years, and 18% were 75 years of age and older) to evaluate the effects of PREMPRO (0.625 mg conjugated estrogens plus 2.5 mg medroxyprogesterone acetate) on the incidence of probable dementia (primary outcome) compared with placebo.

After an average follow-up of 4 years, 40 women in the estrogen/progestin group (45 per 10,000 women-years) and 21 in the placebo group (22 per 10,000 women-years) were diagnosed with probable dementia. The relative risk of probable dementia in the hormone therapy group was 2.05

(95% CI, 1.21 to 3.48) compared to placebo. Differences between groups became apparent in the first year of treatment. It is unknown whether these findings apply to younger postmenopausal women. (See **BOXED WARNINGS, WARNINGS, Dementia** and **PRECAUTIONS, Geriatric Use**.)

INDICATIONS AND USAGE

Premarin therapy is indicated in the:
1. Treatment of moderate to severe vasomotor symptoms associated with the menopause.
2. Treatment of moderate to severe symptoms of vulvar and vaginal atrophy associated with the menopause. When prescribing solely for the treatment of symptoms of vulvar and vaginal atrophy, topical vaginal products should be considered.
3. Treatment of hypoestrogenism due to hypogonadism, castration or primary ovarian failure.
4. Treatment of breast cancer (for palliation only) in appropriately selected women and men with metastatic disease.
5. Treatment of advanced androgen-dependent carcinoma of the prostate (for palliation only).
6. Prevention of postmenopausal osteoporosis. When prescribing solely for the prevention of postmenopausal osteoporosis, therapy should only be considered for women at significant risk of osteoporosis and for whom non-estrogen medications are not considered to be appropriate. (See **CLINICAL PHARMACOLOGY, Clinical Studies**.)
The mainstays for decreasing the risk of postmenopausal osteoporosis are weight-bearing exercise, adequate calcium and vitamin D intake, and when indicated, pharmacologic therapy. Postmenopausal women require an average of 1500 mg/day of elemental calcium. Therefore, when not contraindicated, calcium supplementation may be helpful for women with suboptimal dietary intake. Vi-

tamin D supplementation of 400-800 IU/day may also be required to ensure adequate daily intake in postmenopausal women.

CONTRAINDICATIONS

Estrogens should not be used in individuals with any of the following conditions:
1. Undiagnosed abnormal genital bleeding.
2. Known, suspected, or history of cancer of the breast except in appropriately selected patients being treated for metastatic disease.
3. Known or suspected estrogen-dependent neoplasia.
4. Active deep vein thrombosis, pulmonary embolism or a history of these conditions.
5. Active or recent (e.g., within past year) arterial thromboembolic disease (e.g., stroke, myocardial infarction).
6. Liver dysfunction or disease.
7. Premarin tablets should not be used in patients with known hypersensitivity to their ingredients.
8. Known or suspected pregnancy. There is no indication for Premarin in pregnancy. There appears to be little or no increased risk of birth defects in children born to women who have used estrogen and progestins from oral contraceptives inadvertently during pregnancy. (See **PRECAUTIONS**.)

WARNINGS

See **BOXED WARNINGS**.
1. **Cardiovascular disorders.** Estrogen and estrogen/progestin therapy have been associated with an increased risk of cardiovascular events such as myocardial infarction and stroke, as well as venous thrombosis and pulmonary embolism (venous thromboembolism or VTE). Should any of these occur or be suspected, estrogens should be discontinued immediately.

Continued on next page

TABLE 3. PERCENT CHANGE IN BONE MINERAL DENSITY: COMPARISON BETWEEN ACTIVE AND PLACEBO GROUPS IN THE INTENT-TO-TREAT POPULATION, LAST OBSERVATION CARRIED FORWARD

Region Evaluated Treatment Group[a]	No. of Subjects	Baseline (g/cm²) Mean ± SD	Change from Baseline (%) Adjusted Mean ± SE	p-Value vs Placebo
L₂ to L₄ BMD				
0.625	83	1.17 ± 0.15	2.46 ± 0.37	<0.001
0.45	91	1.13 ± 0.15	2.26 ± 0.35	<0.001
0.3	87	1.14 ± 0.15	1.13 ± 0.36	<0.001
Placebo	85	1.14 ± 0.14	-2.45 ± 0.36	
Total Body BMD				
0.625	84	1.15 ± 0.08	0.68 ± 0.17	<0.001
0.45	91	1.14 ± 0.08	0.74 ± 0.16	<0.001
0.3	87	1.14 ± 0.07	0.40 ± 0.17	<0.001
Placebo	85	1.13 ± 0.08	-1.50 ± 0.17	
Femoral Neck BMD				
0.625	84	0.91 ± 0.14	1.82 ± 0.45	<0.001
0.45	91	0.89 ± 0.13	1.84 ± 0.44	<0.001
0.3	87	0.86 ± 0.11	0.62 ± 0.45	<0.001
Placebo	85	0.88 ± 0.14	-1.72 ± 0.45	
Femoral Trochanter BMD				
0.625	84	0.78 ± 0.13	3.82 ± 0.58	<0.001
0.45	91	0.76 ± 0.12	3.16 ± 0.56	0.003
0.3	87	0.75 ± 0.10	3.05 ± 0.57	0.005
Placebo	85	0.75 ± 0.12	0.81 ± 0.58	

a: Identified by dosage (mg) of Premarin or placebo.

TABLE 4. RELATIVE AND ABSOLUTE RISK SEEN IN THE ESTROGEN ALONE SUBSTUDY OF WHI[a]

Event[c]	Relative Risk* Premarin vs Placebo at 6.8 Years (95% CI)	Placebo n = 5429	Premarin n = 5310
		Absolute Risk per 10,000 Women-years	
CHD events	0.91 (0.75-1.12)	54	49
Non-fatal MI	*0.89 (0.70-1.12)*	*41*	*37*
CHD death	*0.94 (0.65-1.36)*	*16*	*15*
Invasive breast cancer	0.77 (0.59-1.01)	33	26
Stroke	1.39 (1.10-1.77)	32	44
Pulmonary embolism	1.34 (0.87-2.06)	10	13
Colorectal cancer	1.08 (0.75-1.55)	16	17
Hip fracture	0.61 (0.41-0.91)	17	11
Death due to other causes than the events above	1.08 (0.88-1.32)	50	53
Global Index[b]	1.01 (0.91-1.12)	190	192
Deep vein thrombosis[c]	1.47 (1.04-2.08)	15	21
Vertebral fractures[c]	0.62 (0.42-0.93)	17	11
Total fractures[c]	0.70 (0.63-0.79)	195	139

a: adapted from JAMA, 2004; 291:1701-1712
b: a subset of the events was combined in a "global index," defined as the earliest occurrence of CHD events, invasive breast cancer, stroke, pulmonary embolism, endometrial cancer, colorectal cancer, hip fracture, or death due to other causes
c: not included in Global Index
* nominal confidence intervals unadjusted for multiple looks and multiple comparisons.

Premarin—Cont.

Risk factors for arterial vascular disease (e.g., hypertension, diabetes mellitus, tobacco use, hypercholesterolemia, and obesity) and/or venous thromboembolism (e.g., personal history or family history of VTE, obesity, and systemic lupus erythematosus) should be managed appropriately.

a. ***Coronary heart disease and stroke.*** In the estrogen alone substudy of the Women's Health Initiative (WHI) study, an increased risk of stroke was observed in women receiving Premarin (0.625 mg conjugated estrogens) per day compared to women receiving placebo (44 vs 32 per 10,000 women-years). The increase in risk was observed in year one and persisted. (See **CLINICAL PHARMACOLOGY, Clinical Studies.**)

In the estrogen plus progestin substudy of WHI, an increased risk of coronary heart disease (CHD) events (defined as nonfatal myocardial infarction and CHD death) was observed in women receiving PREMPRO (0.625 mg conjugated estrogens plus 2.5 mg medroxyprogesterone acetate) per day compared to women receiving placebo (37 vs 30 per 10,000 women-years). The increase in risk was observed in year one and persisted.

In the same estrogen plus progestin substudy of WHI, an increased risk of stroke was observed in women receiving PREMPRO compared to women receiving placebo (29 vs 21 per 10,000 women-years). The increase in risk was observed after the first year and persisted.

In postmenopausal women with documented heart disease (n = 2,763, average age 66.7 years) a controlled clinical trial of secondary prevention of cardiovascular disease (Heart and Estrogen/progestin Replacement Study; HERS) treatment with PREMPRO (0.625 mg conjugated estrogen plus 2.5 mg medroxyprogesterone acetate per day) demonstrated no cardiovascular benefit. During an average follow-up of 4.1 years, treatment with PREMPRO did not reduce the overall rate of CHD events in postmenopausal women with established coronary heart disease. There were more CHD events in the PREMPRO-treated group than in the placebo group in year 1, but not during the subsequent years. Two thousand three hundred and twenty one women from the original HERS trial agreed to participate in an open label extension of HERS, HERS II. Average follow-up in HERS II was an additional 2.7 years, for a total of 6.8 years overall. Rates of CHD events were comparable among women in the PREMPRO group and the placebo group in HERS, HERS II, and overall.

Large doses of estrogen (5 mg conjugated estrogens per day), comparable to those used to treat cancer of the prostate and breast, have been shown in a large prospective clinical trial in men to increase the risk of nonfatal myocardial infarction, pulmonary embolism, and thrombophlebitis.

b. ***Venous thromboembolism (VTE).*** In the estrogen alone substudy of the Women's Health Initiative (WHI) study, an increased risk of deep vein thrombosis was observed in women receiving Premarin compared to placebo (21 vs 15 per 10,000 women-years). The increase in VTE risk was observed during the first year. (See **CLINICAL PHARMACOLOGY, Clinical Studies.**)

In the estrogen plus progestin substudy of WHI, a 2-fold greater rate of VTE, including deep venous thrombosis and pulmonary embolism, was observed in women receiving PREMPRO compared to women receiving placebo. The rate of VTE was 34 per 10,000 women-years in the PREMPRO group compared to 16 per 10,000 women-years in the placebo group. The increase in VTE risk was observed during the first year and persisted.

If feasible, estrogens should be discontinued at least 4 to 6 weeks before surgery of the type associated with an increased risk of thromboembolism, or during periods of prolonged immobilization.

2. **Malignant neoplasms.**

a. ***Endometrial cancer.*** The use of unopposed estrogens in women with intact uteri has been associated with an increased risk of endometrial cancer. The reported endometrial cancer risk among unopposed estrogen users with an intact uterus is about 2- to 12-fold greater than in non-users, and appears dependent on duration of treatment and on estrogen dose. Most studies show no significant increased risk associated with the use of estrogens for less than one year. The greatest risk appears associated with prolonged use, with increased risks of 15- to 24-fold for five to ten years or more, and this risk has been shown to persist for at least 8 to 15 years after estrogen therapy is discontinued.

Clinical surveillance of all women taking estrogen/progestin combinations is important. Adequate diagnostic measures, including endometrial sampling when indicated, should be undertaken to rule out malignancy in all cases of undiagnosed persistent or recurring abnormal vaginal bleeding. There is no evidence that the use of natural estrogens results in a different endometrial risk profile than synthetic estrogens of equivalent estrogen dose. Adding a progestin to postmenopausal estrogen therapy has been shown to reduce the risk of endometrial hyperplasia, which may be a precursor to endometrial cancer.

b. ***Breast cancer.*** In some studies, the use of estrogens and progestins by postmenopausal women has been reported to increase the risk of breast cancer. The most important randomized clinical trial providing information about this issue is the Women's Health Initiative (WHI) trial of estrogen plus progestin (see **CLINICAL PHARMACOLOGY, Clinical Studies**). The results from observational studies are generally consistent with those of the WHI clinical trial.

TABLE 5. RELATIVE AND ABSOLUTE RISK SEEN IN THE ESTROGEN PLUS PROGESTIN SUBSTUDY OF WHI[a]

Event[c]	Relative Risk Prempro vs Placebo at 5.2 Years (95% CI*)	Placebo n = 8102	Prempro n = 8506
		Absolute Risk per 10,000 Women-years	
CHD events	1.29 (1.02-1.63)	30	37
Non-fatal MI	*1.32 (1.02-1.72)*	*23*	*30*
CHD death	*1.18 (0.70-1.97)*	*6*	*7*
Invasive breast cancer[b]	1.26 (1.00-1.59)	30	38
Stroke	1.41 (1.07-1.85)	21	29
Pulmonary embolism	2.13 (1.39-3.25)	8	16
Colorectal cancer	0.63 (0.43-0.92)	16	10
Endometrial cancer	0.83 (0.47-1.47)	6	5
Hip fracture	0.66 (0.45-0.98)	15	10
Death due to causes other than the events above	0.92 (0.74-1.14)	40	37
Global Index[c]	1.15 (1.03-1.28)	151	170
Deep vein thrombosis[d]	2.07 (1.49-2.87)	13	26
Vertebral fractures[d]	0.66 (0.44-0.98)	15	9
Other osteoporotic fractures[d]	0.77 (0.69-0.86)	170	131

a: adapted from JAMA, 2002; 288:321-333
b: includes metastatic and non-metastatic breast cancer with the exception of in situ breast cancer
c: a subset of the events was combined in a "global index," defined as the earliest occurrence of CHD events, invasive breast cancer, stroke, pulmonary embolism, endometrial cancer, colorectal cancer, hip fracture, or death due to other causes
d: not included in Global Index
* nominal confidence intervals unadjusted for multiple looks and multiple comparisons.

After a mean follow-up of 5.6 years, the WHI trial reported an increased risk of breast cancer in women who took estrogen plus progestin. Observational studies have also reported an increased risk for estrogen/progestin combination therapy, and a smaller increased risk for estrogen alone therapy, after several years of use. For both findings, the excess risk increased with duration of use, and appeared to return to baseline over about five years after stopping treatment (only the observational studies have substantial data on risk after stopping). In these studies, the risk of breast cancer was greater, and became apparent earlier, with estrogen/progestin combination therapy as compared to estrogen alone therapy. However, these studies have not found significant variation in the risk of breast cancer among different estrogens or among different estrogen/progestin combinations, doses, or routes of administration.

In the WHI trial of estrogen plus progestin, 26% of the women reported prior use of estrogen alone and/or estrogen/progestin combination hormone therapy. After a mean follow-up of 5.6 years during the clinical trial, the overall relative risk of invasive breast cancer was 1.24 (95% confidence interval 1.01-1.54), and the overall absolute risk was 41 vs. 33 cases per 10,000 women-years, for estrogen plus progestin compared with placebo. Among women who reported prior use of hormone therapy, the relative risk of invasive breast cancer was 1.86, and the absolute risk was 46 vs. 25 cases per 10,000 women-years, for estrogen plus progestin compared with placebo. Among women who reported no prior use of hormone therapy, the relative risk of invasive breast cancer was 1.09, and the absolute risk was 40 vs. 36 cases per 10,000 women-years for estrogen plus progestin compared with placebo. In the WHI trial, invasive breast cancers were larger and diagnosed at a more advanced stage in the estrogen plus progestin group compared with the placebo group. Metastatic disease was rare with no apparent difference between the two groups. Other prognostic factors such as histologic subtype, grade and hormone receptor status did not differ between the groups.

The observational Million Women Study in Europe reported an increased risk of mortality due to breast cancer among current users of estrogens alone or estrogens plus progestins compared to never users, while the estrogen plus progestin sub-study of WHI showed no effect on breast cancer mortality with a mean follow-up of 5.6 years.

The use of estrogen plus progestin has been reported to result in an increase in abnormal mammograms requiring further evaluation. All women should receive yearly breast examinations by a healthcare provider and perform monthly breast self-examinations. In addition, mammography examinations should be scheduled based on patient age, risk factors, and prior mammogram results.

3. **Dementia.** In the estrogen alone Women's Health Initiative Memory Study (WHIMS), a substudy of WHI, a population of 2,947 hysterectomized women aged 65 to 79 years was randomized to Premarin (0.625 mg) or placebo. In the estrogen plus progestin WHIMS substudy, a population of 4,532 postmenopausal women aged 65 to 79 years was randomized to PREMPRO (0.625 mg/2.5 mg) or placebo.

In the estrogen alone substudy, after an average follow-up of 5.2 years, 28 women in the estrogen alone group and 19 women in the placebo group were diagnosed with probable dementia. The relative risk of probable dementia for Premarin alone versus placebo was 1.49 (95% CI 0.83-2.66). The absolute risk of probable dementia for Premarin alone versus placebo was 37 versus 25 cases per 10,000 women-years.

In the estrogen plus progestin substudy, after an average follow-up of 4 years, 40 women in the estrogen plus progestin group and 21 women in the placebo group were diagnosed with probable dementia. The relative risk of probable dementia for estrogen plus progestin versus placebo was 2.05 (95% CI 1.21-3.48). The absolute risk of probable dementia for PREMPRO versus placebo was 45 versus 22 cases per 10,000 women-years.

Since both substudies were conducted in women aged 65 to 79 years, it is unknown whether these findings apply to younger postmenopausal women. (See **BOXED WARNINGS** and **PRECAUTIONS, Geriatric Use.**)

4. **Gallbladder Disease.** A 2- to 4-fold increase in the risk of gallbladder disease requiring surgery in postmenopausal women receiving estrogens has been reported.

5. **Hypercalcemia.** Estrogen administration may lead to severe hypercalcemia in patients with breast cancer and bone metastases. If hypercalcemia occurs, use of the drug should be stopped and appropriate measures taken to reduce the serum calcium level.

6. **Visual abnormalities.** Retinal vascular thrombosis has been reported in patients receiving estrogens. Discontinue medication pending examination if there is sudden partial or complete loss of vision, or a sudden onset of proptosis, diplopia, or migraine. If examination reveals papilledema or retinal vascular lesions, estrogens should be discontinued.

PRECAUTIONS

A. General

1. ***Addition of a progestin when a woman has not had a hysterectomy.***

Studies of the addition of a progestin for 10 or more days of a cycle of estrogen administration, or daily with estrogen in a continuous regimen, have reported a lowered incidence of endometrial hyperplasia than would be induced by estrogen treatment alone. Endometrial hyperplasia may be a precursor to endometrial cancer.

There are, however, possible risks that may be associated with the use of progestins with estrogens compared to estrogen-alone regimens. These include: a possible increased risk of breast cancer, adverse effects on lipoprotein metabolism (e.g., lowering HDL, raising LDL) and impairment of glucose tolerance.

2. ***Elevated blood pressure.***

In a small number of case reports, substantial increases in blood pressure have been attributed to idiosyncratic reactions to estrogens. In a large, randomized, placebo-controlled clinical trial, a generalized effect of estrogen therapy on blood pressure was not seen. Blood pressure should be monitored at regular intervals during estrogen use.

3. ***Hypertriglyceridemia.***
In patients with pre-existing hypertriglyceridemia, estrogen therapy may be associated with elevations of plasma triglycerides leading to pancreatitis and other complications. In the HOPE study, the mean percent increase from baseline in serum triglycerides after one year of treatment with Premarin 0.625 mg, 0.45 mg, and 0.3 mg compared with placebo were 34.3, 30.2, 25.1, and 10.7, respectively. After two years of treatment, the mean percent changes were 47.6, 32.5, 19.0, and 5.5, respectively.
4. ***Impaired liver function and past history of cholestatic jaundice.***
Estrogens may be poorly metabolized in patients with impaired liver function. For patients with a history of cholestatic jaundice associated with past estrogen use or with pregnancy, caution should be exercised and in the case of recurrence, medication should be discontinued.
5. ***Hypothyroidism.***
Estrogen administration leads to increased thyroid-binding globulin (TBG) levels. Patients with normal thyroid function can compensate for the increased TBG by making more thyroid hormone, thus maintaining free T_4 and T_3 serum concentrations in the normal range. Patients dependent on thyroid hormone replacement therapy who are also receiving estrogens may require increased doses of their thyroid replacement therapy. These patients should have their thyroid function monitored in order to maintain their free thyroid hormone levels in an acceptable range.
6. ***Fluid retention.***
Because estrogens may cause some degree of fluid retention, patients with conditions that might be influenced by this factor, such as cardiac or renal dysfunction, warrant careful observation when estrogens are prescribed.
7. ***Hypocalcemia.***
Estrogens should be used with caution in individuals with severe hypocalcemia.
8. ***Ovarian cancer.***
The estrogen plus progestin substudy of WHI reported that after an average follow-up of 5.6 years, the relative risk for ovarian cancer for estrogen plus progestin versus placebo was 1.58 (95% confidence interval 0.77 – 3.24) but was not statistically significant. The absolute risk of estrogen plus progestin versus placebo was 4.2 versus 2.7 cases per 10,000 women-years. In some epidemiologic studies, the use of estrogen-only products, in particular for ten or more years, has been associated with an increased risk of ovarian cancer. Other epidemiologic studies have not found these associations.
9. ***Exacerbation of endometriosis.***
Endometriosis may be exacerbated with administration of estrogen therapy.
A few cases of malignant transformation of residual endometrial implants have been reported in women treated post-hysterectomy with estrogen alone therapy. For patients known to have residual endometriosis post-hysterectomy, the addition of progestin should be considered.
10. ***Exacerbation of other conditions.***
Estrogen therapy may cause an exacerbation of asthma, diabetes mellitus, epilepsy, migraine, porphyria, systemic lupus erythematosus, and hepatic hemangiomas and should be used with caution in patients with these conditions.

B. Patient Information
Physicians are advised to discuss the contents of the PATIENT INFORMATION leaflet with patients for whom they prescribe Premarin.

C. Laboratory Tests
Estrogen administration should be initiated at the lowest dose for the treatment of postmenopausal moderate to severe vasomotor symptoms and moderate to severe symptoms of postmenopausal vulvar and vaginal atrophy and then guided by clinical response rather than by serum hormone levels (e.g., estradiol, FSH). Laboratory parameters may be useful in guiding dosage for the treatment of hypoestrogenism due to hypogonadism, castration and primary ovarian failure.

D. Drug/Laboratory Test Interactions
1. Accelerated prothrombin time, partial thromboplastin time, and platelet aggregation time; increased platelet count; increased factors II, VII antigen, VIII antigen, VIII coagulant activity, IX, X, XII, VII-X complex, II-VII-X complex, and beta-thromboglobulin; decreased levels of anti-factor Xa and antithrombin III, decreased antithrombin III activity; increased levels of fibrinogen and fibrinogen activity; increased plasminogen antigen and activity.
2. Increased thyroid binding globulin (TBG) levels leading to increased circulating total thyroid hormone levels as measured by protein-bound iodine (PBI), T_4 levels (by column or by radioimmunoassay) or T_3 levels by radioimmunoassay. T_3 resin uptake is decreased, reflecting the elevated TBG. Free T_4 and free T_3 concentrations are unaltered. Patients on thyroid replacement therapy may require higher doses of thyroid hormone.
3. Other binding proteins may be elevated in serum, i.e., corticosteroid binding globulin (CBG), sex hormone binding globulin (SHBG), leading to increased total circulating corticosteroids and sex steroids, respectively. Free hormone concentrations may be decreased. Other plasma proteins may be increased (angiotensinogen/renin substrate, alpha-1-antitrypsin, ceruloplasmin).

TABLE 6. NUMBER (%) OF PATIENTS REPORTING ≥ 5% TREATMENT EMERGENT ADVERSE EVENTS

Body System Adverse event	--Conjugated Estrogens Treatment Group-- 0.625 mg (n = 348)	0.45 mg (n = 338)	0.3 mg (n = 326)	Placebo (n = 332)
Any adverse event	323 (93%)	305 (90%)	292 (90%)	281 (85%)
Body as a Whole				
Abdominal pain	56 (16%)	50 (15%)	54 (17%)	37 (11%)
Accidental injury	21 (6%)	41 (12%)	20 (6%)	29 (9%)
Asthenia	25 (7%)	23 (7%)	25 (8%)	16 (5%)
Back pain	49 (14%)	43 (13%)	43 (13%)	39 (12%)
Flu syndrome	37 (11%)	38 (11%)	33 (10%)	35 (11%)
Headache	90 (26%)	109 (32%)	96 (29%)	93 (28%)
Infection	61 (18%)	75 (22%)	74 (23%)	74 (22%)
Pain	58 (17%)	61 (18%)	66 (20%)	61 (18%)
Digestive System				
Diarrhea	21 (6%)	25 (7%)	19 (6%)	21 (6%)
Dyspepsia	33 (9%)	32 (9%)	36 (11%)	46 (14%)
Flatulence	24 (7%)	23 (7%)	18 (6%)	9 (3%)
Nausea	32 (9%)	21 (6%)	21 (6%)	30 (9%)
Musculoskeletal System				
Arthralgia	47 (14%)	42 (12%)	22 (7%)	39 (12%)
Leg cramps	19 (5%)	23 (7%)	11 (3%)	7 (2%)
Myalgia	18 (5%)	18 (5%)	29 (9%)	25 (8%)
Nervous System				
Depression	25 (7%)	27 (8%)	17 (5%)	22 (7%)
Dizziness	19 (5%)	20 (6%)	12 (4%)	17 (5%)
Insomnia	21 (6%)	25 (7%)	24 (7%)	33 (10%)
Nervousness	12 (3%)	17 (5%)	6 (2%)	7 (2%)
Respiratory System				
Cough increased	13 (4%)	22 (7%)	14 (4%)	14 (4%)
Pharyngitis	35 (10%)	35 (10%)	40 (12%)	38 (11%)
Rhinitis	21 (6%)	30 (9%)	31 (10%)	42 (13%)
Sinusitis	22 (6%)	36 (11%)	24 (7%)	24 (7%)
Upper respiratory infection	42 (12%)	34 (10%)	28 (9%)	35 (11%)
Skin and Appendages				
Pruritus	14 (4%)	17 (5%)	16 (5%)	7 (2%)
Urogenital System				
Breast pain	38 (11%)	41 (12%)	24 (7%)	29 (9%)
Leukorrhea	18 (5%)	22 (7%)	13 (4%)	9 (3%)
Vaginal hemorrhage	47 (14%)	14 (4%)	7 (2%)	0
Vaginal moniliasis	20 (6%)	18 (5%)	17 (5%)	6 (2%)
Vaginitis	24 (7%)	20 (6%)	16 (5%)	4 (1%)

4. Increased plasma HDL and HDL_2 cholesterol subfraction concentrations, reduced LDL cholesterol concentrations, increased triglyceride levels.
5. Impaired glucose tolerance.
6. Reduced response to metyrapone test.

E. Carcinogenesis, Mutagenesis, Impairment of Fertility
(See **BOXED WARNINGS, WARNINGS,** and **PRECAUTIONS**.)
Long term continuous administration of natural and synthetic estrogens in certain animal species increases the frequency of carcinomas of the breast, uterus, cervix, vagina, testis, and liver.

F. Pregnancy
Premarin should not be used during pregnancy. (See **CONTRAINDICATIONS**).

G. Nursing Mothers
Estrogen administration to nursing mothers has been shown to decrease the quantity and quality of the milk. Detectable amounts of estrogens have been identified in the milk of mothers receiving this drug. Caution should be exercised when Premarin is administered to a nursing woman.

H. Pediatric Use
Estrogen therapy has been used for the induction of puberty in adolescents with some forms of pubertal delay. Safety and effectiveness in pediatric patients have not otherwise been established.
Large and repeated doses of estrogen over an extended time period have been shown to accelerate epiphyseal closure, which could result in short stature if treatment is initiated before the completion of physiologic puberty in normally developing children. If estrogen is administered to patients whose bone growth is not complete, periodic monitoring of bone maturation and effects on epiphyseal centers is recommended during estrogen administration.
Estrogen treatment of prepubertal girls also induces premature breast development and vaginal cornification, and may induce vaginal bleeding. In boys, estrogen treatment may modify the normal pubertal process and induce gynecomastia. See **INDICATIONS** and **DOSAGE AND ADMINISTRATION** sections.

I. Geriatric Use
Of the total number of subjects in the estrogen alone substudy of the Women's Health Initiative (WHI) study, 46% (n=4,943) were 65 years and over, while 7.1% (n=767) were 75 years and over. There was a higher relative risk (Premarin vs. placebo) of stroke in women less than 75 years of age compared to women 75 years and over.
In the estrogen alone substudy of the Women's Health Initiative Memory Study (WHIMS), a substudy of WHI, a population of 2,947 hysterectomized women, aged 65 to 79 years, was randomized to Premarin (0.625 mg) or placebo. In the estrogen alone group, after an average follow-up of 5.2 years, the relative risk (Premarin versus placebo) of probable dementia was 1.49 (95% CI 0.83-2.66).
Of the total number of subjects in the estrogen plus progestin substudy of the Women's Health Initiative study, 44% (n=7,320) were 65 years and over, while 6.6% (n=1,095) were 75 years and over. There was a higher relative risk (PREMPRO vs placebo) of stroke and invasive breast cancer in women 75 and over compared to women less than 75 years of age.
In the estrogen plus progestin substudy of WHIMS, a population of 4,532 postmenopausal women, aged 65 to 79 years, was randomized to PREMPRO (0.625 mg/2.5 mg) or placebo. In the estrogen plus progestin group, after an average follow-up of 4 years, the relative risk (PREMPRO versus placebo) of probable dementia was 2.05 (95% CI 1.21-3.48).
Pooling the events in women receiving Premarin or PREMPRO in comparison to those in women on placebo, the overall relative risk for probable dementia was 1.76 (95% CI 1.19-2.60). Since both substudies were conducted in women aged 65 to 79 years, it is unknown whether these findings apply to younger postmenopausal women. (See **BOXED WARNINGS** and **WARNINGS, Dementia.**)
With respect to efficacy in the approved indications, there have not been sufficient numbers of geriatric patients involved in studies utilizing Premarin to determine whether those over 65 years of age differ from younger subjects in their response to Premarin.

ADVERSE REACTIONS

See **BOXED WARNINGS, WARNINGS,** and **PRECAUTIONS**.
Because clinical trials are conducted under widely varying conditions, adverse reaction rates observed in the clinical trials of a drug cannot be directly compared to rates in the clinical trials of another drug and may not reflect the rates observed in practice. The adverse reaction information from clinical trials does, however, provide a basis for identifying the adverse events that appear to be related to drug use and for approximating rates.
During the first year of a 2-year clinical trial with 2333 postmenopausal women between 40 and 65 years of age (88% Caucasian), 1012 women were treated with conjugated estrogens and 332 were treated with placebo. Table 6 summarizes adverse events that occurred at a rate of ≥ 5%.
[See table 6 above]
The following additional adverse reactions have been reported with estrogen and/or progestin therapy:
1. *Genitourinary system*
Changes in vaginal bleeding pattern and abnormal withdrawal bleeding or flow; breakthrough bleeding, spotting, dysmenorrhea
Increase in size of uterine leiomyomata
Vaginitis, including vaginal candidiasis
Change in amount of cervical secretion
Change in cervical ectropion
Ovarian cancer
Endometrial hyperplasia
Endometrial cancer
2. *Breasts*
Tenderness, enlargement, pain, discharge, galactorrhea
Fibrocystic breast changes
Breast cancer

Continued on next page

Premarin—Cont.

3. *Cardiovascular*
Deep and superficial venous thrombosis
Pulmonary embolism
Thrombophlebitis
Myocardial infarction
Stroke
Increase in blood pressure
4. *Gastrointestinal*
Nausea, vomiting
Abdominal cramps, bloating
Cholestatic jaundice
Increased incidence of gallbladder disease
Pancreatitis
Enlargement of hepatic hemangiomas
5. *Skin*
Chloasma or melasma that may persist when drug is discontinued
Erythema multiforme
Erythema nodosum
Hemorrhagic eruption
Loss of scalp hair
Hirsutism
Pruritus, rash
6. *Eyes*
Retinal vascular thrombosis
Intolerance to contact lenses
7. *Central Nervous System*
Headache
Migraine
Dizziness
Mental depression
Chorea
Nervousness
Mood disturbances
Irritability
Exacerbation of epilepsy
Dementia
8. *Miscellaneous*
Increase or decrease in weight
Reduced carbohydrate tolerance
Aggravation of porphyria
Edema
Arthralgias
Leg cramps
Changes in libido
Urticaria, angioedema, anaphylactoid/anaphylactic reactions
Hypocalcemia
Exacerbation of asthma
Increased triglycerides

OVERDOSAGE

Serious ill effects have not been reported following acute ingestion of large doses of estrogen-containing drug products by young children. Overdosage of estrogen may cause nausea and vomiting, and withdrawal bleeding may occur in females.

DOSAGE AND ADMINISTRATION

When estrogen is prescribed for a postmenopausal woman with a uterus, progestin should also be initiated to reduce the risk of endometrial cancer. A woman without a uterus does not need progestin. Use of estrogen, alone or in combination with a progestin, should be with the lowest effective dose and for the shortest duration consistent with treatment goals and risks for the individual woman. Patients should be re-evaluated periodically as clinically appropriate (e.g., at 3-month to 6-month intervals) to determine if treatment is still necessary (see **BOXED WARNINGS** and **WARNINGS**). For women with a uterus, adequate diagnostic measures, such as endometrial sampling, when indicated, should be undertaken to rule out malignancy in cases of undiagnosed persistent or recurring abnormal vaginal bleeding.

1. For treatment of moderate to severe vasomotor symptoms and/or moderate to severe symptoms of vulvar and vaginal atrophy associated with the menopause. When prescribing solely for the treatment of moderate to severe symptoms of vulvar and vaginal atrophy, topical vaginal products should be considered.
   Patients should be treated with the lowest effective dose. Generally women should be started at 0.3 mg Premarin daily. Subsequent dosage adjustment may be made based upon the individual patient response. This dose should be periodically reassessed by the healthcare provider.
   Premarin therapy may be given continuously with no interruption in therapy, or in cyclical regimens (regimens such as 25 days on drug followed by five days off drug) as is medically appropriate on an individualized basis.
2. For prevention of postmenopausal osteoporosis:
   When prescribing solely for the prevention of postmenopausal osteoporosis, therapy should be considered only for women at significant risk of osteoporosis and for whom non-estrogen medications are not considered to be appropriate. Patients should be treated with the lowest effective dose. Generally women should be started at 0.3 mg Premarin daily. Subsequent dosage adjustment may be made based upon the individual clinical and bone mineral density responses. This dose should be periodically reassessed by the healthcare provider.
   Premarin therapy may be given continuously with no interruption in therapy, or in cyclical regimens (regimens such as 25 days on drug followed by five days off drug) as is medically appropriate on an individualized basis.
3. For treatment of female hypoestrogenism due to hypogonadism, castration, or primary ovarian failure:
   Female hypogonadism—0.3 mg or 0.625 mg daily, administered cyclically (e.g., three weeks on and one week off). Doses are adjusted depending on the severity of symptoms and responsiveness of the endometrium.
   In clinical studies of delayed puberty due to female hypogonadism, breast development was induced by doses as low as 0.15 mg. The dosage may be gradually titrated upward at 6 to 12 month intervals as needed to achieve appropriate bone age advancement and eventual epiphyseal closure. Clinical studies suggest that doses of 0.15 mg, 0.3 mg, and 0.6 mg are associated with mean ratios of bone age advancement to chronological age progression (ΔBA/ΔCA) of 1.1, 1.5, and 2.1, respectively. (Premarin in the dose strength of 0.15 mg is not available commercially). Available data suggest that chronic dosing with 0.625 mg is sufficient to induce artificial cyclic menses with sequential progestin treatment and to maintain bone mineral density after skeletal maturity is achieved.
   Female castration or primary ovarian failure—1.25 mg daily, cyclically. Adjust dosage, upward or downward, according to severity of symptoms and response of the patient. For maintenance, adjust dosage to lowest level that will provide effective control.
4. For treatment of breast cancer, for palliation only, in appropriately selected women and men with metastatic disease:
   Suggested dosage is 10 mg three times daily for a period of at least three months.
5. For treatment of advanced androgen-dependent carcinoma of the prostate, for palliation only:
   1.25 mg to 2 × 1.25 mg three times daily. The effectiveness of therapy can be judged by phosphatase determinations as well as by symptomatic improvement of the patient.

HOW SUPPLIED

Premarin (conjugated estrogens tablets, USP)
— Each oval yellow tablet contains 1.25 mg, in bottles of 100 (NDC 0046-1104-81); and 1,000 (NDC 0046-1104-91).
— Each oval white tablet contains 0.9 mg, in bottles of 100 (NDC 0046-0864-81).
— Each oval maroon tablet contains 0.625 mg, in bottles of 100 (NDC 0046-0867-81); 1,000 (NDC 0046-0867-91); and Unit-Dose Packages of 100 (NDC 0046-0867-99).
— Each oval blue tablet contains 0.45 mg, in bottles of 100 (NDC 0046-0936-81).
— Each oval green tablet contains 0.3 mg, in bottles of 100 (NDC 0046-0868-81) and 1,000 (NDC 0046-0868-91).

The appearance of these tablets is a trademark of Wyeth Pharmaceuticals.

Store at 20-25° C (68-77° F); excursions permitted to 15-30° C (59-86° F) [see USP Controlled Room Temperature].

Dispense in a well-closed container as defined in the USP.

PATIENT INFORMATION

(Updated April 2005)
Premarin®
(conjugated estrogens tablets, USP)

Read this PATIENT INFORMATION before you start taking Premarin and read what you get each time you refill Premarin. There may be new information. This information does not take the place of talking to your healthcare provider about your medical condition or your treatment.

What is the most important information I should know about Premarin (an estrogen mixture)?

- Estrogens increase the chances of getting cancer of the uterus.
  Report any unusual vaginal bleeding right away while you are taking Premarin. Vaginal bleeding after menopause may be a warning sign of cancer of the uterus (womb). Your healthcare provider should check any unusual vaginal bleeding to find out the cause.
- Do not use estrogens with or without progestins to prevent heart disease, heart attacks, strokes, or dementia.
  Using estrogens with or without progestins may increase your chances of getting heart attacks, strokes, breast cancer, and blood clots. Using estrogens, with or without progestins, may increase your risk of dementia, based on a study of women age 65 years or older. You and your healthcare provider should talk regularly about whether you still need treatment with Premarin.

What is Premarin?

Premarin is a medicine that contains a mixture of estrogen hormones.

Premarin is used after menopause to:

- **reduce moderate to severe hot flashes.** Estrogens are hormones made by a woman's ovaries. The ovaries normally stop making estrogens when a woman is between 45 and 55 years old. This drop in body estrogen levels causes the "change of life" or menopause (the end of monthly menstrual periods). Sometimes both ovaries are removed during an operation before natural menopause takes place. The sudden drop in estrogen levels causes "surgical menopause."
  When the estrogen levels begin dropping, some women get very uncomfortable symptoms, such as feelings of warmth in the face, neck, and chest, or sudden strong feelings of heat and sweating ("hot flashes" or "hot flushes"). In some women the symptoms are mild, and they will not need to take estrogens. In other women, symptoms can be more severe. You and your healthcare provider should talk regularly about whether you still need treatment with Premarin.
- **treat moderate to severe dryness, itching, and burning, in and around the vagina.** You and your healthcare provider should talk regularly about whether you still need treatment with Premarin to control these problems. If you use Premarin only to treat your dryness, itching, and burning in and around your vagina, talk with your healthcare provider about whether a topical vaginal product would be better for you.
- **help reduce your chances of getting osteoporosis (thin weak bones).** Osteoporosis from menopause is a thinning of the bones that makes them weaker and easier to break. If you use Premarin only to prevent osteoporosis from menopause, talk with your healthcare provider about whether a different treatment or medicine without estrogens might be better for you. You and your healthcare provider should talk regularly about whether you should continue with Premarin.
  Weight-bearing exercise, like walking or running, and taking calcium and vitamin D supplements may also lower your chances for getting postmenopausal osteoporosis. It is important to talk about exercise and supplements with your healthcare provider before starting them.

Premarin is also used to:

- **treat certain conditions in women before menopause if their ovaries do not make enough estrogen naturally.**
- **ease symptoms of certain cancers that have spread through the body, in men and women.**

Who should not take Premarin?

Do not start taking Premarin if you:

- **have unusual vaginal bleeding.**
- **currently have or have had certain cancers.** Estrogens may increase the chances of getting certain types of cancers, including cancer of the breast or uterus. If you have or have had cancer, talk with your healthcare provider about whether you should take Premarin.
- **had a stroke or heart attack in the past year.**
- **currently have or have had blood clots.**
- **currently have liver problems.**
- **are allergic to Premarin tablets or any of its ingredients.** See the end of this leaflet for a list of all the ingredients in Premarin.
- **think you may be pregnant.**

Tell your healthcare provider:

- **if you are breast feeding.** The hormones in Premarin can pass into your milk.
- **about all of your medical problems.** Your healthcare provider may need to check you more carefully if you have certain conditions, such as asthma (wheezing), epilepsy (seizures), migraine, endometriosis, lupus, problems with your heart, liver, thyroid, kidneys, or have high calcium levels in your blood.
- **about all the medicines you take,** including prescription and nonprescription medicines, vitamins, and herbal supplements. Some medicines may affect how Premarin works. Premarin may also affect how your other medicines work.
- **if you are going to have surgery or will be on bedrest.** You may need to stop taking estrogens.

How should I take Premarin?

- Take one Premarin tablet at the same time each day.
- If you miss a dose, take it as soon as possible. If it is almost time for your next dose, skip the missed dose and go back to your normal schedule. Do not take 2 doses at the same time.
- Estrogens should be used at the lowest dose possible for your treatment only as long as needed. You and your healthcare provider should talk regularly (for example, every 3 to 6 months) about the dose you are taking and whether you still need treatment with Premarin.

What are the possible side effects of Premarin?

Less common but serious side effects include:

- Breast cancer
- Cancer of the uterus
- Stroke
- Heart attack
- Blood clots
- Dementia
- Gallbladder disease
- Ovarian cancer

These are some of the warning signs of serious side effects:

- Breast lumps
- Unusual vaginal bleeding
- Dizziness and faintness
- Changes in speech
- Severe headaches
- Chest pain
- Shortness of breath
- Pains in your legs
- Changes in vision
- Vomiting

Call your healthcare provider right away if you get any of these warning signs, or any other unusual symptom that concerns you.

Common side effects include:

- Headache
- Breast pain

- Irregular vaginal bleeding or spotting
- Stomach/abdominal cramps, bloating
- Nausea and vomiting
- Hair loss

Other side effects include:
- High blood pressure
- Liver problems
- High blood sugar
- Fluid retention
- Enlargement of benign tumors of the uterus ("fibroids")
- Vaginal yeast infections

These are not all the possible side effects of Premarin. For more information, ask your healthcare provider or pharmacist.

What can I do to lower my chances of getting a serious side effect with Premarin?
- Talk with your healthcare provider regularly about whether you should continue taking Premarin.
- If you have a uterus, talk to your healthcare provider about whether the addition of a progestin is right for you. In general, the addition of a progestin is recommended for women with a uterus to reduce the chance of getting cancer of the uterus.
- See your healthcare provider right away if you get vaginal bleeding while taking Premarin.
- Have a breast exam and mammogram (breast X-ray) every year unless your healthcare provider tells you something else. If members of your family have had breast cancer or if you have ever had breast lumps or an abnormal mammogram, you may need to have breast exams more often.
- If you have high blood pressure, high cholesterol (fat in the blood), diabetes, are overweight, or if you use tobacco, you may have higher chances for getting heart disease. Ask your healthcare provider for ways to lower your chances for getting heart disease.

General information about the safe and effective use of Premarin

Medicines are sometimes prescribed for conditions that are not mentioned in patient information leaflets. Do not take Premarin for conditions for which it was not prescribed. Do not give Premarin to other people, even if they have the same symptoms you have. It may harm them.

Keep Premarin out of the reach of children.

This leaflet provides a summary of the most important information about Premarin. If you would like more information, talk with your healthcare provider or pharmacist. You can ask for information about Premarin that is written for health professionals. You can get more information by calling the toll free number 800-934-5556.

What are the ingredients in Premarin?

Premarin contains a mixture of conjugated estrogens, which are a mixture of sodium estrone sulfate and sodium equilin sulfate and other components including sodium sulfate conjugates, 17 α-dihydroequilin, 17 α-estradiol, and 17 β-dihydroequilin. Premarin 0.3 mg, 0.45 mg, 0.625 mg, and 0.9 mg tablets also contain the following inactive ingredients: calcium phosphate tribasic, calcium sulfate, carnauba wax, microcrystalline cellulose, powdered cellulose, glyceryl monooleate, lactose monohydrate, magnesium stearate, methylcellulose, pharmaceutical glaze, polyethylene glycol, stearic acid (not present in 0.45 mg tablet), sucrose, and titanium dioxide.

Premarin 1.25 mg tablets contain the following inactive ingredients: calcium phosphate tribasic, hydroxypropyl cellulose, microcrystalline cellulose, powdered cellulose, hypromellose, lactose monohydrate, magnesium stearate, polyethylene glycol, sucrose and titanium dioxide.

The tablets come in different strengths and each strength tablet is a different color. The color ingredients are:
— 0.3 mg tablet (green color): D&C Yellow No. 10, FD&C Blue No. 1, FD&C Blue No. 2, and FD&C Yellow No. 6.
— 0.45 mg tablet (blue color): FD&C Blue No. 2.
— 0.625 mg tablet (maroon color): FD&C Blue No. 2, D&C Red No. 27, and FD&C Red No. 40.
— 0.9 mg tablet (white color): D&C Red No. 6 and D&C Red No. 7.
— 1.25 mg tablet (yellow color): black iron oxide, D&C Yellow No. 10, and FD&C Yellow No. 6.

The appearance of these tablets is a trademark of Wyeth Pharmaceuticals.

This product's label may have been revised after this insert was used in production. For further product information and current package insert, please visit www.wyeth.com or call our medical communications department toll-free at 1-800-934-5556.

Wyeth®
Wyeth Pharmaceuticals Inc.
Philadelphia, PA 19101   W10405C012
                                     ET01
                            Rev 04/05

PREMARIN®   ℞
[prĕm'ă-rĭn]
(conjugated estrogens)
Vaginal Cream in a nonliquefying base
℞ only

Prescribing information for this product, which appears on pages 3371–3375 of the 2005 PDR, has been completely revised as follows. Please write "See Supplement A" next to the product heading.

NOTE: PATIENT INFORMATION LEAFLET ATTACHED.

> **ESTROGENS INCREASE THE RISK OF ENDOMETRIAL CANCER**
>
> Close clinical surveillance of all women taking estrogens is important. Adequate diagnostic measures, including endometrial sampling when indicated, should be undertaken to rule out malignancy in all cases of undiagnosed persistent or recurring abnormal vaginal bleeding. There is no evidence that the use of "natural" estrogens results in a different endometrial risk profile than synthetic estrogens of equivalent estrogen dose.
>
> **CARDIOVASCULAR AND OTHER RISKS**
>
> Estrogens with or without progestins should not be used for the prevention of cardiovascular disease or dementia.
>
> The Women's Health Initiative (WHI) study reported increased risks of stroke and deep vein thrombosis in postmenopausal women (50 to 79 years of age) during 6.8 years of treatment with conjugated estrogens (0.625 mg) relative to placebo.
>
> The WHI study reported increased risks of myocardial infarction, stroke, invasive breast cancer, pulmonary emboli, and deep vein thrombosis in postmenopausal women (50 to 79 years of age) during 5 years of treatment with oral conjugated estrogens (0.625 mg) combined with medroxyprogesterone acetate (2.5 mg) relative to placebo. (See **CLINICAL PHARMACOLOGY, Clinical Studies.**)
>
> The Women's Health Initiative Memory Study (WHIMS), a substudy of WHI, reported increased risk of developing probable dementia in postmenopausal women 65 years of age or older during 4 to 5.2 years of treatment with oral conjugated estrogens, with or without medroxyprogesterone acetate, relative to placebo. It is unknown whether this finding applies to younger postmenopausal women.
>
> Other doses of conjugated estrogens and medroxyprogesterone acetate, and other combinations and dosage forms of estrogens and progestins were not studied in the WHI clinical trials and, in the absence of comparable data, these risks should be assumed to be similar. Because of these risks, estrogens with or without progestins should be prescribed at the lowest effective doses and for the shortest duration consistent with treatment goals and risks for the individual woman.

DESCRIPTION

Each gram of Premarin® (conjugated estrogens) Vaginal Cream contains 0.625 mg conjugated estrogens, USP in a nonliquefying base containing cetyl esters wax, cetyl alcohol, white wax, glyceryl monostearate, propylene glycol monostearate, methyl stearate, benzyl alcohol, sodium lauryl sulfate, glycerin, and mineral oil. Premarin Vaginal Cream is applied intravaginally.

Premarin (conjugated estrogens) Vaginal Cream contains a mixture of conjugated estrogens obtained exclusively from natural sources, occurring as the sodium salts of water-soluble estrogen sulfates blended to represent the average composition of material derived from pregnant mares' urine. It is a mixture of sodium estrone sulfate and sodium equilin sulfate. It contains as concomitant components, as sodium sulfate conjugates, 17 α-dihydroequilin, 17 α-estradiol, and 17 β-dihydroequilin.

CLINICAL PHARMACOLOGY

Endogenous estrogens are largely responsible for the development and maintenance of the female reproductive system and secondary sexual characteristics. Although circulating estrogens exist in a dynamic equilibrium of metabolic interconversions, estradiol is the principal intracellular human estrogen and is substantially more potent than its metabolites, estrone and estriol, at the receptor level.

The primary source of estrogen in normally cycling adult women is the ovarian follicle, which secretes 70 to 500 mcg of estradiol daily, depending on the phase of the menstrual cycle. After menopause, most endogenous estrogen is produced by conversion of androstenedione, secreted by the adrenal cortex, to estrone by peripheral tissues. Thus, estrone and the sulfate-conjugated form, estrone sulfate, are the most abundant circulating estrogen in postmenopausal women.

Estrogens act through binding to nuclear receptors in estrogen-responsive tissues. To date, two estrogen receptors have been identified. These vary in proportion from tissue to tissue.

Circulating estrogens modulate the pituitary secretion of the gonadotropins, luteinizing hormone (LH) and follicle stimulating hormone (FSH) through a negative feedback mechanism. Estrogens act to reduce the elevated levels of these gonadotropins seen in postmenopausal women.

Pharmacokinetics

Absorption

Conjugated estrogens are soluble in water and are well absorbed through the skin, mucous membranes, and the gastrointestinal tract after release from the drug formulation.

Distribution

The distribution of exogenous estrogens is similar to that of endogenous estrogens. Estrogens are widely distributed in the body and are generally found in higher concentration in the sex hormone target organs. Estrogens circulate in the blood largely bound to sex hormone-binding globulin (SHBG) and albumin.

Metabolism

Exogenous estrogens are metabolized in the same manner as endogenous estrogens. Circulating estrogens exist in a dynamic equilibrium of metabolic interconversions. These transformations take place mainly in the liver. Estradiol is converted reversibly to estrone, and both can be converted to estriol, which is the major urinary metabolite. Estrogens also undergo enterohepatic recirculation via sulfate and glucuronide conjugation in the liver, biliary secretion of conjugates into the intestine, and hydrolysis in the gut followed by reabsorption. In postmenopausal women a significant proportion of the circulating estrogens exists as sulfate conjugates, especially estrone sulfate, which serves as a circulating reservoir for the formation of more active estrogens.

Excretion

Estradiol, estrone, and estriol are excreted in the urine along with glucuronide and sulfate conjugates.

Special Populations

No pharmacokinetic studies were conducted in special populations, including patients with renal or hepatic impairment.

Drug Interactions

Data from a single-dose drug-drug interaction study involving oral conjugated estrogens and medroxyprogesterone acetate indicate that the pharmacokinetic dispositions of both drugs are not altered when the drugs are coadministered. No other clinical drug-drug interaction studies have been conducted with conjugated estrogens.

In vitro and in vivo studies have shown that estrogens are metabolized partially by cytochrome P450 3A4 (CYP3A4). Therefore, inducers or inhibitors of CYP3A4 may affect estrogen drug metabolism. Inducers of CYP3A4 such as St. John's Wort preparations (Hypericum perforatum), phenobarbital, carbamazepine, and rifampin may reduce plasma concentrations of estrogens, possibly resulting in a decrease in therapeutic effects and/or changes in the uterine bleeding profile. Inhibitors of CYP3A4 such as erythromycin, clarithromycin, ketoconazole, itraconazole, ritonavir and grapefruit juice may increase plasma concentrations of estrogens and may result in side effects.

Clinical Studies

Women's Health Initiative Studies.

The Women's Health Initiative (WHI) enrolled a total of 27,000 predominantly healthy postmenopausal women to assess the risks and benefits of either the use of Premarin tablets (0.625 mg conjugated estrogens per day) alone or the use of PREMPRO™ tablets (0.625 mg conjugated estrogens plus 2.5 mg medroxyprogesterone acetate per day) compared to placebo in the prevention of certain chronic diseases. The primary endpoint was the incidence of coronary heart disease (CHD) (nonfatal myocardial infarction and CHD death), with invasive breast cancer as the primary adverse outcome studied. A "global index" included the earliest occurrence of CHD, invasive breast cancer, stroke, pulmonary embolism (PE), endometrial cancer, colorectal cancer, hip fracture, or death due to other cause. The study did not evaluate the effects of Premarin tablets or PREMPRO on menopausal symptoms.

The estrogen plus progestin substudy was stopped early because, according to the predefined stopping rule, the increased risk of breast cancer and cardiovascular events exceeded the specified benefits included in the "global index." Results of the estrogen plus progestin substudy, which included 16,608 women (average age of 63 years, range 50 to 79; 83.9% White, 6.5% Black, 5.5% Hispanic), after an average follow-up of 5.2 years are presented in Table 1 below.

[See table 1 at top of next page]

For those outcomes included in the "global index," the absolute excess risks per 10,000 women-years in the group treated with PREMPRO were 7 more CHD events, 8 more strokes, 8 more PEs, and 8 more invasive breast cancers, while the absolute risk reductions per 10,000 women-years were 6 fewer colorectal cancers and 5 fewer hip fractures. The absolute excess risk of events included in the "global index" was 19 per 10,000 women-years. There was no difference between the groups in terms of all-cause mortality. (See **BOXED WARNINGS, WARNINGS**, and **PRECAUTIONS**.)

Women's Health Initiative Memory Study.

The Women's Health Initiative Memory Study (WHIMS), a substudy of WHI, enrolled 4,532 predominantly healthy postmenopausal women 65 years of age and older (47% were age 65 to 69 years, 35% were 70 to 74 years, and 18% were 75 years of age and older) to evaluate the effects of PREMPRO (0.625 mg conjugated estrogens plus 2.5 mg medroxyprogesterone acetate) on the incidence of probable dementia (primary outcome) compared with placebo.

After an average follow-up of 4 years, 40 women in the estrogen/progestin group (45 per 10,000 women-years) and 21 in the placebo group (22 per 10,000 women-years) were diagnosed with probable dementia. The relative risk of probable dementia in the hormone therapy group was 2.05 (95% CI, 1.21 to 3.48) compared to placebo. Differences between groups became apparent in the first year of treatment. It is unknown whether these findings apply to younger postmenopausal women. (See **BOXED WARNING** and **WARNINGS, Dementia.**)

INDICATIONS AND USAGE

Premarin (conjugated estrogens) Vaginal Cream is indicated in the treatment of atrophic vaginitis and kraurosis vulvae.

Continued on next page

Premarin Vaginal Cream—Cont.

CONTRAINDICATIONS

Premarin Vaginal Cream should not be used in women with any of the following conditions:

1. Undiagnosed abnormal genital bleeding.
2. Known, suspected, or history of cancer of the breast.
3. Known or suspected estrogen-dependent neoplasia.
4. Active deep vein thrombosis, pulmonary embolism or a history of these conditions.
5. Active or recent (e.g., within past year) arterial thromboembolic disease (e.g., stroke, myocardial infarction).
6. Liver dysfunction or disease.
7. Premarin Vaginal Cream should not be used in patients with known hypersensitivity to its ingredients.
8. Known or suspected pregnancy. There is no indication for Premarin Vaginal Cream in pregnancy. There appears to be little or no increased risk of birth defects in children born to women who have used estrogen and progestins from oral contraceptives inadvertently during pregnancy. (See **PRECAUTIONS**.)

WARNINGS

See **BOXED WARNINGS**.

Systemic absorption may occur with the use of Premarin Vaginal Cream. The warnings, precautions, and adverse reactions associated with oral Premarin treatment should be taken into account.

1. **Cardiovascular disorders.**

Estrogen and estrogen/progestin therapy have been associated with an increased risk of cardiovascular events such as myocardial infarction and stroke, as well as venous thrombosis and pulmonary embolism (venous thromboembolism or VTE). Should any of these occur or be suspected, estrogens should be discontinued immediately.

Risk factors for arterial vascular disease (e.g., hypertension, diabetes mellitus, tobacco use, hypercholesterolemia, and obesity) and/or venous thromboembolism (e.g., personal history or family history of VTE, obesity, and systemic lupus erythematosus) should be managed appropriately.

a. Coronary heart disease and stroke. In the Premarin tablets substudy of the Women's Health Initiative (WHI) study, an increase in the number of myocardial infarctions and strokes has been observed in women receiving Premarin compared to placebo. (See **CLINICAL PHARMACOLOGY, Clinical Studies.**)

In the estrogen plus progestin substudy of WHI, an increased risk of coronary heart disease (CHD) events (defined as nonfatal myocardial infarction and CHD death) was observed in women receiving PREMPRO (0.625 mg conjugated estrogens plus 2.5 mg medroxyprogesterone acetate) per day compared to women receiving placebo (37 vs 30 per 10,000 women-years). The increase in risk was observed in year one and persisted.

In the same substudy of the WHI, an increased risk of stroke was observed in women receiving PREMPRO compared to women receiving placebo (29 vs 21 per 10,000 women-years). The increase in risk was observed after the first year and persisted.

In postmenopausal women with documented heart disease (n = 2,763, average age 66.7 years) a controlled clinical trial of secondary prevention of cardiovascular disease (Heart and Estrogen/progestin Replacement Study; HERS) treatment with PREMPRO (0.625 mg conjugated estrogen plus 2.5 mg medroxyprogesterone acetate per day) demonstrated no cardiovascular benefit. During an average follow-up of 4.1 years, treatment with PREMPRO did not reduce the overall rate of CHD events in postmenopausal women with established coronary heart disease. There were more CHD events in the PREMPRO-treated group than in the placebo group in year 1, but not during the subsequent years. Two thousand three hundred and twenty one women from the original HERS trial agreed to participate in an open label extension of HERS, HERS II. Average follow-up in HERS II was an additional 2.7 years, for a total of 6.8 years overall. Rates of CHD events were comparable among women in the PREMPRO group and the placebo group in HERS, HERS II, and overall.

Large doses of estrogen (5 mg conjugated estrogens per day), comparable to those used to treat cancer of the prostate and breast, have been shown in a large prospective clinical trial in men to increase the risks of nonfatal myocardial infarction, pulmonary embolism, and thrombophlebitis.

b. Venous thromboembolism (VTE). In the Premarin tablets substudy of the Women's Health Initiative (WHI), an increase in VTE has been observed in women receiving Premarin compared to placebo. (See **CLINICAL PHARMACOLOGY, Clinical Studies.**)

In the estrogen plus progestin substudy of WHI, a 2-fold greater rate of VTE, including deep venous thrombosis and pulmonary embolism, was observed in women receiving PREMPRO compared to women receiving placebo. The rate of VTE was 34 per 10,000 women-years in the Prempro group compared to 16 per 10,000 women-years in the placebo group. The increase in VTE risk was observed during the first year and persisted.

If feasible, estrogens should be discontinued at least 4 to 6 weeks before surgery of the type associated with an increased risk of thromboembolism, or during periods of prolonged immobilization.

2. **Malignant neoplasms.**

a. Endometrial cancer. The use of unopposed estrogens in women with intact uteri has been associated with an increased risk of endometrial cancer. The reported endometrial cancer risk among unopposed estrogen users is about 2- to 12-fold greater than in non-users, and appears dependent on duration of treatment and on estrogen dose. Most studies show no significant increased risk associated with use of estrogens for less than one year. The greatest risk appears associated with prolonged use, with increased risks of 15- to 24-fold for five to ten years or more and this risk has been shown to persist for at least 8 to 15 years after estrogen therapy is discontinued.

Table 1. RELATIVE AND ABSOLUTE RISK SEEN IN THE ESTROGEN PLUS PROGESTIN SUBSTUDY OF WHI[a]

Event[c]	Relative Risk Prempro vs Placebo at 5.2 Years (95% CI*)	Placebo n = 8102	Prempro n = 8506
		Absolute Risk per 10,000 Women-years	
CHD events	1.29 (1.02-1.63)	30	37
Non-fatal MI	*1.32 (1.02-1.72)*	*23*	*30*
CHD death	*1.18 (0.70-1.97)*	*6*	*7*
Invasive breast cancer[b]	1.26 (1.00-1.59)	30	38
Stroke	1.41 (1.07-1.85)	21	29
Pulmonary embolism	2.13 (1.39-3.25)	8	16
Colorectal cancer	0.63 (0.43-0.92)	16	10
Endometrial cancer	0.83 (0.47-1.47)	6	5
Hip fracture	0.66 (0.45-0.98)	15	10
Death due to causes other than the events above	0.92 (0.74-1.14)	40	37
Global Index[c]	1.15 (1.03-1.28)	151	170
Deep vein thrombosis[d]	2.07 (1.49-2.87)	13	26
Vertebral fractures[d]	0.66 (0.44-0.98)	15	9
Other osteoporotic fractures[d]	0.77 (0.69-0.86)	170	131

[a] adapted from JAMA, 2002; 288:321-333
[b] includes metastatic and non-metastatic breast cancer with the exception of in situ breast cancer
[c] a subset of the events was combined in a "global index", defined as the earliest occurrence of CHD events, invasive breast cancer, stroke, pulmonary embolism, endometrial cancer, colorectal cancer, hip fracture, or death due to other causes
[d] not included in Global Index
* nominal confidence intervals unadjusted for multiple looks and multiple comparisons

Clinical surveillance of all women taking estrogen/progestin combinations is important. Adequate diagnostic measures, including endometrial sampling when indicated, should be undertaken to rule out malignancy in all cases of undiagnosed persistent or recurring abnormal vaginal bleeding. There is no evidence that the use of natural estrogens results in a different endometrial risk profile than synthetic estrogens of equivalent estrogen dose. Adding a progestin to postmenopausal estrogen therapy has been shown to reduce the risk of endometrial hyperplasia, which may be a precursor to endometrial cancer.

b. Breast cancer. The use of estrogens and progestins by postmenopausal women has been reported to increase the risk of breast cancer. The most important randomized clinical trial providing information about this issue is the Women's Health Initiative (WHI) trial of estrogen plus progestin (See **CLINICAL PHARMACOLOGY, Clinical Studies**). The results from observational studies are generally consistent with those of the WHI trial.

After a mean follow-up of 5.6 years, the WHI trial reported an increased risk of breast cancer in women who took estrogen plus progestin. Observational studies have also reported an increased risk for estrogen/progestin combination therapy, and a smaller increased risk for estrogen alone therapy, after several years of use. For both findings, the excess risk increased with duration of use, and appeared to return to baseline over about five years after stopping treatment (only the observational studies have substantial data on risk after stopping). In these studies, the risk of breast cancer was greater, and became apparent earlier, with estrogen/progestin combination therapy as compared to estrogen alone therapy. However, these studies have not found significant variation in the risk of breast cancer among different estrogens or among different estrogen/progestin combinations, doses, or routes of administration.

In the WHI trial of estrogen plus progestin, 26% of the women reported prior use of estrogen alone and/or estrogen/progestin combination hormone therapy. After a mean follow-up of 5.6 years during the clinical trial, the overall relative risk of invasive breast cancer was 1.24 (95% confidence interval 1.01-1.54), and the overall absolute risk was 41 vs. 33 cases per 10,000 women-years, for estrogen plus progestin compared with placebo. Among women who reported prior use of hormone therapy, the relative risk of invasive breast cancer was 1.86, and the absolute risk was 46 vs. 25 cases per 10,000 women-years, for estrogen plus progestin compared with placebo. Among women who reported no prior use of hormone therapy, the relative risk of invasive breast cancer was 1.09, and the absolute risk was 40 vs. 36 cases per 10,000 women-years for estrogen plus progestin compared with placebo. In the WHI trial, invasive breast cancers were larger and diagnosed at a more advanced stage in the estrogen plus progestin group compared with the placebo group. Metastatic disease was rare with no apparent difference between the two groups. Other prognostic factors such as histologic subtype, grade and hormone receptor status did not differ between the groups. The observational Million Women Study in Europe reported an increased risk of mortality due to breast cancer among current users of hormone therapy compared to never users, while the estrogen plus progestin sub-study of WHI showed no effect on breast cancer mortality with a mean follow-up of 5.6 years.

The observational Million Women Study in Europe reported an increased risk of mortality due to breast cancer among current users of estrogens alone or estrogens plus progestins compared to never users, while the estrogen plus progestin sub-study of WHI showed no effect on breast cancer mortality with a mean follow-up of 5.6 years.

The use of estrogen plus progestin has been reported to result in an increase in abnormal mammograms requiring further evaluation. All women should receive yearly breast examinations by a healthcare provider and perform monthly breast self-examinations. In addition, mammography examinations should be scheduled based on patient age, risk factors, and prior mammogram results.

3. **Dementia.**

In the Women's Health Initiative Memory Study (WHIMS), an ancillary study of WHI, a population of 4,532 women aged 65 to 79 years was randomized to PREMPRO (0.625 mg/2.5 mg) or placebo. A population of 2,947 hysterectomized women, aged 65 to 79 years, was randomized to Premarin (0.625 mg) or placebo. In the planned analysis, pooling the events in women receiving Premarin or PREMPRO in comparison to those in women on placebo, the overall relative risk (RR) for probable dementia was 1.76 (95% CI 1.19-2.60. In the estrogen-alone group, after an average follow-up of 5.2 years a RR of 1.49 (95% CI 0.83-2.66) for probable dementia was observed compared to placebo. In the estrogen-plus-progestin group, after an average follow-up of 4 years, a RR of 2.05 (95% CI 1.21-3.48) for probable dementia was observed compared to placebo. Since this study was conducted in women aged 65 to 79 years, it is unknown whether these findings apply to younger postmenopausal women. (See **PRECAUTIONS, Geriatric Use.**)

4. **Gallbladder disease.**

A 2- to 4-fold increase in the risk of gallbladder disease requiring surgery in postmenopausal women receiving postmenopausal estrogens has been reported.

5. **Hypercalcemia.**

Estrogen administration may lead to severe hypercalcemia in patients with breast cancer and bone metastases. If hypercalcemia occurs, use of the drug should be stopped and appropriate measures taken to reduce the serum calcium level.

6. **Visual abnormalities.**

Retinal vascular thrombosis has been reported in patients receiving estrogens. Discontinue medication pending examination if there is sudden partial or complete loss of vision, or a sudden onset of proptosis, diplopia, or migraine. If examination reveals papilledema or retinal vascular lesions, estrogens should be discontinued.

PRECAUTIONS

A. General

1. ***Addition of a progestin when a woman has not had a hysterectomy.***

Studies of the addition of a progestin for 10 or more days of a cycle of estrogen administration or daily with estrogen in a continuous regimen have reported a lowered incidence of endometrial hyperplasia than would be induced by estrogen treatment alone. Endometrial hyperplasia may be a precursor to endometrial cancer.

There are, however, possible risks that may be associated with the use of progestins with estrogens compared to estrogen-alone regimens. These include a possible increased risk of breast cancer, adverse effects on lipoprotein metabolism (e.g., lowering HDL, raising LDL) and impairment of glucose tolerance.

2. Elevated blood pressure.
In a small number of case reports, substantial increases in blood pressure have been attributed to idiosyncratic reactions to estrogens. In a large, randomized, placebo-controlled clinical trial, a generalized effect of estrogen therapy on blood pressure was not seen. Blood pressure should be monitored at regular intervals with estrogen use.

3. Hypertriglyceridemia.
In patients with pre-existing hypertriglyceridemia, estrogen therapy may be associated with elevations of plasma triglycerides leading to pancreatitis and other complications.

4. Impaired liver function and past history of cholestatic jaundice.
Estrogens may be poorly metabolized in patients with impaired liver function. For patients with a history of cholestatic jaundice associated with past estrogen use or with pregnancy, caution should be exercised and in the case of recurrence, medication should be discontinued.

5. Hypothyroidism.
Estrogen administration leads to increased thyroid-binding globulin (TBG) levels. Patients with normal thyroid function can compensate for the increased TBG by making more thyroid hormone, thus maintaining free T_4 and T_3 serum concentrations in the normal range. Patients dependent on thyroid hormone replacement therapy who are also receiving estrogens may require increased doses of their thyroid replacement therapy. These patients should have their thyroid function monitored in order to maintain their free thyroid hormone levels in an acceptable range.

6. Fluid retention.
Because estrogens may cause some degree of fluid retention, patients with conditions that might be influenced by this factor, such as cardiac or renal dysfunction, warrant careful observation when estrogens are prescribed.

7. Hypocalcemia.
Estrogens should be used with caution in individuals with severe hypocalcemia.

8. Ovarian cancer.
The estrogen plus progestin substudy of WHI reported that after an average follow-up of 5.6 years, the relative risk for ovarian cancer for estrogen plus progestin versus placebo was 1.58 (95% confidence interval 0.77 – 3.24) but was not statistically significant. The absolute risk for estrogen plus progestin versus placebo was 4.2 versus 2.7 cases per 10,000 women-years. In some epidemiologic studies, the use of estrogen-only products, in particular for ten or more years, has been associated with an increased risk of ovarian cancer. Other epidemiologic studies have not found these associations.

9. Exacerbation of endometriosis.
Endometriosis may be exacerbated with administration of estrogen therapy.
A few cases of malignant transformation of residual endometrial implants have been reported in women treated post-hysterectomy with estrogen alone therapy. For patients known to have residual endometriosis post-hysterectomy, the addition of progestin should be considered.

10. Exacerbation of other conditions.
Estrogen therapy may cause an exacerbation of asthma, diabetes mellitus, epilepsy, migraine, porphyria, systemic lupus erythematosus, and hepatic hemangiomas and should be used with caution in women with these conditions.

11. Barrier contraceptives.
Premarin Vaginal Cream exposure has been reported to weaken latex condoms. The potential for Premarin Vaginal Cream to weaken and contribute to the failure of condoms, diaphragms, or cervical caps made of latex or rubber should be considered.

B. Patient Information
Physicians are advised to discuss the contents of the PATIENT INFORMATION leaflet with patients for whom they prescribe Premarin Vaginal Cream.

C. Laboratory Tests
Estrogen administration should be guided by clinical response at the lowest dose for the treatment of postmenopausal vulvar and vaginal atrophy.

D. Drug/Laboratory Test Interactions
1. Accelerated prothrombin time, partial thromboplastin time, and platelet aggregation time; increased platelet count; increased factors II, VII antigen, VIII antigen, VIII coagulant activity, IX, X, XII, VII-X complex, II-VII-X complex, and beta-thromboglobulin; decreased levels of antifactor Xa and antithrombin III, decreased antithrombin III activity; increased levels of fibrinogen and fibrinogen activity; increased plasminogen antigen and activity.
2. Increased thyroid-binding globulin (TBG) leading to increased circulating total thyroid hormone, as measured by protein-bound iodine (PBI), T_4 levels (by column or by radioimmunoassay) or T_3 levels by radioimmunoassay. T_3 resin uptake is decreased, reflecting the elevated TBG. Free T_4 and free T_3 concentrations are unaltered. Patients on thyroid replacement therapy may require higher doses of thyroid hormone.

3. Other binding proteins may be elevated in serum, i.e., corticosteroid binding globulin (CBG), sex hormone-binding globulin (SHBG), leading to increased total circulating corticosteroids and sex steroids, respectively. Free hormone concentrations may be decreased. Other plasma proteins may be increased (angiotensinogen/renin substrate, alpha-1-antitrypsin, ceruloplasmin).
4. Increased plasma HDL and HDL_2 cholesterol subfraction concentrations, reduced LDL cholesterol concentration, increased triglyceride levels.
5. Impaired glucose tolerance.
6. Reduced response to metyrapone test.

E. Carcinogenesis, Mutagenesis, Impairment of Fertility
(See **BOXED WARNINGS**, **WARNINGS**, and **PRECAUTIONS**.)
Long-term continuous administration of natural and synthetic estrogens in certain animal species increases the frequency of carcinomas of the breast, uterus, cervix, vagina, testis, and liver.

F. Pregnancy
Premarin Vaginal Cream should not be used during pregnancy. (See **CONTRAINDICATIONS**.)

G. Nursing Mothers
Estrogen administration to nursing mothers has been shown to decrease the quantity and quality of breast milk. Detectable amounts of estrogens have been identified in the milk of mothers receiving the drug. Caution should be exercised when Premarin Vaginal Cream is administered to a nursing woman.

H. Pediatric Use
Estrogen therapy has been used for the induction of puberty in adolescents with some forms of pubertal delay. Safety and effectiveness in pediatric patients have not otherwise been established.

Large and repeated doses of estrogen over an extended time period have been shown to accelerate epiphyseal closure, which could result in short adult stature if treatment is initiated before the completion of physiologic puberty in normally developing children. If estrogen is administered to patients whose bone growth is not complete, periodic monitoring of bone maturation and effects on epiphyseal centers is recommended during estrogen administration.

Estrogen treatment of prepubertal girls also induces premature breast development and vaginal cornification, and may induce vaginal bleeding. In boys, estrogen treatment may modify the normal pubertal process and induce gynecomastia. See **INDICATIONS** and **DOSAGE AND ADMINISTRATION** sections.

I. Geriatric Use
Of the total number of subjects in the estrogen plus progestin substudy of the Women's Health Initiative study, 44% (n = 7,320) were 65 years and over, while 6.6% (n = 1,095) were 75 years and over (See **CLINICAL PHARMACOLOGY, Clinical Studies**). There was a higher incidence of stroke and invasive breast cancer in women 75 and over compared to women less than 75 years of age.

In the Women's Health Initiative Memory Study (WHIMS), an ancillary study of WHI, a population of 4,532 women aged 65 to 79 years was randomized to PREMPRO (0.625 mg/2.5 mg) or placebo. A population of 2,947 hysterectomized women, aged 65 to 79 years, was randomized to Premarin (0.625 mg) or placebo. In the planned analysis, pooling the events in women receiving Premarin or PREMPRO in comparison to those in women on placebo, the overall relative risk (RR) for probable dementia was 1.76 (95% CI 1.19-2.60). In the estrogen-alone group, after an average follow-up of 5.2 years a RR of 1.49 (95% CI 0.83-2.66) for probable dementia was observed compared to placebo. In the estrogen-plus-progestin group, after an average follow-up of 4 years, a RR of 2.05 (95% CI 1.21-3.48) for probable dementia was observed compared to placebo. Since this study was conducted in women aged 65 to 79 years, it is unknown whether these findings apply to younger postmenopausal women. (See **WARNINGS, Dementia**).
There have not been sufficient numbers of geriatric patients involved in studies utilizing Premarin Vaginal Cream to determine whether those over 65 years of age differ from younger subjects in their response to Premarin Vaginal Cream.

ADVERSE REACTIONS
See **BOXED WARNINGS**, **WARNINGS**, and **PRECAUTIONS**.
Systemic absorption may occur with the use of Premarin Vaginal Cream. Warnings, precautions, and adverse reactions associated with oral Premarin treatment should be taken into account.
The following additional adverse reactions have been reported with estrogen and/or progestin therapy:
1. *Genitourinary system:* Breakthrough bleeding, spotting, change in menstrual flow; dysmenorrhea; premenstrual-like syndrome; amenorrhea during and after treatment; increase in size of uterine fibromyomata; vaginitis, including vaginal candidiasis; change in cervical erosion and in degree of cervical secretion; cystitis-like syndrome; application site reactions of vulvovaginal discomfort including burning and irritation; genital pruritus; ovarian cancer; endometrial hyperplasia; endometrial cancer; precocious puberty.
2. *Breasts:* Tenderness, pain, enlargement, secretion; breast cancer; fibrocystic breast changes.

3. *Cardiovascular:* Deep and superficial venous thrombosis; pulmonary embolism, myocardial infarction, stroke; increase in blood pressure.
4. *Gastrointestinal:* Nausea, vomiting, abdominal cramps, bloating; cholestatic jaundice; pancreatitis; increased incidence of gallbladder disease; enlargement of hepatic hemangiomas.
5. *Skin:* Chloasma or melasma which may persist when drug is discontinued; erythema multiforme; erythema nodosum; hemorrhagic eruption; loss of scalp hair; hirsutism; pruritis; rash; urticaria.
6. *Eyes:* Retinal vascular thrombosis; intolerance to contact lenses.
7. *Central Nervous System:* Headache; migraine; dizziness; nervousness; mood disturbances; irritability; mental depression; chorea; exacerbation of epilepsy; dementia.
8. *Miscellaneous:* Increase or decrease in weight; reduced carbohydrate tolerance; glucose intolerance; aggravation of porphyria; edema; changes in libido; anaphylactoid/anaphylactic reactions; hypocalcemia; exacerbation of asthma; angioedema; hypersensitivity; increased triglycerides; arthralgias; leg cramps.

OVERDOSAGE
Serious ill effects have not been reported following acute ingestion of large doses of estrogen/progestin containing drug products by young children. Overdosage of estrogens may cause nausea and vomiting, and withdrawal bleeding may occur in females.

DOSAGE AND ADMINISTRATION
Use of Premarin Vaginal Cream, alone or in combination with a progestin, should be limited to the shortest duration consistent with treatment goals and risks for the individual woman. Patients should be re-evaluated periodically as clinically appropriate (e.g., at 3-month to 6-month intervals) to determine if treatment is still necessary (See **BOXED WARNINGS** and **WARNINGS**). For women who have a uterus, adequate diagnostic measures, such as endometrial sampling, when indicated, should be undertaken to rule out malignancy in cases of undiagnosed persistent or recurring abnormal vaginal bleeding.
Given cyclically for short-term use only:
For treatment of atrophic vaginitis, or kraurosis vulvae. The lowest dose that will control symptoms should be chosen and medication should be discontinued as promptly as possible. Administration should be cyclic (e.g., three weeks on and one week off).
Usual Dosage Range:
½ to 2 g daily, intravaginally, depending on the severity of the condition.
Instructions For Use Of Gentle Measure™ Applicator
1. Remove cap from tube.
2. Screw nozzle end of applicator onto tube.
3. *Gently* squeeze tube from the *bottom* to force sufficient cream into the barrel to provide the prescribed dose. Use the marked stopping points on the applicator as a guideline to measure the correct dose.
4. Unscrew applicator from tube.
5. Lie on back with knees drawn up. To deliver medication, gently insert applicator deeply into vagina and press plunger downward to its original position.
To Cleanse: Pull plunger to remove it from barrel. Wash with mild soap and warm water.
DO NOT BOIL OR USE HOT WATER.

HOW SUPPLIED
Premarin® (conjugated estrogens) Vaginal Cream—Each gram contains 0.625 mg conjugated estrogens, USP.
Combination package: Each contains Net Wt. 1 ½ oz (42.5 g) tube with one plastic applicator calibrated in ½ g increments to a maximum of 2 g (NDC 0046-0872-93).
Also Available—Refill package: Each contains Net Wt. 1 ½ oz (42.5 g) tube (NDC 0046-0872-01).
Store at room temperature (approximately 25° C).

PATIENT INFORMATION
(Updated February 16, 2005)
Premarin® (conjugated estrogens) **Vaginal Cream**
Read this PATIENT INFORMATION before you start using Premarin Vaginal Cream and read what you get each time you refill Premarin Vaginal Cream. There may be new information. This information does not take the place of talking to your healthcare provider about your medical condition or your treatment.

What is the most important information I should know about Premarin (an estrogen mixture)?

• Estrogens increase the chances of getting cancer of the uterus.
Report any unusual vaginal bleeding right away while you are taking Premarin. Vaginal bleeding after menopause may be a warning sign of cancer of the uterus (womb). Your healthcare provider should check any unusual vaginal bleeding to find out the cause.
• Do not use estrogens with or without progestins to prevent heart disease, heart attacks, strokes, or dementia.
Using estrogens with or without progestins may increase your chances of getting heart attacks, strokes, breast cancer, and blood clots. Using estrogens, with or without progestins, may increase your risk of de-

Continued on next page

Premarin Vaginal Cream—Cont.

mentia based on a study of women age 65 years or older. You and your healthcare provider should talk regularly about whether you still need treatment with Premarin Vaginal Cream.

What is Premarin Vaginal Cream?

Premarin Vaginal Cream is a medicine that contains a mixture of estrogen hormones.

Premarin Vaginal Cream is used to:

• treat dryness, itching, and burning, in and around the vagina due to menopause. You and your healthcare provider should talk regularly about whether you still need treatment with Premarin Vaginal Cream to control these problems.

Who should not use Premarin Vaginal Cream?

Do not start using Premarin Vaginal Cream if you:

• **have unusual vaginal bleeding.**

• **currently have or have had certain cancers.**
Estrogens may increase the chances of getting certain types of cancers, including cancer of the breast or uterus. If you have or have had cancer, talk with your healthcare provider about whether you should use Premarin Vaginal Cream.

• **had a stroke or heart attack in the past year.**

• **currently have or had blood clots.**

• **currently have liver problems.**

• **are allergic to Premarin Vaginal Cream or any of its ingredients.**
See the end of this leaflet for a list of all the ingredients in Premarin Vaginal Cream.

• **think you may be pregnant.**

Tell your healthcare provider:

• **if you are breast feeding.** The hormones in Premarin Vaginal Cream can pass into your milk.

• **about all of your medical problems.** Your healthcare provider may need to check you more carefully if you have certain conditions, such as asthma (wheezing), epilepsy (seizures), migraine, endometriosis, lupus, or problems with your heart, liver, thyroid, kidneys, or have high calcium levels in your blood.

• **about all the medicines you take,** including prescription and nonprescription medicines, vitamins, and herbal supplements. Some medicines may affect how Premarin Vaginal Cream works. Premarin Vaginal Cream may also affect how your other medicines work.

• **if you are going to have surgery or will be on bedrest.** You may need to stop using Premarin Vaginal Cream.

How should I use Premarin Vaginal Cream?

The Gentle Measure™ Applicator has been specifically designed for comfortable, easy use.

1. Remove cap from tube.
2. Screw nozzle end of applicator onto tube.
3. *Gently* squeeze tube from the *bottom* to force sufficient cream into the barrel to provide the prescribed dose. Use the marked stopping points on the applicator as a guideline to measure the correct dose, as prescribed by your healthcare provider.
4. Unscrew applicator from tube.
5. Lie on back with knees drawn up. To deliver medication, gently insert applicator deeply into vagina and press plunger downward to its original position.

TO CLEANSE: Pull plunger to remove it from barrel. Wash with mild soap and warm water.

DO NOT BOIL OR USE HOT WATER.

Premarin Vaginal Cream should be used at the lowest possible dose for your treatment and only as long as needed. You and your healthcare provider should talk regularly (for example, every 3 to 6 months) about the dose you are taking and whether you still need treatment with Premarin Vaginal Cream.

What are the possible side effects of Premarin Vaginal Cream?

Although Premarin Vaginal Cream is only used in and around the vagina, the risks associated with Premarin tablets should be taken into account.

Less common but serious side effects of estrogens include:

• Breast cancer
• Cancer of the uterus
• Stroke
• Heart attack
• Blood clots
• Dementia
• Gallbladder disease
• Ovarian cancer

These are some of the warning signs of serious side effects:

• Breast lumps
• Unusual vaginal bleeding
• Dizziness and faintness
• Changes in speech
• Severe headaches
• Chest pain
• Shortness of breath
• Pains in your legs
• Changes in vision
• Vomiting

Call your healthcare provider right away if you get any of these warning signs, or any other unusual symptom that concerns you.

Common side effects of estrogens include:

• Headache
• Breast tenderness

• Irregular vaginal bleeding or spotting
• Stomach/abdominal cramps, bloating
• Nausea and vomiting
• Hair loss
• Reactions from inserting Premarin Vaginal Cream such as vaginal burning, irritation, and itching

Other side effects of estrogens include:

• High blood pressure
• Liver problems
• High blood sugar
• Fluid retention
• Enlargement of benign tumors of the uterus ("fibroids")
• Vaginal yeast infections
• Allergic Reactions

These are not all the possible side effects of Premarin Vaginal Cream. For more information, ask your healthcare provider or pharmacist.

What can I do to lower my chances of getting a serious side effect with Premarin Vaginal Cream?

• Talk with your healthcare provider regularly about whether you should continue using Premarin Vaginal Cream.

• See your healthcare provider right away if you get vaginal bleeding while using Premarin Vaginal Cream.

• Have a breast exam and mammogram (breast X-ray) every year unless your healthcare provider tells you something else. If members of your family have had breast cancer or if you have ever had breast lumps or an abnormal mammogram, you may need to have breast exams more often.

• If you have high blood pressure, high cholesterol (fat in the blood), diabetes, are overweight, or if you use tobacco, you may have higher chances for getting heart disease. Ask your health care provider for ways to lower your chances for getting heart disease.

General information about the safe and effective use of Premarin Vaginal Cream

Medicines are sometimes prescribed for conditions that are not mentioned in patient information leaflets. Do not use Premarin Vaginal Cream for conditions for which it was not prescribed. Do not give Premarin Vaginal Cream to other people, even if they have the same symptoms you have. It may harm them. **Keep Premarin Vaginal Cream out of the reach of children.**

This leaflet provides a summary of the most important information about Premarin Vaginal Cream. If you would like more information, talk with your healthcare provider or pharmacist. You can ask for information about Premarin Vaginal Cream that is written for health professionals. You can get more information by calling the toll free number 1-800-934-5556.

What are the ingredients in Premarin Vaginal Cream?

Premarin Vaginal Cream contains a mixture of conjugated estrogens, which are a mixture of sodium estrone sulfate and sodium equilin sulfate and other components including sodium sulfate conjugates: 17 α-dihydroequilin, 17 α-estradiol, and 17 β-dihydroequilin. Premarin Vaginal Cream also contains cetyl esters wax, cetyl alcohol, white wax, glyceryl monostearate, propylene glycol monostearate, methyl stearate, benzyl alcohol, sodium lauryl sulfate, glycerin, and mineral oil.

Premarin® (conjugated estrogens) Vaginal Cream—Each gram contains 0.625 mg conjugated estrogens, USP.

Combination package: Each contains Net Wt. 1 ½ oz (42.5 g) tube with one plastic applicator calibrated in ½ g increments to a maximum of 2 g (NDC 0046-0872-93).

Also Available—Refill package: Each contains Net Wt. 1 ½ oz (42.5 g) tube (NDC 0046-0872-01).

Store at room temperature (approximately 25° C).

Wyeth®

Wyeth Pharmaceuticals Inc.

Philadelphia, PA 19101

W10413C006
ET01
Revised February 16, 2005

Premarin® (conjugated estrogens)

Vaginal Cream in a nonliquefying base

℞ only

◄TEAR HERE

PATIENT INFORMATION

Read this PATIENT INFORMATION before you start using Premarin Vaginal Cream and read what you get each time you refill Premarin Vaginal Cream. There may be new information. This information does not take the place of talking to your healthcare provider about your medical condition or your treatment.

What is the most important information I should know about Premarin (an estrogen mixture)?

• Estrogens increase the chances of getting cancer of the uterus.
Report any unusual vaginal bleeding right away while you are taking Premarin. Vaginal bleeding after menopause may be a warning sign of cancer of the uterus (womb). Your healthcare provider should check any unusual vaginal bleeding to find out the cause.

• Do not use estrogens with or without progestins to prevent heart disease, heart attacks, strokes, or dementia.
Using estrogens with or without progestins may increase your chances of getting heart attacks, strokes, breast cancer, and blood clots. Using estrogens, with or without progestins, may increase your risk of dementia based on a study of women age 65 years or

---

older. You and your healthcare provider should talk regularly about whether you still need treatment with Premarin Vaginal Cream.

What is Premarin Vaginal Cream?

Premarin Vaginal Cream is a medicine that contains a mixture of estrogen hormones.

Premarin Vaginal Cream is used to:

• treat dryness, itching, and burning, in and around the vagina due to menopause.

You and your healthcare provider should talk regularly about whether you still need treatment with Premarin Vaginal Cream to control these problems.

Who should not use Premarin Vaginal Cream?

Do not start using Premarin Vaginal Cream if you:

• **have unusual vaginal bleeding.**

• **currently have or have had certain cancers.**
Estrogens may increase the chances of getting certain types of cancers, including cancer of the breast or uterus. If you have or have had cancer, talk with your healthcare provider about whether you should use Premarin Vaginal Cream.

• **had a stroke or heart attack in the past year.**

• **currently have or had blood clots.**

• **currently have liver problems.**

• **are allergic to Premarin Vaginal Cream or any of its ingredients.**
See the end of this leaflet for a list of all the ingredients in Premarin Vaginal Cream.

• **think you may be pregnant.**

Tell your healthcare provider:

• **if you are breast feeding.** The hormones in Premarin Vaginal Cream can pass into your milk.

• **about all of your medical problems.** Your healthcare provider may need to check you more carefully if you have certain conditions, such as asthma (wheezing), epilepsy (seizures), migraine, endometriosis, lupus, problems with your heart, liver, thyroid, kidneys, or have high calcium levels in your blood.

• **about all the medicines you take,** including prescription and nonprescription medicines, vitamins, and herbal supplements. Some medicines may affect how Premarin Vaginal Cream works. Premarin Vaginal Cream may also affect how your other medicines work.

• **if you are going to have surgery or will be on bedrest.** You may need to stop using Premarin Vaginal Cream.

How should I use Premarin Vaginal Cream?

The Gentle Measure™ Applicator has been specifically designed for comfortable, easy use.

1. Remove cap from tube.
2. Screw nozzle end of applicator onto tube.
3. *Gently* squeeze tube from the *bottom* to force sufficient cream into the barrel to provide the prescribed dose. Use the marked stopping points on the applicator as a guideline to measure the correct dose.
4. Unscrew nozzle end of applicator onto tube.
5. Lie on back with knees drawn up. To deliver medication, gently insert applicator deeply into vagina and press plunger downward to its original position.

TO CLEANSE: Pull plunger to remove it from barrel. Wash with mild soap and warm water.

DO NOT BOIL OR USE HOT WATER.

Premarin Vaginal Cream should be used at the lowest dose possible for your treatment and only as long as needed. You and your healthcare provider should talk regularly (for example, every 3 to 6 months) about the dose you are taking and about whether you still need treatment with Premarin Vaginal Cream.

What are the possible side effects of Premarin Vaginal Cream?

Although Premarin Vaginal Cream is only used in and around vagina, the risks associated with Premarin tablets should be taken into account.

Less common but serious side effects of estrogens include:

• Breast cancer
• Cancer of the uterus
• Stroke
• Heart attack
• Dementia
• Blood clots
• Gallbladder disease
• Ovarian cancer

These are some of the warning signs of serious side effects:

• Breast lumps
• Unusual vaginal bleeding
• Dizziness and faintness
• Changes in speech
• Severe headaches
• Chest pain
• Shortness of breath
• Pains in your legs
• Changes in vision
• Vomiting

Call your healthcare provider right away if you get any of these warning signs, or any other unusual symptom that concerns you.

Common side effects of estrogens include:

• Headache
• Breast tenderness
• Irregular vaginal bleeding or spotting
• Stomach/abdominal cramps, bloating
• Nausea and vomiting
• Hair loss

- Reactions from inserting Premarin Vaginal Cream such as vaginal burning, irritation, and itching

Other side effects of estrogens include:

- High blood pressure
- Liver problems
- High blood sugar
- Fluid retention
- Enlargement of benign tumors of the uterus ("fibroids")
- Vaginal yeast infections
- Allergic reactions

These are not all the possible side effects of Premarin Vaginal Cream. For more information, ask your healthcare provider or pharmacist.

What can I do to lower my chances of getting a serious side effect with Premarin Vaginal Cream?

- Talk with your healthcare provider regularly about whether you should continue using Premarin Vaginal Cream.
- See your healthcare provider right away if you get vaginal bleeding while using Premarin Vaginal Cream.
- Have a breast exam and mammogram (breast X-ray) every year unless your healthcare provider tells you something else. If members of your family have had breast cancer or if you have ever had breast lumps or an abnormal mammogram, you may need to have breast exams more often.
- If you have high blood pressure, high cholesterol (fat in the blood), diabetes, are overweight, or if you use tobacco, you may have higher chances for getting heart disease. Ask your health care provider for ways to lower your chances for getting heart disease.

General information about the safe and effective use of Premarin Vaginal Cream

Medicines are sometimes prescribed for conditions that are not mentioned in patient information leaflets. Do not use Premarin Vaginal Cream for conditions for which it was not prescribed. Do not give Premarin Vaginal Cream to other people, even if they have the same symptoms you have. It may harm them. **Keep Premarin Vaginal Cream out of the reach of children.**

This leaflet provides a summary of the most important information about Premarin Vaginal Cream. If you would like more information, talk with your healthcare provider or pharmacist. You can ask for information about Premarin Vaginal Cream that is written for health professionals. You can get more information by calling the toll free number 800-934-5556.

What are the ingredients in Premarin Vaginal Cream?

Premarin Vaginal Cream contains a mixture of conjugated estrogens, which are a mixture of sodium estrone sulfate and sodium equilin sulfate and other components including sodium sulfate conjugates: 17 α-dihydroequilin, 17 α-estradiol, and 17 β-dihydroequilin. Premarin Vaginal Cream also contains cetyl esters wax, cetyl alcohol, white wax, glyceryl monostearate, propylene glycol monostearate, methyl stearate, benzyl alcohol, sodium lauryl sulfate, glycerin, and mineral oil.

Premarin® (conjugated estrogens) Vaginal Cream—Each gram contains 0.625 mg conjugated estrogens, USP.

Combination package: Each contains Net Wt. 1 ½ oz (42.5 g) tube with one plastic applicator calibrated in ½ g increments to a maximum of 2 g (NDC 0046-0872-93).

Also Available—Refill package: Each contains Net Wt. 1 ½ oz (42.5 g) tube (NDC 0046-0872-01).

Store at room temperature (approximately 25° C).

This product's label may have been revised after this insert was used in production. For further product information and current package insert, please visit www.wyeth.com or call our medical communications department toll-free at 1-800-934-5556.

Wyeth®

Wyeth Pharmaceuticals Inc. W10413C006
Philadelphia, PA 19101 ET01
Revised February 16, 2005

PREMPRO™ ℞

[*prěm-prō*]

(conjugated estrogens/medroxyprogesterone acetate tablets)

PREMPHASE®

[*prěm-fāz*]

(conjugated estrogens/medroxyprogesterone acetate tablets)

℞ only

Prescribing information for this product, which appears on pages 3375–3382 of the 2005 PDR, has been completely revised as follows. Please write "See Supplement A" next to the product heading.

WARNING

Estrogens and progestins should not be used for the prevention of cardiovascular disease or dementia.

The Women's Health Initiative (WHI) study reported increased risks of myocardial infarction, stroke, invasive breast cancer, pulmonary emboli, and deep vein thrombosis in postmenopausal women (50 to 79 years of age) during 5 years of treatment with conjugated estrogens (0.625 mg) combined with medroxyprogesterone acetate (2.5 mg) relative to placebo. (See **CLINICAL PHARMACOLOGY, Clinical Studies.**)

The WHI study reported increased risks of stroke and deep vein thrombosis in postmenopausal women (50 to 79 years of age) during 6.8 years of treatment with conjugated estrogens (0.625 mg) relative to placebo.

The Women's Health Initiative Memory Study (WHIMS), a substudy of WHI, reported increased risk of developing probable dementia in postmenopausal women 65 years of age or older during 4 to 5.2 years of treatment with conjugated estrogens, with or without medroxyprogesterone acetate, relative to placebo. It is unknown whether this finding applies to younger postmenopausal women.

Other doses of conjugated estrogens and medroxyprogesterone acetate, and other combinations and dosage forms of estrogens and progestins were not studied in the WHI clinical trials and, in the absence of comparable data, these risks should be assumed to be similar. Because of these risks, estrogens with or without progestins should be prescribed at the lowest effective doses and for the shortest duration consistent with treatment goals and risks for the individual woman.

TABLE 1. PHARMACOKINETIC PARAMETERS FOR UNCONJUGATED AND CONJUGATED ESTROGENS (CE) AND MEDROXYPROGESTERONE ACETATE (MPA)

DRUG	2 × 0.625 mg CE/2.5 mg MPA Combination Tablets (n=54)				2 × 0.625 mg CE/5 mg MPA Combination Tablets (n=51)			
PK Parameter Arithmetic Mean (%CV)	C_{max} (pg/mL)	t_{max} (h)	$t_{1/2}$ (h)	AUC (pg•h/mL)	C_{max} (pg/mL)	t_{max} (h)	$t_{1/2}$ (h)	AUC (pg•h/mL)
Unconjugated Estrogens								
Estrone	175 (23)	7.6 (24)	31.6 (23)	5358 (34)	124 (43)	10 (35)	62.2 (137)	6303 (40)
BA* -Estrone	159 (26)	7.6 (24)	16.9 (34)	3313 (40)	104 (49)	10 (35)	26.0 (100)	3136 (51)
Equilin	71 (31)	5.8 (34)	9.9 (35)	951 (43)	54 (43)	8.9 (34)	15.5 (53)	1179 (56)
PK Parameter Arithmetic Mean (%CV)	C_{max} (ng/mL)	t_{max} (h)	$t_{1/2}$ (h)	AUC (ng•h/mL)	C_{max} (ng/mL)	t_{max} (h)	$t_{1/2}$ (h)	AUC (ng•h/mL)
Conjugated Estrogens								
Total Estrone	6.6 (38)	6.1 (28)	20.7 (34)	116 (59)	6.3 (48)	9.1 (29)	23.6 (36)	151 (42)
BA* -Total Estrone	6.4 (39)	6.1 (28)	15.4 (34)	100 (57)	6.2 (48)	9.1 (29)	20.6 (35)	139 (40)
Total Equilin	5.1 (45)	4.6 (35)	11.4 (25)	50 (70)	4.2 (52)	7.0 (36)	17.2 (131)	72 (50)
PK Parameter Arithmetic Mean (%CV)	C_{max} (ng/mL)	t_{max} (h)	$t_{1/2}$ (h)	AUC (ng•h/mL)	C_{max} (ng/mL)	t_{max} (h)	$t_{1/2}$ (h)	AUC (ng•h/mL)
Medroxyprogesterone Acetate								
MPA	1.5 (40)	2.8 (54)	37.6 (30)	37 (30)	4.8 (31)	2.4 (50)	46.3 (39)	102 (28)

BA* = Baseline adjusted
C_{max} = peak plasma concentration
t_{max} = time peak concentration occurs
$t_{1/2}$ = apparent terminal-phase disposition half-life ($0.693/\lambda_z$)
AUC = total area under the concentration-time curve

DESCRIPTION

PREMPRO™ 0.3 mg/1.5 mg therapy consists of a single tablet containing 0.3 mg of the conjugated estrogens (CE) found in Premarin® tablets and 1.5 mg of medroxyprogesterone acetate (MPA) for oral administration.

PREMPRO 0.45 mg/1.5 mg therapy consists of a single tablet containing 0.45 mg of the conjugated estrogens found in Premarin tablets and 1.5 mg of medroxyprogesterone acetate for oral administration.

PREMPRO 0.625 mg/2.5 mg therapy consists of a single tablet containing 0.625 mg of the conjugated estrogens found in Premarin tablets and 2.5 mg of medroxyprogesterone acetate for oral administration.

PREMPRO 0.625 mg/5 mg therapy consists of a single tablet containing 0.625 mg of the conjugated estrogens found in Premarin tablets and 5 mg of medroxyprogesterone acetate for oral administration.

PREMPHASE® therapy consists of two separate tablets, a maroon Premarin tablet containing 0.625 mg of conjugated estrogens that is taken orally on days 1 through 14 and a light-blue tablet containing 0.625 mg of the conjugated estrogens found in Premarin tablets and 5 mg of medroxyprogesterone acetate that is taken orally on days 15 through 28.

The conjugated estrogens found in Premarin tablets are a mixture of sodium estrone sulfate and sodium equilin sulfate, obtained exclusively from natural sources and blended to represent the average composition of materials derived from pregnant mares' urine. They contain as concomitant components, as sodium sulfate conjugates, 17 α-dihydroequilin, 17 α-estradiol and 17 β-dihydroequilin.

Medroxyprogesterone acetate is a derivative of progesterone. It is a white to off-white, odorless, crystalline powder, stable in air, melting between 200°C and 210°C. It is freely soluble in chloroform, soluble in acetone and in dioxane, sparingly soluble in alcohol and in methanol, slightly soluble in ether, and insoluble in water. The chemical name for MPA is pregn-4-ene-3, 20-dione, 17-(acetyloxy)-6-methyl-, (6α)-. Its molecular formula is $C_{24}H_{34}O_4$, with a molecular weight of 386.53. Its structural formula is:

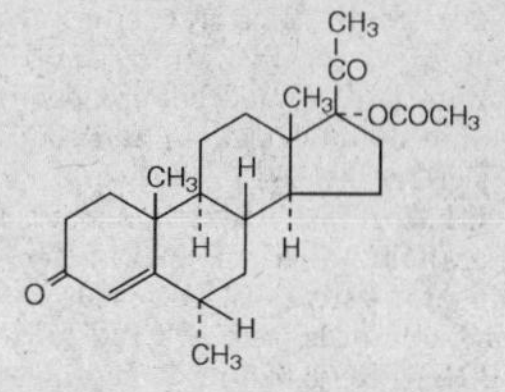

PREMPRO 0.3 mg/1.5 mg

Each cream tablet for oral administration contains 0.3 mg conjugated estrogens, 1.5 mg medroxyprogesterone acetate, and the following inactive ingredients: calcium phosphate tribasic, calcium sulfate, carnauba wax, cellulose, glyceryl monooleate, lactose, magnesium stearate, methylcellulose, pharmaceutical glaze, polyethylene glycol, sucrose, povidone, titanium dioxide, yellow ferric oxide.

PREMPRO 0.45 mg/1.5 mg

Each gold tablet for oral administration contains 0.45 mg conjugated estrogens, 1.5 mg medroxyprogesterone acetate and the following inactive ingredients: calcium phosphate tribasic, calcium sulfate, carnauba wax, cellulose, glyceryl monooleate, lactose, magnesium stearate, methylcellulose, pharmaceutical glaze, polyethylene glycol, sucrose, povidone, titanium dioxide, yellow ferric oxide.

PREMPRO 0.625 mg/2.5 mg

Each peach tablet for oral administration contains 0.625 mg conjugated estrogens, 2.5 mg of medroxyprogesterone acetate and the following inactive ingredients: calcium phosphate tribasic, calcium sulfate, carnauba wax, cellulose, glyceryl monooleate, lactose, magnesium stearate, methylcellulose, pharmaceutical glaze, polyethylene glycol, sucrose, povidone, titanium dioxide, red ferric oxide.

PREMPRO 0.625 mg/5 mg

Each light-blue tablet for oral administration contains 0.625 mg conjugated estrogens, 5 mg of medroxyprogesterone acetate and the following inactive ingredients: calcium phosphate tribasic, calcium sulfate, carnauba wax, cellulose, glyceryl monooleate, lactose, magnesium stearate, methylcellulose, pharmaceutical glaze, polyethylene glycol, sucrose, povidone, titanium dioxide, FD&C Blue No. 2.

PREMPHASE

Each maroon Premarin tablet for oral administration contains 0.625 mg of conjugated estrogens and the following inactive ingredients: calcium phosphate tribasic, calcium sulfate, carnauba wax, cellulose, glyceryl monooleate, lactose, magnesium stearate, methylcellulose, pharmaceutical glaze, polyethylene glycol, stearic acid, sucrose, titanium dioxide, FD&C Blue No. 2, D&C Red No. 27, FD&C Red No. 40. These tablets comply with USP Drug Release Test 1.

Each light-blue tablet for oral administration contains 0.625 mg of conjugated estrogens and 5 mg of medroxyprogesterone acetate and the following inactive ingredients: calcium phosphate tribasic, calcium sulfate, carnauba wax, cellulose, glyceryl monooleate, lactose, magnesium stearate, methylcellulose, pharmaceutical glaze, polyethylene glycol, sucrose, povidone, titanium dioxide, FD&C Blue No. 2.

Continued on next page

Prempro/Premphase—Cont.

CLINICAL PHARMACOLOGY

Endogenous estrogens are largely responsible for the development and maintenance of the female reproductive system and secondary sexual characteristics. Although circulating estrogens exist in a dynamic equilibrium of metabolic interconversions, estradiol is the principal intracellular human estrogen and is substantially more potent than its metabolites, estrone and estriol, at the receptor level.

The primary source of estrogen in normally cycling adult women is the ovarian follicle, which secretes 70 to 500 mcg of estradiol daily, depending on the phase of the menstrual cycle. After menopause, most endogenous estrogen is produced by conversion of androstenedione, secreted by the adrenal cortex, to estrone by peripheral tissues. Thus, estrone and the sulfate-conjugated form, estrone sulfate, are the most abundant circulating estrogens in postmenopausal women.

Estrogens act through binding to nuclear receptors in estrogen-responsive tissues. To date, two estrogen receptors have been identified. These vary in proportion from tissue to tissue.

Circulating estrogens modulate the pituitary secretion of the gonadotropins, luteinizing hormone (LH) and follicle stimulating hormone (FSH) through a negative feedback mechanism. Estrogens act to reduce the elevated levels of these gonadotropins seen in postmenopausal women.

Parenterally administered medroxyprogesterone acetate (MPA) inhibits gonadotropin production, which in turn prevents follicular maturation and ovulation, although available data indicate that this does not occur when the usually recommended oral dosage is given as single daily doses. MPA may achieve its beneficial effect on the endometrium in part by decreasing nuclear estrogen receptors and suppression of epithelial DNA synthesis in endometrial tissue. Androgenic and anabolic effects of MPA have been noted, but the drug is apparently devoid of significant estrogenic activity.

Pharmacokinetics

Absorption

Conjugated estrogens are soluble in water and are well absorbed from the gastrointestinal tract after release from the drug formulation. However, PREMPRO and PREMPHASE contain a formulation of medroxyprogesterone acetate (MPA) that is immediately released and conjugated estrogens that are slowly released over several hours. MPA is well absorbed from the gastrointestinal tract. Table 1 summarizes the mean pharmacokinetic parameters for unconjugated and conjugated estrogens, and medroxyprogesterone acetate following administration of 2 PREMPRO 0.625 mg/2.5 mg and 2 PREMPRO 0.625 mg/5 mg tablets to healthy postmenopausal women.

[See table 1 at top of previous page]

Table 2 summarizes the mean pharmacokinetic parameters for unconjugated and conjugated estrogens and medroxyprogesterone acetate following administration of 2 PREMPRO 0.45 mg/1.5 mg and 2 PREMPRO 0.3 mg/1.5 mg tablets to healthy, postmenopausal women.

[See table 2 above]

TABLE 2. PHARMACOKINETIC PARAMETERS FOR UNCONJUGATED AND CONJUGATED ESTROGENS (CE) AND MEDROXYPROGESTERONE ACETATE (MPA)

DRUG	2 × 0.3 mg CE/1.5 mg MPA Combination (n = 30)				2 × 0.45 mg CE/1.5 mg MPA Combination (n = 61)			
PK Parameter Arithmetic Mean (%CV)	C_{max} (pg/mL)	t_{max} (h)	$t_{1/2}$ (h)	AUC (pg•h/mL)	C_{max} (pg/mL)	t_{max} (h)	$t_{1/2}$ (h)	AUC (pg•h/mL)
Unconjugated Estrogens								
Estrone	79 (35)	9.4 (86)	51.3 (30)	5029 (45)	91 (30)	9.8 (47)	48.9 (28)	5786 (42)
BA* -Estrone	56 (46)	9.4 (86)	19.8 (39)	1429 (49)	67 (37)	9.8 (47)	21.5 (49)	2042 (52)
Equilin	30 (43)	7.9 (42)	14.0 (75)	590 (42)	35 (40)	8.5 (34)	16.4 (49)	825 (44)
PK Parameter Arithmetic Mean (%CV)	C_{max} (ng/mL)	t_{max} (h)	$t_{1/2}$ (h)	AUC (ng•h/mL)	C_{max} (ng/mL)	t_{max} (h)	$t_{1/2}$ (h)	AUC (ng•h/mL)
Conjugated Estrogens								
Total Estrone	2.4 (38)	7.1 (27)	26.5 (33)	62 (48)	3.0 (37)	8.2 (39)	25.9 (23)	78 (40)
BA* -Total Estrone	2.2 (36)	7.1 (27)	16.3 (32)	41 (44)	2.8 (36)	8.2 (39)	16.9 (36)	56 (39)
Total Equilin	1.5 (47)	5.5 (29)	11.5 (24)	22 (41)	1.9 (42)	7.2 (33)	12.2 (25)	31 (52)
PK Parameter Arithmetic Mean (%CV)	C_{max} (ng/mL)	t_{max} (h)	$t_{1/2}$ (h)	AUC (ng•h/mL)	C_{max} (ng/mL)	t_{max} (h)	$t_{1/2}$ (h)	AUC (ng•h/mL)
Medroxyprogesterone Acetate								
MPA	1.2 (42)	2.8 (61)	42.3 (34)	29.4 (30)	1.2 (42)	2.7 (52)	47.2 (41)	32.0 (36)

BA* = Baseline adjusted
C_{max} = peak plasma concentration
t_{max} = time peak concentration occurs
$t_{1/2}$ = apparent terminal-phase disposition half-life ($0.693/\lambda_z$)
AUC = total area under the concentration-time curve

TABLE 3. SUMMARY TABULATION OF THE NUMBER OF HOT FLUSHES PER DAY – MEAN VALUES AND COMPARISONS BETWEEN THE ACTIVE TREATMENT GROUPS AND THE PLACEBO GROUP – PATIENTS WITH AT LEAST 7 MODERATE TO SEVERE FLUSHES PER DAY OR AT LEAST 50 PER WEEK AT BASELINE, LOCF

Treatment[a] (No. of Patients) Time Period (week)	No. of Hot Flushes/Day: Baseline Mean ± SD	Observed Mean ± SD	Mean Change ± SD	p-Values vs. Placebo[b]
0.625 mg/2.5 mg (n=34)				
4	11.98 ± 3.54	3.19 ± 3.74	-8.78 ± 4.72	<0.001
12	11.98 ± 3.54	1.16 ± 2.22	-10.82 ± 4.61	<0.001
0.45 mg/1.5 mg (n=29)				
4	12.61 ± 4.29	3.64 ± 3.61	-8.98 ± 4.74	<0.001
12	12.61 ± 4.29	1.69 ± 3.36	-10.92 ± 4.63	<0.001
0.3 mg/1.5 mg (n=33)				
4	11.30 ± 3.13	3.70 ± 3.29	-7.60 ± 4.71	<0.001
12	11.30 ± 3.13	1.31 ± 2.82	-10.00 ± 4.60	<0.001
Placebo (n=28)				
4	11.69 ± 3.87	7.89 ± 5.28	-3.80 ± 4.71	–
12	11.69 ± 3.87	5.71 ± 5.22	-5.98 ± 4.60	–

a: Identified by dosage (mg) of Premarin/MPA or placebo.
b: There were no statistically significant differences between the 0.625 mg/2.5 mg, 0.45 mg/1.5 mg, and 0.3 mg/1.5 mg groups at any time period.

Food-Effect: Single dose studies in healthy, postmenopausal women were conducted to investigate any potential drug interaction when PREMPRO or PREMPHASE is administered with a high fat breakfast. Administration with food decreased the C_{max} of total estrone by 18 to 34% and increased total equilin C_{max} by 38% compared to the fasting state, with no other effect on the rate or extent of absorption of other conjugated or unconjugated estrogens. Administration with food approximately doubles MPA C_{max} and increases MPA AUC by approximately 20 to 30%.

Dose Proportionality: The C_{max} and AUC values for MPA observed in two separate pharmacokinetic studies conducted with 2 PREMPRO 0.625 mg/2.5 mg or 2 PREMPRO or PREMPHASE 0.625 mg/5 mg tablets exhibited nonlinear dose proportionality; doubling the MPA dose from 2 × 2.5 to 2 × 5.0 mg increased the mean C_{max} and AUC by 3.2 and 2.8 folds, respectively.

The dose proportionality of estrogens and medroxyprogesterone acetate was assessed by combining pharmacokinetic data across another two studies totaling 61 healthy, postmenopausal women. Single conjugated estrogens doses of 2 × 0.3 mg, 2 × 0.45 mg, or 2 × 0.625 mg were administered either alone or in combination with medroxyprogesterone acetate doses of 2 × 1.5 mg or 2 × 2.5 mg. Most of the estrogen components demonstrated dose proportionality; however, several estrogen components did not. Medroxyprogesterone acetate pharmacokinetic parameters increased in a dose-proportional manner.

Distribution

The distribution of exogenous estrogens is similar to that of endogenous estrogens. Estrogens are widely distributed in the body and are generally found in higher concentrations in the sex hormone target organs. Estrogens circulate in the blood largely bound to sex hormone binding globulin (SHBG) and albumin. MPA is approximately 90% bound to plasma proteins but does not bind to SHBG.

Metabolism

Exogenous estrogens are metabolized in the same manner as endogenous estrogens. Circulating estrogens exist in a dynamic equilibrium of metabolic interconversions. These transformations take place mainly in the liver. Estradiol is converted reversibly to estrone, and both can be converted to estriol, which is the major urinary metabolite. Estrogens also undergo enterohepatic recirculation via sulfate and glucuronide conjugation in the liver, biliary secretion of conjugates into the intestine, and hydrolysis in the gut followed by reabsorption. In postmenopausal women a significant proportion of the circulating estrogens exists as sulfate conjugates, especially estrone sulfate, which serves as a circulating reservoir for the formation of more active estrogens. Metabolism and elimination of MPA occur primarily in the liver via hydroxylation, with subsequent conjugation and elimination in the urine.

Excretion

Estradiol, estrone, and estriol are excreted in the urine along with glucuronide and sulfate conjugates. Most metabolites of MPA are excreted as glucuronide conjugates with only minor amounts excreted as sulfates.

Special Populations

No pharmacokinetic studies were conducted in special populations, including patients with renal or hepatic impairment.

Drug Interactions

Data from a single-dose drug-drug interaction study involving conjugated estrogens and medroxyprogesterone acetate indicate that the pharmacokinetic disposition of both drugs is not altered when the drugs are coadministered. No other clinical drug-drug interaction studies have been conducted with conjugated estrogens.

In vitro and in vivo studies have shown that estrogens are metabolized partially by cytochrome P450 3A4 (CYP3A4). Therefore, inducers or inhibitors of CYP3A4 may affect estrogen drug metabolism. Inducers of CYP3A4 such as St. John's Wort preparations (Hypericum perforatum), phenobarbital, carbamazepine, and rifampin may reduce plasma concentrations of estrogens, possibly resulting in a decrease in therapeutic effects and/or changes in the uterine bleeding profile. Inhibitors of CYP3A4 such as erythromycin, clarithromycin, ketoconazole, itraconazole, ritonavir and grapefruit juice may increase plasma concentrations of estrogens and may result in side effects.

Clinical Studies

Effects on vasomotor symptoms.

In the first year of the Health and Osteoporosis, Progestin and Estrogen (HOPE) Study, a total of 2805 postmenopausal women (average age 53.3 ± 4.9 years) were randomly assigned to one of eight treatment groups of either placebo or conjugated estrogens with or without medroxyprogesterone acetate. Efficacy for vasomotor symptoms was assessed during the first 12 weeks of treatment in a subset of symptomatic women (n = 241) who had at least 7 moderate to severe hot flushes daily or at least 50 moderate to severe hot flushes during the week before randomization. PREMPRO 0.625 mg/2.5 mg, 0.45 mg/1.5 mg, and 0.3 mg/1.5 mg were shown to be statistically better than placebo at weeks 4 and 12 for relief of both the frequency and severity of moderate to severe vasomotor symptoms. Table 3 shows the adjusted mean number of hot flushes in the PREMPRO 0.625 mg/2.5 mg, 0.45 mg/1.5 mg, 0.3 mg/1.5 mg, and placebo groups during the initial 12-week period.

[See table 3 above]

Effects on vulvar and vaginal atrophy.

Results of vaginal maturation indexes at cycles 6 and 13 showed that the differences from placebo were statistically significant ($p < 0.001$) for all treatment groups (conjugated estrogens alone and conjugated estrogens/medroxyprogesterone acetate treatment groups).

Effects on the endometrium.

In a 1-year clinical trial of 1376 women (average age 54.0 ± 4.6 years) randomized to PREMPRO 0.625 mg/2.5 mg (n=340), PREMPRO 0.625 mg/5 mg (n=338), PREMPHASE 0.625 mg/5 mg (n=351), or Premarin 0.625 mg alone (n=347), results of evaluable biopsies at 12 months (n=279, 274, 277, and 283, respectively) showed a reduced risk of endometrial hyperplasia in the two PREMPRO treatment groups (less than 1%) and in the PREMPHASE treatment

group (less than 1%; 1% when focal hyperplasia was included) compared to the Premarin group (8%; 20% when focal hyperplasia was included). See Table 4.
[See table 4 at right]

In the first year of the Health and Osteoporosis, Progestin and Estrogen (HOPE) Study, 2001 women (average age 53.3 ± 4.9 years) of whom 88% were Caucasian were treated with either Premarin 0.625 mg alone (n = 348), Premarin 0.45 mg alone (n = 338), Premarin 0.3 mg alone (n = 326) or PREMPRO 0.625 mg/2.5 mg (n = 331), PREMPRO 0.45 mg/ 1.5 mg (n = 331) or PREMPRO 0.3 mg/1.5 mg (n = 327). Results of evaluable endometrial biopsies at 12 months showed a reduced risk of endometrial hyperplasia or cancer in the PREMPRO treatment groups compared with the corresponding Premarin alone treatment groups, except for the PREMPRO 0.3 mg/1.5 mg and Premarin 0.3 mg alone groups, in each of which there was only 1 case. See Table 5. No endometrial hyperplasia or cancer was noted in those patients treated with the continuous combined regimens who continued for a second year in the osteoporosis and metabolic substudy of the HOPE study. See Table 6.
[See table 5 at right]
[See table 6 below]

Effects on uterine bleeding or spotting.

The effects of PREMPRO on uterine bleeding or spotting, as recorded on daily diary cards, were evaluated in 2 clinical trials. Results are shown in Figures 1 and 2.

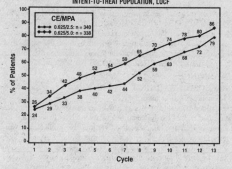

FIGURE 1. PATIENTS WITH CUMULATIVE AMENORRHEA OVER TIME PERCENTAGES OF WOMEN WITH NO BLEEDING OR SPOTTING AT A GIVEN CYCLE THROUGH CYCLE 13 INTENT-TO-TREAT POPULATION, LOCF

Note: The percentage of patients who were amenorrheic in a given cycle and through cycle 13 is shown. If data were missing, the bleeding value from the last reported day was carried forward (LOCF).

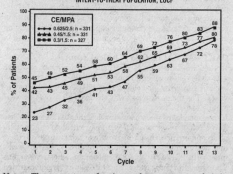

FIGURE 2. PATIENTS WITH CUMULATIVE AMENORRHEA OVER TIME PERCENTAGES OF WOMEN WITH NO BLEEDING OR SPOTTING AT A GIVEN CYCLE THROUGH CYCLE 13 INTENT-TO-TREAT POPULATION, LOCF

Note: The percentage of patients who were amenorrheic in a given cycle and through cycle 13 is shown. If data were missing, the bleeding value from the last reported day was carried forward (LOCF).

Effects on bone mineral density.
Health and Osteoporosis, Progestin and Estrogen (HOPE) Study

The HOPE study was a double-blind, randomized, placebo/ active-drug-controlled, multicenter study of healthy postmenopausal women with an intact uterus. Subjects (mean age 53.3 ± 4.9 years) were 2.3 ± 0.9 years, on average, since menopause, and took one 600-mg tablet of elemental calcium (Caltrate) daily. Subjects were not given vitamin D supplements. They were treated with PREMPRO 0.625 mg/ 2.5 mg, 0.45 mg/1.5 mg or 0.3 mg/1.5 mg, comparable doses of Premarin alone, or placebo. Prevention of bone loss was assessed by measurement of bone mineral density (BMD), primarily at the anteroposterior lumbar spine (L_2 to L_4). Secondarily, BMD measurements of the total body, femoral neck, and trochanter were also analyzed. Serum osteocalcin, urinary calcium, and N-telopeptide were used as bone turnover markers (BTM) at cycles 6, 13, 19, and 26.

Intent-to-treat subjects

All active treatment groups showed significant differences from placebo in each of the 4 BMD endpoints. These significant differences were seen at cycles 6, 13, 19, and 26. With PREMPRO, the mean percent increases in the primary efficacy measure (L_2 to L_4 BMD) at the final on-therapy evaluation (cycle 26 for those who completed and the last available evaluation for those who discontinued early) were 3.28% with 0.625 mg/2.5 mg, 2.18% with 0.45 mg/1.5 mg, and 1.71% with 0.3 mg/1.5 mg. The placebo group showed a

mean percent decrease from baseline at the final evaluation of 2.45%. These results show that the lower dose regimens of PREMPRO were effective in increasing L_2 to L_4 BMD compared with placebo and, therefore, support the efficacy of lower doses of PREMPRO.

The analysis for the other 3 BMD endpoints yielded mean percent changes from baseline in femoral trochanter that were generally larger than those seen for L_2 to L_4 and changes in femoral neck and total body that were generally smaller than those seen for L_2 to L_4. Significant differences between groups indicated that each of the PREMPRO treatment groups was more effective than placebo for all 3 of

these additional BMD endpoints. With regard to femoral neck and total body, the continuous combined treatment groups all showed mean percent increases in BMD while the placebo group showed mean percent decreases. For femoral trochanter, each of the PREMPRO groups showed a mean percent increase that was significantly greater than the small increase seen in the placebo group. The percent changes from baseline to final evaluation are shown in Table 7.
[See table 7 above]

TABLE 4. INCIDENCE OF ENDOMETRIAL HYPERPLASIA AFTER ONE YEAR OF TREATMENT

	PREMPRO 0.625 mg/2.5 mg	PREMPRO 0.625 mg/5 mg	PREMPHASE 0.625 mg/5 mg	Premarin 0.625 mg
Total number of patients	340	338	351	347
Number of patients with evaluable biopsies	279	274	277	283
No. (%) of patients with biopsies				
• all focal and non-focal hyperplasia	2 (<1)*	0 (0)*	3 (1)*	57 (20)
• excluding focal cystic hyperplasia	2 (<1)*	0 (0)*	1 (<1)*	25 (8)

*Significant (p<0.001) in comparison with Premarin (0.625 mg) alone.

TABLE 5. INCIDENCE OF ENDOMETRIAL HYPERPLASIA/CANCER[a] AFTER ONE YEAR OF TREATMENT[b]

Patient	Prempro 0.625 mg/ 2.5 mg	Premarin 0.625 mg	Prempro 0.45 mg/ 1.5 mg	Premarin 0.45 mg	Prempro 0.3 mg/ 1.5 mg	Premarin 0.3 mg
Total number of patients	331	348	331	338	327	326
Number of patients with evaluable biopsies	278	249	272	279	271	269
No. (%) of patients with biopsies						
• hyperplasia/cancer[a] (consensus[c])	0 (0)[d]	20 (8)	1 (<1)[a,d]	9 (3)	1 (<1)[e]	1 (<1)[a]

a: All cases of hyperplasia/cancer were endometrial hyperplasia except for 1 patient in the Premarin 0.3 mg group diagnosed with endometrial cancer based on endometrial biopsy and 1 patient in the Premarin/MPA 0.45 mg/1.5 mg group diagnosed with endometrial cancer based on endometrial biopsy.
b: Two (2) primary pathologists evaluated each endometrial biopsy. Where there was lack of agreement on the presence or absence of hyperplasia/cancer between the two, a third pathologist adjudicated (consensus).
c: For an endometrial biopsy to be counted as consensus endometrial hyperplasia or cancer, at least 2 pathologists had to agree on the diagnosis.
d: Significant (p <0.05) in comparison with corresponding dose of Premarin alone.
e: Non-significant in comparison with corresponding dose of Premarin alone.

TABLE 6. OSTEOPOROSIS AND METABOLIC SUBSTUDY, INCIDENCE OF ENDOMETRIAL HYPERPLASIA/CANCER[a] AFTER TWO YEARS OF TREATMENT[b]

Patient	Prempro 0.625 mg/ 2.5 mg	Premarin 0.625 mg	Prempro 0.45 mg/ 1.5 mg	Premarin 0.45 mg	Prempro 0.3 mg/ 1.5 mg	Premarin 0.3 mg
Total number of patients	75	65	75	74	79	73
Number of patients with evaluable biopsies	62	55	69	67	75	63
No. (%) of patients with biopsies						
• hyperplasia/cancer[a] (consensus[c])	0 (0)[d]	15 (27)	0 (0)[d]	10 (15)	0 (0)[d]	2 (3)

a: All cases of hyperplasia/cancer were endometrial hyperplasia in patients who continued for a second year in the osteoporosis and metabolic substudy of the HOPE study.
b: Two (2) primary pathologists evaluated each endometrial biopsy. Where there was lack of agreement on the presence or absence of hyperplasia/cancer between the two, a third pathologist adjudicated (consensus).
c: For an endometrial biopsy to be counted as consensus endometrial hyperplasia or cancer, at least 2 pathologists had to agree on the diagnosis.
d: Significant (p <0.05) in comparison with corresponding dose of Premarin alone.

TABLE 7. PERCENT CHANGE IN BONE MINERAL DENSITY: COMPARISON BETWEEN ACTIVE AND PLACEBO GROUPS IN THE INTENT-TO-TREAT POPULATION, LAST OBSERVATION CARRIED FORWARD

Region Evaluated Treatment Group[a]	No. of Subjects	Baseline (g/cm²) Mean ± SD	Change from Baseline (%) Adjusted Mean ± SE	p-Value vs Placebo
L_2 to L_4 BMD				
0.625/2.5	81	1.14 ± 0.16	3.28 ± 0.37	<0.001
0.45/1.5	89	1.16 ± 0.14	2.18 ± 0.35	<0.001
0.3/1.5	90	1.14 ± 0.15	1.71 ± 0.35	<0.001
Placebo	85	1.14 ± 0.14	-2.45 ± 0.36	
Total body BMD				
0.625/2.5	81	1.14 ± 0.08	0.87 ± 0.17	<0.001
0.45/1.5	89	1.14 ± 0.07	0.59 ± 0.17	<0.001
0.3/1.5	91	1.13 ± 0.08	0.60 ± 0.16	<0.001
Placebo	85	1.13 ± 0.08	-1.50 ± 0.17	
Femoral neck BMD				
0.625/2.5	81	0.89 ± 0.14	1.62 ± 0.46	<0.001
0.45/1.5	89	0.89 ± 0.12	1.48 ± 0.44	<0.001
0.3/1.5	91	0.86 ± 0.11	1.31 ± 0.43	<0.001
Placebo	85	0.88 ± 0.14	-1.72 ± 0.45	
Femoral trochanter BMD				
0.625/2.5	81	0.77 ± 0.14	3.35 ± 0.59	0.002
0.45/1.5	89	0.76 ± 0.12	2.84 ± 0.57	0.011
0.3/1.5	91	0.76 ± 0.12	3.93 ± 0.56	<0.001
Placebo	85	0.75 ± 0.12	0.81 ± 0.58	

a: Identified by dosage (mg/mg) of Premarin/MPA or placebo.

Continued on next page

Prempro/Premphase—Cont.

Figure 3 shows the cumulative percentage of subjects with percent changes from baseline in spine BMD equal to or greater than the percent change shown on the x-axis.

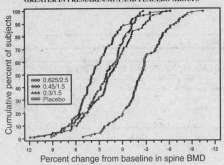

FIGURE 3. CUMULATIVE PERCENT OF SUBJECTS WITH CHANGES FROM BASELINE IN SPINE BMD OF GIVEN MAGNITUDE OR GREATER IN PREMARIN/MPA AND PLACEBO GROUPS

The mean percent changes from baseline in L_2 to L_4 BMD for women who completed the bone density study are shown with standard error bars by treatment group in Figure 4. Significant differences between each of the PREMPRO dosage groups and placebo were found at cycles 6, 13, 19, and 26.

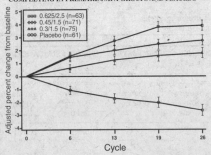

FIGURE 4. ADJUSTED MEAN (SE) PERCENT CHANGE FROM BASELINE AT EACH CYCLE IN SPINE BMD: SUBJECTS COMPLETING IN PREMARIN/MPA GROUPS AND PLACEBO

The bone turnover markers, serum osteocalcin and urinary N-telopeptide, significantly decreased (p < 0.001) in all active-treatment groups at cycles 6, 13, 19, and 26 compared with the placebo group. Larger mean decreases from baseline were seen with the active groups than with the placebo group. Significant differences from placebo were seen less frequently in urine calcium; only with PREMPRO 0.625 mg/2.5 mg and 0.45 mg/1.5 mg were there significantly larger mean decreases than with placebo at 3 or more of the 4 time points.

Women's Health Initiative Studies.

A substudy of the Women's Health Initiative (WHI) enrolled 16,608 predominantly healthy postmenopausal women (average age of 63 years, range 50 to 79; 83.9% White, 6.5% Black, 5.5% Hispanic) to assess the risks and benefits of the use of PREMPRO (0.625 mg conjugated estrogens plus 2.5 mg medroxyprogesterone acetate per day) compared to placebo in the prevention of certain chronic diseases. The primary endpoint was the incidence of coronary heart disease (CHD) (nonfatal myocardial infarction and CHD death), with invasive breast cancer as the primary adverse outcome studied. A "global index" included the earliest occurrence of CHD, invasive breast cancer, stroke, pulmonary embolism (PE), endometrial cancer, colorectal cancer, hip fracture, or death due to other cause. The study did not evaluate the effects of PREMPRO on menopausal symptoms. The estrogen plus progestin substudy was stopped early because, according to the predefined stopping rule, the increased risk of breast cancer and cardiovascular events exceeded the specified benefits included in the "global index." Results are presented in Table 8 below:
[See table 8 below]

For those outcomes included in the "global index", the absolute excess risks per 10,000 women-years in the group treated with PREMPRO were 7 more CHD events, 8 more strokes, 8 more PEs, and 8 more invasive breast cancers, while the absolute risk reductions per 10,000 women-years were 6 fewer colorectal cancers and 5 fewer hip fractures. The absolute excess risk of events included in the "global index" was 19 per 10,000 women-years. There was no difference between the groups in terms of all-cause mortality. (See **BOXED WARNING, WARNINGS,** and **PRECAUTIONS.**)

Women's Health Initiative Memory Study.

The Women's Health Initiative Memory Study (WHIMS), a substudy of WHI, enrolled 4,532 predominantly healthy postmenopausal women 65 years of age and older (47% were age 65 to 69 years, 35% were 70 to 74 years, and 18% were 75 years of age and older) to evaluate the effects of PREMPRO (0.625 mg conjugated estrogens plus 2.5 mg medroxyprogesterone acetate) on the incidence of probable dementia (primary outcome) compared with placebo.

After an average follow-up of 4 years, 40 women in the estrogen/progestin group (45 per 10,000 women-years) and 21 in the placebo group (22 per 10,000 women-years) were diagnosed with probable dementia. The relative risk of probable dementia in the hormone therapy group was 2.05 (95% CI, 1.21 to 3.48) compared to placebo. Differences between groups became apparent in the first year of treatment. It is unknown whether these findings apply to younger postmenopausal women. (See **BOXED WARNING** and **WARNINGS, Dementia.**)

INDICATIONS AND USAGE

PREMPRO or PREMPHASE therapy is indicated in women who have a uterus for the:
1. Treatment of moderate to severe vasomotor symptoms associated with the menopause.
2. Treatment of moderate to severe symptoms of vulvar and vaginal atrophy associated with the menopause. When prescribing solely for the treatment of symptoms of vulvar and vaginal atrophy, topical vaginal products should be considered.

3. Prevention of postmenopausal osteoporosis. When prescribing solely for the prevention of postmenopausal osteoporosis, therapy should only be considered for women at significant risk of osteoporosis and for whom non-estrogen medications are not considered to be appropriate. (See **CLINICAL PHARMACOLOGY, Clinical Studies.**)

The mainstays for decreasing the risk of postmenopausal osteoporosis are weight-bearing exercise, adequate calcium and vitamin D intake, and when indicated, pharmacologic therapy. Postmenopausal women require an average of 1500 mg/day of elemental calcium. Therefore, when not contraindicated, calcium supplementation may be helpful for women with suboptimal dietary intake. Vitamin D supplementation of 400-800 IU/day may also be required to ensure adequate daily intake in postmenopausal women.

CONTRAINDICATIONS

Estrogens/progestins combined should not be used in women with any of the following conditions:
1. Undiagnosed abnormal genital bleeding.
2. Known, suspected, or history of cancer of the breast.
3. Known or suspected estrogen-dependent neoplasia.
4. Active deep vein thrombosis, pulmonary embolism or a history of these conditions.
5. Active or recent (e.g., within past year) arterial thromboembolic disease (e.g., stroke, myocardial infarction).
6. Liver dysfunction or disease.
7. PREMPRO or PREMPHASE therapy should not be used in patients with known hypersensitivity to their ingredients.
8. Known or suspected pregnancy. There is no indication for PREMPRO or PREMPHASE in pregnancy. There appears to be little or no increased risk of birth defects in children born to women who have used estrogen and progestins from oral contraceptives inadvertently during pregnancy. (See **PRECAUTIONS.**)

WARNINGS

See **BOXED WARNING.**

1. Cardiovascular disorders.

Estrogen/progestin therapy has been associated with an increased risk of cardiovascular events such as myocardial infarction and stroke, as well as venous thrombosis and pulmonary embolism (venous thromboembolism or VTE). Should any of these occur or be suspected, estrogen/progestin therapy should be discontinued immediately.

Risk factors for arterial vascular disease (e.g., hypertension, diabetes mellitus, tobacco use, hypercholesterolemia, and obesity) and/or venous thromboembolism (e.g., personal history or family history of VTE, obesity, and systemic lupus erythematosus) should be managed appropriately.

a. Coronary heart disease and stroke. In the estrogen plus progestin substudy of the Women's Health Initiative (WHI) study, an increased risk of coronary heart disease (CHD) events (defined as nonfatal myocardial infarction and CHD death) was observed in women receiving PREMPRO (0.625 mg conjugated estrogens plus 2.5 mg medroxyprogesterone acetate) per day compared to women receiving placebo (37 vs 30 per 10,000 women-years). The increase in risk was observed in year one and persisted. (See **CLINICAL PHARMACOLOGY, Clinical Studies.**)

In the same substudy of WHI, an increased risk of stroke was observed in women receiving PREMPRO compared to women receiving placebo (29 vs 21 per 10,000 women-years). The increase in risk was observed after the first year and persisted.

In postmenopausal women with documented heart disease (n = 2,763, average age 66.7 years) a controlled clinical trial of secondary prevention of cardiovascular disease (Heart and Estrogen/progestin Replacement Study; HERS) treatment with PREMPRO (0.625 mg conjugated estrogens plus 2.5 mg medroxyprogesterone acetate per day) demonstrated no cardiovascular benefit. During an average follow-up of 4.1 years, treatment with PREMPRO did not reduce the overall rate of CHD events in postmenopausal women with established coronary heart disease. There were more CHD events in the PREMPRO-treated group than in the placebo group in year 1, but not during the subsequent years. Two thousand three hundred and twenty one women from the original HERS trial agreed to participate in an open label extension of HERS, HERS II. Average follow-up in HERS II was an additional 2.7 years, for a total of 6.8 years overall. Rates of CHD events were comparable among women in the PREMPRO group and the placebo group in HERS, HERS II, and overall.

Large doses of estrogen (5 mg conjugated estrogens per day), comparable to those used to treat cancer of the prostate and breast, have been shown in a large prospective clinical trial in men to increase the risk of nonfatal myocardial infarction, pulmonary embolism, and thrombophlebitis.

b. Venous thromboembolism (VTE). In the estrogen plus progestin substudy of WHI, a 2-fold greater rate of VTE, including deep venous thrombosis and pulmonary embolism, was observed in women receiving PREMPRO compared to women receiving placebo. The rate of VTE was 34 per 10,000 women-years in the PREMPRO group compared to 16 per 10,000 women-years in the placebo group. The increase in VTE risk was observed during the first year and persisted. (See **CLINICAL PHARMACOLOGY, Clinical Studies.**)

If feasible, estrogens should be discontinued at least 4 to 6 weeks before surgery of the type associated with an increased risk of thromboembolism, or during periods of prolonged immobilization.

TABLE 8. RELATIVE AND ABSOLUTE RISK SEEN IN THE ESTROGEN PLUS PROGESTIN SUBSTUDY OF WHI[a]

Event[c]	Relative Risk PREMPRO vs Placebo at 5.2 Years (Nominal 95% CI*)	Placebo n=8102	PREMPRO n=8506
		Absolute Risk per 10,000 Women-years	
CHD events	1.29 (1.02-1.63)	30	37
Non-fatal MI	*1.32 (1.02-1.72)*	*23*	*30*
CHD death	*1.18 (0.70-1.97)*	*6*	*7*
Invasive breast cancer[b]	1.26 (1.00-1.59)	30	38
Stroke	1.41 (1.07-1.85)	21	29
Pulmonary embolism	2.13 (1.39-3.25)	8	16
Colorectal cancer	0.63 (0.43-0.92)	16	10
Endometrial cancer	0.83 (0.47-1.47)	6	5
Hip fracture	0.66 (0.45-0.98)	15	10
Death due to causes other than the events above	0.92 (0.74-1.14)	40	37
Global Index[c]	1.15 (1.03-1.28)	151	170
Deep vein thrombosis[d]	2.07 (1.49-2.87)	13	26
Vertebral fractures[d]	0.66 (0.44-0.98)	15	9
Other osteoporotic fractures[d]	0.77 (0.69-0.86)	170	131

a: adapted from JAMA, 2002; 288:321-333
b: includes metastatic and non-metastatic breast cancer with the exception of in situ breast cancer
c: a subset of the events was combined in a "global index," defined as the earliest occurrence of CHD events, invasive breast cancer, stroke, pulmonary embolism, endometrial cancer, colorectal cancer, hip fracture, or death due to other causes
d: not included in Global Index
*: nominal confidence intervals unadjusted for multiple looks and multiple comparisons. Except for deep vein thrombosis and other osteoporotic fractures, the relative risks were not statistically significant.

2. Malignant neoplasms.

a. Breast cancer.

The use of estrogens and progestins by postmenopausal women has been reported to increase the risk of breast cancer. The most important randomized clinical trial providing information about this issue is the Women's Health Initiative (WHI) trial of estrogen plus progestin (see **CLINICAL PHARMACOLOGY, Clinical Studies.**) The results from observational studies are generally consistent with those of the WHI clinical trial.

After a mean follow-up of 5.6 years, the WHI trial reported an increased risk of breast cancer in women who took estrogen plus progestin. Observational studies have also reported an increased risk for estrogen/progestin combination therapy, and a smaller increased risk for estrogen alone therapy, after several years of use. For both findings, the excess risk increased with duration of use, and appeared to return to baseline over about five years after stopping treatment (only the observational studies have substantial data on risk after stopping). In these studies, the risk of breast cancer was greater, and became apparent earlier, with estrogen/progestin combination therapy as compared to estrogen alone therapy. However, these studies have not found significant variation in the risk of breast cancer among different estrogens or among different estrogen/progestin combinations, doses, or routes of administration.

In the WHI trial of estrogen plus progestin, 26% of the women reported prior use of estrogen alone and/or estrogen/progestin combination hormone therapy. After a mean follow-up of 5.6 years during the clinical trial, the overall relative risk of invasive breast cancer was 1.24 (95% confidence interval 1.01-1.54), and the overall absolute risk was 41 vs. 33 cases per 10,000 women-years, for estrogen plus progestin compared with placebo. Among women who reported prior use of hormone therapy, the relative risk of invasive breast cancer was 1.86, and the absolute risk was 46 vs. 25 cases per 10,000 women-years, for estrogen plus progestin compared with placebo. Among women who reported no prior use of hormone therapy, the relative risk of invasive breast cancer was 1.09, and the absolute risk was 40 vs. 36 cases per 10,000 women-years for estrogen plus progestin compared with placebo. In the WHI trial, invasive breast cancers were larger and diagnosed at a more advanced stage in the estrogen plus progestin group compared with the placebo group. Metastatic disease was rare with no apparent difference between the two groups. Other prognostic factors such as histologic subtype, grade and hormone receptor status did not differ between the groups.

The observational Million Women Study in Europe reported an increased risk of mortality due to breast cancer among current users of estrogens alone or estrogens plus progestins compared to never users, while the estrogen plus progestin sub-study of WHI showed no effect on breast cancer mortality with a mean follow-up of 5.6 years.

The use of estrogen plus progestin has been reported to result in an increase in abnormal mammograms requiring further evaluation. All women should receive yearly breast examinations by a healthcare provider and perform monthly breast self-examinations. In addition, mammography examinations should be scheduled based on patient age, risk factors, and prior mammogram results.

b. Endometrial cancer. The reported endometrial cancer risk among unopposed estrogen users is about 2- to 12-fold greater than in nonusers, and appears dependent on duration of treatment and on estrogen dose. Most studies show no significant increased risk associated with the use of estrogens for less than one year. The greatest risk appears associated with prolonged use, with increased risks of 15- to 24-fold for five to ten years or more, and this risk has been shown to persist for at least 8 to 15 years after estrogen therapy is discontinued.

Clinical surveillance of all women taking estrogen/progestin combinations is important. Adequate diagnostic measures, including endometrial sampling when indicated, should be undertaken to rule out malignancy in all cases of undiagnosed persistent or recurring abnormal vaginal bleeding. There is no evidence that the use of natural estrogens results in a different endometrial risk profile than synthetic estrogens of equivalent estrogen dose.

Endometrial hyperplasia (a possible precursor of endometrial cancer) has been reported to occur at a rate of approximately 1% or less with PREMPRO or PREMPHASE in two large clinical trials. In the two large clinical trials described above, two cases of endometrial cancer were reported to occur among women taking combination Premarin/medroxyprogesterone acetate therapy.

3. Dementia.

In the Women's Health Initiative Memory Study (WHIMS), an ancillary study of WHI, a population of 4,532 women aged 65 to 79 years was randomized to PREMPRO (0.625 mg/2.5 mg) or placebo. A population of 2,947 hysterectomized women, aged 65 to 79 years, was randomized to Premarin (0.625 mg) or placebo. In the planned analysis, pooling the events in women receiving Premarin or PREMPRO in comparison to those in women on placebo, the overall relative risk (RR) for probable dementia was 1.76 (95% CI 1.19-2.60). In the estrogen-alone group, after an average follow-up of 5.2 years a RR of 1.49 (95% CI 0.83-2.66) for probable dementia was observed compared to placebo. In the estrogen-plus-progestin group, after an average follow-up of 4 years, a RR of 2.05 (95% CI 1.21-3.48) for probable dementia was observed compared to placebo. Since this study was conducted in women aged 65 to 79 years, it is unknown whether these findings apply to younger postmenopausal women. (See **PRECAUTIONS, Geriatric Use.**)

4. Gallbladder Disease.

A 2- to 4-fold increase in the risk of gallbladder disease requiring surgery in postmenopausal women receiving estrogens has been reported.

5. Hypercalcemia.

Estrogen administration may lead to severe hypercalcemia in patients with breast cancer and bone metastases. If hypercalcemia occurs, use of the drug should be stopped and appropriate measures taken to reduce the serum calcium level.

6. Visual Abnormalities.

Retinal vascular thrombosis has been reported in patients receiving estrogens. Discontinue medication pending examination if there is sudden partial or complete loss of vision, or a sudden onset of proptosis, diplopia, or migraine. If examination reveals papilledema or retinal vascular lesions, estrogens should be discontinued.

PRECAUTIONS

A. General

1. Addition of a progestin when a woman has not had a hysterectomy.

Studies of the addition of a progestin for 10 or more days of a cycle of estrogen administration, or daily with estrogen in a continuous regimen, have reported a lowered incidence of endometrial hyperplasia than would be induced by estrogen treatment alone. Endometrial hyperplasia may be a precursor to endometrial cancer.

There are, however, possible risks that may be associated with the use of progestins with estrogens compared with estrogen-alone regimens. These include a possible increased risk of breast cancer, adverse effects on lipoprotein metabolism (e.g., lowering HDL, raising LDL) and impairment of glucose tolerance.

2. Elevated blood pressure.

In a small number of case reports, substantial increases in blood pressure have been attributed to idiosyncratic reactions to estrogens. In a large, randomized, placebo-controlled clinical trial, a generalized effect of estrogen therapy on blood pressure was not seen. Blood pressure should be monitored at regular intervals with estrogen use.

3. Hypertriglyceridemia.

In patients with pre-existing hypertriglyceridemia, estrogen therapy may be associated with elevations of plasma triglycerides leading to pancreatitis and other complications. In the HOPE study, the mean percent increase from baseline in serum triglycerides after one year of treatment with PREMPRO 0.625 mg/2.5 mg, 0.45 mg/1.5 mg, and 0.3 mg/1.5 mg compared with placebo were 32.8, 24.8, 23.3, and 10.7, respectively. After two years of treatment, the mean percent changes were 33.0, 17.1, 21.6, and 5.5, respectively.

4. Impaired liver function and past history of cholestatic jaundice.

Estrogens may be poorly metabolized in patients with impaired liver function. For patients with a history of cholestatic jaundice associated with past estrogen use or with pregnancy, caution should be exercised and in the case of recurrence, medication should be discontinued.

5. Hypothyroidism.

Estrogen administration leads to increased thyroid-binding globulin (TBG) levels. Patients with normal thyroid function can compensate for the increased TBG by making more thyroid hormone, thus maintaining free T_4 and T_3 serum concentrations in the normal range. Patients dependent on thyroid hormone replacement therapy who are also receiving estrogens may require increased doses of their thyroid replacement therapy. These patients should have their thyroid function monitored in order to maintain their free thyroid hormone levels in an acceptable range.

6. Fluid retention.

Because estrogens/progestins may cause some degree of fluid retention, patients with conditions that might be influenced by this factor, such as cardiac or renal dysfunction, warrant careful observation when estrogens are prescribed.

7. Hypocalcemia.

Estrogens should be used with caution in individuals with severe hypocalcemia.

8. Ovarian cancer.

The estrogen plus progestin substudy of WHI reported that after an average follow-up of 5.6 years, the relative risk of ovarian cancer for estrogen plus progestin versus placebo was 1.58 (95% confidence interval 0.77–3.24) but was not statistically significant. The absolute risk for estrogen plus progestin versus placebo was 4.2 versus 2.7 cases per 10,000 women-years. In some epidemiologic studies, the use of estrogen-only products, in particular for ten or more years, has been associated with an increased risk of ovarian cancer. Other epidemiologic studies have not found these associations.

9. Exacerbation of endometriosis.

Endometriosis may be exacerbated with administration of estrogen therapy.

10. Exacerbation of other conditions.

Estrogen therapy may cause an exacerbation of asthma, diabetes mellitus, epilepsy, migraine, porphyria, systemic lupus erythematosus, and hepatic hemangiomas and should be used with caution in women with these conditions.

B. Patient Information

Physicians are advised to discuss the contents of the PATIENT INFORMATION leaflet with patients for whom they prescribe PREMPRO or PREMPHASE.

C. Laboratory Tests

Estrogen administration should be initiated at the lowest dose approved for the indication and then guided by clinical response rather than by serum hormone levels (e.g., estradiol, FSH).

D. Drug/Laboratory Test Interactions

1. Accelerated prothrombin time, partial thromboplastin time, and platelet aggregation time; increased platelet count; increased factors II, VII antigen, VIII coagulant activity, IX, X, XII, VII-X complex, II-VII-X complex, and beta-thromboglobulin; decreased levels of anti-factor Xa and antithrombin III, decreased antithrombin III activity; increased levels of fibrinogen and fibrinogen activity; increased plasminogen antigen and activity.
2. Increased thyroid binding globulin (TBG) levels leading to increased circulating total thyroid hormone levels as measured by protein-bound iodine (PBI), T_4 levels (by column or by radioimmunoassay), or T_3 levels by radioimmunoassay. T_3 resin uptake is decreased, reflecting the elevated TBG. Free T_4 and free T_3 concentrations are unaltered. Patients on thyroid replacement therapy may require higher doses of thyroid hormone.
3. Other binding proteins may be elevated in serum, i.e., corticosteroid binding globulin (CBG), sex hormone binding globulin (SHBG), leading to increased total circulating corticosteroids and sex steroids, respectively. Free hormone concentrations may be decreased. Other plasma proteins may be increased (angiotensinogen/renin substrate, alpha-1-antitrypsin, ceruloplasmin).
4. Increased plasma HDL and HDL_2 cholesterol subfraction concentrations, reduced LDL cholesterol concentration, increased triglyceride levels.
5. Impaired glucose tolerance.
6. Reduced response to metyrapone test.
7. Aminoglutethimide administered concomitantly with medroxyprogesterone acetate (MPA) may significantly depress the bioavailability of MPA.

E. Carcinogenesis, Mutagenesis, Impairment of Fertility

(See **BOXED WARNINGS, WARNINGS,** and **PRECAUTIONS.**)

Long-term continuous administration of natural and synthetic estrogens in certain animal species increases the frequency of carcinomas of the breasts, uterus, cervix, vagina, testis, and liver.

In a two-year oral study of medroxyprogesterone acetate (MPA) in which female rats were exposed to dosages of up to 5000 mcg/kg/day in their diets (50 times higher – based on AUC values – than the level observed experimentally in women taking 10 mg of MPA), a dose-related increase in pancreatic islet cell tumors (adenomas and carcinomas) occurred. Pancreatic tumor incidence was increased at 1000 and 5000 mcg/kg/day, but not at 200 mcg/kg/day.

A decreased incidence of spontaneous mammary gland tumors was observed in all three MPA-treated groups, compared with controls, in the two-year rat study. The mechanism for the decreased incidence of mammary gland tumors observed in the MPA-treated rats may be linked to the significant decrease in serum prolactin concentration observed in rats.

Beagle dogs treated with MPA developed mammary nodules, some of which were malignant. Although nodules occasionally appeared in control animals, they were intermittent in nature, whereas the nodules in the drug-treated animals were larger, more numerous, persistent, and there were some breast malignancies with metastases. It is known that progestogens stimulate synthesis and release of growth hormone in dogs. The growth hormone, along with the progestogen, stimulates mammary growth and tumors. In contrast, growth hormone in humans is not increased, nor does growth hormone have any significant mammotrophic role. No pancreatic tumors occurred in dogs.

F. Pregnancy

PREMPRO and PREMPHASE should not be used during pregnancy. (See **CONTRAINDICATIONS.**)

G. Nursing Mothers

Estrogen administration to nursing mothers has been shown to decrease the quantity and quality of the milk. Detectable amounts of estrogen and progestin have been identified in the milk of mothers receiving these drugs. Caution should be exercised when PREMPRO or PREMPHASE are administered to a nursing woman.

H. Pediatric Use

PREMPRO and PREMPHASE are not indicated in children.

I. Geriatric Use

Of the total number of subjects in the estrogen plus progestin substudy of the Women's Health Initiative study, 44% (n = 7320) were 65 years and over, while 6.6% (n = 1,095) were 75 years and over (see **CLINICAL PHARMACOLOGY, Clinical Studies**). There was a higher incidence of stroke and invasive breast cancer in women 75 and over compared to women less than 75 years of age.

In the Women's Health Initiative Memory Study (WHIMS), an ancillary study of WHI, a population of 4,532 women aged 65 to 79 years was randomized to PREMPRO (0.625 mg/2.5 mg) or placebo. A population of 2,947 hysterectomized women, aged 65 to 79 years, was randomized to Premarin (0.625 mg) or placebo. In the planned analysis, pooling the events in women receiving Premarin or PREMPRO in comparison to those in women on placebo, the overall relative risk (RR) for probable dementia was 1.76 (95% CI 1.19-2.60). In the estrogen-alone group, after an average follow-up of 5.2 years a RR of 1.49 (95% CI 0.83-2.66) for probable dementia was observed compared to placebo. In the estrogen-plus-progestin group, after an average follow-up of 4 years, a RR of 2.05 (95% CI 1.21-3.48) for probable dementia was observed compared to placebo. Since this study was conducted in women aged 65 to 79

Continued on next page

Prempro/Premphase—Cont.

years, it is unknown whether these findings apply to younger postmenopausal women. (See **WARNINGS, Dementia.**)

With respect to efficacy in the approved indications, there have not been sufficient numbers of geriatric patients involved in studies utilizing Premarin and medroxyprogesterone acetate to determine whether those over 65 years of age differ from younger subjects in their response to PREMPRO or PREMPHASE.

ADVERSE REACTIONS

See **BOXED WARNING, WARNINGS,** and **PRECAUTIONS.**

Because clinical trials are conducted under widely varying conditions, adverse reaction rates observed in the clinical trials of a drug cannot be directly compared with rates in the clinical trials of another drug and may not reflect the rates observed in practice. The adverse reaction information from clinical trials does, however, provide a basis for identifying the adverse events that appear to be related to drug use and for approximating rates.

In a 1-year clinical trial that included 678 postmenopausal women treated with PREMPRO, 351 postmenopausal women treated with PREMPHASE, and 347 postmenopausal women treated with Premarin, the following adverse events occurred at a rate ≥ 5% (see Table 9):

[See table 9 at right]

During the first year of a 2-year clinical trial with 2333 postmenopausal women between 40 and 65 years of age (88% Caucasian), 2001 women received continuous regimens of either 0.625 mg of CE with or without 2.5 mg MPA, or 0.45 mg or 0.3 mg of CE with or without 1.5 mg MPA, and 332 received placebo tablets. Table 10 summarizes adverse events that occurred at a rate ≥ 5% in at least 1 treatment group.

[See table 10 at right]

The following additional adverse reactions have been reported with estrogen and/or progestin therapy:

1. *Genitourinary system*

Changes in vaginal bleeding pattern and abnormal withdrawal bleeding or flow, breakthrough bleeding, spotting, dysmenorrhea, change in amount of cervical secretion, premenstrual-like syndrome, cystitis-like syndrome, increase in size of uterine leiomyomata, vaginal candidiasis, amenorrhea, changes in cervical erosion, ovarian cancer, endometrial hyperplasia, endometrial cancer.

2. *Breasts*

Tenderness, enlargement, pain, nipple discharge, galactorrhea, fibrocystic breast changes, breast cancer.

3. *Cardiovascular*

Deep and superficial venous thrombosis, pulmonary embolism, thrombophlebitis, myocardial infarction, stroke, increase in blood pressure.

4. *Gastrointestinal*

Nausea, cholestatic jaundice, changes in appetite, vomiting, abdominal cramps, bloating, increased incidence of gallbladder disease, pancreatitis, enlargement of hepatic hemangiomas.

5. *Skin*

Chloasma or melasma that may persist when drug is discontinued, erythema multiforme, erythema nodosum, hemorrhagic eruption, loss of scalp hair, hirsutism, itching, urticaria, pruritus, generalized rash, rash (allergic) with and without pruritus, acne.

6. *Eyes*

Neuro-ocular lesions, e.g., retinal vascular thrombosis and optic neuritis, intolerance of contact lenses.

7. *Central Nervous System (CNS)*

Headache, dizziness, mental depression, mood disturbances, anxiety, irritability, nervousness, migraine, chorea, insomnia, somnolence, exacerbation of epilepsy, dementia.

8. *Miscellaneous*

Increase or decrease in weight, edema, changes in libido, fatigue, backache, reduced carbohydrate tolerance, aggravation of porphyria, pyrexia, urticaria, angioedema, anaphylactoid/anaphylactic reactions, hypocalcemia, exacerbation of asthma, increased triglycerides.

OVERDOSAGE

Serious ill effects have not been reported following acute ingestion of large doses of estrogen/progestin-containing drug products by young children. Overdosage of estrogen/progestin may cause nausea and vomiting, and withdrawal bleeding may occur in females.

DOSAGE AND ADMINISTRATION

Use of estrogens, alone or in combination with a progestin, should be with the lowest effective dose and for the shortest duration consistent with treatment goals and risks for the individual woman. Patients should be re-evaluated periodically as clinically appropriate (e.g., at 3-month to 6-month intervals) to determine if treatment is still necessary (see **BOXED WARNING** and **WARNINGS.**) For women who have a uterus, adequate diagnostic measures, such as endometrial sampling, when indicated, should be undertaken to rule out malignancy in cases of undiagnosed persistent or recurring abnormal vaginal bleeding.

PREMPRO therapy consists of a single tablet to be taken once daily.

1. For treatment of moderate to severe vasomotor symptoms and/or moderate to severe symptoms of vulvar and vaginal atrophy associated with the menopause. When

prescribing solely for the treatment of symptoms of vulvar and vaginal atrophy, topical vaginal products should be considered.
- PREMPRO 0.3 mg/1.5 mg
- PREMPRO 0.45 mg/1.5 mg
- PREMPRO 0.625 mg/2.5 mg
- PREMPRO 0.625 mg/5 mg
- PREMPHASE

Patients should be treated with the lowest effective dose. Generally women should be started at 0.3 mg/1.5 mg PREMPRO daily. Subsequent dosage adjustment may be made based upon the individual patient response. In pa-

TABLE 9: ALL TREATMENT EMERGENT STUDY EVENTS REGARDLESS OF DRUG RELATIONSHIP REPORTED AT A FREQUENCY ≥ 5%

Body System Adverse event	PREMPRO 0.625 mg/2.5 mg continuous (n=340)	PREMPRO 0.625 mg/5.0 mg continuous (n=338)	PREMPHASE 0.625 mg/5.0 mg sequential (n=351)	PREMARIN 0.625 mg daily (n=347)
Body as a whole				
abdominal pain	16%	21%	23%	17%
accidental injury	5%	4%	5%	5%
asthenia	6%	8%	10%	8%
back pain	14%	13%	16%	14%
flu syndrome	10%	13%	12%	14%
headache	36%	28%	37%	38%
infection	16%	16%	18%	14%
pain	11%	13%	12%	13%
pelvic pain	4%	5%	5%	5%
Digestive system				
diarrhea	6%	6%	5%	10%
dyspepsia	6%	6%	5%	5%
flatulence	8%	9%	8%	5%
nausea	11%	9%	11%	11%
Metabolic and Nutritional				
peripheral edema	4%	4%	3%	5%
Musculoskeletal system				
arthralgia	9%	7%	9%	7%
leg cramps	3%	4%	5%	4%
Nervous system				
depression	6%	11%	11%	10%
dizziness	5%	3%	4%	6%
hypertonia	4%	3%	3%	7%
Respiratory system				
pharyngitis	11%	11%	13%	12%
rhinitis	8%	6%	8%	7%
sinusitis	8%	7%	7%	5%
Skin and appendages				
pruritus	10%	8%	5%	4%
rash	4%	6%	4%	3%
Urogenital system				
breast pain	33%	38%	32%	12%
cervix disorder	4%	4%	5%	5%
dysmenorrhea	8%	5%	13%	5%
leukorrhea	6%	5%	9%	8%
vaginal hemorrhage	2%	1%	3%	6%
vaginitis	7%	7%	5%	3%

TABLE 10. PERCENT OF PATIENTS WITH TREATMENT EMERGENT STUDY EVENTS REGARDLESS OF DRUG RELATIONSHIP REPORTED AT A FREQUENCY ≥ 5% DURING STUDY YEAR 1

Body System Adverse event	Premarin 0.625 mg daily (n=348)	Prempro 0.625 mg/ 2.5 mg continuous (n=331)	Premarin 0.45 mg daily (n=338)	Prempro 0.45 mg/ 1.5 mg continuous (n=331)	Premarin 0.3 mg daily (n=326)	Prempro 0.3 mg/ 1.5 mg continuous (n=327)	Placebo daily (n=332)
Any adverse event	93%	92%	90%	89%	90%	90%	85%
Body as a whole							
abdominal pain	16%	17%	15%	16%	17%	13%	11%
accidental injury	6%	10%	12%	9%	6%	9%	9%
asthenia	7%	8%	7%	8%	8%	6%	5%
back pain	14%	12%	13%	13%	13%	12%	12%
flu syndrome	11%	8%	11%	11%	10%	10%	11%
headache	26%	28%	32%	29%	29%	33%	28%
infection	18%	21%	22%	19%	23%	18%	22%
pain	17%	14%	18%	15%	20%	20%	18%
Digestive system							
diarrhea	6%	7%	7%	7%	6%	6%	6%
dyspepsia	9%	8%	9%	8%	11%	6%	14%
flatulence	7%	7%	7%	8%	6%	5%	3%
nausea	9%	7%	7%	10%	6%	8%	9%
Musculoskeletal system							
arthralgia	14%	9%	12%	13%	7%	10%	12%
leg cramps	5%	7%	7%	5%	3%	4%	2%
myalgia	5%	5%	5%	5%	9%	4%	8%
Nervous system							
anxiety	5%	4%	4%	5%	4%	2%	4%
depression	7%	11%	8%	5%	5%	8%	7%
dizziness	6%	3%	6%	5%	4%	5%	5%
insomnia	6%	6%	7%	7%	7%	6%	10%
nervousness	3%	3%	5%	2%	2%	2%	2%
Respiratory system							
cough increased	4%	8%	7%	5%	4%	6%	4%
pharyngitis	10%	11%	10%	8%	12%	9%	11%
rhinitis	6%	8%	9%	9%	10%	10%	13%
sinusitis	6%	8%	11%	8%	7%	10%	7%
upper respiratory infection	12%	10%	10%	9%	9%	11%	11%
Skin and appendages							
pruritus	4%	4%	5%	5%	5%	5%	2%
Urogenital system							
breast enlargement	<1%	5%	1%	3%	2%	2%	<1%
breast pain	11%	26%	12%	21%	7%	13%	9%
dysmenorrhea	4%	5%	3%	6%	1%	3%	<1%
leukorrhea	5%	4%	7%	5%	4%	3%	3%
vaginal hemorrhage	14%	6%	4%	4%	2%	2%	0%
vaginal moniliasis	6%	8%	5%	7%	5%	4%	2%
vaginitis	7%	5%	6%	6%	5%	4%	1%

tients where bleeding or spotting remains a problem, after appropriate evaluation, consideration should be given to changing the dose level. This dose should be periodically reassessed by the healthcare provider.

2. For prevention of postmenopausal osteoporosis. When prescribing solely for the prevention of postmenopausal osteoporosis, therapy should be considered only for women at significant risk of osteoporosis and for whom non-estrogen medications are not considered to be appropriate.

- PREMPRO 0.3 mg/1.5 mg
- PREMPRO 0.45 mg/1.5 mg
- PREMPRO 0.625 mg/2.5 mg
- PREMPRO 0.625 mg/5 mg
- PREMPHASE

Patients should be treated with the lowest effective dose. Generally women should be started at 0.3 mg/1.5 mg PREMPRO daily. Dosage may be adjusted depending on individual clinical and bone mineral density responses. This dose should be periodically reassessed by the healthcare provider.

In patients where bleeding or spotting remains a problem, after appropriate evaluation, consideration should be given to changing the dose level. This dose should be periodically reassessed by the healthcare provider.

PREMPHASE therapy consists of two separate tablets; one maroon 0.625 mg Premarin tablet taken daily on days 1 through 14 and one light-blue tablet, containing 0.625 mg conjugated estrogens and 5 mg of medroxyprogesterone acetate, taken on days 15 through 28.

HOW SUPPLIED

PREMPRO therapy consists of a single tablet to be taken once daily.

PREMPRO 0.3 mg/1.5 mg

Each carton contains 3 EZ DIAL® dispensers containing 28 tablets. One EZ DIAL dispenser contains 28 oval, cream tablets containing 0.3 mg of the conjugated estrogens found in Premarin tablets and 1.5 mg medroxyprogesterone acetate for oral administration (NDC 0046-0938-09).

PREMPRO 0.45 mg/1.5 mg

Each carton includes 3 EZ DIAL dispensers containing 28 tablets. One EZ DIAL dispenser contains 28 oval, gold tablets containing 0.45 mg of the conjugated estrogens found in Premarin tablets and 1.5 mg medroxyprogesterone acetate for oral administration (NDC 0046-0937-09).

PREMPRO 0.625 mg/2.5 mg

Each carton includes 3 EZ DIAL dispensers containing 28 tablets. One EZ DIAL dispenser contains 28 oval, peach tablets containing 0.625 mg of the conjugated estrogens found in Premarin tablets and 2.5 mg of medroxyprogesterone acetate for oral administration (NDC 0046-0875-06).

PREMPRO 0.625 mg/5 mg

Each carton includes 3 EZ DIAL dispensers containing 28 tablets. One EZ DIAL dispenser contains 28 oval, light-blue tablets containing 0.625 mg of the conjugated estrogens found in Premarin tablets and 5 mg of medroxyprogesterone acetate for oral administration (NDC 0046-0975-06).

PREMPHASE therapy consists of two separate tablets; one maroon Premarin tablet taken daily on days 1 through 14 and one light-blue tablet taken on days 15 through 28.

Each carton includes 3 EZ DIAL dispensers containing 28 tablets. One EZ DIAL dispenser contains 14 oval, maroon Premarin tablets containing 0.625 mg of conjugated estrogens and 14 oval, light-blue tablets that contain 0.625 mg of the conjugated estrogens found in Premarin tablets and 5 mg of medroxyprogesterone acetate for oral administration (NDC 0046-2573-06).

The appearance of PREMPRO tablets is a trademark of Wyeth Pharmaceuticals.

The appearance of Premarin tablets is a trademark of Wyeth Pharmaceuticals. The appearance of the conjugated estrogens/medroxyprogesterone acetate combination tablets is a registered trademark.

Store at 20–25°C (68–77°F); excursions permitted to 15–30°C (59–86°F) [see USP Controlled Room Temperature].

PATIENT INFORMATION

(Updated August 9, 2004)

PREMPRO™

(conjugated estrogens/medroxyprogesterone acetate tablets)

PREMPHASE®

(conjugated estrogens/medroxyprogesterone acetate tablets)

Read this PATIENT INFORMATION before you start taking PREMPRO or PREMPHASE and read what you get each time you refill PREMPRO or PREMPHASE. There may be new information. This information does not take the place of talking to your healthcare provider about your medical condition or your treatment.

What is the most important information I should know about PREMPRO and PREMPHASE (combinations of estrogens and a progestin)?

Do not use estrogens and progestins to prevent heart disease, heart attacks, strokes, or dementia.

Using estrogens and progestins may increase your chances of getting heart attacks, strokes, breast cancer, or blood clots. Using estrogens, with or without progestins, may increase your risk of dementia, based on a study of women age 65 years or older. You and your

---

healthcare provider should talk regularly about whether you still need treatment with PREMPRO or PREMPHASE.

What is PREMPRO or PREMPHASE?

PREMPRO or PREMPHASE are medicines that contain two kinds of hormones, estrogens and a progestin.

PREMPRO or PREMPHASE is used after menopause to:

- **reduce moderate to severe hot flashes.** Estrogens are hormones made by a woman's ovaries. The ovaries normally stop making estrogens when a woman is between 45 and 55 years old. This drop in body estrogen levels causes the "change of life" or menopause (the end of monthly menstrual periods). Sometimes, both ovaries are removed during an operation before natural menopause takes place. The sudden drop in estrogen levels causes "surgical menopause."

When the estrogen levels begin dropping, some women get very uncomfortable symptoms, such as feelings of warmth in the face, neck, and chest, or sudden strong feelings of heat and sweating ("hot flashes" or "hot flushes"). In some women the symptoms are mild, and they will not need to take estrogens. In other women, symptoms can be more severe. You and your healthcare provider should talk regularly about whether you still need treatment with PREMPRO or PREMPHASE.

- **treat moderate to severe dryness, itching, and burning, in and around the vagina.** You and your healthcare provider should talk regularly about whether you still need treatment with PREMPRO or PREMPHASE to control these problems. If you use Premarin only to treat your dryness, itching, and burning in and around your vagina, talk with your healthcare provider about whether a topical vaginal product would be better for you.

- **help reduce your chances of getting osteoporosis (thin weak bones).** Osteoporosis from menopause is a thinning of the bones that makes them weaker and easier to break. If you use PREMPRO or PREMPHASE only to prevent osteoporosis from menopause, talk with your healthcare provider about whether a different treatment or medicine without estrogens might be better for you. You and your healthcare provider should talk regularly about whether you should continue with PREMPRO or PREMPHASE. Weight-bearing exercise, like walking or running, and taking calcium and vitamin D supplements may also lower your chances of getting postmenopausal osteoporosis. It is important to talk about exercise and supplements with your healthcare provider before starting them.

Who should not take PREMPRO or PREMPHASE?

Do not take PREMPRO or PREMPHASE if you have had your uterus removed (hysterectomy).

PREMPRO and PREMPHASE contain a progestin to decrease the chances of getting cancer of the uterus. If you do not have a uterus, you do not need a progestin and you should not take PREMPRO or PREMPHASE.

Do not start taking PREMPRO or PREMPHASE if you:

- **have unusual vaginal bleeding.**
- **currently have or have had certain cancers.** Estrogens may increase the chances of getting certain types of cancers, including cancer of the breast or uterus. If you have or had cancer, talk with your healthcare provider about whether you should take PREMPRO or PREMPHASE.
- **had a stroke or heart attack in the past year.**
- **currently have or have had blood clots.**
- **currently have liver problems.**
- **are allergic to PREMPRO or PREMPHASE or any of their ingredients.** See the end of this leaflet for a list of all the ingredients in PREMPRO and PREMPHASE.
- **think you may be pregnant.**

Tell your healthcare provider:

- **if you are breastfeeding.** The hormones in PREMPRO and PREMPHASE can pass into your milk.
- **about all of your medical problems.** Your healthcare provider may need to check you more carefully if you have certain conditions, such as asthma (wheezing), epilepsy (seizures), migraine, endometriosis, lupus, problems with your heart, liver, thyroid, kidneys, or have high calcium levels in your blood.
- **about all the medicines you take,** including prescription and nonprescription medicines, vitamins, and herbal supplements. Some medicines may affect how PREMPRO or PREMPHASE works. PREMPRO or PREMPHASE may also affect how your other medicines work.
- **if you are going to have surgery or will be on bedrest.** You may need to stop taking estrogens and progestins.

How should I take PREMPRO or PREMPHASE?

- Take one PREMPRO or PREMPHASE tablet at the same time each day.
- If you miss a dose, take it as soon as possible. If it is almost time for your next dose, skip the missed dose and go back to your normal schedule. Do not take 2 doses at the same time.
- Estrogens should be used at the lowest dose possible for your treatment only as long as needed. You and your healthcare provider should talk regularly (for example, every 3 to 6 months) about the dose you are taking and whether you still need treatment with PREMPRO or PREMPHASE.

What are the possible side effects of PREMPRO or PREMPHASE?

Less common but serious side effects include:

- Breast cancer
- Cancer of the uterus

- Stroke
- Heart attack
- Blood clots
- Dementia
- Gallbladder disease
- Ovarian cancer

These are some of the warning signs of serious side effects:

- Breast lumps
- Unusual vaginal bleeding
- Dizziness and faintness
- Changes in speech
- Severe headaches
- Chest pain
- Shortness of breath
- Pains in your legs
- Changes in vision
- Vomiting

Call your healthcare provider right away if you get any of these warning signs, or any other unusual symptoms that concerns you.

Common side effects include:

- Headache
- Breast pain
- Irregular vaginal bleeding or spotting
- Stomach/abdominal cramps/bloating
- Nausea and vomiting
- Hair loss

Other side effects include:

- High blood pressure
- Liver problems
- High blood sugar
- Fluid retention
- Enlargement of benign tumors of the uterus ("fibroids")
- Vaginal yeast infections
- Mental depression

These are not all the possible side effects of PREMPRO or PREMPHASE. For more information, ask your healthcare provider or pharmacist.

What can I do to lower my chances of getting a serious side effect with PREMPRO or PREMPHASE?

- Talk with your healthcare provider regularly about whether you should continue taking PREMPRO or PREMPHASE.
- See your healthcare provider right away if you get vaginal bleeding while taking PREMPRO or PREMPHASE.
- Have a breast exam and mammogram (breast X-ray) every year unless your healthcare provider tells you something else. If members of your family have had breast cancer or if you have ever had breast lumps or an abnormal mammogram, you may need to have breast exams more often.
- If you have high blood pressure, high cholesterol (fat in the blood), diabetes, are overweight, or if you use tobacco, you may have higher chances for getting heart disease. Ask your healthcare provider for ways to lower your chances of getting heart attacks.

General Information about the safe and effective use of PREMPRO and PREMPHASE

Medicines are sometimes prescribed for conditions that are not mentioned in patient information leaflets. Do not take PREMPRO or PREMPHASE for conditions for which it was not prescribed. Do not give PREMPRO or PREMPHASE to other people, even if they have the same symptoms you have. It may harm them.

Keep PREMPRO and PREMPHASE out of the reach of children.

This leaflet provides a summary of the most important information about PREMPRO and PREMPHASE. If you would like more information, talk with your healthcare provider or pharmacist. You can ask for information about PREMPRO and PREMPHASE that is written for health professionals. You can get more information by calling the toll free number 800-934-5556.

What are the ingredients in PREMPRO and PREMPHASE?

PREMPRO contains the same conjugated estrogens found in Premarin which are a mixture of sodium estrone sulfate and sodium equilin sulfate and other components including sodium sulfate conjugates, 17α-dihydroequilin, 17α-estradiol and 17β-dihydroequilin. PREMPRO also contains either 1.5, 2.5, or 5 mg of medroxyprogesterone acetate. PREMPRO also contains calcium phosphate tribasic, calcium sulfate, carnauba wax, cellulose, glyceryl monooleate, lactose, magnesium stearate, methylcellulose, pharmaceutical glaze, polyethylene glycol, sucrose, povidone, titanium dioxide, and yellow ferric oxide or red ferric oxide or FD&C Blue No. 2.

PREMPHASE is two separate tablets. One tablet (maroon color) is 0.625 mg of Premarin which is a mixture of sodium estrone sulfate and sodium equilin sulfate and other components including sodium sulfate conjugates, 17 α-dihydroequilin, 17 α-estradiol and 17 β-dihydroequilin. The maroon tablet also contains calcium phosphate tribasic, calcium sulfate, carnauba wax, cellulose, glyceryl monooleate, lactose, magnesium stearate, methylcellulose, pharmaceutical glaze, polyethylene glycol, stearic acid, sucrose, titanium dioxide, FD&C Blue No. 2, D&C Red No. 27, FD&C Red No. 40. The second tablet (light blue color) contains 0.625 mg of the same ingredients as the maroon color tablet plus 5 mg of medroxyprogesterone acetate. The light blue tablet also contains calcium phosphate tribasic, calcium sulfate, carnauba wax, cellulose, glyceryl monooleate,

Continued on next page

Prempro/Premphase—Cont.

lactose, magnesium stearate, methylcellulose, pharmaceutical glaze, polyethylene glycol, sucrose, povidone, titanium dioxide, FD&C Blue No. 2.

PREMPRO therapy consists of a single tablet to be taken once daily.

PREMPRO 0.3 mg/1.5 mg

Each carton includes 3 EZ DIAL® dispensers containing 28 tablets. One EZ DIAL dispenser contains 28 oval, cream tablets containing 0.3 mg of the conjugated estrogens found in Premarin tablets and 1.5 mg of medroxyprogesterone acetate for oral administration.

PREMPRO 0.45 mg/1.5 mg

Each carton includes 3 EZ DIAL dispensers containing 28 tablets. One EZ DIAL dispenser contains 28 oval, gold tablets containing 0.45 mg of the conjugated estrogens found in Premarin tablets and 1.5 mg of medroxyprogesterone acetate for oral administration.

PREMPRO 0.625 mg/2.5 mg

Each carton includes 3 EZ DIAL dispensers containing 28 tablets. One EZ DIAL dispenser contains 28 oval, peach tablets containing 0.625 mg of the conjugated estrogens found in Premarin tablets and 2.5 mg of medroxyprogesterone acetate for oral administration.

PREMPRO 0.625 mg/5 mg

Each carton includes 3 EZ DIAL dispensers containing 28 tablets. One EZ DIAL dispenser contains 28 oval, light-blue tablets containing 0.625 mg of the conjugated estrogens found in Premarin tablets and 5 mg of medroxyprogesterone acetate for oral administration.

PREMPHASE therapy consists of two separate tablets; one maroon Premarin tablet taken daily on days 1 through 14 and one light-blue tablet taken on days 15 through 28.

Each carton includes 3 EZ DIAL dispensers containing 28 tablets. One EZ DIAL dispenser contains 14 oval, maroon Premarin tablets containing 0.625 mg of conjugated estrogens and 14 oval, light-blue tablets that contain 0.625 mg of the conjugated estrogens found in Premarin tablets and 5 mg of medroxyprogesterone acetate for oral administration.

The appearance of PREMPRO tablets is a trademark of Wyeth Pharmaceuticals.

The appearance of Premarin tablets is a trademark of Wyeth Pharmaceuticals. The appearance of the conjugated estrogens/medroxyprogesterone acetate combination tablets is a registered trademark.

Store at 20–25°C (68–77°F); excursions permitted to 15–30°C (59–86°F) [see USP Controlled Room Temperature].

This product's label may have been revised after this insert was used in production. For further product information and current package insert, please visit www.wyeth.com or call our medical communications department toll-free at 1-800-934-5556.

Wyeth®

Wyeth Pharmaceuticals Inc.
Philadelphia, PA 19101

W10407C012
ET01
Revised August 9, 2004

PREVNAR® ℞

[prĕv′năr]

Pneumococcal 7-valent Conjugate Vaccine
(Diphtheria CRM_{197} Protein)
FOR PEDIATRIC USE ONLY
℞ only
For Intramuscular Injection Only

Prescribing Information for this product, which appears on pages 3382–3389 of the 2005 PDR, has been completely revised as follows. Please write "See Supplement A" next to the product heading.

This product's label may have been revised after this insert was used in production. For further product information and current package insert, please visit www.wyeth.com or call our medical communications department toll-free at 1-800-934-5556.

DESCRIPTION

Pneumococcal 7-valent Conjugate Vaccine (Diphtheria CRM_{197} Protein), Prevnar®, is a sterile solution of saccharides of the capsular antigens of *Streptococcus pneumoniae* serotypes 4, 6B, 9V, 14, 18C, 19F, and 23F individually conjugated to diphtheria CRM_{197} protein. Each serotype is grown in soy peptone broth. The individual polysaccharides are purified through centrifugation, precipitation, ultrafiltration, and column chromatography. The polysaccharides are chemically activated to make saccharides which are directly conjugated to the protein carrier CRM_{197} to form the glycoconjugate. This is effected by reductive amination. CRM_{197} is a nontoxic variant of diphtheria toxin isolated from cultures of *Corynebacterium diphtheriae* strain C7 (β197) grown in a casamino acids and yeast extract-based medium. CRM_{197} is purified through ultrafiltration, ammonium sulfate precipitation, and ion-exchange chromatography. The individual glycoconjugates are purified by ultrafiltration and column chromatography and are analyzed for saccharide to protein ratios, molecular size, free saccharide, and free protein.

The individual glycoconjugates are compounded to formulate the vaccine, Prevnar®. Potency of the formulated vaccine is determined by quantification of each of the saccharide antigens, and by the saccharide to protein ratios in the individual glycoconjugates.

Prevnar® is manufactured as a liquid preparation. Each 0.5 mL dose is formulated to contain: 2 µg of each saccharide for serotypes 4, 9V, 14, 18C, 19F, and 23F, and 4 µg of serotype 6B per dose (16 µg total saccharide); approximately 20 µg of CRM_{197} carrier protein; and 0.125 mg of aluminum per 0.5 mL dose as aluminum phosphate adjuvant.

After shaking, the vaccine is a homogeneous, white suspension.

TABLE 1
Efficacy of Prevnar® Against Invasive Disease Due to *S. pneumoniae* in Cases Accrued From October 15, 1995 Through August 20, 1998[20,21]

	Prevnar® Number of Cases	Control* Number of Cases	Efficacy	95% CI
Vaccine serotypes				
Per protocol	**0**	**17**	**100%**	**75.4, 100**
Intent-to-treat	**0**	**22**	**100%**	**81.7, 100**
All pneumococcal serotypes				
Per protocol	2	20	90.0%	58.3, 98.9
Intent-to-treat	3	27†	88.9%	63.8, 97.9

* Investigational meningococcal group C conjugate vaccine (MnCC).
† Includes one case in an immunocompromised subject.

TABLE 2
Efficacy of Prevnar® Against Otitis Media in the Finnish and NCKP Trials[20,21,22,23]

	Per Protocol		Intent-to-Treat	
	Vaccine Efficacy Estimate*	95% Confidence Interval	Vaccine Efficacy Estimate*	95% Confidence Interval
Finnish Trial	N=1632		N=1662	
AOM due to Vaccine Serotypes	**57%**	**44, 67**	**54%**	**41, 64**
All culture-confirmed pneumococcal AOM regardless of serotype	34%	21, 45	32%	19, 42
NCKP Trial	N=23,746		N=34,146	
All Otitis Media Episodes regardless of etiology†	**7%**	**4, 10**	**6%**	**4, 9**

* All vaccine efficacy estimates in the table are statistically significant.
† The vaccine efficacy against all AOM episodes in the Finnish trial, while not reaching statistical significance, was 6% (95% CI: -4, 16) in the per protocol population and 4% (95% CI: -7, 14) in the intent-to-treat population.

CLINICAL PHARMACOLOGY

S. pneumoniae is an important cause of morbidity and mortality in persons of all ages worldwide. The organism causes invasive infections, such as bacteremia and meningitis, as well as pneumonia and upper respiratory tract infections including otitis media and sinusitis. In children older than 1 month, *S. pneumoniae* is the most common cause of invasive disease.[1] Data from community-based studies performed between 1986 and 1995, indicate that the overall annual incidence of invasive pneumococcal disease in the United States (US) is an estimated 10 to 30 cases per 100,000 persons, with the highest risk in children aged less than or equal to 2 years of age (140 to 160 cases per 100,000 persons).[2,3] Children in group child care have an increased risk for invasive pneumococcal disease.[4,5] Immunocompromised individuals with neutropenia, asplenia, sickle cell disease, disorders of complement and humoral immunity, human immunodeficiency virus (HIV) infections or chronic underlying disease are also at increased risk for invasive pneumococcal disease.[5] *S. pneumoniae* is the most common cause of bacterial meningitis in the US.[1] The annual incidence of pneumococcal meningitis in children between 1 to 23 months of age is approximately 7 cases per 100,000 persons.[1] Pneumococcal meningitis in childhood has been associated with 8% mortality and may result in neurological sequelae (25%) and hearing loss (32%) in survivors.[6]

Acute otitis media (AOM) is a common childhood disease, with more than 60% of children experiencing an episode by one year of age, and more than 90% of children experiencing an episode by age 5. Prior to the US introduction of Prevnar® in the year 2000, approximately 24.5 million ambulatory care visits and 490,000 procedures for myringotomy with tube placement were attributed to otitis media annually.[7,8] The peak incidence of AOM is 6 to 18 months of age.[9] Otitis media is less common, but occurs, in older children. In a 1990 surveillance by the Centers for Disease Control and Prevention (CDC), otitis media was the most common principal illness diagnosis in children 2-10 years of age.[10] Complications of AOM include persistent middle ear effusion, chronic otitis media, transient hearing loss, or speech delays and, if left untreated, may lead to more serious diseases such as mastoiditis and meningitis. *S. pneumoniae* is an important cause of AOM. It is the bacterial pathogen most commonly isolated from middle ear fluid, identified in 20% to 40% of middle ear fluid cultures in AOM.[11,12] Pneumococcal otitis media is associated with higher rates of fever, and is less likely to resolve spontaneously than AOM due to either nontypeable *H. influenzae* or *M. catarrhalis*.[13,14] Prior to the introduction of Prevnar®, the seven serotypes contained in the vaccine accounted for approximately 60% of AOM due to *S. pneumoniae* (12%-24% of all AOM).[15]

The exact contribution of *S. pneumoniae* to childhood pneumonia is unknown, as it is often not possible to identify the causative organisms. In studies of children less than 5 years of age with community-acquired pneumonia, where diagnosis was attempted using serological methods, antigen testing, or culture data, 30% of cases were classified as bacterial pneumonia, and 70% of these (21% of total community-acquired pneumonia) were found to be due to *S. pneumoniae*.[16]

In the past decade the proportion of *S. pneumoniae* isolates resistant to antibiotics has been on the rise in the US and worldwide. In a multi-center US surveillance study, the prevalence of penicillin and cephalosporin-nonsusceptible (intermediate or high level resistance) invasive disease isolates from children was 21% (range <5% to 38% among centers), and 9.3% (range 0%-18%), respectively. Over the 3-year surveillance period (1993-1996), there was a 50% increase in penicillin-nonsusceptible *S. pneumoniae* (PNSP) strains and a three-fold rise in cephalosporin-nonsusceptible strains.[5] Although generally less common than PNSP, pneumococci resistant to macrolides and trimethoprim-sulfamethoxazole have also been observed. Day care attendance, a history of ear infection, and a recent history of antibiotic exposure, have also been associated with invasive infections with PNSP in children 2 months to 59 months of age.[4,5] There has been no difference in mortality associated with PNSP strains.[5,6] However, the American Academy of Pediatrics (AAP) revised the antibiotic treatment guidelines in 1997 in response to the increased prevalence of antibiotic-resistant pneumococci.[17]

Approximately 90 serotypes of *S. pneumoniae* have been identified based on antigenic differences in their capsular polysaccharides. The distribution of serotypes responsible for disease differ with age and geographic location.[18]

Serotypes 4, 6B, 9V, 14, 18C, 19F, and 23F have been responsible for approximately 80% of invasive pneumococcal disease in children <6 years of age in the US.[15] These 7 serotypes also accounted for 74% of PNSP and 100% of pneumococci with high level penicillin resistance isolated from children <6 years with invasive disease during a 1993-1994 surveillance by the CDC.[19]

Results of Clinical Evaluations

Efficacy Against Invasive Disease

Efficacy was assessed in a randomized, double-blinded clinical trial in a multiethnic population at Northern California Kaiser Permanente (NCKP) from October 1995 through August 20, 1998, in which 37,816 infants were randomized to receive either Prevnar® or a control vaccine (an investigational meningococcal group C conjugate vaccine [MnCC]) at 2, 4, 6, and 12-15 months of age. Prevnar® was administered to 18,906 children and the control vaccine to 18,910 children. Routinely recommended vaccines were also administered which changed during the trial to reflect changing AAP and Advisory Committee on Immunization Practices (ACIP) recommendations. A planned interim analysis was performed upon accrual of 17 cases of invasive disease due to vaccine-type *S. pneumoniae* (August 1998). Ancillary endpoints for evaluation of efficacy against pneumococcal disease were also assessed in this trial.

Invasive disease was defined as isolation and identification of *S. pneumoniae* from normally sterile body sites in children presenting with an acute illness consistent with pneumococcal disease. Weekly surveillance of listings of cultures from the NCKP Regional Microbiology database was conducted to assure ascertainment of all cases. The primary endpoint was efficacy against invasive pneumococcal disease due to vaccine serotypes. The per protocol analysis of the primary endpoint included cases which occurred ≥14 days after the third dose. The intent-to-treat (ITT) analysis included all cases of invasive pneumococcal disease due to vaccine serotypes in children who received at least one dose of vaccine. Secondary analyses of efficacy against all invasive pneumococcal disease, regardless of serotype, were also performed according to these same per protocol and ITT definitions. Results of these analyses are presented in Table 1.

[See table 1 at top of previous page]

All 22 cases of invasive disease due to vaccine serotype strains in the ITT population were bacteremic. In addition, the following diagnoses were also reported: meningitis (2), pneumonia (2), and cellulitis (1).

Data accumulated through an extended follow-up period to April 20, 1999, resulted in a similar efficacy estimate (Per protocol: 1 case in Pneumococcal 7-valent Conjugate Vaccine (Diphtheria CRM$_{197}$ Protein), Prevnar® group, 39 cases in control group; ITT: 3 cases in Prevnar® group, 49 cases in the control group).[21]

Efficacy Against Otitis Media

The efficacy of Prevnar® against otitis media was assessed in two clinical trials: a trial in Finnish infants at the National Public Health Institute and the invasive disease efficacy trial in US infants at Northern California Kaiser Permanente (NCKP).

The trial in Finland was a randomized, double-blind trial in which 1,662 infants were equally randomized to receive either Prevnar® or a control vaccine (Hepatitis B vaccine [Hep B]) at 2, 4, 6, and 12–15 months of age. All infants received a Diphtheria Tetanus Pertussis Vaccine - *Haemophilus influenzae* type b vaccine (DTP-Hib) combination vaccine concurrently at 2, 4, and 6 months of age, and Inactivated Poliovirus Vaccine (IPV) concurrently at 12 months of age. Parents of study participants were asked to bring their children to the study clinics if the child had respiratory infections or symptoms suggesting acute otitis media (AOM). If AOM was diagnosed, tympanocentesis was performed, and the middle ear fluid was cultured. If *S. pneumoniae* was isolated, serotyping was performed.

AOM was defined as a visually abnormal tympanic membrane suggesting effusion in the middle ear cavity, concomitantly with at least one of the following symptoms of acute infection: fever, ear ache, irritability, diarrhea, vomiting, acute otorrhea not caused by external otitis, or other symptoms of respiratory infection. A new visit or "episode" was defined as a visit with a study physician at which time a diagnosis of AOM was made and at least 30 days had elapsed since any previous visit for otitis media. The primary endpoint was efficacy against AOM episodes caused by vaccine serotypes in the per protocol population.

In the NCKP invasive disease efficacy trial, the effectiveness of Prevnar® in reducing the incidence of otitis media was assessed from the beginning of the trial in October 1995 through April 1998. During this time, 34,146 infants were randomized to receive either Prevnar® (N=17,070), or the control, an investigational meningococcal group C conjugate vaccine (N=17,076), at 2, 4, 6, and 12-15 months of age.

Physician visits for otitis media were identified by physician coding of outpatient encounter forms. Because visits may have included both acute and follow-up care, a new visit or "episode" was defined as a visit that was at least 21 days following a previous visit for otitis media (at least 42 days, if the visit appointment was made > 3 days in advance). Data on placement of ear tubes were collected from automated databases. No routine tympanocentesis was performed, and no standard definition of otitis media was used by study physicians. The primary otitis media endpoint was efficacy against all otitis media episodes in the per protocol population.

Table 2 presents the per protocol and intent-to-treat results of key otitis media analyses for both studies. The per protocol analyses include otitis media episodes that occurred ≥14 days after the third dose. The intent-to-treat analyses include all otitis media episodes in children who received at least one dose of vaccine.

[See table 2 at top of previous page]

The vaccine efficacy against AOM episodes due to vaccine-related serotypes (6A, 9N, 18B, 19A, 23A), also assessed in the Finnish trial, was 51% (95% CI: 27, 67) in the per protocol population and 44% (95% CI: 20, 62) in the intent-to-treat population. The vaccine efficacy against AOM episodes caused by serotypes unrelated to the vaccine was -33% (95% CI: -80, 1) in the per protocol population and -39% (95% CI: -86, -3) in the intent-to-treat population, indicating that children who received Prevnar® appear to be at increased risk of otitis media due to pneumococcal serotypes not represented in the vaccine, compared to children who received the control vaccine. However, vaccination with Prevnar® reduced pneumococcal otitis media episodes overall.

Several other otitis media endpoints were also assessed in the two trials. Recurrent AOM, defined as 3 episodes in 6 months or 4 episodes in 12 months, was reduced by 9% in both the per protocol and intent-to-treat populations (95% CI: 3, 15 in per protocol and 95% CI: 4, 14 in intent-to-treat) in the NCKP trial. This observation was supported by a similar trend, although not statistically significant, seen in the Finnish trial. The NCKP trial also demonstrated a 20% reduction (95% CI: 2, 35) in the placement of tympanostomy tubes in the per protocol population and a 21% reduction (95% CI: 4, 34) in the intent-to-treat population.

Data from the NCKP trial accumulated through an extended follow-up period to April 20, 1999, in which a total of 37,866 children were included (18,925 in Prevnar® group and 18,941 in MnCC control group), resulted in similar otitis media efficacy estimates for all endpoints.[24]

Immunogenicity

Routine Schedule

Subjects from a subset of selected study sites in the NCKP efficacy study were approached for participation in the immunogenicity portion of the study on a volunteer basis. Immune responses following three or four doses of Prevnar® or the control vaccine were evaluated in children who received either concurrent Diphtheria and Tetanus Toxoids and Pertussis Vaccine Adsorbed and Haemophilus b Conjugate Vaccine (Diphtheria CRM$_{197}$ Protein Conjugate), (DTP-HbOC), or Diphtheria and Tetanus Toxoids and Acellular Pertussis Vaccine Adsorbed (DTaP), and Haemophilus b Conjugate Vaccine (Diphtheria CRM$_{197}$ Protein Conjugate), (HbOC) vaccines at 2, 4, and 6 months of age. The use of Hepatitis B (Hep B), Oral Polio Vaccine (OPV), Inactivated Polio Vaccine (IPV), Measles-Mumps-Rubella (MMR), and Varicella vaccines were permitted according to the AAP and ACIP recommendations.

Table 3 presents the geometric mean concentrations (GMC) of pneumococcal antibodies following the third and fourth doses of Prevnar® or the control vaccine when administered concurrently with DTP-HbOC vaccine in the efficacy study.

[See table 3 above]

In another randomized study (Manufacturing Bridging Study, 118-16), immune responses were evaluated following three doses of Pneumococcal 7-valent Conjugate Vaccine

TABLE 3
Geometric Mean Concentrations (µg/mL) of Pneumococcal Antibodies Following the Third and Fourth Doses of Prevnar® or Control* When Administered Concurrently With DTP-HbOC in the Efficacy Study[20,21]

Serotype	Post dose 3 GMC[†] (95% CI for Prevnar®)		Post dose 4 GMC[‡] (95% CI for Prevnar®)	
	Prevnar®[§]	Control*	Prevnar®[§]	Control*
	N=88	N=92	N=68	N=61
4	1.46 (1.19, 1.78)	0.03	2.38 (1.88, 3.03)	0.04
6B	4.70 (3.59, 6.14)	0.08	14.45 (11.17, 18.69)	0.17
9V	1.99 (1.64, 2.42)	0.05	3.51 (2.75, 4.48)	0.06
14	4.60 (3.70, 5.74)	0.05	6.52 (5.18, 8.21)	0.06
18C	2.16 (1.73, 2.69)	0.04	3.43 (2.70, 4.37)	0.07
19F	1.39 (1.16, 1.68)	0.09	2.07 (1.66, 2.57)	0.18
23F	1.85 (1.46, 2.34)	0.05	3.82 (2.85, 5.11)	0.09

*Control was investigational meningococcal group C conjugate vaccine (MnCC).
[†] Mean age of Prevnar® group was 7.8 months and of control group was 7.7 months. N is slightly less for some serotypes in each group.
[‡] Mean age of Prevnar® group was 14.2 months and of control group was 14.4 months. N is slightly less for some serotypes in each group.
[§] p<0.001 when Prevnar® compared to control for each serotype using a Wilcoxon's test.

TABLE 4
Geometric Mean Concentrations (µg/mL) of Pneumococcal Antibodies Following the Third Dose of Prevnar® or Control* When Administered Concurrently With DTaP and HbOC in the Efficacy Study[†] and Manufacturing Bridging Study[20,21,25]

Serotype	Efficacy Study Post dose 3 GMC[‡] (95% CI for Prevnar®)		Manufacturing Bridging Study Post dose 3 GMC[§] (95% CI for Prevnar®)	
	Prevnar®[‖]	Control*	Prevnar®[‖]	Control*
	N=32	N=32	N=159	N=83
4	1.47 (1.08, 2.02)	0.02	2.03 (1.75, 2.37)	0.02
6B	2.18 (1.20, 3.96)	0.06	2.97 (2.43, 3.65)	0.07
9V	1.52 (1.04, 2.22)	0.04	1.18 (1.01, 1.39)	0.04
14	5.05 (3.32, 7.70)	0.04	4.64 (3.80, 5.66)	0.04
18C	2.24 (1.65, 3.02)	0.04	1.96 (1.66, 2.30)	0.04
19F	1.54 (1.09, 2.17)	0.10	1.91 (1.63, 2.25)	0.08
23F	1.48 (0.97, 2.25)	0.05	1.71 (1.44, 2.05)	0.05

*Control in efficacy study was investigational meningococcal group C conjugate vaccine (MnCC) and in Manufacturing Bridging Study was concomitant vaccines only.
[†] Sufficient data are not available to reliably assess GMCs following 4 doses of Prevnar® when administered with DTaP in the NCKP efficacy study.
[‡] Mean age of the Prevnar® study group was 7.4 months and of the control group was 7.6 months. N is slightly less for some serotypes in each group.
[§] Mean age of the Prevnar® study group and the control group was 7.2 months.
[‖] p<0.001 when Prevnar® compared to control for each serotype using a Wilcoxon's test in the efficacy study and two-sample t-test in the Manufacturing Bridging Study.

Continued on next page

Prevnar—Cont.

(Diphtheria CRM$_{197}$ Protein), Prevnar® administered concomitantly with DTaP and HbOC vaccines at 2, 4, and 6 months of age, IPV at 2 and 4 months of age, and Hep B at 2 and 6 months of age. The control group received concomitant vaccines only. Table 4 presents the immune responses to pneumococcal polysaccharides observed in both this study and in the subset of subjects from the efficacy study that received concomitant DTaP and HbOC vaccines.
[See table 4 on previous page]
In all studies in which the immune responses to Prevnar® were contrasted to control, a significant antibody response was seen to all vaccine serotypes following three or four doses, although geometric mean concentrations of antibody varied among serotypes.[20,21,23,25,26,27,28,29,30] The minimum serum antibody concentration necessary for protection against invasive pneumococcal disease or against pneumococcal otitis media has not been determined for any serotype. Prevnar® induces functional antibodies to all vaccine serotypes, as measured by opsonophagocytosis following three doses.[30]

Previously Unvaccinated Older Infants and Children
To determine an appropriate schedule for children 7 months of age or older at the time of the first immunization with Prevnar®, 483 children in 4 ancillary studies received Prevnar® at various schedules and were evaluated for immunogenicity. GMCs attained using the various schedules among older infants and children were comparable to immune responses of children, who received concomitant DTaP, in the NCKP efficacy study (118-8) after 3 doses for most serotypes, as shown in Table 5. These data support the schedule for previously unvaccinated older infants and children who are beyond the age of the infant schedule. For usage in older infants and children, see **DOSAGE AND ADMINISTRATION**.
[See table 5 above]

INDICATIONS AND USAGE

Prevnar® is indicated for active immunization of infants and toddlers against invasive disease caused by *S. pneumoniae* due to capsular serotypes included in the vaccine (4, 6B, 9V, 14, 18C, 19F, and 23F). The routine schedule is 2, 4, 6, and 12–15 months of age.
The decision to administer Pneumococcal 7-valent Conjugate Vaccine (Diphtheria CRM$_{197}$ Protein), Prevnar® should be based primarily on its efficacy in preventing invasive pneumococcal disease. As with any vaccine, Prevnar® may not protect all individuals receiving the vaccine from invasive pneumococcal disease.
Prevnar® is also indicated for active immunization of infants and toddlers against otitis media caused by serotypes included in the vaccine. However, for vaccine serotypes, protection against otitis media is expected to be substantially lower than protection against invasive disease. Additionally, because otitis media is caused by many organisms other than serotypes of *S. pneumoniae* represented in the vaccine, protection against all causes of otitis media is expected to be low.
(See **CLINICAL PHARMACOLOGY** for estimates of efficacy against invasive disease and otitis media).
For additional information on usage, see **DOSAGE AND ADMINISTRATION**.
This vaccine is not intended to be used for treatment of active infection.

CONTRAINDICATIONS

Hypersensitivity to any component of the vaccine, including diphtheria toxoid, is a contraindication to use of this vaccine.

WARNINGS

THIS VACCINE WILL NOT PROTECT AGAINST *S. PNEUMONIAE* DISEASE CAUSED BY SEROTYPES UNRELATED TO THOSE IN THE VACCINE, NOR WILL IT PROTECT AGAINST OTHER MICROORGANISMS THAT CAUSE INVASIVE INFECTIONS SUCH AS BACTEREMIA AND MENINGITIS OR NON-INVASIVE INFECTIONS SUCH AS OTITIS MEDIA.
This vaccine should not be given to infants or children with thrombocytopenia or any coagulation disorder that would contraindicate intramuscular injection unless the potential benefit clearly outweighs the risk of administration. If the decision is made to administer this vaccine to children with coagulation disorders, it should be given with caution. (See **DRUG INTERACTIONS**.)
Immunization with Prevnar® does not substitute for routine diphtheria immunization.
The vial stopper contains dry natural rubber that may cause hypersensitivity reactions when handled by or when the product is injected into persons with known or possible latex sensitivity.

PRECAUTIONS

Prevnar® is for intramuscular use only. Prevnar® SHOULD UNDER NO CIRCUMSTANCES BE ADMINISTERED INTRAVENOUSLY. The safety and immunogenicity for other routes of administration (eg, subcutaneous) have not been evaluated.
Fever, and rarely febrile seizure, have been reported in children receiving Prevnar®. For children at higher risk of seizures than the general population, appropriate antipyretics (dosed according to respective prescribing information) may be administered around the time of vaccination, to reduce the possibility of post-vaccination fever.

TABLE 5
Geometric Mean Concentrations (µg/mL) of Pneumococcal Antibodies Following Immunization of Children From 7 Months Through 9 Years of Age With Prevnar®[31]

Age group, Vaccinations	Study	Sample Size(s)	4	6B	9V	14	18C	19F	23F
7-11 mo. 3 doses	118-12	22	2.34	3.66	2.11	9.33	2.31	1.60	2.50
	118-16	39	3.60	4.63	2.04	5.48	1.98	2.15	1.93
12-17 mo. 2 doses	118-15*	82-84†	3.91	4.67	1.94	6.92	2.25	3.78	3.29
	118-18	33	7.02	4.25	3.26	6.31	3.60	3.29	2.92
18-23 mo. 2 doses	118-15*	52-54†	3.36	4.92	1.80	6.69	2.65	3.17	2.71
	118-18	45	6.85	3.71	3.86	6.48	3.42	3.86	2.75
24-35 mo. 1 dose	118-18	53	5.34	2.90	3.43	1.88	3.03	4.07	1.56
36-59 mo. 1 dose	118-18	52	6.27	6.40	4.62	5.95	4.08	6.37	2.95
5-9 yrs. 1 dose	118-18	101	6.92	20.84	7.49	19.32	6.72	12.51	11.57
118-8, DTaP	Post dose 3	31-32†	1.47	2.18	1.52	5.05	2.24	1.54	1.48

Bold = GMC not inferior to 118-8, DTaP post dose 3 (one-sided lower limit of the 95% CI of GMC ratio ≥0.50).
* Study in Navajo and Apache populations.
† Numbers vary with serotype.

TABLE 6
Percentage of Subjects Reporting Local Reactions Within 2 Days Following Immunization With Prevnar®* and DTaP Vaccines† at 2, 4, 6, and 12-15 Months of Age[20,21]

Reaction	Dose 1		Dose 2		Dose 3		Dose 4	
	Prevnar® Site	DTaP Site	Prevnar® Site	DTaP Site	Prevnar® Site	DTaP Site	Prevnar® Site	DTaP Site‡
	N=693	N=693	N=526	N=526	N=422	N=422	N=165	N=165
Erythema								
Any	10.0	6.7§	11.6	10.5	13.8	11.4	10.9	3.6§
>2.4 cm	1.3	0.4§	0.6	0.6	1.4	1.0	3.6	0.6
Induration								
Any	9.8	6.6§	12.0	10.5	10.4	10.4	12.1	5.5§
>2.4 cm	1.6	0.9	1.3	1.7	2.4	1.9	5.5	1.8
Tenderness								
Any	17.9	16.0	19.4	17.3	14.7	13.1	23.3	18.4
Interfered with limb movement	3.1	1.8§	4.1	3.3	2.9	1.9	9.2	8.0

* HbOC was administered in the same limb as Pneumococcal 7-valent Conjugate Vaccine (Diphtheria CRM$_{197}$ Protein), Prevnar®. If reactions occurred at either or both sites on that limb, the more severe reaction was recorded.
† If Hep B vaccine was administered simultaneously, it was administered into the same limb as DTaP. If reactions occurred at either or both sites on that limb, the more severe reaction was recorded.
‡ Subjects may have received DTP or a mixed DTP/DTaP regimen for the primary series. Thus, this is the 4th dose of a pertussis vaccine, but not a 4th dose of DTaP.
§ p<0.05 when Prevnar® site compared to DTaP site using the sign test.

Minor illnesses, such as a mild respiratory infection with or without low-grade fever, are not generally contraindications to vaccination. The decision to administer or delay vaccination because of a current or recent febrile illness depends largely on the severity of the symptoms and their etiology. The administration of Prevnar should be postponed in subjects suffering from acute severe febrile illness.[32,33]

General
CARE IS TO BE TAKEN BY THE HEALTHCARE PROFESSIONAL FOR THE SAFE AND EFFECTIVE USE OF THIS PRODUCT.
1. PRIOR TO ADMINISTRATION OF ANY DOSE OF THIS VACCINE, THE PARENT OR GUARDIAN SHOULD BE ASKED ABOUT THE PERSONAL HISTORY, FAMILY HISTORY, AND RECENT HEALTH STATUS OF THE VACCINE RECIPIENT. THE HEALTHCARE PROFESSIONAL SHOULD ASCERTAIN PREVIOUS IMMUNIZATION HISTORY, CURRENT HEALTH STATUS, AND OCCURRENCE OF ANY SYMPTOMS AND/OR SIGNS OF AN ADVERSE EVENT AFTER PREVIOUS IMMUNIZATIONS IN THE CHILD TO BE IMMUNIZED, IN ORDER TO DETERMINE THE EXISTENCE OF ANY CONTRAINDICATION TO IMMUNIZATION WITH THIS VACCINE AND TO ALLOW AN ASSESSMENT OF RISKS AND BENEFITS.
2. BEFORE THE ADMINISTRATION OF ANY BIOLOGICAL, THE HEALTHCARE PROFESSIONAL SHOULD TAKE ALL PRECAUTIONS KNOWN FOR THE PREVENTION OF ALLERGIC OR ANY OTHER ADVERSE REACTIONS. This should include a review of the patient's history regarding possible sensitivity; the ready availability of epinephrine 1:1000 and other appropriate agents used for control of immediate allergic reactions; and a knowledge of the recent literature pertaining to use of the biological concerned, including the nature of side effects and adverse reactions that may follow its use.

3. Children with impaired immune responsiveness, whether due to the use of immunosuppressive therapy (including irradiation, corticosteroids, antimetabolites, alkylating agents, and cytotoxic agents), a genetic defect, HIV infection, or other causes, may have reduced antibody response to active immunization.[32,33,34] (See **DRUG INTERACTIONS**.)
4. The use of pneumococcal conjugate vaccine does not replace the use of 23-valent pneumococcal polysaccharide vaccine in children ≥ 24 months of age with sickle cell disease, asplenia, HIV infection, chronic illness or who are immunocompromised. Data on sequential vaccination with Prevnar® followed by 23-valent pneumococcal polysaccharide vaccine are limited. In a randomized study, 23 children ≥ 2 years of age with sickle cell disease were administered either 2 doses of Prevnar® followed by a dose of polysaccharide vaccine or a single dose of polysaccharide vaccine alone. In this small study, safety and immune responses with the combined schedule were similar to polysaccharide vaccine alone.[35]
5. Since this product is a suspension containing an aluminum adjuvant, shake vigorously immediately prior to use to obtain a uniform suspension prior to withdrawing the dose.
6. A separate sterile syringe and needle or a sterile disposable unit should be used for each individual to prevent transmission of hepatitis or other infectious agents from one person to another. Needles should be disposed of properly and should not be recapped.
7. The vaccine is to be administered immediately after being drawn up into a syringe. Use one dose per vial; do not re-enter vial. Discard unused portions.
8. Special care should be taken to prevent injection into or near a blood vessel or nerve.
9. The vial stopper contains dry natural rubber that may cause hypersensitivity reactions when handled by or when the product is injected into persons with known or possible latex sensitivity.

Information for Parents or Guardians

Prior to administration of this vaccine, the healthcare professional should inform the parent, guardian, or other responsible adult of the potential benefits and risks to the patient (see **ADVERSE REACTIONS** and **WARNINGS** sections), and the importance of completing the immunization series unless contraindicated. Parents or guardians should be instructed to report any suspected adverse reactions to their healthcare professional. The healthcare professional should provide vaccine information statements prior to each vaccination.

DRUG INTERACTIONS

Children receiving therapy with immunosuppressive agents (large amounts of corticosteroids, antimetabolites, alkylating agents, cytotoxic agents) may not respond optimally to active immunization.[33,34] (See **PRECAUTIONS, General.**) As with other intramuscular injections, Prevnar® should be given with caution to children on anticoagulant therapy.

Simultaneous Administration with Other Vaccines

During clinical studies, Prevnar® was administered simultaneously with DTaP and HbOC, IPV, Hep B vaccines, MMR, and Varicella vaccine. Thus, the safety experience with Prevnar® reflects the use of this product as part of the routine immunization schedule.[20,21,25,27,28,30]

The immune response to routine vaccines when administered with Prevnar® (at separate sites) was assessed in 3 clinical studies in which there was a control group for comparison. Higher antibody levels (GMC) to Hib were observed after 3 doses of HbOC given with Prevnar in the infant series, compared to HbOC without Prevnar. After the 4th dose, Hib GMCs were lower when HbOC was given with Prevnar compared to control; however, over 97% of children receiving HbOC with Prevnar achieved a serum antibody concentration of ≥1 µg/mL. Although some inconsistent differences in response to pertussis antigens were observed, the clinical relevance is unknown. The response to 2 doses of IPV given concomitantly with Prevnar®, assessed 3 months after the second dose, was equivalent to controls for poliovirus Types 2 and 3, but lower for Type 1. In another study, over 98% of subjects achieved neutralizing antibody titers ≥1:8 for all polio types, following a third dose of IPV given concomitantly with Prevnar at 12 months of age.[36] Seroresponse rates to measles, mumps and rubella were similar after MMR was given concomitantly with Prevnar at 12 months of age compared to seroresponse rates after MMR was given without Prevnar at 12 months of age.[37] Varicella immunogenicity data from controlled clinical trials with concurrent administration of Prevnar® are not available.

CARCINOGENESIS, MUTAGENESIS, IMPAIRMENT OF FERTILITY

Prevnar® has not been evaluated for any carcinogenic or mutagenic potential, or impairment of fertility.

PREGNANCY

Pregnancy Category C

Animal reproductive studies have not been conducted with this product. It is not known whether Prevnar® can cause fetal harm when administered to a pregnant woman or whether it can affect reproductive capacity. This vaccine is not recommended for use in pregnant women.

Nursing Mothers

It is not known whether vaccine antigens or antibodies are excreted in human milk. This vaccine is not recommended for use in a nursing mother.

PEDIATRIC USE

Prevnar® has been shown to be usually well-tolerated and immunogenic in infants. The safety and effectiveness of Prevnar® in children below the age of 6 weeks or on or after the 10th birthday have not been established. Immune responses elicited by Prevnar® among infants born prematurely have not been adequately studied. See **DOSAGE AND ADMINISTRATION** for the recommended pediatric dosage.

GERIATRIC USE

This vaccine is NOT recommended for use in adult populations. It is not to be used as a substitute for the pneumococcal polysaccharide vaccine in geriatric populations.

ADVERSE REACTIONS

Pre-Licensure Clinical Trial Experience

The majority of the safety experience with Prevnar® comes from the NCKP Efficacy Trial in which 17,066 infants received 55,352 doses of Prevnar®, along with other routine childhood vaccines through April 1998 (see **CLINICAL PHARMACOLOGY** section). The number of Prevnar® recipients in the safety analysis differs from the number included in the efficacy analysis due to the different lengths of follow-up for these study endpoints. Safety was monitored in this study using several modalities. Local reactions and systemic events occurring within 48 hours of each dose of vaccine were ascertained by scripted telephone interview on a randomly selected subset of approximately 3,000 children in each vaccine group. The rate of relatively rare events requiring medical attention was evaluated across all doses in all study participants using automated databases. Specifically, rates of hospitalizations within 3, 14, 30, and 60 days of immunization, and of emergency room visits within 3, 14, and 30 days of immunization were assessed and compared between vaccine groups for each diagnosis. Seizures within 3 and 30 days of immunization were ascertained across multiple settings (hospitalizations, emergency room or clinic visits, telephone interviews). Deaths and SIDS were ascertained through April 1999. Hospitalizations due to diabetes, autoimmune disorders, and blood disorders were ascertained through August 1999.

TABLE 7
Percentage of Subjects Reporting Local Reactions Within 3 Days of Immunization With Prevnar® in Infants and Children from 7 Months Through 9 Years of Age[31]

Age at 1st Vaccination	7-11 Mos.						12-23 Mos.			24-35 Mos.	36-59 Mos.	5-9 Yrs.
Study No.	118-12			118-16			118-9*	118-18		118-18	118-18	118-18
Dose Number	1	2	3[†]	1	2	3[†]	1	1	2	1	1	1
Number of Subjects	54	51	24	81	76	50	60	114	117	46	48	49
Reaction												
Erythema												
Any	16.7	11.8	20.8	7.4	7.9	14.0	48.3	10.5	9.4	6.5	29.2	24.2
>2.4 cm[‡]	1.9	0.0	0.0	0.0	0.0	0.0	6.7	1.8	1.7	0.0	8.3	7.1
Induration												
Any	16.7	11.8	8.3	7.4	3.9	10.0	48.3	8.8	6.0	10.9	22.9	25.5
>2.4 cm[‡]	3.7	0.0	0.0	0.0	0.0	0.0	3.3	0.9	0.9	2.2	6.3	9.3
Tenderness												
Any	13.0	11.8	12.5	8.6	10.5	12.0	46.7	25.7	26.5	41.3	58.3	82.8
Interfered with limb movement[§]	1.9	2.0	4.2	1.2	1.3	0.0	3.3	6.2	8.5	13.0	20.8	39.4

* For 118-9, 2 of 60 subjects were ≥24 months of age.
† For 118-12, dose 3 was administered at 15-18 mos. of age. For 118-16, dose 3 was administered at 12-15 mos. of age.
‡ For 118-16 and 118-18, ≥2 cm.
§ Tenderness interfering with limb movement.

TABLE 8
Percentage of Subjects* Reporting Systemic Events Within 2 Days Following Immunization With Prevnar® or Control[†] Vaccine Concurrently With DTaP Vaccine at 2, 4, 6, and 12-15 Months of Age[20,21]

Reaction	Dose 1		Dose 2		Dose 3		Dose 4[‡]	
	Prevnar®	Control[†]	Prevnar®	Control[†]	Prevnar®	Control[†]	Prevnar®	Control[†]
	N=710	N=711	N=559	N=508	N=461	N=414	N=224	N=230
Fever								
≥38.0°C	15.1	9.4[§]	23.9	10.8[§]	19.1	11.8[§]	21.0	17.0
>39.0°C	0.9	0.3	2.5	0.8[§]	1.7	0.7	1.3	1.7
Irritability	48.0	48.2	58.7	45.3[§]	51.2	44.8	44.2	42.6
Drowsiness	40.7	42.0	25.6	22.8	19.5	21.9	17.0	16.5
Restless Sleep	15.3	15.1	20.2	19.3	25.2	19.0[§]	20.2	19.1
Decreased Appetite	17.0	13.5	17.4	13.4	20.7	13.8[§]	20.5	23.1
Vomiting	14.6	14.5	16.8	14.4	10.4	11.6	4.9	4.8
Diarrhea	11.9	8.4[§]	10.2	9.3	8.3	9.4	11.6	9.2
Urticaria-like Rash	1.4	0.3[§]	1.3	1.4	0.4	0.5	0.5	1.7

* Approximately 75% of subjects received prophylactic or therapeutic antipyretics within 48 hours of each dose.
† Investigational meningococcal group C conjugate vaccine (MnCC).
‡ Most of these children had received DTP for the primary series. Thus, this is a 4th dose of a pertussis vaccine, but not of DTaP.
§ p<0.05 when Prevnar® compared to control group using a Chi-Square test.

In Table 6 the rate of local reactions at the Prevnar® injection site is compared at each dose to the DTaP injection site in the same children.
[See table 6 on previous page]
Table 7 presents the rates of local reactions in previously unvaccinated older infants and children.
[See table 7 above]
Table 8 presents the rate of systemic events observed in the efficacy study when Prevnar® was administered concomitantly with DTaP.
[See table 8 above]
Table 9 presents results from a second study (Manufacturing Bridging Study) conducted at Northern California and Denver Kaiser sites, in which children were randomized to receive one of three lots of Pneumococcal 7-valent Conjugate Vaccine (Diphtheria CRM$_{197}$ Protein), Prevnar®, with concomitant vaccines including DTaP, or the same concomitant vaccines alone. Information was ascertained by scripted telephone interview, as described above.
[See table 9 at top of next page]
Fever (≥38.0°C) within 48 hours of a vaccine dose was reported by a greater proportion of subjects who received Prevnar®, compared to control (investigational meningococcal group C conjugate vaccine [MnCC]), after each dose when administered concurrently with DTP-HbOC or DTaP in the efficacy study. In the Manufacturing Bridging Study, fever within 48-72 hours was also reported more commonly after each dose compared to infants in the control group who received only recommended vaccines. When adminis-

tered concurrently with DTaP in either study, fever rates among Prevnar® recipients ranged from 15% to 34%, and were greatest after the 2nd dose.
Table 10 presents the frequencies of systemic reactions in previously unvaccinated older infants and children.
[See table 10 at top of next page]
Of the 17,066 subjects who received at least one dose of Prevnar® in the efficacy trial, there were 24 hospitalizations (for 29 diagnoses) within 3 days of a dose from October 1995 through April 1998. Diagnoses were as follows: bronchiolitis (5); congenital anomaly (4); elective procedure, UTI (3 each); acute gastroenteritis, asthma, pneumonia (2 each); aspiration, breath holding, influenza, inguinal hernia repair, otitis media, febrile seizure, viral syndrome, well child/reassurance (1 each). There were 162 visits to the emergency room (for 182 diagnoses) within 3 days of a dose from October 1995 through April 1998. Diagnoses were as follows: febrile illness (20); acute gastroenteritis (19); trauma, URI (16 each); otitis media (15); well child (13); irritable child, viral syndrome (10 each); rash (8); croup, pneumonia (6 each); poisoning/ingestion (5); asthma, bronchiolitis (4 each); febrile seizure, UTI (3 each); thrush, wheezing, breath holding, choking, conjunctivitis, inguinal hernia repair, pharyngitis (2 each); colic, colitis, congestive heart failure, elective procedure, hives, influenza, ingrown toenail, local swelling, roseola, sepsis (1 each).[20,21]
In the large-scale efficacy study, urticaria-like rash was reported in 0.4%-1.4% of children within 48 hours following

Continued on next page

TABLE 9
Percentage of Subjects* Reporting Systemic Reactions Within 3 Days Following Immunization With Prevnar®, DTaP, HbOC, Hep B, and IPV vs. Control† in Manufacturing Bridging Study[25]

Reaction	Dose 1		Dose 2		Dose 3	
	Prevnar®	Control†	Prevnar®	Control†	Prevnar®	Control†
	N=498	N=108	N=452	N=99	N=445	N=89
Fever						
≥38.0°C	21.9	10.2‡	33.6	17.2‡	28.1	23.6
>39.0°C	0.8	0.9	3.8	0.0	2.2	0.0
Irritability	59.7	60.2	65.3	52.5‡	54.2	50.6
Drowsiness	50.8	38.9‡	30.3	31.3	21.2	20.2
Decreased Appetite	19.1	15.7	20.6	11.1‡	20.4	9.0‡

* Approximately 72% of subjects received prophylactic or therapeutic antipyretics within 48 hours of each dose.
† Control group received concomitant vaccines only in the same schedule as the Prevnar® group (DTaP, HbOC at dose 1, 2, 3; IPV at doses 1 and 2; Hep B at doses 1 and 3).
‡ p<0.05 when Prevnar® compared to control group using Fisher's Exact test.

TABLE 10
Percentage of Subjects Reporting Systemic Reactions Within 3 Days of Immunization With Prevnar® in Infants and Children from 7 Months Through 9 Years of Age[31]

Age at 1st Vaccination	7-11 Mos.						12-23 Mos.			24-35 Mos.	36-59 Mos.	5-9 Yrs.
Study No.	118-12			118-16			118-9*	118-18		118-18	118-18	118-18
Dose Number	1	2	3†	1	2	3†	1	1	2	1	1	1
Number of Subjects	54	51	24	85	80	50	60	120	117	47	52	100
Reaction												
Fever												
≥38.0°C	20.8	21.6	25.0	17.6	18.8	22.0	36.7	11.7	6.8	14.9	11.5	7.0
>39.0°C	1.9	5.9	0.0	1.6	3.9	2.6	0.0	4.4	0.0	4.2	2.3	1.2
Fussiness	29.6	39.2	16.7	54.1	41.3	38.0	40.0	37.5	36.8	46.8	34.6	29.3
Drowsiness	11.1	17.6	16.7	24.7	16.3	14.0	13.3	18.3	11.1	12.8	17.3	11.0
Decreased Appetite	9.3	15.7	0.0	15.3	15.0	30.0	25.0	20.8	16.2	23.4	11.5	9.0

* For 118-9, 2 of 60 subjects were ≥24 months of age.
† For 118-12, dose 3 was administered at 15-18 mos. of age. For 118-16, dose 3 was administered at 12-15 mos. of age.

TABLE 11
Age and Season-Adjusted Comparison of SIDS Rates in the NCKP Efficacy Trial With the Expected Rate from the California State Data for 1995-1997[20,21]

Vaccine	<One Week After Immunization		≤Two Weeks After Immunization		≤One Month After Immunization		≤One Year After Immunization	
	Exp	Obs	Exp	Obs	Exp	Obs	Exp	Obs
Prevnar®	1.06	1	2.09	2	4.28	2	8.08	4
Control*	1.06	2	2.09	3†	4.28	3†	8.08	8†

* Investigational meningococcal group C conjugate vaccine (MnCC).
† Does not include one additional case of SIDS-like death in a child older than the usual SIDS age (448 days).

Prevnar—Cont.

immunization with Prevnar® administered concurrently with other routine childhood vaccines. Urticaria-like rash was reported in 1.3%-6% of children in the period from 3 to 14 days following immunization, and was most often reported following the fourth dose when it was administered concurrently with MMR vaccine. Based on limited data, it appears that children with urticaria-like rash after a dose of Prevnar® may be more likely to report urticaria-like rash following a subsequent dose of Prevnar®.

One case of a hypotonic-hyporesponsive episode (HHE) was reported in the efficacy study following Prevnar® and concurrent DTP vaccines in the study period from October 1995 through April 1998. Two additional cases of HHE were reported in four other studies and these also occurred in children who received Prevnar® concurrently with DTP vaccine.

In the Kaiser efficacy study in which 17,066 children received a total of 55,352 doses of Prevnar® and 17,080 children received a total of 55,387 doses of the control vaccine (investigational meningococcal group C conjugate vaccine [MnCC]), seizures were reported in 8 Prevnar® recipients and 4 control vaccine recipients within 3 days of immunization from October 1995 through April 1998. Of the 8 Prevnar® recipients, 7 received concomitant DTP-containing vaccines and one received DTaP. Of the 4 control vaccine recipients, 3 received concomitant DTP-containing vaccines and one received DTaP.[20,21] In the other 4 studies combined,

in which 1,102 children were immunized with 3,347 doses of Prevnar® and 408 children were immunized with 1,310 doses of control vaccine (either investigational meningococcal group C conjugate vaccine [MnCC] or concurrent vaccines), there was one seizure event reported within 3 days of immunization.[28] This subject received Prevnar® concurrent with DTaP vaccine.

Twelve deaths (5 SIDS and 7 with clear alternative cause) occurred among subjects receiving Prevnar®, of which 11 (4 SIDS and 7 with clear alternative cause) occurred in the Kaiser efficacy study from October 1995 until April 20, 1999. In comparison, 21 deaths (8 SIDS, 12 with clear alternative cause and one SIDS-like death in an older child), occurred in the control vaccine group during the same time period in the efficacy study.[20,21,25] The number of SIDS deaths in the efficacy study from October 1995 until April 20, 1999 was similar to or lower than the age and season-adjusted expected rate from the California State data from 1995–1997 and are presented in Table 11.
[See table 11 above]

In a review of all hospitalizations that occurred between October 1995 and August 1999 in the efficacy study for the specific diagnoses of aplastic anemia, autoimmune disease, autoimmune hemolytic anemia, diabetes mellitus, neutropenia, and thrombocytopenia, the numbers of such cases were equal to or less than the expected numbers based on the 1995 Kaiser Vaccine Safety Data Link (VSD) data set.

Overall, the safety of Prevnar® was evaluated in a total of five clinical studies in the US in which 18,168 infants and

children received a total of 58,699 doses of vaccine at 2, 4, 6, and 12-15 months of age. In addition, the safety of Prevnar® was evaluated in 831 Finnish infants using the same schedule, and the overall safety profile was similar to that in US infants. The safety of Prevnar® was also evaluated in 560 children from 4 ancillary studies in the US who started immunization at 7 months to 9 years of age. Tables 12 and 13 summarize systemic reactogenicity data within 2 or 3 days across 4,748 subjects in US studies (3,848 infant doses and 997 toddler doses) for whom these data were collected and according to the pertussis vaccine administered concurrently.

TABLE 12
Overall Percentage of Doses Associated With Systemic Events Within 2 or 3 Days For The US Efficacy Study and All US Ancillary Studies When Prevnar® Administered To Infants As a Primary Series at 2, 4, and 6 Months of Age[20,21,25,27,28,29]

Systemic Event	Prevnar® Concurrently With DTaP and HbOC (3,848 Doses)†	DTaP and HbOC Control (538 Doses)‡
Fever		
≥38.0°C	21.1	14.2
>39.0°C	1.8	0.4
Irritability	52.5	45.2
Drowsiness	32.9	27.7
Restless Sleep	20.6	22.3
Decreased Appetite	18.1	13.6
Vomiting	13.4	9.8
Diarrhea	9.8	4.4
Urticaria-like Rash	0.6	0.3

† Total from which reaction data are available varies between reactions from 3,121-3,848 doses. Data from studies 118-8, 118-12, 118-16.
‡ Total from which reaction data are available varies between reactions from 295-538 doses. Data from studies 118-12 and 118-16.

TABLE 13
Overall Percentage of Doses Associated With Systemic Events Within 2 or 3 Days For The US Efficacy Study and All US Ancillary Studies When Prevnar® Administered To Toddlers as a Fourth Dose At 12 to 15 Months of Age[20,21,27]

Systemic Event	Prevnar® Concurrently With DTaP and HbOC (270 Doses)†	Prevnar® Only No Concurrent Vaccines (727 Doses)‡
Fever		
≥38.0°C	19.6	13.4
>39.0°C	1.5	1.2
Irritability	45.9	45.8
Drowsiness	17.5	15.9
Restless Sleep	21.2	21.2
Decreased Appetite	21.1	18.3
Vomiting	5.6	6.3
Diarrhea	13.7	12.8
Urticaria-like Rash	0.7	1.2

† Total from which reaction data are available varies between reactions from 269-270 doses. Data from studies 118-7 and 118-8.
‡ Total from which reaction data are available varies between reactions from 725-727 doses. Data from studies 118-7 and 118-8.

With vaccines in general, including Pneumococcal 7-valent Conjugate Vaccine (Diphtheria CRM_{197} Protein), Prevnar®, it is not uncommon for patients to note within 48 to 72 hours at or around the injection site the following minor reactions: edema; pain or tenderness; redness, inflammation or skin discoloration; mass; or local hypersensitivity reaction. Such local reactions are usually self-limited and require no therapy.

As with other aluminum-containing vaccines, a nodule may occasionally be palpable at the injection site for several weeks.[38]

Postmarketing Experience

Additional adverse reactions identified from postmarketing experience are listed below:

Administration site conditions: injection site dermatitis, injection site urticaria, injection site pruritus

Blood and lymphatic system disorders: lymphadenopathy localized to the region of the injection site

Immune system disorders: hypersensitivity reaction including face edema, dyspnea, bronchospasm; anaphylactic/anaphylactoid reaction including shock

Skin and subcutaneous tissue disorders: angioneurotic edema, erythema multiforme

There have been spontaneous reports of apnea in temporal association with the administration of Prevnar. In most cases Prevnar was administered concomitantly with other vaccines including DTP, DTaP, hepatitis B vaccines, IPV, Hib, MMR, and/or varicella vaccine. In addition, in most of the reports existing medical conditions such as history of apnea, infection, prematurity, and/or seizure were present.

ADVERSE EVENT REPORTING

Any suspected adverse events following immunization should be reported by the healthcare professional to the US Department of Health and Human Services (DHHS). The National Vaccine Injury Compensation Program requires that the manufacturer and lot number of the vaccine administered be recorded by the healthcare professional in the vaccine recipient's permanent medical record (or in a permanent office log or file), along with the date of administration of the vaccine and the name, address, and title of the person administering the vaccine.

The US DHHS has established the Vaccine Adverse Event Reporting System (VAERS) to accept all reports of suspected adverse events after the administration of any vaccine including, but not limited to, the reporting of events required by the National Childhood Vaccine Injury Act of 1986. The FDA VAERS web site is: http://www.fda.gov/cber/vaers/vaers.htm.

The VAERS toll-free number for VAERS forms and information is 800-822-7967.[39]

OVERDOSAGE

There have been reports of overdose with Prevnar®, including cases of administration of a higher than recommended dose and cases of subsequent doses administered closer than recommended to the previous dose. Most individuals were asymptomatic. In general, adverse events reported with overdose have also been reported with recommended single doses of Prevnar®.

DOSAGE AND ADMINISTRATION

For intramuscular injection only. *Do not inject intravenously.*

The dose is 0.5 mL to be given intramuscularly.

Since this product is a suspension containing an adjuvant, shake vigorously immediately prior to use to obtain a uniform suspension in the vaccine container. The vaccine should not be used if it cannot be resuspended.

After shaking, the vaccine is a homogeneous, white suspension.

Parenteral drug products should be inspected visually for particulate matter and discoloration prior to administration (see **DESCRIPTION**). This product should not be used if particulate matter or discoloration is found.

The vaccine should be injected intramuscularly. The preferred sites are the anterolateral aspect of the thigh in infants or the deltoid muscle of the upper arm in toddlers and young children. The vaccine should not be injected in the gluteal area or areas where there may be a major nerve trunk and/or blood vessel. Before injection, the skin at the injection site should be cleansed and prepared with a suitable germicide. After insertion of the needle, aspirate and wait to see if any blood appears in the syringe, which will help avoid inadvertent injection into a blood vessel. If blood appears, withdraw the needle and prepare for a new injection at another site.

The vaccine is to be administered immediately after being drawn up into a syringe. Use one dose per vial; do not re-enter vial. Discard unused portions.

Vaccine Schedule

For infants, the immunization series of Prevnar® consists of three doses of 0.5 mL each, at approximately 2-month intervals, followed by a fourth dose of 0.5 mL at 12-15 months of age. The customary age for the first dose is 2 months of age, but it can be given as young as 6 weeks of age. The recommended dosing interval is 4 to 8 weeks. The fourth dose should be administered at approximately 12-15 months of age, and at least 2 months after the third dose.

Vaccination schedule for infants and toddlers

Dose:	Dose 1*†	Dose 2†	Dose 3†	Dose 4‡
Age at Dose:	2 months	4 months	6 months	12-15 months

* Dose 1 may be given as early as 6 weeks of age
† The recommended dosing interval is 4 to 8 weeks.
‡ The fourth dose should be administered at approximately 12-15 months of age, and at least 2 months after the third dose.

Previously Unvaccinated Older Infants and Children

For previously unvaccinated older infants and children, who are beyond the age of the routine infant schedule, the following schedule applies:[31]

Vaccine schedule for previously unvaccinataed children ≥7 months of age

Age at First Dose	Total Number of 0.5 mL Doses
7-11 months of age	3*
12-23 months of age	2†
≥24 months through 9 years of age	1

* 2 doses at least 4 weeks apart; third dose after the one-year birthday, separated from the second dose by at least 2 months.
† 2 doses at least 2 months apart.

(See **CLINICAL PHARMACOLOGY** section for the limited available immunogenicity data and **ADVERSE REACTIONS** section for limited safety data corresponding to the previously noted vaccination schedule for older children). Safety and immunogenicity data are either limited or not available for children in specific high risk groups for invasive pneumococcal disease (eg, persons with sickle cell disease, asplenia, HIV-infected).

HOW SUPPLIED

24 Vial, 1 Dose (5 per package) - NDC 0005-1970-67

CPT Code 90669

STORAGE

DO NOT FREEZE. STORE REFRIGERATED, AWAY FROM FREEZER COMPARTMENT, AT 2°C TO 8°C (36°F TO 46°F).

REFERENCES

1. Schuchat A, Robinson K, Wenger JD, et al. Bacterial meningitis in the United States in 1995. N Engl J Med. 1997; 337:970-6.
2. Zangwill KM, Vadheim CM, Vannier AM, et al. Epidemiology of invasive pneumococcal disease in Southern California: implications for the design and conduct of a pneumococcal conjugate vaccine efficacy trial. J Infect Dis. 1996; 174:752-9.
3. Breiman R, Spika J, Navarro V, et al. Pneumococcal bacteremia in Charleston County, South Carolina. Arch Intern Med. 1990; 150:1401-5.
4. Levine O, Farley M, Harrison LH, et al. Risk factors for invasive pneumococcal disease in children: a population-based case-control study in North America. Pediatrics. 1999; 103:1-5.
5. Kaplan SL, Mason EO, Barson WJ, et al. Three-year multicenter surveillance of systemic pneumococcal infections in children. Pediatrics. 1998; 102:538-44.
6. Arditi M, Mason E, Bradley J, et al. Three-year multicenter surveillance of pneumococcal meningitis in children: clinical characteristics and outcome related to penicillin susceptibility and dexamethasone use. Pediatrics. 1998; 102:1087-97.
7. Shappert SM. Ambulatory care visits to physician offices, hospital outpatient departments, and emergency departments: United States, 1997. National Center for Health Statistics. Vital Health Sat. 1999; 13(143):1-41.
8. Hall MJ, Lawrence L. Ambulatory surgery in the United States, 1996. Adv Data Vital Health Stat. 1998; 300:1-16.
9. Teele DW, Klein JO, Rosner B, et al. Epidemiology of otitis media during the first seven years of life in children in greater Boston: a prospective, cohort study. J Infect Dis. 1989; 160:83-94.
10. Shappert, SM. Office visits for otitis media: United States, 1975-1990. Adv Data Vital Health Stat. 1992; 214:1-20.
11. Bluestone CD, Stephenson BS, Martin LM. Ten-year review of otitis media pathogens. Pediatr Infect Dis J. 1992; 11:S7-S11.
12. Giebink GS. The microbiology of otitis media. Pediatr Infect Dis J. 1989; 8:S18-S20.
13. Rodriguez WJ, Schwartz RH. *Streptococcus pneumoniae* causes otitis media with higher fever and more redness of tympanic membrane than *Haemophilus influenzae* or *Moraxella catarrhalis*. Pediatr Infect Dis J. 1999; 18:942-4.
14. Barnett ED, Klein JO. The problem of resistant bacteria for the management of acute otitis media. Ped Clin North Am. 1995; 42:509-17.
15. Butler JC, Breiman RF, Lipman HB, et al. Serotype distribution of *Streptococcus pneumoniae* infections among preschool children in the United States, 1978-1994: implications for development of a conjugate vaccine. J Infect Dis. 1995; 171:885-9.
16. Paisley JW, Lauer BA, McIntosh K, et al. Pathogens associated with acute lower respiratory tract infection in young children. Pediatr Infect Dis J. 1984; 3:14-9.
17. American Academy of Pediatrics Committee on Infectious Diseases. Therapy for children with invasive pneumococcal infections. Pediatrics. 1997; 99:289-300.
18. Hausdorff WP, Bryant J, Paradiso PR, Siber GR. Which pneumococcal serogroups cause the most invasive disease: implications for conjugate vaccine formulation and use, part I. Clin Infect Dis. 2000; 30:100-21.
19. Butler JC, Hoffman J, Cetron MS, et al. The continued emergence of drug-resistant *Streptococcus pneumoniae* in the United States. An Update from the Centers for Disease Control and Prevention's Pneumococcal Sentinel Surveillance System. J Infect Dis. 1996; 174:986-93.
20. Lederle Laboratories, Data on File: D118-P8.
21. Black S, Shinefield H, Ray P, et al. Efficacy, safety and immunogenicity of heptavalent pneumococcal conjugate vaccine in children. Pediatr Infect Dis J. 2000; 19:187-195.
22. Lederle Laboratories, Data on File: D118-P809.
23. Eskola J, Kilpi T, Palma A, et al. Efficacy of a pneumococcal conjugate vaccine against acute otitis media. N Engl J Med. 2001; 344:403-409.
24. Fireman B, Black S, Shinefield H, et al. The impact of the pneumococcal conjugate vaccine on otitis media. Pediatr Infect Dis J. 2003;22:10-16.
25. Lederle Laboratories, Data on File: D118-P16.
26. Lederle Laboratories, Data on File: D118-P8 Addendum DTaP Immunogenicity.
27. Shinefield HR, Black S, Ray P. Safety and immunogenicity of heptavalent pneumococcal CRM197 conjugate vaccine in infants and toddlers. Pediatr Infect Dis J. 1999; 18:757-63.
28. Lederle Laboratories, Data on File: D118-P12.
29. Rennels MD, Edwards KM, Keyserling HL, et al. Safety and immunogenicity of heptavalent pneumococcal vaccine conjugated to CRM$_{197}$ in United States infants. Pediatrics. 1998; 101(4):604-11.
30. Lederle Laboratories, Data on File: D118-P3.
31. Lederle Laboratories, Data on File: Integrated Summary on Catch-Up.
32. Report of the Committee on Infectious Diseases 24th Edition. Elk Grove Village, IL: American Academy of Pediatrics. 1997; 31-3.
33. Update: Vaccine Side Effects, Adverse Reactions, Contraindications, and Precautions. MMWR. 1996; 45 (RR-12):1-35.
34. Centers for Disease Control and Prevention. General recommendations on immunization. Recommendations of the Advisory Committee on Immunization Practices (ACIP) and the American Academy of Family Physicians (AAFP). MMWR. 2002; 51(RR-2):1-36.
35. Vernacchio L, Neufeld EJ, MacDonald K, et al. Combined schedule of 7-valent pneumococcal conjugate vaccine followed by 23-valent pneumococcal vaccine in children and young adults with sickle cell disease. J Pediatr. 1998; 103:275-8.
36. Wyeth, Data on file: Final clinical study report D140-P1.
37. Wyeth, Data on file: Final clinical study report MMR100495.
38. Fawcett HA, Smith NP. Injection-site granuloma due to aluminum. Archives Dermatology. 1984; 120:1318-22.
39. Vaccines Adverse Event Reporting System – United States. MMWR. 1990; 39:730-3.

Wyeth®
Manufactured by:
Wyeth Pharmaceuticals Inc.
Philadelphia, PA 19101
US Govt. License No. 3

W10430C004
ET01
Rev 02/05

PROTONIX® ℞

[prō'tŏn-ĭks]
(pantoprazole sodium)
Delayed-Release Tablets
℞ only

Prescribing information for this product, which appears on pages 3389–3393 of the 2005 PDR, has been revised as follows. Please write "See Supplement A" next to the product heading.

This product's label may have been revised after this insert was used in production. For further product information and current package insert, please visit www.wyeth.com or call our medical communications department toll-free at 1-800-934-5556.

In the **Adverse Reactions** section, the *"Postmarketing Reports"* subsection was revised as follows:

Postmarketing Reports

There have been spontaneous reports of adverse events with the postmarketing use of pantoprazole. These reports include the following:

BODY AS A WHOLE: anaphylaxis (including anaphylactic shock), angioedema (Quincke's edema).

DIGESTIVE SYSTEM: increased salivation, nausea, pancreatitis.

HEMIC AND LYMPHATIC SYSTEM: pancytopenia.

HEPATO-BILIARY SYSTEM: hepatocellular damage leading to jaundice and hepatic failure.

MUSCULOSKELETAL SYSTEM: elevated CPK (creatine phosphokinase), rhabdomyolysis.

NERVOUS SYSTEM: confusion, hypokinesia, speech disorder, vertigo.

SKIN AND APPENDAGES: severe dermatologic reactions, including erythema multiforme, Stevens-Johnson syndrome, and toxic epidermal necrolysis (TEN, some fatal).

SPECIAL SENSES: anterior ischemic optic neuropathy, blurred vision, tinnitus.

UROGENITAL SYSTEM: interstitial nephritis.

Continued on next page

Protonix Tablets—Cont.

Packaged by
Wyeth Pharmaceuticals, Inc.
Philadelphia, PA 19101
under license from
ALTANA Pharma
D78467 Konstanz, Germany
W10438C010
ET01
Rev12/04

PROTONIX® I.V. ℞

[*prō'tō-nĭks*]
(pantoprazole sodium)
for Injection
℞ only

Prescribing information for this product, which appears on pages 3392–3395 of the 2005 PDR, has been completely revised as follows. Please write "See Supplement A" next to the product heading.

DESCRIPTION

The active ingredient in PROTONIX® I.V. (pantoprazole sodium) for Injection is a substituted benzimidazole, sodium 5-(difluoromethoxy)-2-[[(3,4-dimethoxy-2-pyridinyl)methyl] sulfinyl]-1H-benzimidazole, a compound that inhibits gastric acid secretion. Its empirical formula is $C_{16}H_{14}F_2N_3NaO_4S$, with a molecular weight of 405.4. The structural formula is:

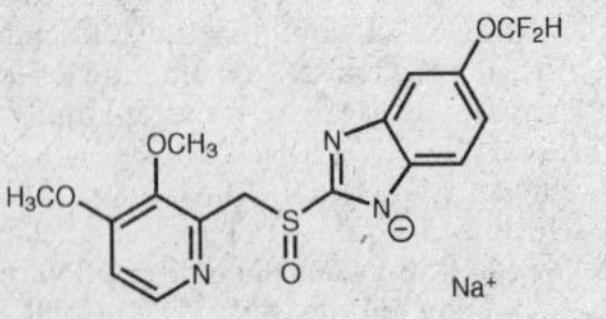

Pantoprazole sodium is a white to off-white crystalline powder and is racemic. Pantoprazole has weakly basic and acidic properties. Pantoprazole sodium is freely soluble in water, very slightly soluble in phosphate buffer at pH 7.4, and practically insoluble in n-hexane. The stability of the compound in aqueous solution is pH-dependent. The rate of degradation increases with decreasing pH. The reconstituted solution of PROTONIX I.V. for Injection is in the pH range 9.0 to 10.5.
PROTONIX I.V. for Injection is supplied as a freeze-dried powder in a clear glass vial fitted with a rubber stopper and crimp seal containing pantoprazole sodium, equivalent to 40 mg of pantoprazole, edetate disodium (1 mg), and sodium hydroxide to adjust pH.

CLINICAL PHARMACOLOGY

Pharmacokinetics

Pantoprazole peak serum concentration (C_{max}) and area under the serum concentration-time curve (AUC) increase in a manner proportional to intravenous doses from 10 mg to 80 mg. Pantoprazole does not accumulate and its pharmacokinetics are unaltered with multiple daily dosing. Following the administration of PROTONIX I.V. for Injection, the serum concentration of pantoprazole declines biexponentially with a terminal elimination half-life of approximately one hour. In extensive metabolizers (see **CLINICAL PHARMACOLOGY, Metabolism**) with normal liver function receiving a 40 mg dose of PROTONIX I.V. for Injection by constant rate over 15 minutes, the peak concentration (C_{max}) is 5.52 µg/mL and the total area under the plasma concentration versus time curve (AUC) is 5.4 µg · hr/mL. The total clearance is 7.6-14.0 L/h and the apparent volume of distribution is 11.0-23.6 L.

Distribution

The apparent volume of distribution of pantoprazole is approximately 11.0-23.6 L, distributing mainly in extracellular fluid. The serum protein binding of pantoprazole is about 98%, primarily to albumin.

Metabolism

Pantoprazole is extensively metabolized in the liver through the cytochrome P450 (CYP) system. Pantoprazole metabolism is independent of the route of administration (intravenous or oral). The main metabolic pathway is demethylation, by CYP2C19, with subsequent sulfation; other metabolic pathways include oxidation by CYP3A4. There is no evidence that any of the pantoprazole metabolites have significant pharmacologic activity. CYP2C19 displays a known genetic polymorphism due to its deficiency in some sub-populations (e.g., 3% of Caucasians and African-Americans and 17-23% of Asians). Although these sub-populations of slow pantoprazole metabolizers have elimination half-life values from 3.5 to 10.0 hours, they still have minimal accumulation (≤23%) with once daily dosing.

Elimination

After administration of a single intravenous dose of ^{14}C-labeled pantoprazole to healthy, normal metabolizer subjects, approximately 71% of the dose was excreted in the urine with 18% excreted in the feces through biliary excretion. There was no renal excretion of unchanged pantoprazole.

Gastric Acid Output (mEq/hr, Mean ± SD) and Percent Inhibition[a] (Mean ± SD) of Pentagastrin-Stimulated Acid Output Over 24 Hours Following a Single Dose of PROTONIX I.V. for Injection[b] in Healthy Subjects

Treatment Dose	—2 hours— Acid Output	% Inhibition	—4 hours— Acid Output	% Inhibition	—12 hours— Acid Output	% Inhibition	—24 hours— Acid Output	% Inhibition
0 mg (Placebo, n=4)	39 ± 21	NA	26 ± 14	NA	32 ± 20	NA	38 ± 24	NA
20 mg (n=4-6)	13 ± 18	47 ± 27	6 ± 8	83 ± 21	20 ± 20	54 ± 44	30 ± 23	45 ± 43
40 mg (n=8)	5 ± 5	82 ± 11	4 ± 4	90 ± 11	11 ± 10	81 ± 13	16 ± 12	52 ± 36
80 mg (n=8)	0.1 ± 0.2	96 ± 6	0.3 ± 0.4	99 ± 1	2 ± 2	90 ± 7	7 ± 4	63 ± 18

a: Compared to individual subject baseline prior to treatment with PROTONIX I.V. for Injection.
NA = not applicable.
b: Inhibition of gastric acid output and the percent inhibition of stimulated acid output in response to PROTONIX I.V. for Injection may be higher after repeated doses.

Special Populations

Geriatric

After repeated I.V. administration in elderly subjects (65 to 76 years of age), pantoprazole AUC and elimination half-life values were similar to those observed in younger subjects. No dosage adjustment is recommended based on age.

Pediatric

The pharmacokinetics of pantoprazole have not been investigated in patients <18 years of age.

Gender

After oral administration there is a modest increase in pantoprazole AUC and C_{max} in women compared to men. However, weight-normalized clearance values are similar in women and men. No dosage adjustment is warranted based on gender (also see **Use in Women**).

Renal Impairment

In patients with severe renal impairment, pharmacokinetic parameters for pantoprazole were similar to those of healthy subjects. No dosage adjustment is necessary in patients with renal impairment or in patients undergoing hemodialysis.

Hepatic Impairment

Oral administration studies (absolute bioavailability is approximately 70%) were performed in patients with mild to severe hepatic impairment. Maximum pantoprazole concentrations increased only slightly (1.5-fold) relative to healthy subjects. Although serum elimination half-life values increased to 7-9 hours and AUC values increased by 5- to 7-fold in hepatic-impaired patients, these increases were no greater than those observed in slow CYP2C19 metabolizers, where no dosage adjustment is warranted. These pharmacokinetic changes in hepatic-impaired patients result in minimal drug accumulation following once daily multiple-dose administration equal to or less than 21%. No dosage adjustment is needed in patients with mild to severe hepatic impairment. Doses higher than 40 mg/day have not been studied in hepatically-impaired patients.

Drug-Drug Interactions

Pantoprazole is metabolized mainly by CYP2C19 and to minor extents by CYPs 3A4, 2D6 and 2C9. In *in vivo* drug-drug interaction studies with CYP2C19 substrates (diazepam [also a CYP3A4 substrate] and phenytoin [also a CYP3A4 inducer]), nifedipine, midazolam, and clarithromycin (CYP3A4 substrates), metoprolol (a CYP2D6 substrate), diclofenac, naproxen and piroxicam (CYP2C9 substrates) and theophylline (a CYP1A2 substrate) in healthy subjects, the pharmacokinetics of pantoprazole were not significantly altered. It is, therefore, expected that other drugs metabolized by CYPs 2C19, 3A4, 2D6, 2C9 and 1A2 would not significantly affect the pharmacokinetics of pantoprazole. *In vivo* studies also suggest that pantoprazole does not significantly affect the kinetics of other drugs (cisapride, theophylline, diazepam [and its active metabolite, desmethyldiazepam], phenytoin, warfarin, metoprolol, nifedipine, carbamazepine, midazolam, clarithromycin, naproxen, piroxicam and oral contraceptives [levonorgestrel/ethinyl estradiol]) metabolized by CYPs 2C19, 3A4, 2D6, 2C9 and 1A2. Therefore, it is expected that pantoprazole would not significantly affect the pharmacokinetics of other drugs metabolized by these isozymes. Dosage adjustment of such drugs is not necessary when they are co-administered with pantoprazole. In other *in vivo* studies, digoxin, ethanol, glyburide, antipyrine, caffeine, metronidazole, and amoxicillin had no clinically relevant interactions with pantoprazole. Although no significant drug-drug interactions have been observed in clinical studies, the potential for significant drug-drug interactions with more than once daily dosing with high doses of pantoprazole has not been studied in poor metabolizers or individuals who are hepatically impaired.

Pharmacodynamics

Mechanism of Action

Pantoprazole is a proton pump inhibitor (PPI) that suppresses the final step in gastric acid production by covalently binding to the (H^+, K^+)-ATPase enzyme system at the secretory surface of the gastric parietal cell. This effect leads to inhibition of both basal and stimulated gastric acid secretion irrespective of the stimulus. The binding to the (H^+, K^+)-ATPase results in a duration of antisecretory effect that persists longer than 24 hours for all doses tested.

Antisecretory Activity

The magnitude and time course for inhibition of pentagastrin-stimulated acid output (PSAO) by single doses (20 to 120 mg) of PROTONIX I.V. for Injection were assessed in a single-dose, open-label, placebo-controlled, dose-response study. The results of this study are shown in the table below. Healthy subjects received a continuous infusion for 25 hours of pentagastrin (PG) at 1 µg/kg/h, a dose known to produce submaximal gastric acid secretion. The placebo group showed a sustained, continuous acid output for 25 hours, validating the reliability of the testing model. PROTONIX I.V. for Injection had an onset of antisecretory activity within 15 to 30 minutes of administration. Doses of 20 to 80 mg of PROTONIX I.V. for Injection substantially reduced the 24-hour cumulative PSAO in a dose-dependent manner, despite a short plasma elimination half-life. Complete suppression of PSAO was achieved with 80 mg within approximately 2 hours and no further significant suppression was seen with 120 mg. The duration of action of PROTONIX I.V. for Injection was 24 hours.
[See table above]
In one study of gastric pH in healthy subjects, pantoprazole was administered orally (40 mg enteric coated tablets) or intravenously (40 mg) once daily for 5 days and pH was measured for 24 hours following the fifth dose. The outcome measure was median percent of time that pH was ≥ 4 and the results were similar for intravenous and oral medications; however, the clinical significance of this parameter is unknown.

Serum Gastrin Effects

Serum gastrin concentrations were assessed in two placebo-controlled studies.
In a 5-day study of oral pantoprazole with 40 and 60 mg doses in healthy subjects, following the last dose on day 5, median 24-hour serum gastrin concentrations were elevated by 3-4 fold compared to placebo in both 40 and 60 mg dose groups. However, by 24 hours following the last dose, median serum gastrin concentrations for both groups returned to normal levels.
In another placebo-controlled, 7-day study of 40 mg intravenous or oral pantoprazole in patients with GERD and a history of erosive esophagitis, the mean serum gastrin concentration increased approximately 50% from baseline and as compared with placebo, but remained within the normal range.
During 6 days of repeated administration of PROTONIX I.V. for Injection in patients with Zollinger-Ellison Syndrome, consistent changes of serum gastrin concentrations from baseline were not observed.

Enterochromaffin-Like (ECL) Cell Effects

There are no data available on the effects of intravenous pantoprazole on ECL cells.
In a nonclinical study in Sprague-Dawley rats, lifetime exposure (24 months) to pantoprazole at doses of 0.5 to 200 mg/kg/day resulted in dose-related increases in gastric ECL-cell proliferation and gastric neuroendocrine (NE)-cell tumors. Gastric NE-cell tumors in rats may result from chronic elevation of serum gastrin concentrations. The high density of ECL cells in the rat stomach makes this species highly susceptible to the proliferative effects of elevated gastrin concentrations produced by proton pump inhibitors. However, there were no observed elevations in serum gastrin following the administration of pantoprazole at a dose of 0.5 mg/kg/day. In a separate study, a gastric NE-cell tumor without concomitant ECL-cell proliferative changes was observed in 1 female rat following 12 months of dosing with pantoprazole at 5 mg/kg/day and a 9 month off-dose recovery (see **PRECAUTIONS, Carcinogenesis, Mutagenesis, Impairment of Fertility**).

Other Effects

No clinically relevant effects of pantoprazole on cardiovascular, respiratory, ophthalmic, or central nervous system function have been detected. In a clinical pharmacology study, pantoprazole 40 mg given orally once daily for 2 weeks had no effect on the levels of the following hormones: cortisol, testosterone, triiodothyronine (T3), thyroxine (T4), thyroid-stimulating hormone, thyronine-binding protein, parathyroid hormone, insulin, glucagon, renin, aldosterone, follicle-stimulating hormone, luteinizing hormone, prolactin and growth hormone.

Clinical Studies

Gastroesophageal Reflux Disease (GERD) Associated With a History of Erosive Esophagitis

A multicenter, double-blind, two-period placebo-controlled study was conducted to assess the ability of PROTONIX® I.V. (pantoprazole sodium) for Injection to maintain gastric acid suppression in patients switched from the oral dosage form of pantoprazole to the intravenous dosage form. Gastroesophageal reflux disease (GERD) patients (n=65, 26 to 64 years; 35 female; 9 black, 11 Hispanic, 44 white, 1 other) with a history of erosive esophagitis were randomized to receive either 20 or 40 mg of oral pantoprazole once per day for 10 days (period 1) and, then were switched in period 2 to either daily intravenous pantoprazole or placebo for 7 days, matching their respective dose level from period 1. Patients were administered all test medication with a light meal. Maximum acid output (MAO) and basal acid output (BAO) were determined 24 hours following the last day of oral medication (day 10), the first day (day 1) of intravenous administration and the last day of intravenous administration (day 7). MAO was estimated from a 1 hour continuous collection of gastric contents following subcutaneous injection of 6.0 μg/kg of pentagastrin. This study demonstrated that, after 10 days of repeated oral administration followed by 7 days of intravenous administration, the oral and intravenous dosage forms of PROTONIX 40 mg are similar in their ability to suppress MAO and BAO in patients with GERD and a history of erosive esophagitis (see table below). Also, patients on oral PROTONIX who were switched to intravenous placebo experienced a significant increase in acid output within 48 hours of their last oral dose. However, at 48 hours after their last oral dose, patients treated with PROTONIX I.V. for Injection had a significantly lower mean basal acid output than those treated with placebo.

[See first table at right]

ANTISECRETORY EFFECTS (mEq/h) OF 40 mg PROTONIX I.V. for INJECTION AND 40 mg ORAL PROTONIX IN GERD PATIENTS WITH A HISTORY OF EROSIVE ESOPHAGITIS

Parameter	PROTONIX Delayed-Release Tablets DAY 10	PROTONIX I.V. for Injection DAY 7	Placebo I.V. DAY 7
Mean maximum acid output	6.49 n=30	6.62 n=23	29.19* n=7
Mean basal acid output	0.80 n=30	0.53 n=23	4.14* n=7

*P<0.0001 Significantly different from PROTONIX I.V. for Injection.

To evaluate the effectiveness of PROTONIX I.V. (pantoprazole sodium) for Injection as an initial treatment to suppress gastric acid secretion, two studies were conducted.

Study 1 was a multicenter, double-blind, placebo controlled, study of the pharmacodynamic effects of PROTONIX I.V. for Injection and oral PROTONIX. Patients with GERD and a history of erosive esophagitis (n=78, 20-67 years; 39 females; 7 black, 19 Hispanic, 52 white) were randomized to receive either 40 mg intravenous pantoprazole, 40 mg oral pantoprazole, or placebo once daily for 7 days. Following an overnight fast, test medication was administered and patients were given a light meal within 15 minutes. MAO and BAO were determined 24 hours following the last day of study medication. MAO was estimated from a 1 hour continuous collection of gastric contents following subcutaneous injection of 6.0 μg/kg of pentagastrin to stimulate acid secretion. This study demonstrated that, after treatment for 7 days, patients treated with PROTONIX I.V. for Injection had a significantly lower MAO and BAO than those treated with placebo (p <0.001), and results were comparable to those of patients treated with oral PROTONIX (see table below).

[See second table above]

ANTISECRETORY EFFECTS (mEq/h) OF INITIAL TREATMENT WITH 40 mg PROTONIX I.V. for INJECTION AND 40 mg ORAL PROTONIX IN GERD PATIENTS WITH A HISTORY OF EROSIVE ESOPHAGITIS

Parameter	PROTONIX I.V. for Injection DAY 7	PROTONIX Delayed-Release Tablets DAY 7	Placebo DAY 7
Maximum acid output (mean ± SD)	8.4 ± 5.9 n=25	6.3 ± 6.6 n=22	20.9 ± 14.5* n=24
Basal acid output (mean ± SD)	0.4 ± 0.5 n=25	0.6 ± 0.8 n=22	2.8 ± 3.0* n=23

*P<0.0001 Significantly different from PROTONIX I.V. for Injection.

Study 2 was a single-center, double-blind, parallel-group study to compare the clinical effects of PROTONIX I.V. for Injection and oral PROTONIX. Patients (n=45, median age 56 years, 21 males and 24 females) with acute endoscopically proven reflux esophagitis (Savary/Miller Stage II or III) with at least 1 of 3 symptoms typical for reflux esophagitis (acid eructation, heartburn, or pain on swallowing) were randomized to receive either 40 mg intravenous pantoprazole or 40 mg oral pantoprazole daily for 5 days. After the initial 5 days, all patients were treated with 40 mg oral pantoprazole daily to complete a total of 8 weeks of treatment. Symptom relief was assessed by calculating the daily mean of the sums of the average scores for these 3 symptoms and the daily mean of the average score for each of the symptoms separately. There was no significant difference in symptom relief between PROTONIX I.V. and oral PROTONIX therapy within the first 5 days. A repeat endoscopy after 8 weeks of treatment revealed that 20 out of 23 (87%) of the PROTONIX I.V. plus oral PROTONIX patients and 19 out of 22 (86%) of the oral PROTONIX patients had endoscopically proven healing of their esophageal lesions.

Data comparing PROTONIX I.V. for Injection to other proton pump inhibitors (oral or I.V.) or H2 receptor antagonists (oral or I.V.) are limited, and therefore, are inadequate to support any conclusions regarding comparative efficacy.

Pathological Hypersecretion Associated with Zollinger-Ellison Syndrome

Two studies measured the pharmacodynamic effects of 6 day treatment with PROTONIX I.V. for Injection in patients with Zollinger-Ellison Syndrome (with and without multiple endocrine neoplasia type I). In one of these studies, an initial treatment with PROTONIX I.V. for Injection in 21 patients (29 to 75 years; 8 female; 4 black, 1 Hispanic, 16 white) reduced acid output to the target level (≤ 10 mEq/h) and significantly reduced H+ concentration and the volume of gastric secretions; target levels were achieved within 45 minutes of drug administration.

In the other study of 14 patients (38 to 67 years; 5 female; 2 black, 12 white) with Zollinger-Ellison Syndrome, treatment was switched from an oral proton pump inhibitor to PROTONIX I.V. for Injection. PROTONIX I.V. for Injection maintained or improved control of gastric acid secretion.

In both studies, PROTONIX I.V. for Injection 160 or 240 mg per day in divided doses maintained basal acid secretion below target levels in all patients. Target levels were 10 mEq/h in patients without prior gastric surgery, and 5 mEq/h in all patients with prior gastric acid-reducing surgery. Once gastric acid secretion was controlled, there was no evidence of tolerance during this 7 day study. Basal acid secretion was maintained below target levels for at least 24 hours in all patients and through the end of treatment in these studies (3 to 7 days) in all but 1 patient who required a dose adjustment guided by acid output measurements until acid control was achieved. In both studies, doses were adjusted to the individual patient need, but gastric acid secretion was controlled in greater than 80% of patients by a starting regimen of 80 mg q12h.

INDICATIONS AND USAGE

Treatment of Gastroesophageal Reflux Disease Associated With a History of Erosive Esophagitis

PROTONIX I.V. for Injection is indicated for short-term treatment (7 to 10 days) of patients with gastroesophageal reflux disease (GERD) and a history of erosive esophagitis.

Pathological Hypersecretion Associated with Zollinger-Ellison Syndrome

PROTONIX I.V. for Injection is indicated for the treatment of pathological hypersecretory conditions associated with Zollinger-Ellison Syndrome or other neoplastic conditions.

CONTRAINDICATIONS

PROTONIX I.V. for Injection is contraindicated in patients with known hypersensitivity to the formulation.

PRECAUTIONS

General

Immediate hypersensitivity reactions: Anaphylaxis has been reported with use of intravenous pantoprazole. This may require emergency medical treatment.

Injection site reactions: Thrombophlebitis was associated with the administration of intravenous pantoprazole.

Hepatic effects: Mild, transient transaminase elevations have been observed in clinical studies. The clinical significance of this finding in a large population of subjects administered intravenous pantoprazole is unknown. (See **ADVERSE REACTIONS** section).

Symptomatic response to therapy with pantoprazole does not preclude the presence of gastric malignancy.

As with any other intravenous product containing edetate disodium (the salt form of EDTA) which is a potent chelator of metal ions including zinc, zinc supplementation should be considered in patients treated with PROTONIX I.V. for Injection who are prone to zinc deficiency. Caution should be used when other EDTA containing products are also co-administered intravenously.

Treatment with PROTONIX® I.V. (pantoprazole sodium) for Injection should be discontinued as soon as the patient is able to resume treatment with PROTONIX Delayed-Release Tablets.

Drug Interactions

Pantoprazole is metabolized through the cytochrome P450 system, primarily the CYP2C19 and CYP3A4 isozymes, and subsequently undergoes Phase II conjugation. (See **CLINICAL PHARMACOLOGY, Drug-Drug Interactions.**)

Based on studies evaluating possible interactions of pantoprazole with other drugs, no dosage adjustment is needed with concomitant use of the following: theophylline, cisapride, antipyrine, caffeine, carbamazepine, diazepam (and its active metabolite, desmethyldiazepam), diclofenac, naproxen, piroxicam, digoxin, ethanol, glyburide, an oral contraceptive (levonorgestrel/ethinyl estradiol), metoprolol, nifedipine, phenytoin, warfarin (see below), midazolam, clarithromycin, metronidazole, or amoxicillin. Clinically relevant interactions of pantoprazole with other drugs with the same metabolic pathways are not expected. Therefore, when co-administered with pantoprazole, adjustment of the dosage of pantoprazole or of such drugs may not be necessary. There was also no interaction with concomitantly administered antacids. There have been postmarketing reports of increased INR and prothrombin time in patients receiving proton pump inhibitors, including pantoprazole, and warfarin concomitantly. Increases in INR and prothrombin time may lead to abnormal bleeding and even death. Patients treated with proton pump inhibitors and warfarin concomitantly should be monitored for increases in INR and prothrombin time.

Because of profound and long lasting inhibition of gastric acid secretion, pantoprazole may interfere with absorption of drugs where gastric pH is an important determinant of their bioavailability (e.g., ketoconazole, ampicillin esters, and iron salts).

Carcinogenesis, Mutagenesis, Impairment of Fertility

In a 24-month carcinogenicity study, Sprague-Dawley rats were treated orally with doses of 0.5 to 200 mg/kg/day, about 0.1 to 40 times the exposure on a body surface area basis, of a 50-kg person dosed at 40 mg/day. In the gastric fundus, treatment at 0.5 to 200 mg/kg/day produced enterochromaffin-like (ECL) cell hyperplasia and benign and malignant neuroendocrine cell tumors in a dose-related manner. In the forestomach, treatment at 50 and 200 mg/kg/day (about 10 and 40 times the recommended human dose on a body surface area basis) produced benign squamous cell papillomas and malignant squamous cell carcinomas. Rare gastrointestinal tumors associated with pantoprazole treatment included an adenocarcinoma of the duodenum at 50 mg/kg/day, and benign polyps and adenocarcinomas of the gastric fundus at 200 mg/kg/day. In the liver, treatment at 0.5 to 200 mg/kg/day produced dose-related increases in the incidences of hepatocellular adenomas and carcinomas. In the thyroid gland, treatment at 200 mg/kg/day produced increased incidences of follicular cell adenomas and carcinomas for both male and female rats.

Sporadic occurrences of hepatocellular adenomas and a hepatocellular carcinoma were observed in Sprague-Dawley rats exposed to pantoprazole in 6-month and 12-month oral toxicity studies.

In a 24-month carcinogenicity study, Fischer 344 rats were treated orally with doses of 5 to 50 mg/kg/day, approximately 1 to 10 times the recommended human dose based on body surface area. In the gastric fundus, treatment at 5 to 50 mg/kg/day produced enterochromaffin-like (ECL) cell hyperplasia and benign and malignant neuroendocrine cell tumors. Dose selection for this study may not have been adequate to comprehensively evaluate the carcinogenic potential of pantoprazole.

In a 24-month carcinogenicity study, B6C3F1 mice were treated orally with doses of 5 to 150 mg/kg/day, 0.5 to 15 times the recommended human dose based on body surface area. In the liver, treatment at 150 mg/kg/day produced increased incidences of hepatocellular adenomas and carcinomas in female mice. Treatment at 5 to 150 mg/kg/day also produced gastric fundic ECL cell hyperplasia.

Pantoprazole was positive in the *in vitro* human lymphocyte chromosomal aberration assays, in one of two mouse micronucleus tests for clastogenic effects, and in the *in vitro* Chinese hamster ovarian cell/HGPRT forward mutation assay for mutagenic effects. Equivocal results were observed in the *in vivo* rat liver DNA covalent binding assay. Pantoprazole was negative in the *in vitro* Ames mutation assay, the *in vitro* unscheduled DNA synthesis (UDS) assay with rat hepatocytes, the *in vitro* AS52/GPT mammalian cell-forward gene mutation assay, the *in vitro* thymidine kinase mutation test with mouse lymphoma L5178Y cells, and the *in vivo* rat bone marrow cell chromosomal aberration assay. A 26-week p53 +/− transgenic mouse carcinogenicity study was not positive.

Pantoprazole at oral doses up to 500 mg/kg/day in male rats (98 times the recommended human dose based on body surface area) and 450 mg/kg/day in female rats (88 times the recommended human dose based on body surface area) was found to have no effect on fertility and reproductive performance.

Pregnancy

Teratogenic Effects

Pregnancy Category B

Teratology studies have been performed in rats at intravenous doses up to 20 mg/kg/day (4 times the recommended human dose based on body surface area) and rabbits at intravenous doses up to 15 mg/kg/day (6 times the recom-

Continued on next page

Protonix I.V.—Cont.

mended human dose based on body surface area) and have revealed no evidence of impaired fertility or harm to the fetus due to pantoprazole. There are, however, no adequate and well-controlled studies in pregnant women. Because animal reproduction studies are not always predictive of human response, this drug should be used during pregnancy only if clearly needed.

Nursing Mothers

Pantoprazole and its metabolites are excreted in the milk of rats. Pantoprazole excretion in human milk has been detected in a study of a single nursing mother after a single 40 mg oral dose. The clinical relevance of this finding is not known. Many drugs which are excreted in human milk have a potential for serious adverse reactions in nursing infants. Based on the potential for tumorigenicity shown for pantoprazole in rodent carcinogenicity studies, a decision should be made whether to discontinue nursing or to discontinue the drug, taking into account the benefit of the drug to the mother.

Pediatric Use

Safety and effectiveness in pediatric patients have not been established.

Use in Women

No gender-related differences in the safety profile of intravenous pantoprazole were seen in international trials involving 166 men and 120 women with erosive esophagitis associated with GERD. Erosive esophagitis healing rates in the 221 women treated with oral pantoprazole in U.S. clinical trials were similar to those found in men. The incidence rates of adverse events were also similar between men and women.

Use in Elderly

No age-related differences in the safety profile of intravenous pantoprazole were seen in international trials involving 86 elderly (≥ 65 years old) and 200 younger (< 65 years old) patients with erosive esophagitis associated with GERD. Erosive esophagitis healing rates in the 107 elderly patients (≥ 65 years old) treated with oral pantoprazole in U.S. clinical trials were similar to those found in patients under the age of 65. The incidence rates of adverse events and laboratory abnormalities in patients aged 65 years and older were similar to those associated with patients younger than 65 years of age.

Laboratory Tests

There have been reports of false-positive urine screening tests for tetrahydrocannabinol (THC) in patients receiving most proton pump inhibitors, including pantoprazole. An alternative confirmatory method should be considered to verify positive results.

ADVERSE REACTIONS

Safety Experience with Intravenous Pantoprazole

Intravenous pantoprazole has been studied in clinical trials in several populations including patients with GERD and a history of erosive esophagitis, patients with Zollinger-Ellison Syndrome, patients involved in clinical trials for other disorders which may respond to proton pump inhibitor therapy, and healthy subjects. Adverse experiences occurring in >1% of patients treated with intravenous pantoprazole (n=836) in domestic or international clinical trials are shown below by body system. In most instances, the relationship to pantoprazole was unclear.

BODY AS A WHOLE: abdominal pain, headache, injection site reaction (including thrombophlebitis and abscess).

DIGESTIVE SYSTEM: constipation, dyspepsia, nausea, diarrhea.

NERVOUS SYSTEM: insomnia, dizziness.

RESPIRATORY SYSTEM: rhinitis.

Head-to-head comparative studies between PROTONIX I.V. for Injection and oral PROTONIX, other proton pump inhibitors (oral or I.V.), or H2 receptor antagonists (oral or I.V.) have been limited. The available information does not provide sufficient evidence to distinguish the safety profile of these regimens.

Safety Experience with Oral Pantoprazole

In clinical trials in patients with erosive esophagitis associated with GERD treated with oral pantoprazole, the following adverse events, regardless of causality, occurred at a rate of ≥1%.

BODY AS A WHOLE: headache, asthenia, back pain, chest pain, neck pain, flu syndrome, infection, pain.

CARDIOVASCULAR SYSTEM: migraine.

DIGESTIVE SYSTEM: diarrhea, flatulence, abdominal pain, eructation, constipation, dyspepsia, gastroenteritis, gastrointestinal disorder, nausea, rectal disorder, vomiting.

HEPATO-BILIARY SYSTEM: liver function tests abnormal, SGPT increased.

METABOLIC AND NUTRITIONAL: hyperglycemia, hyperlipemia.

MUSCULOSKELETAL SYSTEM: arthralgia.

NERVOUS SYSTEM: insomnia, anxiety, dizziness, hypertonia.

RESPIRATORY SYSTEM: bronchitis, cough increased, dyspnea, pharyngitis, rhinitis, sinusitis, upper respiratory tract infection.

SKIN AND APPENDAGES: rash.

UROGENITAL SYSTEM: urinary frequency, and urinary tract infection.

Additional adverse experiences occurring in <1% of patients with erosive esophagitis associated with GERD receiving oral pantoprazole based on pooled results from either domestic or international trials are shown below within each body system. In most instances, the relationship to pantoprazole was unclear.

BODY AS A WHOLE: abscess, allergic reaction, chills, cyst, face edema, fever, generalized edema, heat stroke, hernia, laboratory test abnormal, malaise, moniliasis, neoplasm, non-specified drug reaction, photosensitivity reaction.

CARDIOVASCULAR SYSTEM: abnormal electrocardiogram, angina pectoris, arrhythmia, atrial fibrillation/flutter, cardiovascular disorder, chest pain substernal, congestive heart failure, hemorrhage, hypertension, hypotension, myocardial infarction, myocardial ischemia, palpitation, retinal vascular disorder, syncope, tachycardia, thrombophlebitis, thrombosis, vasodilatation.

DIGESTIVE SYSTEM: anorexia, aphthous stomatitis, cardiospasm, colitis, dry mouth, duodenitis, dysphagia, enteritis, esophageal hemorrhage, esophagitis, gastrointestinal carcinoma, gastrointestinal hemorrhage, gastrointestinal moniliasis, gingivitis, glossitis, halitosis, hematemesis, increased appetite, melena, mouth ulceration, oral moniliasis, periodontal abscess, periodontitis, rectal hemorrhage, stomach ulcer, stomatitis, stools abnormal, tongue discoloration, ulcerative colitis.

ENDOCRINE SYSTEM: diabetes mellitus, glycosuria, goiter.

HEPATO-BILIARY SYSTEM: biliary pain, hyperbilirubinemia, cholecystitis, cholelithiasis, cholestatic jaundice, hepatitis, alkaline phosphatase increased, gamma glutamyl transpeptidase increased, SGOT increased.

HEMIC AND LYMPHATIC SYSTEM: anemia, ecchymosis, eosinophilia, hypochromic anemia, iron deficiency anemia, leukocytosis, leukopenia, thrombocytopenia.

METABOLIC AND NUTRITIONAL: dehydration, edema, gout, peripheral edema, thirst, weight gain, weight loss.

MUSCULOSKELETAL SYSTEM: arthritis, arthrosis, bone disorder, bone pain, bursitis, joint disorder, leg cramps, neck rigidity, myalgia, tenosynovitis.

NERVOUS SYSTEM: abnormal dreams, confusion, convulsion, depression, dry mouth, dysarthria, emotional lability, hallucinations, hyperkinesia, hypesthesia, libido decreased, nervousness, neuralgia, neuritis, neuropathy, paresthesia, reflexes decreased, sleep disorder, somnolence, thinking abnormal, tremor, vertigo.

RESPIRATORY SYSTEM: asthma, epistaxis, hiccup, laryngitis, lung disorder, pneumonia, voice alteration.

SKIN AND APPENDAGES: acne, alopecia, contact dermatitis, dry skin, eczema, fungal dermatitis, hemorrhage, herpes simplex, herpes zoster, lichenoid dermatitis, maculopapular rash, pruritus, skin disorder, skin ulcer, sweating, urticaria.

SPECIAL SENSES: abnormal vision, amblyopia, cataract specified, deafness, diplopia, ear pain, extraocular palsy, glaucoma, otitis externa, taste perversion, tinnitus.

UROGENITAL SYSTEM: albuminuria, balanitis, breast pain, cystitis, dysmenorrhea, dysuria, epididymitis, hematuria, impotence, kidney calculus, kidney pain, nocturia, prostatic disorder, pyelonephritis, scrotal edema, urethral pain, urethritis, urinary tract disorder, urination impaired, vaginitis.

Postmarketing Reports

The postmarketing safety profile of intravenous pantoprazole is not substantially different from that of oral pantoprazole (described below).

There have been spontaneous reports of adverse events with postmarketing use of intravenous or oral pantoprazole. These reports include the following:

BODY AS A WHOLE: anaphylaxis (including anaphylactic shock), angioedema (Quincke's edema).

DIGESTIVE SYSTEM: increased salivation, nausea, pancreatitis.

HEMIC AND LYMPHATIC SYSTEM: pancytopenia.

HEPATO-BILIARY SYSTEM: hepatocellular damage leading to jaundice and hepatic failure.

MUSCULOSKELETAL SYSTEM: elevated CPK (creatine phosphokinase), rhabdomyolysis.

NERVOUS SYSTEM: confusion, hypokinesia, speech disorder, vertigo.

SKIN AND APPENDAGES: severe dermatologic reactions, including erythema multiforme, Stevens-Johnson syndrome, and toxic epidermal necrolysis (TEN, some fatal).

SPECIAL SENSES: anterior ischemic optic neuropathy, blurred vision, tinnitus.

UROGENITAL SYSTEM: interstitial nephritis.

Laboratory Values

In U.S. clinical trials of patients with GERD and a history of erosive esophagitis and international clinical trials of patients with erosive esophagitis associated with GERD, the overall percentages of transaminase elevations did not increase during treatment with intravenous pantoprazole. For other laboratory parameters, there were no clinically important changes identified.

In two U.S. controlled trials of oral pantoprazole in patients with erosive esophagitis associated with GERD, 0.4% of the patients on 40 mg oral pantoprazole experienced SGPT elevations of greater than three times the upper limit of normal at the final treatment visit. Except in those patients where there was a clear alternative explanation for a laboratory value change, such as intercurrent illness, the elevations tended to be mild and sporadic. The following changes in laboratory parameters were reported as adverse events: creatinine increased, hypercholesterolemia, and hyperuricemia.

OVERDOSAGE

Experience in patients taking very high doses of pantoprazole is limited. There have been spontaneous reports of overdosage with pantoprazole, including a suicide in which pantoprazole 560 mg and undetermined amounts of chloroquine and zopiclone were also ingested. There have also been spontaneous reports of patients taking similar amounts of pantoprazole (400 and 600 mg) with no adverse effects.

Pantoprazole is not removed by hemodialysis. In case of overdose, treatment should be symptomatic and supportive. Single intravenous doses of pantoprazole at 378, 230, and 266 mg/kg (38, 46, and 177 times the recommended human dose based on body surface area) were lethal to mice, rats and dogs, respectively. The symptoms of acute toxicity were hypoactivity, ataxia, hunched sitting, limb-splay, lateral position, segregation, absence of ear reflex, and tremor.

DOSAGE AND ADMINISTRATION

PROTONIX I.V. for Injection may be administered intravenously through a dedicated line or through a Y-site. The intravenous line should be flushed before and after administration of PROTONIX I.V. for Injection with either 5% Dextrose Injection, USP, 0.9% Sodium Chloride Injection, USP, or Lactated Ringer's Injection, USP. When administered through a Y-site, PROTONIX I.V. for Injection is compatible with the following solutions: 5% Dextrose Injection, USP, 0.9% Sodium Chloride Injection, USP, or Lactated Ringer's Injection, USP.

Midazolam HCl has been shown to be incompatible with Y-site administration of PROTONIX I.V. for Injection. PROTONIX I.V. for Injection may not be compatible with products containing zinc. When PROTONIX I.V. for Injection is administered through a Y-site, immediately stop use if precipitation or discoloration occurs.

Parenteral drug products should be inspected visually for particulate matter and discoloration prior to and during administration whenever solution and container permit.

Treatment with PROTONIX I.V. for Injection should be discontinued as soon as the patient is able to be treated with PROTONIX Delayed-Release Tablets. Also, data on the safe and effective dosing for conditions other than those described in **INDICATIONS AND USAGE**, such as life-threatening upper gastrointestinal bleeds, are not available. PROTONIX I.V. 40 mg once daily does not raise gastric pH to levels sufficient to contribute to the treatment of such life-threatening conditions.

Parenteral routes of administration other than intravenous are not recommended.

No dosage adjustment is necessary in patients with renal impairment, hepatic impairment, or for elderly patients. Doses higher than 40 mg/day have not been studied in hepatically-impaired patients. No dosage adjustment is necessary in patients undergoing hemodialysis.

Treatment of Gastroesophageal Reflux Disease Associated With a History of Erosive Esophagitis

The recommended adult dose is 40 mg pantoprazole given once daily by intravenous infusion for 7 to 10 days. Safety and efficacy of PROTONIX I.V. for Injection as a treatment of patients with GERD and a history of erosive esophagitis for more than 10 days have not been demonstrated (see **INDICATIONS AND USAGE**).

Fifteen Minute Infusion

PROTONIX I.V. for Injection should be reconstituted with 10 mL of 0.9% Sodium Chloride Injection, USP, and further diluted (admixed) with 100 mL of 5% Dextrose Injection, USP, 0.9% Sodium Chloride Injection, USP, or Lactated Ringer's Injection, USP, to a final concentration of approximately 0.4 mg/mL. The reconstituted solution may be stored for up to 2 hours at room temperature prior to further dilution; the admixed solution may be stored for up to 22 hours at room temperature prior to intravenous infusion. Both the reconstituted solution and the admixed solution do not need to be protected from light.

PROTONIX I.V. for Injection admixtures should be administered intravenously over a period of approximately 15 minutes at a rate of approximately 7 mL/min.

Two Minute Infusion

PROTONIX I.V. for Injection should be reconstituted with 10 mL of 0.9% Sodium Chloride Injection, USP, to a final concentration of approximately 4 mg/mL. The reconstituted solution may be stored for up to 2 hours at room temperature prior to intravenous infusion and does not need to be protected from light. PROTONIX I.V. for Injection should be administered intravenously over a period of at least 2 minutes.

Pathological Hypersecretion Associated with Zollinger-Ellison Syndrome

The dosage of PROTONIX I.V. for Injection in patients with pathological hypersecretory conditions associated with Zollinger-Ellison Syndrome or other neoplastic conditions varies with individual patients. The recommended adult dosage is 80 mg q12h. The frequency of dosing can be adjusted to individual patient needs based on acid output measurements. In those patients who need a higher dosage, 80 mg q8h is expected to maintain acid output below 10 mEq/h. Daily doses higher than 240 mg or administered for more than 6 days have not been studied. (See **Clinical Studies** section.) Transition from oral to I.V. and from I.V. to oral formulations of gastric acid inhibitors should be performed in such a manner to ensure continuity of effect of suppression of acid secretion. Patients with Zollinger-Ellison Syndrome may be vulnerable to serious clinical complications of increased acid production even after a short period of loss of effective inhibition.

Fifteen Minute Infusion

Each vial of PROTONIX I.V. for Injection should be reconstituted with 10 mL of 0.9% Sodium Chloride Injection, USP. The contents of the two vials should be combined and further diluted (admixed) with 80 mL of 5% Dextrose Injection, USP, 0.9% Sodium Chloride Injection, USP, or Lactated Ringer's Injection, USP, to a total volume of 100 mL with a final concentration of approximately 0.8 mg/mL. The reconstituted solution may be stored for up to 2 hours at room temperature prior to further dilution; the admixed solution may be stored for up to 22 hours at room temperature prior to intravenous infusion. Both the reconstituted solution and the admixed solution do not need to be protected from light.

PROTONIX I.V. for Injection should be administered intravenously over a period of approximately 15 minutes at a rate of approximately 7 mL/min.

Two Minute Infusion

PROTONIX I.V. for Injection should be reconstituted with 10 mL of 0.9% Sodium Chloride Injection, USP, per vial to a final concentration of approximately 4 mg/mL. The reconstituted solution may be stored for up to 2 hours at room temperature prior to intravenous infusion and does not need to be protected from light. The total volume from both vials should be administered intravenously over a period of at least 2 minutes.

HOW SUPPLIED

PROTONIX® I.V. (pantoprazole sodium) for Injection is supplied as a freeze-dried powder containing 40 mg of pantoprazole per vial.

PROTONIX I.V. for Injection is available as follows:

NDC 0008-0923-51 One carton containing 1 vial of PROTONIX I.V. for Injection (each vial containing 40-mg pantoprazole).

Storage

Store PROTONIX I.V. for Injection vials at 20°-25°C (68°-77°F); excursions permitted to 15°-30°C (59°-86°F). [See USP Controlled Room Temperature.] Protect from light.

Caution: the reconstituted product should not be frozen.

U.S. Patent No. 4,758,579

Marketed by Wyeth Pharmaceuticals Inc.
Philadelphia, PA 19101
under license from
ALTANA Pharma
D78467 Konstanz, Germany

W10447C012
ET01
Rev 02/05

RAPAMUNE® ℞

[răp-ă-mūn]
(sirolimus)
Oral Solution and Tablets
℞ only

Prescribing information for this product, which appears on pages 3395-3402 of the 2005 PDR, has been completely revised as follows. Please write "See Supplement A" next to the product heading.

This product's label may have been revised after this insert was used in production. For further product information and current package insert, please visit www.wyeth.com or call our medical communications department toll-free at 1-800-934-5556.

> WARNING:
> Increased susceptibility to infection and the possible development of lymphoma may result from immunosuppression. Only physicians experienced in immunosuppressive therapy and management of renal transplant patients should use Rapamune®. Patients receiving the drug should be managed in facilities equipped and staffed with adequate laboratory and supportive medical resources. The physician responsible for maintenance therapy should have complete information requisite for the follow-up of the patient.

DESCRIPTION

Rapamune® (sirolimus) is an immunosuppressive agent. Sirolimus is a macrocyclic lactone produced by *Streptomyces hygroscopicus*. The chemical name of sirolimus (also known as rapamycin) is (3*S*,6*R*,7*E*,9*R*,10*R*,12*R*,14*S*,15*E*,17*E*,19*E*,21*S*,23*S*,26*R*,27*R*,34a*S*)-9,10,12,13,14,21,22,23,24,25,26,27,32,33,34, 34a-hexadecahydro-9,27-dihydroxy-3-[(1*R*)-2-[(1*S*,3*R*,4*R*)-4-hydroxy-3-methoxycyclohexyl]-1-methylethyl]-10,21-dimethoxy-6,8,12,14,20,26-hexamethyl-23,27-epoxy-3*H*-pyrido[2,1-c][1,4] oxaazacyclohentriacontine-1,5,11,28,29 (4*H*,6*H*,31*H*)-pentone. Its molecular formula is $C_{51}H_{79}NO_{13}$ and its molecular weight is 914.2. The structural formula of sirolimus is shown below.

[See chemical structure at top of next column]

Sirolimus is a white to off-white powder and is insoluble in water, but freely soluble in benzyl alcohol, chloroform, acetone, and acetonitrile.

Rapamune® is available for administration as an oral solution containing 1 mg/mL sirolimus. Rapamune is also available as a white, triangular-shaped tablet containing 1-mg sirolimus, and as a yellow to beige triangular-shaped tablet containing 2-mg sirolimus.

The inactive ingredients in Rapamune® Oral Solution are Phosal 50 PG® (phosphatidylcholine, propylene glycol, mono- and di-glycerides, ethanol, soy fatty acids, and ascorbyl palmitate) and polysorbate 80. Rapamune Oral Solution contains 1.5% - 2.5% ethanol.

SIROLIMUS PHARMACOKINETIC PARAMETERS (MEAN ± SD) IN RENAL TRANSPLANT PATIENTS (MULTIPLE DOSE ORAL SOLUTION)[a,b]

N	Dose	$C_{max,ss}$[c] (ng/mL)	$t_{max,ss}$ (h)	$AUC_{\tau,ss}$[c] (ng•h/mL)	CL/F/WT[d] (mL/h/kg)
19	2 mg	12.2 ± 6.2	3.01 ± 2.40	158 ± 70	182 ± 72
23	5 mg	37.4 ± 21	1.84 ± 1.30	396 ± 193	221 ± 143

a: Sirolimus administered four hours after cyclosporine oral solution (MODIFIED) (e.g., Neoral® Oral Solution) and/or cyclosporine capsules (MODIFIED) (e.g., Neoral® Soft Gelatin Capsules).
b: As measured by the Liquid Chromatographic/Tandem Mass Spectrometric Method (LC/MS/MS).
c: These parameters were dose normalized prior to the statistical comparison.
d: CL/F/WT = oral dose clearance.

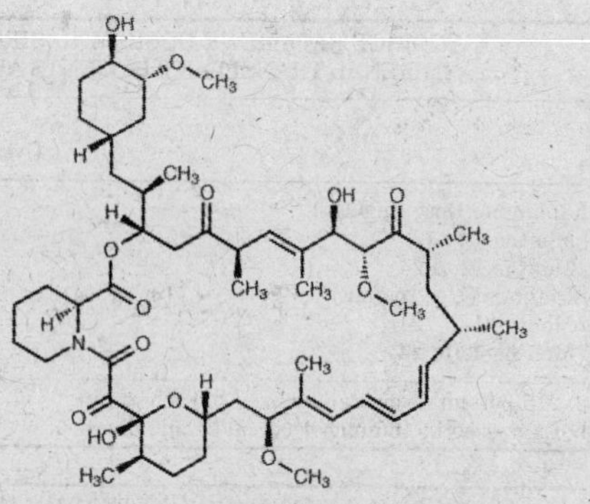

The inactive ingredients in Rapamune® Tablets include sucrose, lactose, polyethylene glycol 8000, calcium sulfate, microcrystalline cellulose, pharmaceutical glaze, talc, titanium dioxide, magnesium stearate, povidone, poloxamer 188, polyethylene glycol 20,000, glyceryl monooleate, carnauba wax, and other ingredients. The 2 mg dosage strength also contains iron oxide yellow 10 and iron oxide brown 70.

CLINICAL PHARMACOLOGY

Mechanism of Action

Sirolimus inhibits T lymphocyte activation and proliferation that occurs in response to antigenic and cytokine (Interleukin [IL]-2, IL-4, and IL-15) stimulation by a mechanism that is distinct from that of other immunosuppressants. Sirolimus also inhibits antibody production. In cells, sirolimus binds to the immunophilin, FK Binding Protein-12 (FKBP-12), to generate an immunosuppressive complex. The sirolimus:FKBP-12 complex has no effect on calcineurin activity. This complex binds to and inhibits the activation of the mammalian Target Of Rapamycin (mTOR), a key regulatory kinase. This inhibition suppresses cytokine-driven T-cell proliferation, inhibiting the progression from the G_1 to the S phase of the cell cycle.

Studies in experimental models show that sirolimus prolongs allograft (kidney, heart, skin, islet, small bowel, pancreatico-duodenal, and bone marrow) survival in mice, rats, pigs, and/or primates. Sirolimus reverses acute rejection of heart and kidney allografts in rats and prolongs the graft survival in presensitized rats. In some studies, the immunosuppressive effect of sirolimus lasts up to 6 months after discontinuation of therapy. This tolerization effect is alloantigen specific.

In rodent models of autoimmune disease, sirolimus suppresses immune-mediated events associated with systemic lupus erythematosus, collagen-induced arthritis, autoimmune type I diabetes, autoimmune myocarditis, experimental allergic encephalomyelitis, graft-versus-host disease, and autoimmune uveoretinitis.

Pharmacokinetics

Sirolimus pharmacokinetic activity has been determined following oral administration in healthy subjects, pediatric patients, hepatically-impaired patients, and renal transplant patients.

Absorption

Following administration of Rapamune® Oral Solution, sirolimus is rapidly absorbed, with a mean time-to-peak concentration (t_{max}) of approximately 1 hour after a single dose in healthy subjects and approximately 2 hours after multiple oral doses in renal transplant recipients. The systemic availability of sirolimus was estimated to be approximately 14% after the administration of Rapamune Oral Solution. The mean bioavailability of sirolimus after administration of the tablet is about 27% higher relative to the oral solution. Sirolimus oral tablets are not bioequivalent to the oral solution; however, clinical equivalence has been demonstrated at the 2-mg dose level. (See **Clinical Studies** and **DOSAGE AND ADMINISTRATION**).

Sirolimus concentrations, following the administration of Rapamune Oral Solution to stable renal transplant patients, are dose proportional between 3 and 12 mg/m^2.

Food effects: In 22 healthy volunteers receiving Rapamune Oral Solution, a high-fat meal (861.8 kcal, 54.9% kcal from fat) altered the bioavailability characteristics of sirolimus. Compared with fasting, a 34% decrease in the peak blood sirolimus concentration (C_{max}), a 3.5-fold increase in the time-to-peak concentration (t_{max}), and a 35% increase in total exposure (AUC) was observed. After administration of Rapamune Tablets and a high-fat meal in 24 healthy volunteers, C_{max}, t_{max}, and AUC showed increases of 65%, 32%, and 23%, respectively. To minimize variability, both Rapamune Oral Solution and Tablets should be taken consistently with or without food (See **DOSAGE AND ADMINISTRATION**).

Distribution

The mean (± SD) blood-to-plasma ratio of sirolimus was 36 ± 18 in stable renal allograft recipients after administration of oral solution, indicating that sirolimus is extensively partitioned into formed blood elements. The mean volume of distribution (V_{ss}/F) of sirolimus is 12 ± 8 L/kg. Sirolimus is extensively bound (approximately 92%) to human plasma proteins. In man, the binding of sirolimus was shown mainly to be associated with serum albumin (97%), α_1-acid glycoprotein, and lipoproteins.

Metabolism

Sirolimus is a substrate for both cytochrome P450 IIIA4 (CYP3A4) and P-glycoprotein (P-gp). Sirolimus is extensively metabolized by the CYP3A4 isozyme in the intestinal wall and liver and undergoes counter-transport from enterocytes of the small intestine into the gut lumen by the P-gp drug efflux pump. Sirolimus is potentially recycled between enterocytes and the gut lumen to allow continued metabolism by CYP3A4. Therefore, absorption and subsequent elimination of systemically absorbed sirolimus may be influenced by drugs that affect these proteins. Inhibitors of CYP3A4 and P-gp increase sirolimus concentrations. Inducers of CYP3A4 and P-gp decrease sirolimus concentrations. (See **WARNINGS** and **PRECAUTIONS, Drug Interactions and Other drug interactions**). Sirolimus is extensively metabolized by O-demethylation and/or hydroxylation. Seven (7) major metabolites, including hydroxy, demethyl, and hydroxydemethyl, are identifiable in whole blood. Some of these metabolites are also detectable in plasma, fecal, and urine samples. Glucuronide and sulfate conjugates are not present in any of the biologic matrices. Sirolimus is the major component in human whole blood and contributes to more than 90% of the immunosuppressive activity.

Excretion

After a single dose of [^{14}C]sirolimus oral solution in healthy volunteers, the majority (91%) of radioactivity was recovered from the feces, and only a minor amount (2.2%) was excreted in urine.

Pharmacokinetics in renal transplant patients

Rapamune Oral Solution: Pharmacokinetic parameters for sirolimus oral solution given daily in combination with cyclosporine and corticosteroids in renal transplant patients are summarized below based on data collected at months 1, 3, and 6 after transplantation (Studies 1 and 2; see **CLINICAL STUDIES**). There were no significant differences in any of these parameters with respect to treatment group or month.

[See table above]

Whole blood sirolimus trough concentrations (mean ± SD), as measured by immunoassay, for the 2 mg/day and 5 mg/day dose groups were 8.6 ± 4.0 ng/mL (n = 226) and 17.3 ± 7.4 ng/mL (n = 219), respectively. Whole blood trough sirolimus concentrations, as measured by LC/MS/MS, were significantly correlated (r^2=0.96) with $AUC_{\tau,ss}$. Upon repeated twice daily administration without an initial loading dose in a multiple-dose study, the average trough concentration of sirolimus increases approximately 2 to 3-fold over the initial 6 days of therapy at which time steady state is reached. A loading dose of 3 times the maintenance dose will provide near steady-state concentrations within 1 day in most patients. The mean ± SD terminal elimination half life ($t_{1/2}$) of sirolimus after multiple dosing in stable renal transplant patients was estimated to be about 62 ± 16 hours.

Rapamune Tablets: Pharmacokinetic parameters for sirolimus tablets administered daily in combination with cyclosporine and corticosteroids in renal transplant patients are summarized below based on data collected at months 1 and 3 after transplantation (Study 3; see **CLINICAL STUDIES**).

[See first table at top of next page]

Whole blood sirolimus trough concentrations (mean ± SD), as measured by immunoassay, for 2 mg of oral solution and 2 mg of tablets over 6 months, were 8.9 ± 4.4 ng/mL (n = 172) and 9.5 ± 3.9 ng/mL (n = 179), respectively. Whole blood trough sirolimus concentrations, as measured by LC/MS/MS, were significantly correlated (r^2 = 0.85) with $AUC_{\tau,ss}$. Mean whole blood sirolimus trough concentrations in patients receiving either Rapamune Oral Solution or Rapamune Tablets with a loading dose of three times the maintenance dose achieved steady-state concentrations within 24 hours after the start of dose administration.

Average Rapamune doses and sirolimus whole blood trough concentrations for tablets administered daily in combina-

Continued on next page

Rapamune—Cont.

tion with cyclosporine and following cyclosporine withdrawal, in combination with corticosteroids in renal transplant patients (Study 4; see **CLINICAL STUDIES**) are summarized in the table below.
[See second table at right]
The withdrawal of cyclosporine and concurrent increases in sirolimus trough concentrations to steady-state required approximately 6 weeks. Larger Rapamune® doses were required due to the absence of the inhibition of sirolimus metabolism and transport by cyclosporine and to achieve higher target concentrations during concentration-controlled administration following cyclosporine withdrawal.

Special Populations

Hepatic impairment: Sirolimus oral solution (15 mg) was administered as a single oral dose to 18 subjects with normal hepatic function and to 18 patients with Child-Pugh classification A or B hepatic impairment, in which hepatic impairment was primary and not related to an underlying systemic disease. Shown below are the mean ± SD pharmacokinetic parameters following the administration of sirolimus oral solution.
[See third table at right]
Compared with the values in the normal hepatic group, the hepatic impairment group had higher mean values for sirolimus AUC (61%) and $t_{1/2}$ (43%) and had lower mean values for sirolimus CL/F/WT (33%). The mean $t_{1/2}$ increased from 79 ± 12 hours in subjects with normal hepatic function to 113 ± 41 hours in patients with impaired hepatic function. The rate of absorption of sirolimus was not altered by hepatic disease, as evidenced by C_{max} and t_{max} values. However, hepatic diseases with varying etiologies may show different effects and the pharmacokinetics of sirolimus in patients with severe hepatic dysfunction is unknown. Dosage adjustment is recommended for patients with mild to moderate hepatic impairment (see **DOSAGE AND ADMINISTRATION**).

Renal impairment: The effect of renal impairment on the pharmacokinetics of sirolimus is not known. However, there is minimal (2.2%) renal excretion of the drug or its metabolites.

Pediatric: Sirolimus pharmacokinetic data were collected in concentration-controlled trials of pediatric renal transplant patients who were also receiving cyclosporine and corticosteroids. The target ranges for trough concentrations were either 10-20 ng/mL for the 21 children receiving tablets, or 5-15 ng/mL for the one child receiving oral solution. The children aged 6-11 years (n = 8) received mean ± SD doses of 1.75 ± 0.71 mg/day (0.064 ± 0.018 mg/kg, 1.65 ± 0.43 mg/m²). The children aged 12-18 years (n = 14) received mean ± SD doses of 2.79 ± 1.25 mg/day (0.053 ± 0.0150 mg/kg, 1.86 ± 0.61 mg/m²). At the time of sirolimus blood sampling for pharmacokinetic evaluation, the majority (80%) of these pediatric patients received the sirolimus dose at 16 hours after the once daily cyclosporine dose.
[See fourth table at right]
The table below summarizes pharmacokinetic data obtained in pediatric dialysis patients with chronically impaired renal function.
[See fifth table at right]

Geriatric: Clinical studies of Rapamune did not include a sufficient number of patients >65 years of age to determine whether they will respond differently than younger patients. After the administration of Rapamune Oral Solution, sirolimus trough concentration data in 35 renal transplant patients >65 years of age were similar to those in the adult population (n = 822) 18 to 65 years of age. Similar results were obtained after the administration of Rapamune Tablets to 12 renal transplant patients >65 years of age compared with adults (n = 167) 18 to 65 years of age.

Gender: After the administration of Rapamune Oral Solution, sirolimus oral dose clearance in males was 12% lower than that in females; male subjects had a significantly longer $t_{1/2}$ than did female subjects (72.3 hours versus 61.3 hours). A similar trend in the effect of gender on sirolimus oral dose clearance and $t_{1/2}$ was observed after the administration of Rapamune Tablets. Dose adjustments based on gender are not recommended.

Race: In large phase 3 trials (Studies 1 and 2) using Rapamune Oral Solution and cyclosporine oral solution (MODIFIED) (e.g., Neoral® Oral Solution) and/or cyclosporine capsules (MODIFIED) (e.g., Neoral® Soft Gelatin Capsules), there were no significant differences in mean trough sirolimus concentrations over time between black (n = 139) and non-black (n = 724) patients during the first 6 months after transplantation at sirolimus doses of 2 mg/day and 5 mg/day. Similarly, after administration of Rapamune Tablets (2 mg/day) in a phase III trial, mean sirolimus trough concentrations over 6 months were not significantly different among black (n = 51) and non-black (n = 128) patients.

CLINICAL STUDIES

Rapamune® Oral Solution: The safety and efficacy of Rapamune® Oral Solution for the prevention of organ rejection following renal transplantation were assessed in two randomized, double-blind, multicenter, controlled trials. These studies compared two dose levels of Rapamune Oral Solution (2 mg and 5 mg, once daily) with azathioprine (Study 1) or placebo (Study 2) when administered in combination with cyclosporine and corticosteroids. Study 1 was conducted in the United States at 38 sites.

SIROLIMUS PHARMACOKINETIC PARAMETERS (MEAN ± SD) IN RENAL TRANSPLANT PATIENTS (MULTIPLE DOSE TABLETS)[a,b]

n	Dose (2 mg/day)	$C_{max,ss}$[c] (ng/mL)	$t_{max,ss}$ (h)	$AUC_{\tau,ss}$[c] (ng•h/mL)	CL/F/WT[d] (mL/h/kg)
17	Oral solution	14.4 ± 5.3	2.12 ± 0.84	194 ± 78	173 ± 50
13	Tablets	15.0 ± 4.9	3.46 ± 2.40	230 ± 67	139 ± 63

a: Sirolimus administered four hours after cyclosporine oral solution (MODIFIED) (e.g., Neoral® Oral Solution) and/or cyclosporine capsules (MODIFIED) (e.g., Neoral® Soft Gelatin Capsules).
b: As measured by the Liquid Chromatographic/Tandem Mass Spectrometric Method (LC/MS/MS).
c: These parameters were dose normalized prior to the statistical comparison.
d: CL/F/WT = oral dose clearance.

AVERAGE RAPAMUNE DOSES AND SIROLIMUS TROUGH CONCENTRATIONS (MEAN ± SD) IN RENAL TRANSPLANT PATIENTS AFTER MULTIPLE DOSE TABLET ADMINISTRATION

	Rapamune with Cyclosporine Therapy[a]	Rapamune Following Cyclosporine Withdrawal[a]
Rapamune Dose (mg/day)		
Months 4 to 12	2.1 ± 0.7	8.2 ± 4.2
Months 12 to 24	2.0 ± 0.8	6.4 ± 3.0
Sirolimus C_{min}, (ng/mL)[b]		
Months 4 to 12	10.7 ± 3.8	23.3 ± 5.0
Months 12 to 24	11.2 ± 4.1	22.5 ± 4.8

a: 215 patients were randomized to each group.
b: Expressed by immunoassay and equivalence.

SIROLIMUS PHARMACOKINETIC PARAMETERS (MEAN ± SD) IN 18 HEALTHY SUBJECTS AND 18 PATIENTS WITH HEPATIC IMPAIRMENT (15 MG SINGLE DOSE – ORAL SOLUTION)

Population	$C_{max,ss}$[a] (ng/mL)	t_{max} (h)	$AUC_{0-\infty}$ (ng•h/mL)	CL/F/WT (mL/h/kg)
Healthy subjects	78.2 ± 18.3	0.82 ± 0.17	970 ± 272	215 ± 76
Hepatic impairment	77.9 ± 23.1	0.84 ± 0.17	1567 ± 616	144 ± 62

a: As measured by LC/MS/MS.

SIROLIMUS PHARMACOKINETIC PARAMETERS (MEAN ± SD) IN PEDIATRIC RENAL TRANSPLANT PATIENTS (MULTIPLE DOSE CONCENTRATION CONTROL)[a,b]

Age (y)	n	Body weight (kg)	$C_{max,ss}$ (ng/mL)	$t_{max,ss}$ (h)	$C_{min, ss}$ (ng/ml)	$AUC_{\tau,ss}$ (ng•h/mL)	CL/F[c] (mL/h/kg)	CL/F[c] (L/h/m²)
6-11	8	27 ± 10	22.1 ± 8.9	5.88 ± 4.05	10.6 ± 4.3	356 ± 127	214 ± 129	5.4 ± 2.8
12-18	14	52 ± 15	34.5 ± 12.2	2.7 ± 1.5	14.7 ± 8.6	466 ± 236	136 ± 57	4.7 ± 1.9

a: Sirolimus co-administered with cyclosporine oral solution (MODIFIED) (e.g., Neoral Oral Solution) and/or cyclosporine capsules (MODIFIED) (e.g., Neoral Soft Gelatin Capsules).
b: As measured by Liquid Chromatographic/Tandem Mass Spectrometric Method (LC/MS/MS).
c: Oral-dose clearance adjusted by either body weight (kg) or body surface area (m²).

SIROLIMUS PHARMACOKINETIC PARAMETERS (MEAN ± SD) IN PEDIATRIC PATIENTS WITH STABLE CHRONIC RENAL FAILURE MAINTAINED ON HEMODIALYSIS OR PERITONEAL DIALYSIS (1, 3, 9, 15 MG/M² SINGLE DOSE)*

Age Group (y)	n	t_{max} (h)	$t_{1/2}$ (h)	CL/F (mL/h/kg)
5-11	9	1.1 ±-0.5	71 ± 40	580 ± 450
12-18	11	0.79 ± 0.17	55 ± 18	450 ± 232

* All subjects received sirolimus oral solution

INCIDENCE (%) OF EFFICACY FAILURE AT 6 AND 24 MONTHS FOR STUDY 1[a,b]

Parameter	Rapamune® Oral Solution 2 mg/day (n = 284)	Rapamune® Oral Solution 5 mg/day (n = 274)	Azathioprine 2-3 mg/kg/day (n = 161)
Efficacy failure at 6 months[c]	18.7	16.8	32.3
Components of efficacy failure			
Biopsy-proven acute rejection	16.5	11.3	29.2
Graft loss	1.1	2.9	2.5
Death	0.7	1.8	0
Lost to follow-up	0.4	0.7	0.6
Efficacy failure at 24 months	32.8	25.9	36.0
Components of efficacy failure			
Biopsy-proven acute rejection	23.6	17.5	32.3
Graft loss	3.9	4.7	3.1
Death	4.2	3.3	0
Lost to follow-up	1.1	0.4	0.6

a: Patients received cyclosporine and corticosteroids.
b: Includes patients who prematurely discontinued treatment.
c: Primary endpoint.

Seven hundred nineteen (719) patients were enrolled in this trial and randomized following transplantation; 284 were randomized to receive Rapamune Oral Solution 2 mg/day, 274 were randomized to receive Rapamune Oral Solution 5 mg/day, and 161 to receive azathioprine 2-3 mg/kg/day. Study 2 was conducted in Australia, Canada, Europe, and the United States, at a total of 34 sites. Five hundred seventy-six (576) patients were enrolled in this trial and randomized before transplantation; 227 were randomized to receive Rapamune Oral Solution 2 mg/day, 219 were randomized to receive Rapamune Oral Solution 5 mg/day, and 130 to receive placebo. In both studies, the use of antilymphocyte antibody induction therapy was prohibited. In both studies, the primary efficacy endpoint was the rate of efficacy failure in the first 6 months after transplantation. Efficacy failure was defined as the first occurrence of an acute rejection episode (confirmed by biopsy), graft loss, or death. The tables below summarize the results of the primary efficacy analyses from these trials. Rapamune Oral Solution, at doses of 2 mg/day and 5 mg/day, significantly reduced the

incidence of efficacy failure (statistically significant at the <0.025 level; nominal significance level adjusted for multiple [2] dose comparisons) at 6 months following transplantation compared with both azathioprine and placebo.
[See sixth table on previous page]
[See first table at right]
Patient and graft survival at 1 year were co-primary endpoints. The table below shows graft and patient survival at 1 and 2 years in Study 1 and 1 and 3 years in Study 2. The graft and patient survival rates were similar in patients treated with Rapamune and comparator-treated patients.
[See second table at right]
The reduction in the incidence of first biopsy-confirmed acute rejection episodes in patients treated with Rapamune compared with the control groups included a reduction in all grades of rejection.
In Study 1, which was prospectively stratified by race within center, efficacy failure was similar for Rapamune Oral Solution 2 mg/day and lower for Rapamune Oral Solution 5 mg/day compared with azathioprine in black patients. In Study 2, which was not prospectively stratified by race, efficacy failure was similar for both Rapamune Oral Solution doses compared with placebo in black patients. The decision to use the higher dose of Rapamune Oral Solution in black patients must be weighed against the increased risk of dose-dependent adverse events that were observed with the Rapamune Oral Solution 5-mg dose (see **ADVERSE REACTIONS**).
[See third table at right]
Mean glomerular filtration rates (GFR) post transplant were calculated by using the Nankivell equation at 12 and 24 months for Study 1, and 12 and 36 months for Study 2. Mean GFR was lower in patients treated with cyclosporine and Rapamune Oral Solution compared with those treated with cyclosporine and the respective azathioprine or placebo control.
[See fourth table at right]
Within each treatment group in Studies 1 and 2, mean GFR at one year post transplant was lower in patients who experienced at least 1 episode of biopsy-proven acute rejection, compared with those who did not.
Renal function should be monitored and appropriate adjustment of the immunosuppression regimen should be considered in patients with elevated or increasing serum creatinine levels (see **PRECAUTIONS**).
Rapamune® Tablets: The safety and efficacy of Rapamune Oral Solution and Rapamune Tablets for the prevention of organ rejection following renal transplantation were compared in a randomized multicenter controlled trial (Study 3). This study compared a single dose level (2 mg, once daily) of Rapamune Oral Solution and Rapamune Tablets when administered in combination with cyclosporine and corticosteroids. The study was conducted at 30 centers in Australia, Canada, and the United States. Four hundred seventy-seven (477) patients were enrolled in this study and randomized before transplantation; 238 patients were randomized to receive Rapamune Oral Solution 2 mg/day and 239 patients were randomized to receive Rapamune Tablets 2 mg/day. In this study, the use of antilymphocyte antibody induction therapy was prohibited. The primary efficacy endpoint was the rate of efficacy failure in the first 3 months after transplantation. Efficacy failure was defined as the first occurrence of an acute rejection episode (confirmed by biopsy), graft loss, or death.
The table below summarizes the result of the efficacy failure analysis at 3 and 6 months from this trial. The overall rate of efficacy failure at 3 months, the primary endpoint, in the tablet treatment group was equivalent to the rate in the oral solution treatment group.
[See table at top of next page]
Graft and patient survival at 12 months were co-primary endpoints. There was no significant difference between the oral solution and tablet formulations for both graft and patient survival. Graft survival was 92.0% and 88.7% for the oral solution and tablet treatment groups, respectively. The patient survival rates in the oral solution and tablet treatment groups were 95.8% and 96.2%, respectively.
The mean GFR at 12 months, calculated by the Nankivell equation, were not significantly different for the oral solution group and for the tablet group.
The table below summarizes the mean GFR at one-year post-transplantation for all patients in Study 3 who had serum creatinine measured at 12 months.

OVERALL CALCULATED GLOMERULAR FILTRATION RATES (CC/MIN) BY NANKIVELL EQUATION AT 12 MONTHS POST TRANSPLANT: STUDY 3[a,b]

	Rapamune® Oral Solution	Rapamune® Tablets
Mean ± SEM	53.1 ± 1.7 (n = 229)	51.7 ± 1.7 (n = 225)

a: Includes patients who prematurely discontinued treatment.
b: Patients who had a graft loss were included in the analysis with GFR set to 0.0.

In Study 4, the safety and efficacy of Rapamune as a maintenance regimen were assessed following cyclosporine withdrawal at 3 to 4 months post renal transplantation. Study 4 was a randomized, multicenter, controlled trial conducted at 57 centers in Australia, Canada, and Europe. Five hundred twenty-five (525) patients were enrolled. All patients in this study received the tablet formulation. This study compared patients who were administered Rapamune, cyclosporine, and corticosteroids continuously with patients who received the same standardized therapy for the first 3 months after transplantation (prerandomization period) followed by the withdrawal of cyclosporine. During cyclosporine withdrawal the Rapamune dosages were adjusted to achieve targeted sirolimus whole blood trough concentration ranges (20 to 30 ng/mL, experimental immunoassay). At 3 months, 430 patients were equally randomized to either Rapamune with cyclosporine therapy or Rapamune as a maintenance regimen following cyclosporine withdrawal. Eligibility for randomization included no Banff Grade 3 acute rejection episode or vascular rejection in the 4 weeks before random assignment; serum creatinine ≤ 4.5 mg/dL; and adequate renal function to support cyclosporine withdrawal (in the opinion of the investigator). The primary efficacy endpoint was graft survival at 12 months after transplantation. Secondary efficacy endpoints were the rate of biopsy-confirmed acute rejection, patient survival, incidence of efficacy failure (defined as the first occurrence of either biopsy-proven acute rejection, graft loss, or death), and treatment failure (defined as the first occurrence of either discontinuation, acute rejection, graft loss, or death).
The safety and efficacy of cyclosporine withdrawal in high-risk patients have not been adequately studied and it is therefore not recommended. This includes patients with Banff grade III acute rejection or vascular rejection prior to cyclosporine withdrawal, those who are dialysis-dependent, serum creatinine > 4.5 mg/dL, black patients, re-

INCIDENCE (%) OF EFFICACY FAILURE AT 6 AND 36 MONTHS FOR STUDY 2[a,b]

Parameter	Rapamune® Oral Solution 2 mg/day (n = 227)	Rapamune® Oral Solution 5 mg/day (n = 219)	Placebo (n = 130)
Efficacy failure at 6 months[c]	30.0	25.6	47.7
Components of efficacy failure			
Biopsy-proven acute rejection	24.7	19.2	41.5
Graft loss	3.1	3.7	3.9
Death	2.2	2.7	2.3
Lost to follow-up	0	0	0
Efficacy failure at 36 months	44.1	41.6	54.6
Components of efficacy failure			
Biopsy-proven acute rejection	32.2	27.4	43.9
Graft loss	6.2	7.3	4.6
Death	5.7	5.9	5.4
Lost to follow-up	0	0.9	0.8

a: Patients received cyclosporine and corticosteroids.
b: Includes patients who prematurely discontinued treatment.
c: Primary endpoint.

GRAFT AND PATIENT SURVIVAL (%) FOR STUDY 1 (12 AND 24 MONTHS) AND STUDY 2 (12 AND 36 MONTHS)[a,b]

Parameter	Rapamune® Oral Solution 2 mg/day	Rapamune® Oral Solution 5 mg/day	Azathioprine 2-3 mg/kg/day	Placebo
Study 1	(n = 284)	(n = 274)	(n = 161)	
Graft survival				
Month 12	94.7	92.7	93.8	
Month 24	85.2	89.1	90.1	
Patient survival				
Month 12	97.2	96.0	98.1	
Month 24	92.6	94.9	96.3	
Study 2	(n = 227)	(n = 219)		(n = 130)
Graft survival				
Month 12	89.9	90.9		87.7
Month 36	81.1	79.9		80.8
Patient survival				
Month 12	96.5	95.0		94.6
Month 36	90.3	89.5		90.8

a: Patients received cyclosporine and corticosteroids.
b: Includes patients who prematurely discontinued treatment.

PERCENTAGE OF EFFICACY FAILURE BY RACE AT 6 MONTHS[a,b]

Parameter	Rapamune® Oral Solution 2 mg/day	Rapamune® Oral Solution 5 mg/day	Azathioprine 2-3 mg/kg/day	Placebo
Study 1				
Black (n = 166)	34.9 (n = 63)	18.0 (n = 61)	33.3 (n = 42)	
Non-black (n = 553)	14.0 (n = 221)	16.4 (n = 213)	31.9 (n = 119)	
Study 2				
Black (n = 66)	30.8 (n = 26)	33.7 (n = 27)		38.5 (n = 13)
Non-black (n = 510)	29.9 (n = 201)	24.5 (n = 192)		48.7 (n = 117)

a: Patients received cyclosporine and corticosteroids.
b: Includes patients who prematurely discontinued treatment.

OVERALL CALCULATED GLOMERULAR FILTRATION RATES (Mean ± SEM, cc/min) BY NANKIVELL EQUATION POST TRANSPLANT[a,b]

Parameter	Rapamune® Oral Solution 2 mg/day	Rapamune® Oral Solution 5 mg/day	Azathioprine 2-3 mg/kg/day	Placebo
Study 1				
Month 12	57.4 ± 1.3 (n = 269)	54.6 ± 1.3 (n = 248)	64.1 ± 1.6 (n = 149)	
Month 24	58.4 ± 1.5 (n = 221)	52.6 ± 1.5 (n = 222)	62.4 ± 1.9 (n = 132)	
Study 2				
Month 12	52.4 ± 1.5 (n = 211)	51.5 ± 1.5 (n = 199)		58.0 ± 2.1 (n = 117)
Month 36	48.1 ± 1.8 (n = 183)	46.1 ± 2.0 (n = 177)		53.4 ± 2.7 (n = 102)

a: Includes patients who prematurely discontinued treatment.
b: Patients who had a graft loss were included in the analysis with GFR set to 0.0.

Continued on next page

Rapamune—Cont.

transplants, multi-organ transplants, or patients with high panel of reactive antibodies (See **INDICATIONS AND USAGE**).

The table below summarizes the resulting graft and patient survival at 12, 24, and 36 months for this trial. At 12, 24, and 36 months, graft and patient survival were similar for both groups.

GRAFT AND PATIENT SURVIVAL (%): STUDY 4[a]

Parameter	Rapamune with Cyclosporine Therapy (n = 215)	Rapamune Following Cyclosporine Withdrawal (n = 215)
Graft Survival		
Month 12[b]	95.8	97.2
Month 24	91.2	93.5
Month 36	85.1	91.2
Patient Survival		
Month 12	97.2	98.1
Month 24	94.0	95.3
Month 36	88.4	93.5

a: Includes patients who prematurely discontinued treatment.
b: Primary efficacy endpoint.

The table below summarizes the results of first biopsy-proven acute rejection at 12 and 36 months. There was a significant difference in first biopsy-proven rejection between the two groups during post-randomization through 12 months. Most of the post-randomization acute rejections occurred in the first 3 months following randomization.

INCIDENCE OF FIRST BIOPSY-PROVEN
ACUTE REJECTION (%) BY TREATMENT GROUP AT
36 MONTHS: STUDY 4[a]

Period	Rapamune with Cyclosporine Therapy (n = 215)	Rapamune Following Cyclosporine withdrawal (n = 215)
Prerandomization[b]	9.3	10.2
Postrandomization through 12 months[b]	4.2	9.8
Postrandomization from 12 to 36 months	1.4	0.5
Postrandomization through 36 months	5.6	10.2
Total at 36 months	14.9	20.5

a: Includes patients who prematurely discontinued treatment.
b: Randomization occurred at 3 months ± 2 weeks.

Patients receiving renal allografts with ≥ 4 HLA mismatches experienced significantly higher rates of acute rejection following randomization to the cyclosporine withdrawal group compared with patients who continued cyclosporine (15.3% vs 3.0%). Patients receiving renal allografts with ≤ 3 HLA mismatches, demonstrated similar rates of acute rejection between treatment groups (6.8% vs 7.7%) following randomization.

The table below summarizes the mean calculated GFR in Study 4.

CALCULATED GLOMERULAR FILTRATION RATES
(mL/min) BY NANKIVELL EQUATION AT 12, 24,
AND 36 MONTHS POST TRANSPLANT: STUDY 4[a,b]

Parameter	Rapamune with Cyclosporine Therapy	Rapamune Following Cyclosporine Withdrawal
Month 12		
Mean ± SEM	53.2 ± 1.5 n = 208	59.3 ± 1.5 n = 203
Month 24		
Mean ± SEM	48.4 ± 1.7 n = 203	58.4 ± 1.6 n = 201
Month 36		
Mean ± SEM	47.3 ± 1.8 (n = 194)	59.4 ± 1.8 (n = 194)

a: Includes patients who prematurely discontinued treatment.
b: Patients who had a graft loss were included in the analysis and had their GFR set to 0.0.

The mean GFR at 12, 24, and 36 months, calculated by the Nankivell equation, was significantly higher for patients receiving Rapamune as a maintenance regimen following cyclosporine withdrawal than for those in the Rapamune with cyclosporine therapy group. Patients who had an acute rejection prior to randomization had a significantly higher GFR following cyclosporine withdrawal compared to those in the Rapamune with cyclosporine group. There was no significant difference in GFR between groups for patients who experienced acute rejection postrandomization.

INCIDENCE (%) OF EFFICACY FAILURE AT 3 AND 6 MONTHS: STUDY 3[a,b]

	Rapamune® Oral Solution (n = 238)	Rapamune® Tablets (n = 239)
Efficacy Failure at 3 months[c]	23.5	24.7
Components of efficacy failure		
Biopsy-proven acute rejection	18.9	17.6
Graft loss	3.4	6.3
Death	1.3	0.8
Efficacy Failure at 6 months	26.1	27.2
Components of efficacy failure		
Biopsy-proven acute rejection	21.0	19.2
Graft loss	3.4	6.3
Death	1.7	1.7

a: Patients received cyclosporine and corticosteroids.
b: Includes patients who prematurely discontinued treatment.
c: Efficacy failure at 3 months was the primary endpoint.

Pediatrics: Rapamune® was evaluated in a 36-month, open-label, randomized, controlled clinical trial at 14 North American centers in pediatric (aged 3 to < 18 years) renal transplant recipients considered to be at high immunologic risk for developing chronic allograft nephropathy, defined as a history of one or more acute allograft rejection episodes and/or the presence of chronic allograft nephropathy on a renal biopsy. Seventy-eight (78) subjects were randomized in a 2:1 ratio to Rapamune® (sirolimus target concentrations of 5 to 15 ng/mL, by chromatographic assay, n = 53) in combination with a calcineurin inhibitor and corticosteroids or to continue calcineurin-inhibitor-based immunosuppressive therapy (n = 25). The primary endpoint of the study was efficacy failure as defined by the first occurrence of biopsy confirmed acute rejection, graft loss, or death, and the trial was designed to show superiority of Rapamune® added to a calcineurin-inhibitor-based immunosuppressive regimen compared to a calcineurin-inhibitor-based regimen. The cumulative incidence of efficacy failure up to 36 months was 45.3% in the Rapamune® group compared to 44.0% in the control group, and did not demonstrate superiority. There was one death in each group. The use of Rapamune® in combination with calcineurin inhibitors and corticosteroids was associated with an increased risk of deterioration of renal function, serum lipid abnormalities (including but not limited to increased serum triglycerides and cholesterol), and urinary tract infections. This study does not support the addition of Rapamune® to calcineurin-inhibitor-based immunosuppressive therapy in this subpopulation of pediatric renal transplant patients.

INDICATIONS AND USAGE

Rapamune® (sirolimus) is indicated for the prophylaxis of organ rejection in patients aged 13 years or older receiving renal transplants. It is recommended that Rapamune be used initially in a regimen with cyclosporine and corticosteroids. In patients at low to moderate immunologic risk cyclosporine should be withdrawn 2 to 4 months after transplantation and Rapamune® dose should be increased to reach recommended blood concentrations (See **DOSAGE AND ADMINISTRATION**).

The safety and efficacy of cyclosporine withdrawal in high-risk patients have not been adequately studied and it is therefore not recommended. This includes patients with Banff grade III acute rejection or vascular rejection prior to cyclosporine withdrawal, those who are dialysis-dependent, or with serum creatinine > 4.5 mg/dL, black patients, retransplants, multi-organ transplants, patients with high panel of reactive antibodies (See **CLINICAL STUDIES**).

The safety and efficacy of Rapamune® have not been established in pediatric patients less than 13 years old, or in pediatric (< 18 years) renal transplant recipients considered at high immunologic risk (see **PRECAUTIONS, Pediatric use**, and **CLINICAL STUDIES, Pediatrics**).

CONTRAINDICATIONS

Rapamune is contraindicated in patients with a hypersensitivity to sirolimus or its derivatives or any component of the drug product.

WARNINGS

Increased susceptibility to infection and the possible development of lymphoma and other malignancies, particularly of the skin, may result from immunosuppression (see **ADVERSE REACTIONS**). Oversuppression of the immune system can also increase susceptibility to infection including opportunistic infections, fatal infections, and sepsis. Only physicians experienced in immunosuppressive therapy and management of organ transplant patients should use Rapamune. Patients receiving the drug should be managed in facilities equipped and staffed with adequate laboratory and supportive medical resources. The physician responsible for maintenance therapy should have complete information requisite for the follow-up of the patient.

Hypersensitivity reactions, including anaphylactic/anaphylactoid reactions, have been associated with the administration of sirolimus (see **ADVERSE REACTIONS**).

As usual for patients with increased risk for skin cancer, exposure to sunlight and UV light should be limited by wearing protective clothing and using a sunscreen with a high protection factor.

Increased serum cholesterol and triglycerides, that may require treatment, occurred more frequently in patients treated with Rapamune compared with azathioprine or placebo controls (see **PRECAUTIONS**).

In Studies 1 and 2, from month 6 through months 24 and 36, respectively, mean serum creatinine was increased and mean glomerular filtration rate was decreased in patients treated with Rapamune and cyclosporine compared with those treated with cyclosporine and placebo or azathioprine controls. The rate of decline in renal function was greater in patients receiving Rapamune and cyclosporine compared with control therapies (see **CLINICAL STUDIES**).

Renal function should be closely monitored during the administration of Rapamune® in combination with cyclosporine since long-term administration can be associated with deterioration of renal function. Appropriate adjustment of the immunosuppression regimen, including discontinuation of Rapamune and/or cyclosporine, should be considered in patients with elevated or increasing serum creatinine levels. Caution should be exercised when using other drugs which are known to impair renal function. In patients at low to moderate immunologic risk continuation of combination therapy with cyclosporine beyond 4 months following transplantation should only be considered when the benefits outweigh the risks of this combination for the individual patients (see **PRECAUTIONS**).

In clinical trials, Rapamune has been administered concurrently with corticosteroids and with the following formulations of cyclosporine:

Sandimmune® Injection (cyclosporine injection)
Sandimmune® Oral Solution (cyclosporine oral solution)
Sandimmune® Soft Gelatin Capsules (cyclosporine capsules)
Neoral® Soft Gelatin Capsules (cyclosporine capsules [MODIFIED])
Neoral® Oral Solution (cyclosporine oral solution [MODIFIED])

The efficacy and safety of the use of Rapamune in combination with other immunosuppressive agents has not been determined.

Liver Transplantation – Excess Mortality, Graft Loss, and Hepatic Artery Thrombosis (HAT):
The use of sirolimus in combination with tacrolimus was associated with excess mortality and graft loss in a study in de novo liver transplant recipients. Many of these patients had evidence of infection at or near the time of death.
In this and another study in de novo liver transplant recipients, the use of sirolimus in combination with cyclosporine or tacrolimus was associated with an increase in HAT; most cases of HAT occurred within 30 days post-transplantation and most led to graft loss or death.
Lung Transplantation – Bronchial Anastomotic Dehiscence:
Cases of bronchial anastomotic dehiscence, most fatal, have been reported in de novo lung transplant patients when sirolimus has been used as part of an immunosuppressive regimen.
The safety and efficacy of Rapamune® (sirolimus) as immunosuppressive therapy have not been established in liver or lung transplant patients, and therefore, such use is not recommended.

Co-administration of sirolimus with strong inhibitors of CYP3A4 and/or P-gp (such as ketoconazole, voriconazole, itraconazole, erythromycin, telithromycin, or clarithromycin) or strong inducers of CYP3A4 and/or P-gp (such as rifampin or rifabutin) is not recommended (see **CLINICAL PHARMACOLOGY, Metabolism**, and **PRECAUTIONS, Drug Interactions** and **Other drug interactions**).

PRECAUTIONS
General
Rapamune is intended for oral administration only.
Lymphocele, a known surgical complication of renal transplantation, occurred significantly more often in a dose-related fashion in patients treated with Rapamune. Appropriate operative measures should be considered to minimize this complication.

Lipids
The use of Rapamune® in renal transplant patients was associated with increased serum cholesterol and triglycerides that may require treatment.
In Studies 1 and 2, in *de novo* renal transplant recipients who began the study with normal, fasting, total serum cholesterol (<200 mg/dL) or normal, fasting, total serum tri-

glycerides (<200 mg/dL), there was an increased incidence of hypercholesterolemia (fasting serum cholesterol >240 mg/dL) or hypertriglyceridemia (fasting serum triglycerides >500 mg/dL), respectively, in patients receiving both Rapamune® 2 mg and Rapamune® 5 mg compared with azathioprine and placebo controls.

Treatment of new-onset hypercholesterolemia with lipid-lowering agents was required in 42-52% of patients enrolled in the Rapamune arms of Studies 1 and 2 compared with 16% of patients in the placebo arm and 22% of patients in the azathioprine arm.

In Study 4 during the prerandomization period, mean fasting serum cholesterol and triglyceride values rapidly increased, and peaked at 2 months with mean cholesterol values > 240 mg/dL and triglycerides > 250 mg/dL. After randomization mean cholesterol and triglyceride values remained higher in the cyclosporine withdrawal arm compared to the Rapamune® and cyclosporine combination.

Renal transplant patients have a higher prevalence of clinically significant hyperlipidemia. Accordingly, the risk/benefit should be carefully considered in patients with established hyperlipidemia before initiating an immunosuppressive regimen including Rapamune.

Any patient who is administered Rapamune should be monitored for hyperlipidemia using laboratory tests and if hyperlipidemia is detected, subsequent interventions such as diet, exercise, and lipid-lowering agents, as outlined by the National Cholesterol Education Program guidelines, should be initiated.

In clinical trials, the concomitant administration of Rapamune and HMG-CoA reductase inhibitors and/or fibrates appeared to be well tolerated.

During Rapamune therapy with cyclosporine, patients administered an HMG-CoA reductase inhibitor and/or fibrate should be monitored for the possible development of rhabdomyolysis and other adverse effects as described in the respective labeling for these agents.

Renal Function

Patients treated with cyclosporine and Rapamune were noted to have higher serum creatinine levels and lower glomerular filtration rates compared with patients treated with cyclosporine and placebo or azathioprine controls (Studies 1 and 2). The rate of decline in renal function in these studies was greater in patients receiving Rapamune and cyclosporine compared with control therapies. In patients at low to moderate immunologic risk (See **CLINICAL STUDIES**) continuation of combination therapy with cyclosporine beyond 4 months following transplantation should only be considered when the benefits outweigh the risks of this combination for the individual patients. (see **WARNINGS**).

Renal function should be monitored during the administration of Rapamune® in combination with cyclosporine. Appropriate adjustment of the immunosuppression regimen, including discontinuation of Rapamune and/or cyclosporine, should be considered in patients with elevated or increasing serum creatinine levels. Caution should be exercised when using agents (e.g., aminoglycosides, and amphotericin B) that are known to have a deleterious effect on renal function.

Antimicrobial Prophylaxis

Cases of *Pneumocystis carinii* pneumonia have been reported in patients not receiving antimicrobial prophylaxis. Therefore, antimicrobial prophylaxis for *Pneumocystis carinii* pneumonia should be administered for 1 year following transplantation.

Cytomegalovirus (CMV) prophylaxis is recommended for 3 months after transplantation, particularly for patients at increased risk for CMV disease.

Interstitial Lung Disease

Cases of interstitial lung disease (including pneumonitis, and infrequently bronchiolitis obliterans organizing pneumonia [BOOP] and pulmonary fibrosis), some fatal, with no identified infectious etiology have occurred in patients receiving immunosuppressive regimens including Rapamune. In some cases, the interstitial lung disease has resolved upon discontinuation or dose reduction of Rapamune. The risk may be increased as the trough Rapamune concentration increases (see **ADVERSE REACTIONS, Other clinical experience**).

Information for Patients

Patients should be given complete dosage instructions (see **Patient Instructions**). Women of childbearing potential should be informed of the potential risks during pregnancy and that they should use effective contraception prior to initiation of Rapamune therapy, during Rapamune therapy and for 12 weeks after Rapamune therapy has been stopped (see **PRECAUTIONS: Pregnancy**).

Patients should be told that exposure to sunlight and UV light should be limited by wearing protective clothing and using a sunscreen with a high protection factor because of the increased risk for skin cancer (see **WARNINGS**).

Laboratory Tests

Whole blood sirolimus concentrations should be monitored in patients receiving concentration-controlled Rapamune. Monitoring is also necessary in patients likely to have altered drug metabolism, in patients ≥13 years who weigh less than 40 kg, in patients with hepatic impairment, and during concurrent administration of potent CYP3A4 inducers and inhibitors (see **PRECAUTIONS: Drug Interactions**).

Drug Interactions

Sirolimus is known to be a substrate for both cytochrome CYP3A4 and P-gp. The pharmacokinetic interaction between sirolimus and concomitantly administered drugs is discussed below. Drug interaction studies have not been conducted with drugs other than those described below.

Cyclosporine capsules MODIFIED:

Cyclosporine is a substrate and inhibitor of CYP3A4 and P-gp.

Because of the effect of cyclosporine capsules (MODIFIED), it is recommended that sirolimus should be taken 4 hours after administration of cyclosporine oral solution (MODIFIED) and/or cyclosporine capsules (MODIFIED) (see DOSAGE AND ADMINISTRATION).

Studies assessing the effect of concomitant administration of cyclosporine capsules (MODIFIED) with sirolimus oral solution and with sirolimus tablets are summarized below.

Rapamune Oral Solution: In a single dose drug-drug interaction study, 24 healthy volunteers were administered 10 mg sirolimus either simultaneously or 4 hours after a 300 mg dose of Neoral® Soft Gelatin Capsules (cyclosporine capsules [MODIFIED]). For simultaneous administration, the mean C_{max} and AUC of sirolimus were increased by 116% and 230%, respectively, relative to administration of sirolimus alone. However, when given 4 hours after Neoral® Soft Gelatin Capsules (cyclosporine capsules [MODIFIED]) administration, sirolimus C_{max} and AUC were increased by 37% and 80%, respectively, compared with administration of sirolimus alone.

In a single-dose cross-over drug-drug interaction study, 33 healthy volunteers received 5 mg sirolimus alone, 2 hours before, and 2 hours after a 300 mg dose of Neoral® Soft Gelatin Capsules (cyclosporine capsules [MODIFIED]). When given 2 hours before Neoral® Soft Gelatin Capsules (cyclosporine capsules [MODIFIED]) administration, sirolimus C_{max} and AUC were comparable to those with administration of sirolimus alone. However, when given 2 hours after, the mean C_{max} and AUC of sirolimus were increased by 126% and 141%, respectively, relative to administration of sirolimus alone.

Mean cyclosporine C_{max} and AUC were not significantly affected when sirolimus was given simultaneously or when administered 4 hours after Neoral® Soft Gelatin Capsules (cyclosporine capsules [MODIFIED]). However, after multiple-dose administration of sirolimus given 4 hours after Neoral® in renal post-transplant patients over 6 months, cyclosporine oral-dose clearance was reduced, and lower doses of Neoral® Soft Gelatin Capsules (cyclosporine capsules [MODIFIED]) were needed to maintain target cyclosporine concentration.

Rapamune Tablets: In a single-dose drug-drug interaction study, 24 healthy volunteers were administered 10 mg sirolimus (Rapamune Tablets) either simultaneously or 4 hours after a 300-mg dose of Neoral® Soft Gelatin Capsules (cyclosporine capsules [MODIFIED]). For simultaneous administration, mean C_{max} and AUC were increased by 512% and 148%, respectively, relative to administration of sirolimus alone. However, when given 4 hours after cyclosporine administration, sirolimus C_{max} and AUC were both increased by only 33% compared with administration of sirolimus alone.

Cyclosporine oral solution: In a multiple-dose study in 150 psoriasis patients, sirolimus 0.5, 1.5, and 3 mg/m²/day was administered simultaneously with Sandimmune® Oral Solution (cyclosporine Oral Solution) 1.25 mg/kg/day. The increase in average sirolimus trough concentrations ranged between 67% to 86% relative to when sirolimus was administered without cyclosporine. The intersubject variability (%CV) for sirolimus trough concentrations ranged from 39.7% to 68.7%. There was no significant effect of multiple-dose sirolimus on cyclosporine trough concentrations following Sandimmune® Oral Solution (cyclosporine oral solution) administration. However, the %CV was higher (range 85.9%-165%) than those from previous studies.

Sandimmune® Oral Solution (cyclosporine oral solution) is not bioequivalent to Neoral® Oral Solution (cyclosporine oral solution MODIFIED), and should not be used interchangeably. Although there is no published data comparing Sandimmune® Oral Solution (cyclosporine oral solution) to SangCya® Oral Solution (cyclosporine oral solution [MODIFIED]), they should not be used interchangeably. Likewise, Sandimmune® Soft Gelatin Capsules (cyclosporine capsules) are not bioequivalent to Neoral® Soft Gelatin Capsules (cyclosporine capsules [MODIFIED]) and should not be used interchangeably.

Diltiazem: Diltiazem is a substrate and inhibitor of CYP3A4 and P-gp; sirolimus concentrations should be monitored and a dose adjustment may be necessary. The simultaneous oral administration of 10 mg of sirolimus oral solution and 120 mg of diltiazem to 18 healthy volunteers significantly affected the bioavailability of sirolimus. Sirolimus C_{max}, t_{max}, and AUC were increased 1.4-, 1.3-, and 1.6-fold, respectively. Sirolimus did not affect the pharmacokinetics of either diltiazem or its metabolites desacetyldiltiazem and desmethyldiltiazem.

Erythromycin: Erythromycin is a substrate and inhibitor of CYP3A4 and P-gp; co-administration of sirolimus oral solution or tablets and erythromycin is not recommended (see **WARNINGS**). The simultaneous oral administration of 2 mg daily of sirolimus oral solution and 800 mg q 8h of erythromycin as erythromycin ethylsuccinate tablets at steady state to 24 healthy volunteers significantly affected the bioavailability of sirolimus and erythromycin. Sirolimus C_{max} and AUC were increased 4.4- and 4.2-fold respectively and t_{max} was increased by 0.4 hr. Erythromycin C_{max} and AUC were increased 1.6- and 1.7-fold, respectively, and t_{max} was increased by 0.3 hr.

Ketoconazole: Ketoconazole is a strong inhibitor of CYP3A4 and P-gp; co-administration of sirolimus oral solution or tablets and ketoconazole is not recommended (see **WARNINGS**). Multiple-dose ketoconazole administration significantly affected the rate and extent of absorption and sirolimus exposure after administration of Rapamune® Oral Solution, as reflected by increases in sirolimus C_{max}, t_{max}, and AUC of 4.3-fold, 38%, and 10.9-fold, respectively. However, the terminal $t_{1/2}$ of sirolimus was not changed. Single-dose sirolimus did not affect steady-state 12-hour plasma ketoconazole concentrations.

Rifampin: Rifampin is a strong inducer of CYP3A4 and P-gp; co-administration of sirolimus oral solution or tablets and rifampin is not recommended (see **WARNINGS**). Pretreatment of 14 healthy volunteers with multiple doses of rifampin, 600 mg daily for 14 days, followed by a single 20-mg dose of sirolimus oral solution, greatly increased sirolimus oral-dose clearance by 5.5-fold (range = 2.8 to 10), which represents mean decreases in AUC and C_{max} of about 82% and 71%, respectively. In patients where rifampin is indicated, alternative therapeutic agents with less enzyme induction potential should be considered.

Verapamil: Verapamil is a substrate and inhibitor of CYP3A4 and P-gp; sirolimus concentrations should be monitored and a dose adjustment may be necessary. The simultaneous oral administration of 2 mg daily of sirolimus oral solution and 180 mg q 12h of verapamil at steady state to 26 healthy volunteers significantly affected the bioavailability of sirolimus and verapamil. Sirolimus C_{max} and AUC were increased 2.3- and 2.2-fold, respectively, without substantial change in t_{max}. The C_{max} and AUC of the pharmacologically active S(-) enantiomer of verapamil were both increased 1.5-fold and t_{max} was decreased by 1.2 hr.

Drugs which may be coadministered without dose adjustment

Clinically significant pharmacokinetic drug-drug interactions were not observed in studies of drugs listed below. A synopsis of the type of study performed for each drug is provided. Sirolimus and these drugs may be coadministered without dose adjustments.

Acyclovir: Acyclovir, 200 mg, was administered once daily for 3 days followed by a single 10-mg dose of sirolimus oral solution on day 3 in 20 adult healthy volunteers.

Digoxin: Digoxin, 0.25 mg, was administered daily for 8 days and a single 10-mg dose of sirolimus oral solution was given on day 8 to 24 healthy volunteers.

Glyburide: A single 5-mg dose of glyburide and a single 10-mg dose of sirolimus oral solution were administered to 24 healthy volunteers. Sirolimus did not affect the hypoglycemic action of glyburide.

Nifedipine: A single 60-mg dose of nifedipine and a single 10-mg dose of sirolimus oral solution were administered to 24 healthy volunteers.

Norgestrel/ethinyl estradiol (Lo/Ovral®): Sirolimus oral solution, 2 mg, was given daily for 7 days to 21 healthy female volunteers on norgestrel/ethinyl estradiol.

Prednisolone: Pharmacokinetic information was obtained from 42 stable renal transplant patients receiving daily doses of prednisone (5-20 mg/day) and either single or multiple doses of sirolimus oral solution (0.5-5 mg/m² q 12h).

Sulfamethoxazole/trimethoprim (Bactrim®): A single oral dose of sulfamethoxazole (400 mg)/trimethoprim (80 mg) was given to 15 renal transplant patients receiving daily oral doses of sirolimus (8 to 25 mg/m²).

Other drug interactions

Co-administration of sirolimus with strong inhibitors of CYP3A4 and/or P-gp (such as ketoconazole, voriconazole, itraconazole, erythromycin, telithromycin, or clarithromycin) or strong inducers of CYP3A4 and/or P-gp (such as rifampin or rifabutin) is not recommended (see **WARNINGS**). Sirolimus is extensively metabolized by the CYP3A4 isoenzyme in the intestinal wall and liver and undergoes counter-transport from enterocytes of the small intestine into the gut lumen by the P-gp drug efflux pump. Sirolimus is potentially recycled between enterocytes and the gut lumen to allow continued metabolism by CYP3A4. Therefore, absorption and the subsequent elimination of systemically absorbed sirolimus may be influenced by drugs that affect these proteins. Strong inhibitors of CYP3A4 and P-gp significantly decrease the metabolism of sirolimus and increase sirolimus concentrations, while strong inducers of CYP3A4 and P-gp significantly increase the metabolism of sirolimus and decrease sirolimus concentrations.

In patients in whom strong inhibitors or inducers of CYP3A4 are indicated, alternative therapeutic agents with less potential for inhibition or induction of CYP3A4 should be considered.

Sirolimus is a substrate for the multidrug efflux pump, P-gp in the small intestine. Therefore, absorption of sirolimus may be influenced by drugs that affect P-gp.

Aside from those mentioned above, other drugs that increase sirolimus blood concentrations include (but are not limited to):

- Calcium channel blockers: nicardipine.
- Antifungal agents: clotrimazole, fluconazole.
- Antibiotics: troleandomycin.
- Gastrointestinal prokinetic agents: cisapride, metoclopramide.
- Other drugs: bromocriptine, cimetidine, danazol, HIV-protease inhibitors (e.g., ritonavir, indinavir).

Aside from those mentioned above, other drugs that decrease sirolimus concentrations include (but are not limited to):

Continued on next page

Rapamune—Cont.

Anticonvulsants: carbamazepine, phenobarbital, phenytoin.
Antibiotics: rifapentine.

Care should be exercised when drugs or other substances that are metabolized by CYP3A4 are administered concomitantly with Rapamune. Grapefruit juice reduces CYP3A4-mediated metabolism of Rapamune and must not be used for dilution (see **DOSAGE AND ADMINISTRATION**).

Herbal Preparations

St. John's Wort (*hypericum perforatum*) induces CYP3A4 and P-gp. Since sirolimus is a substrate for both cytochrome CYP3A4 and P-gp, there is the potential that the use of St. John's Wort in patients receiving Rapamune could result in reduced sirolimus concentrations.

Vaccination

Immunosuppressants may affect response to vaccination. Therefore, during treatment with Rapamune, vaccination may be less effective. The use of live vaccines should be avoided; live vaccines may include, but are not limited to measles, mumps, rubella, oral polio, BCG, yellow fever, varicella, and TY21a typhoid.

Drug-Laboratory Test Interactions

There are no studies on the interactions of sirolimus in commonly employed clinical laboratory tests.

Carcinogenesis, Mutagenesis, and Impairment of Fertility

Sirolimus was not genotoxic in the in vitro bacterial reverse mutation assay, the Chinese hamster ovary cell chromosomal aberration assay, the mouse lymphoma cell forward mutation assay, or the in vivo mouse micronucleus assay.

Carcinogenicity studies were conducted in mice and rats. In an 86-week female mouse study at dosages of 0, 12.5, 25 and 50/6 (dosage lowered from 50 to 6 mg/kg/day at week 31 due to infection secondary to immunosuppression) there was a statistically significant increase in malignant lymphoma at all dose levels (approximately 16 to 135 times the clinical doses adjusted for body surface area) compared with controls. In a second mouse study at dosages of 0, 1, 3 and 6 mg/kg (approximately 3 to 16 times the clinical dose adjusted for body surface area), hepatocellular adenoma and carcinoma (males), were considered Rapamune related. In the 104-week rat study at dosages of 0, 0.05, 0.1, and 0.2 mg/kg/day (approximately 0.4 to 1 times the clinical dose adjusted for body surface area), there was a statistically significant increased incidence of testicular adenoma in the 0.2 mg/kg/day group.

There was no effect on fertility in female rats following the administration of sirolimus at dosages up to 0.5 mg/kg (approximately 1 to 3 times the clinical doses adjusted for body surface area). In male rats, there was no significant difference in fertility rate compared to controls at a dosage of 2 mg/kg (approximately 4 to 11 times the clinical doses adjusted for body surface area). Reductions in testicular weights and/or histological lesions (e.g., tubular atrophy and tubular giant cells) were observed in rats following dosages of 0.65 mg/kg (approximately 1 to 3 times the clinical doses adjusted for body surface area) and above and in a monkey study at 0.1 mg/kg (approximately 0.4 to 1 times the clinical doses adjusted for body surface area) and above. Sperm counts were reduced in male rats following the administration of sirolimus for 13 weeks at a dosage of 6 mg/kg (approximately 12 to 32 times the clinical doses adjusted for body surface area), but showed improvement by 3 months after dosing was stopped.

Pregnancy

Pregnancy Category C: Sirolimus was embryo/feto toxic in rats at dosages of 0.1 mg/kg and above (approximately 0.2 to 0.5 the clinical doses adjusted for body surface area). Embryo/feto toxicity was manifested as mortality and reduced fetal weights (with associated delays in skeletal ossification). However, no teratogenesis was evident. In combination with cyclosporine, rats had increased embryo/feto mortality compared with Rapamune alone. There were no effects on rabbit development at the maternally toxic dosage of 0.05 mg/kg (approximately 0.3 to 0.8 times the clinical doses adjusted for body surface area). There are no adequate and well controlled studies in pregnant women. Effective contraception must be initiated before Rapamune therapy, during Rapamune therapy, and for 12 weeks after Rapamune therapy has been stopped. Rapamune should be used during pregnancy only if the potential benefit outweighs the potential risk to the embryo/fetus.

Use during lactation

Sirolimus is excreted in trace amounts in milk of lactating rats. It is not known whether sirolimus is excreted in human milk. The pharmacokinetic and safety profiles of sirolimus in infants are not known. Because many drugs are excreted in human milk and because of the potential for adverse reactions in nursing infants from sirolimus, a decision should be made whether to discontinue nursing or to discontinue the drug, taking into account the importance of the drug to the mother.

Pediatric use

The safety and efficacy of Rapamune® in pediatric patients below the age of 13 years have not been established.

The safety and efficacy of Rapamune® Oral Solution and Rapamune® Tablets have been established in children aged 13 or older judged to be at low to moderate immunologic risk. Use of Rapamune® Oral Solution and Rapamune® Tablets in this subpopulation of children aged 13 or older is supported by evidence from adequate and well-controlled trials of Rapamune® Oral Solution in adults with additional pharmacokinetic data in pediatric renal transplantation recipients (see **CLINICAL PHARMACOLOGY, Special Populations, *Pediatric***).

Safety and efficacy information from a controlled clinical trial in pediatric and adolescent (< 18 years of age) renal transplant recipients judged to be at high immunologic risk, defined as a history of one or more acute rejection episodes and/or the presence of chronic allograft nephropathy, do not support the chronic use of Rapamune® Oral Solution or Tablets in combination with calcineurin inhibitors and corticosteroids, due to the increased risk of lipid abnormalities and deterioration of renal function associated with these immunosuppressive regimens, without increased benefit with respect to acute rejection, graft survival, or patient survival (see **CLINICAL STUDIES, Pediatrics**).

Geriatric use

Clinical studies of Rapamune Oral Solution or Tablets did not include sufficient numbers of patients aged 65 years and over to determine whether safety and efficacy differ in this population from younger patients. Data pertaining to sirolimus trough concentrations suggest that dose adjustments based upon age in geriatric renal patients are not necessary.

ADVERSE REACTIONS

Rapamune® Oral Solution: The incidence of adverse reactions was determined in two randomized, double-blind, multicenter controlled trials in which 499 renal transplant patients received Rapamune Oral Solution 2 mg/day, 477 received Rapamune Oral Solution 5 mg/day, 160 received azathioprine, and 124 received placebo. All patients were treated with cyclosporine and corticosteroids. Data (≥ 12 months post-transplant) presented in the table below show the adverse reactions that occurred in any treatment group with an incidence of ≥ 20%.

Specific adverse reactions associated with the administration of Rapamune (sirolimus) Oral Solution occurred at a significantly higher frequency than in the respective control group. For both Rapamune Oral Solution 2 mg/day and 5 mg/day these include hypercholesterolemia, hyperlipemia, hypertension, and rash; for Rapamune Oral Solution 2 mg/day acne; and for Rapamune Oral Solution 5 mg/day anemia, arthralgia, diarrhea, hypokalemia, and thrombocytopenia. The elevations of triglycerides and cholesterol and decreases in platelets and hemoglobin occurred in a dose-related manner in patients receiving Rapamune.

Patients maintained on Rapamune Oral Solution 5 mg/day, when compared with patients on Rapamune Oral Solution 2 mg/day, demonstrated an increased incidence of the following adverse events: anemia, leukopenia, thrombocytopenia, hypokalemia, hyperlipemia, fever, and diarrhea.

In general, adverse events related to the administration of Rapamune were dependent on dose/concentration.

[See table below]

With longer term follow-up, the adverse event profile remained similar. Some new events became significantly different among the treatment groups. For events which occurred at a frequency of ≥ 20% by 24 months for Study 1 and 36 months for Study 2, only the incidence of edema became significantly higher in both Rapamune groups as compared with the control group. The incidence of headache became significantly more common in the Rapamune 5mg/day group as compared with control therapy.

At 24 months for Study 1, the following treatment-emergent infections were significantly different among the treatment groups: bronchitis, Herpes simplex, pneumonia, pyelonephritis, and upper respiratory infections. In each instance, the incidence was highest in the Rapamune 5 mg/day group, lower in the Rapamune 2 mg/day group and lowest in the azathioprine group. Except for upper respiratory infections in the Rapamune 5 mg/day cohort, the remainder of events occurred with a frequency of < 20%.

At 36 months in Study 2 only the incidence of treatment-emergent Herpes simplex was significantly different among the treatment groups, being higher in the Rapamune 5 mg/day group than either of the other groups.

The table below summarizes the incidence of malignancies in the two controlled trials for the prevention of acute rejection. At 24 (Study 1) and 36 months (Study 2) there were no significant differences among treatment groups.

[See first table at top of next page]

Among the adverse events that were reported at a rate of ≥3% and <20% at 12 months, the following were more prominent in patients maintained on Rapamune 5 mg/day, when compared with patients on Rapamune 2 mg/day: epistaxis, lymphocele, insomnia, thrombotic thrombocytopenic purpura (hemolytic-uremic syndrome), skin ulcer, increased LDH, hypotension, facial edema.

The following adverse events were reported with ≥3% and <20% incidence in patients in any Rapamune treatment

ADVERSE EVENTS OCCURRING AT A FREQUENCY OF ≥ 20% IN ANY TREATMENT GROUP IN PREVENTION OF ACUTE RENAL REJECTION TRIALS (%) AT ≥ 12 MONTHS POST-TRANSPLANTATION FOR STUDIES 1 AND 2[a]

Body System	Rapamune® Oral Solution -------2 mg/day-------		Rapamune® Oral Solution -------5 mg/day-------		Azathioprine 2-3 mg/kg/day	Placebo
Adverse Event	Study 1 (n = 281)	Study 2 (n = 218)	Study 1 (n = 269)	Study 2 (n = 208)	Study 1 (n = 160)	Study 2 (n = 124)
Body As A Whole						
Abdominal pain	28	29	30	36	29	30
Asthenia	38	22	40	28	37	28
Back pain	16	23	26	22	23	20
Chest pain	16	18	19	24	16	19
Fever	27	23	33	34	33	35
Headache	23	34	27	34	21	31
Pain	24	33	29	29	30	25
Cardiovascular System						
Hypertension	43	45	39	49	29	48
Digestive System						
Constipation	28	36	34	38	37	31
Diarrhea	32	25	42	35	28	27
Dyspepsia	17	23	23	25	24	34
Nausea	31	25	36	31	39	29
Vomiting	21	19	25	25	31	21
Hemic And Lymphatic System						
Anemia	27	23	37	33	29	21
Leukopenia	9	9	15	13	20	8
Thrombocytopenia	13	14	20	30	9	9
Metabolic And Nutritional						
Creatinine increased	35	39	37	40	28	38
Edema	24	20	16	18	23	15
Hypercholesteremia (See **WARNINGS** and **PRECAUTIONS**)	38	43	42	46	33	23
Hyperkalemia	15	17	12	14	24	27
Hyperlipemia (See **WARNINGS** and **PRECAUTIONS**)	38	45	44	57	28	23
Hypokalemia	17	11	21	17	11	9
Hypophosphatemia	20	15	23	19	20	19
Peripheral edema	60	54	64	58	58	48
Weight gain	21	11	15	8	19	15
Musculoskeletal System						
Arthralgia	25	25	27	31	21	18
Nervous System						
Insomnia	14	13	22	14	18	8
Tremor	31	21	30	22	28	19
Respiratory System						
Dyspnea	22	24	28	30	23	30
Pharyngitis	17	16	16	21	17	22
Upper respiratory infection	20	26	24	23	13	23
Skin And Appendages						
Acne	31	22	20	22	17	19
Rash	12	10	13	20	6	6
Urogenital System						
Urinary tract infection	20	26	23	33	31	26

a: Patients received cyclosporine and corticosteroids.

group in the two controlled clinical trials for the prevention of acute rejection, BODY AS A WHOLE: abdomen enlarged, abscess, ascites, cellulitis, chills, face edema, flu syndrome, generalized edema, hernia, *Herpes zoster* infection, lymphocele, malaise, pelvic pain, peritonitis, sepsis; CARDIOVASCULAR SYSTEM: atrial fibrillation, congestive heart failure, hemorrhage, hypervolemia, hypotension, palpitation, peripheral vascular disorder, postural hypotension, syncope, tachycardia, thrombophlebitis, thrombosis, vasodilatation, venous thromboembolism; DIGESTIVE SYSTEM: anorexia, dysphagia, eructation, esophagitis, flatulence, gastritis, gastroenteritis, gingivitis, gum hyperplasia, ileus, liver function tests abnormal, mouth ulceration, oral moniliasis, stomatitis; ENDOCRINE SYSTEM: Cushing's syndrome, diabetes mellitus, glycosuria; HEMIC AND LYMPHATIC SYSTEM: ecchymosis, leukocytosis, lymphadenopathy, polycythemia, thrombotic thrombocytopenic purpura (hemolytic-uremic syndrome); METABOLIC AND NUTRITIONAL: acidosis, alkaline phosphatase increased, BUN increased, creatine phosphokinase increased, dehydration, healing abnormal, hypercalcemia, hyperglycemia, hyperphosphatemia, hypocalcemia, hypoglycemia, hypomagnesemia, hyponatremia, lactic dehydrogenase increased, AST/SGOT increased, ALT/SGPT increased, weight loss; MUSCULOSKELETAL SYSTEM: arthrosis, bone necrosis, leg cramps, myalgia, osteoporosis, tetany; NERVOUS SYSTEM: anxiety, confusion, depression, dizziness, emotional lability, hypertonia, hypesthesia, hypotonia, insomnia, neuropathy, paresthesia, somnolence; RESPIRATORY SYSTEM: asthma, atelectasis, bronchitis, cough increased, epistaxis, hypoxia, lung edema, pleural effusion, pneumonia, rhinitis, sinusitis; SKIN AND APPENDAGES: fungal dermatitis, hirsutism, pruritus, skin hypertrophy, skin ulcer, sweating; SPECIAL SENSES: abnormal vision, cataract, conjunctivitis, deafness, ear pain, otitis media, tinnitus; UROGENITAL SYSTEM: albuminuria, bladder pain, dysuria, hematuria, hydronephrosis, impotence, kidney pain, kidney tubular necrosis, nocturia, oliguria, pyelonephritis, pyuria, scrotal edema, testis disorder, toxic nephropathy, urinary frequency, urinary incontinence, urinary retention.

Less frequently occurring adverse events included: mycobacterial infections, Epstein-Barr virus infections, and pancreatitis.

Among the events which were reported at an incidence of ≥ 3% and < 20% by 24 months for Study 1 and 36 months for Study 2, tachycardia and Cushing's syndrome were reported significantly more commonly in both Rapamune groups as compared with the control therapy. Events that were reported more commonly in the Rapamune 5 mg/day group than either the Rapamune 2 mg/day group and/or control group were: abnormal healing, bone necrosis, chills, congestive heart failure, dysuria, hernia, hirsutism, urinary frequency, and lymphadenopathy.

Rapamune® Tablets: The safety profile of the tablet did not differ from that of the oral solution formulation. The incidence of adverse reactions up to 12 months was determined in a randomized, multicenter controlled trial (Study 3) in which 229 renal transplant patients received Rapamune Oral Solution 2 mg once daily and 228 patients received Rapamune Tablets 2 mg once daily. All patients were treated with cyclosporine and corticosteroids. The adverse reactions that occurred in either treatment group with an incidence of ≥ 20% in Study 3 are similar to those reported for Studies 1 and 2. There was no notable difference in the incidence of these adverse events between treatment groups (oral solution versus tablets) in Study 3, with the exception of acne, which occurred more frequently in the oral solution group, and tremor which occurred more frequently in the tablet group, particularly in Black patients. The adverse events that occurred in patients with an incidence of ≥3% and <20% in either treatment group in Study 3 were similar to those reported in Studies 1 and 2. There was no notable difference in the incidence of these adverse events between treatment groups (oral solution versus tablets) in Study 3, with the exception of hypertonia, which occurred more frequently in the oral solution group and diabetes mellitus which occurred more frequently in the tablet group. Hispanic patients in the tablet group experienced hyperglycemia more frequently than Hispanic patients in the oral solution group. In Study 3 alone, menorrhagia, metrorrhagia, and polyuria occurred with an incidence of ≥3% and <20%.

The clinically important opportunistic or common transplant-related infections were identical in all three studies and the incidences of these infections were similar in Study 3 compared with Studies 1 and 2. The incidence rates of these infections were not significantly different between the oral solution and tablet treatment groups in Study 3.

In Study 3 (at 12 months), there were two cases of lymphoma/lymphoproliferative disorder in the oral solution treatment group (0.8%) and two reported cases of lymphoma/lymphoproliferative disorder in the tablet treatment group (0.8%). These differences were not statistically significant and were similar to the incidences observed in Studies 1 and 2.

Rapamune following cyclosporine withdrawal: The incidence of adverse reactions was determined through 36 months in a randomized, multicenter controlled trial (Study 4) in which 215 renal transplant patients received Rapamune as a maintenance regimen following cyclosporine withdrawal and 215 patients received Rapamune with cyclosporine therapy. All patients were treated with corticosteroids. The safety profile prior to randomization (start of cyclosporine withdrawal) was similar to that of the 2-mg Rapamune groups in Studies 1, 2, and 3. Following randomization (at 3 months) patients who had cyclosporine eliminated from their therapy experienced significantly higher incidences of abnormal liver function tests (including increased AST/SGOT and increased ALT/SGPT), hypokalemia, thrombocytopenia, abnormal healing, ileus, and rectal disorder. Conversely, the incidence of hypertension, cyclosporine toxicity, increased creatinine, abnormal kidney function, toxic nephropathy, edema, hyperkalemia, hyperuricemia, and gum hyperplasia was significantly higher in patients who remained on cyclosporine than those who had cyclosporine withdrawn from therapy. Mean systolic and diastolic blood pressure improved significantly following cyclosporine withdrawal.

In Study 4, at 36 months, the incidence of Herpes zoster infection was significantly lower in patients receiving Rapamune following cyclosporine withdrawal compared with patients who continued to receive Rapamune and cyclosporine.

The incidence of malignancies in Study 4 is presented in the table below. In Study 4, the incidence of lymphoma/lymphoproliferative disease was similar in all treatment groups. The overall incidence of malignancy was higher in patients receiving Rapamune plus cyclosporine compared with patients who had cyclosporine withdrawn.

[See second table above]

INCIDENCE (%) OF MALIGNANCIES IN STUDIES 1 (24 MONTHS) AND STUDY 2 (36 MONTHS) POST-TRANSPLANT[a,b]

Malignancy	Rapamune® Oral Solution 2 mg/day Study 1 (n = 284)	Rapamune® Oral Solution 2 mg/day Study 2 (n = 227)	Rapamune® Oral Solution 5 mg/day Study 1 (n = 274)	Rapamune® Oral Solution 5 mg/day Study 2 (n = 219)	Azathioprine 2-3 mg/kg/day Study 1 (n = 161)	Placebo Study 2 (n = 130)
Lymphoma/ lymphoproliferative disease	**0.7**	**1.8**	**1.1**	**3.2**	**0.6**	**0.8**
Skin Carcinoma						
Any Squamous Cell[c]	0.4	2.7	2.2	0.9	3.8	3.0
Any Basal Cell[c]	0.7	2.2	1.5	1.8	2.5	5.3
Melanoma	0.0	0.4	0.0	1.4	0.0	0.0
Miscellaneous/Not Specified	0.0	0.0	0.0	0.0	0.0	0.8
Total	**1.1**	**4.4**	**3.3**	**4.1**	**4.3**	**7.7**
Other Malignancy	**1.1**	**2.2**	**1.5**	**1.4**	**0.6**	**2.3**

a: Patients received cyclosporine and corticosteroids.
b: Includes patients who prematurely discontinued treatment.
c: Patients may be counted in more than one category.

INCIDENCE (%) OF MALIGNANCIES IN STUDY 4 AT 36 MONTHS POST-TRANSPLANT[a,b]

Malignancy	Nonrandomized (n = 95)	Rapamune with Cyclosporine Therapy (n = 215)	Rapamune Following Cyclosporine Withdrawal (n = 215)
Lymphoma/lymphoproliferative disease	**1.1**	**1.4**	**0.5**
Skin Carcinoma			
Any Squamous Cell[c]	1.1	1.9	2.3
Any Basal Cell[c]	3.2	4.7	2.3
Melanoma	0.0	0.5	0.0
Miscellaneous/Not Specified	1.1	0.9	0.0
Total	**4.2**	**6.5**	**3.7**
Other Malignancy	**1.1**	**3.3**	**1.4**

a: Patients received cyclosporine and corticosteroids.
b: Includes patients who prematurely discontinued treatment.
c: Patients may be counted in more than one category.

Pediatrics: Safety was assessed in the controlled clinical trial in pediatric (< 18 years of age) renal transplant patients considered high immunologic risk, defined as a history of one or more acute allograft rejection episodes and/or the presence of chronic allograft nephropathy on a renal biopsy (see **CLINICAL STUDIES**). The use of Rapamune® in combination with calcineurin inhibitors and corticosteroids was associated with an increased risk of deterioration of renal function, serum lipid abnormalities (including but not limited to increased serum triglycerides and cholesterol), and urinary tract infections.

Other clinical experience: Cases of interstitial lung disease (including pneumonitis, and infrequently bronchiolitis obliterans organizing pneumonia [BOOP] and pulmonary fibrosis), some fatal, with no identified infectious etiology have occurred in patients receiving immunosuppressive regimens including Rapamune. In some cases, the interstitial lung disease has resolved upon discontinuation or dose reduction of Rapamune. The risk may be increased as the sirolimus trough concentration increases (see **PRECAUTIONS, General, *Interstitial Lung Disease***). There have been reports of neutropenia and rare reports of pancytopenia. Hypersensitivity reactions, including anaphylactic/anaphylactoid reactions, have been associated with the administration of sirolimus (see **WARNINGS**). Hepatotoxicity has been reported, including fatal hepatic necrosis with elevated sirolimus trough concentrations. There have been rare reports of lymphedema. Abnormal healing following transplant surgery has been reported, including fascial dehiscence and anastomotic disruption (e.g., wound, vascular, airway, ureteral, biliary).

The safety and efficacy of conversion from calcineurin inhibitors to sirolimus in maintenance renal transplant population has not been established. In an ongoing study evaluating the safety and efficacy of conversion from calcineurin inhibitors to sirolimus (target concentrations of 12-20 ng/mL) in maintenance renal transplant patients; enrollment was stopped in the subset of patients (n=90) with a baseline glomerular filtration rate of less than 40 mL/min. There was a higher rate of serious adverse events including pneumonia, acute rejection, graft loss and death in this sirolimus treatment arm.

OVERDOSAGE

Reports of overdose with Rapamune have been received; however, experience has been limited. In general, the adverse effects of overdose are consistent with those listed in the **ADVERSE REACTIONS** section (see **ADVERSE REACTIONS**).

General supportive measures should be followed in all cases of overdose. Based on the poor aqueous solubility and high erythrocyte and plasma protein binding of sirolimus, it is anticipated that sirolimus is not dialyzable to any significant extent. In mice and rats, the acute oral lethal dose was greater than 800 mg/kg.

DOSAGE AND ADMINISTRATION

It is recommended that Rapamune Oral Solution and Tablets be used initially in a regimen with cyclosporine and corticosteroids. Cyclosporine withdrawal is recommended 2 to 4 months after transplantation in patients at low to moderate immunologic risk.

The safety and efficacy of cyclosporine withdrawal in high-risk patients have not been adequately studied and it is therefore not recommended. This includes patients with Banff grade III acute rejection or vascular rejection prior to cyclosporine withdrawal, those who are dialysis-dependent, or with serum creatinine > 4.5 mg/dL, black patients, retransplants, multi-organ transplants, patients with high panel of reactive antibodies (See **INDICATIONS AND USAGE** and **CLINICAL STUDIES**).

Two-mg of Rapamune oral solution has been demonstrated to be clinically equivalent to 2-mg Rapamune oral tablets and hence, are interchangeable on a mg to mg basis. However, it is not known if higher doses of Rapamune oral solution are clinically equivalent to higher doses of tablets on a mg to mg basis. (See **CLINICAL PHARMACOLOGY: Absorption**). Rapamune is to be administered orally once daily.

Rapamune and cyclosporine combination therapy: The initial dose of Rapamune should be administered as soon as possible after transplantation. For *de novo* transplant recipients, a loading dose of Rapamune of 3 times the maintenance dose should be given. A daily maintenance dose of 2-mg is recommended for use in renal transplant patients, with a loading dose of 6 mg. Although a daily maintenance dose of 5 mg, with a loading dose of 15 mg was used in clinical trials of the oral solution and was shown to be safe and effective, no efficacy advantage over the 2-mg dose could be established for renal transplant patients. Patients receiving 2 mg of Rapamune Oral Solution per day demonstrated an overall better safety profile than did patients receiving 5 mg of Rapamune Oral Solution per day.

Continued on next page

Rapamune—Cont.

Rapamune following cyclosporine withdrawal: Initially, patients considered for cyclosporine withdrawal should be receiving Rapamune and cyclosporine combination therapy. At 2 to 4 months following transplantation, cyclosporine should be progressively discontinued over 4 to 8 weeks and the Rapamune® dose should be adjusted to obtain whole blood trough concentrations within the range of 12 to 24 ng/mL (chromatographic method). Therapeutic drug monitoring should not be the sole basis for adjusting Rapamune therapy. Careful attention should be made to clinical signs/symptoms, tissue biopsy, and laboratory parameters. Cyclosporine inhibits the metabolism and transport of sirolimus, and consequently, sirolimus concentrations will decrease when cyclosporine is discontinued unless the Rapamune dose is increased. The Rapamune® dose will need to be approximately 4-fold higher to account for both the absence of the pharmacokinetic interaction (approximately 2-fold increase) and the augmented immunosuppressive requirement in the absence of cyclosporine (approximately 2-fold increase).

Frequent Rapamune® dose adjustments based on non-steady-state sirolimus concentrations can lead to overdosing or underdosing because sirolimus has a long half-life. Once Rapamune® maintenance dose is adjusted, patients should be retained on the new maintenance dose at least for 7 to 14 days before further dosage adjustment with concentration monitoring. In most patients dose adjustments can be based on simple proportion: new Rapamune® dose = current dose x (target concentration/current concentration). A loading dose should be considered in addition to a new maintenance dose when it is necessary to considerably increase sirolimus trough concentrations: Rapamune® loading dose = 3 × (new maintenance dose - current maintenance dose). The maximum Rapamune® dose administered on any day should not exceed 40 mg. If an estimated daily dose exceeds 40 mg due to the addition of a loading dose, the loading dose should be administered over 2 days. Sirolimus trough concentrations should be monitored at least 3 to 4 days after a loading dose(s).

To minimize the variability of exposure to Rapamune, this drug should be taken consistently with or without food. Grapefruit juice reduces CYP3A4-mediated drug metabolism and potentially enhances P-gp mediated drug countertransport from enterocytes of the small intestine. This juice must not be administered with Rapamune or used for dilution.

It is recommended that sirolimus be taken 4 hours after administration of cyclosporine oral solution (MODIFIED) and/or cyclosporine capsules (MODIFIED).

Dosage Adjustments

The initial dosage in patients ≥13 years who weigh less than 40 kg should be adjusted, based on body surface area, to 1 mg/m^2/day. The loading dose should be 3 mg/m^2.

Patients with Hepatic Impairment:

It is recommended that the maintenance dose of Rapamune be reduced by approximately one third in patients with hepatic impairment.

Patients with Renal Impairment:

It is not necessary to modify the Rapamune loading dose. Dosage need not be adjusted because of impaired renal function.

Blood Concentration Monitoring

Whole blood trough concentrations of sirolimus should be monitored in patients receiving concentration-controlled Rapamune®. Monitoring is also necessary in pediatric patients, in patients with hepatic impairment, during concurrent administration of CYP3A4 and/or P-gp inducers and inhibitors, and/or if cyclosporine dosage is markedly changed or discontinued (see **DOSAGE AND ADMINISTRATION**).

In controlled clinical trials with concomitant cyclosporine (Studies 1 and 2), mean sirolimus whole blood trough concentrations through month 12 following transplantation, as measured by immunoassay, were 9 ng/mL (range 4.5-14 ng/mL [10th to 90th percentile]) for the 2 mg/day treatment group, and 17 ng/mL (range 10-28 ng/mL [10th to 90th percentile]) for the 5 mg/day dose.

In a controlled clinical trial with cyclosporine withdrawal (Study 4), the mean sirolimus whole blood trough concentrations during months 4 through 12 following transplantation, as measured by immunoassay, were 10.7 ng/mL (range 6.3-16.0 ng/mL [10th to 90th percentile]) in the concomitant Rapamune and cyclosporine treatment group (n = 205) and were 23.3 ng/mL (range 17.0-29.0 ng/mL [10th to 90th percentile]) in the cyclosporine withdrawal treatment group (n = 200).

Results from other assays may differ from those with an immunoassay. On average, chromatographic methods (HPLC UV or LC/MS/MS) yield results that are approximately 20% lower than the immunoassay for whole blood concentration determinations. Adjustments to the targeted range should be made according to the assay utilized to determine sirolimus trough concentrations. Therefore, comparison between concentrations in the published literature and an individual patient concentration using current assays must be made with detailed knowledge of the assay methods employed. A discussion of the different assay methods is contained in *Clinical Therapeutics*, Volume 22, Supplement B, April 2000.

Instructions for Dilution and Administration of Rapamune® Oral Solution Bottles

The amber oral dose syringe should be used to withdraw the prescribed amount of Rapamune® Oral Solution from the bottle. Empty the correct amount of Rapamune from the syringe into only a glass or plastic container holding at least two (2) ounces (1/4 cup, 60 mL) of water or orange juice. No other liquids, including grapefruit juice, should be used for dilution. Stir vigorously and drink at once. Refill the container with an additional volume (minimum of four [4] ounces [1/2 cup, 120 mL]) of water or orange juice, stir vigorously, and drink at once.

Rapamune Oral Solution contains polysorbate-80, which is known to increase the rate of di-(2-ethylhexyl)phthalate (DEHP) extraction from polyvinyl chloride (PVC). This should be considered during the preparation and administration of Rapamune Oral Solution. It is important that the recommendations in **DOSAGE AND ADMINISTRATION** be followed closely.

Handling and Disposal

Since Rapamune is not absorbed through the skin, there are no special precautions. However, if direct contact with the skin or mucous membranes occurs, wash thoroughly with soap and water; rinse eyes with plain water.

HOW SUPPLIED

Rapamune® Oral Solution is supplied at a concentration of 1 mg/mL in:

Cartons:

NDC # 0008-1030-06 containing a 2 oz (60 mL fill) amber glass bottle.

In addition to the bottles, each carton is supplied with an oral syringe adapter for fitting into the neck of the bottle, sufficient disposable amber oral syringes and caps for daily dosing, and a carrying case.

Rapamune® Tablets are available as follows:

1 mg, white, triangular-shaped tablets marked "RAPAMUNE 1 mg" on one side.

NDC # 0008-1031-05, bottle of 100 tablets.

NDC # 0008-1031-10, Redipak® cartons of 100 tablets (10 blister cards of 10 tablets each).

2 mg, yellow to beige triangular-shaped tablets marked "RAPAMUNE 2 mg" on one side.

NDC # 0008-1032-05, bottle of 100 tablets.

NDC # 0008-1032-10, Redipak® cartons of 100 tablets (10 blister cards of 10 tablets each [2 x 5]).

Storage

Rapamune® Oral Solution bottles should be stored protected from light and refrigerated at 2°C to 8°C (36°F to 46°F). Once the bottle is opened, the contents should be used within one month. If necessary, the patient may store the bottles at room temperatures up to 25°C (77°F) for a short period of time (e.g., not more than 15 days for the bottles).

An amber syringe and cap are provided for dosing and the product may be kept in the syringe for a maximum of 24 hours at room temperatures up to 25°C (77°F) or refrigerated at 2°C to 8°C (36°F to 46°F). The syringe should be discarded after one use. After dilution, the preparation should be used immediately.

Rapamune Oral Solution provided in bottles may develop a slight haze when refrigerated. If such a haze occurs allow the product to stand at room temperature and shake gently until the haze disappears. The presence of this haze does not affect the quality of the product.

Rapamune® Tablets should be stored at 20° to 25°C (USP Controlled Room Temperature) (68° to 77°F). Use cartons to protect blister cards and strips from light. Dispense in a tight, light-resistant container as defined in the USP.

US Pat. Nos.: 5,100,899; 5,212,155; 5,308,847; 5,403,833; 5,536,729.

PATIENT INSTRUCTIONS FOR RAPAMUNE® (SIROLIMUS) ORAL SOLUTION

Bottles

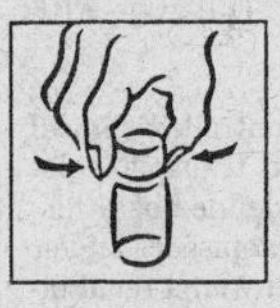

1. Open the solution bottle. Remove the safety cap by squeezing the tabs on the cap and twisting counter-clockwise.

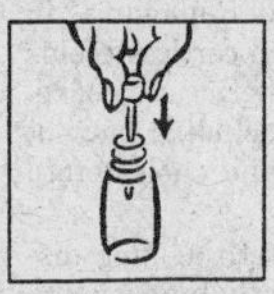

2. On first use, insert the adapter assembly (plastic tube with stopper) tightly into the bottle until it is even with the top of the bottle. Do not remove the adapter assembly from the bottle once inserted.

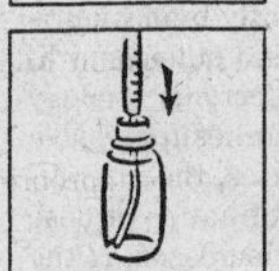

3. For each use, tightly insert one of the amber syringes with the plunger fully depressed into the opening in the adapter.

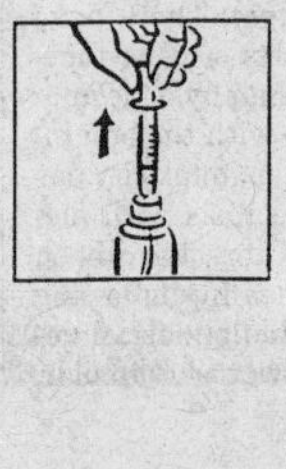

4. Withdraw the prescribed amount of Rapamune® Oral Solution by gently pulling out the plunger of the syringe until the bottom of the black line of the plunger is even with the appropriate mark on the syringe. Always keep the bottle in an upright position. If bubbles form in the syringe, empty the syringe into the bottle and repeat the procedure.

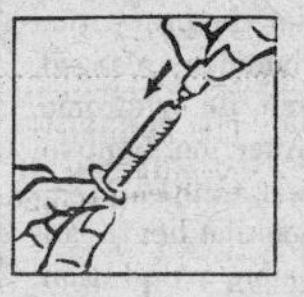

5. You may have been instructed to carry your medication with you. If it is necessary to carry the filled syringe, place a cap securely on the syringe – the cap should snap into place.

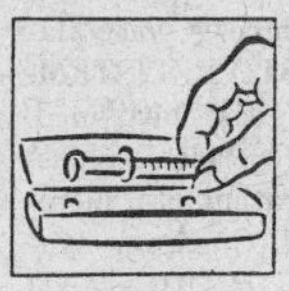

6. Then place the capped syringe in the enclosed carrying case. Once in the syringe, the medication may be kept at room temperature or refrigerated and should be used within 24 hours. Extreme temperatures (below 36°F and above 86°F) should be avoided. Remember to keep this medication out of the reach of children.

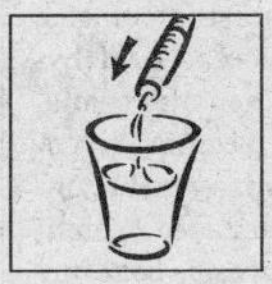

7. Empty the syringe into a glass or plastic cup containing at least 2 ounces (1/4 cup, 60 mL) of water or orange juice, stir vigorously for one (1) minute and drink immediately. Refill the container with at least 4 ounces (1/2 cup, 120 mL) of water or orange juice, stir vigorously again and drink the rinse solution. Apple juice, grapefruit juice, or other liquids are NOT to be used. Only glass or plastic cups should be used to dilute Rapamune® Oral Solution. The syringe and cap should be used once and then discarded.

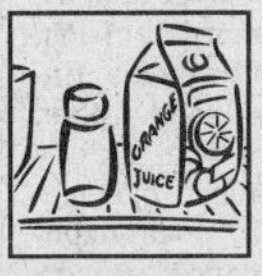

8. Always store the bottles of medication in the refrigerator. When refrigerated, a slight haze may develop in the solution. The presence of a haze does not affect the quality of the product. If this happens, bring the Rapamune® Oral Solution to room temperature and shake until the haze disappears. If it is necessary to wipe clean the mouth of the bottle before returning the product to the refrigerator, wipe with a dry cloth to avoid introducing water, or any other liquid, into the bottle.

Wyeth®
Wyeth Pharmaceuticals Inc. W10431C010
Philadelphia, PA 19101 ET01
Rev 03/05

REFACTO® ℞

[rē-făk'tō]

Antihemophilic Factor, Recombinant

℞ only

Prescribing information for this product, which appears on pages 3402–3404 of the 2005 PDR, has been completely revised as follows. Please write "See Supplement A" next to the product heading.

This product's label may have been revised after this insert was used in production. For further product information and current package insert, please visit www.wyeth.com or call our medical communications department toll-free at 1-800-934-5556.

DESCRIPTION

ReFacto® Antihemophilic Factor (Recombinant) is a purified protein produced by recombinant DNA technology for use in therapy of factor VIII deficiency. ReFacto is a glycoprotein with an approximate molecular mass of 170 kDa consisting of 1438 amino acids. It has an amino acid sequence that is comparable to the 90 + 80 kDa form of factor VIII, and post-translational modifications that are similar to those of the plasma-derived molecule. ReFacto has *in vitro* functional characteristics comparable to those of endogenous factor VIII.

ReFacto is produced by a genetically engineered Chinese hamster ovary (CHO) cell line. The CHO cell line secretes B-domain deleted recombinant factor VIII into a defined cell culture medium that contains human serum albumin and recombinant insulin, but does not contain any proteins derived from animal sources. The protein is purified by a chromatography purification process that yields a high-purity, active product. The potency expressed in international units (IU) is determined using the European Pharmacopoeial chromogenic assay against the WHO standard. The specific activity of ReFacto is 9110-13700 IU per milligram of protein. ReFacto is not purified from human blood and contains no preservatives or added human components in the final formulation.

ReFacto is formulated as a sterile, nonpyrogenic, lyophilized powder preparation for intravenous (IV) injection. It is available in single-use vials containing the labeled amount of factor VIII activity (IU). Each vial contains nominally 250, 500, 1000 or 2000 IU of ReFacto per vial. The formulated product is a clear colorless solution upon reconstitution and contains sodium chloride, sucrose, L-histidine, calcium chloride, and polysorbate 80.

CLINICAL PHARMACOLOGY

Factor VIII is the specific clotting factor deficient in patients with hemophilia A (classical hemophilia). The administration of ReFacto® Antihemophilic Factor (Recombinant) increases plasma levels of factor VIII activity and can temporarily correct the *in vitro* coagulation defect in these patients.

Activated factor VIII acts as a cofactor for activated factor IX accelerating the conversion of factor X to activated factor X. Activated factor X converts prothrombin into thrombin. Thrombin then converts fibrinogen into fibrin and a clot is formed. Factor VIII activity is greatly reduced in patients with hemophilia A and therefore replacement therapy is necessary.

In a crossover pharmacokinetic study of eighteen (18) previously treated patients **using the chromogenic assay,** the circulating mean half-life for ReFacto was 14.5 ± 5.3 hours (ranged from 7.6-27.7 hours), which was not statistically significantly different from plasma-derived Antihemophilic Factor (Human) (pdAHF), which had a mean half-life of 13.7 ± 3.4 hours (ranged from 8.8-23.7 hours). Mean incremental recovery (K-value) of ReFacto in plasma was 2.4 ± 0.4 IU/dL per IU/kg (ranged from 1.9-3.3 IU/dL per IU/kg). This was comparable to the mean incremental recovery observed in plasma for pdAHF which was 2.3 ± 0.3 IU/dL per IU/kg (ranged from 1.7-2.9 IU/dL per IU/kg). **Results obtained from this controlled pharmacokinetic study, which used a central laboratory for the analysis of all plasma samples, showed that the one-stage factor VIII clotting assay gave results which were approximately 50% of the values obtained with the chromogenic assay** (see **DOSAGE AND ADMINISTRATION**).

In two additional clinical studies, pharmacokinetic parameters were evaluated for previously treated patients [PTPs] and previously untreated patients [PUPs]. In PTPs (n=87) ReFacto had a mean incremental recovery of 2.4 ± 0.4 IU/dL per IU/kg (ranged from 1.1-3.8 IU/dL per IU/kg) and an elimination half-life (n=67) of 10.7 ± 2.8 hours. In PUPs (n=45) ReFacto had a lower mean incremental recovery of 1.7 ± 0.4 IU/dL per IU/kg (ranged from 0.2-2.8 IU/dL per IU/kg) as compared to PTPs. Population pharmacokinetic modeling using data from 44 PUPs led to a mean estimated half-life of ReFacto in PUPs of 8.0 ± 2.2 hours. These parameters did not change over time (12 months) for PTPs or PUPs.

In clinical studies of ReFacto involving a total of 218 patients (117 PTPs including 4 who participated in the surgery study only, and 101 PUPs), more than 84 million IU were administered over a period of up to 54 months. The 117 PTPs were given a median of 230 injections (range of 4-1530 injections) over a median of 1200 days (range of 31-1640 days). The 101 PUPs were given a median of 26 injections (range of 1-490 injections) over a median of 830 days (range of 1-1298 days). One hundred thirteen PTPs and 99 PUPs were evaluated for efficacy in bleeding episodes. The 113 PTPs experienced a median of 54 bleeding episodes and the 99 PUPs experienced a median of 12 bleeding episodes. All were treated successfully on an on-demand basis or for the reduction of bleeding episodes except for one PTP and two PUPs who discontinued ReFacto treatment and switched to another product after the development of inhibitors. Bleeding episodes included hemarthroses, and bleeding in soft tissue, muscle, and other anatomical sites.

One of 113 previously treated patients (PTPs) who were evaluated for efficacy in bleeding episodes developed a high titer inhibitor. The patient was noted initially to have low titer inhibitor (1.2 BU) at a local laboratory at 98 exposure days and 2 BU at the central laboratory at 113 exposure days. **After 18 months on continued treatment with ReFacto, the inhibitor level rose to nearly 13 BU and a bleeding episode failed to respond to ReFacto treatment.** In this study the incidence of inhibitor development to factor VIII using ReFacto is similar to that reported for other factor VIII products[1-4].

ReFacto has been studied in short-term routine prophylaxis. In uncontrolled clinical trials, an average dose of 27 ± 10 IU/kg in PTPs (n=77) and an average dose of 57 ± 20 IU/kg in PUPs (n=17) was given repeatedly at variable intervals longer than 2 weeks. In 64 patients who had both on-demand and prophylactic periods during their time on study, the mean rate of spontaneous musculoskeletal bleeding episodes was less during periods of routine prophylaxis. There were an average of 10 bleeding episodes per year during the prophylactic periods compared to an average of 37 bleeding episodes per year during the on-demand periods. The clinical trial experience with routine prophylaxis in PUPs is limited (n=17). These non-randomized trial results should be interpreted with caution, as the investigators exercised their own discretion in deciding when and in whom prophylaxis was to be initiated and terminated.

Management of hemostasis was evaluated in the surgical setting where 28 surgical procedures have been performed in 25 patients. The average preoperative dose in PTPs was 59 IU/kg. Procedures included orthopedic procedures, inguinal hernia repair, epidural hematoma evacuation, transposition ulnar nerve, and other minor procedures (e.g., venous access catheter placement and explantation, toenail removal). Circulatory factor VIII levels targeted to restore and maintain hemostasis were achieved. While the one-stage clotting assay was used most frequently in the surgical setting (24 versus 4 surgeries), hemostasis was maintained throughout the surgical period regardless of which assay was used. Hemostatic efficacy was rated as excellent or good in all procedures.

The occurrence of neutralizing antibody (inhibitors) is well known in the treatment of patients with hemophilia A[5,6,7]. Thirty-two out of 101 PUPs (32%) developed an inhibitor: 16 out of 101 (16%) with a high titer (> 5 BU) (12 of the 16 patients had peak values ≥ 10 BU) and 16 out of 101 (16%) with a low titer (≤ 5 BU). In this study the incidence of inhibitor development to factor VIII using ReFacto is similar to that reported for other factor VIII products[5-10].

INDICATIONS AND USAGE

ReFacto® Antihemophilic Factor (Recombinant) is indicated for the control and prevention of hemorrhagic episodes and for surgical prophylaxis in patients with hemophilia A (congenital factor VIII deficiency or classic hemophilia).

ReFacto is indicated for short-term routine prophylaxis to reduce the frequency of spontaneous bleeding episodes. The effect of regular routine prophylaxis on long-term morbidity and mortality is unknown.

ReFacto can be of a significant therapeutic value for treatment of hemophilia A in certain patients with inhibitors to factor VIII[11]. In clinical studies of ReFacto, patients who developed inhibitors on study continued to manifest a clinical response when inhibitor titers were < 10 BU. When an inhibitor is present, the dosage requirement of factor VIII is variable. The dosage can be determined only by a clinical response and by monitoring of circulating factor VIII levels after treatment (see **DOSAGE AND ADMINISTRATION**).

ReFacto does not contain von Willebrand factor and therefore is not indicated in von Willebrand's disease.

CONTRAINDICATIONS

Known hypersensitivity to mouse, hamster, or bovine proteins may be a contraindication to the use of ReFacto® Antihemophilic Factor (Recombinant).

WARNINGS

As with any intravenous protein product, allergic type hypersensitivity reactions are possible. Patients should be informed of the early signs of hypersensitivity reactions including hives, generalized urticaria, tightness of the chest, wheezing, hypotension, and anaphylaxis. Patients should be advised to discontinue use of the product and contact their physicians if these symptoms occur.

PRECAUTIONS

General

Activity-neutralizing antibodies (inhibitors) have been detected in patients receiving factor VIII-containing products. Low titer inhibitors are common in previously untreated patients and in previously treated patients on factor VIII products, as are high titer inhibitors in previously untreated patients. High titer inhibitors, which are generally rare in previously treated patients, have been reported in previously treated patients on ReFacto. As with all coagulation factor VIII products, patients should be monitored for the development of inhibitors that should be titrated in Bethesda Units using appropriate biological testing.

Reports of lack of effect, mainly in prophylaxis patients, have been received in the clinical trials and in the post-marketing setting. The reported lack of effect has been described as bleeding into target joints, bleeding into new joints or a subjective feeling by the patient of new onset bleeding. When switching to ReFacto it is important to individually titrate and monitor each patient's dose in order to ensure an adequate therapeutic response (see **DOSAGE AND ADMINISTRATION**).

Formation of Antibodies to Mouse and Hamster Protein

As Antihemophilic Factor (Recombinant), ReFacto contains trace amounts of mouse protein (maximum of 5 ng/1000 IU) and hamster protein (maximum of 30 ng/1000 IU), the remote possibility exists that patients treated with this product may develop hypersensitivity to these non-human mammalian proteins.

Carcinogenicity, Mutagenicity, Impairment of Fertility

ReFacto® Antihemophilic Factor (Recombinant) has been shown to be nonmutagenic in the mouse micronucleus assay. No other mutagenicity studies and no investigations on carcinogenesis or impairment of fertility have been conducted.

Pregnancy Category C

Animal reproduction and lactation studies have not been conducted with ReFacto® Antihemophilic Factor (Recombinant). It is not known whether ReFacto can affect reproductive capacity or cause fetal harm when given to pregnant women. ReFacto should be administered to pregnant and lactating women only if clearly indicated.

Pediatric Use

ReFacto® Antihemophilic Factor (Recombinant) is appropriate for use in children of all ages, including newborns. Safety and efficacy studies have been performed both in previously treated children and adolescents (N=22, ages 8-15 years) and in previously untreated neonates, infants, and children (N=101, ages 0-52 months) (see **CLINICAL PHARMACOLOGY** and **PRECAUTIONS**).

Geriatric Use

Clinical studies of ReFacto did not include sufficient numbers of subjects aged 65 and over to determine whether they respond differently from younger subjects. Other reported clinical experience has not identified differences in responses between the elderly and younger patients. As with any patient receiving ReFacto, dose selection for an elderly patient should be individualized.

ADVERSE REACTIONS

As with the intravenous administration of any protein product, the following reactions may be observed after administration: headache, fever, chills, flushing, nausea, vomiting, lethargy, or manifestations of allergic reactions. During clinical studies with ReFacto® Antihemophilic Factor (Recombinant), 77 adverse reactions in 43 of 218 patients (20%) probably or possibly-related to therapy were reported for 64,363 infusions (0.12%). These were anaphylaxis (1), dyspnea (6), urticaria (1), nausea (11), headache (4), vasodilation (5), dizziness (4), permanent venous access catheter complications (3), asthenia (3), fever (3), taste perversion [altered taste] (3), bleeding/hematoma (3), infected hematoma (1), anorexia (2), diarrhea (2), injection site reaction (2), somnolence (2), rash (2), pruritus (2), angina pectoris (1), tachycardia (1), perspiration increased (1), chills (1), increased amino transferase (1), increased bilirubin (1), pain in finger (1), muscle weakness (1), CPK increase (1), cold sensation (1), eye disorder-vision abnormal (1), coughing (1), myalgia (1), gastroenteritis (1), abdominal pain (1), acne (1), and forehead bruises (1). If any adverse reaction takes place that is thought to be related to administration of ReFacto, the rate of infusion should be decreased or stopped.

Inhibitor development is a known adverse event associated with the treatment of patients with hemophilia A. In addition to the one report of high titer inhibitors in the clinical study of PTPs (see **CLINICAL PHARMACOLOGY**), there have been reports of high titer inhibitors in PTPs in the post-marketing setting. High and low titer inhibitors have been reported in PUPs in both clinical trials and the post-marketing setting (see **PRECAUTIONS, General**).

A total of 182 adverse reactions in 54 of 218 patients (25%) who received 32,013 infusions (0.6%) were reported by the investigator to have an "unlikely" or "not assessable" relationship to ReFacto administration. The study sponsor considered that the events may be of possible or of unknown relationship to therapy because of the temporal relationship to the infusion and/or the frequency of the event for a given patient and/or because insufficient information was available to assign another causality. In this category, 25 patients experienced the following 38 events which are different from the events described above: pain (10), rhinitis (10), vomiting (4), insomnia (3), constipation (2), pharyngitis (2), flushing (1), palpitation (1), sinusitis (1), gastritis (1), dyspepsia (1), hypotension (1), and URI (1).

Other adverse experiences that were reported during the clinical trials, but which were assessed by both the investigator and the sponsor as "unlikely" to be related to ReFacto administration included: dyspnea (3), rash (2), pruritus (1), neuropathy (1), arm weakness (1), and thrombophlebitis of upper arm (1).

DOSAGE AND ADMINISTRATION

Treatment with ReFacto® Antihemophilic Factor (Recombinant) should be initiated under the supervision of a physician experienced in the treatment of hemophilia A.

The labeled potency of ReFacto is based on the European Pharmacopoeial chromogenic substrate assay, whereas other factor VIII products are labeled based on the one-stage clotting assay. With recombinant factor VIII products, the chromogenic assay typically yields results which are higher than the results obtained with the one-stage clotting assay. When switching between products it is important to individually titrate each patient's dose in order to ensure an adequate therapeutic response (see **PRECAUTIONS, General**). Results obtained from a controlled pharmacokinetic study, which used one central laboratory for the analysis of all plasma samples, showed that the one-stage factor VIII clotting assay gave results that were approximately 50% of those obtained with the chromogenic substrate assay (see **CLINICAL PHARMACOLOGY**). In addition, in clinical trials of ReFacto use in the surgical setting in which multiple laboratories were used for plasma sample analysis, the ratio of factor VIII activity results obtained by the one-stage clotting and chromogenic substrate assays ranged between 20 and 80%.

When monitoring patients' factor VIII activity levels during treatment, the available clinical data suggest that either assay may be used. Most patients in clinical trials were monitored with the one-stage clotting assay (see **CLINICAL PHARMACOLOGY**). It is necessary to adhere to the incubation/activation times and other test conditions as specified by the assay manufacturers.

Dosage and duration of treatment depend on the severity of the factor VIII deficiency, the location and extent of bleeding, and the patient's clinical condition. Doses administered should be titrated to the patient's clinical response. In the presence of an inhibitor, higher doses may be required.

Precise monitoring of the replacement therapy by means of coagulation analysis (plasma factor VIII activity) is recommended, particularly for surgical intervention.

One international unit (IU) of factor VIII activity corresponds approximately to the quantity of factor VIII in one mL of normal human plasma. The calculation of the required dosage of factor VIII is based upon the empirical finding that, on average, 1 IU of factor VIII per kg body weight raises the plasma factor VIII activity by approximately 2 IU/dL per IU/kg administered. The required dosage is determined using the following formula:

Required units = body weight (kg)
× desired factor VIII rise (IU/dL or % of normal)
× 0.5 (IU/kg per IU/dL)

Continued on next page

Type of Hemorrhage	Factor VIII Level Required (IU/dL or % of normal)	Frequency of Doses (h)/ Duration of Therapy (d)
Minor Early hemarthrosis, minor muscle or oral bleeds.	20–40	Repeat every 12 to 24 hours as necessary until resolved. At least 1 day, depending upon the severity of the hemorrhage.
Moderate Hemorrhages into muscles. Mild trauma capitis. Minor operations including tooth extraction. Hemorrhages into the oral cavity.	30–60	Repeat infusion every 12–24 hours for 3–4 days or until adequate local hemostasis is achieved. For tooth extraction a single infusion plus oral antifibrinolytic therapy within 1 hour may be sufficient.
Major Gastrointestinal bleeding. Intracranial, intra-abdominal or intrathoracic hemorrhages. Fractures. Major operations.	60–100	Repeat infusion every 8–24 hours until threat is resolved or in the case of surgery, until adequate local hemostasis is achieved.

Refacto—Cont.

The following chart can be used to guide dosing in bleeding episodes and surgery:
[See table above]
For short-term routine prophylaxis to prevent or reduce the frequency of spontaneous musculoskeletal hemorrhage in patients with hemophilia A, ReFacto should be given at least twice a week. In some cases, especially pediatric patients, shorter dosage intervals or higher doses may be necessary. Pharmacokinetic/pharmacodynamic modeling, based on pharmacokinetic data from 185 infusions in 102 PTPs, predicts that routine prophylactic dosing 3 times per week may be associated with a lower bleeding risk than with dosing twice weekly. No randomized comparison of different doses or frequency regimens of ReFacto for routine prophylaxis has been performed. In clinical studies in PTPs (ages 8-73 years) and PUPs (ages 9-52 months), the mean dose used for routine prophylaxis was 27 ± 10 IU/kg and 57 ± 20 IU/kg, respectively.
Patients using ReFacto should be monitored for the development of factor VIII inhibitors. If expected factor VIII activity plasma levels are not attained, or if bleeding is not controlled with an appropriate dose, an assay should be performed to determine if a factor VIII inhibitor is present. If the inhibitor is present at levels less than 5 Bethesda Units, administration of additional antihemophilic factor may neutralize the inhibitor.
ReFacto is administered by IV infusion after reconstitution of the lyophilized powder with Sodium Chloride Diluent (provided).
ReFacto, when reconstituted, contains polysorbate-80, which is known to increase the rate of di-(2-ethylhexyl) phthalate (DEHP) extraction from polyvinyl chloride (PVC). This should be considered during the preparation and administration of ReFacto, including storage time elapsed in a PVC container following reconstitution. It is important that the recommendations in **DOSAGE AND ADMINISTRATION** be followed closely.

INSTRUCTIONS FOR USE

Patients should follow the specific reconstitution and administration procedures provided by their physicians. The procedures below are provided as general guidelines for the reconstitution and administration of ReFacto.

Reconstitution
Always wash your hands before performing the following procedures. Aseptic technique (meaning clean and germ free) should be used during the reconstitution procedure. All components used in the reconstitution and administration of this product should be used as soon as possible after opening their sterile containers to minimize unnecessary exposure to the atmosphere.
ReFacto® Antihemophilic Factor (Recombinant) is administered by intravenous (IV) infusion after reconstitution with the supplied diluent (0.9% Sodium Chloride Diluent, 4 mL disposable syringe for drug diluent use with ReFacto Antihemophilic Factor [Recombinant]) syringe.
1. Allow the vials of lyophilized ReFacto and the pre-filled diluent syringe to reach room temperature.
2. Remove the plastic flip-top cap from the ReFacto vial to expose the central portions of the rubber stopper.

3. Wipe the top of the vial with the alcohol swab provided, or use another antiseptic solution, and allow to dry. After cleaning, do not touch the rubber stopper with your hand or allow it to touch any surface.
4. Peel back the cover from the clear plastic vial adapter package. **Do not remove the adapter from the package.**
5. While holding the adapter package, place the vial adapter over the vial and press down firmly on the pack-

age until the adapter spike penetrates the vial stopper. Leave the adapter package in place.

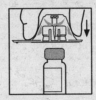

6. Grasp the plunger rod per the diagram. Avoid contact with the shaft of the plunger rod. Attach the threaded end of the plunger rod to the diluent syringe plunger by pushing and turning firmly.

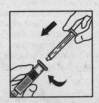

7. Remove the tamper-resistant plastic tip cap from the diluent syringe by bending down and up to break the perforation. Do not touch the inside of the cap or the syringe tip. Place the cap on its side on a clean surface in a spot where it would be least likely to become environmentally contaminated.

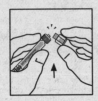

8. Lift the package away from the adapter and discard.

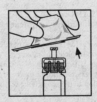

9. Connect the diluent syringe to the vial adapter by inserting the tip into the adapter opening while firmly pushing and turning the syringe clockwise until secured.

10. Inject all the diluent into the ReFacto vial.

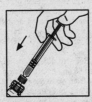

11. Without removing the syringe, **gently** swirl the contents of the vial until the powder is dissolved.

12. Inspect the final solution for specks before administration. The solution should appear clear and colorless.
    Note: If you use more than one vial of ReFacto per infusion, reconstitute each vial as per the previous instructions.
13. Invert the vial and draw the solution into the syringe.
    Note: If you prepared more than one vial of ReFacto, remove the diluent syringe from the vial adapter, leaving the vial adapter attached to the vial. Quickly attach a separate large luer lock syringe and draw back the reconstituted contents as instructed above. Repeat this procedure with each vial in turn. Do not detach the diluent syringes or the large luer lock syringe until you are ready to attach the large luer lock syringe to the next vial adapter.

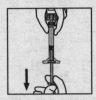

14. Detach the syringe from the vial adapter by gently pulling and turning the syringe counter-clockwise. Discard the vial with the adapter attached.
    Note: If the solution is not to be used immediately, the syringe cap should be carefully replaced. Do not touch the syringe tip or the inside of the cap.
ReFacto should be administered within 3 hours after reconstitution. The reconstituted solution may be stored at room temperature prior to administration.

Administration (Intravenous Injection)
ReFacto® Antihemophilic Factor (Recombinant) should be administered using the tubing provided in this kit, and the pre-filled diluent syringe provided or a single sterile disposable plastic syringe. In addition, the solution should be withdrawn from the vial using the vial adapter.
1. Attach the syringe to the luer end of the infusion set tubing provided and perform venipuncture as instructed by your physician.
After reconstitution, ReFacto should be injected intravenously over several minutes. The rate of administration should be determined by the patient's comfort level.
Following completion of ReFacto treatment, remove the infusion set and discard. The amount of drug product remaining in the infusion set is not clinically significant.
Dispose of all unused solution, the empty vial(s), and the used needles and syringes in an appropriate container for throwing away waste that might hurt others if not handled properly.

Storage
Product as packaged for sale: ReFacto® Antihemophilic Factor (Recombinant) should be stored under refrigeration at a temperature of 2° to 8°C (36° to 46°F). ReFacto may also be stored at room temperature not to exceed 25°C (77°F) for up to 3 months, until the expiration date. The patient should write in the space provided on the outer carton the date the product was placed at room temperature. At the end of the 3-month period, the product should not be put back into the refrigerator, but should be used immediately or discarded. Freezing should be avoided to prevent damage to the pre-filled diluent syringe. During storage, avoid prolonged exposure of ReFacto® vial to light. Do not use ReFacto after the expiry date on the label.
Product after reconstitution: The product does not contain a preservative and should be used within 3 hours.

HOW SUPPLIED
ReFacto® Antihemophilic Factor (Recombinant) is supplied in single-use (4mL size, dried) vials which contain nominally 250, 500, 1000 or 2000 IU per vial (NDC 58394-007-02, 58394-006-02, 58394-005-02, 58394-011-02, respectively) with one pre-filled syringe (0.9% Sodium Chloride Diluent, 4 mL disposable syringe for drug diluent use with ReFacto Antihemophilic Factor [Recombinant]) for reconstitution, one vial adapter, one sterile infusion set, and two (2) alcohol swabs. Actual factor VIII activity in IU is stated on the label of each vial.

REFERENCES
1. Kessler C, Sachse K. Factor VIII:C inhibitor associated with monoclonal-antibody purified FVIII concentrate. Lancet 1990; 335:1403.
2. Schwartz RS, Abildgaard CF, Aledort LM, et al. Human recombinant DNA-derived antihemophilic factor (factor VIII) in the treatment of hemophilia A. N Engl J Med 1990;323:1800–1805.
3. White GC II, Courter S, Bray GL, et al. A multicenter study of recombinant factor VIII (recombinate) in previously treated patients with hemophilia A. Thromb Haemost 1997;77(4):660–667.
4. Abshire TC, Brackmann HH, Scharrer I, et al. Sucrose formulated recombinant human antihemophilic Factor VIII is safe and efficacious for treatment of hemophilia A

in home therapy: Results of a multicenter, international, clinical investigation. Thromb Haemost 2000;83(6):811–816.

5. Ehrenforth S, Kreuz W, Scharrer I, et al. Incidence of development of factor VIII and factor IX inhibitors in hemophiliacs. Lancet. 1992;339:594-598.

6. Bray GL, Gomperts ED, Courter S, et al. A multicenter study of recombinant factor VIII (Recombinate): safety, efficacy, and inhibitor risk in previously untreated patients with hemophilia A. Blood. 1994;83(9):2428-2435.

7. Lusher J, Arkin S, Abildgaard CF, Schwartz RS, Group TKPUPS. Recombinant factor VIII for the treatment of previously untreated patients with hemophilia A. N Engl J Med. 1993;328:453-459.

8. Scharrer I, Bray G. Incidence of inhibitors in haemophilia A patients - a review of recent studies of recombinant and plasma-derived factor VIII concentrates. Hemophilia 1999;5:145.

9. Gruppo R, Chen H, Schroth P, et al. Safety and immunogenicity of recombinant factor VIII (Recombinate) in previously untreated patients: A 7.3 year update. Haemophilia 1998;4:228 (abstract no. 291, XXIII Congress of the WFH, The Hague).

10. Lusher J, Abildgaard C, Arkin S, et al. Human recombinant DNA-derived antihemophilic factor in the treatment of previously untreated patients with hemophilia A: Final report on a hallmark clinical investigation. J Thromb Haemost 2004;2:574-83.

11. Kessler CM. An Introduction to Factor VIII Inhibitors: The Detection and Quantitation. American Journal of Medicine 91 1991, (Supplement 5A): 1S-5S.

Wyeth®
Wyeth Pharmaceuticals Inc.
Philadelphia, PA 19101
US Govt. License No. 3
Telephone: 1-800-934-5556

W10403C008
ET01
Rev 02/05

MedWatch

The FDA Safety Information and Adverse Event Reporting Program

For VOLUNTARY reporting of adverse events and product problems

Form Approved: OMB No. 0910-0291, Expires: 03/31/05
See OMB statement on reverse.

Page _____ of _____

FDA USE ONLY
Triage unit sequence #

A. PATIENT INFORMATION

1. Patient Identifier	2. Age at Time of Event:	3. Sex	4. Weight
In confidence	or _____ Date of Birth:	☐ Female ☐ Male	_____ lbs or _____ kgs

B. ADVERSE EVENT OR PRODUCT PROBLEM

1. ☐ **Adverse Event** and/or ☐ **Product Problem** (e.g., defects/malfunctions)

2. Outcomes Attributed to Adverse Event (Check all that apply)

☐ Death: _____ (mo/day/yr)
☐ Life-threatening
☐ Hospitalization - initial or prolonged

☐ Disability
☐ Congenital Anomaly
☐ Required Intervention to Prevent Permanent Impairment/Damage
☐ Other: _____

3. Date of Event (mo/day/year)

4. Date of This Report (mo/day/year)

5. Describe Event or Problem

6. Relevant Tests/Laboratory Data, Including Dates

7. Other Relevant History, Including Preexisting Medical Conditions (e.g., allergies, race, pregnancy, smoking and alcohol use, hepatic/renal dysfunction, etc.)

PLEASE TYPE OR USE BLACK INK

C. SUSPECT MEDICATION(S)

1. Name (Give labeled strength & mfr/labeler, if known)

#1

#2

2. Dose, Frequency & Route Used

#1

#2

3. Therapy Dates (If unknown, give duration) from/to (or best estimate)

#1

#2

4. Diagnosis for Use (Indication)

#1

#2

5. Event Abated After Use Stopped or Dose Reduced?

#1 ☐ Yes ☐ No ☐ Doesn't Apply
#2 ☐ Yes ☐ No ☐ Doesn't Apply

6. Lot # (if known)

#1

#2

7. Exp. Date (if known)

#1

#2

8. Event Reappeared After Reintroduction?

#1 ☐ Yes ☐ No ☐ Doesn't Apply
#2 ☐ Yes ☐ No ☐ Doesn't Apply

9. NDC# (For product problems only)

_ - _ - _

10. Concomitant Medical Products and Therapy Dates (Exclude treatment of event)

D. SUSPECT MEDICAL DEVICE

1. Brand Name

2. Type of Device

3. Manufacturer Name, City and State

4. Model #	Lot #	5. Operator of Device
Catalog #	Expiration Date (mo/day/yr)	☐ Health Professional ☐ Lay User/Patient
Serial #	Other #	☐ Other: _____

6. If Implanted, Give Date (mo/day/yr)

7. If Explanted, Give Date (mo/day/yr)

8. Is this a Single-use Device that was Reprocessed and Reused on a Patient?
☐ Yes ☐ No

9. If Yes to Item No. 8, Enter Name and Address of Reprocessor

10. Device Available for Evaluation? (Do not send to FDA)
☐ Yes ☐ No ☐ Returned to Manufacturer on: _____ (mo/day/yr)

11. Concomitant Medical Products and Therapy Dates (Exclude treatment of event)

E. REPORTER (See confidentiality section on back)

1. Name and Address

Phone #

2. Health Professional?
☐ Yes ☐ No

3. Occupation

4. Also Reported to:
☐ Manufacturer
☐ User Facility
☐ Distributor/Importer

5. If you do NOT want your identity disclosed to the manufacturer, place an "X" in this box: ☐

FDA

Mail to: **MedWatch**
5600 Fishers Lane
Rockville, MD 20852-9787

-or-

FAX to:
1-800-FDA-0178

FORM FDA 3500 (12/03) Submission of a report does not constitute an admission that medical personnel or the product caused or contributed to the event.

ADVICE ABOUT VOLUNTARY REPORTING

Report adverse experiences with:

- Medications *(drugs or biologics)*
- Medical devices *(including in-vitro diagnostics)*
- Special nutritional products *(dietary supplements, medical foods, infant formulas)*
- Cosmetics
- Medication errors

Report product problems - quality, performance or safety concerns such as:

- Suspected counterfeit product
- Suspected contamination
- Questionable stability
- Defective components
- Poor packaging or labeling
- Therapeutic failures

Report SERIOUS adverse events. An event is serious when the patient outcome is:

- Death
- Life-threatening *(real risk of dying)*
- Hospitalization *(initial or prolonged)*
- Disability *(significant, persistent or permanent)*
- Congenital anomaly
- Required intervention to prevent permanent impairment or damage

Report even if:

- You're not certain the product caused the event
- You don't have all the details

How to report:

- Just fill in the sections that apply to your report
- Use section C for all products except medical devices
- Attach additional blank pages if needed
- Use a separate form for each patient
- Report either to FDA or the manufacturer *(or both)*

Confidentiality: The patient's identity is held in strict confidence by FDA and protected to the fullest extent of the law. FDA will not disclose the reporter's identity in response to a request from the public, pursuant to the Freedom of Information Act. The reporter's identity, including the identity of a self-reporter, may be shared with the manufacturer unless requested otherwise.

If your report involves a serious adverse event with a device and it occurred in a facility outside a doctor's office, that facility may be legally required to report to FDA and/or the manufacturer. Please notify the person in that facility who would handle such reporting.

Important numbers:

- 1-800-FDA-0178 -- To FAX report
- 1-800-FDA-1088 -- To report by phone or for more information
- 1-800-822-7967 -- For a VAERS form for vaccines

To Report via the Internet:

http://www.fda.gov/medwatch/report.htm

-Fold Here-

FORM FDA 3500 (12/03) (Back)   Please Use Address Provided Below -- Fold in Thirds, Tape and Mail

DEPARTMENT OF HEALTH & HUMAN SERVICES

Public Health Service
Food and Drug Administration
Rockville, MD 20857

Official Business
Penalty for Private Use $300

BUSINESS REPLY MAIL
FIRST CLASS MAIL   PERMIT NO. 946   ROCKVILLE MD

POSTAGE WILL BE PAID BY FOOD AND DRUG ADMINISTRATION

MEDWATCH
The FDA Safety Information and Adverse Event Reporting Program
Food and Drug Administration
5600 Fishers Lane
Rockville, MD 20852-9787

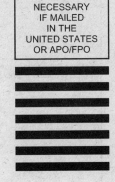

NO POSTAGE
NECESSARY
IF MAILED
IN THE
UNITED STATES
OR APO/FPO

VACCINE ADVERSE EVENT REPORTING SYSTEM
24 Hour Toll-Free Information 1-800-822-7967
P.O. Box 1100, Rockville, MD 20849-1100
PATIENT IDENTITY KEPT CONFIDENTIAL

VAERS

For CDC/FDA Use Only

VAERS Number _____

Date Received _____

Patient Name:	Vaccine administered by (Name):	Form completed by (Name):
_____ Last First M.I. Address _____ _____ _____ _____ City State Zip Telephone no. (___) _____	_____ Responsible Physician _____ Facility Name/Address _____ _____ _____ _____ City State Zip Telephone no. (___) _____	_____ Relation ☐ Vaccine Provider ☐ Patient/Parent to Patient ☐ Manufacturer ☐ Other Address *(if different from patient or provider)* _____ _____ _____ City State Zip Telephone no. (___) _____

1. State	2. County where administered	3. Date of birth __/__/__ mm dd yy	4. Patient age	5. Sex ☐ M ☐ F	6. Date form completed __/__/__ mm dd yy

7. Describe adverse events(s) (symptoms, signs, time course) and treatment, if any	8. Check all appropriate: ☐ Patient died (date __/__/__) mm dd yy ☐ Life threatening illness ☐ Required emergency room/doctor visit ☐ Required hospitalization (_____days) ☐ Resulted in prolongation of hospitalization ☐ Resulted in permanent disability ☐ None of the above

9. Patient recovered ☐ YES ☐ NO ☐ UNKNOWN	10. Date of vaccination	11. Adverse event onset
12. Relevant diagnostic tests/laboratory data	__/__/__ mm dd yy AM Time _____ PM	__/__/__ mm dd yy AM Time _____ PM

13. Enter all vaccines given on date listed in no. 10

	Vaccine (type)	Manufacturer	Lot number	Route/Site	No. Previous Doses
a.	_____	_____	_____	_____	_____
b.	_____	_____	_____	_____	_____
c.	_____	_____	_____	_____	_____
d.	_____	_____	_____	_____	_____

14. Any other vaccinations within 4 weeks prior to the date listed in no. 10

	Vaccine (type)	Manufacturer	Lot number	Route/Site	No. Previous doses	Date given
a.	_____	_____	_____	_____	_____	_____
b.	_____	_____	_____	_____	_____	_____

15. Vaccinated at: ☐ Private doctor's office/hospital ☐ Military clinic/hospital ☐ Public health clinic/hospital ☐ Other/unknown	16. Vaccine purchased with: ☐ Private funds ☐ Military funds ☐ Public funds ☐ Other/unknown	17. Other medications

18. Illness at time of vaccination (specify)	19. Pre-existing physician-diagnosed allergies, birth defects, medical conditions (specify)

20. Have you reported this adverse event previously?	☐ No ☐ To health department ☐ To doctor ☐ To manufacturer	***Only for children 5 and under***

22. Birth weight _____ lb. _____ oz.	23. No. of brothers and sisters

21. Adverse event following prior vaccination (check all applicable, specify)

	Adverse Event	Onset Age	Type Vaccine	Dose no. in series
☐ In patient	_____	_____	_____	_____
☐ In brother or sister	_____	_____	_____	_____

Only for reports submitted by manufacturer/immunization project

24. Mfr./imm. proj. report no.	25. Date received by mfr./imm.proj.
26. 15 day report? ☐ Yes ☐ No	27. Report type ☐ Initial ☐ Follow-Up

Health care providers and manufacturers are required by law (42 USC 300aa-25) to report reactions to vaccines listed in the Table of Reportable Events Following Immunization. Reports for reactions to other vaccines are voluntary except when required as a condition of immunization grant awards.

Form VAERS-1(FDA)

BUSINESS REPLY MAIL
FIRST-CLASS MAIL   PERMIT NO. 1895   ROCKVILLE, MD

POSTAGE WILL BE PAID BY ADDRESSEE

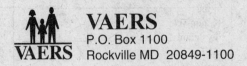

VAERS
P.O. Box 1100
Rockville MD 20849-1100

DIRECTIONS FOR COMPLETING FORM
(Additional pages may be attached if more space is needed.)

GENERAL

- Use a separate form for each patient. Complete the form to the best of your abilities. Items 3, 4, 7, 8, 10, 11, and 1 essential and should be completed whenever possible. Parents/Guardians may need to consult the facility where administered for some of the information (such as manufacturer, lot number or laboratory data.)
- Refer to the Reportable Events Table (RET) for events mandated for reporting by law. Reporting for other serious related but not on the RET is encouraged.
- Health care providers other than the vaccine administrator (VA) treating a patient for a suspected adverse event sl VA and provide the information about the adverse event to allow the VA to complete the form to meet the VA's leg
- These data will be used to increase understanding of adverse events following vaccination and will become part of Act System 09-20-0136, "Epidemiologic Studies and Surveillance of Disease Problems". Information identifying th received the vaccine or that person's legal representative will not be made available to the public, but may be avail vaccinee or legal representative.
- Postage will be paid by addressee. Forms may be photocopied (must be front & back on same sheet).

SPECIFIC INSTRUCTIONS

Form Completed By: To be used by parents/guardians, vaccine manufacturers/distributors, vaccine administrators, a completing the form on behalf of the patient or the health professional who administered the vaccine.

Item 7:   Describe the suspected adverse event. Such things as temperature, local and general signs and symptor duration of symptoms, diagnosis, treatment and recovery should be noted.

Item 9:   Check "YES" if the patient's health condition is the same as it was prior to the vaccine, "NO" if the patient to the pre-vaccination state of health, or "UNKNOWN" if the patient's condition is not known.

Item 10:   Give dates and times as specifically as you can remember. If you do not know the exact time, please
and 11:   indicate "AM" or "PM" when possible if this information is known. If more than one adverse event, give th time for the most serious event.

Item 12:   Include "negative" or "normal" results of any relevant tests performed as well as abnormal findings.

Item 13:   List ONLY those vaccines given on the day listed in Item 10.

Item 14:   List any other vaccines that the patient received within 4 weeks prior to the date listed in Item 10.

Item 16:   This section refers to how the person who gave the vaccine purchased it, not to the patient's insurance.

Item 17:   List any prescription or non-prescription medications the patient was taking when the vaccine(s) was give

Item 18:   List any short term illnesses the patient had on the date the vaccine(s) was given (i.e., cold, flu, ear infect

Item 19:   List any pre-existing physician-diagnosed allergies, birth defects, medical conditions (including developm neurologic disorders) for the patient.

Item 21:   List any suspected adverse events the patient, or the patient's brothers or sisters, may have had to previc If more than one brother or sister, or if the patient has reacted to more than one prior vaccine, use additional pag explain completely. For the onset age of a patient, provide the age in months if less than two years old.

Item 26:   This space is for manufacturers' use only.